# Access the BNF *your* way

The *British National Formulary* (BNF) and *BNF for Children* are updated monthly online via MedicinesComplete; ensuring healthcare professionals always have the latest prescribing advice.

You can be alerted to all the latest updates, by signing up to the BNF eNewsletter at: www.bnf.org/newsletter

## ONLINE

 MedicinesComplete

**BNF on MedicinesComplete**
Access BNF and *BNF for Children* on MedicinesComplete and receive the very latest drug information through monthly online updates.

**BNF** on FormularyComplete

**BNF on FormularyComplete**
Allowing you to create, edit and manage local formulary content built upon the trusted prescribing advice of the BNF and *BNF for Children*.

**BNF on Evidence Search**
Search the BNF and *BNF for Children* alongside other authoritative clinical and non-clinical evidence and best practice at http://evidence.nhs.uk from NICE.

## MOBILE

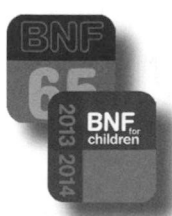

**BNF app** – Stay up to date anywhere with the BNF app available for iOS, Android and Blackberry.

**BNF PDA version** – Full content of the BNF is available for use via a PDA.

## PRINT

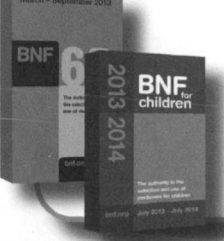

**BNF subscription** – if print is your preferred access method, take advantage of our subscription option and be assured that the latest BNF will be with you as soon as the book is published. One or two year packages (including or excluding BNFC) are available. Discounted pricing also available on bulk sales.

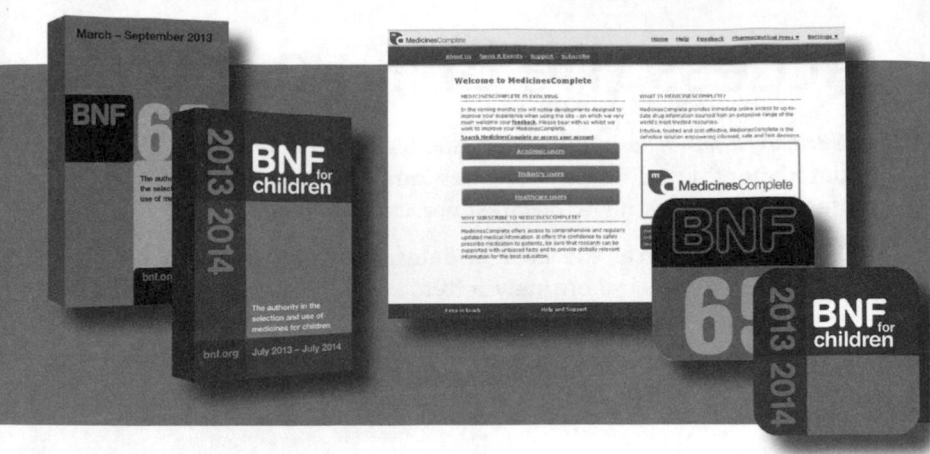

If you are entitled to a free NHS copy of *BNF for Children*, please refer to page ii for full details on distribution or tel: **01268 495 609** / email: **bnf@binleys.com**

# How to purchase

**Purchase direct from Pharmaceutical Press** by visiting **www.pharmpress.com/bnf**

For enquiries about the BNF or BNFC in print contact:
**direct@macmillan.co.uk**
**+44 (0) 1256 302 699**

For enquiries concerning MedicinesComplete, BNF on FormularyComplete, or bulk orders of 20 copies or more of the print edition: **pharmpress@rpharms.com**
**+44 (0) 20 7572 2266**

Download mobile apps by visiting your appropriate app store. Available for iOS, Android and Blackberry

For pricing information please visit the website
**www.pharmpress.com/bnf**

Stay up-to-date, sign up to the BNF eNewsletter at:
**www.bnf.org/newsletter**

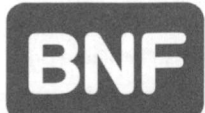
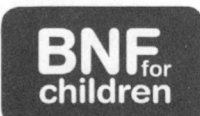

# Contents

# Preface

*BNF for Children* aims to provide prescribers, pharmacists, and other healthcare professionals with sound up-to-date information on the use of medicines for treating children.

A joint publication of the British Medical Association, the Royal Pharmaceutical Society, the Royal College of Paediatrics and Child Health, and the Neonatal and Paediatric Pharmacists Group, *BNF for Children* ('BNFC') is published under the authority of a Paediatric Formulary Committee which comprises representatives of these bodies, the Department of Health for England, and the Medicines and Healthcare products Regulatory Agency.

Many areas of paediatric practice have suffered from inadequate information on effective medicines. BNFC addresses this significant knowledge gap by providing practical information on the use of medicines in children of all ages from birth to adolescence. Information in BNFC has been validated against emerging evidence, best-practice guidelines, and crucially, advice from a network of clinical experts.

Drawing information from manufacturers' literature where appropriate, BNFC also includes a great deal of advice that goes beyond marketing authorisations (product licences). This is necessary because licensed indications frequently do not cover the clinical needs of children; in some cases, products for use in children need to be specially manufactured or imported. Careful consideration has been given to establishing the clinical need for unlicensed interventions with respect to the evidence and experience of their safety and efficacy; local paediatric formularies, clinical literature and national information resources have been invaluable in this process.

BNFC has been designed for rapid reference and the information presented has been carefully selected to aid decisions on prescribing, dispensing and administration of medicines. Less detail is given on areas such as malignant disease and the very specialist use of medicines generally undertaken in tertiary centres. BNFC should be interpreted in the light of professional knowledge and it should be supplemented as necessary by specialised publications. Information is also available from Medicines Information Services (see inside front cover).

It is **important** to use the most recent BNFC information for making clinical decisions. The print edition of *BNF for Children* is updated in July each year. Monthly updates are provided online via the BNF Publications website bnfc.org, MedicinesComplete, and the NHS Evidence portal. The more important changes for this edition are listed on p. xvii; changes listed online are cumulative (from one print edition to the next), and can be printed off each month to show the main changes since the last print edition as an aide memoire for those using print copies.

The website (bnfc.org) includes additional information of relevance to healthcare professionals. Other digital formats of BNFC—including versions for mobile devices and integration into local formularies—are also available.

BNF Publications welcomes comments from healthcare professionals. Comments and constructive criticism should be sent to:
British National Formulary,
Royal Pharmaceutical Society,
1 Lambeth High Street, London SE1 7JN.
bnfc@bnf.org

The contact email for manufacturers or pharmaceutical companies wishing to contact BNF Publications is manufacturerinfo@bnf.org

# Acknowledgements

The Paediatric Formulary Committee is grateful to individuals and organisations that have provided advice and information to the *BNF for Children* (BNFC).

The principal contributors for this edition were:

M.N. Badminton, S. Bailey, G.D.L. Bates, H. Bedford, M.W. Beresford, R.M. Bingham, L. Brook, K.G. Brownlee, M. Burch, I.F. Burgess, A. Cant, L.J. Carr, R. Carr, E.A. Chalmers, T.D. Cheetham, A.G. Cleary, A.J. Cotgrove, J.B.S. Coulter, B.G. Craig, S.M. Creighton, J.H. Cross, A. Dhawan, P.N. Durrington, A. Durward, A.B. Edgar, J.A. Edge, D.A.C. Elliman, N.D. Embleton, P.J. Goadsby, P.W. Golightly, J. Gray, J.W. Gregory, P. Gringras, J.P. Harcourt, P.J. Helms, C. Hendriksz, R.F. Howard, R.G. Hull, H.R. Jenkins, S. Jones, B.A. Judd, P.T. Khaw, J.M.W. Kirk, P.J. Lee, T.H. Lee, E.G.H. Lyall, A. MacDonald, P.S. Malone, S.D. Marks, D.F. Marsh, P.J. McKiernan, L.M. Melvin, E. Miller, R.E. Morton, C. Moss, P. Mulholland, M.S. Murphy, C. Nelson-Piercy, J.M. Neuberger, K.K. Nischal, C.Y. Ng, L.P. Omerod, J.Y. Paton, G.A. Pearson, M.M. Ramsay, J. Rogers, K.E. Rogstad, P.C. Rubin, J.W. Sander, N.J. Scolding, M.R. Sharland, N.J. Shaw, O.F.W. Stumper, A.G. Sutcliffe, A.M. Szarewski, E.A. Taylor, S. Thomas, A.H. Thomson, M.A. Thomson, J.A. Vale, S. Vijay, J.O. Warner, D.A. Warrell, N.J.A. Webb, A.D. Weeks, R. Welbury, W.P. Whitehouse, C.E. Willoughby, C. Wren, A. Wright, M.M. Yaqoob, Z. Zaiwalla, and S.M. Zuberi.

Members of the British Association of Dermatologists' Therapy & Guidelines Subcommittee, D.A. Buckley, R. Davis, E. Duarte Williams, J. Hughes, N.J. Levell, A.J. McDonagh, P. McHenry, I. Nasr, S. Punjabi, A. Sahota, V. Swale, S.E. Haveron (Secretariat), and M.F. Mohd Mustapa (Secretariat) have provided valuable advice.

Members of the Advisory Committee on Malaria Prevention, R.H. Behrens, D. Bell, P.L. Chiodini, S. Clarke, V.Field, F. Genasi, L. Goodyer, A. Green, J. Jones, G. Kassianos, D.G. Lalloo, G. Pasvol, M. Powell, D.V. Shingadia, N.O. Subair, C.J.M. Whitty, M. Blaze (Secretariat), and V. Smith (Secretariat) have provided valuable advice.

Members of the UK Ophthalmic Pharmacy Group have also provided valuable advice.

R. Suvarna and colleagues at the MHRA have provided valuable assistance.

Correspondents in the pharmaceutical industry have provided information on new products and commented on products in BNFC . NHS Prescription Services has supplied the prices of products in the BNFC.

Numerous doctors, pharmacists, nurses, and others have sent comments and suggestions.

Invaluable contribution to BNFC interactions provided by C.L. Preston, S.Z. Khan, D.M. McGuirk, J.M. Sharp, and N. Virani.

The BNFC has valuable access to the *Martindale* data banks by courtesy of A. Brayfield and staff.

F. Gibson and staff provided valuable technical assistance.

A. Holmes and E. Laughton provided considerable assistance during the production of this edition of BNFC.

Typesetting services were provided by Data Standards Ltd.

# BNF Staff

**Managing Editor**

Suhas Khanderia *BPharm, MSc, MBA, MRPharmS*

**Managing Editor: Knowledge Creation**

Rachel S. M. Ryan *BPharm, MRPharmS* (acting until April 2013)

**Lead Editors**

Bryony Jordan *BSc, DipPharmPract, MRPharmS*

John Martin *BPharm, PhD, MRPharmS*

Shama M. S. Wagle *BPharm, DipPharmPract, MRPharmS*

**Senior Clinical Writers**

Sejal Amin *BPharm, MSc*

Susan E. Clarke *BPharm, DipClinPharm, MRPharmS*

**Clinical Writers**

Kristina Fowlie *MPharm, CertPharmPract, MRPharmS*

Belén Granell Villén *BSc, DipClinPharm*

Manjula Halai *BScChem, MPharm*

Angela M. G. McFarlane *BSc, DipClinPharm, MRPharmS*

Sarah Mohamad *MPharm, MRPharmS*

Heenaben Patel *MPharm, DipClinPharm, MRPharmS*

Barbara Schneider *MPharm, DipClinPharm, MRPharmS*

Vinaya K. Sharma *BPharm, MSc, DipPIM, MRPharmS*

Anna Sparshatt *MPharm, CertPharmPract, CertPsychTherap*

Kate Towers *BPharm* (AU), *GCClinPharm*

Katie E. Walters *MPharm, CertPharmPract, MRPharmS*

**Editorial Assistants**

Rhiannon Howe *BMedSc*

Cristina Lopez-Bueno *BA*

**Senior BNF Administrator**

Heidi Homar *BA*

**Clinical Decision Support Product Manager**

Ferenc P. Wórum *MD* (HU), *MSc*

**Terminologist**

Sarah Peck *BSc*

**Production Manager**

Tamsin Cousins *BSc*

**Senior Production Editor**

Linda Paulus *MA*

**BNF Publishing Director**

Duncan S. T. Enright *MA, PGCE, MInstP*

**Managing Director, Pharmaceutical Press**

Alina Lourie *B.Ed, MSc*

**Senior Medical Adviser**

Derek G. Waller *BSc, MB, BS, DM, FRCP*

# Paediatric Formulary Committee 2012–2013

**Chair**

Warren Lenney
*MD, FRCP, FRCPCH, DCH*

**Committee Members**

Indraneel Banerjee
*MB BS, MD, FRCPCH*

Neil A. Caldwell
*BSc, MSc, MRPharmS*

Martin G. Duerden
*BMedSci, MB BS, DRCOG, MRCGP, DipTher, DPH*

Julia Dunne
*BA, MB BS, FRCP*

James H. Larcombe
*MB, ChB, FRCGP, DipAdvGP*

John Marriott
*BSc, PhD, MRPharmS, FHEA*

E. David G. McIntosh
*MB BS, MPH, PhD, FAFPHM, FRACP, FRCPCH, FFPM, DRCOG, DCH, DipPharmMed*

Neena Modi
*MB, ChB, MD, FRCP, FRCPCH*

Julia Simmons
*BSc, MRPharmS*

Adam Sutherland
*MPharm, MSc*

David Tuthill
*MB, BCh, FRCPCH*

Edward R. Wozniack
*BSc, MB BS, FRCP, FRCPCH, DCH*

**Executive Secretary**

Heidi Homar
*BA*

# Dental Advisory Group 2012–2013

**Chair**

David Wray
*MD, BDS, MB ChB, FDSRCPS, FDSRCS Ed, F MedSci*

**Committee Members**

Christine Arnold
*BDS, DDPHRCS, MCDH*

Andrew K. Brewer
*BSc, BchD*

Barry Cockcroft
*BDS, FFDS (Eng)*

Duncan S.T. Enright
*MA, PGCE, MInstP*

Lesley P. Longman
*BSc, BDS, FDSRCS Ed, PhD*

Sarah Manton
*BDS, FDSRCS Ed, FHEA, PhD*

John Martin
*BPharm, PhD, MRPharmS*

Michelle Moffat
*BDS, MFDS RCS Ed, M Paed Dent RPCS, FDS (Paed Dent) RSC Ed*

Sarah Mohamad
*MPharm, MRPharmS*

Rachel S.M. Ryan
*BPharm, MRPharmS*

**Secretary**

Arianne J. Matlin
*MA, MSc, PhD*

**Executive Secretary**

Heidi Homar
*BA*

> **Advice on dental practice**
> The **British Dental Association** has contributed to the advice on medicines for dental practice through its representatives on the Dental Advisory Group.

# Nurse Prescribers' Advisory Group 2012–2013

# How *BNF for Children* is constructed

*BNF for Children* (BNFC) is unique in bringing together authoritative, independent guidance on best practice with clinically validated drug information, enabling healthcare professionals to select safe and effective medicines for individual children.

Information in BNFC has been validated against emerging evidence, best-practice guidelines, and advice from a network of clinical experts. BNFC includes a great deal of advice that goes beyond marketing authorisations (product licences or summaries of product characteristics). This is necessary because licensed indications frequently do not cover the clinical needs of children; in some cases, products for use in children need to be specially manufactured or imported. Careful consideration has been given to establishing the clinical need for unlicensed interventions with respect to the evidence and experience of their safety and efficacy.

Hundreds of changes are made between print editions, and are published monthly online. The most clinically significant changes are listed at the front of each edition (p. xvii).

## Paediatric Formulary Committee

The Paediatric Formulary Committee (PFC) is responsible for the content of BNFC. The PFC includes a neonatologist and paediatricians appointed by the Royal College of Paediatrics and Child Health, paediatric pharmacists appointed by the Royal Pharmaceutical Society and the Neonatal and Paediatric Pharmacists Group, doctors appointed by the BMJ Group, a GP appointed by the Royal College of General Practitioners, and representatives from the Medicines and Healthcare products Regulatory Agency (MHRA) and the Department of Health for England. The PFC decides on matters of policy and reviews amendments to BNFC in the light of new evidence and expert advice.

## Dental Advisory Group

The Dental Advisory Group oversees the preparation of advice on the drug management of dental and oral conditions; the group includes representatives from the British Dental Association and a representative from the UK Health Departments.

## Editorial team

BNFC clinical writers have all worked as pharmacists and have a sound understanding of how drugs are used in clinical practice, including paediatrics. Each clinical writer is responsible for editing, maintaining, and updating specific chapters of BNFC. During the publication cycle the clinical writers review information in BNFC against a variety of sources (see below).

Amendments to the text are drafted when the clinical writers are satisfied that any new information is reliable and relevant. The draft amendments are passed to expert advisers for comment and then presented to the Paediatric Formulary Committee for consideration. Additionally, sections are regularly chosen from every chapter for thorough review. These planned reviews aim to verify all the information in the selected sections and to draft any amendments to reflect current best practice.

Clinical writers prepare the text for publication and undertake a number of checks on the knowledge at various stages of the production.

## Expert advisers

BNFC uses about 80 expert clinical advisers (including doctors, pharmacists, nurses, and dentists) throughout the UK to help with the clinical content. The role of these expert advisers is to review existing text and to comment on amendments drafted by the clinical writers. These clinical experts help to ensure that BNFC remains reliable by:

- commenting on the relevance of the text in the context of best clinical practice in the UK;

- checking draft amendments for appropriate interpretation of any new evidence;

- providing expert opinion in areas of controversy or when reliable evidence is lacking;

- advising on areas where BNFC diverges from summaries of product characteristics;

- advising on the use of unlicensed medicines or of licensed medicines for unlicensed uses ('off-label' use);

- providing independent advice on drug interactions, prescribing in hepatic impairment, renal impairment, pregnancy, breast-feeding, neonatal care, palliative care, and the emergency treatment of poisoning.

In addition to consulting with regular advisers, BNFC calls on other clinical specialists for specific developments when particular expertise is required.

BNFC also works closely with a number of expert bodies that produce clinical guidelines. Drafts or pre-publication copies of guidelines are routinely received for comment and for assimilation into BNFC.

## Sources of BNFC information

BNFC uses a variety of sources for its information; the main ones are shown below.

**Summaries of product characteristics**  BNFC receives summaries of product characteristics (SPCs) of all new products as well as revised SPCs for existing products. The SPCs are a key source of product information and are carefully processed, despite the ever-increasing volume of information being issued by the pharmaceutical industry. Such processing involves:

- verifying the approved names of all relevant ingredients including 'non-active' ingredients (BNFC is committed to using approved names and descriptions as laid down by the Human Medicines Regulations 2012);

- comparing the indications, cautions, contra-indications, and side-effects with similar existing drugs. Where these are different from the expected pattern, justification is sought for their inclusion or exclusion;

- seeking independent data on the use of drugs in pregnancy and breast-feeding;

- incorporating the information into BNFC using established criteria for the presentation and inclusion of the data;

- checking interpretation of the information by a second clinical writer before submitting to a lead editor; changes relating to doses receive an extra check;

- identifying potential clinical problems or omissions and seeking further information from manufacturers or from expert advisers;

- careful validation of any areas of divergence of BNFC from the SPC before discussion by the Committee (in the light of supporting evidence);

- constructing, with the help of expert advisers, a comment on the role of the drug in the context of similar drugs.Much of this processing is applicable to the following sources as well.

**Expert advisers**   The role of expert clinical advisers in providing the appropriate clinical context for all BNFC information is discussed above.

**Literature**   Clinical writers monitor core medical, paediatric, and pharmaceutical journals. Research papers and reviews relating to drug therapy are carefully processed. When a difference between the advice in BNFC and the paper is noted, the new information is assessed for reliability and relevance to UK clinical practice. If necessary, new text is drafted and discussed with expert advisers and the Paediatric Formulary Committee. BNFC enjoys a close working relationship with a number of national information providers.

**Systematic reviews**   BNFC has access to various databases of systematic reviews (including the Cochrane Library and various web-based resources). These are used for answering specific queries, for reviewing existing text, and for constructing new text. Clinical writers receive training in critical appraisal, literature evaluation, and search strategies. Reviews published in Clinical Evidence are used to validate BNFC advice.

**Consensus guidelines**   The advice in BNFC is checked against consensus guidelines produced by expert bodies. A number of bodies make drafts or pre-publication copies of the guidelines available to BNFC; it is therefore possible to ensure that a consistent message is disseminated. BNFC routinely processes guidelines from the National Institute for Health and Clinical Excellence (NICE), the Scottish Medicines Consortium (SMC), and the Scottish Intercollegiate Guidelines Network (SIGN).

**Reference sources**   Paediatric formularies and reference sources are used to provide background information for the review of existing text or for the construction of new text. The BNFC team works closely with the editorial team that produces *Martindale: The Complete Drug Reference*. BNFC has access to *Martindale* information resources and each team keeps the other informed of significant developments and shifts in the trends of drug usage.

**Statutory information**   BNFC routinely processes relevant information from various Government bodies including Statutory Instruments and regulations affecting the Prescription only Medicines Order. Official

compendia such as the British Pharmacopoeia and its addenda are processed routinely to ensure that BNFC complies with the relevant sections of the Human Medicines Regulations 2012.

BNFC maintains close links with the Home Office (in relation to controlled drug regulations) and the Medicines and Healthcare products Regulatory Agency (including the British Pharmacopoeia Commission). Safety warnings issued by the Commission on Human Medicines (CHM) and guidelines on drug use issued by the UK health departments are processed as a matter of routine.

Relevant professional statements issued by the Royal Pharmaceutical Society are included in BNFC as are guidelines from bodies such as the Royal College of Paediatrics and Child Health.

BNFC reflects information from the Drug Tariff, the Scottish Drug Tariff, and the Northern Ireland Drug Tariff.

**Pricing information**   NHS Prescription Services (from the NHS Business Services Authority) provides information on prices of medicinal products and appliances in BNFC.

**Comments from readers**   Readers of BNFC are invited to send in comments. Numerous letters and emails are received by the BNF team. Such feedback helps to ensure that BNFC provides practical and clinically relevant information. Many changes in the presentation and scope of BNFC have resulted from comments sent in by users.

**Comments from industry**   Close scrutiny of BNFC by the manufacturers provides an additional check and allows them an opportunity to raise issues about BNFC's presentation of the role of various drugs; this is yet another check on the balance of BNFC advice. All comments are looked at with care and, where necessary, additional information and expert advice are sought.

**Virtual user groups**   BNFC has set up virtual user groups across various healthcare professions (e.g. doctors, pharmacists, nurses). The aim of these groups will be to provide feedback to the editors and publishers to ensure that BNF publications continue to serve the needs of its users.

**Market research**   Market research is conducted at regular intervals to gather feedback on specific areas of development, such as drug interactions or changes to the way information is presented in digital formats.

> BNFC is an independent professional publication that is kept up-to-date and addresses the day-to-day prescribing information needs of healthcare professionals treating children. Use of this resource throughout the health service helps to ensure that medicines are used safely, effectively, and appropriately in children.

# How to use *BNF for Children*

*BNF for Children* (BNFC) provides information on the use of medicines in children ranging from neonates (including preterm neonates) to adolescents. The terms infant, child, and adolescent are not used consistently in the literature; to avoid ambiguity actual ages are used in the dose statements in BNFC. The term neonate is used to describe a newborn infant aged 0–28 days. The terms child or children are used generically to describe the entire range from infant to adolescent in BNFC.

In order to achieve the safe, effective, and appropriate use of medicines in children, healthcare professionals must be able to use BNFC effectively, and keep up to date with significant changes in BNFC that are relevant to their clinical practice. *How to Use BNF for Children* is aimed as a quick refresher for all healthcare professionals involved with prescribing, monitoring, supplying, and administering medicines for children, and as a learning aid for students training to join these professions. While *How to Use BNF for Children* is linked to the main elements of rational prescribing, the generic structure of this section means that it can be adapted for teaching and learning in different clinical settings.

## Structure of BNFC

The Contents list (on p. iii) shows that information in BNFC is divided into:

- *How BNF for Children is Constructed* (p. ix);
- *Changes* (p. xvii);
- *General Guidance* (p. 1), which provides practical information on many aspects of prescribing from writing a prescription to prescribing in palliative care;
- *Emergency Treatment of Poisoning* (p. 23), which provides an overview on the management of acute poisoning;
- *Classified notes on clinical conditions, drugs, and preparations*, these notes are divided into 15 chapters, each of which is related to a particular system of the body (e.g. chapter 3, Respiratory System) or to an aspect of paediatric care (e.g. chapter 5, Infections). Each chapter is further divided into classified sections. Each section usually begins with *prescribing notes* followed by relevant drug *monographs* and *preparations* (see fig. 1). Drugs are classified in a section according to their pharmacology and therapeutic use;
- *Appendices and Indices*, includes 4 Appendices (providing information on drug interactions, borderline substances, cautionary and advisory labels for dispensed medicines, and intravenous infusions for neonatal intensive care), the Dental Practitioners' Formulary, the Nurse Prescribers' Formulary, Nonmedical Prescribing, Index of Manufacturers, and the main Index. The information in the Appendices should be used in conjunction with relevant information in the chapters.

## Finding information in BNFC

BNFC includes a number of aids to help access relevant information:

- *Index*, where entries are included in alphabetical order of non-proprietary drug names, proprietary drug names, clinical conditions, and prescribing topics. A specific entry for 'Dental Prescribing' brings together topics of relevance to dentists. The page reference to the drug monograph is shown in **bold** type. References to drugs in Appendices 1 and 3 are not included in the main Index;
- *Contents* (p. iii), provides a hierarchy of how information in BNFC is organised;
- The beginning of each chapter includes *a classified hierarchy* of how information is organised in that chapter;
- *Running heads*, located next to the page number on the top of each page, show the section of BNFC that is being used;
- *Thumbnails*, on the outer edge of each page, show the chapter of BNFC that is being used;
- *Cross-references*, lead to additional relevant information in other parts of BNFC.

## Finding dental information in BNFC

Extra signposts have been added to help access dental information in BNFC:

- *Prescribing in Dental Practice* (p. 21), includes a contents list dedicated to drugs and topics of relevance to dentists, together with cross-references to the prescribing notes in the appropriate sections of BNFC. For example, a review of this list shows that information on the local treatment of oral infections is located in chapter 12 (Ear, Nose, and Oropharynx) while information on the systemic treatment of these infections is found in chapter 5 (Infections). Further guidance for dental practice can be found in the BNF.
- *Side-headings*, in the prescribing notes, side-headings facilitate the identification of advice on oral conditions (e.g. Dental and Orofacial Pain, p. 199);
- *Dental prescribing on NHS*, in the body of BNFC, preparations that can be prescribed using NHS form FP10D (GP14 in Scotland, WP10D in Wales) can be identified by means of a note headed 'Dental prescribing on NHS' (e.g. Aciclovir Oral Suspension, p. 326).

## Identifying effective drug treatments

The prescribing notes in BNFC provide an overview of the drug management of common conditions and facilitate rapid appraisal of treatment options (e.g. epilepsy, p. 216). For ease of use, information on the management of certain conditions has been tabulated (e.g. acute asthma, p. 134).

Advice issued by the National Institute for Health and Clinical Excellence (NICE) is integrated within BNFC prescribing notes if appropriate. Summaries of NICE technology appraisals, and relevant short guidelines, are included in pink panels. BNFC also includes advice issued by the Scottish Medicines Consortium (SMC) when a medicine is restricted or not recommended for use within NHS Scotland.

In order to select safe and effective medicines for individual children, information in the prescribing notes must be used in conjunction with other prescribing details about the drugs and knowledge of the child's medical and drug history.

A brief description of the clinical uses of a drug can usually be found in the Indication and Dose section of its monograph (e.g. ibuprofen, p. 504); a cross-reference is provided to any indications for that drug that are covered in other sections of BNFC.

The symbol ◢ is used to denote preparations that are considered to be less suitable for prescribing. Although

## Figure 1   Illustrates the typical layout of a drug monograph and preparation records in BNFC

**DRUG NAME** ◢ ←

**Cautions**  details of precautions required and also any monitoring required
  **Counselling**  Verbal explanation to the patient of specific details of the drug treatment (e.g. posture when taking a medicine)
**Contra-indications**  circumstances when a drug should be avoided
**Hepatic impairment**  advice on the use of a drug in hepatic impairment
**Renal impairment**  advice on the use of a drug in renal impairment
**Pregnancy**  advice on the use of a drug during pregnancy
**Breast-feeding**  advice on the use of a drug during breast-feeding
**Side-effects**  very common (greater than 1 in 10) and common (1 in 100 to 1 in 10); *less commonly* (1 in 1000 to 1 in 100); *rarely* (1 in 10 000 to 1 in 1000); *very rarely* (less than 1 in 10 000); also reported, frequency not known
**Licensed use**  shows if a drug unlicensed in the UK, or 'off-label' use of drug licensed in the UK

**Indication and dose**
  Details of uses and indications
  • By route
  Child dose and frequency of administration (max. dose) for specific age group
  • By alternative route
  Child dose and frequency
**Administration**  practical advice on the administration of a drug

[1]**Approved Name** (Non-proprietary) [PoM] ←
  Pharmaceutical form, sugar-free, active ingredient mg/mL, net price, pack size = basic NHS price. Label: (as in Appendix 3)
1. Exceptions to the prescribing status are indicated by a note or footnote.

**Proprietary Name** (Manufacturer) [PoM] [NHS] ←
  Pharmaceutical form, colour, coating, active ingredient and amount in dosage form, net price, pack size = basic NHS price. Label: (as in Appendix 3)
  **Excipients**  include clinically important excipients
  **Electrolytes**  clinically significant quantities of electrolytes
  **Note**  Specific notes about the product e.g. handling

In the case of compound preparations, the indications, cautions, contra-indications, side-effects and interactions of all constituents should be taken into account for prescribing.

When no suitable licensed preparation is available, details of preparations that may be imported or formulations available as manufactured specials or extemporaneous preparations are included.

### Drugs
Drugs appear under pharmacopoeial or other non-proprietary titles. When there is an *appropriate current monograph* (Human Medicines Regulations 2012) preference is given to a name at the head of that monograph; otherwise a British Approved Name (BAN), if available, is used.

The symbol ◢ is used to denote those preparations considered to be less suitable for prescribing. Although such preparations may not be considered as drugs of first choice, their use may be justifiable in certain circumstances.

### Prescription-only medicines [PoM]
This symbol has been placed against preparations that are available only on a prescription from an appropriate practitioner. For more detailed information see *Medicines, Ethics and Practice*, London, Pharmaceutical Press (always consult latest edition).

The symbols [CD2] [CD3] [CD4-1] [CD4-2] indicate that the preparations are subject to the prescription requirements of the Misuse of Drugs Act. For advice on prescribing such preparations see Prescribing Controlled Drugs.

### Preparations not available for NHS prescription [NHS]
This symbol has been placed against preparations that are not prescribable under the NHS. Those prescribable only for specific disorders have a footnote specifying the condition(s) for which the preparation remains available. Some preparations which are not *prescribable* by brand name under the NHS may nevertheless be *dispensed* using the brand name provided that the prescription shows an appropriate non-proprietary name.

### Preparations
Preparations are included under a non-proprietary title, if they are marketed under such a title, if they are not otherwise prescribable under the NHS, or if they may be prepared extemporaneously.

### Prices
Prices have been calculated from the basic cost used in pricing NHS prescriptions, see also Prices in BNFC.

such preparations may not be considered as drugs of first choice, their use may be justifiable in certain circumstances.

## Drug management of medical emergencies

Guidance on the drug management of medical emergencies can be found in the relevant BNFC chapters (e.g. treatment of anaphylaxis is included in section 3.4.3). A summary of drug doses used for Medical Emergencies in the Community can be found in the glossy pages at the back of BNFC. Algorithms for Newborn, Paediatric Basic, and Paediatric Advanced Life Support can also be found within these pages.

## Minimising harm in children with co-morbidities

The drug chosen to treat a particular condition should have minimal detrimental effects on the child's other diseases and minimise the child's susceptibility to adverse effects. To achieve this, the *Cautions*, *Contra-indications*, and *Side-effects* of the relevant drug should be reviewed, and can usually be found in the drug monograph. However, if a class of drugs (e.g. tetracyclines, p. 276) share the same cautions, contra-indications, and side-effects, these are amalgamated in the prescribing notes while those unique to a particular drug in that class are included in its individual drug monograph. Occasionally, the cautions, contra-indications, and side-effects may be included within a preparation record if they are specific to that preparation or if the preparation is not accompanied by a monograph.

The information under Cautions can be used to assess the risks of using a drug in a child who has co-morbidities that are also included in the Cautions for that drug—if a safer alternative cannot be found, the drug may be prescribed while monitoring the child for adverse-effects or deterioration in the co-morbidity. Contra-indications are far more restrictive than Cautions and mean that the drug should be avoided in a child with a condition that is contra-indicated.

The impact that potential side-effects may have on a child's quality of life should also be assessed. For instance, in a child who has constipation, it may be preferable to avoid a drug that frequently causes constipation. The prescribing notes in BNFC may highlight important safety concerns and differences between drugs in their ability to cause certain side-effects.

## Prescribing for children with hepatic or renal impairment

Drug selection should aim to minimise the potential for drug accumulation, adverse drug reactions, and exacerbation of pre-existing hepatic or renal disease. If it is necessary to prescribe drugs whose effect is altered by hepatic or renal disease, appropriate drug dose adjustments should be made, and the child should be monitored adequately. The general principles for prescribing are outlined under *Prescribing in Hepatic Impairment* (p. 13) and *Prescribing in Renal Impairment* (p. 13). Information about drugs that should be avoided or used with caution in hepatic disease or renal impairment can be found in drug monographs under *Hepatic Impairment* and *Renal Impairment* (e.g. fluconazole, p. 304). However, if a class of drugs (e.g. tetracyclines, p. 276) share

the same recommendations for use in hepatic disease or renal impairment, this advice is presented in the prescribing notes under *Hepatic Impairment* and *Renal Impairment* and any advice that is unique to a particular drug in that class is included in its individual drug monograph.

## Prescribing for patients who are pregnant or breast-feeding

Drug selection should aim to minimise harm to the fetus, nursing infant, and mother. The infant should be monitored for potential side-effects of drugs used by the mother during pregnancy or breast-feeding. The general principles for prescribing are outlined under *Prescribing in Pregnancy* (p. 15) and *Prescribing in Breast-feeding* (p. 15). The prescribing notes in BNFC chapters provide guidance on the drug treatment of common conditions that can occur during pregnancy and breast-feeding (e.g. asthma, p. 131). Information about the use of specific drugs during pregnancy and breast-feeding can be found in their drug monographs under *Pregnancy* and *Breast-feeding* (e.g. fluconazole, p. 304). However, if a class of drugs (e.g. tetracyclines, p. 276) share the same recommendations for use during pregnancy or breast-feeding, this advice is amalgamated in the prescribing notes under *Pregnancy* and *Breast-feeding* while any advice that is unique to a particular drug in that class is included in its individual drug monograph.

## Minimising drug interactions

Drug selection should aim to minimise drug interactions. If it is necessary to prescribe a potentially serious combination of drugs, children should be monitored appropriately. The mechanisms underlying drug interactions are explained in Appendix 1 (p. 655).

Details of drug interactions can be found in Appendix 1 of BNFC (p. 655). Drugs and their interactions are listed in alphabetical order of the non-proprietary drug name, and cross-references to drug classes are provided where appropriate. Each drug or drug class is listed twice: in the alphabetical list and also against the drug or class with which it interacts. The symbol • is placed against interactions that are potentially serious and where combined administration of drugs should be avoided (or only undertaken with caution and appropriate monitoring). Interactions that have no symbol do not usually have serious consequences.

If a drug or drug class has interactions, a cross reference to where these can be found in Appendix 1 is provided under the Cautions of the drug monograph or prescribing notes.

## Selecting the dose

The drug dose is usually located in pink panels within the *Indication and Dose* section of the drug monograph or within the *Dose* section of the preparation record. Doses are linked to specific indications and routes of administration. The dose of a drug may vary according to different indications, routes of administration, age, body-weight, and body-surface area. When the dose of a drug varies according to different indications, each indication and its accompanying dose is included in a separate pink panel (e.g. aciclovir, p. 324). The dose is located within the preparation record when the dose varies according to different formulations of that drug (e.g. amphotericin, p. 308) or when a preparation has a dose different to that in its monograph. Occasionally, drug doses may be included in the prescribing notes for practical reasons (e.g. doses of drugs in *Helicobacter pylori* eradication regimens, p. 41). The right dose should be selected for the right age and body-weight (or body surface area) of the child, as well as for the right indication, route of administration, and preparation.

> Doses in BNFC are usually assigned to specific age ranges; neonatal doses are preceded by the word Neonate, all other doses are preceded by the word Child. Age ranges in BNFC are described as shown in the following example:
> Child 1 month–4 years refers to a child from 1 month old up to their 4th birthday;
> Child 4–10 years refers to a child from the day of their 4th birthday up to their 10th birthday.
> However, a pragmatic approach should be applied to these cut-off points depending on the child's physiological development, condition, and if weight is appropriate for the child's age.

For some drugs (e.g. gentamicin, p. 280) the neonatal dose varies according to the *postmenstrual* age of the neonate. Postmenstrual age is the neonate's total age expressed in weeks from the start of the mother's last menstrual period. For example, a 3 week old baby born at 27 weeks gestation is treated as having a postmenstrual age of 30 weeks. A term baby has a postmenstrual age of 37–42 weeks when born. For most other drugs, the dose can be based on the child's actual date of birth irrespective of postmenstrual age. However, the degree of prematurity, the maturity of renal and hepatic function, and the clinical properties of the drug need to be considered on an individual basis.

Many children's doses in BNFC are standardised by *body-weight*. To calculate the dose for a given child the weight-standardised dose is multiplied by the child's weight (or occasionally by the child's ideal weight for height). The calculated dose should not normally exceed the maximum recommended dose for an adult. For example, if the dose is 8 mg/kg (max. 300 mg), a child of 10 kg body-weight should receive 80 mg, but a child of 40 kg body-weight should receive 300 mg (rather than 320 mg). Calculation by body-weight in the overweight child may result in much higher doses being administered than necessary; in such cases, the dose should be calculated from an ideal weight for height.

Occasionally, some doses in BNFC are standardised by *body surface area* because many physiological phenomena correlate better with body surface area. In these cases, to calculate the dose for a given child, the body surface area-standardised dose is multiplied by the child's body surface area. The child's body surface area can be estimated from his or her weight using the tables for Body Surface Area in Children located in the glossy pages at the back of the print version of BNFC.

The doses of some drugs may need to be adjusted if their effects are altered by concomitant use with other drugs, or in patients with hepatic or renal impairment (see Minimising Drug Interactions, and Prescribing for Children with Hepatic or Renal Impairment).

Wherever possible, doses are expressed in terms of a definite frequency (e.g. if the dose is 1 mg/kg twice daily, a child of body-weight 9 kg would receive 9 mg twice daily). Occasionally, it is necessary to include doses in the total daily dose format (e.g. 10 mg/kg daily in 3 divided doses); in these cases the total daily dose should be divided into individual doses (in this example a child of body-weight 9 kg would receive 30 mg 3 times daily).

Most drugs can be administered at slightly irregular intervals during the day. Some drugs, e.g. antimicrobials, are best given at regular intervals. Some flexibility should be allowed in children to avoid waking them during the night. For example, the night-time dose may be given at the child's bedtime.

Special care should be taken when converting doses from one metric unit to another, and when calculating infusion rates or the volume of a preparation to administer. Conversions for imperial to metric measures can be found in the glossy pages at the back of BNFC. Where possible, doses should be rounded to facilitate administration of suitable volumes of liquid preparations, or an appropriate strength of tablet or capsule.

## Selecting a suitable preparation

Children should be prescribed a preparation that complements their daily routine, and that provides the right dose of drug for the right indication and route of administration.

In BNFC, preparations usually follow immediately after the monograph for the drug which is their main ingredient. The preparation record (see fig. 1) provides information on the type of formulation (e.g. tablet), the amount of active drug in a solid dosage form, and the concentration of active drug in a liquid dosage form. The legal status is shown for prescription only medicines and controlled drugs; any exception to the legal status is shown by a Note immediately after the preparation record or a footnote. If a proprietary preparation has a distinct colour, coating, scoring, or flavour, this is shown in the preparation record. If a proprietary preparation includes excipients usually specified in BNFC (see p. 2), these are shown in the *Excipients* statement, and if it contains clinically significant quantities of electrolytes, these are usually shown in the *Electrolytes* statement.

Branded oral liquid preparations that do not contain fructose, glucose, or sucrose are described as 'sugar-free' in BNFC. Preparations containing hydrogenated glucose syrup, mannitol, maltitol, sorbitol, or xylitol are also marked 'sugar-free' since there is evidence that they do not cause dental caries. Children receiving medicines containing cariogenic sugars, or their carers, should be advised of appropriate dental hygiene measures to prevent caries. Sugar-free preparations should be used whenever possible.

Where a drug has several preparations, those of a similar type may be grouped together under a heading (e.g. 'Modified-release' for theophylline preparations, p. 141). Where there is good evidence to show that the preparations for a particular drug are not interchangeable, this is stated in a Note either in the Dose section of the monograph or by the group of preparations affected. When the dose of a drug varies according to different formulations of that drug, the right dose should be prescribed for the preparation selected.

In the case of compound preparations, the prescribing information of all constituents should be taken into account for prescribing.

Unlicensed preparations that are available from 'Special order' manufacturers and specialist importing companies are included (e.g. betaine tablets, p. 496).

## Writing prescriptions

Guidance is provided on writing prescriptions that will help to reduce medication errors, see p. 4. Prescription requirements for controlled drugs are also specified on p. 8.

## Administering drugs

Basic information on the route of administration is provided in the Indication and Dose section of a drug monograph or the Dose section of a preparation record. Further details, such as masking the bitter taste of some medicines, may be provided in the *Administration* section of a drug monograph (e.g. proguanil, p. 338). Practical information is also provided on the preparation of intravenous drug infusions, including compatibility of drugs with standard intravenous infusion fluids, method of dilution or reconstitution, and administration rates (e.g. co-amoxiclav, p. 264). The *Administration* section is located within preparation records when this information varies according to different preparations of that drug (e.g. amphotericin, p. 308). If a class of drugs (e.g. topical corticosteroids, p. 561) share the same administration advice, this may be presented in the prescribing notes.

Whenever possible, intramuscular injections should be **avoided** in children because they are painful.

Information on intravenous infusions for neonatal intensive care can also be found in Appendix 4, p. 807.

## Advising children (and carers)

The prescriber, the child's carer, and the child (if appropriate) should agree on the health outcomes desired and on the strategy for achieving them (see Taking Medicines to Best Effect, p. 1). Taking the time to explain to the child (and carers) the rationale and the potential adverse effects of treatment may improve adherence. For some medicines there is a special need for counselling (e.g. recognising signs of blood, liver, or skin disorders with carbamazepine); this is shown in *Counselling* statements, usually in the Cautions or Indication and Dose section of a monograph, or within a preparation record if it is specific to that preparation.

Children and their carers should be advised if treatment is likely to affect their ability to perform skilled tasks (e.g. driving).

Cautionary and advisory labels that pharmacists are recommended to add when dispensing are included in the preparation record (see fig. 1). Details of these labels can be found in Appendix 3 (p. 804).

## Monitoring drug treatment

Children should be monitored to ensure they are achieving the expected benefits from drug treatment without any unwanted side-effects. The prescribing notes or the Cautions in the drug monograph specify any special monitoring requirements. Further information on monitoring the plasma concentration of drugs with a narrow therapeutic index can be found in the Pharmacokinetics section or as a Note under the Dose section of the drug monograph.

## Identifying and reporting adverse drug reactions

Clinically relevant *Side-effects* for most drugs are included in the monographs. However, if a class of drugs (e.g. tetracyclines, p. 276) share the same side-effects, these are presented in the prescribing notes while those unique to a particular drug in that class are included in its individual drug monograph. Occasionally, side-effects may be included within a preparation record if they are specific to that preparation or if the preparation is not accompanied by a monograph.

Side-effects are generally listed in order of frequency and arranged broadly by body systems. Occasionally a rare side-effect might be listed first if it is considered to be particularly important because of its seriousness. The frequency of side-effects is described in fig. 1.

An exhaustive list of side-effects is not included for drugs that are used by specialists (e.g. cytotoxic drugs and drugs used in anaesthesia). Recognising that hypersensitivity reactions can occur with virtually all medicines, this effect is generally not listed, unless the drug carries an increased risk of such reactions. BNFC also omits effects that are likely to have little clinical consequence (e.g. transient increase in liver enzymes).

The prescribing notes in BNFC may highlight important safety concerns and differences between drugs in their ability to cause certain side-effects. Safety warnings issued by the Commission on Human Medicines (CHM) or Medicines and Healthcare products Regulatory Agency (MHRA) can also be found here or in the drug monographs.

Adverse Reactions to Drugs (p. 11) provides advice on preventing adverse drug reactions, and guidance on reporting adverse drug reactions to the MHRA. The black triangle symbol ▼ identifies those preparations in BNFC that are monitored intensively by the MHRA; however, in light of new EU legislation this will change, for latest information see www.mhra.gov.uk.

## Finding significant changes in BNFC

The print edition of BNFC is published in July each year, and monthly updates are provided online via bnfc.org, MedicinesComplete, and the NHS Evidence portal. BNFC includes lists of changes that are relevant to clinical practice:

- *Changes* (p. xvii), provides a list of significant changes, dose changes, classification changes, new names, and new preparations that have been incorporated into BNFC, as well as a list of preparations that have been discontinued and removed from BNFC. For ease of identification, the margins of these pages are marked in pink. Changes listed online are cumulative (from one print edition to the next), and can be printed off each month to show the main changes since the last print edition as an aide memoire for those using print copies;

- *E-newsletter*, the BNF & BNFC e-newsletter service is available free of charge. It alerts healthcare professionals to details of significant changes in the clinical content of these publications and to the way that this information is delivered. Newsletters also review clinical case studies and provide tips on using these publications effectively. To sign up for e-newsletters go to bnf.org/newsletter. To visit the e-newsletter archive, go to bnf.org/bnf/org_450066.htm.

So many changes are made for each update of BNFC, that not all of them can be accommodated in the *Changes* section. We encourage healthcare professionals to review regularly the prescribing information on drugs that they encounter frequently.

## Nutrition

Appendix 2 (p. 757) includes tables of ACBS-approved enteral feeds and nutritional supplements based on their energy and protein content. There are separate tables for specialised formulae for specific clinical conditions. Classified sections on foods for special diets and nutritional supplements for metabolic diseases are also included.

## Licensed status of medicines

BNFC includes advice on the use of unlicensed medicines or of licensed medicines for unlicensed applications ('off-label' use). Such advice reflects careful consideration of the options available to manage a given condition and the weight of evidence and experience of the unlicensed intervention. Limitations of the marketing authorisation should not preclude unlicensed use where clinically appropriate.

The *Licensed Use* statement in a drug monograph is used to indicate that:

* a drug is not licensed in the UK (e.g. potassium canrenoate, p. 80);

* a drug is licensed in the UK, but not for use in children (e.g. lansoprazole, p. 44);

* BNFC advice for certain indications, age groups of children, routes of administration, or preparations falls outside a drug's marketing authorisation (e.g. naproxen, p. 506).

The absence of the *Licensed Use* statement from a drug monograph indicates that the drug is licensed for all indications given in the monograph (e.g. zanamivir, p. 330).

Prescribing unlicensed medicines or medicines outside their marketing authorisation alters (and probably increases) the prescriber's professional responsibility and potential liability. The prescriber should be able to justify and feel competent in using such medicines. Further information can be found in *BNF for Children* and Marketing Authorisation, p. 2.

## Prices in BNFC

Basic NHS **net prices** are given in BNFC to provide an indication of relative cost. Where there is a choice of suitable preparations for a particular disease or condition the relative cost may be used in making a selection. Cost-effective prescribing must, however, take into account other factors (such as dose frequency and duration of treatment) that affect the total cost. The use of more expensive drugs is justified if it will result in better treatment of the patient, or a reduction of the length of an illness, or the time spent in hospital. Prices generally reflect whole dispensing packs; prices for injections are stated per ampoule, vial, or syringe. The price for an extemporaneously prepared preparation has been omitted where the net cost of the ingredients

used to make it would give a misleadingly low impression of the final price.

BNFC prices are not suitable for quoting to patients seeking private prescriptions or contemplating over-the-counter purchases because they do not take into account VAT, professional fees, and other overheads.

A fuller explanation of costs to the NHS may be obtained from the Drug Tariff. Separate drug tariffs are applicable to England and Wales, Scotland, and Northern Ireland; prices in the different tariffs may vary.

## Extra resources on the BNFC website

While the BNFC website (bnfc.org) provides online access to BNFC content, it also provides additional resources such as *Frequently Asked Questions* and online calculators.

# Changes

Monthly updates are provided online via bnfc.org, MedicinesComplete, and the NHS Evidence portal. The changes listed below are cumulative (from one print edition to the next).

## Significant changes

Significant changes have been made in the following sections for *BNF for Children 2013–2014*:

Prices in BNFC [No price update for print edition of BNFC 2013–2014]

Palliative Care [section re-organised and new equivalence dose tables added]

Paracetamol poisoning [updated advice on management], Emergency Treatment of Poisoning

Gastro-oesophageal reflux in pregnancy, section 1.1

Omalizumab for severe persistent allergic asthma [NICE guidance], section 3.4.2

Adrenaline auto-injectors for anaphylaxis [brand prescribing recommended], section 3.4.3

Treatment of hereditary angioedema updated, section 3.4.3

Caffeine monographs reviewed; caffeine doses expressed in terms of caffeine citrate only, section 3.5.1

Septicaemia in neonates, section 5.1, Table 1

Tobramycin by dry powder inhalation for pseudomonal lung infection in cystic fibrosis [NICE guidance], section 5.1.4

Standard regimen for the treatment of tuberculosis [updated doses of rifampicin and ethambutol], section 5.1.9

Oral tacrolimus products: prescribe and dispense by brand name only, to minimise the risk of inadvertent switching between products, which has been associated with reports of toxiciy and graft rejection [MHRA/CHM advice], section 8.2.2

Treatment of glaucoma updated, section 11.6

Pertussis vaccine [immunisation of pregnant women], section 14.4

Label 30 [updated in line with Human Medicines Regulations 2012], appendix 3, recommended label wordings

## Dose changes

Changes in dose statements introduced into *BNF for Children 2013–2014*:

Aciclovir [treatment of herpes simplex, chickenpox and herpes zoster], p. 324

Adalimumab [licensed age], p. 512

Azyter® [licensed age], p. 521

Benzylpenicillin [neonatal dose], p. 260

Budesonide [croup], p. 147

Ciprofloxacin [prevention of secondary case of meningococcal meningitis], p. 256

Clindamycin [oral dose], p. 285

Cycloserine [dose in renal impairment], p. 295

*Easyhaler*® Salbutamol, p. 138

Ethambutol [standard treatment regimen and dose in renal impairment], p. 293 and p. 295

Fenofibrate, p. 129

*Foradil*®, p. 136

Formoterol [dose for children under 12 years], p. 136

Human papilloma virus vaccine [schedule updated], p. 611

Influenza vaccine, p. 612

Isoniazid [dose in renal impairment], p. 295

*Lipantil*®, p. 129

Nevirapine, p. 322

Oseltamivir [dose in renal impairment], p. 329

Penicillamine, p. 489

Pyrazinamide [dose in renal impairment], p. 296

Pizotifen, p. 215

Rifampicin [paediatric dose for standard treatment regimen of tuberculosis], p. 293

Teicoplanin [renal dose], p. 288

Voriconazole [oral dose], p. 306

## Classification changes

Classification changes have been made in the following sections of *BNF for Children 2013–2014*:

General information and changes [title change]

Changes [title change]

Section 4.2.3 Drugs used for mania and hypomania [title change]

Section 8.2.3 Anti-lymphocyte monoclonal antibodies [title change]

## New Names

Name changes introduced in *BNF for Children 2013–2014*:

Betamethasone Soluble Tablets [formerly *Betnesol*® Soluble Tablets], p. 546

Betamethasone and clioquinol cream or ointment [formerly *Betnovate-C*® cream or ointment], p. 565

Betamethasone and neomycin cream or ointment [formerly *Betnovate-N*® cream or ointment], p. 565

*Cystine500*® [formerly Cystine Amino Acid Supplement], p. 798

*Isoleucine50*® [formerly Isoleucine Amino Acid Supplement], p. 799

*Leucine100*® [formerly Leucine Amino Acid Supplement], p. 799

*Phenylalanine50*® [formerly Phenylalanine Amino Acid Supplement], p. 799

*Tyrosine1000*® [formerly Tyrosine Amino Acid Supplement], p. 799

*Valine50*® [formerly Valine Amino Acid Supplement], p. 799

## Deleted preparations

Preparations listed below have been discontinued during the compilation of *BNF for Children 2013–2014*:

*Alphosyl HC*®
*Asilone*®
*Aveeno Colloidal*® bath additive
*Begrivac*®
*Burinex*®
*Carbalax*®
*Eucardic*®
*Fersamal*® tablets
*Fibrelief*®
*Flagyl S*® suspension
Halothane
Hydrocortisone eye drops
*MabCampath*®
*Merbentyl*®
Methionine
*Miacalcic*® nasal spray
*Mobic*®
Neomycin eye drops and eye ointment
*Nutrizym 10*®
*Nyogel*®
*Periogard*®
*Predenema*®
*Retin-A*®
*Sandocal*®+D
*Synflex*®
*Tamiflu*® (oseltamivir) 60 mg/5 mL oral suspension
*Toradol*® tablets
*Trandate*® injection
*Urdox*®
*Viracept*®
*Xamiol*®

*Flutiform*® [fluticasone propionate and formoterol fumarate], p. 148
*Fycompa*® [perampanel], p. 225
*Hidrasec*® [racecadotril], p. 47
*Nimenrix*® [meningococcal A, C, W135, and Y conjugate vaccine], p. 616
*Peyona*® [caffeine citrate], p. 161
*Revatio*® oral solution [sildenafil], p. 96
*Soliris*® [eculizumab], p. 455
*Sorbisterit*® [calcium polystyrene sulfonate], p. 460
*Tamiflu*® (oseltamivir) 30 mg/5 mL oral suspension, p. 330
*Tear-Lac*® [hypromellose], p. 533
*Tepadina*® [thiotepa], p. 421
*Viread*® granules [tenofovir disoproxil (as fumarate)], p. 316
*Xaluprine*® [mercaptopurine], p. 424
*Zinamide*® [pyrazinamide], p. 296

## New preparations

Preparations included in the relevant sections of *BNF for Children 2013–2014*:

*Aquamax*® cream, p. 554
*Aquamax*® cream wash, p. 557
*Capexion*® [tacrolimus], p. 437
*Carmize*® [carmellose sodium], p. 532
*Cayston*® [aztreonam powder for nebuliser solution], p. 276
*Clasteon*® tablets [sodium clodronate], p. 390
*DigiFab*® [digoxin-specific antibody], p. 74
*Dymista*® [fluticasone propionate with azelastine hydrochloride], p. 543
*Elvanse*® [lisdexamfetamine dimesylate], p. 190
*Flexitol*® Heel Balm, p. 556
*Fluenz*® [influenza vaccine], p. 613

# General guidance

## General guidance

Medicines should be given to children only when they are necessary, and in all cases the potential benefit of administering the medicine should be considered in relation to the risk involved. This is particularly important during pregnancy, when the risk to both mother and fetus must be considered (for further details see Prescribing in Pregnancy, p. 15).

It is important to discuss treatment options carefully with the child and the child's carer (see also Taking Medicines to Best Effect, below). In particular, the child and the child's carer should be helped to distinguish the adverse effects of prescribed drugs from the effects of the medical disorder. When the beneficial effects of the medicine are likely to be delayed, this should be highlighted.

**Taking medicines to best effect** Difficulties in adherence to drug treatment occur regardless of age. Factors that contribute to poor compliance with prescribed medicines include:

- difficulty in taking the medicine (e.g. inability to swallow the medicine);
- unattractive formulation (e.g. unpleasant taste);
- prescription not collected or not dispensed;
- purpose of medicine not clear;
- perceived lack of efficacy;
- real or perceived adverse effects;
- carers' or child's perception of the risk and severity of side-effects may differ from that of the prescriber;
- instructions for administration not clear.

The prescriber, the child's carer, and the child (if appropriate) should agree on the health outcomes desired and on the strategy for achieving them ('concordance'). The prescriber should be sensitive to religious, cultural, and personal beliefs of the child's family that can affect acceptance of medicines.

Taking the time to explain to the child (and carers) the rationale and the potential adverse effects of treatment may improve adherence. Reinforcement and elaboration of the physician's instructions by the pharmacist and other members of the healthcare team can be important. Giving advice on the management of adverse effects and the possibility of alternative treatments may encourage carers and children to seek advice rather than merely abandon unacceptable treatment.

Simplifying the drug regimen may help; the need for frequent administration may reduce adherence, although there appears to be little difference in adherence between once-daily and twice-daily administration. Combination products reduce the number of drugs taken but at the expense of the ability to titrate individual doses.

**Drug treatment in children** Children, and particularly neonates, differ from adults in their response to drugs. Special care is needed in the neonatal period (first 28 days of life) and doses should always be calculated with care; the risk of toxicity is increased by a reduced rate of drug clearance and differing target organ sensitivity.

For guidance on selecting doses of drugs in children see How to Use *BNF for Children*, p. xiii.

**Administration of medicines to children** Children should be involved in decisions about taking medicines and encouraged to take responsibility for using them correctly. The degree of such involvement will depend on the child's age, understanding, and personal circumstances.

Occasionally a medicine or its taste has to be disguised or masked with small quantities of food. However, unless specifically permitted (e.g. some formulations of pancreatin), a medicine should **not** be mixed with large quantities of food because the full dose might not be taken and the child might develop an aversion to food if the medicine imparts an unpleasant taste. Medicines should **not** be mixed or administered in a baby's feeding bottle.

Children under 5 years (and some older children) find a liquid formulation more acceptable than tablets or capsules. However, for long-term treatment it may be possible for a child to be taught to take tablets or capsules.

An oral syringe (see below) should be used for accurate measurement and controlled administration of an oral liquid medicine. The unpleasant taste of an oral liquid can be disguised by flavouring it or by giving a favourite food or drink immediately afterwards, but the potential for food-drug interactions should be considered.

Advice should be given on dental hygiene to those receiving medicines containing cariogenic sugars for long-term treatment; sugar-free medicines should be provided whenever possible.

Children with nasal feeding tubes in place for prolonged periods should be encouraged to take medicines by mouth if possible; enteric feeding should generally be interrupted before the medicine is given (particularly if enteral feeds reduce the absorption of a particular drug). Oral liquids can be given through the tube provided that precautions are taken to guard against blockage; the dose should be washed down with warm water. When a medicine is given through a nasogastric tube to a neonate, **sterile water** must be used to accompany the medicine or to wash it down.

The intravenous route is generally chosen when a medicine cannot be given by mouth; reliable access, often a central vein, should be used for children whose treatment involves irritant or inotropic drugs or who need to receive the medicine over a long period or for home therapy. The subcutaneous route is used most commonly for insulin administration. Intramuscular injections should preferably be **avoided** in children, particularly neonates, infants, and young children. However, the intramuscular route may be advantageous for administration of single doses of medicines when intravenous cannulation would be more problematic or painful to the child. Certain drugs, e.g. some vaccines, are only administered intramuscularly.

The intrathecal, epidural and intraosseous routes should be used **only** by staff specially trained to administer medicines by these routes. Local protocols for the management of intrathecal injections must be in place (section 8.1).

**Managing medicines in school** Administration of a medicine during schooltime should be avoided if possible; medicines should be prescribed for once or twice-daily administration whenever practicable. If the medicine needs to be taken in school, this should be discussed with parents or carers and the necessary arrangements made in advance; where appropriate, involvement of a school nurse should be sought. *Managing Medicines in Schools and Early Years Settings* produced by the Department of Health provides guidance on using medicines in schools (www.dh.gov.uk).

**Patient information leaflets** Manufacturers' patient information leaflets that accompany a medicine, cover only the licensed use of the medicine (see *BNF for Children* and Marketing Authorisation, below). Therefore, when a medicine is used outside its licence, it may be appropriate to advise the child and the child's parent or carer that some of the information in the leaflet might not apply to the child's treatment. Where necessary, inappropriate advice in the patient information leaflet should be identified and reassurance provided about the correct use in the context of the child's condition.

**Biosimilar medicines** A biosimilar medicine is a new biological product that is similar to a medicine that has already been authorised to be marketed (the biological reference medicine) in the European Union. The active substance of a biosimilar medicine is similar, but not identical, to the biological reference medicine. Biological products are different from standard chemical products in terms of their complexity and although theoretically there should be no important differences between the biosimilar and biological reference medicine in terms of safety or efficacy, when prescribing biological products, it is good practice to use the brand name. This will ensure that substitution of a biosimilar medicine does not occur when the medicine is dispensed.

Biosimilar medicines have black triangle status (▼, see p. 12) at the time of initial marketing; however, in light of new EU legislation this will change, for latest information see www.mhra.gov.uk. It is important to report suspected adverse reactions to biosimilar medicines using the Yellow Card Scheme (p. 11). For biosimilar medicines, adverse reaction reports should clearly state the brand name and the batch number of the suspected medicine.

**Complementary and alternative medicine** An increasing amount of information on complementary and alternative medicine is becoming available. Where appropriate, the child and the child's carers should be asked about the use of their medicines, including dietary supplements and topical products. The scope of *BNF for Children* is restricted to the discussion of conventional medicines but reference is made to complementary

treatments if they affect conventional therapy (e.g. interactions with St John's wort—see Appendix 1). Further information on herbal medicines is available at www.mhra.gov.uk.

**BNF for Children and marketing authorisation** Where appropriate the *doses, indications, cautions, contra-indications,* and *side-effects* in *BNF for Children* reflect those in the manufacturers' Summaries of Product Characteristics (SPCs) which, in turn, reflect those in the corresponding marketing authorisations (formerly known as Product Licences). *BNF for Children* does not generally include proprietary medicines that are not supported by a valid Summary of Product Characteristics or when the marketing authorisation holder has not been able to supply essential information. When a preparation is available from more than one manufacturer, *BNF for Children* reflects advice that is the most clinically relevant regardless of any variation in the marketing authorisation. Unlicensed products can be obtained from 'special-order' manufacturers or specialist importing companies, see p. 823.

As far as possible, medicines should be prescribed within the terms of the marketing authorisation. However, many children require medicines not specifically licensed for paediatric use. Although medicines cannot be promoted outside the limits of the licence, the Medicines Act does not prohibit the use of unlicensed medicines.

*BNF for Children* includes advice involving the use of unlicensed medicines or of licensed medicines for unlicensed uses ('off-label' use). Such advice reflects careful consideration of the options available to manage a given condition and the weight of evidence and experience of the unlicensed intervention (see also Unlicensed Medicines, p. 6). Where the advice falls outside a drug's marketing authorisation, *BNF for Children* shows the licensing status in the drug monograph. However, limitations of the marketing authorisation should not preclude unlicensed use where clinically appropriate.

> **Prescribing unlicensed medicines**
> Prescribing unlicensed medicines or medicines outside the recommendations of their marketing authorisation alters (and probably increases) the prescriber's professional responsibility and potential liability. The prescriber should be able to justify and feel competent in using such medicines.

**Drugs and skilled tasks** Prescribers and other healthcare professionals should advise children and their carers if treatment is likely to affect their ability to perform skilled tasks (e.g. driving). This applies especially to drugs with sedative effects; patients should be warned that these effects are increased by alcohol. General information about a patient's fitness to drive is available from the Driver and Vehicle Licensing Agency at www.dvla.gov.uk.

**Oral syringes** An **oral syringe** is supplied when oral liquid medicines are prescribed in doses other than multiples of 5 mL. The oral syringe is marked in 0.5-mL divisions from 1 to 5 mL to measure doses of less than 5 mL (other sizes of oral syringe may also be available). It is provided with an adaptor and an instruction leaflet. The *5-mL spoon* is used for doses of 5 mL (or multiples thereof).

**Excipients** Branded oral liquid preparations that do not contain *fructose, glucose,* or *sucrose* are described as 'sugar-free' in *BNF for Children*. Preparations containing hydrogenated glucose syrup, mannitol, maltitol, sorbitol, or xylitol are also marked 'sugar-free' since they do not cause dental caries. Children receiving medicines containing cariogenic sugars, or their carers, should be advised of dental hygiene measures to prevent caries. Sugar-free preparations should be used whenever possible, particularly if treatment is required for a long period.

Where information on the presence of *alcohol, aspartame, gluten, sulfites, tartrazine, arachis (peanut) oil* or *sesame oil* is available, this is indicated in *BNF for Children* against the relevant preparation.

Information is provided on *selected excipients* in skin preparations (section 13.1.3), in vaccines (section 14.1), and on *selected preservatives* and *excipients* in eye drops and injections.

The presence of *benzyl alcohol* and *polyoxyl castor oil* (polyethoxylated castor oil) in injections is indicated in *BNF for Children*. Benzyl alcohol has been associated with a fatal toxic syndrome in preterm neonates, and therefore, parenteral preparations containing the preservative should not be used in neonates. Polyoxyl castor oils, used as vehicles in intravenous injections, have been associated with severe anaphylactoid reactions.

The presence of *propylene glycol* in oral or parenteral medicines is indicated in *BNF for Children*; it can cause adverse effects if its elimination is impaired, e.g. in renal failure, in neonates and young children, and in slow metabolisers of the substance. It may interact with metronidazole.

The *lactose* content in most medicines is too small to cause problems in most lactose-intolerant children. However in severe lactose intolerance, the lactose content should be determined before prescribing. The amount of lactose varies according to manufacturer, product, formulation, and strength.

> **Important**
> In the absence of information on excipients in *BNF for Children* and in the product literature (available at www.medicines.org.uk/emc/), contact the manufacturer (see Index of Manufacturers) if it is essential to check details.

**Health and safety** When handling chemical or biological materials particular attention should be given to the possibility of allergy, fire, explosion, radiation, or poisoning. Care is required to avoid sources of heat (including hair dryers) when flammable substances are used on the skin or hair. Substances, such as corticosteroids, some antimicrobials, phenothiazines, and many cytotoxics, are irritant or very potent and should be handled with caution; contact with the skin and inhalation of dust should be avoided. Healthcare professionals and carers should guard against exposure to sensitising, toxic or irritant substances if it is necessary to crush tablets or open capsules.

**EEA and Swiss prescriptions** Pharmacists can dispense prescriptions issued by doctors and dentists from the European Economic Area (EEA) or Switzerland (except prescriptions for controlled drugs in Schedules 1, 2, or 3, or for drugs without a UK marketing authorisation). Prescriptions should be written in ink or otherwise so as to be indelible, should be dated, should state the name of the patient, should state the address of the prescriber, should contain particulars indicating whether the prescriber is a doctor or dentist, and should be signed by the prescriber.

**Security and validity of prescriptions** The Councils of the British Medical Association and the Royal Pharmaceutical Society have issued a joint statement on the security and validity of prescriptions.

In particular, prescription forms should:

- not be left unattended at reception desks;
- not be left in a car where they may be visible; and
- when not in use, be kept in a locked drawer within the surgery and at home.

Where there is any doubt about the authenticity of a prescription, the pharmacist should contact the prescriber. If this is done by telephone, the number should be obtained from the directory rather than relying on the information on the prescription form, which may be false.

**Patient group direction (PGD)** In most cases, the most appropriate clinical care will be provided on an individual basis by a prescriber to a specific child. However, a Patient Group Direction for supply and administration of medicines by other healthcare professionals can be used where it would benefit the child's care without compromising safety.

A Patient Group Direction is a written direction relating to the supply and administration (or administration only) of a licensed prescription-only medicine (including some Controlled Drugs in specific circumstances) by certain classes of healthcare professionals; the Direction is signed by a doctor (or dentist) and by a pharmacist. Further information on Patient Group Directions is available in Health Service Circular HSC 2000/026 (England), HDL (2001) 7 (Scotland), and WHC (2000) 116 (Wales) and at www.nelm.nhs.uk/en/Communities/NeLM/PGDs; see also the Human Medicines Regulations 2012.

**NICE and Scottish Medicines Consortium** Advice issued by the National Institute for Health and Care Excellence (NICE) is included in *BNF for Children* when relevant. *BNF for Children* also includes advice issued by the Scottish Medicines Consortium (SMC) when a medicine is restricted or not recommended for use within NHS Scotland. If advice within a NICE Single Technology Appraisal differs from SMC advice, the Scottish Executive expects NHS Boards within NHS Scotland to comply with the SMC advice. Details of the advice together with updates can be obtained from www.nice.org.uk and from www.scottishmedicines.org.uk.

# Prescription writing

> **Shared care**
> In its guidelines on responsibility for prescribing (circular EL (91) 127) between hospitals and general practitioners, the Department of Health has advised that legal responsibility for prescribing lies with the doctor who signs the prescription.

Prescriptions[1] should be written legibly in ink or otherwise so as to be indelible[2], should be dated, should state the full name and address of the patient, the address of the prescriber, an indication of the type of prescriber, and should be signed in ink by the prescriber[3]. The age and the date of birth of the child should preferably be stated, and it is a legal requirement in the case of prescription-only medicines to state the age for children under 12 years.

Wherever appropriate the prescriber should state the current weight of the child to enable the dose prescribed to be checked. Consideration should also be given to including the dose per unit mass e.g. mg/kg or the dose per m$^2$ body-surface area e.g. mg/m$^2$ where this would reduce error.

The following should be noted:

(a) The strength or quantity to be contained in capsules, lozenges, tablets, etc. should be stated by the prescriber. In particular, strengths of liquid preparations should be clearly stated (e.g. 125 mg/5 mL).

(b) The unnecessary use of decimal points should be avoided, e.g. 3 mg, not 3.0 mg.
   Quantities of 1 gram or more should be written as 1 g, etc.
   Quantities less than 1 gram should be written in milligrams, e.g. 500 mg, not 0.5 g.
   Quantities less than 1 mg should be written in micrograms, e.g. 100 micrograms, not 0.1 mg.
   When decimals are unavoidable a zero should be written in front of the decimal point where there is no other figure, e.g. 0.5 mL, not .5 mL.
   Use of the decimal point is acceptable to express a range, e.g. 0.5 to 1 g.

(c) 'Micrograms' and 'nanograms' should **not** be abbreviated. Similarly 'units' should **not** be abbreviated.

(d) The term 'millilitre' (ml or mL)[4] is used in medicine and pharmacy, and cubic centimetre, c.c., or cm$^3$ should not be used.

(e) Dose and dose frequency should be stated; in the case of preparations to be taken 'as required' a **minimum dose interval** should be specified.
   Care should be taken to ensure the child receives the correct dose of the active drug. Therefore, the dose should normally be stated in terms of the mass of the active drug (e.g. '125 mg 3 times daily'); terms

such as '5 mL' or '1 tablet' should be avoided except for compound preparations.
When doses other than multiples of 5 mL are prescribed for *oral liquid preparations* the dose-volume will be provided by means of an **oral syringe**, see p. 2 (except for preparations intended to be measured with a pipette).

(f) For suitable quantities of dermatological preparations, see section 13.1.2.

(g) The names of drugs and preparations should be written clearly and **not** abbreviated, using approved titles **only** (see also advice in box on p. 5 to **avoid** creating generic titles for modified-release preparations).

(h) The quantity to be supplied may be stated by indicating the number of days of treatment required in the box provided on NHS forms. In most cases the exact amount will be supplied. This does not apply to items directed to be used as required—if the dose and frequency are not given then the quantity to be supplied needs to be stated.
   When several items are ordered on one form the box can be marked with the number of days of treatment provided the quantity is added for any item for which the amount cannot be calculated.

(i) Although directions should preferably be in **English without abbreviation**, it is recognised that some Latin abbreviations are used (for details see Inside Back Cover).

For a sample prescription, see below.

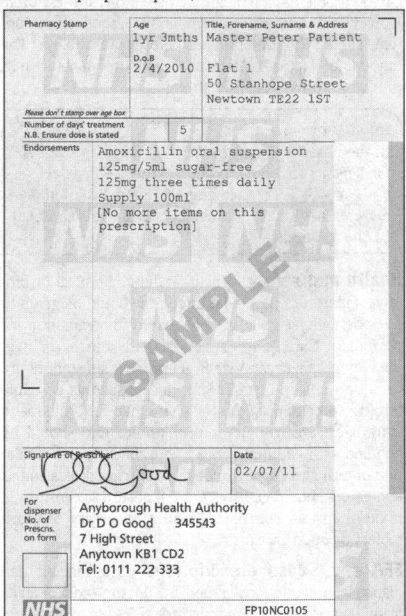

1. These recommendations are acceptable for **prescription-only medicines** (PoM). For items marked CD2, CD3, CD4-1, and CD4-2, see also Prescribing Controlled Drugs, p. 8.
2. It is permissible to issue carbon copies of NHS prescriptions as long as they are signed in ink.
3. Computer-generated facsimile signatures do not meet the legal requirement.
4. The use of capital 'L' in mL is a printing convention throughout *BNF for Children*; both 'mL' and 'ml' are recognised SI abbreviations.

**Abbreviation of titles**  In general, titles of drugs and preparations should be written *in full*. Unofficial abbreviations should **not** be used as they may be misinterpreted.

**Non-proprietary titles** Where non-proprietary ('generic') titles are given, they should be used for prescribing. This will enable any suitable product to be dispensed, thereby saving delay to the patient and sometimes expense to the health service. The only exception is where there is a demonstrable difference in clinical effect between each manufacturer's version of the formulation, making it important that the child should always receive the same brand; in such cases, the brand name or the manufacturer should be stated.

---

### Non-proprietary names of compound preparations

Non-proprietary names of **compound preparations** which appear in *BNF for Children* are those that have been compiled by the British Pharmacopoeia Commission or another recognised body; whenever possible they reflect the names of the active ingredients. Prescribers should avoid creating their own compound names for the purposes of generic prescribing; such names do not have an approved definition and can be misinterpreted.

Special care should be taken to avoid errors when prescribing compound preparations; in particular the hyphen in the prefix 'co-' should be retained.

Special care should also be taken to avoid creating generic names for **modified-release** preparations where the use of these names could lead to confusion between formulations with different duration of action.

---

# Supply of medicines

When supplying a medicine for a child, the pharmacist should ensure that the child and the child's carer understand the nature and identity of the medicine and how it should be used. The child and the carer should be provided with appropriate information (e.g. how long the medicine should be taken for and what to do if a dose is missed or the child vomits soon after the dose is given).

**Safety in the home**  Carers and relatives of children must be warned to keep all medicines out of the reach and sight of children. Tablets, capsules and oral and external liquid preparations must be dispensed in a reclosable *child-resistant container* unless:

- the medicine is in an original pack or patient pack such as to make this inadvisable;
- the child's carer will have difficulty in opening a child-resistant container;
- a specific request is made that the product shall not be dispensed in a child-resistant container;
- no suitable child-resistant container exists for a particular liquid preparation.

All patients should be advised to dispose of *unwanted medicines* by returning them to a pharmacy for destruction.

**Labelling of prescribed medicines**  There is a legal requirement for the following to appear on the label of any prescribed medicine:

- name of the patient;
- name and address of the person dispensing the medicine;
- date of dispensing;
- name of the medicine;
- directions for use of the medicine;
- precautions relating to the use of the medicine;
- the words 'Keep out of the reach of children' (or a similar warning);
- where applicable, the words 'For external use only'.

A pharmacist can exercise professional skill and judgement to amend or include more appropriate wording for the name of the medicine, the directions for use, or the precautions relating to the use of the medicine. The Royal Pharmaceutical Society advises that the labels of dispensed medicines should indicate the total quantity of the product dispensed in the container to which the label refers. This requirement applies equally to solid, liquid, internal, and external preparations. If a product is dispensed in more than one container, the reference should be to the amount in each container.

**Unlicensed medicines**  A drug or formulation that is not covered by a marketing authorisation (see also *BNF for Children* and Marketing Authorisation) may be obtained from a pharmaceutical company, imported by a specialist importer, manufactured by a commercial or hospital licensed manufacturing unit (see Special-order Manufacturers, p. 823), or prepared extemporaneously (see below) against a prescription.

The safeguards that apply to products with marketing authorisation should be extended, as far as possible, to the use of unlicensed medicines. The safety, efficacy, and quality (including labelling) of unlicensed medicines should be assured by means of clear policies on their prescribing, purchase, supply, and administration. Extra care is required with unlicensed medicines because less information may be available on the drug and any formulation of the drug.

The following should be agreed with the supplier when ordering an unlicensed or extemporaneously prepared medicine:

- the specification of the formulation;
- documentation confirming the specification and quality of the product supplied (e.g. a certificate of conformity or of analysis);
- for imported preparations product and licensing information should be supplied in English.

**Extemporaneous preparations**  A product should be dispensed extemporaneously only when no product with a marketing authorisation is available. Every effort should be made to ensure that an extemporaneously prepared product is stable and that it delivers the requisite dose reliably; the child should be provided with a consistent formulation regardless of where the medicine is supplied to minimise variations in quality. Where there is doubt about the formulation, advice should be sought from a medicines information centre, the pharmacy at a children's hospital, a hospital production unit, a hospital quality control department, or the manufacturer.

In many cases it is preferable to give a licensed product by an unlicensed route (e.g. an injection solution given by mouth) than to prepare a special formulation. When tablets or capsules are cut, dispersed, or used for preparing liquids immediately before administration, it is important to confirm uniform dispersal of the active ingredient, especially if only a portion of the solid content (e.g. a tablet segment) is used or if only an aliquot of the liquid is to be administered.

In some cases the child's clinical condition may require a dose to be administered in the absence of full information on the method of administration. It is important to ensure that the appropriate supporting information is available at the earliest opportunity.

Preparation of products that produce harmful dust (e.g. cytotoxic drugs, hormones, or potentially sensitising drugs such as neomycin) should be **avoided** or undertaken with appropriate precautions to protect staff and carers (see also Safety in the Home, above).

The BP direction that a preparation must be *freshly prepared* indicates that it must be made not more than 24 hours before it is issued for use. The direction that a preparation should be *recently prepared* indicates that deterioration is likely if the preparation is stored for longer than about 4 weeks at 15–25° C.

The term **water** used without qualification means either potable water freshly drawn direct from the public supply and suitable for drinking or freshly boiled and cooled purified water. The latter should be used if the public supply is from a local storage tank or if the potable water is unsuitable for a particular preparation. See also Water for Injections, section 9.2.2.

# Emergency supply of medicines

## Emergency supply requested by member of the public

Pharmacists are sometimes called upon by members of the public to make an emergency supply of medicines. The Human Medicines Regulations 2012 allow exemptions from the Prescription Only requirements for emergency supply to be made by a person lawfully conducting a retail pharmacy business provided:

(a) that the pharmacist has interviewed the person requesting the prescription-only medicine and is satisfied:

  (i) that there is immediate need for the prescription-only medicine and that it is impracticable in the circumstances to obtain a prescription without undue delay;

  (ii) that treatment with the prescription-only medicine has on a previous occasion been prescribed for the person requesting it;

  (iii) as to the dose that it would be appropriate for the person to take;

(b) that no greater quantity shall be supplied than will provide 5 days' treatment of phenobarbital, phenobarbital sodium, or Controlled Drugs in Schedules 4 or 5,[1] or 30 days' treatment for other prescription-only medicines, except when the prescription-only medicine is:

  (i) insulin, an ointment or cream, or a preparation for the relief of asthma in an aerosol dispenser when the smallest pack can be supplied;

  (ii) an oral contraceptive when a full cycle may be supplied;

  (iii) an antibiotic in liquid form for oral administration when the smallest quantity that will provide a full course of treatment can be supplied;

(c) that an entry shall be made by the pharmacist in the prescription book stating:

  (i) the date of supply;

  (ii) the name, quantity, and, where appropriate, the pharmaceutical form and strength;

  (iii) the name and address of the patient;

  (iv) the nature of the emergency;

(d) that the container or package must be labelled to show:

  (i) the date of supply;

  (ii) the name, quantity, and, where appropriate, the pharmaceutical form and strength;

  (iii) the name of the patient;

  (iv) the name and address of the pharmacy;

  (v) the words 'Emergency supply';

  (vi) the words 'Keep out of the reach of children' (or similar warning);

(e) that the prescription-only medicine is not a substance specifically excluded from the emergency supply provision, and does not contain a Controlled Drug specified in Schedules 1, 2, or 3 to the Misuse of Drugs Regulations 2001 except for phenobarbital or phenobarbital sodium for the treatment of epilepsy: for details see *Medicines, Ethics and Practice*, London, Pharmaceutical Press (always consult latest edition).[1]

## Emergency supply requested by prescriber

Emergency supply of a prescription-only medicine may also be made at the request of a doctor, a dentist, a supplementary prescriber, a community practitioner nurse prescriber, a nurse, pharmacist or optometrist independent prescriber, or a doctor or dentist from the European Economic Area or Switzerland, provided:

(a) that the pharmacist is satisfied that the prescriber by reason of some emergency is unable to furnish a prescription immediately;

(b) that the prescriber has undertaken to furnish a prescription within 72 hours;

(c) that the medicine is supplied in accordance with the directions of the prescriber requesting it;

(d) that the medicine is not a Controlled Drug specified in Schedules 1, 2, or 3 to the Misuse of Drugs Regulations 2001 except for phenobarbital or phenobarbital sodium for the treatment of epilepsy: for details see *Medicines, Ethics and Practice*, London, Pharmaceutical Press (always consult latest edition);[1]

(e) that an entry shall be made in the prescription book stating:

  (i) the date of supply;

  (ii) the name, quantity, and, where appropriate, the pharmaceutical form and strength;

  (iii) the name and address of the practitioner requesting the emergency supply;

  (iv) the name and address of the patient;

  (v) the date on the prescription;

  (vi) when the prescription is received the entry should be amended to include the date on which it is received.

## Royal Pharmaceutical Society's guidelines

1. The pharmacist should consider the medical consequences of *not* supplying a medicine in an emergency.

2. If the pharmacist is unable to make an emergency supply of a medicine the pharmacist should advise the patient how to obtain essential medical care.

For conditions that apply to supplies made at the request of a patient, see *Medicines, Ethics and Practice*, London, Pharmaceutical Press (always consult latest edition).

---

1. Doctors or dentists from the European Economic Area and Switzerland, or their patients, cannot request an emergency supply of Controlled Drugs in schedules 1, 2, or 3, or drugs that do not have a UK marketing authorisation.

# Prescribing Controlled Drugs

The Misuse of Drugs Act, 1971 prohibits certain activities in relation to 'Controlled Drugs', in particular their manufacture, supply, and possession. The penalties applicable to offences involving the different drugs are graded broadly according to the *harmfulness attributable to a drug when it is misused* and for this purpose the drugs are defined in the following three classes:

**Class A** includes: alfentanil, cocaine, diamorphine (heroin), dipipanone, lysergide (LSD), methadone, methylenedioxymethamfetamine (MDMA, 'ecstasy'), morphine, opium, pethidine, phencyclidine, remifentanil, and class B substances when prepared for injection

**Class B** includes: oral amfetamines, barbiturates, cannabis, cannabis resin, codeine, ethylmorphine, glutethimide, nabilone, pentazocine, phenmetrazine, and pholcodine

**Class C** includes: certain drugs related to the amfetamines such as benzfetamine and chlorphentermine, buprenorphine, diethylpropion, mazindol, meprobamate, pemoline, pipradrol, most benzodiazepines, zolpidem, androgenic and anabolic steroids, clenbuterol, chorionic gonadotrophin (HCG), non-human chorionic gonadotrophin, somatotropin, somatrem, and somatropin

The Misuse of Drugs Regulations 2001 (and subsequent amendments) define the classes of person who are authorised to supply and possess controlled drugs while acting in their professional capacities and lay down the conditions under which these activities may be carried out. In the regulations drugs are divided into five schedules each specifying the requirements governing such activities as import, export, production, supply, possession, prescribing, and record keeping which apply to them.

**Schedule 1** includes drugs such as lysergide which is not used medicinally. Possession and supply are prohibited except in accordance with Home Office authority.

**Schedule 2** includes drugs such as diamorphine (heroin), morphine, nabilone, remifentanil, pethidine, secobarbital, glutethimide, amfetamine, and cocaine and are subject to the full controlled drug requirements relating to prescriptions, safe custody (except for secobarbital), the need to keep registers, etc. (unless exempted in Schedule 5).

**Schedule 3** includes the barbiturates (except secobarbital, now Schedule 2), buprenorphine, diethylpropion, mazindol, meprobamate, midazolam, pentazocine, phentermine, and temazepam. They are subject to the special prescription requirements (except for temazepam) and to the safe custody requirements (except for any 5,5 disubstituted barbituric acid (e.g. phenobarbital), mazindol, meprobamate, midazolam, pentazocine, phentermine, or any stereoisomeric form or salts of the above). Records in registers do not need to be kept (although there are requirements for the retention of invoices for 2 years).

**Schedule 4** includes in Part I benzodiazepines (except temazepam and midazolam which are in Schedule 3) and zolpidem, which are subject to minimal control. Part II includes androgenic and anabolic steroids, clenbuterol, chorionic gonadotrophin (HCG), non-human chorionic gonadotrophin, somatotropin, somatrem, and somatropin. Controlled Drug prescription requirements do not apply (but see Department of Health Guidance, p. 9) and Schedule 4 Controlled Drugs are not subject to safe custody requirements.

**Schedule 5** includes those preparations which, because of their strength, are exempt from virtually all Controlled Drug requirements other than retention of invoices for two years.

**Prescriptions** Preparations in Schedules 2, 3, and 4 of the Misuse of Drugs Regulations 2001 (and subsequent amendments) are identified throughout *BNF for Children* using the following symbols:

- CD2 for preparations in Schedule 2;
- CD3 for preparations in Schedule 3;
- CD4-1 for preparations in Schedule 4 (Part I);
- CD4-2 for preparations in Schedule 4 (Part II). The principal legal requirements relating to medical prescriptions are listed below (see also Department of Health Guidance, p. 9).

---

**Prescription requirements**

Prescriptions for Controlled Drugs that are subject to prescription requirements[1] must be indelible[2] and must be *signed* by the prescriber, *be dated*, and specify the prescriber's *address*. The prescription must always state:

- The name and address of the patient;
- In the case of a preparation, the form[3] and where appropriate the strength[4] of the preparation;
- either the total quantity (in both words and figures) of the preparation,[5] or the number (in both words and figures) of dosage units, as appropriate, to be supplied; in any other case, the total quantity (in both words and figures) of the Controlled Drug to be supplied;
- The dose;[6]
- The words 'for dental treatment only' if issued by a dentist.

---

A pharmacist is **not** allowed to dispense a Controlled Drug unless all the information required by law is given on the prescription. In the case of a prescription for a Controlled Drug in Schedule 2 or 3, a pharmacist can amend the prescription if it specifies the total quantity only in words or in figures or if it contains minor typographical errors, provided that such amendments

1. All preparations in Schedules 2 and 3, except temazepam.
2. A machine-written prescription is acceptable. The prescriber's signature must be handwritten.
3. The dosage form (e.g. tablets) must be included on a Controlled Drugs prescription irrespective of whether it is implicit in the proprietary name (e.g. *MST Continus*) or whether only one form is available.
4. When more than one strength of a preparation exists the strength required must be specified.
5. The Home Office has advised that quantities of liquid preparations such as methadone mixture should be written in millilitres.
6. The instruction 'one as directed' constitutes a dose but 'as directed' does not.

are indelible and clearly attributable to the pharmacist.[1] Failure to comply with the regulations concerning the writing of prescriptions will result in inconvenience to patients and carers and delay in supply of the necessary medicine. A prescription for a Controlled Drug in Schedules 2, 3, or 4 is valid for 28 days from the date stated thereon.[2]

**Instalments and 'repeats'** A prescription may order a Controlled Drug to be dispensed by instalments; the amount of instalments and the intervals to be observed must be specified.[3]

Instalment prescriptions must be dispensed in accordance with the directions in the prescription. However, the Home Office has approved specific wording which may be included in an instalment prescription to cover certain situations; for example, if a pharmacy is closed on the day when an instalment is due. For details see *Medicines, Ethics and Practice*, London, Pharmaceutical Press (always consult latest edition) or see *Drug Misuse and Dependence: UK Guidelines on Clinical Management* (2007), available at www.nta.nhs.uk/uploads/clinical_-guidelines_2007.pdf.

Prescriptions ordering 'repeats'on the same form are **not** permitted for Controlled Drugs in Schedules 2 or 3.

**Private prescriptions** Private prescriptions for Controlled Drugs in Schedules 2 and 3 must be written on specially designated forms provided by Primary Care Trusts in England, Health Boards in Scotland, Local Health Boards in Wales or the Northern Ireland Central Services Agency; in addition, prescriptions must specify the *prescriber's identification number*. Prescriptions to be supplied by a pharmacist in hospital are exempt from the requirement for private prescriptions.

**Department of Health guidance** Guidance (June 2006) issued by the Department of Health in England on prescribing and dispensing of Controlled Drugs requires:

- in general, prescriptions for Controlled Drugs in Schedules 2, 3, and 4 to be limited to a supply of up to 30 days' treatment; exceptionally, to cover a justifiable clinical need and after consideration of any risk, a prescription can be issued for a longer period, but the reasons for the decision should be recorded on the patient's notes;

- the patient's identifier to be shown on NHS and private prescriptions for Controlled Drugs in Schedules 2 and 3.

Further information is available at www.gov.uk/dh.

---

1. Implementation date for *N. Ireland* not confirmed.
2. The prescriber may forward-date the prescription; the start date may also be specified in the body of the prescription.
3. A total of 14 days' treatment by instalment of any drug listed in Schedule 2 of the Misuse of Drugs Regulations, buprenorphine and diazepam may be prescribed in England. In *England*, forms FP10(MDA) (blue) and FP10H (MDA) (blue) should be used. In *Scotland*, forms GP10 (peach), HBP (blue), or HBPA (pink) should be used. In *Wales* a total of 14 days' treatment by instalment of any drug listed in Schedules 2–5 of the Misuse of Drugs Regulations may be prescribed. In Wales, form WP10(MDA) or form WP10HP(AD) should be used.

For a sample prescription, see below..

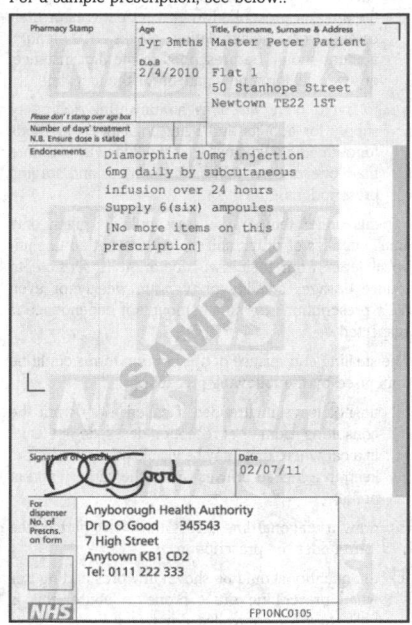

**Dependence and misuse** The most serious drugs of addiction are **cocaine**, **diamorphine** (heroin), **morphine**, and the **synthetic opioids**.

Despite marked reduction in the prescribing of **amfetamines** there is concern that abuse of illicit amfetamine and related compounds is widespread.

**Benzodiazepines** are commonly misused. However, the misuse of **barbiturates** is now uncommon because of their declining medicinal use and consequent availability.

**Cannabis** (Indian hemp) has no approved medicinal use and cannot be prescribed by doctors. Its use is illegal but widespread. Cannabis is a mild hallucinogen seldom accompanied by a desire to increase the dose; withdrawal symptoms are unusual. **Lysergide** (lysergic acid diethylamide, LSD) is a much more potent hallucinogen; its use can lead to severe psychotic states which can be life-threatening.

There are concerns over increases in the availability and the misuse of other drugs with variously combined hallucinogenic, anaesthetic, or sedative properties. These include ketamine and gamma-hydroxybutyrate (sodium oxybate, GHB).

**Prescribing drugs likely to cause dependence or misuse** The prescriber has three main responsibilities:

- to avoid creating dependence by introducing drugs to patients without sufficient reason. In this context, the proper use of the morphine-like drugs is well understood. The dangers of other Controlled Drugs are less clear because recognition of dependence is not easy and its effects, and those of withdrawal, are less obvious;

- to see that the patient does not gradually increase the dose of a drug, given for good medical reasons, to the point where dependence becomes more likely. The prescriber should keep a close eye on the amount prescribed to prevent patients or their carers from accumulating stocks. A minimal amount should be prescribed in the first instance, or when seeing a new patient for the first time;

- to avoid being used as an unwitting source of supply for addicts and being vigilant to methods for obtaining medicines which include visiting more than one doctor, fabricating stories, and forging prescriptions.

Patients under temporary care should be given only small supplies of drugs unless they present an unequivocal letter from their own doctor. It is sensible to reduce dosages steadily or to issue weekly or even daily prescriptions for small amounts if dependence is suspected.

The stealing and misuse of prescription forms could be minimised by the following precautions:

(a) do not leave unattended if called away from the consulting room or at reception desks; do not leave in a car where they may be visible; when not in use, keep in a locked drawer within the surgery and at home;

(b) draw a diagonal line across the blank part of the form under the prescription;

(c) the quantity should be shown in words and figures when prescribing drugs prone to abuse; this is obligatory for controlled drugs (see Prescriptions, above);

(d) alterations are best avoided but if any are made they should be clear and unambiguous; add initials against altered items;

(e) if prescriptions are left for collection they should be left in a safe place in a sealed envelope.

**Travelling abroad**  Prescribed drugs listed in Schedule 4 Part II (CD Anab) and Schedule 5 of the Misuse of Drugs Regulations 2001 are not subject to export or import licensing. However, patients intending to travel abroad for more than 3 months carrying any amount of drugs listed in Schedules 2, 3, or 4 Part I (CD Benz) will require a personal export/import licence. Further details can be obtained at www.homeoffice.gov.uk/drugs/licensing/personal, or from the Home Office by contacting licensing_enquiry.aadu@homeoffice.gsi.gov.uk (in cases of emergency, telephone (020) 7035 6330).

Applications must be supported by a covering letter from the prescriber and should give details of:

- the patient's name and current address;

- the quantities of drugs to be carried;

- the strength and form in which the drugs will be dispensed;

- the country or countries of destination;

- the dates of travel to and from the United Kingdom.

Applications for licences should be sent to the Home Office, Drugs Licensing, Peel Building, 2 Marsham Street, London, SW1P 4DF. Alternatively, completed application forms can be emailed to licensing_enquiry.aadu@homeoffice.gsi.gov.uk with a scanned copy of the covering letter from the prescriber. A minimum of two weeks should be allowed for processing the application.

Patients travelling for less than 3 months do not require a personal export/import licence for carrying Controlled Drugs, but are advised to carry a letter from the prescribing doctor. Those travelling for more than 3 months are advised to make arrangements to have their medication prescribed by a practitioner in the country they are visiting.

Doctors who wish to take Controlled Drugs abroad while accompanying patients may similarly be issued with licences. Licences are not normally issued to doctors who wish to take Controlled Drugs abroad solely in case a family emergency should arise.

Personal export/import licences do not have any legal status outside the UK and are issued only to comply with the Misuse of Drugs Act and facilitate passage through UK Customs and Excise control. For clearance in the country to be visited it would be necessary to approach that country's consulate in the UK.

## Notification of drug misusers

Doctors should report cases of drug misuse to their regional or national drug misuse database or centre—for further advice and contact telephone numbers consult the BNF.

# Adverse reactions to drugs

Any drug may produce unwanted or unexpected adverse reactions. Rapid detection and recording of adverse drug reactions is of vital importance so that unrecognised hazards are identified promptly and appropriate regulatory action is taken to ensure that medicines are used safely. Healthcare professionals and coroners (see also Self-reporting, below) are urged to report suspected adverse drug reactions directly to the Medicines and Healthcare products Regulatory Agency (MHRA) through the Yellow Card Scheme using the electronic form at www.mhra.gov.uk/yellowcard. Alternatively, prepaid Yellow Cards for reporting are available from the address below and are also bound in this book (inside back cover).

Send Yellow Cards to:
FREEPOST YELLOW CARD
(No other address details required)
Tel: 0800 731 6789

Suspected adverse drug reactions to *any* therapeutic agent should be reported, including drugs *(self-medication* as well as those *prescribed)*, blood products, vaccines, radiographic contrast media, complementary and herbal products. For biosimilar medicines and vaccines, adverse reaction reports should clearly state the brand name and the batch number of the suspected medicine or vaccine.

The reporting of **all** suspected adverse drug reactions, no matter how minor, in children under 18 years, including those relating to unlicensed or off-label use of medicines, is **strongly encouraged** through the Yellow Card Scheme even if the intensive monitoring symbol (▼, see below) has been removed. This is because experience in children may still be limited.

The identification and reporting of adverse reactions to drugs in children is particularly important because:

- the action of the drug and its pharmacokinetics in children (especially in the very young) may be different from that in adults;

- drugs may not be extensively tested in children;

- children may be more susceptible to developmental disorders or they may have delayed adverse reactions which do not occur in adults;

- many drugs are not specifically licensed for use in children and are used 'off-label';

- suitable formulations may not be available to allow precise dosing in children;

- the nature and course of illnesses and adverse drug reactions may differ between adults and children.

Spontaneous reporting is particularly valuable for recognising possible new hazards rapidly. An adverse reaction should be reported even if it is not certain that the drug has caused it, or if the reaction is well recognised, or if other drugs have been given at the same time. Reports of overdoses (deliberate or accidental) can complicate the assessment of adverse drug reactions, but provide important information on the potential toxicity of drugs.

A 24-hour Freephone service is available to all parts of the UK for advice and information on suspected adverse drug reactions; contact the National Yellow Card Information Service at the MHRA on 0800 731 6789. Outside office hours a telephone-answering machine will take messages.

The following Yellow Card Centres can be contacted for further information:

Yellow Card Centre Northwest
2nd Floor
70 Pembroke Place
Liverpool L69 3GF
Tel: (0151) 794 8122

Yellow Card Centre Northern & Yorkshire
Wolfson Unit
Claremont Place
Newcastle upon Tyne NE2 4HH
Tel: (0191) 260 6182

Yellow Card Centre Wales
Cardiff University
Department of Pharmacology, Therapeutics and Toxicology
Heath Park
Cardiff CF14 4XN
Tel: (029) 2074 4181

Yellow Card Centre West Midlands
City Hospital
Dudley Road
Birmingham B18 7QH
Tel: (0121) 507 5672

Yellow Card Centre Scotland
CARDS, Royal Infirmary of Edinburgh
51 Little France Crescent
Old Dalkeith Road
Edinburgh EH16 4SA
Tel: (0131) 242 2919

The MHRA's database facilitates the monitoring of adverse drug reactions.

More detailed information on reporting and a list of products currently under intensive monitoring can be found on the MHRA website: www.mhra.gov.uk.

> **MHRA Drug Safety Update**
> Drug Safety Update is a monthly newsletter from the MHRA and the Commission on Human Medicines (CHM); it is available at www.mhra.gov.uk/drugsafetyupdate.

**Self-reporting** Patients and their carers can also report suspected adverse drug reactions to the MHRA. Reports can be submitted directly to the MHRA through the Yellow Card Scheme using the electronic form at www.mhra.gov.uk/yellowcard or by telephone on 0808 100 3352. Alternatively, patient Yellow Cards are available from pharmacies and GP surgeries, or can be downloaded from www.mhra.gov.uk, where more detailed information on patient reporting is available. Information for patients about the Yellow Card Scheme is available in other languages at www.mhra.gov.uk/yellowcard.

**Prescription-event monitoring** In addition to the MHRA's Yellow Card Scheme, an independent scheme monitors the safety of new medicines using a different approach. The Drug Safety Research Unit identifies patients who have been prescribed selected new med-

Adverse reactions to drugs

icines and collects data on clinical events in these patients. The data are submitted on a voluntary basis by general practitioners on green forms. More information about the scheme and the Unit's educational material is available from www.dsru.org.

**Newer drugs and vaccines** Only limited information is available from clinical trials on the safety of new medicines. Further understanding about the safety of medicines depends on the availability of information from routine clinical practice.

The black triangle symbol (▼) identifies newly licensed medicines that are monitored intensively by the MHRA; however, in light of new EU legislation this will change, for latest information see www.mhra.gov.uk. Such medicines include new active substances, biosimilar medicines, medicines that have been licensed for administration by a new route or drug delivery system, or for significant new indications which may alter the established risks and benefits of that drug, or that contain a new combination of active substances. There is no standard time for which products retain a black triangle; safety data are usually reviewed after 2 years.

**Adverse reactions to medical devices** Suspected adverse reactions to medical devices including dental or surgical materials, intra-uterine devices, and contact lens fluids should be reported. Information on reporting these can be found at: www.mhra.gov.uk.

**Side-effects in the *BNF for Children*** The *BNF for Children* includes clinically relevant side-effects for most drugs; an exhaustive list is not included for drugs that are used by specialists (e.g. cytotoxic drugs and drugs used in anaesthesia). Where causality has not been established, side-effects in the manufacturers' literature may be omitted from the *BNF for Children*.

In the product literature the frequency of side-effects is generally described as follows:

| | |
|---|---|
| Very common | greater than 1 in 10 |
| Common | 1 in 100 to 1 in 10 |
| Uncommon ['less commonly' in BNF for Children] | 1 in 1000 to 1 in 100 |
| Rare | 1 in 10 000 to 1 in 1000 |
| Very rare | less than 1 in 10 000 |

## Special problems

**Symptoms** Children may be poor at expressing the symptoms of an adverse drug reaction and parental opinion may be required.

**Delayed drug effects** Some reactions (e.g. cancers and effects on development) may become manifest months or years after exposure. Any suspicion of such an association should be reported directly to the MHRA through the Yellow Card Scheme.

**Congenital abnormalities** When an infant is born with a congenital abnormality or there is a malformed aborted fetus doctors are asked to consider whether this might be an adverse reaction to a drug and to report all drugs (including self-medication) taken during pregnancy.

## Prevention of adverse reactions

Adverse reactions may be prevented as follows:

- never use any drug unless there is a good indication. If the patient is pregnant do not use a drug unless the need for it is imperative;

- allergy and idiosyncrasy are important causes of adverse drug reactions. Ask if the child has had previous reactions to the drug or formulation;

- prescribe as few drugs as possible and give very clear instructions to the child, parent, or carer;

- whenever possible use a familiar drug; with a new drug be particularly alert for adverse reactions or unexpected events;

- consider if excipients (e.g. colouring agents) may be contributing to the adverse reaction. If the reaction is minor, a trial of an alternative formulation of the same drug may be considered before abandoning the drug;

- obtain a full drug history including asking if the child is already taking other drugs *including over-the-counter medicines*; interactions may occur;

- age and hepatic or renal disease may alter the metabolism or excretion of drugs, particularly in neonates, which can affect the potential for adverse effects. Genetic factors may also be responsible for variations in metabolism, and therefore for the adverse effects of the drug;

- warn the child, parent, or carer if serious adverse reactions are liable to occur.

## Defective medicines

During the manufacture or distribution of a medicine an error or accident may occur whereby the finished product does not conform to its specification. While such a defect may impair the therapeutic effect of the product and could adversely affect the health of a patient, it should **not** be confused with an Adverse Drug Reaction where the product conforms to its specification.

The Defective Medicines Report Centre assists with the investigation of problems arising from licensed medicinal products thought to be defective and co-ordinates any necessary protective action. Reports on suspect defective medicinal products should include the brand or the non-proprietary name, the name of the manufacturer or supplier, the strength and dosage form of the product, the product licence number, the batch number or numbers of the product, the nature of the defect, and an account of any action already taken in consequence. The Centre can be contacted at:

The Defective Medicines Report Centre
Medicines and Healthcare products Regulatory Agency
151 Buckingham Palace Road
London, SW1W 9SZ
Tel: (020) 3080 6588
info@mhra.gsi.gov.uk

# Prescribing in hepatic impairment

Children have a large reserve of hepatic metabolic capacity and modification of the choice and dosage of drugs is usually unnecessary even in apparently severe liver disease. However, special consideration is required in the following situations:

- liver failure characterised by severe derangement of liver enzymes and profound jaundice; the use of sedative drugs, opioids, and drugs such as diuretics and amphotericin which produce hypokalaemia may precipitate hepatic encephalopathy;

- impaired coagulation, which can affect response to oral anticoagulants;

- in cholestatic jaundice elimination may be impaired of drugs such as fusidic acid and rifampicin which are excreted in the bile;

- in hypoproteinaemia, the effect of highly protein-bound drugs such as phenytoin, prednisolone, warfarin, and benzodiazepines may be increased;

- use of hepatotoxic drugs is more likely to cause toxicity in children with liver disease; such drugs should be avoided if possible;

- in neonates, particularly preterm neonates, and also in infants metabolic pathways may differ from older children and adults because liver enzyme pathways may be immature.

Where care is needed when prescribing in hepatic impairment, this is indicated under the relevant drug in *BNF for Children*.

# Prescribing in renal impairment

The use of drugs in children with reduced renal function can give rise to problems for several reasons:

- reduced renal excretion of a drug or its metabolites may produce toxicity;

- sensitivity to some drugs is increased even if elimination is unimpaired;

- many side-effects are tolerated poorly by children with renal impairment;

- some drugs are not effective when renal function is reduced;

- neonates, particularly preterm, may have immature renal function.

Many of these problems can be avoided by reducing the dose or by using alternative drugs.

## Principles of dose adjustment in renal impairment

The level of renal function below which the dose of a drug must be reduced depends on the proportion of the drug eliminated by renal excretion and its toxicity.

For many drugs with only minor or no dose-related side-effects, very precise modification of the dose regimen is unnecessary and a simple scheme for dose reduction is sufficient

For more toxic drugs with a small safety margin dose regimens based on glomerular filtration rate should be used. When both efficacy and toxicity are closely related to plasma-drug concentration, recommended regimens should be regarded only as a guide to initial treatment; subsequent doses must be adjusted according to clinical response and plasma-drug concentration.

The total daily maintenance dose of a drug can be reduced either by reducing the size of the individual doses or by increasing the interval between doses. For some drugs, although the size of the maintenance dose is reduced it is important to give a loading dose if an immediate effect is required. This is because it takes

about five times the half-life of the drug to achieve steady-state plasma concentration. Because the plasma half-life of drugs excreted by the kidney is prolonged in renal impairment, it can take many doses at the reduced dosage to achieve a therapeutic plasma concentration. The loading dose should usually be the same as the initial dose for a child with normal renal function.

**Nephrotoxic drugs** should, if possible, be avoided in children with renal disease because the consequences of nephrotoxicity are likely to be more serious when the renal reserve is already reduced.

Glomerular filtration rate is low at birth and increases rapidly during the first 6 months. Thereafter, glomerular filtration rate increases gradually to reach adult levels by 1–2 years of age, when standardised to a typical adult body surface area ($1.73\,m^2$). In the first weeks after birth, serum creatinine falls; a single measure of serum creatinine provides only a crude estimate of renal function and observing the change over days is of more use. In the neonate, a sustained rise in serum creatinine or a lack of the expected postnatal decline, is indicative of a reduced glomerular filtration rate.

Dose recommendations are based on the severity of renal impairment. This is expressed in terms of **glomerular filtration rate** ($mL/minute/1.73\,m^2$).

The following equations provide a guide to glomerular filtration rate.

Child over 1 year:
Estimated glomerular filtration rate ($mL/minute/1.73\,m^2$)= $40^1$ × height (cm)/serum creatinine (micromol/litre)

Neonate:
Estimated glomerular filtration rate ($mL/minute/1.73\,m^2$)= $30^1$ × height (cm)/serum creatinine (micromol/litre)

---

1. The values used in these formulas may differ according to locality or laboratory.

The serum-creatinine concentration is sometimes used as a measure of renal function but is only a **rough guide** even when corrected for age, weight, and sex.

> **Important**
> The information on dose adjustment in *BNF for Children* is expressed in terms of estimated glomerular filtration rate.
> Renal function in adults is increasingly being reported as estimated glomerular filtration rate (eGFR) normalised to a body surface area of 1.73 m$^2$; however, eGFR is derived from the MDRD (Modification of Diet in Renal Disease) formula which is not validated for use in children. eGFR derived from the MDRD formula should **not** be used to adjust drug doses in children with renal impairment.

In *BNF for Children*, values for measures of renal function are included where possible. However, where such values are not available, the *BNF for Children* reflects the terms used in the published information.

*Chronic kidney disease in **adults**: UK guidelines for identification, management and referral* (March 2006) defines renal function as follows:

| Degree of impairment | eGFR[1] mL/minute/1.73 m$^2$ |
|---|---|
| Normal: Stage 1 | More than 90 (with other evidence of kidney damage) |
| Mild: Stage 2 | 60–89 (with other evidence of kidney damage) |
| Moderate[2]: Stage 3 | 30–59 |
| Severe: Stage 4 | 15–29 |
| Established renal failure: Stage 5 | Less than 15 |

1. Estimated glomerular filtration rate (eGFR) derived from the Modification of Diet in Renal Disease (MDRD) formula for use in patients over 18 years
2. NICE clinical guideline 73 (September 2008)—Chronic kidney disease: Stage 3A eGFR = 45–59, Stage 3B eGFR = 30–44

> **Dialysis**
> For prescribing in children on renal replacement therapy consult specialist literature.

Drug prescribing should be kept to the minimum in all children with severe renal disease.

If even mild renal impairment is considered likely on clinical grounds, renal function should be checked before prescribing **any** drug which requires dose modification.

Where care is needed when prescribing in renal impairment, this is indicated under the relevant drug in *BNF for Children*.

# Prescribing in pregnancy

Drugs can have harmful effects on the fetus at any time during pregnancy. It is important to bear this in mind when prescribing for a female of *childbearing age* or for men *trying to father* a child.

During the *first trimester* drugs may produce congenital malformations (teratogenesis), and the period of greatest risk is from the third to the eleventh week of pregnancy.

During the *second* and *third trimesters* drugs may affect the growth and functional development of the fetus or have toxic effects on fetal tissues; and drugs given shortly before term or during labour may have adverse effects on labour or on the neonate after delivery.

*BNF for Children* identifies drugs which:

- may have harmful effects in pregnancy and indicates the trimester of risk;
- are not known to be harmful in pregnancy.

The information is based on human data but information on *animal* studies has been included for some drugs when its omission might be misleading. Maternal drug doses may require adjustment during pregnancy due to changes in maternal physiology but this is beyond the scope of *BNF for Children*.

Where care is needed when prescribing in pregnancy, this is indicated under the relevant drug in *BNF for Children*.

> **Important**
> Drugs should be prescribed in pregnancy only if the expected benefit to the mother is thought to be greater than the risk to the fetus, and all drugs should be avoided if possible during the first trimester. Drugs which have been extensively used in pregnancy and appear to be usually safe should be prescribed in preference to new or untried drugs; and the smallest effective dose should be used.
>
> Few drugs have been shown conclusively to be teratogenic in humans but no drug is safe beyond all doubt in early pregnancy. Screening procedures are available where there is a known risk of certain defects.
>
> **Absence of information does not imply safety.**
> It should be noted that *BNF for Children* provides independent advice and may not always agree with the product literature.
>
> Information on drugs and pregnancy is also available from the UK Teratology Information Service, www. uktis.org
>
> Tel: 0844 892 0909 (09:00–17:00 Monday to Friday; urgent enquiries only outside these hours).

# Prescribing in breast-feeding

Breast-feeding is beneficial; the immunological and nutritional value of breast milk to the infant is greater than that of formula feeds.

Although there is concern that drugs taken by the mother might affect the infant, there is very little information on this. In the absence of evidence of an effect, the potential for harm to the infant can be inferred from:

- the amount of drug or active metabolite of the drug delivered to the infant (dependent on the pharmacokinetic characteristics of the drug in the mother);
- the efficiency of absorption, distribution and elimination of the drug by the infant (infant pharmacokinetics);
- the nature of the effect of the drug on the infant (pharmacodynamic properties of the drug in the infant).

Most medicines given to a mother cause no harm to breast-fed infants and there are few contra-indications to breast-feeding when maternal medicines are necessary. However, administration of some drugs to nursing mothers can harm the infant. In the first week of life, some such as preterm or jaundiced infants are at a slightly higher risk of toxicity.

Toxicity to the infant can occur if the drug enters the milk in pharmacologically significant quantities. The concentration in milk of some drugs (e.g. fluvastatin) may exceed the concentration in maternal plasma so that therapeutic doses in the mother can cause toxicity to the infant. Some drugs inhibit the infant's sucking reflex (e.g. phenobarbital) while others can affect lactation (e.g. bromocriptine). Drugs in breast milk may, at least theoretically, cause hypersensitivity in the infant even when concentration is too low for a pharmacological effect. *BNF for Children* identifies drugs:

- which should be used with caution or which are contra-indicated in breast-feeding for the reasons given above;
- which, on present evidence, may be given to the mother during breast-feeding, because they appear in milk in amounts which are too small to be harmful to the infant;
- which are not known to be harmful to the infant although they are present in milk in significant amounts.

Where care is needed when prescribing in breast-feeding, this is indicated under the relevant drug in *BNF for Children*.

> **Important**
> For many drugs insufficient evidence is available to provide guidance and it is advisable to administer only essential drugs to a mother during breast-feeding. Because of the inadequacy of information on drugs in breast milk information in *BNF for Children* should be used only as a guide; absence of information does not imply safety.

# Prescribing in palliative care

Palliative care is the active total care of children and young adults who have incurable, life-limiting conditions and are not expected to survive beyond young adulthood.

The child may be cared for in a hospice or at home according to the needs of the child and the child's family. In all cases, children should receive total care of their physical, emotional, social, and spiritual needs, and their families should be supported throughout. In particular, specialist palliative care is essential for end-of-life care of the child and for supporting the family through death and bereavement.

**Drug treatment** The number of drugs should be as few as possible. Oral medication is usually appropriate unless there is severe nausea and vomiting, dysphagia, weakness, or coma, when parenteral medication may be necessary.

## Pain

Pain management in palliative care is focused on achieving control of pain by administering the right drug in the right dose at the right time. Analgesics can be divided into three broad classes: non-opioid (paracetamol, NSAID), opioid (e.g. codeine 'weak', morphine 'strong') and adjuvant (e.g. antidepressants, antiepileptics). Drugs from the different classes are used alone or in combination according to the type of pain and response to treatment. Analgesics are more effective in preventing pain than in the relief of established pain; it is important that they are given regularly.

Paracetamol (p. 200) or a NSAID (p. 500) given regularly will often be sufficient to manage mild pain. If non-opioid analgesics alone are not sufficient, then an opioid analgesic alone or in combination with a non-opioid analgesic at an adequate dosage, may be helpful in the control of moderate pain. Codeine (p. 205) or tramadol (p. 211) can be considered for moderate pain. If these preparations do not control the pain then morphine (p. 208) is the most useful opioid analgesic. Alternatives to morphine, including transdermal buprenorphine (p. 205), transdermal fentanyl (p. 207), hydromorphone (p. 208), methadone (p. 208), or oxycodone (p. 210), should be initiated by those with experience in palliative care. Initiation of an opioid analgesic should not be delayed by concern over a theoretical likelihood of psychological dependence (addiction).

**Bone metastases** In addition to the above approach, radiotherapy and bisphosphonates, (p. 388), may be useful for pain due to bone metastases.

**Neuropathic pain** Patients with neuropathic pain (p. 213) may benefit from a trial of a tricyclic antidepressant, most commonly amitriptyline (p. 185), for several weeks. An antiepileptic such as carbamazepine (p. 219), may be added or substituted if pain persists. Ketamine is sometimes used under specialist supervision for neuropathic pain that responds poorly to opioid analgesics. Pain due to nerve compression may be reduced by a corticosteroid such as dexamethasone, which reduces oedema around the tumour, thus reducing compression. Nerve blocks can be considered when pain is localised to a specific area. Transcutaneous electrical nerve stimulation (TENS) may also help.

## Pain management with opioids

**Oral route** Treatment with morphine is given by mouth as immediate-release or modified-release preparations. During the titration phase the initial dose is based on the previous medication used, the severity of the pain, and other factors such as presence of renal impairment or frailty. The dose is given either as an immediate-release preparation 4-hourly (for starting doses, see Morphine, p. 208), or as a 12-hourly modified-release preparation, in addition to rescue doses. The starting dose of 12-hourly modified-release preparations is usually 200–800 micrograms/kg every 12 hours. If replacing a weaker opioid analgesic (such as codeine), starting doses are usually higher.

If pain occurs between regular doses of morphine ('breakthrough pain'), an additional dose ('rescue dose') of immediate-release morphine should be given. An additional dose should also be given 30 minutes before an activity that causes pain, such as wound dressing. The standard dose of a strong opioid for breakthrough pain is usually one-tenth to one-sixth of the regular 24-hour dose, repeated every 2–4 hours as required (up to hourly may be needed if pain is severe or in the last days of life). Review pain management if rescue analgesic is required frequently (twice daily or more). Each child should be assessed on an individual basis. Formulations of fentanyl that are administered nasally, buccally or sublingually are not licensed for use in children; their usefulness in children is also limited by dose availability.

Children often require a higher dose of morphine in proportion to their body-weight compared to adults. Children are more susceptible to certain adverse effects of opioids such as urinary retention (which can be eased by bethanechol), and opioid-induced pruritus.

When adjusting the dose of morphine, the number of rescue doses required and the response to them should be taken into account; increments of morphine should not exceed one-third to one-half of the total daily dose every 24 hours. Thereafter, the dose should be adjusted with careful assessment of the pain, and the use of adjuvant analgesics should also be considered. Upward titration of the dose of morphine stops when either the pain is relieved or unacceptable adverse effects occur, after which it is necessary to consider alternative measures.

Once their pain is controlled, children started on 4-hourly immediate-release morphine can be transferred to the same total 24-hour dose of morphine given as the modified-release preparation for 12-hourly or 24-hourly administration. The first dose of the modified-release preparation is given with, or within 4 hours of the last dose of the immediate-release preparation. For preparations suitable for 12-hourly or 24-hourly administration see modified-release preparations under Morphine, (p. 208). Increments should be made to the dose, not to the frequency of administration. The patient must be monitored closely for efficacy and side-effects, particularly constipation, and nausea and vomiting. A suitable laxative (p. 56) should be prescribed routinely.

Oxycodone (p. 210) can be used in children who require an opioid but cannot tolerate morphine. If the child is already receiving an opioid, oxycodone should be started at a dose equivalent to the current analgesic (see below). Oxycodone immediate-release preparations can be given for breakthrough pain.

## Equivalent doses of opioid analgesics

This is only an **approximate** guide (doses may not correspond with those given in clinical practice); children should be carefully monitored after any change in medication and dose titration may be required

| Analgesic | Route | Dose |
|---|---|---|
| Codeine | PO | 100 mg |
| Diamorphine | IM, IV, SC | 3 mg |
| Dihydrocodeine | PO | 100 mg |
| Hydromorphone | PO | 2 mg |
| Morphine | PO | 10 mg |
| Morphine | IM, IV, SC | 5 mg |
| Oxycodone | PO | 6.6 mg |
| Tramadol | PO | 100 mg |

PO = by mouth; IM = intramuscular, IV = intravenous, SC= subcutaneous

**Parenteral route** Diamorphine (p. 206) is preferred for injection because, being more soluble, it can be given in a smaller volume. The equivalent subcutaneous dose is approximately a third of the oral dose of morphine. Subcutaneous infusion of diamorphine via a continuous infusion device can be useful (for details, see Continuous Subcutaneous Infusions), (p. 19).

If the child can resume taking medicines by mouth, then oral morphine may be substituted for subcutaneous infusion of diamorphine. See table of Approximate Equivalent doses of Morphine and Diamorphine, (p. 20).

**Rectal route** Morphine is also available for rectal administration as suppositories.

**Transdermal route** Transdermal preparations of fentanyl (p. 207) and buprenorphine [not licensed for use in children] are available; they are not suitable for acute pain or in those children whose analgesic requirements are changing rapidly because the long time to steady state prevents rapid titration of the dose. Prescribers should ensure that they are familiar with the correct use of transdermal preparations (see under fentanyl) because inappropriate use has caused fatalities.

The following 24-hour oral doses of morphine are considered to be *approximately* equivalent to the buprenorphine and fentanyl patches shown, however when switching due to possible opioid-induced hyperalgesia, reduce the calculated equivalent dose of the new opioid by one-quarter to one-half.

## Buprenorphine patches are *approximately* equivalent to the following 24-hour doses of oral morphine

| | | |
|---|---|---|
| morphine salt 12 mg daily | ≡ *BuTrans*® '5' patch | 7-day patches |
| morphine salt 24 mg daily | ≡ *BuTrans*® '10' patch | 7-day patches |
| morphine salt 48 mg daily | ≡ *BuTrans*® '20' patch | 7-day patches |
| morphine salt 84 mg daily | ≡ *Transtec*® '35' patch | 4-day patches |
| morphine salt 126 mg daily | ≡ *Transtec*® '52.5' patch | 4-day patches |
| morphine salt 168 mg daily | ≡ *Transtec*® '70' patch | 4-day patches |

Note Conversion ratios vary and these figures are a guide only. Morphine equivalences for transdermal opioid preparations have been approximated to allow comparison with available preparations of oral morphine

## 72-hour Fentanyl patches are *approximately* equivalent to the following 24-hour doses of oral morphine

| | |
|---|---|
| morphine salt 30 mg daily | ≡ fentanyl '12' patch |
| morphine salt 60 mg daily | ≡ fentanyl '25' patch |
| morphine salt 120 mg daily | ≡ fentanyl '50' patch |
| morphine salt 180 mg daily | ≡ fentanyl '75' patch |
| morphine salt 240 mg daily | ≡ fentanyl '100' patch |

Note Fentanyl equivalences in this table are for children on well-tolerated opioid therapy for long periods, see Transdermal Route above, and section 4.7.2; fentanyl patches should not be used in opioid naive children. Conversion ratios vary and these figures are a guide only. Morphine equivalences for transdermal opioid preparations have been approximated to allow comparison with available preparations of oral morphine

## Symptom control

**Unlicensed indications or routes**
Several recommendations in this section involve unlicensed indications or routes.

**Anorexia** Anorexia may be helped by prednisolone or dexamethasone.

**Anxiety** Anxiety can be treated with a long-acting benzodiazepine such as diazepam, or by continuous infusion of the short-acting benzodiazepine midazolam. Interventions for more acute episodes of anxiety (such as panic attacks) include short-acting benzodiazepines such as lorazepam given sublingually or midazolam given subcutaneously. Temazepam provides useful night-time sedation in some children.

**Capillary bleeding** Capillary bleeding can be treated with tranexamic acid (p. 121) by mouth; treatment is usually continued for one week after the bleeding has stopped but it can be continued at a reduced dose if bleeding persists. Alternatively, gauze soaked in tranexamic acid 100 mg/mL or adrenaline (epinephrine) solution 1 mg/mL (1 in 1000) can be applied to the affected area.

Vitamin K may be useful for the treatment and prevention of bleeding associated with prolonged clotting in liver disease. In severe chronic cholestasis, absorption of vitamin K may be impaired; either parenteral or water-soluble oral vitamin K should be considered (section 9.6.6).

**Constipation** Constipation is a common cause of distress and is almost invariable after administration of an opioid analgesic. It should be prevented if possible by the regular administration of laxatives. Suitable laxatives include osmotic laxatives (p. 60) (such as lactulose or macrogols), stimulant laxatives (p. 58) (such as co-danthramer and senna) or the combination of lactulose and a senna preparation. Naloxone given by mouth may help relieve opioid-induced constipation; it is poorly absorbed but opioid withdrawal reactions have been reported.

**Convulsions** Intractable seizures are relatively common in children dying from non-malignant conditions. Phenobarbital by mouth or as a continuous subcutaneous infusion may be beneficial; continuous infusion of midazolam is an alternative. Both cause drowsiness, but this is rarely a concern in the context of intractable seizures. For breakthrough convulsions diazepam (p. 234) given rectally (as a solution), buccal midazolam (p. 236), or paraldehyde (p. 236) as an enema may be appropriate.

For the use of midazolam by subcutaneous infusion using a continuous infusion device, see p. 19 .

**Dry mouth** Dry mouth may be caused by certain medications including opioid analgesics, antimuscarinic drugs (e.g. hyoscine), antidepressants and some antiemetics; if possible, an alternative preparation should be considered. Dry mouth may be relieved by good mouth care and measures such as chewing sugar-free gum, sucking ice or pineapple chunks, or the use of artificial saliva (p. 550); dry mouth associated with candidiasis can be treated by oral preparations of nystatin (p. 548) or miconazole (p. 548); alternatively, fluconazole (p. 304) can be given by mouth.

**Dysphagia** A corticosteroid such as dexamethasone may help, temporarily, if there is an obstruction due to tumour. See also Dry Mouth, above.

**Dyspnoea** Breathlessness at rest may be relieved by regular oral morphine in carefully titrated doses. Diazepam may be helpful for dyspnoea associated with anxiety. Sublingual lorazepam or subcutaneous or buccal midazolam are alternatives. A nebulised short-acting beta$_2$ agonist (section 3.1.1.1) or a corticosteroid (section 3.2), such as dexamethasone or prednisolone, may also be helpful for bronchospasm or partial obstruction.

**Excessive respiratory secretion** Excessive respiratory secretion (death rattle) may be reduced by hyoscine hydrobromide patches (p. 198) or by subcutaneous or intravenous injection of hyoscine hydrobromide 10 micrograms/kg (max. 600 micrograms) every 4 to 8 hours; however, care must be taken to avoid the discomfort of dry mouth. Alternatively, glycopyrronium (p. 636) may be given.

For the administration of hyoscine hydrobromide by subcutaneous or intravenous infusion using a continuous infusion device, see p. 19.

**Fungating tumours** Fungating tumours can be treated by regular dressing and antibacterial drugs; systemic treatment with metronidazole (p. 298) is often required to reduce malodour, but topical metronidazole (p. 589) is also used.

**Gastro-intestinal pain** The pain of bowel colic may be reduced by loperamide (p. 46). Hyoscine hydrobromide (p. 38) may also be helpful in reducing the frequency of spasms; it is given sublingually at a dose of 10 micrograms/kg (max. 300 micrograms) 3 times daily as *Kwells*® tablets. For the dose by subcutaneous infusion, see p. 19.

Gastric distension pain due to pressure on the stomach may be helped by a preparation incorporating an antacid with an antiflatulent (p. 35) and a prokinetic such as domperidone (p. 40) before meals.

**Hiccup** Hiccup due to gastric distension may be helped by a preparation incorporating an antacid with an antiflatulent (p. 35)

**Hypercalcaemia** See section 9.5.1.2.

**Insomnia** Children with advanced cancer may not sleep because of discomfort, cramps, night sweats, joint stiffness, or fear. There should be appropriate treatment of these problems before hypnotics (p. 168) are used. Benzodiazepines, such as temazepam, may be useful.

**Intractable cough** Intractable cough may be relieved by moist inhalations or by regular administration of oral morphine every 4 hours. Methadone linctus should be avoided because it has a long duration of action and tends to accumulate.

**Mucosal bleeding** Mucosal bleeding from the mouth and nose occurs commonly in the terminal phase, particularly in a child suffering from haemopoietic malignancy. Bleeding from the nose caused by a single bleeding point can be arrested by cauterisation or by dressing it. Tranexamic acid (p. 121) may be effective applied topically or given systemically.

**Muscle spasm** The pain of muscle spasm can be helped by a muscle relaxant such as diazepam (p. 517) or baclofen (p. 516).

**Nausea and vomiting** Nausea and vomiting are common in children with advanced cancer. Ideally, the cause should be determined before treatment with an antiemetic (section 4.6) is started.

Nausea and vomiting with opioid therapy are less common in children than in adults but may occur particularly in the initial stages and can be prevented by giving an antiemetic. An antiemetic is usually necessary only for the first 4 or 5 days and therefore combined preparations containing an opioid with an antiemetic are not recommended because they lead to unnecessary antiemetic therapy (and associated side-effects when used long-term).

Metoclopramide has a prokinetic action and is used by mouth for nausea and vomiting associated with gastritis, gastric stasis, and functional bowel obstruction. Drugs with antimuscarinic effects antagonise prokinetic drugs and, if possible, should not therefore be used concurrently.

Haloperidol (p. 174) is used by mouth or by continuous intravenous or subcutaneous infusion for most metabolic causes of vomiting (e.g. hypercalcaemia, renal failure).

Cyclizine (p. 193) is used for nausea and vomiting due to mechanical bowel obstruction, raised intracranial pressure, and motion sickness.

Ondansetron (p. 197) is most effective when the vomiting is due to damaged or irritated gut mucosa (e.g. after chemotherapy or radiotherapy).

Antiemetic therapy should be reviewed every 24 hours; it may be necessary to substitute the antiemetic or to add another one.

Levomepromazine (p. 175) can be used if first-line antiemetics are inadequate. Dexamethasone by mouth can be used as an adjunct.

For the administration of antiemetics by subcutaneous infusion using a continuous infusion device, see below.

For the treatment of nausea and vomiting associated with cancer chemotherapy, see section 8.1.

**Pruritus** Pruritus, even when associated with obstructive jaundice, often responds to simple measures such as application of emollients (p. 554). Ondansetron may be effective in some children. Where opioid analgesics cause pruritus it may be appropriate to review the dose or to switch to an alternative opioid analgesic. In the case of obstructive jaundice, further measures include administration of colestyramine (p. 69).

**Raised intracranial pressure** Headache due to raised intracranial pressure often responds to a high dose of a corticosteroid, such as dexamethasone, for 4 to 5 days, subsequently reduced if possible; dexamethasone should be given before 6 p.m. to reduce the risk of insomnia. Treatment of headache and of associated nausea and vomiting should also be considered.

**Restlessness and confusion** Restlessness and confusion may require treatment with haloperidol (p. 174) 10–20 micrograms/kg by mouth every 8–12 hours. Levomepromazine (p. 175) is also used occasionally for restlessness. See also below.

---

# Continuous subcutaneous infusions

Although drugs can usually be administered *by mouth* to control symptoms in palliative care, the parenteral route may sometimes be necessary. Repeated administration of *intramuscular injections* should be avoided in children, particularly if cachectic. This has led to the use of portable continuous infusion devices such as syringe drivers to give a *continuous subcutaneous infusion*, which can provide good control of symptoms with little discomfort or inconvenience to the patient.

> **Syringe driver rate settings**
> Staff using syringe drivers should be **adequately trained** and different rate settings should be **clearly identified** and **differentiated**; incorrect use of syringe drivers is a common cause of medication errors.

Indications for the **parenteral route** are:

- inability to take medicines by mouth owing to *nausea and vomiting, dysphagia, severe weakness,* or *coma;*

- *malignant bowel obstruction* for which surgery is inappropriate (avoiding the need for an intravenous infusion or for insertion of a nasogastric tube);

- refusal by the child to take regular medication by mouth.

**Bowel colic and excessive respiratory secretions** Hyoscine hydrobromide (p. 198) effectively reduces respiratory secretions and is sedative (but occasionally causes paradoxical agitation); it is given in a *subcutaneous* or *intravenous infusion dose* of 40–60 micrograms/kg/24 hours. Glycopyrronium (p. 636) may also be used.

Hyoscine butylbromide (p. 38) is effective in bowel colic, is less sedative than hyoscine hydrobromide, but is not always adequate for the control of respiratory secretions; it is given by *subcutaneous infusion* (**important:** *hyoscine butylbromide* must not be confused with *hyoscine hydrobromide*, above).

**Convulsions** If a child has previously been receiving an antiepileptic drug *or* has a primary or secondary cerebral tumour *or* is at risk of convulsion (e.g. owing to uraemia) antiepileptic medication should not be stopped. Midazolam (p. 236) is the benzodiazepine antiepileptic of choice for *continuous subcutaneous infusion*.

**Nausea and vomiting** Levomepromazine (p. 175) causes sedation in about 50% of patients. Haloperidol (p. 174) has little sedative effect.

Cyclizine (p. 193) is particularly likely to precipitate if mixed with diamorphine or other drugs (see under Mixing and Compatibility); it is given by *subcutaneous infusion*.

**Pain control** Diamorphine (p. 206) is the preferred opioid since its high solubility permits a large dose to be given in a small volume (see under Mixing and Compatibility). The table on p. 20 shows approximate equivalent doses of morphine and diamorphine.

**Restlessness and confusion** Haloperidol has little sedative effect. Levomepromazine (p. 175) has a sedative effect. Midazolam is a sedative and an antiepileptic that may be suitable for a very restless patient.

**Mixing and compatibility** The general principle that injections should be given into separate sites (and should not be mixed) does not apply to the use of syringe drivers in palliative care. Provided that there is evidence of compatibility, selected injections can be mixed in syringe drivers. Not all types of medication can be used in a subcutaneous infusion. In particular, chlorpromazine, prochlorperazine, and diazepam are **contra-indicated** as they cause skin reactions at the injection site; to a lesser extent cyclizine and levomepromazine also sometimes cause local irritation.

In theory injections dissolved in water for injections are more likely to be associated with pain (possibly owing to their hypotonicity). The use of physiological saline (sodium chloride 0.9%) however increases the likelihood of precipitation when more than one drug is used; moreover subcutaneous infusion rates are so slow (0.1–0.3 mL/hour) that pain is not usually a problem when water is used as a diluent.

Diamorphine can be given by subcutaneous infusion in a strength of up to 250 mg/mL; up to a strength of 40 mg/mL either *water for injections* or *physiological saline* (sodium chloride 0.9%) is a suitable diluent—

above that strength only *water for injections* is used (to avoid precipitation).

The following can be mixed with *diamorphine*:

Cyclizine[1]            Hyoscine hydrobromide
Dexamethasone[2]       Levomepromazine
Haloperidol[3]         Metoclopramide[4]
Hyoscine butylbromide  Midazolam

Subcutaneous infusion solution should be monitored regularly both to check for precipitation (and discoloration) and to ensure that the infusion is running at the correct rate.

## Problems encountered with syringe drivers

The following are problems that may be encountered with syringe drivers and the action that should be taken:

- if the subcutaneous infusion runs *too quickly* check the rate setting and the calculation;

- if the subcutaneous infusion runs *too slowly* check the start button, the battery, the syringe driver, the cannula, and make sure that the injection site is not inflamed;

- if there is an *injection site reaction* make sure that the site does not need to be changed—firmness or swelling at the site of injection is not in itself an indication for change, but pain or obvious inflammation is.

### Equivalent doses of morphine sulfate and diamorphine hydrochloride given over 24 hours

These equivalences are *approximate only* and may need to be adjusted according to response

| MORPHINE | | PARENTERAL DIAMORPHINE |
|---|---|---|
| Oral morphine sulphate | Subcutaneous infusion of morphine sulphate | Subcutaneous infusion of diamorphine hydrochloride |
| over 24 hours | over 24 hours | over 24 hours |
| 30 mg | 15 mg | 10 mg |
| 60 mg | 30 mg | 20 mg |
| 90 mg | 45 mg | 30 mg |
| 120 mg | 60 mg | 40 mg |
| 180 mg | 90 mg | 60 mg |
| 240 mg | 120 mg | 80 mg |
| 360 mg | 180 mg | 120 mg |
| 480 mg | 240 mg | 160 mg |
| 600 mg | 300 mg | 200 mg |
| 780 mg | 390 mg | 260 mg |
| 960 mg | 480 mg | 320 mg |
| 1200 mg | 600 mg | 400 mg |

If breakthrough pain occurs give a subcutaneous injection equivalent to one-tenth to one-sixth of the total 24-hour subcutaneous infusion dose. With an intermittent subcutaneous injection absorption is smoother so that the risk of adverse effects at peak absorption is avoided (an even better method is to use a subcutaneous butterfly needle).

To minimise the risk of infection no subcutaneous infusion solution should be used for longer than 24 hours.

---

1. Cyclizine may precipitate at concentrations above 10 mg/mL *or* in the presence of sodium chloride 0.9% *or* as the concentration of diamorphine relative to cyclizine increases; mixtures of diamorphine and cyclizine are also likely to precipitate after 24 hours.
2. Special care is needed to avoid precipitation of dexamethasone when preparing it.
3. Mixtures of haloperidol and diamorphine are likely to precipitate after 24 hours if haloperidol concentration is above 2 mg/mL.
4. Under some conditions, infusions containing metoclopramide become discoloured; such solutions should be discarded.

# Prescribing in dental practice

Advice on the drug management of dental and oral conditions is covered in the main text. For ease of access, guidance on such conditions is usually identified by means of a relevant heading (e.g. Dental and Orofacial Pain) in the appropriate sections.

The following is a list of topics of particular relevance to dentists.

**General guidance**
  Prescribing by dentists, see BNF
  Oral side-effects of drugs, see BNF
  Medical emergencies in dental practice, see BNF
  Medical problems in dental practice, see BNF
**Drug management of dental and oral conditions**
  **Dental and orofacial pain, p. 199**
  Neuropathic pain, p. 213
  Non-opioid analgesics and compound analgesic preparations, p. 199
  Opioid analgesics, p. 205
  Non-steroidal anti-inflammatory drugs, p. 501

**Oral infections**
  Bacterial infections, p. 245
    Phenoxymethylpenicillin, p. 260
    Broad-spectrum penicillins (amoxicillin and ampicillin), p. 263
    Cephalosporins (cefalexin and cefradine), p. 268
    Tetracyclines, p. 276
    Macrolides (clarithromycin, erythromycin and azithromycin), p. 282
    Clindamycin, p. 285
    Metronidazole, p. 298
    Fusidic acid p. 589
  Fungal infections, p. 548
    Local treatment, p. 548
    Systemic treatment, p. 303
  Viral infections, p. 547
    Herpetic gingivostomatitis, local treatment, p. 547
    Herpetic gingivostomatitis, systemic treatment, p. 324 and p. 547
    Herpes labialis, p. 593

**Anaesthetics, anxiolytics and hypnotics**
  Anaesthesia, sedation, and resuscitation in dental practice, p. 630
  Hypnotics, p. 169
  Sedation for dental procedures, p. 637
  Local anaesthesia, p. 649

**Oral ulceration and inflammation, p. 545**
**Mouthwashes and gargles, p. 549**
**Dry mouth, p. 550**
**Minerals**
  Fluorides, p. 477
**Aromatic inhalations, p. 165**
**Nasal decongestants, p. 544**

**Dental Practitioners' Formulary, p. 810**

Prescribing in dental practice

# Drugs and sport

UK Anti-Doping, the national body responsible for the UK's anti-doping policy, advises that athletes are personally responsible should a prohibited substance be detected in their body. An advice card listing examples of permitted and prohibited substances is available from:

UK Anti-Doping
Oceanic House
1a Cockspur Street
London SW1Y 5BG
Tel: (020) 7766 7350
information@ukad.org.uk
www.ukad.org.uk

> **General Medical Council's advice**
> Doctors who prescribe or collude in the provision of drugs or treatment with the intention of improperly enhancing an individual's performance in sport contravene the GMC's guidance, and such actions would usually raise a question of a doctor's continued registration. This does not preclude the provision of any care or treatment where the doctor's intention is to protect or improve the patient's health.

# Emergency treatment of poisoning

These notes provide only an overview of the treatment of poisoning and it is strongly recommended that either **TOXBASE** or the **UK National Poisons Information Service** (see below) be consulted when there is doubt about the degree of risk or about appropriate management.

Most childhood poisoning is accidental. Other causes include intentional overdose, drug abuse, iatrogenic and deliberate poisoning. The drugs most commonly involved in childhood poisoning are paracetamol, ibuprofen, orally ingested creams, aspirin, iron preparations, cough medicines, and the contraceptive pill.

**Hospital admission** Children who have features of poisoning should generally be admitted to hospital. Children who have taken poisons with delayed actions should also be admitted, even if they appear well. Delayed-action poisons include aspirin, iron, paracetamol, tricyclic antidepressants, and co-phenotrope (diphenoxylate with atropine, *Lomotil®*); the effects of modified-release preparations are also delayed. A note of all relevant information, including what treatment has been given, should accompany the patient to hospital.

## Further information and advice

**TOXBASE**, the primary clinical toxicology database of the National Poisons Information Service, is available on the Internet to registered users at www.toxbase.org (a backup site is available at www.toxbasebackup.org if the main site cannot be accessed). It provides information about routine diagnosis, treatment, and management of patients exposed to drugs, household products, and industrial and agricultural chemicals.

> Specialist information and advice on the treatment of poisoning is available day and night from the **UK National Poisons Information Service** on the following number:
> Tel: 0844 892 0111

Advice on laboratory analytical services can be obtained from TOXBASE or from the National Poisons Information Service.

Help with identifying capsules or tablets may be available from a regional medicines information centre (see inside front cover) or (out of hours) from the National Poisons Information Service.

## General care

It is often impossible to establish with certainty the identity of the poison and the size of the dose. This is not usually important because a few poisons (such as opioids, paracetamol, and iron) have specific antidotes; few children require active removal of the poison. In most children, treatment is directed at managing symptoms as they arise. Nevertheless, knowledge of the type and timing of poisoning can help in anticipating the course of events. All relevant information should be sought from the poisoned child and from their carers.

However, such information should be interpreted with care because it may not be complete or entirely reliable. Sometimes symptoms arise from other illnesses, and children should be assessed carefully. Accidents may involve a number of domestic and industrial products (the contents of which are not generally known). The **National Poisons Information Service** should be consulted when there is doubt about any aspect of suspected poisoning.

## Respiration

Respiration is often impaired in unconscious children. An obstructed airway requires immediate attention. In the absence of trauma, the airway should be opened with simple measures such as chin lift or jaw thrust. An oropharyngeal or nasopharyngeal airway may be useful in children with reduced consciousness to prevent obstruction, provided ventilation is adequate. Intubation and ventilation should be considered in children whose airway cannot be protected or who have respiratory acidosis because of inadequate ventilation; such children should be monitored in a critical care area.

Most poisons that impair consciousness also depress respiration. Assisted ventilation (either mouth-to-mouth or using a bag-valve-mask device) may be needed. Oxygen is not a substitute for adequate ventilation, although it should be given in the highest concentration possible in poisoning with carbon monoxide and irritant gases.

The potential for pulmonary aspiration of gastric contents should be considered.

## Blood pressure

Hypotension is common in severe poisoning with central nervous system depressants; if severe, this may lead to irreversible brain damage or renal tubular necrosis. Hypotension should be corrected initially by raising the foot of the bed and administration of either sodium chloride intravenous infusion or a colloidal infusion. Vasoconstrictor sympathomimetics (section 2.7.2) are rarely required and their use may be discussed with a paediatric intensive care unit.

Fluid depletion without hypotension is common after prolonged coma and after aspirin poisoning due to vomiting, sweating, and hyperpnoea.

Hypertension, often transient, occurs less frequently than hypotension in poisoning; it may be associated with sympathomimetic drugs such as amfetamines, phencyclidine, and cocaine.

## Heart

Cardiac conduction defects and arrhythmias can occur in acute poisoning, notably with tricyclic antidepressants, some antipsychotics, and some antihistamines. Arrhythmias often respond to correction of underlying hypoxia, acidosis, or other biochemical abnormalities, but ventricular arrhythmias that cause serious hypotension may require treatment (section 2.3.1). If the QT interval is prolonged, specialist advice should be sought because the use of some anti-arrhythmic drugs may be inappropriate. Supraventricular arrhythmias are seldom life-threatening and drug treatment is best withheld until the child reaches hospital.

## Body temperature

Hypothermia may develop in patients of any age who have been deeply unconscious for some hours, particularly following overdose with barbiturates or phenothiazines. It may be missed unless core temperature is measured using a low-reading rectal thermometer or by some other means. Hypothermia should be managed by prevention of further heat loss and appropriate rewarming as clinically indicated.

Hyperthermia can develop in children taking CNS stimulants; children are also at risk when taking therapeutic doses of drugs with antimuscarinic properties. Hyperthermia is initially managed by removing all unnecessary clothing and using a fan. Sponging with **tepid** water will promote evaporation. Advice should be sought from the National Poisons Information Service on the management of severe hyperthermia resulting from conditions such as the serotonin syndrome.

Both hypothermia and hyperthermia require **urgent** hospitalisation for assessment and supportive treatment.

## Convulsions

Single short-lived convulsions (lasting less than 5 minutes) do not require treatment. If convulsions are protracted or recur frequently, lorazepam 100 micrograms/kg (max. 4 mg) or diazepam (preferably as emulsion) 300–400 micrograms/kg (max. 10 mg) should be given by slow intravenous injection into a large vein. Benzodiazepines should not be given by the intramuscular route for convulsions. If the intravenous route is not readily available, midazolam can be given by the buccal route or diazepam can be administered as a rectal solution (section 4.8.2).

## Methaemoglobinaemia

Drug- or chemical-induced methaemoglobinaemia should be treated with **methylthioninium chloride** if the methaemoglobin concentration is 30% or higher, *or* if symptoms of tissue hypoxia are present despite oxygen therapy. Methylthioninium chloride reduces the ferric iron of methaemoglobin back to the ferrous iron of haemoglobin; in high doses, methylthioninium can itself cause methaemoglobinaemia.

### ▌ METHYLTHIONINIUM CHLORIDE
(Methylene blue)

**Cautions** children under 3 months more susceptible to methaemoglobinaemia from high doses of methylthioninium; G6PD deficiency (seek advice from National Poisons Information Service); chlorate poisoning (reduces efficacy of methylthioninium); methaemoglobinaemia due to treatment of cyanide poisoning with sodium nitrite (seek advice from National Poisons Information Service); pulse oximetry may give false estimation of oxygen saturation; **interactions:** Appendix 1 (methylthioninium)

**Renal impairment**   use with caution in severe impairment (dose reduction may be required)

**Pregnancy**   no information available, but risk to fetus of untreated methaemoglobinaemia likely to be significantly higher than risk of treatment

**Breast-feeding**   manufacturer advises avoid breast-feeding for up to 6 days after administration—no information available

**Side-effects**   nausea, vomiting, abdominal pain, hyperbilirubinaemia (in infants), chest pain, arrhythmia, hypertension, hypotension, dyspnoea, tachypnoea, headache, dizziness, tremor, confusion, anxiety, agitation, fever, haemolytic anaemia, methaemoglobinaemia, blue-green discoloration of urine, faeces, and skin, mydriasis, sweating

**Indications and dose**

**Drug- or chemical-induced methaemoglobinaemia** (see notes above)

* By slow intravenous injection over 5 minutes

**Neonate** seek advice from National Poisons Information Service

**Child 1–3 months** seek advice from National Poisons Information Service

**Child 3 months–18 years** 1–2 mg/kg, repeated after 30–60 minutes if necessary; seek advice from National Poisons Information Service if further repeat doses required (max. cumulative dose per course 7 mg/kg, or if aniline- or dapsone-induced methaemoglobinaemia, 4 mg/kg)

**Administration**   for *intravenous injection*, may be diluted with Glucose 5% to minimise injection-site pain; not compatible with Sodium Chloride 0.9%

**Proveblue®** (Martindale) PoM
Injection, methylthioninium chloride 5 mg/mL, net price 10-mL amp = £39.38

## Removal and elimination

**Prevention of absorption** Given by mouth, **activated charcoal** can adsorb many poisons in the gastro-intestinal system, thereby reducing their absorption. The **sooner** it is given the **more effective** it is, but it may still be effective up to 1 hour after ingestion of the poison—longer in the case of modified-release preparations or of drugs with antimuscarinic (anticholinergic) properties. It is particularly useful for the prevention of absorption of poisons that are toxic in small amounts such as antidepressants.

A second dose may occasionally be required when blood-drug concentration continues to rise suggesting delayed drug release or delayed gastric emptying.

For the use of charcoal in active elimination techniques, see below.

**Active elimination techniques** Repeated doses of **activated charcoal** by mouth may *enhance the elimination* of some drugs after they have been absorbed; repeated doses are given after overdosage with:

Carbamazepine

Dapsone

Phenobarbital

Quinine

Theophylline

Vomiting should be treated (e.g. with an antiemetic drug) since it may reduce the efficacy of charcoal treatment. In cases of intolerance, the dose may be reduced and the frequency increased but this may compromise efficacy.

Other techniques intended to enhance the elimination of poisons after absorption are only practicable in hospital and are only suitable for a small number of severely poisoned patients. Moreover, they only apply to a limited number of poisons. Examples include:

- haemodialysis for ethylene glycol, lithium, methanol, phenobarbital, salicylates, and sodium valproate
- alkalinisation of the urine for salicylates.

**Removal from the gastro-intestinal tract** Gastric lavage is rarely required as benefit rarely outweighs risk; advice should be sought from the National Poisons Information Service if a significant quantity of iron or lithium has been ingested within the previous hour.

*Whole bowel irrigation* (by means of a bowel cleansing preparation) has been used in poisoning with certain modified-release or enteric-coated formulations, in severe poisoning with lithium salts, and if illicit drugs are carried in the gastro-intestinal tract ('body-packing'). However, it is not clear that the procedure improves outcome and advice should be sought from the National Poisons Information Service.

The administration of **laxatives** alone has no role in the management of the poisoned child and is not a recommended method of gut decontamination. The routine use of a laxative in combination with activated charcoal has mostly been abandoned. Laxatives should not be administered to young children because of the likelihood of fluid and electrolyte imbalance.

## ▎ CHARCOAL, ACTIVATED

**Cautions** drowsy or comatose child (risk of aspiration—ensure airway protected); reduced gastrointestinal motility (risk of obstruction); **not** for poisoning with petroleum distillates, corrosive substances, alcohols, malathion, cyanides, and metal salts including iron and lithium salts

**Side-effects** black stools

**Indications and dose**

### Reduction of absorption of poisons
- By mouth
  - **Neonate** 1 g/kg
  - **Child 1 month–12 years** 1 g/kg (max. 50 g)
  - **Child 12–18 years** 50 g

### Active elimination of poisons
- By mouth
  - **Neonate** 1 g/kg every 4 hours
  - **Child 1 month–12 years** 1 g/kg (max. 50 g) every 4 hours
  - **Child 12–18 years** 50 g every 4 hours

**Administration** suspension or reconstituted powder may be mixed with soft drinks (e.g. caffeine-free diet cola) or fruit juices to mask the taste

**Actidose-Aqua® Advance** (Alliance)
Oral suspension, activated charcoal 1.04 g/5 mL, net price 50-g pack (240 mL) = £8.69

**Carbomix®** (Beacon)
Granules, activated charcoal, net price 50-g pack = £11.90

**Charcodote®** (TEVA UK)
Oral suspension, activated charcoal 1 g/5 mL, net price 50-g pack = £11.88

## Specific drugs

## Alcohol

Features of acute intoxication with alcohol (ethanol) in children include ataxia, dysarthria, nystagmus, and drowsiness, which may progress to coma, with hypotension and acidosis. Aspiration of vomit is a special hazard and hypoglycaemia may occur. Patients are managed supportively, with particular attention to maintaining a clear airway and measures to reduce the risk of aspiration of gastric contents. The blood glucose is measured and glucose given if indicated.

> The **National Poisons Information Service** (Tel: 0844 892 0111) will provide specialist advice on all aspects of poisoning day and night

## Analgesics (non-opioid)

**Aspirin** The main features of salicylate poisoning are hyperventilation, tinnitus, deafness, vasodilatation, and sweating. Coma is uncommon but indicates very severe poisoning. The associated acid-base disturbances are complex.

Treatment must be in hospital, where plasma salicylate, pH, and electrolytes (particularly potassium) can be measured; absorption of aspirin may be slow and the plasma-salicylate concentration may continue to rise for several hours, requiring repeated measurement. Plasma-salicylate concentration may not correlate with clinical severity in children, and clinical and biochemical assessment is necessary. Generally, the clinical severity of poisoning is less below a plasma-salicylate concentration of 500 mg/litre (3.6 mmol/litre) unless there is evidence of metabolic acidosis. Activated charcoal should be given within 1 hour of ingesting more than 125 mg/kg aspirin. Fluid losses should be replaced and intravenous sodium bicarbonate may be given (ensuring plasma-potassium concentration is maintained within the reference range) to enhance urinary salicylate excretion (optimum urinary pH 7.5–8.5); treatment should be given in a high dependency unit.

Plasma-potassium concentration should be corrected before giving sodium bicarbonate as hypokalaemia may complicate alkalinisation of the urine.

Haemodialysis is the treatment of choice for severe salicylate poisoning and should be considered when the plasma-salicylate concentration exceeds 700 mg/litre (5.1 mmol/litre) or in the presence of severe metabolic acidosis, convulsions, renal failure, pulmonary oedema or persistently high plasma-salicylate concentrations unresponsive to urinary alkalinisation.

**NSAIDs** Mefenamic acid has important consequences in overdosage because it can cause convulsions, which if prolonged or recurrent, require treatment with intravenous lorazepam or diazepam.

Emergency treatment of poisoning

Emergency treatment of poisoning

Overdosage with ibuprofen may cause nausea, vomiting, epigastric pain, and tinnitus, but more serious toxicity is very uncommon. Activated charcoal followed by symptomatic measures are indicated if more than 100 mg/kg has been ingested within the preceding hour.

## Paracetamol

> In cases of **intravenous paracetamol** poisoning contact the National Poisons Information Service for advice on risk assessment and management.

Toxic doses of paracetamol may cause severe hepatocellular necrosis and, much less frequently, renal tubular necrosis. Nausea and vomiting, the only early features of poisoning, usually settle within 24 hours. Persistence beyond this time, often associated with the onset of right subcostal pain and tenderness, usually indicates development of hepatic necrosis. Liver damage is maximal 3–4 days after paracetamol overdose and may lead to encephalopathy, haemorrhage, hypoglycaemia, cerebral oedema, and death. Therefore, despite a lack of significant early symptoms, children who have taken an overdose of paracetamol should be transferred to hospital urgently.

To avoid underestimating the potentially toxic paracetamol dose ingested by obese children who weigh more than 110 kg, use a body-weight of 110 kg (rather than their actual body-weight) when calculating the total dose of paracetamol ingested (in mg/kg).

**Acetylcysteine** protects the liver if infused up to, and possibly beyond, 24 hours of ingesting paracetamol. It is most effective if given within 8 hours of ingestion, after which effectiveness declines. Very rarely, giving acetylcysteine by mouth [unlicensed route] is an alternative if intravenous access is not possible—contact the National Poisons Information Service for advice.

**Acute overdose** Hepatotoxicity may occur after a single ingestion of more than 150 mg/kg paracetamol taken in less than 1 hour. Rarely, hepatotoxicity may develop with single ingestions as low as 75 mg/kg of paracetamol taken in less than 1 hour. Children who have ingested 75 mg/kg or more of paracetamol in less than 1 hour should be referred to hospital. Administration of activated charcoal should be considered if paracetamol in excess of 150 mg/kg is thought to have been ingested within the previous hour.

Children at risk of liver damage and, therefore, requiring acetylcysteine, can be identified from a single measurement of the plasma-paracetamol concentration, related to the time from ingestion, provided this time interval is not less than 4 hours; earlier samples may be misleading. The concentration is plotted on a paracetamol treatment graph, with a reference line ('treatment

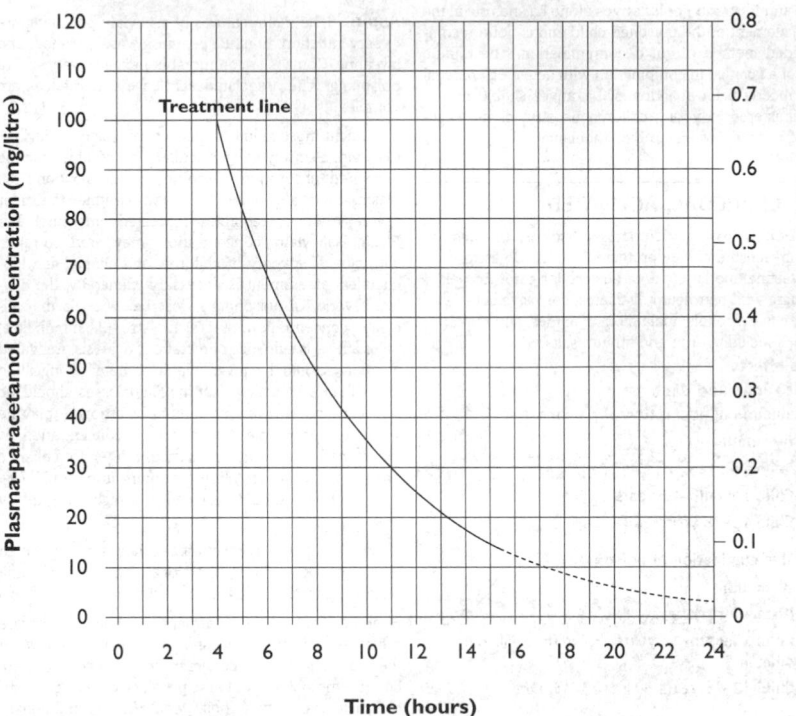

Patients whose plasma-paracetamol concentrations are on or above the **treatment line** should be treated with acetylcysteine by intravenous infusion.

The prognostic accuracy after 15 hours is uncertain, but a plasma-paracetamol concentration on or above the treatment line should be regarded as carrying a serious risk of liver damage.

Graph reproduced courtesy of Medicines and Healthcare products Regulatory Agency line') joining plots of 100 mg/litre (0.66 mmol/litre) at 4 hours and 3.13 mg/litre (0.02 mmol/litre) at 24 hours (see p. 26). Acetylcysteine treatment should commence immediately in children:

- whose plasma-paracetamol concentration falls on or above the *treatment line* on the paracetamol treatment graph (see p. 26);

- who present 8–24 hours after taking an acute overdose of more than 150 mg/kg of paracetamol, even if the plasma-paracetamol concentration is not yet available; acetylcysteine can be discontinued if the plasma-paracetamol concentration is later reported to be below the *treatment line* on the paracetamol treatment graph (see p. 26), provided that the child is asymptomatic and liver function tests, serum creatinine and INR are normal.

The prognostic accuracy of a plasma-paracetamol concentration taken after 15 hours is uncertain, but a concentration on or above the *treatment line* on the paracetamol treatment graph (see p. 26) should be regarded as carrying a serious risk of liver damage. If more than 15 hours have elapsed since ingestion, or there is doubt about appropriate management, advice should be sought from the National Poisons Information Service.

**'Staggered' overdose, uncertain time of overdose, or therapeutic excess** A 'staggered' overdose involves ingestion of a potentially toxic dose of paracetamol over more than one hour. Therapeutic excess is the inadvertent ingestion of a potentially toxic dose of paracetamol during its clinical use. The paracetamol treatment graph is unreliable if a 'staggered' overdose is taken, if there is uncertainty about the time of the overdose, or if there is therapeutic excess. In these cases, children who have taken more than 150 mg/kg of paracetamol in any 24-hour period are at risk of toxicity and should be commenced on acetylcysteine immediately, unless it is more than 24 hours since the last ingestion, the patient is asymptomatic, the plasma-paracetamol concentration is undetectable, and liver function tests, serum creatinine and INR are normal.

Rarely, toxicity can occur with paracetamol doses between 75–150 mg/kg in any 24-hour period; for some children this may be within the licensed dose, but ingestion of a licensed dose of paracetamol is not considered an overdose. Clinical judgement of the individual case is necessary to determine whether to treat those who have ingested this amount of paracetamol.

Although there is some evidence suggesting that factors such as the use of liver enzyme-inducing drugs (e.g. carbamazepine, efavirenz, nevirapine, phenobarbital, phenytoin, primidone, rifabutin, rifampicin, St John's wort), chronic alcoholism, and starvation may increase the risk of hepatotoxicity, the CHM has advised that these should no longer be used in the assessment of paracetamol toxicity.

Significant toxicity is unlikely if, 24 hours or longer after the last paracetamol ingestion, the patient is asymptomatic, the plasma-paracetamol concentration is undetectable, and liver function tests, serum creatinine and INR are normal. Children with clinical features of hepatic injury such as jaundice or hepatic tenderness should be treated urgently with acetylcysteine. If there is uncertainty about a patient's risk of toxicity after paracetamol overdose, treatment with acetylcysteine should be commenced. Advice should be sought from the National Poisons Information Service whenever necessary.

## ◢ ACETYLCYSTEINE

**Cautions** atopy, asthma (see Side-effects below, but do not delay acetylcysteine treatment); acetylcysteine may mildly increase INR and prothrombin time

**Side-effects** hypersensitivity-like reactions managed by reducing infusion rate or suspending until reaction settled (rash also managed by giving antihistamine; acute asthma managed by giving nebulised short-acting beta$_2$ agonist)—contact the National Poisons Information Service if reaction severe; mild increase in INR and prothrombin time

### Indications and dose

**Paracetamol overdosage** see notes above

- **By intravenous infusion**

  **Neonate** initially 150 mg/kg in 3 mL/kg glucose 5% and given over 1 hour, followed by 50 mg/kg in 7 mL/kg glucose 5% and given over 4 hours, then 100 mg/kg in 14 mL/kg glucose 5% and given over 16 hours

  **Child 1 month–18 years**

  **Body-weight under 20 kg** initially 150 mg/kg in 3 mL/kg glucose 5% and given over 1 hour, followed by 50 mg/kg in 7 mL/kg glucose 5% and given over 4 hours, then 100 mg/kg in 14 mL/kg glucose 5% and given over 16 hours

  **Body-weight 20–40 kg** initially 150 mg/kg in 100 mL glucose 5% and given over 1 hour, followed by 50 mg/kg in 250 mL glucose 5% and given over 4 hours, then 100 mg/kg in 500 mL glucose 5% and given over 16 hours

  **Body-weight over 40 kg** see Acetylcysteine Dose and Administration in the *BNF*

**Note** Glucose 5% is preferred infusion fluid; Sodium Chloride 0.9% is an alternative if Glucose 5% unsuitable

**Acetylcysteine** (Non-proprietary) ▣PoM▣
Concentrate for intravenous infusion, acetylcysteine 200 mg/mL, net price 10-mL amp = £1.96

**Parvolex®** (UCB Pharma) ▣PoM▣
Concentrate for intravenous infusion, acetylcysteine 200 mg/mL, net price 10-mL amp = £2.25
Electrolytes Na$^+$ 14 mmol/10-mL amp

> The **National Poisons Information Service** (Tel: 0844 892 0111) will provide specialist advice on all aspects of poisoning day and night

## Analgesics (opioid)

Opioids (narcotic analgesics) cause varying degrees of coma, respiratory depression, and pinpoint pupils. The specific antidote **naloxone** is indicated if there is coma or bradypnoea. Since naloxone has a shorter duration of action than many opioids, close monitoring and repeated injections are necessary according to the respiratory rate and depth of coma. When repeated administration of naloxone is required, it can be given by continuous intravenous infusion instead and the rate of infusion adjusted according to vital signs. All children should be observed for at least 6 hours after the last dose of naloxone. The effects of some opioids, such as buprenorphine, are only partially reversed by naloxone. Dextropropoxyphene and methadone have very long durations of action; patients may need to be monitored for long periods following large overdoses.

Naloxone reverses the opioid effects of dextropropoxyphene; the long duration of action of dextropropoxyphene calls for prolonged monitoring and further doses of naloxone may be required. Norpropoxyphene, a metabolite of dextropropoxyphene, also has cardiotoxic effects which may require treatment with **sodium bicarbonate**, or **magnesium sulfate**, or both; arrhythmias may occur for up to 12 hours.

[1] **Naloxone** (Non-proprietary) (PoM)
Injection, naloxone hydrochloride 20 micrograms/mL, net price 2-mL amp = £5.50; 400 micrograms/mL, net price 1-mL amp = £4.10; 1 mg/mL, 2-mL prefilled syringe = £8.36

[1] **Minijet® Naloxone** (UCB Pharma) (PoM)
Injection, naloxone hydrochloride 400 micrograms/mL, net price 1-mL disposable syringe = £20.40, 2-mL disposable syringe = £12.96, 5-mL disposable syringe = £12.68

## NALOXONE HYDROCHLORIDE

**Cautions** physical dependence on opioids; cardiac irritability; naloxone is short-acting, see notes above
**Pregnancy** section 15.1.7
**Breast-feeding** section 15.1.7
**Indications and dose**

> **Safe Practice**
> Doses used in acute opioid overdosage may not be appropriate for the management of opioid-induced respiratory depression and sedation in those receiving palliative care and in chronic opioid use; see also section 15.1.7 for management of postoperative respiratory depression

> **Overdosage with opioids**
> • **By intravenous injection**
> **Neonate** 10 micrograms/kg; if no response, give subsequent dose of 100 micrograms/kg (then review diagnosis); further doses may be required if respiratory function deteriorates
> **Child 1 month–12 years** 10 micrograms/kg; if no response, give subsequent dose of 100 micrograms/kg (then review diagnosis); further doses may be required if respiratory function deteriorates
> **Child 12–18 years** 0.4–2 mg; if no response, repeat at intervals of 2–3 minutes to a max. of 10 mg (then review diagnosis); further doses may be required if respiratory function deteriorates
> • **By subcutaneous or intramuscular injection**
> As intravenous injection but only if intravenous route not feasible (onset of action slower)
> • **By continuous intravenous infusion using an infusion pump**
> **Neonate** rate adjusted according to response (initially, rate may be set at 60% of the initial resuscitative *intravenous injection* dose per hour)
> **Child 1 month–18 years** rate adjusted according to response (initially, rate may be set at 60% of the initial resuscitative *intravenous injection* dose per hour)
> **Note** The initial resuscitative *intravenous injection* dose is that which maintained satisfactory ventilation for at least 15 minutes

> **Reversal of postoperative respiratory depression, reversal of respiratory and CNS depression in neonate following maternal opioid use during labour** section 15.1.7

**Administration** for *continuous intravenous infusion*, dilute to a concentration of up to 200 micrograms/mL with Glucose 5% *or* Sodium Chloride 0.9%

## Antidepressants

**Tricyclic and related antidepressants** Tricyclic and related antidepressants cause dry mouth, coma of varying degree, hypotension, hypothermia, hyperreflexia, extensor plantar responses, convulsions, respiratory failure, cardiac conduction defects, and arrhythmias. Dilated pupils and urinary retention also occur. Metabolic acidosis may complicate severe poisoning; delirium with confusion, agitation, and visual and auditory hallucinations, are common during recovery.

Assessment in hospital is strongly advised in case of poisoning by *tricyclic and related antidepressants* but symptomatic treatment can be given before transfer. Supportive measures to ensure a clear airway and adequate ventilation during transfer are mandatory. Intravenous lorazepam or diazepam (preferably in emulsion form) may be required to treat convulsions. Activated charcoal given within 1 hour of the overdose reduces absorption of the drug. Although arrhythmias are worrying, some will respond to correction of hypoxia and acidosis. The use of anti-arrhythmic drugs is best avoided, but intravenous infusion of sodium bicarbonate can arrest arrhythmias or prevent them in those with an extended QRS duration. Diazepam given by mouth is usually adequate to sedate delirious children but large doses may be required.

**Selective serotonin re-uptake inhibitors (SSRIs)** Symptoms of poisoning by selective serotonin re-uptake inhibitors include nausea, vomiting, agitation, tremor, nystagmus, drowsiness, and sinus tachycardia; convulsions may occur. Rarely, severe poisoning results in the serotonin syndrome, with marked neuropsychiatric effects, neuromuscular hyperactivity, and autonomic instability; hyperthermia, rhabdomyolysis, renal failure, and coagulopathies may develop.

Management of SSRI poisoning is supportive. Activated charcoal given within 1 hour of the overdose reduces absorption of the drug. Convulsions can be treated with lorazepam, diazepam, or buccal midazolam (see p. 24). Contact the National Poisons Information Service for the management of hyperthermia or the serotonin syndrome.

## Antimalarials

Overdosage with quinine, chloroquine, or hydroxychloroquine is extremely hazardous and difficult to treat. Urgent advice from the National Poisons Information Service is essential. Life-threatening features include arrhythmias (which can have a very rapid onset) and convulsions (which can be intractable).

---

1. (PoM) restriction does not apply where administration is for saving life in emergency

## Beta-blockers

Therapeutic overdosages with beta-blockers may cause lightheadedness, dizziness, and possibly syncope as a result of bradycardia and hypotension; heart failure may be precipitated or exacerbated. These complications are most likely in children with conduction system disorders or impaired myocardial function. Bradycardia is the most common arrhythmia caused by beta-blockers, but sotalol may induce ventricular tachyarrhythmias (sometimes of the torsade de pointes type). The effects of massive overdosage can vary from one beta-blocker to another; propranolol overdosage in particular may cause coma and convulsions.

*Acute massive overdosage* must be managed in hospital and expert advice should be obtained. Maintenance of a clear airway and adequate ventilation is mandatory. An intravenous injection of atropine is required to treat bradycardia (40 micrograms/kg, max. 3 mg). Cardiogenic shock unresponsive to atropine is probably best treated with an intravenous injection of glucagon (50–150 micrograms/kg, max. 10 mg) [unlicensed indication and dose] in glucose 5% (with precautions to protect the airway in case of vomiting) followed by an intravenous infusion of 50 micrograms/kg/hour. If glucagon is not available, intravenous isoprenaline (available from 'special-order' manufacturers or specialist importing companies, see p. 823) is an alternative. A cardiac pacemaker can be used to increase the heart rate.

## Calcium-channel blockers

Features of calcium-channel blocker poisoning include nausea, vomiting, dizziness, agitation, confusion, and coma in severe poisoning. Metabolic acidosis and hyperglycaemia may occur. Verapamil and diltiazem have a profound cardiac depressant effect causing hypotension and arrhythmias, including complete heart block and asystole. The dihydropyridine calcium-channel blockers cause severe hypotension secondary to profound peripheral vasodilatation.

Activated charcoal should be considered if the child presents within 1 hour of overdosage with a calcium-channel blocker; repeated doses of activated charcoal are considered if a modified-release preparation is involved (although activated charcoal may be effective beyond 1 hour with modified-release preparations). In children with significant features of poisoning, calcium chloride or calcium gluconate (section 9.5.1.1) is given by injection; atropine is given to correct symptomatic bradycardia. In severe cases, an insulin and glucose infusion may be required in the management of hypotension and myocardial failure. For the management of hypotension, the choice of inotropic sympathomimetic depends on whether hypotension is secondary to vasodilatation or to myocardial depression—advice should be sought from the National Poisons Information Service (p. 23).

## Hypnotics and anxiolytics

**Benzodiazepines** Benzodiazepines taken alone cause drowsiness, ataxia, dysarthria, nystagmus, and occasionally respiratory depression, and coma. They potentiate the effects of other central nervous system depressants taken concomitantly. Activated charcoal can be given within 1 hour of ingesting a significant quantity of benzodiazepine, provided the child is awake and the airway is protected. Use of the benzodiazepine antagonist flumazenil [unlicensed indication] can be hazardous, particularly in mixed overdoses involving tricyclic antidepressants or in benzodiazepine-dependent patients. Flumazenil may prevent the need for ventilation, particularly in children with severe respiratory disorders; it should be used on expert advice and not as a diagnostic test in children with a reduced level of consciousness.

## Iron salts

Iron poisoning in childhood is usually accidental. The symptoms are nausea, vomiting, abdominal pain, diarrhoea, haematemesis, and rectal bleeding. Hypotension and hepatocellular necrosis can occur later. Coma, shock and metabolic acidosis indicate severe poisoning.

Advice should be sought from the National Poisons Information Service if a significant quantity of iron has been ingested within the previous hour.

Mortality is reduced by intensive and specific therapy with **desferrioxamine**, which chelates iron. The serum-iron concentration is measured as an emergency and intravenous desferrioxamine given to chelate absorbed iron in excess of the expected iron binding capacity. In **severe toxicity** intravenous desferrioxamine should be given *immediately* without waiting for the result of the serum-iron measurement.

> The **National Poisons Information Service** (Tel: 0844 892 0111) will provide specialist advice on all aspects of poisoning day and night

### ◢ DESFERRIOXAMINE MESILATE
(Deferoxamine Mesilate)

**Cautions** section 9.1.3
**Renal impairment** section 9.1.3
**Pregnancy** section 9.1.3
**Breast-feeding** section 9.1.3
**Side-effects** section 9.1.3
**Licensed use** licensed for use in children (age range not specified by manufacturer)
**Indications and dose**
Iron poisoning
• **By continuous intravenous infusion**
  **Neonate** up to 15 mg/kg/hour, reduced after 4–6 hours; max. 80 mg/kg in 24 hours (in severe cases, higher doses on advice from the National Poisons Information Service)

  **Child 1 month–18 years** up to 15 mg/kg/hour, reduced after 4–6 hours; max. 80 mg/kg in 24 hours (in severe cases, higher doses on advice from the National Poisons Information Service)

Chronic iron overload section 9.1.3

◢**Preparations**
Section 9.1.3

## Lithium

Lithium intoxication can occur as a complication of long-term therapy and is caused by reduced excretion of the drug because of a variety of factors including dehydration, deterioration of renal function, infections, and co-administration of diuretics or NSAIDs (or other drugs that interact). Acute deliberate overdoses may also occur with delayed onset of symptoms (12 hours or more) due to slow entry of lithium into the tissues and continuing absorption from modified-release formulations.

The early clinical features are non-specific and may include apathy and restlessness which could be confused with mental changes due to the child's depressive illness. Vomiting, diarrhoea, ataxia, weakness, dysarthria, muscle twitching, and tremor may follow. Severe poisoning is associated with convulsions, coma, renal failure, electrolyte imbalance, dehydration, and hypotension.

Therapeutic serum-lithium concentrations are within the range of 0.4–1 mmol/litre; concentrations in excess of 2 mmol/litre are usually associated with serious toxicity and such cases may need treatment with haemodialysis if neurological symptoms or renal failure are present. In acute overdosage, much higher serum-lithium concentrations may be present without features of toxicity and all that is usually necessary is to take measures to increase urine output (e.g. by increasing fluid intake, but avoiding diuretics). Otherwise, treatment is supportive with special regard to electrolyte balance, renal function, and control of convulsions. Whole-bowel irrigation should be considered for significant ingestion, but advice should be sought from the National Poisons Information Service (p. 23).

> The **National Poisons Information Service** (Tel: 0844 892 0111) will provide specialist advice on all aspects of poisoning day and night

## Phenothiazines and related drugs

Phenothiazines cause less depression of consciousness and respiration than other sedatives. Hypotension, hypothermia, sinus tachycardia, and arrhythmias may complicate poisoning. Dystonic reactions can occur with therapeutic doses (particularly with prochlorperazine and trifluoperazine), and convulsions may occur in severe cases. Arrhythmias may respond to correction of hypoxia, acidosis, and other biochemical abnormalities, but specialist advice should be sought if arrhythmias result from a prolonged QT interval; the use of some anti-arrhythmic drugs can worsen such arrhythmias. Dystonic reactions are rapidly abolished by injection of drugs such as procyclidine (section 4.9.2) or diazepam (section 4.8.2, emulsion preferred).

## Second-generation antipsychotic drugs

Features of poisoning by second-generation antipsychotic drugs (section 4.2.1) include drowsiness, convulsions, extrapyramidal symptoms, hypotension, and ECG abnormalities (including prolongation of the QT interval). Management is supportive. Activated charcoal can be given within 1 hour of ingesting a significant quantity of a second-generation antipsychotic drug.

## Stimulants

**Amfetamines** Amfetamines cause wakefulness, excessive activity, paranoia, hallucinations, and hypertension followed by exhaustion, convulsions, hyperthermia, and coma. The early stages can be controlled by diazepam or lorazepam; advice should be sought from the National Poisons Information Service (p. 23) on the management of hypertension. Later, tepid spong-

ing, anticonvulsants, and artificial respiration may be needed.

**Cocaine** Cocaine stimulates the central nervous system, causing agitation, dilated pupils, tachycardia, hypertension, hallucinations, hyperthermia, hypertonia, and hyperreflexia; cardiac effects include chest pain, myocardial infarction, and arrhythmias.

Initial treatment of cocaine poisoning involves cooling measures for hyperthermia (see p. 24); agitation, hypertension, and cardiac effects require specific treatment and expert advice should be sought.

**Ecstasy** Ecstasy (methylenedioxymethamfetamine, MDMA) may cause severe reactions, even at doses that were previously tolerated. The most serious effects are delirium, coma, convulsions, ventricular arrhythmias, hyperthermia, rhabdomyolysis, acute renal failure, acute hepatitis, disseminated intravascular coagulation, adult respiratory distress syndrome, hyperreflexia, hypotension and intracerebral haemorrhage; hyponatraemia has also been associated with ecstasy use and syndrome of inappropriate antidiuretic hormone secretion (SIADH) can occur.

Treatment of methylenedioxymethamfetamine poisoning is supportive, with diazepam to control persistent convulsions and close monitoring including ECG. For the management of agitation, seek specialist advice. Self-induced water intoxication should be considered in patients with ecstasy poisoning.

'Liquid ecstasy' is a term used for sodium oxybate (gamma-hydroxybutyrate, GHB), which is a sedative.

## Theophylline

Theophylline and related drugs are often prescribed as modified-release formulations and toxicity can therefore be delayed. They cause vomiting (which may be severe and intractable), agitation, restlessness, dilated pupils, sinus tachycardia, and hyperglycaemia. More serious effects are haematemesis, convulsions, and supraventricular and ventricular arrhythmias. Severe hypokalaemia may develop rapidly.

Repeated doses of activated charcoal can be used to eliminate theophylline even if more than 1 hour has elapsed after ingestion and especially if a modified-release preparation has been taken (see also under Active Elimination Techniques). Ondansetron (section 4.6) may be effective for severe vomiting that is resistant to other antiemetics. Hypokalaemia is corrected by intravenous infusion of potassium chloride (section 9.2.2.1) in 0.9% sodium chloride and may be so severe as to require high doses under ECG monitoring. Convulsions should be controlled by intravenous administration of lorazepam or diazepam (see Convulsions, p. 24). For the management of agitation associated with theophylline overdosage, seek specialist advice.

Provided the child does **not** suffer from asthma, a short-acting beta-blocker (section 2.4) can be administered intravenously to reverse severe tachycardia, hypokalaemia, and hyperglycaemia.

## Other poisons

Consult either the National Poisons Information Service day and night or TOXBASE, see p. 23.

# Cyanides

Oxygen should be administered to children with cyanide poisoning. The choice of antidote depends on the severity of poisoning, certainty of diagnosis, and the cause. **Dicobalt edetate** is the antidote of choice when there is a strong clinical suspicion of severe cyanide poisoning. Dicobalt edetate itself is toxic, associated with anaphylactoid reactions, and is potentially fatal if administered in the absence of cyanide poisoning. A regimen of **sodium nitrite** followed by **sodium thiosulfate** is an alternative if dicobalt edetate is not available.

**Hydroxocobalamin** (*Cyanokit*®—no other preparation of hydroxocobalamin is suitable) can be considered for use in victims of smoke inhalation who show signs of significant cyanide poisoning.

## ▌ DICOBALT EDETATE

**Cautions** owing to toxicity to be used only for definite cyanide poisoning when patient tending to lose, or has lost, consciousness; **not** to be used as a precautionary measure

**Side-effects** hypotension, tachycardia, and vomiting; anaphylactoid reactions including facial and laryngeal oedema and cardiac abnormalities

**Indications and dose**

Severe poisoning with cyanides

* By intravenous injection

  Consult the National Poisons Information Service

**¹Dicobalt Edetate** (Non-proprietary) PoM
Injection, dicobalt edetate 15 mg/mL, net price 20-mL (300-mg) amp = £13.75

## ▌ HYDROXOCOBALAMIN

**Side-effects** gastro-intestinal disturbances, transient hypertension, peripheral oedema, dyspnoea, throat disorders, hot flush, dizziness, headache, restlessness, memory impairment, red coloration of urine, lymphocytopenia, eye disorders, pustular rashes, pruritus, reversible red coloration of skin and mucous membranes

**Indications and dose**

Poisoning with cyanides  see notes above

* By intravenous infusion

  **Child body-weight 5 kg and over** 70 mg/kg (max. 5 g) over 15 minutes; a second dose of 70 mg/kg (max. 5 g) can be given over 15 minutes–2 hours depending on severity of poisoning and patient stability

**Administration** for *intravenous infusion*, reconstitute 5-g vial with 200 mL Sodium Chloride 0.9%; gently invert vial for at least 1 minute to mix (do not shake)

**Cyanokit**® (Swedish Orphan) PoM
Intravenous infusion, powder for reconstitution, hydroxocobalamin, net price 5-g vial = £772.00
**Note** Deep red colour of hydroxocobalamin may interfere with laboratory tests (see Side-effects, above) and haemodialysis

---

1. PoM restriction does not apply where administration is for saving life in emergency

## ▌ SODIUM NITRITE

**Side-effects** flushing and headache due to vasodilatation

**Indications and dose**

Poisoning with cyanides (used in conjunction with sodium thiosulfate)

  See under preparation

**¹Sodium Nitrite** PoM
Injection, sodium nitrite 3% (30 mg/mL) in water for injections
**Dose**

* By intravenous injection over 5–20 minutes

  **Child 1 month–18 years** 4–10 mg/kg max. 300 mg (0.13–0.33 mL/kg, max. 10 mL, of 3% solution) followed by sodium thiosulfate injection 400 mg/kg, max. 12.5 g (0.8 mL/kg, max. 25 mL, of 50% solution) over 10 minutes

Available from 'special-order' manufacturers or specialist importing companies, see p. 823

## ▌ SODIUM THIOSULFATE

**Indications and dose**

Poisoning with cyanides (used in conjunction with sodium nitrite)

  See above under Sodium Nitrite

**¹Sodium Thiosulfate** PoM
Injection, sodium thiosulfate 50% (500 mg/mL) in water for injections
Available from 'special-order' manufacturers or specialist importing companies, see p. 823

## Ethylene glycol and methanol

**Fomepizole** (available from 'special-order' manufacturers or specialist importing companies, see p. 823) is the treatment of choice for ethylene glycol and methanol (methyl alcohol) poisoning. If necessary, **ethanol** (by mouth or by intravenous infusion) can be used, but with caution. Advice on the treatment of ethylene glycol and methanol poisoning should be obtained from the National Poisons Information Service. It is important to start antidote treatment promptly in cases of suspected poisoning with these agents.

## Heavy metals

Heavy metal antidotes include succimer (DMSA) [unlicensed], unithiol (DMPS) [unlicensed], sodium calcium edetate [unlicensed], and dimercaprol. Dimercaprol in the management of heavy metal poisoning has been superseded by other chelating agents. In all cases of heavy metal poisoning, the advice of the National Poisons Information Service should be sought.

## Noxious gases

**Carbon monoxide** Carbon monoxide poisoning is usually due to inhalation of smoke, car exhaust, or fumes caused by blocked flues or incomplete combustion of fuel gases in confined spaces.

Immediate treatment of carbon monoxide poisoning is essential. The child should be moved to fresh air, the airway cleared, and high-flow **oxygen** 100% administered as soon as available. Artificial respiration should be given as necessary and continued until adequate

Emergency treatment of poisoning

spontaneous breathing starts, or stopped only after persistent and efficient treatment of cardiac arrest has failed. The child should be admitted to hospital because complications may arise after a delay of hours or days. Cerebral oedema may occur in severe poisoning and is treated with an intravenous infusion of mannitol (section 2.2.5). Referral for hyperbaric oxygen treatment should be discussed with the National Poisons Information Service if the patient is pregnant or in cases of severe poisoning such as if the child is or has been unconscious, or has psychiatric or neurological features other than a headache or has myocardial ischaemia or an arrhythmia, or has a blood carboxyhaemoglobin concentration of more than 20%.

**Sulfur dioxide, chlorine, phosgene, ammonia** All of these gases can cause upper respiratory tract and conjunctival irritation. Pulmonary oedema, with severe breathlessness and cyanosis may develop suddenly up to 36 hours after exposure. Death may occur. Children are kept under observation and those who develop pulmonary oedema are given oxygen. Assisted ventilation may be necessary in the most serious cases.

## CS Spray

CS spray, which is used for riot control, irritates the eyes (hence 'tear gas') and the respiratory tract; symptoms normally settle spontaneously within 15 minutes. If symptoms persist, the patient should be removed to a well-ventilated area, and the exposed skin washed with soap and water after removal of contaminated clothing. Contact lenses should be removed and rigid ones washed (soft ones should be discarded). Eye symptoms should be treated by irrigating the eyes with physiological saline (or water if saline is not available) and advice sought from an ophthalmologist. Patients with features of severe poisoning, particularly respiratory complications, should be admitted to hospital for symptomatic treatment.

## Nerve agents

Treatment of nerve agent poisoning is similar to organophosphorus insecticide poisoning (see below), but advice must be sought from the National Poisons Information Service. The risk of cross-contamination is significant; adequate decontamination and protective clothing for healthcare personnel are essential. In emergencies involving the release of nerve agents, kits ('NAAS pods') containing **pralidoxime** can be obtained through the Ambulance Service from the National Blood Service (or the Welsh Blood Service in South Wales or designated hospital pharmacies in Northern Ireland and Scotland—see TOXBASE for list of designated centres).

## Pesticides

**Organophosphorus insecticides** Organophosphorus insecticides are usually supplied as powders or dissolved in organic solvents. All are absorbed through the bronchi and intact skin as well as through the gut and inhibit cholinesterase activity, thereby prolonging and intensifying the effects of acetylcholine. Toxicity between different compounds varies considerably, and onset may be delayed after skin exposure.

Anxiety, restlessness, dizziness, headache, miosis, nausea, hypersalivation, vomiting, abdominal colic, diarrhoea, bradycardia, and sweating are common features of organophosphorus poisoning. Muscle weakness and fasciculation may develop and progress to generalised flaccid paralysis, including the ocular and respiratory muscles. Convulsions, coma, pulmonary oedema with copious bronchial secretions, hypoxia, and arrhythmias occur in severe cases. Hyperglycaemia and glycosuria without ketonuria may also be present.

Further absorption of the organophosphorus insecticide should be prevented by moving the child to fresh air, removing soiled clothing, and washing contaminated skin. In severe poisoning it is vital to ensure a clear airway, frequent removal of bronchial secretions, and adequate ventilation and oxygenation; gastric lavage may be considered provided that the airway is protected. **Atropine** will reverse the muscarinic effects of acetylcholine and is given by intravenous injection in a dose of 20 micrograms/kg (max. 2 mg) as atropine sulfate every 5 to 10 minutes (according to the severity of poisoning) until the skin becomes flushed and dry, the pupils dilate, and bradycardia is abolished.

**Pralidoxime chloride**, a cholinesterase reactivator, is used as an adjunct to atropine in moderate or severe poisoning. It improves muscle tone within 30 minutes of administration. Pralidoxime chloride is continued until the patient has not required atropine for 12 hours. Pralidoxime chloride can be obtained from designated centres, the names of which are held by the National Poisons Information Service (see p. 23).

> The **National Poisons Information Service** (Tel: 0844 892 0111) will provide specialist advice on all aspects of poisoning day and night

## ◼ PRALIDOXIME CHLORIDE

**Cautions** myasthenia gravis

**Contra-indications** poisoning with carbamates or organophosphorus compounds without anticholinesterase activity

**Renal impairment** use with caution

**Side-effects** drowsiness, dizziness, disturbances of vision, nausea, tachycardia, headache, hyperventilation, and muscular weakness

**Licensed use** licensed for use in children (age range not specified by manufacturer)

**Indications and dose**

Adjunct to atropine in the treatment of poisoning by organophosphorus insecticide or nerve agent

• **By intravenous infusion over 20 minutes**

**Child under 18 years** initially 30 mg/kg, followed by 8 mg/kg/hour; usual max. 12 g in 24 hours

Note The loading dose may be administered by intravenous injection (diluted to a concentration of 50 mg/mL with water for injections) over at least 5 minutes if pulmonary oedema is present or if it is not practical to administer an intravenous infusion; pralidoxime chloride doses may differ from those in product literature

**Administration** for *intravenous infusion*, reconstitute each vial with 20 mL Water for Injections, then dilute to a concentration of 10–20 mg/mL with Sodium Chloride 0.9%

**[1]Pralidoxime chloride** ~~PoM~~

Injection, powder for reconstitution, pralidoxime chloride 1 g/vial

Available as *Protopam* ® (from designated centres for organophosphorus insecticide poisoning or from the National Blood Service (or Welsh Ambulance Services for Mid West and South East Wales)—see TOXBASE for list of designated centres)

---

## Snake bites and animal stings

**Snake bites** Envenoming from snake bite is uncommon in the UK. Many exotic snakes are kept, some illegally, but the only indigenous venomous snake is the adder (*Vipera berus*). The bite may cause local and systemic effects. Local effects include pain, swelling, bruising, and tender enlargement of regional lymph nodes. Systemic effects include early anaphylactic symptoms (transient hypotension with syncope, angio-edema, urticaria, abdominal colic, diarrhoea, and vomiting), with later persistent or recurrent hypotension, ECG abnormalities, spontaneous systemic bleeding, coagulopathy, adult respiratory distress syndrome, and acute renal failure. Fatal envenoming is rare but the potential for severe envenoming must not be underestimated.

Early anaphylactic symptoms should be treated with **adrenaline (epinephrine)** (section 3.4.3). Indications for antivenom treatment include *systemic envenoming*, especially hypotension (see above), ECG abnormalities, vomiting, haemostatic abnormalities, and marked local envenoming such that after bites on the hand or foot, swelling extends beyond the wrist or ankle within 4 hours of the bite. The contents of one vial (10 mL) of **European viper venom antiserum** (to order, email immform@dh.gsi.gov.uk) is given *by intravenous injection* over 10–15 minutes or *by intravenous infusion* over 30 minutes after diluting in sodium chloride 0.9% (use 5 mL diluent/kg body-weight). The **same dose** should be used for **adults** and **children**. The dose can be repeated after 1–2 hours if symptoms of *systemic envenoming* persist. However, for those children who present with clinical features of *severe envenoming* (e.g. shock, ECG abnormalities, or local swelling that has advanced from the foot to above the knee or from the hand to above the elbow within 2 hours of the bite), an initial dose of 2 vials (20 mL) of the antiserum is recommended; if symptoms of *systemic envenoming* persist contact the National Poisons Information Service. Adrenaline (epinephrine) injection must be immediately to hand for treatment of anaphylactic reactions to the antivenom (for the management of anaphylaxis see section 3.4.3).

Antivenom is available for bites by certain foreign snakes and spiders, stings by scorpions and fish. For information on identification, management, and for supply in an emergency, telephone the National Poisons Information Service. Whenever possible the TOXBASE entry should be read, and relevant information collected, before telephoning the National Poisons Information Service (see p. 23).

**Insect stings** Stings from ants, wasps, hornets, and bees cause local pain and swelling but seldom cause severe direct toxicity unless many stings are inflicted at the same time. If the sting is in the mouth or on the tongue local swelling may threaten the upper airway.

The stings from these insects are usually treated by cleaning the area with a topical antiseptic. Bee stings should be removed as quickly as possible. Anaphylactic reactions require immediate treatment with intramuscular **adrenaline (epinephrine)**; self-administered (or administered by a carer) intramuscular adrenaline (e.g. *EpiPen* ®) is the best first-aid treatment for children with severe hypersensitivity. An inhaled bronchodilator should be used for asthmatic reactions. For the management of anaphylaxis, see section 3.4.3. A short course of an **oral antihistamine** or a **topical corticosteroid** may help to reduce inflammation and relieve itching. A vaccine containing extracts of bee and wasp venom can be used to reduce the risk of severe anaphylaxis and systemic reactions in children with systemic hypersensitivity to bee or wasp stings (section 3.4.2).

**Marine stings** The severe pain of weeverfish (*Trachinus vipera*) and Portuguese man-o'-war stings can be relieved by immersing the stung area immediately in uncomfortably hot, but not scalding, water (not more than 45° C). Children stung by jellyfish and Portuguese man-o'-war around the UK coast should be removed from the sea as soon as possible. Adherent tentacles should be lifted off carefully (wearing gloves or using tweezers) or washed off with seawater. Alcoholic solutions, including suntan lotions, should **not** be applied because they can cause further discharge of stinging hairs. Ice packs can be used to reduce pain.

---

1. ~~PoM~~ restriction does not apply where administration is for saving life in emergency

# 1 Gastro-intestinal system

This chapter includes advice on the drug management of the following:

*Clostridium difficile* infection, p. 49
constipation, p. 56
Crohn's disease, p. 47
food allergy, p. 55
*Helicobacter pylori* infection, p. 41
irritable bowel syndrome, p. 48
malabsorption syndromes, p. 49
NSAID-associated ulcers, p. 41
ulcerative colitis, p. 47

## 1.1 Dyspepsia and gastro-oesophageal reflux disease

**1.1.1** Antacids and simeticone

**1.1.2** Compound alginate preparations

### Dyspepsia

Dyspepsia covers upper abdominal pain, fullness, early
satiety, bloating, and nausea. It can occur with gastric
and duodenal ulceration (section 1.3), gastro-oesophageal reflux disease, gastritis, and upper gastro-intestinal motility disorders, but most commonly it is of
uncertain origin.

Children with dyspepsia should be advised about lifestyle changes (see Gastro-oesophageal reflux disease,
below). Some medications may cause dyspepsia—these
should be stopped, if possible.

A compound alginate preparation (section 1.1.2) may
provide relief from dyspepsia; persistent dyspepsia
requires investigation. Treatment with a H₂-receptor
antagonist (section 1.3.1) or a proton pump inhibitor
(section 1.3.5) should be initiated only on the advice of a
hospital specialist.

*Helicobacter pylori* may be present in children with dyspepsia. *H. pylori* eradication therapy (section 1.3) should
be considered for persistent dyspepsia if it is ulcer-like.
However, most children with functional (investigated,
non-ulcer) dyspepsia do not benefit symptomatically
from *H. pylori* eradication.

### Gastro-oesophageal reflux disease

Gastro-oesophageal reflux disease includes non-erosive
gastro-oesophageal reflux and erosive oesophagitis.
Uncomplicated gastro-oesophageal reflux is common
in infancy and most symptoms, such as intermittent
vomiting or repeated, effortless regurgitation, resolve
without treatment between 12 and 18 months of age.

Older children with gastro-oesophageal reflux disease may have heartburn, acid regurgitation and dysphagia. Oesophageal inflammation (oesophagitis), ulceration or stricture formation may develop in early childhood; gastro-oesophageal reflux disease may also be associated with chronic respiratory disorders including asthma.

Parents and carers of *neonates* and *infants* should be reassured that most symptoms of uncomplicated gastro-oesophageal reflux resolve without treatment. An increase in the frequency and a decrease in the volume of feeds may reduce symptoms. A feed thickener or pre-thickened formula feed (Appendix 2) can be used on the advice of a dietician. If necessary, a suitable alginate-containing preparation (section 1.1.2) can be used instead of thickened feeds.

*Older children* should be advised about life-style changes such as weight reduction if overweight, and the avoidance of alcohol and smoking. An alginate-containing antacid (section 1.1.2) can be used to relieve symptoms.

Children who do not respond to these measures or who have problems such as respiratory disorders or suspected oesophagitis need to be referred to hospital. On the advice of a paediatrician, a **histamine H$_2$-receptor antagonist** (section 1.3.1) can be used to relieve symptoms of gastro-oesophageal reflux disease, promote mucosal healing and permit reduction in antacid consumption. A **proton pump inhibitor** (section 1.3.5) can be used for the treatment of moderate, non-erosive oesophagitis that is unresponsive to an H$_2$-receptor antagonist. Endoscopically confirmed *erosive*, *ulcerative*, or *stricturing* disease in children is usually treated with a proton pump inhibitor. Reassessment is necessary if symptoms persist despite 4–6 weeks of treatment; long-term use of an H$_2$-receptor antagonist or proton pump inhibitor should not be undertaken without full assessment of the underlying condition. For endoscopically confirmed *erosive, ulcerative*, or *stricturing* disease, the proton pump inhibitor usually needs to be maintained at the minimum effective dose.

Motility stimulants (section 1.2), such as domperidone or erythromycin may improve gastro-oesophageal sphincter contraction and accelerate gastric emptying. Evidence for the long-term efficacy of motility stimulants in the management of gastro-oesophageal reflux in children is unconvincing.

For advice on specialised formula feeds, see section 9.4.2.

**Pregnancy** If dietary and lifestyle changes (see notes above) fail to control gastro-oesophageal reflux disease in pregnancy, an antacid (section 1.1.1) or an alginate (section 1.1.2) can be tried. If this is ineffective, ranitidine (section 1.3.1) can be tried. Omeprazole (section 1.3.5) is reserved for women with severe or complicated reflux disease.

## 1.1.1 Antacids and simeticone

Antacids (usually containing aluminium or magnesium compounds) can be used for short-term relief of intermittent symptoms of *ulcer dyspepsia* and *non-erosive gastro-oesophageal reflux* (see section 1.1) in children; they are also used in functional (non-ulcer) dyspepsia, but the evidence of benefit is uncertain.

**Aluminium-** and **magnesium-containing** antacids, being relatively insoluble in water, are long-acting if retained in the stomach. Magnesium-containing antacids tend to be laxative whereas aluminium-containing antacids may be constipating; antacids containing both magnesium and aluminium may reduce these colonic side-effects. Aluminium-containing antacids should not be used in children with renal impairment, or in neonates and infants because accumulation may lead to increased plasma-aluminium concentrations.

Complexes such as **hydrotalcite** confer no special advantage.

**Calcium-containing** antacids can induce rebound acid secretion; with modest doses the clinical significance of this is doubtful, but prolonged high doses also cause hypercalcaemia and alkalosis.

**Simeticone** (activated dimeticone) is used to treat infantile colic, but the evidence of benefit is uncertain. Simeticone is added to an antacid as an antifoaming agent to relieve flatulence; such preparations may also be useful for the relief of hiccup in palliative care (see Prescribing in Palliative Care, p. 18).

**Alginates** act as mucosal protectants in gastro-oesophageal reflux disease (section 1.1.2). The amount of additional ingredient or antacid in individual preparations varies widely, as does their sodium content, so that preparations may not be freely interchangeable.

**Hepatic impairment** In children with fluid retention, avoid antacids containing large amounts of sodium. Avoid antacids that cause constipation because this can precipitate coma. Avoid antacids containing magnesium salts in hepatic coma if there is a risk of renal failure.

**Renal impairment** In children with fluid retention, avoid antacids containing large amounts of sodium. There is a risk of accumulation and aluminium toxicity with antacids containing aluminium salts. Absorption of aluminium from aluminium salts is increased by citrates, which are contained in many effervescent preparations (such as effervescent analgesics). Antacids containing magnesium salts should be avoided or used at a reduced dose because there is an increased risk of toxicity.

**Interactions** Antacids should preferably not be taken at the same time as other drugs since they may impair absorption. Antacids may also damage enteric coatings designed to prevent dissolution in the stomach. See also **Appendix 1** (antacids, calcium salts).

**Low Na$^+$**
The words 'low Na$^+$' added after some preparations indicate a sodium content of less than 1 mmol per tablet or 10-mL dose.

## Aluminium- and magnesium-containing antacids

### ALUMINIUM HYDROXIDE

**Cautions** see notes above; **interactions**: Appendix 1 (antacids)
**Contra-indications** hypophosphataemia; neonates and infants
**Hepatic impairment** see notes above
**Renal impairment** see notes above
**Side-effects** see notes above
**Indications and dose**
  Dyspepsia for dose see preparations

  Hyperphosphataemia section 9.5.2.2

◢ **Co-magaldrox**

Co-magaldrox is a mixture of aluminium hydroxide and magnesium hydroxide; the proportions are expressed in the form $x/y$ where $x$ and $y$ are the strengths in milligrams per unit dose of magnesium hydroxide and aluminium hydroxide respectively

**Maalox**® (Sanofi-Aventis)

Suspension, sugar-free, co-magaldrox 195/220 (magnesium hydroxide 195 mg, dried aluminium hydroxide 220 mg/5 mL (low $Na^+$)). Net price 500 mL = £2.79

Dose
- By mouth
  **Child 14–18 years** 10–20 mL 20–60 minutes after meals and at bedtime, or when required

**Mucogel**® (Chemidex)

Suspension, sugar-free, co-magaldrox 195/220 (magnesium hydroxide 195 mg, dried aluminium hydroxide 220 mg/5 mL (low $Na^+$)). Net price 500 mL = £1.71

Dose
- By mouth
  **Child 12–18 years** 10–20 mL 3 times daily, 20–60 minutes after meals and at bedtime, or when required

## ◼ MAGNESIUM TRISILICATE

**Cautions** heart failure, hypertension; metabolic or respiratory alkalosis, hypermagnesaemia; **interactions**: Appendix 1 (antacids)
**Contra-indications** severe renal failure; hypophosphataemia
**Hepatic impairment** see notes above
**Renal impairment** see notes above; magnesium trisilicate mixture has a high sodium content
**Side-effects** see notes above; silica-based renal stones reported on long-term treatment
**Indications and dose**
  Dyspepsia for dose see under preparation

**Magnesium Trisilicate Mixture, BP**
(Magnesium Trisilicate Oral Suspension)
Oral suspension, 5% each of magnesium trisilicate, light magnesium carbonate, and sodium bicarbonate in a suitable vehicle with a peppermint flavour. Contains about 6 mmol $Na^+/10$ mL

Dose
- By mouth
  **Child 5–12 years** 5–10 mL with water 3 times daily or as required
  **Child 12–18 years** 10–20 mL with water 3 times daily or as required

## Aluminium-magnesium complexes

### ◼ HYDROTALCITE

Aluminium magnesium carbonate hydroxide hydrate

**Cautions** see notes above; **interactions**: Appendix 1 (antacids)
**Hepatic impairment** see notes above
**Renal impairment** see notes above
**Side-effects** see notes above
**Indications and dose**
  Dyspepsia for dose see under preparation

◢ **With simeticone**
**Altacite Plus**®
  see below

## Antacid preparations containing simeticone

**Altacite Plus**® (Peckforton)

Suspension, sugar-free, co-simalcite 125/500 (simeticone 125 mg, hydrotalcite 500 mg)/5 mL (low $Na^+$). Net price 500 mL = £2.79

Dose
- By mouth
  **Child 8–12 years** 5 mL 4 times daily (between meals and at bedtime) when required
  **Child 12–18 years** 10 mL 4 times daily (between meals and at bedtime) when required

**Maalox Plus**® (Sanofi-Aventis)

Suspension, sugar-free, dried aluminium hydroxide 220 mg, simeticone 25 mg, magnesium hydroxide 195 mg/5 mL (low $Na^+$). Net price 500 mL = £2.79

Dose
- By mouth
  **Child 2–5 years** 5 mL 3 times daily
  **Child 5–12 years** 5–10 mL 3–4 times daily
  **Child 12–18 years** 5–10 mL 4 times daily (after meals and at bedtime) or when required

## Simeticone alone

### ◼ SIMETICONE

Activated dimeticone

**Indications and dose**

Colic or wind pain for dose see under individual preparations

**Dentinox**® (DDD)

Colic drops (= emulsion), simeticone 21 mg/2.5-mL dose. Net price 100 mL = £1.73

Dose
- By mouth
  **Neonate** 2.5 mL with or after each feed (max. 6 doses in 24 hours); may be added to bottle feed
  **Child 1 month–2 years** 2.5 mL with or after each feed (max. 6 doses in 24 hours); may be added to bottle feed

**Note** The brand name *Dentinox*® is also used for other preparations including teething gel

**Infacol**® (Forest)

Liquid, sugar-free, simeticone 40 mg/mL (low $Na^+$). Net price 50 mL = £2.26. Counselling, use of dropper

Dose
- By mouth
  **Neonate** 0.5–1 mL before feeds
  **Child 1 month–2 years** 0.5–1 mL before feeds

## 1.1.2 Compound alginate preparations

Alginate taken in combination with an antacid increases the viscosity of stomach contents and can protect the oesophageal mucosa from acid reflux. Some alginate-containing preparations form a viscous gel ('raft') that floats on the surface of the stomach contents, thereby reducing symptoms of reflux. Alginate-containing preparations are used in the management of mild symptoms of dyspepsia and gastro-oesophageal reflux disease (see section 1.1). Antacids may damage enteric coatings designed to prevent dissolution in the stomach. For **interactions**, see Appendix 1 (antacids, calcium salts).

Preparations containing aluminium should not be used in children with renal impairment, or in neonates and infants.

## Alginate raft-forming oral suspensions

The following preparations contain sodium alginate, sodium bicarbonate, and calcium carbonate in a suitable flavoured vehicle, and conform to the specification for Alginate Raft-forming Oral Suspension, BP.

### Acidex® (Pinewood)

Liquid, sugar-free, sodium alginate 250 mg, sodium bicarbonate 133.5 mg, calcium carbonate 80 mg/5 mL. Contains about 3 mmol Na⁺/5 mL, net price 500 mL (aniseed- or peppermint-flavour) = £2.30

**Dose**
- By mouth

    **Child 6–12 years** 5–10 mL after meals and at bedtime
    **Child 12–18 years** 10–20 mL after meals and at bedtime

### Gaviscon® (Reckitt Benckiser)

Suspension, sugar-free, aniseed- or peppermint flavour, sodium alginate 250 mg, sodium bicarbonate 133.5 mg, calcium carbonate 80 mg/5 mL. Contains 3.1 mmol Na⁺/5 mL. Net price 300 mL = £3.84, 600 mL = £6.29

**Dose**
- By mouth

    **Child 6–12 years** 5–10 mL after meals and at bedtime
    **Child 12–18 years** 10–20 mL after meals and at bedtime

### Peptac® (IVAX)

Suspension, sugar-free, sodium bicarbonate 133.5 mg, sodium alginate 250 mg, calcium carbonate 80 mg/5 mL. Contains 3.1 mmol Na⁺/5 mL. Net price 500 mL (aniseed- or peppermint-flavoured) = £2.16

**Dose**
- By mouth

    **Child 6–12 years** 5–10 mL after meals and at bedtime
    **Child 12–18 years** 10–20 mL after meals and at bedtime

## Other compound alginate preparations

### Gastrocote® (Actavis)

Tablets, alginic acid 200 mg, dried aluminium hydroxide 80 mg, magnesium trisilicate 40 mg, sodium bicarbonate 70 mg. Contains about 1 mmol Na⁺/tablet. Net price 100-tab pack = £3.51

**Cautions** diabetes mellitus (high sugar content)

**Dose**
- By mouth

    **Child 6–18 years** 1–2 tablets chewed 4 times daily (after meals and at bedtime)

Liquid, sugar-free, peach-coloured, dried aluminium hydroxide 80 mg, magnesium trisilicate 40 mg, sodium alginate 220 mg, sodium bicarbonate 70 mg/5 mL. Contains 2.13 mmol Na⁺/5 mL. Net price 500 mL = £2.67

**Dose**
- By mouth

    **Child 6–12 years** 5–10 mL 4 times daily (after meals and at bedtime)
    **Child 12–18 years** 5–15 mL 4 times daily (after meals and at bedtime)

### Gaviscon® Advance (Reckitt Benckiser)

Chewable tablets, sugar-free, sodium alginate 500 mg, potassium bicarbonate 100 mg. Contains 2.25 mmol Na⁺, 1 mmol K⁺/tablet. Net price 60-tab pack (peppermint-flavour) = £3.07

**Excipients** include aspartame (section 9.4.1)

**Dose**
- By mouth

    **Child 6–12 years** 1 tablet to be chewed after meals and at bedtime (under medical advice only)
    **Child 12–18 years** 1–2 tablets to be chewed after meals and at bedtime

Suspension, sugar-free, aniseed- or peppermint-flavour, sodium alginate 500 mg, potassium bicarbonate 100 mg/5 mL. Contains 2.3 mmol Na⁺, 1 mmol K⁺/5 mL, net price 250 mL = £2.56, 500 mL = £5.12

**Dose**
- By mouth

    **Child 2–12 years** 2.5–5 mL after meals and at bedtime (under medical advice only)
    **Child 12–18 years** 5–10 mL after meals and at bedtime

### Gaviscon® Infant (Reckitt Benckiser)

Oral powder, sugar-free, sodium alginate 225 mg, magnesium alginate 87.5 mg, with colloidal silica and mannitol/dose. Contains 0.92 mmol Na⁺/dose. Net price 30 doses = £2.46

**Dose**
- By mouth

    **Neonate body-weight under 4.5 kg** 1 'dose' mixed with feeds (or water, for breast-fed infants) when required (max. 6 times in 24 hours)
    **Neonate body-weight over 4.5 kg** 2 'doses' mixed with feeds (or water, for breast-fed infants) when required (max. 6 times in 24 hours)
    **Child 1 month–2 years**
    **Body-weight under 4.5 kg** dose as for neonate
    **Body-weight over 4.5 kg** 2 'doses' mixed with feeds (or water, for breast-fed infants) when required (max. 6 times in 24 hours)

**Note** Not to be used in preterm neonates, or where excessive water loss likely (e.g. fever, diarrhoea, vomiting, high room temperature), or if intestinal obstruction. Not to be used with other preparations containing thickening agents

### Safe Practice

Each half of the dual sachet is identified as 'one dose'. To avoid errors prescribe with directions in terms of 'dose'

### Topal® (Fabre)

Tablets, alginic acid 200 mg, dried aluminium hydroxide 200 mg, light magnesium carbonate 40 mg with lactose 220 mg, sucrose 880 mg, sodium bicarbonate 40 mg (low Na⁺). Net price 42-tab pack = £1.67

**Cautions** diabetes mellitus (high sugar content)

**Dose**
- By mouth

    **Child 12–18 years** 1–3 tablets chewed 4 times daily (after meals and at bedtime)

**1**

**Gastro-intestinal system**

## 1.2 Antispasmodics and other drugs altering gut motility

Drugs in this section include antimuscarinic compounds and drugs believed to be direct relaxants of intestinal smooth muscle. The smooth muscle relaxant properties of antimuscarinic and other antispasmodic drugs may be useful in *irritable bowel syndrome*.

The dopamine-receptor antagonist **domperidone** stimulates transit in the gut.

## Antimuscarinics

Antimuscarinics (formerly termed 'anticholinergics') reduce intestinal motility. They are occasionally used for the management of *irritable bowel syndrome* but the evidence of their value has not been established and response varies. Other indications for antimuscarinic drugs include asthma and airways disease (section 3.1.2), motion sickness (section 4.6), urinary frequency and enuresis (section 7.4.2), mydriasis and cycloplegia (section 11.5), premedication (section 15.1.3), palliative care (p. 18), and as an antidote to organophosphorus poisoning (p. 32).

Antimuscarinics that are used for gastro-intestinal smooth muscle spasm include the tertiary amine **dicycloverine hydrochloride** and the quaternary ammonium compounds **propantheline bromide** and **hyoscine butylbromide**. The quaternary ammonium compounds are less lipid soluble than atropine and so are less likely to cross the blood–brain barrier; they are also less well absorbed from the gastro-intestinal tract.

Dicycloverine hydrochloride may also have some direct action on smooth muscle. Hyoscine butylbromide is advocated as a gastro-intestinal antispasmodic, but it is poorly absorbed; the injection may be useful in endoscopy and radiology.

**Cautions**   Antimuscarinics should be used with caution in children (especially children with Down's syndrome) due to increased risk of side-effects; they should also be used with caution in autonomic neuropathy, hypertension, conditions characterised by tachycardia (including hyperthyroidism, cardiac insufficiency, cardiac surgery), pyrexia, and in children susceptible to angle-closure glaucoma. Antimuscarinics are not used in children with gastro-oesophageal reflux disease, diarrhoea or ulcerative colitis. **Interactions:** Appendix 1 (antimuscarinics).

**Contra-indications**   Antimuscarinics are contra-indicated in myasthenia gravis (but may be used to decrease muscarinic side-effects of anticholinesterases—section 10.2.1), paralytic ileus, pyloric stenosis, and toxic megacolon.

**Side-effects**   Side-effects of antimuscarinics include constipation, transient bradycardia (followed by tachycardia, palpitation and arrhythmias), reduced bronchial secretions, urinary urgency and retention, dilatation of the pupils with loss of accommodation, photophobia, dry mouth, flushing and dryness of the skin. Side-effects that occur occasionally include nausea, vomiting, and giddiness; very rarely, angle closure glaucoma may occur.

## DICYCLOVERINE HYDROCHLORIDE
(Dicyclomine hydrochloride)

**Cautions**   see notes above
**Contra-indications**   see notes above; child under 6 months
**Pregnancy**   not known to be harmful; manufacturer advises use only if essential
**Breast-feeding**   avoid—present in milk; apnoea reported in infant
**Side-effects**   see notes above
**Indications and dose**

Symptomatic relief of gastro-intestinal disorders characterised by smooth muscle spasm
* By mouth
    Child 6 months–2 years 5–10 mg 3–4 times daily 15 minutes before feeds
    Child 2–12 years 10 mg 3 times daily
    Child 12–18 years 10–20 mg 3 times daily

**Dicycloverine** (Non-proprietary) PoM
Tablets, dicycloverine hydrochloride 10 mg, net price 100-tab pack = £16.25; 20 mg, 84-tab pack = £19.95
Syrup, dicycloverine hydrochloride 10 mg/5 mL, net price 120 mL = £28.75
Note Dicycloverine hydrochloride can be sold to the public provided that max. single dose is 10 mg and max. daily dose is 60 mg

**Compound preparations**
**Kolanticon®** (Peckforton)
Gel, sugar-free, dicycloverine hydrochloride 2.5 mg, dried aluminium hydroxide 200 mg, light magnesium oxide 100 mg, simeticone 20 mg/5 mL, net price 200 mL = £2.21, 500 mL = £3.35
Dose
    Child 12–18 years 10–20 mL every 4 hours when required

## HYOSCINE BUTYLBROMIDE

**Cautions**   see notes above; also intestinal and urinary outlet obstruction
**Contra-indications**   see notes above
**Pregnancy**   manufacturer advises avoid
**Breast-feeding**   amount too small to be harmful
**Side-effects**   see notes above
**Licensed use**   *tablets* not licensed for use in children under 6 years; *injection* not licensed for use in children (age range not specified by manufacturer)
**Indications and dose**

Symptomatic relief of gastro-intestinal or genitourinary disorders characterised by smooth muscle spasm
* By mouth
    Child 6–12 years 10 mg 3 times daily
    Child 12–18 years 20 mg 4 times daily

Excessive respiratory secretions and bowel colic in palliative care (see also p. 19)
* By mouth
    Child 1 month–2 years 300–500 micrograms/kg (max. 5 mg) 3–4 times daily
    Child 2–5 years 5 mg 3–4 times daily
    Child 5–12 years 10 mg 3–4 times daily
    Child 12–18 years 10–20 mg 3–4 times daily

- By intramuscular or intravenous injection

  **Child 1 month–4 years** 300–500 micrograms/kg (max. 5 mg) 3–4 times daily

  **Child 5–12 years** 5–10 mg 3–4 times daily

  **Child 12–18 years** 10–20 mg 3–4 times daily

---

Acute spasm, spasm in diagnostic procedures

- By intramuscular or intravenous injection

  **Child 2–6 years** 5 mg repeated after 30 minutes if necessary (may be repeated more frequently in endoscopy), max. 15 mg daily

  **Child 6–12 years** 5–10 mg repeated after 30 minutes if necessary (may be repeated more frequently in endoscopy), max. 30 mg daily

  **Child 12–18 years** 20 mg repeated after 30 minutes if necessary (may be repeated more frequently in endoscopy), max. 80 mg daily

**Administration** for *intravenous injection*, may be diluted with Glucose 5% *or* Sodium Chloride 0.9%; give over at least 1 minute.

For administration *by mouth*, injection solution may be used; content of ampoule may be stored in a refrigerator for up to 24 hours after opening

**Buscopan®** (Boehringer Ingelheim) [PoM]
Tablets, coated, hyoscine butylbromide 10 mg, net price 56-tab pack = £2.25
**Note** Hyoscine butylbromide tablets can be sold to the public for medically confirmed irritable bowel syndrome, provided single dose does not exceed 20 mg, daily dose does not exceed 80 mg, and pack does not contain a total of more than 240 mg

Injection, hyoscine butylbromide 20 mg/mL. Net price 1-mL amp = 22p

## ▌ PROPANTHELINE BROMIDE

**Cautions**  see notes above
**Contra-indications**  see notes above
**Hepatic impairment**  manufacturer advises caution
**Renal impairment**  manufacturer advises caution
**Pregnancy**  manufacturer advises avoid unless essential
**Breast-feeding**  may suppress lactation
**Side-effects**  see notes above
**Licensed use**  *tablets* not licensed for use in children under 12 years

**Indications and dose**

Symptomatic relief of gastro-intestinal disorders characterised by smooth muscle spasm

- By mouth

  **Child 1 month–12 years** 300 micrograms/kg (max. 15 mg) 3–4 times daily at least one hour before food

  **Child 12–18 years** 15 mg 3 times daily at least one hour before meals and 30 mg at night (max. 120 mg daily)

**Pro-Banthine®** (Archimedes) [PoM]
Tablets, pink, s/c, propantheline bromide 15 mg, net price 112-tab pack = £14.40. Label: 23

---

## Other antispasmodics

**Alverine**, **mebeverine**, and **peppermint oil** are believed to be direct relaxants of intestinal smooth muscle and may relieve pain in *irritable bowel syndrome*

and primary dysmenorrhoea. They have no serious adverse effects; peppermint oil occasionally causes heartburn.

## ▌ ALVERINE CITRATE

**Contra-indications**  paralytic ileus
**Pregnancy**  use with caution
**Breast-feeding**  manufacturer advises avoid—limited information available
**Side-effects**  nausea; dyspnoea; headache, dizziness; pruritus, rash; hepatitis also reported

**Indications and dose**

Adjunct in gastro-intestinal disorders characterised by smooth muscle spasm, dysmenorrhoea

- By mouth

  **Child 12–18 years** 60–120 mg 1–3 times daily

**Spasmonal®** (Meda)
Capsules, alverine citrate 60 mg (blue/grey), net price 100-cap pack = £9.47; 120 mg (*Spasmonal® Forte*, blue/grey), 60-cap pack = £10.94

## ▌ MEBEVERINE HYDROCHLORIDE

**Contra-indications**  paralytic ileus
**Pregnancy**  not known to be harmful—manufacturers advise avoid
**Breast-feeding**  manufacturers advise avoid—no information available
**Side-effects**  allergic reactions (including rash, urticaria, angioedema) reported
**Licensed use**  *tablets and liquid* not licensed for use in children under 10 years; *granules* not licensed for use in children under 12 years; *modified-release capsules* not licensed for use in children under 18 years

**Indications and dose**

Adjunct in gastro-intestinal disorders characterised by smooth muscle spasm

- By mouth

  **Child 3–4 years** 25 mg 3 times daily, preferably 20 minutes before meals

  **Child 4–8 years** 50 mg 3 times daily, preferably 20 minutes before meals

  **Child 8–10 years** 100 mg 3 times daily, preferably 20 minutes before meals

  **Child 10–18 years** 135–150 mg 3 times daily, preferably 20 minutes before meals

**Mebeverine Hydrochloride** (Non-proprietary) [PoM]
Tablets, mebeverine hydrochloride 135 mg, net price 100-tab pack = £4.21. Counselling, administration

Oral suspension, mebeverine hydrochloride (as mebeverine embonate) 50 mg/5 mL, net price 300 mL = £137.00. Counselling, administration

**Colofac®** (Abbott Healthcare) [PoM]
Tablets, s/c, mebeverine hydrochloride 135 mg, net price 100-tab pack = £7.52. Counselling, administration

**Gastro-intestinal system** *(side margin)*
**1** *(side margin)*

◢Modified release

**Colofac® MR** (Abbott Healthcare) [PoM]
Capsules, m/r, mebeverine hydrochloride 200 mg, net price 60-cap pack = £6.67. Label: 25

**Dose**
**Irritable bowel syndrome**
- By mouth
  **Child 12–18 years** 1 capsule twice daily

◢Compound preparations

[1]**Fybogel® Mebeverine** (Reckitt Benckiser) [PoM]
Granules, buff, effervescent, ispaghula husk 3.5 g, mebeverine hydrochloride 135 mg/sachet, net price 10 sachets = £2.50. Label: 13, 22, counselling, see below

**Excipients** include aspartame (section 9.4.1)
**Electrolytes** $K^+$ 7 mmol/sachet

**Dose**
**Irritable bowel syndrome**
- By mouth
  **Child 12–18 years** 1 sachet in water, morning and evening 30 minutes before food; an additional sachet may also be taken before the midday meal if necessary

**Counselling** Preparations that swell in contact with liquid should always be carefully swallowed with water and should not be taken immediately before going to bed

## PEPPERMINT OIL

**Cautions** sensitivity to menthol
**Pregnancy** not known to be harmful
**Breast-feeding** significant levels of menthol in breast milk unlikely
**Side-effects** heartburn, perianal irritation; *rarely*, allergic reactions (including rash, headache, bradycardia, muscle tremor, ataxia)
**Local irritation** Capsules should not be broken or chewed because peppermint oil may irritate mouth or oesophagus

**Indications and dose**
**Relief of abdominal colic and distension, particularly in irritable bowel syndrome**
- By mouth
  **Child 15–18 years** 1–2 capsules, swallowed whole with water, 3 times daily for up to 3 months if necessary

**Colpermin®** (McNeil)
Capsules, e/c, light blue/dark blue, blue band, peppermint oil 0.2 mL. Net price 100-cap pack = £12.05. Label: 5, 25
**Excipients** include arachis (peanut) oil

## Motility stimulants

**Domperidone** and **metoclopramide** (section 4.6) are dopamine receptor antagonists which stimulate gastric emptying and small intestinal transit, and enhance the strength of oesophageal sphincter contraction. Metoclopramide and occasionally domperidone can cause acute dystonic reactions—for further details of this and other side-effects, see section 4.6.

A low dose of **erythromycin** stimulates gastro-intestinal motility and may be used on the advice of a paediatric gastroenterologist to promote tolerance of enteral feeds; erythromycin may be less effective as a prokinetic drug in preterm neonates than in older children.

1. 10-sachet pack of *Fybogel® Mebeverine* can be sold to the public for use in children over 12 years

## DOMPERIDONE

**Cautions** see under Domperidone (section 4.6)
**Side-effects** see under Domperidone (section 4.6); also QT-interval prolongation reported
**Licensed use** not licensed for use in gastro-intestinal stasis; not licensed for use in children for gastro-oesophageal reflux disease

**Indications and dose**
**Gastro-oesophageal reflux disease (but efficacy not proven, see section 1.1), gastro-intestinal stasis**
- By mouth
  **Neonate** 100–300 micrograms/kg 4–6 times daily before feeds
  **Child 1 month–12 years** 200–400 micrograms/kg (max. 20 mg) 3–4 times daily before food
  **Child 12–18 years** 10–20 mg, 3–4 times daily before food

**Nausea and vomiting** section 4.6

◢Preparations
Section 4.6

## ERYTHROMYCIN

**Cautions** see section 5.1.5; **interactions:** Appendix 1 (macrolides)
**Side-effects** see section 5.1.5
**Licensed use** not licensed for use in gastro-intestinal stasis

**Indications and dose**
**Gastro-intestinal stasis**
- By mouth
  **Neonate** 3 mg/kg 4 times daily
  **Child 1 month–18 years** 3 mg/kg 4 times daily
- By intravenous infusion
  **Neonate** 3 mg/kg 4 times daily
  **Child 1 month–1 year** 3 mg/kg 4 times daily

◢Preparations
Section 5.1.5

## 1.3 Antisecretory drugs and mucosal protectants

**1.3.1** H₂-receptor antagonists
**1.3.2** Selective antimuscarinics
**1.3.3** Chelates and complexes
**1.3.4** Prostaglandin analogues
**1.3.5** Proton pump inhibitors

Peptic ulceration commonly involves the stomach, duodenum, and lower oesophagus; after gastric surgery it involves the gastro-enterostomy stoma.

Healing can be promoted by general measures, stopping smoking and taking antacids and by antisecretory drug treatment, but relapse is common when treatment ceases. Nearly all duodenal ulcers and most gastric ulcers not associated with NSAIDs are caused by *Helicobacter pylori*.

The management of *H. pylori* infection and of NSAID-associated ulcers is discussed below.

## *Helicobacter pylori* infection

Eradication of *Helicobacter pylori* reduces the recurrence of gastric and duodenal ulcers and the risk of rebleeding. The presence of *H. pylori* should be confirmed before starting eradication treatment. If possible, the antibacterial sensitivity of the organism should be established at the time of endoscopy and biopsy. Acid inhibition combined with antibacterial treatment is highly effective in the eradication of *H. pylori*; reinfection is rare. Antibiotic-associated colitis is an uncommon risk.

Treatment to eradicate *H. pylori* infection in children should be initiated under specialist supervision. One-week triple-therapy regimens that comprise omeprazole, amoxicillin, and either clarithromycin or metronidazole are recommended. Resistance to clarithromycin or to metronidazole is much more common than to amoxicillin and can develop during treatment. A regimen containing amoxicillin and clarithromycin is therefore recommended for initial therapy and one containing amoxicillin and metronidazole is recommended for eradication failure or for a child who has been treated with a macrolide for other infections. There is usually no need to continue antisecretory treatment (with a proton pump inhibitor or $H_2$-receptor antagonist); however, if the ulcer is large, or complicated by haemorrhage or perforation then antisecretory treatment is continued for a further 3 weeks. Lansoprazole may be considered if omeprazole is unsuitable. Treatment failure usually indicates antibacterial resistance or poor compliance.

Two-week triple-therapy regimens offer the possibility of higher eradication rates compared to one-week regimens, but adverse effects are common and poor compliance is likely to offset any possible gain.

Two-week dual-therapy regimens using a proton pump inhibitor and a single antibacterial produce low rates of *H. pylori* eradication and are **not** recommended.

For the role of *H. pylori* eradication therapy in children starting or taking NSAIDs, see NSAID-associated ulcers, below.

### Test for *Helicobacter pylori*

$^{13}$C-Urea breath test kits are available for confirming the presence of gastro-duodenal infection with *Helicobacter pylori*. The test involves collection of breath samples before and after ingestion of an oral solution of $^{13}$C-urea; the samples are sent for analysis by an appropriate laboratory. The test should not be performed within 4 weeks of treatment with an antibacterial or within 2 weeks of treatment with an antisecretory drug. A specific $^{13}$C-Urea breath test kit for children is available (*Helicobacter Test INFAI for children of the age 3–11*®). However the appropriateness of testing for *H. pylori* infection in children has not been established. Breath, saliva, faecal, and urine tests for *H. pylori* are frequently unreliable in children; the most accurate method of diagnosis is endoscopy with biopsy.

### Helicobacter Test INFAI for children of the age 3–11® (Infai) PoM

Oral powder, $^{13}$C-urea 45 mg, net price 1 kit (including 4 breath sample containers, straws) = £19.20 (spectrometric analysis included)

### Helicobacter Test INFAI® (Infai) PoM

Oral powder, $^{13}$C-urea 75 mg, net price 1 kit (including 4 breath-sample containers, straws) = £19.20 (spectrometric analysis included); 1 kit (including 2 breath bags) = £14.20 (spectroscopic analysis not included); 50-test set = £855.00 (spectrometric analysis included)

## NSAID-associated ulcers

Gastro-intestinal bleeding and ulceration can occur with NSAID use (section 10.1.1). In adults, the risk of serious upper gastro-intestinal side-effects varies between individual NSAIDs (see Gastro-intestinal side-effects, p. 502). Whenever possible, NSAIDs should be **withdrawn** if an ulcer occurs.

Children at high risk of developing gastro-intestinal complications with a NSAID include those with a history of peptic ulcer disease or serious upper gastro-intestinal complication, those taking other medicines that increase the risk of upper gastro-intestinal side-effects, or those with serious co-morbidity. In children at risk of ulceration, a proton pump inhibitor (section 1.3.5) can be considered for protection against gastric and duodenal ulcers associated with non-selective NSAIDs; high dose ranitidine is an alternative .

### Recommended regimens for *Helicobacter pylori* eradication

| Eradication therapy | Age range | Oral dose (to be used in combination with omeprazole, section 1.3.5) |
|---|---|---|
| Amoxicillin | 1–6 years | 250 mg twice daily (with clarithromycin) |
| | | 125 mg 3 times daily (with metronidazole) |
| | 6–12 years | 500 mg twice daily (with clarithromycin) |
| | | 250 mg 3 times daily (with metronidazole) |
| | 12–18 years | 1 g twice daily (with clarithromycin) |
| | | 500 mg 3 times daily (with metronidazole) |
| Clarithromycin | 1–12 years | 7.5 mg/kg (max. 500 mg) twice daily (with metronidazole or amoxicillin) |
| | 12–18 years | 500 mg twice daily (with metronidazole or amoxicillin) |
| Metronidazole | 1–6 years | 100 mg twice daily (with clarithromycin) |
| | | 100 mg 3 times daily (with amoxicillin) |
| | 6–12 years | 200 mg twice daily (with clarithromycin) |
| | | 200 mg 3 times daily (with amoxicillin) |
| | 12–18 years | 400 mg twice daily (with clarithromycin) |
| | | 400 mg 3 times daily (with amoxicillin) |

**1**

**Gastro-intestinal system**

NSAID use and *H. pylori* infection are independent risk factors for gastro-intestinal bleeding and ulceration. In children already taking a NSAID, eradication of *H. pylori* is unlikely to reduce the risk of NSAID-induced bleeding or ulceration. However, in children about to start long-term NSAID treatment who are *H. pylori* positive and have dyspepsia or a history of gastric or duodenal ulcer, eradication of *H. pylori* may reduce the overall risk of ulceration.

If the *NSAID can be discontinued* in a child who has developed an ulcer, a proton pump inhibitor usually produces the most rapid healing; alternatively the ulcer can be treated with an H$_2$-receptor antagonist.

If *NSAID treatment needs to continue*, the ulcer is treated with a proton pump inhibitor (section 1.3.5).

### 1.3.1 H$_2$-receptor antagonists

Histamine H$_2$-receptor antagonists heal *gastric* and *duodenal ulcers* by reducing gastric acid output as a result of histamine H$_2$-receptor blockade; they are also used to relieve symptoms of *dyspepsia* and *gastro-oesophageal reflux disease* (section 1.1). H$_2$-receptor antagonists should not normally be used for *Zollinger–Ellison syndrome* because proton pump inhibitors (section 1.3.5) are more effective.

Maintenance treatment with low doses has largely been replaced in *Helicobacter pylori* positive children by eradication regimens (section 1.3).

H$_2$-receptor antagonist therapy can promote healing of *NSAID-associated ulcers* (section 1.3).

Treatment with a H$_2$-receptor antagonist has not been shown to be beneficial in haematemesis and melaena, but prophylactic use reduces the frequency of bleeding from *gastroduodenal erosions in hepatic coma*, and possibly in other conditions requiring intensive care. Treatment also reduces the risk of *acid aspiration* in obstetric patients at delivery (Mendelson's syndrome).

H$_2$-receptor antagonists are also used to reduce the degradation of pancreatic enzyme supplements (section 1.9.4) in children with cystic fibrosis.

**Side-effects**   Side-effects of H$_2$-receptor antagonists include diarrhoea, headache, and dizziness. Rash (including erythema multiforme and toxic epidermal necrolysis) occurs less frequently. Other side-effects reported rarely or very rarely include hepatitis, cholestatic jaundice, bradycardia, psychiatric reactions (including confusion, depression, and hallucinations) particularly in the very ill, blood disorders (including leucopenia, thrombocytopenia, and pancytopenia), arthralgia, and myalgia. There are isolated reports of gynaecomastia and impotence.

### ▌ RANITIDINE

**Cautions**   interactions: Appendix 1 (histamine H$_2$-antagonists)

**Renal impairment**   use half normal dose if estimated glomerular filtration rate less than 50 mL/minute/1.73 m$^2$

**Pregnancy**   manufacturer advises avoid unless essential, but not known to be harmful

**Breast-feeding**   significant amount present in milk, but not known to be harmful

**Side-effects**   see notes above; also *less commonly* blurred vision; also reported pancreatitis, involuntary movement disorders, interstitial nephritis, alopecia

**Licensed use**   *oral* preparations not licensed for use in children under 3 years; *injection* not licensed for use in children under 6 months

### Indications and dose

**Reflux oesophagitis, benign gastric and duodenal ulceration, prophylaxis of stress ulceration, other conditions where gastric acid reduction is beneficial** (see notes above and section 1.9.4)

- By mouth

  **Neonate** 2 mg/kg 3 times daily but absorption unreliable; max. 3 mg/kg 3 times daily

  **Child 1–6 months** 1 mg/kg 3 times daily; max. 3 mg/kg 3 times daily

  **Child 6 months–3 years** 2–4 mg/kg twice daily

  **Child 3–12 years** 2–4 mg/kg (max. 150 mg) twice daily; increased up to 5 mg/kg (max. 300 mg) twice daily in severe gastro-oesophageal reflux disease

  **Child 12–18 years** 150 mg twice daily *or* 300 mg at night; increased if necessary, to 300 mg twice daily *or* 150 mg 4 times daily for up to 12 weeks in moderate to severe gastro-oesophageal reflux disease

  **Note** In fat malabsorption syndrome, give 1–2 hours before food to enhance effects of pancreatic enzyme replacement

- By slow intravenous injection

  **Neonate** 0.5–1 mg/kg every 6–8 hours

  **Child 1 month–18 years** 1 mg/kg (max. 50 mg) every 6–8 hours (may be given as an intermittent infusion at a rate of 25 mg/hour)

**Administration**   For *slow intravenous injection* dilute to a concentration of 2.5 mg/mL with Glucose 5% *or* Sodium Chloride 0.9%; give over at least 3 minutes

**Ranitidine** (Non-proprietary)  PoM
Tablets, ranitidine (as hydrochloride) 150 mg, net price 60-tab pack = £1.97; 300 mg, 30-tab pack = £2.17
Brands include *Ranitic*®

Effervescent tablets, ranitidine (as hydrochloride) 150 mg, net price 60-tab pack = £18.04; 300 mg, 30-tab pack = £17.03. Label: 13
Excipients   may include sodium (check with supplier)

Oral solution, ranitidine (as hydrochloride) 75 mg/5 mL, 100 mL = £7.44, 300 mL = £19.61
Excipients   may include alcohol (check with supplier)
Note   Ranitidine can be sold to the public for children over 16 years (provided packs do not contain more than 2 weeks' supply) for the short-term symptomatic relief of heartburn, dyspepsia, and hyperacidity, and for the prevention of these symptoms when associated with consumption of food or drink (max. single dose 75 mg, max. daily dose 300 mg)

Injection, ranitidine (as hydrochloride) 25 mg/mL, net price 2-mL amp = 57p

**Zantac**® (GSK)  PoM
Tablets, f/c, ranitidine (as hydrochloride) 150 mg, net price 60-tab pack = £1.30; 300 mg, 30-tab pack = £1.30

Syrup, sugar-free, ranitidine (as hydrochloride) 75 mg/5 mL. Net price 300 mL = £20.76
Excipients   include alcohol 8%

Injection, ranitidine (as hydrochloride) 25 mg/mL. Net price 2-mL amp = 57p

## 1.3.2 Selective antimuscarinics

Classification not used in *BNF for Children*.

## 1.3.3 Chelates and complexes

**Sucralfate** is a complex of aluminium hydroxide and sulfated sucrose that appears to act by protecting the mucosa from acid-pepsin attack; it has minimal antacid properties. Sucralfate can be used to prevent stress ulceration in children receiving intensive care. It should be used with caution in this situation (**important:** reports of bezoar formation, see Bezoar Formation below).

## ▌SUCRALFATE

**Cautions** administration of sucralfate and enteral feeds should be separated by 1 hour; **interactions:** Appendix 1 (sucralfate)

> **Bezoar formation** Following reports of bezoar formation associated with sucralfate, caution is advised in seriously ill patients, especially those receiving concomitant enteral feeds or those with predisposing conditions such as delayed gastric emptying

**Renal impairment** use with caution; aluminium is absorbed and may accumulate

**Pregnancy** no evidence of harm; absorption from gastro-intestinal tract negligible

**Breast-feeding** amount probably too small to be harmful

**Side-effects** constipation; *less frequently* diarrhoea, nausea, indigestion, flatulence, gastric discomfort, back pain, dizziness, headache, drowsiness, bezoar formation (see above), dry mouth, and rash

**Licensed use** not licensed for use in children under 15 years; tablets not licensed for prophylaxis of stress ulceration

**Indications and dose**

> **Prophylaxis of stress ulceration in child under intensive care**
> * By mouth
>> **Child 1 month–2 years** 250 mg 4–6 times daily
>> **Child 2–12 years** 500 mg 4–6 times daily
>> **Child 12–15 years** 1 g 4–6 times daily
>> **Child 15–18 years** 1 g 6 times daily; max. 8 g daily

> **Benign gastric and duodenal ulceration**
> * By mouth
>> **Child 1 month–2 years** 250 mg 4–6 times daily
>> **Child 2–12 years** 500 mg 4–6 times daily
>> **Child 12–15 years** 1 g 4–6 times daily
>> **Child 15–18 years** 2 g twice daily (on rising and at bedtime) *or* 1 g 4 times daily (1 hour before meals and at bedtime) taken for 4–6 weeks, or in resistant cases up to 12 weeks; max. 8 g daily

**Administration** for administration *by mouth*, sucralfate should be given 1 hour before meals, see also Cautions, above; *oral suspension* blocks fine-bore feeding tubes; crushed *tablets* may be dispersed in water.

**Antepsin®** (Chugai) (PoM)
Tablets, scored, sucralfate 1 g, net price 50-tab pack = £5.77. Label: 5
Suspension, sucralfate, 1 g/5 mL, net price 250 mL (aniseed- and caramel-flavoured) = £5.77. Label: 5

## 1.3.4 Prostaglandin analogues

Classification not used in *BNF for Children*.

## 1.3.5 Proton pump inhibitors

Proton pump inhibitors inhibit gastric acid secretion by blocking the hydrogen-potassium adenosine triphosphatase enzyme system (the 'proton pump') of the gastric parietal cell. **Omeprazole** is an effective short-term treatment for *gastric* and *duodenal ulcers*; it is also used in combination with antibacterials for the eradication of *Helicobacter pylori* (see p. 41 for specific regimens). An initial short course of omeprazole is the treatment of choice in *gastro-oesophageal reflux disease* with severe symptoms; children with endoscopically confirmed *erosive*, *ulcerative*, or *stricturing oesophagitis* usually need to be maintained on omeprazole.

Omeprazole is also used for the prevention and treatment of NSAID-associated ulcers (see p. 41). In children who need to continue NSAID treatment after an ulcer has healed, the dose of omeprazole should not normally be reduced because asymptomatic ulcer deterioration may occur.

Omeprazole is effective in the treatment of the *Zollinger-Ellison syndrome* (including cases resistant to other treatment). It is also used to reduce the degradation of pancreatic enzyme supplements (section 1.9.4) in children with cystic fibrosis.

**Lansoprazole** is not licensed for use in children, but may be considered when the available formulations of omeprazole are unsuitable.

**Esomeprazole** can be used for the management of gastro-oesophageal reflux disease when the available formulations of omeprazole and lansoprazole are unsuitable.

**Cautions** Measurement of serum-magnesium concentrations should be considered before and during prolonged treatment with a proton pump inhibitor, especially when used with other drugs that cause hypomagnesaemia or with digoxin. A proton pump inhibitor should be prescribed for appropriate indications at the lowest effective dose for the shortest period; the need for long-term treatment should be reviewed periodically.

**Side-effects** Side-effects of the proton pump inhibitors include gastro-intestinal disturbances (including nausea, vomiting, abdominal pain, flatulence, diarrhoea, constipation), and headache. Less frequent side-effects include dry mouth, peripheral oedema, dizziness, sleep disturbances, fatigue, paraesthesia, arthralgia, myalgia, rash, and pruritus. Other side-effects reported *rarely* or *very rarely* include taste disturbance, stomatitis, hepatitis, jaundice, hypersensitivity reactions (including anaphylaxis, bronchospasm), fever, depression, hallucinations, confusion, gynaecomastia, interstitial nephritis, hyponatraemia, hypomagnesaemia (usually after 1 year of treatment, but sometimes after 3 months of treatment), blood disorders (including leucopenia, leucocytosis, pancytopenia, thrombocytopenia), visual disturbances, sweating, photosensitivity, alopecia, Stevens-Johnson syndrome, and toxic epidermal necrolysis. By decreasing gastric acidity, proton pump inhibitors may increase the risk of gastro-intestinal infections (including *Clostridium difficile* infection).

**1 Gastro-intestinal system**

Rebound acid hypersecretion and protracted dyspepsia may occur after stopping prolonged treatment with a proton pump inhibitor.

### ■ ESOMEPRAZOLE

**Cautions** interactions: Appendix 1 (proton pump inhibitors)

**Hepatic impairment** child 1–12 years max. 10 mg daily in severe impairment; child 12–18 years max. 20 mg daily in severe impairment

**Renal impairment** manufacturer advises caution in severe renal insufficiency

**Pregnancy** manufacturer advises caution—no information available

**Breast-feeding** manufacturer advises avoid—no information available

**Side-effects** see notes above

**Licensed use** tablets and capsules not licensed for use in children 1–12 years

**Indications and dose**

> **Gastro-oesophageal reflux disease (in the presence of erosive reflux oesophagitis)**
> - By mouth
>   **Child 1–12 years**
>   **Body-weight 10–20 kg** 10 mg once daily for 8 weeks
>   **Body-weight over 20 kg** 10–20 mg once daily for 8 weeks
>   **Child 12–18 years** 40 mg once daily for 4 weeks, continued for further 4 weeks if not fully healed or symptoms persist; maintenance 20 mg daily
> - By intravenous injection over at least 3 minutes *or* by intravenous infusion
>   **Child 1–12 years**
>   **Body-weight under 20 kg** 10 mg once daily
>   **Body-weight over 20 kg** 10–20 mg once daily
>   **Child 12–18 years** 40 mg once daily

> **Symptomatic treatment of gastro-oesophageal reflux disease (in the absence of oesophagitis)**
> - By mouth
>   **Child 1–12 years, body-weight over 10 kg** 10 mg once daily for up to 8 weeks
>   **Child 12–18 years** 20 mg once daily for up to 4 weeks
> - By intravenous injection over at least 3 minutes *or* by intravenous infusion
>   **Child 1–12 years** 10 mg once daily
>   **Child 12–18 years** 20 mg once daily

**Administration** for *intravenous infusion*, dilute reconstituted solution to a concentration not exceeding 800 micrograms/mL with Sodium Chloride 0.9%; give over 10–30 minutes

**Esomeprazole** (Non-proprietary) [PoM]
Capsules, enclosing e/c pellets, esomeprazole (as magnesium salt) 20 mg, net price 28-cap pack = £12.95; 40 mg, 28-cap pack = £17.63. Counselling, administration
Brands include *Emozul®*
Administration Do not chew or crush capsules; swallow whole *or* mix capsule contents in water and drink within 30 minutes; for administration through a gastric tube, consult product literature

Tablets, e/c, esomeprazole (as magnesium salt) 20 mg, net price 28-tab pack = £15.95; 40 mg, 28-tab pack = £20.30. Counselling, administration
Administration Do not chew or crush tablets; swallow whole *or* disperse in water and drink within 30 minutes; for administration through a gastric tube, consult product literature
Injection, powder for reconstitution, esomeprazole (as sodium salt), net price 40-mg vial = £3.10

**Nexium®** (AstraZeneca) [PoM]
Tablets, e/c, f/c, esomeprazole (as magnesium trihydrate) 20 mg (light pink), net price 28-tab pack = £18.50; 40 mg (pink), 28-tab pack = £25.19. Counselling, administration
Administration Do not chew or crush tablets; swallow whole *or* disperse in water and drink within 30 minutes; for administration through a gastric tube, consult product literature
Granules, yellow, e/c, esomeprazole (as magnesium trihydrate) 10 mg/sachet, net price 28-sachet pack = £25.19. Label: 25, counselling, administration
Administration Disperse the contents of each sachet in approx. 15 mL water. Stir and leave to thicken for a few minutes; stir again before administration and use within 30 minutes; rinse container with 15 mL water to obtain full dose; for administration through gastric tube, consult product literature
Injection, powder for reconstitution, esomeprazole (as sodium salt), net price 40-mg vial = £3.13

### ■ LANSOPRAZOLE

**Cautions** interactions: Appendix 1 (proton pump inhibitors)

**Hepatic impairment** use half normal dose in moderate to severe liver disease

**Pregnancy** manufacturer advises avoid

**Breast-feeding** avoid —present in milk in *animal* studies

**Side-effects** see notes above; also glossitis, pancreatitis, anorexia, restlessness, tremor, impotence, petechiae, and purpura; *very rarely* colitis, raised serum cholesterol or triglycerides

**Licensed use** not licensed for use in children

**Indications and dose**

> **Gastro-oesophageal reflux disease, acid-related dyspepsia, treatment of duodenal and benign gastric ulcer including those complicating NSAID therapy, fat malabsorption despite pancreatic enzyme replacement therapy in cystic fibrosis**
> - By mouth
>   **Child body-weight under 30 kg** 0.5–1 mg/kg (max. 15 mg) once daily in the morning
>   **Child body-weight over 30 kg** 15–30 mg once daily in the morning

**Administration** for administration by a *nasogastric tube* or an *oral syringe*, *Zoton FasTab®* can be dispersed in a small amount of water

**Zoton®** (Pfizer) [PoM]
FasTab® (= orodispersible tablet), lansoprazole 15 mg, net price 28-tab pack = £2.99; 30 mg, 28-tab pack = £5.50. Label: 5, 22, counselling, administration
Excipients include aspartame (section 9.4.1)
Counselling Tablets should be placed on the tongue, allowed to disperse and swallowed, or may be swallowed whole with a glass of water.

## ▲ OMEPRAZOLE

**Cautions** interactions: Appendix 1 (proton pump inhibitors)

**Hepatic impairment** no more than 700 micrograms/kg (max. 20 mg) once daily

**Pregnancy** not known to be harmful

**Breast-feeding** present in milk but not known to be harmful

**Side-effects** see notes above; also agitation and impotence

**Licensed use** *capsules* and *tablets* not licensed for use in children except for severe ulcerating reflux oesophagitis in children over 1 year; *injection* not licensed for use in children under 12 years

### Indications and dose

Gastro-oesophageal reflux disease, acid-related dyspepsia, treatment of duodenal and benign gastric ulcers including those complicating NSAID therapy, prophylaxis of acid aspiration, Zollinger-Ellison syndrome, fat malabsorption despite pancreatic enzyme replacement therapy in cystic fibrosis

- By mouth

  **Neonate** 700 micrograms/kg once daily, increased if necessary after 7–14 days to 1.4 mg/kg; some neonates may require up to 2.8 mg/kg once daily

  **Child 1 month–2 years** 700 micrograms/kg once daily, increased if necessary to 3 mg/kg (max. 20 mg) once daily

  **Child body-weight 10–20 kg** 10 mg once daily increased if necessary to 20 mg once daily (in severe ulcerating reflux oesophagitis, max. 12 weeks at higher dose)

  **Child body-weight over 20 kg** 20 mg once daily increased if necessary to 40 mg once daily (in severe ulcerating reflux oesophagitis, max. 12 weeks at higher dose)

- By intravenous injection over 5 minutes *or* by intravenous infusion

  **Child 1 month–12 years** initially 500 micrograms/kg (max. 20 mg) once daily, increased to 2 mg/kg (max. 40 mg) once daily if necessary

  **Child 12–18 years** 40 mg once daily

*Helicobacter pylori* **eradication** (in combination with antibacterials see p. 41)

- By mouth

  **Child 1–12 years** 1–2 mg/kg (max. 40 mg) once daily

  **Child 12–18 years** 40 mg once daily

**Administration** for administration *by mouth*, swallow whole, *or* disperse *Losec MUPS®* tablets in water, *or* mix capsule contents or *Losec MUPS®* tablets with fruit juice or yoghurt. Preparations consisting of an e/c tablet within a capsule should **not** be opened.

For administration through an *enteral feeding tube*, use *Losec MUPS®* or the contents of a capsule containing omeprazole dispersed in a large volume of water, or in 10 mL Sodium Bicarbonate 8.4% (1 mmol Na⁺/mL) (allow to stand for 10 minutes before administration).

For *intermittent intravenous infusion*, dilute reconstituted solution to a concentration of 400 micrograms/mL with Glucose 5% *or* Sodium Chloride 0.9%; give over 20–30 minutes

**Omeprazole** (Non-proprietary) (PoM)

Capsules, enclosing e/c granules, omeprazole 10 mg, net price 28-cap pack = £1.81; 20 mg, 28-cap pack = £1.92; 40 mg, 7-cap pack = £1.95, 28-cap pack = £21.65. Counselling, administration

Note Some preparations consist of an e/c tablet within a capsule

Dental prescribing on NHS Gastro-resistant omeprazole capsules may be prescribed

Tablets, e/c, omeprazole 10 mg, net price 28-tab pack = £5.84; 20 mg, 28-tab pack = £5.71; 40 mg, 7-tab pack = £5.15. Label: 25

Intravenous infusion, powder for reconstitution, omeprazole (as sodium salt), net price 40-mg vial = £5.18

**Losec®** (AstraZeneca) (PoM)

MUPS® (multiple-unit pellet system = dispersible tablets), f/c, omeprazole 10 mg (light pink), net price 28-tab pack = £7.75; 20 mg (pink), 28-tab pack = £11.60; 40 mg (red-brown), 7-tab pack = £5.80. Counselling, administration

Capsules, enclosing e/c granules, omeprazole 10 mg (pink), net price 28-cap pack = £7.75; 20 mg (pink/brown), 28-cap pack = £11.60; 40 mg (brown), 7-cap pack = £5.80. Counselling, administration

Intravenous infusion, powder for reconstitution, omeprazole (as sodium salt), net price 40-mg vial = £5.41

Injection, powder for reconstitution, omeprazole (as sodium salt), net price 40-mg vial (with solvent) = £5.41

## 1.4 Acute diarrhoea

**1.4.1 Adsorbents and bulk-forming drugs**

**1.4.2 Antimotility drugs**

**1.4.3 Enkephalinase inhibitors**

The priority in acute diarrhoea, as in gastro-enteritis, is the prevention or reversal of fluid and electrolyte depletion—this is particularly important in infants. For details of **oral rehydration preparations**, see section 9.2.1.2. Severe dehydration requires immediate admission to hospital and urgent replacement of fluid and electrolytes.

**Antimotility drugs** (section 1.4.2) relieve symptoms of diarrhoea. They are used in the management of uncomplicated acute diarrhoea in adults, but are **not** recommended for use in children under 12 years. Fluid and electrolyte replacement (section 9.2.1.2) are of prime importance in the treatment of acute diarrhoea.

**Racecadotril** (section 1.4.3) is licensed, as an adjunct to rehydration, for the symptomatic treatment of uncomplicated acute diarrhoea; however, it should only be used when usual supportive measures, including oral rehydration, are insufficient to control the condition.

**Antispasmodics** (section 1.2) are occasionally of value in treating abdominal cramp associated with diarrhoea but they should **not** be used for primary treatment. Antispasmodics and antiemetics should be **avoided** in young children with gastro-enteritis since they are rarely effective and have troublesome side-effects.

Antibacterial drugs are generally unnecessary in simple gastro-enteritis because the complaint usually resolves quickly without such treatment, and infective diarrhoeas in the UK often have a viral cause. Systemic bacterial infection does, however, need appropriate systemic treatment; for drugs used in campylobacter enteritis, shigellosis, and salmonellosis, see p. 246

**Colestyramine** (section 1.9.2) binds unabsorbed bile salts and provides symptomatic relief of diarrhoea following ileal disease or resection.

## 1.4.1 Adsorbents and bulk-forming drugs

Adsorbents such as kaolin are **not** recommended for *acute diarrhoeas*. Bulk-forming drugs, such as ispaghula, methylcellulose, and sterculia (section 1.6.1) are rarely effective in controlling faecal consistency in ileostomy and colostomy.

## 1.4.2 Antimotility drugs

Antimotility drugs prolong the duration of intestinal transit by binding to opioid receptors in the gastrointestinal tract. Loperamide does not cross the blood-brain barrier readily. Antimotility drugs have a role in the management of uncomplicated *acute diarrhoea* in adults but not in children under 12 years; see also section 1.4. However, in the case of dehydration, fluid and electrolyte replacement (section 9.2.1.2) are of primary importance.

For comments on their role in *chronic bowel disorders* see section 1.5. Antimotility drugs are also used in children with *stoma* (section 1.8).

### CODEINE PHOSPHATE

**Cautions**   see section 4.7.2; tolerance and dependence may occur with prolonged use; **interactions:** Appendix 1 (opioid analgesics)

**Contra-indications**   see section 4.7.2; also conditions where inhibition of peristalsis should be avoided, where abdominal distension develops, or in acute diarrhoeal conditions such as acute ulcerative colitis or antibiotic-associated colitis

**Hepatic impairment**   section 4.7.2

**Renal impairment**   section 4.7.2

**Pregnancy**   section 4.7.2

**Breast-feeding**   section 4.7.2

**Side-effects**   section 4.7.2

**Indications and dose**

> **Diarrhoea** (but see notes above)
>
> • By mouth
>
> **Child 12–18 years** 30 mg (range 15–60 mg) 3–4 times daily

> **Pain** section 4.7.2

◀**Preparations**
Section 4.7.2

### CO-PHENOTROPE

A mixture of diphenoxylate hydrochloride and atropine sulfate in the mass proportions 100 parts to 1 part respectively

**Cautions**   section 4.7.2; also young children are particularly susceptible to **overdosage** and symptoms

may be delayed and observation is needed for at least 48 hours after ingestion; presence of subclinical doses of atropine may give rise to atropine side-effects in susceptible individuals or in overdosage (section 1.2); **interactions:** Appendix 1 (antimuscarinics, opioid analgesics)

**Contra-indications**   section 4.7.2 and also see under Antimuscarinics (section 1.2)

**Hepatic impairment**   section 4.7.2; also avoid in jaundice

**Renal impairment**   section 4.7.2

**Pregnancy**   section 4.7.2

**Breast-feeding**   may be present in milk

**Side-effects**   section 4.7.2 and also see under Antimuscarinics (section 1.2); also abdominal pain, anorexia, fever

**Licensed use**   not licensed for use in children under 4 years

**Indications and dose**

> See preparations

**Administration**   for administration *by mouth* tablets may be crushed

**Co-phenotrope** (Non-proprietary) PoM
Tablets, co-phenotrope 2.5/0.025 (diphenoxylate hydrochloride 2.5 mg, atropine sulfate 25 micrograms), net price 100 = £8.95
**Brands include** *Lomotil®*
Dose

> **Control of faecal consistency after colostomy or ileostomy, adjunct to rehydration in acute diarrhoea** (but see notes above)
>
> • By mouth
>
> **Child 2–4 years** half tablet 3 times daily
>
> **Child 4–9 years** 1 tablet 3 times daily
>
> **Child 9–12 years** 1 tablet 4 times daily
>
> **Child 12–16 years** 2 tablets 3 times daily
>
> **Child 16–18 years** initially 4 tablets then 2 tablets 4 times daily

> **Note** Co-phenotrope 2.5/0.025 can be sold to the public for children over 16 years (provided packs do not contain more than 20 tablets) as an adjunct to rehydration in acute diarrhoea (max. daily dose 10 tablets)

### LOPERAMIDE HYDROCHLORIDE

**Cautions**   see notes above; **interactions:** Appendix 1 (loperamide)

**Contra-indications**   conditions where inhibition of peristalsis should be avoided, where abdominal distension develops, or in conditions such as active ulcerative colitis or antibiotic-associated colitis

**Hepatic impairment**   risk of accumulation—manufacturer advises caution

**Pregnancy**   manufacturer advises avoid—no information available

**Breast-feeding**   amount probably too small to be harmful

**Side-effects**   nausea, flatulence, headache, dizziness; *less commonly* dyspepsia, vomiting, abdominal pain, dry mouth, drowsiness, rash (rarely Stevens-Johnson syndrome, toxic epidermal necrolysis); *rarely* paralytic ileus, fatigue, hypertonia, urinary retention

**Licensed use**   *capsules* not licensed for use in children under 8 years; *syrup* not licensed for use in children under 4 years; not licensed for use in children for chronic diarrhoea

**Indications and dose**

Chronic diarrhoea

- By mouth

  **Child 1 month–1 year** 100–200 micrograms/kg twice daily, 30 minutes before feeds; up to 2 mg/kg daily in divided doses occasionally required

  **Child 1–12 years** 100–200 micrograms/kg (max. 2 mg) 3–4 times daily; up to 1.25 mg/kg daily in divided doses may be required (max. 16 mg daily)

  **Child 12–18 years** 2–4 mg 2–4 times daily (max. 16 mg daily)

Acute diarrhoea (but see notes above)

- By mouth

  **Child 4–8 years** 1 mg 3–4 times daily for *up to 3 days only*

  **Child 8–12 years** 2 mg 4 times daily for up to 5 days

  **Child 12–18 years** initially 4 mg, then 2 mg after each loose stool for up to 5 days (usual dose 6–8 mg daily; max. 16 mg daily)

**Loperamide** (Non-proprietary) (PoM)

Capsules, loperamide hydrochloride 2 mg, net price 30-cap pack = £1.07

Tablets, loperamide hydrochloride 2 mg, net price 30-tab pack = £2.15

Brands include *Norimode*®

Note Loperamide can be sold to the public, for use in children over 12 years, provided it is licensed and labelled for the treatment of acute diarrhoea

**Imodium**® (Janssen) (PoM)

Syrup, sugar-free, red, loperamide hydrochloride 1 mg/5 mL. Net price 100 mL = £1.17

◀ Compound preparations

**Imodium**® **Plus** (McNeil)

Caplets (= tablets), loperamide hydrochloride 2 mg, simeticone 125 mg, net price 6-tab pack = £2.27, 12-tab pack = £3.58

Dose

Acute diarrhoea with abdominal colic

   **Child 12–18 years** initially 1 caplet, then 1 caplet after each loose stool; max. 4 caplets daily for up to 2 days

---

## 1.4.3 Enkephalinase inhibitors

**Racecadotril** is a pro-drug of thiorphan. Thiorphan is an enkephalinase inhibitor that inhibits the breakdown of endogenous opioids, thereby reducing intestinal secretions. Racecadotril is licensed, as an adjunct to rehydration, for the symptomatic treatment of uncomplicated acute diarrhoea; it should only be used in children over 3 months of age when usual supportive measures, including oral rehydration, are insufficient to control the condition. Racecadotril does not affect the duration of intestinal transit.

The *Scottish Medicines Consortium*, p. 3 has advised (November 2012) that racecadotril (*Hidrasec*®) is **not** recommended for use within NHS Scotland for the treatment of acute diarrhoea because there is insufficient evidence that it improves the recovery rate.

---

### ■ RACECADOTRIL

**Hepatic impairment** manufacturer advises avoid

**Renal impairment** manufacturer advises avoid

**Pregnancy** manufacturer advises avoid—no information available

**Breast-feeding** manufacturer advises avoid—no information available

**Side-effects** headache; *less commonly* rash

**Indications and dose**

Acute uncomplicated diarrhoea (but see notes above)

- By mouth

  **Child 3 months–18 years**

  **Body-weight less than 9 kg** 10 mg 3 times daily until diarrhoea stops (max. duration of treatment 7 days)

  **Body-weight 9–13 kg** 20 mg 3 times daily until diarrhoea stops (max. duration of treatment 7 days)

  **Body-weight 13–27 kg** 30 mg 3 times daily until diarrhoea stops (max. duration of treatment 7 days)

  **Body-weight over 27 kg** 60 mg 3 times daily until diarrhoea stops (max. duration of treatment 7 days)

**Hidrasec**® (Abbott Healthcare) ▼ (PoM)

Granules, racecadotril 10 mg/sachet, net price 20-sachet pack = £8.42; 30 mg/sachet, 20-sachet pack = £8.42. Counselling, administration

Excipients include sucrose 970 mg/10 mg sachet (2.9 g/30 mg sachet)

Administration granules may be added to food or mixed with water or bottle feeds and then taken immediately

---

## 1.5   Chronic bowel disorders

| | |
|---|---|
| **1.5.1** | Aminosalicylates |
| **1.5.2** | Corticosteroids |
| **1.5.3** | Drugs affecting the immune response |
| **1.5.4** | Food allergy |

Individual symptoms of chronic bowel disorders need specific treatment including dietary manipulation as well as drug treatment and the maintenance of a liberal fluid intake.

### Inflammatory bowel disease

Chronic inflammatory bowel diseases include *ulcerative colitis* and *Crohn's disease*. The treatment of inflammatory bowel disease in children should be initiated and supervised by a paediatric gastroenterologist. Effective management requires drug therapy, attention to nutrition, and in severe or chronic active disease, surgery.

**Aminosalicylates** (balsalazide, mesalazine, olsalazine, and sulfasalazine), **corticosteroids** (hydrocortisone, budesonide, and prednisolone), and **drugs that affect the immune response** are used in the treatment of inflammatory bowel disease.

**Treatment of acute ulcerative colitis and Crohn's disease** Acute mild to moderate disease affecting the rectum (proctitis) or the recto-sigmoid (distal colitis) is treated initially with local application of an aminosalicylate (section 1.5.1); alternatively a local corticosteroid (section 1.5.2) can be used but it is less effective. Foam preparations and suppositories are useful for children who have difficulty retaining liquid enemas.

Diffuse inflammatory bowel disease or disease that does not respond to local therapy requires oral treatment. Mild disease affecting the proximal colon can be treated with an oral aminosalicylate alone; a combination of a local and an oral aminosalicylate can be used in proctitis or distal colitis. Refractory or moderate inflammatory bowel disease usually requires adjunctive use of an oral corticosteroid such as **prednisolone** (section 1.5.2) for 4–8 weeks. Modified-release **budesonide** is used for children with Crohn's disease affecting the ileum and the ascending colon; it causes fewer systemic side-effects than oral prednisolone, but may be less effective. As an alternative to an oral corticosteroid, **enteral nutrition** (Appendix 2) may be used for 6–8 weeks in children with active Crohn's disease.

Severe inflammatory bowel disease or disease that is not responding to an oral corticosteroid requires hospital admission and treatment with an intravenous corticosteroid such as **hydrocortisone** (p. 375) or **methylprednisolone** (p. 376); other therapy may include intravenous fluid and electrolyte replacement, and possibly parenteral nutrition. Children with ulcerative colitis that fails to respond adequately to these measures may benefit from a short course of ciclosporin. Children with unresponsive or chronically active Crohn's disease may benefit from azathioprine, mercaptopurine, or once-weekly methotrexate; these drugs have a slow onset of action.

**Infliximab** (section 1.5.3) is used in specialist centres for children with severe active Crohn's disease or severe active ulcerative colitis whose condition has not responded adequately to treatment with a corticosteroid and a conventional drug that affects the immune response, or who are intolerant of them. There are concerns about the long-term safety of infliximab in children; hepatosplenic T-cell lymphoma has been reported.

Crohn's disease of the mouth or of the perineum is more common in children than in adults and it is difficult to treat; elimination diets and the use of a topical corticosteroid (section 13.4) may be beneficial, but a systemic corticosteroid (section 6.3.2) and occasionally azathioprine may be required in severe cases.

**NICE guidance**
**Infliximab for Crohn's disease (May 2010)**
In children over 6 years of age, infliximab is recommended for the treatment of severe active Crohn's disease that has not responded to conventional therapy (including corticosteroids, other drugs affecting the immune response, and primary nutrition therapy) or when conventional therapy cannot be used because of intolerance or contra-indications. Infliximab should be given as a planned course of treatment for 12 months or until treatment failure, whichever is shorter. Treatment should be continued beyond 12 months only if there is evidence of active disease—in these cases the need for treatment should be reviewed at least annually. If the disease relapses after stopping treatment, infliximab can be restarted [but see Hypersensitivity Reactions under Infliximab, p. 55].
www.nice.org.uk/TA187

**NICE guidance**
**Infliximab for subacute manifestations of ulcerative colitis (April 2008)**
Infliximab is **not** recommended for the treatment of subacute manifestations of moderate to severe active ulcerative colitis that would normally be managed in an outpatient setting.
www.nice.org.uk/TA140

**Maintenance of remission of acute ulcerative colitis and Crohn's disease**  Children should be advised not to smoke because smoking increases the risk of relapse in Crohn's disease. Smoking cessation (section 4.10.2) should be encouraged when necessary. **Aminosalicylates** are efficacious in the maintenance of remission of ulcerative colitis, but there is no evidence of efficacy in the maintenance of remission of Crohn's disease. Corticosteroids are **not** suitable for maintenance treatment because of their side-effects. In resistant or frequently relapsing cases either **azathioprine** (section 1.5.3) or **mercaptopurine** (section 1.5.3) may be helpful. **Methotrexate** (section 1.5.3) is used in Crohn's disease when azathioprine or mercaptopurine are ineffective or not tolerated. Infliximab (p. 55) can be used for maintenance therapy in Crohn's disease or ulcerative colitis in children who respond to the initial induction course of this drug. There are concerns about the long-term safety of infliximab in children.

**Fistulating Crohn's disease**  Treatment may not be necessary for simple, asymptomatic perianal fistulas. **Metronidazole** (section 5.1.11) or **ciprofloxacin** (section 5.1.12) may be beneficial for the treatment of fistulating Crohn's disease [both unlicensed for this indication]. Metronidazole by mouth is used at a dose of 7.5 mg/kg 3 times daily, usually for 1 month; it should not be used for longer than 3 months because of concerns about peripheral neuropathy. Ciprofloxacin by mouth is given at a dose of 5 mg/kg twice daily. Other antibacterials should be given if specifically indicated (e.g. sepsis associated with fistulas and perianal disease) and for managing bacterial overgrowth in the small bowel. Fistulas may also require surgical exploration and local drainage.

Either **azathioprine** or **mercaptopurine** is used as a second-line treatment for fistulating Crohn's disease and continued for maintenance. **Infliximab** is used for fistulating Crohn's disease refractory to conventional treatments; maintenance therapy with infliximab should be considered for patients who respond to the initial induction course.

**Adjunctive treatment of inflammatory bowel disease**  Due attention should be paid to diet; high-fibre or low-residue diets should be used as appropriate.

Antimotility drugs such as codeine phosphate and loperamide, and antispasmodic drugs may precipitate paralytic ileus and megacolon in active ulcerative colitis; treatment of the inflammation is more logical. Laxatives may be required in proctitis. Diarrhoea resulting from the loss of bile-salt absorption (e.g. in terminal ileal disease or bowel resection) may improve with **colestyramine** (section 1.9.2), which binds bile salts.

## Irritable bowel syndrome

Irritable bowel syndrome can present with pain, constipation, or diarrhoea. Some children have important psychological aggravating factors which respond to reassurance. The **fibre** intake of children with irritable bowel syndrome should be reviewed. If an increase in dietary fibre is required, soluble fibre (e.g. oats, ispaghula husk, or sterculia) is recommended; insoluble fibre (e.g. bran) should be avoided. A **laxative** (section 1.6) can be used to treat constipation. An osmotic laxative, such as a macrogol, is preferred; lactulose may cause bloating. **Loperamide** (section 1.4.2) may relieve diarrhoea and antispasmodic drugs (section 1.2) may relieve pain. Opioids with a central action, such as codeine, are better avoided because of the risk of dependence.

## Clostridium difficile infection

*Clostridium difficile* infection is caused by colonisation of the colon with *Clostridium difficile* and production of toxin. It often follows antibiotic therapy and is usually of acute onset, but may become chronic. It is a particular hazard of ampicillin, amoxicillin, co-amoxiclav, second- and third-generation cephalosporins, clindamycin, and quinolones, but few antibacterials are free of this side-effect. Oral **metronidazole** (section 5.1.11) or oral **vancomycin** (section 5.1.7) are used as specific treatment; vancomycin may be preferred for very sick patients. Metronidazole can be given by intravenous infusion if oral treatment is inappropriate.

## Malabsorption syndromes

Individual conditions need specific management and also general nutritional consideration. Coeliac disease (gluten enteropathy) usually needs a gluten-free diet (Appendix 2) and pancreatic insufficiency needs pancreatin supplements (section 1.9.4).

For further information on foods for special diets (ACBS), see Appendix 2.

## 1.5.1 Aminosalicylates

**Sulfasalazine** is a combination of 5-aminosalicylic acid ('5-ASA') and sulfapyridine; sulfapyridine acts only as a carrier to the colonic site of action but still causes side-effects. In the newer aminosalicylates, **mesalazine** (5-aminosalicylic acid), **balsalazide** (a prodrug of 5-aminosalicylic acid) and **olsalazine** (a dimer of 5-aminosalicylic acid which cleaves in the lower bowel), the sulfonamide-related side-effects of sulfasalazine are avoided, but 5-aminosalicylic acid alone can still cause side-effects including blood disorders (see recommendation below) and lupus-like syndrome also seen with sulfasalazine.

**Cautions** Renal function should be monitored before starting an oral aminosalicylate, at 3 months of treatment, and then annually during treatment (more frequently in renal impairment). Blood disorders can occur with aminosalicylates (see recommendation below).

> **Blood disorders**
> Children receiving aminosalicylates and their carers should be advised to report any unexplained bleeding, bruising, purpura, sore throat, fever or malaise that occurs during treatment. A blood count should be performed and the drug stopped immediately if there is suspicion of a blood dyscrasia.

**Contra-indications** Aminosalicylates should be avoided in salicylate hypersensitivity.

**Side-effects** Side-effects of the aminosalicylates include diarrhoea, nausea, vomiting, abdominal pain, exacerbation of symptoms of colitis, headache, hypersensitivity reactions (including rash and urticaria); side-effects that occur rarely include acute pancreatitis, hepatitis, myocarditis, pericarditis, lung disorders (including eosinophilia and fibrosing alveolitis), peripheral neuropathy, blood disorders (including agranulocytosis, aplastic anaemia, leucopenia, methaemoglobinaemia, neutropenia, and thrombocytopenia—see also recommendation above), renal dysfunction (interstitial nephritis, nephrotic syndrome), myalgia, arthralgia, skin reactions (including lupus erythematosus-like syndrome, Stevens-Johnson syndrome), alopecia.

## ▌ BALSALAZIDE SODIUM

**Cautions** see notes above; also history of asthma; **interactions:** Appendix 1 (aminosalicylates)
Blood disorders see recommendation above
**Contra-indications** see notes above
**Hepatic impairment** avoid in severe impairment
**Renal impairment** manufacturer advises avoid in moderate to severe impairment
**Pregnancy** manufacturer advises avoid
**Breast-feeding** monitor infant for diarrhoea
**Side-effects** see notes above; also cholelithiasis
**Licensed use** not licensed for use in children under 18 years

### Indications and dose

> **Treatment of mild to moderate ulcerative colitis and maintenance of remission**
> • By mouth
> **Child 12–18 years** acute attack, 2.25 g 3 times daily until remission occurs or for up to max. 12 weeks; maintenance, 1.5 g twice daily, adjusted according to response (max. 3 g twice daily)

**Colazide®** (Almirall) [PoM]
Capsules, beige, balsalazide sodium 750 mg, net price 130-cap pack = £30.42. Label: 21, 25, counselling, blood disorder symptoms (see recommendation above)

## ▌ MESALAZINE

**Cautions** see notes above; **interactions:** Appendix 1 (aminosalicylates)
Blood disorders see recommendation above
**Contra-indications** see notes above; blood clotting abnormalities
**Hepatic impairment** avoid in severe impairment
**Renal impairment** use with caution; avoid if estimated glomerular filtration rate less than 20 mL/minute/1.73 m$^2$
**Pregnancy** negligible quantity crosses placenta
**Breast-feeding** diarrhoea reported but negligible amounts detected in breast milk; monitor infant for diarrhoea
**Side-effects** see notes above
**Licensed use** *Asacol®* (all preparations) and *Salofalk®* enema not licensed for use in children under 18 years; *Salofalk®* suppositories, *Pentasa®* tablets and suppositories not licensed for use in children under 15 years; *Pentasa®* granules not licensed for use in chil-

dren under 6 years; *Salofalk*® rectal foam no dose recommendations for children (age range not specified by manufacturer)

**Indications and dose**

**Treatment of mild to moderate ulcerative colitis and maintenance of remission** for dose see under preparations below

> The delivery characteristics of oral mesalazine preparations may vary; these preparations should not be considered interchangeable

**Asacol**® (Warner Chilcott) [PoM]

Foam enema, mesalazine 1 g/metered application, net price 14-application canister with disposable applicators and plastic bags = £26.72. Counselling, blood disorder symptoms (see recommendation above)

**Excipients** include disodium edetate, hydroxybenzoates (parabens), polysorbate 20, sodium metabisulfite

**Dose**

**Acute attack affecting the rectosigmoid region**

- By rectum

  **Child 12–18 years** 1 metered application (mesalazine 1 g) into the rectum daily for 4–6 weeks

**Acute attack affecting the descending colon**

- By rectum

  **Child 12–18 years** 2 metered applications (mesalazine 2 g) once daily for 4–6 weeks

Suppositories, mesalazine 250 mg, net price 20-suppos pack = £4.82; 500 mg, 10-suppos pack = £4.82. Counselling, blood disorder symptoms (see recommendation above)

**Dose**

**Treatment and maintenance of remission of ulcerative colitis affecting the rectosigmoid region**

- By rectum

  **Child 12–18 years** 250–500 mg 3 times daily, with last dose at bedtime

**Asacol**® **MR** (Warner Chilcott) [PoM]

Tablets, red, e/c, mesalazine 400 mg, net price 90-tab pack = £29.41, 120-tab pack = £39.21. Label: 5, 25, counselling, blood disorder symptoms (see recommendation above)

**Dose**

**Acute attack**

- By mouth

  **Child 12–18 years** 800 mg 3 times daily

**Maintenance of remission of ulcerative colitis and Crohn's ileo-colitis**

- By mouth

  **Child 12–18 years** 400–800 mg 2–3 times daily

**Note** Preparations that lower stool pH (e.g. lactulose) may prevent release of mesalazine

**Ipocol**® (Sandoz) [PoM]

Tablets, e/c, mesalazine 400 mg, net price 120-tab pack = £41.62. Label: 5, 25, counselling, blood disorder symptoms (see recommendation above)

**Dose**

**Acute attack**

- By mouth

  **Child 12–18 years** 800 mg 3 times daily

**Maintenance of remission**

- By mouth

  **Child 12–18 years** 400–800 mg 3 times daily

**Mesren MR**® (IVAX) [PoM]

Tablets, red-brown, e/c, mesalazine 400 mg, net price 90-tab pack = £19.50, 120-tab pack = £26.00. Label: 5, 25, counselling, blood disorder symptoms (see recommendation above)

**Dose**

**Acute attack**

- By mouth

  **Child 12–18 years** 800 mg 3 times daily

**Maintenance of remission of ulcerative colitis and Crohn's ileo-colitis**

- By mouth

  **Child 12–18 years** 400–800 mg 3 times daily

**Pentasa**® (Ferring) [PoM]

Tablets, m/r, mesalazine 500 mg (grey, scored), net price 100-tab pack = £24.21; 1 g, 60-tab pack = £36.89. Counselling, administration (see dose), blood disorder symptoms (see recommendation above)

**Dose**

**Acute attack**

- By mouth

  **Child 5–15 years** 15–20 mg/kg (max. 1 g) 3 times daily

  **Child 15–18 years** 1–2 g twice daily; total daily dose may alternatively be given in 3 divided doses

**Maintenance of remission**

- By mouth

  **Child 5–15 years** 10 mg/kg (max. 500 mg) 2–3 times daily

  **Child 15–18 years** 2 g once daily

**Administration** tablets may be halved, quartered, or dispersed in water, but should not be chewed

Granules, m/r, pale grey-brown, mesalazine 1 g/sachet, net price 50-sachet pack = £28.82; 2 g/sachet, 60-sachet pack = £72.05. Counselling, administration (see dose), blood disorder symptoms (see recommendation above)

**Dose**

**Acute attack**

- By mouth

  **Child 5–12 years** 15–20 mg/kg (max. 1 g) 3 times daily

  **Child 12–18 years** 1–2 g twice daily; total daily dose may alternatively be given in 3–4 divided doses

**Maintenance of remission**

- By mouth

  **Child 5–12 years** 10 mg/kg (max. 500 mg) 2–3 times daily

  **Child 12–18 years** 2 g once daily

**Administration** contents of one sachet should be weighed and divided immediately before use; discard any remaining granules. Granules should be placed on tongue and washed down with water or orange juice without chewing

Retention enema, mesalazine 1 g in 100-mL pack, net price 7 enemas = £17.73. Counselling, blood disorder symptoms (see recommendation above)

**Dose**

**Acute attack affecting the rectosigmoid region**

- By rectum

  **Child 12–18 years** 1 g at bedtime

Suppositories, mesalazine 1 g, net price 28-suppos pack = £40.01. Counselling, blood disorder symptoms (see recommendation above)

**Dose**

**Acute attack, ulcerative proctitis**

- By rectum

  **Child 12–18 years** 1 g daily for 2–4 weeks

**Maintenance, ulcerative proctitis**

- By rectum

  **Child 12–18 years** 1 g daily

**Salofalk®** (Dr Falk) PoM

Tablets, e/c, yellow, mesalazine 250 mg, net price 100-tab pack = £16.19; 500 mg, 100-tab pack = £32.38. Label: 5, 25, counselling, blood disorder symptoms (see recommendation above)

**Dose**

**Acute attack**

- By mouth

  **Child 6–18 years and body-weight under 40 kg** 10–20 mg/kg 3 times daily

  **Child 6–18 years and body-weight over 40 kg** 0.5–1 g 3 times daily

**Maintenance of remission**

- By mouth

  **Child 6–18 years and body-weight under 40 kg** 5–10 mg/kg 3 times daily; total daily dose may alternatively be given in 2 divided doses

  **Child 6–18 years and body-weight over 40 kg** 500 mg 3 times daily

Granules, m/r, grey, e/c, vanilla-flavoured, mesalazine 500 mg/sachet, net price 100-sachet pack = £28.74; 1 g/sachet, 50-sachet pack = £28.74; 1.5 g/sachet, 60-sachet pack = £48.85; 3 g/sachet, 60-sachet pack = £97.70. Label: 25, counselling, administration (see dose), blood disorder symptoms (see recommendation above)

Excipients include aspartame (section 9.4.1)

**Dose**

**Acute attack**

- By mouth

  **Child 6–18 years and body-weight under 40 kg** 10–20 mg/kg 3 times daily

  **Child 6–18 years and body-weight over 40 kg** 1.5–3 g once daily (preferably in the morning) *or* 0.5–1 g 3 times daily

**Maintenance of remission**

- By mouth

  **Child 6–18 years and body-weight under 40 kg** 5–10 mg/kg 3 times daily; total daily dose may alternatively be given in 2 divided doses

  **Child 6–18 years and body-weight over 40 kg** 500 mg 3 times daily

**Administration** Granules should be placed on the tongue and washed down with water without chewing

**Note** Preparations that lower stool pH (e.g. lactulose) may prevent release of mesalazine

Suppositories, mesalazine 500 mg. Net price 30-suppos pack = £14.81. Counselling, blood disorder symptoms (see recommendation above)

**Dose**

**Acute attack**

- By rectum

  **Child 12–18 years** 0.5–1 g 2–3 times daily adjusted according to response

Enema, mesalazine 2 g in 59-mL pack. Net price 7 enemas = £29.92. Counselling, blood disorder symptoms (see recommendation above)

**Dose**

**Acute attack *or* maintenance**

- By rectum

  **Child 12–18 years** 2 g once daily at bedtime

Rectal foam, mesalazine 1 g/metered application, net price 14-application canister with disposable applicators and plastic bags = £30.17. Counselling, blood disorder symptoms (see recommendation above)

Excipients include cetostearyl alcohol, disodium edetate, polysorbate 60, propylene glycol, sodium metabisulfite

**Dose**

**Mild ulcerative colitis affecting sigmoid colon and rectum**

- By rectum

  **Child 12–18 years** 2 metered applications (mesalazine 2 g) into the rectum at bedtime or in 2 divided doses

## OLSALAZINE SODIUM

**Cautions** see notes above; **interactions:** Appendix 1 (aminosalicylates)

**Blood disorders** see recommendation above

**Contra-indications** see notes above

**Renal impairment** use with caution; manufacturer advises avoid in significant impairment

**Pregnancy** manufacturer advises avoid unless potential benefit outweighs risk

**Breast-feeding** monitor infant for diarrhoea

**Side-effects** see notes above; watery diarrhoea common; also reported, tachycardia, palpitation, pyrexia, blurred vision, and photosensitivity

**Licensed use** not licensed for use in children under 12 years

**Indications and dose**

**Treatment of acute attack of mild ulcerative colitis**

- By mouth

  **Child 2–18 years** 500 mg twice daily after food increased if necessary over 1 week to max. 1 g 3 times daily

**Maintenance of remission of mild ulcerative colitis**

- By mouth

  **Child 2–18 years** 250–500 mg twice daily after food

**Administration** Capsules can be opened and contents sprinkled on food

**Dipentum®** (UCB Pharma) PoM

Capsules, brown, olsalazine sodium 250 mg. Net price 112-cap pack = £19.77. Label: 21, counselling, blood disorder symptoms (see recommendation above)

Tablets, yellow, scored, olsalazine sodium 500 mg. Net price 60-tab pack = £21.18. Label: 21, counselling, blood disorder symptoms (see recommendation above)

**1**

**Gastro-intestinal system**

## ■ SULFASALAZINE
(Sulphasalazine)

**Cautions** see notes above; also history of allergy or asthma; G6PD deficiency (section 9.1.5); slow acetylator status; risk of haematological and hepatic toxicity (differential white cell, red cell, and platelet counts initially and at monthly intervals for first 3 months; liver function tests at monthly intervals for first 3 months); maintain adequate fluid intake; upper gastro-intestinal side-effects common with doses over 4 g daily; acute porphyria (section 9.8.2); **interactions:** Appendix 1 (aminosalicylates)
**Blood disorders** see recommendation above

**Contra-indications** see notes above; also sulfonamide hypersensitivity; child under 2 years of age

**Hepatic impairment** use with caution

**Renal impairment** risk of toxicity, including crystalluria, in moderate impairment—ensure high fluid intake; avoid in severe impairment

**Pregnancy** theoretical risk of neonatal haemolysis in third trimester; adequate folate supplements should be given to mother

**Breast-feeding** small amount in milk (1 report of bloody diarrhoea); theoretical risk of neonatal haemolysis especially in G6PD-deficient infants

**Side-effects** see notes above; also cough, insomnia, dizziness, fever, blood disorders (including Heinz body anaemia, megaloblastic anaemia), proteinuria, tinnitus, stomatitis, taste disturbances, and pruritus; *less commonly* dyspnoea, depression, convulsions, vasculitis, and alopecia; also reported loss of appetite, hypersensitivity reactions (including exfoliative dermatitis, epidermal necrolysis, photosensitivity, anaphylaxis, serum sickness), ataxia, hallucinations, aseptic meningitis, oligospermia, crystalluria, disturbances of smell, and parotitis; yellow-orange discoloration of skin, urine, and other body fluids; some soft contact lenses may be stained

**Indications and dose**

> **Treatment of acute attack of mild to moderate and severe ulcerative colitis, active Crohn's disease**
> - By mouth
>   **Child 2–12 years** 10–15 mg/kg (max. 1 g) 4–6 times daily until remission occurs; increased to max. 60 mg/kg daily in divided doses, if necessary
>   **Child 12–18 years** 1–2 g 4 times daily until remission occurs

> **Maintenance of remission of mild to moderate and severe ulcerative colitis**
> - By mouth
>   **Child 2–12 years** 5–7.5 mg/kg (max. 500 mg) 4 times daily
>   **Child 12–18 years** 500 mg 4 times daily

> **Treatment of mild to moderate or severe ulcerative colitis and maintenance of remission, active Crohn's disease**
> - By rectum as suppositories
>   **Child 5–8 years** 500 mg twice daily
>   **Child 8–12 years** 500 mg in the morning and 1 g at night
>   **Child 12–18 years** 0.5–1 g twice daily

> **Juvenile idiopathic arthritis** section 10.1.3

**Sulfasalazine** (Non-proprietary) PoM
Tablets, sulfasalazine 500 mg, net price 112 = £6.74. Label: 14, counselling, blood disorder symptoms (see recommendation above), contact lenses may be stained

Tablets, e/c, sulfasalazine 500 mg. Net price 112-tab pack = £14.46. Label: 5, 14, 25, counselling, blood disorder symptoms (see recommendation above), contact lenses may be stained
**Brands include** *Sulazine EC*®

Suspension, sulfasalazine 250 mg/5 mL, net price 500 mL = £29.50. Label: 14, counselling, blood disorder symptoms (see recommendation above), contact lenses may be stained
**Excipients** may include alcohol

**Salazopyrin**® (Pharmacia) PoM
Tablets, yellow, scored, sulfasalazine 500 mg. Net price 112-tab pack = £6.97. Label: 14, counselling, blood disorder symptoms (see recommendation above), contact lenses may be stained

EN-Tabs® (= tablets e/c), yellow, f/c, sulfasalazine 500 mg. Net price 112-tab pack = £8.43. Label: 5, 14, 25, counselling, blood disorder symptoms (see recommendation above), contact lenses may be stained

Suppositories, yellow, sulfasalazine 500 mg. Net price 10 = £3.30. Label: 14, counselling, blood disorder symptoms (see recommendation above), contact lenses may be stained

## ■ 1.5.2 Corticosteroids

For the role of corticosteroids in acute ulcerative colitis and Crohn's disease, see Inflammatory Bowel Disease, p. 47.

## ■ BUDESONIDE

**Cautions** section 6.3.2; **interactions:** Appendix 1 (corticosteroids)

**Contra-indications** section 6.3.2

**Hepatic impairment** section 6.3.2

**Pregnancy** section 6.3.2

**Breast-feeding** section 6.3.2

**Side-effects** section 6.3.2

**Licensed use** not licensed for use in children

**Indications and dose**
> See preparations

**Administration** Capsules can be opened and the contents mixed with apple or orange juice

**Budenofalk**® (Dr Falk) PoM
Capsules, pink, enclosing e/c granules, budesonide 3 mg, net price 100-cap pack = £75.05. Label: 5, 10, steroid card, 22, 25
**Dose**
> **Mild to moderate Crohn's disease affecting ileum or ascending colon, chronic diarrhoea due to collagenous colitis**
> - By mouth
>   **Child 12–18 years** 3 mg 3 times daily for up to 8 weeks; reduce dose for the last 2 weeks of treatment. See also section 6.3.2

**Entocort®** (AstraZeneca) [PoM]
CR Capsules, grey/pink, enclosing e/c, m/r granules, budesonide 3 mg, net price 100-cap pack = £99.00. Label: 5, 10, steroid card, 22, 25
**Note** Dispense in original container (contains desiccant)
**Dose**

### Mild to moderate Crohn's disease affecting the ileum or ascending colon
- By mouth
  **Child 12–18 years** 9 mg once daily in the morning before breakfast for up to 8 weeks; reduce dose for the last 2–4 weeks of treatment. See also section 6.3.2

Enema, budesonide 2 mg/100 mL when dispersible tablet reconstituted in isotonic saline vehicle, net price pack of 7 dispersible tablets and bottles of vehicle = £33.00
**Dose**

### Ulcerative colitis involving rectal and recto-sigmoid disease
- By rectum
  **Child 12–18 years** 1 enema at bedtime for 4 weeks

## ▌ HYDROCORTISONE

**Cautions** section 6.3.2; systemic absorption may occur; prolonged use should be avoided
**Contra-indications** intestinal obstruction, bowel perforation, recent intestinal anastomoses, extensive fistulas; untreated infection
**Side-effects** section 6.3.2; also local irritation
**Indications and dose**

### Inflammatory bowel disease
- By intravenous administration
  See p. 375
- By rectum
  See preparations

**Colifoam®** (Meda) [PoM]
Foam in aerosol pack, hydrocortisone acetate 10%, net price 14-application cannister with applicator = £9.28
**Excipients** include cetyl alcohol, hydroxybenzoates (parabens), propylene glycol
**Dose**

### Ulcerative colitis, proctitis, proctosigmoiditis
- By rectum
  **Child 2–18 years** initially 1 metered application (125 mg hydrocortisone acetate) inserted into the rectum once or twice daily for 2–3 weeks, then once on alternate days

## ▌ PREDNISOLONE

**Cautions** section 6.3.2; systemic absorption may occur; prolonged use should be avoided
**Contra-indications** section 6.3.2; intestinal obstruction, bowel perforation, recent intestinal anastomoses, extensive fistulas; untreated infection
**Hepatic impairment** section 6.3.2
**Renal impairment** section 6.3.2
**Pregnancy** section 6.3.2
**Breast-feeding** section 6.3.2
**Side-effects** section 6.3.2
**Licensed use** prednisolone rectal foam not licensed for use in children (age range not specified by manufacturer)

**Indications and dose**

### Ulcerative colitis, Crohn's disease see also under preparations, below
- By mouth
  **Child 2–18 years** 2 mg/kg (max. 60 mg) once daily until remission occurs, followed by reducing doses
- By rectum
  See under preparations

**Other indications** section 6.3.2

### ▌ Oral preparations
Section 6.3.2

### ▌ Rectal preparations
**Prednisolone** (Non-proprietary) [PoM]
Rectal foam in aerosol pack, prednisolone 20 mg (as metasulfobenzoate sodium)/metered application, net price 14-application cannister with disposable applicators = £48.00
**Dose**

### Proctitis and distal ulcerative colitis
- By rectum
  **Child 12–18 years** 1 metered application (20 mg prednisolone) inserted into the rectum once or twice daily for 2 weeks, continued for further 2 weeks if good response

**Predsol®** (UCB Pharma) [PoM]
Suppositories, prednisolone 5 mg (as sodium phosphate). Net price 10 = £1.35
**Dose**

### Proctitis and rectal complications of Crohn's disease
- By rectum
  **Child 2–18 years** 5 mg inserted night and morning after a bowel movement

## 1.5.3 Drugs affecting the immune response

Azathioprine, mercaptopurine, or once weekly methotrexate are used to induce remission in unresponsive or chronically active Crohn's disease. Azathioprine or mercaptopurine may also be helpful for retaining remission in frequently relapsing inflammatory bowel disease; once weekly methotrexate is used in Crohn's disease when azathioprine or mercaptopurine are ineffective or not tolerated. Response to azathioprine or mercaptopurine may not become apparent for several months. Folic acid (section 9.1.2) should be given to reduce the possibility of methotrexate toxicity. Folic acid is usually given at a dose of 5 mg weekly on a different day to the methotrexate; alternative regimens may be used in some settings.

Ciclosporin (cyclosporin) is a potent immunosuppressant and is markedly nephrotoxic. In children with severe ulcerative colitis unresponsive to other treatment, ciclosporin may reduce the need for urgent colorectal surgery.

## ▌ AZATHIOPRINE

**Cautions** section 8.2.1; **interactions**: Appendix 1 (azathioprine)
**Contra-indications** section 8.2.1
**Hepatic impairment** section 8.2.1

**Renal impairment** section 8.2.1
**Pregnancy** section 8.2.1
**Breast-feeding** section 8.2.1
**Side-effects** section 8.2.1
**Indications and dose**

Severe ulcerative colitis and Crohn's disease
- By mouth
  **Child 2–18 years** initially 2 mg/kg once daily, then increased if necessary up to 2.5 mg/kg once daily

Transplantation rejection section 8.2.1

Rheumatic diseases section 10.1.3

◢ **Preparations**
Section 8.2.1

## ▊ CICLOSPORIN

**Cautions** section 8.2.2; **interactions:** Appendix 1 (ciclosporin)
**Hepatic impairment** section 8.2.2
**Renal impairment** section 8.2.2
**Pregnancy** section 8.2.2
**Breast-feeding** section 8.2.2
**Side-effects** section 8.2.2
**Licensed use** not licensed for use in ulcerative colitis
**Indications and dose**

Refractory ulcerative colitis
- By mouth
  **Child 2–18 years** initially 2 mg/kg twice daily, dose adjusted according to blood-ciclosporin concentration and response; max. 5 mg/kg twice daily
  **Important** For advice on counselling and conversion between preparations, see section 8.2.2
- By intravenous infusion
  **Child 3–18 years** initially 0.5–1 mg/kg twice daily, dose adjusted according to blood-ciclosporin concentration and response

Nephrotic syndrome section 8.2.2

Transplantation rejection and auto-immune conditions section 8.2.2

Atopic dermatitis and psoriasis section 13.5.3

**Administration** for *intermittent intravenous infusion*, dilute to a concentration of 0.5–2.5 mg/mL with Glucose 5% *or* Sodium Chloride 0.9% and give over 2–6 hours; not to be used with PVC equipment; observe patient for signs of anaphylaxis for at least 30 minutes after starting infusion and at frequent intervals thereafter

◢ **Preparations**
Section 8.2.2

## ▊ MERCAPTOPURINE
(6-Mercaptopurine)

**Cautions** section 8.1.3; see also Azathioprine, section 8.2.1
**Contra-indications** section 8.1.3
**Hepatic impairment** section 8.1.3
**Renal impairment** section 8.1.3
**Pregnancy** section 8.1.3
**Breast-feeding** section 8.1.3

**Side-effects** section 8.1.3
**Licensed use** not licensed for use in severe ulcerative colitis and Crohn's disease; for other indications, see section 8.1.3
**Indications and dose**

Severe ulcerative colitis and Crohn's disease
- By mouth
  **Child 2–18 years** 1–1.5 mg/kg once daily (initial max. 50 mg; may be increased to 75 mg once daily)

Acute leukaemias section 8.1.3

◢ **Preparations**
Section 8.1.3

## ▊ METHOTREXATE

**Cautions** section 10.1.3
**Contra-indications** section 10.1.3
**Hepatic impairment** section 10.1.3
**Renal impairment** section 8.1.3
**Pregnancy** section 8.1.3
**Breast-feeding** section 8.1.3
**Side-effects** section 10.1.3
**Licensed use** not licensed for use in children for non-malignant conditions
**Indications and dose**

Severe acute Crohn's disease
- By subcutaneous or intramuscular injection
  **Child 7–18 years** 15 mg/m$^2$ (max. 25 mg) once weekly

Maintenance of remission of severe Crohn's disease
- By mouth or by subcutaneous or intramuscular injection
  **Child 7–18 years** 15 mg/m$^2$ (max. 25 mg) once weekly; dose reduced according to response to lowest effective dose

---

### Safe Practice
Note that the above dose is a **weekly** dose. To avoid error with low-dose methotrexate, it is recommended that:
- the child or their carer is carefully advised of the **dose** and **frequency** and the reason for taking methotrexate and any other prescribed medicine (e.g. folic acid);
- only one strength of methotrexate tablet (usually 2.5 mg) is prescribed and dispensed;
- the prescription and the dispensing label clearly show the dose and frequency of methotrexate administration;
- the child or their carer is warned to report immediately the onset of any feature of blood disorders (e.g. sore throat, bruising, and mouth ulcers), liver toxicity (e.g. nausea, vomiting, abdominal discomfort, and dark urine), and respiratory effects (e.g. shortness of breath).

---

Malignant disease section 8.1.3

Rheumatic disease section 10.1.3

Psoriasis section 13.5.3

◢ **Preparations**
Section 10.1.3

## Cytokine modulators

**Infliximab** is a monoclonal antibody which inhibits the pro-inflammatory cytokine, tumour necrosis factor alpha. It should be administered under specialist supervision where adequate resuscitation facilities are available. It is used in the treatment of severe refractory Crohn's disease or ulcerative colitis. Infliximab should be used only when treatment with other immunomodulating drugs has failed or is not tolerated and for children in whom surgery is inappropriate.

### ■ INFLIXIMAB

**Cautions** monitor for infections before, during, and for 6 months after treatment (see also Tuberculosis below); predisposition to infection; chronic hepatitis B—monitor for active infection; mild heart failure (discontinue if symptoms develop or worsen); demyelinating CNS disorders (risk of exacerbation); history or development of malignancy; history of prolonged immunosuppressant or PUVA treatment in patients with psoriasis; **interactions:** Appendix 1 (infliximab)

**Tuberculosis** Children should be evaluated for tuberculosis before treatment. Active tuberculosis should be treated with standard treatment (section 5.1.9) for at least 2 months before starting infliximab. Children who have previously received adequate treatment for tuberculosis can start infliximab but should be monitored every 3 months for possible recurrence. In those without active tuberculosis but who were previously not treated adequately, chemoprophylaxis should ideally be completed before starting infliximab. In children at high risk of tuberculosis who cannot be assessed by tuberculin skin test, chemoprophylaxis can be given concurrently with infliximab. Children and their carers should be advised to seek medical attention if symptoms suggestive of tuberculosis (e.g. persistent cough, weight loss, and fever) develop

**Blood disorders** Children and their carers should be advised to seek medical attention if symptoms suggestive of blood disorders (such as fever, sore throat, bruising, or bleeding) develop

**Hypersensitivity reactions** Hypersensitivity reactions (including fever, chest pain, hypotension, hypertension, dyspnoea, transient visual loss, pruritus, urticaria, serum sickness-like reactions, angioedema, anaphylaxis) reported during or within 1–2 hours after infusion (risk greatest during first or second infusion or in children who discontinue other immunosuppressants). All children should be observed carefully for 1–2 hours after infusion and resuscitation equipment should be available for immediate use. Prophylactic antipyretics, antihistamines, or hydrocortisone may be administered. Readministration not recommended after infliximab-free interval of more than 16 weeks—risk of delayed hypersensitivity reactions. Children and carers should be advised to keep Alert card with them at all times and seek medical advice if symptoms of delayed hypersensitivity develop

**Contra-indications** severe infections (see also under Cautions); moderate or severe heart failure

**Pregnancy** use only if essential; manufacturer advises adequate contraception during and for at least 6 months after last dose

**Breast-feeding** amount probably too small to be harmful

**Side-effects** see under Cytokine Modulators (section 10.1.3) and Cautions above; also constipation, diarrhoea, dyspepsia, gastro-intestinal haemorrhage, gastro-oesophageal reflux, flushing, hypotension, hypertension, palpitation, tachycardia, sleep disturbances, dizziness, paraesthesia, hypoaesthesia, arthralgia, myalgia, epistaxis, alopecia, rash, ecchymosis, hyperhydrosis, new onset or worsening psoriasis, dry

skin; *less commonly* hepatitis, cholecystitis, intestinal perforation, pancreatitis, heart failure, arrhythmia, bradycardia, syncope, peripheral ischaemia, pleurisy, pulmonary oedema, amnesia, agitation, confusion, nervousness, neuropathy, seizures, vaginitis, eye disorders, bullous eruption, cheilitis, seborrhoea, impaired healing, rosacea, hyperkeratosis, abnormal skin pigmentation; *rarely* pericardial effusion, vasospasm, interstitial lung disease, leukaemia, lymphoma, demyelinating disorders, Stevens-Johnson Syndrome, toxic epidermal necrolysis; also reported hepatic failure

**Licensed use** not licensed for fistulating Crohn's disease in children

**Indications and dose**

**Severe active Crohn's disease**

• **By intravenous infusion**

**Child 6–18 years** initially 5 mg/kg, then 5 mg/kg 2 weeks and 6 weeks after initial dose, then 5 mg/kg every 8 weeks; interval between maintenance doses adjusted according to response; discontinue if no response within 10 weeks of initial dose

**Fistulating Crohn's disease**

• **By intravenous infusion**

**Child 6–18 years** initially 5 mg/kg, then 5 mg/kg 2 weeks and 6 weeks after initial dose, then if condition has responded, consult literature for guidance on further doses

**Severe active ulcerative colitis**

• **By intravenous infusion**

**Child 6–18 years** initially 5 mg/kg, then 5 mg/kg 2 weeks and 6 weeks after initial dose, then 5 mg/kg every 8 weeks; discontinue if no response within 8 weeks of initial dose

**Administration** for *intravenous infusion* reconstitute each 100-mg vial of powder with 10 mL Water for Injections; to dissolve, gently swirl vial without shaking; allow to stand for 5 minutes; dilute required dose with Sodium Chloride 0.9% to a final volume of 250 mL and give through a low protein-binding filter (1.2 micron or less) over at least 2 hours; start infusion within 3 hours of reconstitution

**Remicade®** (MSD) ⒫ⓞⓜ
Intravenous infusion, powder for reconstitution, infliximab, net price 100-mg vial = £419.62. Label: 10, alert card, counselling, tuberculosis, blood disorders, and hypersensitivity reactions

### 1.5.4  Food allergy

Allergy with classical symptoms of vomiting, colic and diarrhoea caused by specific foods such as cow's milk should be managed by strict avoidance. The condition should be distinguished from symptoms of occasional food intolerance in children with irritable bowel syndrome. **Sodium cromoglicate** (sodium cromoglycate) may be helpful as an adjunct to dietary avoidance.

### ■ SODIUM CROMOGLICATE
(Sodium cromoglycate)

**Pregnancy** not known to be harmful
**Breast-feeding** unlikely to be present in milk
**Side-effects** occasional nausea, rashes, and joint pain

**1** Gastro-intestinal system

Gastro-intestinal system

1

### Indications and dose

**Food allergy (in conjunction with dietary restriction)**

- **By mouth**

  **Child 2–14 years** 100 mg 4 times daily before meals, dose may be increased after 2–3 weeks to a max. 40 mg/kg daily and then reduced according to response

  **Child 14–18 years** 200 mg 4 times daily before meals, dose may be increased after 2–3 weeks to max. 40 mg/kg daily and then reduced according to response

**Asthma** section 3.3.1

**Allergic conjunctivitis** section 11.4.2

**Allergic rhinitis** section 12.2.1

**Administration** capsules may be swallowed whole or the contents dissolved in hot water and diluted with cold water before taking

**Nalcrom®** (Sanofi-Aventis) PoM
Capsules, sodium cromoglicate 100 mg. Net price 100-cap pack = £59.75. Label: 22, counselling, administration

## 1.6  Laxatives

|       |                                          |
|-------|------------------------------------------|
| 1.6.1 | **Bulk-forming laxatives**               |
| 1.6.2 | **Stimulant laxatives**                  |
| 1.6.3 | **Faecal softeners**                     |
| 1.6.4 | **Osmotic laxatives**                    |
| 1.6.5 | **Bowel cleansing preparations**         |
| 1.6.6 | **Peripheral opioid-receptor antagonists** |

Before prescribing laxatives it is important to be sure that the child *is* constipated and that the constipation is *not* secondary to an underlying undiagnosed complaint.

Laxatives should be prescribed by a healthcare professional experienced in the management of constipation in children. Delays of greater than 3 days between stools may increase the likelihood of pain on passing hard stools leading to anal fissure, anal spasm and eventually to a learned response to avoid defaecation.

In *infants*, increased intake of fluids, particularly fruit juice containing sorbitol (e.g. prune, pear, or apple), may be sufficient to soften the stool. In infants under 1 year of age with mild constipation, **lactulose** (section 1.6.4) can be used to soften the stool; either an oral preparation containing **macrogols** or, rarely, **glycerol** suppositories can be used to clear faecal impaction. The infant should be referred to a hospital paediatric specialist if these measures fail.

The diet of *children over 1 year of age* should be reviewed to ensure that it includes an adequate intake of fibre and fluid. An osmotic laxative containing **macrogols** (section 1.6.4) can also be used, particularly in children with chronic constipation; **lactulose** is an alternative in children who cannot tolerate a macrogol. If there is an inadequate response to the osmotic laxative, a **stimulant laxative** (section 1.6.2) can be added.

Treatment of faecal impaction may initially increase symptoms of soiling and abdominal pain. In children

over 1 year of age with faecal impaction, an oral preparation containing **macrogols** (section 1.6.4) is used to clear faecal mass and to establish and maintain soft well-formed stools. If disimpaction does not occur after 2 weeks, a **stimulant laxative** (section 1.6.2) can be added. If the impacted mass is not expelled following treatment with macrogols and a stimulant laxative, a **sodium citrate** enema can be administered. Although rectal administration of laxatives may be effective, this route is frequently distressing for the child and may lead to persistence of withholding. A **phosphate enema** may be administered under specialist supervision if disimpaction does not occur after a sodium citrate enema; a **bowel cleansing preparation** (section 1.6.5) is an alternative. Manual evacuation under anaesthetic may be necessary if disimpaction does not occur after oral and rectal treatment, or if the child is afraid.

Long-term regular use of laxatives is essential to maintain well-formed stools and prevent recurrence in children with chronic constipation or a history of faecal impaction; intermittent use may provoke relapses. In children with chronic constipation, laxatives should be continued for several weeks after a regular pattern of bowel movements or toilet training is established. The dose of laxatives should then be tapered gradually, over a period of months, according to response. Some children may require laxative therapy for several years.

> For children with chronic constipation, it may be necessary to exceed the licensed doses of some laxatives. Parents and carers of children should be advised to adjust the dose of laxative in order to establish a regular pattern of bowel movements in which stools are soft, well-formed, and passed without discomfort.
>
> Laxatives should be administered at a time that produces an effect that is likely to fit in with the child's toilet routine.

For the role of laxatives in the treatment of irritable bowel syndrome, see p. 48. For the prevention of opioid-induced constipation in palliative care, see p. 18.

**Pregnancy** If dietary and lifestyle changes fail to control constipation in pregnancy, moderate doses of poorly absorbed laxatives may be used. A bulk-forming laxative should be tried first. An osmotic laxative, such as lactulose, can also be used. Bisacodyl or senna may be suitable, if a stimulant effect is necessary.

Laxatives are also of value in *drug-induced constipation* (see Prescribing in Palliative Care, p. 18), in *distal intestinal obstruction syndrome* in children with cystic fibrosis, for the expulsion of *parasites* after anthelmintic treatment, and to clear the alimentary tract before *surgery and radiological procedures* (section 1.6.5).

> The laxatives that follow have been divided into 5 main groups (sections 1.6.1–1.6.5). This simple classification disguises the fact that some laxatives have a complex action.

## 1.6.1  Bulk-forming laxatives

Bulk-forming laxatives are of value if the diet is deficient in fibre. They relieve constipation by increasing faecal mass which stimulates peristalsis; children and their carers should be advised that the full effect may take some days to develop.

During treatment with bulk-forming laxatives, adequate fluid intake must be maintained to avoid intestinal obstruction. Proprietary preparations containing a bulking agent such as ispaghula husk are often difficult to administer to children.

Bulk-forming laxatives may be used in the management of children with *haemorrhoids*, *anal fissure*, and *irritable bowel syndrome*.

## ISPAGHULA HUSK

**Cautions** adequate fluid intake should be maintained to avoid intestinal obstruction

**Contra-indications** difficulty in swallowing, intestinal obstruction, colonic atony, faecal impaction

**Side-effects** flatulence and abdominal distension (especially during the first few days of treatment), gastro-intestinal obstruction or impaction; hypersensitivity reported

**Licensed use** *Isogel*® licensed for use in children (age range not specified by manufacturer)

### Indications and dose

See under preparations

**Counselling** Preparations that swell in contact with liquid should always be carefully swallowed with water and should not be taken immediately before going to bed

**Fybogel**® (Reckitt Benckiser)

Granules, buff, effervescent, sugar- and gluten-free, ispaghula husk 3.5 g/sachet (low Na$^+$), net price 30 sachets (plain, lemon, or orange flavour) = £1.84. Label: 13, counselling, see above

Excipients include aspartame 16 mg/sachet (see section 9.4.1)

Dose

**Constipation**

● **By mouth**

**Child 6–12 years** ½–1 level 5-mL spoonful in water twice daily, preferably after meals

**Child 12–18 years** 1 sachet (or 2 level 5-mL spoonfuls) in water twice daily, preferably after meals

**Isogel**® (Potters)

Granules, brown, sugar- and gluten-free, ispaghula husk 90%. Net price 200 g = £2.67. Label: 13, counselling, see above

Dose

**Constipation**

● **By mouth**

**Child 6–12 years** 1 level 5-mL spoonful in water once or twice daily, preferably at mealtimes

**Child 12–18 years** 2 level 5-mL spoonfuls in water once or twice daily, preferably at mealtimes

Note May be difficult to obtain

**Ispagel Orange**® (LPC)

Granules, beige, effervescent, sugar- and gluten-free, ispaghula husk 3.5 g/sachet, net price 30 sachets = £2.10. Label: 13, counselling, see above

Excipients include aspartame (section 9.4.1)

Dose

**Constipation**

● **By mouth**

**Child 6–12 years** ½–1 level 5-mL spoonful in water twice daily, preferably after meals

**Child 12–18 years** 1 sachet (or 2 level 5-mL spoonfuls) in water 1–3 times daily, preferably after meals

**Regulan**® (Procter & Gamble)

Powder, beige, sugar- and gluten-free, ispaghula husk 3.4 g/5.85-g sachet (orange or lemon/lime flavour). Net price 30 sachets = £2.44. Label: 13, counselling, see above

Excipients include aspartame (section 9.4.1)

Dose

**Constipation**

● **By mouth**

**Child 6–12 years** ½–1 level 5-mL spoonful in water 1–3 times daily, preferably after meals

**Child 12–18 years** 1 sachet in 150 mL water 1–3 times daily, preferably after meals

## METHYLCELLULOSE

**Cautions** see under Ispaghula Husk

**Contra-indications** see under Ispaghula Husk; also infective bowel disease

**Side-effects** see under Ispaghula Husk

**Licensed use** no age limit specified by manufacturer

### Indications and dose

See under preparation below

**Counselling** Preparations that swell in contact with liquid should always be carefully swallowed with water and should not be taken immediately before going to bed

**Celevac**® (Amdipharm)

Tablets, pink, scored, methylcellulose '450' 500 mg, net price 112-tab pack = £3.22. Counselling, see above and dose

Dose

**Constipation, diarrhoea** (see notes above)

● **By mouth**

**Child 7–12 years** 2 tablets twice daily

**Child 12–18 years** 3–6 tablets twice daily

Administration In constipation the dose should be taken with at least 300 mL liquid. In diarrhoea, ileostomy, and colostomy control, avoid liquid intake for 30 minutes before and after dose

## STERCULIA

**Cautions** see under Ispaghula Husk

**Contra-indications** see under Ispaghula Husk

**Pregnancy** manufacturer of *Normacol Plus*® advises avoid

**Breast-feeding** manufacturer of *Normacol Plus*® advises avoid

**Side-effects** see under Ispaghula Husk

### Indications and dose

**Constipation** for dose see under preparation

**Counselling** Preparations that swell in contact with liquid should always be carefully swallowed with water and should not be taken immediately before going to bed

**Normacol**® (Norgine)

Granules, coated, gluten-free, sterculia 62%. Net price 500 g = £5.94; 60 × 7-g sachets = £4.99. Label: 25, 27, counselling, see above

Dose

● **By mouth**

**Child 6–12 years** ½–1 heaped 5-mL spoonful *or* the contents of ½–1 sachet, washed down without chewing with plenty of liquid once or twice daily after meals

**Child 12–18 years** 1–2 heaped 5-mL spoonfuls *or* the contents of 1–2 sachets, washed down without chewing with plenty of liquid once or twice daily after meals

Administration May be mixed with soft food (e.g. yoghurt) before swallowing, followed by plenty of liquid

**1** Gastro-intestinal system

**Normacol Plus®** (Norgine)

Granules, brown, coated, gluten-free, sterculia 62%, frangula (standardised) 8%. Net price 500 g = £6.34; 60 × 7 g sachets = £5.34. Label: 25, 27, Counselling, see above

**Dose**

• By mouth

**Child 6–12 years** ½-1 heaped 5-mL spoonful or the contents of ½-1 sachet, washed down without chewing with plenty of liquid, once or twice daily after meals

**Child 12–18 years** 1–2 heaped 5-mL spoonfuls or the contents of 1–2 sachets, washed down without chewing with plenty of liquid, once or twice daily after meals

## 1.6.2   Stimulant laxatives

Stimulant laxatives include **bisacodyl**, **sodium picosulfate**, and members of the **anthraquinone** group, **senna** and **dantron**. The indications for dantron are limited (see below) by its potential carcinogenicity (based on *rodent* carcinogenicity studies) and evidence of genotoxicity. Powerful stimulants such as **cascara** (an anthraquinone) and **castor oil** are obsolete. **Docusate sodium** probably acts both as a stimulant and as a softening agent.

Stimulant laxatives increase intestinal motility and often cause abdominal cramp; they should be avoided in intestinal obstruction. Stools should be softened by increasing dietary fibre and liquid or with an osmotic laxative (section 1.6.4) before giving a stimulant laxative. In chronic constipation, especially where withholding of stool occurs, additional doses of a stimulant laxative may be required. Long-term use of stimulant laxatives is sometimes necessary (see section 1.6), but excessive use can cause diarrhoea and related effects such as hypokalaemia.

**Glycerol** suppositories act as a lubricant and as a rectal stimulant by virtue of the mildly irritant action of glycerol.

## ◼ BISACODYL

**Cautions**   prolonged use (risk of electrolyte imbalance)

**Contra-indications**   intestinal obstruction, acute abdominal conditions, acute inflammatory bowel disease, severe dehydration

**Pregnancy**   see Pregnancy, p. 56

**Side-effects**   see notes above; nausea and vomiting; colitis also reported; *suppositories* local irritation

**Indications and dose**

**Constipation** (tablets act in 10–12 hours; suppositories act in 20–60 minutes)

• By mouth

**Child 4–18 years** 5–20 mg once daily, adjusted according to response

• By rectum (suppositories)

**Child 2–18 years** 5–10 mg once daily, adjusted according to response

**Bowel clearance before radiological procedures and surgery**

• By mouth and by rectum

**Child 4–10 years** *by mouth*, 5 mg at bedtime for 2 days before procedure and, if necessary, *by rectum*, 5 mg suppository 1 hour before procedure

**Child 10–18 years** *by mouth*, 10 mg at bedtime for 2 days before procedure and, if necessary, *by rectum*, 10 mg suppository 1 hour before procedure

**Bisacodyl** (Non-proprietary)

Tablets, e/c, bisacodyl 5 mg, net price 100 = £3.27. Label: 5, 25

Suppositories, bisacodyl 10 mg, net price 12 = £1.11

Paediatric suppositories, bisacodyl 5 mg, net price 5 = 94p

**Note** The brand name *Dulcolax®* 〔NHS〕 (Boehringer Ingelheim) is used for bisacodyl tablets, net price 10-tab pack = 74p; suppositories (10 mg), 10 = £1.57; paediatric suppositories (5 mg), 5 = 94p

The brand names *Dulcolax®* Pico Liquid and *Dulcolax®* Pico Perles are used for sodium picosulfate preparations

## ◼ DANTRON
### (Danthron)

**Cautions**   avoid prolonged contact with skin (as in incontinent patients or infants wearing nappies)—risk of irritation and excoriation; *rodent* studies indicate potential carcinogenic risk

**Contra-indications**   see Bisacodyl above

**Pregnancy**   manufacturers of co-danthramer and co-danthrusate advise avoid—no information available

**Breast-feeding**   manufacturers of co-danthramer and co-danthrusate advise avoid—limited information available

**Side-effects**   see notes above; also urine may be coloured red

**Indications and dose**

**Constipation in terminally ill children** for dose see under preparations

◢**With poloxamer '188' (as co-danthramer)**

**Note** Co-danthramer suspension 5 mL = one co-danthramer capsule, **but** strong co-danthramer suspension 5 mL = two strong co-danthramer capsules

**Co-danthramer** (Non-proprietary)  〔PoM〕

Capsules, co-danthramer 25/200 (dantron 25 mg, poloxamer '188' 200 mg). Net price 60-cap pack = £12.86. Label: 14, (urine red)

**Dose**

• By mouth

**Child 6–12 years** 1 capsule at night (restricted indications, see notes above)

**Child 12–18 years** 1–2 capsules at night (restricted indications, see notes above)

Strong capsules, co-danthramer 37.5/500 (dantron 37.5 mg, poloxamer '188' 500 mg). Net price 60-cap pack = £15.55. Label: 14, (urine red)

**Dose**

• By mouth

**Child 12–18 years** 1–2 capsules at night (restricted indications, see notes above)

Suspension, co-danthramer 25/200 in 5 mL (dantron 25 mg, poloxamer '188' 200 mg/5 mL). Net price 300 mL = £11.27, 1 litre = £37.57. Label: 14, (urine red)

**Brands include** *Codalax®* 〔NHS〕, *Danlax®*

**Dose**

• By mouth

**Child 2–12 years** 2.5–5 mL at night (restricted indications, see notes above)

**Child 12–18 years** 5–10 mL at night (restricted indications, see notes above)

Strong suspension, co-danthramer 75/1000 in 5 mL (dantron 75 mg, poloxamer '188' 1 g/5 mL). Net price 300 mL = £30.13. Label: 14, (urine red)
Brands include *Codalax Forte*® [JHS]
**Dose**

- **By mouth**
  **Child 12–18 years** 5 mL at night (restricted indications, see notes above)

◢ **With docusate sodium (as co-danthrusate)**

**Co-danthrusate** (Non-proprietary) [PoM]
Capsules, co-danthrusate 50/60 (dantron 50 mg, docusate sodium 60 mg). Net price 63-cap pack = £15.87. Label: 14, (urine red)
Brands include *Normax*® [JHS]
**Dose**

- **By mouth**
  **Child 6–12 years** 1 capsule at night (restricted indications, see notes above)
  **Child 12–18 years** 1–3 capsules at night (restricted indications, see notes above)

Suspension, yellow, co-danthrusate 50/60 (dantron 50 mg, docusate sodium 60 mg/5 mL). Net price 200 mL = £8.75. Label: 14, (urine red)
Brands include *Normax*®
**Dose**

- **By mouth**
  **Child 6–12 years** 5 mL at night (restricted indications, see notes above)
  **Child 12–18 years** 5–15 mL at night (restricted indications, see notes above)

## ◼ DOCUSATE SODIUM
(Dioctyl sodium sulphosuccinate)

**Cautions** see notes above; do not give with liquid paraffin

**Contra-indications** see notes above; also for *rectal preparations*, haemorrhoids or anal fissure

**Pregnancy** not known to be harmful—manufacturer advises caution

**Breast-feeding** present in milk following oral administration—manufacturer advises caution; rectal administration not known to be harmful

**Side-effects** see notes above; also rash

**Licensed use** *adult oral solution and capsules* not licensed for use in children under 12 years

**Indications and dose**

Constipation

- **By mouth**
  **Child 6 months–2 years** 12.5 mg 3 times daily, adjusted according to response (use paediatric oral solution)
  **Child 2–12 years** 12.5–25 mg 3 times daily, adjusted according to response (use paediatric oral solution)
  **Child 12–18 years** up to 500 mg daily in divided doses, adjusted according to response
  **Note** Oral preparations act within 1–2 days; response to rectal administration usually occurs within 20 minutes

Adjunct in abdominal radiological procedures

- **By mouth**
  **Child 12–18 years** 400 mg with barium meal

**Administration** for administration *by mouth*, solution may be mixed with milk or squash

**Dioctyl**® (UCB Pharma)
Capsules, yellow/white, docusate sodium 100 mg, net price 30-cap pack = £1.92, 100-cap pack = £6.40

**Docusol**® (Typharm)
Adult oral solution, sugar-free, docusate sodium 50 mg/5 mL, net price 300 mL = £5.49
Paediatric oral solution, sugar-free, docusate sodium 12.5 mg/5 mL, net price 300 mL = £5.29

◢ **Rectal preparations**

**Norgalax Micro-enema**® (Norgine)
Enema, docusate sodium 120 mg in 10-g single-dose disposable packs. Net price 10-g unit = 57p
**Dose**

- **By rectum**
  **Child 12–18 years** 1 enema as a single dose

## ◼ GLYCEROL
(Glycerin)

**Indications and dose**

Constipation

- **By rectum**
  **Child 1 month–1 year** 1-g suppository as required
  **Child 1–12 years** 2-g suppository as required
  **Child 12–18 years** 4-g suppository as required

**Glycerol Suppositories, BP**
(Glycerin Suppositories)
Suppositories, gelatin 140 mg, glycerol 700 mg, purified water to 1 g, net price 12 = £1.27 (1 g), £1.29 (2 g), £1.48 (4 g)
**Administration** Moisten with water before insertion

## ◼ SENNA

**Cautions** see notes above
**Contra-indications** see notes above
**Pregnancy** see Pregnancy, p. 56
**Breast-feeding** not known to be harmful
**Side-effects** see notes above
**Licensed use** *tablets* not licensed for use in children under 6 years; *syrup* not licensed for use in children under 2 years

**Indications and dose**

Constipation for dose see under preparations
**Note** Onset of action 8–12 hours; initial dose should be low

**Senna** (Non-proprietary)
Tablets, total sennosides (calculated as sennoside B) 7.5 mg. Net price 60 = £1.47
Brands include *Senokot*® [JHS]
**Dose**

- **By mouth**
  **Child 2–4 years** ½–2 tablets once daily, adjusted according to response
  **Child 4–6 years** ½–4 tablets once daily, adjusted according to response
  **Child 6–18 years** 1–4 tablets once daily, adjusted according to response

1 Gastro-intestinal system

**Manevac®** (HFA Healthcare)
Granules, coated, senna fruit 12.4%, ispaghula 54.2%, net price 400 g = £7.45. Label: 25, counselling, administration
Excipients include sucrose 800 mg per level 5-mL spoonful of granules
**Dose**
- By mouth
    **Child 12–18 years** 1–2 level 5-mL spoonfuls at night with at least 150 mL water, fruit juice, milk, or warm drink

Counselling Preparations that swell in contact with liquid should always be carefully swallowed with water or appropriate fluid and should not be taken immediately before going to bed

**Senokot®** (Reckitt Benckiser)
Tablets ⓃⒽⓈ, see above

Syrup, sugar-free, brown, total sennosides (calculated as sennoside B) 7.5 mg/5 mL. Net price 500 mL = £2.69
**Dose**
- By mouth
    **Child 1 month–4 years** 2.5–10 mL once daily, adjusted according to response
    **Child 4–18 years** 2.5–20 mL once daily, adjusted according to response

## SODIUM PICOSULFATE
(Sodium picosulphate)

**Cautions** see notes above; active inflammatory bowel disease (avoid if fulminant)
**Contra-indications** see notes above; severe dehydration
**Pregnancy** see Pregnancy, p. 56
**Breast-feeding** not known to be present in milk but manufacturer advises avoid unless potential benefit outweighs risk
**Side-effects** see notes above; also nausea and vomiting
**Licensed use** elixir, licensed for use in children (age range not specified by manufacturer); Perles® not licensed for use in children under 4 years
**Indications and dose**
Constipation
- By mouth
    **Child 1 month–4 years** 2.5–10 mg once daily, adjusted according to response
    **Child 4–18 years** 2.5–20 mg once daily, adjusted according to response
    Note onset of action 6–12 hours

Bowel evacuation before abdominal radiological and endoscopic procedures on the colon, and surgery section 1.6.5

**Sodium Picosulfate** (Non-proprietary)
Elixir, sodium picosulfate 5 mg/5 mL, net price 100 mL = £1.85
Note The brand name Dulcolax® Pico Liquid (Boehringer Ingelheim) is used for sodium picosulfate elixir 5 mg/5 mL

**Dulcolax® Pico** (Boehringer Ingelheim)
Perles® (= capsules), sodium picosulfate 2.5 mg, net price 20-cap pack = £1.93, 50-cap pack = £2.73
Note The brand name Dulcolax® is also used for bisacodyl tablets and suppositories

◢**Bowel cleansing preparations**
Section 1.6.5

## 1.6.3  Faecal softeners

Enemas containing **arachis oil** (ground-nut oil, peanut oil) lubricate and soften impacted faeces and promote a bowel movement.

Bulk laxatives (section 1.6.1) and non-ionic surfactant 'wetting' agents e.g. docusate sodium (section 1.6.2) also have softening properties. Such drugs are useful for oral administration in the management of anal fissure; glycerol suppositories (section 1.6.2) are useful for rectal use.

### ARACHIS OIL

**Cautions** intestinal obstruction; hypersensitivity to soya
**Contra-indications** inflammatory bowel disease, hypersensitivity to arachis oil or peanuts
**Licensed use** licensed for use in children (age range not specified by manufacturer
**Indications and dose**
Impacted faeces
- By rectum
    **Child 3–7 years** 45–65 mL as required
    **Child 7–12 years** 65–100 mL as required
    **Child 12–18 years** 100–130 mL as required

**Administration** warm enema in warm water before use

**Arachis Oil Enema** (Non-proprietary)
Enema, arachis (peanut) oil in 130-mL single-dose disposable packs. Net price 130 mL = £7.98

## 1.6.4  Osmotic laxatives

Osmotic laxatives increase the amount of water in the large bowel, either by drawing fluid from the body into the bowel or by retaining the fluid they were administered with.

**Lactulose** is a semi-synthetic disaccharide which is not absorbed from the gastro-intestinal tract. It produces an osmotic diarrhoea of low faecal pH, and discourages the proliferation of ammonia-producing organisms. It is therefore useful in the treatment of hepatic encephalopathy.

**Macrogols** are inert polymers of ethylene glycol which sequester fluid in the bowel; giving fluid with macrogols may reduce the dehydrating effect sometimes seen with osmotic laxatives. Macrogols are an effective non-traumatic means of evacuation in children with faecal impaction and can be used in the long-term management of chronic constipation.

Saline purgatives such as **magnesium hydroxide** are commonly abused but are satisfactory for occasional use; adequate fluid intake should be maintained. **Magnesium salts** are useful where rapid bowel evacuation is required. **Sodium salts** should be avoided as they may give rise to sodium and water retention in susceptible individuals. **Phosphate enemas** are useful in bowel clearance before radiology, endoscopy, and surgery. Enemas containing **phosphate** or **sodium citrate**, and oral **bowel cleansing preparations** (section 1.6.5) should only be used on the advice of a specialist practitioner.

# ■ LACTULOSE

**Cautions**  lactose intolerance; **interactions**: Appendix 1 (lactulose)

**Contra-indications**  galactosaemia, intestinal obstruction

**Pregnancy**  not known to be harmful; see also Pregnancy, p. 56

**Side-effects**  nausea (can be reduced by administration with water, fruit juice or with meals), vomiting, flatulence, cramps, and abdominal discomfort

**Licensed use**  not licensed for use in children for hepatic encephalopathy

**Indications and dose**

> Constipation (may take up to 48 hours to act)
> - **By mouth**
>   > **Child 1 month–1 year** 2.5 mL twice daily, adjusted according to response
>   > **Child 1–5 years** 2.5–10 mL twice daily, adjusted according to response
>   > **Child 5–18 years** 5–20 mL twice daily, adjusted according to response
>
> Hepatic encephalopathy
> - **By mouth**
>   > **Child 12–18 years** 30–50 mL 3 times daily; adjust dose to produce 2–3 soft stools per day

**Lactulose** (Non-proprietary)
Solution, lactulose 3.1–3.7 g/5 mL with other ketoses. Net price 300-mL = £2.10, 500-mL = £2.59; 10 × 15 mL sachet pack = £2.50
Brands include *Duphalac®* ⓌⓘⓈ, *Lactugal®*, *Laevolac®*

# ■ MACROGOLS
(Polyethylene glycols)

**Cautions**  discontinue if symptoms of fluid and electrolyte disturbance; see also preparations below

**Contra-indications**  intestinal perforation or obstruction, paralytic ileus, severe inflammatory conditions of the intestinal tract (such as Crohn's disease, ulcerative colitis, and toxic megacolon); see also preparations below

**Pregnancy**  manufacturers advise use only if essential—no information available

**Breast-feeding**  manufacturer of *Movicol®* oral concentrate advises avoid—no information available

**Side-effects**  abdominal distension and pain, nausea, flatulence

**Licensed use**  *Movicol® Paediatric Plain* not licensed for use in faecal impaction in children under 5 years, or for chronic constipation in children under 2 years

**Indications and dose**

> See under preparations below

**Macrogol Oral Powder, Compound** (Non-proprietary)
Oral powder, macrogol '3350' (polyethylene glycol '3350') 13.125 g, sodium bicarbonate 178.5 mg, sodium chloride 350.7 mg, potassium chloride 46.6 mg/sachet, net price 20-sachet pack = £4.45, 30-sachet pack = £6.68. Label: 13, counselling, administration
Brands include *Laxido® Orange*, *Molaxole®*
Cautions  patients with cardiovascular impairment should not take more than 2 sachets in any 1 hour

**Dose**
> Chronic constipation
> - **By mouth**
>   > **Child 12–18 years** 1–3 sachets daily in divided doses usually for up to 2 weeks; maintenance, 1–2 sachets daily
>   > Administration  Mix contents of each sachet in half a glass (approx. 125 mL) of water
>
> Faecal impaction
> - **By mouth**
>   > **Child 12–18 years** 4 sachets on first day, then increased in steps of 2 sachets daily to max. 8 sachets daily; total daily dose to be drunk within a 6 hour period. After disimpaction, switch to maintenance therapy
>   > Administration  Mix contents of 2 sachets in a glass (approx. 250 mL) of water. After reconstitution the solution should be kept in a refrigerator and discarded if unused after 6 hours

**Movicol®** (Norgine)
Oral powder, macrogol '3350' (polyethylene glycol '3350') 13.125 g, sodium bicarbonate 178.5 mg, sodium chloride 350.7 mg, potassium chloride 46.6 mg/sachet, net price 20-sachet pack (lime- and lemon-flavoured) = £4.45, 30-sachet pack (lime- and lemon- or chocolate- or plain- flavoured) = £6.68, 50-sachet pack (lime- and lemon- or plain- flavoured) = £11.13. Label: 13, counselling, administration
Note  Amount of potassium chloride varies according to flavour of *Movicol®* as follows: plain-flavour (sugar-free) = 50.2 mg/sachet; lime and lemon flavour = 46.6 mg/sachet; chocolate flavour = 31.7 mg/sachet. 1 sachet when reconstituted with 125 mL water provides $K^+$ 5.4 mmol/litre
Cautions  patients with cardiovascular impairment should not take more than 2 sachets in any 1 hour

**Dose**
> Chronic constipation
> - **By mouth**
>   > **Child 12–18 years** 1–3 sachets daily in divided doses usually for up to 2 weeks; maintenance, 1–2 sachets daily
>   > Administration  Mix contents of each sachet in half a glass (approx. 125 mL) of water
>
> Faecal impaction
> - **By mouth**
>   > **Child 12–18 years** 4 sachets on first day, then increased in steps of 2 sachets daily to max. 8 sachets daily; total daily dose to be drunk within a 6 hour period. After disimpaction, switch to maintenance laxative therapy
>   > Administration  Mix contents of 2 sachets in a glass (approx. 250 mL) of water. After reconstitution the solution should be kept in a refrigerator and discarded if unused after 6 hours

Oral concentrate, macrogol '3350' (polyethylene glycol '3350') 13.125 g, sodium bicarbonate 178.5 mg, sodium chloride 350.7 mg, potassium chloride 46.6 mg/25 mL, net price 500 mL (orange-flavoured) = £4.45. Label: 13, counselling, administration
Note  25 mL of oral concentrate when diluted with 100 mL water provides $K^+$ 5.4 mmol/litre

**Dose**
> Chronic constipation
> - **By mouth**
>   > **Child 12–18 years** 25 mL 1–3 times daily, usually for up to 2 weeks; maintenance, 25 mL 1–2 times daily
>   > Administration  25 mL of oral concentrate to be diluted with half a glass (approx. 100 mL) of water. After dilution the solution should be discarded if unused after 24 hours

1 Gastro-intestinal system

Gastro-intestinal system

**Movicol®-Half** (Norgine)
Oral powder, sugar-free, macrogol '3350' (polyethylene glycol '3350') 6.563 g, sodium bicarbonate 89.3 mg, sodium chloride 175.4 mg, potassium chloride 23.3 mg/sachet, net price 20-sachet pack (lime and lemon flavour) = £2.67, 30-sachet pack = £4.01. Label: 13, counselling, administration
Cautions  patients with impaired cardiovascular function should not take more than 4 sachets in any 1 hour

**Dose**

**Chronic constipation**

- By mouth
  **Child 12–18 years** 2–6 sachets daily in divided doses usually for up to 2 weeks; maintenance, 2–4 sachets daily
  **Administration** Mix contents of each sachet in quarter of a glass (approx. 60–65 mL) of water

**Faecal impaction**

- By mouth
  **Child 12–18 years** 8 sachets on first day, then increased in steps of 4 sachets daily to max. 16 sachets daily; total daily dose to be drunk within 6 hours. After disimpaction, switch to maintenance laxative therapy
  **Administration** Mix contents of 4 sachets in a glass (approx. 250 mL) of water. After reconstitution the solution should be kept in a refrigerator and discarded if unused after 6 hours.

**Movicol® Paediatric** (Norgine) PoM
Oral powder, macrogol '3350' (polyethylene glycol '3350') 6.563 g, sodium bicarbonate 89.3 mg, sodium chloride 175.4 mg, potassium chloride 25.1 mg/sachet, net price 30-sachet pack (chocolate- or plain-flavoured) = £4.38. Label: 13, counselling, administration
Note  Amount of potassium chloride varies according to flavour of *Movicol® Paediatric* as follows: chocolate flavour = 15.9 mg/sachet; plain flavour (sugar-free) = 25.1 mg/sachet. 1 sachet when reconstituted with 62.5 mL water provides K⁺ 5.4 mmol/litre.
Cautions  *with high doses*, impaired gag reflex, reflux oesophagitis, impaired consciousness
Contra-indications  cardiovascular impairment, renal impairment——no information available

**Dose**

**Chronic constipation, prevention of faecal impaction**

- By mouth
  **Child under 1 year** ½–1 sachet daily
  **Child 1–6 years** 1 sachet daily; adjust dose to produce regular soft stools (max. 4 sachets daily)
  **Child 6–12 years** 2 sachets daily; adjust dose to produce regular soft stools (max. 4 sachets daily)
  **Administration** Mix contents of each sachet in quarter of a glass (approx. 60–65 mL) of water

**Faecal impaction**

- By mouth
  **Child under 1 year** ½–1 sachet daily
  **Child 1–5 years** 2 sachets on first day, then 4 sachets daily for 2 days, then 6 sachets daily for 2 days, then 8 sachets daily. After disimpaction, switch to maintenance laxative therapy
  **Child 5–12 years** 4 sachets on first day, then increased in steps of 2 sachets daily to max. 12 sachets daily. After disimpaction, switch to maintenance laxative therapy
  **Administration** Mix contents of each sachet in quarter of a glass (approx. 60–65 mL) of water; total daily dose to be taken over a 12-hour period

## ■ MAGNESIUM SALTS

Cautions  see also notes above; interactions: Appendix 1 (antacids)
Contra-indications  acute gastro-intestinal conditions
Hepatic impairment  avoid in hepatic coma if risk of renal failure
Renal impairment  avoid or reduce dose; increased risk of toxicity
Side-effects  colic
Indications and dose
  Constipation see under preparations below

■ Magnesium hydroxide

**Magnesium Hydroxide Mixture, BP**
Aqueous suspension containing about 8% hydrated magnesium oxide. Do not store in cold place
Dose

- By mouth
  **Child 3–12 years** 5–10 mL with water at bedtime when required
  **Child 12–18 years** 30–45 mL with water at bedtime when required

■ Bowel cleansing preparations
Section 1.6.5

## ■ PHOSPHATES (RECTAL)

Cautions  see also notes above; *with enema*, electrolyte disturbances, congestive heart failure, ascites, uncontrolled hypertension, maintain adequate hydration
Contra-indications  acute gastro-intestinal conditions (including gastro-intestinal obstruction, inflammatory bowel disease, and conditions associated with increased colonic absorption)
Renal impairment  use enema with caution
Side-effects  local irritation; *with enema*, electrolyte disturbances
Indications and dose
  Constipation, bowel evacuation before abdominal radiological procedures, endoscopy, and surgery
    For dose see preparations

**Fleet® Ready-to-use Enema** (Casen-Fleet)
Enema, sodium acid phosphate 21.4 g, sodium phosphate 9.4 g/118 mL, net price 133-mL pack (delivers 118 mL dose) with standard tube = 57p
Dose

- By rectum
  **Child 3–7 years** 40–60 mL once daily
  **Child 7–12 years** 60–90 mL once daily
  **Child 12–18 years** 90–118 mL once daily

**Phosphates Enema BP Formula B**
Enema, sodium dihydrogen phosphate dihydrate 12.8 g, disodium phosphate dodecahydrate 10.24 g, purified water, freshly boiled and cooled, to 128 mL. Net price 128 mL with standard tube = £2.98, with long rectal tube = £3.98
Dose

- By rectum
  **Child 3–7 years** 45–65 mL once daily
  **Child 7–12 years** 65–100 mL once daily
  **Child 12–18 years** 100–128 mL once daily

## ◼ SODIUM CITRATE (RECTAL)

**Cautions** see notes above

**Contra-indications** acute gastro-intestinal conditions

**Indications and dose**

Constipation for dose see under preparations

**Micolette Micro-enema®** (Pinewood)

Enema, sodium citrate 450 mg, sodium lauryl sulfoacetate 45 mg, glycerol 625 mg, together with citric acid, potassium sorbate, and sorbitol in a viscous solution, in 5-mL single-dose disposable packs with nozzle. Net price 5 mL = 38p

**Dose**

* By rectum
   **Child 3–18 years** 5–10 mL as a single dose

**Micralax Micro-enema®** (UCB Pharma)

Enema, sodium citrate 450 mg, sodium alkylsulfoacetate 45 mg, sorbic acid 5 mg, together with glycerol and sorbitol in a viscous solution in 5-mL single-dose disposable packs with nozzle. Net price 5 mL = 41p

**Dose**

* By rectum
   **Child 3–18 years** 5 mL as a single dose

**Relaxit Micro-enema®** (Crawford)

Enema, sodium citrate 450 mg, sodium lauryl sulfate 75 mg, sorbic acid 5 mg, together with glycerol and sorbitol in a viscous solution in 5-mL single-dose disposable packs with nozzle. Net price 5 mL = 32p

**Dose**

* By rectum
   **Child 1 month–18 years** 5 mL as a single dose (insert only half nozzle length in child under 3 years)

## 1.6.5 Bowel cleansing preparations

Bowel cleansing preparations are used before colonic surgery, colonoscopy, or radiological examination to ensure the bowel is free of solid contents. They are **not** treatments for constipation.

**Cautions** Bowel cleansing preparations should be used with caution in children, particularly in those with fluid and electrolyte disturbances. Renal function should be measured before starting treatment in patients at risk of fluid and electrolyte disturbances. Hypovolaemia should be corrected before administration of bowel cleansing preparations. Adequate hydration should be maintained during treatment. Bowel cleansing preparations should be used with caution in colitis (avoid if acute severe colitis), or in those who are debilitated. Other oral drugs should not be taken one hour before or after administration of bowel cleansing preparations because absorption may be impaired.

**Contra-indications** Bowel cleansing preparations are contra-indicated in patients with gastro-intestinal obstruction or perforation, gastric retention, acute severe colitis, or toxic megacolon.

**Side-effects** Side-effects of bowel cleansing preparations include nausea, vomiting, abdominal pain (usually transient—reduced by taking more slowly), and abdominal distention. Less frequent side-effects include headache, dizziness, dehydration, and electrolyte disturbances.

## ◼ MACROGOLS

**Cautions** see notes above; also heart failure

**Contra-indications** see notes above; also gastro-intestinal ulceration

**Pregnancy** manufacturers advise use only if essential—no information available

**Breast-feeding** manufacturers advise use only if essential—no information available

**Side-effects** see notes above; also anal discomfort

**Licensed use** *Klean-Prep®* not licensed for use in children

**Indications and dose**

See preparations

**Klean-Prep®** (Norgine)

Oral powder, sugar-free, macrogol '3350' (polyethylene glycol '3350') 59 g, anhydrous sodium sulfate 5.685 g, sodium bicarbonate 1.685 g, sodium chloride 1.465 g, potassium chloride 743 mg/sachet, net price 4 sachets = £8.23. Label: 10, patient information leaflet, counselling

**Excipients** include aspartame (section 9.4.1)

**Electrolytes** 1 sachet when reconstituted with 1 litre water provides Na$^+$ 125 mmol, K$^+$ 10 mmol, Cl$^-$ 35 mmol, HCO$_3^-$ 20 mmol

**Dose**

**Bowel cleansing before radiological examination, colonoscopy, or surgery**

* By mouth
   **Child 12–18 years** 2 litres of reconstituted solution on the evening before procedure and 2 litres of reconstituted solution on the morning of procedure; alternatively, a glass (approx. 250 mL) of reconstituted solution every 10–15 minutes, or by nasogastric tube 20–30 mL/minute, starting on the day before procedure until 4 litres have been consumed. Treatment can be stopped if bowel motions become watery and clear. To facilitate gastric emptying, domperidone (section 1.2) may be given 30 minutes before starting

**Distal intestinal obstruction syndrome**

* By mouth, nasogastric or gastrostomy tube
   **Child 1–18 years** 10 mL/kg/hour for 30 minutes, then 20 mL/kg/hour for 30 minutes, then increase to 25 mL/kg/hour if tolerated; max. 100 mL/kg (or 4 litres) over 4 hours; repeat 4-hour treatment if necessary

**Administration** 1 sachet should be reconstituted with 1 litre of water. Flavouring such as clear fruit cordials may be added if required. Solid food should not be taken for at least 2 hours before starting treatment. After reconstitution the solution should be kept in a refrigerator and discarded if unused after 24 hours.

## ◼ MAGNESIUM CITRATE

Reconstitution of a sachet containing 11.57 g magnesium carbonate and 17.79 g anhydrous citric acid produces a solution containing magnesium citrate

**Cautions** see notes above

**Contra-indications** see notes above

**Hepatic impairment** avoid in hepatic coma if risk of renal failure

**Renal impairment** avoid if estimated glomerular filtration rate less than 30 mL/minute/1.73 m$^2$—risk of hypermagnesaemia

**Pregnancy** caution

**Breast-feeding** caution

**Side-effects** see notes above

**Indications and dose**

See preparations

 **1 Gastro-intestinal system**

**Citramag®** (Sanochemia)
Oral powder, sugar-free, effervescent, magnesium carbonate 11.57 g, anhydrous citric acid 17.79 g/sachet, net price 10-sachet pack (lemon and lime flavour) = £17.20. Label: 10, patient information leaflet, 13, counselling, see below
**Electrolytes** Mg$^{2+}$ 118 mmol/sachet

**Dose**

Bowel evacuation on day before radiological examination, colonoscopy, or surgery

* By mouth

**Child 5–10 years** on day before procedure, one-third of a sachet at 8 a.m. and one-third of a sachet between 2 and 4 p.m.

**Child 10–18 years** on day before procedure, ½–1 sachet at 8 a.m. and ½–1 sachet between 2 and 4 p.m.

**Counselling** One sachet should be reconstituted with 200 mL of hot water; the solution should be allowed to cool for approx. 30 minutes before drinking. Low residue or fluid only diet (e.g. water, fruit squash, lemonade, clear soup, black tea or coffee) recommended before procedure (according to hospital advice) and copious intake of clear fluids recommended until procedure

## ■ SODIUM PICOSULFATE WITH MAGNESIUM CITRATE

**Cautions** see notes above; also recent gastro-intestinal surgery; cardiac disease (avoid in congestive cardiac failure)

**Contra-indications** see notes above; also gastro-intestinal ulceration; ascites; congestive cardiac failure

**Hepatic impairment** avoid in hepatic coma if risk of renal failure

**Renal impairment** avoid if estimated glomerular filtration rate less than 30 mL/minute/1.73 m$^2$—risk of hypermagnesaemia

**Pregnancy** caution

**Breast-feeding** caution

**Side-effects** see notes above; also anal discomfort, sleep disturbances, fatigue, and rash

**Indications and dose**

See preparations

**Picolax®** (Ferring)
Oral powder, sugar-free, sodium picosulfate 10 mg/sachet, with magnesium citrate, net price 20-sachet pack = £33.90. Label: 10, patient information leaflet, 13, counselling, see below
**Electrolytes** K$^+$ 5 mmol, Mg$^{2+}$ 87 mmol/sachet

**Dose**

Bowel evacuation on day before radiological procedure, endoscopy, or surgery

* By mouth

**Child 1–2 years** ¼ sachet before 8 a.m. then ¼ sachet 6–8 hours later

**Child 2–4 years** ½ sachet before 8 a.m. then ½ sachet 6–8 hours later

**Child 4–9 years** 1 sachet before 8 a.m. then ½ sachet 6–8 hours later

**Child 9–18 years** 1 sachet before 8 a.m. then 1 sachet 6–8 hours later

**Note** Acts within 3 hours of first dose. Low residue diet recommended on the day before procedure and copious intake of water or other clear fluids recommended during treatment

**Counselling** One sachet should be reconstituted with 150 mL (approx. half a glass) of cold water; children and carers should be warned that heat is generated during reconstitution and that the solution should be allowed to cool before drinking

## Amidotrizoates

*Gastrografin®* is an **amidotrizoate** radiological contrast medium with high osmolality; it is used in the treatment of meconium ileus in neonates and in the management of distal intestinal obstruction syndrome in children with cystic fibrosis.

## ■ AMIDOTRIZOATES
### Diatrizoates

**Cautions** asthma or history of allergy, latent hyperthyroidism, dehydration and electrolyte disturbance (correct first); in children with oesophageal fistulae (aspiration may lead to pulmonary oedema); benign nodular goitre; enteritis; risk of anaphylactoid reactions increased by concomitant administration of beta-blockers

**Contra-indications** hypersensitivity to iodine, hyperthyroidism

**Pregnancy** manufacturer advises caution

**Breast-feeding** amount probably too small to be harmful

**Side-effects** diarrhoea, nausea, vomiting; also reported, abdominal pain, intestinal perforation, bowel necrosis, oral mucosal blistering, hypersensitivity reactions, pyrexia, headache, dizziness, disturbances in consciousness, hyperthyroidism, electrolyte disturbances, and skin reactions (including toxic epidermal necrolysis)

**Licensed use** not licensed for use in distal intestinal obstruction syndrome

**Indications and dose**

Uncomplicated meconium ileus

* By rectum

**Neonate** 15–30 mL as a single dose

Distal intestinal obstruction syndrome

* By mouth or by rectum

**Child 1 month–2 years** 15–30 mL as a single dose

**Child body-weight 15–25 kg** 50 mL as a single dose

**Child body-weight over 25 kg** 100 mL as a single dose

**Administration** Intravenous prehydration is essential in neonates and infants. Fluid intake should be encouraged for 3 hours after administration. *By mouth*, for child bodyweight under 25 kg, dilute *Gastrografin®* with 3 times its volume of water or fruit juice; for child bodyweight over 25 kg, dilute *Gastrografin®* with twice its volume of water or fruit juice. *By rectum*, administration must be carried out slowly under radiological supervision to ensure required site is reached. For child under 5 years, dilute *Gastrografin®* with 5 times its volume of water; for child over 5 years dilute *Gastrografin®* with 4 times its volume of water.

Radiological investigations dose to be recommended by radiologist

**Gastrografin®** (Bayer Schering)
Solution, sodium amidotrizoate 100 mg, meglumine amidotrizoate 660 mg/mL, net price 100-mL bottle = £14.69
**Excipients** include disodium edetate

## 1.6.6 Peripheral opioid-receptor antagonists

Classification not used in *BNF for Children*.

## 1.7 Local preparations for anal and rectal disorders

**1.7.1** Soothing anal and rectal preparations

**1.7.2** Compound anal and rectal preparations with corticosteroids

**1.7.3** Rectal sclerosants

**1.7.4** Management of anal fissures

In children with perianal soreness or pruritus ani, good toilet hygiene is essential; the use of alcohol-free 'wet-wipes' after each bowel motion, regular bathing and the avoidance of local irritants such as bath additives is recommended. Excoriated skin is best treated with a protective barrier emollient (section 13.2.2); in children over 1 month, **hydrocortisone** ointment or cream (section 13.4) or a compound rectal preparation (section 1.7.2) may be used for a short period of time, up to a maximum of 7 days.

*Pruritus ani* caused by threadworm infection requires treatment with an anthelmintic (section 5.5.1). Topical application of **white soft paraffin** or other bland emollient (section 13.2.1) may reduce anal irritation caused by threadworms.

*Perianal erythema* caused by streptococcal infection should be treated initially with an oral antibacterial such as **phenoxymethylpenicillin** (section 5.1.1.1) or **erythromycin** (section 5.1.5), while awaiting results of culture and sensitivity testing.

*Perianal candidiasis* (thrush) requires treatment with a topical antifungal preparation (section 13.10.2). For treatment of vulvovaginal candidiasis, see section 7.2.2.

*Proctitis* associated with inflammatory bowel disease in children is treated with corticosteroids and aminosalicylates (section 1.5).

For the management of anal fissures, see section 1.7.4.

## 1.7.1 Soothing anal and rectal preparations

Haemorrhoids in children are rare, but may occur in infants with portal hypertension. Soothing rectal preparations containing mild astringents such as bismuth subgallate, zinc oxide, and hammamelis may provide symptomatic relief, but proprietary preparations which also contain lubricants, vasoconstrictors, or mild antiseptics may cause further perianal irritation.

**Local anaesthetics** may be used to relieve pain in children with anal fissures or pruritus ani, but local anaesthetics are absorbed through the rectal mucosa and may cause sensitisation of the anal skin. Excessive use of local anaesthetics may result in systemic effects, see section 15.2. Preparations containing local anaesthetics should be used for no longer than 2–3 days.

**Lidocaine** ointment (section 15.2) may be applied before defaecation to relieve pain associated with anal fissure, but local anaesthetics can cause stinging initially and this may aggravate the child's fear of pain.

Other local anaesthetics such as tetracaine, cinchocaine (dibucaine), and pramocaine (pramoxine) may be included in rectal preparations, but these are more irritant than lidocaine.

**Corticosteroids** are often combined with local anaesthetics and soothing agents in topical preparations for haemorrhoids and proctitis. Topical preparations containing corticosteroids (section 1.7.2) should not be used long-term or if infection (such as herpes simplex) is present. For further information on the use of topical corticosteroids, see section 13.4.

## 1.7.2 Compound anal and rectal preparations with corticosteroids

**Anugesic-HC®** (Pfizer) PoM
Cream, benzyl benzoate 1.2%, bismuth oxide 0.875%, hydrocortisone acetate 0.5%, Peru balsam 1.85%, pramocaine hydrochloride 1%, zinc oxide 12.35%. Net price 30 g (with rectal nozzle) = £3.71
**Dose**

**Haemorrhoids, pruritus ani**

- By rectum

   **Child 12–18 years** apply night and morning and after a bowel movement; do not use for longer than 7 days

Suppositories, buff, benzyl benzoate 33 mg, bismuth oxide 24 mg, bismuth subgallate 59 mg, hydrocortisone acetate 5 mg, Peru balsam 49 mg, pramocaine hydrochloride 27 mg, zinc oxide 296 mg, net price 12 = £2.69
**Dose**

**Haemorrhoids, pruritus ani**

- By rectum

   **Child 12–18 years** insert 1 suppository night and morning and after a bowel movement; do not use for longer than 7 days

**Anusol-HC®** (McNeil) PoM
Ointment, benzyl benzoate 1.25%, bismuth oxide 0.875%, bismuth subgallate 2.25%, hydrocortisone acetate 0.25%, Peru balsam 1.875%, zinc oxide 10.75%. Net price 30 g (with rectal nozzle) = £3.29
**Dose**

**Haemorrhoids, pruritus ani**

- By rectum

   **Child 12–18 years** apply night and morning and after a bowel movement; do not use for longer than 7 days

Suppositories, benzyl benzoate 33 mg, bismuth oxide 24 mg, bismuth subgallate 59 mg, hydrocortisone acetate 10 mg, Peru balsam 49 mg, zinc oxide 296 mg. Net price 12 = £2.31
**Dose**

**Haemorrhoids, pruritus ani**

- By rectum

   **Child 12–18 years** insert 1 suppository night and morning and after a bowel movement; do not use for longer than 7 days

1 Gastro-intestinal system

**Gastro-intestinal system**
**1**

**Perinal®** (Dermal)
Spray application, hydrocortisone 0.2%, lidocaine hydrochloride 1%. Net price 30-mL pack = £6.11
Dose
**Haemorrhoids, pruritus ani**
• By rectum
  **Child 2–18 years** spray once over the affected area up to 3 times daily; do not use for longer than 7 days without medical advice (child under 14 years, on medical advice only)

**Proctofoam HC®** (Meda) [PoM]
Foam in aerosol pack, hydrocortisone acetate 1%, pramocaine hydrochloride 1%. Net price 21.2-g pack (approx. 40 applications) with applicator = £5.06
Dose
**Pain and irritation associated with local, non-infected anal or perianal conditions**
• By rectum
  **Child 12–18 years** 1 applicatorful (4–6 mg hydrocortisone acetate, 4–6 mg pramocaine hydrochloride) by rectum 2–3 times daily and after a bowel movement (max. 4 times daily); do not use for longer than 7 days

**Proctosedyl®** (Sanofi-Aventis) [PoM]
Ointment, cinchocaine (dibucaine) hydrochloride 0.5%, hydrocortisone 0.5%, net price 30 g = £10.34 (with cannula)
Dose
**Haemorrhoids, pruritus ani**
• By rectum
  **Child 1 month–18 years** apply morning and night and after a bowel movement, externally or by rectum; do not use for longer than 7 days

Suppositories, cinchocaine (dibucaine) hydrochloride 5 mg, hydrocortisone 5 mg, net price 12 = £4.66
Dose
**Haemorrhoids, pruritus ani**
• By rectum
  **Child 12–18 years** insert 1 suppository night and morning and after a bowel movement; do not use for longer than 7 days

**Scheriproct®** (Bayer) [PoM]
Ointment, cinchocaine (dibucaine) hydrochloride 0.5%, prednisolone hexanoate 0.19%, net price 30 g = £2.94
Dose
**Haemorrhoids, pruritus ani**
• By rectum
  **Child 1 month–18 years** apply twice daily for 5–7 days (3–4 times daily on 1st day if necessary), then once daily for a few days after symptoms have cleared

Suppositories, cinchocaine (dibucaine) hydrochloride 1 mg, prednisolone hexanoate 1.3 mg, net price 12 = £1.38
Dose
**Haemorrhoids, pruritus ani**
• By rectum
  **Child 12–18 years** insert 1 suppository daily after a bowel movement, for 5–7 days (in severe cases initially 2–3 times daily)

**Ultraproct®** (Meadow) [PoM]
Ointment, cinchocaine (dibucaine) hydrochloride 0.5%, fluocortolone caproate 0.095%, fluocortolone pivalate 0.092%, net price 30 g (with rectal nozzle) = £4.57

Dose
**Haemorrhoids, pruritus ani**
  **Child 1 month–18 years** apply twice daily for 5–7 days (3–4 times daily on 1st day if necessary), then once daily for a few days after symptoms have cleared

Suppositories, cinchocaine (dibucaine) hydrochloride 1 mg, fluocortolone caproate 630 micrograms, fluocortolone pivalate 610 micrograms, net price 12 = £2.15
Dose
**Haemorrhoids, pruritus ani**
• By rectum
  **Child 12–18 years** insert 1 suppository daily after a bowel movement, for 5–7 days (in severe cases initially 2–3 times daily) then 1 suppository every other day for 1 week

**Uniroid-HC®** (Chemidex) [PoM]
Ointment, cinchocaine (dibucaine) hydrochloride 0.5%, hydrocortisone 0.5%, net price 30 g (with applicator) = £4.23
Dose
**Haemorrhoids, pruritus ani**
• By rectum
  **Child 1 month–18 years** apply twice daily and after a bowel movement, externally or by rectum; do not use for longer than 7 days (child under 12 years, on medical advice only)

Suppositories, cinchocaine (dibucaine) hydrochloride 5 mg, hydrocortisone 5 mg, net price 12 = £1.91
Dose
**Haemorrhoids, pruritus ani**
• By rectum
  **Child 12–18 years** insert 1 suppository twice daily and after a bowel movement; do not use for longer than 7 days

**Xyloproct®** (AstraZeneca) [PoM]
Ointment (water-miscible), aluminium acetate 3.5%, hydrocortisone acetate 0.275%, lidocaine 5%, zinc oxide 18%, net price 20 g (with applicator) = £2.26
Dose
**Haemorrhoids, pruritus ani**
• By rectum
  **Child 1 month–18 years** apply several times daily; short-term use only

### 1.7.3 Rectal sclerosants

Classification not used in *BNF for Children*.

### 1.7.4 Management of anal fissures

The management of anal fissures includes stool softening (section 1.6) and the short-term use of a topical preparation containing a local anaesthetic (section 1.7.1). If these measures are inadequate, children with chronic anal fissures should be referred for specialist treatment in hospital. Topical **glyceryl trinitrate**, 0.05% or 0.1% ointment, may be used in children to relax the anal sphincter, relieve pain and aid healing of anal fissures. Excessive application of topical nitrates causes side-effects such as headache, flushing, dizziness, and postural hypotension.

Before considering surgery, **diltiazem** 2% ointment may be used in children with chronic anal fissures resistant to topical nitrates.

Ointments containing glyceryl trinitrate in a range of strengths or diltiazem 2% are available as manufactured specials (see Special-order Manufacturers, p. 823).

## 1.8 Stoma and enteral feeding tubes

### Stoma

Prescribing for children with stoma calls for special care. The following is a brief account of some of the main points to be borne in mind.

When a solid-dose formulation such as a capsule or a tablet is given the contents of the ostomy bag should be checked for any remnants; response to treatment should be carefully monitored because of the possibility of incomplete absorption. *Enteric-coated* and *modified-release* preparations are **unsuitable**, particularly in children with an ileostomy, as there may not be sufficient release of the active ingredient.

**Laxatives**   Enemas and washouts should be used in children with stoma only under specialist supervision; they should **not** be prescribed for those with an ileostomy as they may cause rapid and severe loss of water and electrolytes.

Children with colostomy may suffer from constipation and whenever possible it should be treated by increasing fluid intake or dietary fibre. If a laxative (section 1.6) is required, it should generally be used for short periods only.

**Antidiarrhoeals**   Loperamide, codeine phosphate, and **co-phenotrope** (section 1.4.2) are effective for controlling excessive stool losses. Bulk-forming drugs (section 1.6.1) may be tried but it is often difficult to adjust the dose appropriately.

**Antibacterials** should **not** be given for an episode of acute diarrhoea.

**Antacids**   The tendency to diarrhoea from magnesium salts or constipation from aluminium salts may be increased in children with stoma.

**Diuretics**   Diuretics should be used with caution in children with an ileostomy because they may become excessively dehydrated and potassium depletion may easily occur. It is usually advisable to use a **potassium-sparing** diuretic (section 2.2.3).

**Digoxin**   Children with stoma are particularly susceptible to hypokalaemia. This predisposes children on digoxin to digoxin toxicity; potassium supplements (section 9.2.1.1) or a potassium-sparing diuretic (section 2.2.3) may be advisable.

**Analgesics**   Opioid analgesics (section 4.7.2) may cause troublesome constipation in children with colostomy. When a non-opioid analgesic is required **paracetamol** is usually suitable; anti-inflammatory analgesics may cause gastric irritation and bleeding.

**Iron preparations**   Iron supplements may cause loose stools and sore skin at the stoma site. If this is troublesome and if iron is definitely indicated a parenteral iron preparation (section 9.1.1.2) should be used. Modified-release iron preparations should be **avoided**.

**Care of stoma**   Children and carers are usually given advice about the use of *cleansing agents, protective creams, lotions, deodorants,* or *sealants* whilst in hospital, either by the surgeon or by a stoma-care nurse. Voluntary organisations offer help and support to patients with stoma.

### Enteral feeding tubes

Care is required in choosing an appropriate formulation of a drug for administration through a nasogastric narrow-bore feeding tube or through a percutaneous endoscopic gastrostomy (PEG) or jejunostomy tube. Liquid preparations (or soluble tablets) are preferred; injection solutions may also be suitable for administration through an enteral tube.

If a solid formulation of a medicine needs to be given, it should be given as a suspension of particles fine enough to pass through the tube. It is possible to crush many immediate-release tablets but enteric-coated or modified-release preparations should **not** be crushed.

Enteral feeds may affect the absorption of drugs and it is therefore important to consider the timing of drug administration in relation to feeds. If more than one drug needs to be given, they should be given separately and the tube should be flushed with water after each drug has been given.

**Clearing blockages**   Carbonated (sugar-free) drinks may be marginally more effective than water in unblocking feeding tubes, but mildly acidic liquids (such as pineapple juice or cola-based drinks) can coagulate protein in feeds, causing further blockage. If these measures fail to clear the enteral feeding tube, an alkaline solution containing pancreatic enzymes may be introduced into the tube (followed after at least 5 minutes by water). Specific products designed to break up blockages caused by formula feeds are also available.

## 1.9 Drugs affecting intestinal secretions

1.9.1   **Drugs affecting biliary composition and flow**

1.9.2   **Bile acid sequestrants**

1.9.3   **Aprotinin**

1.9.4   **Pancreatin**

### 1.9.1 Drugs affecting biliary composition and flow

Bile acids (**ursodeoxycholic** and **chenodeoxycholic acid**) may be used as dietary supplements in children with inborn errors of bile acid synthesis. Ursodeoxycholic acid is used to improve the flow of bile in children with cholestatic conditions such as familial intrahepatic cholestasis, biliary atresia in infants, cystic-fibrosis-related liver disease, and cholestasis caused by total parenteral nutrition or following liver transplantation.

1 Gastro-intestinal system

Ursodeoxycholic acid may also relieve the severe itching associated with cholestasis.

In sclerosing cholangitis, ursodeoxycholic acid is used to lower liver enzyme and serum-bilirubin concentrations.

Ursodeoxycholic acid is also used in the treatment of intrahepatic cholestasis in pregnancy.

**Smith-Lemli-Opitz syndrome**  Chenodeoxycholic and ursodeoxycholic acid have been used with cholesterol in children with Smith-Lemli-Opitz syndrome. Chenodeoxycholic acid is also used in combination with cholic acid to treat bile acid synthesis defects but cholic acid is difficult to obtain. Chenodeoxycholic acid and cholesterol are available from 'special-order' manufacturers or specialist importing companies, see p. 823.

## URSODEOXYCHOLIC ACID

**Cautions**  interactions: Appendix 1 (bile acids)

**Contra-indications**  radio-opaque stones; non-functioning gall bladder (in patients with radiolucent gallstones)

**Hepatic impairment**  avoid in chronic liver disease (but used in primary biliary cirrhosis)

**Pregnancy**  no evidence of harm but manufacturer advises avoid

**Breast-feeding**  not known to be harmful but manufacturer advises avoid

**Side-effects**  rarely, diarrhoea

**Licensed use**  not licensed for use in children for indications shown below

**Indications and dose**

Cholestasis
- By mouth

  **Neonate** 5 mg/kg 3 times daily, adjust dose and frequency according to response, max. 10 mg/kg 3 times daily

  **Child 1 month–2 years** 5 mg/kg 3 times daily, adjust dose and frequency according to response, max. 10 mg/kg 3 times daily

Improvement of hepatic metabolism of essential fatty acids and bile flow, in children with cystic fibrosis
- By mouth

  **Child 1 month–18 years** 10–15 mg/kg twice daily; total daily dose may alternatively be given in 3 divided doses

Cholestasis associated with total parenteral nutrition
- By mouth

  **Neonate** 10 mg/kg 3 times daily

  **Child 1 month–18 years** 10 mg/kg 3 times daily

Sclerosing cholangitis
- By mouth

  **Child 1 month–18 years** 5–10 mg/kg 2–3 times daily, adjusted according to response, max. 15 mg/kg 3 times daily

**Ursodeoxycholic Acid** (Non-proprietary) PoM
Tablets, ursodeoxycholic acid 150 mg, net price 60-tab pack = £20.48; 300 mg, 60-tab pack = £38.86. Label: 21

Capsules, ursodeoxycholic acid 250 mg, net price 60-cap pack = £38.86. Label: 21

**Destolit®** (Norgine) PoM
Tablets, scored, ursodeoxycholic acid 150 mg, net price 60-tab pack = £17.67. Label: 21

**Ursofalk®** (Dr Falk) PoM
Capsules, ursodeoxycholic acid 250 mg, net price 60-cap pack = £30.17, 100-cap pack = £31.88. Label: 21

Suspension, sugar-free, ursodeoxycholic acid 250 mg/5 mL, net price 250 mL = £26.98. Label: 21

**Ursogal®** (Galen) PoM
Tablets, scored, ursodeoxycholic acid 150 mg, net price 60-tab pack = £17.05. Label: 21

Capsules, ursodeoxycholic acid 250 mg, net price 60-cap pack = £30.50. Label: 21

# Other preparations for bile synthesis defects

## CHENODEOXYCHOLIC ACID

**Cautions**  see under Ursodeoxycholic Acid; interactions: Appendix 1 (bile acids)

**Contra-indications**  see under Ursodeoxycholic Acid

**Pregnancy**  avoid—fetotoxicity reported in *animal* studies

**Side-effects**  see under Ursodeoxycholic Acid

**Licensed use**  not licensed

**Indications and dose**

Cerebrotendinous xanthomatosis
- By mouth

  **Neonate** 5 mg/kg 3 times daily

  **Child 1 month–18 years** 5 mg/kg 3 times daily

Defective synthesis of bile acid
- By mouth

  **Neonate** initially 5 mg/kg 3 times daily, reduced to 2.5 mg/kg 3 times daily

  **Child 1 month–18 years** initially 5 mg/kg 3 times daily, reduced to 2.5 mg/kg 3 times daily

Smith-Lemli-Opitz syndrome see notes above
- By mouth

  **Neonate** 7 mg/kg once daily or in divided doses

  **Child 1 month–18 years** 7 mg/kg once daily or in divided doses

**Administration**  for administration *by mouth*, add the contents of a 250-mg capsule to 25 mL of sodium bicarbonate solution 8.4% (1 mmol/mL) to produce a suspension containing chenodeoxycholic acid 10 mg/mL; use immediately after preparation, discard any remaining suspension

**Chenodeoxycholic acid** (Non-proprietary) PoM
Capsules, chenodeoxycholic acid 250 mg
Available from 'special-order' manufacturers or specialist importing companies, see p. 823

Gastro-intestinal system

1

## CHOLESTEROL

**Cautions**   consult product literature
**Contra-indications**   consult product literature
**Licensed use**   not licensed
**Indications and dose**

> Smith-Lemli-Opitz syndrome
> * By mouth
> > **Neonate** 5–10 mg/kg 3–4 times daily
> >
> > **Child 1 month–18 years** 5–10 mg/kg 3–4 times daily (doses up to 15 mg/kg 4 times daily have been used)

**Administration**   cholesterol powder can be mixed with a vegetable oil before administration

**Cholesterol Powder** (Non-proprietary)
  Available from 'special-order' manufacturers or specialist importing companies, see p. 823

## 1.9.2 Bile acid sequestrants

**Colestyramine** is an anion-exchange resin that forms an insoluble complex with bile acids in the gastro-intestinal tract; it is used to relieve diarrhoea associated with surgical procedures such as ileal resection, or following radiation therapy. Colestyramine is also used in the treatment of familial hypercholesterolaemia (see section 2.12), and to relieve pruritus in children with partial biliary obstruction, (for treatment of pruritus, see section 3.4.1). Colestyramine is not absorbed from the gastro-intestinal tract, but will interfere with the absorption of a number of drugs, so timing of administration is important.

## COLESTYRAMINE
(Cholestyramine)

**Cautions**   section 2.12
**Contra-indications**   section 2.12
**Pregnancy**   section 2.12
**Breast-feeding**   section 2.12
**Side-effects**   section 2.12
**Licensed use**   not licensed for use in children under 6 years
**Indications and dose**

> Pruritus associated with partial biliary obstruction and primary biliary cirrhosis, diarrhoea associated with Crohn's disease, ileal resection, vagotomy, diabetic vagal neuropathy, and radiation
> * By mouth
> > **Child 1 month–1 year** 1 g once daily in a suitable liquid, adjusted according to response; total daily dose may alternatively be given in 2–4 divided doses (max. 9 g daily)
> >
> > **Child 1–6 years** 2 g once daily in a suitable liquid, adjusted according to response; total daily dose may alternatively be given in 2–4 divided doses (max. 18 g daily)
> >
> > **Child 6–12 years** 4 g once daily in a suitable liquid, adjusted according to response; total daily dose may alternatively be given in 2–4 divided doses (max. 24 g daily)
> >
> > **Child 12–18 years** 4–8 g once daily in a suitable liquid, adjusted according to response; total daily

> dose may alternatively be given in 2–4 divided doses (max. 36 g daily)
>
> **Counselling** Other drugs should be taken at least 1 hour before or 4–6 hours after colestyramine to reduce possible interference with absorption
>
> **Note** For treatment of diarrhoea induced by bile acid malabsorption, if no response within 3 days an alternative therapy should be initiated

> Hypercholesterolaemia   section 2.12

**Administration**   The contents of one sachet should be mixed with at least 150 mL of water or other suitable liquid such as fruit juice, skimmed milk, thin soups, or pulpy fruits with a high moisture content

◢**Preparations**
Section 2.12

## 1.9.3 Aprotinin

Classification not used in *BNF for Children.*

## 1.9.4 Pancreatin

Pancreatin, containing a mixture of protease, lipase and amylase in varying proportions, aids the digestion of starch, fat, and protein. Supplements of pancreatin are given by mouth to compensate for reduced or absent exocrine secretion in cystic fibrosis, and following pancreatectomy, total gastrectomy, or chronic pancreatitis.

The dose of pancreatin is adjusted according to size, number, and consistency of stools, and the nutritional status of the child; extra allowance will be needed if snacks are taken between meals. Daily dose should not exceed 10 000 lipase units per kg body-weight per day, (**important**: see advice on Higher-strength preparations below).

### Pancreatin preparations

| Preparation | Protease units | Amylase units | Lipase units |
|---|---|---|---|
| Creon® 10 000 capsule, e/c granules | 600 | 8000 | 10 000 |
| Creon® Micro e/c granules (per 100 mg) | 200 | 3600 | 5000 |
| Pancrex® granules (per gram) | 300 | 4000 | 5000 |
| Pancrex V® capsule, powder | 430 | 9000 | 8000 |
| Pancrex V '125'® capsule, powder | 160 | 3300 | 2950 |
| Pancrex V® e/c tablet | 110 | 1700 | 1900 |
| Pancrex V® Forte e/c tablet | 330 | 5000 | 5600 |
| Pancrex V® powder (per gram) | 1400 | 30 000 | 25 000 |

**Higher-strength pancreatin preparations** *Pancrease HL*® and *Nutrizym 22*® have been associated with the development of large bowel strictures (fibrosing colonopathy) in children with cystic fibrosis aged between 2 and 13 years. The following is recommended:

* *Pancrease HL*®, *Nutrizym 22*® should not be used in children under 16 years with cystic fibrosis;

**1**   Gastro-intestinal system

- the total dose of pancreatic enzyme supplements used in patients with cystic fibrosis should not usually exceed 10 000 units of lipase per kg body-weight daily;

- if a patient on any pancreatin preparation develops new abdominal symptoms (or any change in existing abdominal symptoms) the patient should be reviewed to exclude the possibility of colonic damage.

Possible risk factors are gender (boys at greater risk than girls), more severe cystic fibrosis, and concomitant use of laxatives. The peak age for developing fibrosing colonopathy is between 2 and 8 years.

### Higher-strength pancreatin preparations

| Preparation | Protease units | Amylase units | Lipase units |
|---|---|---|---|
| Creon® 25 000 capsule, e/c pellets | 1000 | 18 000 | 25 000 |
| Creon® 40 000 capsule, e/c granules | 1600 | 25 000 | 40 000 |
| Nutrizym 22® capsule, e/c minitablets | 1100 | 19 800 | 22 000 |
| Pancrease HL® capsule, e/c minitablets | 1250 | 22 500 | 25 000 |

Pancreatin is inactivated by gastric acid therefore pancreatin preparations are best taken with food (or immediately before or after food). In children with cystic fibrosis with persistent fat malabsorption despite optimal use of enzyme replacement, an $H_2$-receptor antagonist (section 1.3.1), or a proton pump inhibitor (section 1.3.5) may improve fat digestion and absorption. Enteric-coated preparations are designed to deliver a higher enzyme concentration in the duodenum (provided the capsule contents are swallowed whole without chewing). If the capsules are opened the enteric-coated granules should be mixed with milk, slightly acidic soft food or liquid such as apple juice, and then swallowed immediately without chewing. Any left-over food or liquid containing pancreatin should be discarded. Since pancreatin is also inactivated by heat, excessive heat should be avoided if preparations are mixed with liquids or food.

Pancreatin can irritate the perioral skin and buccal mucosa if retained in the mouth, and excessive doses can cause perianal irritation. Hypersensitivity reactions may occur particularly if the powder is handled.

### ■ PANCREATIN

**Cautions** see notes above; hyperuricaemia and hyperuricosuria have been associated with very high doses; **interactions:** Appendix 1 (pancreatin)

**Pregnancy** not known to be harmful

**Side-effects** nausea, vomiting, abdominal discomfort; skin and mucosal irritation (see notes above)

**Indications and dose**

Pancreatic insufficiency for dose see individual preparations, below

**Creon® 10 000** (Abbott Healthcare)

Capsules, brown/clear, enclosing buff-coloured e/c granules of pancreatin (pork), providing: protease 600 units, lipase 10 000 units, amylase 8000 units, net price 100-cap pack = £12.93. Counselling, see dose

**Dose**

- By mouth

Child 1 month–18 years initially 1–2 capsules with each meal either taken whole or contents mixed with acidic fluid or soft food (then swallowed immediately without chewing), see notes above

**Creon® Micro** (Abbott Healthcare)

Gastro-resistant granules, brown, pancreatin (pork), providing: protease 200 units, lipase 5000 units, amylase 3600 units per 100 mg, net price 20 g = £31.50. Counselling, see dose

**Dose**

- By mouth

Neonate initially 100 mg before each feed; granules can be mixed with a small amount of breast milk or formula feed and administered immediately (manufacturer recommends mixing with a small amount of apple juice before administration)

Child 1 month–18 years initially 100 mg before each feed or meal; granules can be mixed with a small amount of milk or soft food and administered immediately (manufacturer recommends mixing with acidic liquid or pureed fruit before administration); see notes above

Note 100 mg granules = one measured scoopful (scoop supplied with product). Granules should not be chewed before swallowing.

**Pancrex®** (Essential)

Granules, pancreatin (pork), providing minimum of: protease 300 units, lipase 5000 units, amylase 4000 units/g. Net price 300 g = £20.39. Label: 25, counselling, see dose

Excipients include lactose (7 g per 10 g dose)

**Dose**

- By mouth

Child 2–18 years 5–10 g just before meals washed down or mixed with milk or water

**Pancrex V®** (Essential)

Capsules, pancreatin (pork), providing minimum of: protease 430 units, lipase 8000 units, amylase 9000 units, net price 300-cap pack = £15.80. Counselling, see dose

**Dose**

- By mouth

Child 1 month–1 year contents of 1–2 capsules mixed with feeds

Child 1–18 years 2–6 capsules with meals, swallowed whole or sprinkled on food

Capsules '125', pancreatin (pork), providing minimum of: protease 160 units, lipase 2950 units, amylase 3300 units, net price 300-cap pack = £9.72. Counselling, see dose

**Dose**

- By mouth

Neonate contents of 1–2 capsules in each feed (or mix with feed and give by spoon)

Tablets, e/c, pancreatin (pork), providing minimum of: protease 110 units, lipase 1900 units, amylase 1700 units, net price 300-tab pack = £4.51. Label: 5, 25, counselling, see dose

**Dose**

- By mouth

Child 2–18 years 5–15 tablets before meals

Tablets forte, e/c, pancreatin (pork), providing minimum of: protease 330 units, lipase 5600 units, amylase 5000 units, net price 300-tab pack = £13.74. Label: 5, 25, counselling, see dose

**Dose**

- By mouth

  **Child 2–18 years** 6–10 tablets before meals

Powder, pancreatin (pork), providing minimum of: protease 1400 units, lipase 25 000 units, amylase 30 000 units/g, net price 300 g = £24.28. Counselling, see dose

**Dose**

- By mouth

  **Neonate** 250–500 mg with each feed

  **Child 1 month–18 years** 0.5–2 g with meals, washed down or mixed with milk or water

◢ **Higher-strength preparations**

See warning above

**Counselling** It is important to ensure adequate hydration at all times in children receiving higher-strength pancreatin preparations.

**Creon® 25 000** (Abbott Healthcare) [PoM]

Capsules, orange/clear, enclosing brown-coloured e/c pellets of pancreatin (pork), providing: protease (total) 1000 units, lipase 25 000 units, amylase 18 000 units, net price 100-cap pack = £28.25. Counselling, see above and under dose

**Dose**

- By mouth

  **Child 2–18 years** initially 1–2 capsules with meals either taken whole or contents mixed with acidic fluid or soft food (then swallowed immediately without chewing), see notes above

**Creon® 40 000** (Abbott Healthcare) [PoM]

Capsules, brown/clear, enclosing brown-coloured e/c granules of pancreatin (pork), providing: protease (total) 1600 units, lipase 40 000 units, amylase 25 000 units, net price 100-cap pack = £60.00. Counselling, see above and under dose

**Dose**

- By mouth

  **Child 2–18 years** initially 1–2 capsules with meals either taken whole or contents mixed with acidic fluid or soft food (then swallowed immediately without chewing), see notes above

**Nutrizym 22®** (Merck Serono) [PoM]

Capsules, red/yellow, enclosing e/c minitablets of pancreatin (pork), providing minimum of: protease 1100 units, lipase 22 000 units, amylase 19 800 units, net price 100-cap pack = £33.33. Counselling, see above and under dose

**Dose**

- By mouth

  **Child 15–18 years** 1–2 capsules with meals and 1 capsule with snacks, swallowed whole or contents taken with water or mixed with soft food (then swallowed immediately without chewing), see notes above

**Pancrease HL®** (Janssen) [PoM]

Capsules, enclosing light brown e/c minitablets of pancreatin (pork), providing minimum of: protease 1250 units, lipase 25 000 units, amylase 22 500 units. Net price 100 = £31.70. Counselling, see above and under dose

**Dose**

- By mouth

  **Child 15–18 years** 1–2 capsules during each meal and 1 capsule with snacks swallowed whole or contents mixed with slightly acidic liquid or soft food (then swallowed immediately without chewing), see notes above

**1 Gastro-intestinal system**

# 2 Cardiovascular system

This chapter also includes advice on the drug management of the following:

## 2.1 Positive inotropic drugs

**2.1.1 Cardiac glycosides**

**2.1.2 Phosphodiesterase type-3 inhibitors**

Positive inotropic drugs increase the force of contraction of the myocardium. Drugs which produce inotropic effects include cardiac glycosides, phosphodiesterase inhibitors, and some sympathomimetics (section 2.7.1).

### 2.1.1 Cardiac glycosides

The cardiac glycoside digoxin increases the force of myocardial contraction and reduces conductivity within the atrioventricular (AV) node.

Digoxin is most useful in the treatment of supraventricular tachycardias, especially for controlling ventricular response in persistent atrial fibrillation (section 2.3.1). Digoxin has a limited role in children with chronic heart failure; for reference to the role of digoxin in heart failure, see section 2.2.

For the management of atrial fibrillation, the maintenance dose of digoxin is determined on the basis of the ventricular rate at rest, which should not be allowed to fall below an acceptable level for the child.

Digoxin is now rarely used for rapid control of heart rate (see section 2.3.2), even with intravenous administration, response may take many hours; persistence of tachycardia is therefore not an indication for exceeding the recommended dose. The intramuscular route is **not** recommended.

In children with heart failure who are in sinus rhythm, a loading dose may not be required.

Unwanted effects depend both on the concentration of digoxin in the plasma and on the sensitivity of the conducting system or of the myocardium, which is often increased in heart disease. It can sometimes be difficult to distinguish between toxic effects and clinical deterioration because the symptoms of both are similar. The plasma-digoxin concentration alone cannot indicate toxicity reliably, but the likelihood of toxicity increases progressively through the range 1.5 to 3 micrograms/litre for digoxin. Renal function is very important in determining digoxin dosage.

Hypokalaemia predisposes the child to digitalis toxicity and should be avoided; it is managed by giving a potassium-sparing diuretic or, if necessary, potassium supplements.

If toxicity occurs, digoxin should be withdrawn; serious manifestations require urgent specialist management. **Digoxin-specific antibody fragments** are available for reversal of life-threatening overdosage (see Digoxin-specific Antibody, p. 74).

## DIGOXIN

**Cautions**   sick sinus syndrome; thyroid disease; hypoxia; severe respiratory disease; avoid hypokalaemia, hypomagnesaemia, hypercalcaemia, and hypoxia (risk of digitalis toxicity); monitor serum electrolytes and renal function; avoid rapid intravenous administration (risk of hypertension and reduced coronary flow); **interactions:** Appendix 1 (cardiac glycosides)

**Contra-indications**   intermittent complete heart block, second degree AV block; supraventricular arrhythmias associated with accessory conducting pathways e.g. Wolff-Parkinson-White syndrome (although can be used in infancy); ventricular tachycardia or fibrillation; hypertrophic cardiomyopathy (unless concomitant atrial fibrillation and heart failure—but use with caution); myocarditis; constrictive pericarditis (unless to control atrial fibrillation or improve systolic dysfunction—but use with caution)

**Renal impairment**   use half normal dose if estimated glomerular filtration rate is 10–50 mL/minute/1.73 m$^2$ and use a quarter normal dose if estimated glomerular filtration rate is less than 10 mL/minute/1.73 m$^2$; monitor plasma-digoxin concentration; toxicity increased by electrolyte disturbances

**Pregnancy**   may need dosage adjustment

**Breast-feeding**   amount too small to be harmful

**Side-effects**   see notes above; also nausea, vomiting, diarrhoea; arrhythmias, conduction disturbances; dizziness; blurred or yellow vision; rash, eosinophilia; *less commonly* depression; *very rarely* anorexia, intestinal ischaemia and necrosis, psychosis, apathy, confusion, headache, fatigue, weakness, gynaecomastia on long-term use, and thrombocytopenia

**Pharmacokinetics**   For plasma-digoxin concentration assay, blood should be taken at least 6 hours after a dose; plasma-digoxin concentration should be maintained in the range 0.8–2 micrograms/litre (see also notes above)

**Licensed use**   heart failure, supraventricular arrhythmias

### Indications and dose

**Supraventricular arrhythmias and chronic heart failure** (see also notes above) consult product literature for details

• **By mouth**

**Neonate under 1.5 kg** initially 25 micrograms/kg in 3 divided doses for 24 hours then 4–6 micrograms/kg daily in 1–2 divided doses

**Neonate 1.5–2.5 kg** initially 30 micrograms/kg in 3 divided doses for 24 hours then 4–6 micrograms/kg daily in 1–2 divided doses

**Neonate over 2.5 kg** initially 45 micrograms/kg in 3 divided doses for 24 hours then 10 micrograms/kg daily in 1–2 divided doses

**Child 1 month–2 years** initially 45 micrograms/kg in 3 divided doses for 24 hours then 10 micrograms/kg daily in 1–2 divided doses

**Child 2–5 years** initially 35 micrograms/kg in 3 divided doses for 24 hours then 10 micrograms/kg daily in 1–2 divided doses

**Child 5–10 years** initially 25 micrograms/kg (max. 750 micrograms) in 3 divided doses for 24 hours then 6 micrograms/kg daily (max. 250 micrograms daily) in 1–2 divided doses

**Child 10–18 years** initially 0.75–1.5 mg in 3 divided doses for 24 hours then 62.5–250 micrograms daily in 1–2 divided doses (higher doses may be necessary)

• **By intravenous infusion (but rarely necessary)**

**Neonate under 1.5 kg** initially 20 micrograms/kg in 3 divided doses for 24 hours then 4–6 micrograms/kg daily in 1–2 divided doses

**Neonate 1.5–2.5 kg** initially 30 micrograms/kg in 3 divided doses for 24 hours then 4–6 micrograms/kg daily in 1–2 divided doses

**Neonate over 2.5 kg** initially 35 micrograms/kg in 3 divided doses for 24 hours then 10 micrograms/kg daily in 1–2 divided doses

**Child 1 month–2 years** initially 35 micrograms/kg in 3 divided doses for 24 hours then 10 micrograms/kg daily in 1–2 divided doses

**Child 2–5 years** initially 35 micrograms/kg in 3 divided doses for 24 hours then 10 micrograms/kg daily in 1–2 divided doses

**Child 5–10 years** initially 25 micrograms/kg (max. 500 micrograms) in 3 divided doses for 24 hours then 6 micrograms/kg daily (max. 250 micrograms daily) in 1–2 divided doses

**Child 10–18 years** initially 0.5–1 mg in 3 divided doses for 24 hours then 62.5–250 micrograms daily in 1–2 divided doses (higher doses may be necessary)

**Note** The above doses may need to be reduced if digoxin (or another cardiac glycoside) has been given in the preceding 2 weeks. When switching from intravenous to oral route may need to increase dose by 20–30% to maintain the same

2

Cardiovascular system

plasma-digoxin concentration. Plasma monitoring may be required when changing formulation to take account of varying bioavailabilities. For plasma concentration monitoring, blood should ideally be taken at least 6 hours after a dose

**Administration** for *intravenous infusion*, dilute with Sodium Chloride 0.9% *or* Glucose 5% to a max. concentration of 62.5 micrograms/mL; loading doses should be given over 30–60 minutes and maintenance dose over 10–20 minutes.

For *oral* administration, oral solution must **not** be diluted

**Digoxin** (Non-proprietary) [PoM]
Tablets, digoxin 62.5 micrograms, net price 28-tab pack = £2.03; 125 micrograms, 28-tab pack = £1.12; 250 micrograms, 28-tab pack = £1.13

Injection, digoxin 250 micrograms/mL, net price 2-mL amp = 70p
Excipients  include alcohol, propylene glycol (see Excipients, p. 2)

Paediatric injection, digoxin 100 micrograms/mL
Available from 'special-order' manufacturers or specialist importing companies, see p. 823

**Lanoxin®** (Aspen) [PoM]
Tablets, digoxin 125 micrograms, net price 500-tab pack = £8.09; 250 micrograms (scored), 500-tab pack = £8.09

Injection, digoxin 250 micrograms/mL, net price 2-mL amp = 66p

**Lanoxin-PG®** (Aspen) [PoM]
Tablets, blue, digoxin 62.5 micrograms, net price 500-tab pack = £8.09

Elixir, yellow, digoxin 50 micrograms/mL. Do not dilute, measure with pipette. Net price 60 mL = £5.35. Counselling, use of pipette

## Digoxin-specific antibody

Serious cases of digoxin toxicity should be discussed with the National Poisons Information Service, p. 23. **Digoxin-specific antibody fragments** are indicated for the treatment of known or strongly suspected life-threatening digoxin toxicity associated with ventricular arrhythmias or bradyarrhythmias unresponsive to atropine and when measures beyond the withdrawal of digoxin and correction of any electrolyte abnormalities are considered necessary (see also notes above).

**DigiFab®** (BTG) ▼ [PoM]
Intravenous infusion, powder for reconstitution, digoxin-specific antibody fragments (F(ab)), net price 40-mg vial = £750.00 (hosp. only)
Dose
Consult product literature

## 2.1.2  Phosphodiesterase type-3 inhibitors

**Enoximone** and **milrinone** are phosphodiesterase type-3 inhibitors that exert most of their effect on the myocardium. They possess positive inotropic and vasodilator activity and are useful in infants and children with low cardiac output especially after cardiac surgery. Phosphodiesterase type-3 inhibitors should be limited to short-term use because long-term oral administration has been associated with increased mortality in adults with congestive heart failure.

## ENOXIMONE

**Cautions**  heart failure associated with hypertrophic cardiomyopathy, stenotic or obstructive valvular disease or other outlet obstruction; monitor blood pressure, heart rate, ECG, central venous pressure, fluid and electrolyte status, renal function, platelet count, hepatic enzymes; avoid extravasation; **interactions:** Appendix 1 (phosphodiesterase type-3 inhibitors)
**Hepatic impairment**  dose reduction may be required
**Renal impairment**  consider dose reduction
**Pregnancy**  manufacturer advises use only if potential benefit outweighs risk
**Breast-feeding**  manufacturer advises caution—no information available
**Side-effects**  ectopic beats; less frequently ventricular tachycardia or supraventricular arrhythmias (more likely in children with pre-existing arrhythmias); hypotension; also headache, insomnia, nausea and vomiting, diarrhoea; occasionally, chills, oliguria, fever, urinary retention; upper and lower limb pain
**Licensed use**  not licensed for use in children
**Indications and dose**

> **Congestive heart failure, low cardiac output following cardiac surgery**
> * **By intravenous injection and continuous intravenous infusion**
>    **Neonate** initial loading dose of 500 micrograms/kg *by slow intravenous injection*, followed by 5–20 micrograms/kg/minute *by continuous intravenous infusion* over 24 hours adjusted according to response; max 24 mg/kg over 24 hours
>    **Child 1 month–18 years** initial loading dose of 500 micrograms/kg *by slow intravenous injection*, followed by 5–20 micrograms/kg/minute *by continuous intravenous infusion* over 24 hours adjusted according to response; max. 24 mg/kg over 24 hours

**Administration**  for *intravenous administration*, dilute to concentration of 2.5 mg/mL with Sodium Chloride 0.9% *or* Water for Injections; the initial loading dose should be given by slow intravenous injection over at least 15 minutes. Use plastic apparatus—crystal formation if glass used

**Perfan®** (INCA-Pharm) [PoM]
Injection, enoximone 5 mg/mL. For dilution before use. Net price 20-mL amp = £15.02
Excipients  include alcohol, propylene glycol (see Excipients, p. 2)

## MILRINONE

**Cautions**  see under Enoximone; also correct hypokalaemia; monitor renal function; **interactions:** Appendix 1 (phosphodiesterase type-3 inhibitors)
**Contra-indications**  severe hypovolaemia
**Renal impairment**  use half to three-quarters normal dose and monitor response if estimated glomerular filtration rate less than 50 mL/minute/1.73 m$^2$
**Pregnancy**  manufacturer advises use only if potential benefit outweighs risk
**Breast-feeding**  manufacturer advises avoid—no information available
**Side-effects**  ectopic beats, ventricular tachycardia, supraventricular arrhythmias (more likely in children with pre-existing arrhythmias), hypotension; head-

ache; *less commonly* ventricular fibrillation, chest pain, tremor, hypokalaemia, thrombocytopenia; *very rarely* bronchospasm, anaphylaxis, and rash

**Licensed use** not licensed for use in children under 18 years

**Indications and dose**

Congestive heart failure, low cardiac output following cardiac surgery, shock

• **By intravenous infusion**

**Neonate** initially 50–75 micrograms/kg over 30–60 minutes (reduce or omit initial dose if at risk of hypotension) then 30–45 micrograms/kg/hour by *continuous intravenous infusion* for 2–3 days (usually for 12 hours after cardiac surgery)

**Child 1 month–18 years** initially 50–75 micrograms/kg over 30–60 minutes (reduce or omit initial dose if at risk of hypotension) then 30–45 micrograms/kg/hour by *continuous intravenous infusion* for 2–3 days (usually for 12 hours after cardiac surgery)

**Administration** for *intravenous infusion* dilute with Glucose 5% *or* Sodium Chloride 0.9% *or* Sodium Chloride and Glucose intravenous infusion to a concentration of 200 micrograms/mL (higher concentrations of 400 micrograms/mL have been used); loading dose may be given undiluted if fluid-restricted

**Primacor**® (Sanofi-Aventis) ⒫ₒₘ
Injection, milrinone (as lactate) 1 mg/mL, net price 10-mL amp = £16.61

## 2.2  Diuretics

| 2.2.1 | Thiazides and related diuretics |
| 2.2.2 | Loop diuretics |
| 2.2.3 | Potassium-sparing diuretics and aldosterone antagonists |
| 2.2.4 | Potassium-sparing diuretics with other diuretics |
| 2.2.5 | Osmotic diuretics |
| 2.2.6 | Mercurial diuretics |
| 2.2.7 | Carbonic anhydrase inhibitors |
| 2.2.8 | Diuretics with potassium |

Diuretics are used for a variety of conditions in children including pulmonary oedema (caused by conditions such as respiratory distress syndrome and bronchopulmonary dysplasia), congestive heart failure, and hypertension. Hypertension in children is often resistant to therapy and may require the use of several drugs in combination (see section 2.5). Maintenance of fluid and electrolyte balance can be difficult in children on diuretics, particularly neonates whose renal function may be immature.

**Loop diuretics** (section 2.2.2) are used for pulmonary oedema, congestive heart failure, and in renal disease.

**Thiazides** (section 2.2.1) are used less commonly than loop diuretics but are often used in combination with loop diuretics or spironolactone in the management of pulmonary oedema and, in lower doses, for hypertension associated with cardiac disease.

**Aminophylline infusion** has been used with intravenous furosemide to relieve fluid overload in critically ill children.

**Heart failure**   Heart failure is less common in children than in adults; it can occur as a result of congenital heart disease (e.g. septal defects), dilated cardiomyopathy, myocarditis, or cardiac surgery. Drug treatment of heart failure due to left ventricular systolic dysfunction is covered below; optimal management of heart failure with preserved left ventricular function has not been established.

**Acute heart failure** can occur after cardiac surgery or as a complication in severe acute infections with or without myocarditis. Therapy consists of volume loading, vasodilator or inotropic drugs.

**Chronic heart failure** is initially treated with a **loop diuretic** (section 2.2.2), usually furosemide supplemented with **spironolactone, amiloride, or potassium.**

If diuresis with furosemide is insufficient, the addition of **metolazone** or a **thiazide diuretic** (section 2.2.1) can be considered. With metolazone, the resulting diuresis can be profound and care is needed to avoid potentially dangerous electrolyte disturbance.

If diuretics are insufficient an ACE inhibitor, titrated to the maximum tolerated dose, can be used. **ACE inhibitors** (section 2.5.5.1) are used for the treatment of all grades of heart failure in adults and can also be useful for children with heart failure. Addition of **digoxin** (section 2.1.1) can be considered in children who remain symptomatic despite treatment with a diuretic and an ACE inhibitor.

Some beta-blockers improve outcome in adults with heart failure, but data on beta-blockers in children are limited. **Carvedilol** (section 2.4) has vasodilatory properties and therefore (like ACE inhibitors) also lowers afterload.

In children receiving specialist cardiology care, the phosphodiesterase type-3 inhibitor **enoximone** is sometimes used by mouth for its inotropic and vasodilator effects. Spironolactone (section 2.2.3) is usually used as a potassium-sparing drug with a loop diuretic; in adults low doses of spironolactone are effective in the treatment of heart failure. Careful monitoring of serum potassium is necessary if spironolactone is used in combination with an ACE inhibitor.

**Potassium loss**   Hypokalaemia can occur with both thiazide and loop diuretics. The risk of hypokalaemia depends on the duration of action as well as the potency and is thus greater with thiazides than with an equipotent dose of a loop diuretic.

Hypokalaemia is particularly dangerous in children being treated with cardiac glycosides. In hepatic failure hypokalaemia caused by diuretics can precipitate encephalopathy.

The use of potassium-sparing diuretics (section 2.2.3) avoids the need to take potassium supplements.

### 2.2.1  Thiazides and related diuretics

Thiazides and related compounds are moderately potent diuretics; they inhibit sodium reabsorption at the beginning of the distal convoluted tubule. They are usually administered early in the day so that the diuresis does not interfere with sleep.

**2  Cardiovascular system**

In the management of *hypertension* a low dose of a thiazide produces a maximal or near-maximal blood pressure lowering effect, with very little biochemical disturbance. Higher doses cause more marked changes in plasma potassium, sodium, uric acid, glucose, and lipids, with little advantage in blood pressure control. For reference to the use of thiazides in chronic heart failure see section 2.2.

**Bendroflumethiazide** is licensed for use in children; **chlorothiazide** is also used.

**Chlortalidone**, a thiazide-related compound, has a longer duration of action than the thiazides and may be given on alternate days in younger children.

**Metolazone** is particularly effective when combined with a loop diuretic (even in renal failure) and is most effective when given 30–60 minutes before furosemide; profound diuresis can occur and the child should therefore be monitored carefully.

**Cautions** See also section 2.2. Thiazides and related diuretics can exacerbate diabetes, gout, and systemic lupus erythematosus. Electrolytes should be monitored particularly with high doses, long-term use, or in renal impairment. Thiazides and related diuretics should also be used with caution in nephrotic syndrome, hyperaldosteronism, and malnourishment; **interactions:** Appendix 1 (diuretics).

**Contra-indications** Thiazides and related diuretics should be avoided in refractory hypokalaemia, hyponatraemia, and hypercalcaemia, symptomatic hyperuricaemia, and Addison's disease.

**Hepatic impairment** Thiazides and related diuretics should be used with caution in mild to moderate impairment and avoided in severe impairment. Hypokalaemia may precipitate coma, although hypokalaemia can be prevented by using a potassium-sparing diuretic.

**Renal impairment** Thiazides and related diuretics should be used with caution because they can further reduce renal function. They are ineffective if estimated glomerular filtration rate is less than 30 mL/minute/1.73 m$^2$ and should be avoided; metolazone remains effective but with a risk of excessive diuresis.

**Pregnancy** Thiazides and related diuretics should not be used to treat gestational hypertension. They may cause neonatal thrombocytopenia, bone marrow suppression, jaundice, electrolyte disturbances, and hypoglycaemia; placental perfusion may also be reduced. Stimulation of labour, uterine inertia, and meconium staining have also been reported.

**Breast-feeding** The amount of bendroflumethiazide, chlorothiazide, chlortalidone, and metolazone present in milk is too small to be harmful; large doses may suppress lactation.

**Side-effects** Side-effects of thiazides and related diuretics include mild gastro-intestinal disturbances, postural hypotension, altered plasma-lipid concentrations, metabolic and electrolyte disturbances including hypokalaemia (see also notes above), hyponatraemia, hypomagnesaemia, hypercalcaemia, hyperglycaemia, hypochloraemic alkalosis, and hyperuricaemia, and gout. Less common side-effects include blood disorders including agranulocytosis, leucopenia and thrombocytopenia, and impotence. Pancreatitis, intrahepatic cholestasis, cardiac arrhythmias, headache, dizziness, paraesthesia, visual disturbances, and hypersensitivity reactions (including pneumonitis, pulmonary oedema, photosensitivity, and severe skin reactions) have also been reported.

## BENDROFLUMETHIAZIDE
(Bendrofluazide)

**Cautions** see notes above
**Contra-indications** see notes above
**Hepatic impairment** see notes above
**Renal impairment** see notes above
**Pregnancy** see notes above
**Breast-feeding** see notes above
**Side-effects** see notes above
**Indications and dose**

> Oedema in heart failure, renal disease, and hepatic disease; pulmonary oedema; hypertension
> - By mouth
>   **Child 1 month–2 years** 50–100 micrograms/kg daily adjusted according to response
>   **Child 2–12 years** initially 50–400 micrograms/kg (max. 10 mg) daily then 50–100 micrograms/kg daily adjusted according to response (max. 10 mg daily)
>   **Child 12–18 years** initially 5–10 mg daily or on alternate days (2.5 mg daily in hypertension) as a single morning dose, adjusted according to response (max. 10 mg daily)

**Bendroflumethiazide** (Non-proprietary) [PoM]
Tablets, bendroflumethiazide 2.5 mg, net price 28-tab pack = 79p; 5 mg, 28-tab pack = 86p
Brands include *Aprinox®*, *Neo-NaClex®*

## CHLOROTHIAZIDE

**Cautions** see notes above; also neonate (theoretical risk of kernicterus if very jaundiced)
**Contra-indications** see notes above
**Hepatic impairment** see notes above
**Renal impairment** see notes above
**Pregnancy** see notes above
**Breast-feeding** see notes above
**Side-effects** see notes above
**Licensed use** not licensed
**Indications and dose**

> Heart failure, hypertension, ascites
> - By mouth
>   **Neonate** 10–20 mg/kg twice daily
>   **Child 1–6 months** 10–20 mg/kg twice daily
>   **Child 6 months–12 years** 10 mg/kg twice daily (max. 1 g daily)
>   **Child 12–18 years** 0.25–1 g once daily *or* 125–500 mg twice daily

> Chronic hypoglycaemia section 6.1.4

> Diabetes insipidus section 6.5.2

**◢Preparations**
Chlorothiazide oral suspension 250 mg/5 mL is
available from 'special-order' manufacturers or specialist importing companies, see p. 823

## ◼ CHLORTALIDONE
(Chlorthalidone)

**Cautions** see notes above
**Contra-indications** see notes above
**Hepatic impairment** see notes above
**Renal impairment** see notes above
**Pregnancy** see notes above
**Breast-feeding** see notes above
**Side-effects** see notes above; also *rarely* jaundice
**Indications and dose**

Hypertension
* By mouth
  **Child 5–12 years** 0.5–1 mg/kg in the morning
  every 48 hours; max. 1.7 mg/kg every 48 hours
  **Child 12–18 years** 25 mg daily in the morning,
  increased to 50 mg daily if necessary (but see
  notes above)

Stable heart failure
* By mouth
  **Child 5–12 years** 0.5–1 mg/kg in the morning
  every 48 hours; max. 1.7 mg/kg every 48 hours
  **Child 12–18 years** 25–50 mg daily in the morning,
  increased if necessary to 100–200 mg daily
  (reduce to lowest effective dose for maintenance)

Ascites, oedema in nephrotic syndrome
* By mouth
  **Child 5–12 years** 0.5–1 mg/kg in the morning
  every 48 hours; max. 1.7 mg/kg every 48 hours
  **Child 12–18 years** up to 50 mg daily

**Hygroton®** (Alliance) PoM
Tablets, yellow, scored, chlortalidone 50 mg, net
price 28-tab pack = £1.64

## ◼ METOLAZONE

**Cautions** see notes above; also acute porphyria (sec-
tion 9.8.2)
**Contra-indications** see notes above
**Hepatic impairment** see notes above
**Renal impairment** see notes above
**Pregnancy** see notes above
**Breast-feeding** see notes above
**Side-effects** see notes above; also chills, chest pain
**Licensed use** not licensed for use in children
**Indications and dose**

Oedema resistant to loop diuretics in heart failure, renal disease, and hepatic disease; pulmonary oedema; adjunct to loop diuretics to induce
diuresis
* By mouth
  **Child 1 month–12 years** 100–200 micrograms/kg
  once or twice daily
  **Child 12–18 years** 5–10 mg once daily in the
  morning, increased to 5–10 mg twice daily in
  resistant oedema

**Administration** tablets may be crushed and mixed
with water immediately before use

**Metolazone** (Non-Proprietary) PoM
Tablets, metolazone 2.5 mg and 5 mg
Available from 'special-order' manufacturers or
specialist importing companies, see p. 823

## ◼ 2.2.2 Loop diuretics

Loop diuretics inhibit reabsorption of sodium, potassium, and chloride from the ascending limb of the loop
of Henlé in the renal tubule and are powerful diuretics.

**Furosemide** and **bumetanide** are similar in activity;
they produce dose-related diuresis. Furosemide is
used extensively in children. It can be used for pulmonary oedema (e.g. in respiratory distress syndrome and
bronchopulmonary dysplasia), congestive heart failure,
and in renal disease.

**Cautions** Hypovolaemia and hypotension should be
corrected before initiation of treatment with loop diuretics; electrolytes should be monitored during treatment
(see also Potassium Loss, section 2.2). Loop diuretics
should be used with caution in comatose and precoma-
tose states associated with liver cirrhosis. Loop diuretics
can exacerbate diabetes (but hyperglycaemia less likely
than with thiazides) and gout; they can also cause acute
urinary retention in children with obstruction of urinary
outflow, therefore adequate urinary output should be
established before initiating treatment.

**Contra-indications** Loop diuretics should be
avoided in severe hypokalaemia, severe hyponatraemia,
anuria, and in renal failure due to nephrotoxic or hepatotoxic drugs.

**Hepatic impairment** Hypokalaemia induced by
loop diuretics may precipitate hepatic encephalopathy
and coma—potassium-sparing diuretics can be used to
prevent this.

**Renal impairment** High doses of loop diuretics
may occasionally be needed; high doses or rapid intravenous administration can cause tinnitus and deafness;
high doses of bumetanide can also cause musculoskeletal pain.

**Pregnancy** Furosemide and bumetanide should not
be used to treat gestational hypertension because of the
maternal hypovolaemia associated with this condition.

**Side-effects** Side-effects of loop diuretics include
mild gastro-intestinal disturbances, pancreatitis, hepatic
encephalopathy, postural hypotension, temporary
increase in serum-cholesterol and triglyceride concentration, hyperglycaemia (less common than with thiazides), acute urinary retention, electrolyte disturbances
(including hyponatraemia, hypokalaemia (see section
2.2), increased calcium excretion (nephrocalcinosis
and nephrolithiasis reported with long-term use of furosemide in preterm infants), hypochloraemia, and hypomagnesaemia), metabolic alkalosis, blood disorders
(including bone marrow depression, thrombocytopenia,
and leucopenia), hyperuricaemia, visual disturbances,
tinnitus and deafness (usually with high doses and rapid
intravenous administration, and in renal impairment),
rash, and photosensitivity.

**2**

**Cardiovascular system**

## 2 Cardiovascular system

## BUMETANIDE

**Cautions** see notes above
**Contra-indications** see notes above
**Hepatic impairment** see notes above
**Renal impairment** see notes above
**Pregnancy** see notes above
**Breast-feeding** no information available; may inhibit lactation
**Side-effects** see notes above; also gynaecomastia, breast pain, musculoskeletal pain (associated with high doses in renal failure)
**Licensed use** not licensed for use in children under 12 years

### Indications and dose

Oedema in heart failure, renal disease, and hepatic disease; pulmonary oedema

* By mouth

  **Child 1 month–12 years** 15–50 micrograms/kg 1–4 times daily (max. single dose 2 mg); do not exceed 5 mg daily

  **Child 12–18 years** 1 mg in the morning, repeated after 6–8 hours if necessary; severe cases, 5 mg daily increased by 5 mg every 12–24 hours according to response

* By intravenous injection

  **Child 12–18 years** 1–2 mg, repeated after 20 minutes if necessary

* By intravenous infusion over 30–60 minutes

  **Child 1 month–12 years** 25–50 micrograms/kg

  **Child 12–18 years** 1–5 mg

**Administration** for *intravenous infusion*, dilute with Glucose 5% *or* Sodium Chloride 0.9%; concentrations above 25 micrograms/mL may cause precipitation

**Bumetanide** (Non-proprietary) PoM
Tablets, bumetanide 1 mg, net price 28-tab pack = £1.12; 5 mg, 28-tab pack = £4.33
Oral liquid, bumetanide 1 mg/5 mL, net price 150 mL = £128.00
Injection, bumetanide 500 micrograms/mL, net price 4-mL amp = £1.79

## FUROSEMIDE
(Frusemide)

**Cautions** see notes above; also hypoproteinaemia may reduce effect and increase risk of side-effects; hepatorenal syndrome; risk of ototoxicity may be reduced by giving high oral doses in 2 or more divided doses; effect may be prolonged in neonates; some liquid preparations contain alcohol, caution especially in neonates; **interactions:** Appendix 1 (diuretics)
**Contra-indications** see notes above
**Hepatic impairment** see notes above
**Renal impairment** see notes above; also lower rate of infusion may be necessary
**Pregnancy** see notes above
**Breast-feeding** amount too small to be harmful; may inhibit lactation
**Side-effects** see notes above; also intrahepatic cholestasis and gout

### Indications and dose

Oedema in heart failure, renal disease, and hepatic disease; pulmonary oedema

* By mouth

  **Neonate** 0.5–2 mg/kg every 12–24 hours (every 24 hours if postmenstrual age under 31 weeks)

  **Child 1 month–12 years** 0.5–2 mg/kg 2–3 times daily (every 24 hours if postmenstrual age under 31 weeks); higher doses may be required in resistant oedema; max. 12 mg/kg daily, not to exceed 80 mg daily

  **Child 12–18 years** 20–40 mg daily, increased in resistant oedema to 80–120 mg daily

* By slow intravenous injection

  **Neonate** 0.5–1 mg/kg every 12–24 hours (every 24 hours if postmenstrual age under 31 weeks)

  **Child 1 month–12 years** 0.5–1 mg/kg repeated every 8 hours as necessary; max. 2 mg/kg (max. 40 mg) every 8 hours

  **Child 12–18 years** 20–40 mg repeated every 8 hours as necessary; higher doses may be required in resistant cases

* By continuous intravenous infusion

  **Child 1 month–18 years** 0.1–2 mg/kg/hour (following cardiac surgery, initially 100 micrograms/kg/hour, doubled every 2 hours until urine output exceeds 1 mL/kg/hour)

Oliguria

* By mouth

  **Child 12–18 years** initially 250 mg daily; if necessary, dose increased in steps of 250 mg given every 4–6 hours; max. single dose 2 g

* By intravenous infusion

  **Child 1 month–12 years** 2–5 mg/kg up to 4 times daily (max. 1 g daily)

  **Child 12–18 years** initially 250 mg over 1 hour, increase to 500 mg over 2 hours if satisfactory urine output not obtained, then give a further 1 g over 4 hours if no satisfactory response within subsequent hour, if no response obtained dialysis probably required; effective dose (up to 1 g, max. rate 4 mg/minute) can be repeated every 24 hours

**Administration** for administration *by mouth*, tablets can be crushed and mixed with water *or* injection solution diluted and given by mouth.
For *intravenous injection*, give over 5–10 minutes at a usual rate of 100 micrograms/kg/minute (not exceeding 500 micrograms/kg/minute), max. 4 mg/minute.
For *intravenous infusion*, dilute with Sodium Chloride 0.9% to a concentration of 1–2 mg/mL; glucose solutions unsuitable (infusion pH must be above 5.5)

**Furosemide** (Non-proprietary) PoM
Tablets, furosemide 20 mg, net price 28-tab pack = 81p; 40 mg, 28-tab pack = 84p; 500 mg, 28-tab pack = £4.05
Brands include *Rusyde*®
Oral solution, sugar-free, furosemide, net price 20 mg/5 mL, 150 mL = £13.97; 40 mg/5 mL, 150 mL = £18.19; 50 mg/5 mL, 150 mL = £19.35
Brands include *Frusol*® (contains alcohol 10%)
Injection, furosemide 10 mg/mL, net price 2-mL amp = 30p; 5-mL amp = 38p; 25-mL amp = £2.50

**Lasix®** (Sanofi-Aventis) PoM
Injection, furosemide 10 mg/mL, net price 2-mL amp = 75p
**Note** Large-volume furosemide injections also available; brands include *Minijet®*

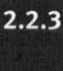

### 2.2.3  Potassium-sparing diuretics and aldosterone antagonists

**Spironolactone** is the most commonly used potassium-sparing diuretic in children; it is an aldosterone antagonist and enhances potassium retention and sodium excretion in the distal tubule. Spironolactone is combined with other diuretics to reduce urinary potassium loss. It is also used in nephrotic syndrome, the long-term management of Bartter's syndrome, and high doses can help to control ascites in babies with chronic neonatal hepatitis. The clinical value of spironolactone in the management of pulmonary oedema in preterm neonates with chronic lung disease is uncertain.

**Potassium canrenoate**, given intravenously, is an alternative aldosterone antagonist that may be useful if a potassium-sparing diuretic is required and the child is unable to take oral medication. It is metabolised to canrenone, which is also a metabolite of spironolactone.

**Amiloride** on its own is a weak diuretic. It causes retention of potassium and is therefore given with thiazide or loop diuretics as an alternative to giving potassium supplements (see section 2.2.4 for compound preparations with thiazides or loop diuretics).

A potassium-sparing diuretic such as spironolactone or amiloride may also be used in the management of amphotericin-induced hypokalaemia.

Potassium supplements must **not** be given with potassium-sparing diuretics. Administration of a potassium-sparing diuretic to a child receiving an ACE inhibitor or an angiotensin-II receptor antagonist (section 2.5.5) can also cause severe hyperkalaemia.

### AMILORIDE HYDROCHLORIDE

**Cautions** monitor electrolytes; diabetes mellitus; interactions: Appendix 1 (diuretics)
**Contra-indications** hyperkalaemia; anuria; Addison's disease
**Renal impairment** monitor plasma-potassium concentration (high risk of hyperkalaemia in renal impairment); manufacturers advise avoid in severe impairment
**Pregnancy** not to be used for treating hypertension in pregnancy
**Breast-feeding** manufacturer advises avoid—no information available
**Side-effects** abdominal pain, gastro-intestinal bleeding, dry mouth, thirst, diarrhoea, constipation, anorexia, jaundice, dyspepsia, flatulence, vomiting, nausea, angina, arrhythmias, palpitation, postural hypotension, dyspnoea, cough, nasal congestion, confusion, headache, insomnia, weakness, tremor, agitation, dizziness, malaise, paraesthesia, encephalopathy, urinary disturbances, sexual dysfunction, hyperkalaemia, muscle cramp, arthralgia, visual disturbances, raised intra-ocular pressure, tinnitus, alopecia, pruritus, rash
**Licensed use** not licensed for use in children

**Indications and dose**

> **Adjunct to thiazide or loop diuretics for oedema in heart failure, and hepatic disease (where potassium conservation desirable)**
> • By mouth
> > **Neonate** 100–200 micrograms/kg twice daily
> > **Child 1 month–12 years** 100–200 micrograms/kg twice daily; max. 20 mg daily
> > **Child 12–18 years** 5–10 mg twice daily

**Amiloride** (Non-proprietary) PoM
Tablets, amiloride hydrochloride 5 mg, net price 28-tab pack = 96p
Oral solution, sugar-free, amiloride hydrochloride 5 mg/5 mL, net price 150 mL = £39.73
**Brands include** *Amilamont®* (*excipients include* propylene glycol, see Excipients p. 2)

◢**Compound preparations with thiazide or loop diuretics**
See section 2.2.4

---

## Aldosterone antagonists

### SPIRONOLACTONE

**Cautions** potential metabolic products carcinogenic in *rodents*; monitor electrolytes (discontinue if hyperkalaemia); acute porphyria (section 9.8.2); **interactions:** Appendix 1 (diuretics)
**Contra-indications** hyperkalaemia; anuria; Addison's disease
**Renal impairment** monitor plasma-potassium concentration (high risk of hyperkalaemia in renal impairment); avoid in acute renal insufficiency or severe impairment
**Pregnancy** use only if potential benefit outweighs risk—feminisation of male fetus in *animal* studies
**Breast-feeding** metabolites present in milk but amount probably too small to be harmful
**Side-effects** gastro-intestinal disturbances, hepatotoxicity, malaise, confusion, drowsiness, dizziness, gynaecomastia, benign breast tumour, breast pain, menstrual disturbances, changes in libido, hypertrichosis, electrolyte disturbances including hyperkalaemia (discontinue) and hyponatraemia, acute renal failure, hyperuricaemia, leucopenia, agranulocytosis, thrombocytopenia, leg cramps, alopecia, rash, Stevens-Johnson syndrome
**Licensed use** not licensed for reduction of hypokalaemia induced by diuretics or amphotericin
**Indications and dose**

> **Oedema in heart failure and in ascites, nephrotic syndrome, reduction of hypokalaemia induced by diuretics or amphotericin**
> • By mouth
> > **Neonate** 1–2 mg/kg daily in 1–2 divided doses; up to 7 mg/kg daily in resistant ascites
> > **Child 1 month–12 years** 1–3 mg/kg daily in 1–2 divided doses; up to 9 mg/kg daily in resistant ascites
> > **Child 12–18 years** 50–100 mg daily in 1–2 divided doses; up to 9 mg/kg daily (max. 400 mg daily) in resistant ascites

**2**

**Cardiovascular system**

**Spironolactone** (Non-proprietary) PoM
Tablets, spironolactone 25 mg, net price 28 = £1.50;
50 mg, 28 = £2.11; 100 mg, 28 = £2.46. Label: 21

Oral suspensions, spironolactone 5 mg/5 mL,
10 mg/5 mL, 25 mg/5 mL, 50 mg/5 mL, and
100 mg/5 mL
Available from 'special-order' manufacturers or specialist
importing companies, see p. 823

**Aldactone**® (Pharmacia) PoM
Tablets, f/c, spironolactone 25 mg (buff), net price
100-tab pack = £8.89; 50 mg (white), 100-tab pack =
£17.78; 100 mg (buff), 28-tab pack = £9.96. Label:
21

### POTASSIUM CANRENOATE

**Cautions** potential metabolic products carcinogenic in
*rodents*; monitor electrolytes (discontinue if hyperkalaemia); hypotension; acute porphyria (section
9.8.2); interactions: Appendix 1 (diuretics)
**Contra-indications** hyperkalaemia; hyponatraemia
**Renal impairment** use with caution and monitor
plasma-potassium concentration if estimated glomerular filtration rate 30–60 mL/minute/1.73 m²; avoid
if estimated glomerular filtration rate less than 30 mL/
minute/1.73 m²
**Pregnancy** crosses placenta; feminisation and undes-
cended testes in male fetus in *animal* studies—manufacturer advises avoid
**Breast-feeding** present in breast milk—manufacturer
advises avoid
**Side-effects** drowsiness, headache, ataxia; menstrual
irregularities; hyperuricaemia; pain at injection site on
rapid administration; *less commonly* thrombocytopenia, eosinophilia, and hyperkalaemia; *rarely* hepatotoxicity, agranulocytosis, osteomalacia, hoarseness
and deepening of voice, hypersensitivity reactions
(including urticaria and erythema), and alopecia; also
gastro-intestinal disturbances, hypotension, transient
confusion with high doses, hyponatraemia, hypochloraemic acidosis, mastalgia, gynaecomastia, and
hirsutism
**Licensed use** not licensed for use in the UK
**Indications and dose**

Short-term diuresis for oedema in heart failure
and in ascites

• By intravenous injection over at least 3 minutes
or intravenous infusion
**Neonate** 1–2 mg/kg twice daily
**Child 1 month–12 years** 1–2 mg/kg twice daily
**Child 12–18 years** 1–2 mg/kg (max. 200 mg)
twice daily
Note To convert to equivalent oral spironolactone dose,
multiply potassium canrenoate dose by 0.7

**Administration** consult product literature

### Preparations
Potassium canrenoate injection is available from
'special-order' manufacturers or specialist importing
companies, see p. 823

## 2.2.4 Potassium-sparing diuretics with other diuretics

Although it is preferable to prescribe diuretics separately in children, the use of fixed combinations may
be justified in older children if compliance is a problem.
The most commonly used preparations are listed below
(but they may not be licensed for use in children—
consult product literature), for other preparations see
the BNF. For interactions, see Appendix 1 (diuretics).

### Amiloride with thiazides
**Co-amilozide** (Non-proprietary) PoM
Tablets, co-amilozide 2.5/25 (amiloride hydro-
chloride 2.5 mg, hydrochlorothiazide 25 mg), net
price 28-tab pack = £3.73
Brands include *Moduret 25*®

### Amiloride with loop diuretics
**Co-amilofruse** (Non-proprietary) PoM
Tablets, co-amilofruse 2.5/20 (amiloride hydro-
chloride 2.5 mg, furosemide 20 mg). Net price 28-tab
pack = £1.18, 56-tab pack = £1.83
Brands include *Frumil LS*®

Tablets, co-amilofruse 5/40 (amiloride hydrochloride
5 mg, furosemide 40 mg). Net price 28-tab pack =
£1.17, 56-tab pack = £1.42
Brands include *Frumil*®

Tablets, co-amilofruse 10/80 (amiloride hydrochloride 10 mg, furosemide 80 mg), net price 28-tab
pack = £11.51

## 2.2.5 Osmotic diuretics

**Mannitol** is used to treat cerebral oedema, raised intra-
ocular pressure, peripheral oedema, and ascites.

### MANNITOL
**Cautions** extravasation causes inflammation and
thrombophlebitis; monitor fluid and electrolyte balance, serum osmolality, and pulmonary and renal
function; assess cardiac function before and during
treatment; interactions: Appendix 1 (mannitol)
**Contra-indications** severe heart failure; severe
pulmonary oedema; intracranial bleeding (except
during craniotomy); anuria; severe dehydration
**Renal impairment** use with caution in severe
impairment
**Pregnancy** manufacturer advises avoid unless essential—no information available
**Breast-feeding** manufacturer advises avoid unless
essential—no information available
**Side-effects** *less commonly* hypotension, thrombophlebitis, fluid and electrolyte imbalance; *rarely* dry
mouth, thirst, nausea, vomiting, oedema, raised
intracranial pressure, arrhythmia, hypertension,
pulmonary oedema, chest pain, headache, convulsions, dizziness, chills, fever, urinary retention,
focal osmotic nephrosis, dehydration, cramp, blurred
vision, rhinitis, skin necrosis, and hypersensitivity
reactions (including urticaria and anaphylaxis); *very
rarely* congestive heart failure and acute renal failure
**Licensed use** not licensed for use in children under 12
years

**Indications and dose**

> Cerebral oedema, raised intra-ocular pressure
> * **By intravenous infusion over 30-60 minutes**
>   **Child 1 month-12 years** 0.25-1.5 g/kg repeated if necessary 1-2 times after 4-8 hours
>   **Child 12-18 years** 0.25-2 g/kg repeated if necessary 1-2 times after 4-8 hours

> Peripheral oedema and ascites
> * **By intravenous infusion over 2-6 hours**
>   **Child 1 month-18 years** 1-2 g/kg

**Administration** examine infusion for crystals; if crystals present, dissolve by warming infusion fluid (allow to cool to body temperature before administration); for mannitol 20%, an in-line filter is recommended (15-micron filters have been used)

**Mannitol** (Baxter) PoM
Intravenous infusion, mannitol 10%, net price 500-mL *Viaflex*® bag = £2.26, 500-mL *Viaflo*® bag = £2.15; 20%, 250-mL *Viaflex*® bag = £3.27, 250-mL *Viaflo*® bag = £3.27, 500-mL *Viaflex*® bag = £3.29, 500-mL *Viaflo*® bag = £3.12

## 2.2.6  Mercurial diuretics

Classification not used in *BNF for Children*.

## 2.2.7  Carbonic anhydrase inhibitors

The carbonic anhydrase inhibitor **acetazolamide** is a weak diuretic although it is little used for its diuretic effect. Acetazolamide and eye drops of dorzolamide and brinzolamide inhibit the formation of aqueous humour and are used in glaucoma (section 11.6). In children, acetazolamide is also used in the treatment of epilepsy (section 4.8.1), and raised intracranial pressure (section 11.6).

## 2.2.8  Diuretics with potassium

Diuretics and potassium supplements should be prescribed separately for children.

## 2.3  Anti-arrhythmic drugs

2.3.1  **Management of arrhythmias**
2.3.2  **Drugs for arrhythmias**

## 2.3.1  Management of arrhythmias

Management of an arrhythmia requires precise diagnosis of the type of arrhythmia; electrocardiography and referral to a paediatric cardiologist is essential; underlying causes such as heart failure require appropriate treatment.

Arrhythmias may be broadly divided into bradycardias, supraventricular tachycardias, and ventricular arrhythmias.

**Bradycardia** Adrenaline (epinephrine) is useful in the treatment of symptomatic bradycardia in an infant or child.

## Supraventricular tachycardias

In supraventricular tachycardia adenosine is given by rapid intravenous injection. If adenosine is ineffective, intravenous amiodarone, flecainide, or a beta-blocker (such as esmolol, see section 2.4) can be tried; verapamil can also be considered in children over 1 year. Atenolol, sotalol (section 2.4), and flecainide are used for the prophylaxis of paroxysmal supraventricular tachycardias.

The use of d.c. shock and vagal stimulation also have a role in the treatment of supraventricular tachycardia.

**Syndromes associated with accessory conducting pathways** Amiodarone, flecainide, or a beta-blocker is used to prevent recurrence of supraventricular tachycardia in infants and young children with these syndromes (e.g. Wolff-Parkinson-White syndrome).

**Atrial flutter** In atrial flutter without structural heart defects, sinus rhythm is restored with d.c. shock or cardiac pacing; drug treatment is usually not necessary. Amiodarone is used in atrial flutter when structural heart defects are present or after heart surgery. Sotalol (section 2.4) may also be considered.

**Atrial fibrillation** Atrial fibrillation is very rare in children. To restore sinus rhythm d.c. shock is used; beta-blockers, alone or together with digoxin, may be useful for ventricular rate control.

**Ectopic tachycardia** Intravenous amiodarone is used in conjunction with body cooling and synchronised pacing in *postoperative* junctional ectopic tachycardia. Oral amiodarone or flecainide are used in *congenital* junctional ectopic tachycardia.

Amiodarone, flecainide, or a beta-blocker are used in atrial ectopic tachycardia; amiodarone is preferred in those with poor ventricular function.

## Ventricular tachycardia and ventricular fibrillation

Pulseless ventricular tachycardia or ventricular fibrillation require resuscitation, see Paediatric Advanced Life Support algorithm (inside back cover). Amiodarone is used in resuscitation for pulseless ventricular tachycardia or ventricular fibrillation unresponsive to d.c. shock; lidocaine can be used as an alternative only if amiodarone is not available.

Amiodarone is also used in a haemodynamically stable child when drug treatment is required; lidocaine can be used as an alternative only if amiodarone is not available.

**Torsade de pointes** Torsade de pointes is a form of ventricular tachycardia associated with long QT syndrome, which may be congenital or drug induced. Episodes may be self-limiting, but are frequently recurrent and can cause impairment or loss of consciousness. If not controlled, the arrhythmia can progress to ventricular fibrillation and sometimes death. Intravenous magnesium sulfate (section 9.5.1.3) can be used to treat torsade de pointes (dose recommendations vary—consult local guidelines). Anti-arrhythmics can further prolong the QT interval, thus worsening the condition.

**2 Cardiovascular system**

**2 Cardiovascular system**

## 2.3.2 Drugs for arrhythmias

Anti-arrhythmic drugs can be classified clinically as those acting on supraventricular arrhythmias (adenosine, digoxin, and verapamil), those acting on both supraventricular and ventricular arrhythmias (amiodarone, beta-blockers, flecainide, and procainamide), and those acting on ventricular arrhythmias (lidocaine). For the treatment of bradycardia, see section 2.3.1.

Anti-arrhythmic drugs can also be classified according to their effects on the electrical behaviour of myocardial cells during activity (the Vaughan Williams classification) although this classification is of less clinical significance:

Class I: membrane stabilising drugs (e.g. lidocaine, flecainide)

Class II: beta-blockers

Class III: amiodarone; sotalol (also Class II)

Class IV: calcium-channel blockers (includes verapamil but not dihydropyridines)

**Cautions** The negative inotropic effects of anti-arrhythmic drugs tend to be additive. Therefore special care should be taken if two or more are used, especially if myocardial function is impaired. Most drugs that are effective in countering arrhythmias can also provoke them in some circumstances; moreover, hypokalaemia enhances the arrhythmogenic (pro-arrhythmic) effect of many drugs.

**Adenosine** is the treatment of choice for terminating supraventricular tachycardias, including those associated with accessory conducting pathways (e.g. Wolff-Parkinson-White syndrome). It is also used in the diagnosis of supraventricular arrhythmias. It is not negatively inotropic and does not cause significant hypotension; it can be used safely in children with impaired cardiac function or postoperative arrhythmias. The injection should be administered by rapid intravenous injection into a central or large peripheral vein.

**Amiodarone** is useful in the management of both supraventricular and ventricular tachyarrhythmias. It can be given by intravenous infusion and by mouth, and causes little or no myocardial depression. Unlike oral amiodarone, intravenous amiodarone acts relatively rapidly. Intravenous amiodarone is also used in cardiopulmonary resuscitation for ventricular fibrillation or pulseless ventricular tachycardia unresponsive to d.c. shock (see algorithm, inside back cover).

Amiodarone has a very long half-life (extending to several weeks) and only needs to be given once daily (but high doses may cause nausea unless divided). Many weeks or months may be required to achieve steady-state plasma-amiodarone concentration; this is particularly important when drug interactions are likely (see also Appendix 1).

Most patients taking amiodarone develop corneal microdeposits (reversible on withdrawal of treatment); these rarely interfere with vision, but drivers may be dazzled by headlights at night. However, if vision is impaired or if optic neuritis or optic neuropathy occur, amiodarone must be stopped to prevent blindness and expert advice sought. Because of the possibility of phototoxic reactions, children and carers should be advised to shield the child's skin from light during treatment and for several months after discontinuing

amiodarone; a wide-spectrum sunscreen (section 13.8.1) should be used to protect against both long-wave ultraviolet and visible light.

Amiodarone contains iodine and can cause disorders of thyroid function; both hypothyroidism and hyperthyroidism can occur. Clinical assessment alone is unreliable, and laboratory tests should be performed before treatment and every 6 months. Thyroxine (T4) may be raised in the absence of hyperthyroidism; therefore tri-iodothyronine (T3), T4, and thyroid-stimulating hormone (TSH) should all be measured. A raised T3 and T4 with a very low or undetectable TSH concentration suggests the development of thyrotoxicosis. The thyrotoxicosis may be very refractory, and amiodarone should usually be withdrawn at least temporarily to help achieve control; treatment with carbimazole may be required. Hypothyroidism can be treated with replacement therapy without withdrawing amiodarone if it is essential; careful supervision is required.

Pneumonitis should always be suspected if new or progressive shortness of breath or cough develops in a patient taking amiodarone. Fresh neurological symptoms should raise the possibility of peripheral neuropathy. Amiodarone is also associated with hepatotoxicity (see under amiodarone, below).

**Beta-blockers** act as anti-arrhythmic drugs principally by attenuating the effects of the sympathetic system on automaticity and conductivity within the heart, for details see section 2.4. For special reference to the role of **sotalol** in ventricular arrhythmias, see section 2.4.

Oral administration of **digoxin** (section 2.1.1) slows the ventricular rate in atrial fibrillation and in atrial flutter. However, intravenous infusion of digoxin is rarely effective for rapid control of ventricular rate.

**Flecainide** is useful for the treatment of resistant re-entry supraventricular tachycardia, ventricular tachycardia, ventricular ectopic beats, arrhythmias associated with accessory conducting pathways (e.g. Wolff-Parkinson-White syndrome), and paroxysmal atrial fibrillation. Flecainide crosses the placenta and can be used to control fetal supraventricular arrhythmias.

**Lidocaine** can be used in cardiopulmonary resuscitation in children with ventricular fibrillation or pulseless ventricular tachycardia unresponsive to d.c. shock, but only if amiodarone is not available. Doses may need to be reduced in children with persistently poor cardiac output and hepatic or renal failure (see under lidocaine, below).

**Verapamil** (section 2.6.2) can cause severe haemodynamic compromise (refractory hypotension and cardiac arrest) when used for the acute treatment of arrhythmias in neonates and infants; it is contra-indicated in children under 1 year. It is also contra-indicated in those with congestive heart failure, syndromes associated with accessory conducting pathways (e.g. Wolff-Parkinson-White syndrome) and in most receiving concomitant beta-blockers. It can be useful in older children with supraventricular tachycardia.

## ADENOSINE

**Cautions** monitor ECG and have resuscitation facilities available; atrial fibrillation or flutter with accessory pathway (conduction down anomalous pathway may increase); first degree AV block; bundle branch block; left main coronary artery stenosis; uncorrected hypovolaemia; stenotic valvular heart disease; left to right shunt; pericarditis; pericardial effusion; autonomic dysfunction; stenotic carotid artery disease with cerebrovascular insufficiency; recent myocardial infarction; heart failure; heart transplant (see dose); **interactions**: Appendix 1 (adenosine)

**Contra-indications** second- or third-degree AV block and sick sinus syndrome (unless pacemaker fitted); long QT syndrome; severe hypotension; decompensated heart failure; asthma

**Pregnancy** large doses may produce fetal toxicity; manufacturer advises use only if potential benefit outweighs risk

**Breast-feeding** no information available—unlikely to be present in milk owing to short half-life

**Side-effects** nausea; arrhythmia (discontinue if asystole or severe bradycardia occur), sinus pause, AV block, flushing, angina (discontinue), dizziness; dyspnoea; headache; *less commonly* metallic taste, palpitation, hyperventilation, weakness, blurred vision, sweating; *very rarely* transient worsening of intracranial hypertension, bronchospasm, injection-site reactions; *also reported* vomiting, syncope, hypotension (discontinue if severe), cardiac arrest, respiratory failure (discontinue), and convulsions

**Licensed use** not licensed for use in children

**Indications and dose**

Arrhythmias (see also section 2.3.1), diagnosis of arrhythmias

- By rapid intravenous injection

**Neonates** 150 micrograms/kg; if necessary repeat injection every 1–2 minutes increasing dose by 50–100 micrograms/kg until tachycardia terminated or max. single dose of 300 micrograms/kg given

**Child 1 month–1 year** 150 micrograms/kg; if necessary repeat injection every 1–2 minutes increasing the dose by 50–100 micrograms/kg until tachycardia terminated or max. single dose of 500 micrograms/kg given

**Child 1–12 years** 100 micrograms/kg; if necessary repeat injection every 1–2 minutes increasing dose by 50–100 micrograms/kg until tachycardia terminated or max. single dose of 500 micrograms/kg (max. 12 mg) given

**Child 12–18 years** initially 3 mg; if necessary followed by 6 mg after 1–2 minutes, and then by 12 mg after a further 1–2 minutes

**Note** In some children over 12 years 3-mg dose ineffective (e.g. if a small peripheral vein is used for administration) and higher initial dose sometimes used; however, those with *heart transplant* are **very sensitive** to the effects of adenosine, and should **not** receive higher initial doses. In children receiving dipyridamole reduce dose to a quarter of usual dose of adenosine

**Administration** by *rapid intravenous injection* over 2 seconds into central or large peripheral vein followed by rapid Sodium Chloride 0.9% flush; Injection solution may be diluted with Sodium Chloride 0.9% if required

**Adenosine** (Non-proprietary) PoM
Injection, adenosine 3 mg/mL, net price 2-mL vial = £4.45 (hosp. only)
Intravenous infusion, adenosine 3 mg/mL, net price 10-mL vial = £11.67 (hosp.only)

**Adenocor®** (Sanofi-Aventis) PoM
Injection, adenosine 3 mg/mL, net price 2-mL vial = £4.45 (hosp. only)

**Adenoscan®** (Sanofi-Aventis) PoM
Intravenous infusion, adenosine 3 mg/mL, net price 10-mL vial = £14.26 (hosp. only)
**Note** *Adenoscan®* may be used in conjunction with radionuclide myocardial perfusion imaging in patients who cannot exercise adequately or for whom exercise is inappropriate—consult product literature

## AMIODARONE HYDROCHLORIDE

**Cautions** liver-function and thyroid-function tests required before treatment and then every 6 months (see notes above for tests of thyroid function); hypokalaemia (measure serum-potassium concentration before treatment); pulmonary function tests and chest x-ray required before treatment; heart failure; severe bradycardia and conduction disturbances in excessive dosage; intravenous use may cause moderate and transient fall in blood pressure (circulatory collapse precipitated by rapid administration or overdosage) or severe hepato-cellular toxicity (monitor transaminases closely); ECG monitoring and resuscitation facilities must be available during intravenous use; acute porphyria (section 9.8.2); avoid benzyl alcohol containing injections in neonates (see Excipients, p. 2); **interactions**: Appendix 1 (amiodarone)

**Contra-indications** *except in cardiac arrest*: sinus bradycardia, sino-atrial heart block; unless pacemaker fitted avoid in severe conduction disturbances or sinus node disease; thyroid dysfunction; iodine sensitivity; avoid *intravenous use* in severe respiratory failure, circulatory collapse, or severe arterial hypotension; avoid bolus injection in congestive heart failure or cardiomyopathy; avoid rapid loading after cardiac surgery

**Pregnancy** possible risk of neonatal goitre; use only if no alternative

**Breast-feeding** avoid; significant amount present in milk—risk of neonatal hypothyroidism from release of iodine

**Side-effects** nausea, vomiting, taste disturbances, raised serum transaminases (may require dose reduction or withdrawal if accompanied by acute liver disorders), jaundice; bradycardia (see Cautions); pulmonary toxicity (including pneumonitis and fibrosis); tremor, sleep disorders; hypothyroidism, hyperthyroidism; reversible corneal microdeposits (sometimes with night glare); phototoxicity, persistent slate-grey skin discoloration (see also notes above); *less commonly* onset or worsening of arrhythmia, conduction disturbances (see Cautions), peripheral neuropathy and myopathy (usually reversible on withdrawal); *very rarely* chronic liver disease including cirrhosis, sinus arrest, bronchospasm (in patients with severe respiratory failure), ataxia, benign intracranial hypertension, headache, vertigo, epididymo-orchitis, impotence, haemolytic or aplastic anaemia, thrombocytopenia, rash (including exfoliative dermatitis), hypersensitivity including vasculitis, alopecia, impaired vision due to optic neuritis or optic neuropathy (including blindness), anaphylaxis on rapid injection, also hypotension, respiratory distress syndrome, sweating, and hot flushes

**Licensed use** not licensed for use in children under 3 years

**2 Cardiovascular system**

### Indications and dose

**Supraventricular and ventricular arrhythmias** see notes above (initiated in hospital or under specialist supervision)

- **By mouth**

**Neonate** initially 5–10 mg/kg twice daily for 7–10 days, then reduced to maintenance dose of 5–10 mg/kg once daily

**Child 1 month–12 years** initially 5–10 mg/kg (max. 200 mg) twice daily for 7–10 days, then reduced to maintenance dose of 5–10 mg/kg once daily (max. 200 mg daily)

**Child 12–18 years** 200 mg 3 times daily for 1 week then 200 mg twice daily for 1 week then usually 200 mg daily adjusted according to response

- **By intravenous infusion**

**Neonate** initially 5 mg/kg over 30 minutes then 5 mg/kg over 30 minutes every 12–24 hours

**Child 1 month–18 years** initially 5–10 mg/kg over 20 minutes–2 hours then *by continuous infusion* 300 micrograms/kg/hour, increased according to response to max. 1.5 mg/kg/hour; do not exceed 1.2 g in 24 hours

**Ventricular fibrillation or pulseless ventricular tachycardia refractory to defibrillation** (see also section 2.3.1)

- **By intravenous injection**

**Neonate** 5 mg/kg over at least 3 minutes

**Child 1 month–18 years** 5 mg/kg (max. 300 mg) over at least 3 minutes

**Administration** intravenous administration via central venous catheter recommended if repeated or continuous infusion required, as infusion via peripheral veins may cause pain and inflammation.

For *intravenous infusion*, dilute to a concentration of not less than 600 micrograms/mL with Glucose 5%; incompatible with Sodium Chloride infusion; avoid equipment containing the plasticizer di-2-ethyl-hexphthalate (DEHP).

For administration *by mouth*, tablets may be crushed and dispersed in water; injection solution should **not** be given orally (irritant)

**Amiodarone** (Non-proprietary) PoM
Tablets, amiodarone hydrochloride 100 mg, net price 28-tab pack = £1.75; 200 mg, 28-tab pack = £2.22. Label: 11

Injection, amiodarone hydrochloride 30 mg/mL, net price 10-mL prefilled syringe = £19.60
Excipients may include benzyl alcohol (avoid in neonates unless no safer alternative available, see Excipients, p. 2)

Sterile concentrate, amiodarone hydrochloride 50 mg/mL, net price 3-mL amp = £1.33, 6-mL amp = £2.86. For dilution and use as an infusion
Excipients may include benzyl alcohol (avoid in neonates unless no safer alternative available, see Excipients, p. 2)

**Cordarone X**® (Sanofi-Aventis) PoM
Tablets, scored, amiodarone hydrochloride 100 mg, net price 28-tab pack = £4.28; 200 mg, 28-tab pack = £6.99. Label: 11

Sterile concentrate, amiodarone hydrochloride 50 mg/mL, net price 3-mL amp = £1.33. For dilution and use as an infusion
Excipients include benzyl alcohol (avoid in neonates unless no safer alternative available, see Excipients, p. 2)

### FLECAINIDE ACETATE

**Cautions** children with pacemakers (especially those who may be pacemaker dependent because stimulation threshold may rise appreciably); atrial fibrillation following heart surgery; monitor ECG and have resuscitation facilities available during intravenous use; **interactions:** Appendix 1 (flecainide)

**Contra-indications** heart failure; abnormal left ventricular function; long-standing atrial fibrillation where conversion to sinus rhythm not attempted; haemodynamically significant valvular heart disease; avoid in sinus node dysfunction, atrial conduction defects, second-degree or greater AV block, bundle branch block or distal block unless pacing rescue available

**Hepatic impairment** avoid or reduce dose in severe impairment; monitor plasma concentration (see pharmacokinetics below)

**Renal impairment** reduce dose by 25–50% if estimated glomerular filtration rate less than 35 mL/minute/1.73 m$^2$ and monitor plasma-flecainide concentration (see pharmacokinetics below)

**Pregnancy** used in pregnancy to treat maternal and fetal arrhythmias in specialist centres; toxicity reported in *animal* studies; infant hyperbilirubinaemia also reported

**Breast-feeding** significant amount present in milk but not known to be harmful

**Side-effects** oedema, pro-arrhythmic effects; dyspnoea; dizziness, asthenia, fatigue, fever; visual disturbances; *rarely* pneumonitis, hallucinations, depression, confusion, amnesia, dyskinesia, convulsions, peripheral neuropathy; *also reported* gastrointestinal disturbances, anorexia, hepatic dysfunction, flushing, syncope, drowsiness, tremor, vertigo, headache, anxiety, insomnia, ataxia, paraesthesia, hypoaesthesia, anaemia, leucopenia, thrombocytopenia, corneal deposits, tinnitus, increased antinuclear antibodies, hypersensitivity reactions (including rash, urticaria, and photosensitivity), increased sweating

**Pharmacokinetics** plasma-flecainide concentration for optimal response 200–800 micrograms/litre; blood sample should be taken immediately before next dose

**Licensed use** not licensed for use in children under 12 years

### Indications and dose

**Resistant re-entry supraventricular tachycardia, ventricular ectopic beats or ventricular tachycardia, arrhythmias associated with accessory conduction pathways (e.g. Wolff-Parkinson-White syndrome), paroxysmal atrial fibrillation**

- **By mouth**

**Neonate** 2 mg/kg 2–3 times daily adjusted according to response and plasma-flecainide concentration

**Child 1 month–12 years** 2 mg/kg 2–3 times daily adjusted according to response and plasma-flecainide concentration (max. 8 mg/kg/day or 300 mg daily)

**Child 12–18 years** initially 50–100 mg twice daily; max. 300 mg daily (max. 400 mg daily for ventricular arrhythmias in heavily built children)

- **By slow intravenous injection or intravenous infusion**

**Neonate** 1–2 mg/kg over 10–30 minutes; if necessary followed by continuous infusion at a rate of 100–250 micrograms/kg/hour until arrhythmia controlled; transfer to *oral* treatment as above

**Child 1 month–12 years** 2 mg/kg over 10–30 minutes; if necessary followed by continuous infusion at a rate of 100–250 micrograms/kg/hour until arrhythmia controlled (max. cumulative dose 600 mg in 24 hours); transfer to *oral* treatment as above

**Child 12–18 years** 2 mg/kg (max. 150 mg) over 10–30 minutes; if necessary followed by continuous infusion at a rate of 1.5 mg/kg/hour for 1 hour, then reduced to 100–250 micrograms/kg/hour until arrhythmia controlled (max. cumulative dose 600 mg in first 24 hours); transfer to *oral* treatment as above

**Administration**  for administration *by mouth*, milk, infant formula, and dairy products may reduce absorption of flecainide—separate doses from feeds. Liquid has a local anaesthetic effect and should be given at least 30 minutes before or after food. Do not store liquid in refrigerator as precipitation occurs.

For *intravenous administration*, give initial dose over 30 minutes in children with sustained ventricular tachycardia or cardiac failure.

Dilute injection using Glucose 5%; concentrations of more than 300 micrograms/mL are unstable in chloride-containing solutions

**Flecainide** (Non-proprietary) PoM
Tablets, flecainide acetate 50 mg, net price 60-tab pack = £6.04; 100 mg, 60-tab pack = £8.95

Liquid, available from 'special-order' manufacturers or specialist importing companies, see p. 823

**Tambocor**® (Meda) PoM
Tablets, flecainide acetate 50 mg, net price 60-tab pack = £11.57; 100 mg (scored), 60-tab pack = £16.53

Injection, flecainide acetate 10 mg/mL, net price 15-mL amp = £4.40

◢**Modified release**
**Tambocor**® **XL** (Meda) PoM
Capsules, m/r, grey/pink, flecainide acetate 200 mg, net price 30-cap pack = £14.77. Label: 25
**Dose**
**Supraventricular arrhythmias**

- **By mouth**
**Child 12–18 years** 200 mg once daily
**Note** Not to be used to control arrhythmias in acute situations; children stabilised on 200 mg daily of immediate-release flecainide may be transferred to *Tambocor*® *XL*

## LIDOCAINE HYDROCHLORIDE
(Lignocaine hydrochloride)

**Cautions**  lower doses in congestive heart failure and following cardiac surgery; monitor ECG; resuscitation facilities should be available; **interactions:** Appendix 1 (lidocaine)

**Contra-indications**  sino-atrial disorders, all grades of atrioventricular block, severe myocardial depression; acute porphyria (section 9.8.2)

**Hepatic impairment**  caution—increased risk of side-effects

**Renal impairment**  possible accumulation of lidocaine and active metabolite; caution in severe impairment

**Pregnancy**  crosses the placenta but not known to be harmful in *animal* studies—use if benefit outweighs risk

**Breast-feeding**  present in milk but amount too small to be harmful

**Side-effects**  dizziness, paraesthesia, or drowsiness (particularly if injection too rapid); other CNS effects include confusion, respiratory depression and convulsions; hypotension and bradycardia (may lead to cardiac arrest); *rarely* hypersensitivity reactions including anaphylaxis

**Licensed use**  not licensed for use in children under 1 year

**Indications and dose**

Ventricular arrhythmias, pulseless ventricular tachycardia or ventricular fibrillation

- **By intravenous or intraosseous injection, and intravenous infusion**

**Neonate** 0.5–1 mg/kg by injection followed by infusion of 0.6–3 mg/kg/hour; if infusion not immediately available following initial injection, injection of 0.5–1 mg/kg may be repeated at intervals of not less than 5 minutes (to max. total dose 3 mg/kg) until infusion can be initiated

**Child 1 month–12 years** 0.5–1 mg/kg by injection followed by infusion of 0.6–3 mg/kg/hour; if infusion not immediately available following initial injection, injection of 0.5–1 mg/kg may be repeated at intervals of not less than 5 minutes (to max. total dose 3 mg/kg) until infusion can be initiated

**Child 12–18 years** 50–100 mg by injection followed by infusion of 120 mg over 30 minutes *then* 240 mg over 2 hours *then* 60 mg/hour; reduce dose further if infusion continued beyond 24 hours; if infusion not immediately available following initial injection, injection of 50–100 mg may be repeated at intervals of not less than 5 minutes (to max. 300 mg in 1 hour) until infusion can be initiated

Neonatal seizures (section 4.8.1)

- **By intravenous infusion**

**Neonate** initially 2 mg/kg over 10 minutes, followed by 6 mg/kg/hour for 6 hours; reduce dose over the following 24 hours (4 mg/kg/hour for 12 hours, then 2 mg/kg/hour for 12 hours)
**Note** Preterm neonates may require lower doses

Eye section 11.7

Local anaesthesia section 15.2

**Administration**  for *intravenous infusion*, dilute with Glucose 5% or Sodium Chloride 0.9%

**Lidocaine** (Non-proprietary) [PoM]
Injection 1%, lidocaine hydrochloride 10 mg/mL, net price 2-mL amp = 21p; 5-mL amp = 26p; 10-mL amp = 39p; 20-mL amp = 78p

Injection 2%, lidocaine hydrochloride 20 mg/mL, net price 2-mL amp = 32p; 5-mL amp = 31p; 10-mL amp = 60p; 20-mL amp = 80p

Infusion, lidocaine hydrochloride 0.1% (1 mg/mL) and 0.2% (2 mg/mL) in glucose intravenous infusion 5%. 500-mL containers

**Minijet® Lidocaine** (UCB Pharma) [PoM]
Injection, lidocaine hydrochloride 1% (10 mg/mL), net price 10-mL disposable syringe = £8.48; 2% (20 mg/mL), 5-mL disposable syringe = £8.18

# 2.4 Beta-adrenoceptor blocking drugs

Beta-adrenoceptor blocking drugs (beta-blockers) block the beta-adrenoceptors in the heart, peripheral vasculature, bronchi, pancreas, and liver.

Many beta-blockers are available but experience in children is limited to the use of only a few.

Differences between beta-blockers may affect choice. The water-soluble beta-blockers, atenolol and sotalol, are less likely to enter the brain and may therefore cause less sleep disturbance and nightmares. Water-soluble beta-blockers are excreted by the kidneys and dosage reduction is often necessary in renal impairment.

Some beta-blockers, such as atenolol, have an intrinsically longer duration of action and can be given only once daily. Carvedilol and labetalol are beta-blockers which have, in addition, an arteriolar vasodilating action and thus lower peripheral resistance. Although carvedilol and labetalol possess both alpha- and beta-blocking properties, these drugs have no important advantages over other beta-blockers in the treatment of hypertension.

Beta-blockers slow the heart and can depress the myocardium; they are contra-indicated in children with second- or third-degree heart block. Sotalol may prolong the QT interval, and it occasionally causes life-threatening ventricular arrhythmias (**important:** particular care is required to avoid hypokalaemia in children taking sotalol).

Beta-blockers can precipitate asthma and should usually be avoided in children with a history of asthma or bronchospasm. If there is no alternative, a child with well-controlled asthma can be treated for a co-existing condition (e.g. arrhythmia) with a cardioselective beta-blocker, which should be initiated with caution at a low dose by a specialist and the child monitored closely for adverse effects. Atenolol and metoprolol have less effect on the $beta_2$ (bronchial) receptors and are, therefore, relatively *cardioselective*, but they are not *cardiospecific*; they have a lesser effect on airways resistance but are not free of this side-effect.

Beta-blockers are also associated with fatigue, coldness of the extremities, and sleep disturbances with nightmares (may be less common with the water-soluble beta-blockers, see above).

Beta-blockers can affect carbohydrate metabolism causing hypoglycaemia or hyperglycaemia in children with or without diabetes; they can also interfere with metabolic and autonomic responses to hypoglycaemia thereby masking symptoms such as tachycardia. However, beta-blockers are not contra-indicated in diabetes, although the cardioselective beta-blockers (e.g. atenolol and metoprolol) may be preferred. Beta-blockers should be avoided altogether in those with frequent episodes of hypoglycaemia.

**Pregnancy** Beta-blockers may cause intra-uterine growth restriction, neonatal hypoglycaemia, and bradycardia; the risk is greater in severe hypertension. The use of labetalol in maternal hypertension is not known to be harmful, except possibly in the first trimester. Information on the safety of carvedilol during pregnancy is lacking. If beta-blockers are used close to delivery, infants should be monitored for signs of beta-blockade (and alpha-blockade with labetalol or carvedilol). For the treatment of hypertension in pregnancy, see section 2.5.

**Breast-feeding** Infants should be monitored as there is a risk of possible toxicity due to beta-blockade (and alpha-blockade with labetalol or carvedilol), but the amount of most beta-blockers present in milk is too small to affect infants. Atenolol and sotalol are present in milk in greater amounts than other beta-blockers. The manufacturer of esmolol advises avoidance if breast-feeding.

**Hypertension** Beta-blockers are effective for reducing blood pressure (section 2.5), but their mode of action is not understood; they reduce cardiac output, alter baroceptor reflex sensitivity, and block peripheral adrenoceptors. Some beta-blockers depress plasma renin secretion. It is possible that a central effect may also partly explain their mode of action. Blood pressure can usually be controlled with relatively few side-effects. In general the dose of beta-blocker does not have to be high.

**Labetalol** may be given intravenously for *hypertensive emergencies* in children (section 2.5); however, care is needed to avoid dangerous hypotension or beta-blockade, particularly in neonates. **Esmolol** is also used intravenously for the treatment of hypertension particularly in the peri-operative period.

Beta-blockers can be used to control the pulse rate in children with *phaeochromocytoma* (section 2.5.4). However, they should never be used alone as beta-blockade without concurrent alpha-blockade may lead to a hypertensive crisis; phenoxybenzamine should always be used together with the beta-blocker.

**Arrhythmias** In arrhythmias (section 2.3), beta-blockers act principally by attenuating the effects of the sympathetic system on automaticity and conductivity within the heart. They can be used alone or in conjunction with digoxin to control the ventricular rate in *atrial fibrillation*. Beta-blockers are also useful in the management of *supraventricular tachycardias* and *ventricular tachycardias* particularly to prevent recurrence of the tachycardia.

**Esmolol** is a relatively cardioselective beta-blocker with a very short duration of action, used intravenously for the short-term treatment of supraventricular arrhythmias and sinus tachycardia, particularly in the peri-operative period.

**Sotalol** is a non-cardioselective beta-blocker with additional class III anti-arrhythmic activity. Atenolol and sotalol suppress ventricular ectopic beats and non-sustained ventricular tachycardia (section 2.3.1). However, the pro-arrhythmic effects of sotalol, particularly in children with sick sinus syndrome, may prolong the QT interval and induce torsade de pointes.

**Heart failure**  Beta-blockers may produce benefit in heart failure by blocking sympathetic activity and the addition of a beta-blocker such as **carvedilol** to other treatment for heart failure may be beneficial. Treatment should be initiated by those experienced in the management of heart failure (see section 2.2 for details on heart failure).

**Thyrotoxicosis**  Beta-blockers are used in the management of *thyrotoxicosis* including neonatal thyrotoxicosis; **propranolol** can reverse clinical symptoms within 4 days. Beta-blockers are also used for the pre-operative preparation for thyroidectomy; the thyroid gland is rendered less vascular, thus facilitating surgery (section 6.2.2).

**Other uses**  In tetralogy of Fallot, esmolol or propranolol may be given intravenously in the initial management of *cyanotic spells*; propranolol is given by mouth for preventing cyanotic spells. If a severe cyanotic spell in a child with congenital heart disease persists despite optimal use of 100% oxygen, propranolol is given by intravenous infusion (for dose, see below). If cyanosis is still present after 10 minutes, sodium bicarbonate intravenous infusion is given in a dose of 1 mmol/kg to correct acidosis (or dose calculated according to arterial blood gas results); sodium bicarbonate 4.2% intravenous infusion is appropriate for a child under 1 year and sodium bicarbonate 8.4% intravenous infusion in children over 1 year. If blood-glucose concentration is less than 3 mmol/litre, glucose 10% intravenous infusion is given in a dose of 2 mL/kg (glucose 200 mg/kg) over 10 minutes, followed by morphine in a dose of 100 micrograms/kg by intravenous or intramuscular injection.

Beta-blockers are also used in the *prophylaxis of migraine* (section 4.7.4.2). Betaxolol, carteolol, levobunolol, and timolol are used topically in *glaucoma* (section 11.6).

## PROPRANOLOL HYDROCHLORIDE

**Cautions**  see notes above; also avoid abrupt withdrawal; first-degree AV block; portal hypertension (risk of deterioration in liver function); diabetes (see also notes above); history of obstructive airways disease (introduce cautiously and monitor lung function—see also notes above); myasthenia gravis; symptoms of thyrotoxicosis may be masked (see also notes above); psoriasis; history of hypersensitivity—may increase sensitivity to allergens and result in more serious hypersensitivity response, also may reduce response to adrenaline (epinephrine); **interactions**: Appendix 1 (beta-blockers), **important**: verapamil interaction, see also p. 107

**Contra-indications**  asthma (but see notes above), uncontrolled heart failure, marked bradycardia, hypotension, sick sinus syndrome, second- or third-degree AV block, cardiogenic shock, metabolic acidosis, severe peripheral arterial disease; phaeochromocytoma (apart from specific use with alphablockers, see also notes above)

Bronchospasm Beta-blockers, including those considered to be cardioselective, should usually be avoided in children with a history of asthma or bronchospasm. However, where there is no alternative a cardioselective beta-blocker can be given with caution under specialist supervision

**Hepatic impairment**  reduce oral dose
**Renal impairment**  manufacturer advises caution—dose reduction may be required
**Pregnancy**  see notes above
**Breast-feeding**  see notes above
**Side-effects**  see notes above; also gastro-intestinal disturbances; bradycardia, heart failure, hypotension, conduction disorders, peripheral vasoconstriction (including exacerbation of intermittent claudication and Raynaud's phenomenon); bronchospasm (see above), dyspnoea; headache, fatigue, sleep disturbances, paraesthesia, dizziness, psychoses; sexual dysfunction; purpura, thrombocytopenia; visual disturbances; exacerbation of psoriasis, alopecia; *rarely* rashes and dry eyes (reversible on withdrawal); **overdosage**: see Emergency Treatment of Poisoning, p. 29
**Licensed use**  not licensed for treatment of hypertension in children under 12 years

### Indications and dose

#### Arrhythmias

- **By mouth**

  **Neonate** 250–500 micrograms/kg 3 times daily, adjusted according to response

  **Child 1 month–18 years** 250–500 micrograms/kg 3–4 times daily, adjusted according to response; max. 1 mg/kg 4 times daily, total daily dose not to exceed 160 mg daily

- **By slow intravenous injection, with ECG monitoring**

  **Neonate** 20–50 micrograms/kg repeated if necessary every 6–8 hours

  **Child 1 month–18 years** 25–50 micrograms/kg repeated every 6–8 hours if necessary

#### Hypertension

- **By mouth**

  **Neonate** initially 250 micrograms/kg 3 times daily, increased if necessary to max. 2 mg/kg 3 times daily

  **Child 1 month–12 years** 0.25–1 mg/kg 3 times daily, increased at weekly intervals to max. 5 mg/kg daily in divided doses

  **Child 12–18 years** initially 80 mg twice daily; increased at weekly intervals as required; maintenance 160–320 mg daily; slow-release preparations may be used for once daily administration

#### Tetralogy of Fallot

- **By mouth**

  **Neonate** 0.25–1 mg/kg 2–3 times daily, max. 2 mg/kg 3 times daily

  **Child 1 month–12 years** 0.25–1 mg/kg 3–4 times daily, max. 5 mg/kg daily in divided doses

- **By slow intravenous injection with ECG monitoring**

  **Neonate** initially 15–20 micrograms/kg (max. 100 micrograms/kg), repeated every 12 hours if necessary

  **Child 1 month–12 years** initially 15–20 micrograms/kg (max. 100 micrograms/kg), repeated every 6–8 hours if necessary; higher doses rarely necessary

**2**

**Cardiovascular system**

**Migraine prophylaxis**
- By mouth

  **Child 2–12 years** initially 200–500 micrograms/kg twice daily; usual dose 10–20 mg twice daily; max. 2 mg/kg twice daily

  **Child 12–18 years** initially 20–40 mg twice daily; usual dose 40–80 mg twice daily; max. 2 mg/kg (max. 120 mg) twice daily

**Administration** for *slow intravenous injection*, give over at least 3–5 minutes; rate of administration should not exceed 1 mg/minute. May be diluted with Sodium Chloride 0.9% or Glucose 5%. Incompatible with bicarbonate.

**Note** Excessive bradycardia can be countered with intravenous injection of atropine sulfate; for **overdosage** see Emergency Treatment of Poisoning, p. 29

**Propranolol** (Non-proprietary) PoM
Tablets, propranolol hydrochloride 10 mg, net price 28-tab pack = 92p; 40 mg, 28-tab pack = 93p; 80 mg, 56-tab pack = £1.54; 160 mg, 56-tab pack = £4.02. Label: 8
Brands include *Angilol*®

Oral solution, propranolol hydrochloride 5 mg/5 mL, net price 150 mL = £12.50; 10 mg/5 mL, 150 mL = £16.45; 40 mg/5 mL, 150 mL = £31.50; 50 mg/5 mL, 150 mL = £19.98. Label: 8
Brands include *Syprol*®

Injection, propranolol hydrochloride 1 mg/mL Available from 'special-order' manufacturers or specialist importing companies, see p. 823

**◢ Modified release**
**Note** Modified-release preparations for once daily administration; use in older children only

**Half-Inderal LA**® (AstraZeneca) PoM
Capsules, m/r, lavender/pink, propranolol hydrochloride 80 mg, net price 28-cap pack = £5.40. Label: 8, 25
**Note** Modified-release capsules containing propranolol hydrochloride 80 mg also available; brands include *Bedranol SR*®, *Half Beta Prograne*®

**Inderal-LA** (AstraZeneca) PoM
Capsules, m/r, lavender/pink, propranolol hydrochloride 160 mg, net price 28-cap pack = £1.91. Label: 8, 25
**Note** Modified-release capsules containing propranolol hydrochloride 160 mg also available; brands include *Bedranol SR*®, *Beta-Prograne*®, *Slo-Pro*®

## ▌ ATENOLOL

**Cautions** see under Propranolol Hydrochloride
**Contra-indications** see under Propranolol Hydrochloride
**Renal impairment** initially use 50% of usual dose if estimated glomerular filtration rate 10–35 mL/minute/1.73 m$^2$; initially use 30–50% of usual dose if estimated glomerular filtration rate less than 10 mL/minute/1.73 m$^2$
**Pregnancy** see notes above
**Breast-feeding** see notes above
**Side-effects** see under Propranolol Hydrochloride
**Licensed use** not licensed for use in children under 12 years

**Indications and dose**
**Hypertension**
- By mouth

  **Neonate** 0.5–2 mg/kg once daily; may be given in 2 divided doses

  **Child 1 month–12 years** 0.5–2 mg/kg once daily (doses higher than 50 mg daily rarely necessary); may be given in 2 divided doses

  **Child 12–18 years** 25–50 mg once daily (higher doses rarely necessary); may be given in 2 divided doses

**Arrhythmias**
- By mouth

  **Neonate** 0.5–2 mg/kg once daily; may be given in 2 divided doses

  **Child 1 month–12 years** 0.5–2 mg/kg once daily (max. 100 mg daily); may be given in 2 divided doses

  **Child 12–18 years** 50–100 mg once daily; may be given in 2 divided doses

**Atenolol** (Non-proprietary) PoM
Tablets, atenolol 25 mg, net price 28-tab pack = 83p; 50 mg, 28-tab pack = 86p; 100 mg, 28-tab pack = 91p. Label: 8

**Tenormin**® (AstraZeneca) PoM
LS tablets, orange, f/c, scored, atenolol 50 mg, net price 28-tab pack = £2.04. Label: 8

Tablets, orange, f/c, scored, atenolol 100 mg, net price 28-tab pack = £3.46. Label: 8

Syrup, sugar-free, atenolol 25 mg/5 mL, net price 300 mL = £8.55. Label: 8

## ▌ CARVEDILOL

**Cautions** see under Propranolol Hydrochloride; monitor renal function during dose titration in children with heart failure who also have low blood pressure, renal impairment, ischaemic heart disease, or diffuse vascular disease
**Contra-indications** see under Propranolol Hydrochloride; acute or decompensated heart failure requiring intravenous inotropes
**Hepatic impairment** avoid
**Pregnancy** see notes above
**Breast-feeding** see notes above
**Side-effects** postural hypotension, dizziness, headache, fatigue, gastro-intestinal disturbances, bradycardia; occasionally diminished peripheral circulation, peripheral oedema and painful extremities, dry mouth, dry eyes, eye irritation or disturbed vision, impotence, disturbances of micturition, influenza-like symptoms; rarely angina, AV block, exacerbation of intermittent claudication or Raynaud's phenomenon; allergic skin reactions, exacerbation of psoriasis, nasal stuffiness, wheezing, depressed mood, sleep disturbances, paraesthesia, heart failure, changes in liver enzymes, thrombocytopenia, leucopenia also reported
**Licensed use** not licensed for use in children under 18 years

## Indications and dose

**Adjunct in heart failure** (limited information available)

- **By mouth**

  **Child 2–18 years** initially 50 micrograms/kg (max. 3.125 mg) twice daily, double dose at intervals of at least 2 weeks up to 350 micrograms/kg (max. 25 mg) twice daily

**Carvedilol** (Non-proprietary) [PoM]
Tablets, carvedilol 3.125 mg, net price 28-tab pack = £1.10; 6.25 mg, 28-tab pack = £1.25; 12.5 mg, 28-tab pack = £1.37; 25 mg, 28-tab pack = £1.84. Label: 8

## ▌ ESMOLOL HYDROCHLORIDE

**Cautions** see under Propranolol Hydrochloride

**Contra-indications** see under Propranolol Hydrochloride

**Renal impairment** manufacturer advises caution

**Pregnancy** see notes above

**Breast-feeding** see notes above

**Side-effects** see under Propranolol Hydrochloride; infusion causes venous irritation and thrombophlebitis

**Licensed use** not licensed for use in children

## Indications and dose

**Arrhythmias, hypertensive emergencies** (see also notes above and section 2.5)

- **By intravenous administration**

  **Child 1 month–18 years** initially by *intravenous injection* over 1 minute 500 micrograms/kg then by *intravenous infusion* 50 micrograms/kg/minute for 4 minutes (rate reduced if low blood pressure or low heart rate); if inadequate response, repeat loading dose and increase maintenance infusion by 50 micrograms/kg/minute increments; repeat until effective or max. infusion of 200 micrograms/kg/minute reached; doses over 300 micrograms/kg/minute not recommended

**Tetralogy of Fallot**

- **By intravenous administration**

  **Neonate** initially by *intravenous injection* over 1–2 minutes 600 micrograms/kg then if necessary by *intravenous infusion* 300–900 micrograms/kg/minute

**Administration** give through a central venous catheter; incompatible with bicarbonate

**Brevibloc**® (Baxter) [PoM]
Injection, esmolol hydrochloride 10 mg/mL, net price 10-mL vial = £7.79, 250-mL infusion bag = £89.69

## ▌ LABETALOL HYDROCHLORIDE

**Cautions** see under Propranolol Hydrochloride; interferes with laboratory tests for catecholamines; liver damage (see below)

**Liver damage** Severe hepatocellular damage reported after both short-term and long-term treatment. Appropriate laboratory testing needed at first symptom of liver dysfunction and if laboratory evidence of damage (or if jaundice) labetalol should be stopped and not restarted

**Contra-indications** see under Propranolol Hydrochloride

**Renal impairment** dose reduction may be required

**Pregnancy** see notes above

**Breast-feeding** see notes above

**Side-effects** postural hypotension (avoid upright position during and for 3 hours after intravenous administration), tiredness, weakness, headache, rashes, scalp tingling, difficulty in micturition, epigastric pain, nausea, vomiting; liver damage (see above); rarely lichenoid rash

**Licensed use** not licensed for use in children

## Indications and dose

**Hypertensive emergencies** see also section 2.5

- **By intravenous infusion**

  **Neonate** 500 micrograms/kg/hour adjusted at intervals of at least 15 minutes according to response; max. 4 mg/kg/hour

  **Child 1 month–12 years** initially 0.5–1 mg/kg/hour adjusted at intervals of at least 15 minutes according to response; max. 3 mg/kg/hour

  **Child 12–18 years** 30–120 mg/hour adjusted at intervals of at least 15 minutes according to response

  **Note** Consult local guidelines. In hypertensive encephalopathy reduce blood pressure to normotensive level over 24–48 hours (more rapid reduction may lead to cerebral infarction, blindness, and death). If child fitting, reduce blood pressure rapidly, but not to normal levels

**Hypertension**

- **By mouth**

  **Child 1 month–12 years** 1–2 mg/kg 3–4 times a day

  **Child 12–18 years** initially 50–100 mg twice daily increased if required at intervals of 3–14 days to usual dose of 200–400 mg twice daily (3–4 divided doses if higher); max. 2.4 g daily

- **By intravenous injection**

  **Child 1 month–12 years** 250–500 micrograms/kg as a single dose; max. 20 mg

  **Child 12–18 years** 50 mg over at least 1 minute, repeated after 5 minutes if necessary; max. total dose 200 mg

**Note** Excessive bradycardia can be countered with intravenous injection of atropine sulfate; for **overdosage** see p. 29

**Administration** for *intravenous infusion*, dilute to a concentration of 1 mg/mL in Glucose 5% *or* Sodium Chloride and Glucose 5%; if fluid restricted may be given undiluted, preferably through a central venous catheter.

For administration *by mouth*, injection may be given orally with squash or juice

**Labetalol Hydrochloride** (Non-proprietary) [PoM]
Tablets, f/c, labetalol hydrochloride 100 mg, net price 56 = £7.85; 200 mg, 56 = £11.49; 400 mg, 56 = £20.60. Label: 8, 21

Injection, labetalol hydrochloride 5 mg/mL, net price 20-mL amp = £4.91

**Trandate**® (PharSafer) [PoM]
Tablets, all orange, f/c, labetalol hydrochloride 50 mg, net price 56-tab pack = £3.64; 100 mg, 56-tab pack = £4.01; 200 mg, 56-tab pack = £6.51; 400 mg, 56-tab pack = £9.05. Label: 8, 21

**Cardiovascular system**

**2**

## ▊ METOPROLOL TARTRATE

**Cautions** see under Propranolol Hydrochloride

**Contra-indications** see under Propranolol Hydrochloride

**Hepatic impairment** reduce dose in severe impairment

**Pregnancy** see notes above

**Breast-feeding** see notes above

**Side-effects** see under Propranolol Hydrochloride

**Licensed use** not licensed for use in children

**Indications and dose**

#### Hypertension

- By mouth

  **Child 1 month–12 years** initially 1 mg/kg twice daily, increased if necessary to max. 8 mg/kg (max. 400 mg) daily in 2–4 divided doses

  **Child 12–18 years** initially 50–100 mg daily increased if necessary to 200 mg daily in 1–2 divided doses; max. 400 mg daily (but high doses rarely necessary)

#### Arrhythmias

- By mouth

  **Child 12–18 years** usually 50 mg 2–3 times daily; up to 300 mg daily in divided doses if necessary

**Metoprolol Tartrate** (Non-proprietary) ⒫ₒₘ
Tablets, metoprolol tartrate 50 mg, net price 28-tab pack = £1.31, 56-tab pack = £1.74; 100 mg, 28-tab pack = £1.59, 56-tab pack = £2.51. Label: 8

**Lopresor®** (Recordati) ⒫ₒₘ
Tablets, f/c, scored, metoprolol tartrate 50 mg (pink), net price 56-tab pack = £2.57; 100 mg (blue), 56-tab pack = £6.68. Label: 8

#### ◀ Modified release

**Lopresor SR®** (Recordati) ⒫ₒₘ
Tablets, m/r, yellow, f/c, metoprolol tartrate 200 mg, net price 28-tab pack = £9.80. Label: 8, 25

**Dose**

#### Hypertension

- By mouth

  **Child 12–18 years** 200 mg once daily

## ▊ SOTALOL HYDROCHLORIDE

**Cautions** see under Propranolol Hydrochloride; correct hypokalaemia, hypomagnesaemia, or other electrolyte disturbances; severe or prolonged diarrhoea; reduce dose or discontinue if corrected QT interval exceeds 550 msec

**Contra-indications** see under Propranolol Hydrochloride; congenital or acquired long QT syndrome; torsade de pointes

**Renal impairment** halve normal dose if estimated glomerular filtration rate 30–60 mL/minute/1.73 m²; use one-quarter normal dose if estimated glomerular filtration rate 10–30 mL/minute/1.73 m²; avoid if estimated glomerular filtration rate less than 10 mL/minute/1.73 m²

**Pregnancy** see notes above

**Breast-feeding** see notes above

**Side-effects** see under Propranolol Hydrochloride; arrhythmogenic (pro-arrhythmic) effect (torsade de pointes—increased risk in females)

**Licensed use** not licensed for use in children under 12 years

**Indications and dose**

#### Ventricular arrhythmias, life-threatening ventricular tachyarrhythmia and supraventricular arrhythmias initiated under specialist supervision and ECG monitoring and measurement of corrected QT interval

- By mouth

  **Neonate** initially 1 mg/kg twice daily, increased as necessary every 3–4 days to max. 4 mg/kg twice daily

#### Atrial flutter, ventricular arrhythmias, life-threatening ventricular tachyarrhythmia and supraventricular arrhythmias initiated under specialist supervision and ECG monitoring and measurement of corrected QT interval

- By mouth

  **Child 1 month–12 years** initially 1 mg/kg twice daily, increased as necessary every 2–3 days to max. 4 mg/kg twice daily (max. 80 mg twice daily)

  **Child 12–18 years** initially 80 mg once daily *or* 40 mg twice daily, increased gradually at intervals of 2–3 days to usual dose 80–160 mg twice daily; higher doses of 480–640 mg daily for life-threatening ventricular arrhythmias under specialist supervision

**Administration** for administration *by mouth*, tablets may be crushed and dispersed in water

**Sotalol** (Non-proprietary) ⒫ₒₘ
Tablets, sotalol hydrochloride 40 mg, net price 56-tab pack = £1.29; 80 mg, 56-tab pack = £1.91; 160 mg, 28-tab pack = £2.32. Label: 8

**Beta-Cardone®** (UCB Pharma) ⒫ₒₘ
Tablets, scored, sotalol hydrochloride 40 mg (green), net price 56-tab pack = £1.29; 80 mg (pink), 56-tab pack = £1.91; 200 mg, 28-tab pack = £2.40. Label: 8

**Sotacor®** (Bristol-Myers Squibb) ⒫ₒₘ
Tablets, scored, sotalol hydrochloride 80 mg, net price 28-tab pack = £3.06. Label: 8

## ▊ 2.5 Hypertension

Hypertension in children and adolescents can have a substantial effect on long-term health. Possible causes of hypertension (e.g. congenital heart disease, renal disease and endocrine disorders) and the presence of any complications (e.g. left ventricular hypertrophy) should be established. Treatment should take account of contributory factors and any factors that increase the risk of cardiovascular complications.

Serious hypertension is rare in *neonates* but it can present with signs of congestive heart failure; the cause is often renal and can follow embolic arterial damage.

Children (or their parents or carers) should be given advice on lifestyle changes to reduce blood pressure or cardiovascular risk; these include weight reduction (in obese children), reduction of dietary salt, reduction of total and saturated fat, increasing exercise, increasing fruit and vegetable intake, and not smoking.

Indications for antihypertensive therapy in children include symptomatic hypertension, secondary hypertension, hypertensive target-organ damage, diabetes mellitus, persistent hypertension despite lifestyle measures (see above), and pulmonary hypertension (section 2.5.1.2). The effect of antihypertensive treatment on growth and development is not known; treatment should be started only if benefits are clear.

Antihypertensive therapy should be initiated with a single drug at the lowest recommended dose; the dose can be increased until the target blood pressure is achieved. Once the highest recommended dose is reached, or sooner if the patient begins to experience side-effects, a second drug may be added if blood pressure is not controlled. If more than one drug is required, these should be given as separate products to allow dose adjustment of individual drugs, but fixed-dose combination products may be useful in adolescents if compliance is a problem.

Acceptable drug classes for use in children with hypertension include **ACE inhibitors** (section 2.5.5.1), **alpha-blockers** (section 2.5.4), **beta-blockers** (section 2.4), **calcium-channel blockers** (section 2.6.2), and **thiazide diuretics** (section 2.2.1). There is limited information on the use of **angiotensin-II receptor antagonists** (section 2.5.5.2) in children. Diuretics and beta-blockers have a long history of safety and efficacy in children. The newer classes of antihypertensive drugs, including ACE inhibitors and calcium-channel blockers have been shown to be safe and effective in short-term studies in children. Refractory hypertension may require additional treatment with agents such as **minoxidil** (section 2.5.1.1) or **clonidine** (section 2.5.2).

**Other measures to reduce cardiovascular risk**   Aspirin (section 2.9) may be used to reduce the risk of cardiovascular events; however, concerns about an increased risk of bleeding and Reye's syndrome need to be considered.

A **statin** can be of benefit in older children who have a high risk of cardiovascular disease and have hypercholesterolaemia (see section 2.12).

**Hypertension in diabetes**   Hypertension can occur in type 2 diabetes and treatment prevents both macrovascular and microvascular complications. ACE inhibitors (section 2.5.5.1) may be considered in children with diabetes and microalbuminaemia or proteinuric renal disease (see also section 6.1.5). Beta-blockers are best avoided in children with, or at a high risk of developing, diabetes, especially when combined with a thiazide diuretic.

**Hypertension in renal disease**   ACE inhibitors may be considered in children with micro-albuminuria or proteinuric renal disease (see also section 6.1.5). High doses of loop diuretics may be required. Specific cautions apply to the use of ACE inhibitors in renal impairment, see section 2.5.5.1, but ACE inhibitors may be

effective. Dihydropyridine calcium-channel blockers may be added.

**Hypertension in pregnancy**   High blood pressure in pregnancy may usually be due to pre-existing essential hypertension or to pre-eclampsia. **Methyldopa** (BNF section 2.5.2) is safe in pregnancy. Beta-blockers are effective and safe in the third trimester. Modified-release preparations of **nifedipine** [unlicensed] are also used for hypertension in pregnancy. Intravenous administration of **labetalol** (section 2.4) can be used to control hypertensive crises; alternatively **hydralazine** (section 2.5.1.1) can be given by the intravenous route.

**Hypertensive emergencies**   Hypertensive emergencies in children may be accompanied by signs of hypertensive encephalopathy, including seizures. Controlled reduction in blood pressure over 72–96 hours is essential; rapid reduction can reduce perfusion leading to organ damage. Treatment should be initiated with intravenous drugs; once blood pressure is controlled, oral therapy can be started. It may be necessary to infuse fluids particularly during the first 12 hours to expand plasma volume should the blood pressure drop too rapidly.

Controlled reduction of blood pressure is achieved by intravenous administration of labetalol (section 2.4) or **sodium nitroprusside** (section 2.5.1.1). **Esmolol** (section 2.4) is useful for short-term use and has a short duration of action. **Nicardipine** (section 2.6.2) can be administered as a continuous intravenous infusion but it is not licensed for this use. In less severe cases, nifedipine capsules (section 2.6.2) can be used.

In resistant cases, **diazoxide** (section 2.5.1.1) is given intravenously, but it can cause sudden hypotension. Other antihypertensive drugs which can be given intravenously include hydralazine (section 2.5.1.1) and **clonidine** (section 2.5.2).

Hypertension in acute nephritis occurs as a result of sodium and water retention; it should be treated with sodium and fluid restriction, and with furosemide (section 2.2.2); antihypertensive drugs may be added if necessary.

For advice on short-term management of hypertensive episodes in phaeochromocytoma, see under Phaeochromocytoma, section 2.5.4.

### 2.5.1   Vasodilator antihypertensive drugs and pulmonary hypertension

**2.5.1.1**   Vasodilator antihypertensives

**2.5.1.2**   Pulmonary hypertension

### 2.5.1.1   Vasodilator antihypertensives

Vasodilators have a potent hypotensive effect, especially when used in combination with a beta-blocker and a thiazide. **Important:** for a warning on the hazards of a very rapid fall in blood pressure, see Hypertensive Emergencies, above.

**Sodium nitroprusside** is given by intravenous infusion to control severe hypertensive crisis when parenteral treatment is necessary. At low doses it reduces systemic vascular resistance and increases cardiac output; at high doses it can produce profound systemic hypotension—continuous blood pressure monitoring is therefore essential. Sodium nitroprusside may also be used to control paradoxical hypertension after surgery for coarctation of the aorta.

**Diazoxide** has also been used by intravenous injection in hypertensive emergencies; however it is not first-line therapy.

**Hydralazine** is given by mouth as an adjunct to other antihypertensives for the treatment of resistant hypertension but is rarely used; when used alone it causes tachycardia and fluid retention. The incidence of side-effects is lower if the dose is kept low, but systemic lupus erythematosus should be suspected if there is unexplained weight loss, arthritis, or any other unexplained ill health.

**Minoxidil** should be reserved for the treatment of severe hypertension resistant to other drugs. Vasodilatation is accompanied by increased cardiac output and tachycardia and children develop fluid retention. For this reason the addition of a beta-blocker and a diuretic (usually furosemide, in high dosage) are mandatory. Hypertrichosis is troublesome and renders this drug unsuitable for females.

**Prazosin** and **doxazosin** (section 2.5.4) have alpha-blocking and vasodilator properties.

## ◼ DIAZOXIDE

**Cautions** during prolonged use monitor white cell and platelet count, and regularly assess growth, bone, and psychological development; **interactions**: Appendix 1 (diazoxide)

**Renal impairment** dose reduction may be required

**Pregnancy** prolonged use may produce alopecia, hypertrichosis, and impaired glucose tolerance in neonate; inhibits uterine activity during labour

**Breast-feeding** manufacturer advises avoid—no information available

**Side-effects** tachycardia, hypotension, hyperglycaemia, sodium and water retention; *rarely* cardiomegaly, hyperosmolar non-ketotic coma, leucopenia, thrombocytopenia, and hirsuitism

**Licensed use** tablets not licensed for resistant hypertension

**Indications and dose**

> **Hypertensive emergencies** initiated on specialist advice
> ● By intravenous injection
>> **Child 1 month–18 years** 1–3 mg/kg (max. 150 mg) as a single dose, repeat dose after 5–15 minutes until blood pressure controlled; max. 4 doses in 24 hours
>
> **Resistant hypertension**
> ● By mouth
>> **Neonate** initially 1.7 mg/kg 3 times daily, adjusted according to response; usual max. 15 mg/kg daily
>> **Child 1 month–18 years** initially 1.7 mg/kg 3 times daily, adjusted according to response; usual max. 15 mg/kg daily
>
> **Intractable hypoglycaemia** section 6.1.4

**Administration** intravenous injection over 30 seconds. Do not dilute

**Eudemine®** (Mercury) ⒫ᴼᴹ ◣
Injection, diazoxide 15 mg/mL, net price 20-mL amp = £30.00

Tablets, see section 6.1.4

## ◼ HYDRALAZINE HYDROCHLORIDE

**Cautions** cerebrovascular disease; occasionally blood pressure reduction too rapid even with low parenteral doses; manufacturer advises test for antinuclear factor and for proteinuria every 6 months and check acetylator status before increasing dose, but evidence of clinical value unsatisfactory; **interactions**: Appendix 1 (hydralazine)

**Contra-indications** idiopathic systemic lupus erythematosus, severe tachycardia, high output heart failure, myocardial insufficiency due to mechanical obstruction, cor pulmonale; acute porphyria (section 9.8.2)

**Hepatic impairment** reduce dose

**Renal impairment** reduce dose if estimated glomerular filtration rate less than 30 mL/minute/1.73 m²

**Pregnancy** neonatal thrombocytopenia reported, but risk should be balanced against risk of uncontrolled maternal hypertension; manufacturer advises avoid before third trimester

**Breast-feeding** present in milk but not known to be harmful; monitor infant

**Side-effects** tachycardia, palpitation, flushing, hypotension, fluid retention, gastro-intestinal disturbances; headache, dizziness; systemic lupus erythematosus-like syndrome after long-term therapy (especially in slow acetylator individuals); rarely rashes, fever, peripheral neuritis, polyneuritis, paraesthesia, arthralgia, myalgia, increased lacrimation, nasal congestion, dyspnoea, agitation, anxiety, anorexia; blood disorders (including leucopenia, thrombocytopenia, haemolytic anaemia), abnormal liver function, jaundice, raised plasma creatinine, proteinuria and haematuria reported

**Licensed use** not licensed for use in children

**Indications and dose**

> **Hypertension**
> ● By mouth
>> **Neonate** 250–500 micrograms/kg every 8–12 hours increased as necessary to max. 2–3 mg/kg every 8 hours
>> **Child 1 month–12 years** 250–500 micrograms/kg every 8–12 hours increased as necessary to max. 7.5 mg/kg daily (not exceeding 200 mg daily)
>> **Child 12–18 years** 25 mg twice daily, increased to usual max. 50–100 mg twice daily
> ● By slow intravenous injection
>> **Neonate** 100–500 micrograms/kg repeated every 4–6 hours as necessary; max. 3 mg/kg daily
>> **Child 1 month–12 years** 100–500 micrograms/kg repeated every 4–6 hours as necessary; max. 3 mg/kg daily (not exceeding 60 mg daily)
>> **Child 12–18 years** 5–10 mg repeated every 4–6 hours as necessary

- By continuous intravenous infusion (preferred route in cardiac patients)

  **Neonate** 12.5–50 micrograms/kg/hour; max. 2 mg/kg daily

  **Child 1 month–12 years** 12.5–50 micrograms/kg/hour; max. 3 mg/kg daily

  **Child 12–18 years** 3–9 mg/hour; max. 3 mg/kg daily

**Administration** for *intravenous injection*, initially reconstitute 20 mg with 1 mL Water for Injections, then dilute to a concentration of 0.5–1 mg/mL with Sodium Chloride 0.9% and administer over 5–20 minutes.

For *continuous intravenous infusion*, initially reconstitute 20 mg with 1 mL Water for Injections, then dilute with Sodium Chloride 0.9%. Incompatible with Glucose intravenous infusion.

For administration *by mouth*, diluted injection may be given orally

**Hydralazine** (Non-proprietary) [PoM]
Tablets, hydralazine hydrochloride 25 mg, net price 56-tab pack = £9.32; 50 mg, 56-tab pack = £16.84

**Apresoline**® (Amdipharm) [PoM]
Tablets, yellow, s/c, hydralazine hydrochloride 25 mg, net price 84-tab pack = £3.38
Excipients include gluten, propylene glycol (see Excipients, p. 2)

Injection, powder for reconstitution, hydralazine hydrochloride, net price 20-mg amp = £2.22

---

### ■ MINOXIDIL

**Cautions** see notes above; acute porphyria (section 9.8.2); **interactions:** Appendix 1 (vasodilator antihypertensives)

**Contra-indications** phaeochromocytoma

**Renal impairment** use with caution in significant impairment

**Pregnancy** avoid—possible toxicity including reduced placental perfusion; neonatal hirsutism reported

**Breast-feeding** present in milk but not known to be harmful

**Side-effects** sodium and water retention; weight gain, peripheral oedema, tachycardia, hypertrichosis; reversible rise in creatinine and blood urea nitrogen; occasionally, gastro-intestinal disturbances, breast tenderness, rashes

**Indications and dose**

Severe hypertension

- By mouth

  **Child 1 month–12 years** initially 200 micrograms/kg daily in 1–2 divided doses, increased in steps of 100–200 micrograms/kg daily at intervals of at least 3 days; max. 1 mg/kg daily

  **Child 12–18 years** initially 5 mg daily in 1–2 divided doses, increased in steps of 5–10 mg at intervals of at least 3 days; max. 100 mg daily (seldom necessary to exceed 50 mg daily)

**Loniten**® (Pharmacia) [PoM]
Tablets, scored, minoxidil 2.5 mg, net price 60-tab pack = £8.88; 5 mg, 60-tab pack = £15.83; 10 mg, 60-tab pack = £30.68

---

### ■ SODIUM NITROPRUSSIDE

**Cautions** hypothyroidism, hyponatraemia, impaired cerebral circulation, hypothermia; monitor blood pressure and blood-cyanide concentration, and if treatment exceeds 3 days also blood-thiocyanate concentration; avoid sudden withdrawal—terminate infusion over 15–30 minutes; **interactions:** Appendix 1 (nitroprusside)

**Contra-indications** severe vitamin $B_{12}$ deficiency; Leber's optic atrophy; compensatory hypertension

**Hepatic impairment** use with caution; avoid in hepatic failure—cyanide or thiocyanate metabolites may accumulate

**Renal impairment** avoid prolonged use—cyanide or thiocyanate metabolites may accumulate

**Pregnancy** avoid prolonged use—potential for accumulation of cyanide in fetus

**Breast-feeding** no information available; caution advised due to thiocyanate metabolite

**Side-effects** associated with over rapid reduction in blood pressure (reduce infusion rate): headache, dizziness, nausea, retching, abdominal pain, perspiration, palpitation, anxiety, retrosternal discomfort; occasionally reduced platelet count, acute transient phlebitis

Cyanide Side-effects caused by excessive plasma concentration of the cyanide metabolite include tachycardia, sweating, hyperventilation, arrhythmias, marked metabolic acidosis (discontinue and give antidote, see p. 31)

**Licensed use** not licensed for use in the UK

**Indications and dose**

Hypertensive emergencies

- By continuous infusion

  **Neonate** 500 nanograms/kg/minute then increased in steps of 200 nanograms/kg/minute as necessary to max. 8 micrograms/kg/minute (max. 4 micrograms/kg/minute if used for longer than 24 hours)

  **Child 1 month–18 years** 500 nanograms/kg/minute then increased in steps of 200 nanograms/kg/minute as necessary to max. 8 micrograms/kg/minute (max. 4 micrograms/kg/minute if used for longer than 24 hours)

**Administration** for *continuous intravenous infusion* in Glucose 5%, infuse *via* infusion device to allow precise control; protect infusion from light. For further details, consult product literature.

**Sodium Nitroprusside** (Non-proprietary) [PoM]
Intravenous infusion, powder for reconstitution, sodium nitroprusside 10 mg/mL. For dilution and use as an infusion. Available from 'special-order' manufacturers or specialist importing companies, see p. 823

---

### 2.5.1.2 Pulmonary hypertension

Only pulmonary *arterial* hypertension is currently suitable for drug treatment. Pulmonary arterial hypertension includes persistent pulmonary hypertension of the newborn, idiopathic pulmonary arterial hypertension in children, and pulmonary hypertension related to congenital heart disease and cardiac surgery.

Some types of pulmonary hypertension are treated with vasodilator antihypertensive therapy and oxygen. Diur-

**2** Cardiovascular system

etics (section 2.2) may also have a role in children with right-sided heart failure.

Initial treatment of *persistent pulmonary hypertension of the newborn* involves the administration of **nitric oxide**; **epoprostenol** can be used until nitric oxide is available. Oral sildenafil may be helpful in less severe cases. Epoprostenol and sildenafil can cause profound systemic hypotension. In rare circumstances either **tolazoline** or **magnesium sulfate** can be given by intravenous infusion when nitric oxide and epoprostenol have failed.

Treatment of *idiopathic pulmonary arterial hypertension* is determined by acute vasodilator testing; drugs used for treatment include calcium-channel blockers (usually **nifedipine**, section 2.6.2), long-term intravenous **epoprostenol**, nebulised **iloprost**, **bosentan**, or **sildenafil**. Anticoagulation (usually with warfarin) may also be required to prevent secondary thrombosis.

**Inhaled nitric oxide** is a potent and selective pulmonary vasodilator. It acts on cyclic guanosine monophosphate (cGMP) resulting in smooth muscle relaxation. Inhaled nitric oxide is used in the treatment of persistent pulmonary hypertension of the newborn, and may also be useful in other forms of arterial pulmonary hypertension. Dependency can occur with high doses and prolonged use; to avoid rebound pulmonary hypertension the drug should be withdrawn gradually, often with the aid of sildenafil.

Excess nitric oxide can cause methaemoglobinaemia; therefore, methaemoglobin concentration should be measured regularly, particularly in neonates.

Nitric oxide increases the risk of haemorrhage by inhibiting platelet aggregation, but it does not usually cause bleeding.

**Epoprostenol** (prostacyclin) is a prostaglandin and a potent vasodilator. It is used in the treatment of persistent pulmonary hypertension of the newborn, idiopathic pulmonary arterial hypertension, and in the acute phase following cardiac surgery. It is given by continuous 24-hour intravenous infusion.

Epoprostenol is a powerful inhibitor of platelet aggregation and there is a possible risk of haemorrhage. It is sometimes used as an antiplatelet in renal dialysis when heparins are unsuitable or contra-indicated. It can also cause serious systemic hypotension and, if withdrawn suddenly, can cause pulmonary hypertensive crisis.

Children on prolonged treatment can become tolerant to epoprostenol, and therefore require an increase in dose.

**Iloprost** is a synthetic analogue of epoprostenol and is efficacious when nebulised in adults with pulmonary arterial hypertension, but experience in children is limited. It is more stable than epoprostenol and has a longer half-life.

**Bosentan** is a dual endothelin receptor antagonist used orally in the treatment of pulmonary arterial hypertension. The concentration of endothelin, a potent vasoconstrictor, is raised in sustained pulmonary hypertension.

**Sildenafil**, a vasodilator developed for the treatment of erectile dysfunction, is also used for pulmonary arterial hypertension. It is used either alone or as an adjunct to other drugs.

Sildenafil is a selective phosphodiesterase type-5 inhibitor. Inhibition of this enzyme in the lungs enhances the vasodilatory effects of nitric oxide and promotes relaxation of vascular smooth muscle.

Sildenafil has also been used in pulmonary hypertension for weaning children off inhaled nitric oxide following cardiac surgery, and less successfully in idiopathic pulmonary arterial hypertension.

The *Scottish Medicines Consortium* (p. 3) has advised (October 2012) that sildenafil (*Revatio ®*) is accepted for restricted use within NHS Scotland for the treatment of pulmonary arterial hypertension in children aged 1–17 years; sildenafil should only be prescribed on the advice of specialists in the Scottish Pulmonary Vascular Unit or the Scottish Adult Congenital Cardiac Service.

**Tolazoline** is now rarely used to correct pulmonary artery vasospasm in pulmonary hypertension of the newborn as better alternatives are available (see above). Tolazoline is an alpha-blocker and produces both pulmonary and systemic vasodilation.

## ▌ BOSENTAN

**Cautions** not to be initiated if systemic systolic blood pressure is below 85 mmHg; monitor liver function before and at monthly intervals during treatment, and 2 weeks after dose increase (reduce dose or suspend treatment if liver enzymes raised significantly)—discontinue if symptoms of liver impairment (see Contra-indications below); monitor haemoglobin before and during treatment (monthly for first 4 months, then 3-monthly thereafter), withdraw treatment gradually; **interactions:** Appendix 1 (bosentan)

**Contra-indications** acute porphyria (section 9.8.2)

**Hepatic impairment** avoid in moderate and severe impairment

**Pregnancy** avoid (teratogenic in *animal* studies); effective contraception required during administration (hormonal contraception not considered effective); monthly pregnancy tests advised

**Breast-feeding** manufacturer advises avoid—no information available

**Side-effects** diarrhoea, gastro-oesophageal reflux, flushing, hypotension, palpitation, oedema, syncope, headache, anaemia; *less commonly* thrombocytopenia, neutropenia, leucopenia; *rarely* liver cirrhosis, liver failure (see cautions above)

### Indications and dose

#### Pulmonary arterial hypertension

- **By mouth**

  **Child 2–18 years and body-weight 10–20 kg**
  initially 31.25 mg once daily increased after 4 weeks to 31.25 mg twice daily

  **Child 2–18 years and body-weight 20–40 kg**
  initially 31.25 mg twice daily increased after 4 weeks to 62.5 mg twice daily

  **Child 12–18 years and body-weight over 40 kg**
  initially 62.5 mg twice daily increased after 4 weeks to 125 mg twice daily; max. 250 mg twice daily

**Administration** tablets may be cut, or suspended in water or non-acidic liquid. Suspension is stable at room-temperature (max. 25˚C) for 24 hours

**Tracleer®** (Actelion) [PoM]
Tablets, f/c, orange, bosentan (as monohydrate)
62.5 mg, net price 56-tab pack = £1510.21; 125 mg,
56-tab pack = £1510.21

**Flolan®** (GSK) [PoM]
Infusion, powder for reconstitution, epoprostenol (as
sodium salt), net price 500-microgram vial (with
diluent) = £62.05; 1.5-mg vial (▼) (with diluent) =
£125.00

# ■ EPOPROSTENOL

**Cautions** anticoagulant monitoring required when
given with anticoagulants; haemorrhagic diathesis;
concomitant use of drugs that increase risk of bleeding; monitor blood pressure; avoid abrupt withdrawal
(risk of rebound pulmonary hypertension, see notes
above)

**Contra-indications** severe left ventricular dysfunction; pulmonary veno-occlusive disease

**Pregnancy** manufacturer advises caution—no information available

**Breast-feeding** manufacturer advises avoid—no
information available

**Side-effects** see notes above; also nausea, vomiting,
diarrhoea, abdominal pain, bleeding, bradycardia,
tachycardia, flushing, chest pain, anxiety, headache,
sepsis, jaw pain, arthralgia; *less commonly* dry mouth,
pulmonary oedema, sweating; *rarely* agitation, pallor

**Licensed use** not licensed for use in children

**Indications and dose**

> Persistent pulmonary hypertension of the new-
> born
>
> • By continuous intravenous infusion
>
> **Neonate** initially 2 nanograms/kg/minute
> adjusted according to response; usual max.
> 20 nanograms/kg/minute (rarely up to 40 nan-
> ograms/kg/minute)

> Idiopathic pulmonary arterial hypertension
>
> • By continuous intravenous infusion
>
> **Child 1 month–18 years** initially 2 nanograms/
> kg/minute increased as necessary up to 40 nan-
> ograms/kg/minute

**Administration** reconstitute using the glycine buffer
diluent provided to make a concentrate (pH 10.5);
filter the concentrate using the filter provided. The
concentrate can be administered via a central venous
catheter, alternatively it may be diluted further either
with the glycine buffer diluent *or* to a minimum
concentration of 1.43 micrograms/mL with Sodium
Chloride 0.9%. Solution stable for 12 hours at room
temperature, although some units use for 24 hours
and allow for loss of potency; solution stable for 24
hours if prepared in glycine buffer diluent only and
administered via an ambulatory cold pouch system
(to maintain solution at 2–8°C).

*Neonatal intensive care*, prepare a filtered concentrate
of 10 micrograms/mL using the 500-microgram vial.
*Neonate body-weight under 2 kg*, using the concentrate,
dilute 150 micrograms/kg body-weight to a final
volume of 50 mL with Sodium Chloride 0.9%; an
intravenous infusion rate of 0.1 mL/hour provides a
dose of 5 nanograms/kg/minute. *Neonate body-weight
over 2 kg*, using the concentrate, dilute 60 micr-
ograms/kg body-weight to a final volume of 50 mL
with Sodium Chloride 0.9%; an intravenous infusion
rate of 0.1 mL/hour provides a dose of 2 nanograms/
kg/minute

# ■ ILOPROST

**Cautions** unstable pulmonary hypertension with
advanced right heart failure; hypotension (do not
initiate if systolic blood pressure below 85 mmHg);
acute pulmonary infection; severe asthma; **interactions**: Appendix 1 (iloprost)

**Contra-indications** decompensated cardiac failure
(unless under medical supervision); severe coronary
heart disease; severe arrhythmias; congenital or
acquired valvular defects of the myocardium; pulmonary veno-occlusive disease; conditions which
increase risk of haemorrhage

**Hepatic impairment** dose may need to be halved in
liver cirrhosis—initially 2.5 micrograms at intervals of
at least 3 hours (max. 6 times daily), adjusted
according to response (consult product literature)

**Pregnancy** manufacturer advises avoid (toxicity in
*animal* studies); effective contraception must be used
during treatment

**Breast-feeding** manufacturer advises avoid—no
information available

**Side-effects** vasodilatation, hypotension, syncope,
cough, headache, throat or jaw pain; nausea, vomiting, diarrhoea, chest pain, dyspnoea, bronchospasm,
and wheezing also reported

**Licensed use** not licensed for use in children under 18
years

**Indications and dose**

> Idiopathic or familial pulmonary arterial hyper-
> tension
>
> • By inhalation of nebulised solution
>
> **Child 8–18 years** initial dose 2.5 micrograms
> increased to 5 micrograms for second dose, if tol-
> erated maintain at 5 micrograms 6–9 times daily
> according to response; reduce to 2.5 micrograms
> 6–9 times daily if higher dose not tolerated

> **Raynaud's syndrome** section 2.6.4.1

**Ventavis®** (Bayer) [PoM]
Nebuliser solution, iloprost (as trometamol) 10 micr-
ograms/mL, net price 30 × 1-mL (10 microgram)
unit-dose vials = £400.19, 168 × 1-mL = £2241.08.
For use with *Prodose®* [NHS] or *Venta-Neb®* [NHS] nebuliser

# ■ MAGNESIUM SULFATE

**Note** Magnesium Sulfate Injection BP is a sterile solution of
Magnesium Sulfate Heptahydrate

**Cautions** see section 9.5.1.3

**Hepatic impairment** see section 9.5.1.3

**Renal impairment** see section 9.5.1.3

**Side-effects** see section 9.5.1.3

**2**

**Cardiovascular system**

**2 Cardiovascular system**

### Indications and dose

**Persistent pulmonary hypertension of the newborn**

• By intravenous infusion

**Neonate** initially 200 mg/kg magnesium sulfate heptahydrate over 20–30 minutes; if response occurs, then by continuous intravenous infusion of 20–75 mg/kg/hour (to maintain plasma-magnesium concentration between 3.5–5.5 mmol/litre), given for up to 5 days

**Severe acute asthma** section 3.1

**Torsade de pointes** section 9.5.1.3

**Neonatal hypocalcaemia** section 9.5.1.3

**Hypomagnesaemia** section 9.5.1.3

**Administration** for *intravenous infusion*, dilute to a max. concentration of 100 mg/mL (10%) magnesium sulfate heptahydrate (200 mg/mL if fluid restricted) with Glucose 5% *or* Sodium Chloride 0.9%

**Magnesium Sulfate Injection, BP** (Non-proprietary) [PoM]

Injection, magnesium sulfate heptahydrate 50% ($Mg^{2+}$ approx. 2 mmol/mL), net price 2-mL (1-g) amp= £2.39, 5-mL (2.5-g) amp = £3.00, 10-mL (5-g) amp = 69p; prefilled 10-mL (5-g) syringe = £4.95

**Note** The BP directs that the label states the strength as the % w/v of magnesium sulfate heptahydrate and as the approximate concentration of magnesium ions ($Mg^{2+}$) in mmol/mL

## SILDENAFIL

**Cautions** hypotension (avoid if severe); intravascular volume depletion; left ventricular outflow obstruction; autonomic dysfunction; other cardiovascular disease; pulmonary veno-occlusive disease; predisposition to priapism; anatomical deformation of the penis; bleeding disorders or active peptic ulceration; ocular disorders; avoid abrupt withdrawal; initiate cautiously if child also on epoprostenol, iloprost, bosentan or nitric oxide; **interactions:** Appendix 1 (sildenafil)

**Contra-indications** recent history of stroke; history of non-arteritic anterior ischaemic optic neuropathy; hereditary degenerative retinal disorders; sickle-cell anaemia; avoid concomitant use of nitrates

**Hepatic impairment** reduce dose if not tolerated in mild to moderate impairment; manufacturer advises avoid in severe impairment

**Renal impairment** reduce dose if not tolerated

**Pregnancy** use only if potential benefit outweighs risk—no evidence of harm in *animal* studies

**Breast-feeding** manufacturer advises avoid—no information available

**Side-effects** diarrhoea, dyspepsia, gastritis, abdominal distension, gastro-oesophageal reflux, haemorrhoids, dry mouth, flushing, oedema, bronchitis, cough, headache, migraine, night sweats, paraesthesia, insomnia, anxiety, tremor, vertigo, fever, influenza-like symptoms, anaemia, back and limb pain, myalgia, visual disturbances, retinal haemorrhage, photophobia, painful red eyes, nasal congestion, epistaxis, alopecia; *less commonly* gynaecomastia, priapism, haematuria, penile haemorrhage; *also reported* rash, retinal vascular occlusion, non-arteritic anterior ischaemic optic

neuropathy (discontinue if sudden visual impairment occurs), and sudden hearing loss (advise patient to seek medical help)

**Licensed use** not licensed for use in children under 1 year

### Indications and dose

**Pulmonary arterial hypertension**

• By mouth

**Neonate** initially 250–500 micrograms/kg every 4–8 hours, adjusted according to response; max. 30 mg daily; start with lower dose and frequency especially if used with other vasodilators (see Cautions above)

**Child 1 month–1 year** initially 250–500 micrograms/kg every 4–8 hours, adjusted according to response; max. 30 mg daily; start with lower dose and frequency especially if used with other vasodilators (see Cautions above)

**Child 1–18 years**

**Body-weight under 20 kg** 10 mg three times daily

**Body-weight over 20 kg** 20 mg three times daily

**Revatio®** (Pfizer) [PoM]

Tablets, f/c, sildenafil (as citrate), 20 mg, net price 90-tab pack = £373.50

Oral suspension, sildenafil (as citrate) 10 mg/mL when reconstituted with water, net price 112-mL = £186.75

## TOLAZOLINE

**Cautions** mitral stenosis; cardiotoxic accumulation may occur with continuous infusion, particularly in renal impairment—monitor blood pressure regularly for sustained systemic hypotension; **interactions:** Appendix 1 (alpha-blockers)

**Contra-indications** peptic ulcer disease

**Renal impairment** accumulates in renal impairment; risk of cardiotoxicity; lower doses may be necessary

**Side-effects** nausea, vomiting, diarrhoea, epigastric pain; flushing, tachycardia, cardiac arrhythmias; headache, shivering, sweating; oliguria, metabolic alkalosis, haematuria, blood dyscrasias (including thrombocytopenia); blotchy skin; at high doses severe hypotension, marked hypertension, renal failure, and haemorrhage reported

**Licensed use** not licensed for use in children

### Indications and dose

**Correction of pulmonary vasospasm in neonates**

• By intravenous injection and continuous intravenous infusion (maintenance)

**Neonate** initially 1 mg/kg *by intravenous injection* over 2–5 minutes, followed if necessary *by continuous intravenous infusion* of 200 micrograms/kg/hour with careful blood pressure monitoring; doses above 300 micrograms/kg/hour associated with cardiotoxicity and renal failure

• By endotracheal administration

**Neonate** 200 micrograms/kg

**Administration** for *continuous intravenous infusion*, dilute with Glucose 5% *or* Sodium Chloride 0.9%. Prepare a fresh solution every 24 hours.
For *endotracheal administration*, dilute with 0.5–1 mL of Sodium Chloride 0.9%

**Tolazoline** (Non-proprietary)

Injection, tolazoline 25 mg/mL

Available from 'special-order' manufacturers or specialist importing companies, see p. 823

## 2.5.2 Centrally acting antihypertensive drugs

**Methyldopa**, a centrally acting antihypertensive, is of little value in the management of refractory sustained hypertension in infants and children. On prolonged use it is associated with fluid retention (which may be alleviated by concomitant use of diuretics).

Methyldopa is effective for the management of hypertension in pregnancy (see BNF section 2.5.2).

**Clonidine** is also a centrally acting antihypertensive but has the disadvantage that sudden withdrawal may cause a hypertensive crisis. Clonidine is also used under specialist supervision for pain management, sedation, and opioid withdrawal, attention deficit hyperactivity disorder, and Tourette syndrome.

### ■ CLONIDINE HYDROCHLORIDE

**Cautions** must be withdrawn gradually to avoid hypertensive crisis; mild to moderate bradyarrhythmia; constipation; polyneuropathy; Raynaud's syndrome or other occlusive peripheral vascular disease; history of depression; **interactions:** Appendix 1 (clonidine)

Skilled tasks Drowsiness may affect performance of skilled tasks (e.g. driving); effects of alcohol may be enhanced

**Contra-indications** severe bradyarrhythmia secondary to second- or third-degree AV block or sick sinus syndrome

**Renal impairment** use with caution

**Pregnancy** may lower fetal heart rate, but risk should be balanced against risk of uncontrolled maternal hypertension; avoid intravenous injection

**Breast-feeding** avoid—present in milk

**Side-effects** constipation, nausea, dry mouth, vomiting, salivary gland pain, postural hypotension, dizziness, sleep disturbances, headache, malaise, drowsiness, depression, sexual dysfunction; *less commonly* bradycardia, Raynaud's syndrome, delusion, hallucination, paraesthesia, pruritus, rash, urticaria; *rarely* colonic pseudo-obstruction, AV block, gynaecomastia, decreased lacrimation, nasal dryness, alopecia; *also reported* hepatitis, fluid retention, bradyarrhythmia, confusion, impaired visual accommodation

**Licensed use** not licensed for use in children

**Indications and dose**

Severe hypertension

• By mouth

**Child 2–18 years** initially 0.5–1 microgram/kg 3 times daily, increased gradually if necessary; max. 25 micrograms/kg daily in divided doses (not exceeding 1.2 mg daily)

• By slow intravenous injection

**Child 2–18 years** 2–6 micrograms/kg (max. 300 micrograms) as a single dose

**Administration** for *intravenous injection*, give over 10–15 minutes; compatible with Sodium Chloride 0.9% *or* Glucose 5%.

For administration *by mouth*, tablets may be crushed and dissolved in water

---

**Catapres**® (Boehringer Ingelheim) PoM

Tablets, scored, clonidine hydrochloride 100 micrograms, net price 100-tab pack = £5.32. Label: 3, 8

Injection, clonidine hydrochloride 150 micrograms/mL, net price 1-mL amp = 28p

## 2.5.3 Adrenergic neurone blocking drugs

Adrenergic neurone blocking drugs prevent the release of noradrenaline from postganglionic adrenergic neurones. These drugs do not control supine blood pressure and may cause postural hypotension. For this reason they have largely fallen from use in adults and are rarely used in children.

## 2.5.4 Alpha-adrenoceptor blocking drugs

**Doxazosin** and **prazosin** have post-synaptic alpha-blocking and vasodilator properties and rarely cause tachycardia. They can, however, reduce blood pressure rapidly after the first dose and should be introduced with caution.

Alpha-blockers can be used with other antihypertensive drugs in the treatment of resistant hypertension.

### ■ DOXAZOSIN

**Cautions** care with initial dose (postural hypotension); pulmonary oedema due to aortic or mitral stenosis; cataract surgery (risk of intra-operative floppy iris syndrome); heart failure; **interactions:** Appendix 1 (alpha-blockers)

Driving May affect performance of skilled tasks e.g. driving

**Contra-indications** history of postural hypotension

**Hepatic impairment** use with caution; manufacturer advises avoid in severe impairment—no information available

**Pregnancy** no evidence of teratogenicity; manufacturers advise use only when potential benefit outweighs risk

**Breast-feeding** accumulates in milk in *animal* studies—manufacturer advises avoid

**Side-effects** gastro-intestinal disturbances; oedema, hypotension, postural hypotension, palpitation, tachycardia; dyspnoea, rhinitis, coughing; asthenia, fatigue, vertigo, dizziness, headache, paraesthesia, sleep disturbance, anxiety, depression; influenza-like symptoms; back pain, myalgia; *less commonly* weight changes; angina, myocardial infarction; hypoaesthesia, syncope, tremor, agitation, micturition disturbances, impotence, epistaxis, arthralgia, gout, tinnitus, hypersensitivity reactions (including pruritus, purpura, rash); *very rarely* cholestasis, hepatitis, jaundice, bradycardia, arrhythmias, bronchospasm, hot flushes, gynaecomastia, priapism, abnormal ejaculation, leucopenia, thrombocytopenia, blurred vision, and alopecia

**Licensed use** not licensed for use in children

**Indications and dose**

**Hypertension** (see notes above)

● **By mouth**

**Child 6–12 years** 500 micrograms once daily, increased at 1-week intervals to 2–4 mg daily

**Child 12–18 years** 1 mg daily, increased after 1–2 weeks to 2 mg once daily, and thereafter to 4 mg once daily if necessary; usual max. 4 mg daily (rarely up to 16 mg daily may be required)

**Dysfunctional voiding** section 7.4.1

**Doxazosin** (Non-proprietary) PoM
Tablets, doxazosin (as mesilate) 1 mg, net price 28-tab pack = 93p; 2 mg, 28-tab pack = 99p; 4 mg, 28-tab pack = £1.39. Counselling, initial dose, driving
Brands include *Doxadura*®

**Cardura**® (Pfizer) PoM
Tablets, doxazosin (as mesilate) 1 mg, net price 28-tab pack = £10.56; 2 mg, 28-tab pack = £14.08. Counselling, initial dose, driving

◢**Modified-release**
Note Children stabilised on immediate-release doxazosin can be transferred to the equivalent dose of modified-release doxazosin

**Doxazosin** (Non-proprietary) PoM
Tablets, m/r, doxazosin (as mesilate) 4 mg, net price 28-tab pack = £6.33. Label: 25, counselling, initial dose, driving
Brands include *Doxadura*® *XL, Doxzogen*® *XL, Raporsin*® *XL, Slocinx*® *XL*

**Cardura**® **XL** (Pfizer) PoM
Tablets, m/r, doxazosin (as mesilate) 4 mg, net price 28-tab pack = £5.70; 8 mg, 28-tab pack = £9.98. Label: 25, counselling, initial dose, driving

# ▮ PRAZOSIN

**Cautions** first dose may cause collapse due to hypotension (therefore should be taken on retiring to bed); cataract surgery (risk of intra-operative floppy iris syndrome); **interactions:** Appendix 1 (alpha-blockers)
Driving May affect performance of skilled tasks e.g. driving

**Contra-indications** not recommended for congestive heart failure due to mechanical obstruction (e.g. aortic stenosis)

**Hepatic impairment** start with low doses and adjust according to response

**Renal impairment** start with low doses in moderate to severe impairment; increase with caution

**Pregnancy** no evidence of teratogenicity; manufacturer advises use only when potential benefit outweighs risk

**Breast-feeding** present in milk; manufacturer advises use with caution

**Side-effects** gastro-intestinal disturbances; postural hypotension, oedema, palpitation; dyspnoea, nasal congestion; drowsiness, headache, depression, nervousness, vertigo; urinary frequency; weakness; blurred vision; *less commonly* tachycardia, insomnia, paraesthesia, sweating, impotence, arthralgia, eye disorders, tinnitus, epistaxis, allergic reactions including rash, pruritus, and urticaria; *rarely* pancreatitis, flushing, vasculitis, bradycardia, hallucinations, worsening of narcolepsy, gynaecomastia, priapism, urinary incontinence, and alopecia

**Licensed use** not licensed for use in children under 12 years

**Indications and dose**

**Hypertension** (see notes above)

● **By mouth**

**Child 1 month–12 years** 10–15 micrograms/kg 2–4 times daily (initial dose at bedtime) increased gradually to max. 500 micrograms/kg daily in divided doses (not exceeding 20 mg daily)

**Child 12–18 years** 500 micrograms 2–3 times daily (initial dose at bedtime), increased after 3–7 days to 1 mg 2–3 times daily for a further 3–7 days; further increased gradually if necessary to max. 20 mg daily in divided doses

**Congestive heart failure** (but rarely used, see section 2.2)

● **By mouth**

**Child 1 month–12 years** 5 micrograms/kg twice daily (initial dose at bedtime), increased gradually to max. 100 micrograms/kg daily in divided doses

**Child 12–18 years** 500 micrograms 2–4 times daily (initial dose at bedtime), increasing to 4 mg daily in divided doses; maintenance 4–20 mg daily in divided doses

**Administration** for administration *by mouth*, tablets may be dispersed in water

**Prazosin** (Non-proprietary) PoM
Tablets, prazosin (as hydrochloride) 500 micrograms, net price 56-tab pack = £2.51; 1 mg, 56-tab pack = £3.23; 2 mg, 56-tab pack = £4.39; 5 mg, 56-tab pack = £8.75. Counselling, initial dose, driving

**Hypovase**® (Pfizer) PoM
Tablets, prazosin (as hydrochloride) 500 micrograms, net price 60-tab pack = £2.69; 1 mg, scored, 60-tab pack = £3.46. Counselling, initial dose, driving

## Phaeochromocytoma

Long-term management of phaeochromocytoma involves surgery. However, surgery should not take place until there is adequate blockade of both alpha- and beta-adrenoceptors. Alpha-blockers are used in the short-term management of hypertensive episodes in phaeochromocytoma. Once alpha blockade is established, tachycardia can be controlled by the cautious addition of a beta-blocker (section 2.4); a cardioselective beta-blocker is preferred. There is no nationwide consensus on the optimal drug regimen or doses used for the management of phaeochromocytoma.

**Phenoxybenzamine**, a powerful alpha-blocker, is effective in the management of phaeochromocytoma but it has many side-effects.

# ▮ PHENOXYBENZAMINE HYDROCHLORIDE

**Cautions** congestive heart failure; severe ischaemic heart disease (see also Contra-indications); cerebrovascular disease (avoid if history of cerebrovascular accident); monitor blood pressure regularly during infusion; carcinogenic in *animals*; avoid in acute porphyria (section 9.8.2); avoid extravasation (irritant to tissues); avoid contact with skin (risk of contact sensitisation)

2 Cardiovascular system

**Contra-indications**  history of cerebrovascular accident; avoid infusion in hypovolaemia

**Renal impairment**  use with caution

**Pregnancy**  hypotension in newborn may occur

**Breast-feeding**  may be present in milk

**Side-effects**  postural hypotension with dizziness and marked compensatory tachycardia, lassitude, nasal congestion, miosis, inhibition of ejaculation; *rarely* gastro-intestinal disturbances; decreased sweating and dry mouth after intravenous infusion; idiosyncratic profound hypotension within few minutes of starting infusion; convulsions following rapid intravenous infusion also reported

**Licensed use**  not licensed for use in children

### Indications and dose

**Hypertension in phaeochromocytoma**

- By mouth

  **Child 1 month–18 years** 0.5–1 mg/kg twice daily adjusted according to response

- By intravenous infusion

  **Child 1 month–18 years** 0.5–1 mg/kg daily adjusted according to response; occasionally up to 2 mg/kg daily may be required; do not repeat dose within 24 hours

**Administration**  for administration *by mouth*, capsules may be opened.

For *intravenous infusion*, dilute with Sodium Chloride 0.9% and give over at least 2 hours; max. 4 hours between dilution and completion of infusion

**Phenoxybenzamine** (Non-proprietary) PoM
Injection concentrate, phenoxybenzamine hydrochloride 50 mg/mL, to be diluted before use. Net price 2-mL amp = £57.14 (hosp. only)

**Dibenyline®** (Mercury) PoM
Capsules, red/white, phenoxybenzamine hydrochloride 10 mg, net price 30-cap pack = £10.84

## 2.5.5  Drugs affecting the renin-angiotensin system

**2.5.5.1  Angiotensin-converting enzyme inhibitors**

**2.5.5.2  Angiotensin-II receptor antagonists**

### 2.5.5.1  Angiotensin-converting enzyme inhibitors

ACE Angiotensin-converting enzyme inhibitors (ACE inhibitors) inhibit the conversion of angiotensin I to angiotensin II. The main indications of ACE inhibitors in children are shown below. In infants and young children, captopril is often considered first.

**Initiation under specialist supervision**  Treatment with ACE inhibitors should be initiated under specialist supervision and with careful clinical monitoring in children.

**Heart failure**  ACE inhibitors have a valuable role in all grades of heart failure, usually combined with a loop diuretic (section 2.2). Potassium supplements and potassium-sparing diuretics should be discontinued before introducing an ACE inhibitor because of the risk of hyperkalaemia. In adults, a low dose of spironolactone may be beneficial in severe heart failure and can

be used with an ACE inhibitor provided serum potassium is monitored carefully. Profound first-dose hypotension can occur when ACE inhibitors are introduced to children with heart failure who are already taking a high dose of a loop diuretic (see Cautions below). Temporary withdrawal of the loop diuretic reduces the risk, but can cause severe rebound pulmonary oedema.

**Hypertension**  ACE inhibitors may be considered for hypertension when thiazides and beta-blockers are contra-indicated, not tolerated, or fail to control blood pressure; they may be considered for hypertension in children with type 1 diabetes with nephropathy (see also section 6.1.5). ACE inhibitors can reduce blood pressure very rapidly in some patients particularly in those receiving diuretic therapy (see Cautions, below); the first dose should preferably be given at bedtime.

**Diabetic nephropathy**  For comment on the role of ACE inhibitors in the management of diabetic nephropathy, see section 6.1.5.

**Renal effects**  Renal function and electrolytes should be checked before starting ACE inhibitors (or increasing the dose) and monitored during treatment (more frequently if features mentioned below are present). Hyperkalaemia and other side-effects of ACE inhibitors are more common in children with impaired renal function and the dose may need to be reduced (see Renal Impairment, below).

Concomitant treatment with NSAIDs increases the risk of renal damage, and potassium-sparing diuretics (or potassium-containing salt substitutes) increase the risk of hyperkalaemia.

In children with severe bilateral renal artery stenosis (or severe stenosis of the artery supplying a single functioning kidney), ACE inhibitors reduce or abolish glomerular filtration and are likely to cause severe and progressive renal failure. They are therefore contra-indicated in children known to have these forms of critical renovascular disease.

ACE inhibitor treatment is unlikely to have an adverse effect on overall renal function in children with severe unilateral renal artery stenosis and a normal contralateral kidney, but glomerular filtration is likely to be reduced (or even abolished) in the affected kidney and the long-term consequences are unknown.

ACE inhibitors are therefore best avoided in those with known or suspected renovascular disease, unless the blood pressure cannot be controlled by other drugs. If they are used in these circumstances renal function needs to be monitored.

ACE inhibitors should also be used with particular caution in children who may have undiagnosed and clinically silent renovascular disease. ACE inhibitors are useful for the management of hypertension and proteinuria in children with nephritis. They are thought to have a beneficial effect by reducing intra-glomerular hypertension and protecting the glomerular capillaries and membrane.

**Cautions**  ACE inhibitors need to be initiated with care in children receiving diuretics (**important:** see Concomitant Diuretics, below); first doses can cause hypotension especially in children taking high doses of diuretics, on a low-sodium diet, on dialysis, dehydrated, or with heart failure (see above). Discontinue if marked elevation of hepatic enzymes or jaundice (risk of hepatic necrosis). Renal function should be monitored before

*2 Cardiovascular system*

and during treatment. For use in pre-existing renovascular disease, see Renal Effects above. The risk of agranulocytosis is possibly increased in collagen vascular disease (blood counts recommended). ACE inhibitors should be used with care in children with severe or symptomatic aortic stenosis (risk of hypotension) and in hypertrophic cardiomyopathy. They should be used with care (or avoided) in those with a history of idiopathic or hereditary angioedema. Children with primary aldosteronism and Afro-Caribbean children may respond less well to ACE inhibitors. **Interactions:** Appendix 1 (ACE inhibitors).

**Anaphylactoid reactions** To prevent anaphylactoid reactions, ACE inhibitors should be avoided during dialysis with high-flux polyacrylonitrile membranes and during low-density lipoprotein apheresis with dextran sulfate; they should also be withheld before desensitisation with wasp or bee venom.

**Concomitant diuretics** ACE inhibitors can cause a very rapid fall in blood pressure in volume-depleted children; treatment should therefore be initiated with very low doses. In some children the diuretic dose may need to be reduced or the diuretic discontinued at least 24 hours beforehand (may not be possible in heart failure—risk of pulmonary oedema). If high-dose diuretic therapy cannot be stopped, close observation is recommended after administration of the first dose of ACE inhibitor, for at least 2 hours or until the blood pressure has stabilised.

**Contra-indications** ACE inhibitors are contra-indicated in children with hypersensitivity to ACE inhibitors (including angioedema) and in bilateral renovascular disease (see also above).

**Renal impairment** See Renal Effects above; start with low dose and adjust according to response.

**Pregnancy** ACE inhibitors should be avoided in pregnancy unless essential—they may adversely affect fetal and neonatal blood pressure control and renal function; skull defects and oligohydramnios have also been reported.

**Side-effects** ACE inhibitors can cause profound hypotension (see Cautions), renal impairment (see Renal Effects above), and a persistent dry cough. They can also cause angioedema (onset may be delayed; higher incidence reported in Afro-Caribbean patients), rash (which may be associated with pruritus and urticaria), pancreatitis, and upper respiratory-tract symptoms such as sinusitis, rhinitis, and sore throat. Gastrointestinal effects reported with ACE inhibitors include nausea, vomiting, dyspepsia, diarrhoea, constipation, and abdominal pain. Altered liver function tests, cholestatic jaundice, hepatitis, fulminant hepatic necrosis, and hepatic failure have been reported—discontinue if marked elevation of hepatic enzymes or jaundice. Hyperkalaemia, hypoglycaemia and blood disorders including thrombocytopenia, leucopenia, neutropenia, and haemolytic anaemia have also been reported. Other reported side-effects include headache, dizziness, fatigue, malaise, taste disturbance, paraesthesia, bronchospasm, fever, serositis, vasculitis, myalgia, arthralgia, positive antinuclear antibody, raised erythrocyte sedimentation rate, eosinophilia, leucocytosis, and photosensitivity.

**Neonates** The neonatal response to treatment with ACE inhibitors is very variable, and some neonates develop profound hypotension with even small doses; a test-dose should be used initially and increased cautiously. Adverse effects such as apnoea, seizures, renal failure, and severe unpredictable hypotension are very common in the first month of life and it is therefore recommended that ACE inhibitors are avoided whenever possible, particularly in preterm neonates.

---

## ▌ CAPTOPRIL

**Cautions** see notes above; acute porphyria (section 9.8.2)

**Contra-indications** see notes above

**Renal impairment** see notes above

**Pregnancy** see notes above

**Breast-feeding** avoid in first few weeks after delivery, particularly in preterm infants—risk of profound neonatal hypotension; can be used in older infant if essential but monitor infant's blood pressure

**Side-effects** see notes above; tachycardia, serum sickness, weight loss, stomatitis, maculopapular rash, photosensitivity, flushing and acidosis

**Licensed use** not licensed for use in children under 18 years

**Indications and dose**

**Hypertension, heart failure, proteinuria in nephritis** (under specialist supervision)

- **By mouth**

  **Neonate** (caution, see neonatal information above) test dose, 10–50 micrograms/kg (10 micrograms/kg in neonate less than 37 weeks postmenstrual age), monitor blood pressure carefully for 1–2 hours; if tolerated give 10–50 micrograms/kg 2–3 times daily increased as necessary to max. 2 mg/kg daily in divided doses (max. 300 micrograms/kg daily in divided doses in neonate less than 37 weeks postmenstrual age)

  **Child 1 month–12 years** test dose, 100 micrograms/kg (max. 6.25 mg), monitor blood pressure carefully for 1–2 hours; if tolerated give 100–300 micrograms/kg 2–3 times a day, increased as necessary to max. 6 mg/kg daily in divided doses (max. 4 mg/kg daily in divided doses for child 1 month–1 year)

  **Child 12–18 years** test dose, 100 micrograms/kg or 6.25 mg, monitor blood pressure carefully for 1–2 hours; if tolerated give 12.5–25 mg 2–3 times a day, increased as necessary to max. 150 mg daily in divided doses

**Diabetic nephropathy** (under specialist supervision)

- **By mouth**

  **Child 12–18 years** test dose, 100 micrograms/kg or 6.25 mg, monitor blood pressure carefully for 1–2 hours; if tolerated, give 12.5–25 mg 2–3 times a day, increased as necessary to max. 150 mg daily in divided doses

**Administration** Administer under close supervision, see notes above. Give test dose whilst child supine. Tablets can be dispersed in water

**Captopril** (Non-proprietary) ℗oM

Tablets, captopril 12.5 mg, net price 56-tab pack = £1.51; 25 mg, 56-tab pack = £1.56; 50 mg, 56-tab pack = £1.96

Brands include *Ecopace*®, *Kaplon*®

Liquid, various strengths available from 'special-order' manufacturers or specialist importing companies, see p. 823

**Capoten®** (Squibb) [PoM]
Tablets, captopril 25 mg, net price 28-tab pack = £5.26; 50 mg (scored), 28-tab pack = £8.98

# ■ ENALAPRIL MALEATE

**Cautions** see notes above
**Contra-indications** see notes above
**Hepatic impairment** monitor closely
**Renal impairment** see notes above
**Pregnancy** see notes above
**Breast-feeding** avoid in first few weeks after delivery, particularly in preterm infants—risk of profound neonatal hypotension; can be used in older infant if essential but monitor infant's blood pressure
**Side-effects** see notes above; also dyspnoea; depression, asthenia; blurred vision; *less commonly* dry mouth, peptic ulcer, anorexia, ileus; arrhythmias, palpitation, flushing; confusion, nervousness, drowsiness, insomnia, vertigo; impotence; muscle cramps; tinnitus; alopecia, sweating; hyponatraemia; *rarely* stomatitis, glossitis, Raynaud's syndrome, pulmonary infiltrates, allergic alveolitis, abnormal dreams, gynaecomastia, Stevens-Johnson syndrome, toxic epidermal necrolysis, exfoliative dermatitis, pemphigus; *very rarely* gastro-intestinal angioedema
**Licensed use** not licensed for use in children for congestive heart failure, proteinuria in nephritis or diabetic nephropathy; not licensed for use in children less than 20 kg for hypertension

**Indications and dose**

**Hypertension, congestive heart failure, proteinuria in nephritis** (under specialist supervision)
• **By mouth**
    **Neonate** (limited information) initially 10 micrograms/kg once daily, monitor blood pressure carefully for 1–2 hours, increased as necessary up to 500 micrograms/kg daily in 1–3 divided doses
    **Child 1 month–12 years** initially 100 micrograms/kg once daily, monitor blood pressure carefully for 1–2 hours, increased as necessary up to max. 1 mg/kg daily in 1–2 divided doses
    **Child 12–18 years** initially 2.5 mg once daily, monitor blood pressure carefully for 1–2 hours, usual maintenance dose 10–20 mg daily in 1–2 divided doses; max. 40 mg daily in 1–2 divided doses if body-weight over 50 kg

**Diabetic nephropathy** (under specialist supervision)
• **By mouth**
    **Child 12–18 years** initially 2.5 mg once daily, monitor blood pressure carefully for 1–2 hours, usual maintenance dose 10–20 mg daily in 1–2 divided doses; max. 40 mg daily in 1–2 divided doses if body-weight over 50 kg

**Administration** tablets may be crushed and suspended in water immediately before use

**Enalapril Maleate** (Non-proprietary) [PoM]
Tablets, enalapril maleate 2.5 mg, net price 28-tab pack = £1.05; 5 mg, 28-tab pack = 96p; 10 mg, 28-tab pack = £1.05; 20 mg, 28-tab pack = £1.24
**Brands include** *Ednyt®*

Liquid, various strengths available from 'special-order' manufacturers or specialist importing companies, see p. 823

**Innovace®** (MSD) [PoM]
Tablets, enalapril maleate 2.5 mg, net price 28-tab pack = £5.35; 5 mg (scored), 28-tab pack = £7.51; 10 mg (red), 28-tab pack = £10.53; 20 mg (peach), 28-tab pack = £12.51

# ■ LISINOPRIL

**Cautions** see notes above
**Contra-indications** see notes above
**Renal impairment** see notes above
**Pregnancy** see notes above
**Breast-feeding** avoid—no information available
**Side-effects** see notes above; also *less commonly* tachycardia, palpitation, cerebrovascular accident, Raynaud's syndrome, confusion, mood changes, vertigo, sleep disturbances, asthenia, impotence; *rarely* dry mouth, gynaecomastia, alopecia, psoriasis; *very rarely* allergic alveolitis, pulmonary infiltrates, profuse sweating, pemphigus, Stevens-Johnson syndrome, and toxic epidermal necrolysis
**Licensed use** not licensed for use in children

**Indications and dose**

**Hypertension, proteinuria in nephritis** (under specialist supervision)
• **By mouth**
    **Child 6–12 years** initially 70 micrograms/kg (max. 5 mg) once daily, increased in intervals of 1–2 weeks to max. 600 micrograms/kg (*or* 40 mg) once daily
    **Child 12–18 years** initially 5 mg once daily; usual maintenance dose 10–20 mg once daily; max. 80 mg once daily

**Diabetic nephropathy** (under specialist supervision)
• **By mouth**
    **Child 12–18 years** initially 5 mg once daily; usual maintenance dose 10–20 mg once daily; max. 80 mg once daily

**Heart failure (adjunct)** (under specialist supervision)
• **By mouth**
    **Child 12–18 years** initially 2.5 mg once daily; increased in steps no greater than 10 mg at intervals of at least 2 weeks up to max. 35 mg once daily if tolerated

**Lisinopril** (Non-proprietary) [PoM]
Tablets, lisinopril (as dihydrate) 2.5 mg, net price 28-tab pack = 87p; 5 mg, 28-tab pack = 93p; 10 mg, 28-tab pack = £1.01; 20 mg, 28-tab pack = £1.19

Liquid, various strengths available from 'special-order' manufacturers or specialist importing companies, see p. 823

**Zestril®** (AstraZeneca) [PoM]
Tablets, lisinopril (as dihydrate) 5 mg (pink), net price 28-tab pack = £1.31; 10 mg (pink), 28-tab pack = £2.05; 20 mg (pink), 28-tab pack = £2.17

**2.5.5.2 Angiotensin-II receptor antagonists**

**Losartan** and valsartan are specific angiotensin-II receptor antagonists with many properties similar to those of the ACE inhibitors. However, unlike ACE inhi-

**2 Cardiovascular system**

bitors, they do not inhibit the breakdown of bradykinin and other kinins, and thus are less likely to cause the persistent dry cough which can complicate ACE inhibitor therapy. They are therefore a useful alternative for children who have to discontinue an ACE inhibitor because of persistent cough.

Losartan or valsartan can be used as an alternative to an ACE inhibitor in the management of hypertension.

**Cautions**  Angiotensin-II receptor antagonists should be used with caution in renal artery stenosis (see also Renal Effects under ACE Inhibitors, section 2.5.5.1). Monitoring of plasma-potassium concentration is advised, particularly in children with renal impairment. Angiotensin-II receptor antagonists should be used with caution in aortic or mitral valve stenosis and in hypertrophic cardiomyopathy. They should be used with caution in those with a history of angioedema. Children with primary aldosteronism, and Afro-Caribbean children (particularly those with left ventricular hypertrophy), may not benefit from an angiotensin-II receptor antagonist. **Interactions**: Appendix 1 (angiotensin-II receptor antagonists).

**Pregnancy**  Angiotensin-II receptor antagonists should be avoided in pregnancy, unless essential. They may adversely affect fetal and neonatal blood pressure and renal function; oligohydramnios and neonatal skull defects have also been reported.

**Breast-feeding**  Information on the use of angiotensin-II receptor antagonists in breast-feeding patients is limited, so they are not recommended in these patients. Alternative treatment options, with more established safety information during breast-feeding, are available.

**Side-effects**  Side-effects of angiotensin-II receptor antagonists include symptomatic hypotension (including dizziness), particularly in children with hyponatraemia or intravascular volume depletion (e.g. those taking high-dose diuretics). Hyperkalaemia occurs occasionally; angioedema has also been reported (sometimes with delayed onset).

## ■ LOSARTAN POTASSIUM

**Cautions**  see notes above; also severe heart failure
**Hepatic impairment**  avoid—no information available
**Renal impairment**  see notes above; also avoid if estimated glomerular filtration rate less than 30 mL/minute/1.73m$^2$—no information available
**Pregnancy**  see notes above
**Breast-feeding**  see notes above
**Side-effects**  see notes above; also malaise, anaemia; *less commonly* abdominal pain, constipation, diarrhoea, nausea, vomiting, angina, palpitation, oedema, dyspnoea, cough, headache, sleep disorders, drowsiness, urticaria, pruritus, rash; *rarely* hepatitis, atrial fibrillation, cerebrovascular accident, and paraesthesia; *also reported* pancreatitis, depression, erectile dysfunction, thrombocytopenia, hyponatraemia, arthralgia, myalgia, rhabdomyolysis, tinnitus, photosensitivity, and vasculitis (including Henoch-Schönlein purpura)

**Indications and dose**
**Hypertension** (under specialist supervision)
- By mouth
  **Child 6–18 years**
  **Body-weight 20–50 kg** initially 700 micrograms/kg (max. 25 mg) once daily (lower dose in intravascular volume depletion), adjusted according to response; max. 50 mg once daily
  **Body-weight 50 kg and over** initially 50 mg daily (initially 25 mg once daily in intravascular volume depletion), adjusted according to response; max. 1.4 mg/kg (max. 100 mg) once daily

**Losartan Potassium** (Non-proprietary) ▣PoM▣
Tablets, losartan potassium 12.5 mg, net price 28-tab pack = £7.70; 25 mg, 28-tab pack = £2.64; 50 mg, 28-tab pack = £2.38; 100 mg, 28-tab pack = £2.84

**Cozaar**® (MSD) ▣PoM▣
Tablets, f/c, losartan potassium 12.5 mg (blue), net price 28-tab pack = £8.09; 25 mg (white), 28-tab pack = £16.18; 50 mg (white, scored), 28-tab pack = £12.80; 100 mg (white), 28-tab pack = £16.18
Oral suspension, losartan potassium 12.5 mg/5 mL when reconstituted with solvent provided, net price 200 mL (berry-citrus flavour) = £53.68

## ■ VALSARTAN

**Cautions**  see notes above
**Contra-indications**  biliary cirrhosis, cholestasis
**Hepatic impairment**  max. 80 mg daily in mild to moderate impairment; avoid in severe impairment
**Renal impairment**  see notes above; also avoid if estimated glomerular filtration rate less than 30 mL/minute/1.73m$^2$—no information available
**Pregnancy**  see notes above
**Breast-feeding**  see notes above
**Side-effects**  see notes above; also *less commonly* abdominal pain, nausea, diarrhoea, cough, malaise, headache; *also reported* anaemia, renal failure, neutropenia, thrombocytopenia, myalgia, vasculitis, serum sickness, rash, pruritus
**Licensed use**  capsules not licensed for use in children
**Indications and dose**
**Hypertension** (under specialist supervision)
- By mouth
  **Child 6–18 years**
  **Body-weight 18–35 kg** initially 40 mg once daily, adjusted according to response; max. 80 mg daily
  **Body-weight 35–80 kg** initially 80 mg once daily, adjusted according to response; max. 160 mg daily
  **Body-weight 80 kg and over** initially 80 mg once daily, adjusted according to response; max. 320 mg daily

**Valsartan** (Non-proprietary) ▼ ▣PoM▣
Tablets, valsartan 40 mg, net price 7-tab pack = £2.55; 80 mg, 28-tab pack = £13.97; 160 mg, 28-tab pack = £18.41; 320 mg, 28-tab pack = £20.23

**Diovan®** (Novartis) ▼ PoM
Capsules, valsartan 40 mg (grey), net price 28-cap pack = £13.97; 80 mg (grey/pink), 28-cap pack = £13.97; 160 mg (grey/pink), 28-cap pack = £18.41
Tablets, f/c, scored, valsartan 40 mg (yellow), net price 7-tab pack = £3.49; 320 mg (dark grey-violet), 28-tab pack = £20.23

## 2.6 Nitrates, calcium-channel blockers, and other antianginal drugs

2.6.1 **Nitrates**

2.6.2 **Calcium-channel blockers**

2.6.3 **Other antianginal drugs**

2.6.4 **Peripheral vasodilators and related drugs**

Nitrates and calcium-channel blockers have a vasodilating and, consequently, blood-pressure lowering effect. Vasodilators can act in heart failure by arteriolar dilation, which reduces both peripheral vascular resistance and left ventricular pressure during systole resulting in improved cardiac output. They can also cause venous dilatation, which results in dilatation of capacitance vessels, increase of venous pooling, and diminution of venous return to the heart (decreasing left ventricular end-diastolic pressure).

## 2.6.1 Nitrates

Nitrates are potent coronary vasodilators, but their principal benefit follows from a reduction in venous return which reduces left ventricular work. Unwanted effects such as flushing, headache, and postural hypotension may limit therapy, especially if the child is unusually sensitive to the effects of nitrates or is hypovolaemic.

For the use of glyceryl trinitrate in extravasation, see section 10.3.

Children receiving nitrates continuously throughout the day can develop tolerance (with reduced therapeutic effects). Reduction of blood-nitrate concentrations to low levels for 4 to 8 hours each day usually maintains effectiveness in such patients.

### GLYCERYL TRINITRATE

**Cautions** hypothyroidism; malnutrition; hypothermia; recent history of myocardial infarction; heart failure due to obstruction; hypoxaemia or other ventilation and perfusion abnormalities; susceptibility to angle-closure glaucoma; metal-containing transdermal systems should be removed before magnetic resonance imaging procedures, cardioversion, or diathermy; avoid abrupt withdrawal; monitor blood pressure and heart rate during infusion; tolerance (see notes above); **interactions:** Appendix 1 (nitrates)

**Contra-indications** hypersensitivity to nitrates; hypotensive conditions and hypovolaemia; hypertrophic cardiomyopathy; aortic stenosis; cardiac tamponade; constrictive pericarditis; mitral stenosis; toxic pulmonary oedema; raised intracranial pressure due to cerebral haemorrhage or head trauma; marked anaemia

**Hepatic impairment**   caution in severe impairment
**Renal impairment**   manufacturers advise use with caution in severe impairment
**Pregnancy**   not known to be harmful
**Breast-feeding**   no information available—manufacturers advise use only if potential benefit outweighs risk

**Side-effects**   postural hypotension, tachycardia (but paradoxical bradycardia also reported); throbbing headache, dizziness; *less commonly* nausea, vomiting, heartburn, flushing, syncope, temporary hypoxaemia, rash, application-site reactions with transdermal patches; *very rarely* angle-closure glaucoma
**Injection** Specific side-effects following injection (particularly if given too rapidly) include severe hypotension, diaphoresis, apprehension, restlessness, muscle twitching, retrosternal discomfort, palpitation, abdominal pain; prolonged administration has been associated with methaemoglobinaemia

**Licensed use**   not licensed for use in children
**Indications and dose**

> **Hypertension during and after cardiac surgery, heart failure after cardiac surgery, coronary vasoconstriction in myocardial ischaemia, vasoconstriction in shock**
>
> • **By continuous intravenous infusion**
>
>   **Neonate** 0.2–0.5 micrograms/kg/minute, dose adjusted according to response; usual dose 1–3 micrograms/kg/minute; max. 10 micrograms/kg/minute
>
>   **Child 1 month–18 years** initially 0.2–0.5 micrograms/kg/minute, dose adjusted according to response, usual dose 1–3 micrograms/kg/minute; max. 10 micrograms/kg/minute (do not exceed 200 micrograms/minute)

**Administration**   for *continuous intravenous infusion*, dilute to max. concentration of 400 micrograms/mL (but concentration of 1 mg/mL has been used via a central venous catheter) with Glucose 5% *or* Sodium Chloride 0.9%.
Glass or polyethylene apparatus is preferable; loss of potency will occur if PVC is used.
*Neonatal intensive care*, dilute 3 mg/kg body-weight to a final volume of 50 mL with infusion fluid; an intravenous infusion rate of 1 mL/hour provides a dose of 1 microgram/kg/minute

**Glyceryl Trinitrate** (Non-proprietary) PoM
Injection, glyceryl trinitrate 1 mg/mL, net price 50-mL vial = £15.90
Note To be diluted before use or given undiluted with syringe pump

Injection, glyceryl trinitrate 5 mg/mL, net price 5-mL amp = £6.49; 10-mL amp =£12.98
Excipients may include ethanol, propylene glycol
Note To be diluted before use

**Nitrocine®** (UCB Pharma) PoM
Injection, glyceryl trinitrate 1 mg/mL, net price 10-mL amp = £5.88
Excipients include propylene glycol
Note To be diluted before use or given undiluted with syringe pump

**Nitronal®** (Merck Serono) PoM
Injection, glyceryl trinitrate 1 mg/mL, net price 5-mL vial = £1.80; 50-mL vial = £14.76
Note To be diluted before use or given undiluted with syringe pump

**2**

**Cardiovascular system**

## 2.6.2 Calcium-channel blockers

Calcium-channel blockers (less correctly called 'calcium-antagonists') interfere with the inward displacement of calcium ions through the slow channels of active cell membranes. They influence the myocardial cells, the cells within the specialised conducting system of the heart, and the cells of vascular smooth muscle. Thus, myocardial contractility may be reduced, the formation and propagation of electrical impulses within the heart may be depressed, and coronary or systemic vascular tone may be diminished.

Calcium-channel blockers differ in their predilection for the various possible sites of action and, therefore, their therapeutic effects are disparate, with much greater variation than those of beta-blockers. There are important differences between verapamil, diltiazem, and the dihydropyridine calcium-channel blockers (amlodipine, nicardipine, nifedipine, and nimodipine). Verapamil and diltiazem should usually be avoided in heart failure because they may further depress cardiac function and cause clinically significant deterioration.

**Verapamil** is used for the treatment of hypertension (section 2.5) and arrhythmias (section 2.3.2). However, it is no longer first-line treatment for arrhythmias in children because it has been associated with fatal collapse especially in infants under 1 year; adenosine is now recommended for first-line use.

Verapamil is a highly negatively inotropic calcium channel-blocker and it reduces cardiac output, slows the heart rate, and may impair atrioventricular conduction. It may precipitate heart failure, exacerbate conduction disorders, and cause hypotension at high doses and should **not** be used with beta-blockers (see p. 107). Constipation is the most common side-effect.

**Nifedipine** relaxes vascular smooth muscle and dilates coronary and peripheral arteries. It has more influence on vessels and less on the myocardium than does verapamil, and unlike verapamil has no anti-arrhythmic activity. It rarely precipitates heart failure because any negative inotropic effect is offset by a reduction in left ventricular work. Short-acting formulations of nifedipine are not recommended for long-term management of hypertension; their use may be associated with large variations in blood pressure and reflex tachycardia. However, they may be used if a modified-release preparation delivering the appropriate dose is not available or if a child is unable to swallow (a liquid preparation may be prepared using capsules). Nifedipine may also be used for the management of angina due to coronary artery disease in Kawasaki disease or progeria and in the management of Raynaud's syndrome.

**Nicardipine** has similar effects to those of nifedipine and may produce less reduction of myocardial contractility; it is used to treat hypertensive crisis.

**Amlodipine** also resembles nifedipine and nicardipine in its effects and does not reduce myocardial contractility or produce clinical deterioration in heart failure. It has a longer duration of action and can be given once daily. Nifedipine and amlodipine are used for the treatment of hypertension. Side-effects associated with vasodilatation such as flushing and headache (which become less obtrusive after a few days), and ankle swelling (which may respond only partially to diuretics) are common.

**Nimodipine** is related to nifedipine but the smooth muscle relaxant effect preferentially acts on cerebral arteries. Its use is confined to prevention and treatment of vascular spasm following aneurysmal subarachnoid haemorrhage.

**Diltiazem** is a peripheral vasodilator and also has mild depressor effects on the myocardium. It is used in the treatment of Raynaud's syndrome.

**Withdrawal**  There is some evidence that sudden withdrawal of calcium-channel blockers may be associated with an exacerbation of myocardial ischaemia.

## ▌ AMLODIPINE

**Cautions**  acute porphyria (but see section 9.8.2); **interactions:** Appendix 1 (calcium-channel blockers)

**Contra-indications**  cardiogenic shock, significant aortic stenosis

**Hepatic impairment**  may need dose reduction—half-life prolonged

**Pregnancy**  no information available—manufacturer advises avoid, but risk to fetus should be balanced against risk of uncontrolled maternal hypertension

**Breast-feeding**  manufacturer advises avoid—no information available

**Side-effects**  abdominal pain, nausea; palpitation, flushing, oedema; headache, dizziness, sleep disturbances, fatigue; *less commonly* gastro-intestinal disturbances, dry mouth, taste disturbances, hypotension, syncope, chest pain, dyspnoea, rhinitis, mood changes, asthenia, tremor, paraesthesia, urinary disturbances, impotence, gynaecomastia, weight changes, myalgia, muscle cramps, back pain, arthralgia, visual disturbances, tinnitus, pruritus, rashes (including isolated reports of erythema multiforme), sweating, alopecia, purpura, and skin discolouration; *very rarely* gastritis, pancreatitis, hepatitis, jaundice, cholestasis, gingival hyperplasia, myocardial infarction, arrhythmias, tachycardia, vasculitis, coughing, peripheral neuropathy, hyperglycaemia, thrombocytopenia, angioedema, and urticaria; **overdosage:** see Emergency Treatment of Poisoning, p. 29

**Licensed use**  not licensed for use in children under 6 years

### Indications and dose

> **Hypertension**
>
> ● **By mouth**
>
> **Child 1 month–12 years** initially 100–200 micrograms/kg once daily; if necessary increase at intervals of 1–2 weeks up to 400 micrograms/kg once daily; max. 10 mg once daily
>
> **Child 12–18 years** initially 5 mg once daily; if necessary increase at intervals of 1–2 weeks to max. 10 mg once daily

**Administration**  tablets may be dispersed in water
**Note** Tablets from various suppliers may contain different salts (e.g. amlodipine besilate, amlodipine maleate, and amlodipine mesilate) but the strength is expressed in terms of amlodipine (base); tablets containing different salts are considered interchangeable

**Amlodipine** (Non-proprietary) [PoM]
Tablets, amlodipine (as maleate or as mesilate) 5 mg, net price 28-tab pack = £1.05; 10 mg, 28-tab pack = £1.20
**Brands include** Amlostin®

**Istin®** (Pfizer) (PoM)
Tablets, amlodipine (as besilate) 5 mg, net price 28-tab pack = £11.08; 10 mg, 28-tab pack = £16.55

## DILTIAZEM HYDROCHLORIDE

**Cautions** heart failure or significantly impaired left ventricular function, bradycardia (avoid if severe), first degree AV block, or prolonged PR interval; **interactions:** Appendix 1 (calcium-channel blockers)

**Contra-indications** severe bradycardia, significant aortic stenosis, cardiogenic shock, left ventricular failure with pulmonary congestion, second- or third-degree AV block (unless pacemaker fitted), sick sinus syndrome; acute porphyria (section 9.8.2)

**Hepatic impairment** reduce dose

**Renal impairment** start with smaller dose

**Pregnancy** avoid

**Breast-feeding** significant amount present in milk—no evidence of harm but avoid unless no safer alternative

**Side-effects** bradycardia, sino-atrial block, AV block, palpitation, dizziness, hypotension, malaise, asthenia, headache, hot flushes, gastro-intestinal disturbances, oedema (notably of ankles); rarely rashes (including erythema multiforme and exfoliative dermatitis), photosensitivity; hepatitis, gynaecomastia, gum hyperplasia, extrapyramidal symptoms, depression reported; **overdosage:** see Emergency Treatment of Poisoning, p. 29

**Licensed use** not licensed for use in children

**Indications and dose**

Raynaud's syndrome

• By mouth

**Child 12–18 years** 30–60 mg 2–3 times daily

◢Standard formulations
**Note** These formulations are licensed as generics and there is no requirement for brand name dispensing. Although their means of formulation has called for the strict designation 'modified-release' their duration of action corresponds to that of tablets requiring administration more frequently

**Diltiazem** (Non-proprietary) (PoM)
Tablets, m/r (but see note above), diltiazem hydrochloride 60 mg, net price 84-tab pack = £2.93. Label: 25

**Tildiem®** (Sanofi-Aventis) (PoM)
Tablets, m/r (but see note above), off-white, diltiazem hydrochloride 60 mg, net price 90-tab pack = £7.96. Label: 25

## NICARDIPINE HYDROCHLORIDE

**Cautions** congestive heart failure or significantly impaired left ventricular function; **interactions:** Appendix 1 (calcium-channel blockers)

**Contra-indications** cardiogenic shock; significant aortic stenosis; acute porphyria (section 9.8.2)

**Hepatic impairment** half-life prolonged in severe impairment—may need dose reduction

**Renal impairment** start with smaller dose

**Pregnancy** may inhibit labour; toxicity in *animal* studies; manufacturer advises avoid, but risk to fetus should be balanced against risk of uncontrolled maternal hypertension

**Breast-feeding** manufacturer advises avoid—no information available

**Side-effects** dizziness, headache, peripheral oedema, flushing, palpitation, nausea; also gastro-intestinal disturbances, drowsiness, insomnia, tinnitus, hypotension, rashes, dyspnoea, paraesthesia, frequency of micturition; thrombocytopenia, depression and impotence reported; **overdosage:** see Emergency Treatment of Poisoning, p. 29

**Licensed use** not licensed for use in children

**Indications and dose**

Hypertensive crisis

• By continuous intravenous infusion

**Neonate** initially 500 nanograms/kg/minute, adjusted according to response; usual maintenance of 1–4 micrograms/kg/minute

**Child 1 month–18 years** initially 500 nanograms/kg/minute, adjusted according to response; usual maintenance of 1–4 micrograms/kg/minute (max. 250 micrograms/minute)

**Administration** for *intravenous infusion*, dilute to a concentration of 100 micrograms/mL with Glucose 5% *or* Sodium Chloride 0.9%; to minimise peripheral venous irritation, change site of infusion every 12 hours

**Cardene IV®** (PoM)
Injection, nicardipine 2.5 mg/mL (10-mL ampoule)
Available from 'special-order' manufacturers or specialist importing companies, see p. 823

## NIFEDIPINE

**Cautions** see notes above; also poor cardiac reserve; heart failure or significantly impaired left ventricular function (heart failure deterioration observed); severe hypotension; diabetes mellitus; acute porphyria (but see section 9.8.2); **interactions:** Appendix 1 (calcium-channel blockers)

**Contra-indications** cardiogenic shock; significant aortic stenosis

**Hepatic impairment** dose reduction may be required in severe liver disease

**Pregnancy** may inhibit labour; manufacturer advises avoid before week 20, but risk to fetus should be balanced against risk of uncontrolled maternal hypertension; use only if other treatment options are not indicated or have failed

**Breast-feeding** amount too small to be harmful but manufacturer advises avoid

**Side-effects** gastro-intestinal disturbance; hypotension, oedema, vasodilatation, palpitation; headache, dizziness, lethargy, asthenia; *less commonly* tachycardia, hypotension, syncope, chills, nasal congestion, dyspnoea, anxiety, sleep disturbance, vertigo, migraine, paraesthesia, tremor, polyuria, dysuria, nocturia, erectile dysfunction, epistaxis, myalgia, joint swelling, visual disturbance, sweating, and hypersensitivity reactions (including angioedema, jaundice, pruritus, urticaria, and rash); *rarely* gum hyperplasia, mood disturbances, hyperglycaemia, male infertility, purpura, and photosensitivity reactions; also reported dysphagia, intestinal obstruction, intestinal ulcer, bezoar formation, gynaecomastia, agranulocytosis, and anaphylaxis; **overdosage:** see Emergency Treatment of Poisoning, p. 29

**Licensed use** not licensed for use in children

**Indications and dose**

**Hypertensive crisis, acute angina in Kawasaki disease or progeria**
- By mouth (see Administration, below)
  Child 1 month–18 years 250–500 micrograms/kg (max. 20 mg) as a single dose

**Hypertension, angina in Kawasaki disease or progeria**
- By mouth
  Child 1 month–12 years 200–300 micrograms/kg 3 times daily; max. 3 mg/kg daily or 90 mg daily
  Child 12–18 years 5–20 mg 3 times daily; max. 90 mg daily
  Note Dose frequency depends on preparation used

**Raynaud's syndrome**
- By mouth
  Child 2–18 years 2.5–10 mg 2–4 times daily; start with low doses at night and increase gradually to avoid postural hypotension
  Note Dose frequency depends on preparation used

**Persistent hyperinsulinaemic hypoglycaemia** see also section 6.1.4
- By mouth
  Neonate 100–200 micrograms/kg (max. 600 micrograms/kg) 4 times daily

**Administration** for rapid effect in *hypertensive crisis* or *acute angina*, bite capsules and swallow liquid or use liquid preparation if 5-mg or 10-mg dose inappropriate; if liquid unavailable, extract contents of capsule via a syringe and use immediately—cover syringe with foil to protect contents from light; capsule contents may be diluted with water if necessary.

Modified-release tablets may be crushed—this may alter the release profile; crushed tablets should be administered within 30–60 seconds to avoid significant loss of potency of drug

**Nifedipine** (Non-proprietary) PoM
Capsules, nifedipine 5 mg, net price 84-cap pack = £2.97; 10 mg, 84-cap pack = £4.00
**Dose**
> Give 3 times daily

Oral liquid, available from 'special-order' manufacturers or specialist importing companies, see p. 823

**Adalat®** (Bayer) PoM
Capsules, orange, nifedipine 5 mg, net price 90-cap pack = £5.73; 10 mg, 90-cap pack = £7.30
Note Adalat liquid gel capsules contain 5 mg nifedipine in 0.17 mL and 10 mg nifedipine in 0.34 mL
**Dose**
> Give 3 times daily

◀ **Modified release**
Note Different versions of modified-release preparations may not have the same clinical effect. To avoid confusion between these different formulations of nifedipine, prescribers should specify the brand to be dispensed. Modified-release formulations may not be suitable for dose titration in hepatic disease

**Adalat® LA** (Bayer) PoM
LA 20 tablets, m/r, f/c, pink, nifedipine 20 mg, net price 28-tab pack = £4.97. Label: 25
LA 30 tablets, m/r, f/c, pink, nifedipine 30 mg, net price 28-tab pack = £6.85. Label: 25

LA 60 tablets, m/r, f/c, pink, nifedipine 60 mg, net price 28-tab pack = £9.03. Label: 25
Counselling Tablet membrane may pass through gastro-intestinal tract unchanged, but being porous has no effect on efficacy
Cautions dose form not appropriate for use in hepatic impairment or where there is a history of oesophageal or gastro-intestinal obstruction, decreased lumen diameter of the gastro-intestinal tract, or inflammatory bowel disease (including Crohn's disease)
**Dose**
> Give once daily

**Adalat® Retard** (Bayer) PoM
Retard 10 tablets, m/r, f/c, grey-pink, nifedipine 10 mg, net price 56-tab pack = £7.34. Label: 25
Retard 20 tablets, m/r, f/c, grey-pink, nifedipine 20 mg, net price 56-tab pack = £8.81. Label: 25
**Dose**
> Give twice daily

**Adipine® MR** (Chiesi) PoM
Tablets, m/r, nifedipine 10 mg (pink), net price 56-tab pack = £3.73; 20 mg (pink), 56-tab pack = £5.21. Label: 25
**Dose**
> Give twice daily

**Adipine® XL** (Chiesi) PoM
Tablets, m/r, red, nifedipine 30 mg, net price 28-tab pack = £4.70; 60 mg, 28-tab pack = £7.10. Label: 25
**Dose**
> Give once daily

**Coracten SR®** (UCB Pharma) PoM
Capsules, m/r, nifedipine 10 mg (grey/pink, enclosing yellow pellets), net price 60-cap pack = £3.90; 20 mg (pink/brown, enclosing yellow pellets), 60-cap pack = £5.41. Label: 25
**Dose**
> Give twice daily

**Coracten XL®** (UCB Pharma) PoM
Capsules, m/r, nifedipine 30 mg (brown), net price 28-cap pack = £4.89; 60 mg (orange), 28-cap pack = £7.34. Label: 25
**Dose**
> Give once daily

**Fortipine LA 40®** (Mercury) PoM
Tablets, m/r, red, nifedipine 40 mg, net price 30-tab pack = £9.60. Label: 21, 25
**Dose**
> Give 1–2 times daily

**Nifedipress® MR** (Dexcel) PoM
Tablets, m/r, pink, nifedipine 10 mg, net price 56-tab pack = £9.23; 20 mg, 56-tab pack = £10.06. Label: 25
**Dose**
> Give twice daily

Note Also available as *Calchan®* MR

**Tensipine MR®** (Genus) PoM
Tablets, m/r, pink-grey, nifedipine 10 mg, net price 56-tab pack = £4.30; 20 mg, 56-tab pack = £5.49. Label: 21, 25
**Dose**
> Give twice daily

*(side text)* 2 Cardiovascular system

**Valni XL®** (Winthrop) PoM
Tablets, m/r, red, nifedipine 30 mg, net price 28-tab pack = £7.29; 60 mg, 28-tab pack = £9.13. Label: 25
**Cautions** dose form not appropriate for use in hepatic impairment, or where there is a history of oesophageal or gastro-intestinal obstruction, decreased lumen diameter of the gastro-intestinal tract, inflammatory bowel disease, or ileostomy after proctocolectomy
**Dose**

> Give once daily

# ▉ NIMODIPINE

**Cautions** cerebral oedema or severely raised intracranial pressure; hypotension; avoid concomitant administration of nimodipine tablets and infusion, other calcium-channel blockers, or beta-blockers; concomitant nephrotoxic drugs; **interactions:** Appendix 1 (calcium-channel blockers, alcohol (infusion only))
**Contra-indications** acute porphyria (section 9.8.2)
**Hepatic impairment** elimination reduced in cirrhosis—monitor blood pressure
**Renal impairment** manufacturer advises monitor renal function closely with intravenous administration
**Pregnancy** manufacturer advises use only if potential benefit outweighs risks
**Breast-feeding** manufacturer advises avoid—present in milk
**Side-effects** hypotension, variation in heart-rate, flushing, headache, gastro-intestinal disorders, nausea, sweating and feeling of warmth; thrombocytopenia and ileus reported; **overdosage:** see Emergency Treatment of Poisoning, p. 29
**Licensed use** not licensed for use in children
**Indications and dose**

> **Treatment of vasospasm following subarachnoid haemorrhage** under specialist advice only
> • **By intravenous infusion**
>> **Child 1 month–12 years** initially 15 micrograms/kg/hour (max. 500 micrograms/hour) or initially 7.5 micrograms/kg/hour if blood pressure unstable; increase after 2 hours to 30 micrograms/kg/hour (max. 2 mg/hour) if no severe decrease in blood pressure; continue for at least 5 days (max. 14 days)
>> **Child 12–18 years** initially 500 micrograms/hour (up to 1 mg/hour if body-weight over 70 kg and blood pressure stable), increase after 2 hours to 1–2 mg/hour if no severe fall in blood pressure; continue for at least 5 days (max. 14 days)

> **Prevention of vasospasm following subarachnoid haemorrhage**
> • **By mouth**
>> **Child 1 month–18 years** 0.9–1.2 mg/kg (max. 60 mg) 6 times daily, starting within 4 days of haemorrhage and continued for 21 days

**Administration** for continuous intravenous infusion, administer undiluted via a Y-piece on a central venous catheter connected to a running infusion of Glucose 5%, or Sodium Chloride 0.9%; not to be added to an infusion container; incompatible with polyvinyl chloride giving sets or containers; protect infusion from light.
For administration by mouth, tablets may be crushed or halved but are light sensitive—administer immediately

**Nimotop®** (Bayer) PoM
Tablets, yellow, f/c, nimodipine 30 mg, net price 100-tab pack = £33.60

Intravenous infusion, nimodipine 200 micrograms/mL; also contains ethanol 20% and macrogol '400' 17%. Net price 50-mL vial (with polyethylene infusion catheter) = £11.46
**Note** Polyethylene, polypropylene, or glass apparatus should be used; PVC should be avoided

# ▉ VERAPAMIL HYDROCHLORIDE

**Cautions** first-degree AV block; patients taking beta-blockers (**important:** see below); **interactions:** Appendix 1 (calcium-channel blockers)
**Verapamil and beta-blockers Verapamil** injection should not be given to patients recently treated with beta-blockers because of the risk of hypotension and asystole. The suggestion that when verapamil injection has been given first, an interval of 30 minutes before giving a beta-blocker is sufficient has not been confirmed.
It may also be hazardous to give verapamil and a beta-blocker together by mouth (should only be contemplated if myocardial function well preserved).
**Contra-indications** hypotension, bradycardia, second- and third-degree AV block, sick sinus syndrome, cardiogenic shock, sino-atrial block; history of heart failure or significantly impaired left ventricular function, even if controlled by therapy; atrial flutter or fibrillation complicating syndromes associated with accessory conducting pathways (e.g. Wolff-Parkinson-White syndrome); acute porphyria (section 9.8.2)
**Hepatic impairment** oral dose may need to be reduced
**Pregnancy** may reduce uterine blood flow with fetal hypoxia; manufacturer advises avoid during first trimester unless absolutely necessary; may inhibit labour
**Breast-feeding** amount too small to be harmful
**Side-effects** constipation; less commonly nausea, vomiting, flushing, headache, dizziness, fatigue, ankle oedema; rarely allergic reactions (erythema, pruritus, urticaria, angioedema, Stevens-Johnson syndrome); myalgia, arthralgia, paraesthesia, erythromelalgia; increased prolactin concentration; gynaecomastia and gingival hyperplasia after long-term treatment; after intravenous administration or high doses, hypotension, heart failure, bradycardia, heart block, and asystole; hypersensitivity reactions involving reversibly raised liver function tests; **overdosage:** see Emergency Treatment of Poisoning, p. 29
**Licensed use** Modified release preparation not licensed for use in children
**Indications and dose**

> **Hypertension, prophylaxis of supraventricular arrhythmias** under specialist advice only
> • **By mouth**
>> **Child 1–2 years** 20 mg 2–3 times daily
>> **Child 2–18 years** 40–120 mg 2–3 times daily

> **Treatment of supraventricular arrhythmias**
> • **By intravenous injection over 2–3 minutes (with ECG and blood-pressure monitoring and under specialist advice)**
>> **Child 1–18 years** 100–300 micrograms/kg (max. 5 mg) as a single dose, repeated after 30 minutes if necessary

**2**

**Cardiovascular system**

**Administration** for *intravenous injection*, may be diluted with Glucose 5% *or* Sodium Chloride 0.9%; incompatible with solutions of pH greater than 6

### Verapamil (Non-proprietary) PoM

Tablets, coated, verapamil hydrochloride 40 mg, net price 84-tab pack = £1.55; 80 mg, 84-tab pack = £1.91; 120 mg, 28-tab pack = £1.54; 160 mg, 56-tab pack = £28.20

Oral solution, verapamil hydrochloride 40 mg/5 mL, net price 150 mL = £36.90
**Brands include** *Zolvera* ®

### Cordilox® (Dexcel) PoM

Tablets, yellow, f/c, verapamil hydrochloride 40 mg, net price 84-tab pack = £1.50; 80 mg, 84-tab pack = £2.05; 120 mg, 28-tab pack = £1.15; 160 mg, 56-tab pack = £2.80

Injection, verapamil hydrochloride 2.5 mg/mL, net price 2-mL amp = £1.11

### Securon® (Abbott Healthcare) PoM

Injection, verapamil hydrochloride 2.5 mg/mL, net price 2-mL amp = £1.08

◢**Modified release**

### Half Securon SR® (Abbott Healthcare) PoM

Tablets, m/r, f/c, verapamil hydrochloride 120 mg, net price 28-tab pack = £7.71. Label: 25
**Dose**
> Give once daily (doses above 240 mg daily, give 2–3 times daily)

### Securon SR® (Abbott Healthcare) PoM

Tablets, m/r, pale green, f/c, scored, verapamil hydrochloride 240 mg, net price 28-tab pack = £5.00. Label: 25
**Dose**
> Give once daily (doses above 240 mg daily, give 2–3 times daily)

### Univer® (Cephalon) PoM

Capsules, m/r, verapamil hydrochloride 120 mg (yellow/dark blue), net price 28-cap pack = £4.86; 180 mg (yellow), 56-cap pack = £11.38; 240 mg (yellow/dark blue), 28-cap pack = £7.67. Label: 25
**Excipients** include propylene glycol (see Excipients, p. 2)
**Dose**
> Give once daily

### Verapress MR® (Dexcel) PoM

Tablets, m/r, pale green, f/c, verapamil hydrochloride 240 mg, net price 28-tab pack = £6.04. Label: 25
**Dose**
> Give 1–2 times daily

**Note** Also available as *Cordilox* ® MR

### Vertab® SR 240 (Chiesi) PoM

Tablets, m/r, pale green, f/c, scored, verapamil hydrochloride 240 mg, net price 28-tab pack = £5.45. Label: 25
**Dose**
> Give 1–2 times daily

## 2.6.3 Other antianginal drugs

Classification not used in *BNF for Children*.

## 2.6.4 Peripheral vasodilators and related drugs

*Raynaud's syndrome* consists of recurrent, long-lasting, and episodic vasospasm of the fingers and toes often associated with exposure to cold. Management includes avoidance of exposure to cold and stopping smoking (if appropriate). More severe symptoms may require vasodilator treatment, which is most often successful in primary Raynaud's syndrome. **Nifedipine and diltiazem** (section 2.6.2) are useful for reducing the frequency and severity of vasospastic attacks. In very severe cases, where digital infarction is likely, intravenous infusion of the prostacyclin analogue **iloprost** may be helpful.

Vasodilator therapy is not established as being effective for *chilblains* (section 13.13).

### ILOPROST

**Cautions** see section 2.5.1.2
**Contra-indications** see section 2.5.1.2
**Hepatic impairment** dose may need to be halved in liver cirrhosis
**Side-effects** see section 2.5.1.2
**Licensed use** not licensed for use in children
**Indications and dose**

**Raynaud's syndrome** see notes above
• **By intravenous infusion**
> **Child 12–18 years** initially 30 nanograms/kg/hour, increased gradually to 60–120 nanograms/kg/hour given over 6 hours daily for 3–5 days

**Pulmonary hypertension** section 2.5.1.2

**Administration** for *intravenous infusion*, dilute to a concentration of 200 nanograms/mL with Glucose 5% or Sodium Chloride 0.9%; alternatively, may be diluted to a concentration of 2 micrograms/mL and given via syringe driver

### Iloprost (Non-proprietary)

Concentrate for infusion, iloprost (as trometamol) 100 micrograms/mL
For dilution and use as an intravenous infusion
**Note** available on a named patient basis from Bayer Schering in 0.5 mL and 1 mL ampoules

## 2.7 Sympathomimetics

### 2.7.1 Inotropic sympathomimetics
### 2.7.2 Vasoconstrictor sympathomimetics
### 2.7.3 Cardiopulmonary resuscitation

The properties of sympathomimetics vary according to whether they act on alpha or on beta adrenergic receptors. Response to sympathomimetics can also vary considerably in children, particularly neonates. It is important to titrate the dose to the desired effect and to monitor the child closely.

## 2.7.1 Inotropic sympathomimetics

The cardiac stimulants **dobutamine** and **dopamine** act on beta$_1$ receptors in cardiac muscle and increase contractility with little effect on rate.

Dopamine has a variable, unpredictable, and dose dependent impact on vascular tone. Low dose infusion (2 micrograms/kg/minute) normally causes vasodilatation, but there is little evidence that this is clinically beneficial; moderate doses increase myocardial contractility and cardiac output in older children, but in neonates moderate doses may cause a reduction in cardiac output. High doses cause vasoconstriction and increase vascular resistance, and should therefore be used with caution following cardiac surgery, or where there is co-existing neonatal pulmonary hypertension.

In neonates the response to inotropic sympathomimetics varies considerably, particularly in those born prematurely; careful dose titration and monitoring are necessary.

**Isoprenaline** injection is available from 'special-order' manufacturers or specialist importing companies, see p. 823.

**Shock**  Shock is a medical emergency associated with a high mortality. The underlying causes of shock such as haemorrhage, sepsis or myocardial insufficiency should be corrected. Additional treatment is dependent on the type of shock.

*Septic shock* is associated with severe hypovolaemia (due to vasodilation and capillary leak) which should be corrected with crystalloids or colloids (section 9.2.2). If hypotension persists despite volume replacement, **dopamine** should be started. For shock refractory to treatment with dopamine, if cardiac output is high and peripheral vascular resistance is low (warm shock), **noradrenaline** (norepinephrine) (section 2.7.2) should be added *or* if cardiac output is low and peripheral vascular resistance is high (cold shock), **adrenaline** (epinephrine) (section 2.7.2) should be added. Additionally, in cold shock, a vasodilator such as **milrinone** (section 2.1.2), **glyceryl trinitrate** (section 2.6.1), or **sodium nitroprusside** (on specialist advice only) (section 2.5.1.1) can be used to reduce vascular resistance.

If the shock is resistant to volume expansion and catecholamines, and there is suspected or proven adrenal insufficiency, low dose **hydrocortisone** (section 6.3.2) can be used. ACTH-stimulated plasma-cortisol concentration should be measured; however, hydrocortisone can be started without such information.

Alternatively, if the child is resistant to catecholamines, and vascular resistance is low, **vasopressin** (section 6.5.2) can be added.

*Neonatal septic shock* can be complicated by the transition from fetal to neonatal circulation. Treatment to reverse right ventricular failure, by decreasing pulmonary artery pressures, is commonly needed in neonates with fluid-refractory shock and persistent pulmonary hypertension of the newborn (section 2.5.1.2). Rapid administration of fluid in neonates with patent ductus arteriosus may cause left-to-right shunting and congestive heart failure induced by ventricular overload.

In *cardiogenic shock*, the aim is to improve cardiac output and to reduce the afterload on the heart. If central venous pressure is low, cautious volume expansion with a colloid or crystalloid can be used. An inotrope such as **adrenaline** (epinephrine) (section 2.7.2) or **dopamine** should be given to increase cardiac output. **Dobutamine** is a peripheral vasodilator and is an alternative if hypotension is not significant.

**Milrinone** (section 2.1.2) has both inotropic and vasodilatory effects and can be used when vascular resistance is high. Alternatively, **glyceryl trinitrate** (2.6.1) or **sodium nitroprusside** (on specialist advice only) (section 2.5.1.1) can be used to reduce vasoconstriction.

*Hypovolaemic shock* should be treated with a crystalloid or colloid solution (or whole or reconstituted blood if source of hypovolaemia is haemorrhage) and further steps to improve cardiac output and decrease vascular resistance can be taken, as in cardiogenic shock.

The use of sympathomimetic inotropes and vasoconstrictors should preferably be confined to the intensive care setting and undertaken with invasive haemodynamic monitoring.

For advice on the management of anaphylactic shock, see section 3.4.3.

---

### ▌ DOBUTAMINE

**Cautions**  arrhythmias, acute myocardial infarction, acute heart failure, severe hypotension, marked obstruction of cardiac ejection (such as idiopathic hypertrophic subaortic stenosis); correct hypovolaemia before starting treatment; tolerance may develop with continuous infusions longer than 72 hours; hyperthyroidism; **interactions:** Appendix 1 (sympathomimetics)

**Contra-indications**  phaeochromocytoma

**Pregnancy**  no evidence of harm in *animal* studies—manufacturers advise use only if benefit outweighs risk

**Breast-feeding**  manufacturers advise avoid—no information available

**Side-effects**  nausea; hypotension, hypertension (marked increase in systolic blood pressure indicates overdose), arrhythmias, palpitation, chest pain; dyspnoea, bronchospasm; headache; fever; increased urinary urgency; eosinophilia; rash, phlebitis; *very rarely* myocardial infarction, hypokalaemia; *also reported* coronary artery spasm and thrombocytopenia

**Licensed use**  strong sterile solution not licensed for use in children

#### Indications and dose

> **Inotropic support in low cardiac output states, after cardiac surgery, cardiomyopathies, shock**
>
> • **By continuous intravenous infusion**
>
>> **Neonate** initially 5 micrograms/kg/minute, adjusted according to response to 2–15 micrograms/kg/minute; max. 20 micrograms/kg/minute
>>
>> **Child 1 month–18 years** initially 5 micrograms/kg/minute adjusted according to response to 2–20 micrograms/kg/minute

**Administration**  for *continuous intravenous infusion*, using infusion pump, dilute to a concentration of 0.5–1 mg/mL (max. 5 mg/mL if fluid restricted) with Glucose 5% or Sodium Chloride 0.9%; infuse higher concentration solutions through central venous catheter only. Incompatible with bicarbonate and other strong alkaline solutions.

*Neonatal intensive care*, dilute 30 mg/kg body-weight to a final volume of 50 mL with infusion fluid; an intravenous infusion rate of 0.5 mL/hour provides a dose of 5 micrograms/kg/minute

**Dobutamine** (Non-proprietary) [PoM]
Injection, dobutamine (as hydrochloride) 5 mg/mL,
net price 50-mL vial = £7.50
Excipients  may include sulfites
Note  To be diluted before use or given undiluted with
syringe pump

Concentrate for intravenous infusion, dobutamine
(as hydrochloride) 12.5 mg/mL, net price 20-mL
amp = £5.20
Excipients  may include sulfites
Note  To be diluted before use

## DOPAMINE HYDROCHLORIDE

**Cautions**  correct hypovolaemia; hyperthyroidism;
interactions: Appendix 1 (sympathomimetics)
**Contra-indications**  tachyarrhythmia, phaeochromocytoma
**Pregnancy**  no evidence of harm in *animal* studies—
manufacturer advises use only if potential benefit
outweighs risk
**Breast-feeding**  may suppress lactation—not known
to be harmful
**Side-effects**  nausea, vomiting, chest pain, palpitation,
tachycardia, vasoconstriction, hypotension, dyspnoea, headache; *less commonly* bradycardia, hypertension, gangrene, mydriasis; *rarely* fatal ventricular
arrhythmias
**Licensed use**  not licensed for use in children under 12
years

### Indications and dose

To correct the haemodynamic imbalance due to
acute hypotension, shock, cardiac failure, adjunct
following cardiac surgery

• By continuous intravenous infusion

  **Neonate** initially 3 micrograms/kg/minute,
  adjusted according to response (max. 20 micr-
  ograms/kg/minute)

  **Child 1 month–18 years** initially 5 micrograms/
  kg/minute adjusted according to response (max.
  20 micrograms/kg/minute)

**Administration**  for *continuous intravenous infusion*,
dilute to a max. concentration of 3.2 mg/mL with
Glucose 5% *or* Sodium Chloride 0.9%. Infuse higher
concentrations through central venous catheter using
a syringe pump to avoid extravasation and fluid
overload. Incompatible with bicarbonate and other
alkaline solutions.
*Neonatal intensive care*, dilute 30 mg/kg body-weight
to a final volume of 50 mL with infusion fluid; an
intravenous infusion rate of 0.3 mL/hour provides a
dose of 3 micrograms/kg/minute

**Dopamine** (Non-proprietary) [PoM]
Concentrate for intravenous infusion, dopamine
hydrochloride 40 mg/mL, net price 5-mL amp =
90p; 160 mg/mL, 5-mL amp = £3.40.
Note  To be diluted before use

Intravenous infusion, dopamine hydrochloride
1.6 mg/mL in glucose 5% intravenous infusion
Available from 'special-order' manufacturers or specialist
importing companies, see p. 823

## 2.7.2 Vasoconstrictor sympathomimetics

Vasoconstrictor sympathomimetics raise blood pressure
transiently by acting on alpha-adrenergic receptors to
constrict peripheral vessels. They are sometimes used as
an emergency method of elevating blood pressure where
other measures have failed (see also section 2.7.1).

The danger of vasoconstrictors is that although they
raise blood pressure they also reduce perfusion of vital
organs such as the kidney.

**Ephedrine** is used to reverse hypotension caused by
spinal and epidural anaesthesia.

**Metaraminol** is used as a vasopressor during cardiopulmonary bypass.

**Phenylephrine** causes peripheral vasoconstriction and
increases arterial pressure.

Ephedrine, metaraminol and phenylephrine are rarely
needed in children and should be used under specialist
supervision.

**Noradrenaline** (norepinephrine) is reserved for children
with low systemic vascular resistance that is unresponsive to fluid resuscitation following septic shock, spinal
shock, and anaphylaxis.

**Adrenaline** (epinephrine) is mainly used for its inotropic
action. Low doses (acting on beta receptors) cause systemic and pulmonary vasodilation, with some increase in
heart rate and stroke volume and also an increase in
contractility; high doses act predominantly on alpha
receptors causing intense systemic vasoconstriction.

## EPHEDRINE HYDROCHLORIDE

**Cautions**  hyperthyroidism, diabetes mellitus, hypertension, susceptibility to angle-closure glaucoma,
interactions: Appendix 1 (sympathomimetics)
**Renal impairment**  use with caution
**Pregnancy**  increased fetal heart rate reported with
parenteral ephedrine
**Breast-feeding**  irritability and disturbed sleep
reported
**Side-effects**  nausea, vomiting, anorexia; tachycardia
(sometimes bradycardia), arrhythmias, anginal pain,
vasoconstriction with hypertension, vasodilation with
hypotension, dizziness and flushing; dyspnoea; headache, anxiety, restlessness, confusion, psychoses,
insomnia, tremor; difficulty in micturition, urine
retention; sweating, hypersalivation; changes in
blood-glucose concentration; *very rarely* angle-closure
glaucoma

### Indications and dose

Reversal of hypotension from epidural and spinal
anaesthesia

• By slow intravenous injection of a solution containing ephedrine hydrochloride 3 mg/mL

  **Child 1–12 years** 500–750 micrograms/kg *or* 17–
  25 mg/m$^2$ every 3–4 minutes according to
  response; max. 30 mg during episode

  **Child 12–18 years** 3–7.5 mg (max. 9 mg) repeated
  every 3–4 minutes according to response, max.
  30 mg during episode

Nasal congestion section 12.2.2

**Administration**  for *slow intravenous injection*, give via
central venous catheter

**Ephedrine Hydrochloride** (Non-proprietary) [PoM]
Injection, ephedrine hydrochloride 3 mg/mL, net price 10-mL amp = £3.25; 30 mg/mL, net price 1-mL amp = 41p

## ■ METARAMINOL

**Cautions** see under Noradrenaline; longer duration of action than noradrenaline (norepinephrine), see below; cirrhosis; **interactions:** Appendix 1 (sympathomimetics)
**Hypertensive response** Metaraminol has a longer duration of action than noradrenaline, and an excessive vasopressor response may cause a prolonged rise in blood pressure

**Contra-indications** see under Noradrenaline

**Pregnancy** may reduce placental prefusion—manufacturer advises use only if potential benefit outweighs risk

**Breast-feeding** manufacturer advises caution—no information available

**Side-effects** see under Noradrenaline; also tachycardia; fatal ventricular arrhythmia reported in Laennec's cirrhosis

**Licensed use** not licensed for use in children

### Indications and dose

Acute hypotension

● By intravenous infusion

     **Child 12–18 years** 15–100 mg adjusted according to response

Emergency treatment of acute hypotension

● By intravenous administration

     **Child 12–18 years** initially by *intravenous injection* 0.5–5 mg, then by *intravenous infusion* 15–100 mg adjusted according to response

**Administration** for *intravenous infusion*, dilute to a concentration of 30–200 micrograms/mL with Glucose 5% or Sodium Chloride 0.9% and give through a central venous catheter

**Metaraminol** (Non-proprietary) [PoM]
Injection, metaraminol 10 mg (as tartrate)/mL.
Available from 'special-order' manufacturers or specialist importing companies, see p. 823

## ■ NORADRENALINE/NOREPINEPHRINE

**Cautions** coronary, mesenteric, or peripheral vascular thrombosis; following myocardial infarction; Prinzmetal's variant angina, hyperthyroidism, diabetes mellitus; hypoxia or hypercapnia; uncorrected hypovolaemia; extravasation at injection site may cause necrosis; susceptibility to angle-closure glaucoma **interactions:** Appendix 1 (sympathomimetics)

**Contra-indications** hypertension (monitor blood pressure and rate of flow frequently)

**Pregnancy** avoid—may reduce placental perfusion

**Side-effects** anorexia, nausea, vomiting, hypoxia, arrhythmias, peripheral ischaemia, palpitation, hypertension, bradycardia, tachycardia, dyspnoea, headache, insomnia, confusion, anxiety, psychosis, weakness, tremor, urinary retention, angle-closure glaucoma

**Licensed use** not licensed for use in children

### Indications and dose

Acute hypotension (septic shock) or shock secondary to excessive vasodilation (as noradrenaline)

● By continuous intravenous infusion

     **Neonate** 20–100 nanograms (base)/kg/minute adjusted according to response; max. 1 microgram (base)/kg/minute

     **Child 1 month–18 years** 20–100 nanograms (base)/kg/minute adjusted according to response; max. 1 microgram (base)/kg/minute
     **Note** 1 mg of noradrenaline base is equivalent to 2 mg of noradrenaline acid tartrate. Dose expressed as the base

**Administration** for *continuous intravenous infusion*, dilute to a max. concentration of noradrenaline (base) 40 micrograms/mL (higher concentrations can be used if fluid-restricted) with Glucose 5% or Sodium Chloride and Glucose. Infuse through central venous catheter; discard if discoloured. Incompatible with bicarbonate or alkaline solutions.

*Neonatal intensive care*, dilute 600 micrograms (base)/kg body-weight to a final volume of 50 mL with infusion fluid; an intravenous infusion rate of 0.1 mL/hour provides a dose of 20 nanograms (base)/kg/minute

**Noradrenaline/Norepinephrine** (Non-proprietary) [PoM]
Injection, noradrenaline base 1 mg/mL (as noradrenaline acid tartrate 2 mg/mL). For dilution before use. Net price 2-mL amp = £2.40, 4-mL amp = £4.40, 20-mL amp = £6.35
**Note** For a period of time preparations on the UK market may be described as *either* noradrenaline base or noradrenaline acid tartrate; doses above are expressed as the base

## ■ PHENYLEPHRINE HYDROCHLORIDE

**Cautions** see under Noradrenaline; longer duration of action than noradrenaline (norepinephrine), see below; coronary disease
**Hypertensive response** Phenylephrine has a longer duration of action than noradrenaline, and an excessive vasopressor response may cause a prolonged rise in blood pressure

**Contra-indications** see under Noradrenaline; severe hyperthyroidism

**Pregnancy** avoid if possible; malformations reported following use in first trimester; fetal hypoxia and bradycardia reported in late pregnancy and labour

**Side-effects** see under Noradrenaline; also tachycardia or reflex bradycardia

**Licensed use** not licensed for use in children by intravenous infusion or injection

### Indications and dose

Acute hypotension

● By subcutaneous or intramuscular injection (but intravenous injection preferred, see below)

     **Child 1–12 years** 100 micrograms/kg every 1–2 hours as needed (max. 5 mg)

     **Child 12–18 years** 2–5 mg, followed if necessary after at least 15 minutes by further doses of 1–10 mg (max. initial dose 5 mg)

● By slow intravenous injection

     **Child 1–12 years** 5–20 micrograms/kg (max. 500 micrograms) repeated as necessary after at least 15 minutes

     **Child 12–18 years** 100–500 micrograms repeated as necessary after at least 15 minutes

**2** Cardiovascular system

**2 Cardiovascular system**

- By intravenous infusion

  **Child 1–16 years** 100–500 nanograms/kg/minute, adjusted according to response

  **Child 16–18 years** initially up to 180 micrograms/minute reduced to 30–60 micrograms/minute according to response

**Administration** for *intravenous injection*, dilute to a concentration of 1 mg/mL with Water for Injections and administer slowly.

For *intravenous infusion*, dilute to a concentration of 20 micrograms/mL with Glucose 5% or Sodium Chloride 0.9% and administer as a continuous infusion via a central venous catheter using a controlled infusion device

**Phenylephrine** (Sovereign) PoM
Injection, phenylephrine hydrochloride 10 mg/mL (1%), net price 1-mL amp = £5.50

## ADRENALINE/EPINEPHRINE

**Cautions** ischaemic heart disease, severe angina, obstructive cardiomyopathy, hypertension, arrhythmias, cerebrovascular disease; occlusive vascular disease, monitor blood pressure and ECG; cor pulmonale; organic brain damage, psychoneurosis; phaeochromocytoma; diabetes mellitus, hyperthyroidism; hypokalaemia, hypercalcaemia; susceptibility to angle-closure glaucoma; **interactions:** Appendix 1 (sympathomimetics)

**Renal impairment** manufacturers advise use with caution in severe impairment

**Pregnancy** may reduce placental perfusion and can delay second stage of labour; manufacturers advise use only if benefit outweighs risk

**Breast-feeding** present in milk but unlikely to be harmful as poor oral bioavailability

**Side-effects** nausea, vomiting, dry mouth, anorexia, hypersalivation; arrhythmias, palpitation, tachycardia, syncope, angina, hypertension (risk of cerebral haemorrhage), cold extremities, pallor; dyspnoea, pulmonary oedema (on excessive dosage or extreme sensitivity); anxiety, tremor, restlessness, headache, insomnia, confusion, weakness, dizziness, hallucinations, psychosis; hyperglycaemia; difficulty in micturition, urinary retention; metabolic acidosis; hypokalaemia; mydriasis, angle-closure glaucoma; tissue necrosis at injection site and of extremities, liver and kidneys, sweating

**Indications and dose**

**Acute hypotension**

- By continuous intravenous infusion

  **Neonate** initially 100 nanograms/kg/minute adjusted according to response; higher doses up to 1.5 micrograms/kg/minute have been used in acute hypotension

  **Child 1 month–18 years** initially 100 nanograms/kg/minute adjusted according to response; higher doses up to 1.5 micrograms/kg/minute have been used in acute hypotension

**Anaphylaxis** section 3.4.3

**Cardiopulmonary arrest** section 2.7.3

**Administration** for *continuous intravenous infusion*, dilute with Glucose 5% or Sodium Chloride 0.9% and give through a central venous catheter. Incompatible with bicarbonate and alkaline solutions.

*Neonatal intensive care*, dilute 3 mg/kg body-weight to a final volume of 50 mL with infusion fluid; an intravenous infusion rate of 0.1 mL/hour provides a dose of 100 nanograms/kg/minute

**Note** These infusions are usually made up with adrenaline 1 in 1000 (1 mg/mL) solution; this concentration of adrenaline is not licensed for intravenous administration

◢**Preparations**
Section 3.4.3

## 2.7.3 Cardiopulmonary resuscitation

The algorithms for cardiopulmonary resuscitation (see inside back cover) reflect the recommendations of the Resuscitation Council (UK); they cover paediatric basic life support, paediatric advanced life support, and newborn life support. The guidelines are available at www.resus.org.uk.

**Paediatric advanced life support** Cardiopulmonary (cardiac) arrest in children is rare and frequently represents the terminal event of progressive shock or respiratory failure.

During cardiopulmonary arrest in children without intravenous access, the intraosseous route is chosen because it provides rapid and effective response; if circulatory access cannot be gained, the endotracheal tube can be used. When the endotracheal route is used ten times the intravenous dose should be used; the drug should be injected quickly down a narrow bore suction catheter beyond the tracheal end of the tube and then flushed in with 1 or 2 mL of sodium chloride 0.9%. The endotracheal route is useful for lipid-soluble drugs, including lidocaine, adrenaline, atropine, and naloxone. Drugs that are not lipid-soluble (e.g. sodium bicarbonate and calcium chloride) should **not** be administered by this route because they will injure the airways.

For the management of acute anaphylaxis see section 3.4.3.

## 2.8 Anticoagulants and protamine

**2.8.1** Parenteral anticoagulants
**2.8.2** Oral anticoagulants
**2.8.3** Protamine sulfate

Although thrombotic episodes are uncommon in childhood, anticoagulants may be required in children with congenital heart disease; in children undergoing haemodialysis; for preventing thrombosis in children requiring chemotherapy and following surgery; and for systemic venous thromboembolism secondary to inherited thrombophilias, systemic lupus erythematosus, or indwelling central venous catheters.

## 2.8.1 | Parenteral anticoagulants

heparin is required, protamine sulfate (section 2.8.3) is a specific antidote (but only partially reverses the effects of low molecular weight heparins).

## Heparin

**Heparin** initiates anticoagulation rapidly but has a short duration of action. It is now often referred to as being **standard** or **unfractionated heparin** to distinguish it from the **low molecular weight heparins** (see p. 114), which have a longer duration of action. For children at high risk of bleeding, unfractionated heparin is more suitable than low molecular weight heparin because its effect can be terminated rapidly by stopping the infusion.

Heparins are used in both the treatment and prophylaxis of thromboembolic disease, mainly to prevent further clotting rather than to lyse existing clots—surgery or a thrombolytic drug may be necessary if a thrombus obstructs major vessels.

**Treatment** For the initial treatment of thrombotic episodes unfractionated heparin is given as an intravenous loading dose, followed by continuous intravenous infusion (using an infusion pump) or by intermittent subcutaneous injection; the use of intermittent intravenous injection is no longer recommended. Alternatively, a low molecular weight heparin may be given for initial treatment. If an oral anticoagulant (usually warfarin, section 2.8.2) is also required, it may be started at the same time as the heparin (the heparin needs to be continued for at least 5 days and until the INR has been in the therapeutic range for 2 consecutive days). Laboratory monitoring of coagulation activity, preferably on a daily basis, involves determination of the activated partial thromboplastin time (APTT) (for unfractionated heparin only) or of the anti-Factor Xa concentration (for low molecular weight heparins). Local guidelines on recommended APTT for neonates and children should be followed; monitoring of APTT should be discussed with a specialist prior to treatment for thrombotic episodes in neonates.

**Prophylaxis** Low-dose unfractionated heparin by subcutaneous injection is used to prevent thrombotic episodes in 'high-risk' patients; laboratory monitoring of APTT or anti-Factor Xa concentration is also required in prophylactic regimens in children. Low molecular weight heparins, **aspirin** (section 2.9), and **warfarin** (section 2.8.2) can also be used for prophylaxis.

**Pregnancy** Heparins are used for the management of thromboembolic disease in pregnancy because they do not cross the placenta. Low molecular weight heparins are preferred because they have a lower risk of osteoporosis and of heparin-induced thrombocytopenia. Low molecular weight heparins are eliminated more rapidly in pregnancy, requiring alteration of the dosage regimen for drugs such as dalteparin, enoxaparin, and tinzaparin. Treatment should be stopped at the onset of labour and advice sought from a specialist on continuing therapy after birth.

**Extracorporeal circuits** Unfractionated heparin is also used in the maintenance of extracorporeal circuits in cardiopulmonary bypass and haemodialysis.

**Haemorrhage** If haemorrhage occurs it is usually sufficient to withdraw unfractionated or low molecular weight heparin, but if rapid reversal of the effects of the

## ■ HEPARIN

**Cautions** see notes above; concomitant use of drugs that increase risk of bleeding; **interactions**: Appendix 1 (heparin)

**Heparin-induced thrombocytopenia** Clinically important heparin-induced thrombocytopenia is immune-mediated and does not usually develop until after 5–10 days; it can be complicated by thrombosis. Platelet counts should be measured just before treatment with unfractionated or low molecular weight heparin, and regular monitoring of platelet counts may be required if given for longer than 4 days[1]. Signs of heparin-induced thrombocytopenia include a 30% reduction of platelet count, thrombosis, or skin allergy. If heparin-induced thrombocytopenia is strongly suspected or confirmed, the heparin should be **stopped** and an alternative anticoagulant, such as danaparoid, should be given. Ensure platelet counts return to normal range in those who require warfarin

**Hyperkalaemia** Inhibition of aldosterone secretion by unfractionated or low molecular weight heparin can result in hyperkalaemia; patients with diabetes mellitus, chronic renal failure, acidosis, raised plasma-potassium concentration, or those taking potassium-sparing drugs seem to be more susceptible. The risk appears to increase with duration of therapy and plasma-potassium concentration should be measured in children at risk of hyperkalaemia before starting the heparin and monitored regularly thereafter, particularly if treatment is to be continued for longer than 7 days

**Contra-indications** haemophilia and other haemorrhagic disorders, thrombocytopenia (including history of heparin-induced thrombocytopenia), recent cerebral haemorrhage, severe hypertension; peptic ulcer; after major trauma or recent surgery to eye or nervous system; acute bacterial endocarditis; spinal or epidural anaesthesia with treatment doses of unfractionated or low molecular weight heparin; hypersensitivity to unfractionated or low molecular weight heparin

**Hepatic impairment** risk of bleeding increased—reduce dose or avoid in severe impairment (including oesophageal varices)

**Renal impairment** risk of bleeding increased in severe impairment—dose may need to be reduced

**Pregnancy** does not cross the placenta; maternal osteoporosis reported after prolonged use; multidose vials may contain benzyl alcohol—some manufacturers advise avoid; see also notes above

**Breast-feeding** not excreted in milk due to high molecular weight

**Side-effects** haemorrhage (see notes above), thrombocytopenia (see Cautions); *rarely* rebound hyperlipidaemia following unfractionated heparin withdrawal, priapism, hyperkalaemia (see Cautions), osteoporosis (risk lower with low molecular weight heparins), alopecia on prolonged use, injection-site reactions, skin necrosis, and hypersensitivity reactions (including urticaria, angioedema, and anaphylaxis)

**Licensed use** some preparations licensed for use in children

---

1. See the British Society for Haematology's Guidelines on the diagnosis and management of heparin-induced thrombocytopenia: second edition. *Br J Haematol* 2012; 159: 528-540

2

Cardiovascular system

### Indications and dose

**Maintenance of neonatal umbilical arterial catheter**

* By intravenous infusion

  **Neonate** 0.5 units/hour

**Treatment of thrombotic episodes**

* By intravenous administration

  **Neonate** initially 75 units/kg (50 units/kg if under 35 weeks postmenstrual age) *by intravenous injection*, then *by continuous intravenous infusion* 25 units/kg/hour, adjusted according to APTT

  **Child 1 month–1 year** initially 75 units/kg *by intravenous injection*, then *by continuous intravenous infusion* 25 units/kg/hour, adjusted according to APTT

  **Child 1–18 years** initially 75 units/kg *by intravenous injection*, then *by continuous intravenous infusion* 20 units/kg/hour, adjusted according to APTT

* By subcutaneous injection

  **Child 1 month–18 years** 250 units/kg twice daily, adjusted according to APTT

**Prophylaxis of thrombotic episodes**

* By subcutaneous injection

  **Child 1 month–18 years** 100 units/kg (max. 5000 units) twice daily, adjusted according to APTT

**Prevention of clotting in extracorporeal circuits** consult product literature

**Maintenance of cardiac shunts and critical stents** consult local protocol

**Administration** for *continuous intravenous infusion*, dilute with Glucose 5% or Sodium Chloride 0.9%. *Maintenance of neonatal umbilical arterial catheter*, dilute 50 units to a final volume of 50 mL with Sodium Chloride 0.45% or use ready-made bag containing 500 units in 500 mL Sodium Chloride 0.9%; infuse at 0.5 mL/hour. *Neonatal intensive care (treatment of thrombosis)*, dilute 1250 units/kg body-weight to a final volume of 50 mL with infusion fluid; an intravenous infusion rate of 1 mL/hour provides a dose of 25 units/kg/hour

**Heparin Sodium** (Non-proprietary) PoM
Injection, heparin sodium 1000 units/mL, net price 1-mL amp = 99p, 5-mL amp = £2.50, 5-mL vial = £2.50, 10-mL amp = £4.31, 20-mL amp = £7.09; 5000 units/mL, 1-mL amp = £1.94, 5-mL amp = £5.06, 5-mL vial = £5.64; 25 000 units/mL, 0.2-mL amp = £2.49, 1-mL amp = £5.13, 5-mL vial = £11.11
Excipients may include benzyl alcohol (avoid in neonates, see Excipients, p. 2)

**Heparin Calcium** (Non-proprietary) PoM
Injection, heparin calcium 25 000 units/mL, net price 0.2-mL amp = £2.61

## Low molecular weight heparins

**Dalteparin, enoxaparin,** and **tinzaparin** are low molecular weight heparins used for treatment and prophylaxis of thrombotic episodes in children (see also Heparin, p. 113). Their duration of action is longer than that of unfractionated heparin and in adults and older children *once-daily subcutaneous* dosage is sometimes possible; however, younger children require relatively higher doses (possibly due to larger volume of distribution, altered heparin pharmacokinetics, or lower plasma concentrations of antithrombin) and twice daily dosage is sometimes necessary. Low molecular weight heparins are convenient to use, especially in children with poor venous access. Routine monitoring of anti-Factor Xa activity is not usually required except in neonates; monitoring may also be necessary in severely ill children and those with renal or hepatic impairment.

**Haemorrhage** See under Heparin.

**Hepatic impairment** Reduce dose in severe impairment—risk of bleeding may be increased.

**Pregnancy** Not known to be harmful, low molecular weight heparins do not cross the placenta; see also Heparin, p. 113.

**Breast-feeding** Due to the relatively high molecular weight of these drugs and inactivation in the gastrointestinal tract, passage into breast-milk and absorption by the nursing infant are likely to be negligible; however manufacturers advise avoid.

## DALTEPARIN SODIUM

**Cautions** see under Heparin and notes above
**Contra-indications** see under Heparin
**Hepatic impairment** see notes above
**Renal impairment** risk of bleeding may be increased—dose reduction and monitoring of anti-Factor Xa may be required; unfractionated heparin may be preferable
**Pregnancy** see notes above; also multidose vial contains benzyl alcohol—manufacturer advises avoid
**Breast-feeding** see notes above
**Side-effects** see under Heparin
**Licensed use** not licensed for use in children

### Indications and dose

**Treatment of thrombotic episodes**

* By subcutaneous injection

  **Neonate** 100 units/kg twice daily

  **Child 1 month–12 years** 100 units/kg twice daily

  **Child 12–18 years** 200 units/kg (max. 18 000 units) once daily, if increased risk of bleeding reduced to 100 units/kg twice daily

**Treatment of venous thromboembolism in pregnancy**

* By subcutaneous injection

  **Child 12–18 years** early pregnancy body-weight under 50 kg, 5000 units twice daily; body-weight 50–70 kg, 6000 units twice daily; body-weight 70–90 kg, 8000 units twice daily; body-weight over 90 kg, 10 000 units twice daily

**Prophylaxis of thrombotic episodes**

* By subcutaneous injection

  **Neonate** 100 units/kg once daily

  **Child 1 month–12 years** 100 units/kg once daily

  **Child 12–18 years** 2500–5000 units once daily

**Fragmin**® (Pfizer) [PoM]

Injection (single-dose syringe), dalteparin sodium 12 500 units/mL, net price 2500-unit (0.2-mL) syringe = £1.86; 25 000 units/mL, 5000-unit (0.2-mL) syringe = £2.82, 7500-unit (0.3-mL) syringe = £4.23, 10 000-unit (0.4-mL) syringe = £5.65, 12 500-unit (0.5-mL) syringe = £7.06, 15 000-unit (0.6-mL) syringe = £8.47, 18 000-unit (0.72-mL) syringe = £10.16

Injection, dalteparin sodium 2500 units/mL (for subcutaneous or intravenous use), net price 4-mL (10 000-unit) amp = £5.12; 10 000-units/mL (for subcutaneous or intravenous use), 1-mL (10 000-unit) amp = £5.12; 25 000 units/mL (for subcutaneous use only), 4-mL (100 000-unit) vial = £48.66
**Excipients** include benzyl alcohol (in 100 000-unit/4 mL multidose vial) (avoid in neonates, see, p. 2)

Injection (graduated syringe), dalteparin sodium 10 000 units/mL, net price 1-mL (10 000-unit) syringe = £5.65

## ENOXAPARIN SODIUM

**Cautions** see under Heparin and notes above
**Contra-indications** see under Heparin
**Hepatic impairment** see notes above
**Renal impairment** risk of bleeding may be increased; reduce dose if estimated glomerular filtration rate less than 30 mL/minute/1.73 m²; monitoring of anti-Factor Xa may be required; unfractionated heparin may be preferable
**Pregnancy** see notes above; also multidose vial contains benzyl alcohol—avoid
**Breast-feeding** see notes above
**Side-effects** see under Heparin
**Licensed use** not licensed for use in children
**Indications and dose**

> Treatment of thrombotic episodes
> • By subcutaneous injection
>> **Neonate** 1.5–2 mg/kg twice daily
>> **Child 1–2 months** 1.5 mg/kg twice daily
>> **Child 2 months–18 years** 1 mg/kg twice daily

> Treatment of venous thromboembolism in pregnancy
> • By subcutaneous injection
>> **Child 12–18 years** early pregnancy body-weight under 50 kg, 40 mg (4000 units) twice daily; body-weight 50–70 kg, 60 mg (6000 units) twice daily; body-weight 70–90 kg, 80 mg (8000 units) twice daily; body-weight over 90 kg, 100 mg (10 000 units) twice daily

> Prophylaxis of thrombotic episodes
> • By subcutaneous injection
>> **Neonate** 750 micrograms/kg twice daily
>> **Child 1–2 months** 750 micrograms/kg twice daily
>> **Child 2 months–18 years** 500 micrograms/kg twice daily; max. 40 mg daily

**Clexane**® (Sanofi-Aventis) [PoM]

Injection, enoxaparin sodium 100 mg/mL, net price 20-mg (0.2-mL, 2000-units) syringe = £3.03, 40-mg (0.4-mL, 4000-units) syringe = £4.04, 60-mg (0.6-mL, 6000-units) syringe = £4.57, 80-mg (0.8-mL, 8000-units) syringe = £6.49, 100-mg (1-mL,

10 000-units) syringe = £8.04, 300-mg (3-mL, 30 000-units) vial (*Clexane*® *Multi-Dose*) = £21.33; 150 mg/mL (*Clexane*® *Forte*), 120-mg (0.8-mL, 12 000-units) syringe = £9.77, 150-mg (1-mL, 15 000-units) syringe = £11.10
**Excipients** include benzyl alcohol (in 300 mg multidose vials) (avoid in neonates, see, p. 2)

## TINZAPARIN SODIUM

**Cautions** see under Heparin and notes above
**Contra-indications** see under Heparin
**Hepatic impairment** see notes above
**Renal impairment** risk of bleeding may be increased—monitoring of anti-Factor Xa may be required if estimated glomerular filtration rate less than 30 mL/minute/1.73m²; dose reduction may be required if estimated glomerular filtration rate less than 20 mL/minute/1.73m²; unfractionated heparin may be preferable
**Pregnancy** see notes above; also vials contain benzyl alcohol—manufacturer advises avoid
**Breast-feeding** see notes above
**Side-effects** see under Heparin; also *less commonly* headache
**Licensed use** not licensed for use in children
**Indications and dose**

> Treatment of thrombotic episodes
> • By subcutaneous injection
>> **Child 1–2 months** 275 units/kg once daily
>> **Child 2 months–1 year** 250 units/kg once daily
>> **Child 1–5 years** 240 units/kg once daily
>> **Child 5–10 years** 200 units/kg once daily
>> **Child 10–18 years** 175 units/kg once daily

> Treatment of venous thromboembolism in pregnancy
> • By subcutaneous injection
>> **Child 12–18 years** 175 units/kg once daily (based on early pregnancy body-weight)

> Prophylaxis of thrombotic episodes
> • By subcutaneous injection
>> **Child 1 month–18 years** 50 units/kg once daily

**Innohep**® (LEO) [PoM]

Injection, tinzaparin sodium 10 000 units/mL, net price 2500-unit (0.25-mL) syringe = £1.98, 3500-unit (0.35-mL) syringe = £2.77, 4500-unit (0.45-mL) syringe = £3.56, 20 000-unit (2-mL) vial = £10.56

Injection, tinzaparin sodium 20 000 units/mL, net price 0.5-mL (10 000-unit) syringe = £8.46, 0.7-mL (14 000-unit) syringe = £11.85, 0.9-mL (18 000-unit) syringe = £15.23, 2-mL (40 000-unit) vial = £34.20
**Excipients** include benzyl alcohol (in vials) (avoid in neonates, see Excipients, p. 2), sulfites (in 20 000 units/mL vial and syringe)

## Heparinoids

**Danaparoid** is a heparinoid that has a role in children who develop heparin-induced thrombocytopenia, providing they have no evidence of cross-reactivity.

## DANAPAROID SODIUM

**Cautions** recent bleeding or risk of bleeding; concomitant use of drugs that increase risk of bleeding; antibodies to heparins (risk of antibody-induced thrombocytopenia)

**Contra-indications** haemophilia and other haemorrhagic disorders, thrombocytopenia (unless patient has heparin-induced thrombocytopenia), recent cerebral haemorrhage, severe hypertension, active peptic ulcer (unless this is the reason for operation), diabetic retinopathy, acute bacterial endocarditis, spinal or epidural anaesthesia with treatment doses of danaparoid

**Hepatic impairment** caution in moderate impairment (increased risk of bleeding); avoid in severe impairment unless the child has heparin-induced thrombocytopenia and no alternative available

**Renal impairment** use with caution in moderate impairment; increased risk of bleeding (monitor anti-Factor Xa activity); avoid in severe impairment unless child has heparin-induced thrombocytopenia and no alternative available

**Pregnancy** manufacturer advises avoid—limited information available but not known to be harmful

**Breast-feeding** amount probably too small to be harmful but manufacturer advises avoid

**Side-effects** haemorrhage; hypersensitivity reactions (including rash)

**Licensed use** not licensed for use in children

**Indications and dose**

> **Thromboembolic disease in children with history of heparin-induced thrombocytopenia**
>
> • By intravenous administration
>
> **Neonate** initially 30 units/kg *by intravenous injection* then *by continuous intravenous infusion* 1.2–2 units/kg/hour adjusted according to coagulation activity
>
> **Child 1 month–16 years** initially 30 units/kg (max. 1250 units if body-weight under 55 kg, 2500 units if over 55 kg) *by intravenous injection* then *by continuous intravenous infusion* 1.2–2 units/kg/hour adjusted according to coagulation activity
>
> **Child 16–18 years** initially 2500 units (1250 units if body-weight under 55 kg, 3750 units if over 90 kg) *by intravenous injection* then *by continuous intravenous infusion* 400 units/hour for 2 hours, *then* 300 units/hour for 2 hours, *then* 200 units/hour for 5 days adjusted according to coagulation activity

**Administration** for *intravenous infusion*, dilute with Glucose 5% *or* Sodium Chloride 0.9%

**Organan®** (Organon) [PoM]
Injection, danaparoid sodium 1250 units/mL, net price 0.6-mL amp (750 units) = £26.68

## Heparin flushes

The use of heparin flushes should be kept to a minimum. For maintaining patency of peripheral venous catheters, sodium chloride 0.9% injection is as effective as heparin flushes. The role of heparin flushes in maintaining patency of arterial and central venous catheters is unclear.

**Heparin Sodium** (Non-proprietary) [PoM]
Solution, heparin sodium 10 units/mL, net price 5-mL amp = £1.00; 100 units/mL, 2-mL amp = £1.05
**Excipients** may include benzyl alcohol (avoid in neonates, see Excipients, p. 2)

## Epoprostenol

Epoprostenol (prostacyclin) can be given to inhibit platelet aggregation during renal dialysis when heparins are unsuitable or contra-indicated. For its use in pulmonary hypertension, see section 2.5.1.2. It is a potent vasodilator and therefore its side-effects include flushing, headache, and hypotension.

## 2.8.2 Oral anticoagulants

Oral anticoagulants antagonise the effects of vitamin K and take at least 48 to 72 hours for the anticoagulant effect to develop fully; if an immediate effect is required, unfractionated or low molecular weight heparin must be given concomitantly.

**Uses** Warfarin is the drug of choice for the treatment of systemic thromboembolism in children (not neonates) after initial heparinisation. It may also be used occasionally for the treatment of intravascular or intracardiac thrombi. Warfarin is used prophylactically in those with chronic atrial fibrillation, dilated cardiomyopathy, certain forms of reconstructive heart surgery, mechanical prosthetic heart valves, and some forms of hereditary thrombophilia (e.g. homozygous protein C deficiency).

Unfractionated or a low molecular weight heparin (section 2.8.1) is usually preferred for the prophylaxis of venous thromboembolism in children undergoing surgery; alternatively warfarin can be continued in selected children currently taking warfarin and who are at a high risk of thromboembolism (seek expert advice).

**Dose** The base-line prothrombin time should be determined but the initial dose should not be delayed whilst awaiting the result.

An induction dose is usually given over 4 days (see under Warfarin Sodium below). The subsequent maintenance dose depends on the prothrombin time, reported as INR (international normalised ratio) and should be taken at the same time each day.

**Target INR** The following indications and target INRs[1] for **adults** take into account recommendations of the British Society for Haematology[2]:

INR 2.5 for:

• treatment of deep-vein thrombosis or pulmonary embolism (including those associated with antiphospholipid syndrome or for recurrence in patients no longer receiving warfarin)

• atrial fibrillation

• cardioversion—target INR should be achieved at least 3 weeks before cardioversion and anticoagulation should continue for at least 4 weeks after the procedure (higher target values, such as an

---

1. An INR which is within 0.5 units of the target value is generally satisfactory; larger deviations require dosage adjustment. Target values (rather than ranges) are now recommended.
2. Guidelines on Oral Anticoagulation with Warfarin—fourth edition. *Br J Haematol* 2011; **154**: 311–324.

INR of 3, can be used for up to 4 weeks before the procedure to avoid cancellations due to low INR)

- dilated cardiomyopathy

- mitral stenosis or regurgitation in patients with either atrial fibrillation, a history of systemic embolism, a left atrial thrombus, or an enlarged left atrium

- bioprosthetic heart valves in the mitral position (treat for 3 months), or in patients with a history of systemic embolism (treat for at least 3 months), or with a left atrial thrombus at surgery (treat until clot resolves), or with other risk factors (e.g. atrial fibrillation or a low ventricular ejection fraction)

- acute arterial embolism requiring embolectomy (consider long-term treatment)

- myocardial infarction;

INR 3.5 for:

- recurrent deep-vein thrombosis or pulmonary embolism in patients currently receiving anticoagulation with INR above 2;

Mechanical prosthetic heart valves:

- the recommended target INR depends on the type and location of the valve, and patient-related risk factors

- consider increasing the INR target, or adding an antiplatelet drug, if an embolic event occurs whilst anticoagulated at the target INR.

**Monitoring** It is essential that the INR be determined daily or on alternate days in early days of treatment, *then* at longer intervals (depending on response[1]) *then* up to every 12 weeks.

**Haemorrhage** The main adverse effect of all oral anticoagulants is haemorrhage. Checking the INR and omitting doses when appropriate is essential; if the anticoagulant is stopped but not reversed, the INR should be measured 2–3 days later to ensure that it is falling. The cause of an elevated INR should be investigated. The following recommendations (which take into account the recommendations of the British Society for Haematology[2]) are based on the result of the INR and whether there is major or minor bleeding; the recommendations apply to **adults** taking warfarin:

- Major bleeding—stop warfarin; give phytomenadione (vitamin K₁) 5 mg by slow intravenous injection; give dried prothrombin complex (factors II, VII, IX, and X—section 2.11) 25–50 units/kg (if dried prothrombin complex unavailable, fresh frozen plasma 15 mL/kg can be given but is less effective); recombinant factor VIIa is not recommended for emergency anticoagulation reversal

- INR > 8.0, minor bleeding—stop warfarin; give phytomenadione (vitamin K₁) 1–3 mg by slow intravenous injection; repeat dose of phytomenadione if INR still too high after 24 hours; restart warfarin when INR < 5.0

- INR > 8.0, no bleeding—stop warfarin; give phytomenadione (vitamin K₁) 1–5 mg by mouth [unlicensed use]; repeat dose of phytomenadione if INR still too high after 24 hours; restart warfarin when INR < 5.0

- INR 5.0–8.0, minor bleeding—stop warfarin; give phytomenadione (vitamin K₁) 1–3 mg by slow intravenous injection; restart warfarin when INR < 5.0

- INR 5.0–8.0, no bleeding—withhold 1 or 2 doses of warfarin and reduce subsequent maintenance dose

- Unexpected bleeding at therapeutic levels—always investigate possibility of underlying cause e.g. unsuspected renal or gastro-intestinal tract pathology

**Pregnancy** Oral anticoagulants are teratogenic and should not be given in the first trimester of pregnancy. Adolescents at risk of pregnancy should be warned of this danger since stopping warfarin before the sixth week of gestation may largely avoid the risk of fetal abnormality. Oral anticoagulants cross the placenta with risk of congenital malformations, and placental, fetal, or neonatal haemorrhage, especially during the last few weeks of pregnancy and at delivery. Therefore, if at all possible, oral anticoagulants should be avoided in pregnancy, especially in the first and third trimesters. Difficult decisions may have to be made, particularly in those with prosthetic heart valves or with a history of recurrent venous thrombosis, pulmonary embolism, or atrial fibrillation.

Babies of mothers taking warfarin at the time of delivery need to be offered immediate prophylaxis with at least 100 micrograms/kg of intramuscular phytomenadione (vitamin K₁), see section 9.6.6

**Breast-feeding** With warfarin, there is a risk of haemorrhage which is increased by vitamin-K deficiency. Warfarin is not present in milk in significant amounts and appears safe.

**Dietary differences** Infant formula is supplemented with vitamin K, which makes formula-fed infants resistant to warfarin; they may therefore need higher doses. In contrast breast milk contains low concentrations of vitamin K making breast-fed infants more sensitive to warfarin.

**Treatment booklets** Anticoagulant treatment booklets should be issued to children or their carers; these booklets include advice for children or their carers on anticoagulant treatment, an alert card to be carried by the patient at all times, and a section for recording of INR results and dosage information. In **England, Wales**, and **Northern Ireland**, they are available for purchase from:

3M Security Print and Systems Limited
Gorse Street, Chadderton
Oldham,
OL9 9QH
Tel: 0845 610 1112

GP practices can obtain supplies through their Primary Care Trust (PCT) or Agency stores. NHS Hospitals can order supplies from www.nhsforms.co.uk or by emailing nhsforms@mmm.com.

In **Scotland**, treatment booklets and starter information packs can be obtained by emailing stockorders.dppas@apsgroup.co.uk.

Electronic copies of the booklets and further advice are also available at www.npsa.nhs.uk/nrls/alerts-and-directives/alerts/anticoagulant.

---

1. Change in child's clinical condition, particularly associated with liver disease, intercurrent illness, or drug administration, necessitates more frequent testing. See also **interactions**, Appendix 1 (warfarin). Major changes in diet (especially involving salads and vegetables) and in alcohol consumption may also affect warfarin control.
2. Guidelines on Oral Anticoagulation with Warfarin—fourth edition. *Br J Haematol* 2011; **154**: 311–324.

# WARFARIN SODIUM

**Cautions** see notes above; also conditions in which risk of bleeding is increased, e.g. history of gastro-intestinal bleeding, peptic ulcer, recent surgery, recent ischaemic stroke, postpartum (delay warfarin until risk of haemorrhage is low—usually 5–7 days after delivery), bacterial endocarditis (use only if warfarin otherwise indicated); uncontrolled hypertension; concomitant use of drugs that increase risk of bleeding; avoid cranberry juice; **interactions:** Appendix 1 (warfarin)

**Contra-indications** haemorrhagic stroke; significant bleeding; avoid use within 48 hours postpartum

**Hepatic impairment** avoid in severe impairment, especially if prothrombin time already prolonged

**Renal impairment** use with caution (avoid in severe impairment)

**Pregnancy** see notes above

**Breast-feeding** see notes above

**Side-effects** haemorrhage—see notes above; also nausea, vomiting, diarrhoea, jaundice, hepatic dysfunction, pancreatitis, pyrexia, alopecia, purpura, rash, 'purple toes', skin necrosis (increased risk in patients with protein C or protein S deficiency)

**Licensed use** not licensed for use in children

**Indications and dose**

> **Treatment and prophylaxis of thrombotic episodes**
> - By mouth
>
> **Neonate (under specialist advice)** 200 micrograms/kg as a single dose on first day, reduced to 100 micrograms/kg once daily for following 3 days (but if INR still below 1.4 use 200 micrograms/kg once daily, or if INR above 3 use 50 micrograms/kg once daily, if INR above 3.5 omit dose); then adjusted according to INR, usual maintenance 100–300 micrograms/kg once daily (may need up to 400 micrograms/kg once daily especially if bottle fed—see notes above)
>
> **Child 1 month–18 years** 200 micrograms/kg (max. 10 mg) as a single dose on first day, reduced to 100 micrograms/kg (max. 5 mg) once daily for following 3 days (but if INR still below 1.4 use 200 micrograms/kg (max. 10 mg) once daily, or if INR above 3 use 50 micrograms/kg (max. 2.5 mg) once daily, or if INR above 3.5 omit dose); then adjusted according to INR, usual maintenance 100–300 micrograms/kg once daily (may need up to 400 micrograms/kg once daily especially if bottle fed—see notes above)
>
> **Note** Induction dose may need to be altered according to condition (e.g. abnormal liver function tests, cardiac failure), concomitant interacting drugs, and if baseline INR above 1.3

**Warfarin** (Non-proprietary) (PoM)

Tablets, warfarin sodium 500 micrograms (white), net price 28-tab pack = £1.49; 1 mg (brown), 28-tab pack = 93p; 3 mg (blue), 28-tab pack = 95p; 5 mg (pink), 28-tab pack = £1.03. Label: 10, anticoagulant card

**Brands include** *Marevan*®

Oral suspension, warfarin sodium 5 mg/5 mL, net price 150-mL = £90.00. Label: 10, anticoagulant card

**Protamine sulfate** is used to treat overdosage of unfractionated or low molecular weight heparin. The long half-life of low molecular weight heparins should be taken into consideration when determining the dose of protamine sulfate; the effects of low molecular weight heparins can persist for up to 24 hours after administration. Excessive doses of protamine sulfate can have an anticoagulant effect.

# PROTAMINE SULFATE

**Cautions** see above; also monitor activated partial thromboplastin time or other appropriate blood clotting parameters; if increased risk of allergic reaction to protamine (includes previous treatment with protamine or protamine insulin, allergy to fish, and adolescent males who are infertile)

**Side-effects** nausea, vomiting, lassitude, flushing, hypotension, hypertension, bradycardia, dyspnoea, rebound bleeding, back pain; hypersensitivity reactions (including angioedema, anaphylaxis) and pulmonary oedema reported

**Indications and dose**

> **Overdosage with intravenous injection or intravenous infusion of unfractionated heparin**
> - By intravenous injection (rate not exceeding 5 mg/minute)
>
> **Child 1 month–18 years** *to neutralise each 100 units of unfractionated heparin,* 1 mg if less than 30 minutes lapsed since overdose, 500–750 micrograms if 30–60 minutes lapsed, 375–500 micrograms if 60–120 minutes lapsed, 250–375 micrograms if over 120 minutes lapsed; max. 50 mg

> **Overdosage with subcutaneous injection of unfractionated heparin**
> - By intravenous injection and intravenous infusion
>
> **Child 1 month–18 years** 1 mg neutralises approx. 100 units of unfractionated heparin; give 50–100% of the total dose by *intravenous injection* (rate not exceeding 5 mg/minute), then give any remainder of dose by *intravenous infusion* over 8–16 hours; max. total dose 50 mg

> **Overdosage with subcutaneous injection of low molecular weight heparin**
> - By intermittent intravenous injection (rate not exceeding 5 mg/minute) or by continuous intravenous infusion
>
> **Child 1 month–18 years** 1 mg neutralises approx. 100 units low molecular weight heparin (consult product literature of low molecular weight heparin for details); max. 50 mg

**Administration** may be diluted if necessary with Sodium Chloride 0.9%

**Protamine Sulfate** (Non-proprietary) (PoM)

Injection, protamine sulfate 10 mg/mL, net price 5-mL amp = £1.43; 10-mL amp = £4.15

Antiplatelet drugs decrease platelet aggregation and inhibit thrombus formation in the arterial circulation, because in faster-flowing vessels, thrombi are composed mainly of platelets with little fibrin.

**Aspirin** has limited use in children because it has been associated with Reye's syndrome. Aspirin-containing preparations should not be given to children and adolescents under 16 years, unless specifically indicated, such as for Kawasaki syndrome (see below), for prophylaxis of clot formation after cardiac surgery, or for prophylaxis of stroke in children at high risk.

If aspirin causes dyspepsia, or if the child is at a high risk of gastro-intestinal bleeding, a proton pump inhibitor (section 1.3.5) or a H₂-receptor antagonist (section 1.3.1) can be added.

**Dipyridamole** is also used as an antiplatelet drug to prevent clot formation after cardiac surgery and may be used with specialist advice for treatment of persistent coronary artery aneurysms in Kawasaki syndrome.

**Kawasaki syndrome**    Initial treatment is with high-dose aspirin and a single dose of intravenous normal immunoglobulin (p. 623); this combination has an additive anti-inflammatory effect resulting in faster resolution of fever and a decreased incidence of coronary artery complications. After the acute phase, when the patient is afebrile, aspirin is continued at a lower dose to prevent coronary artery abnormalities.

---

### ■ ASPIRIN (antiplatelet)
(Acetylsalicylic Acid)

**Cautions**  asthma; uncontrolled hypertension; previous peptic ulceration (but manufacturers may advise avoidance of low-dose aspirin in history of peptic ulceration); concomitant use of drugs that increase risk of bleeding; G6PD deficiency (section 9.1.5); dehydration; **interactions:** Appendix 1 (aspirin)

**Contra-indications**  children under 16 years (risk of Reye's syndrome) unless for indications below; active peptic ulceration; haemophilia and other bleeding disorders

**Hypersensitivity**  Aspirin and other NSAIDs are **contra-indicated** in history of hypersensitivity to aspirin or any other NSAID—which includes those in whom attacks of asthma, angioedema, urticaria, or rhinitis have been precipitated by aspirin or any other NSAID

**Hepatic impairment**  avoid in severe impairment—increased risk of gastro-intestinal bleeding

**Renal impairment**  use with caution (avoid in severe impairment); sodium and water retention; deterioration in renal function; increased risk of gastro-intestinal bleeding

**Pregnancy**  use with caution during third trimester; impaired platelet function and risk of haemorrhage; delayed onset and increased duration of labour with increased blood loss; avoid analgesic doses if possible in last few weeks (low doses probably not harmful); with high doses, closure of fetal ductus arteriosus *in utero* and possibly persistent pulmonary hypertension of newborn; kernicterus in jaundiced neonates

**Breast-feeding**  avoid—possible risk of Reye's syndrome; regular use of high doses could impair platelet function and produce hypoprothrombinaemia in infant if neonatal vitamin K stores low

**Side-effects**  bronchospasm; gastro-intestinal haemorrhage (occasionally major), also other haemorrhage (e.g. subconjunctival)

**Licensed use**  not licensed for use in children under 16 years

### Indications and dose
#### Kawasaki syndrome
● By mouth

> **Neonate** initially 8 mg/kg 4 times daily for 2 weeks *or* until afebrile, followed by 5 mg/kg once daily for 6–8 weeks; if no evidence of coronary lesions after 8 weeks, discontinue treatment or seek expert advice

> **Child 1 month–12 years** initially 7.5–12.5 mg/kg 4 times daily for 2 weeks or until afebrile, then 2–5 mg/kg once daily for 6–8 weeks; if no evidence of coronary lesions after 8 weeks, discontinue treatment or seek expert advice

#### Antiplatelet, prevention of thrombus formation after cardiac surgery
● By mouth

> **Neonate** 1–5 mg/kg once daily

> **Child 1 month–12 years** 1–5 mg/kg (usual max. 75 mg) once daily

> **Child 12–18 years** 75 mg once daily

**Aspirin** (Non-proprietary) ℗ₒₘ
Dispersible tablets, aspirin 75 mg, net price 28 = 83p; 300 mg, 100-tab pack = £2.88 Label: 13, 21, 32
Tablets, e/c, aspirin 75 mg, net price 28-tab pack = 93p; 56-tab pack = £1.03; 300 mg, 100-tab pack = £5.29. Label: 5, 25, 32
Brands include *Caprin®*, *Micropirin®*
Suppositories, available from 'special-order' manufacturers or specialist importing companies, see p. 823

**Nu-Seals® Aspirin** (Alliance) ℗ₒₘ
Tablets, e/c, aspirin 75 mg, net price 56-tab pack = £3.12; 300 mg, 100-tab pack = £4.15. Label: 5, 25, 32

---

### ■ DIPYRIDAMOLE

**Cautions**  aortic stenosis, left ventricular outflow obstruction, heart failure; may exacerbate migraine; hypotension; myasthenia gravis (risk of exacerbation); concomitant use of drugs that increase risk of bleeding; coagulation disorders; **interactions:** Appendix 1 (dipyridamole)

**Pregnancy**  not known to be harmful

**Breast-feeding**  manufacturers advise use only if essential—small amount present in milk

**Side-effects**  gastro-intestinal effects, dizziness, myalgia, throbbing headache, hypotension, hot flushes and tachycardia; hypersensitivity reactions such as rash, urticaria, severe bronchospasm and angioedema; increased bleeding during or after surgery; thrombocytopenia reported

**Licensed use**  not licensed for use in children

### Indications and dose
#### Kawasaki syndrome
● By mouth

> **Child 1 month–12 years** 1 mg/kg 3 times daily

#### Prevention of thrombus formation after cardiac surgery
● By mouth

> **Child 1 month–12 years** 2.5 mg/kg twice daily

> **Child 12–18 years** 100–200 mg 3 times daily

**Administration**  injection solution can be given orally

**2 Cardiovascular system**

**2 Cardiovascular system**

**Dipyridamole** (Non-proprietary) PoM
Tablets, coated, dipyridamole 25 mg, net price 84 = £3.11; 100 mg, 84 = £2.80. Label: 22

Oral suspension, dipyridamole 50 mg/5 ml, net price 150 mL = £40.63

**Persantin**® (Boehringer Ingelheim) PoM
Tablets, s/c, dipyridamole, 100 mg, net price 84-tab pack = £4.16. Label: 22

Injection, dipyridamole 5 mg/mL, net price 2-mL amp = 12p

## 2.10 Myocardial infarction and fibrinolysis

2.10.1 Management of myocardial infarction

2.10.2 Fibrinolytic drugs

## 2.10.1 Management of myocardial infarction

This section is not included in *BNF for Children*.

## 2.10.2 Fibrinolytic drugs

Fibrinolytic drugs act as thrombolytics by activating plasminogen to form plasmin, which degrades fibrin and so breaks up thrombi.

**Alteplase**, **streptokinase**, and **urokinase** are used in children to dissolve intravascular thrombi and unblock occluded arteriovenous shunts, catheters, and indwelling central lines blocked with fibrin clots. Treatment should be started as soon as possible after a clot has formed and discontinued once a pulse in the affected limb is detected, or the shunt or catheter unblocked.

The safety and efficacy of treatment remains uncertain, especially in neonates. A fibrinolytic drug is probably only appropriate where arterial occlusion threatens ischaemic damage; an anticoagulant may stop the clot getting bigger. Alteplase is the preferred fibrinolytic in children and neonates; there is less risk of adverse effects including allergic reactions.

**Cautions**   Thrombolytic drugs should be used with caution if there is a risk of bleeding including that from venepuncture or invasive procedures. They should also be used with caution in conditions with an increased risk of haemorrhage, or where there has been recent or concomitant use of drugs that increase the risk of bleeding.

**Contra-indications**   Thrombolytic drugs are contra-indicated in recent haemorrhage, trauma, or surgery (including dental extraction), coagulation defects, bleeding diatheses, severe hypertension, arteriovenous malformation, aneurysm, neoplasm with risk of haemorrhage, pericarditis, bacterial endocarditis, and acute pancreatitis.

Prolonged persistence of antibodies to streptokinase can reduce the effectiveness of subsequent treatment; therefore, streptokinase should not be used again beyond 4 days of first administration. Streptokinase should also be avoided in children who have had streptococcal infection in the last 12 months.

**Hepatic impairment**   Thrombolytic drugs should be avoided in severe hepatic impairment as there is an increased risk of bleeding.

**Pregnancy**   Thrombolytic drugs can possibly lead to premature separation of the placenta in the first 18 weeks of pregnancy. There is also a risk of maternal haemorrhage throughout pregnancy and post-partum, and also a theoretical risk of fetal haemorrhage throughout pregnancy.

**Side-effects**   Side-effects of thrombolytics are mainly bleeding, nausea, and vomiting. Reperfusion can cause cerebral and pulmonary oedema. Hypotension can also occur and can usually be controlled by elevating the patient's legs, or by reducing the rate of infusion or stopping it temporarily. Back pain, fever, and convulsions have been reported. Bleeding is usually limited to the site of injection, but intracerebral haemorrhage or bleeding from other sites can occur. Serious bleeding calls for discontinuation of the thrombolytic and may require administration of coagulation factors and antifibrinolytic drugs (e.g. tranexamic acid). Thrombolytics can cause allergic reactions (including rash, flushing and uveitis) and anaphylaxis has been reported (for details of management see Allergic Emergencies, section 3.4.3). Guillain-Barré syndrome has been reported rarely after streptokinase treatment.

### ALTEPLASE
(rt-PA, tissue-type plasminogen activator)

**Cautions**   see notes above

**Contra-indications**   see notes above; also recent ulcerative gastro-intestinal disease; oesophageal varices; stroke; concomitant treatment with oral anticoagulants; recent delivery

**Hepatic impairment**   see notes above

**Pregnancy**   see notes above

**Side-effects**   see notes above; also risk of cerebral bleeding increased in acute stroke

**Licensed use**   *Actilyse*® not licensed for use in children

**Indications and dose**

See under preparations, below

**Actilyse**® (Boehringer Ingelheim) PoM
Injection, powder for reconstitution, alteplase 10 mg (5.8 million units)/vial, net price per vial (with diluent) = £120.00; 20 mg (11.6 million units)/vial (with diluent and transfer device) = £180.00; 50 mg (29 million units)/vial (with diluent and transfer device) = £300.00

**Dose**

**Intravascular thrombosis** doses may vary—consult local guidelines

• **By intravenous infusion**

**Neonate** 100–500 micrograms/kg/hour for 3–6 hours; use ultrasound assessment to monitor effect before considering a second course of treatment

**Child 1 month–18 years** 100–500 micrograms/kg/hour for 3–6 hours; max. 100 mg total daily dose; use ultrasound assessment to monitor effect before considering a second course of treatment

**Administration** for *intravenous infusion*, dissolve in Water for Injections to a concentration of 1 mg/mL or 2 mg/mL and infuse intravenously; alternatively dilute further in Sodium Chloride 0.9% to a concentraton of not less than 200 micrograms/mL; not to be diluted in Glucose

**Actlyse Cathflo**® (Boehringer Ingelheim) [PoM]
Injection, powder for reconstitution, alteplase 2 mg
(1.16 million units)/vial, net price vial (with diluent)
= £45.00

**Dose**

**Thrombolytic treatment of occluded central venous access devices (including those used for haemodialysis)** consult product literature

## ◢ STREPTOKINASE

**Cautions** see notes above; also cerebrovascular disease; mitral valve defect; atrial fibrillation; septic thrombotic disease; cavernous pulmonary disease; recent delivery or abortion

**Contra-indications** see notes above; also concomitant treatment with oral anticoagulants

**Hepatic impairment** see notes above

**Pregnancy** see notes above

**Side-effects** see notes above

**Licensed use** not licensed for use in children under 18 years

**Indications and dose**

Intravascular thrombosis

• By intravenous infusion

**Child 1 month–12 years** initially 2500–4000 units/ kg over 30 minutes, followed by *continuous intravenous infusion* of 500–1000 units/kg/hour for up to 3 days until reperfusion occurs

**Child 12–18 years** initially 250 000 units over 30 minutes, followed by *continuous intravenous infusion* of 100 000 units/hour for up to 3 days until reperfusion occurs

**Administration** reconstitute with Sodium Chloride 0.9%, then dilute further with Glucose 5% or Sodium Chloride 0.9% after reconstitution. Monitor fibrinogen concentration closely; if fibrinogen concentration less than 1 g/litre, stop streptokinase infusion and start unfractionated heparin; restart streptokinase once fibrinogen concentration reaches 1 g/litre

**Streptase**® (CSL Behring) [PoM]
Injection, powder for reconstitution, streptokinase, net price 250 000-unit vial = £15.91; 1.5 million-unit vial = £83.44 (hosp. only)

## ◢ UROKINASE

**Cautions** see notes above; also severe cerebrovascular disease; mitral valve defect; atrial fibrillation; septic thrombotic disease; cavernous pulmonary disease; recent delivery

**Contra-indications** see notes above; also recent stroke; concomitant treatment with oral anticoagulants or heparin

**Hepatic impairment** see notes above

**Pregnancy** see notes above

**Side-effects** see notes above

**Indications and dose**

Occluded arteriovenous shunts, catheters, and indwelling central lines

• By injection directly into catheter or central line

**Neonate** 5000–25 000 units in sodium chloride 0.9% to fill catheter dead-space **only**; leave for 20–60 minutes then aspirate the lysate; flush with sodium chloride 0.9%

**Child 1 month–18 years** 5000–25 000 units in sodium chloride 0.9% to fill catheter dead-space **only**; leave for 20–60 minutes then aspirate the lysate; flush with sodium chloride 0.9%

**Administration** may be diluted, after reconstitution, with Sodium Chloride 0.9%

**Urokinase** (Non-Proprietary) [PoM]
Injection, powder for reconstitution, urokinase, net price 10 000-unit vial = £33.79; 50 000-unit vial = £69.70; 100 000-unit vial = £106.17; 250 000-unit vial = £185.65; 500 000-unit vial = £365.00

**Syner-KINASE**® (Syner-Med) [PoM]
Injection, powder for reconstitution, urokinase, net price 10 000-unit vial = £35.95; 25 000-unit vial = £45.95; 100 000-unit vial = £112.95

## 2.11 Antifibrinolytic drugs and haemostatics

Fibrin dissolution can be impaired by the administration of **tranexamic acid**, which inhibits fibrinolysis. It can be used to prevent bleeding or treat bleeding associated with excessive fibrinolysis (e.g. in surgery, dental extraction, obstetric disorders, and traumatic hyphaema) and in the management of menorrhagia; it may also be used in hereditary angioedema (section 3.4.3), epistaxis, and thrombolytic overdose. Tranexamic acid can also be used in cardiac surgery to reduce blood loss and to reduce the need for use of blood products.

**Desmopressin** (section 6.5.2) is used in the management of mild to moderate haemophilia and von Willebrands' disease. It is also used for testing fibrinolytic response.

## ◢ TRANEXAMIC ACID

**Cautions** massive haematuria (avoid if risk of ureteric obstruction); before initiating treatment for menorrhagia, exclude structural or histological causes or fibroids causing distortion of uterine cavity; irregular menstrual bleeding (establish cause before initiating therapy); patients receiving oral contraceptives (increased risk of thrombosis); regular liver function tests in long-term treatment of hereditary angioedema

**Contra-indications** thromboembolic disease; fibrinolytic conditions following disseminated intravascular coagulation (unless predominant activation of fibrinolytic system with severe bleeding); history of convulsions

**Renal impairment** reduce dose in mild to moderate impairment; avoid in severe impairment

**Pregnancy** no evidence of teratogenicity in *animal* studies; manufacturer advises use only if potential benefit outweighs risk—crosses the placenta

**Breast-feeding** small amount present in milk—antifibrinolytic effect in infant unlikely

**2**

**Cardiovascular system**

Side-effects nausea, vomiting, diarrhoea (reduce dose); *less commonly* dermatitis; *rarely* thromboembolic events, visual disturbances including impairment of colour vision (discontinue); *also reported* malaise and hypotension on rapid intravenous injection, convulsions (usually with high doses)

**Licensed use** not licensed for reduction of blood loss during cardiac surgery; injection not licensed for use in children under 1 year or for administration by intravenous infusion

### Indications and dose

Inhibition of fibrinolysis, hereditary angioedema
- By mouth

  **Child 1 month–18 years** 15–25 mg/kg (max. 1.5 g) 2–3 times daily
- By intravenous injection over at least 10 minutes

  **Child 1 month–18 years** 10 mg/kg (max. 1 g) 2–3 times daily
- By continuous intravenous infusion

  **Child 1 month–18 years** 45 mg/kg over 24 hours

Prevention of excessive bleeding after dental procedures (e.g. in haemophilia)
- By intravenous injection pre-operatively

  **Child 6–18 years** 10 mg/kg (max. 1.5 g)
- By mouth pre-operatively

  **Child 6–18 years** 15–25 mg/kg (max. 1.5 g)
- By mouth postoperatively

  **Child 6–18 years** 15–25 mg/kg (max. 1.5 g) 2–3 times daily for up to 8 days
- Mouthwash 5% solution (specialist use only)

  **Child 6–18 years** rinse mouth with 5–10 mL 4 times daily for 2 days; not to be swallowed

  Note Mouthwash available only as extemporaneously prepared preparation, see Extemporaneous Preparations, p. 6

Menorrhagia
- By mouth

  **Child 12–18 years** 1 g 3 times daily for up to 4 days; max. 4 g daily (initiate when menstruation has started)

Reduction of blood loss during cardiac surgery
consult local protocol

**Administration** for *intravenous administration*, dilute with Glucose 5% *or* Sodium Chloride 0.9%

**Tranexamic acid** (Non-proprietary) PoM
Tablets, tranexamic acid 500 mg, net price 60-tab pack = £5.27

**Cyklokapron**® (Meda) PoM
Tablets, f/c, scored, tranexamic acid 500 mg, net price 60-tab pack = £14.30

**Cyklokapron**® (Pfizer) PoM
Injection, tranexamic acid 100 mg/mL, net price 5-mL amp = £1.55

## Blood products

These products should be used on the advice of a haematologist.

## DRIED PROTHROMBIN COMPLEX
(Human Prothrombin Complex)

Dried prothrombin complex is prepared from human plasma by a suitable fractionation technique, and contains factor IX, together with variable amounts of factors II, VII, and X

**Cautions** risk of thrombosis; disseminated intravascular coagulation; history of myocardial infarction or coronary heart disease; postoperative use; vaccination against hepatitis A (p. 608) and hepatitis B (p. 610) may be required

**Contra-indications** angina; recent myocardial infarction (except in life-threatening haemorrhage following overdosage of oral anticoagulants, and before induction of fibrinolytic therapy); history of heparin-induced thrombocytopenia

**Hepatic impairment** monitor closely (risk of thromboembolic complications)

**Side-effects** thrombotic events (including disseminated intravascular coagulation); *rarely* headache; *very rarely* pyrexia, antibody formation, hypersensitivity reactions (including anaphylaxis); nephrotic syndrome also reported

### Indications and dose

Treatment and peri-operative prophylaxis of haemorrhage in congenital deficiency of factors II, VII, IX, or X if purified specific coagulation factors not available, treatment and peri-operative prophylaxis of haemorrhage in acquired deficiency of factors II, VII, IX, or X (e.g. during warfarin treatment—see section 2.8.2)

Consult haematologist

Available from CSL Behring (*Beriplex*® *P/N*), Octapharma (*Octaplex*®)

## FACTOR VIIa (RECOMBINANT)
Eptacog alfa (activated)

**Cautions** risk of thrombosis or disseminated intravascular coagulation

**Side-effects** *very rarely* nausea, thrombotic events (including myocardial infarction and cerebrovascular accident), coagulation disorders, fever, pain, and allergic reactions including rash

### Indications and dose

Treatment and prophylaxis of haemorrhage in haemophilia A or B with inhibitors to factors VIII or IX, acquired haemophilia, factor VII deficiency, or Glanzmann's thrombasthenia

Consult haematologist

Available from Novo Nordisk (*NovoSeven*®)

## FACTOR VIII FRACTION, DRIED
(Human Coagulation Factor VIII, Dried)

Dried factor VIII fraction is prepared from human plasma by a suitable fractionation technique; it may also contain varying amounts of von Willebrand factor

**Cautions** monitor for development of factor VIII inhibitors; intravascular haemolysis after large or frequently repeated doses in patients with blood groups A, B, or AB—less likely with high potency concentrates; vaccination against hepatitis A (p. 608) and hepatitis B (p. 610) may be required (not necessary with recombinant preparation)

**Side-effects** gastro-intestinal disturbances, taste disturbances; flushing, palpitation; dyspnoea, coughing; headache, dizziness, paraesthesia, drowsiness; blurred vision; antibody formation; hypersensitivity reactions including hypotension, angioedema, chills, fever, urticaria, and anaphylaxis

**Indications and dose**

> Treatment and prophylaxis of haemorrhage in congenital factor VIII deficiency (haemophilia A), acquired factor VIII deficiency, or von Willebrand's disease
>
>> Consult haematologist

Available from Biotest UK (*Haemoctin*®), CSL Behring (*Haemate*® *P*), BPL (*Optivate*®; *8Y*®), Grifols (*Alphanate*®; *Fanhdi*®), Octapharma (*Octanate*®; *Wilate*®); *Haemoctin*®, *Optivate*®, *Fanhdi*®, and *Octanate*® are not indicated for use in von Willebrand's disease

**Note** Preparation of recombinant human coagulation factor VIII (octocog alfa) available from CSL Behring (*Helixate*® *NexGen*), Baxter (*Advate*®), Bayer (*Kogenate*® *Bayer*); preparation of recombinant human coagulation factor VIII (moroctocog alfa) available from Wyeth (*ReFacto AF*®); octocog alfa and moroctocog alfa not indicated for use in von Willebrand's disease

## FACTOR VIII INHIBITOR BYPASSING FRACTION

Preparations with factor VIII inhibitor bypassing activity are prepared from human plasma

**Cautions** vaccination against hepatitis A (p. 608) and hepatitis B (p. 610) may be required

**Contra-indications** disseminated intravascular coagulation

**Side-effects** thrombosis, disseminated intravascular coagulation, myocardial infarction; paraesthesia; pyrexia; hypersensitivity reactions including hypotension, flushing, urticaria, rash, and anaphylaxis

**Indications and dose**

> Treatment and prophylaxis of haemorrhage in congenital factor VIII deficiency (haemophilia A) and factor VIII inhibitors; treatment of haemorrhage in non-haemophiliac children with acquired factor VIII inhibitors
>
>> Consult haematologist

Available from Baxter (*FEIBA*®)

## FACTOR IX FRACTION, DRIED

Dried factor IX fraction is prepared from human plasma by a suitable fractionation technique; it may also contain clotting factors II, VII, and X

**Cautions** risk of thrombosis—principally with former low purity products; vaccination against hepatitis A (p. 608) and hepatitis B (p. 610) may be required (not necessary with recombinant preparation)

**Contra-indications** disseminated intravascular coagulation

**Side-effects** gastro-intestinal disturbances; headache, dizziness; allergic reactions including chills, fever

**Indications and dose**

> Treatment and prophylaxis of haemorrhage in congenital factor IX deficiency (haemophilia B)
>
>> Consult haematologist

Available from CSL Behring (*Mononine*®), BPL (*Replenine*®-*VF*, Dried Factor IX Fraction), Grifols ( *AlphaNine*®), Biotest UK (*Haemonine*®)

**Note** Preparation of recombinant coagulation factor IX (nonacog alfa) available from Pfizer (*BeneFIX*®)

## FACTOR XIII FRACTION, DRIED
(Human Fibrin-stabilising Factor, Dried)

**Cautions** vaccination against hepatitis A (p. 608) and hepatitis B (p. 610) may be required

**Side-effects** *rarely* allergic reactions and fever

**Indications and dose**

> Congenital factor XIII deficiency
>
>> Consult haematologist

Available from CSL Behring (*Fibrogammin*® *P*)

## FIBRINOGEN, DRIED
(Human Fibrinogen)

Fibrinogen is prepared from human plasma

**Cautions** risk of thrombosis

**Pregnancy** manufacturer advises not known to be harmful—no information available

**Breast-feeding** manufacturer advises avoid—no information available

**Side-effects** *rarely* fever, allergic reactions; *very rarely* thromboembolic events (including myocardial infarction and pulmonary embolism)

**Indications and dose**

> Treatment of haemorrhage in congenital hypofibrinogenaemia or afibrinogenaemia
>
>> Consult haematologist

Available from CSL Behring (*Riastap*®)

## FRESH FROZEN PLASMA

Fresh frozen plasma is prepared from the supernatant liquid obtained by centrifugation of one donation of whole blood

**Cautions** need for compatibility; cardiac decompensation; pulmonary oedema; severe protein S deficiency (avoid products with low protein S activity e.g. *Octaplas*® or *OctaplasLG*®); vaccination against hepatitis A (p. 608) and hepatitis B (p. 610) may be required

**Contra-indications** avoid use as a volume expander; IgA deficiency with confirmed antibodies to IgA

**Side-effects** nausea, rash, pruritus; *less commonly* vomiting, oedema; *rarely* tachycardia, agitation, allergic reactions (including chills, fever, bronchospasm, cardiorespiratory collapse); *very rarely* arrhythmia, thromboembolism, hypertension

**Indications and dose**

> Replacement of coagulation factors or other plasma proteins where their concentration or functional activity is critically reduced
>
>> Consult haematologist

Available from Regional Blood Transfusion Services

**Note** Children under 16 years should only receive virucidally inactivated preparations of fresh frozen plasma, sourced from 'low prevalence BSE regions' such as the USA

**Note** Preparations of solvent/detergent treated human plasma (frozen) from pooled donors are available from Octapharma (*Octaplas*®; *OctaplasLG*®)

## PROTEIN C CONCENTRATE

Protein C is prepared from human plasma

**Cautions** hypersensitivity to heparins; vaccination against hepatitis A (p. 608) and hepatitis B (p. 610) may be required

**Side-effects** *very rarely* fever, bleeding, dizziness, and hypersensitivity reactions

**Indications and dose**

> Congenital protein C deficiency
>
>> Consult haematologist

Available from Baxter (*Ceprotin*®)

**2 Cardiovascular system**

## 2.12 Lipid-regulating drugs

Atherosclerosis begins in childhood and raised serum-cholesterol in children is associated with cardiovascular disease in adulthood. Lowering the cholesterol, without hindering growth and development in children and adolescents, should reduce the risk of cardiovascular disease in later life.

The risk factors for developing cardiovascular disease include raised serum cholesterol concentration, smoking, hypertension, impaired glucose tolerance, male sex, ethnicity, obesity, triglyceride concentration, chronic kidney disease, and a family history of cardiovascular disease. Heterozygous familial hypercholesterolaemia is the most common cause of raised serum cholesterol in children; homozygous familial hypercholesterolaemia is very rare and its specialised management is not covered in *BNF for Children*. Familial hypercholesterolaemia can lead to a greater risk of early coronary heart disease and should be managed by a specialist.

Secondary causes of hypercholesterolaemia should be addressed, these include obesity, diet, diabetes mellitus, hypothyroidism (see below), nephrotic syndrome, obstructive biliary disease, glycogen storage disease, and drugs such as corticosteroids.

**Management**   The aim of management of hypercholesterolaemia is to reduce the risk of atherosclerosis while ensuring adequate growth and development. Children with hypercholesterolaemia (or their carers) should receive advice on appropriate lifestyle changes such as improved diet, increased exercise, weight reduction, and not smoking; hypertension should also be managed appropriately (section 2.5). Drug therapy may also be necessary and is discussed below.

**Hypothyroidism**   Children with hypothyroidism should receive adequate thyroid replacement therapy before their requirement for lipid-regulating treatment is assessed because correction of hypothyroidism itself may resolve the lipid abnormality. Untreated hypothyroidism increases the risk of myositis with lipid-regulating drugs.

**Drug treatment in heterozygous familial hypercholesterolaemia**   Lifestyle modifications alone are unlikely to lower cholesterol concentration adequately in heterozygous familial hypercholesterolaemia and drug treatment is often required. Lipid-regulating drugs should be considered by the age of 10 years. The decision to initiate drug treatment will depend on the child's age, the age of onset of coronary heart disease within the family, and the presence of other cardiovascular risk factors. In children with a family history of coronary heart disease in early adulthood, drug treatment before the age of 10 years, and a combination of lipid-regulating drugs may be necessary.

**Drug treatment in secondary hypercholesterolaemia**   If 6–12 months of dietary and other lifestyle interventions has failed to lower cholesterol concentration adequately, drug treatment may be indicated in children 10 years and older (rarely necessary in younger children) who are at a high risk of developing cardiovascular disease.

**Choice of drugs**   Experience in the use of lipid-regulating drugs in children is limited and they should be initiated on specialist advice.

Statins are the drugs of first choice in children and are generally well tolerated; atorvastatin and simvastatin are the preferred statins. Other lipid-regulating drugs can be used if statins are ineffective or are not tolerated.

**Ezetimibe** can be used alone when statins are not tolerated, or in combination with a statin when a high-dose statin fails to control cholesterol concentration adequately.

**Bile acid sequestrants** are also available but tolerability of and compliance with these drugs is poor, and their use is declining.

Evidence for the use of a fibrate (**bezafibrate** or **fenofibrate**) in children is limited; fibrates should be considered only if dietary intervention and treatment with a statin and a bile acid sequestrant is unsuccessful or contra-indicated.

In hypertriglyceridaemia which cannot be controlled by very strict diet, omega-3 fatty acid compounds can be considered.

## Statins

The statins (**atorvastatin**, **fluvastatin**, **pravastatin**, **rosuvastatin** and **simvastatin**) competitively inhibit 3-hydroxy-3-methylglutaryl coenzyme A (HMG CoA) reductase, an enzyme involved in cholesterol synthesis, especially in the liver. They are more effective than other classes of drugs in lowering LDL-cholesterol but less effective than the fibrates in reducing triglycerides. Statins also increase concentrations of HDL-cholesterol.

Statins reduce cardiovascular disease events and total mortality in adults, irrespective of the initial cholesterol concentration.

**Cautions**   Hypothyroidism should be managed adequately before starting treatment with a statin (see Hypothyroidism, above). Statins should be used with caution in those with a history of liver disease or with a high alcohol intake—see also Hepatic Impairment, below. There is little information available on a rational approach to liver-function monitoring; however, a NICE guideline[1] suggests that liver enzymes should be measured before treatment, and repeated within 3 months and at 12 months of starting treatment, unless indicated at other times by signs or symptoms suggestive of hepatotoxicity. Those with serum transaminases that are raised, but less than 3 times the upper limit of the reference range, should **not** be routinely excluded from statin therapy. Those with serum transaminases of more than 3 times the upper limit of the reference range should discontinue statin therapy. Statins should be used with caution in those with risk factors for myopathy or rhabdomyolysis; children or their carers should be advised to report unexplained muscle pain (see Muscle Effects below). Creatine kinase concentration should be measured in children before treatment and if unexplained muscle pain occurs. Statins should be avoided in acute porphyria (section 9.8.2). **Interactions**: Appendix 1 (statins).

**Hepatic impairment**   Statins should be used with caution in those with a history of liver disease and avoided in active liver disease or when there are unexplained persistent elevations in serum transaminases.

1. NICE clinical guideline 67 (May 2008). Lipid Modification—Cardiovascular risk assessment and the modification of blood lipids for the primary and secondary prevention of cardiovascular disease

**Pregnancy** Statins should be avoided in pregnancy as congenital anomalies have been reported and the decreased synthesis of cholesterol possibly affects fetal development. Adequate contraception is required during treatment and for 1 month afterwards.

**Breast-feeding** The manufacturers of atorvastatin, fluvastatin, rosuvastatin, and simvastatin advise avoiding use in mothers who are breast-feeding as there is no information available. The manufacturers of pravastatin advise against use in breast-feeding mothers as a small amount of drug is present in breast milk.

**Side-effects** The statins have been associated with myalgia, myopathy, myositis, and rhabdomyolysis (see Muscle Effects below). Statins can alter liver function tests, and rarely cause hepatitis and jaundice; pancreatitis and hepatic failure have been reported very rarely. Other side-effects include gastro-intestinal disturbances, sleep disturbance, headache, dizziness, depression, paraesthesia, asthenia, peripheral neuropathy, amnesia, fatigue, sexual dysfunction, thrombocytopenia, arthralgia, visual disturbance, alopecia, and hypersensitivity reactions (including rash, pruritus, urticaria, and very rarely lupus erythematosus-like reactions). In very rare cases, statins can cause interstitial lung disease; if children develop symptoms such as dyspnoea, cough, and weight loss, they should seek medical attention. Statins can cause hyperglycaemia and may be associated with the development of diabetes mellitus, particularly in those already at risk of the condition.

Muscle effects The risk of myopathy, myositis, and rhabdomyolysis associated with statin use is rare. Although myalgia has been reported commonly in those receiving statins, muscle toxicity truly attributable to statin use is rare. Muscle toxicity can occur with all statins, however the likelihood increases with higher doses and in certain individuals (see below). Statins should be used with caution in children at increased risk of muscle toxicity, including those with a personal or family history of muscular disorders, previous history of muscular toxicity, a high alcohol intake, renal impairment, or hypothyroidism. There is an increased incidence of myopathy if a statin is given at a high dose, or if it is given with a fibrate (the combination of a statin and gemfibrozil should preferably be avoided), with lipid-lowering doses of nicotinic acid, with fusidic acid (risk of rhabdomyolysis—the combination of a statin and fusidic acid should be avoided; temporarily discontinue statin and restart 7 days after last fusidic acid dose), or with drugs that increase the plasma-statin concentration, such as macrolide antibiotics, imidazole and triazole antifungals, and ciclosporin—see **interactions**: Appendix 1 (statins); close monitoring of liver function and, if muscular symptoms occur, of creatine kinase is necessary. In children at increased risk of muscle effects, a statin should not usually be started if the baseline creatine kinase concentration is more than 5 times the upper limit of normal (some children may present with an extremely elevated baseline creatine kinase concentration, due to e.g. rigorous exercise—specialist advice should be sought regarding consideration of statin therapy in these children.

If muscular symptoms or raised creatine kinase occur during treatment, other possible causes (e.g. rigorous physical activity, hypothyroidism, infection, recent trauma, and drug or alcohol addiction) should be excluded before statin therapy is implicated. When a statin is suspected to be the cause of myopathy, and creatine kinase concentration is markedly elevated (more than 5 times upper limit of normal), or if muscular symptoms are severe, treatment should be discontinued. If symptoms resolve and creatine kinase concentrations return to normal, the statin should be reintroduced at a lower dose and the child monitored closely; an alternative statin should be prescribed if unacceptable side-effects are experienced with a particular statin. Statins should not be discontinued in the event of small, asymptomatic elevations of creatine kinase. Routine monitoring of creatine kinase is unnecessary in asymptomatic children.

**Counselling** Advise children or their carers to report promptly unexplained muscle pain, tenderness, or weakness.

## ATORVASTATIN

**Cautions** see notes above; also haemorrhagic stroke

**Hepatic impairment** see notes above

**Pregnancy** see notes above

**Breast-feeding** see notes above

**Side-effects** see notes above; also nasopharyngitis, epistaxis, pharyngeolaryngeal pain, back pain, hyperglycaemia; *less commonly* blurred vision, pyrexia, anorexia, malaise, chest pain, weight gain, hypoglycaemia, tinnitus, peripheral oedema, neck pain; *rarely* cholestasis, Stevens-Johnson syndrome, toxic epidermal necrolysis; *very rarely* gynaecomastia, hearing loss

**Indications and dose**

Hyperlipidaemia including familial hypercholesterolaemia

- By mouth

    **Child 10–18 years** initially 10 mg once daily, increased if necessary at intervals of at least 4 weeks to usual max. 20 mg once daily (max. 80 mg once daily in homozygous familial hypercholesterolaemia)

    **Note** Reduced dose required (max. 10 mg daily) with concomitant ciclosporin, or tipranavir combined with ritonavir—seek specialist advice (see also Appendix 1)

**Atorvastatin** (Non-proprietary) PoM

Tablets, atorvastatin (as calcium trihydrate) 10 mg, net price 28-tab pack = £1.89; 20 mg, 28-tab pack = £2.71; 40 mg, 28-tab pack = £2.90; 80 mg, 28-tab pack = £6.07. Counselling, muscle effects, see notes above

**Lipitor®** (Pfizer) PoM

Chewable tablets ▼, atorvastatin (as calcium trihydrate) 10 mg, net price 30-tab pack = £13.80; 20 mg, 30-tab pack = £26.40. Label: 24, counselling, muscle effects, see notes above

Tablets, all f/c, atorvastatin (as calcium trihydrate) 10 mg, net price 28-tab pack = £13.00; 20 mg, 28-tab pack = £24.64; 40 mg, 28-tab pack = £24.64; 80 mg, 28-tab pack = £28.21. Counselling, muscle effects, see notes above

## FLUVASTATIN

**Cautions** see notes above

**Hepatic impairment** see notes above

**Renal impairment** manufacturer advises doses above 40 mg daily should be initiated with caution if estimated glomerular filtration rate is less than 30 mL/minute/1.73 m$^2$

**Pregnancy** see notes above

**Breast-feeding** see notes above

**Side-effects** see notes above; also *very rarely* vasculitis

**Indications and dose**

Heterozygous familial hypercholesterolaemia

- By mouth

    **Child 9–18 years** initially 20 mg daily in the evening, adjusted in steps of 20 mg daily at intervals of at least 6 weeks; max. 80 mg daily (40 mg twice daily)

**2 Cardiovascular system**

**Fluvastatin** (Non-proprietary) PoM
Capsules, fluvastatin (as sodium salt) 20 mg, net price 28-cap pack = £5.03; 40 mg, 28-cap pack = £5.36. Counselling, muscle effects, see notes above

**Lescol**® (Novartis) PoM
Capsules, fluvastatin (as sodium salt) 20 mg (brown/yellow), net price 28-cap pack = £15.26; 40 mg (brown/orange), 28-cap pack = £15.26, 56-cap pack = £30.53. Counselling, muscle effects, see notes above

◢ **Modified release**

**Fluvastatin** (Non-proprietary) PoM
Tablets, m/r, fluvastatin (as sodium salt) 80 mg, net price 28-tab pack = £19.20. Label: 25, counselling, muscle effects, see notes above

**Dose**

> **Child 9–18 years** 80 mg once daily (dose form not appropriate for initial dose titration)

**Brands include** *Dorisin*® *XL*, *Luvinsta*® *XL*, *Pinmactil*®, *Stefluvin*® *XL*

**Lescol**® **XL** (Novartis) PoM
Tablets, m/r, yellow, fluvastatin (as sodium salt) 80 mg, net price 28-tab pack = £19.20. Label: 25, counselling, muscle effects, see notes above

**Dose**

> **Child 9–18 years** 80 mg once daily (dose form not appropriate for initial dose titration)

## ■ PRAVASTATIN SODIUM

**Cautions** see notes above
**Hepatic impairment** see notes above
**Renal impairment** start with lower doses in moderate to severe impairment
**Pregnancy** see notes above
**Breast-feeding** see notes above
**Side-effects** see notes above; *less commonly* abnormal urination (including dysuria, nocturia, and frequency); *very rarely* fulminant hepatic necrosis

**Indications and dose**

> Hyperlipidaemia including familial hyper-cholesterolaemia
> • By mouth
> **Child 8–14 years** 10 mg once daily at night, adjusted at intervals of at least 4 weeks to max. 20 mg once daily at night
> **Child 14–18 years** 10 mg once daily at night, adjusted at intervals of at least 4 weeks to max. 40 mg once daily at night

**Pravastatin** (Non-proprietary) PoM
Tablets, pravastatin sodium 10 mg, net price 28-tab pack = £1.72; 20 mg, 28-tab pack = £2.02; 40 mg, 28-tab pack = £2.78. Counselling, muscle effects, see notes above

**Lipostat**® (Squibb) PoM
Tablets, all yellow, pravastatin sodium 10 mg, net price 28-tab pack = £14.18; 20 mg, 28-tab pack = £26.01; 40 mg, 28-tab pack = £26.01. Counselling, muscle effects, see notes above

## ■ ROSUVASTATIN

**Cautions** see notes above; children of Asian origin; use lower max. dose in children with risk factors for myopathy or rhabdomyolysis (including personal or family history of muscular disorders or toxicity)
**Hepatic impairment** see notes above
**Renal impairment** reduce dose if estimated glomerular filtration rate less than 60 mL/minute/1.73 m²; avoid if estimated glomerular filtration rate less than 30 mL/minute/1.73 m²
**Pregnancy** see notes above
**Breast-feeding** see notes above
**Side-effects** see notes above; also diabetes mellitus, proteinuria; *very rarely* haematuria; *also reported* oedema

**Indications and dose**

> Hyperlipidaemia including familial hyper-cholesterolaemia
> • By mouth
> **Child 10–18 years** initially 5 mg daily, increased if necessary at intervals of at least 4 weeks to usual max. 20 mg once daily
> **Note** Reduced dose required with concomitant fibrate—seek specialist advice

**Crestor**® (AstraZeneca) PoM
Tablets, f/c, rosuvastatin (as calcium salt) 5 mg (yellow), net price 28-tab pack = £18.03; 10 mg (pink), 28-tab pack = £18.03; 20 mg (pink), 28-tab pack = £26.02. Counselling, muscle effects, see notes above

## ■ SIMVASTATIN

**Cautions** see notes above
**Hepatic impairment** see notes above
**Renal impairment** doses above 10 mg daily should be used with caution if estimated glomerular filtration rate less than 30 mL/minute/1.73 m²
**Pregnancy** see notes above
**Breast-feeding** see notes above
**Side-effects** see notes above; also *rarely* anaemia; *also reported* tendinopathy
**Licensed use** not licensed for use in children under 10 years

**Indications and dose**

> Hyperlipidaemia including familial hyper-cholesterolaemia
> • By mouth
> **Child 5–10 years** initially 10 mg at night increased, if necessary, at intervals of at least 4 weeks to max. 20 mg at night
> **Child 10–18 years** initially 10 mg at night increased, if necessary, at intervals of at least 4 weeks to max. 40 mg at night
> **Note** Reduced dose required with concomitant amiodarone, bezafibrate, amlodipine, diltiazem, or verapamil—seek specialist advice

**Simvastatin** (Non-proprietary) ▼ PoM
Tablets, simvastatin 10 mg, net price 28-tab pack = 90p; 20 mg, 28-tab pack = £1.01; 40 mg, 28-tab pack = £1.32; 80 mg, 28-tab pack = £2.29. Counselling, muscle effects, see notes above
**Brands include** *Simvador*®

Oral suspension, simvastatin 20 mg/5 mL, net price 150-mL = £99.50, 40 mg/5 mL, 150-mL = £152.00. Counselling, muscle effects, see notes above
**Excipients** may include propylene glycol

**Zocor®** (MSD) ▼ [PoM]

Tablets, all f/c, simvastatin 10 mg (peach), net price 28-tab pack = £18.03; 20 mg (tan), 28-tab pack = £29.69; 40 mg (red), 28-tab pack = £29.69; 80 mg (red), 28-tab pack = £29.69. Counselling, muscle effects, see notes above

◀**With ezetimibe**

**Note** For homozygous familial hypercholesterolaemia, primary hypercholesterolaemia, and mixed hyperlipidaemia in children over 10 years stabilised on the individual components in the same proportions, or for children not adequately controlled by statin alone. Treatment should be initiated by a specialist. For prescribing information on ezetimibe, see Ezetimibe

**Inegy®** (MSD) [PoM]

Tablets, simvastatin 20 mg, ezetimibe 10 mg, net price 28-tab pack = £33.42; simvastatin 40 mg, ezetimibe 10 mg, 28-tab pack = £38.98; simvastatin 80 mg, ezetimibe 10 mg, 28-tab pack = £14.21. Counselling, muscle effects, see notes above

---

# Bile acid sequestrants

**Colestyramine** (cholestyramine) and **colestipol** are bile acid sequestrants used in the management of hypercholesterolaemia. They act by binding bile acids, preventing their reabsorption; this promotes hepatic conversion of cholesterol into bile acids; the resultant increased LDL-receptor activity of liver cells increases the clearance of LDL-cholesterol from the plasma. Thus both compounds effectively reduce LDL-cholesterol but can aggravate hypertriglyceridaemia. Bile acid sequestrants are not well tolerated and compliance with treatment is poor, therefore they are rarely used in children.

**Cautions** Bile acid sequestrants interfere with the absorption of fat-soluble vitamins; supplements of vitamins A, D, K, and folic acid may be required when treatment is prolonged and the child's growth and development should be monitored. **Interactions:** Appendix 1 (bile acid sequestrants).

**Pregnancy and breast-feeding** Bile acid sequestrants should be used with caution as although the drugs are not absorbed, they may cause fat-soluble vitamin deficiency on prolonged use.

**Side-effects** As bile acid sequestrants are not absorbed, gastro-intestinal side-effects predominate. Constipation is common, but diarrhoea has occurred, as have nausea, vomiting, and gastro-intestinal discomfort. Hypertriglyceridaemia may be aggravated. An increased bleeding tendency has been reported due to hypoprothrombinaemia associated with vitamin K deficiency.

**Counselling** Other drugs should be taken at least 1 hour before or 4–6 hours after bile acid sequestrants to reduce possible interference with absorption.

## ▌ COLESTYRAMINE
(Cholestyramine)

**Cautions** see notes above

**Contra-indications** complete biliary obstruction (not likely to be effective)

**Pregnancy** see notes above

**Breast-feeding** see notes above

**Side-effects** see notes above; intestinal obstruction reported rarely and hyperchloraemic acidosis reported on prolonged use

**Licensed use** licensed in children over 6 years to reduce cholesterol; see also section 1.9.2

**Indications and dose**

**Familial hypercholesterolaemia**

• **By mouth**

**Child 6–12 years** initially 4 g once daily increased to 4 g up to 3 times daily according to response

**Child 12–18 years** initially 4 g once daily increased by 4 g at weekly intervals to 12–24 g daily in 1–4 divided doses, then adjusted according to response; max. 36 g daily

**Cholestatic pruritus** section 1.9.2

**Diarrhoea** section 1.9.2

**Administration** The contents of each sachet should be mixed with at least 150 mL of water or other suitable liquid such as fruit juice, skimmed milk, thin soups, and pulpy fruits with a high moisture content; total daily dose may be given as a single dose if tolerated

**Colestyramine** (Non-proprietary) [PoM]

Powder, sugar-free, colestyramine (anhydrous) 4 g/sachet, net price 50-sachet pack = £18.34. Label: 13, counselling, avoid other drugs at same time (see notes above)

Excipients may include aspartame (section 9.4.1)

**Questran®** (Bristol-Myers Squibb) [PoM]

Powder, colestyramine (anhydrous) 4 g/sachet, net price 50-sachet pack = £10.76. Label: 13, counselling, avoid other drugs at same time (see notes above)

Excipients include sucrose 3.79 g/sachet

**Questran Light®** (Bristol-Myers Squibb) [PoM]

Powder, sugar-free, colestyramine (anhydrous) 4 g/sachet, net price 50-sachet pack = £16.15. Label: 13, counselling, avoid other drugs at same time (see notes above)

Excipients include aspartame (section 9.4.1)

## ▌ COLESTIPOL HYDROCHLORIDE

**Cautions** see notes above

**Pregnancy** see notes above

**Breast-feeding** see notes above

**Side-effects** see notes above

**Licensed use** not licensed for use in children

**Indications and dose**

**Familial hypercholesterolaemia**

• **By mouth**

**Child 12–18 years** initially 5 g 1–2 times daily increased if necessary in 5-g increments at intervals of 1 month to max. of 30 g daily in 1–2 divided doses

**Administration** the contents of each sachet should be mixed with at least 100 mL of water or other suitable liquid such as fruit juice or skimmed milk; alternatively it can be mixed with thin soups, cereals, yoghurt, or pulpy fruits ensuring at least 100 mL of liquid is provided; total daily dose may be given as a single dose if tolerated

**Colestid**® (Pharmacia) [PoM]
Granules, yellow, colestipol hydrochloride 5 g/
sachet, net price 30 sachets = £15.05. Label: 13,
counselling, avoid other drugs at same time (see
notes above)

Colestid Orange, granules, yellow/orange, colestipol
hydrochloride 5 g/sachet, with aspartame, net price
30 sachets = £15.05. Label: 13, counselling, avoid
other drugs at same time (see notes above)

## Ezetimibe

Ezetimibe inhibits the intestinal absorption of cholesterol. It is given in combination with a statin or alone if a
statin is inappropriate. If ezetimibe is used in combination with a statin, there is an increased risk of rhabdomyolysis (see also Muscle Effects, p. 125)

### EZETIMIBE

**Cautions** interactions: Appendix 1 (ezetimibe)
**Hepatic impairment** avoid in moderate and severe
impairment—may accumulate
**Pregnancy** manufacturer advises use only if potential
benefit outweighs risk—no information available
**Breast-feeding** manufacturer advises avoid—present
in milk in *animal* studies
**Side-effects** gastro-intestinal disturbances; headache,
fatigue; myalgia; *rarely* arthralgia, hypersensitivity
reactions (including rash, angioedema, and anaphylaxis), hepatitis; *very rarely* pancreatitis, cholelithiasis,
cholecystitis, thrombocytopenia, raised creatine
kinase, myopathy, and rhabdomyolysis
**Indications and dose**
> Adjunct to dietary measures and statin treatment
> in primary hypercholesterolaemia and homozy-
> gous familial hypercholesterolaemia (ezetimibe
> alone in primary hypercholesterolaemia if statin
> inappropriate or not tolerated); adjunct to dietary
> measures in homozygous sitosterolaemia
> • By mouth
>   Child 10–18 years 10 mg once daily

**Ezetrol**® (MSD) [PoM]
Tablets, ezetimibe 10 mg, net price 28-tab pack =
£26.31

◢With simvastatin
See under Simvastatin

## Fibrates

Bezafibrate and fenofibrate act mainly by decreasing
serum triglycerides; they have variable effects on LDL-
cholesterol. Fibrates may reduce the risk of coronary
heart disease in those with low HDL-cholesterol or with
raised triglycerides.

Fibrates can cause a myositis-like syndrome, especially
in children with impaired renal function. Also, combination of a fibrate with a statin increases the risk of muscle
effects (especially rhabdomyolysis) and should be used
with caution (see Muscle Effects, p. 125).

There is limited evidence to support their use in children
and they should only be considered if treatment with a
statin and a bile acid sequestrant is unsuccessful or
contra-indicated.

### BEZAFIBRATE

**Cautions** correct hypothyroidism before initiating
treatment (see Hypothyroidism, p. 124); see under
Myotoxicity below; **interactions**: Appendix 1
(fibrates)
**Contra-indications** hypoalbuminaemia, primary
biliary cirrhosis, gall bladder disease, nephrotic
syndrome
**Hepatic impairment** avoid in severe liver disease
**Renal impairment** reduce dose if estimated glomerular filtration rate 15–60 mL/minute/1.73 m²; avoid
if estimated glomerular filtration rate less than 15 mL/
minute/1.73 m²
Myotoxicity Special care needed in children with renal
disease, as progressive increases in serum-creatinine
concentration or failure to follow dosage guidelines may
result in myotoxicity (rhabdomyolysis); discontinue if
myotoxicity suspected or creatine kinase concentration
increases significantly
**Pregnancy** manufacturers advise avoid—embryotoxicity in *animal* studies
**Breast-feeding** manufacturer advises avoid—no
information available
**Side-effects** gastro-intestinal disturbances, anorexia;
*less commonly* cholestasis, weight gain, dizziness,
headache, fatigue, drowsiness, renal impairment,
raised serum creatinine (unrelated to renal impairment), erectile dysfunction, myotoxicity (with myasthenia or myalgia)—particular risk in renal impairment (see Cautions), urticaria, pruritus,
photosensitivity reactions; *very rarely* gallstones,
hypoglycaemia, anaemia, leucopenia, thrombocytopenia, increased platelet count, alopecia, Stevens-
Johnson syndrome, and toxic epidermal necrolysis
**Licensed use** not licensed for use in children
**Indications and dose**
> Hyperlipidaemia including familial hyper-
> cholesterolaemia (on specialist advice only)
> • By mouth
>   Child 10–18 years 200 mg once daily adjusted
>   according to response to max. 200 mg 3 times
>   daily

**Bezafibrate** (Non-proprietary) [PoM]
Tablets, bezafibrate 200 mg, net price 100-tab pack
= £6.86. Label: 21

**Bezalip**® (Actavis) [PoM]
Tablets, f/c, bezafibrate 200 mg, net price 100-tab
pack = £8.63. Label: 21

### FENOFIBRATE

**Cautions** see under Bezafibrate; liver function tests
recommended every 3 months for first year (discontinue treatment if significantly raised)
**Contra-indications** gall bladder disease; pancreatitis
(unless due to severe hypertriglyceridaemia); photosensitivity to ketoprofen
**Hepatic impairment** avoid
**Renal impairment** reduce dose if estimated glomerular filtration rate less than 60 mL/minute/1.73 m²;
avoid if estimated glomerular filtration rate less than
15 mL/minute/1.73 m²
Myotoxicity Special care needed in patients with renal
disease, as progressive increases in serum-creatinine
concentration or failure to follow dosage guidelines may
result in myotoxicity (rhabdomyolysis); discontinue if
myotoxicity suspected or creatine kinase concentration
increases significantly

**Pregnancy** avoid—embryotoxicity in animal studies

**Breast-feeding** manufacturer advises avoid—no information available

**Side-effects** see under Bezafibrate; *also less commonly* pancreatitis, pulmonary embolism; *rarely* hepatitis; *also reported* interstitial pneumopathies

**Indications and dose**

See under preparations

**Fenofibrate** (Non-proprietary) ᴾᵒᴹ
Capsules, fenofibrate (micronised) 67 mg, net price 90-cap pack = £23.30. Label: 21

Dose

**Hyperlipidaemias including familial hyper-cholesterolaemia (on specialist advice only)**

• By mouth

**Child 4–15 years** 1 capsule/20 kg body-weight (max. 4 capsules) daily

**Child 15–18 years** initially 3 capsules daily, increased if necessary to 4 capsules daily

**Lipantil®** (Abbott Healthcare) ᴾᵒᴹ
Lipantil® Micro 67 capsules, yellow, fenofibrate (micronised) 67 mg, net price 90-cap pack = £23.30. Label: 21

Dose

**Hyperlipidaemias including familial hyper-cholesterolaemia (on specialist advice only)**

• By mouth

**Child 4–15 years** 1 capsule/20 kg body-weight (max. 4 capsules) daily

**Child 15–18 years** initially 3 capsules daily, increased if necessary to 4 capsules daily

## 2.13 Local sclerosants

Classification not used in *BNF for Children*.

## 2.14 Drugs affecting the ductus arteriosus

## Closure of the ductus arteriosus

Patent ductus arteriosus is a frequent problem in premature neonates with respiratory distress syndrome. Substantial left-to-right shunting through the ductus arteriosus may increase the risk of intraventricular haemorrhage, necrotising enterocolitis, bronchopulmonary dysplasia, and possibly death.

Indometacin or ibuprofen can be used to close the ductus arteriosus. **Indometacin** has been used for many years and is effective but it reduces cerebral blood flow, and causes a transient fall in renal and gastro-intestinal blood flow. **Ibuprofen** may also be used; it has little effect on renal function (there may be a small reduction in sodium excretion) when used in doses for closure of the ductus arteriosus; gastro-intestinal problems are uncommon.

If drug treatment fails to close the ductus arteriosus, surgery may be indicated.

### ▌IBUPROFEN

**Cautions** may mask symptoms of infection; monitor for bleeding; monitor gastro-intestinal function; allergic disorders; **interactions:** Appendix 1 (NSAIDs)

**Contra-indications** life-threatening infection; active bleeding especially intracranial or gastro-intestinal; thrombocytopenia or coagulation defects; marked unconjugated hyperbilirubinaemia; known or suspected necrotising enterocolitis; pulmonary hypertension

**Hepatic impairment** increased risk of gastro-intestinal bleeding and fluid retention; avoid in severe liver disease

**Renal impairment** use lowest effective dose and monitor renal function; sodium and water retention; deterioration in renal function possibly leading to renal failure; avoid if possible in severe impairment

**Side-effects** intestinal perforation; intraventricular haemorrhage; ischaemic brain injury; bronchopulmonary dysplasia, pulmonary haemorrhage; thrombocytopenia, neutropenia, oliguria, haematuria, fluid retention, hyponatraemia; *less commonly* gastro-intestinal haemorrhage; hypoxaemia

**Licensed use** Orphan licence for the injection for closure of ductus arteriosus in premature neonates less than 34 weeks postmenstrual age

**Indications and dose**

**Closure of ductus arteriosus**

• By slow intravenous injection

**Neonate** initially 10 mg/kg as a single dose followed at 24-hour intervals by 2 doses of 5 mg/kg; course may be repeated after 48 hours if necessary

Mild to moderate pain, pain and inflammation of soft tissue injuries and rheumatic disease, pyrexia section 10.1.1

**Administration** for *slow intravenous injection*, give over 15 minutes, preferably undiluted. May be diluted with Glucose 5% *or* Sodium Chloride 0.9%

**Pedea®** (Orphan Europe) ᴾᵒᴹ
Intravenous solution, ibuprofen 5 mg/mL, net price 4 × 2-mL vials = £288.00

### ▌INDOMETACIN

**Cautions** see notes above; also may mask symptoms of infection; may reduce urine output by 50% or more (monitor carefully—see also under Anuria or Oliguria, below) and precipitate renal impairment especially if extracellular volume depleted, heart failure, sepsis, or concomitant use of nephrotoxic drugs; may induce hyponatraemia; inhibition of platelet aggregation (monitor for bleeding); **interactions:** Appendix 1 (NSAIDs)

**Contra-indications** untreated infection, bleeding (especially with active intracranial haemorrhage or gastro-intestinal bleeding); thrombocytopenia, coagulation defects, necrotising enterocolitis

**Hepatic impairment** increased risk of gastro-intestinal bleeding and fluid retention; avoid in severe impairment

**Renal impairment** use lowest effective dose and monitor renal function; sodium and water retention; deterioration in renal function possibly leading to renal failure; avoid if possible in severe impairment
**Anuria or oliguria** If anuria or marked oliguria (urinary output less than 0.6 mL/kg/hour), delay further doses until renal function returns to normal

**2 Cardiovascular system**

**Side-effects** haemorrhagic, renal, gastro-intestinal, metabolic, and coagulation disorders; pulmonary hypertension, intracranial bleeding, fluid retention, and exacerbation of infection

### Indications and dose

Symptomatic ductus arteriosus

• By intravenous infusion over 20–30 minutes

Neonate initially 100–200 micrograms/kg as a single dose followed by 2 doses of 100 micrograms/kg at 24-hour intervals; if residual patency present, give 100 micrograms/kg for a further 3 doses at 24-hour intervals

Note Monitor carefully to ensure adequate urine output, see Anuria or Oliguria above

Pain and inflammation in rheumatic disease section 10.1.1

**Administration** for *intravenous infusion*, dilute each vial with 1–2 mL Sodium Chloride 0.9% *or* Water for Injections

**Indometacin** (Non-proprietary) PoM
Injection, indometacin
Available from 'special-order' manufacturers or specialist importing companies, see p. 823

## Maintenance of patency

In the newborn with duct-dependent congenital heart disease it is often necessary to maintain the patency of the ductus arteriosus whilst awaiting surgery.

Alprostadil (prostaglandin E1) and dinoprostone (prostaglandin E2) are potent vasodilators that are effective for maintaining the patency of the ductus arteriosus. They are usually given by continuous intravenous infusion, but oral dosing of dinoprostone is still used in some centres.

During the infusion of a prostaglandin, the newborn requires careful monitoring of heart rate, blood pressure, respiratory rate, and core body temperature. In the event of complications such as apnoea, profound bradycardia, or severe hypotension, the infusion should be temporarily stopped and the complication dealt with; the infusion should be restarted at a lower dose. Recurrent or prolonged apnoea may require ventilatory support in order for the prostaglandin infusion to continue.

### ALPROSTADIL

**Cautions** see notes above; also history of haemorrhage; avoid in hyaline membrane disease; monitor arterial pressure, respiratory rate, heart rate, temperature, and venous blood pressure in arm and leg; facilities for intubation and ventilation must be immediately available; **interactions:** Appendix 1 (alprostadil)

**Side-effects** apnoea (particularly in neonates under 2 kg), flushing, bradycardia, hypotension, tachycardia, cardiac arrest, oedema, diarrhoea, fever, convulsions, disseminated intravascular coagulation, hypokalaemia; cortical proliferation of long bones; weakening of the wall of the ductus arteriosus and pulmonary artery may follow prolonged use; gastric-outlet obstruction reported

### Indications and dose

Maintaining patency of the ductus arteriosus

• By continuous intravenous infusion

Neonate initially 5 nanograms/kg/minute, adjusted according to response in steps of 5 nanograms/kg/minute; max. 100 nanograms/kg/minute (but associated with increased side-effects)

Note Alprostadil doses in BNFC may differ from those in product literature

**Administration** dilute 150 micrograms/kg body-weight to a final volume of 50 mL with Glucose 5% *or* Sodium Chloride 0.9%; an intravenous infusion rate of 0.1 mL/hour provides a dose of 5 nanograms/kg/minute. Undiluted solution must not come into contact with the barrel of the plastic syringe; add the required volume of alprostadil to a volume of infusion fluid in the syringe and then make up to final volume

**Prostin VR®** (Pharmacia) PoM
Intravenous solution, alprostadil 500 micrograms/mL in alcohol. For dilution and use as an infusion. Net price 1-mL amp = £75.19 (hosp.only)

### DINOPROSTONE

**Cautions** see notes above; also history of haemorrhage; avoid in hyaline membrane disease; monitor arterial oxygenation, heart rate, temperature, and blood pressure in arm and leg; facilities for intubation and ventilation must be immediately available; **interactions:** Appendix 1 (prostaglandins)

**Hepatic impairment** manufacturer advises avoid

**Renal impairment** manufacturer advises avoid

**Side-effects** nausea, vomiting, diarrhoea; flushing, bradycardia, hypotension, cardiac arrest; respiratory depression and apnoea, particularly with high doses and in low birth-weight neonates, bronchospasm; pyrexia and raised white blood cell count, shivering; local reactions, erythema; if used for longer than 5 days, gastric outlet obstruction; cortical hyperostosis (prolonged use)

**Licensed use** not licensed for use in children

### Indications and dose

Maintaining patency of the ductus arteriosus

• By continuous intravenous infusion

Neonate initially 5 nanograms/kg/minute, increased as necessary in 5 nanogram/kg/minute increments to 20 nanograms/kg/minute

Note Doses up to 100 nanograms/kg/minute have been used but are associated with increased side-effects

• By mouth

Neonate 20–25 micrograms/kg every 1–2 hours doubled if necessary; if treatment continues for more than 1 week gradually reduce the dose

**Administration** for *continuous intravenous infusion*, dilute to a concentration of 1 microgram/mL with Glucose 5% *or* Sodium Chloride 0.9%.
For administration *by mouth*, injection solution can be given orally; dilute with water

**Prostin® E2** (Pharmacia) PoM
Intravenous solution, for dilution and use as an infusion, dinoprostone 1 mg/mL, net price 0.75-mL amp = £8.52; 10 mg/mL, 0.5-mL amp = £18.40 (both hosp. only)

# 131

# 3 Respiratory system

This chapter includes advice on the drug management of the following:
acute asthma, p. 132
anaphylaxis, p. 157
angioedema, p. 160
chronic asthma, p. 133
croup, p. 135

## 3.1 Bronchodilators

### Asthma

Drugs used in the management of asthma include beta$_2$ agonists (section 3.1.1), antimuscarinic bronchodilators (section 3.1.2), theophylline (section 3.1.3), corticosteroids (section 3.2), cromoglicate and nedocromil (section 3.3.1), leukotriene receptor antagonists (section 3.3.2), and in specialist centres, omalizumab (section 3.4.2).

For tables outlining the management of chronic asthma and management of acute asthma, see p. 133 and p. 134.

### Administration of drugs for asthma

**Inhalation** This route delivers the drug directly to the airways; the dose required is smaller than when given by mouth and side-effects are reduced. See Inhaler devices, section 3.1.5.

*Solutions for nebulisation* for use in acute severe asthma are administered over 5–10 minutes from a nebuliser, usually driven by oxygen in hospital. See Nebulisers, section 3.1.5.

**Oral** Systemic side-effects occur more frequently when a drug is given orally rather than by inhalation. Oral corticosteroids, theophylline, and leukotriene receptor antagonists are sometimes required for the management of asthma. Oral administration of a beta$_2$ agonist is generally not recommended for children, but may be necessary in infants and young children who are unable or unwilling to use an inhaler device.

**Parenteral** Drugs such as beta$_2$ agonists, corticosteroids, and aminophylline can be given by injection in acute severe asthma when drug administration by nebulisation is inadequate or inappropriate; in these circumstances the child should generally be treated in a high-dependency or intensive care unit.

### Pregnancy and breast-feeding

Women with asthma should be closely monitored during pregnancy. Well-controlled asthma has no important effects on pregnancy, labour, or the fetus. Drugs for asthma should preferably be administered by inhalation to minimise fetal drug exposure. Inhaled drugs, theophylline, and prednisolone can be taken as normal during pregnancy and breast-feeding. For the use of leukotriene receptor antagonists during pregnancy see section 3.3.2. Women planning to become pregnant should be counselled about the importance of taking their asthma medication regularly to maintain good control.

Severe acute exacerbations of asthma can have an adverse effect on pregnancy and should be treated promptly in hospital with conventional therapy, including nebulisation of a beta$_2$ agonist, and oral or parenteral administration of a corticosteroid; prednisolone is the preferred corticosteroid for oral administration since very little of the drug reaches the fetus. Oxygen should be given immediately to maintain an arterial oxygen saturation of 94–98% and prevent maternal and fetal hypoxia. An intravenous beta$_2$ agonist, aminophylline, or magnesium sulfate can be used during pregnancy if necessary; parenteral beta$_2$ agonists can affect the myometrium, see BNF section 7.1.3.

## Management of acute asthma[1]

> **Important**
>
> Regard each emergency consultation as being for **severe acute asthma** until shown otherwise.
>
> Failure to respond adequately **at any time** requires immediate transfer to hospital.

Severe acute asthma can be fatal and must be treated promptly. Treatment of severe acute asthma is safer in hospital where resuscitation facilities are immediately available. Treatment should **never** be delayed for investigations, children should **never** be sedated, and the possibility of a pneumothorax should be considered. If the child's condition deteriorates despite pharmacological treatment, urgent transfer to a paediatric intensive care unit should be arranged. For a table outlining the management of severe acute asthma, see Management of acute asthma table, p. 134.

**Mild to moderate acute asthma**   Administer a **short-acting beta$_2$ agonist** using a pressurised metered-dose inhaler with a spacer device; for a child under 3 years use a close-fitting facemask. Give 1 puff every 15–30 seconds up to a maximum of 10 puffs; repeat dose after 10–20 minutes if necessary.

Give **prednisolone** by mouth, child under 12 years 1–2 mg/kg (max. 40 mg) once daily for up to 3 days, or longer if necessary; if the child has been taking an oral corticosteroid for more than a few days, give prednisolone 2 mg/kg (max. 60 mg) once daily. For children 12–18 years, give prednisolone 40–50 mg daily for at least 5 days.

1. Advice on the management of acute asthma is based on the recommendations of the British Thoracic Society and Scottish Intercollegiate Guidelines Network (updated January 2012); updates available at www.brit-thoracic.org.uk

If response is poor or if a relapse occurs within 3–4 hours, transfer child **immediately** to hospital for assessment and further treatment.

Children under 18 months often respond poorly to bronchodilators; nebulised beta$_2$ agonists have been associated with mild (but occasionally severe) paradoxical bronchospasm and transient worsening of oxygen saturation; response to prednisolone may also be poor in this age group.

**Severe or life-threatening acute asthma**   Start treatment below and transfer **immediately** to hospital. Administer high-flow **oxygen** (section 3.6) using a close-fitting face mask or nasal prongs.

Treat severe or life-threatening acute exacerbations of asthma with an inhaled **short-acting beta$_2$ agonist** (as above). Treatment of life-threatening asthma should be initiated with nebulised salbutamol 2.5 mg or terbutaline 5 mg (via an oxygen-driven nebuliser if available); nebulised doses may be doubled for children over 5 years. Repeat the dose every 20–30 minutes or as necessary, then reduce the frequency on improvement.

Give **prednisolone** by mouth, child under 12 years 1–2 mg/kg (max. 40 mg) once daily for up to 3 days, or longer if necessary; if the child has been taking an oral corticosteroid for more than a few days, give prednisolone 2 mg/kg (max. 60 mg) once daily. For children 12–18 years, give prednisolone 40–50 mg daily for at least 5 days. If oral administration is not possible, use intravenous **hydrocortisone** (preferably as sodium succinate) 4 mg/kg (max. 100 mg) every 6 hours (alternatively, if weight unavailable, child under 2 years 25 mg every 6 hours, 2–5 years 50 mg every 6 hours, 5–18 years 100 mg every 6 hours).

If response is poor, add nebulised **ipratropium bromide**, child under 12 years give 250 micrograms every 20–30 minutes for the first 2 hours, then every 4–6 hours as necessary. For children 12–18 years, give ipratropium bromide 500 micrograms every 4–6 hours as necessary.

If the condition does not respond or is life-threatening, transfer the child to an intensive care unit and treat with a parenteral **short-acting beta$_2$ agonist** (e.g. salbutamol, section 3.1.1.1) or parenteral **aminophylline** (section 3.1.3). Children over 2 years with severe acute asthma may be helped by intravenous infusion of **magnesium sulfate injection** 40 mg/kg (max. 2 g) over 20 minutes (section 9.5.1.3), but evidence of benefit is limited.

**Follow-up in all cases**   Episodes of acute asthma should be regarded as a failure of preventive therapy. A careful history should be taken to establish the reason for the exacerbation. Inhaler technique should be checked and regular treatment should be reviewed in accordance with the Management of Chronic Asthma table, p. 133. Children or their carers should be given an asthma action plan aimed at preventing relapse, optimising treatment, and preventing delay in seeking assistance in future exacerbations. If possible, follow-up within 48 hours should be arranged with the general practitioner or appropriate primary care health professional. Children should also be reviewed in a paediatric asthma clinic within 1–2 months of the exacerbation, and referred to a paediatric respiratory specialist if the exacerbation included life-threatening features.

## Management of chronic asthma

**Important**    Start at **step most appropriate** to initial severity; before initiating a new drug consider whether diagnosis is correct, check compliance and inhaler technique, and eliminate trigger factors for acute exacerbations

### Child 5–18 years

**Step 1: occasional relief bronchodilator**

Inhaled short-acting beta$_2$ agonist as required (up to once daily)

**Note** Move to step 2 if needed more than twice a week, or if night-time symptoms at least once a week, or if exacerbation in the last 2 years

**Step 2: regular inhaled preventer therapy**

Inhaled short-acting beta$_2$ agonist as required
*plus*
Regular standard-dose[1] inhaled corticosteroid (alternatives[2] are considerably less effective)

**Step 3: inhaled corticosteroid + inhaled long-acting beta$_2$ agonist**

Inhaled short-acting beta$_2$ agonist as required
*plus*
Regular standard-dose[1] inhaled corticosteroid
*plus*
Regular inhaled long-acting beta$_2$ agonist (salmeterol *or* formoterol)
*If asthma not controlled*
Increase dose of inhaled corticosteroid to upper end of standard dose range[1]
*and*
*Either* stop long-acting beta$_2$ agonist if of no benefit
*Or* continue long-acting beta$_2$ agonist if of some benefit
*If asthma still not controlled and long-acting beta$_2$ agonist stopped*, add one of

    Leukotriene receptor antagonist

    Modified-release oral theophylline

**Step 4: high-dose inhaled corticosteroid + regular bronchodilators**

Inhaled short-acting beta$_2$ agonist as required
*with*
Regular high-dose[3] inhaled corticosteroid
*plus*
Inhaled long-acting beta$_2$ agonist (if of benefit)
*plus*
A 6-week sequential therapeutic trial of one or more of

    Leukotriene receptor antagonist

    Modified-release oral theophylline

    Modified-release oral beta$_2$ agonist

**Step 5: regular corticosteroid tablets**

Refer to respiratory paediatrician
Inhaled short-acting beta$_2$ agonist as required
*with*
Regular high-dose[3] inhaled corticosteroid
*and*
One or more long-acting bronchodilators (see step 4)
*plus*
Regular prednisolone tablets (as single daily dose)
**Note** In addition to regular prednisolone, continue high-dose inhaled corticosteroid (in exceptional cases may exceed licensed doses)

**Stepping down**

Review treatment every 3 months; if control achieved, step-wise reduction may be possible; reduce dose of *inhaled* corticosteroid slowly (consider reduction every 3 months, decreasing dose by up to 50% each time) to the lowest dose which controls asthma

### Child under 5 years[4]

**Step 1: occasional relief bronchodilator**

Short-acting beta$_2$ agonist as required (not more than once daily)

**Note** Preferably by inhalation (less effective and more side-effects when given as tablets or syrup)
Move to step 2 if needed more than twice a week, or if night-time symptoms at least once a week, or if exacerbation in the last 2 years

**Step 2: regular preventer therapy**

Inhaled short-acting beta$_2$ agonist as required
*plus*
Regular standard-dose[1] inhaled corticosteroid
*Or* leukotriene receptor antagonist if inhaled corticosteroid cannot be used

**Step 3: add-on therapy**

Child under 2 years:
Refer to respiratory paediatrician
Child 2–5 years:
Inhaled short-acting beta$_2$ agonist as required
*plus*
Regular standard-dose[1] inhaled corticosteroid
*plus*
Leukotriene receptor antagonist

**Step 4: persistent poor control**

Refer to respiratory paediatrician

**Stepping down**

Regularly review need for treatment

1. **Standard doses** of inhaled corticosteroids

    **Beclometasone dipropionate or budesonide:**
    Child under 12 years 100–200 micrograms twice daily;
    Child 12–18 years 100–400 micrograms twice daily.

    **Fluticasone propionate:**
    Child 4–12 years 50–100 micrograms twice daily;
    Child 12–18 years 50–200 micrograms twice daily.

    **Mometasone furoate:**
    Child 12–18 years 400 micrograms as a single dose in the evening or in 2 divided doses.

    **Note** Dose adjustments may be required for some inhaler devices, see under individual preparations, section 3.2

2. Alternatives to inhaled corticosteroid are leukotriene receptor antagonists, theophylline, inhaled nedocromil, or inhaled cromoglicate.

3. **High doses** of inhaled corticosteroids

    **Beclometasone dipropionate or budesonide:**
    Child 5–12 years 200–400 micrograms twice daily;
    Child 12–18 years 0.4–1 mg twice daily.

    **Fluticasone propionate:**
    Child 5–12 years 100–200 micrograms twice daily;
    Child 12–18 years 200–500 micrograms twice daily.

    **Mometasone furoate:**
    Child 12–18 years 400 micrograms twice daily.

    **Note** Dose adjustments may be required for some inhaler devices, see under individual preparations, section 3.2.

    Failure to achieve control with these doses is unusual, see also Side-effects of Inhaled Corticosteroids, section 3.2

4. Lung-function measurements cannot be used to guide management in those under 5 years

**3**

**Respiratory system**

Advice on the management of chronic asthma is based on the recommendations of the British Thoracic Society and Scottish Intercollegiate Guidelines Network (updated January 2012); updates available at www.brit-thoracic.org.uk

Respiratory system

3

## Management of acute asthma

**Important**  The assessment of acute asthma in early childhood can be difficult. Children with severe or life-threatening acute asthma may not be distressed and may not have all of these abnormalities; the presence of any should alert the doctor. Regard each emergency consultation as being for **severe acute asthma** until shown otherwise

| Moderate acute asthma | Severe acute asthma | Life-threatening acute asthma |
|---|---|---|
| • Able to talk<br>• Respiration (breaths/minute) Child 2–5 years ≤ 40, 5–12 years ≤ 30, 12–18 years < 25<br>• Pulse (beats/minute) Child 2–5 years ≤ 140, 5–12 years ≤ 125, 12–18 years < 110<br>• Arterial oxygen saturation ≥ 92%<br>• Peak flow Child 5–12 years ≥ 50% of predicted or best, 12–18 years > 50%<br><br>*Treat at home or in surgery and assess response to treatment* | • Child under 12 years too breathless to talk or feed, 12–18 years cannot complete sentences in one breath<br>• Use of accessory breathing muscles<br>• Respiration (breaths/minute) Child 2–5 years > 40; 5–12 years > 30, 12–18 years ≥ 25<br>• Pulse (beats/minute) Child 2–5 years > 140; 5–12 years > 125, 12–18 years ≥ 110<br>• Arterial oxygen saturation Child under 12 years < 92%, 12–18 years ≥ 92%<br>• Peak flow Child 5–12 years <50% of predicted or best, 12–18 years 33–50%<br><br>*Start treatment below and send immediately to hospital* | • Silent chest, cyanosis, poor respiratory effort<br>• Arrhythmia, hypotension<br>• Exhaustion, altered consciousness, agitation, confusion<br>• Arterial oxygen saturation < 92%<br>• Peak flow < 33% of predicted or best<br><br>*Start treatment below and send immediately to hospital; consult with senior medical staff and refer to paediatric intensive care* |
| **Treatment**<br>• Inhaled **short-acting beta₂ agonist** via a large-volume spacer (and a close-fitting face mask if child under 3 years) or oxygen-driven nebuliser (if available); give 2–10 puffs of **salbutamol** 100 micrograms/metered inhalation each inhaled separately, and repeat at 10–20 minute intervals if necessary *or* give nebulised **salbutamol**, Child under 5 years 2.5 mg, 5–12 years 2.5–5 mg, 12–18 years 5 mg *or* **terbutaline**, Child under 5 years 5 mg, 5–12 years 5–10 mg, 12–18 years 10 mg, and repeat at 20–30 minute intervals as necessary<br>• **Prednisolone** by mouth Child under 12 years 1–2 mg/kg (max. 40 mg) daily for up to 3 days or longer if necessary; if the child has been taking an oral corticosteroid for more than a few days, give prednisolone 2 mg/kg (max. 60 mg); Child 12–18 years 40–50 mg daily for at least 5 days<br><br>*Monitor response for 15–30 minutes*<br><br>*If response is poor or a relapse occurs in 3–4 hours, send immediately to hospital for assessment and further treatment* | **Treatment**<br>• High-flow **oxygen** (if available)<br>• Inhaled **short-acting beta₂ agonist** via a large-volume spacer (and a close-fitting face mask if child under 3 years) or oxygen-driven nebuliser (if available) as for moderate acute asthma<br>• **Prednisolone** by mouth as for moderate acute asthma *or* intravenous **hydrocortisone** (preferably as sodium succinate) 4 mg/kg (max. 100 mg) every 6 hours (alternatively, if weight unavailable, Child under 2 years 25 mg, 2–5 years 50 mg, 5–18 years 100 mg, every 6 hours) until conversion to oral prednisolone is possible<br><br>*Monitor response for 15–30 minutes*<br><br>*If response is poor:*<br>• Inhaled **ipratropium bromide** via oxygen-driven nebuliser (if available), Child under 12 years 250 micrograms repeated every 20–30 minutes for the first 2 hours, then every 4–6 hours as necessary; Child 12–18 years, 500 micrograms every 4–6 hours as necessary<br><br>*Refer those who fail to respond and require ventilatory support to a paediatric intensive care or high-dependency unit*<br>• Consider intravenous **beta₂ agonist**, **aminophylline**, or **magnesium sulfate** [unlicensed indication] only after consultation with senior medical staff | **Treatment**<br>• High-flow **oxygen** (if available)<br>• Inhaled **short-acting beta₂ agonist** via oxygen-driven nebuliser (if available); give **salbutamol**, Child under 5 years 2.5 mg, 5–12 years 2.5–5 mg, 12–18 years 5 mg, *or* **terbutaline**, Child under 5 years 5 mg, 5–12 years 5–10 mg, 12–18 years 10 mg, and repeat as necessary; reserve **intravenous beta₂ agonists** for those in whom inhaled therapy cannot be used reliably or there is no current effect<br>• **Prednisolone** by mouth as for moderate acute asthma *or* intravenous **hydrocortisone** as for severe acute asthma<br>• Inhaled **ipratropium bromide** via oxygen-driven nebuliser (if available) as for severe acute asthma<br><br>*Monitor response for 15–30 minutes*<br><br>*If response is poor:*<br>• Consider intravenous **beta₂ agonists, aminophylline**, or **magnesium sulfate** [unlicensed indication] only after consultation with senior medical staff |

**Follow up in all cases**

Monitor symptoms and peak flow. Set up asthma action plan and check inhaler technique with child and carer
Review by general practitioner or appropriate primary care health professional within 48 hours, see also p. 132

Advice on the management of acute asthma is based on the recommendations of the British Thoracic Society and Scottish Intercollegiate Guidelines Network (updated January 2012); updates available at www.brit-thoracic.org.uk

## Croup

Mild croup is largely self-limiting, but treatment with a single dose of a corticosteroid (e.g. **dexamethasone** 150 micrograms/kg) by mouth is of benefit.

Severe croup (or mild croup that might cause complications) calls for hospital admission—a single dose of either dexamethasone 150 micrograms/kg or prednisolone 1–2 mg/kg, can be administered by mouth before transfer to hospital. In hospital, dexamethasone 150 micrograms/kg (by mouth or by injection) or budesonide 2 mg by nebulisation (section 3.2) will often reduce symptoms; the dose may be repeated after 12 hours if necessary.

For severe croup not effectively controlled with corticosteroid treatment, nebulised **adrenaline** (section 3.4.3) solution 1 in 1000 (1 mg/mL) can be given with close clinical monitoring in a dose of 400 micrograms/kg (max. 5 mg) repeated after 30 minutes if necessary (the dose may be diluted with sterile sodium chloride 0.9% solution). The effects of nebulised adrenaline last 2–3 hours; the child needs to be carefully monitored for recurrence of the obstruction.

## 3.1.1  Adrenoceptor agonists
### (Sympathomimetics)
#### 3.1.1.1  Selective beta$_2$ agonists
#### 3.1.1.2  Other adrenoceptor agonists

The selective beta$_2$ agonists (selective beta$_2$-adrenoceptor agonists, selective beta$_2$ stimulants) such as salbutamol or terbutaline are the safest and most effective short-acting beta$_2$ agonists for the treatment of asthma.

Adrenaline (epinephrine), which has both alpha- and beta-adrenoceptor agonist properties, is used in the emergency management of acute allergic and anaphylactic reactions (section 3.4.3); it is also used as a nebuliser solution to treat severe croup.

### 3.1.1.1  Selective beta$_2$ agonists

Selective beta$_2$ agonists produce bronchodilation. A short-acting beta$_2$ agonist is used for immediate relief of asthma symptoms while a long-acting beta$_2$ agonist is used in addition to an inhaled corticosteroid in children requiring prophylactic treatment.

Management of Chronic Asthma table, see p. 133
Management of Acute Asthma table, see p. 134
For guidance on the use of inhalers and spacer devices, see section 3.1.5

**Short-acting beta$_2$ agonists**  Mild to moderate symptoms of asthma respond rapidly to the inhalation of a selective short-acting beta$_2$ agonist such as **salbutamol** or **terbutaline**. If beta$_2$ agonist inhalation is needed more often than twice a week, or if night-time symptoms occur at least once a week, or if there has been an exacerbation in the last 2 years, prophylactic treatment should be considered, using a stepped approach as outlined in the Management of Chronic Asthma table, p. 133.

A short-acting beta$_2$ agonist inhaled immediately before exertion reduces *exercise-induced asthma*; however, frequent exercise-induced asthma probably reflects poor overall control and calls for reassessment of asthma treatment.

**Long-acting beta$_2$ agonists**  Formoterol and salmeterol are longer-acting beta$_2$ agonists which are administered by inhalation. They should be used for asthma only in children who regularly use an inhaled corticosteroid (see CHM advice below). They have a role in the long-term control of chronic asthma (see Management of Chronic Asthma table, p. 133) and they can be useful in nocturnal asthma. Salmeterol should not be used for the relief of an asthma attack; it has a slower onset of action than salbutamol or terbutaline. Formoterol is licensed for short-term symptom relief and for the prevention of exercise-induced bronchospasm; its speed of onset of action is similar to that of salbutamol.

Combination inhalers that contain a long-acting beta$_2$ agonist and a corticosteroid (section 3.2) ensure that long-acting beta$_2$ agonists are not used without concomitant corticosteroids, but reduce the flexibility to adjust the dose of each component.

### CHM advice
To ensure safe use, the CHM has advised that for the management of chronic asthma, long-acting beta$_2$ agonists (formoterol and salmeterol) should:
- be added only if regular use of standard-dose inhaled corticosteroids has failed to control asthma adequately;
- not be initiated in patients with rapidly deteriorating asthma;
- be introduced at a low dose and the effect monitored before considering dose increase;
- be discontinued in the absence of benefit;
- not be used for the relief of exercise-induced asthma symptoms unless regular inhaled corticosteroids are also used;
- be reviewed as clinically appropriate: stepping down therapy should be considered when good long-term asthma control has been achieved.

A daily dose of 24 micrograms of formoterol should be sufficient for the majority of children, particularly for younger age-groups; higher doses should be used rarely, and only when control is not maintained on the lower dose.

Children and their carers should be advised to report any deterioration in symptoms following initiation of treatment with a long-acting beta$_2$ agonist, see Management of Chronic Asthma table, p. 133.

**Inhalation**  A *pressurised metered-dose inhaler* is an effective method of drug administration in mild to moderate chronic asthma; to deliver the drug effectively particularly in children under 12 years, a spacer device should be used (see also NICE guidance, section 3.1.5). When a pressurised metered-dose inhaler with a spacer is unsuitable or inconvenient, a *dry-powder inhaler* or *breath-actuated inhaler* may be used instead if the child is able to use the device effectively. At recommended inhaled doses the duration of action of salbutamol and terbutaline is about 3 to 5 hours and for salmeterol and formoterol is about 12 hours. The **dose**, the frequency, and the maximum number of inhalations in 24 hours of the beta$_2$ agonist should be **stated explicitly** to the child and the child's carer. High doses of beta$_2$ agonists can be dangerous in some children (see Cautions, below). Excessive use is usually an indication of **inadequately controlled** asthma and should be managed with a prophylactic drug such as an inhaled corticosteroid. The child and the child's carer should be advised to seek medical advice when the prescribed dose of beta$_2$ agonist fails to provide the usual degree of symptomatic relief because this usually indicates a worsening of the asthma and the child may require alternative medication (see Management of Chronic Asthma table, p. 133).

Children and their carers should be advised to follow manufacturers' instructions on the care and cleansing of inhaler devices.

*Nebuliser (or respirator) solutions* of salbutamol and terbutaline are used for the treatment of severe acute asthma both in hospital and in general practice. Children with a severe attack of asthma should have oxygen if possible during nebulisation since beta$_2$ agonists can increase arterial hypoxaemia, see also section 3.1.5.

**Oral**   Oral preparations of beta$_2$ agonists may be used for children if an inhaler device cannot be used but inhaled beta$_2$ agonists are more effective and have fewer side-effects. A modified-release formulation of salbutamol may be of value in nocturnal asthma as an alternative to modified-release theophylline preparations (section 3.1.3), but an inhaled long-acting beta$_2$ agonist is preferable.

**Parenteral**   Beta$_2$ agonists can be given intravenously in children with severe or life-threatening acute asthma. Chronic asthma unresponsive to stepwise treatment (see Management of Chronic Asthma, p. 133) may benefit from continuous subcutaneous infusion of a beta$_2$ agonist, but this should be used only under the supervision of a respiratory specialist; the evidence of benefit is uncertain and it may be difficult to withdraw such treatment once started.

**Cautions**   Beta$_2$ agonists should be used with caution in diabetes—monitor blood glucose (risk of ketoacidosis, especially when a beta$_2$ agonist is given intravenously). Beta$_2$ agonists should also be used with caution in hyperthyroidism, cardiovascular disease, arrhythmias, susceptibility to QT-interval prolongation, and hypertension. **Interactions:** Appendix 1 (sympathomimetics, beta$_2$).

**Hypokalaemia** Potentially serious hypokalaemia may result from beta$_2$ agonist therapy. Particular caution is required in severe asthma, because this effect may be potentiated by concomitant treatment with theophylline and its derivatives, corticosteroids, and diuretics, and by hypoxia. Plasma-potassium concentration should therefore be monitored in severe asthma.

**Side-effects**   Side-effects of the beta$_2$ agonists include fine tremor (particularly in the hands), nervous tension, headache, peripheral dilatation and palpitation. Other side-effects include tachycardia, arrhythmias, peripheral vasodilation, myocardial ischaemia, and disturbances of sleep and behaviour. Muscle cramps and hypersensitivity reactions including paradoxical bronchospasm (occasionally severe), urticaria, angioedema, hypotension, and collapse have also been reported. High doses of beta$_2$ agonists are associated with hypokalaemia (see Hypokalaemia, above).

## FORMOTEROL FUMARATE
(Eformoterol fumarate)

**Note** For use in asthma only in children who regularly use an inhaled corticosteroid, see notes above

**Cautions**   see notes above

**Pregnancy**   see p. 131

**Breast-feeding**   see p. 131

**Side-effects**   see notes above; nausea, dizziness, rash, taste disturbances, and pruritus also reported

### Indications and dose

> **Reversible airways obstruction (including nocturnal asthma and prevention of exercise-induced bronchospasm) in patients requiring long-term regular bronchodilator therapy** see also Management of Chronic Asthma table, p. 133; for dose see preparations below
>
> **Counselling** Advise children and carers not to exceed prescribed dose, and to follow manufacturer's directions; if a previously effective dose of inhaled formoterol fails to provide adequate relief, a doctor's advice should be obtained as soon as possible

**Formoterol** (Non-proprietary) ꟼoMꟽ
Dry powder for inhalation, formoterol fumarate 12 micrograms/metered inhalation, net price 120-dose unit = £23.75. Counselling, administration
Brands include *Easyhaler® Formoterol*

**Dose**

> **Chronic asthma**
> - **By inhalation of powder**
>   Child 6–12 years 12 micrograms twice daily
>   Child 12–18 years 12 micrograms twice daily, increased to 24 micrograms twice daily in more severe airways obstruction

**Atimos Modulite®** (Chiesi) ꟼoMꟽ
Aerosol inhalation, formoterol fumarate 12 micrograms/metered inhalation, net price 100-dose unit = £30.06. Counselling, administration

**Dose**

> **Chronic asthma**
> - **By aerosol inhalation**
>   Child 12–18 years 12 micrograms twice daily, increased to max. 24 micrograms twice daily in more severe airways obstruction

**Foradil®** (Novartis) ꟼoMꟽ
Dry powder for inhalation, formoterol fumarate 12 micrograms/capsule, net price 60-cap pack (with inhaler device) = £23.38. Counselling, administration

**Dose**

> **Chronic asthma**
> - **By inhalation of powder**
>   Child 6–12 years 12 micrograms twice daily
>   Child 12–18 years 12 micrograms twice daily, increased to 24 micrograms twice daily in more severe airways obstruction

**Oxis®** (AstraZeneca) ꟼoMꟽ
Turbohaler®(= dry powder inhaler), formoterol fumarate 6 micrograms/inhalation, net price 60-dose unit = £24.80; 12 micrograms/inhalation, 60-dose unit = £24.80. Counselling, administration

**Dose**

> **Chronic asthma**
> - **By inhalation of powder**
>   Child 6–18 years 6–12 micrograms 1–2 times daily; occasionally up to 48 micrograms daily may be needed (max. single dose 12 micrograms); reassess treatment if

additional doses required on more than 2 days a week
(see also CHM advice above)

**Relief of bronchospasm**

- **By inhalation of powder**
  **Child 6–18 years** 6–12 micrograms

**Prevention of exercise-induced bronchospasm**

- **By inhalation of powder**
  **Child 6–18 years** 6–12 micrograms before exercise

◢**Compound preparations**

For **compound preparations** containing formoterol,
see *Flutiform*® and *Symbicort*®, section 3.2

---

◢■ **SALBUTAMOL**
(Albuterol)

**Cautions** see notes above

**Pregnancy** see p. 131

**Breast-feeding** see p. 131

**Side-effects** see notes above; also lactic acidosis with
high doses

**Licensed use** not licensed for use in hyperkalaemia;
syrup and tablets not licensed for use in children
under 2 years; modified-release tablets not licensed
for use in children under 3 years; injection not
licensed for use in children

**Indications and dose**

Acute asthma

- **By aerosol or nebulised solution inhalation**
  See Management of Acute Asthma, p. 132

- **By intravenous injection over 5 minutes (see also
  Management of Acute Asthma, p. 132)**
  **Child 1 month–2 years** 5 micrograms/kg as a
  single dose
  **Child 2–18 years** 15 micrograms/kg (max.
  250 micrograms) as a single dose

- **By continuous intravenous infusion**
  **Child 1 month–18 years** 1–2 micrograms/kg/
  minute, adjusted according to response and heart
  rate up to 5 micrograms/kg/minute; doses above
  2 micrograms/kg/minute should be given in an
  intensive care setting

Exacerbations of reversible airways obstruction
(including nocturnal asthma) and prevention of
allergen- or exercise-induced bronchospasm, see
also Management of Chronic Asthma, p. 133

- **By aerosol inhalation**
  **Child 1 month–18 years** 100–200 micrograms (1–
  2 puffs); for persistent symptoms up to 4 times
  daily

- **By inhalation of powder**
  See under preparations

- **By mouth (but use by inhalation preferred)**
  **Child 1 month–2 years** 100 micrograms/kg (max.
  2 mg) 3–4 times daily
  **Child 2–6 years** 1–2 mg 3–4 times daily
  **Child 6–12 years** 2 mg 3–4 times daily
  **Child 12–18 years** 2–4 mg 3–4 times daily

**Severe hyperkalaemia (section 9.2.1.1)**

- **By intravenous injection over 5 minutes**
  **Neonate** 4 micrograms/kg as a single dose; repeat
  if necessary
  **Child 1 month–18 years** 4 micrograms/kg as a
  single dose; repeat if necessary

- **By inhalation of nebulised solution (but intravenous injection preferred)**
  **Neonate** 2.5–5 mg as a single dose; repeat if
  necessary
  **Child 1 month–18 years** 2.5–5 mg as a single dose;
  repeat if necessary

**Administration** for *continuous intravenous infusion*,
dilute to a concentration of 200 micrograms/mL with
Glucose 5% *or* Sodium Chloride 0.9%; if fluid-
restricted, can be given undiluted through central
venous catheter

For *intravenous injection*, dilute to a concentration of
50 micrograms/mL with Glucose 5%, Sodium Chloride 0.9%, *or* Water for injections

For *nebulisation*, dilute nebuliser solution with a suitable volume of sterile Sodium Chloride 0.9% solution
according to nebuliser type and duration of administration; salbutamol and ipratropium bromide solutions are compatible and can be mixed for nebulisation

◢**Oral**

**Salbutamol** (Non-proprietary) PoM

Tablets, salbutamol (as sulfate) 2 mg, net price 28-
tab pack = £17.74; 4 mg, 28-tab pack = £16.40

Oral solution, salbutamol (as sulfate) 2 mg/5 mL, net
price 150 mL = £1.55
Brands include *Salapin*® (sugar-free)

**Ventmax**® **SR** (Chiesi) PoM

Capsules, m/r, salbutamol (as sulfate) 4 mg (green/
grey), net price 56-cap pack = £8.08; 8 mg (white),
56-cap pack = £9.69. Label: 25
Dose
**Chronic asthma** (but see notes above)

- **By mouth**
  **Child 3–12 years** 4 mg twice daily
  **Child 12–18 years** 8 mg twice daily

**Ventolin**® (A&H) PoM

Syrup, sugar-free, salbutamol (as sulfate) 2 mg/5 mL,
net price 150 mL = 60p

◢**Parenteral**

**Ventolin**® (A&H) PoM

Injection, salbutamol (as sulfate) 500 micrograms/
mL, net price 1-mL amp = 38p

Solution for intravenous infusion, salbutamol (as
sulfate) 1 mg/mL. Dilute before use. Net price 5-mL
amp = £2.48

**3**

**Respiratory system**

**3 Respiratory system**

◢Inhalation

**Counselling** Advise children and carers not to exceed prescribed dose and to follow manufacturer's directions; if a previously effective dose of inhaled salbutamol fails to provide at least 3 hours relief, a doctor's advice should be obtained as soon as possible.

**Salbutamol** (Non-proprietary) (PoM)

Aerosol inhalation, salbutamol (as sulfate) 100 micrograms/metered inhalation, net price 200-dose unit = £3.19. Counselling, administration

Brands include *AirSalb®*, *Salamol®*

Nebuliser solution, salbutamol (as sulfate) 1 mg/mL, net price 20 × 2.5 mL (2.5 mg) = £1.91; 2 mg/mL, 20 × 2.5 mL (5 mg) = £3.82. May be diluted with sterile sodium chloride 0.9%

Brands include *Salamol Steri-Neb®*

**Airomir®** (IVAX) (PoM)

Aerosol inhalation, salbutamol (as sulfate) 100 micrograms/metered inhalation, net price 200-dose unit = £1.97. Counselling, administration

Autohaler (breath-actuated aerosol inhalation), salbutamol (as sulfate) 100 micrograms/metered inhalation, net price 200-dose unit = £6.02. Counselling, administration

**Asmasal Clickhaler®** (UCB Pharma) (PoM)

Dry powder for inhalation, salbutamol (as sulfate) 95 micrograms/metered inhalation, net price 200-dose unit = £5.65. Counselling, administration

**Dose**

**Acute bronchospasm**

- By inhalation of powder

  **Child 5–18 years** 1–2 puffs; for persistent symptoms up to 4 times daily (but see also Management of Chronic Asthma, p. 133)

**Prophylaxis of allergen- or exercise-induced bronchospasm**

- By inhalation of powder

  **Child 5–18 years** 1–2 puffs

**Easyhaler® Salbutamol** (Orion) (PoM)

Dry powder for inhalation, salbutamol (as sulfate) 100 micrograms/metered inhalation, net price 200-dose unit = £3.31; 200 micrograms/metered inhalation, 200-dose unit = £6.63. Counselling, administration,

**Dose**

**Acute bronchospasm**

- By inhalation of powder

  **Child 5–12 years** 100–200 micrograms; max. 800 micrograms daily (but see also Management of Chronic Asthma, p. 133)

  **Child 12–18 years** initially 100–200 micrograms, increased to 400 micrograms if necessary; max. 800 micrograms daily (but see also Management of Chronic Asthma, p. 133)

**Prophylaxis of allergen- or exercise-induced bronchospasm**

- By inhalation of powder

  **Child 5–12 years** 100–200 micrograms

  **Child 12–18 years** 200 micrograms

**Pulvinal® Salbutamol** (Chiesi) (PoM)

Dry powder for inhalation, salbutamol 200 micrograms/metered inhalation, net price 100-dose unit = £4.85. Counselling, administration

**Dose**

**Acute bronchospasm**

- By inhalation of powder

  **Child 5–18 years** 200 micrograms; for persistent symptoms up to 800 micrograms daily (but see also Management of Chronic Asthma, p. 133)

**Prophylaxis of allergen- or exercise- induced bronchospasm**

- By inhalation of powder

  **Child 5–18 years** 200 micrograms

**Salamol Easi-Breathe®** (IVAX) (PoM)

Aerosol inhalation, salbutamol 100 micrograms/metered inhalation, net price 200-dose breath-actuated unit = £6.30. Counselling, administration

**Salbulin Novolizer®** (Meda) (PoM)

Dry powder for inhalation, salbutamol (as sulfate) 100 micrograms/metered inhalation, net price refillable 200-dose unit = £4.95; 200-dose refill = £2.75. Counselling, administration

**Dose**

**Acute bronchospasm**

- By inhalation of powder

  **Child 6–12 years** 100–200 micrograms; for persistent symptoms up to 400 micrograms daily (but see also Management of Chronic Asthma, p. 133)

  **Child 12–18 years** 100–200 micrograms; for persistent symptoms up to 800 micrograms daily (but see also Management of Chronic Asthma, p. 133)

**Prophylaxis of allergen- or exercise-induced bronchospasm**

- By inhalation of powder

  **Child 6–12 years** 100–200 micrograms

  **Child 12–18 years** 200 micrograms

**Ventolin®** (A&H) (PoM)

Accuhaler® (dry powder for inhalation), disk containing 60 blisters of salbutamol (as sulfate) 200 micrograms/blister with *Accuhaler®* device, net price = £4.92. Counselling, administration

**Dose**

**Acute bronchospasm**

- By inhalation of powder

  **Child 5–18 years** 200 micrograms; for persistent symptoms up to 4 times daily but see also Management of Chronic Asthma, p. 133

**Prophylaxis of allergen- or exercise-induced bronchospasm**

- By inhalation of powder

  **Child 5–18 years** 200 micrograms

Evohaler® (aerosol inhalation), salbutamol (as sulfate) 100 micrograms/metered inhalation, net price 200-dose unit = £1.50. Counselling, administration

Nebules® (for use with nebuliser), salbutamol (as sulfate) 1 mg/mL, net price 20 × 2.5 mL (2.5 mg) = £1.68; 2 mg/mL, 20 × 2.5 mL (5 mg) = £2.83. May be diluted with sterile sodium chloride 0.9%

Respirator solution (for use with a nebuliser or ventilator), salbutamol (as sulfate) 5 mg/mL. Net price 20 mL = £2.18 (hosp. only). May be diluted with sterile sodium chloride 0.9%

## ◢ SALMETEROL

**Note** Not for immediate relief of acute attacks; for use in asthma only in children who regularly use an inhaled corticosteroid, see notes above

**Cautions**  see notes above

**Pregnancy**  see p. 131

**Breast-feeding**  see p. 131

**Side-effects** see notes above; nausea, dizziness, arthralgia, and rash also reported

**Licensed use** *Neovent®* not licensed for use in children under 12 years

**Indications and dose**

Reversible airways obstruction (including nocturnal asthma and prevention of exercise-induced bronchospasm) in patients requiring long-term regular bronchodilator therapy see also Management of Chronic Asthma, p. 133

- **By inhalation**

  **Child 5–12 years** 50 micrograms (2 puffs or 1 blister) twice daily

  **Child 12–18 years** 50 micrograms (2 puffs or 1 blister) twice daily; up to 100 micrograms (4 puffs or 2 blisters) twice daily in more severe airways obstruction

  **Counselling** Advise children and carers that salmeterol should **not** be used for relief of acute attacks, not to exceed prescribed dose, and to follow manufacturer's directions; if a previously effective dose of inhaled salmeterol fails to provide adequate relief, a doctor's advice should be obtained as soon as possible

**Salmeterol** (Non-proprietary) [PoM]

Aerosol inhalation, salmeterol (as xinafoate) 25 micrograms/metered inhalation, net price 120-dose unit = £27.80. Counselling, administration
**Brands include** *Neovent®*

**Serevent®** (A&H) [PoM]

Accuhaler® (dry powder for inhalation), disk containing 60 blisters of salmeterol (as xinafoate) 50 micrograms/blister with *Accuhaler®* device, net price = £29.26. Counselling, administration

Evohaler® (aerosol inhalation), salmeterol (as xinafoate) 25 micrograms/metered inhalation, net price 120-dose unit = £29.26. Counselling, administration

Diskhaler® (dry powder for inhalation), disks containing 4 blisters of salmeterol (as xinafoate) 50 micrograms/blister, net price 15 disks with *Diskhaler®* device = £35.79, 15-disk refill = £35.15. Counselling, administration

◢**Compound preparations**

For **compound preparations** containing salmeterol, see section 3.2

---

## ■ TERBUTALINE SULFATE

**Cautions** see notes above
**Pregnancy** see p. 131
**Breast-feeding** see p. 131
**Side-effects** see notes above
**Licensed use** tablets not licensed for use in children under 7 years; injection not licensed for use in children under 2 years

**Indications and dose**

Acute asthma

- **By inhalation of nebulised solution**
  See Management of Acute Asthma, p. 132

- **By subcutaneous or slow intravenous injection**
  **Child 2–15 years** 10 micrograms/kg (max. 300 micrograms) up to 4 times daily
  **Child 15–18 years** 250–500 micrograms up to 4 times daily

- **By continuous intravenous infusion**
  **Child 1 month–18 years** initially 2–4 micrograms/kg as a loading dose, then 1–10 micrograms/hour according to response and heart rate (doses above 10 micrograms/kg/hour with close monitoring)

Exacerbations of reversible airways obstruction (including nocturnal asthma) and prevention of exercise-induced bronchospasm see Management of Chronic Asthma table, p. 133

- **By inhalation of powder**
  **Child 5–18 years** 500 micrograms (1 inhalation) up to 4 times daily (for occasional use only)

- **By mouth (but not recommended)**
  **Child 1 month–7 years** 75 micrograms/kg (max. 2.5 mg) 3 times daily
  **Child 7–15 years** 2.5 mg 2–3 times daily
  **Child 15–18 years** initially 2.5 mg 3 times daily, increased if necessary to 5 mg 3 times daily

**Administration** For *continuous intravenous infusion*, dilute to a concentration of 5 micrograms/mL with Glucose 5% *or* Sodium Chloride 0.9%; if fluid-restricted, dilute to a concentration of 100 micrograms/mL

For *nebulisation*, dilute nebuliser solution with sterile Sodium Chloride 0.9% solution according to nebuliser type and duration of administration; terbutaline and ipratropium bromide solutions are compatible and may be mixed for nebulisation.

◢**Oral and parenteral**

**Bricanyl®** (AstraZeneca) [PoM]

Tablets, scored, terbutaline sulfate 5 mg, net price 100-tab pack = £4.09

Syrup, sugar-free, terbutaline sulfate 1.5 mg/5 mL, net price 100 mL = £2.00

Injection, terbutaline sulfate 500 micrograms/mL, net price 1-mL amp = 30p; 5-mL amp = £1.40

◢**Inhalation**

**Counselling** Advise children and carers not to exceed prescribed dose and to follow manufacturer's directions; if a previously effective dose of inhaled terbutaline fails to provide at least 3 hours relief, a doctor's advice should be obtained as soon as possible

**Bricanyl®** (AstraZeneca) [PoM]

Turbohaler® (= dry powder inhaler), terbutaline sulfate 500 micrograms/metered inhalation, net price 100-dose unit = £6.92. Counselling, administration

Respules® (= single-dose units for nebulisation), terbutaline sulfate 2.5 mg/mL, net price 20 × 2-mL units (5 mg) = £4.04

---

**3.1.1.2 Other adrenoceptor agonists**

Adrenaline (epinephrine) injection (1 in 1000) is used in the emergency treatment of acute allergic and anaphylactic reactions (section 3.4.3), in angioedema (section 3.4.3), and in cardiopulmonary resuscitation (section 2.7.3). Adrenaline solution (1 in 1000) is used by nebulisation in the management of severe croup (section 3.1).

## 3.1.2 Antimuscarinic bronchodilators

**Ipratropium** by nebulisation can be added to other standard treatment in life-threatening acute asthma or if acute asthma fails to improve with standard therapy (see Management of Acute Asthma, p. 132). Ipratropium can be used to provide short-term relief in chronic asthma, but short-acting beta₂ agonists act more quickly and are preferred.

The aerosol inhalation of ipratropium has a maximum effect 30–60 minutes after use; its duration of action is 3 to 6 hours.

### IPRATROPIUM BROMIDE

**Cautions**   risk of glaucoma (see below), bladder outflow obstruction; cystic fibrosis; **interactions:** Appendix 1 (antimuscarinics)

   Glaucoma  *Acute angle-closure glaucoma* has been reported with nebulised ipratropium, particularly when given with nebulised salbutamol (and possibly other beta₂ agonists); care needed to protect the child's eyes from nebulised drug or from drug powder

**Pregnancy**   see p. 131

**Breast-feeding**   see p. 131

**Side-effects**   dry mouth, nausea, gastro-intestinal motility disorder (including constipation and diarrhoea), throat irritation, cough, headache, dizziness; *less commonly* vomiting, stomatitis, palpitation, tachycardia, bronchospasm (including paradoxical bronchospasm), laryngospasm, pharyngeal oedema, urinary retention, mydriasis, angle-closure glaucoma, pruritus; *rarely* atrial fibrillation, ocular accommodation disorder

**Indications and dose**

Acute asthma

- By inhalation of nebulised solution

   See Management of Acute Asthma, section 3.1

Reversible airways obstruction  see notes above

- By aerosol inhalation

   **Child 1 month–6 years** 20 micrograms 3 times daily

   **Child 6–12 years** 20–40 micrograms 3 times daily

   **Child 12–18 years** 20–40 micrograms 3–4 times daily

   **Counselling**  Advise child and carer not to exceed prescribed dose and to follow manufacturer's directions

Rhinitis section 12.2.2

**Ipratropium Bromide** (Non-proprietary)  ᴾᵒᴹ
   Nebuliser solution, ipratropium bromide 250 micrograms/mL, net price 20 × 1-mL (250-microgram) unit-dose vials = £6.75, 60 × 1-mL = £21.78; 20 × 2-mL (500-microgram) = £7.43, 60 × 2-mL = £26.97

**Atrovent**® (Boehringer Ingelheim)  ᴾᵒᴹ
   Aerosol inhalation, ipratropium bromide 20 micrograms/metered inhalation, net price 200-dose unit = £5.05. Counselling, administration

   Nebuliser solution, isotonic, ipratropium bromide 250 micrograms/mL, net price 20 × 1-mL unit-dose vials = £4.14, 60 × 1-mL vials = £12.44; 20 × 2-mL vials = £4.87, 60 × 2-mL vials = £14.59

**Ipratropium Steri-Neb**® (IVAX)  ᴾᵒᴹ
   Nebuliser solution, isotonic, ipratropium bromide 250 micrograms/mL, net price 20 × 1-mL (250-microgram) unit-dose vials = £8.72; 20 × 2-mL (500-microgram) = £9.94

**Respontin**® (A&H)  ᴾᵒᴹ
   Nebuliser solution, isotonic, ipratropium bromide 250 micrograms/mL, net price 20 × 1-mL (250-microgram) unit-dose vials = £4.78; 20 × 2-mL (500-microgram) = £5.60

## 3.1.3 Theophylline

**Theophylline** is a xanthine used as a bronchodilator in asthma, see Management of Chronic Asthma p. 133. It may have an additive effect when used in conjunction with small doses of beta₂ agonists; the combination may increase the risk of side-effects, including hypokalaemia (see p. 136).

Theophylline is given by injection as **aminophylline**, a mixture of theophylline with ethylenediamine, which is 20 times more soluble than theophylline alone. Aminophylline injection is needed rarely for severe acute asthma (see Management of Acute Asthma p. 134). It must be given by **very slow** intravenous injection (over at least 20 minutes) or by intravenous infusion; it is too irritant for intramuscular use. Measurement of plasma-theophylline concentration may be helpful and is **essential** if a loading dose of aminophylline is to be given to children who are already taking theophylline, because serious side-effects such as convulsions and arrhythmias can occasionally precede other symptoms of toxicity.

Theophylline is metabolised in the liver. The plasma-theophylline concentration is *increased* in heart failure, hepatic impairment, viral infections, and by drugs that inhibit its metabolism. The plasma-theophylline concentration is *decreased* in smokers, by alcohol consumption, and by drugs that induce its metabolism. For interactions of theophylline, see Appendix 1.

**Plasma-theophylline concentration**  In most individuals a plasma-theophylline concentration of 10–20 mg/litre (55–110 micromol/litre) is required for satisfactory bronchodilation, but a lower concentration of 5–15 mg/litre may be effective. Adverse effects can occur within the range 10–20 mg/litre and both the frequency and severity increase if the concentration exceeds 20 mg/litre.

Plasma-theophylline concentration is measured 5 days after starting oral treatment and at least 3 days after any dose adjustment. A blood sample should usually be taken 4–6 hours after an oral dose of a modified-release preparation (sampling times may vary—consult local guidelines). If aminophylline is given intravenously, a blood sample should be taken 4–6 hours after starting treatment.

### THEOPHYLLINE

**Cautions**  see notes above; also cardiac arrhythmias or other cardiac disease, hypertension, hyperthyroidism; peptic ulcer; epilepsy; fever; hypokalaemia risk, p. 136; avoid in acute porphyria (section 9.8.2); monitor plasma-theophylline concentration (see notes above); dose adjustment may be necessary if

*Respiratory system*   *3*

smoking started or stopped during treatment; **interactions:** Appendix 1 (theophylline) and notes above

**Hepatic impairment**  reduce dose

**Pregnancy**  neonatal irritability and apnoea reported; see also p. 131

**Breast-feeding**  present in milk—irritability in infant reported; modified-release preparations preferable; see also p. 131

**Side-effects**  nausea, vomiting, gastric irritation, diarrhoea, palpitation, tachycardia, arrhythmias, headache, CNS stimulation, insomnia, convulsions **overdosage:** see Emergency Treatment of Poisoning, p. 30

**Licensed use**  *Slo-Phyllin*® capsules not licensed for use in children under 2 years

**Indications and dose**

> **Chronic asthma**
>
> See under preparations below and Management of Chronic Asthma table, p. 133
>
> Note  Plasma-theophylline concentration for optimum response 10–20 mg/litre (55–110 micromol/litre); narrow margin between therapeutic and toxic dose, see also notes above

◀ **Modified release**

Note  The rate of absorption from modified-release preparations can vary between different brands. If a prescription for a modified-release oral theophylline preparation does not specify a brand name, the pharmacist should contact the prescriber and agree the brand to be dispensed. Additionally, it is essential that a child discharged from hospital should be maintained on the brand on which that child was stabilised as an in-patient.

**Nuelin SA**®  (Meda)

SA tablets, m/r, theophylline 175 mg. Net price 60-tab pack = £3.19. Label: 21, 25

**Dose**

> **Chronic asthma**
>
> • By mouth
>
> **Child 6–12 years** 175 mg every 12 hours
>
> **Child 12–18 years** 175–350 mg every 12 hours

SA 250 tablets, m/r, scored, theophylline 250 mg. Net price 60-tab pack = £4.46. Label: 21, 25

**Dose**

> **Chronic asthma**
>
> • By mouth
>
> **Child 6–12 years** 125–250 mg every 12 hours
>
> **Child 12–18 years** 250–500 mg every 12 hours

**Slo-Phyllin**®  (Merck Serono)

Capsules, m/r, theophylline 60 mg (white/clear, enclosing white pellets), net price 56-cap pack = £2.76; 125 mg (brown/clear, enclosing white pellets), 56-cap pack = £3.48; 250 mg (purple/clear, enclosing white pellets), 56-cap pack = £4.34. Label: 25, or counselling, see below

**Dose**

> **Chronic asthma**
>
> • By mouth
>
> **Child 6 months–2 years** 12 mg/kg (max. 120 mg) every 12 hours
>
> **Child 2–6 years** 60–120 mg every 12 hours
>
> **Child 6–12 years** 125–250 mg every 12 hours
>
> **Child 12–18 years** 250–500 mg every 12 hours
>
> **Administration**  Contents of the capsule (enteric-coated granules) may be sprinkled on to a spoonful of soft food (e.g. yoghurt) and swallowed without chewing

**Uniphyllin Continus**®  (Napp)

Tablets, m/r, theophylline 200 mg, net price 56-tab pack = £2.94; 300 mg, 56-tab pack = £4.77; 400 mg, 56-tab pack = £5.32. Label: 25

**Dose**

> **Chronic asthma**
>
> • By mouth
>
> **Child 2–12 years** 9 mg/kg (max. 200 mg) every 12 hours; some children with chronic asthma may require 10–16 mg/kg (max. 400 mg) every 12 hours
>
> **Child 12–18 years** 200 mg every 12 hours, increased according to response to 400 mg every 12 hours
>
> Note  May be appropriate to give larger evening or morning dose to achieve optimum therapeutic effect when symptoms most severe; in children whose night or daytime symptoms persist despite other therapy, who are not currently receiving theophylline, total daily requirement may be added as a single evening or morning dose

## ◼ AMINOPHYLLINE

Note  Aminophylline is a stable mixture or combination of theophylline and ethylenediamine; the ethylenediamine confers greater solubility in water

**Cautions**  see under Theophylline; also rapid intravenous injection can cause arrhythmias

**Hepatic impairment**  see under Theophylline

**Pregnancy**  see under Theophylline

**Breast-feeding**  see under Theophylline

**Side-effects**  see under Theophylline; also allergy to ethylenediamine can cause urticaria, erythema, and exfoliative dermatitis; hypotension, arrhythmias, and convulsions, especially if given rapidly by intravenous injection

**Licensed use**  Aminophylline injection not licensed for use in children under 6 months

**Indications and dose**

> To avoid excessive dosage in obese children, dose should be calculated on the basis of ideal weight for height

> **Chronic asthma** (see also Management of Chronic Asthma, p. 133)
>
> • By mouth
>
> See under preparations below

> **Severe acute asthma not previously treated with theophylline** (with close monitoring; see also Management of Acute Asthma, section 3.1)
>
> • By intravenous injection over at least 20 minutes
>
> **Child 1 month–18 years** 5 mg/kg (max. 500 mg) then by intravenous infusion

> **Severe acute asthma** (with close monitoring; see also Management of Acute Asthma, section 3.1)
>
> • By intravenous infusion
>
> **Child 1 month–12 years** 1 mg/kg/hour adjusted according to plasma-theophylline concentration
>
> **Child 12–18 years** 500–700 micrograms/kg/hour adjusted according to plasma-theophylline concentration

> Note  Plasma-theophylline concentration for optimum response in asthma 10–20 mg/litre (55–110 micromol/litre); narrow margin between therapeutic and toxic dose; children taking oral theophylline or aminophylline should not normally receive a loading dose of intravenous aminophylline; it is recommended that plasma-theophylline

3  Respiratory system

concentration is measured in all children receiving intravenous aminophylline (see notes above)

**Administration** For *intravenous infusion*, dilute to a concentration of 1 mg/mL with Glucose 5% or Sodium Chloride 0.9%

**Aminophylline** (Non-proprietary) [PoM]
Injection, aminophylline 25 mg/mL, net price 10-mL amp = 84p

◢**Modified release**
Note Advice about modified-release theophylline preparations on p. 141 also applies to modified-release aminophylline preparations

**Phyllocontin Continus®** (Napp)
Tablets, m/r, yellow, f/c, aminophylline hydrate 225 mg, net price 56-tab pack = £2.39. Label: 25

**Dose**

**Chronic asthma** (see also Management of Chronic Asthma, p. 133)

• By mouth
**Child body-weight over 40 kg** initially 1 tablet twice daily, increased after 1 week to 2 tablets twice daily according to plasma-theophylline concentration

---

## 3.1.4 Compound bronchodilator preparations

In general, children are best treated with single-ingredient preparations, such as a selective beta₂ agonist (section 3.1.1.1) or ipratropium bromide (section 3.1.2), so that the dose of each drug can be adjusted. This flexibility is lost with compound bronchodilator preparations.

---

## 3.1.5 Peak flow meters, inhaler devices, and nebulisers

### Peak flow meters

Peak flow meters may be used to assess lung function in children over 5 years with asthma, but symptom monitoring is the most reliable assessment of asthma control. They are best used for short periods to assess the severity of asthma and to monitor response to treatment; continuous use of peak flow meters may detract from compliance with inhalers.

Peak flow charts should be issued where appropriate, and are available to purchase from:

3M Security Print and Systems Limited
Gorse Street, Chadderton
Oldham,
OL9 9QH
Tel: 0845 610 1112

GP practices can obtain supplies through their Primary Care Trust (PCT) or Agency stores.

NHS Hospitals can order supplies from www.nhsforms.co.uk or by emailing nhsforms@mmm.com.

In Scotland, peak flow charts can be obtained by emailing stockorders.dppas@apsgroup.co.uk.

### Standard Range Peak Flow Meter

Conforms to standard EN ISO 23747: 2007
AirZone®, range 60–720 litres/minute, net price = £4.50, replacement mouthpiece = 38p (Clement Clarke)

Medi®, range 60–800 litres/minute, net price = £4.50 (Medicare)

MicroPeak®, range 60–800 litres/minute, net price = £6.50, replacement mouthpiece = 38p (Micro Medical)

Mini-Wright®, range 60–800 litres/minute, net price = £6.86, replacement mouthpiece = 38p (Clement Clarke)

Personal Best®, range 60–800 litres/minute, net price = £6.86, replacement mouthpiece = 25p (Respironics)

Piko-1®, range 15–999 litres/minute, net price = £9.50, replacement mouthpiece = 38p (nSPIRE Health)

Pinnacle®, range 60–900 litres/minute, net price = £6.50 (Fyne Dynamics)

Pocketpeak®, range 60–800 litres/minute, net price = £6.53, replacement mouthpiece = 38p (nSPIRE Health)

Vitalograph®, range 50–800 litres/minute, net price = £4.75 (a child's peak flow meter is also available), replacement mouthpiece = 40p (Vitalograph)

Note Readings from new peak flow meters are often lower than those obtained from old Wright-scale peak flow meters and the correct recording chart should be used

### Low Range Peak Flow Meter

Compliant to standard EN ISO 23747: 2007 except for scale range

Medi®, range 40–420 litres/minute, net price = £6.50 (Medicare)

Mini-Wright®, range 30–400 litres/minute, net price = £6.90, replacement mouthpiece = 38p (Clement Clarke)

Pocketpeak®, range 50–400 litres/minute, net price = £6.53, replacement mouthpiece = 38p (nSPIRE Health)

Note Readings from new peak flow meters are often lower than those obtained from old Wright-scale peak flow meters and the correct recording chart should be used

---

### Drug delivery devices

**Inhaler devices** A *pressurised metered-dose inhaler* is an effective method of drug administration in mild to moderate chronic asthma; to deliver the drug effectively, a spacer device should also be used (see also NICE guidance, below). By the age of 3 years, a child can usually be taught to use a spacer device without a mask. As soon as a child is able to use the mouthpiece, then this is the preferred delivery system.

*Dry powder inhalers* may be useful in children over 5 years, who are unwilling or unable to use a pressurised metered-dose inhaler with a spacer device; *breath-actuated inhalers* may be useful in older children if they are able to use the device effectively. The child or child's carer should be instructed carefully on the use of the inhaler. It is important to check that the inhaler is being used correctly; poor inhalation technique may be mistaken for a lack of response to the drug.

On changing from a pressurised metered-dose inhaler to a dry powder inhaler, the child may notice a lack of sensation in the mouth and throat previously associated with each actuation; coughing may occur more frequently following use of a dry-powder inhaler.

CFC-free metered-dose inhalers should be cleaned **weekly** according to the manufacturer's instructions.

**Spacer devices**    Spacer devices are particularly useful for infants, for children with poor inhalation technique, or for nocturnal asthma, because the device reduces the need for coordination between actuation of a pressurised metered-dose inhaler and inhalation. The spacer device reduces the velocity of the aerosol and subsequent impaction on the oropharynx and allows more time for evaporation of the propellant so that a larger proportion of the particles can be inhaled and deposited in the lungs. Smaller-volume spacers may be more manageable for pre-school children and infants. The spacer device used must be compatible with the prescribed metered-dose inhaler.

**Use and care of spacer devices**    The suitability of the spacer device should be carefully assessed; opening the one-way valve is dependent on the child's inspiratory flow. Some devices can be tipped to 45° to open the valve during inhaler actuation and inspiration to assist the child.

Inhalation from the spacer device should follow the actuation as soon as possible because the drug aerosol is very short-lived. The total dose (which may be more than a single puff) should be administered as single actuations (with tidal breathing for 10–20 seconds or 5 breaths for each actuation) for children with good inspiratory flow. Larger doses may be necessary for a child with acute bronchospasm; for guidance on the Management of Acute Asthma, see section 3.1.

The device should be cleansed once a month by washing in mild detergent and then allowed to dry in air without rinsing; the mouthpiece should be wiped clean of detergent before use. Some manufacturers recommend more frequent cleaning, but this should be avoided since any electrostatic charge may affect drug delivery. Spacer devices should be replaced every 6–12 months.

**A2A Spacer®** (Clement Clarke)
Spacer device, for use with all pressurised (aerosol) inhalers, net price = £4.15; with small or medium mask = £6.80

**Able Spacer®** (Clement Clarke)
Spacer device, small-volume device. For use with all pressurised (aerosol) inhalers, net price standard device = £4.33; with infant or child mask = £7.06

**AeroChamber® Plus** (GSK)
Spacer device, medium-volume device. For use with all pressurised (aerosol) inhalers, net price standard device (blue) = £4.53, with mask (blue) = £7.56; infant device (orange) with mask = £7.56; child device (yellow) with mask = £7.56

**Babyhaler®** (A&H) ⟨NHS⟩
Spacer device, paediatric use with *Flixotide®*, and *Ventolin®* inhalers, net price = £11.34

**Haleraid®** (A&H)
Inhalation aid, device to place over pressurised (aerosol) inhalers to aid when strength in hands is impaired (e.g. arthritis). For use with *Flixotide®*, *Seretide®*, and *Ventolin®* inhalers. Available as *Haleraid®-120* for 120-dose inhalers and *Haleraid®-200* for 200-dose inhalers, net price = 80p

**OptiChamber®** (Respironics)
Spacer device, for use with all pressurised (aerosol) inhalers, net price = £4.28

**OptiChamber® Diamond** (Respironics)
Spacer device, for use with all pressurised (aerosol) inhalers, net price = £4.49; with small, medium, or large mask = £7.49

**Pocket Chamber®** (nSPIRE Health)
Spacer device, small-volume device. For use with all pressurised (aerosol) inhalers, net price = £4.18; with infant, small, medium, or large mask = £9.75

**Space Chamber Plus®** (Medical Developments)
Spacer device, for use with all pressurised (aerosol) inhalers, net price standard device = £4.26; compact device = £4.26

**Volumatic®** (A&H)
Spacer inhaler, large-volume device. For use with *Clenil Modulite®*, *Flixotide®*, *Seretide®*, *Serevent®*, and *Ventolin®* inhalers, net price = £2.81; with paediatric mask = £2.81

**Vortex®** (Pari)
Spacer device, medium-volume device. For use with all pressurised (aerosol) inhalers, net price with mouthpiece = £6.07; with mask for infant or child = £7.99; with adult mask = £9.97 ⟨NHS⟩

# Nebulisers

In England and Wales nebulisers and compressors are not available on the NHS (but they are free of VAT); some nebulisers (but not compressors) are available on form GP10A in Scotland (for details consult Scottish Drug Tariff).

A nebuliser converts a solution of a drug into an aerosol for inhalation. It is used to deliver higher doses of drug to the airways than is usual with standard inhalers. The main indications for use of a nebuliser are:

- to deliver a beta$_2$ agonist or ipratropium to a child with an *acute exacerbation* of asthma or of airways obstruction;

- to deliver *prophylactic medication* to a child unable to use other conventional devices;

- to deliver an antibacterial (such as colistimethate sodium or tobramycin) to a child with chronic purulent infection (as in cystic fibrosis or bronchiectasis);

- to deliver budesonide to a child with severe croup.

The proportion of a nebuliser solution that reaches the lungs depends on the type of nebuliser and although it can be as high as 30% it is more frequently close to 10% and sometimes below 10%. The remaining solution is left in the nebuliser as residual volume or it is deposited in the mouthpiece and tubing. The extent to which the nebulised solution is deposited in the airways or alveoli depends on particle size. Particles with a median diameter of 1–5 microns are deposited in the airways and are therefore appropriate for asthma whereas a particle size of 1–2 microns is needed for alveolar deposition. The type of nebuliser is therefore chosen according to the deposition required and according to the viscosity of the solution.

Some jet nebulisers are able to increase drug output during inspiration and hence increase efficiency.

Nebulised bronchodilators are appropriate for children with chronic persistent asthma or those with severe acute asthma. In chronic asthma, nebulised bronchodilators should only be used to relieve persistent daily wheeze, however, with the development of spacers with facemasks, it is now unusual for a child to require long-term nebulised asthma therapy (see Management of Chronic Asthma table, p. 133). The use of nebulisers in chronic persistent asthma should be considered only:

- after a review of the diagnosis and use of current inhaler devices;

- if the airflow obstruction is significantly reversible by bronchodilators without unacceptable side-effects;

- if the child does not benefit from use of conventional inhaler device, such as pressurised metered-dose inhaler plus spacer;

- if the child is complying with the prescribed dose and frequency of anti-inflammatory treatment including regular use of high-dose inhaled corticosteroid.

When a nebuliser is prescribed, the child or child's carer must:

- have clear instructions from a doctor, specialist nurse, physiotherapist, or pharmacist on the use of the nebuliser (and on peak-flow monitoring—see notes above);

- be instructed not to treat acute attacks without also seeking medical help;

- have regular follow up with doctor or specialist nurse.

*Jet nebulisers* are more widely used than ultrasonic nebulisers. Most jet nebulisers require an optimum flow rate of 6–8 litres/minute and in hospital can be driven by piped air or oxygen; in acute asthma the nebuliser should always be driven by oxygen. Domiciliary oxygen cylinders do not provide an adequate flow rate therefore an electrical compressor is required for domiciliary use.

---

**Safe practice**

The Department of Health has reminded users of the need to use the correct grade of tubing when connecting a nebuliser to a medical gas supply or compressor.

---

## Nebuliser diluent

Nebulisation may be carried out using an undiluted nebuliser solution or it may require dilution beforehand. The usual diluent is sterile sodium chloride 0.9% (physiological saline).

**Sodium Chloride** (Non-proprietary) [PoM]
Nebuliser solution, sodium chloride 0.9%, net price 20 × 2.5 mL = £11.50
Brands include *Saline Steripoule®*, *Saline Steri-Neb®*

---

## 3.2 Corticosteroids

Corticosteroids are effective in the management of *asthma*; they reduce airway inflammation.

An inhaled corticosteroid is used regularly for prophylaxis of asthma when a child requires a beta$_2$ agonist more than twice a week, or if symptoms disturb sleep at least once a week, or if the child has suffered an exacerbation in the last 2 years requiring a systemic corticosteroid (see Management of Chronic Asthma table, p. 133).

Current or previous smoking reduces the effectiveness of inhaled corticosteroids and higher doses may be necessary.

Corticosteroid inhalers must be used regularly for maximum benefit; alleviation of symptoms usually occurs 3 to 7 days after initiation but may take longer. **Beclometasone dipropionate, budesonide, fluticasone propionate,** and **mometasone furoate** appear to be equally effective. A spacer device should be used for administering inhaled corticosteroids in children under 15 years (see NICE guidance, section 3.1.5); a spacer device is also useful in children over 15 years, particularly if high doses are required.

In children 12–18 years using an inhaled corticosteroid and a long-acting beta$_2$ agonist for the prophylaxis of asthma, but who are poorly controlled, (see step 3 of the Management of Chronic Asthma table, p. 133) *Symbicort®* (budesonide with formoterol) may be used as a reliever (instead of a short-acting beta$_2$ agonist), in addition to its regular use for the prophylaxis of asthma [unlicensed]. *Symbicort®* can also be used in this way in children 12–18 years using an inhaled corticosteroid with a dose greater than 400 micrograms beclometasone dipropionate daily[1], but who are poorly controlled [unlicensed] (see step 2 of the Management of Chronic Asthma table, p. 133). When starting this treatment, the total regular dose of inhaled corticosteroid should not

---

1. For standard doses of other inhaled corticosteroids, see Management of Chronic Asthma table, p. 133

be reduced. Children and their carers must be carefully instructed on the appropriate dose and management of exacerbations before initiating this treatment, preferably by a respiratory specialist. Children using budesonide with formoterol as a reliever once a day or more should have their treatment reviewed regularly; see also Side-effects below. This management approach has not been investigated with combination inhalers containing other corticosteroids and long-acting beta$_2$ agonists.

High doses of inhaled corticosteroids can be prescribed for children who respond only partially to standard doses of an inhaled corticosteroid and a long-acting beta$_2$ agonist or to other long-acting bronchodilators (see Management of Chronic Asthma table, p. 133). High doses should be continued only if there is clear benefit over the lower dose. The recommended maximum dose of an inhaled corticosteroid should not generally be exceeded; however, if a higher dose is required it should be initiated and supervised by a respiratory paediatrician. The use of high doses of an inhaled corticosteroid can minimise the requirement for an oral corticosteroid.

**Cautions of inhaled corticosteroids** Systemic therapy may be required during periods of stress, such as during severe infections, or when airways obstruction or mucus prevent drug access to smaller airways; **interactions:** Appendix 1 (corticosteroids).

**Paradoxical bronchospasm** The potential for paradoxical bronchospasm (calling for discontinuation and alternative therapy) should be borne in mind—mild bronchospasm may be prevented by inhalation of a short-acting beta$_2$ agonist beforehand (or by transfer from an aerosol inhalation to a dry powder inhalation if suitable).

**CFC-free inhalers** Chlorofluorocarbon (CFC) propellants in pressurised aerosol inhalers have been replaced by hydrofluoroalkane (HFA) propellants.

Doses for corticosteroid CFC-free inhalers may be different from traditional CFC-containing inhalers and may differ between brands, see MHRA/CHM advice below.

> **MHRA/CHM advice (July 2008)**
> Beclometasone dipropionate CFC-free pressurised metered-dose inhalers (*Qvar*® and *Clenil Modulite*®) are **not** interchangeable and should be prescribed by brand name; *Qvar*® has extra-fine particles, is more potent than traditional beclometasone dipropionate CFC-containing inhalers, and is approximately twice as potent as *Clenil Modulite*®.

**Side-effects of inhaled corticosteroids** Inhaled corticosteroids have considerably fewer systemic effects than oral corticosteroids, but adverse effects have been reported.

High doses of inhaled corticosteroids (see Management of Chronic Asthma table, p. 133) used for prolonged periods can induce adrenal suppression. Inhaled corticosteroids have occasionally been associated with adrenal crisis and coma in children; excessive doses should be **avoided**. Children using high doses of inhaled corticosteroids should be under the supervision of a paediatrician for the duration of the treatment; they should be

given a 'steroid card' (section 6.3.2) and specific written advice to consider corticosteroid replacement during an episode of stress, such as a severe intercurrent illness or an operation.

In adults, bone mineral density is sometimes reduced following long-term inhalation of higher doses of corticosteroids, predisposing patients to osteoporosis (section 6.6). It is, therefore, sensible to ensure that the dose of an inhaled corticosteroid is no higher than necessary to keep a child's asthma under good control.

Growth restriction associated with systemic corticosteroid therapy does not seem to occur with recommended doses of inhaled corticosteroids; although initial growth velocity may be reduced, there appears to be no effect on achieving normal adult height. However, the height and weight of children receiving prolonged treatment with inhaled corticosteroid should be monitored annually; if growth is slowed, referral to a paediatrician should be considered.

Hoarseness, dysphonia, throat irritation, and candidiasis of the mouth or throat may occur with inhaled corticosteroids (see Candidiasis below). Paradoxical bronchospasm has been reported very rarely. Anxiety, depression, sleep disturbances, behavioural changes including hyperactivity, irritability, and aggression have been reported; hyperglycaemia (usually only with high doses), skin thinning, and bruising have also been reported.

**Candidiasis** The risk of oral candidiasis can be reduced by using a spacer device with the corticosteroid inhaler; rinsing the mouth with water after inhalation of a dose may also be helpful. Antifungal oral suspension or oral gel (section 12.3.2) can be used to treat oral candidiasis while continuing corticosteroid therapy.

**Oral** An acute attack of asthma should be treated with a short course (3–5 days) of oral corticosteroid, see Management of Acute Asthma, p. 132. The dose can usually be stopped abruptly but it should be reduced gradually in children under 12 years who have taken corticosteroids for more than 14 days. Tapering is not needed in children 12–18 years provided the child receives an inhaled corticosteroid in an adequate dose (apart from those on maintenance oral corticosteroid treatment or where oral corticosteroids are required for 3 or more weeks); see also Withdrawal of Corticosteroids, section 6.3.2.

In chronic continuing asthma, when the response to other drugs has been inadequate, longer term administration of an oral corticosteroid may be necessary; in such cases high doses of an inhaled corticosteroid should be continued to minimise oral corticosteroid requirements.

An oral corticosteroid should normally be taken as a single dose in the morning to reduce the disturbance to circadian cortisol secretion. Dosage should always be titrated to the lowest dose that controls symptoms. Some clinicians use alternate-day dosing of an oral corticosteroid.

**Parenteral** For the use of hydrocortisone injection in the emergency treatment of acute severe asthma, see Management of Acute Asthma, p. 132.

**3**

**Respiratory system**

### NICE guidance
### Inhaled corticosteroids for the treatment of chronic asthma (children under 12 years, November 2007; adults and children over 12 years, March 2008)

For children with chronic asthma in whom treatment with an inhaled corticosteroid is considered appropriate, the least costly product that is suitable for an individual child (taking into consideration NICE TAs 38 and 10), within its marketing authorisation, is recommended

For children with chronic asthma in whom treatment with an inhaled corticosteroid and a long-acting beta$_2$ agonist is considered appropriate, the following apply:

- the use of a combination inhaler within its marketing authorisation is recommended as an option;
- the decision to use a combination inhaler or two agents in separate inhalers should be made on an individual basis, taking into consideration therapeutic need and the likelihood of treatment adherence;
- if a combination inhaler is chosen, then the least costly inhaler that is suitable for the individual child is recommended.

www.nice.org.uk/TA131
www.nice.org.uk/TA138

## BECLOMETASONE DIPROPIONATE
### (Beclomethasone Dipropionate)

**Cautions** see notes above
**Pregnancy** see p. 131
**Breast-feeding** see p. 131
**Side-effects** see notes above
**Licensed use** *Becodisk®-400, Clenil Modulite®*-200 and -250, and *Qvar®* are not licensed for use in children under 12 years; *Easyhaler® Beclometasone Dipropionate* is not licensed for use in children under 18 years

### Indications and dose
#### Prophylaxis of asthma
See Management of Chronic Asthma table, p. 133
**Important** for *Asmabec Clickhaler®, Becodisks®*, and *Qvar®* doses, see under preparations below

**Beclometasone** (Non-proprietary) [PoM]
Dry powder for inhalation, beclometasone dipropionate 100 micrograms/metered inhalation, net price 100-dose unit = £5.36; 200 micrograms/metered inhalation, 100-dose unit = £9.89, 200-dose unit = £14.93; 400 micrograms/metered inhalation, 100-dose unit = £19.61. Label: 8, counselling, administration; also 10 and steroid card with high doses
Brands include *Pulvinal® Beclometasone Dipropionate, Easyhaler® Beclometasone Dipropionate*

**Asmabec Clickhaler®** (UCB Pharma) [PoM]
Dry powder for inhalation, beclometasone dipropionate 100 micrograms/metered inhalation, net price 200-dose unit = £9.43; 250 micrograms/metered inhalation, 100-dose unit = £11.83. Label: 8, counselling, administration; also 10 and steroid card with high doses
**Dose**
#### Prophylaxis of asthma
- By inhalation of powder
  **Child 6–12 years** 100–200 micrograms twice daily, adjusted as necessary
  **Child 12–18 years** 100–400 micrograms twice daily, adjusted as necessary; max. 1 mg twice daily

**Becodisks®** (A&H) [PoM]
Dry powder for inhalation, disks containing 8 blisters of beclometasone dipropionate 100 micrograms/blister, net price 15 disks with *Diskhaler®* device = £11.30, 15-disk refill = £10.76; 200 micrograms/blister, 15 disks with *Diskhaler®* device = £21.54, 15-disk refill = £20.99; 400 micrograms/blister, 15 disks with *Diskhaler®* device = £42.52, 15-disk refill = £41.98. Label: 8, counselling, administration; also 10 and steroid card with high doses
**Note** *Becodisks®* preparations are being discontinued; some strengths may no longer be available
**Dose**
#### Prophylaxis of asthma
- By inhalation of powder
  **Child 5–12 years** 100–200 micrograms twice daily, adjusted as necessary
  **Child 12–18 years** 400–800 micrograms twice daily, adjusted as necessary

**Clenil Modulite®** (Chiesi) [PoM]
Aerosol inhalation, beclometasone dipropionate 50 micrograms/metered inhalation, net price 200-dose unit = £3.70; 100 micrograms/metered inhalation = £7.42; 200 micrograms/metered inhalation = £16.17; 250 micrograms/metered inhalation = £16.29. Label: 8, counselling, administration; also 10 and steroid card with high doses
**Dose**
#### Prophylaxis of asthma
- By aerosol inhalation
  **Child 2–12 years** 100–200 micrograms twice daily
  **Child 12–18 years** 200–400 micrograms twice daily adjusted as necessary up to 1 mg twice daily

**Note** *Clenil Modulite®* is not interchangeable with other CFC-free beclometasone dipropionate inhalers; the MHRA has advised (July 2008) that CFC-free beclometasone dipropionate inhalers should be prescribed by brand name, see p. 145
**Dental Prescribing on NHS** *Clenil Modulite®* 50 micrograms/metered inhalation may be prescribed

**Qvar®** (TEVA UK) [PoM]
Aerosol inhalation, beclometasone dipropionate 50 micrograms/metered inhalation, net price 100-dose unit = £7.87; 100 micrograms/metered inhalation, 200-dose unit = £17.21. Label: 8, counselling, administration; also 10 and steroid card with high doses

Autohaler® (breath-actuated aerosol inhalation), beclometasone dipropionate 50 micrograms/metered inhalation, net price 200-dose unit = £7.87; 100 micrograms/metered inhalation, 200-dose unit = £17.21. Label: 8, counselling, administration; also 10 and steroid card with high doses

Easi-Breathe® (breath-actuated aerosol inhalation), beclometasone dipropionate 50 micrograms/metered inhalation, net price 200-dose = £7.74; 100 micrograms/metered inhalation, 200-dose = £16.95. Label: 8, counselling, administration; also 10 and steroid card with high doses
**Dose**
#### Prophylaxis of asthma
- By aerosol inhalation
  **Child 12–18 years** 50–200 micrograms twice daily, increased if necessary to max. 400 micrograms twice daily

**Important** When switching a child with well-controlled

asthma from another corticosteroid inhaler, initially a 100-microgram metered dose of *Qvar*® should be prescribed for:

- 200–250 micrograms of beclometasone dipropionate or budesonide
- 100 micrograms of fluticasone propionate

When switching a child with poorly controlled asthma from another corticosteroid inhaler, initially a 100-microgram metered dose of *Qvar*® should be prescribed for 100 micrograms of beclometasone dipropionate, budesonide, or fluticasone propionate; the dose of *Qvar*® should be adjusted according to response

**Note** *Qvar*® is not interchangeable with other CFC-free beclometasone dipropionate inhalers; the MHRA has advised (July 2008) that beclometasone dipropionate CFC-free inhalers should be prescribed by brand name, see p. 145

## ▌ BUDESONIDE

**Cautions**   see notes above

**Pregnancy**   see p. 131

**Breast-feeding**   see p. 131

**Side-effects**   see notes above

**Licensed use**   *Pulmicort*® *nebuliser solution* not licensed for use in children under 3 months; not licensed for use in bronchopulmonary dysplasia; *Symbicort*® not licensed for use in children for asthma maintenance and reliever therapy

### Indications and dose

**Prophylaxis of asthma** see Management of Chronic Asthma table, p. 133, and preparations below

#### Croup

- **By inhalation of nebuliser suspension**

  **Child over 1 month** 2 mg as single dose or in 2 divided doses separated by 30 minutes; dose may be repeated every 12 hours until clinical improvement

#### Bronchopulmonary dysplasia with spontaneous respiration

- **By inhalation of nebuliser suspension**

  **Neonate** 500 micrograms twice daily

  **Child 1–4 months** 500 micrograms twice daily; for severe symptoms in child body-weight 2.5 kg or over, 1 mg twice daily

**Budesonide** (Non-proprietary) (PoM)

Dry powder for inhalation, budesonide 100 micrograms/metered inhalation, net price 200-dose unit = £8.86; 200 micrograms/metered inhalation 200-dose unit = £17.71; 400 micrograms/metered inhalation 100-dose unit = £17.71. Label: 8, counselling, administration; also 10 and steroid card with high doses

**Brands include** *Easyhaler*® *Budesonide*

**Dose**

##### Prophylaxis of asthma

- **By inhalation of powder**

  **Child 6–12 years** 100–400 micrograms twice daily, adjusted as necessary; alternatively, in mild to moderate asthma, 200–400 micrograms as a single dose each evening if stabilised on daily dose given in 2 divided doses

  **Child 12–18 years** 100–800 micrograms twice daily, adjusted as necessary; alternatively, in mild to moderate asthma, 200–400 micrograms (max. 800 micrograms) as a single dose each evening if stabilised on daily dose given in 2 divided doses

**Budelin Novolizer**® (Meda) (PoM)

Dry powder for inhalation, budesonide 200 micrograms, net price refillable inhaler device and 100-dose cartridge = £14.86; 100-dose refill cartridge = £9.59. Label: 8, counselling, administration; also 10 and steroid card with high doses

**Dose**

##### Prophylaxis of asthma

- **By inhalation of powder**

  **Child 6–12 years** 200–400 micrograms twice daily, adjusted as necessary; alternatively, in mild to moderate asthma, 200–400 micrograms as a single dose each evening if stabilised on daily dose given in 2 divided doses

  **Child 12–18 years** 200–800 micrograms twice daily, adjusted as necessary; alternatively, in mild to moderate asthma, 200–400 micrograms as a single dose each evening if stabilised on daily dose given in 2 divided doses (max. 800 micrograms)

**Pulmicort**® (AstraZeneca) (PoM)

*Turbohaler*® (= dry powder inhaler), budesonide 100 micrograms/metered inhalation, net price 200-dose unit = £11.84; 200 micrograms/metered inhalation, 100-dose unit = £11.84; 400 micrograms/metered inhalation, 50-dose unit = £13.86. Label: 8, counselling, administration; also 10 and steroid card with high doses

**Dose**

##### Prophylaxis of asthma

- **By inhalation of powder**

  **Child 5–12 years** 100–400 micrograms twice daily, adjusted as necessary; alternatively, in mild to moderate asthma, 200–400 micrograms as a single dose each evening if stabilised on daily dose given in 2 divided doses

  **Child 12–18 years** 100–800 micrograms twice daily, adjusted as necessary; alternatively, in mild to moderate asthma, 200–400 micrograms (max. 800 micrograms) as a single dose each evening if stabilised on daily dose given in 2 divided doses

*Respules*® (= single-dose units for nebulisation), budesonide 250 micrograms/mL, net price 20 × 2-mL (500-microgram) unit = £20.02; 500 micrograms/mL, 20 × 2-mL (1-mg) unit = £30.30. May be diluted with sterile sodium chloride 0.9%. Label: 8, counselling, administration, 10, steroid card

**Note** Not suitable for use in ultrasonic nebulisers

**Dose**

##### Prophylaxis of asthma

- **By inhalation of nebuliser suspension**

  **Child 3 months–12 years** initially 0.5–1 mg twice daily, reduced to 250–500 micrograms twice daily

  **Child 12–18 years** initially 1–2 mg twice daily, reduced to 0.5–1 mg twice daily

### ◢ Compound preparations

For prescribing information on formoterol fumarate, see section 3.1.1.1

**Symbicort**® (AstraZeneca) (PoM)

Symbicort 100/6 Turbohaler® (= dry powder inhaler), budesonide 100 micrograms, formoterol fumarate 6 micrograms/metered inhalation, net price 120-dose unit = £33.00. Label: 8, counselling, administration

**Dose**

##### Asthma, maintenance therapy

- **By inhalation of powder**

  **Child 6–12 years** 1–2 puffs twice daily reduced to 1 puff once daily if control maintained

  **Child 12–18 years** 1–2 puffs twice daily reduced to 1 puff once daily if control maintained

**3**

**Respiratory system**

**Asthma, maintenance and reliever therapy** (but see p. 144)

• **By inhalation of powder**

**Child 12–18 years** 2 puffs daily in 1–2 divided doses; for relief of symptoms, 1 puff as needed up to max. 6 puffs at a time; max. 8 puffs daily

**Symbicort 200/6 Turbohaler®** (= dry powder inhaler), budesonide 200 micrograms, formoterol fumarate 6 micrograms/metered inhalation, net price 120-dose unit = £38.00. Label: 8, counselling, administration; also 10 and steroid card with high doses

**Dose**

**Asthma, maintenance therapy**

• **By inhalation of powder**

**Child 12–18 years** 1–2 puffs twice daily reduced in well-controlled asthma to 1 puff once daily

**Asthma, maintenance and reliever therapy** (but see p. 144)

• **By inhalation of powder**

**Child 12–18 years** 2 puffs daily in 1–2 divided doses, increased if necessary to 2 puffs twice daily; for relief of symptoms, 1 puff as needed up to max. 6 puffs at a time; max. 8 puffs daily

**Symbicort 400/12 Turbohaler®** (= dry powder inhaler), budesonide 400 micrograms, formoterol fumarate 12 micrograms/metered inhalation, net price 60-dose unit = £38.00. Label: 8, counselling, administration; also 10 and steroid card with high doses

**Dose**

**Asthma, maintenance therapy**

• **By inhalation of powder**

**Child 12–18 years** 1 puff twice daily; may be reduced in well-controlled asthma to 1 puff once daily

## ◼ CICLESONIDE

**Cautions** see notes above
**Pregnancy** see p. 131
**Breast-feeding** see p. 131
**Side-effects** see notes above; also nausea, taste disturbance

**Indications and dose**

Prophylaxis of asthma

• **By aerosol inhalation**

**Child 12–18 years** 160 micrograms daily as a single dose reduced to 80 micrograms daily if control maintained

**Alvesco®** (Takeda) [PoM]
Aerosol inhalation, ciclesonide 80 micrograms/metered inhalation, net price 120-dose unit = £32.83; 160 micrograms/metered inhalation, 60-dose unit = £19.31, 120-dose unit = £38.62. Label: 8, counselling, administration

## ◼ FLUTICASONE PROPIONATE

**Cautions** see notes above
**Pregnancy** see p. 131
**Breast-feeding** see p. 131
**Side-effects** see notes above; also dyspepsia and arthralgia

**Indications and dose**

Prophylaxis of asthma see Management of Chronic Asthma table, p. 133, and preparations below

**Flixotide®** (A&H) [PoM]
Accuhaler® (dry powder for inhalation), disk containing 60 blisters of *fluticasone propionate* 50 micrograms/blister with *Accuhaler®* device, net price = £6.38; 100 micrograms/blister with *Accuhaler®* device = £8.93; 250 micrograms/blister with *Accuhaler®* device = £21.26; 500 micrograms/blister with *Accuhaler®* device = £36.14. Label: 8, counselling, administration; also 10 and steroid card with high doses

**Dose**

Prophylaxis of asthma

• **By inhalation of powder**

**Child 5–16 years** 50–100 micrograms twice daily adjusted as necessary; max. 200 micrograms twice daily

**Child 16–18 years** 100–500 micrograms twice daily, adjusted as necessary; max. 1 mg twice daily (doses above 500 micrograms twice daily initiated by a specialist)

Evohaler® (aerosol inhalation), fluticasone propionate 50 micrograms/metered inhalation, net price 120-dose unit = £5.44; 125 micrograms/metered inhalation, 120-dose unit = £21.26; 250 micrograms/metered inhalation, 120-dose unit = £36.14. Label: 8, counselling, administration; also 10 and steroid card with high doses

**Dose**

Prophylaxis of asthma

• **By aerosol inhalation**

**Child 4–16 years** 50–100 micrograms twice daily adjusted as necessary; max. 200 micrograms twice daily

**Child 16–18 years** 100–500 micrograms twice daily adjusted as necessary; max. 1 mg twice daily (doses above 500 micrograms twice daily initiated by a specialist)

Nebules® (= single-dose units for nebulisation) fluticasone propionate 250 micrograms/mL, net price 10 × 2-mL (500-microgram) unit = £9.34; 1 mg/mL, 10 × 2-mL (2-mg) unit = £37.35. May be diluted with sterile sodium chloride 0.9%. Label: 8, counselling, administration, 10, steroid card

**Note** Not suitable for use in ultrasonic nebulisers

**Dose**

Prophylaxis of asthma

• **By inhalation of nebuliser suspension**

**Child 4–16 years** 1 mg twice daily

**Child 16–18 years** 0.5–2 mg twice daily

◀**Compound preparations**

For prescribing information on formoterol and salmeterol, see Formoterol Fumarate, and Salmeterol, section 3.1.1.1.

**Flutiform®** (Napp) ▼ [PoM]
Flutiform® 50 micrograms/5 micrograms (aerosol inhalation), fluticasone propionate 50 micrograms, formoterol fumarate 5 micrograms/metered inhalation, net price 120-dose unit = £18.00. Label: 8, counselling, administration

**Dose**

Prophylaxis of asthma

• **By aerosol inhalation**

**Child 12–18 years** 2 puffs twice daily

Flutiform® 125 micrograms/5 micrograms (aerosol inhalation), fluticasone propionate 125 micrograms, formoterol fumarate 5 micrograms/metered inhalation, net price 120-dose unit = £29.26. Label: 8, counselling, administration, 10, steroid card

**Dose**

**Prophylaxis of asthma**

- By aerosol inhalation

    **Child 12–18 years** 2 puffs twice daily

**Seretide®** (A&H) [PoM]

Seretide 100 Accuhaler® (dry powder for inhalation), disk containing 60 blisters of fluticasone propionate 100 micrograms, salmeterol (as xinafoate) 50 micrograms/blister with *Accuhaler®* device, net price = £31.19. Label: 8, counselling, administration

**Dose**

**Prophylaxis of asthma**

- By inhalation of powder

    **Child 5–18 years** 1 inhalation twice daily, reduced to 1 inhalation once daily if control maintained

Seretide 250 Accuhaler® (dry powder for inhalation), disk containing 60 blisters of fluticasone propionate 250 micrograms, salmeterol (as xinafoate) 50 micrograms/blister with *Accuhaler®* device, net price = £35.00. Label: 8, counselling, administration, 10, steroid card

**Dose**

**Prophylaxis of asthma**

- By inhalation of powder

    **Child 12–18 years** 1 inhalation twice daily

Seretide 500 Accuhaler® (dry powder for inhalation), disk containing 60 blisters of fluticasone propionate 500 micrograms, salmeterol (as xinafoate) 50 micrograms/blister with *Accuhaler®* device, net price = £40.92. Label: 8, counselling, administration, 10, steroid card

**Dose**

**Prophylaxis of asthma**

- By inhalation of powder

    **Child 12–18 years** 1 inhalation twice daily

Seretide 50 Evohaler® (aerosol inhalation), fluticasone propionate 50 micrograms, salmeterol (as xinafoate) 25 micrograms/metered inhalation, net price 120-dose unit = £18.00. Label: 8, counselling, administration

**Dose**

**Prophylaxis of asthma**

- By aerosol inhalation

    **Child 5–18 years** 2 puffs twice daily, reduced to 2 puffs once daily if control maintained

Seretide 125 Evohaler® (aerosol inhalation), fluticasone propionate 125 micrograms, salmeterol (as xinafoate) 25 micrograms/metered inhalation, net price 120-dose unit = £35.00. Label: 8, counselling, administration, 10, steroid card

**Dose**

**Prophylaxis of asthma**

- By aerosol inhalation

    **Child 12–18 years** 2 puffs twice daily

Seretide 250 Evohaler® (aerosol inhalation), fluticasone propionate 250 micrograms, salmeterol (as xinafoate) 25 micrograms/metered inhalation, net price 120-dose unit = £59.48. Label: 8, counselling, administration, 10, steroid card

**Dose**

**Prophylaxis of asthma**

- By aerosol inhalation

    **Child 12–18 years** 2 puffs twice daily

## ▌ MOMETASONE FUROATE

**Cautions** see notes above

**Pregnancy** see p. 131

**Breast-feeding** see p. 131

**Side-effects** see notes above; also headache; *less commonly* dyspepsia, weight gain, palpitation

**Indications and dose**

Prophylaxis of asthma see also Management of Chronic Asthma table, p. 133

- By inhalation of powder

    **Child 12–18 years** 400 micrograms as a single dose in the evening or in 2 divided doses, reduced to 200 micrograms once daily if control maintained; dose may be increased to max. 400 micrograms twice daily in severe asthma

**Asmanex®** (MSD) [PoM]

Twisthaler (= dry powder inhaler), mometasone furoate 200 micrograms/metered inhalation, net price 30-dose unit = £15.70, 60-dose unit = £23.54; 400 micrograms/metered inhalation, 30-dose unit = £21.78, 60-dose unit = £36.05. Label: 8, counselling, administration, 10, steroid card

**Note** The *Scottish Medicines Consortium* has advised (November 2003) that *Asmanex®* is restricted for use following failure of first-line inhaled corticosteroids

## 3.3 Cromoglicate and related therapy and leukotriene receptor antagonists

3.3.1 Cromoglicate and related therapy

3.3.2 Leukotriene receptor antagonists

## 3.3.1 Cromoglicate and related therapy

The mode of action of **sodium cromoglicate** and **nedocromil** is not completely understood; they may be of value as *prophylaxis* in asthma with an allergic basis, but the evidence for benefit of sodium cromoglicate in children is contentious. Prophylaxis with cromoglicate or nedocromil is less effective than with inhaled corticosteroids (see Management of Chronic Asthma table). Withdrawal of sodium cromoglicate or nedocromil should be done gradually over a period of one week—symptoms of asthma may recur.

Nedocromil may be of some benefit in the prophylaxis of exercise-induced asthma.

For the use of sodium cromoglicate and nedocromil in allergic conjunctivitis see section 11.4.2; sodium cromo-

3 Respiratory system

glicate is used also in allergic rhinitis (section 12.2.1) and allergy-related diarrhoea (section 1.5.4).

**Paradoxical bronchospasm**  If paradoxical bronchospasm occurs, a short-acting beta₂ agonist such as salbutamol or terbutaline (section 3.1.1.1) should be used to control symptoms; treatment with sodium cromoglicate or nedocromil should be discontinued.

**Side-effects**  Side-effects associated with inhalation of sodium cromoglicate and nedocromil include throat irritation, cough, bronchospasm (including paradoxical bronchospasm—see above), and headache.

## SODIUM CROMOGLICATE
(Sodium Cromoglycate)

**Cautions**  see notes above; also discontinue if eosinophilic pneumonia occurs
**Pregnancy**  see p. 131
**Breast-feeding**  see p. 131
**Side-effects**  see notes above; also rhinitis,eosinophilic pneumonia
**Indications and dose**
Prophylaxis of asthma (see also Management of Chronic Asthma, p. 133)
• By aerosol inhalation
  Child 5–18 years 10 mg (2 puffs) 4 times daily, increased if necessary to 6–8 times daily; an additional dose may also be taken before exercise; maintenance, 5 mg (1 puff) 4 times daily

Food allergy section 1.5.4

Allergic conjunctivitis section 11.4.2

Allergic rhinitis section 12.2.1

**Intal® CFC-free inhaler** (Sanofi-Aventis) [PoM]
Aerosol inhalation, sodium cromoglicate 5 mg/metered inhalation, net price 112-dose unit = £14.84. Label: 8, counselling, administration

## NEDOCROMIL SODIUM

**Cautions**  see notes above
**Pregnancy**  see p. 131
**Breast-feeding**  see p. 131
**Side-effects**  see notes above; also nausea, vomiting, dyspepsia, abdominal pain, pharyngitis; *rarely* taste disturbances
**Licensed use**  not licensed for use in children under 6 years
**Indications and dose**
Prophylaxis of asthma (but see notes above)
• By aerosol inhalation
  Child 5–18 years 4 mg (2 puffs) 4 times daily, when control achieved may be possible to reduce to twice daily
  Counselling Regular use is necessary

Allergic conjunctivitis section 11.4.2

**Tilade® CFC-free inhaler** (Sanofi-Aventis) [PoM]
Aerosol inhalation, mint-flavoured, nedocromil sodium 2 mg/metered inhalation. Net price 112-dose unit = £39.94. Label: 8, counselling, administration

## 3.3.2 Leukotriene receptor antagonists

The leukotriene receptor antagonists, **montelukast** and **zafirlukast**, block the effects of cysteinyl leukotrienes in the airways; they can be used in children for the management of chronic asthma with an inhaled corticosteroid or as an alternative if an inhaled corticosteroid cannot be used (see Management of Chronic Asthma table, p. 133).

Montelukast has not been shown to be more effective than a standard dose of inhaled corticosteroid, but the two drugs appear to have an additive effect. The leukotriene receptor antagonists may be of benefit in exercise-induced asthma and in those with concomitant rhinitis, but they are less effective in children with severe asthma who are also receiving high doses of other drugs.

There is some limited evidence to support the intermittent use of montelukast in children under 12 years with episodic wheeze associated with viral infections [unlicensed use]. Treatment is started at the onset of either asthma symptoms or of coryzal symptoms and continued for 7 days; there is no evidence to support this use in moderate or severe asthma.

**Churg-Strauss syndrome**  Churg-Strauss syndrome has occurred very rarely in association with the use of leukotriene receptor antagonists; in many of the reported cases the reaction followed the reduction or withdrawal of oral corticosteroid therapy. Prescribers should be alert to the development of eosinophilia, vasculitic rash, worsening pulmonary symptoms, cardiac complications, or peripheral neuropathy.

**Pregnancy**  There is limited evidence for the safe use of leukotriene receptor antagonists during pregnancy; however, they can be taken as normal in females who have shown a significant improvement in asthma not achievable with other drugs before becoming pregnant, see also p. 131.

## MONTELUKAST

**Cautions**  interactions: Appendix 1 (leukotriene receptor antagonists)
**Pregnancy**  manufacturer advises avoid unless essential; see also notes above
**Breast-feeding**  manufacturer advises avoid unless essential
**Side-effects**  abdominal pain, thirst, headache, hyperkinesia (in young children); *less commonly* dry mouth, dyspepsia, oedema, dizziness, malaise, sleep disturbances, sleep-walking, abnormal dreams, anxiety, aggression, depression, paraesthesia, hypoaesthesia, seizures, arthralgia, myalgia, epistaxis, bruising, pruritus; *rarely* palpitation, tremor, bleeding; *very rarely* hepatic disorders, hallucinations, suicidal thoughts and behaviour, disorientation, Churg-Strauss syndrome (see notes above), erythema nodosum, erythema multiforme

**Indications and dose**

Prophylaxis of asthma see notes above and Management of Chronic Asthma table, p. 133

● By mouth

Child 6 months–6 years 4 mg once daily in the evening

Child 6–15 years 5 mg once daily in the evening

Child 15–18 years 10 mg once daily in the evening

Symptomatic relief of seasonal allergic rhinitis in children with asthma

● By mouth

Child 15–18 years 10 mg once daily in the evening

**Montelukast** (Non-proprietary) (PoM)
Chewable tablets, montelukast (as sodium salt) 4 mg, net price 28-tab pack = £2.57; 5 mg, 28-tab pack = £2.57. Label: 23, 24
Excipients include aspartame (section 9.4.1)

Granules, montelukast (as sodium salt) 4 mg, net price 28-sachet pack = £24.41. Counselling, administration
Counselling Granules may be swallowed whole or mixed with cold, soft food (but not fluid) and taken immediately

Tablets, montelukast (as sodium salt) 10 mg, net price 28-tab pack = £2.70

**Singulair**® (MSD) (PoM)
Chewable tablets, pink, cherry-flavoured, montelukast (as sodium salt) 4 mg, net price 28-tab pack = £25.69; 5 mg, 28-tab pack = £25.69. Label: 23, 24
Excipients include aspartame equivalent to phenylalanine 674 micrograms/4-mg tablet and 842 micrograms/5-mg tablet (section 9.4.1)

Granules, montelukast (as sodium salt) 4 mg, net price 28-sachet pack = £25.69. Counselling, administration
Counselling Granules may be swallowed whole or mixed with cold, soft food (but not fluid) and taken immediately

Tablets, beige, f/c, montelukast (as sodium salt) 10 mg, net price 28-tab pack = £26.97
Note The *Scottish Medicines Consortium* has advised (June 2007) that *Singulair*® chewable tablets and granules are restricted for use as an alternative to low-dose inhaled corticosteroids for children 2–14 years with mild persistent asthma who have not recently had serious asthma attacks that required oral corticosteroid use, and who are not capable of using inhaled corticosteroids; *Singulair*® chewable tablets and granules should be initiated by a specialist in paediatric asthma

---

### ▲ ZAFIRLUKAST

**Cautions** interactions: Appendix 1 (leukotriene receptor antagonists)
Hepatic disorders Children or their carers should be told how to recognise development of liver disorder and advised to seek medical attention if symptoms or signs such as persistent nausea, vomiting, malaise or jaundice develop

**Hepatic impairment** manufacturer advises avoid

**Renal impairment** manufacturer advises caution

**Pregnancy** manufacturer advises use only if potential benefit outweighs risk; see also notes above

**Breast-feeding** present in milk—manufacturer advises avoid

**Side-effects** gastro-intestinal disturbances; headache; *rarely* bleeding disorders, hypersensitivity reactions including angioedema and skin reactions, arthralgia,

myalgia, hepatitis, hyperbilirubinaemia, thrombocytopenia; *very rarely* Churg-Strauss syndrome (see notes above), agranulocytosis

**Indications and dose**

Prophylaxis of asthma see notes above and Management of Chronic Asthma, p. 133

● By mouth

Child 12–18 years 20 mg twice daily

**Accolate**® (AstraZeneca) (PoM)
Tablets, f/c, zafirlukast 20 mg, net price 56-tab pack = £17.75. Label: 23

## 3.4 Antihistamines, immunotherapy, and allergic emergencies

3.4.1   Antihistamines
3.4.2   Allergen immunotherapy
3.4.3   Allergic emergencies

## 3.4.1 Antihistamines

Antihistamines (histamine $H_1$-receptor antagonists) are classified as *sedating* or *non-sedating*, according to their relative potential for CNS depression. Antihistamines differ in their duration of action, incidence of drowsiness, and antimuscarinic effects; the response to an antihistamine may vary from child to child (see Side-effects, p. 152). Either a sedating or a non-sedating antihistamine may be used to treat an acute allergic reaction; for conditions with more persistent symptoms which require regular treatment, a non-sedating antihistamine should be used to minimise the risk of sedation and psychomotor impairment associated with sedating antihistamines.

Oral antihistamines are used in the treatment of nasal allergies, particularly seasonal allergic rhinitis (hay fever), and may be of some value in vasomotor rhinitis; rhinorrhoea and sneezing is reduced, but antihistamines are usually less effective for nasal congestion. Antihistamines are used topically to treat allergic reactions in the eye (section 11.4.2) and in the nose (section 12.2.1). Topical application of antihistamines to the skin is not recommended (section 13.3).

An oral antihistamine may be used to prevent urticaria, and for the treatment of acute urticarial rashes, pruritus, insect bites, and stings. Antihistamines are also used in the management of nausea and vomiting (section 4.6), of migraine (section 4.7.4.1), and the adjunctive management of anaphylaxis and angioedema (section 3.4.3).

The *non-sedating* antihistamine **cetirizine** is safe and effective in children. Other non-sedating antihistamines that are used include **acrivastine**, **bilastine**, **desloratadine** (an active metabolite of loratadine), **fexofenadine** (an active metabolite of terfenadine), **levocetirizine** (an isomer of cetirizine), **loratadine**, **mizolastine**, and **rupatadine**. Most non-sedating antihistamines are long-acting (usually 12–24 hours). There is little evidence that desloratadine or levocetirizine confer any additional benefit—they should be reserved for children who cannot tolerate other therapies.

*Sedating* antihistamines are occasionally useful when insomnia is associated with urticaria and pruritus (sec-

3
Respiratory system

tion 4.1.1). Most of the sedating antihistamines are relatively short-acting, but promethazine may be effective for up to 12 hours. Alimemazine and promethazine have a more sedative effect than chlorphenamine and cyclizine (section 4.6). Chlorphenamine is used as an adjunct to adrenaline (epinephrine) in the emergency treatment of anaphylaxis and angioedema (section 3.4.3).

**Cautions and contra-indications** Antihistamines should be used with caution in children with epilepsy. Most antihistamines should be avoided in acute porphyria, but some are thought to be safe (see section 9.8.2). Sedating antihistamines have significant antimuscarinic activity—they should **not** be used in neonates and should be used with caution in children with urinary retention, glaucoma, or pyloroduodenal obstruction. Phenothiazine sedating antihistamines, such as alimemazine and promethazine, should not be given to children under 2 years, except on specialist advice, because the safety of such use has not been established. See also MHRA/CHM advice, p. 166. **Interactions:** see Appendix 1 (antihistamines).

**Hepatic impairment** Sedating antihistamines should be avoided in children with severe liver disease—increased risk of coma.

**Pregnancy** Most manufacturers of antihistamines advise avoiding their use during pregnancy; however there is no evidence of teratogenicity, except for hydroxyzine where toxicity has been reported with high doses in *animal* studies. The use of sedating antihistamines in the latter part of the third trimester may cause adverse effects in neonates such as irritability, paradoxical excitability, and tremor.

**Breast-feeding** Most antihistamines are present in breast milk in varying amounts; although not known to be harmful, most manufacturers advise avoiding their use in mothers who are breast-feeding.

**Side-effects** Drowsiness is a significant side-effect with most of the older antihistamines although paradoxical stimulation may occur rarely in children, especially with high doses. Drowsiness may diminish after a few days of treatment and is considerably less of a problem with the newer antihistamines (see also notes above). Side-effects that are more common with the older antihistamines include headache, psychomotor impairment, and antimuscarinic effects such as urinary retention, dry mouth, blurred vision, and gastro-intestinal disturbances. Other rare side-effects of antihistamines include hypotension, palpitation, arrhythmias, extrapyramidal effects, dizziness, confusion, depression, sleep disturbances, tremor, convulsions, hypersensitivity reactions (including bronchospasm, angioedema, anaphylaxis, rashes, and photosensitivity reactions), blood disorders, and liver dysfunction.

## Non-sedating antihistamines

**Skilled tasks** Although drowsiness is rare, children and their carers should be advised that it can occur and may affect performance of skilled tasks (e.g. cycling or driving); alcohol should be avoided.

### ACRIVASTINE

**Cautions** see notes above

**Contra-indications** see notes above; also hypersensitivity to triprolidine

**Renal impairment** avoid in severe impairment

**Pregnancy** see notes above

**Breast-feeding** see notes above

**Side-effects** see notes above

**Indications and dose**

Symptomatic relief of allergy such as hay fever, chronic idiopathic urticaria

- By mouth

  Child 12–18 years 8 mg 3 times daily

**Acrivastine** (Non-proprietary)

Capsules, acrivastine 8 mg, net price 12-cap pack = £2.59, 24-cap pack = £4.49. Counselling, skilled tasks

Brands include *Benadryl® Allergy Relief*

### BILASTINE

**Cautions** see notes above

**Contra-indications** see notes above

**Pregnancy** avoid—limited information available; see also notes above

**Breast-feeding** avoid—no information available; see also notes above

**Side-effects** headache, malaise; *less commonly* abdominal pain, diarrhoea, increased appetite, weight gain, thirst, gastritis, prolongation of the QT interval, dyspnoea, anxiety, insomnia, vertigo, dizziness, pyrexia, oral herpes, tinnitus

**Indications and dose**

Symptomatic relief of allergic rhinoconjunctivitis and urticaria

- By mouth

  Child 12–18 years 20 mg once daily

Counselling Advise carer and child that child should take tablet 1 hour before or 2 hours after food or fruit juice

**Ilaxten®** (Menarini) ▼ PoM

Tablets, scored, bilastine 20 mg, net price 30-tab pack = £15.09. Label: 23, counselling, administration

### CETIRIZINE HYDROCHLORIDE

**Cautions** see notes above

**Contra-indications** see notes above

**Renal impairment** use half normal dose if estimated glomerular filtration rate 30–50 mL/minute/1.73m²; use half normal dose and reduce dose frequency to alternate days if estimated glomerular filtration rate 10–30 mL/minute/1.73m²; avoid if estimated glomerular filtration rate less than 10 mL/minute/1.73m²

**Pregnancy** see notes above

**Breast-feeding** see notes above

**Side-effects** see notes above

**Licensed use** not licensed for use in children under 2 years

**Indications and dose**

Symptomatic relief of allergy such as hay fever, chronic idiopathic urticaria, atopic dermatitis

- By mouth

  Child 1–2 years 250 micrograms/kg twice daily

  Child 2–6 years 2.5 mg twice daily

  Child 6–12 years 5 mg twice daily

  Child 12–18 years 10 mg once daily

**Cetirizine** (Non-proprietary)

Tablets, cetirizine hydrochloride 10 mg, net price 30-tab pack = 95p. Counselling, skilled tasks

**Dental prescribing on NHS** Cetirizine 10 mg Tablets may be prescribed

Oral solution, cetirizine hydrochloride 5 mg/5 mL, net price 200 mL = £2.03. Counselling, skilled tasks

**Note** Sugar-free versions are available and can be ordered by specifying 'sugar-free' on the prescription

**Excipients** may include propylene glycol (see Excipients p. 2)

**Dental prescribing on NHS** Cetirizine Oral Solution 5 mg/5 mL may be prescribed

## DESLORATADINE

**Note** Desloratadine is a metabolite of loratadine

**Cautions** see notes above

**Contra-indications** see notes above; also hypersensitivity to loratadine

**Renal impairment** use with caution in severe impairment

**Pregnancy** see notes above

**Breast-feeding** see notes above

**Side-effects** see notes above; *rarely* myalgia; *very rarely* hallucinations

**Indications and dose**

> Symptomatic relief of allergy such as hay fever, chronic idiopathic urticaria
> * By mouth
>   **Child 1–6 years** 1.25 mg once daily
>   **Child 6–12 years** 2.5 mg once daily
>   **Child 12–18 years** 5 mg once daily

**Desloratadine** (Non-proprietary) [PoM]

Tablets, desloratadine 5 mg, net price 30-tab pack = £6.77. Counselling, skilled tasks

**Neoclarityn**® (MSD) [PoM]

Tablets, blue, f/c, desloratadine 5 mg, net price 30-tab pack = £6.77. Counselling, skilled tasks

Oral solution, desloratadine 2.5 mg/5 mL, net price 100 mL (bubblegum-flavour) = £6.77, 150 mL = £10.15. Counselling, skilled tasks

**Excipients** include propylene glycol (see Excipients p. 2)

## FEXOFENADINE HYDROCHLORIDE

**Note** Fexofenadine is a metabolite of terfenadine

**Cautions** see notes above

**Contra-indications** see notes above

**Pregnancy** see notes above

**Breast-feeding** see notes above

**Side-effects** see notes above

**Indications and dose**

> Symptomatic relief of seasonal allergic rhinitis
> * By mouth
>   **Child 6–12 years** 30 mg twice daily
>   **Child 12–18 years** 120 mg once daily

> Symptomatic relief of chronic idiopathic urticaria
> * By mouth
>   **Child 12–18 years** 180 mg once daily

**Fexofenadine Hydrochloride** (Non-proprietary) [PoM]

Tablets, f/c, fexofenadine hydrochloride 120 mg, net price 30-tab pack = £2.95; 180 mg, 30-tab pack = £3.68. Label: 5, counselling, skilled tasks

**Telfast**® (Sanofi-Aventis) [PoM]

Tablets, f/c, peach, fexofenadine hydrochloride 30 mg, net price 60-tab pack = £5.46; 120 mg, 30-tab pack = £5.99; 180 mg, 30-tab pack = £7.58. Label: 5, counselling, skilled tasks

## LEVOCETIRIZINE HYDROCHLORIDE

**Note** Levocetirizine is an isomer of cetirizine

**Cautions** see notes above

**Contra-indications** see notes above

**Renal impairment** estimated glomerular filtration rate 30–50 mL/minute/1.73 m², reduce dose frequency to alternate days; estimated glomerular filtration rate 10–30 mL/minute/1.73 m², reduce dose frequency to every 3 days; estimated glomerular filtration rate less than 10 mL/minute/1.73 m², avoid

**Pregnancy** see notes above

**Breast-feeding** see notes above

**Side-effects** see notes above; *very rarely* weight gain

**Licensed use** tablets not licensed for use in children under 6 years

**Indications and dose**

> Symptomatic relief of allergy such as hay fever, urticaria
> * By mouth
>   **Child 2–6 years** 1.25 mg twice daily
>   **Child 6–18 years** 5 mg once daily

**Levocetirizine Hydrochloride** (Non-proprietary) [PoM]

Tablets, levocetirizine hydrochloride 5 mg, net price 30-tab pack = £4.39. Counselling, skilled tasks

**Xyzal**® (UCB Pharma) [PoM]

Tablets, f/c, levocetirizine hydrochloride 5 mg, net price 30-tab pack = £4.39. Counselling, skilled tasks

Oral solution, sugar-free, levocetirizine hydrochloride 2.5 mg/5 mL, net price 200 mL = £6.00. Counselling, skilled tasks

## LORATADINE

**Cautions** see notes above

**Contra-indications** see notes above

**Hepatic impairment** reduce dose frequency to alternate days in severe impairment

**Pregnancy** see notes above

**Breast-feeding** see notes above

**Side-effects** see notes above

**Indications and dose**

> Symptomatic relief of allergy such as hay fever, chronic idiopathic urticaria
> * By mouth
>   **Child 2–12 years**
>   **Body-weight under 30 kg** 5 mg once daily
>   **Body-weight over 30 kg** 10 mg once daily
>   **Child 12–18 years** 10 mg once daily

3 Respiratory system

Respiratory system

3

**Loratadine** (Non-proprietary)

Tablets, loratadine 10 mg, net price 30-tab pack = £1.20. Counselling, skilled tasks

**Dental Prescribing on NHS** Loratadine 10 mg Tablets may be prescribed

Syrup, loratadine 5 mg/5 mL, net price 100 mL = £2.65. Counselling, skilled tasks

**Excipients** may include propylene glycol (see Excipients, p. 2)

**Dental Prescribing on NHS** Loratadine Syrup 5 mg/5 mL may be prescribed

## ▮ MIZOLASTINE

**Cautions** see notes above

**Contra-indications** see notes above; also susceptibility to QT-interval prolongation (including cardiac disease and hypokalaemia)

**Hepatic impairment** manufacturer recommends avoid in significant impairment

**Pregnancy** see notes above

**Breast-feeding** see notes above

**Side-effects** see notes above; weight gain; anxiety, asthenia; *less commonly* arthralgia and myalgia

**Indications and dose**

Symptomatic relief of allergy such as hay fever, urticaria

- By mouth

    **Child 12–18 years** 10 mg once daily

**Mizollen**® (Sanofi-Aventis) PoM

Tablets, m/r, scored, mizolastine 10 mg, net price 30-tab pack = £5.77. Label: 25, counselling, skilled tasks

## ▮ RUPATADINE

**Cautions** see notes above; also susceptibility to QT-interval prolongation (including cardiac disease and hypokalaemia)

**Hepatic impairment** manufacturer advises avoid—no information available

**Renal impairment** manufacturer advises avoid—no information available

**Pregnancy** manufacturer advises caution—limited information available; see also notes above

**Breast-feeding** manufacturer advises caution; see also notes above

**Side-effects** see notes above; also asthenia; *less commonly* pyrexia, irritability, increased appetite, arthralgia, and myalgia

**Indications and dose**

Symptomatic relief of allergic rhinitis and urticaria

- By mouth

    **Child 12–18 years** 10 mg once daily

**Rupafin**® (GSK) ▼ PoM

Tablets, salmon, rupatadine (as fumarate) 10 mg, net price 30-tab pack = £5.00. Counselling, skilled tasks

## Sedating antihistamines

**Skilled tasks** Drowsiness may affect performance of skilled tasks (e.g. cycling or driving); sedating effects enhanced by alcohol.

## ▮ ALIMEMAZINE TARTRATE

(Trimeprazine tartrate)

**Cautions** see notes above

**Contra-indications** see notes above

**Hepatic impairment** see notes above

**Renal impairment** avoid

**Pregnancy** see notes above

**Breast-feeding** see notes above

**Side-effects** see notes above

**Licensed use** not licensed for use in children under 2 years

**Indications and dose**

Urticaria, pruritus

- By mouth

    **Child 6 months–2 years** 250 micrograms/kg (max. 2.5 mg) 3–4 times daily—specialist use only

    **Child 2–5 years** 2.5 mg 3–4 times daily

    **Child 5–12 years** 5 mg 3–4 times daily

    **Child 12–18 years** 10 mg 2–3 times daily, in severe cases up to max. 100 mg daily

Premedication section 15.1.4

- By mouth

    **Child 2–7 years** up to max. 2 mg/kg 1–2 hours before operation

**Alimemazine** (Non-proprietary) PoM

Tablets, alimemazine tartrate 10 mg, net price 28-tab pack = £5.99. Label: 2

Oral Solution, alimemazine tartrate 7.5 mg/5 mL, net price 100 mL = £13.71; 30 mg/5 mL, 100-mL = £40.00. Label: 2

## ▮ CHLORPHENAMINE MALEATE

(Chlorpheniramine maleate)

**Cautions** see notes above

**Contra-indications** see notes above

**Hepatic impairment** see notes above

**Pregnancy** see notes above

**Breast-feeding** see notes above

**Side-effects** see notes above; also exfoliative dermatitis and tinnitus reported; injections may cause transient hypotension or CNS stimulation and may be irritant

**Licensed use** *syrup* not licensed for use in children under 1 year; *tablets* not licensed for use in children under 6 years; *injection* not licensed for use in neonates

**Indications and dose**

Symptomatic relief of allergy such as hay fever, urticaria, food allergy, drug reactions, relief of itch associated with chickenpox

- By mouth

    **Child 1 month–2 years** 1 mg twice daily

    **Child 2–6 years** 1 mg every 4–6 hours, max. 6 mg daily

    **Child 6–12 years** 2 mg every 4–6 hours, max. 12 mg daily

    **Child 12–18 years** 4 mg every 4–6 hours, max. 24 mg daily

Emergency treatment of anaphylactic reactions, symptomatic relief of allergy

- By intramuscular or intravenous injection

**Child under 6 months** 250 micrograms/kg (max. 2.5 mg), repeated if required up to 4 times in 24 hours

**Child 6 months–6 years** 2.5 mg, repeated if required up to 4 times in 24 hours

**Child 6–12 years** 5 mg, repeated if required up to 4 times in 24 hours

**Child 12–18 years** 10 mg, repeated if required up to 4 times in 24 hours

**Administration** for *intravenous injection*, give over 1 minute; if small dose required, dilute with Sodium Chloride 0.9%

**Chlorphenamine** (Non-proprietary)

Tablets, chlorphenamine maleate 4 mg, net price 28 = £1.01. Label: 2

**Dental prescribing on NHS** Chlorphenamine tablets may be prescribed

Oral solution, chlorphenamine maleate 2 mg/5 mL, net price 150 mL = £2.51. Label: 2

**Note** Sugar-free versions are available and can be ordered by specifying 'sugar-free' on the prescription

**Dental prescribing on NHS** Chlorphenamine oral solution may be prescribed

Injection 〔PoM〕[1], chlorphenamine maleate 10 mg/mL, net price 1-mL amp = £1.79

**Piriton**® (GSK Consumer Healthcare)

Tablets, yellow, scored, chlorphenamine maleate 4 mg, net price 28 = £1.62. Label: 2

Syrup, chlorphenamine maleate 2 mg/5 mL, net price 150 mL = £2.39. Label: 2

## ▌ HYDROXYZINE HYDROCHLORIDE

**Cautions** see notes above; also susceptibility to QT-interval prolongation

**Contra-indications** see notes above

**Hepatic impairment** reduce daily dose by one-third; see also notes above

**Renal impairment** reduce daily dose by half

**Pregnancy** toxicity in *animal* studies with high doses; see also notes above

**Breast-feeding** see notes above

**Side-effects** see notes above

**Licensed use** *Ucerax*® syrup not licensed for use in children under 1 year

**Indications and dose**

Pruritus

- By mouth

**Child 6 months–6 years** initially 5–15 mg at night, increased if necessary to 50 mg daily in 3–4 divided doses

**Child 6–12 years** initially 15–25 mg at night, increased if necessary to 50–100 mg daily in 3–4 divided doses

**Child 12–18 years** initially 25 mg at night, increased if necessary to 100 mg in 3–4 divided doses

1. 〔PoM〕 restriction does not apply where administration is for saving life in emergency

**Atarax**® (Alliance) 〔PoM〕

Tablets, both f/c, hydroxyzine hydrochloride 10 mg (orange), net price 84-tab pack = £2.18; 25 mg (green), 28-tab pack = £1.17. Label: 2

**Ucerax**® (UCB Pharma) 〔PoM〕

Tablets〔NHS〕, f/c, scored, hydroxyzine hydrochloride 25 mg, net price 25-tab pack = £1.22. Label: 2

Syrup, hydroxyzine hydrochloride 10 mg/5 mL. Net price 200-mL pack = £1.78. Label: 2

## ▌ KETOTIFEN

**Cautions** see notes above

**Contra-indications** see notes above

**Hepatic impairment** see notes above

**Pregnancy** see notes above

**Breast-feeding** see notes above

**Side-effects** see notes above; also irritability, nervousness; *less commonly* cystitis; *rarely* weight gain; *very rarely* Stevens-Johnson syndrome

**Indications and dose**

Symptomatic relief of allergy such as allergic rhinitis

- By mouth

**Child 3–18 years** 1 mg twice daily

**Zaditen**® (Swedish Orphan) 〔PoM〕

Tablets, scored, ketotifen (as hydrogen fumarate) 1 mg, net price 60-tab pack = £7.53. Label: 2, 21

Elixir, ketotifen (as hydrogen fumarate), 1 mg/5 mL, net price 300 mL (strawberry-flavoured) = £8.91. Label: 2, 21

## ▌ PROMETHAZINE HYDROCHLORIDE

**Cautions** see notes above; also severe coronary artery disease

**Contra-indications** see notes above

**Hepatic impairment** see notes above

**Renal impairment** use with caution

**Pregnancy** see notes above

**Breast-feeding** see notes above

**Side-effects** see notes above; also restlessness

**Indications and dose**

Symptomatic relief of allergy such as hay fever, insomnia associated with urticaria and pruritus

- By mouth

**Child 2–5 years** 5 mg twice daily *or* 5–15 mg at night

**Child 5–10 years** 5–10 mg twice daily *or* 10–25 mg at night

**Child 10–18 years** 10–20 mg 2–3 times daily *or* 25 mg at night increased to 25 mg twice daily if necessary

**Sedation** section 4.1.1

**Nausea and vomiting** section 4.6

**3 Respiratory system**

**Phenergan®** (Sanofi-Aventis)

Tablets, both blue, f/c, promethazine hydrochloride 10 mg, net price 56-tab pack = £2.85; 25 mg, 56-tab pack = £4.34. Label: 2

**Dental prescribing on NHS** May be prescribed as Promethazine Hydrochloride Tablets 10 mg or 25 mg

Elixir, golden, promethazine hydrochloride 5 mg/ 5 mL. Net price 100 mL = £2.67. Label: 2

**Excipients** include sulfites

**Electrolytes** Na+ 1.6 mmol/5 mL

**Dental prescribing on NHS** May be prescribed as Promethazine Hydrochloride Oral Solution 5 mg/5 mL

---

## 3.4.2 Allergen immunotherapy

Immunotherapy using allergen vaccines containing house dust mite, animal dander (cat or dog), or extracts of grass and tree pollen can improve symptoms of asthma and allergic rhino-conjunctivitis in children. A vaccine containing extracts of wasp and bee venom is used to reduce the risk of severe anaphylaxis and systemic reactions in children with hypersensitivity to wasp and bee stings. An oral preparation of grass pollen extract (*Grazax®*) is also licensed for grass pollen induced rhinitis and conjunctivitis. Children requiring immunotherapy must be referred to a hospital specialist for accurate allergy diagnosis, assessment, and treatment.

In view of concerns about the safety of desensitising vaccines, it is recommended that they are used by specialists and only for the following indications:

- seasonal allergic hay fever (caused by pollen) that has not responded to anti-allergic drugs;
- hypersensitivity to wasp and bee venoms.

Desensitising vaccines should generally be avoided or used with particular care in children with asthma.

Desensitising vaccines should be avoided in pregnant women, in children under 5 years, and in those taking beta-blockers (adrenaline will be ineffective if a hypersensitivity reaction occurs), or ACE inhibitors (risk of severe anaphylactoid reactions).

Hypersensitivity reactions to immunotherapy (especially to wasp and bee venom extracts) can be life-threatening; bronchospasm usually develops within 1 hour and anaphylaxis within 30 minutes of injection. Therefore, facilities for cardiopulmonary resuscitation must be immediately available and the child needs to be monitored for at least 1 hour after injection. If symptoms or signs of hypersensitivity develop (e.g. rash, urticaria, bronchospasm, faintness), **even when mild**, the child should be observed until these have **resolved completely**. The first dose of oral grass pollen extract (*Grazax®*) should be taken under medical supervision and the child should be monitored for 20–30 minutes.

For details on the management of anaphylaxis, see section 3.4.3.

Each set of allergen extracts usually contains vials for the administration of graded amounts of allergen. Maintenance sets containing vials at the highest strength are also available. Product literature must be consulted for details of allergens, vial strengths, and administration.

## NICE guidance

*Pharmalgen®* for bee and wasp venom allergy (February 2012)

*Pharmalgen®* is an option for the treatment of IgE-mediated bee and wasp venom allergy in those who have had:

- a severe systemic reaction to bee or wasp venom;
- a moderate systemic reaction to bee or wasp venom and who have a raised baseline serum-tryptase concentration, a high risk of future stings, or anxiety about future stings.

Treatment with *Pharmalgen®* should be initiated and monitored in a specialist centre experienced in venom immunotherapy.

www.nice.org.uk/TA246

## ■ BEE AND WASP ALLERGEN EXTRACTS

**Cautions** see notes above and consult product literature

**Contra-indications** see notes above and consult product literature

**Pregnancy** avoid

**Side-effects** consult product literature

**Indications and dose**

**Hypersensitivity to wasp or bee venom** (see notes above)

- By subcutaneous injection

Consult product literature

**Pharmalgen®** (ALK-Abelló) PoM

Bee venom extract (*Apis mellifera*) or wasp venom extract (*Vespula* spp.). Net price initial treatment set = £54.81 (bee), £67.20 (wasp); maintenance treatment set = £63.76 (bee), £82.03 (wasp)

## ■ GRASS AND TREE POLLEN EXTRACTS

**Cautions** see notes above and consult product literature

**Contra-indications** see notes above and consult product literature

**Pregnancy** consult product literature

**Side-effects** consult product literature

**Indications and dose**

**Treatment of seasonal allergic hay fever due to grass or tree pollen** (see notes above)

See under preparations, below

**Pollinex®** (Allergy) PoM

Grasses and rye or tree pollen extract, net price initial treatment set (3 vials) and extension course treatment (1 vial) = £450.00

**Dose**

- By subcutaneous injection

Consult product literature

◀ **Grass pollen extract**

**Grazax®** (ALK-Abelló) PoM

Oral lyophilisates (= freeze-dried tablets), grass pollen extract 75 000 units, net price 30-tab pack = £66.56. Counselling, administration

### Dose

- **By mouth**

  **Child 5–18 years** 1 tablet daily; start treatment at least 4 months before start of pollen season and continue for up to 3 years

  **Counselling** Tablets should be placed under the tongue and allowed to disperse. Advise carer and child that child not to swallow for 1 minute, or eat or drink for 5 minutes, after taking the tablet

## Omalizumab

**Omalizumab** is a monoclonal antibody that binds to immunoglobulin E (IgE). It is licensed for use as additional therapy in children over 6 years with proven IgE-mediated sensitivity to inhaled allergens, whose severe persistent allergic asthma cannot be controlled adequately with high-dose inhaled corticosteroid together with a long-acting beta₂ agonist. Omalizumab should be initiated by physicians experienced in the treatment of severe persistent asthma.

Churg-Strauss syndrome has occurred rarely in patients given omalizumab; the reaction is usually associated with the reduction or withdrawal of oral corticosteroid therapy. Churg-Strauss syndrome can present as eosinophilia, vasculitic rash, cardiac complications, worsening pulmonary symptoms, or peripheral neuropathy. Hypersensitivity reactions can also occur immediately following treatment with omalizumab or sometimes more than 24 hours after the first injection.

For details on the management of anaphylaxis, see section 3.4.3.

The *Scottish Medicines Consortium*, p. 3 has advised (May 2011) that omalizumab is accepted for restricted use within NHS Scotland as add-on therapy to improve asthma control in children (6 to 12 years), adolescents, and adults with severe persistent allergic asthma. Omalizumab is restricted to patients who are prescribed chronic systemic corticosteroids and in whom all other treatments have failed. The response should be assessed at 16 weeks and omalizumab treatment discontinued in patients who have not shown a marked improvement in overall asthma control.

---

**NICE guidance**
**Omalizumab for severe persistent allergic asthma (April 2013)**
Omalizumab is recommended as an option for treating severe persistent confirmed allergic IgE-mediated asthma as an add-on to optimised standard therapy in children aged 6 years and over

- who need continuous or frequent treatment with oral corticosteroids (defined as 4 or more courses in the previous year), **and**
- only if the manufacturer makes omalizumab available with the discount agreed in the patient access scheme.

Optimised standard therapy is defined as a full trial of and, if tolerated, documented compliance with inhaled high-dose corticosteroids, long-acting beta₂ agonists, leukotriene receptor antagonists, theophyllines, oral corticosteroids, and smoking cessation if clinically appropriate.

Children currently receiving omalizumab whose disease does not meet the criteria should be able to continue treatment until they and their clinician consider it appropriate to stop.

www.nice.org.uk/TA278

---

## ▆ OMALIZUMAB

**Cautions** autoimmune disease; susceptibility to helminth infections—discontinue if infection does not respond to anthelmintic

**Hepatic impairment** manufacturer advises caution—no information available

**Renal impairment** manufacturer advises caution—no information available

**Pregnancy** manufacturer advises avoid unless essential; no evidence of teratogenicity in *animal* studies

**Breast-feeding** manufacturer advises avoid—present in milk in *animal* studies

**Side-effects** abdominal pain, headache, pyrexia; *less commonly* dyspepsia, nausea, diarrhoea, weight gain, postural hypotension, flushing, pharyngitis, bronchospasm, cough, syncope, paraesthesia, dizziness, drowsiness, malaise, influenza-like illness, photosensitivity, urticaria, rash, pruritus; *rarely* laryngoedema, parasitic infection, antibody formation; *also reported* arterial thromboembolic events, Churg-Strauss syndrome (see notes above), thrombocytopenia, arthralgia, myalgia, joint swelling, alopecia, serum sickness (including fever and lymphadenopathy)

### Indications and dose

**Prophylaxis of severe persistent allergic asthma** (see notes above)

- **By subcutaneous injection**

  **Child 6–18 years** according to immunoglobulin E concentration and body-weight, consult product literature

**Xolair**® (Novartis) ▣PoM▣
Injection, omalizumab 150 mg/mL, net price 0.5-mL (75-mg) prefilled syringe = £128.07; 1-mL (150-mg) prefilled syringe = £256.15

## ▆ 3.4.3 Allergic emergencies

**Adrenaline** (**epinephrine**) provides physiological reversal of the immediate symptoms associated with hypersensitivity reactions such as *anaphylaxis* and *angioedema*.

## Anaphylaxis

Anaphylaxis is a severe, life-threatening, generalised or systemic hypersensitivity reaction. It is characterised by the rapid onset of respiratory and/or circulatory problems and is usually associated with skin and mucosal changes; prompt treatment is required. Children with pre-existing asthma, especially poorly controlled asthma, are at particular risk of life-threatening reactions. Insect stings are a recognised risk (in particular wasp and bee stings). Latex and certain foods, including eggs, fish, cows' milk protein, peanuts, sesame, shellfish, soy, and tree nuts may also precipitate anaphylaxis. Medicinal products particularly associated with anaphylaxis include blood products, vaccines, allergen immunotherapy preparations, antibacterials, aspirin and other NSAIDs, and neuromuscular blocking drugs. In the case

**3** Respiratory system

of drugs, anaphylaxis is more likely after parenteral administration; resuscitation facilities must always be available when giving injections associated with special risk. Refined arachis (peanut) oil, which may be present in some medicinal products, is unlikely to cause an allergic reaction—nevertheless it is wise to check the full formula of preparations which may contain allergens.

### Treatment of anaphylaxis

*First-line treatment* includes:

- securing the airway, restoration of blood pressure (laying the child flat and raising the legs, or in the recovery position if unconscious or nauseous and at risk of vomiting);

- administering **adrenaline** (epinephrine) by **intramuscular** injection (for doses see Intramuscular Adrenaline, below); the dose should be repeated if necessary at 5-minute intervals according to blood pressure, pulse, and respiratory function [**important**: possible need for *intravenous route using dilute solution* (Adrenaline 1 in 10 000), see Intravenous Adrenaline below];

- administering high-flow **oxygen** (section 3.6) and **intravenous fluids** (section 9.2.2);

- administering an antihistamine, such as **chlorphenamine**, (section 3.4.1) by slow intravenous injection or intramuscular injection as adjunctive treatment given after adrenaline. An intravenous corticosteroid (section 6.3.2) such as **hydrocortisone** (preferably as sodium succinate) is of secondary value in the initial management of anaphylaxis because the onset of action is delayed for several hours, but should be given to prevent further deterioration in severely affected children.

*Continuing respiratory deterioration* requires further treatment with **bronchodilators** including inhaled or intravenous salbutamol (see p. 137), inhaled ipratropium (see p. 140), intravenous aminophylline (see p. 141), or intravenous magnesium sulfate [unlicensed indication] (see Management of Acute Asthma, p. 132). In addition to oxygen, assisted respiration and possibly emergency tracheotomy may be necessary.

When a child is so ill that there is doubt as to the adequacy of the circulation, the initial injection of adrenaline may need to be given as a *dilute solution by the intravenous route*, or by the intraosseous route if venous access is difficult—for details of cautions, dose and strength, see under Intravenous Adrenaline (Epinephrine), below.

On discharge, the child should be considered for further treatment with an oral antihistamine (section 3.4.1) and an oral corticosteroid (section 6.3.2) for up to 3 days to reduce the risk of further reaction. The child, or carer, should be instructed to return to hospital if symptoms recur and to contact their general practitioner for follow-up.

Children who are suspected of having had an anaphylactic reaction should be referred to a specialist for specific allergy diagnosis. Avoidance of the allergen is the principal treatment; if appropriate, an adrenaline auto-injector should be given or a replacement supplied (see Self-administration of Adrenaline, p. 159).

### Intramuscular adrenaline (epinephrine)

The *intramuscular route* is the *first choice route* for the administration of adrenaline in the management of anaphylaxis. Adrenaline is best given as an intramuscular injection into the anterolateral aspect of the middle third of the thigh, it has a rapid onset of action after intramuscular administration and in the shocked patient its absorption from the intramuscular site is faster and more reliable than from the subcutaneous site.

Children with severe allergy, and their carers, should ideally be instructed in the self-administration of adrenaline by intramuscular injection (for details see Self-administration of Adrenaline (Epinephrine), p. 159).

*Prompt injection* of adrenaline is of paramount importance. The following adrenaline doses are recommended for the emergency treatment of anaphylaxis by appropriately trained healthcare professionals, and are based on the revised recommendations of the Working Group of the Resuscitation Council (UK).

**Dose of *intramuscular* injection of adrenaline (epinephrine) for the emergency treatment of anaphylaxis by healthcare professionals**

| Age range | Dose | Volume of adrenaline 1 in 1000 (1 mg/mL) |
|---|---|---|
| Under 6 years | 150 micrograms | 0.15 mL[1] |
| 6–12 years | 300 micrograms | 0.3 mL |
| 12–18 years | 500 micrograms | 0.5 mL[2] |

These doses may be repeated several times if necessary at 5-minute intervals according to blood pressure, pulse, and respiratory function.

1. Use suitable syringe for measuring small volume
2. 300 micrograms (0.3 mL) if child is small or prepubertal

### Intravenous adrenaline (epinephrine)

Intravenous adrenaline should be given only by those experienced in its use, in a setting where patients can be carefully monitored.

Where the child is severely ill and there is real doubt about adequacy of the circulation and absorption from the intramuscular injection site, adrenaline may be given by **slow** *intravenous injection*. Children may respond to as little as 1 microgram/kg (0.01 mL/kg) of the dilute 1 in 10 000 adrenaline injection by **slow** *intravenous injection* repeated according to response. A single dose of adrenaline by intravenous injection should not exceed 50 micrograms; if multiple doses are required consider giving adrenaline by slow intravenous *infusion*. Great vigilance is needed to ensure that the *correct strength* of adrenaline injection is used; anaphylactic shock kits need to make a *very clear distinction* between the 1 in 10 000 strength and the 1 in 1000 strength. It is also important that, where intramuscular injection might still succeed, time should not be wasted seeking intravenous access.

For reference to the use of the intravenous route for *acute hypotension*, see section 2.7.2.

## Self-administration of adrenaline (epinephrine)

Children at considerable risk of anaphylaxis need to carry (or have available) adrenaline at all times and the child, or child's carers, need to be *instructed in advance* when and how to inject it. Packs for self-administration need to be **clearly labelled with instructions** on how to administer adrenaline (intramuscularly, preferably at the midpoint of the outer thigh, through light clothing if necessary). It is important to ensure that an adequate supply is provided to treat symptoms until medical assistance is available.

Adrenaline for administration by intramuscular injection is available in 'auto-injectors' (e.g. *Anapen®*, *EpiPen®* or *Jext®*), pre-assembled syringes fitted with a needle suitable for very rapid administration (if necessary by a bystander or a healthcare provider if it is the only preparation available); injection technique is device specific.

For doses of adrenaline for self-administration, see individual preparations under Adrenaline/Epinephrine (Intramuscular Injection for Self-Administration, below).

# ADRENALINE/EPINEPHRINE

**Cautions** for cautions in non-life-threatening situations, see section 2.7.2

**Interactions** Severe anaphylaxis in children taking beta-blockers may not respond to adrenaline—consider bronchodilator therapy, see intravenous salbutamol (section 3.1.1.1); furthermore, adrenaline may cause severe hypertension and bradycardia in those receiving non-cardioselective beta-blockers. Other **interactions**, see Appendix 1 (sympathomimetics).

**Renal impairment** section 2.7.2

**Pregnancy** section 2.7.2

**Breast-feeding** section 2.7.2

**Side-effects** section 2.7.2

**Licensed use** auto-injector delivering 150-microgram dose of adrenaline not licensed for use in children body-weight under 15 kg

**Indications and dose**

Acute anaphylaxis

- **By intramuscular injection (preferably midpoint in anterolateral thigh) of 1 in 1000 (1 mg/mL) solution for administration by** *healthcare professionals*

  See notes and table above

- **By intramuscular injection for** *self-administration*

  See under preparations

Acute anaphylaxis when there is doubt as to the adequacy of the circulation

- **By slow intravenous injection of 1 in 10 000 (100 micrograms/mL) solution (extreme caution—specialist use only)**

  See notes above

> **Safe Practice**
> Intravenous route should be used with **extreme care** by specialists only, see notes above

**Croup** (section 3.1)

- **By inhalation of nebulised solution of adrenaline 1 in 1000 (1 mg/mL)**

  **Child 1 month–12 years** 400 micrograms/kg (max. 5 mg), repeated after 30 minutes if necessary

  **Administration** For nebulisation, dilute adrenaline 1 in 1000 solution with sterile sodium chloride 0.9% solution

**Acute hypotension, low cardiac output** section 2.7.2

**Cardiopulmonary resuscitation** section 2.7.3

◢**Intramuscular or subcutaneous**

[1]**Adrenaline/Epinephrine 1 in 1000** (Non-proprietary)
Injection, adrenaline (as acid tartrate) 1 mg/mL, net price 0.5-mL amp = 52p; 1-mL amp = 57p
**Excipients** may include sulfites

[1]**Minijet® Adrenaline 1 in 1000** (UCB Pharma) [PoM]
Injection, adrenaline (as hydrochloride) 1 in 1000 (1 mg/mL). Net price 1 mL (with 25 gauge × 0.25 inch needle for subcutaneous injection) = £10.79, 1 mL (with 21 gauge × 1.5 inch needle for intramuscular injection) = £6.36 (both disposable syringes)
**Excipients** include sulfites

◢**Intravenous**

**Extreme caution**, see notes above

**Adrenaline/Epinephrine 1 in 10 000, Dilute** (Non-proprietary) [PoM]
Injection, adrenaline (as acid tartrate) 100 micrograms/mL, 10-mL amp, 1-mL and 10-mL prefilled syringe
**Excipients** may include sulfites

**Minijet® Adrenaline 1 in 10 000** (UCB Pharma) [PoM]
Injection, adrenaline (as hydrochloride) 1 in 10 000 (100 micrograms/mL), net price 3-mL prefilled syringe = £6.27; 10-mL prefilled syringe = £6.15
**Excipients** include sulfites

◢**Intramuscular injection for self-administration**

**Note** Injection technique is device specific. To ensure patients receive the auto-injector device that they have been trained to use, prescribers should specify the brand to be dispensed.

**Anapen®** (Lincoln Medical) [PoM]
Anapen® 150 (delivering a single dose of adrenaline 150 micrograms), adrenaline 500 micrograms/mL (1 in 2000), net price 1.05-mL auto-injector device = £30.67
**Excipients** include sulfites
**Note** 0.75 mL of the solution remains in the auto-injector device after use

**Dose**

Acute anaphylaxis

- **By intramuscular injection**

  **Child body-weight under 15 kg** 150 micrograms repeated after 10–15 minutes as necessary

  **Child body-weight 15–30 kg** 150 micrograms (but on the basis of a dose of 10 micrograms/kg, 300 micrograms may be more appropriate for some children) repeated after 10–15 minutes as necessary

1. [PoM] restriction does not apply to the intramuscular administration of up to 1 mg of adrenaline injection 1 in 1000 (1 mg/mL) for the emergency treatment of anaphylaxis

**Respiratory system**

**3**

[1]Anapen® 300 (delivering a single dose of adrenaline 300 micrograms), adrenaline 1 mg/mL (1 in 1000), net price 1.05-mL auto-injector device = £30.67

Excipients include sulfites

Note 0.75 mL of the solution remains in the auto-injector device after use

Dose

### Acute anaphylaxis

* By intramuscular injection

  **Child body-weight over 30 kg** 300 micrograms repeated after 10–15 minutes as necessary

Anapen® 500 (delivering a single dose of adrenaline 500 micrograms), adrenaline 1.7 mg/mL, net price 1.05-mL auto-injector device = £30.67

Excipients include sulfites

Note 0.75 mL of the solution remains in the auto-injector device after use

Dose

### Acute anaphylaxis

* By intramuscular injection

  **Child 12–18 years body-weight over 60 kg** 500 micrograms repeated after 10–15 minutes if necessary

**EpiPen®** (Meda) PoM

EpiPen® Jr Auto-injector 0.15 mg (delivering a single dose of adrenaline 150 micrograms), adrenaline 500 micrograms/mL (1 in 2000), net price 2-mL auto-injector device = £26.45, 2 × 2-mL auto-injector device = £52.90

Excipients include sulfites

Note 1.7 mL of the solution remains in the auto-injector device after use

Dose

### Acute anaphylaxis

* By intramuscular injection

  **Child body-weight under 15 kg** 150 micrograms repeated after 5–15 minutes as necessary

  **Child body-weight 15–30 kg** 150 micrograms (but on the basis of a dose of 10 micrograms/kg, 300 micrograms may be more appropriate for some children) repeated after 5–15 minutes as necessary

[1]EpiPen® Auto-injector 0.3 mg (delivering a single dose of adrenaline 300 micrograms), adrenaline 1 mg/mL (1 in 1000), net price 2-mL auto-injector device = £26.45, 2 × 2-mL auto-injector device = £52.90

Excipients include sulfites

Note 1.7 mL of the solution remains in the auto-injector device after use

Dose

### Acute anaphylaxis

* By intramuscular injection

  **Child body-weight over 30 kg** 300 micrograms repeated after 5–15 minutes as necessary

**Jext®** (ALK-Abelló) PoM

[1]Jext® 150 micrograms (delivering a single dose of adrenaline (as tartrate) 150 micrograms), adrenaline 1 mg/mL (1 in 1000), net price 1.4-mL auto-injector device = £28.77

Excipients include sulfites

Note 1.25 mL of the solution remains in the auto-injector device after use

Dose

### Acute anaphylaxis

* By intramuscular injection

  **Child body-weight under 15 kg** 150 micrograms repeated after 5–15 minutes as necessary

  **Child body-weight 15–30 kg** 150 micrograms (but on the basis of a dose of 10 micrograms/kg, 300 micrograms may be more appropriate for some children) repeated after 5–15 minutes as necessary

[1]Jext® 300 micrograms (delivering a single dose of adrenaline (as tartrate) 300 micrograms), adrenaline 1 mg/mL (1 in 1000), net price 1.4-mL auto-injector device = £28.77

Excipients include sulfites

Note 1.1 mL of the solution remains in the auto-injector device after use

Dose

### Acute anaphylaxis

* By intramuscular injection

  **Child body-weight over 30 kg** 300 micrograms repeated after 5–15 minutes as necessary

## Angioedema

*Angioedema* is dangerous if *laryngeal oedema* is present. In this circumstance adrenaline (epinephrine) injection and oxygen should be given as described under Anaphylaxis (see above); antihistamines and corticosteroids should also be given (see again above). Tracheal intubation may be necessary. In some children with laryngeal oedema, adrenaline 1 in 1000 (1 mg/mL) solution may be given by nebuliser. However, nebulised adrenaline cannot be relied upon for a systemic effect—intramuscular adrenaline should be used.

**Hereditary angioedema** The treatment of hereditary angioedema should be under specialist supervision. Unlike allergic angioedema, adrenaline, corticosteroids, and antihistamines should not be used for the treatment of acute attacks, including attacks involving laryngeal oedema, as they are ineffective and may delay appropriate treatment—intubation may be necessary. The administration of **C1-esterase inhibitor** (in fresh frozen plasma or in partially purified form) can terminate acute attacks of *hereditary angioedema*; it can also be used for short-term prophylaxis before dental, medical, or surgical procedures. **Tranexamic acid** (section 2.11) is used for short-term or long-term prophylaxis of hereditary angioedema; short-term prophylaxis is started several days before planned procedures which may trigger an acute attack of hereditary angioedema (e.g. dental work) and continued for 2–5 days afterwards. **Danazol** [unlicensed indication, see BNF section 6.7.2] is best avoided in children because of its androgenic effects, but it can be used for short-term prophylaxis of hereditary angioedema.

---

### ▌ C1-ESTERASE INHIBITOR

C1-esterase inhibitor is prepared from human plasma

**Cautions** vaccination against hepatitis A (p. 608) and hepatitis B (p. 610) may be required

**Pregnancy** manufacturer advises avoid unless essential

**Side-effects** thrombosis (with high doses), headache, fever

**Licensed use** *Berinert®* not licensed for short-term prophylaxis of hereditary angioedema

---

1. PoM restriction does not apply to the intramuscular administration of up to 1 mg of adrenaline injection 1 in 1000 (1 mg/mL) for the emergency treatment of anaphylaxis

**Indications and dose**

See preparations

**Berinert®** (CSL Behring) PoM

Injection, powder for reconstitution, C1-esterase inhibitor, net price 500-unit vial (with solvent) = £550.00

Electrolytes Na⁺ approx. 2.1 mmol/vial

**Dose**

**Acute attacks of hereditary angioedema, short-term prophylaxis of hereditary angioedema before surgery or dental procedures** (specialist use only)

• By slow intravenous injection or intravenous infusion

Neonate 20 units/kg

Child 1 month–18 years 20 units/kg

**Cinryze®** (ViroPharma) ▼ PoM

Injection, powder for reconstitution, C1-esterase inhibitor, net price 500-unit vial (with solvent) = £668.00.

Electrolytes Na⁺ approx. 0.5 mmol/vial

**Dose**

**Acute attacks of hereditary angioedema** (specialist use only)

• By slow intravenous injection

Child 12–18 years 1000 units as a single dose; dose may be repeated if necessary

**Short-term prophylaxis of hereditary angioedema before dental, medical, or surgical procedures** (specialist use only)

• By slow intravenous injection

Child 12–18 years 1000 units up to 24 hours before procedure

**Long-term prophylaxis of severe, recurrent attacks of hereditary angioedema where acute treatment is inadequate, or when oral prophylaxis is inadequate or not tolerated** (specialist use only)

• By slow intravenous injection

Child 12–18 years 1000 units every 3–4 days, interval between doses adjusted according to response

**Administration** for slow intravenous injection, reconstitute (with solvent provided) to a concentration of 100 units/mL; give at a rate of 1 mL/minute

## 3.5 Respiratory stimulants and pulmonary surfactants

3.5.1 Respiratory stimulants
3.5.2 Pulmonary surfactants

### 3.5.1 Respiratory stimulants

Respiratory stimulants (analeptic drugs), such as caffeine, reduce the frequency of neonatal apnoea, and the need for mechanical ventilation during the first 7 days of treatment. They are typically used in the management of very preterm neonates, and continued until a postmenstrual age of 34 to 35 weeks is reached (or longer if necessary). They should only be given under **expert supervision** in hospital; it is important to rule out any underlying disorder, such as seizures, hypoglycaemia, or infection, causing respiratory exhaustion before starting treatment with a respiratory stimulant.

**Caffeine citrate** is licensed for the treatment of apnoea in preterm neonates. It is well absorbed when given

orally. The therapeutic range for plasma-caffeine concentration is usually 10–20 mg/litre (50–100 micromol/litre), but a concentration of 25–35 mg/litre (130–180 micromol/litre) may be required.

> **Safe practice**
>
> Some licensed preparations are labelled as caffeine base rather than caffeine citrate. In 2013, there will be a requirement for all preparations to be labelled as caffeine citrate. To minimise confusion and the risk of dosing errors during the changeover period, **always state dose in terms of caffeine citrate when prescribing caffeine**.
>
> Caffeine citrate 2 mg ≡ caffeine base 1 mg

### CAFFEINE CITRATE

**Cautions** gastro-oesophageal reflux; cardiovascular disease; monitor for recurrence of apnoea for 1 week after stopping treatment

**Side-effects** hypertension, tachycardia, irritability, restlessness, hypoglycaemia, hyperglycaemia, fluid and electrolyte imbalance

**Indications and dose**

**Neonatal apnoea**

• By mouth or by intravenous infusion

Neonate initially 20 mg/kg either *by intravenous infusion* over 30 minutes or *by mouth*, then 5 mg/kg once daily either *by intravenous infusion* over 10 minutes or *by mouth*, starting 24 hours after the initial dose; dose may be increased to 10 mg/kg daily if necessary

> **Safe practice**
>
> When prescribing, always state dose in terms of caffeine citrate
>
> Caffeine citrate 2 mg ≡ caffeine base 1 mg

**Administration** caffeine citrate injection may be administered *by mouth* or *by intravenous infusion*

**Caffeine citrate** (Non-proprietary) PoM

Injection, caffeine citrate 10 mg/mL, net price 1-mL amp = £4.89

Note Some stock packaged as caffeine base

Oral solution, caffeine citrate 10 mg/mL, net price 5-mL vial = £24.41

Note Some stock packaged as caffeine base

**Peyona®** (Chiesi) PoM

Injection and oral solution, caffeine citrate 20 mg/mL, net price 1-mL amp = £17.25

### 3.5.2 Pulmonary surfactants

Pulmonary surfactants derived from animal lungs, **beractant** and **poractant alfa** are used to prevent and treat respiratory distress syndrome (hyaline membrane disease) in neonates and preterm neonates. Prophylactic use of a pulmonary surfactant may reduce the need for mechanical ventilation and is more effective than 'rescue treatment' in preterm neonates of 29 weeks or less postmenstrual age.

Pulmonary surfactants may also be of benefit in neonates with meconium aspiration syndrome or intrapartum streptococcal infection.

**3**

Respiratory system

Pulmonary immaturity with surfactant deficit is the commonest reason for respiratory failure in the neonate, especially in those of less than 30 weeks post-menstrual age. Betamethasone (section 6.3.2) given to the mother (at least 12 hours but preferably 48 hours) before delivery substantially enhances pulmonary maturity in the neonate.

**Side-effects** Pulmonary surfactants have been associated with intracranial haemorrhage. Bradycardia, pulmonary haemorrhage, and decreased oxygen saturation have been reported rarely; hyperoxia and obstruction of the endotracheal tube by mucous secretions have also been reported.

## BERACTANT

**Cautions** consult product literature
**Side-effects** see notes above
**Indications and dose**

Treatment of respiratory distress syndrome in preterm neonates, birth-weight over 700 g (specialist use only)
- By endotracheal tube

  **Preterm neonate** phospholipid 100 mg/kg equivalent to a volume of 4 mL/kg, preferably within 8 hours of birth; dose may be repeated within 48 hours at intervals of at least 6 hours for up to 4 doses

Prophylaxis of respiratory distress syndrome in preterm neonates less than 32 weeks post-menstrual age (specialist use only)
- By endotracheal tube

  **Preterm neonate** phospholipid 100 mg/kg equivalent to a volume of 4 ml/kg, preferably within 15 minutes of birth; dose may be repeated within 48 hours at intervals of at least 6 hours for up to 4 doses

**Survanta®** (AbbVie) PoM
Suspension, beractant (bovine lung extract) providing phospholipid 25 mg/mL, with lipids and proteins, net price 8-mL vial = £306.43

## PORACTANT ALFA

**Cautions** consult product literature
**Side-effects** see notes above; also *rarely* hypotension
**Indications and dose**

Treatment of respiratory distress syndrome in neonates, birth-weight over 700 g (specialist use only)
- By endotracheal tube

  **Neonate** 100–200 mg/kg; further doses of 100 mg/kg may be repeated at intervals of 12 hours; max. total dose 300–400 mg/kg

Prophylaxis of respiratory distress syndrome in neonates 24–31 weeks post-menstrual age (specialist use only)
- By endotracheal tube

  **Preterm neonate** 100–200 mg/kg soon after birth, preferably within 15 minutes; further doses of 100 mg/kg may be repeated 6–12 hours later and after a further 12 hours if still intubated; max. total dose 300–400 mg/kg

**Curosurf®** (Chiesi) PoM
Suspension, poractant alfa (porcine lung phospholipid fraction) 80 mg/mL, net price 1.5-mL vial = £281.64; 3-mL vial = £547.40

## 3.6 Oxygen

Oxygen should be regarded as a drug. It is prescribed for hypoxaemic patients to increase alveolar oxygen tension and decrease the work of breathing. The concentration of oxygen required depends on the condition being treated; administration of an inappropriate concentration of oxygen may have serious or even fatal consequences. High concentrations of oxygen can cause pulmonary epithelial damage (bronchopulmonary dysplasia), convulsions, and retinal damage, especially in preterm neonates.

Oxygen is probably the most common drug used in medical emergencies. It should be prescribed initially to achieve a normal or near-normal oxygen saturation. In most acutely ill children with an expected or known normal or low arterial carbon dioxide ($P_aCO_2$), oxygen saturation should be maintained above 92%; some clinicians may aim for a target of 94–98%. In some clinical situations, such as carbon monoxide poisoning, (see also Emergency Treatment of Poisoning, p. 31), it is more appropriate to aim for the highest possible oxygen saturation until the child is stable. Hypercapnic respiratory failure is rare in children; in those children at risk, a lower oxygen saturation target of 88–92% is indicated, see below.

*High concentration oxygen therapy* is safe in uncomplicated cases of conditions such as pneumonia, pulmonary embolism, pulmonary fibrosis, shock, severe trauma, sepsis, or anaphylaxis. In such conditions, low arterial oxygen ($P_aO_2$) is usually associated with low or normal arterial carbon dioxide ($P_aCO_2$) and there is little risk of hypoventilation and carbon dioxide retention.

In severe acute asthma, the arterial carbon dioxide ($P_aCO_2$) is usually subnormal, but as asthma deteriorates it may rise steeply. These patients usually require a high concentration of oxygen and if the arterial carbon dioxide ($P_aCO_2$) remains high despite treatment, intermittent positive pressure ventilation needs to be considered urgently.

Oxygen should not be given to neonates except under expert supervision. Particular care is required in preterm neonates because of the risk of hyperoxia (see above).

*Low concentration oxygen therapy* (controlled oxygen therapy) is reserved for children at risk of hypercapnic respiratory failure, which is more likely in children with:
- advanced cystic fibrosis;
- advanced non-cystic fibrosis bronchiectasis;
- severe kyphoscoliosis or severe ankylosing spondylitis;
- severe lung scarring caused by tuberculosis;
- musculoskeletal disorders with respiratory weakness, especially if on home ventilation;
- an overdose of opioids, benzodiazepines, or other drugs causing respiratory depression.

Until blood gases can be measured, initial oxygen should be given using a controlled concentration of

28% or less, titrated towards a target concentration of 88–92%. The aim is to provide the child with enough oxygen to achieve an acceptable arterial oxygen tension without worsening carbon dioxide retention and respiratory acidosis.

**Domiciliary oxygen**   Oxygen should only be prescribed for use in the home after careful evaluation in hospital by a respiratory care specialist. Carers and children who smoke should be advised of the risks of smoking when receiving oxygen, including the risk of fire. Smoking cessation therapy (section 4.10.2) should be recommended before home oxygen prescription.

## Long-term oxygen therapy

The aim of long-term oxygen therapy is to maintain oxygen saturation of at least 92%. Children (especially those with chronic neonatal oxygen) often require supplemental oxygen, either for 24-hours a day or during periods of sleep; many children are eventually weaned off long-term oxygen therapy as their condition improves.

Long-term oxygen therapy should be considered for children with conditions such as:

- bronchopulmonary dysplasia (chronic neonatal lung disease);
- congenital heart disease with pulmonary hypertension;
- pulmonary hypertension secondary to pulmonary disease;
- idiopathic pulmonary hypertension;
- sickle-cell disease with persistent nocturnal hypoxia;
- interstitial lung disease and obliterative bronchiolitis;
- cystic fibrosis;
- obstructive sleep apnoea syndrome;
- neuromuscular or skeletal disease requiring non-invasive ventilation;
- pulmonary malignancy or other terminal disease with disabling dyspnoea.

Increased respiratory depression is seldom a problem in children with stable respiratory failure treated with low concentrations of oxygen although it may occur during exacerbations; children and their carers should be warned to call for medical help if drowsiness or confusion occurs.

## Short-burst oxygen therapy

Oxygen is occasionally prescribed for short-burst (intermittent) use for episodes of breathlessness.

## Ambulatory oxygen therapy

Ambulatory oxygen is prescribed for children on long-term oxygen therapy who need to be away from home on a regular basis.

## Oxygen therapy equipment

Under the NHS oxygen may be supplied as **oxygen cylinders**. Oxygen flow can be adjusted by means of an oxygen flow meter. Oxygen delivered from a cylinder should be passed through a humidifier if used for long periods.

**Oxygen concentrators** are more economical for children who require oxygen for long periods, and in England and Wales can be ordered on the NHS on a regional tendering basis (see below). A concentrator is recommended for a child who requires oxygen for more than 8 hours a day (or 21 cylinders per month). Exceptionally, if a higher concentration of oxygen is required the output of 2 oxygen concentrators can be combined using a 'Y' connection.

A nasal cannula is usually preferred to a face mask for long-term oxygen therapy from an oxygen concentrator. Nasal cannulas can, however, cause dermatitis and mucosal drying in sensitive individuals.

Giving oxygen by nasal cannula allows the child to talk, eat, and drink, but the concentration is not controlled and the method may not be appropriate for acute respiratory failure. When oxygen is given through a nasal cannula at a rate of 1–2 litres/minute the inspiratory oxygen concentration is usually low, but it varies with ventilation and can be high if the child is underventilating.

## Arrangements for supplying oxygen

The following services may be ordered in England and Wales:

- emergency oxygen;
- short-burst (intermittent) oxygen therapy;
- long-term oxygen therapy;
- ambulatory oxygen.

The type of oxygen service (or combination of services) should be ordered on a Home Oxygen Order Form (HOOF); the amount of oxygen required (hours per day) and flow rate should be specified. The supplier will determine the appropriate equipment to be provided. Special needs or preferences should be specified on the HOOF.

The clinician should obtain the patient's consent to pass on the patient's details to the supplier and the fire brigade. The supplier will contact the patient to make arrangements for delivery, installation, and maintenance of the equipment. The supplier will also train the patient to use the equipment.

The clinician should send order forms to the supplier by facsimile (see below); a copy of the HOOF should be sent to the Primary Care Trust or Local Health Board. The supplier will continue to provide the service until a revised order is received, or until notified that the patient no longer requires the home oxygen service.

HOOF and further instructions are available at www. bprs.co.uk/oxygen.html.

**3**

**Respiratory system**

| | |
|---|---|
| East of England<br>North East | BOC Medical<br>*to order:*<br>Tel: 0800 136 603<br>Fax: 0800 169 9989 |
| South West | Air Liquide<br>*to order:*<br>Tel: 0808 202 2229<br>Fax: 0191 497 4340 |
| London<br>East Midlands<br>North West | Air Liquide<br>*to order:*<br>Tel: 0500 823 773<br>Fax: 0800 781 4610 |
| Yorkshire and Humberside<br>West Midlands<br>Wales | Air Products<br>*to order:*<br>Tel: 0800 373 580<br>Fax: 0800 214 709 |
| South East Coast<br>South Central | Dolby Vivisol<br>*to order:*<br>Tel: 08443 814 402<br>Fax: 0800 781 4610 |

In Scotland, refer the child for assessment by a paediatric respiratory consultant. If the need for a concentrator is confirmed the consultant will arrange for the provision of a concentrator through the Common Services Agency. In **Northern Ireland** oxygen concentrators and cylinders should be prescribed on form HS21; oxygen concentrators are supplied by a local contractor. In **Scotland** and **Northern Ireland**, prescriptions for oxygen cylinders and accessories can be dispensed by pharmacies contracted to provide domiciliary oxygen services.

## 3.7 Mucolytics

Mucolytics, such as **carbocisteine** and **mecysteine**, are used to facilitate mucociliary clearance and expectoration by reducing sputum viscosity but evidence of efficacy is limited.

**Dornase alfa** is a genetically engineered version of a naturally occurring human enzyme which cleaves extracellular deoxyribonucleic acid (DNA); it is used to reduce sputum viscosity in children with cystic fibrosis. Dornase alfa is administered by inhalation using a jet nebuliser (section 3.1.5), usually once daily at least 1 hour before physiotherapy; however, alternate-day therapy may be as effective as daily treatment. Not all children benefit from treatment with dornase alfa; improvement occurs within 2 weeks, but in more severely affected children a trial of 6–12 weeks may be required.

Nebulised **hypertonic sodium chloride** solution may improve mucociliary clearance in children with cystic fibrosis.

Mesna (*Mistabron*®, available from 'special-order' manufacturers or specialist importing companies, see p. 823) is used in some children with cystic fibrosis when other mucolytics have failed to reduce sputum viscosity; 3–6 mL of a 20% solution is nebulised twice daily.

**Acetylcysteine** has been used to treat meconium ileus in neonates and distal intestinal obstruction syndrome in children with cystic fibrosis, but evidence of efficacy is lacking. *Gastrografin*® (section 1.6.5), or a bowel cleansing preparation containing macrogols (section 1.6.5), is usually more effective. Acetylcysteine may be used as a mucolytic to prevent further obstruction.

## ACETYLCYSTEINE

**Cautions**  history of peptic ulceration; asthma

**Side-effects**  hypersensitivity-like reactions including rashes and anaphylaxis

**Licensed use**  not licensed for use in meconium ileus or for distal intestinal obstructive syndrome in children with cystic fibrosis

**Indications and dose**

> **Meconium ileus** (but see notes above)
> * By mouth
>> **Neonate** 200–400 mg up to 3 times daily if necessary

> **Treatment of distal intestinal obstructive syndrome** (but see notes above)
> * By mouth
>> **Child 1 month–2 years** 0.4–3 g as a single dose
>> **Child 2–7 years** 2–3 g as a single dose
>> **Child 7–18 years** 4–6 g as a single dose

> **Prevention of distal intestinal obstruction syndrome**
> * By mouth
>> **Child 1 month–2 years** 100–200 mg 3 times daily
>> **Child 2–12 years** 200 mg 3 times daily
>> **Child 12–18 years** 200–400 mg 3 times daily

**Administration**  For *oral* administration, use oral granules, *or* dilute injection solution (200 mg/mL) to a concentration of 50 mg/mL; orange or blackcurrant juice or cola drink may be used as a diluent to mask the bitter taste

**Acetylcysteine** (Non-proprietary) PoM
Oral granules, acetylcysteine 100 mg/sachet; 200 mg/sachet. Label: 13
Available from 'special-order' manufacturers or specialist importing companies, see p. 823

◢ Injection
See Emergency treatment of poisoning, p. 27

## CARBOCISTEINE

**Cautions**  history of peptic ulceration

**Contra-indications**  active peptic ulceration

**Pregnancy**  manufacturer advises avoid in first trimester

**Breast-feeding**  no information available

**Side-effects**  *rarely* gastro-intestinal bleeding; hypersensitivity reactions (including rash and anaphylaxis) also reported

**Indications and dose**

> **Reduction of sputum viscosity**
> * By mouth
>> **Child 2–5 years** 62.5–125 mg 4 times daily
>> **Child 5–12 years** 250 mg 3 times daily
>> **Child 12–18 years** initially 2.25 g daily in divided doses, then 1.5 g daily in divided doses as condition improves

**Carbocisteine** (Sanofi-Aventis) PoM
Capsules, carbocisteine 375 mg, net price 120-cap pack = £16.03
Brands include *Mucodyne*®

Oral liquid, carbocisteine 125 mg/5 mL, net price 300 mL = £4.39; 250 mg/5 mL, 300 mL = £5.61
Brands include *Mucodyne*® *Paediatric* 125 mg/5 mL (cherry- and raspberry-flavoured) and *Mucodyne*® 250 mg/5 mL (cinnamon- and rum-flavoured)

### ▮ DORNASE ALFA
**Phosphorylated glycosylated recombinant human deoxyribonuclease 1 (rhDNase)**

**Pregnancy** no evidence of teratogenicity; manufacturer advises use only if potential benefit outweighs risk

**Breast-feeding** amount probably too small to be harmful—manufacturer advises caution

**Side-effects** pharyngitis, voice changes, chest pain; occasionally laryngitis, rashes, urticaria, conjunctivitis

**Indications and dose**

> Management of cystic fibrosis patients with a forced vital capacity (FVC) of greater than 40% of predicted to improve pulmonary function
> * By inhalation of nebulised solution (by jet nebuliser)
>   **Child 5–18 years** 2500 units (2.5 mg) once daily

**Pulmozyme**® (Roche) PoM
Nebuliser solution, dornase alfa 1000 units (1 mg)/mL. Net price 2.5-mL (2500 units) vial = £16.55
Note For use undiluted with jet nebulisers only; ultrasonic nebulisers are unsuitable

### ▮ MECYSTEINE HYDROCHLORIDE
**(Methyl Cysteine Hydrochloride)**

**Cautions** history of peptic ulceration

**Pregnancy** manufacturer advises avoid

**Breast-feeding** manufacturer advises avoid

**Indications and dose**

> Reduction of sputum viscosity
> * By mouth
>   **Child 5–12 years** 100 mg 3 times daily
>   **Child 12–18 years** 200 mg 4 times daily for 2 days, then 200 mg 3 times daily for 6 weeks, then 200 mg twice daily

**Visclair**® (Ranbaxy)
Tablets, yellow, s/c, e/c, mecysteine hydrochloride 100 mg, net price 100= £17.65. Label: 5, 22, 25

## Hypertonic sodium chloride

Nebulised hypertonic sodium chloride solution (3–7 %) is used to mobilise lower respiratory tract secretions in mucous consolidation (e.g. cystic fibrosis). Temporary irritation, such as coughing, hoarseness, or reversible bronchoconstriction may occur; an inhaled bronchodilator can be used before treatment with hypertonic sodium chloride to reduce the risk of these adverse effects.

**MucoClear**® **3%** (Pari)
Nebuliser solution, sodium chloride 3%, net price 20 × 4 mL = £12.98; 60 × 4 mL = £27.00
**Dose**
> * By inhalation of nebulised solution
>   **Child** 4 mL 2–4 times daily

**MucoClear**® **6%** (Pari)
Nebuliser solution, sodium chloride 6%, net price 20 × 4 mL = £12.98; 60 × 4 mL = £27.00
**Dose**
> * By inhalation of nebulised solution
>   **Child** 4 mL twice daily

**Nebusal**® **7%** (Forest)
Nebuliser solution, sodium chloride 7%, net price 60 × 4 mL = £27.00
**Dose**
> * By inhalation of nebulised solution
>   **Child** 4 mL up to twice daily

## 3.8 Aromatic inhalations

Inhalations containing volatile substances such as eucalyptus oil are traditionally used to relieve congestion and ease breathing. Although the vapour may contain little of the additive, it encourages deliberate inspiration of warm moist air which is often comforting. Boiling water should not be used for inhalations owing to the risk of scalding.

Strong aromatic decongestants (applied as rubs or to pillows) are not recommended for infants under the age of 3 months. **Sodium chloride 0.9%** solution given as nasal drops can be used to liquefy mucous secretions and relieve nasal congestion in infants and young children; administration before feeds may ease feeding difficulties caused by nasal congestion.

**Benzoin Tincture, Compound, BP**
**(Friars' Balsam)**
Tincture, balsamic acids approx. 4.5%. Label: 15
**Dose**
> **Nasal congestion**
> * By inhalation
>   Add one teaspoonful to a pint of hot, **not** boiling, water and inhale the vapour

**Menthol and Eucalyptus Inhalation, BP 1980**
Inhalation, racementhol or levomenthol 2 g, eucalyptus oil 10 mL, light magnesium carbonate 7 g, water to 100 mL
**Dose**
> **Nasal congestion**
> * By inhalation
>   Add one teaspoonful to a pint of hot, **not** boiling, water and inhale the vapour

**Dental prescribing on the NHS** May be prescribed as Menthol and Eucalyptus Inhalation BP, 1980

## 3.9 Cough preparations

3.9.1 Cough suppressants

3.9.2 Expectorant and demulcent cough preparations

## 3.9.1 Cough suppressants

Cough may be a symptom of an underlying disorder such as asthma (section 3.1), gastro-oesophageal reflux disease (section 1.1), or rhinitis (section 12.2.1), which should be addressed before prescribing cough suppressants. Cough may be associated with smoking or environmental pollutants. Cough can also result from bronchiectasis including that associated with cystic fibrosis; cough can also have a significant habit component. There is little evidence of any significant benefit from the use of cough suppressants in children with acute cough in ambulatory settings. Cough suppressants may cause sputum retention and this can be harmful in children with bronchiectasis.

The use of cough suppressants containing **pholcodine** or similar opioid analgesics is not generally recommended in children and should be avoided in children under 6 years; the use of over-the-counter codeine-containing liquids should be avoided in children under 18 years, see MHRA/CHM advice below.

**Sedating antihistamines** (section 3.4.1) are used as the cough suppressant component of many compound cough preparations on sale to the public; all tend to cause drowsiness which may reflect their main mode of action.

> **MHRA/CHM advice (March 2008 and February 2009)**
> Children under 6 years should not be given over-the-counter cough and cold medicines containing the following ingredients:
> - brompheniramine, chlorphenamine, diphenhydramine, doxylamine, promethazine, or triprolidine (antihistamines);
> - dextromethorphan or pholcodine (cough suppressants);
> - guaifenesin or ipecacuanha (expectorants);
> - phenylephrine, pseudoephedrine, ephedrine, oxymetazoline, or xylometazoline (decongestants).
>
> Over-the-counter cough and cold medicines can be considered for children aged 6–12 years after basic principles of best care have been tried, but treatment should be restricted to five days or less. Children should not be given more than 1 cough or cold preparation at a time because different brands may contain the same active ingredient; care should be taken to give the correct dose.

> **MHRA/CHM advice (October 2010)** Over-the-counter codeine-containing liquid medicines for children
> Children under 18 years should not use codeine-containing over-the-counter liquid medicines for cough suppression

## ▌ PHOLCODINE

**Cautions** asthma; chronic, persistent, or productive cough; **interactions**: Appendix 1 (pholcodine)

**Contra-indications** chronic bronchitis, bronchiectasis, bronchiolitis, children at risk of respiratory failure

**Hepatic impairment** avoid

**Renal impairment** use with caution; avoid in severe impairment

**Pregnancy** manufacturer advises avoid unless potential benefit outweighs risk

**Breast-feeding** manufacturer advises avoid unless potential benefit outweighs risk—no information available

**Side-effects** nausea, vomiting, constipation, sputum retention, drowsiness, dizziness, excitation, confusion, rash

**Indications and dose**

> **Dry cough** (but not generally recommended for children, see notes above)
> - By mouth
> **Child 6–12 years** 2–5 mg 3–4 times daily
> **Child 12–18 years** 5–10 mg 3–4 times daily

**Pholcodine Linctus, BP**
Linctus (= oral solution), pholcodine 5 mg/5 mL in a suitable flavoured vehicle, containing citric acid monohydrate 1%. Net price 100 mL = 31p
**Brands include** *Pavacol-D*® (sugar-free), *Galenphol*® (sugar-free)

**Pholcodine Linctus, Strong, BP**
Linctus (= oral solution), pholcodine 10 mg/5 mL in a suitable flavoured vehicle, containing citric acid monohydrate 2%. Net price 100 mL = 44p
**Brands include** *Galenphol*®

**Galenphol**® (Thornton & Ross)
Paediatric linctus (= oral solution), orange, sugar-free, pholcodine 2 mg/5 mL. Net price 90-mL pack = £1.20

## 3.9.2 Expectorant and demulcent cough preparations

**Simple linctus** and other demulcent cough preparations containing soothing substances, such as syrup or glycerol, may temporarily relieve a dry irritating cough. These preparations have the advantage of being harmless and inexpensive and sugar-free versions are available.

**Expectorants** are claimed to promote expulsion of bronchial secretions but there is no evidence that any drug can specifically facilitate expectoration.

**Compound cough preparations** for children are on sale to the public but should not be used in children under 6 years; the rationale for some is dubious. Care should be taken to give the correct dose and to not use more than one preparation at a time, see MHRA/CHM advice above.

**Simple Linctus, Paediatric, BP**
Linctus (= oral solution), citric acid monohydrate 0.625% in a suitable vehicle with an anise flavour, net price 200 mL = £0.82
A sugar-free version is also available
**Dose**

> **Cough**
> - By mouth
> **Child 1 month–12 years** 5–10 mL 3–4 times daily

**Simple Linctus, BP**

Linctus (= oral solution), citric acid monohydrate 2.5% in a suitable vehicle with an anise flavour, net price 200 mL = £0.76

A sugar-free version is also available

**Dose**

**Cough**

- By mouth

  **Child 12–18 years** 5 mL 3–4 times daily

[1]**Galpseud®** (Thornton & Ross) (PoM) ◢

Tablets, pseudoephedrine hydrochloride 60 mg, net price 24 = £2.25

Linctus, orange, sugar-free, pseudoephedrine hydrochloride 30 mg/5 mL, net price 100 mL = £0.70

**Excipients** include alcohol

[1]**Sudafed®** (McNeil) (PoM) ◢

Tablets, red, f/c, pseudoephedrine hydrochloride 60 mg, net price 24 = £2.12

Elixir, red, pseudoephedrine hydrochloride 30 mg/5 mL, net price 100 mL = £1.05

## 3.11 Antifibrotics

Classification not used in *BNF for Children*

## 3.10 Systemic nasal decongestants

Nasal congestion in children due to allergic or vasomotor rhinitis should be treated with oral antihistamines (section 3.4.1), topical nasal preparations containing corticosteroids (section 12.2.1), or topical decongestants (section 12.2.2).

There is little evidence to support the use of systemic decongestants in children.

**Pseudoephedrine** has few sympathomimetic effects, and is commonly combined with other ingredients (including antihistamines) in preparations intended for the relief of cough and cold symptoms but it should not be used in children under 6 years, see MHRA/CHM advice, p. 166.

### PSEUDOEPHEDRINE HYDROCHLORIDE

**Cautions** hypertension, heart disease, diabetes, hyperthyroidism, raised intra-ocular pressure; **interactions:** Appendix 1 (sympathomimetics)

**Contra-indications** treatment with MAOI within previous 2 weeks

**Hepatic impairment** manufacturer advises caution in severe impairment

**Renal impairment** caution in mild to moderate impairment; manufacturer advises avoid in severe impairment

**Pregnancy** defective closure of the abdominal wall (gastrochisis) reported very rarely in newborns after first trimester exposure

**Breast-feeding** may suppress lactation; avoid if lactation not well established or if milk production insufficient

**Side-effects** nausea, vomiting, hypertension, tachycardia, headache, anxiety, restlessness, insomnia; *rarely* hallucinations, rash; urinary retention also reported

**Indications and dose**

**Congestion of mucous membranes of upper respiratory tract**

- By mouth

  **Child 6–12 years** 30 mg 3–4 times daily

  **Child 12–18 years** 60 mg 3–4 times daily

1. Can be sold to the public provided no more than 720 mg of pseudoephedrine salts are supplied, and ephedrine base (or salts) are not supplied at the same time; for details see *Medicines, Ethics and Practice*, London, Pharmaceutical Press (always consult latest edtion)

# 4 Central nervous system

## 4.1 Hypnotics and anxiolytics

4.1.1 Hypnotics
4.1.2 Anxiolytics
4.1.3 Barbiturates

Most anxiolytics ('sedatives') will induce sleep when given at night and most hypnotics will sedate when given during the day. Hypnotics and anxiolytics should be reserved for short courses to alleviate acute conditions after causal factors have been established.

The role of drug therapy in the management of anxiety disorders in children and adolescents is uncertain; drug therapy should be initiated only by specialists after psychosocial interventions have failed. Benzodiazepines and tricyclic antidepressants have been used but adverse effects may be problematic.

**Skilled tasks**   Hypnotics and anxiolytics may impair judgement and increase reaction time, and so affect ability to drive or perform skilled tasks; they increase the effects of alcohol. Moreover the hangover effects of a night dose may impair performance on the following day.

> **Important**
> 1. Benzodiazepines are indicated for the short-term relief (two to four weeks only) of anxiety that is severe, disabling or causing the child unacceptable distress, occurring alone or in association with insomnia or short-term psychosomatic, organic, or psychotic illness.
> 2. The use of benzodiazepines to treat short-term 'mild' anxiety is inappropriate.
> 3. Benzodiazepines should be used to treat insomnia only when it is severe, disabling, or causing the child extreme distress.

### 4.1.1 Hypnotics

The prescribing of hypnotics to children, except for occasional use such as for sedation for procedures (section 15.1.4), is not justified. There is a risk of habituation with prolonged use. Problems settling children at night should be managed with behavioural therapy.

**Dental procedures**   Some anxious children may benefit from the use of a hypnotic the night before the dental appointment.

## Chloral and derivatives

Chloral hydrate and derivatives were formerly popular hypnotics for children.

Chloral hydrate is now mainly used for sedation during diagnostic procedures (section 15.1.4). It accumulates on prolonged use.

## CHLORAL HYDRATE

**Cautions**   reduce dose in debilitated; avoid prolonged use (and abrupt withdrawal thereafter); avoid contact with skin and mucous membranes; **interactions:** Appendix 1 (anxiolytics and hypnotics)
Skilled tasks Drowsiness may persist the next day and affect performance of skilled tasks (e.g. driving); effects of alcohol enhanced

**Contra-indications**   severe cardiac disease; gastritis; acute porphyria (section 9.8.2)

**Hepatic impairment**   can precipitate coma; reduce dose in mild to moderate hepatic impairment; avoid in severe impairment

**Renal impairment**   avoid in severe impairment

**Pregnancy**   avoid

**Breast-feeding**   risk of sedation in infant—avoid

**Side-effects**   gastric irritation (nausea and vomiting reported), abdominal distention, flatulence, headache, tolerance, dependence, excitement, delirium (especially on abrupt withdrawal), ketonuria, and rash

**Licensed use**   not licensed for sedation for painless procedures

**Indications and dose**

Sedation for painless procedures

• By mouth or by rectum (if oral route not available)

Neonate 30–50 mg/kg 45–60 minutes before procedure; doses up to 100 mg/kg may be used with respiratory monitoring

Child 1 month–12 years 30–50 mg/kg (max. 1 g) 45–60 minutes before procedure; higher doses up to 100 mg/kg (max. 2 g) may be used

Child 12–18 years 1–2 g 45–60 minutes before procedure

**Administration**   for administration *by mouth* dilute liquid with plenty of water or juice to mask unpleasant taste.

**Chloral Mixture, BP 2000** (PoM)
(Chloral Oral Solution)
Mixture, chloral hydrate 500 mg/5 mL in a suitable vehicle. Available from 'special-order' manufacturers or specialist importing companies, see p. 823

**Chloral Elixir, Paediatric, BP 2000** (PoM)
(Chloral Oral Solution, Paediatric)
Elixir, chloral hydrate 200 mg/5 mL (4%) in a suitable vehicle with a black currant flavour. Available from 'special-order' manufacturers or specialist importing companies, see p. 823

**Chloral Hydrate** (Non-proprietary) (PoM)
Suppositories, chloral hydrate 25 mg, 50 mg, 60 mg, 100 mg, 200 mg, 500 mg. Available from 'special-order' manufacturers or specialist importing companies, see p. 823

◢ Cloral betaine

**Welldorm®** (Marlborough) (PoM)
Tablets, blue-purple, f/c, cloral betaine 707 mg (≡ chloral hydrate 414 mg), net price 30-tab pack = £12.10. Label: 19, 27
Dose
Short-term treatment of insomnia
• By mouth
Child 12–18 years 1–2 tablets with water or milk at bedtime, max. 5 tablets (chloral hydrate 2 g) daily

Elixir, red, chloral hydrate 143.3 mg/5 mL, net price 150-mL pack = £8.70. Label: 19, 27
Dose
Short-term treatment of insomnia
• By mouth
Child 2–12 years 1–1.75 mL/kg (chloral hydrate 30–50 mg/kg) with water or milk at bedtime; max. 35 mL (chloral hydrate 1 g) daily
Child 12–18 years 15–45 mL (chloral hydrate 0.4–1.3 g) with water or milk at bedtime; max. 70 mL (chloral hydrate 2 g) daily

## Antihistamines

Some **antihistamines** (section 3.4.1) such as promethazine are used for occasional insomnia in adults; their prolonged duration of action can often cause drowsiness the following day. The sedative effect of antihistamines may diminish after a few days of continued treatment; antihistamines are associated with headache, psychomotor impairment and antimuscarinic effects.

The use of antihistamines as hypnotics in children is not usually justified.

## PROMETHAZINE HYDROCHLORIDE ◢

**Cautions**   see notes in section 3.4.1; also avoid extravasation with intravenous injection

**Contra-indications**   see Promethazine Hydrochloride, section 3.4.1

**Hepatic impairment**   see notes in section 3.4.1

**Renal impairment**   see Promethazine Hydrochloride, section 3.4.1

**Pregnancy**   see notes in section 3.4.1

**Breast-feeding**   see notes in section 3.4.1

**Side-effects**   see Promethazine Hydrochloride, section 3.4.1

**Licensed use**   not licensed for use in children under 2 years

**Indications and dose**

Sedation (short-term use)

• By mouth

Child 2–5 years 15–20 mg

Child 5–10 years 20–25 mg

Child 10–18 years 25–50 mg

**4** Central nervous system

**Sedation in intensive care**

- By mouth or by slow intravenous injection or by deep intramuscular injection

  **Child 1 month–12 years** 0.5–1 mg/kg (max. 25 mg) 4 times daily, adjusted according to response

  **Child 12–18 years** 25–50 mg 4 times daily, adjusted according to response

**Allergy and urticaria** section 3.4.1

**Nausea and vomiting** section 4.6

¹**Promethazine** (Non-proprietary) [PoM]
Injection, promethazine hydrochloride 25 mg/mL, net price 1-mL amp = 68p, 2-mL amp = £1.20

¹**Phenergan**® (Sanofi-Aventis) [PoM]
Injection, promethazine hydrochloride 25 mg/mL, net price 1-mL amp = 67p
**Excipients** include sulfites

◀**Oral preparations**
Section 3.4.1

## Melatonin

Melatonin is a pineal hormone that may affect sleep pattern. Clinical experience suggests that when appropriate behavioural sleep interventions fail, melatonin may be of value for treating sleep onset insomnia and delayed sleep phase syndrome in children with conditions such as visual impairment, cerebral palsy, attention deficit hyperactivity disorder, autism, and learning difficulties. It is also sometimes used before magnetic resonance imaging (MRI), computed tomography (CT), or EEG investigations. Little is known about its long-term effects in children, and there is uncertainty as to the effect on other circadian rhythms including endocrine or reproductive hormone secretion. Treatment with melatonin should be initiated and supervised by a specialist, but may be continued by general practitioners under a shared-care arrangement. The need to continue melatonin therapy should be reviewed every 6 months.

Melatonin is available as a modified-release tablet (*Circadin*®) and also as unlicensed formulations. *Circadin*® is licensed for the short-term treatment of primary insomnia in adults over 55 years. Unlicensed immediate-release preparations are available; the manufacturer should be specified in the shared-care guideline because of variability in clinical effect of unlicensed formulations.

◀ **MELATONIN**

**Cautions** autoimmune disease (manufacturer advises avoid—no information available); **interactions:** Appendix 1 (melatonin)

**Hepatic impairment** clearance reduced—manufacturer advises avoid

**Renal impairment** no information available—caution

**Pregnancy** no information available—avoid

**Breast-feeding** present in milk—avoid

**Side-effects** *less commonly* abdominal pain, dyspepsia, dry mouth, mouth ulceration, weight gain,

hypertension, chest pain, malaise, dizziness, restlessness, nervousness, irritability, anxiety, migraine, proteinuria, glycosuria, pruritus, rash, dry skin; *rarely* thirst, flatulence, halitosis, hypersalivation, vomiting, gastritis, hypertriglyceridaemia, palpitation, syncope, hot flushes, aggression, impaired memory, restless legs syndrome, paraesthesia, mood changes, priapism, increased libido, prostatitis, polyuria, haematuria, leucopenia, thrombocytopenia, electrolyte disturbances, muscle spasm, arthritis, lacrimation, visual disturbances, nail disorder

**Licensed use** not licensed for use in children

**Indications and dose**

**Sleep onset insomnia and delayed sleep phase syndrome** (see notes above)

- By mouth

  **Child 1 month–18 years** initially 2–3 mg daily before bedtime increased if necessary after 1–2 weeks to 4–6 mg daily before bedtime; max. 10 mg daily

**Circadin**® (Flynn) [PoM]
Tablets, m/r, melatonin 2 mg, net price 30-tab pack = £15.39. Label: 2, 21, 25
**Note** Other formulations of melatonin are available from 'special-order' manufacturers or specialist importing companies, see p. 823

### 4.1.2 Anxiolytics

Anxiolytic treatment should be used in children only to relieve acute anxiety (and related insomnia) caused by fear (e.g. before surgery, section 15.1.4.1).

Anxiolytic treatment should be limited to the lowest possible dose for the shortest possible time (see p. 168).

## Buspirone

**Buspirone** is thought to act at specific serotonin (5HT$_{1A}$) receptors; safety and efficacy in children have yet to be determined.

### 4.1.3 Barbiturates

Classification not used in *BNF for Children*.

### 4.2 Drugs used in psychoses and related disorders

4.2.1   Antipsychotic drugs

4.2.2   Antipsychotic depot injections

4.2.3   Drugs used for mania and hypomania

Advice on doses of antipsychotic drugs above *BNF for Children* upper limit

1. Consider alternative approaches including adjuvant therapy.

2. Bear in mind risk factors, including obesity.

3. Consider potential for drug interactions—see **interactions:** Appendix 1 (antipsychotics).

4. Carry out ECG to exclude untoward abnormalities such as prolonged QT interval; repeat ECG periodically and reduce dose if prolonged QT interval or other adverse abnormality develops.

---

1. [PoM] restriction does not apply where administration is for saving life in emergency

5. Increase dose slowly and not more often than once weekly.

6. Carry out regular pulse, blood pressure, and temperature checks; ensure that patient maintains adequate fluid intake.

7. Consider high-dose therapy to be for limited period and review regularly; abandon if no improvement after 3 months (return to standard dosage).

**Important** When prescribing an antipsychotic for administration on an emergency basis, the intramuscular dose should be **lower** than the corresponding oral dose (owing to absence of first-pass effect), particularly if the child is very active (increased blood flow to muscle considerably increases the rate of absorption). The prescription should specify the dose for **each route** and should **not** imply that the same dose can be given by mouth or by intramuscular injection. The dose of antipsychotic for emergency use should be reviewed at least **daily**.

## 4.2.1 Antipsychotic drugs

There is little information on the efficacy and safety of antipsychotic drugs in children and adolescents and much of the information available has been extrapolated from adult data; in particular, little is known about the long-term effects of antipsychotic drugs on the developing nervous system. Antipsychotic drugs should be initiated and managed under the close supervision of an appropriate specialist.

Antipsychotic drugs are also known as 'neuroleptics' and (misleadingly) as 'major tranquillisers'.

In the short term they are used to calm disturbed children whatever the underlying psychopathology, which may be schizophrenia, brain damage, mania, toxic delirium, or agitated depression. Antipsychotic drugs are used to alleviate severe anxiety but this too should be a short-term measure.

**Schizophrenia** The aim of the treatment is to alleviate the suffering of the child (and carer) and to improve social and cognitive functioning. Many children require life-long treatment with antipsychotic medication. Antipsychotic drugs relieve positive psychotic symptoms such as thought disorder, hallucinations, and delusions, and prevent relapse; they are usually less effective on negative symptoms such as apathy and social withdrawal. In many patients, negative symptoms persist between episodes of treated positive symptoms, but earlier treatment of psychotic illness may protect against the development of negative symptoms over time. Children with acute schizophrenia generally respond better than those with chronic symptoms.

Long-term treatment of a child with a definitive diagnosis of schizophrenia is usually required after the first episode of illness in order to prevent relapses. Doses that are effective in acute episodes should generally be continued as prophylaxis.

**First-generation antipsychotic drugs** The first-generation antipsychotic drugs act predominantly by blocking dopamine $D_2$ receptors in the brain. First-generation antipsychotic drugs are not selective for any of the four dopamine pathways in the brain and so can cause a range of side-effects, particularly extrapyramidal symptoms and elevated prolactin. The **phenothiazine** derivatives can be divided into 3 main groups

*Group 1*: chlorpromazine, levomepromazine, and promazine, generally characterised by pronounced sedative effects and moderate antimuscarinic and extrapyramidal side-effects.

*Group 2*: pericyazine and pipotiazine, generally characterised by moderate sedative effects, but fewer extrapyramidal side-effects than groups 1 or 3.

*Group 3*: perphenazine, prochlorperazine, and trifluoperazine, generally characterised by fewer sedative effects and antimuscarinic effects, but more pronounced extrapyramidal side-effects than groups 1 and 2.

**Butyrophenones** (e.g. haloperidol) resemble the *group 3* phenothiazines in their clinical properties. **Diphenylbutylpiperidines** (pimozide) and the **substituted benzamides** (sulpiride) have reduced sedative, antimuscarinic, and extrapyramidal effects.

**Second-generation antipsychotic drugs** The second-generation antipsychotic drugs (also referred as atypical antipsychotic drugs) act on a range of receptors in comparison to first-generation antipsychotic drugs and have more distinct clinical profiles, particularly with regard to side-effects.

**Amisulpride** is a selective dopamine receptor antagonist with high affinity for mesolimbic $D_2$ and $D_3$ receptors; **clozapine** is a dopamine $D_1$, $D_2$, 5-$HT_{2A}$, alpha$_1$-adrenoceptor, and muscarinic receptor antagonist; **olanzapine** is a dopamine $D_1$, $D_2$, $D_4$, 5-$HT_2$, histamine-1, and muscarinic receptor antagonist; **quetiapine** is a dopamine $D_1$, $D_2$, 5-$HT_2$, alpha$_1$-adrenoceptor, and histamine-1 receptor antagonist; and **risperidone** is a dopamine $D_2$, 5-$HT_{2A}$, alpha$_1$-adrenoceptor, and histamine-1 receptor antagonist.

**Aripiprazole** is a dopamine $D_2$ partial agonist with weak 5-$HT_{1a}$ partial agonism and 5-$HT_{2A}$ receptor antagonism. Aripiprazole can cause nausea and, unlike other antipsychotic drugs, lowers prolactin.

> **NICE guidance**
> **Aripiprazole for the treatment of schizophrenia in people aged 15 to 17 years (January 2011)**
> Aripiprazole is recommended as an option for the treatment of schizophrenia in adolescents aged 15 to 17 years who have not responded adequately to, or who are intolerant of, risperidone, or for whom risperidone is contra-indicated.
> www.nice.org.uk/TA213

**Cautions** Antipsychotic drugs should be used with caution in children with cardiovascular disease; an ECG may be required (see individual drug monographs), particularly if physical examination identifies cardiovascular risk factors, if there is a personal history of cardiovascular disease, or if the child is being admitted as an inpatient. Antipsychotic drugs should also be used with caution in children with epilepsy (and conditions predisposing to seizures), depression, myasthenia gravis (avoid chlorpromazine, pericyazine and prochlorperazine) or a susceptibility to angle-closure glaucoma. Caution is also required in severe respiratory disease and in children with a history of jaundice or who have blood dyscrasias (perform blood counts if unexplained infection or fever develops). As photosensitisation may occur with higher dosages, children should avoid direct sunlight. **Interactions:** Appendix 1 (antipsychotics).

**4** Central nervous system

**Contra-indications**    Antipsychotic drugs may be contra-indicated in comatose states, CNS depression, and phaeochromocytoma.

**Skilled tasks**    Drowsiness may affect performance of skilled tasks (e.g. driving or operating machinery), especially at start of treatment; effects of alcohol are enhanced.

**Withdrawal**    There is a high risk of relapse if medication is stopped after 1–2 years. Withdrawal of antipsychotic drugs after long-term therapy should always be gradual and closely monitored to avoid the risk of acute withdrawal syndromes or rapid relapse. Children should be monitored regularly for signs and symptoms of relapse for 2 years after withdrawal of antipsychotic medication.

**Hepatic impairment**    All antipsychotic drugs can precipitate coma if used in hepatic impairment; phenothiazines are hepatotoxic. See also under individual drugs.

**Renal impairment**    Start with small doses of antipsychotic drugs in severe renal impairment because of increased cerebral sensitivity. See also under individual drugs.

**Pregnancy**    Extrapyramidal effects and withdrawal syndrome have been reported occasionally in the neonate when antipsychotic drugs are taken during the third trimester of pregnancy. Following maternal use of antipsychotic drugs in the third trimester, neonates should be monitored for symptoms including agitation, hypertonia, hypotonia, tremor, drowsiness, feeding problems, and respiratory distress. See also under individual drugs.

**Breast-feeding**    There is limited information available on the short- and long-term effects of antipsychotics on the breast-fed infant. *Animal* studies indicate possible adverse effects of antipsychotic medicines on the developing nervous system. Chronic treatment with antipsychotic drugs whilst breast-feeding should be avoided unless absolutely necessary. Phenothiazine derivatives are sometimes used in breast-feeding women for short-term treatment of nausea and vomiting. See also under individual drugs.

**Side-effects**    Side-effects caused by antipsychotic drugs are common and contribute significantly to non-adherence to therapy.

Extrapyramidal symptoms occur most frequently with the group 3 phenothiazine derivatives (perphenazine, prochlorperazine, and trifluoperazine), the butyrophenones (haloperidol), and the first-generation depot preparations. They are easy to recognise but cannot be predicted accurately because they depend on the dose, the type of drug, and on individual susceptibility.

Extrapyramidal symptoms consist of:

- *parkinsonian symptoms* (including tremor), which may appear gradually (but less commonly than in adults);

- *dystonia* (abnormal face and body movements) and *dyskinesia*, which appear after only a few doses;

- *akathisia* (restlessness), which characteristically occurs after large initial doses and may resemble an exacerbation of the condition being treated;

- *tardive dyskinesia* (rhythmic, involuntary movements of tongue, face, and jaw), which usually develops on long-term therapy or with high dosage,

but it may develop on short-term treatment with low doses—short-lived tardive dyskinesia may occur after withdrawal of the drug.

*Parkinsonian symptoms* remit if the drug is withdrawn and may be suppressed by the administration of antimuscarinic drugs (section 4.9.2). However, routine administration of such drugs is not justified because not all children are affected and because they may unmask or worsen tardive dyskinesia.

*Tardive dyskinesia* is the most serious manifestation of extrapyramidal symptoms; it is of particular concern because it may be irreversible on withdrawing therapy and treatment is usually ineffective. In children, tardive dyskinesia is more likely to occur when the antipsychotic drug is withdrawn. However, some manufacturers suggest that drug withdrawal at the earliest signs of tardive dyskinesia (fine vermicular movements of the tongue) may halt its full development. Tardive dyskinesia may occur and treatment must be carefully and regularly reviewed.

Most antipsychotic drugs, both first- and second-generation, increase prolactin concentration to some extent because dopamine inhibits prolactin release. Aripiprazole reduces prolactin because it is a dopamine-receptor partial agonist. Risperidone, amisulpride, and first-generation antipsychotic drugs are most likely to cause symptomatic hyperprolactinaemia. The clinical symptoms of hyperprolactinaemia include sexual dysfunction, reduced bone mineral density, menstrual disturbances, breast enlargement, and galactorrhoea.

Sexual dysfunction is one of the main causes of non-adherence to antipsychotic medication; physical illness, psychiatric illness, and substance misuse are contributing factors. Antipsychotic-induced sexual dysfunction is caused by more than one mechanism. Reduced dopamine transmission and hyperprolactinaemia decrease libido; antimuscarinic effects can cause disorders of arousal; and alpha$_1$-adrenoceptor antagonists are associated with erection and ejaculation problems in males. Risperidone and haloperidol commonly cause sexual dysfunction. If sexual dysfunction is thought to be antipsychotic-induced, dose reduction or switching medication should be considered.

Antipsychotic drugs have been associated with cardiovascular side-effects such as tachycardia, arrhythmias (see under Monitoring), and hypotension (see below). QT-interval prolongation is a particular concern with pimozide (see ECG monitoring in pimozide monograph) and haloperidol. There is also a higher probability of QT-interval prolongation in patients using any intravenous antipsychotic drug, or any antipsychotic drug or combination of antipsychotic drugs with doses exceeding the recommended maximum. Cases of sudden death have occurred.

Hyperglycaemia and sometimes diabetes can occur with antipsychotic drugs, particularly clozapine, olanzapine, quetiapine, and risperidone. All antipsychotic drugs may cause weight gain, but the risk and extent varies. Clozapine and olanzapine commonly cause weight gain.

*Hypotension and interference with temperature regulation* are dose-related side-effects. Clozapine, chlorpromazine, and quetiapine can cause postural hypotension (especially during initial dose titration) which may be associated with syncope or reflex tachycardia in some children.

*Neuroleptic malignant syndrome* (hyperthermia, fluctuating level of consciousness, muscle rigidity, and autonomic dysfunction with pallor, tachycardia, labile blood pressure, sweating, and urinary incontinence) is a rare but potentially fatal side-effect of all antipsychotic drugs. Discontinuation of the antipsychotic drug is essential because there is no proven effective treatment, but bromocriptine, and dantrolene (p. 648) have been used. The syndrome, which usually lasts for 5–7 days after drug discontinuation, may be unduly prolonged if depot preparations have been used.

Hypersalivation associated with clozapine therapy can be treated with hyoscine hydrobromide [unlicensed indication] (p. 198), provided that the patient is not at particular risk from the additive antimuscarinic side-effects of hyoscine and clozapine.

*Other side-effects include:* drowsiness; apathy; agitation, excitement and insomnia; convulsions; dizziness; headache; confusion; gastro-intestinal disturbances; nasal congestion; antimuscarinic symptoms (such as dry mouth, constipation, difficulty with micturition, and blurred vision; *very rarely* precipitation of angle-closure glaucoma); venous thromboembolism; blood dyscrasias (such as agranulocytosis and leucopenia), photosensitisation, contact sensitisation and rashes, and jaundice (including cholestatic); corneal and lens opacities, and purplish pigmentation of the skin, cornea, conjunctiva, and retina.

**Overdosage:** for poisoning with phenothiazines and related compounds and second-generation antipsychotic drugs, see Emergency Treatment of Poisoning, p. 30.

**Choice**  The antipsychotic drugs most commonly used in children are haloperidol, risperidone, and olanzapine. There is little meaningful difference in efficacy between each of the antipsychotic drugs (other than clozapine), and response and tolerability to each antipsychotic drug varies. There is no first-line antipsychotic drug which is suitable for all children. Choice of antipsychotic medication is influenced by the child's medication history, the degree of sedation required (although tolerance to this usually develops), and consideration of individual patient factors such as risk of extrapyramidal side-effects, weight gain, impaired glucose tolerance, QT-interval prolongation, or the presence of negative symptoms.

Second-generation antipsychotic drugs may be better at treating the negative symptoms of schizophrenia. Similarly, second-generation antipsychotic drugs may be prescribed if extrapyramidal side-effects are a particular concern. Of these, aripiprazole, clozapine, olanzapine, and quetiapine are least likely to cause extrapyramidal side-effects. Although amisulpride is a dopamine-receptor antagonist, extrapyramidal side-effects are less common than with the first-generation antipsychotic drugs because amisulpride selectively blocks mesolimbic dopamine receptors, and extrapyramidal symptoms are caused by blockade of the striatal dopamine pathway.

Aripiprazole has negligible effect on the QT-interval. Other antipsychotic drugs with a reduced tendency to prolong QT-interval include amisulpride, clozapine, olanzapine, perphenazine, risperidone, and sulpiride.

Schizophrenia is associated with insulin resistance and diabetes; the risk of diabetes is increased in children with schizophrenia who take antipsychotic drugs. First-generation antipsychotic drugs are less likely to cause diabetes than second-generation antipsychotic drugs, and of the first-generation antipsychotic drugs, haloperidol has the lowest risk. Amisulpride and aripiprazole have the lowest risk of diabetes of the second-generation antipsychotic drugs. Amisulpride, aripiprazole, haloperidol, sulpiride, and trifluoperazine are least likely to cause weight gain.

The antipsychotic drugs with the lowest risk of sexual dysfunction are aripiprazole and quetiapine. Olanzapine may be considered if sexual dysfunction is judged to be secondary to hyperprolactinaemia. Hyperprolactinaemia is usually not clinically significant with aripiprazole, clozapine, olanzapine, and quetiapine treatment. When changing from other antipsychotic drugs a reduction in prolactin concentration may increase fertility.

Children should receive an antipsychotic drug for 4–6 weeks (but see clozapine below) before it is deemed ineffective. Prescribing more than one antipsychotic drug at a time should be avoided except in exceptional circumstances (e.g. clozapine augmentation or when changing medication during titration) because of the increased risk of adverse effects such as extrapyramidal symptoms, QT-interval prolongation, and sudden cardiac death.

Clozapine is used for the treatment of schizophrenia in children unresponsive to, or intolerant of, other antipsychotic drugs. Clozapine should be introduced if schizophrenia is not controlled despite the sequential use of two or more antipsychotic drugs (one of which should be a second-generation antipsychotic drug), each for at least 6–8 weeks. If symptoms do not respond adequately to an optimised dose of clozapine, plasma-clozapine concentration should be checked before adding a second antipsychotic drug to augment clozapine; allow 8–10 weeks' treatment to assess response. Children must be registered with a clozapine patient monitoring service (see under Clozapine).

**Monitoring**  Full blood count, urea and electrolytes, and liver function test monitoring is required at the start of therapy with antipsychotic drugs, and then annually thereafter. Amisulpride and sulpiride do not require liver function test monitoring. Clozapine requires differential white blood cell monitoring weekly for 18 weeks, then fortnightly for up to one year, and then monthly as part of the clozapine patient monitoring service.

Blood lipids and weight should be measured at baseline, at 3 months (weight should be measured at frequent intervals during the first 3 months), and then yearly. Children taking clozapine or olanzapine require more frequent monitoring of these parameters: every 3 months for the first year, then yearly.

Fasting blood glucose should be measured at baseline, at 4–6 months, and then yearly. Children taking clozapine or olanzapine should have fasting blood glucose tested at baseline, after one months' treatment, then every 4–6 months.

Before initiating antipsychotic drugs, an ECG may be required, particularly if physical examination identifies cardiovascular risk factors, if there is a personal history of cardiovascular disease, or if the child is being admitted as an inpatient. ECG monitoring is advised

**4**

**Central nervous system**

for haloperidol and mandatory for pimozide (see individual drug monographs and Side-effects above).

Blood pressure monitoring is advised before starting therapy and frequently during dose titration of antipsychotic drugs. Amisulpride, aripiprazole, trifluoperazine, and sulpiride do not affect blood pressure to the same extent as other antipsychotic drugs and so blood pressure monitoring is not mandatory for these drugs.

It is advisable to monitor prolactin concentration at the start of therapy, at 6 months, and then yearly. Children taking antipsychotic drugs not normally associated with symptomatic hyperprolactinaemia (see Choice above) should be considered for prolactin monitoring if they show symptoms of hyperprolactinaemia (such as breast enlargement and galactorrhoea). Regular clinical monitoring of endocrine function should be considered when children are taking an antipsychotic drug known to increase prolactin levels; this includes measuring weight and height, assessing sexual maturation, and monitoring menstrual function.

Children with schizophrenia should have physical health monitoring (including cardiovascular disease risk assessment) at least once per year.

**Other uses** Nausea and vomiting (section 4.6), choreas, motor tics, and intractable hiccup.

### Equivalent doses of oral antipsychotic drugs

These equivalences are intended **only** as an approximate guide; individual dosage instructions should **also** be checked; children should be carefully monitored after **any** change in medication

| Antipsychotic drug | Daily dose |
|---|---|
| Chlorpromazine | 100 mg |
| Clozapine | 50 mg |
| Haloperidol | 2–3 mg |
| Pimozide | 2 mg |
| Risperidone | 0.5–1 mg |
| Sulpiride | 200 mg |
| Trifluoperazine | 5 mg |

**Important** These equivalences must **not** be extrapolated beyond the max. dose for the drug. Higher doses require careful titration in specialist units and the equivalences shown here may not be appropriate

### Dosage

After an initial period of stabilisation, the total daily oral dose of antipsychotic drugs can be given as a single dose in most children. For advice on doses above the *BNF for Children* upper limit, see p. 170.

## First-generation antipsychotic drugs

### CHLORPROMAZINE HYDROCHLORIDE

**Warning** Owing to the risk of contact sensitisation, pharmacists, nurses, and other health workers should avoid direct contact with chlorpromazine; tablets should not be crushed and solutions should be handled with care

**Cautions** see notes above; also diabetes; children should remain supine, with blood pressure monitoring for 30 minutes after intramuscular injection; dose adjustment may be necessary if smoking started or stopped during treatment

**Contra-indications** see notes above; hypothyroidism

**Hepatic impairment** see notes above

**Renal impairment** see notes above

**Pregnancy** see notes above

**Breast-feeding** see notes above

**Side-effects** see notes above

**Indications and dose**

**Childhood schizophrenia and other psychoses** (under specialist supervision)

- **By mouth**

  **Child 1–6 years** 500 micrograms/kg every 4–6 hours adjusted according to response (max. 40 mg daily)

  **Child 6–12 years** 10 mg 3 times daily, adjusted according to response (max. 75 mg daily)

  **Child 12–18 years** 25 mg 3 times daily (*or* 75 mg at night), adjusted according to response, to usual maintenance dose of 75–300 mg daily (but up to 1 g daily may be required)

**Relief of acute symptoms of psychoses** (under specialist supervision) but see also Cautions and Side-effects

- **By deep intramuscular injection**

  **Child 1–6 years** 500 micrograms/kg every 6–8 hours (max. 40 mg daily)

  **Child 6–12 years** 500 micrograms/kg every 6–8 hours (max. 75 mg daily)

  **Child 12–18 years** 25–50 mg every 6–8 hours

**Chlorpromazine** (Non-proprietary) ℗ℴℳ
Tablets, chlorpromazine hydrochloride 25 mg, net price 28-tab pack = £1.77; 50 mg, 28-tab pack = £2.37; 100 mg, 28-tab pack = £2.31. Label: 2, 11
Brands include *Chloractil*®

Oral solution, chlorpromazine hydrochloride 25 mg/ 5 mL, net price 150 mL = £1.79; 100 mg/5 mL, 150 mL = £4.28. Label: 2, 11

Injection, chlorpromazine hydrochloride 25 mg/mL, net price 1-mL amp = 60p, 2-mL amp = 63p

**Largactil**® (Sanofi-Aventis) ℗ℴℳ
Injection, chlorpromazine hydrochloride 25 mg/mL, net price 2-mL amp = 60p

### HALOPERIDOL

**Cautions** see notes above; also subarachnoid haemorrhage and metabolic disturbances such as hypokalaemia, hypocalcaemia, or hypomagnesaemia; dose adjustment may be necessary if smoking started or stopped during treatment

**Contra-indications** see notes above; QT-interval prolongation (avoid concomitant administration of drugs that prolong QT interval); bradycardia

**Hepatic impairment** see notes above

**Renal impairment** see notes above

**Pregnancy** see notes above

**Breast-feeding** see notes above

**Side-effects** see notes above, but less sedating and fewer antimuscarinic or hypotensive symptoms; depression; weight loss; *less commonly* dyspnoea, oedema; *rarely* bronchospasm, hypoglycaemia, and inappropriate antidiuretic hormone secretion; Stevens-Johnson syndrome and toxic epidermal necrolysis also reported

**Licensed use** not licensed for use in children for nausea and vomiting in palliative care

**Indications and dose**

> **Schizophrenia and other psychoses, mania, short-term adjunctive management of psychomotor agitation, excitement and violent or dangerously impulsive behaviour** (under specialist supervision)
> * By mouth
> **Child 12–18 years** initially 0.5–3 mg 2–3 times daily *or* 3–5 mg 2–3 times daily in severely affected or resistant disease; in resistant schizophrenia up to 30 mg daily may be needed; adjusted according to response to lowest effective maintenance dose (as low as 5–10 mg daily)

> **Motor tics (including Tourette syndrome)** (under specialist supervision)
> * By mouth
> **Child 5–12 years** 12.5–25 micrograms/kg twice daily, adjusted according to response up to 10 mg daily
> **Child 12–18 years** 1.5 mg 3 times daily, adjusted according to response up to 10 mg daily

> **Nausea and vomiting in palliative care**
> * By mouth
> **Child 12–18 years** 1.5 mg once daily at night, increased to 1.5 mg twice daily if necessary; max. 5 mg twice daily
> * By continuous intravenous or subcutaneous infusion
> **Child 1 month–12 years** 25–85 micrograms/kg over 24 hours
> **Child 12–18 years** 1.5–5 mg over 24 hours

**Haloperidol** (Non-proprietary) [PoM]
Tablets, haloperidol 500 micrograms, net price 28-tab pack = 91p; 1.5 mg, 28-tab pack = £1.39; 5 mg, 28-tab pack = £2.15; 10 mg, 28-tab pack = £5.53; 20 mg, 28-tab pack = £14.07. Label: 2

Injection, haloperidol 5 mg/mL, net price 1-mL amp = 49p

**Dozic®** (Rosemont) [PoM]
Oral liquid, sugar-free, haloperidol 1 mg/mL, net price 100-mL pack = £6.86. Label: 2

**Haldol®** (Janssen) [PoM]
Tablets, both scored, haloperidol 5 mg (blue), net price 100-tab pack = £7.21; 10 mg (yellow), 100-tab pack = £14.08. Label: 2

Oral liquid, sugar-free, haloperidol 2 mg/mL, net price 100-mL pack (with pipette) = £4.45. Label: 2

Injection, haloperidol 5 mg/mL, net price 1-mL amp = 37p

**Serenace®** (TEVA UK) [PoM]
Capsules, green, haloperidol 500 micrograms, net price 30-cap pack = 98p. Label: 2

Oral liquid, sugar-free, haloperidol 2 mg/mL, net price 100-mL pack = £7.41, 500-mL pack = £34.48. Label: 2

## LEVOMEPROMAZINE
(Methotrimeprazine)

**Cautions** see notes above; diabetes; children receiving large initial doses should remain supine

**Contra-indications** see notes above

**Hepatic impairment** see notes above

**Renal impairment** see notes above

**Pregnancy** see notes above

**Breast-feeding** see notes above

**Side-effects** see notes above; occasionally raised erythrocyte sedimentation rate occurs; hyperglycaemia also reported

**Indications and dose**

> **Restlessness and confusion in palliative care**
> * By continuous subcutaneous infusion
> **Child 1–12 years** 0.35–3 mg/kg over 24 hours
> **Child 12–18 years** 12.5–200 mg over 24 hours

> **Nausea and vomiting in palliative care**
> * By continuous intravenous or subcutaneous infusion
> **Child 1 month–12 years** 100–400 micrograms/kg over 24 hours
> **Child 12–18 years** 5–25 mg over 24 hours

**Administration** for administration by *subcutaneous infusion* dilute with a suitable volume of Sodium Chloride 0.9%

**Nozinan®** (Sanofi-Aventis) [PoM]
Tablets, scored, levomepromazine maleate 25 mg, net price 84-tab pack = £20.26. Label: 2

Injection, levomepromazine hydrochloride 25 mg/mL, net price 1-mL amp = £2.01

## PERICYAZINE
(Periciazine)

**Cautions** see notes above

**Contra-indications** see notes above

**Hepatic impairment** see notes above

**Renal impairment** see notes above; avoid in renal impairment

**Pregnancy** see notes above

**Breast-feeding** see notes above

**Side-effects** see notes above; more sedating; hypotension common when treatment initiated; respiratory depression

**Licensed use** tablets not licensed for use in children

**Indications and dose**

Schizophrenia, psychoses (severe mental or behavioural disorders only) (under specialist supervision)
- By mouth

  Child 1-12 years initially 500 micrograms daily for 10-kg child, increased by 1 mg for each additional 5 kg to max. total daily dose of 10 mg; dose may be gradually increased according to response but maintenance should not exceed twice initial dose

  Child 12-18 years initially 25 mg 3 times daily increased at weekly intervals by steps of 25 mg according to response; usual max. 100 mg 3 times daily; total daily dose may alternatively be given in 2 divided doses

**Pericyazine** (Non-proprietary) [PoM]
Tablets, pericyazine 2.5 mg, net price 84-tab pack = £9.23; 10 mg, 84-tab pack = £24.95. Label: 2
Syrup, pericyazine 10 mg/5 mL, net price 100-mL pack = £12.08. Label: 2

## PERPHENAZINE

**Cautions** see notes above; hypothyroidism
**Contra-indications** see notes above
**Hepatic impairment** see notes above
**Renal impairment** see notes above
**Pregnancy** see notes above
**Breast-feeding** see notes above
**Side-effects** see notes above; less sedating; dystonia, more frequent (particularly at high dosage); *rarely* systemic lupus erythematosus

**Indications and dose**

Schizophrenia and other psychoses, mania, short-term adjunctive management of anxiety, severe psychomotor agitation, excitement, violent or dangerously impulsive behaviour (under specialist supervision)
- By mouth

  Child 14-18 years initially 4 mg 3 times daily adjusted according to the response; max. 24 mg daily

**Fentazin**® (Mercury) [PoM]
Tablets, both s/c, perphenazine 2 mg, net price 100-tab pack = £22.38; 4 mg, 100-tab pack = £26.34. Label: 2

## PIMOZIDE

**Cautions** see notes above

**ECG monitoring** Following reports of sudden unexplained death, an ECG is recommended before treatment. It is also recommended that patients taking pimozide should have an annual ECG (if the QT interval is prolonged, treatment should be reviewed and either withdrawn or dose reduced under close supervision) and that pimozide should **not** be given with other antipsychotic drugs (including depot preparations), tricyclic antidepressants or other drugs which prolong the QT interval, such as certain antimalarials, antiarrhythmic drugs and certain antihistamines and should **not** be given with drugs which cause electrolyte disturbances (especially diuretics)

**Contra-indications** see notes above; history or family history of congenital QT prolongation; history of arrhythmias

**Hepatic impairment** see notes above

**Renal impairment** see notes above
**Pregnancy** see notes above
**Breast-feeding** see notes above
**Side-effects** see notes above; less sedating; serious arrhythmias, venous thromboembolism, glycosuria, and *rarely*, hyponatraemia reported
**Licensed use** not licensed for use in Tourette syndrome

**Indications and dose**

Schizophrenia (under specialist supervision)
- By mouth

  Child 12-18 years initially 1 mg daily, increased according to response in steps of 2-4 mg at intervals of not less than 1 week; usual dose range 2-20 mg daily

Tourette syndrome (under specialist supervision)
- By mouth

  Child 2-12 years 1-4 mg daily
  Child 12-18 years 2-10 mg daily

**Orap**® (Janssen) [PoM]
Tablets, scored, green, pimozide 4 mg, net price 100-tab pack = £26.87. Label: 2

## SULPIRIDE

**Cautions** see notes above; also excited, agitated, or aggressive children (even low doses may aggravate symptoms)
**Contra-indications** see notes above
**Hepatic impairment** see notes above
**Renal impairment** see notes above
**Pregnancy** see notes above
**Breast-feeding** see notes above
**Side-effects** see notes above; also hepatitis and venous thromboembolism
**Licensed use** not licensed for use in Tourette syndrome

**Indications and dose**

Schizophrenia (under specialist supervision)
- By mouth

  Child 14-18 years 200-400 mg twice daily; max. 800 mg daily in predominantly negative symptoms, dose increased to max. 2.4 g daily in mainly positive symptoms

Tourette syndrome (under specialist supervision)
- By mouth

  Child 2-12 years 50-400 mg twice daily
  Child 12-18 years 100-400 mg twice daily

**Sulpiride** (Non-proprietary) [PoM]
Tablets, sulpiride 200 mg, net price 30-tab pack = £8.09; 56-tab pack = £6.46; 400 mg, 30-tab pack = £18.57. Label: 2

**Dolmatil**® (Sanofi-Aventis) [PoM]
Tablets, both scored, sulpiride 200 mg, net price 100-tab pack = £13.31; 400 mg (f/c), 100-tab pack = £34.87. Label: 2

**Sulpor®** (Rosemont) [PoM]
Oral solution, sugar-free, lemon- and aniseed-fla-
voured, sulpiride 200 mg/5 mL, net price 150 mL =
£25.38. Label: 2

## ▪ TRIFLUOPERAZINE

**Cautions** see notes above
**Contra-indications** see notes above
**Hepatic impairment** see notes above
**Renal impairment** see notes above
**Pregnancy** see notes above
**Breast-feeding** see notes above
**Side-effects** see notes above; extrapyramidal symp-
toms more frequent, especially at doses exceeding
6 mg daily; anorexia; muscle weakness
**Indications and dose**

**Schizophrenia and other psychoses, short-term
adjunctive management of psychomotor agitation, excitement and violent or dangerously
impulsive behaviour** (under specialist supervision)
• By mouth
  **Child 12–18 years** initially 5 mg twice daily,
  increased by 5 mg daily after 1 week, then at
  intervals of 3 days, according to response

**Short-term adjunctive management of severe
anxiety** (under specialist supervision)
• By mouth
  **Child 3–6 years** up to 500 micrograms twice daily
  **Child 6–12 years** up to 2 mg twice daily
  **Child 12–18 years** 1–2 mg twice daily, increased if
  necessary to 3 mg twice daily

**Antiemetic** section 4.6

**Trifluoperazine** (Non-proprietary) [PoM]
Tablets, trifluoperazine (as hydrochloride) 1 mg, net
price 112-tab pack = £7.22; 5 mg, 112-tab pack =
£4.65. Label: 2
Oral solution, trifluoperazine (as hydrochloride)
5 mg/5 mL, net price 150-mL pack = £10.84. Label:
2

**Stelazine®** (Mercury) [PoM]
Tablets, blue, f/c, trifluoperazine (as hydrochloride)
1 mg, net price 112-tab pack = £3.43; 5 mg, 112-tab
pack = £4.89. Label: 2
Syrup, sugar-free, yellow, trifluoperazine (as hydrochloride) 1 mg/5 mL, net price 200-mL pack =
£2.95. Label: 2

## Second-generation antipsychotic drugs

## ▪ AMISULPRIDE

**Cautions** see notes above
**Contra-indications** see notes above; prolactin-
dependent tumours; prepubertal children
**Renal impairment** halve dose if estimated glomerular
filtration rate 30–60 mL/minute/1.73 m²; use one-
third dose if estimated glomerular filtration rate 10–
30 mL/minute/1.73 m²; no information available if

estimated glomerular filtration rate less than 10 mL/
minute/1.73 m²
**Pregnancy** avoid
**Breast-feeding** avoid—no information available
**Side-effects** see notes above; also insomnia, anxiety,
agitation, drowsiness, gastro-intestinal disorders such
as constipation, nausea, vomiting, and dry mouth; *less
commonly* bradycardia; *rarely* seizures; urticaria also
reported
**Licensed use** not licensed for use in children under 18
years
**Indications and dose**

**Acute psychotic episode** (under specialist supervision)
• By mouth
  **Child 15–18 years** 200–400 mg twice daily
  adjusted according to response; max. 1.2 g daily

**Predominantly negative symptoms** (under specia-
list supervision)
• By mouth
  **Child 15–18 years** 50–300 mg daily

**Amisulpride** (Non-proprietary) [PoM]
Tablets, amisulpride 50 mg, net price 60-tab pack =
£7.18; 100 mg, 60-tab pack = £31.74; 200 mg, 60-tab
pack = £16.47; 400 mg, 60-tab pack = £105.68.
Label: 2

**Solian®** (Sanofi-Aventis) [PoM]
Tablets, amisulpride 50 mg, net price 60-tab pack =
£22.76; 100 mg, 60-tab pack = £35.29; 200 mg, 60-
tab pack = £58.99, 400 mg, 60-tab pack = £117.97.
Label: 2
Solution, 100 mg/mL, net price 60 mL (caramel flavour) = £33.76. Label: 2

## ▪ ARIPIPRAZOLE

**Cautions** see notes above; cerebrovascular disease
**Contra-indications** see notes above
**Hepatic impairment** use with caution in severe
impairment
**Pregnancy** see Pregnancy notes, p. 172; also use only
if potential benefit outweighs risk
**Breast-feeding** avoid—present in milk in *animal* studies
**Side-effects** see notes above; gastro-intestinal disturbances; tachycardia; fatigue, insomnia, agitation,
akathesia, drowsiness, restlessness, tremor, headache, asthenia; blurred vision; *less commonly* depression; *very rarely* anorexia, dysphagia, oropharangeal
spasm, laryngospasm, hepatitis, jaundice, hypersalivation, pancreatitis, oedema, thromboembolism,
arrhythmias, bradycardia, hypertension, chest pain,
anxiety, speech disorder, suicidal ideation, seizures,
hyponatraemia, stiffness, myalgia, rhabdomyolysis,
priapism, urinary retention and incontinence, blood
disorders, sweating, alopecia, photosensitivity reactions, rash, and impaired temperature regulation
**Licensed use** not licensed for use in children under 15
years; not licensed for mania in children

**4**

**Central nervous system**

**4 Central nervous system**

## Indications and dose

**Schizophrenia and treatment and recurrence prevention of mania** (under specialist supervision)

- By mouth

  **Child 13–18 years** 2 mg once daily, increased to 5 mg once daily after 2 days, then further increased to 10 mg once daily after a further 2 days; further increased if necessary in steps of 5 mg to max. 30 mg daily

**Abilify®** (Bristol-Myers Squibb) (PoM)

Tablets, aripiprazole 5 mg (blue), net price 28-tab pack = £95.74; 10 mg (pink), 28-tab pack = £95.74; 15 mg (yellow), 28-tab pack = £95.74; 30 mg (pink), 28-tab pack = £191.47. Label: 2

Orodispersible tablets, aripiprazole 10 mg (pink), net price 28-tab pack = £95.74; 15 mg (yellow), 28-tab pack = £95.74. Label: 2, counselling, administration

**Excipients** include aspartame (section 9.4.1)

**Counselling** Tablets should be placed on the tongue and allowed to dissolve, or be dispersed in water and swallowed

Oral solution, aripiprazole 1 mg/mL, net price 150 mL with measuring cup = £102.57. Label: 2

## CLOZAPINE

**Cautions** see notes above; monitor leucocyte and differential blood counts (see Agranulocytosis, below); susceptibility to angle-closure glaucoma; taper off other antipsychotics before starting; close medical supervision during initiation (risk of collapse because of hypotension); dose adjustment may be necessary if smoking started or stopped during treatment

**Withdrawal** On planned withdrawal reduce dose over 1–2 weeks to avoid risk of rebound psychosis. If abrupt withdrawal necessary observe child carefully

**Agranulocytosis** Neutropenia and potentially fatal agranulocytosis reported. Leucocyte and differential blood counts must be normal before starting; monitor counts every week for 18 weeks then at least every 2 weeks and if clozapine continued and blood count stable after 1 year at least every 4 weeks (and 4 weeks after discontinuation); if leucocyte count below 3000/mm³ or if absolute neutrophil count below 1500/mm³ discontinue permanently and refer to haematologist. Patients who have a low white blood cell count because of benign ethnic neutropenia may be started on clozapine with the agreement of a haematologist. Avoid drugs which depress leucopoiesis; children (or carers) should report immediately symptoms of infection, especially influenza-like illness

**Myocarditis and cardiomyopathy** Fatal myocarditis (most commonly in first 2 months) and cardiomyopathy reported.

- Perform physical examination and take full medical history before starting;

- Specialist examination required if cardiac abnormalities or history of heart disease found—clozapine initiated only in absence of severe heart disease and if benefit outweighs risk;

- Persistent tachycardia especially in first 2 months should prompt observation for other indicators for myocarditis or cardiomyopathy;

- If myocarditis or cardiomyopathy suspected clozapine should be stopped and child evaluated urgently by cardiologist;

- Discontinue permanently in clozapine-induced myocarditis or cardiomyopathy

**Gastro-intestinal obstruction** Reactions resembling gastro-intestinal obstruction reported. Clozapine should be used cautiously with drugs which cause constipation (e.g. antimuscarinic drugs) or in children with history of colonic disease or bowel surgery. Monitor for constipation and prescribe laxative if required

**Contra-indications** severe cardiac disorders (e.g. myocarditis; see Cautions); history of neutropenia or agranulocytosis (see Cautions); bone-marrow disorders; paralytic ileus (see Cautions); alcoholic and toxic psychoses; history of circulatory collapse; drug intoxication; coma or severe CNS depression; uncontrolled epilepsy

**Hepatic impairment** monitor hepatic function regularly; avoid in symptomatic or progressive liver disease or hepatic failure

**Renal impairment** avoid in severe impairment

**Pregnancy** see Pregnancy notes, p. 172; use with caution

**Breast-feeding** avoid

**Side-effects** see notes above; also constipation (see Cautions), hypersalivation, dry mouth, nausea, vomiting, anorexia; tachycardia, ECG changes, hypertension; drowsiness, dizziness, headache, dysarthria, tremor, seizures, fatigue, impaired temperature regulation; urinary incontinence and retention; leucopenia, eosinophilia, leucocytosis; blurred vision; sweating; *less commonly* agranulocytosis (**important**: see Cautions); *rarely* dysphagia, hepatitis, cholestatic jaundice, pancreatitis, circulatory collapse, arrhythmia, myocarditis (**important**: see Cautions), pericarditis, agitation, confusion, delirium, pneumonia, anaemia; *very rarely* parotid gland enlargement, intestinal obstruction (see Cautions), cardiomyopathy, myocardial infarction, respiratory depression, obsessive compulsive disorder, priapism, interstitial nephritis, thrombocytopenia, thrombocythaemia, hypertriglyceridaemia, hypercholesterolaemia, hyperlipidaemia, fulminant hepatic necrosis, angle-closure glaucoma, and skin reactions

**Licensed use** not licensed for use in children under 16 years

## Indications and dose

**Schizophrenia in children unresponsive to, or intolerant of, conventional antipsychotic drugs** (under specialist supervision)

- By mouth

  **Child 12–18 years** 12.5 mg once or twice on first day then 25–50 mg on second day then increased gradually (if well tolerated) in steps of 25–50 mg daily over 14–21 days up to 300 mg daily in divided doses (larger dose at night, up to 200 mg daily may be taken as a single dose at bedtime); if necessary may be further increased in steps of 50–100 mg once (preferably) or twice weekly; usual dose 200–450 mg daily (max. 900 mg daily)

  **Note** *Restarting* after *interval of more than 2 days*, 12.5 mg once or twice on first day (but may be feasible to increase more quickly than on initiation)—extreme caution if previous respiratory or cardiac arrest with initial dosing

**Clozaril®** (Novartis) (PoM)

Tablets, yellow, clozapine 25 mg (scored), net price 28-tab pack = £5.40, 84-tab pack (hosp. only) = £16.18, 100-tab pack (hosp. only) = £19.26; 100 mg, 28-tab pack = £21.56, 84-tab pack (hosp. only) = £64.68, 100-tab pack (hosp. only) = £77.00. Label: 2, 10, patient information leaflet

**Note** Child, prescriber, and supplying pharmacist must be registered with the Clozaril Patient Monitoring Service—takes several days to do this

**Denzapine®** (Genus) (PoM)

Tablets, yellow, scored, clozapine 25 mg, net price 84-tab pack = £16.64, 100-tab pack = £19.80;

50 mg, 50-tab pack = £19.80; 100 mg, 84-tab pack = £66.53, 100-tab pack = £79.20; 200 mg, 50-tab pack = £79.20. Label: 2, 10, patient information leaflet

Suspension, clozapine 50 mg/mL, net price 100 mL = £39.60. Label: 2, 10, patient information leaflet, counselling, administration

**Counselling** Shake well for 90 seconds when dispensing or if visibly settled; otherwise shake well for 10 seconds before use

**Note** May be diluted in water

**Note** Child, prescriber, and supplying pharmacist must be registered with the Denzapine Patient Monitoring Service—takes several days to do this

**Zaponex**® (TEVA UK) [PoM]
Tablets, yellow, scored, clozapine 25 mg, net price 84-tab pack = £8.28; 100 mg, 84-tab pack = £33.88. Label: 2, 10, patient information leaflet

**Note** Child, prescriber, and supplying pharmacist must be registered with the Zaponex Treatment Access System—takes several days to do this

## ◼ OLANZAPINE

**Cautions** see notes above; also paralytic ileus, diabetes mellitus (risk of exacerbation or ketoacidosis), low leucocyte or neutrophil count, bone-marrow depression, hyper-eosinophilic disorders, myeloproliferative disease; dose adjustment may be necessary if smoking started or stopped during treatment

**Hepatic impairment** consider initial dose of 5 mg daily

**Renal impairment** consider initial dose of 5 mg daily

**Pregnancy** see Pregnancy notes, p. 172; use only if potential benefit outweighs risk; neonatal lethargy, tremor and hypertonia reported when used in third trimester

**Breast-feeding** avoid—present in milk

**Side-effects** see notes above; also mild, transient antimuscarinic effects; drowsiness, speech difficulty, abnormal gait, hallucinations, akathisia, asthenia, increased appetite, increased body temperature, raised triglyceride concentration, oedema, hyperprolactinaemia (but clinical manifestations uncommon); eosinophilia; *less commonly* hypotension, bradycardia, and urinary incontinence; *rarely* seizures, and leucopenia; *very rarely* hepatitis, pancreatitis, hypercholesterolaemia, hypothermia, urinary retention, priapism, thrombocytopenia, neutropenia, rhabdomyolysis, and angle-closure glaucoma

**Licensed use** not licensed for use in children

**Indications and dose**

> **Schizophrenia, combination therapy for mania** (under specialist supervision)
> • By mouth
>> **Child 12–18 years** initially 5–10 mg daily adjusted to usual range of 5–20 mg daily; doses greater than 10 mg daily only after reassessment; max. 20 mg daily

> **Monotherapy for mania** (under specialist supervision)
> • By mouth
>> **Child 12–18 years** 15 mg daily adjusted to usual range of 5–20 mg daily; doses greater than 15 mg only after reassessment; max. 20 mg daily

**Note** When one or more factors present that might result in slower metabolism (e.g. female gender, non-smoker) consider lower initial dose and more gradual dose increase

**Olanzapine** (Non-proprietary) [PoM]
Tablets, olanzapine 2.5 mg, net price 28-tab pack = £6.56; 5 mg, 28-tab pack = £13.11; 7.5 mg, 56-tab pack = £39.33; 10 mg, 28-tab pack = £26.22; 15 mg, 28-tab pack = £35.75; 20 mg, 28-tab pack = £47.67. Label: 2

Brands include *Zalasta*®

Orodispersible tablets, olanzapine 5 mg, net price 28-tab pack = £38.46; 10 mg, 28-tab pack = £69.92; 15 mg, 28-tab pack = £104.88; 20 mg, 28-tab pack = £139.83. Label: 2, counselling, administration

**Counselling** Olanzapine orodispersible tablet may be placed on the tongue and allowed to dissolve, or dispersed in water, orange juice, apple juice, milk, or coffee

**Zyprexa**® (Lilly) [PoM]
Tablets, f/c, olanzapine 2.5 mg, net price 28-tab pack = £21.85; 5 mg, 28-tab pack = £43.70; 7.5 mg, 56-tab pack = £131.10; 10 mg, 28-tab pack = £87.40; 15 mg (blue), 28-tab pack = £119.18; 20 mg (pink), 28-tab pack = £158.90. Label: 2

Orodispersible tablet (*Velotab*®), yellow, olanzapine 5 mg, net price 28-tab pack = £48.07; 10 mg, 28-tab pack = £87.40; 15 mg, 28-tab pack = £131.10; 20 mg, 28-tab pack = £174.79. Label: 2, counselling, administration

**Excipients** include aspartame (section 9.4.1)

**Counselling** *Velotab*® may be placed on the tongue and allowed to dissolve, or dispersed in water, orange juice, apple juice, milk, or coffee

## ◼ QUETIAPINE

**Cautions** see notes above; cerebrovascular disease; children at risk of aspiration pneumonia

**Hepatic impairment** for *immediate-release tablets*, initially 25 mg daily, increased daily in steps of 25–50 mg

**Pregnancy** see Pregnancy notes, p. 172; use only if potential benefit outweighs risk

**Breast-feeding** avoid—no information available

**Side-effects** see notes above; also dyspepsia, hypertension, elevated plasma-triglyceride and -cholesterol concentrations, peripheral oedema, irritability, dysarthria, asthenia; *less commonly* dysphagia, seizures, restless legs syndrome, hyponatraemia, and eosinophilia; *rarely* priapism; *very rarely* hepatitis, inappropriate secretion of antidiuretic hormone, rhabdomyolysis, angioedema, and Stevens-Johnson syndrome; suicidal behaviour (particularly on initiation) also reported

**Licensed use** not licensed for use in children

**Indications and dose**

> **Schizophrenia** (under specialist supervision)
> • By mouth
>> **Child 12–18 years** initially 25 mg twice daily adjusted in steps of 25–50 mg according to response; max. 750 mg daily

> **Treatment of mania in bipolar disorder** (under specialist supervision)
> • By mouth
>> **Child 12–18 years** 25 mg twice daily on day 1, *then* 50 mg twice daily on day 2, *then* 100 mg twice daily on day 3, *then* 150 mg twice daily on day 4, *then* 200 mg twice daily on day 5; thereafter dose adjusted according to response in steps no greater than 100 mg daily, usual dose 400–600 mg daily in 2 divided doses

**4**

**Central nervous system**

**Quetiapine** (Non-proprietary) [PoM]
Tablets, quetiapine (as fumarate) 25 mg, net price 60-tab pack = £34.59; 100 mg, 60-tab pack = £96.94; 150 mg, 60-tab pack = £96.94; 200 mg, 60-tab pack =£96.94; 300 mg, 60-tab pack = £145.71. Label: 2

**Seroquel®** (AstraZeneca) [PoM]
Tablets, f/c, quetiapine (as fumarate) 25 mg (peach), net price 60-tab pack = £33.83; 100 mg (yellow), 60-tab pack = £113.10; 150 mg (pale yellow), 60-tab pack = £113.10; 200 mg (white), 60-tab pack = £113.10; 300 mg (white), 60-tab pack = £170.00. Label: 2

◢Modified release
**Seroquel® XL** (AstraZeneca) [PoM]
Tablets, m/r, quetiapine (as fumarate) 50 mg (peach), net price 60-tab pack = £67.66; 150 mg (white), 60-tab pack = £113.10; 200 mg (yellow), 60-tab pack = £113.10; 300 mg (pale yellow), 60-tab pack = £170.00; 400 mg (white), 60-tab pack = £226.20. Label: 2, 23, 25

**Dose**

**Schizophrenia** (under specialist supervision)
• By mouth
  **Child 12–18 years** initially 50 mg once daily adjusted in steps of 50 mg daily according to response, usual dose 400–800 mg once daily; max. 800 mg once daily
  **Note** Patients can be switched from immediate-release to modified-release tablets at the equivalent daily dose; to maintain clinical response, dose titration may be required

---

**RISPERIDONE**

**Cautions** see notes above; prolactin-dependent tumours; dehydration; family history of sudden cardiac death (perform ECG); avoid in acute porphyria (section 9.8.2)

**Hepatic impairment** initial and subsequent oral doses should be halved

**Renal impairment** initial and subsequent oral doses should be halved

**Pregnancy** see Pregnancy notes, p. 172; use only if potential benefit outweighs risk

**Breast-feeding** use only if potential benefit outweighs risk—small amount present in milk

**Side-effects** see notes above; also dyspnoea; asthenia, tremor, anxiety; urinary incontinence; arthralgia, myalgia; epistaxis; *less commonly* anorexia, hypoaesthesia, impaired concentration, tinnitus, angioedema; *rarely* intestinal obstruction, pancreatitis, seizures, hyponatraemia; oedema and priapism also reported

**Licensed use** not licensed for use in children for psychosis, mania, or autism

**Indications and dose**

**Acute and chronic psychosis** (under specialist supervision)
• By mouth
  **Child 12–18 years** 2 mg in 1–2 divided doses on first day *then* 4 mg in 1–2 divided doses on second day (slower titration appropriate in some children); usual dose range 4–6 mg daily; doses above 10 mg daily only if benefit considered to outweigh risk (max. 16 mg daily)

**Short-term monotherapy of mania in bipolar disorder** (under specialist supervision)
• By mouth
  **Child 12–18 years** initially 500 micrograms once daily adjusted in steps of 0.5–1 mg daily according to response; usual dose 2.5 mg daily in 1–2 divided doses, max. 6 mg daily

**Short-term treatment (up to 6 weeks) of persistent aggression in conduct disorder** (under specialist supervision)
• By mouth
  **Child 5–18 years and body-weight under 50 kg** initially 250 micrograms once daily increased according to response in steps of 250 micrograms on alternate days; usual dose 500 micrograms daily (up to 750 micrograms once daily has been required)
  **Child 5–18 years and body-weight over 50 kg** initially 500 micrograms once daily increased according to response in steps of 500 micrograms on alternate days; usual dose 1 mg daily (up to 1.5 mg once daily has been required)

**Short-term treatment of severe aggression in autism** (under specialist supervision)
• By mouth
  **Child over 5 years and 15–20 kg** 250 micrograms daily increased if necessary after at least 4 days to 500 micrograms daily; thereafter increased by 250 micrograms daily at 2-week intervals to max. 1 mg daily
  **Child over 5 years and over 20 kg** 500 micrograms daily increased if necessary after at least 4 days to 1 mg daily; thereafter increased by 500 micrograms daily at 2-week intervals; max. daily dose 2.5 mg if under 45 kg; max. daily dose 3 mg if over 45 kg

**Risperidone** (Non-proprietary) [PoM]
Tablets, risperidone 500 micrograms, net price 20-tab pack = 97p; 1 mg, 20-tab pack = £1.18, 60-tab pack = £1.70; 2 mg, 60-tab pack = £2.13; 3 mg, 60-tab pack = £2.71; 4 mg, 60-tab pack = £31.52; 6 mg, 28-tab pack = £24.12. Label: 2

Orodispersible tablets, risperidone 0.5 mg, net price 28-tab pack = £16.88; 1 mg, 28-tab pack = £20.51; 2 mg, 28-tab pack = £37.72; 3 mg, 28-tab pack = £14.39; 4 mg, 28-tab pack = £15.20. Label: 2, counselling, administration
**Counselling** Tablets should be placed on the tongue, allowed to dissolve and swallowed

Liquid, risperidone 1 mg/mL, net price 100-mL pack = £57.40. Label: 2, counselling, use of dose syringe
**Note** Liquid may be diluted with any non-alcoholic drink, except tea

**Risperdal®** (Janssen) [PoM]
Tablets, f/c, scored, risperidone 500 micrograms (brown-red), net price 20-tab pack = £5.08; 1 mg (white), 20-tab pack = £8.36, 60-tab pack = £25.08; 2 mg (orange), 60-tab pack = £49.46; 3 mg (yellow), 60-tab pack = £72.73; 4 mg (green), 60-tab pack = £96.00; 6 mg (yellow), 28-tab pack = £67.88. Label: 2

Orodispersible tablets (*Quicklet*®), pink, risperidone 500 micrograms, net price 28-tab pack = £8.23; 1 mg, 28-tab pack = £17.32; 2 mg, 28-tab pack = £32.65; 3 mg, 28-tab pack = £36.24; 4 mg, 28-tab pack = £46.68. Label: 2, counselling, administration
Excipients include aspartame (section 9.4.1)
Counselling Tablets should be placed on the tongue, allowed to dissolve and swallowed

Liquid, risperidone 1 mg/mL, net price 100-mL pack = £52.87. Label: 2, counselling, use of dose syringe
Note Liquid may be diluted with any non-alcoholic drink, except tea

## 4.2.2 Antipsychotic depot injections

There is limited information on the use of antipsychotic depot injections in children and use should be restricted to specialist centres.

## 4.2.3 Drugs used for mania and hypomania

Antimanic drugs are used in mania to control acute attacks and to prevent recurrence of episodes of mania or hypomania. Long-term treatment of bipolar disorder should continue for at least two years from the last manic episode and up to five years if the patient has risk factors for relapse.

An antidepressant drug (section 4.3) may also be required for the treatment of co-existing depression, but should be avoided in patients with rapid-cycling bipolar disorder, recent history of hypomania, or rapid mood fluctuations.

### Benzodiazepines

Use of benzodiazepines (section 4.1) may be helpful in the initial stages of treatment for behavioural disturbance or agitation; they should not be used for long periods because of the risk of dependence.

### Antipsychotic drugs

Atypical antipsychotic drugs (normally **olanzapine**, **quetiapine**, or **risperidone**) (section 4.2.1) are useful in acute episodes of mania and hypomania; if the response to antipsychotic drugs is inadequate, lithium or valproate may be added. An antipsychotic drug may be used concomitantly with lithium or valproate in the initial treatment of severe acute mania.

Atypical antipsychotics are the treatment of choice for the long-term management of bipolar disorder in children and adolescents; if the patient has frequent relapses or continuing functional impairment, consider concomitant therapy with lithium or valproate. An atypical antipsychotic that causes less weight gain and does not increase prolactin levels is preferred.

When discontinuing antipsychotics, the dose should be reduced gradually over at least 4 weeks if the child is continuing on other antimanic drugs; if the child is not continuing on other antimanic drugs, or has a history of manic relapse, a withdrawal period of up to 3 months is required.

High doses of haloperidol may be hazardous when used with lithium; irreversible toxic encephalopathy has been reported.

### Carbamazepine

Carbamazepine (section 4.8.1) may be used under specialist supervision for the prophylaxis of bipolar disorder (manic-depressive disorder) in children unresponsive to a combination of other prophylactic drugs; it is used in those with rapid-cycling manic-depressive illness (4 or more affective episodes per year). The dose of carbamazepine should not normally be increased if an acute episode of mania occurs. When stopping treatment with carbamazepine, reduce the dose gradually over a period of at least 4 weeks.

### Valproate

Valproic acid (as the semisodium salt) is licensed in adults for the treatment of manic episodes associated with bipolar disorder. Sodium valproate (section 4.8.1) is unlicensed for the treatment of bipolar disorder.

Valproate can be used for the prophylaxis of bipolar disorder [unlicensed use]; however, it should not normally be prescribed for women of child-bearing potential. In patients with frequent relapse or continuing functional impairment, consider switching therapy to lithium or an atypical antipsychotic, or adding lithium or an atypical antipsychotic to valproate. If a patient taking valproate experiences an acute episode of mania that is not ameliorated by increasing the valproate dose, consider concomitant therapy with olanzapine, quetiapine, or risperidone. When stopping valproate reduce the dose gradually over at least 4 weeks.

### Lithium

Lithium salts are used in the prophylaxis and treatment of mania, in the prophylaxis of bipolar disorder (manic-depressive disorder), as concomitant therapy with antidepressant medication in children who have had an incomplete response to treatment for acute depression in bipolar disorder, and in the prophylaxis of recurrent depression (unipolar illness or unipolar depression).

Lithium is used to treat acute episodes of mania in children who have responded to lithium before and whose symptoms are not severe.

The decision to give prophylactic lithium requires specialist advice, and must be based on careful consideration of the likelihood of recurrence in the individual child, and the benefit of treatment weighed against the risks. The full prophylactic effect of lithium may not occur for six to twelve months after the initiation of therapy. An atypical antipsychotic or valproate (given alone or as adjunctive therapy with lithium) are alternative prophylactic treatments in patients who experience frequent relapses or continuing functional impairment. Long-term use of lithium has been associated with thyroid disorders and mild cognitive and memory impairment. Long-term treatment should therefore be undertaken only with careful assessment of risk and benefit, and with monitoring of thyroid function at baseline and every 6 months (more often if there is evidence of deterioration). Renal function should be monitored at baseline and every 6 months thereafter (more often if there is evidence of deterioration or the patient has other risk factors, such as starting ACE inhibitors, NSAIDs, or diuretics). The need for continued therapy should be assessed regularly and children should be maintained on lithium after 3 to 5 years only if benefit persists.

**Serum concentrations**   Lithium salts have a narrow therapeutic/toxic ratio and should not be prescribed unless facilities for monitoring serum-lithium concentrations are available. Samples should be taken 12 hours after the dose to achieve a serum-lithium concentration of 0.4–1 mmol/litre. A target serum-lithium concentration of 0.8–1 mmol/litre is recommended for acute episodes of mania, and for patients who have previously relapsed or have sub-syndromal symptoms. It is important to determine the optimum range for each individual child. Serum-lithium monitoring should be performed weekly after initiation and after each dose change until concentrations are stable, then every 3 months thereafter. Additional serum-lithium measurements should be made if a child develops significant intercurrent disease or if there is a significant change in a child's sodium or fluid intake.

**Overdosage**, usually with serum-lithium concentration of over 1.5 mmol/litre, may be fatal and toxic effects include tremor, ataxia, dysarthria, nystagmus, renal impairment, and convulsions. If these potentially hazardous signs occur, treatment should be stopped, serum-lithium concentrations redetermined, and steps taken to reverse lithium toxicity. In mild cases withdrawal of lithium and administration of sodium and fluid will reverse the toxicity. A serum-lithium concentration in excess of 2 mmol/litre requires urgent treatment as described under Emergency Treatment of Poisoning, p. 29.

**Interactions**   Lithium toxicity is made worse by sodium depletion, therefore concurrent use of diuretics (particularly thiazides) is hazardous and should be avoided. For other **interactions** with lithium, see Appendix 1 (lithium).

**Withdrawal**   While there is no clear evidence of withdrawal or rebound psychosis, abrupt discontinuation of lithium increases the risk of relapse. If lithium is to be discontinued, the dose should be reduced gradually over a period of at least 4 weeks (preferably over a period of up to 3 months). Children and carers should be warned of the risk of relapse if lithium is discontinued abruptly. If lithium is stopped or has to be discontinued abruptly, consider changing therapy to an atypical antipsychotic or valproate.

> **Lithium treatment packs**
> A lithium treatment pack may be given to patients on initiation of treatment with lithium. The pack consists of a patient information booklet, lithium alert card, and a record book for tracking serum-lithium concentration.
> Packs may be purchased from 3M
> Tel: 0845 610 1112
> nhsforms@mmm.uk.com

## ■ LITHIUM CARBONATE

**Cautions**   measure serum-lithium concentration regularly (every 3 months on stabilised regimens), measure renal function and thyroid function every 6 months on stabilised regimens and advise children and carers to seek attention if symptoms of hypothyroidism develop (females are at greater risk) e.g.

lethargy, feeling cold; maintain adequate sodium and fluid intake; test renal function before initiating and if evidence of toxicity; cardiac disease (monitor cardiac function before initiating); QT-interval prolongation; conditions with sodium imbalance such as Addison's disease; reduce dose or discontinue in diarrhoea, vomiting, and intercurrent infection (especially if sweating profusely); psoriasis (risk of exacerbation); diuretic treatment, myasthenia gravis; surgery (section 15.1); if possible avoid abrupt withdrawal (see notes above); **interactions**: Appendix 1 (lithium)
**Counselling**   Children should maintain adequate fluid intake and avoid dietary changes which reduce or increase sodium intake; lithium treatment packs are available (see above)

**Contra-indications**   dehydration, untreated hypothyroidism

**Renal impairment**   avoid if possible or reduce dose and closely monitor serum-lithium concentration

**Pregnancy**   avoid if possible in first trimester (risk of teratogenicity, including cardiac abnormalities); dose requirements increased in second and third trimesters (but on delivery, return abruptly to normal); close monitoring of serum-lithium concentration advised (risk of toxicity in neonate)

**Breast-feeding**   present in milk and risk of toxicity in infant—avoid

**Side-effects**   gastro-intestinal disturbances, fine tremor, renal impairment (particularly impaired urinary concentration and polyuria), polydipsia, leucocytosis; also weight gain and oedema (may respond to dose reduction); hyperparathyroidism and hypercalcaemia reported; signs of intoxication are blurred vision, increasing gastro-intestinal disturbances (anorexia, vomiting, diarrhoea), muscle weakness, arthralgia, myalgia, increased CNS disturbances (mild drowsiness and sluggishness increasing to giddiness with ataxia, coarse tremor, lack of coordination, dysarthria), and require withdrawal of treatment; with severe **overdosage** (serum-lithium concentration above 2 mmol/litre) hyperreflexia and hyperextension of limbs, convulsions, toxic psychoses, syncope, renal failure, circulatory failure, coma, and occasionally, death; goitre, raised antidiuretic hormone concentration, hypothyroidism, hypokalaemia, ECG changes, and kidney changes may also occur; see also Emergency Treatment of Poisoning, p. 29

### Indications and dose

**Treatment and prophylaxis of mania, bipolar disorder, recurrent depression (see also notes above), aggressive or self-mutilating behaviour**

• By mouth

See under preparations below, adjusted to achieve a serum-lithium concentration of 0.4–1 mmol/litre 12 hours after a dose on days 4–7 of treatment, then every week until dosage has remained constant for 4 weeks and every 3 months thereafter; doses are initially divided throughout the day, but once daily administration is preferred when serum-lithium concentration stabilised

**Note** Preparations vary widely in bioavailability; changing the preparation requires the same precautions as initiation of treatment

**Camcolit®** (Norgine) [PoM]
Camcolit 250® tablets, f/c, scored, lithium carbonate 250 mg (Li⁺ 6.8 mmol), net price 100-tab pack = £3.09 Label: 10, lithium card, counselling, see above
Camcolit 400® tablets, m/r, f/c, scored, lithium carbonate 400 mg (Li⁺ 10.8 mmol), net price 100-tab

pack = £4.13. Label: 10, lithium card, 25, counselling, see above

**Dose**

**Treatment**

● By mouth

(see above for advice on bioavailability and serum-lithium monitoring)

**Child 12–18 years** initially 1–1.5 g daily

**Prophylaxis**

● By mouth

(see above for advice on bioavailability and serum-lithium monitoring)

**Child 12–18 years** initially 300–400 mg daily

**Liskonum®** (GSK) [PoM]

Tablets, m/r, f/c, scored, lithium carbonate 450 mg (Li+ 12.2 mmol), net price 60-tab pack = £2.88. Label: 10, lithium card, 25, counselling, see above

**Dose**

**Treatment**

● By mouth

(see above for advice on bioavailability and serum-lithium monitoring)

**Child 12–18 years** initially 225–675 mg twice daily

**Prophylaxis**

● By mouth

(see above for advice on bioavailability and serum-lithium monitoring)

**Child 12–18 years** initially 225–450 mg twice daily

## LITHIUM CITRATE

**Cautions** see Lithium Carbonate and notes above

**Counselling** Patients should maintain an adequate fluid intake and should avoid dietary changes which might reduce or increase sodium intake; lithium treatment cards are available from pharmacies (see above)

**Contra-indications** see Lithium Carbonate

**Renal impairment** see Lithium Carbonate

**Pregnancy** see Lithium Carbonate

**Breast-feeding** see Lithium Carbonate

**Side-effects** see Lithium Carbonate and notes above

**Licensed use** not licensed for use in children

**Indications and dose**

See Lithium Carbonate and notes above

● By mouth

Adjust to achieve serum-lithium concentration of 0.4–1 mmol/litre as described under Lithium Carbonate above

**Note** Preparations vary widely in bioavailability; changing the preparation requires the same precautions as initiation of treatment

**Li-Liquid®** (Rosemont) [PoM]

Oral solution, lithium citrate 509 mg/5 mL (Li+ 5.4 mmol/5 mL), yellow, net price 150-mL pack = £5.79; 1.018 g/5 mL (Li+ 10.8 mmol/5 mL), orange, 150-mL pack = £11.58. Label: 10, lithium card, counselling, see above

**Note** 5-mL dose of 509 mg/5 mL oral solution is equivalent to 200 mg lithium carbonate

**Priadel®** (Sanofi-Aventis) [PoM]

Liquid, sugar-free, lithium citrate 520 mg/5 mL (approx. Li+ 5.4 mmol/5 mL), net price 150-mL pack = £5.61. Label: 10, lithium card, counselling, see above

**Note** 5-mL dose is equivalent to 204 mg lithium carbonate

## **4.3** Antidepressant drugs

4.3.1 Tricyclic antidepressant drugs

4.3.2 Monoamine-oxidase inhibitors

4.3.3 Selective serotonin re-uptake inhibitors

4.3.4 Other antidepressant drugs

> Depression in children should be managed by an appropriate specialist and treatment should involve psychological therapy.

The major classes of antidepressant drugs include the tricyclics and related antidepressant drugs (section 4.3.1), the selective serotonin re-uptake inhibitors (SSRIs) (section 4.3.3), and the monoamine oxidase inhibitors (MAOIs).

Antidepressant drugs should not be used routinely in mild depression, and psychological therapy should be considered initially; however, a trial of antidepressant therapy may be considered in cases refractory to psychological treatments or in those associated with psychosocial or medical problems. Drug treatment of mild depression may also be considered in children with a history of moderate or severe depression.

Choice of antidepressant drug should be based on the individual child's requirements, including the presence of concomitant disease, existing therapy, suicide risk, and previous response to antidepressant therapy.

When drug treatment of depression is considered necessary in children, the SSRIs should be considered first-line treatment; following a safety and efficacy review, **fluoxetine** is licensed to treat depression in children.

Tricyclic antidepressant drugs should be avoided for the treatment of depression in children.

**St John's wort** (*Hypericum perforatum*) is a popular herbal remedy on sale to the public for treating mild depression in adults. It should not be used for the treatment of depression in children because St John's wort can induce drug metabolising enzymes and a number of important interactions with conventional drugs, including conventional antidepressants, have been identified (see Appendix 1, St John's wort). Furthermore, the amount of active ingredient varies between different preparations of St John's wort and switching from one to another can change the degree of enzyme induction. If a child stops taking St John's wort, the concentration of interacting drugs may increase, leading to toxicity.

> **Hyponatraemia and antidepressant therapy**
> Hyponatraemia (possibly due to inappropriate secretion of antidiuretic hormone) has been associated with all types of antidepressants; however, it has been reported more frequently with SSRIs than with other antidepressant drugs. Hyponatraemia should be considered in all children who develop drowsiness, confusion, or convulsions while taking an antidepressant drug.

**4 Central nervous system**

## Suicidal behaviour and antidepressant therapy

The use of antidepressant drugs has been linked with suicidal thoughts and behaviour. Where necessary, children should be monitored for suicidal behaviour, self-harm, and hostility, particularly at the beginning of treatment or if the dose is changed.

**Management**   Children should be reviewed every 1–2 weeks at the start of antidepressant treatment. Treatment should be continued for at least 4 weeks before considering whether to switch antidepressant due to lack of efficacy. In cases of partial response, continue for a further 2–4 weeks. Following remission, antidepressant treatment should be continued at the same dose for at least 6 months. Children with a history of recurrent depression should continue treatment for at least 2 years.

**Withdrawal**   Withdrawal effects may occur within 5 days of stopping treatment with antidepressant drugs; they are usually mild and self-limiting, but in some cases may be severe. The risk of withdrawal symptoms is increased if the antidepressant is stopped suddenly after regular administration for 8 weeks or more. The dose should preferably be reduced gradually over about 4 weeks, or longer if withdrawal symptoms emerge (6 months in children who have been on long-term maintenance treatment). See also section 4.3.1, and section 4.3.3.

**Anxiety**   Management of *acute anxiety* in children with drug treatment is contentious (section 4.1.2). For *chronic anxiety* (of longer than 4 weeks' duration), it may be appropriate to use an antidepressant drug before a benzodiazepine.

## 4.3.1   Tricyclic antidepressant drugs

Tricyclic antidepressants are not effective for treating depression in children.

For reference to the role of some tricyclic antidepressant drugs in some forms of *neuralgia*, see section 4.7.3, and in *nocturnal enuresis* in children, see section 7.4.2.

**Dosage**   It is important to use doses that are sufficiently high for effective treatment but not so high as to cause toxic effects. Low doses should be used for initial treatment.

In most children the long half-life of tricyclic antidepressant drugs allows **once-daily** administration, usually at night; the use of modified-release preparations is therefore unnecessary.

**Cautions**   Tricyclic antidepressant drugs should be used with caution in children with cardiovascular disease (see also Contra-indications, below); because of the risk of arrhythmias, children with concomitant conditions such as hyperthyroidism and phaeochromocytoma should be treated with care. Care is also needed in children with epilepsy and diabetes.

Tricyclic antidepressant drugs have antimuscarinic activity, and therefore caution is needed in children with chronic constipation, urinary retention, or those with a susceptibility to angle-closure glaucoma. Tricyclic antidepressant drugs should be used with caution in children with a significant risk of suicide, or a history of psychosis or bipolar disorder, because antidepressant therapy may aggravate these conditions; treatment should be stopped if the child enters a manic phase.

**Skilled tasks**   Drowsiness may affect the performance of skilled tasks (e.g. driving); effects of alcohol enhanced.

**Contra-indications**   Tricyclic antidepressants are contra-indicated in arrhythmias (particularly heart block), and in the manic phase of bipolar disorder. Avoid treatment with tricyclic antidepressant drugs in acute porphyria (section 9.8.2).

**Hepatic impairment**   The sedative effects of tricyclic antidepressant drugs are increased in children with hepatic impairment. They should be avoided in severe liver disease.

**Breast-feeding**   The amount of tricyclic antidepressants secreted into breast milk is too small to be harmful (but see Doxepin, p. 185).

**Side-effects**   Arrhythmias and heart block occasionally follow the use of tricyclic antidepressants, particularly amitriptyline, and may be a factor in the sudden death of children with cardiac disease; other cardiovascular side-effects include postural hypotension, tachycardia, and ECG changes.

Central nervous system side-effects are common, and include anxiety, dizziness, agitation, confusion, sleep disturbances, irritability, and paraesthesia; drowsiness is associated with some of the tricyclic antidepressants. Convulsions, hallucinations, delusions, mania, and hypomania may occur (see also under Cautions, above), and, *rarely*, extrapyramidal symptoms including tremor and dysarthria.

Antimuscarinic side-effects include dry mouth, blurred vision (*very rarely* precipitation of angle-closure glaucoma), constipation (*rarely* leading to paralytic ileus), and urinary retention.

Endocrine effects include breast enlargement, galactorrhoea, and gynaecomastia. Sexual dysfunction may occur. Changes in blood sugar, increased appetite, and weight gain can accompany treatment with tricyclic antidepressant drugs, but anorexia and weight loss are also seen. Hepatic and haematological reactions may occur. Hyponatraemia has been associated with antidepressant treatment (see Hyponatraemia and Antidepressant Therapy, p. 183). Other class side-effects include nausea, vomiting, taste disturbance, tinnitus, rash, urticaria, pruritus, photosensitivity, alopecia, and sweating.

*Neuroleptic malignant syndrome* (section 4.2.1) may, *very rarely*, occur in the course of antidepressant drug treatment.

*Suicidal behaviour* has been linked with antidepressant drugs (see above).

**Overdosage**   Limited quantities of tricyclic antidepressant drugs should be prescribed at any one time because their cardiovascular and epileptogenic effects are dangerous in overdosage. In particular, overdosage with **amitriptyline** is associated with a relatively high rate of fatality. For advice on overdosage see Emergency Treatment of Poisoning, p. 28.

**Withdrawal**  Withdrawal symptoms include influenza-like symptoms (chills, myalgia, sweating, headache, nausea), insomnia, vivid dreams, and may occasionally include movement disorders and mania. If possible tricyclic antidepressant drugs should be withdrawn slowly (see also section 4.3).

## AMITRIPTYLINE HYDROCHLORIDE

**Cautions**  see notes above; **interactions**: Appendix 1 (antidepressants, tricyclic)

**Contra-indications**  see notes above

**Hepatic impairment**  see notes above

**Pregnancy**  use only if potential benefit outweighs risk

**Breast-feeding**  see notes above

**Side-effects**  see notes above; also abdominal pain, stomatitis, palpitation, oedema, hypertension, restlessness, fatigue, mydriasis, and increased intra-ocular pressure; **overdosage**: see Emergency Treatment of Poisoning, p. 28 (high rate of fatality—see Overdosage, p. 184)

**Licensed use**  not licensed for use in neuropathic pain

**Indications and dose**

Depression (but see notes above)

* By mouth

    **Child 16–18 years** 10–25 mg 3 times daily (total daily dose may alternatively be given as a single dose at bedtime) increased gradually as necessary to 150–200 mg daily

Neuropathic pain

* By mouth

    **Child 2–12 years** initially 200–500 micrograms/kg (max. 10 mg) once daily at night, increased if necessary; max. 1 mg/kg twice daily on specialist advice

    **Child 12–18 years** initially 10 mg once daily at night, increased gradually if necessary to usual dose 75 mg at night; higher doses on specialist advice

**Amitriptyline** (Non-proprietary) ⓟⓞⓜ
Tablets, coated, amitriptyline hydrochloride 10 mg, net price 28 = 90p; 25 mg, 28 = 90p; 50 mg, 28 = £1.00. Label: 2

Oral solution, amitriptyline hydrochloride 25 mg/5 mL, net price 150 mL = £15.47; 50 mg/5 mL, 150 mL = £16.82. Label: 2

## DOXEPIN

**Cautions**  see notes above

**Contra-indications**  see notes above

**Hepatic impairment**  see notes above

**Renal impairment**  use with caution

**Pregnancy**  use with caution—limited information available

**Breast-feeding**  see notes above; accumulation of doxepin metabolite may cause sedation and respiratory depression

**Side-effects**  see notes above; also abdominal pain, stomatitis, diarrhoea, flushing, and oedema

**Indications and dose**

Depressive illness, particularly where sedation is required (but see notes above)

* By mouth

    **Child 12–18 years** initially 75 mg daily in divided doses *or* as a single dose at bedtime, adjusted according to response; usual maintenance 25–300 mg daily (doses above 100 mg given in 3 divided doses)

**Sinepin**® (Marlborough) ⓟⓞⓜ
Capsules, doxepin (as hydrochloride) 25 mg (blue/red), net price 28-cap pack = £3.77; 50 mg (blue), 28-cap pack = £5.71. Label: 2

## IMIPRAMINE HYDROCHLORIDE

**Cautions**  see notes above

**Contra-indications**  see notes above

**Hepatic impairment**  see notes above

**Renal impairment**  use with caution in severe impairment

**Pregnancy**  colic, tachycardia, dyspnoea, irritability, muscle spasms, respiratory depression, and withdrawal symptoms reported in neonates when used in third trimester

**Breast-feeding**  see notes above

**Side-effects**  see notes above; also palpitation, flushing, restlessness, headache, fatigue; *very rarely* abdominal pain, stomatitis, diarrhoea, hypertension, oedema, cardiac decompensation, allergic alveolitis, aggression, myoclonus, peripheral vasospasm, and mydriasis

**Licensed use**  not licensed for use for attention deficit hyperactivity disorder

**Indications and dose**

Nocturnal enuresis

* By mouth

    **Child 6–8 years** 25 mg at bedtime

    **Child 8–11 years** 25–50 mg at bedtime

    **Child 11–18 years** 50–75 mg at bedtime

    **Note**  Initial period of treatment (including gradual withdrawal) 3 months—full physical examination before further course, see also section 7.4.2

Attention deficit hyperactivity disorder (under specialist supervision)

* By mouth

    **Child 6–18 years** 10–30 mg twice daily

**Imipramine** (Non-proprietary) ⓟⓞⓜ
Tablets, coated, imipramine hydrochloride 10 mg, net price 28-tab pack = £1.30; 25 mg, 28-tab pack = £1.24. Label: 2

Oral solution, imipramine hydrochloride 25 mg/5 mL, net price 150-mL = £20.00. Label: 2

## NORTRIPTYLINE

**Cautions**  see notes above; manufacturer advises plasma-nortriptyline concentration monitoring if dose above 100 mg daily, but evidence of practical value uncertain

**Contra-indications**  see notes above

**Hepatic impairment**  see notes above

4 Central nervous system

**Pregnancy** use only if potential benefit outweighs risk

**Breast-feeding** see notes above

**Side-effects** see notes above; also abdominal pain, stomatitis, diarrhoea, hypertension, oedema, flushing, restlessness, fatigue, and mydriasis

**Indications and dose**

**Depression** (but see notes above)

- By mouth

    **Child 12–18 years** low dose initially increased as necessary to 30–50 mg daily in divided doses *or* as a single dose (max. 150 mg daily)

**Allegron®** (King) [PoM]

Tablets, nortriptyline (as hydrochloride) 10 mg, net price 100-tab pack = £12.06; 25 mg (orange, scored), 100-tab pack = £24.02. Label: 2

## 4.3.2 Monoamine-oxidase inhibitors
### (MAOIs)

Classification not used in *BNF for Children.*

## 4.3.3 Selective serotonin re-uptake inhibitors

Citalopram, fluoxetine, fluvoxamine, and sertraline selectively inhibit the re-uptake of serotonin (5-hydroxytryptamine, 5-HT); they are termed selective serotonin re-uptake inhibitors (SSRIs).

### Depressive illness in children and adolescents

The balance of risks and benefits for the treatment of depressive illness in individuals under 18 years is considered unfavourable for the SSRIs **citalopram**, **escitalopram**, **paroxetine**, and **sertraline**, and for **mirtazapine** and **venlafaxine**. Clinical trials have failed to show efficacy and have shown an increase in harmful outcomes. However, it is recognised that specialists may sometimes decide to use these drugs in response to individual clinical need; children and adolescents should be monitored carefully for suicidal behaviour, self-harm or hostility, particularly at the beginning of treatment. Only **fluoxetine** has been shown in clinical trials to be effective for treating depressive illness in children and adolescents. However, it is possible that, in common with the other SSRIs, it is associated with a small risk of self-harm and suicidal thoughts. Overall, the balance of risks and benefits for the treatment of depressive illness in individuals under 18 years is considered favourable for fluoxetine, but children and adolescents must be carefully monitored as above.

**Cautions** SSRIs should be used with caution in children with epilepsy (avoid if poorly controlled, discontinue if convulsions develop), cardiac disease, diabetes mellitus, susceptibility to angle-closure glaucoma, a history of mania or bleeding disorders (especially gastro-intestinal bleeding), and if used together with other drugs that increase the risk of bleeding. They should also be used with caution in those receiving concurrent electroconvulsive therapy (prolonged seizures reported with fluoxetine). SSRIs may also impair performance of skilled tasks (e.g. driving). **Interactions:** Appendix 1 (antidepressants, SSRI).

**Withdrawal** Gastro-intestinal disturbances, headache, anxiety, dizziness, paraesthesia, electric shock sensation in the head, neck, and spine, tinnitus, sleep disturbances, fatigue, influenza-like symptoms, and sweating are the most common features of abrupt withdrawal of an SSRI or marked reduction of the dose; palpitation and visual disturbances can occur less commonly. The dose should be tapered over at least a few weeks to avoid these effects. It may be necessary to withdraw treatment over a longer period; consider obtaining specialist advice if symptoms persist.

**Contra-indications** SSRIs should not be used if the child enters a manic phase.

**Pregnancy** Manufacturers advise that SSRIs should not be used during pregnancy unless the potential benefit outweighs the risk. There is a small increased risk of congenital heart defects when SSRIs are taken during early pregnancy. If SSRIs are used during the third trimester there is a risk of neonatal withdrawal symptoms, and persistent pulmonary hypertension in the newborn has been reported.

**Side-effects** SSRIs are less sedating and have fewer antimuscarinic and cardiotoxic effects than tricyclic antidepressant drugs (section 4.3.1). Side-effects of the SSRIs include gastro-intestinal effects (dose-related and fairly common—include nausea, vomiting, dyspepsia, abdominal pain, diarrhoea, constipation), anorexia with weight loss (increased appetite and weight gain also reported) and hypersensitivity reactions including rash (consider discontinuation—may be sign of impending serious systemic reaction, possibly associated with vasculitis), urticaria, angioedema, anaphylaxis, arthralgia, myalgia and photosensitivity; other side-effects include dry mouth, nervousness, anxiety, headache, insomnia, tremor, dizziness, asthenia, hallucinations, drowsiness, convulsions (see Cautions above), galactorrhoea, sexual dysfunction, urinary retention, sweating, hypomania or mania (see Cautions above), movement disorders and dyskinesias, visual disturbances, hyponatraemia (see Hyponatraemia and Antidepressant Therapy, p. 183), and bleeding disorders including ecchymoses and purpura. Suicidal behaviour has been linked with antidepressants, see p. 184. Angle-closure glaucoma may very rarely be precipitated by treatment with SSRIs.

**Overdosage** for advice on overdosage with SSRIs see Emergency treatment of poisoning, p. 28

## ▌CITALOPRAM

**Cautions** see notes above; susceptibility to QT-interval prolongation

**Contra-indications** see notes above; QT-interval prolongation (avoid concomitant administration of drugs that prolong QT-interval)

**Hepatic impairment** use doses at lower end of range; for *tablets* up to max. 20 mg; for *oral solution* up to max. 16 mg

**Renal impairment** no information available for estimated glomerular filtration rate less than 20 mL/minute/1.73 m$^2$

**Pregnancy** see notes above

**Breast-feeding** present in milk—use with caution

**Side-effects** see notes above; also hepatitis, palpitation, tachycardia, oedema, bradycardia, postural hypotension, haemorrhage, QT-interval prolongation, coughing, yawning, confusion, impaired concentration, aggression, malaise, amnesia, migraine, paraesthesia, abnormal dreams, euphoria, mydriasis, taste disturbance, increased salivation, rhinitis, tinnitus, polyuria, micturition disorders, hypokalaemia, and pruritus

**Licensed use**  not licensed for use in children

**Indications and dose**

> **Major depression** (but see Depressive Illness in Children and Adolescents, above)
>
> • **By mouth as tablets**
>
> **Child 12–18 years** initially 10 mg once daily increased if necessary to 20 mg once daily over 2–4 weeks; max. 40 mg once daily
>
> • **By mouth as oral drops**
>
> **Child 12–18 years** initially 8 mg once daily increased if necessary to 16 mg once daily over 2–4 weeks; max. 32 mg once daily

**Citalopram** (Non-proprietary) ⒫ᴏᴹ

Tablets, citalopram (as hydrobromide) 10 mg, net price 28-tab pack = £1.03; 20 mg, 28-tab pack = £1.30; 40 mg, 28-tab pack = £1.37. Counselling, driving

Oral drops, citalopram (as hydrochloride) 40 mg/mL, net price 15-mL pack = £17.92. Counselling, driving, administration

Note 4 drops (8 mg) can be considered equivalent in therapeutic effect to 10-mg tablet

**Cipramil**® (Lundbeck) ⒫ᴏᴹ

Tablets, f/c, citalopram (as hydrobromide) 10 mg, net price 28-tab pack = £5.38; 20 mg (scored), 28-tab pack = £8.95; 40 mg, 28-tab pack = £15.12. Counselling, driving

Oral drops, sugar-free, citalopram (as hydrochloride) 40 mg/mL, net price 15-mL pack = £10.08. Counselling, driving, administration

Note 4 drops (8 mg) can be considered equivalent in therapeutic effect to 10-mg tablet

Mix with water, orange juice, or apple juice before taking

## FLUOXETINE

**Cautions**  see notes above

**Contra-indications**  see notes above

**Hepatic impairment**  reduce dose or increase dose interval

**Pregnancy**  see notes above

**Breast-feeding**  present in breast milk, avoid

**Side-effects**  see notes above; also dysphagia, vasodilatation, hypotension, flushing, palpitaion, pharyngitis, dyspnoea, chills, taste disturbance, sleep disturbances, malaise, euphoria, confusion, yawning, impaired concentration, changes in blood sugar, alopecia, urinary frequency, haemorrhage, pulmonary inflammation and fibrosis, hepatitis, toxic epidermal necrolysis, priapism, neuroleptic malignant syndrome-like event

**Indications and dose**

> Major depression
>
> • By mouth
>
> **Child 8–18 years** 10 mg daily increased after 1–2 weeks if necessary, max. 20 mg daily
>
> Long duration of action Consider the long half-life of fluoxetine when adjusting dosage (or in overdosage)
>
> Note Daily dose may be administered as a single or divided dose

**Fluoxetine** (Non-proprietary) ⒫ᴏᴹ

Capsules, fluoxetine (as hydrochloride) 20 mg, net price 30-cap pack = £1.90; 60 mg, 30-cap pack = £54.43. Counselling, driving

Brands include *Oxactin*®

Liquid, fluoxetine (as hydrochloride) 20 mg/5 mL, net price 70 mL = £5.04. Counselling, driving

Brands include *Prozep*®

**Prozac**® (Lilly) ⒫ᴏᴹ

Capsules, fluoxetine (as hydrochloride) 20 mg (green/yellow), net price 30-cap pack = £1.50. Counselling, driving

Liquid, fluoxetine (as hydrochloride) 20 mg/5 mL, net price 70 mL = £11.12. Counselling, driving

## FLUVOXAMINE MALEATE

**Cautions**  see notes above

**Contra-indications**  see notes above

**Hepatic impairment**  start with low dose

**Renal impairment**  start with low dose

**Pregnancy**  see notes above

**Breast-feeding**  present in milk—avoid

**Side-effects**  see notes above; palpitation, tachycardia, malaise; *less commonly* postural hypotension, confusion, ataxia; *rarely* abnormal liver function (usually symptomatic—discontinue treatment); *also reported* paraesthesia, taste disturbance, neuroleptic malignant syndrome-like event

**Indications and dose**

> **Obsessive-compulsive disorder**
>
> • By mouth
>
> **Child 8–18 years** initially 25 mg daily increased if necessary in steps of 25 mg every 4–7 days according to response (total daily doses above 50 mg in 2 divided doses); max. 100 mg twice daily
>
> Note If no improvement in obsessive-compulsive disorder within 10 weeks, treatment should be reconsidered

**Fluvoxamine** (Non-proprietary) ⒫ᴏᴹ

Tablets, fluvoxamine maleate 50 mg, net price 60-tab pack = £10.81; 100 mg, 30-tab pack = £11.67. Counselling, driving

**Faverin**® (Abbott Healthcare) ⒫ᴏᴹ

Tablets, f/c, scored, fluvoxamine maleate 50 mg, net price 60-tab pack = £17.10; 100 mg, 30-tab pack = £17.10. Counselling, driving

## SERTRALINE

**Cautions**  see notes above

**Contra-indications**  see notes above

**Hepatic impairment**  reduce dose or increase dose interval in mild or moderate impairment; avoid in severe impairment

**Renal impairment**  use with caution

**Pregnancy**  see notes above

**Breast-feeding**  not known to be harmful but consider discontinuing breast-feeding

**Side-effects**  see notes above; pancreatitis, hepatitis, jaundice, liver failure, stomatitis, palpitation, hypertension, hypercholesterolaemia, tachycardia, postural hypotension, bronchospasm, amnesia, paraesthesia, aggression, hypoglycaemia, hypothyroidism, hyper-

Central nervous system

4

prolactinaemia, urinary incontinence, menstrual irregularities, leucopenia, and tinnitus also reported

**Licensed use** not licensed for use in children for depression

**Indications and dose**

Obsessive-compulsive disorder

● By mouth

**Child 6–12 years** initially 25 mg daily increased to 50 mg daily after 1 week, further increased if necessary in steps of 50 mg at intervals of at least 1 week; max. 200 mg daily

**Child 12–18 years** initially 50 mg daily increased if necessary in steps of 50 mg over several weeks; max. 200 mg daily

Major depression (but see Depressive Illness in Children and Adolescents, above)

● By mouth

**Child 12–18 years** initially 50 mg once daily increased if necessary in steps of 50 mg daily at intervals of at least a week; max. 200 mg once daily

**Sertraline** (Non-proprietary) [PoM]
Tablets, sertraline (as hydrochloride) 50 mg, net price 28-tab pack = £1.15; 100 mg, 28-tab pack = £1.53. Counselling, driving

**Lustral®** (Pfizer) [PoM]
Tablets, both f/c, sertraline (as hydrochloride) 50 mg (scored), net price 28-tab pack = £17.82; 100 mg, 28-tab pack = £29.16. Counselling, driving

## 4.3.4 Other antidepressant drugs

Classification not used in *BNF for Children*.

## 4.4 CNS stimulants and other drugs for attention deficit hyperactivity disorder

CNS stimulants should be prescribed for children with severe and persistent symptoms of *attention deficit hyperactivity disorder* (ADHD), when the diagnosis has been confirmed by a specialist; children with moderate symptoms of ADHD can be treated with CNS stimulants when psychological interventions have been unsuccessful or are unavailable. Prescribing of CNS stimulants may be continued by general practitioners under a shared-care arrangement. Treatment of ADHD often needs to be continued into adolescence, and may need to be continued into adulthood.

Drug treatment of ADHD should be part of a comprehensive treatment programme. The choice of medication should take into consideration co-morbid conditions (such as tic disorders, Tourette syndrome, and epilepsy), the adverse effect profile, potential for drug misuse, tolerance and dependance; and preferences of the child and carers. **Methylphenidate** and **atomoxetine** are used for the management of ADHD; **dexamfetamine** and **lisdexamfetamine** are an alternative in children who do not respond to these drugs. Pulse, blood pressure, psychiatric symptoms, appetite, weight

and height should be recorded at initiation of therapy, following each dose adjustment, and at least every 6 months thereafter.

---

**NICE guidance**
**Methylphenidate, atomoxetine and dexamfetamine for attention deficit hyperactivity disorder (ADHD) (March 2006)**
Methylphenidate, atomoxetine and dexamfetamine are recommended, within their licensed indications, as options for the management of ADHD in children and adolescents.
www.nice.org.uk/TA98

---

The need to continue drug treatment for ADHD should be reviewed at least annually. This may involve suspending treatment.

A tricyclic antidepressant such as **imipramine** (section 4.3.1) is sometimes used in the treatment of ADHD; it should not be prescribed concomitantly with a CNS stimulant.

Dexamfetamine and methylphenidate [both unlicensed] are also used to treat narcolepsy.

## ATOMOXETINE

**Cautions** see notes above; also cerebrovascular or cardiovascular disease (assess for presence of cardiovascular disease before treating); hypertension and tachycardia (monitor heart rate and blood pressure before treatment, after each dose adjustment, and at least every 6 months during treatment); structural cardiac abnormalities; QT-interval prolongation (avoid concomitant use of drugs that prolong QT interval); psychosis or mania; monitor for appearance or worsening of anxiety, depression or tics; history of seizures; aggressive behaviour, hostility, or emotional lability; susceptibility to angle-closure glaucoma; **interactions:** Appendix 1 (atomoxetine)
**Hepatic disorders** Following rare reports of hepatic disorders, children and carers should be advised of the risk and be told how to recognise symptoms; prompt medical attention should be sought in case of abdominal pain, unexplained nausea, malaise, darkening of the urine or jaundice
**Suicidal ideation** Following reports of suicidal thoughts and behaviour, children and carers should be informed about the risk and told to report clinical worsening, suicidal thoughts or behaviour, irritability, agitation, or depression

**Contra-indications** phaeochromocytoma; severe cardiovascular or cerebrovascular disorder

**Hepatic impairment** halve dose in moderate impairment; quarter dose in severe impairment; see also Hepatic Disorders above

**Pregnancy** no information available; avoid unless potential benefit outweighs risk

**Breast-feeding** avoid—present in milk in *animal* studies

**Side-effects** anorexia, dry mouth, nausea, vomiting, abdominal pain, constipation, dyspepsia, flatulence; palpitation, tachycardia, increased blood pressure, postural hypotension, hot flushes; sleep disturbance, dizziness, headache, fatigue, lethargy, drowsiness, irritability, tremor, rigors; urinary retention, prostatitis, sexual dysfunction, menstrual disturbances; conjunctivitis, dermatitis, pruritus, rash, sweating, weight changes; *less commonly* suicidal ideation (see Suicidal ideation, above), aggression, hostility, emotional lability, cold extremities, mydriasis; *very rarely* angle-closure glaucoma; *also reported* hepatic disorders (see Hepatic disorders, above), psychosis, hypoaesthesia, anxiety, depression, seizures, Raynaud's phenomenon, and enuresis

**Licensed use**  doses above 100 mg daily not licensed

**Indications and dose**

**Attention deficit hyperactivity disorder** initiated by specialist

* **By mouth**

    **Child over 6 years (body-weight under 70 kg)** initially 500 micrograms/kg daily for 7 days, increased according to response; usual maintenance dose 1.2 mg/kg daily, but may be increased to 1.8 mg/kg daily (max. 120 mg daily) under the direction of a specialist

    **Child over 6 years (body-weight over 70 kg)** initially 40 mg daily for 7 days, increased according to response; usual maintenance dose 80 mg daily, but may be increased to max. 120 mg daily under the direction of a specialist

**Note**  Total daily dose may be given *either* as a single dose in the morning *or* in 2 divided doses with last dose no later than early evening

**Strattera®** (Lilly)  PoM
Capsules, atomoxetine (as hydrochloride) 10 mg (white), net price 7-cap pack = £15.62, 28-cap pack = £62.46; 18 mg (gold/white), 7-cap pack = £15.62, 28-cap pack = £62.46; 25 mg (blue/white), 7-cap pack = £15.62, 28-cap pack = £62.46; 40 mg (blue), 7-cap pack = £15.62, 28-cap pack = £62.46; 60 mg (blue/gold), 28-cap pack = £62.46; 80 mg (brown/white), 28-cap pack = £83.28; 100 mg (brown), 28-cap pack = £83.28. Label: 3

## ▌ DEXAMFETAMINE SULFATE
(Dexamphetamine sulfate)

**Cautions**  see notes above; also anorexia; mild hypertension (contra-indicated if moderate or severe); psychosis or bipolar disorder; monitor for aggressive behaviour or hostility during initial treatment; history of epilepsy (discontinue if seizures occur); tics and Tourette syndrome (use with caution)—discontinue if tics occur; susceptibility to angle-closure glaucoma; avoid abrupt withdrawal; data on safety and efficacy of long-term use not complete; acute porphyria (see section 9.8.2); **interactions:** Appendix 1 (sympathomimetics)

**Growth restriction**  Monitor height and weight as growth restriction may occur during prolonged therapy (drug-free periods may allow catch-up in growth but withdraw slowly to avoid inducing depression or renewed hyperactivity).

**Contra-indications**  cardiovascular disease including moderate to severe hypertension, structural cardiac abnormalities, hyperexcitability or agitated states, hyperthyroidism, history of drug or alcohol abuse

**Skilled tasks**  May affect performance of skilled tasks (e.g. driving); effects of alcohol unpredictable

**Renal impairment**  use with caution

**Pregnancy**  avoid (retrospective evidence of uncertain significance suggesting possible embryotoxicity)

**Breast-feeding**  significant amount in milk—avoid

**Side-effects**  nausea, diarrhoea, dry mouth, abdominal cramps, anorexia (increased appetite also reported), weight loss, taste disturbance, ischaemic colitis, palpitation, tachycardia, chest pain, hypertension, hypotension, cardiomyopathy, myocardial infarction, cardiovascular collapse, cerebral vasculitis,

stroke, headache, restlessness, depression, hyperreflexia, hyperactivity, impaired concentration, ataxia, anxiety, aggression, dizziness, confusion, sleep disturbances, dysphoria, euphoria, irritability, nervousness, malaise, obsessive-compulsive behaviour, paranoia, psychosis, panic attack, tremor, seizures (see also Cautions), neuroleptic malignant syndrome, anhedonia, growth restriction in children (see also Cautions and notes above), hyperpyrexia, renal impairment, sexual dysfunction, acidosis, rhabdomyolysis, mydriasis, visual disturbances, alopecia, rash, sweating, urticaria; central stimulants have provoked choreoathetoid movements and dyskinesia, tics and Tourette syndrome in predisposed individuals (see also Cautions); *very rarely* angle-closure glaucoma; **overdosage:** see Emergency Treatment of Poisoning, p. 30

**Indications and dose**

**Refractory attention deficit hyperactivity disorder** initiated by specialist

* **By mouth**

    **Child 6–18 years** initially 2.5 mg 2–3 times daily, increased if necessary at weekly intervals by 5 mg; usual max. 1 mg/kg daily, up to 20 mg (40 mg daily has been required in some children); maintenance dose given in 2–4 divided doses

**Administration**  tablets can be halved

**Dexamfetamine** (Non-proprietary)  CD2
Tablets, scored, dexamfetamine sulfate 5 mg, net price 28-tab pack = £15.60. Counselling, driving

## ▌ LISDEXAMFETAMINE MESILATE

**Note**  Lisdexamfetamine is a prodrug of dexamfetamine

**Cautions**  see notes above; also anorexia; history of cardiovascular disease or abnormalities; psychosis or bipolar disorder; monitor for aggressive behaviour or hostility during initial treatment; history of drug or alcohol abuse; may lower seizure threshold (discontinue if seizures occur); tics and Tourette syndrome (use with caution)—discontinue if tics occur; monitor growth in children (see also below); susceptibility to angle-closure glaucoma; avoid abrupt withdrawal; acute porphyria (section 9.8.2); **interactions:** Appendix 1 (sympathomimetics)

**Growth restriction**  Monitor height and weight as growth restriction may occur during prolonged therapy (drug-free periods may allow catch-up in growth but withdraw slowly to avoid inducing depression or renewed hyperactivity)

**Contra-indications**  symptomatic cardiovascular disease including moderate to severe hypertension and advanced arteriosclerosis, hyperexcitability or agitated states, hyperthyroidism

**Renal impairment**  use with caution

**Pregnancy**  manufacturer advises use only if potential benefit outweighs risk

**Breast-feeding**  manufacturer advises avoid—present in human milk

**Side-effects**  nausea, decreased appetite, vomiting, diarrhoea, dry mouth, abdominal cramps, dyspnoea, sleep disturbances, tics, aggression, headache, dizziness, drowsiness, mydriasis, labile mood, weight loss, pyrexia, malaise, growth restriction in children (see also under Cautions and notes above); *less commonly* anorexia, tachycardia, palpitation, hypertension, logorrhoea, anxiety, paranoia, restlessness, depression, dysphoria, dermatillomania, mania, hallucination, sweating, tremor, visual disturbances, sexual

**4**

**Central nervous system**

dysfunction, rash; *very rarely* angle-closure glaucoma; *also reported* cardiomyopathy, euphoria, seizures (see also Cautions), central stimulants have provoked choreoathetoid movements and dyskinesia, and Tourette syndrome in predisposed individuals (see also Cautions); **overdosage:** see Emergency Treatment of Poisoning, p. 30

### Indications and dose

Attention deficit hyperactivity disorder (refractory to methylphenidate treatment) initiated by specialist

- By mouth

    **Child 6–18 years** initially 30 mg once daily in the morning, increased if necessary at weekly intervals by 20 mg; max. 70 mg daily (discontinue if response insufficient after 1 month)

**Administration** Swallow whole or dissolve contents of capsule in a glass of water

**Elvanse®** (Shire) ▼ CD2

Capsule, lisdexamfetamine mesilate 30 mg (white/pink), net price 28-cap pack = £58.24; 50 mg (white/blue), 28-cap pack = £68.60; 70 mg (blue/pink), 28-cap pack = £83.16. Label: 3, 25, counselling, administration

**Counselling** Swallow whole or dissolve contents of capsule in a glass of water

## METHYLPHENIDATE HYDROCHLORIDE

**Cautions** see notes above; also monitor for psychiatric disorders; anxiety or agitation; tics or a family history of Tourette syndrome; drug or alcohol dependence; epilepsy (discontinue if increased seizure frequency); avoid abrupt withdrawal; **interactions:** Appendix 1 (sympathomimetics)

**Contra-indications** severe depression, suicidal ideation; anorexia nervosa; psychosis; uncontrolled bipolar disorder; hyperthyroidism; cardiovascular disease (including heart failure, cardiomyopathy, severe hypertension, and arrhythmias), structural cardiac abnormalities; phaeochromocytoma; vasculitis; cerebrovascular disorders

**Pregnancy** limited experience—avoid unless potential benefit outweighs risk

**Breast-feeding** limited information available—avoid

**Side-effects** abdominal pain, nausea, vomiting, diarrhoea, dyspepsia, dry mouth, anorexia, reduced weight gain; tachycardia, palpitation, arrhythmias, changes in blood pressure; tics (*very rarely* Tourette syndrome), insomnia, nervousness, asthenia, depression, irritability, aggression, headache, drowsiness, dizziness, movement disorders; fever, arthralgia; rash, pruritus, alopecia; growth restriction; *less commonly* constipation, abnormal dreams, confusion, suicidal ideation, urinary frequency, haematuria, muscle cramps, epistaxis; *rarely* sweating and visual disturbances; *very rarely* hepatic dysfunction, cerebral arteritis, psychosis, seizures, neuroleptic malignant syndrome, tolerance and dependence, blood disorders including leucopenia and thrombocytopenia, exfoliative dermatitis, and erythema multiforme; supraventricular tachycardia, bradycardia, and convulsions *also reported*

**Licensed use** not licensed for use in children under 6 years; doses over 60 mg daily not licensed; doses of *Concerta®* XL over 54 mg daily not licensed

### Indications and dose

Attention deficit hyperactivity disorder initiated by specialist

- By mouth

    **Child 4–6 years** 2.5 mg twice daily increased if necessary at weekly intervals by 2.5 mg daily to max. 1.4 mg/kg daily in 2–3 divided doses; discontinue if no response after 1 month

    **Child 6–18 years** initially 5 mg 1–2 times daily, increased if necessary at weekly intervals by 5–10 mg daily; licensed max. 60 mg daily in 2–3 divided doses but may be increased to 2.1 mg/kg daily in 2–3 divided doses (max. 90 mg daily) under the direction of a specialist; discontinue if no response after 1 month

    **Evening dose** If effect wears off in evening (with rebound hyperactivity) a dose at bedtime may be appropriate (establish need with trial bedtime dose)

    **Note** Treatment may be started using a modified-release preparation

**Administration** Contents of *Equasym XL®* capsules, and *Medikinet XL®* capsules, can be sprinkled on a tablespoon of apple sauce, then swallowed immediately without chewing

**Methylphenidate Hydrochloride** (Non-proprietary) CD2

Tablets, methylphenidate hydrochloride 5 mg, net price 30-tab pack = £2.67; 10 mg, 30-tab pack = £6.74; 20 mg, 30-tab pack = £9.59

Brands include *Medikinet®*

**Ritalin®** (Novartis) CD2

Tablets, scored, methylphenidate hydrochloride 10 mg, net price 30-tab pack = £5.57

### ◢Modified release

**Note** Different versions of modified-release preparations may not have the same clinical effect. To avoid confusion between these different formulations of methylphenidate, prescribers should specify the brand to be dispensed.

**Concerta®** XL (Janssen) CD2

Tablets, m/r, methylphenidate hydrochloride 18 mg (yellow), net price 30-tab pack = £31.19; 27 mg (grey), 30-tab pack = £36.81; 36 mg (white), 30-tab pack = £42.45. Label: 25

**Counselling** Tablet membrane may pass through gastrointestinal tract unchanged

**Cautions** dose form not appropriate for use in dysphagia or if gastro-intestinal lumen restricted

### Dose

Attention deficit hyperactivity disorder

- By mouth

    **Child 6–18 years** initially 18 mg once daily (in the morning), increased if necessary at weekly intervals by 18 mg according to response; licensed max. 54 mg once daily, but may be increased to 2.1 mg/kg daily (max. 108 mg daily) under the direction of a specialist; discontinue if no response after 1 month

    **Note** Total daily dose of 15 mg of standard-release formulation is considered equivalent to *Concerta®* XL 18 mg once daily

    **Note** *Concerta®* XL tablets consist of an immediate-release component (22% of the dose) and a modified-release component (78% of the dose)

**Equasym XL®** (Shire) [CD2]

Capsules, m/r, methylphenidate hydrochloride 10 mg (white/green), net price 30-cap pack = £25.00; 20 mg (white/blue), 30-cap pack = £30.00; 30 mg (white/brown), 30-cap pack = £35.00. Label: 25

**Dose**

> **Attention deficit hyperactivity disorder**
>
> • By mouth
>
> **Child 6–18 years** initially 10 mg once daily in the morning before breakfast, increased gradually at weekly intervals if necessary; licensed max. 60 mg daily, but may be increased to 2.1 mg/kg daily (max. 90 mg daily) under the direction of a specialist; discontinue if no response after 1 month
>
> **Note** Contents of capsule can be sprinkled on a tablespoon of apple sauce (then swallowed immediately without chewing)
>
> **Note** *Equasym XL*® capsules consist of an immediate-release component (30% of the dose) and a modified-release component (70% of the dose)

**Medikinet XL®** (Flynn) [CD2]

Capsules, m/r, methylphenidate hydrochloride 5 mg (white), net price 30-cap pack = £24.04; 10 mg (lilac/white), 30-cap pack = £24.04; 20 mg (lilac), 30-cap pack = £28.86; 30 mg (purple/light grey), 30-cap pack = £33.66; 40 mg (purple/grey), 30-cap pack = £57.72. Label: 25

**Dose**

> **Attention deficit hyperactivity disorder**
>
> • By mouth
>
> **Child 6–18 years** 10 mg once daily in the morning with breakfast, adjusted at weekly intervals according to response; licensed max. 60 mg daily, but may be increased to 2.1 mg/kg daily (max. 90 mg daily) under the direction of a specialist; discontinue if no response after 1 month
>
> **Note** Contents of capsule can be sprinkled on a tablespoon of apple sauce, or yoghurt (then swallowed immediately without chewing)
>
> **Note** *Medikinet XL*® capsules consist of an immediate-release component (50% of the dose) and a modified-release component (50% of the dose)

# 4.5 Drugs used in the treatment of obesity

Obesity is associated with many health problems including cardiovascular disease, diabetes mellitus, gallstones, and osteoarthritis. Factors that aggravate obesity may include depression, other psychosocial problems, and some drugs.

The main treatment of the obese individual is a suitable diet, carefully explained to the individual or carer, with appropriate support and encouragement; increased physical activity should also be encouraged. If appropriate, smoking cessation (while maintaining body weight) may be worthwhile before attempting supervised weight loss, since cigarette smoking may be more harmful than obesity.

Obesity should be managed in an appropriate setting by staff who have been trained in the management of obesity in children; the individual or carer should receive advice on diet and lifestyle modification and should be monitored for changes in weight as well as in blood pressure, blood lipids, and other associated conditions.

NICE has recommended (December 2006) that drug treatment should only be considered for obese children after dietary, exercise, and behavioural approaches have been started, and who have associated conditions such as orthopaedic problems or sleep apnoea; treatment is intended both to facilitate weight loss and to maintain reduced weight. Initial treatment should involve a 6–12 month trial of orlistat, with regular reviews of effectiveness, tolerance, and adherence.

**Choice**   Orlistat, a lipase inhibitor, reduces the absorption of dietary fat. Some weight loss in those taking orlistat probably results from a reduction in fat intake to avoid severe gastro-intestinal effects including steatorrhoea. Vitamin supplementation (especially of vitamin D) should be considered.

Thyroid hormones have no place in the treatment of obesity except in biochemically proven hypothyroid children. The use of diuretics, chorionic gonadotrophin, or amfetamines is not appropriate for weight reduction.

## ▮ ORLISTAT

**Cautions** may impair absorption of fat-soluble vitamins; chronic kidney disease or volume depletion; **interactions**: Appendix 1 (orlistat)

> **Multivitamins** If a multivitamin supplement is required, it should be taken at least 2 hours after orlistat dose or at bedtime

**Contra-indications** chronic malabsorption syndrome; cholestasis

**Pregnancy** use with caution

**Breast-feeding** avoid—no information available

**Side-effects** oily leakage from rectum, flatulence, faecal urgency, liquid or oily stools, faecal incontinence, abdominal distension and pain (gastro-intestinal effects minimised by reduced fat intake), tooth and gingival disorders, respiratory infections, malaise, anxiety, headache, menstrual disturbances, urinary-tract infection, hypoglycaemia; *also reported* rectal bleeding, diverticulitis, cholelithiasis, hepatitis, hypothyroidism, oxalate nephropathy, bullous eruptions

**Licensed use** not licensed for use in children

**Indications and dose**

> **Adjunct in obesity** initiated by specialist
>
> • By mouth
>
> **Child 12–18 years** 120 mg taken immediately before, during, or up to 1 hour after each main meal (max. 120 mg 3 times daily); continue treatment beyond 12 weeks only under specialist recommendation
>
> **Note** If a meal is missed or contains no fat, the dose of orlistat should be omitted

**Xenical®** (Roche) [PoM]

Capsules, turquoise, orlistat 120 mg, net price 84-cap pack = £31.63

# 4.6 Drugs used in nausea and vertigo

Antiemetics should be prescribed only when the cause of vomiting is known because otherwise they may delay diagnosis. Antiemetics are unnecessary and sometimes harmful when the cause can be treated, such as in diabetic ketoacidosis, or in digoxin or antiepileptic overdose.

**4 Central nervous system**

If antiemetic drug treatment is indicated, the drug is chosen according to the aetiology of vomiting.

**Antihistamines** are effective against nausea and vomiting resulting from many underlying conditions. There is no evidence that any one antihistamine is superior to another but their duration of action and incidence of adverse effects (drowsiness and antimuscarinic effects) differ.

The **phenothiazines** are dopamine antagonists and act centrally by blocking the chemoreceptor trigger zone. They may be considered for the prophylaxis and treatment of nausea and vomiting associated with diffuse neoplastic disease, radiation sickness, and the emesis caused by drugs such as opioids, general anaesthetics, and cytotoxics. **Prochlorperazine, perphenazine,** and **trifluoperazine** are less sedating than **chlorpromazine**; severe dystonic reactions sometimes occur with phenothiazines (see below). Some phenothiazines are available as rectal suppositories, which can be useful in children with persistent vomiting or with severe nausea; for children over 12 years prochlorperazine can also be administered as a buccal tablet which is placed between the upper lip and the gum.

**Droperidol** is a butyrophenone, structurally related to haloperidol, which blocks dopamine receptors in the chemoreceptor trigger zone.

Other antipsychotic drugs including **haloperidol** and **levomepromazine** (section 4.2.1) are also used for the relief of nausea in palliative care (see Symptom Control, (p. 18) and Continuous Subcutaneous Infusions, (p. 19)).

**Metoclopramide** is an effective antiemetic and its activity closely resembles that of the phenothiazines. Metoclopramide also acts directly on the gastro-intestinal tract and it may be superior to the phenothiazines for emesis associated with gastroduodenal, hepatic, and biliary disease. In postoperative nausea and vomiting, metoclopramide has limited efficacy. For the role of metoclopramide in cytotoxic-induced nausea and vomiting see section 8.1.

> ### Acute dystonic reactions
> Phenothiazines and metoclopramide can all induce acute dystonic reactions such as facial and skeletal muscle spasms and oculogyric crises; children (especially girls, young women, and those under 10 kg) are particularly susceptible. With metoclopramide, dystonic effects usually occur shortly after starting treatment and subside within 24 hours of stopping it. An antimuscarinic drug such as procyclidine (section 4.9.2) is used to abort dystonic attacks.

**Domperidone** acts at the chemoreceptor trigger zone; it has the advantage over metoclopramide and the phenothiazines of being less likely to cause central effects such as sedation and dystonic reactions because it does not readily cross the blood-brain barrier. For the role of domperidone in cytotoxic-induced nausea and vomiting see section 8.1. Domperidone is also used to treat vomiting due to emergency hormonal contraception (section 7.3.5).

**Granisetron** and **ondansetron** are specific 5HT$_3$-receptor antagonists which block 5HT$_3$ receptors in the gastro-intestinal tract and in the CNS. They are of value in the management of nausea and vomiting in children receiving cytotoxics and in postoperative nausea and vomiting.

**Nabilone** is a synthetic cannabinoid with antiemetic properties. It may be used for nausea and vomiting caused by cytotoxic chemotherapy that is unresponsive to conventional antiemetics. Side-effects such as drowsiness and dizziness occur frequently with standard doses.

**Dexamethasone** (section 6.3.2) has antiemetic effects. For the role of dexamethasone in cytotoxic-induced nausea and vomiting see section 8.1.

## Vomiting during pregnancy

Nausea in the first trimester of pregnancy is generally mild and does not require drug therapy. On rare occasions if vomiting is severe, short-term treatment with an antihistamine, such as **promethazine**, may be required. **Prochlorperazine** or **metoclopramide** may be considered as second-line treatments. If symptoms do not settle in 24 to 48 hours then specialist opinion should be sought. Hyperemesis gravidarum is a more serious condition, which requires intravenous fluid and electrolyte replacement and sometimes nutritional support. Supplementation with thiamine must be considered in order to reduce the risk of Wernicke's encephalopathy.

## Postoperative nausea and vomiting

The incidence of postoperative nausea and vomiting depends on many factors including the anaesthetic used, and the type and duration of surgery. Other risk factors include female sex, non-smokers, a history of postoperative nausea and vomiting or motion sickness, and intra-operative and postoperative use of opioids. Therapy to prevent postoperative nausea and vomiting should be based on the assessed risk. Drugs used include **5HT$_3$-receptor antagonists**, **droperidol**, **dexamethasone**, some **phenothiazines** (e.g. prochlorperazine), and **antihistamines** (e.g. cyclizine). A combination of two or more antiemetic drugs that have different mechanisms of action is often indicated in those at high risk of postoperative nausea and vomiting or where postoperative vomiting presents a particular danger (e.g. in some types of surgery). When a prophylactic antiemetic drug has failed, postoperative nausea and vomiting should be treated with one or more drugs from a different class.

## Opioid-induced nausea and vomiting

Cyclizine, ondansetron, and prochlorperazine are used to relieve opioid-induced nausea and vomiting; ondansetron has the advantage of not producing sedation.

## Motion sickness

Antiemetics should be given to prevent motion sickness rather than after nausea or vomiting develop. The most effective drug for the prevention of motion sickness is **hyoscine hydrobromide**. For children over 10 years old, a transdermal hyoscine patch provides prolonged activity but it needs to be applied several hours before travelling. The sedating antihistamines are slightly less effective against motion sickness, but are generally better tolerated than hyoscine. If a sedative effect is desired **promethazine** is useful, but generally a slightly less sedating antihistamine such as **cyclizine** or **cinnarizine** is preferred. Domperidone, metoclopramide, 5HT$_3$-receptor antagonists, and the phenothiazines (except the antihistamine phenothiazine promethazine) are **ineffective** in motion sickness.

## Other vestibular disorders

Management of vestibular diseases is aimed at treating the underlying cause as well as treating symptoms of the balance disturbance and associated nausea and vomiting.

Antihistamines (such as cinnarizine), and **phenothiazines** (such as prochlorperazine) are effective for prophylaxis and treatment of nausea and vertigo resulting from vestibular disorders; however, when nausea and vertigo are associated with middle ear surgery, treatment can be difficult.

## Cytotoxic chemotherapy

For the management of nausea and vomiting induced by cytotoxic chemotherapy, see section 8.1.

## Palliative care

For the management of nausea and vomiting in palliative care, see Symptom Control, (p. 18) and Continuous Subcutaneous Infusions, (p. 19).

## Migraine

For the management of nausea and vomiting associated with migraine, see p. 215.

## Antihistamines

### ◼ CINNARIZINE

**Cautions** section 3.4.1
**Contra-indications** section 3.4.1
**Hepatic impairment** section 3.4.1
**Renal impairment** use with caution—no information available
**Pregnancy** section 3.4.1
**Breast-feeding** section 3.4.1
**Side-effects** section 3.4.1; also *rarely* weight gain, sweating, lichen planus, and lupus-like skin reactions
**Indications and dose**

> Relief of symptoms of vestibular disorders
> • By mouth
> > **Child 5–12 years** 15 mg 3 times daily
> > **Child 12–18 years** 30 mg 3 times daily

> Motion sickness
> • By mouth
> > **Child 5–12 years** 15 mg 2 hours before travel then 7.5 mg every 8 hours during journey if necessary
> > **Child 12–18 years** 30 mg 2 hours before travel then 15 mg every 8 hours during journey if necessary

**Cinnarizine** (Non-proprietary)
Tablets, cinnarizine 15 mg, net price 84-tab pack = £8.84. Label: 2

**Stugeron**® (Janssen)
Tablets, scored, cinnarizine 15 mg, net price 15-tab pack = £1.55, 100-tab pack = £4.18. Label: 2

### ◼ CYCLIZINE

**Cautions** section 3.4.1; severe heart failure; may counteract haemodynamic benefits of opioids; **interactions:** Appendix 1 (antihistamines)
> **Skilled tasks** Drowsiness may affect performance of skilled tasks (e.g. driving); effects of alcohol enhanced
**Contra-indications** section 3.4.1
**Hepatic impairment** section 3.4.1
**Pregnancy** section 3.4.1
**Breast-feeding** no information available
**Side-effects** section 3.4.1
**Licensed use** tablets not licensed for use in children under 6 years; injection not licensed for use in children
**Indications and dose**

> Nausea and vomiting of known cause; nausea and vomiting associated with vestibular disorders and palliative care
> • By mouth or by intravenous injection over 3–5 minutes
> > **Child 1 month–6 years** 0.5–1 mg/kg up to 3 times daily; max. single dose 25 mg
> > **Child 6–12 years** 25 mg up to 3 times daily
> > **Child 12–18 years** 50 mg up to 3 times daily
> > **Note** For motion sickness, take 1–2 hours before departure
> • By rectum
> > **Child 2–6 years** 12.5 mg up to 3 times daily
> > **Child 6–12 years** 25 mg up to 3 times daily
> > **Child 12–18 years** 50 mg up to 3 times daily
> • By continuous intravenous or subcutaneous infusion
> > **Child 1 month–2 years** 3 mg/kg over 24 hours
> > **Child 2–5 years** 50 mg over 24 hours
> > **Child 6–12 years** 75 mg over 24 hours
> > **Child 12–18 years** 150 mg over 24 hours

**Administration** for administration *by mouth*, tablets may be crushed

**Valoid**® (Amdipharm)
Tablets, scored, cyclizine hydrochloride 50 mg, net price 100-tab pack = £7.41. Label: 2

Injection ℗ℴ℧, cyclizine lactate 50 mg/mL, net price 1-mL amp = 51p

**Cyclizine** (Non-proprietary)
Suppositories, 12.5 mg, 25 mg, 50 mg, 100 mg. Available from 'special-order' manufacturers or specialist importing companies, see p. 823

### ◼ PROMETHAZINE HYDROCHLORIDE

**Cautions** see notes in section 3.4.1
**Contra-indications** see Promethazine Hydrochloride, section 3.4.1
**Hepatic impairment** see notes in section 3.4.1
**Renal impairment** see Promethazine Hydrochloride, section 3.4.1
**Pregnancy** see notes in section 3.4.1
**Breast-feeding** see notes in section 3.4.1
**Side-effects** see Promethazine Hydrochloride, section 3.4.1 but more sedating

**4**

**Central nervous system**

**Indications and dose**

**Nausea and vomiting**
- By mouth

   **Child 2–5 years** 5 mg at bedtime on night before travel, repeat following morning if necessary

   **Child 5–10 years** 10 mg at bedtime on night before travel, repeat following morning if necessary

   **Child 10–18 years** 20–25 mg at bedtime on night before travel, repeat following morning if necessary

**Allergy and urticaria** section 3.4.1

**Sedation** section 4.1.1

◀Preparations
Section 3.4.1

## PROMETHAZINE TEOCLATE

**Cautions** section 3.4.1; severe coronary artery disease; asthma, bronchitis, bronchiectasis, Reye's syndrome

**Contra-indications** section 3.4.1

**Hepatic impairment** section 3.4.1

**Renal impairment** use with caution

**Pregnancy** section 3.4.1

**Breast-feeding** section 3.4.1

**Side-effects** section 3.4.1

**Licensed use** not licensed to treat vomiting of pregnancy

**Indications and dose**

**Nausea, vomiting, labyrinthine disorders**
- By mouth

   **Child 5–10 years** 12.5–37.5 mg daily

   **Child 10–18 years** 25–75 mg daily (max. 100 mg)

**Motion sickness prevention**
- By mouth

   **Child 5–10 years** 12.5 mg at bedtime on night before travel *or* 12.5 mg 1–2 hours before travel

   **Child 10–18 years** 25 mg at bedtime on night before travel *or* 25 mg 1–2 hours before travel

**Motion sickness treatment**
- By mouth

   **Child 5–10 years** 12.5 mg at onset, then 12.5 mg at bedtime for 2 days

   **Child 10–18 years** 25 mg at onset, then 25 mg at bedtime for 2 days

**Severe vomiting during pregnancy**
- By mouth

   25 mg at bedtime increased if necessary to max. 100 mg daily (but see also Vomiting During Pregnancy, p. 192)

**Avomine®** (Manx)
Tablets, scored, promethazine teoclate 25 mg, net price 10-tab pack = £1.13; 28-tab pack = £3.13. Label: 2

## Phenothiazines and related drugs

## CHLORPROMAZINE HYDROCHLORIDE

**Cautions** see Chlorpromazine Hydrochloride, section 4.2.1

**Contra-indications** see notes in section 4.2.1

**Hepatic impairment** see notes in section 4.2.1

**Renal impairment** see notes in section 4.2.1

**Pregnancy** see notes in section 4.2.1

**Breast-feeding** see notes in section 4.2.1

**Side-effects** see Chlorpromazine Hydrochloride, section 4.2.1

**Indications and dose**

**Nausea and vomiting of terminal illness (where other drugs are unsuitable)**
- By mouth

   **Child 1–6 years** 500 micrograms/kg every 4–6 hours; max. 40 mg daily

   **Child 6–12 years** 500 micrograms/kg every 4–6 hours; max. 75 mg daily

   **Child 12–18 years** 10–25 mg every 4–6 hours

- By deep intramuscular injection

   **Child 1–6 years** 500 micrograms/kg every 6–8 hours; max. 40 mg daily

   **Child 6–12 years** 500 micrograms/kg every 6–8 hours; max. 75 mg daily

   **Child 12–18 years** initially 25 mg then 25–50 mg every 3–4 hours until vomiting stops

◀Preparations
Section 4.2.1

## DROPERIDOL

**Cautions** section 4.2.1; also chronic obstructive pulmonary disease or respiratory failure; electrolyte disturbances; history of alcohol abuse; continuous pulse oximetry required if risk of ventricular arrhythmia—continue for 30 minutes following administration; **interactions**: Appendix 1 (droperidol)

**Contra-indications** section 4.2.1; QT-interval prolongation (avoid concomitant administration of drugs that prolong QT interval); hypokalaemia; hypomagnesaemia; bradycardia

**Hepatic impairment** max. 625 micrograms repeated every 6 hours as required

**Renal impairment** max. 625 micrograms repeated every 6 hours as required

**Pregnancy** section 4.2.1

**Breast-feeding** limited information available—avoid repeated administration

**Side-effects** section 4.2.1; also anxiety, cardiac arrest, hallucinations, and inappropriate secretion of anti-diuretic hormone

**Indications and dose**

**Prevention and treatment of postoperative nausea and vomiting**
- By intravenous injection

   **Child 2–18 years** 20–50 micrograms/kg (max. 1.25 mg) 30 minutes before the end of surgery, repeated every 6 hours as necessary

**Xomolix®** (ProStrakan) PoM
Injection, droperidol 2.5 mg/mL, net price 1-mL
amp = £3.94

## PERPHENAZINE

**Cautions**  see notes in section 4.2.1
**Contra-indications**  see notes in section 4.2.1
**Hepatic impairment**  see notes in section 4.2.1
**Renal impairment**  see notes in section 4.2.1
**Pregnancy**  see notes in section 4.2.1
**Breast-feeding**  see notes in section 4.2.1
**Side-effects**  see Perphenazine, section 4.2.1
**Indications and dose**

> **Severe nausea and vomiting unresponsive to other antiemetics**
> * By mouth
>> **Child 14–18 years** 4 mg 3 times daily, adjusted according to response, max. 24 mg daily

◀**Preparations**
Section 4.2.1

## PROCHLORPERAZINE

**Cautions**  see notes in section 4.2.1; hypotension more
likely after intramuscular injection
**Contra-indications**  see notes in section 4.2.1
**Hepatic impairment**  see notes in section 4.2.1
**Renal impairment**  see notes in section 4.2.1
**Pregnancy**  see notes in section 4.2.1
**Breast-feeding**  see notes in section 4.2.1
**Side-effects**  see notes in section 4.2.1; respiratory
depression may occur in susceptible children
**Licensed use**  injection not licensed for use in children
**Indications and dose**

> **Prevention and treatment of nausea and vomiting**
> * By mouth
>> **Child 1–12 years and over 10 kg** 250 micrograms/kg 2–3 times daily
>> **Child 12–18 years** 5–10 mg, repeated if necessary up to 3 times daily
> * By intramuscular injection
>> **Child 2–5 years,** 1.25–2.5 mg, repeated if necessary up to 3 times daily
>> **Child 5–12 years** 5–6.25 mg, repeated if necessary up to 3 times daily
>> **Child 12–18 years** 12.5 mg, repeated if necessary up to 3 times daily

> **Note** Doses are expressed as prochlorperazine maleate or mesilate; 1 mg prochlorperazine maleate ≡ 1 mg prochlorperazine mesilate

**Prochlorperazine** (Non-proprietary) PoM
Tablets, prochlorperazine maleate 5 mg, net price
28-tab pack = £1.25, 84-tab pack = £2.28. Label: 2
Injection, prochlorperazine mesilate 12.5 mg/mL,
net price 1-mL amp = 52p

**Stemetil®** (Sanofi-Aventis) PoM
Tablets, prochlorperazine maleate 5 mg (off-white),
net price 28-tab pack = £1.98, 84-tab pack = £5.94.
Label: 2
Syrup, straw-coloured, prochlorperazine mesilate
5 mg/5 mL, net price 100-mL pack = £3.34. Label: 2
Injection, prochlorperazine mesilate 12.5 mg/mL,
net price 1-mL amp = 52p

◀**Buccal preparation**
**Buccastem®** (Alliance) PoM
Tablets (buccal), pale yellow, prochlorperazine maleate 3 mg, net price 5 × 10-tab pack = £6.49.
Label: 2, counselling, administration, see under
Dose below
**Dose**

> * By mouth
>> **Child 12–18 years** 1–2 tablets twice daily; tablets are placed high between upper lip and gum and left to dissolve

## TRIFLUOPERAZINE

**Cautions**  see notes in section 4.2.1
**Contra-indications**  see notes in section 4.2.1
**Hepatic impairment**  see notes in section 4.2.1
**Renal impairment**  see notes in section 4.2.1
**Pregnancy**  see notes in section 4.2.1
**Breast-feeding**  see notes in section 4.2.1
**Side-effects**  see Trifluoperazine section 4.2.1
**Indications and dose**

> **Severe nausea and vomiting unresponsive to other antiemetics**
> * By mouth
>> **Child 3–5 years** up to 500 micrograms twice daily
>> **Child 6–12 years** up to 2 mg twice daily
>> **Child 12–18 years** 1–2 mg twice daily; max. 3 mg twice daily

◀**Preparations**
Section 4.2.1

## Domperidone and metoclopramide

## DOMPERIDONE

**Cautions**  children; cardiac conduction abnormalities
including QT-interval prolongation; electrolyte disturbances; cardiac disease; **interactions:** Appendix 1
(domperidone)
**Contra-indications**  prolactinaemia; if increased gastro-intestinal motility harmful
**Hepatic impairment**  avoid
**Renal impairment**  reduce dose
**Pregnancy**  use only if potential benefit outweighs risk
**Breast-feeding**  amount too small to be harmful
**Side-effects**  rarely gastro-intestinal disturbances
(including cramps), galactorrhoea, gynaecomastia,
amenorrhoea, hyperprolactinaemia; very rarely
ventricular arrhythmias, agitation, drowsiness, nervousness, seizures, extrapyramidal effects, headache;
also reported QT-interval prolongation, sudden cardiac death

**4** Central nervous system

## Indications and dose

**Nausea and vomiting**

- By mouth

  **Child over 1 month and body-weight up to 35 kg** 250–500 micrograms/kg 3–4 times daily; max. 2.4 mg/kg (max. 80 mg) in 24 hours

  **Body-weight 35 kg and over** 10–20 mg 3–4 times daily, max. 80 mg daily

- By rectum

  **Body-weight 15–35 kg** 30 mg twice daily

  **Body-weight over 35 kg** 60 mg twice daily

**Gastro-intestinal stasis** section 1.2

**Domperidone** (Non-proprietary) [PoM]
Tablets, 10 mg (as maleate), net price 30-tab pack = £1.12; 100-tab pack = £1.90. Label: 22

Suspension, domperidone 5 mg/5 mL, net price 200-mL pack = £12.00. Label: 22

**Motilium**® (Zentiva) [PoM]
Tablets, f/c, domperidone 10 mg (as maleate), net price 30-tab pack = £2.71; 100-tab pack = £9.04. Label: 22

Suppositories, domperidone 30 mg, net price 10 = £3.06

## METOCLOPRAMIDE HYDROCHLORIDE

**Cautions** atopic allergy (including asthma); cardiac conduction disturbances (and concomitant use of other drugs affecting cardiac conduction); may mask underlying disorders such as cerebral irritation; epilepsy; acute porphyria (section 9.8.2); **interactions:** Appendix 1 (metoclopramide)

**Contra-indications** gastro-intestinal obstruction, perforation or haemorrhage; 3–4 days after gastro-intestinal surgery; phaeochromocytoma

**Hepatic impairment** reduce dose

**Renal impairment** avoid or use small dose in severe impairment; increased risk of extrapyramidal reactions

**Pregnancy** not known to be harmful

**Breast-feeding** small amount present in milk; avoid

**Side-effects** extrapyramidal effects (see p. 192), hyperprolactinaemia, occasionally tardive dyskinesia on prolonged administration; also reported, dyspnoea, anxiety, confusion, drowsiness, dizziness, tremor, restlessness, diarrhoea, depression, neuroleptic malignant syndrome, visual disturbances, rashes, pruritus, oedema; cardiac conduction abnormalities reported following intravenous administration; *rarely* methaemoglobinaemia (more severe in G6PD deficiency)

**Licensed use** not licensed for use in neonates as a prokinetic

## Indications and dose

**Severe intractable vomiting of known cause, vomiting associated with radiotherapy and cytotoxics, aid to gastro-intestinal intubation, as a prokinetic in neonates**

- By mouth, or by intramuscular injection or by intravenous injection over 1–2 minutes

  **Neonate** 100 micrograms/kg every 6–8 hours (by mouth or by intravenous injection only)

  **Child 1 month–1 year and body-weight up to 10 kg** 100 micrograms/kg (max. 1 mg) twice daily

  **Child 1–3 years and body-weight 10–14 kg** 1 mg 2–3 times daily

  **Child 3–5 years and body-weight 15–19 kg** 2 mg 2–3 times daily

  **Child 5–9 years and body-weight 20–29 kg** 2.5 mg 3 times daily

  **Child 9–18 years and body-weight 30–60 kg** 5 mg 3 times daily

  **Child 15–18 years and body-weight over 60 kg** 10 mg 3 times daily

  **Note** Daily dose of metoclopramide should not normally exceed 500 micrograms/kg

**Premedication in diagnostic procedures**

- By mouth as a single dose 5–10 minutes before examination

  **Child 1 month–3 years and body-weight up to 14 kg** 100 micrograms/kg, max. 1 mg

  **Child 3–5 years and body-weight 15–19 kg** 2 mg

  **Child 5–9 years and body-weight 20–29 kg** 2.5 mg

  **Child 9–15 years and body-weight 30–60 kg** 5 mg

  **Child 15–18 years and body-weight over 60 kg** 10 mg

**Metoclopramide** (Non-proprietary) [PoM]
Tablets, metoclopramide hydrochloride 10 mg, net price 28-tab pack = £1.01

Oral solution, metoclopramide hydrochloride 5 mg/5 mL, net price 150-mL pack = £6.51. Counselling, use of pipette

**Note** Sugar-free versions are available and can be ordered by specifying 'sugar-free' on the prescription

Injection, metoclopramide hydrochloride 5 mg/mL, net price 2-mL amp = 26p

**Maxolon**® (Amdipharm) [PoM]
Tablets, scored, metoclopramide hydrochloride 10 mg, net price 84-tab pack = £5.24

Injection, metoclopramide hydrochloride 5 mg/mL, net price 2-mL amp = 27p

◀**Compound preparations (for migraine)**
Section 4.7.1

## 5HT₃-receptor antagonists

## GRANISETRON

**Cautions** QT-interval prolongation (avoid concomitant use of drugs that prolong QT interval)

**Pregnancy** use only when compelling reasons—no information available

**Breast-feeding** avoid—no information available

**Side-effects** constipation, nausea, diarrhoea, vomiting, abdominal pain; headache, drowsiness, asthenia; fever; *rarely* hepatic dysfunction, chest pain, arrhythmia; *very rarely* anorexia, dizziness, insomnia, agitation, movement disorders, and rash

**Licensed use** sterile solution not licensed for use in children under 2 years

**Indications and dose**

Treatment and prevention of nausea and vomiting induced by cytotoxic chemotherapy or radiotherapy

- **By mouth**

    **Child 12–18 years** 1–2 mg within 1 hour before start of treatment, then 1 mg twice daily during treatment (total daily dose may alternatively be given as a single dose); when intravenous infusion also used, max. combined total 9 mg in 24 hours

- **By intravenous infusion**

    **Child 1 month–12 years** prevention, 40 micrograms/kg (max. 3 mg) before start of cytotoxic therapy; treatment, 40 micrograms/kg (max. 3 mg) repeated within 24 hours if necessary (not less than 10 minutes after initial dose)

- **By intravenous injection or by intravenous infusion**

    **Child 12–18 years** prevention, 3 mg before start of cytotoxic therapy (up to 2 additional 3-mg doses may be given within 24 hours); treatment, 3 mg repeated if necessary (doses must not be given less than 10 minutes apart), max. 9 mg in 24 hours

**Administration** for *intravenous infusion*, dilute up to 3 mL in Glucose 5% *or* Sodium Chloride 0.9% to a total volume of 10–30 mL; give over 5 minutes

**Granisetron** (Non-proprietary) [PoM]
Tablets, granisetron (as hydrochloride) 1 mg, net price 10-tab pack = £51.20

Injection, granisetron (as hydrochloride) 1 mg/mL, for dilution before use, net price 1-mL amp = £1.20, 3-mL amp = £4.80

**Kytril**® (Roche) [PoM]
Tablets, f/c, granisetron (as hydrochloride) 1 mg, net price 10-tab pack = £52.39; 2 mg, 5-tab pack = £52.39

## ■ ONDANSETRON

**Cautions** susceptibility to QT-interval prolongation (including concomitant use of drugs that prolong QT interval, and electrolyte disturbances); subacute intestinal obstruction; adenotonsillar surgery

**Contra-indications** congenital long QT syndrome

**Hepatic impairment** reduce dose in moderate or severe impairment

**Pregnancy** no information available; avoid unless potential benefit outweighs risk

**Breast-feeding** present in milk in *animal* studies—avoid

**Side-effects** constipation; headache; flushing; injection-site reactions; *less commonly* hiccups, hypotension, bradycardia, chest pain, arrhythmias, movement disorders, seizures; *on intravenous administration*, *rarely* dizziness, transient visual disturbances (*very rarely* transient blindness)

**Licensed use** not licensed for radiotherapy-induced nausea and vomiting in children

**Indications and dose**

Prevention and treatment of chemotherapy- and radiotherapy-induced nausea and vomiting

- **By intravenous infusion over at least 15 minutes**

    **Child 6 months–18 years** *either* 5 mg/m$^2$ immediately before chemotherapy (max. single dose 8 mg), then give by mouth, *or* 150 micrograms/kg immediately before chemotherapy (max. single dose 8 mg) repeated every 4 hours for 2 further doses, then give by mouth; max. total daily dose 32 mg

- **By mouth following intravenous administration**

    **Note** Oral dosing can start 12 hours after intravenous administration

    **Child 6 months–18 years**

    **Body surface area less than 0.6 m$^2$ *or* body-weight 10 kg or less** 2 mg every 12 hours for up to 5 days (max. total daily dose 32 mg)

    **Body surface area 0.6 m$^2$ or greater *or* body-weight over 10 kg** 4 mg every 12 hours for up to 5 days (max. total daily dose 32 mg)

Treatment and prevention of postoperative nausea and vomiting

- **By slow intravenous injection over at least 30 seconds**

    **Child 1 month–18 years** 100 micrograms/kg (max. 4 mg) as a single dose before, during, or after induction of anaesthesia

**Administration** for *intravenous infusion*, dilute to a concentration of 320–640 micrograms/mL with Glucose 5% *or* Sodium Chloride 0.9%; give over at least 15 minutes

**Ondansetron** (Non-proprietary) [PoM]
Tablets, ondansetron (as hydrochloride) 4 mg, net price 30-tab pack = £66.85; 8 mg, 10-tab pack = £49.92
**Brands include** *Ondemet*®

Oral solution, ondansetron (as hydrochloride) 4 mg/5 mL, net price 50-mL pack = £35.97
**Brands include** *Demorem*®

Injection, ondansetron (as hydrochloride) 2 mg/mL, net price 2-mL amp = £5.39, 4-mL amp = £10.79
**Brands include** *Ondemet*®

**Zofran**® (GSK) [PoM]
Tablets, yellow, f/c, ondansetron (as hydrochloride) 4 mg, net price 30-tab pack = £107.91; 8 mg, 10-tab pack = £71.94

Oral lyophilisates (*Zofran Melt*®), ondansetron 4 mg, net price 10-tab pack = £35.97; 8 mg, 10-tab pack = £71.94. Counselling, administration
**Excipients** include aspartame (section 9.4.1)
**Counselling** Tablets should be placed on the tongue, allowed to disperse and swallowed

Oral solution, sugar-free, strawberry-flavoured, ondansetron (as hydrochloride) 4 mg/5 mL, net price 50-mL pack = £35.97

Injection, ondansetron (as hydrochloride) 2 mg/mL, net price 2-mL amp = £5.99; 4-mL amp = £11.99

Central nervous system

**4**

# Cannabinoid

## ■ NABILONE

**Cautions** history of psychiatric disorder; hypertension; heart disease; adverse effects on mental state can persist for 48–72 hours after stopping
**Skilled tasks** Drowsiness may affect performance of skilled tasks (e.g. driving); effects of alcohol enhanced

**Hepatic impairment** avoid in severe impairment

**Pregnancy** avoid unless essential

**Breast-feeding** avoid—no information available

**Side-effects** drowsiness, vertigo, euphoria, dry mouth, ataxia, visual disturbance, concentration difficulties, sleep disturbance, dysphoria, hypotension, headache and nausea; also confusion, disorientation, hallucinations, psychosis, depression, decreased coordination, tremors, tachycardia, decreased appetite, and abdominal pain
**Behavioural effects** Children and carers should be made aware of possible changes of mood and other adverse behavioural effects

**Licensed use** not licensed for use in children

**Indications and dose**

**Nausea and vomiting caused by cytotoxic chemotherapy, unresponsive to conventional antiemetics** (under close observation, preferably in hospital setting)

- **By mouth**
  Consult local treatment protocol for details

**Nabilone** (Meda) [CD2]
Capsules, blue/white, nabilone 1 mg, net price 20-cap pack = £125.84. Label: 2, counselling, behavioural effects

# Hyoscine

## ■ HYOSCINE HYDROBROMIDE
(Scopolamine Hydrobromide)

**Cautions** section 1.2; also epilepsy
**Skilled tasks** Drowsiness may affect performance of skilled tasks (e.g. driving) and may persist for up to 24 hours or longer after removal of patch; effects of alcohol enhanced

**Contra-indications** section 1.2

**Hepatic impairment** use with caution

**Renal impairment** use with caution

**Pregnancy** use only if potential benefit outweighs risk; injection may depress neonatal respiration

**Breast-feeding** amount too small to be harmful

**Side-effects** section 1.2

**Licensed use** not licensed for use in excessive respiratory secretions or hypersalivation associated with clozapine therapy

**Indications and dose**

**Motion sickness**

- **By mouth**

  **Child 4–10 years** 75–150 micrograms 30 minutes before start of journey, repeated every 6 hours if required; max. 3 doses in 24 hours

  **Child 10–18 years** 150–300 micrograms 30 minutes before start of journey, repeated every 6 hours if required; max. 3 doses in 24 hours

- **By topical application**

  **Child 10–18 years** apply 1 patch (1 mg) to hairless area of skin behind ear 5–6 hours before journey; replace if necessary after 72 hours, siting replacement patch behind the other ear

**Excessive respiratory secretions**

- **By mouth or by sublingual administration**

  **Child 2–12 years** 10 micrograms/kg, max. 300 micrograms 4 times daily

  **Child 12–18 years** 300 micrograms 4 times daily

- **By transdermal route**

  **Child 1 month–3 years** 250 micrograms every 72 hours (quarter of a patch)

  **Child 3–10 years** 500 micrograms every 72 hours (half a patch)

  **Child 10–18 years** 1 mg every 72 hours (one patch)

- **By subcutaneous injection, intravenous injection, intravenous infusion, or subcutaneous infusion**

  See Continuous Subcutaneous Infusions, (p. 19) and Excessive Respiratory Secretions in Palliative Care, (p. 18).

**Hypersalivation associated with clozapine therapy**

- **By mouth**

  **Child 12–18 years** 300 micrograms up to 3 times daily; max. 900 micrograms daily

**Premedication** section 15.1.3

**Administration** *patch* applied to hairless area of skin behind ear; if less than whole patch required **either** cut with scissors along full thickness ensuring membrane is not peeled away **or** cover portion to prevent contact with skin
For administration *by mouth*, injection solution may be given orally

**Joy-Rides®** (Forest)
Tablets, chewable, hyoscine hydrobromide 150 micrograms, net price 12-tab pack = £1.49. Label: 2, 24

**Kwells®** (Bayer Consumer Care)
Tablets, chewable, hyoscine hydrobromide 150 micrograms (*Kwells® Kids*), net price 12-tab pack = £1.67; 300 micrograms, 12-tab pack = £1.67. Label: 2

**Scopoderm TTS®** (Novartis Consumer Health) [PoM]
Patch, self-adhesive, pink, releasing hyoscine approx. 1 mg/72 hours when in contact with skin, net price 5 = £10.75. Label: 19, counselling, see below
**Counselling** Explain accompanying instructions to child and carer, in particular emphasise advice to wash hands after handling and to wash application site after removing, and to use one patch at a time

## 4.7    Analgesics

| 4.7.1 | Non-opioid analgesics and compound analgesic preparations |
| 4.7.2 | Opioid analgesics |
| 4.7.3 | Neuropathic pain |
| 4.7.4 | Antimigraine drugs |

The non-opioid drugs (section 4.7.1), paracetamol and ibuprofen (and other NSAIDs), are particularly suitable for pain in musculoskeletal conditions, whereas the opioid analgesics (section 4.7.2) are more suitable for moderate to severe pain, particularly of visceral origin.

**Pain in palliative care**   For advice on pain relief in palliative care, see Pain Management With Opioids, (p. 16).

**Pain in sickle-cell disease**   The pain of mild sickle-cell crises is managed with paracetamol, an NSAID (section 10.1.1), codeine, or dihydrocodeine. Severe crises may require the use of morphine or diamorphine; concomitant use of an NSAID may potentiate analgesia and allow lower doses of the opioid to be used. A mixture of nitrous oxide and oxygen (*Entonox®, Equanox®*) may also be used.

**Dental and orofacial pain**   Analgesics should be used judiciously in dental care as a **temporary** measure until the cause of the pain has been dealt with.

Dental pain of inflammatory origin, such as that associated with pulpitis, apical infection, localised osteitis or pericoronitis is usually best managed by treating the infection, providing drainage, restorative procedures, and other local measures. Analgesics provide temporary relief of pain (usually for about 1 to 7 days) until the causative factors have been brought under control. In the case of pulpitis, intra-osseous infection or abscess, reliance on analgesics alone is usually inappropriate.

Similarly the pain and discomfort associated with acute problems of the oral mucosa (e.g. acute herpetic gingivostomatitis, erythema multiforme) may be relieved by **benzydamine** (p. 546) or topical anaesthetics until the cause of the mucosal disorder has been dealt with. However, where a child is febrile, the antipyretic action of **paracetamol** (p. 200) or **ibuprofen** (p. 504) is often helpful.

The *choice* of an analgesic for dental purposes should be based on its suitability for the child. Most dental pain is relieved effectively by non-steroidal anti-inflammatory drugs (NSAIDs) e.g. ibuprofen (section 10.1.1). **Paracetamol** has analgesic and antipyretic effects but no anti-inflammatory effect.

Opioid analgesics (section 4.7.2) such as **dihydrocodeine** act on the central nervous system and are traditionally used for *moderate to severe pain*. However, opioid analgesics are relatively ineffective in dental pain and their side-effects can be unpleasant.

Combining a non-opioid with an opioid analgesic can provide greater relief of pain than either analgesic given alone. However, this applies only when an adequate dose of each analgesic is used. Most combination analgesic preparations have not been shown to provide greater relief of pain than an adequate dose of the non-opioid component given alone. Moreover, combination preparations have the disadvantage of an increased number of side-effects.

Any analgesic given before a dental procedure should have a low risk of increasing postoperative bleeding. In the case of pain after the dental procedure, taking an analgesic before the effect of the local anaesthetic has worn off can improve control. Postoperative analgesia with ibuprofen is usually continued for about 24 to 72 hours.

**Dysmenorrhoea**   Paracetamol or a NSAID (section 10.1.1) will generally provide adequate relief of pain from dysmenorrhoea. Alternatively use of a combined hormonal contraceptive in adolescent girls may prevent the pain.

# 4.7.1 Non-opioid analgesics and compound analgesic preparations

**Paracetamol** has analgesic and antipyretic properties but no demonstrable anti-inflammatory activity; unlike opioid analgesics, it does not cause respiratory depression and is less irritant to the stomach than the NSAIDs. **Overdosage** with paracetamol is particularly dangerous as it may cause hepatic damage which is sometimes not apparent for 4 to 6 days (see Emergency Treatment of Poisoning, p. 26).

**Non-steroidal anti-inflammatory analgesics** (NSAIDs, section 10.1.1) are particularly useful for the treatment of children with chronic disease accompanied by pain and inflammation. Some of them are also used in the short-term treatment of mild to moderate pain including transient musculoskeletal pain but paracetamol is now often preferred. They are also suitable for the relief of pain in *dysmenorrhoea* and to treat pain caused by *secondary bone tumours*, many of which produce lysis of bone and release prostaglandins (see Pain in Palliative Care, (p. 16)). Due to an association with Reye's syndrome (section 2.9), **aspirin** should be avoided in children under 16 years except in Kawasaki syndrome or for its antiplatelet action (section 2.9). NSAIDs are also used for peri-operative analgesia (section 15.1.4.2).

**Dental and orofacial pain**   Most dental pain is relieved effectively by NSAIDs (section 10.1.1).

Paracetamol is less irritant to the stomach than NSAIDs. Paracetamol is a suitable analgesic for children; sugar-free versions can be requested by specifying 'sugar-free' on the prescription.

For further information on the management of dental and orofacial pain, see above.

## Compound analgesic preparations

Compound analgesic preparations that contain a simple analgesic (such as paracetamol) with an opioid component reduce the scope for effective titration of the individual components in the management of pain of varying intensity.

Compound analgesic preparations containing paracetamol with a *low dose* of an opioid analgesic (e.g. 8 mg of codeine phosphate per compound tablet) may be used in older children but the advantages have not been substantiated. The low dose of the opioid may be enough to cause opioid side-effects (in particular, constipation) and can complicate the treatment of **overdosage** (see p. 27) yet may not provide significant additional relief of pain.

A *full dose* of the opioid component (e.g. 60 mg codeine phosphate) in compound analgesic preparations effectively augments the analgesic activity but is associated with the full range of opioid side-effects (including nausea, vomiting, severe constipation, drowsiness, respiratory depression, and risk of dependence on long-term administration). For details of the **side-effects** of opioid analgesics, see p. 204.

In general, when assessing pain, it is necessary to weigh up carefully whether there is a need for a non-opioid and an opioid analgesic to be taken simultaneously.

**4 Central nervous system**

**PARACETAMOL**
(Acetaminophen)

**Cautions**  alcohol dependence; max. daily infusion dose 3 g in patients with hepatocellular insufficiency, chronic alcoholism, chronic malnutrition, or dehydration; high risk of liver toxicity with high doses; before administering, check when paracetamol last administered and cumulative paracetamol dose over previous 24 hours; **interactions**: Appendix 1 (paracetamol)

**Hepatic impairment**  dose-related toxicity—avoid large doses; see also Cautions

**Renal impairment**  increase *infusion* dose interval to every 6 hours if estimated glomerular filtration rate less than 30 mL/minute/1.73m$^2$

**Pregnancy**  not known to be harmful

**Breast-feeding**  amount too small to be harmful

**Side-effects**  side-effects rare, but rashes, blood disorders (including thrombocytopenia, leucopenia, neutropenia) reported; hypotension, flushing, and tachycardia also reported on infusion; **important:** liver damage (and less frequently renal damage) following **overdosage**, see Emergency Treatment of Poisoning, p. 26

**Licensed use**  not licensed for use in children under 2 months by mouth; not licensed for use in preterm neonates by intravenous infusion; doses for severe symptoms not licensed; co-codamol 8/500 tablets not licensed for use in children under 12 years

**Indications and dose**

**Pain; pyrexia with discomfort**

• By mouth

**Neonate 28–32 weeks postmenstrual age** 20 mg/kg as a single dose then 10–15 mg/kg every 8–12 hours as necessary; max. 30 mg/kg daily in divided doses

**Neonate over 32 weeks postmenstrual age** 20 mg/kg as a single dose then 10–15 mg/kg every 6–8 hours as necessary; max. 60 mg/kg daily in divided doses

**Child 1–3 months** 30–60 mg every 8 hours as necessary

**Child 3–6 months** 60 mg every 4–6 hours (max. 4 doses in 24 hours)

**Child 6 months–2 years** 120 mg every 4–6 hours (max. 4 doses in 24 hours)

**Child 2–4 years** 180 mg every 4–6 hours (max. 4 doses in 24 hours)

**Child 4–6 years** 240 mg every 4–6 hours (max. 4 doses in 24 hours)

**Child 6–8 years** 240–250 mg every 4–6 hours (max. 4 doses in 24 hours)

**Child 8–10 years** 360–375 mg every 4–6 hours (max. 4 doses in 24 hours)

**Child 10–12 years** 480–500 mg every 4–6 hours (max. 4 doses in 24 hours)

**Child 12–16 years** 480–750 mg every 4–6 hours (max. 4 doses in 24 hours)

**Child 16–18 years** 500 mg–1 g every 4–6 hours (max. 4 doses in 24 hours)

• By rectum

**Neonate 28–32 weeks postmenstrual age** 20 mg/kg as a single dose then 15 mg/kg every 12 hours as necessary; max. 30 mg/kg daily in divided doses

**Neonate over 32 weeks postmenstrual age** 30 mg/kg as a single dose then 20 mg/kg every 8 hours as necessary; max. 60 mg/kg daily in divided doses

**Child 1–3 months** 30–60 mg every 8 hours as necessary

**Child 3–12 months** 60–125 mg every 4–6 hours as necessary (max. 4 doses in 24 hours)

**Child 1–5 years** 125–250 mg every 4–6 hours as necessary (max. 4 doses in 24 hours)

**Child 5–12 years** 250–500 mg every 4–6 hours as necessary (max. 4 doses in 24 hours)

**Child 12–18 years** 500 mg every 4–6 hours

• By intravenous infusion over 15 minutes

**Preterm neonate over 32 weeks postmenstrual age** 7.5 mg/kg every 8 hours; max. 25 mg/kg daily

**Neonate** 10 mg/kg every 4–6 hours; max. 30 mg/kg daily

**Child body-weight under 50 kg** 15 mg/kg every 4–6 hours; max. 60 mg/kg daily

**Child body-weight over 50 kg** 1 g every 4–6 hours; max. 4 g daily

**Severe postoperative pain (but see Cautions)**

• By mouth

**Child 1 month–6 years** 20–30 mg/kg as a single dose then 15–20 mg/kg every 4–6 hours; max. 90 mg/kg daily in divided doses

**Child 6–12 years** 20–30 mg/kg (max. 1 g) as a single dose then 15–20 mg/kg every 4–6 hours; max. 90 mg/kg (max. 4 g) daily in divided doses

**Child 12–18 years** 1 g every 4–6 hours (max. 4 doses in 24 hours)

• By rectum

**Child 1–3 months** 30 mg/kg as a single dose then 15–20 mg/kg every 4–6 hours; max. 90 mg/kg daily in divided doses

**Child 3 months–6 years** 30–40 mg/kg as a single dose then 15–20 mg/kg every 4–6 hours; max. 90 mg/kg daily in divided doses

**Child 6–12 years** 30–40 mg/kg (max. 1 g) as a single dose then 15–20 mg/kg every 4–6 hours; max. 90 mg/kg (max. 4 g) daily in divided doses

**Child 12–18 years** 1 g every 4–6 hours (max. 4 doses in 24 hours)

**Post-immunisation pyrexia in infants** (see also p. 601)

• By mouth

**Child 2–3 months** 60 mg as a single dose repeated once after 4–6 hours if necessary

**Paracetamol** (Non-proprietary)

Tablets and caplets (PoM)[1], paracetamol 500 mg, net price 16-tab pack = 17p, 32-tab pack = £1.00, 100-tab pack = £1.44. Label: 29, 30

Brands include *Panadol*® JHS,

**Dental prescribing on NHS** Paracetamol Tablets may be prescribed

Capsules (PoM)[1], paracetamol 500 mg, net price 32-cap pack = £1.00, 100-cap pack = £3.34. Label: 29, 30

Brands include *Panadol Capsules*® JHS

Soluble tablets (= Dispersible tablets) (PoM)[2], paracetamol 500 mg, net price 60-tab pack = £4.39. Label: 13, 29, 30

Brands include *Panadol Soluble*® JHS (contains Na+ 18.6 mmol/tablet), *Paracetamol Seltzer*® (contains Na+ 16.9 mmol/tablet)

**Dental prescribing on NHS** Paracetamol Soluble Tablets 500 mg may be prescribed

Paediatric soluble tablets (= Paediatric dispersible tablets), paracetamol 120 mg, net price 16-tab pack = 89p. Label: 13, 30

Brands include *Disprol*® *Soluble Paracetamol* JHS

Oral suspension 120 mg/5 mL (= Paediatric Mixture), paracetamol 120 mg/5 mL, net price 100 mL = 72p, 150 mL = 84p, 200 mL = £1.05, 500 mL = £2.00. Label: 30

**Note** BP directs that when Paediatric Paracetamol Oral Suspension or Paediatric Paracetamol Mixture is prescribed Paracetamol Oral Suspension 120 mg/5 mL should be dispensed; sugar-free versions can be ordered by specifying 'sugar-free' on the prescription

Brands include *Calpol*® *Paediatric*, *Calpol*® *Paediatric* sugar-free, *Disprol*® *Paediatric*, *Medinol*® *Paediatric* sugar-free, *Panadol*® sugar-free

Oral suspension 250 mg/5 mL (= Mixture), paracetamol 250 mg/5 mL, net price 100 mL = 82p, 200 mL = £1.10, 500 mL = £3.29. Label: 30

Brands include *Calpol*® *6 Plus* JHS, *Medinol*® *Over 6* JHS

**Dental prescribing on NHS** Paracetamol Oral Suspension may be prescribed

Suppositories, paracetamol 60 mg, net price 10 = £9.96; 125 mg, 10 = £11.50; 250 mg, 10 = £23.00; 500 mg, 10 = £36.80; 1 g, 12 = £60.00. Label: 30

Brands include *Alvedon*®

**Note** Other strengths available from 'special-order' manufacturers or specialist importing companies, see p. 823

**Panadol OA**® (GSK) (PoM)

Tablets, f/c, paracetamol 1 g, net price 100-tab pack = £3.30. Label: 30

**Dose**

> **Pain, pyrexia**
>
> • By mouth
>
> **Child 12–18 years** 1 tablet up to 4 times daily, not more often than every 4 hours

**Perfalgan**® (Bristol-Myers Squibb) (PoM)

Intravenous infusion, paracetamol 10 mg/mL, net price 50-mL vial = £1.39, 100-mL vial = £1.52

**Administration** give undiluted or dilute to a concentration of 1 mg/mL in Glucose 5% *or* Sodium Chloride 0.9%; use within 1 hour of dilution

---

1. Can be sold to the public provided packs contain no more than 32 capsules or tablets; pharmacists can sell multiple packs up to a total quantity of 100 capsules or tablets in justifiable circumstances; for details see *Medicines, Ethics and Practice*, London, Pharmaceutical Press (always consult latest edition)

2. Can be sold to the public under certain circumstances; for exemptions see *Medicines, Ethics and Practice*, London, Pharmaceutical Press (always consult latest edition)

◢**With codeine phosphate 8 mg**

When co-codamol tablets, dispersible (or effervescent) tablets, or capsules are prescribed and **no strength is stated**, tablets, dispersible (or effervescent) tablets, or capsules, respectively, containing codeine phosphate **8 mg** and paracetamol **500 mg** should be dispensed.

See warnings and notes p. 199

For prescribing information on codeine, see p. 205

[2]**Co-codamol 8/500** (Non-proprietary) (PoM) ◢

Tablets, co-codamol 8/500 (codeine phosphate 8 mg, paracetamol 500 mg), net price 30-tab pack = £1.25, 32-tab pack = 50p, 100-tab pack = £1.35. Label: 29, 30

**Dose**

> **Pain, pyrexia**
>
> • By mouth
>
> **Child 6–12 years** ½–1 tablet every 4–6 hours; max. 4 tablets daily
>
> **Child 12–18 years** 1–2 tablets every 4–6 hours; max. 8 tablets daily

Effervescent *or* dispersible tablets, co-codamol 8/500 (codeine phosphate 8 mg, paracetamol 500 mg), net price 32-tab pack = £1.00, 100-tab pack = £4.32. Label: 13, 29, 30

Brands include *Paracodol*® JHS

**Note** The Drug Tariff allows tablets of co-codamol labelled 'dispersible' to be dispensed against an order for 'effervescent' and *vice versa*

**Dose**

> **Pain, pyrexia**
>
> • By mouth
>
> **Child 6–12 years** ½–1 tablet in water every 4–6 hours; max. 4 tablets daily
>
> **Child 12–18 years** 1–2 tablets in water every 4–6 hours; max. 8 tablets daily

Capsules, co-codamol 8/500 (codeine phosphate 8 mg, paracetamol 500 mg), net price 10-cap pack = £1.10, 20-cap pack = £1.71. Label: 29, 30

Brands include *Paracodol*® JHS

**Dose**

> **Pain, pyrexia**
>
> • By mouth
>
> **Child 12–18 years** 1–2 capsules every 4 hours; max. 8 capsules daily

◢**With codeine phosphate 15 mg**

When co-codamol tablets, dispersible (or effervescent) tablets, or capsules are prescribed and **no strength is stated**, tablets, dispersible (or effervescent) tablets, or capsules, respectively, containing codeine phosphate **8 mg** and paracetamol **500 mg** should be dispensed (see preparations above).

See warnings and notes p. 199

For prescribing information on codeine, see p. 205

**Codipar**® (Mercury) (PoM) ◢

Tablets, co-codamol 15/500 (codeine phosphate 15 mg, paracetamol 500 mg), net price 100-tab pack = £8.25. Label: 2, 29, 30

**Dose**

> **Moderate pain**
>
> • By mouth
>
> **Child 12–18 years** 1–2 tablets every 4 hours; max. 8 tablets daily

Capsules, co-codamol 15/500 (codeine phosphate 15 mg, paracetamol 500 mg), net price 100-cap pack = £7.25. Label: 2, 29, 30

**Dose**

> **Moderate pain**
>
> • By mouth
>
> **Child 12–18 years** 1–2 capsules every 4 hours; max. 8 capsules daily

**4**

**Central nervous system**

**Kapake**® (Galen) [PoM] ◢

Tablets, co-codamol 15/500 (codeine phosphate 15 mg, paracetamol 500 mg), net price 100-tab pack = £8.25. Label: 2, 29, 30

**Dose**

**Moderate pain**

● By mouth

**Child 12–16 years** 1 tablet every 4 hours; max. 4 tablets daily

**Child 16–18 years** 2 tablets every 4 hours; max. 8 tablets daily

◢**With codeine phosphate 30 mg**

When co-codamol tablets, dispersible (or effervescent) tablets, or capsules are prescribed and **no strength is stated**, tablets, dispersible (or effervescent) tablets, or capsules, respectively containing codeine phosphate **8 mg** and paracetamol **500 mg** should be dispensed (see preparations above).

See warnings and notes p. 199

For prescribing information on codeine, see p. 205

**Co-codamol 30/500** (Non-proprietary) [PoM] ◢

Tablets (and caplets) , co-codamol 30/500 (codeine phosphate 30 mg, paracetamol 500 mg), net price 100-tab pack = £3.65. Label: 2, 29, 30

**Dose**

**Severe pain**

● By mouth

**Child 12–18 years** 1–2 tablets every 4 hours; max. 8 tablets daily

Capsules, co-codamol 30/500 (codeine phosphate 30 mg, paracetamol 500 mg), net price 100-cap pack = £5.55. Label: 2, 29, 30

**Brands include** Medocodene®, Zapain®

**Dose**

**Severe pain**

● By mouth

**Child 12–18 years** 1–2 capsules every 4 hours; max. 8 capsules daily

Effervescent tablets, co-codamol 30/500 (codeine phosphate 30 mg, paracetamol 500 mg), net price 100-tab pack = £7.67. Label: 2, 13, 29, 30

**Brands include** Medocodene® Effervescent (contains Na⁺ 13.6 mmol/tablet)

**Dose**

**Severe pain**

● By mouth

**Child 12–18 years** 1–2 tablets in water every 4 hours; max. 8 tablets daily

**Kapake**® (Galen) [PoM] ◢

Tablets, scored, co-codamol 30/500 (codeine phosphate 30 mg, paracetamol 500 mg), net price 30-tab pack = £2.26 (hosp. only), 100-tab pack = £7.10. Label: 2, 29, 30

**Dose**

**Severe pain**

● By mouth

**Child 12–18 years** 1–2 tablets every 4 hours; max. 8 tablets daily

Capsules, co-codamol 30/500 (codeine phosphate 30 mg, paracetamol 500 mg), net price 100-cap pack = £7.10. Label: 2, 29, 30

**Dose**

**Severe pain**

● By mouth

**Child 12–18 years** 1–2 capsules every 4 hours; max. 8 capsules daily

**Solpadol**® (Sanofi-Aventis) [PoM] ◢

Caplets (= tablets), co-codamol 30/500 (codeine phosphate 30 mg, paracetamol 500 mg), net price 100-tab pack = £6.74. Label: 2, 29, 30

**Dose**

**Severe pain**

● By mouth

**Child 12–18 years** 2 tablets every 4 hours; max. 8 tablets daily

Capsules, grey/purple, co-codamol 30/500 (codeine phosphate 30 mg, paracetamol 500 mg), net price 100-cap pack = £6.74. Label: 2, 29, 30

**Dose**

**Severe pain**

● By mouth

**Child 12–18 years** 2 capsules every 4 hours; max. 8 capsules daily

Effervescent tablets, co-codamol 30/500 (codeine phosphate 30 mg, paracetamol 500 mg), net price 32-tab pack = £2.59, 100-tab pack = £8.09. Label: 2, 13, 29, 30

**Electrolytes** Na⁺ 16.9 mmol/tablet

**Dose**

**Severe pain**

● By mouth

**Child 12–18 years** 2 tablets in water every 4 hours; max. 8 tablets daily

**Tylex**® (UCB Pharma) [PoM] ◢

Capsules, co-codamol 30/500 (codeine phosphate 30 mg, paracetamol 500 mg), net price 100-cap pack = £7.70. Label: 2, 29, 30

**Excipients** include sulphites

**Dose**

**Severe pain**

● By mouth

**Child 12–18 years** 1–2 capsules every 4 hours; max. 8 capsules daily

Effervescent tablets, co-codamol 30/500 (codeine phosphate 30 mg, paracetamol 500 mg), net price 100-tab pack = £8.80. Label: 2, 13, 29, 30

**Electrolytes** Na⁺ 14.2 mmol/tablet

**Excipients** include aspartame 25 mg/tablet (section 9.4.1)

**Dose**

**Severe pain**

● By mouth

**Child 12–18 years** 1–2 tablets in water every 4 hours; max. 8 tablets daily

◢**With dihydrocodeine tartrate 10 mg**

When co-dydramol tablets are prescribed and **no strength is stated**, tablets containing dihydrocodeine tartrate **10 mg** and paracetamol **500 mg** should be dispensed.

See warnings and notes on p. 199

For prescribing information on dihydrocodeine, see p. 206

**Co-dydramol** (Non-proprietary) [PoM] ◢

Tablets, co-dydramol 10/500 (dihydrocodeine tartrate 10 mg, paracetamol 500 mg), net price 30-tab pack = £1.21. Label: 29, 30

**Dose**

**Mild to moderate pain**

● By mouth

**Child 12–18 years** 1–2 tablets every 4–6 hours; max. 8 tablets daily

**4 Central nervous system**

◢**With dihydrocodeine tartrate 20 mg**

When co-dydramol tablets are prescribed and **no strength is stated**, tablets containing dihydrocodeine tartrate **10 mg** and paracetamol **500 mg** should be dispensed (see preparation above).

See warnings and notes on p. 199

For prescribing information on dihydrocodeine, see p. 206

**Remedeine**® (Napp) [PoM] ◢

Tablets, paracetamol 500 mg, dihydrocodeine tartrate 20 mg, net price 112-tab pack = £10.57. Label: 2, 30

**Dose**

> **Severe pain**
>
> ● By mouth
>
> **Child 12–18 years** 1–2 tablets every 4–6 hours; max. 8 tablets daily

◢**With dihydrocodeine tartrate 30 mg**

When co-dydramol tablets are prescribed and **no strength is stated**, tablets containing dihydrocodeine tartrate **10 mg** and paracetamol **500 mg** should be dispensed (see preparation above).

See warnings and notes on p. 199

For prescribing information on dihydrocodeine, see p. 206

**Remedeine Forte**® (Napp) [PoM] ◢

Tablets, paracetamol 500 mg, dihydrocodeine tartrate 30 mg, net price 56-tab pack = £6.53. Label: 2, 29, 30

**Dose**

> **Severe pain**
>
> ● By mouth
>
> **Child 12–18 years** 1–2 tablets every 4–6 hours; max. 8 tablets daily

◢**With tramadol**

For prescribing information on tramadol, see section 4.7.2

**Tramacet**® (Grünenthal) [PoM]

Tablets, f/c, yellow, tramadol hydrochloride 37.5 mg, paracetamol 325 mg, net price 60-tab pack = £9.68. Label: 2, 25, 29, 30

**Dose**

> **Moderate to severe pain**
>
> ● By mouth
>
> **Child 12–18 years** 2 tablets not more often than every 6 hours; max. 8 tablets daily

Effervescent tablets, pink, tramadol hydrochloride 37.5 mg, paracetamol 325 mg, net price 60-tab pack = £9.68. Label: 2, 13, 29, 30

Electrolytes  Na⁺ 7.8 mmol/tablet

**Dose**

> **Moderate to severe pain**
>
> ● By mouth
>
> **Child 12–18 years** 2 tablets not more often than every 6 hours; max. 8 tablets daily

◢**With antiemetics**

**Migraleve**® (McNeil) ◢

Tablets, all f/c, *pink tablets*, buclizine hydrochloride 6.25 mg, paracetamol 500 mg, codeine phosphate 8 mg; *yellow tablets*, paracetamol 500 mg, codeine phosphate 8 mg, net price 48-tab *Migraleve* [PoM] (32 pink + 16 yellow) = £4.81; 48 pink (*Migraleve Pink*) = £5.24. Label: 2, (*Migraleve Pink*), 17, 30

**Dose**

> **Treatment of acute migraine**
>
> ● By mouth
>
> **Child under 10 years** only under close medical supervision
>
> **Child 10–14 years** 1 pink tablet at onset of attack, or if it is imminent, then 1 yellow tablet every 4 hours if necessary; max. 1 pink and 3 yellow tablets in 24 hours
>
> **Child 14–18 years** 2 pink tablets at onset of attack, or if it is imminent, then 2 yellow tablets every 4 hours if necessary; max. in 24 hours 2 pink and 6 yellow

**Paramax**® (Sanofi-Aventis) [PoM]

Tablets, scored, paracetamol 500 mg, metoclopramide hydrochloride 5 mg, net price 42-tab pack = £9.64. Label: 17, 30

Sachets, effervescent powder, sugar-free, the contents of 1 sachet = 1 tablet; to be dissolved in ¼ tumblerful of liquid before administration, net price 42-sachet pack = £12.52. Label: 13, 17, 30

**Dose**

> **Treatment of acute migraine**
>
> ● By mouth
>
> **Child 12–18 years** 1 at onset of attack then 1 every 4 hours when necessary to max. of 3 in 24 hours (max. dose of metoclopramide 500 micrograms/kg daily)
>
> **Important** Metoclopramide can cause **severe extrapyramidal effects** (for further details, see p. 192 and p. 196)
>
> **Note** Treatment should not exceed 3 months due to risk of tardive dyskinesia

### 4.7.2  Opioid analgesics

Opioid analgesics are usually used to relieve moderate to severe pain particularly of visceral origin. Repeated administration may cause tolerance, but this is no deterrent in the control of pain in terminal illness, for guidelines see Pain Management with Opioids, (p. 16). Regular use of a potent opioid may be appropriate for certain cases of chronic non-malignant pain; treatment should be supervised by a specialist and the child should be assessed at regular intervals.

**Cautions**  Opioids should be used with caution in children with impaired respiratory function and asthma (avoid during an acute attack), hypotension, shock, myasthenia gravis, obstructive or inflammatory bowel disorders, diseases of the biliary tract, and convulsive disorders. A reduced dose is recommended in hypothyroidism or adrenocortical insufficiency. Repeated use of opioid analgesics is associated with the development of psychological and physical dependence; although this is rarely a problem with therapeutic use, caution is advised if prescribing for patients with a history of drug dependence. Avoid abrupt withdrawal after long-term treatment. Transdermal preparations (fentanyl or buprenorphine patches) are not suitable for acute pain or in those children whose analgesic requirements are changing rapidly, because the long time to steady state prevents rapid titration of the dose.

**Palliative care**  In the control of pain in terminal illness, the cautions listed above should not necessarily be a deterrent to the use of opioid analgesics.

**Contra-indications**  Opioid analgesics should be avoided in children with acute respiratory depression, and when there is a risk of paralytic ileus. They are also contra-indicated in conditions associated with raised intracranial pressure, and in head injury (opioid analgesics interfere with pupillary responses vital for neu-

**4**

**Central nervous system**

rological assessment). Comatose children should not be treated with opioid analgesics.

**Hepatic impairment** Opioid analgesics may precipitate coma in children with hepatic impairment; avoid use or reduce dose.

**Renal impairment** The effects of opioid analgesia are increased and prolonged and there is increased cerebral sensitivity when children with renal impairment are treated with opioid analgesics; avoid use or reduce dose.

**Pregnancy** Respiratory depression and withdrawal symptoms can occur in the neonate if opioid analgesics are used during delivery; also gastric stasis and inhalation pneumonia has been reported in the mother if opioid analgesics are used during labour.

**Side-effects** Opioid analgesics share many side-effects, although qualitative and quantitative differences exist. The most common side-effects include nausea and vomiting (particularly in initial stages), constipation, dry mouth and biliary spasm; larger doses produce muscle rigidity, hypotension and respiratory depression (for reversal of opioid-induced respiratory depression, see section 15.1.7); neonates, particularly if preterm, may be more susceptible. Other common side-effects of opioid analgesics include bradycardia, tachycardia, palpitation, oedema, postural hypotension, hallucinations, vertigo, euphoria, dysphoria, mood changes, dependence, dizziness, confusion, drowsiness, sleep disturbances, headache, sexual dysfunction, difficulty with micturition, urinary retention, ureteric spasm, miosis, visual disturbances, sweating, flushing, rash, urticaria, and pruritus. **Overdosage:** see Emergency Treatment of Poisoning, p. 27.

Long-term use of opioid analgesics can lead to hypogonadism and adrenal insufficiency in both boys and girls. This is thought to be dose related and can lead to amenorrhoea, reduced libido, infertility, depression, and erectile dysfunction. Long-term use of opioid analgesics has also been associated with a state of abnormal pain sensitivity (hyperalgesia). Pain associated with hyperalgesia is usually distinct from pain associated with disease progression or breakthrough pain, and is often more diffuse and less defined. Treatment of hyperalgesia involves reducing the dose of opioid medication or switching therapy; cases of suspected hyperalgesia should be referred to a specialist pain team.

**Interactions** See Appendix 1 (opioid analgesics) (**important:** special hazard with *pethidine and possibly other opioids* and MAOIs).

**Skilled tasks** Drowsiness may affect performance of skilled tasks (e.g. driving); effects of alcohol enhanced. Driving at the start of therapy with opioid analgesics, and following dose changes, should be avoided.

**Strong opioids** Morphine remains the most valuable opioid analgesic for severe pain although it frequently causes nausea and vomiting. It is the standard against which other opioid analgesics are compared. In addition to relief of pain, morphine also confers a state of euphoria and mental detachment.

Morphine is the opioid of choice for the oral treatment of *severe pain in palliative care*. It is given regularly every 4 hours (or every 12 or 24 hours as modified-release preparations). For guidelines on dosage adjustment in palliative care, see Pain Management with Opioids, (p. 16).

**Buprenorphine** has both opioid agonist and antagonist properties and may precipitate withdrawal symptoms,

including pain, in children dependent on other opioids. It has abuse potential and may itself cause dependence. It has a much longer duration of action than morphine and sublingually is an effective analgesic for 6 to 8 hours. Unlike most opioid analgesics, the effects of buprenorphine are only partially reversed by naloxone. It is used rarely in children.

**Diamorphine** (heroin) is a powerful opioid analgesic. It may cause less nausea and hypotension than morphine. In *palliative care* the greater solubility of diamorphine allows effective doses to be injected in smaller volumes and this is important in the emaciated child.

Diamorphine is sometimes given by the intranasal route to treat acute pain in children, for example, in accident and emergency units; however, as yet, there is limited safety and efficacy data to support this practice.

**Alfentanil**, **fentanyl** and **remifentanil** are used by injection for intra-operative analgesia (section 15.1.4.3). Fentanyl is available in a transdermal drug delivery system as a self-adhesive patch which is changed every 72 hours.

**Methadone** is less sedating than morphine and acts for longer periods. In prolonged use, methadone should not be administered more often than twice daily to avoid the risk of accumulation and opioid overdosage. Methadone may be used instead of morphine when excitation (or exacerbation of pain) occurs with morphine. Methadone may also be used to treat children with neonatal abstinence syndrome (section 4.10).

**Papaveretum** should not be used in children; morphine is easier to prescribe and less prone to error with regard to the strength and dose.

**Pethidine** produces prompt but short-lasting analgesia; it is less constipating than morphine, but even in high doses is a less potent analgesic. Its use in children is not recommended. Pethidine is used for analgesia in labour; however, other opioids, such as morphine or diamorphine, are often preferred for obstetric pain.

**Tramadol** is used in older children and produces analgesia by two mechanisms: an opioid effect and an enhancement of serotonergic and adrenergic pathways. It has fewer of the typical opioid side-effects (notably, less respiratory depression, less constipation and less addiction potential); psychiatric reactions have been reported.

**Weak opioids** Codeine is used for the relief of mild to moderate pain but is too constipating for long-term use.

**Dihydrocodeine** has an analgesic efficacy similar to that of codeine; doses may be given every 4 hours.

**Dose** Doses of opioids may need to be **adjusted individually** according to the degree of analgesia and side-effects; response to opioids varies widely, particularly in the neonatal period. Opioid overdosage can have serious consequences and the dose should be calculated and **checked with care**.

**Postoperative analgesia** A combination of opioid and non-opioid analgesics is used to treat postoperative pain (section 15.1.4.2). The use of intra-operative opioids affects the prescribing of postoperative analgesics. A postoperative opioid analgesic should be given with care since it may potentiate any residual respiratory depression (for the treatment of opioid-induced respiratory depression, see section 15.1.7).

**Morphine** is used most widely. **Tramadol** is not as effective in severe pain as other opioid analgesics.

Buprenorphine may antagonise the analgesic effect of previously administered opioids and is generally not recommended. **Pethidine** is unsuitable for postoperative pain because it is metabolised to norpethidine which may accumulate, particularly in neonates and in renal impairment; norpethidine stimulates the central nervous system and may cause convulsions.

Opioids are also given epidurally [unlicensed route] in the postoperative period but are associated with side-effects such as pruritus, urinary retention, nausea and vomiting; respiratory depression can be delayed, particularly with morphine.

For details of patient-controlled analgesia (PCA) and nurse-controlled analgesia (NCA) to relieve postoperative pain, consult hospital protocols.

**Dental and orofacial pain** Opioid analgesics are relatively ineffective in dental pain. Like other opioids, **dihydrocodeine** often causes nausea and vomiting which limits its value in dental pain; if taken for more than a few doses it is also liable to cause constipation. Dihydrocodeine is not very effective in postoperative dental pain.

For the management of dental and orofacial pain, see p. 199.

**Pain management and opioid dependence** Although caution is necessary, patients who are dependent on opioids or have a history of drug dependence may be treated with opioid analgesics when there is a clinical need. Treatment with opioid analgesics in this patient group should normally be carried out with the advice of specialists. However, doctors do not require a special licence to prescribe opioid analgesics to patients with opioid dependence for relief of pain due to organic disease or injury.

**Dependence and withdrawal** Psychological dependence rarely occurs when opioids are used for pain relief but tolerance can develop during long-term treatment; they should be withdrawn gradually to avoid abstinence symptoms. For information on the treatment of neonatal abstinence syndrome, see section 4.10.

## ▮ BUPRENORPHINE

**Cautions** see notes above; also impaired consciousness; effects only partially reversed by naloxone; monitor liver function
**Contra-indications** see notes above
**Hepatic impairment** see notes above
**Renal impairment** see notes above
**Pregnancy** see notes above
**Breast-feeding** present in low levels in breast milk—monitor neonate for drowsiness, adequate weight gain, and developmental milestones
**Side-effects** see notes above; can induce mild withdrawal symptoms in children dependent on opioids; also diarrhoea, abdominal pain, anorexia, dyspepsia; vasodilatation; dyspnoea; paraesthesia, asthenia, fatigue, agitation, anxiety; *less commonly* flatulence, taste disturbance, hypertension, syncope, hypoxia, wheezing, cough, restlessness, depersonalisation, dysarthria, impaired memory, hypoaesthesia, tremor, influenza-like symptoms, pyrexia, rhinitis, rigors, muscle cramp, myalgia, tinnitus, dry eye, and dry skin; *rarely* paralytic ileus, dysphagia, diverticulitis, impaired concentration, and psychosis; *very rarely* retching, hyperventilation, hiccups, and muscle fasciculation; hepatic necrosis and hepatitis also reported

**Licensed use** sublingual tablets not licensed for use in children under 6 years; injection not licensed for use in children under 6 months

### Indications and dose

**Moderate to severe pain**

- By sublingual administration
  **Child body-weight 16–25 kg** 100 micrograms every 6–8 hours
  **Child body-weight 25–37.5 kg** 100–200 micrograms every 6–8 hours
  **Child body-weight 37.5–50 kg** 200–300 micrograms every 6–8 hours
  **Child body-weight over 50 kg** 200–400 micrograms every 6–8 hours

- By intramuscular or by slow intravenous injection
  **Child 6 months–12 years** 3–6 micrograms/kg every 6–8 hours, max. 9 micrograms/kg
  **Child 12–18 years** 300–600 micrograms every 6–8 hours

**Administration** for administration *by mouth*, tablets may be halved

**Temgesic®** (Reckitt Benckiser) ⟨CD3⟩
Tablets (sublingual), buprenorphine (as hydrochloride), 200 micrograms, net price 50-tab pack = £5.13; 400 micrograms, 50-tab pack = £10.26. Label: 2, 26
Injection, buprenorphine (as hydrochloride) 300 micrograms/mL, net price 1-mL amp = 48p

## ▮ CODEINE PHOSPHATE

**Cautions** see notes above; also cardiac arrhythmias; acute abdomen; gallstones
*Variation in metabolism* The capacity to metabolise codeine can vary considerably between individuals and lead to either reduced therapeutic effect or marked increase in side-effects
**Contra-indications** see notes above
**Hepatic impairment** see notes above
**Renal impairment** see notes above
**Pregnancy** see notes above
**Breast-feeding** amount usually too small to be harmful; however, mothers vary considerably in their capacity to metabolise codeine—risk of morphine overdose in infant
**Side-effects** see notes above; also abdominal pain, anorexia, seizures, malaise, hypothermia, antidiuretic effect, and muscle fasciculation; pancreatitis also reported
**Licensed use** tablets not licensed for use in children under 12 years; syrup and injection not licensed for use in children under 1 year

### Indications and dose

**Mild to moderate pain**

- By mouth or by rectum or by subcutaneous injection or by intramuscular injection
  **Neonate** 0.5–1 mg/kg every 4–6 hours
  **Child 1 month–12 years** 0.5–1 mg/kg every 4–6 hours, max. 240 mg daily
  **Child 12–18 years** 30–60 mg every 4–6 hours, max. 240 mg daily

**Codeine Phosphate** (Non-proprietary)
Tablets ⟨PoM⟩, codeine phosphate 15 mg, net price 28-tab pack = £1.14; 30 mg, 28-tab pack = £1.22; 60 mg, 28-tab pack = £1.84. Label: 2

Syrup (PoM), codeine phosphate 25 mg/5 mL, net price 100 mL = 93p. Label: 2

Injection (CD2), codeine phosphate 60 mg/mL, net price 1-mL amp = £2.44

◢With paracetamol
Section 4.7.1

---

## ▌DIAMORPHINE HYDROCHLORIDE
(Heroin Hydrochloride)

**Cautions** see notes above; also severe diarrhoea; toxic psychosis; CNS depression; severe cor pulmonale

**Contra-indications** see notes above; also delayed gastric emptying; phaeochromocytoma

**Hepatic impairment** see notes above

**Renal impairment** see notes above

**Pregnancy** see notes above

**Breast-feeding** therapeutic doses unlikely to affect infant; withdrawal symptoms in infants of dependent mothers; breast-feeding not best method of treating dependence in offspring

**Side-effects** see notes above; also anorexia, taste disturbance; syncope; asthenia, raised intracranial pressure; myocardial infarction also reported

**Licensed use** intranasal route not licensed

**Indications and dose**

> Acute or chronic pain
> - By mouth
>
>> **Child 1 month–12 years** 100–200 micrograms/kg (max. 10 mg) every 4 hours, adjusted according to response
>>
>> **Child 12–18 years** 5–10 mg every 4 hours, adjusted according to response
>
> - By intravenous administration
>
>> **Neonate (ventilated)** initially *by intravenous injection* over 30 minutes, 50 micrograms/kg then *by continuous intravenous infusion*, 15 micrograms/kg/ hour, adjusted according to response
>>
>> **Neonate (non-ventilated)** *by continuous intravenous infusion* 2.5–7 micrograms/kg/hour, adjusted according to response
>>
>> **Child 1 month–12 years** *by continuous intravenous infusion* 12.5–25 micrograms/kg/hour, adjusted according to response
>
> - By intravenous injection
>
>> **Child 1–3 months** 20 micrograms/kg every 6 hours, adjusted according to response
>>
>> **Child 3–6 months** 25–50 micrograms/kg every 6 hours, adjusted according to response
>>
>> **Child 6–12 months** 75 micrograms/kg every 4 hours, adjusted according to response
>>
>> **Child 1–12 years** 75–100 micrograms/kg (max. 5 mg) every 4 hours, adjusted according to response
>>
>> **Child 12–18 years** 2.5–5 mg every 4 hours, adjusted according to response
>
> - By continuous subcutaneous infusion
>
>> See Continuous Subcutaneous Infusions, in Palliative care, (p. 19)
>
> - By subcutaneous or by intramuscular injection
>
>> **Child 12–18 years** 5 mg every 4 hours, adjusted according to response

**Acute pain in an emergency setting; short painful procedures**
- **Intranasally (but see p. 204)**

> **Child over 10 kg** 100 micrograms/kg, max. 10 mg

**Administration** for *intravenous infusion*, dilute in Glucose 5% *or* Sodium Chloride 0.9%; Glucose 5% is preferable

For *intranasal* administration, diamorphine powder should be dissolved in sufficient volume of Water for Injections to provide the requisite dose in 0.2 mL of solution; use solution immediately after preparation

**Diamorphine** (Non-proprietary) (CD2)
Tablets, diamorphine hydrochloride 10 mg, net price 100-tab pack = £16.42. Label: 2

Injection, powder for reconstitution, diamorphine hydrochloride, net price 5-mg amp = £2.57, 10-mg amp = £3.59, 30-mg amp = £3.82, 100-mg amp = £9.34, 500-mg amp = £42.07

---

## ▌DIHYDROCODEINE TARTRATE

**Cautions** see notes above; also pancreatitis; severe cor pulmonale

**Contra-indications** see notes above

**Hepatic impairment** see notes above

**Renal impairment** see notes above

**Pregnancy** see notes above

**Breast-feeding** use only if potential benefit outweighs risk

**Side-effects** see notes above; also paralytic ileus, abdominal pain, diarrhoea, seizures, and paraesthesia

**Licensed use** most preparations not licensed for use in children under 4 years

**Indications and dose**

> Moderate to severe pain
> - By mouth or by intramuscular injection or by subcutaneous injection
>
>> **Child 1–4 years** 500 micrograms/kg every 4–6 hours
>>
>> **Child 4–12 years** 0.5–1 mg/kg (max. 30 mg) every 4–6 hours
>>
>> **Child 12–18 years** 30 mg (max. 50 mg by intramuscular or deep subcutaneous injection) every 4–6 hours

**Dihydrocodeine** (Non-proprietary)
Tablets (PoM), dihydrocodeine tartrate 30 mg, net price 28-tab pack = £1.58. Label: 2
**Dental prescribing on NHS** Dihydrocodeine Tablets 30 mg may be prescribed

Oral solution (PoM), dihydrocodeine tartrate 10 mg/ 5 mL, net price 150 mL = £3.50. Label: 2

Injection (CD2), dihydrocodeine tartrate 50 mg/mL, net price 1-mL amp = £3.17

**DF 118 Forte®** (Martindale) (PoM)
Tablets, dihydrocodeine tartrate 40 mg, net price 100-tab pack = £11.51. Label: 2
**Dose**

> Severe pain
> - By mouth
>
>> **Child 12–18 years** 40–80 mg 3 times daily; max. 240 mg daily

*(side margin)* **4 Central nervous system**

◢Modified release

**DHC Continus®** (Napp) [PoM]

 Tablets, m/r, dihydrocodeine tartrate 60 mg, net price 56-tab pack = £5.18; 90 mg, 56-tab pack = £8.66; 120 mg, 56-tab pack = £10.89. Label: 2, 25

**Dose**

> **Chronic severe pain**
>
> • **By mouth**
>
>   **Child 12–18 years** 60–120 mg every 12 hours

◢With paracetamol

 Section 4.7.1

---

# ▮ FENTANYL

**Cautions**  see notes above; also diabetes mellitus, impaired consciousness, cerebral tumour, see also Transdermal Fentanyl, below

**Contra-indications**  see notes above

**Hepatic impairment**  see notes above

**Renal impairment**  see notes above

**Pregnancy**  see notes above

**Breast-feeding**  monitor infant for opioid-induced side-effects

**Side-effects**  see notes above; also abdominal pain, dyspepsia, diarrhoea, gastro-oesophageal reflux disease, stomatitis, anorexia, hypertension, vasodilatation, dyspnoea, aesthenia, myoclonus, anxiety, tremor, appetite changes, rhinitis, pharyngitis, paraesthesia, application-site reactions; *less commonly* ileus, flatulence, hypoventilation, impaired concentration, impaired coordination, amnesia, speech disorder, malaise, seizure, pyrexia, thirst, blood disorders (including thrombocytopenia), chills; *rarely* hiccups, *very rarely* arrhythmia, apnoea, haemoptysis, ataxia, delusions, bladder pain

**Indications and dose**

**Severe chronic pain**

• **By transdermal route**

  **Child 2–16 years currently treated** with strong opioid analgesic, initial dose based on previous 24-hour opioid requirement (consult product literature)

  **Child 16–18 years** child **not currently treated** with strong opioid analgesic (but see Transdermal Fentanyl, below), one '12' or '25 micrograms/hour' patch replaced after 72 hours; child **currently treated** with strong opioid analgesic, initial dose based on previous 24-hour opioid requirement (consult product literature)

  **Dose adjustment**  When starting, evaluation of the analgesic effect should **not** be made before the system has been worn for **24 hours** (to allow for the gradual increase in plasma-fentanyl concentration)—previous analgesic therapy should be phased out gradually from time of first patch application; if necessary dose should be adjusted at 48–72-hour intervals in steps of 12–25 micrograms/hour. More than one patch may be used at a time (but applied at *same time* to avoid confusion)—consider additional or alternative analgesic therapy if dose required exceeds 300 micrograms/hour (**important:** it takes 17 hours or more for the plasma-fentanyl concentration to decrease by 50%—replacement opioid therapy should be initiated at a low dose and increased gradually)

  **Long duration of action**  In view of the long duration of action, children who have had severe side-effects should be monitored for up to 24 hours after patch removal

> **Breakthrough pain and premedication analgesia** , see under preparation below

**Peri-operative analgesia** section 15.1.4.3

**Conversion** (from oral morphine to transdermal fentanyl), see Pain Management with Opioids, (p. 16)

**Administration**  For *patches*, apply to dry, non-irritated, non-irradiated, non-hairy skin on torso or upper arm, removing after 72 hours and siting replacement patch on a different area (avoid using the same area for several days).

◢Lozenges

**Actiq®** (Flynn) [CD2]

 Lozenge, (with oromucosal applicator), fentanyl (as citrate) 200 micrograms, net price 3 = £17.52, 30 = £175.16; 400 micrograms, 3 = £17.52, 30 = £175.16; 600 micrograms, 3 = £17.52, 30 = £175.16; 800 micrograms, 3 = £17.52, 30 = £175.16; 1.2 mg, 3 = £17.52, 30 = £175.16; 1.6 mg, 3 = £17.52, 30 = £175.16. Label: 2

**Dose**

> **Breakthrough pain**
>
> • **By transmucosal application (lozenge with oromucosal applicator)**
>
>   **Child 16–18 years** initially 200 micrograms (over 15 minutes) repeated if necessary 15 minutes after first dose (no more than 2 dose units for each pain episode); if adequate pain relief not achieved with 1 dose unit for consecutive breakthrough pain episodes, increase the strength of the dose unit until adequate pain relief achieved with 4 lozenges or less daily
>
>   **Note**  If more than 4 episodes of breakthrough pain each day, adjust dose of background analgesic

◢Patches

> **Transdermal fentanyl**
>
> **Fever or external heat**  Monitor patients using patches for increased side-effects if fever present (increased absorption possible); avoid exposing application site to external heat, for example a hot bath or sauna (may also increase absorption)
>
>> Monitor patients using patches for increased side-effects if fever present (increased absorption possible); avoid exposing application site to external heat, for example a hot bath or sauna (may also increase absorption)
>
> **Respiratory depression**  Risk of fatal respiratory depression, particularly in patients not previously treated with a strong opioid analgesic; manufacturer recommends use only in opioid tolerant patients
>
>> Risk of fatal respiratory depression, particularly in patients not previously treated with a strong opioid analgesic; manufacturer recommends use only in opioid tolerant patients
>
> **Counselling**  Patients and carers should be informed about safe use, including correct administration and disposal, strict adherence to dosage instructions, and the symptoms and signs of opioid overdosage. Patches should be removed immediately in case of breathing difficulties, marked drowsiness, confusion, dizziness, or impaired speech, and patients and carers should seek prompt medical attention.

**Prescriptions**  Prescriptions for fentanyl patches can be written to show the strength in terms of the release rate and it is acceptable to write '*Fentanyl 25 patches*' to prescribe patches that release fentanyl 25 micrograms per hour. The dosage should be expressed in terms of the interval between applying a patch and replacing it with a new one, e.g. '*one patch to be applied every 72 hours*'. The total quantity of patches should be written in words and figures.

◢ **4**

**Central nervous system**

**Fentanyl** (Non-proprietary) [CD2]

Patches, self-adhesive, fentanyl, '12' patch (releasing approx. 12 micrograms/hour for 72 hours), net price 5 = £17.76; '25' patch (releasing approx. 25 micrograms/hour for 72 hours), 5 = £25.38; '50' patch (releasing approx. 50 micrograms/hour for 72 hours), 5 = £47.40; '75' patch (releasing approx. 75 micrograms/hour for 72 hours), 5 = £66.08; '100' patch (releasing approx. 100 micrograms/hour for 72 hours), 5 = £81.45. Label: 2, counselling, administration

Brands include *Fencino®*, *Fentalis®*, *Matrifen®*, *Mezolar®*, *Osmanil®*, *Tilofyl®*, *Victanyl®*

**Durogesic DTrans®** (Janssen) [CD2]

Patches, self-adhesive, transparent, fentanyl, '12' patch (releasing approx. 12 micrograms/hour for 72 hours), net price 5 = £17.76; '25' patch (releasing approx. 25 micrograms/hour for 72 hours), 5 = £25.38; '50' patch (releasing approx. 50 micrograms/hour for 72 hours), 5 = £47.40; '75' patch (releasing approx. 75 micrograms/hour for 72 hours), 5 = £66.08; '100' patch (releasing approx. 100 micrograms/hour for 72 hours), 5 = £81.45. Label: 2, counselling, administration

## HYDROMORPHONE HYDROCHLORIDE

**Cautions** see notes above; also pancreatitis; toxic psychosis

**Contra-indications** see notes above; also acute abdomen

**Hepatic impairment** see notes above

**Renal impairment** see notes above

**Pregnancy** see notes above

**Breast-feeding** avoid—no information available

**Side-effects** see notes above; also paralytic ileus, peripheral oedema, seizures, asthenia, dyskinesia, agitation, and tremor

**Indications and dose**

Severe pain in cancer

• By mouth

**Child 12–18 years** 1.3 mg every 4 hours, increased if necessary according to severity of pain

**Administration** Swallow whole capsule or sprinkle contents on soft food

**Palladone®** (Napp) [CD2]

Capsules, hydromorphone hydrochloride 1.3 mg (orange/clear), net price 56-cap pack = £8.82; 2.6 mg (red/clear), 56-cap pack = £17.64. Label: 2, counselling, see below

◢ **Modified release**

**Palladone® SR** (Napp) [CD2]

Capsules, m/r, hydromorphone hydrochloride 2 mg (yellow/clear), net price 56-cap pack = £20.98; 4 mg (pale blue/clear), 56-cap pack = £28.75; 8 mg (pink/clear), 56-cap pack = £56.08; 16 mg (brown/clear), 56-cap pack = £106.53; 24 mg (dark blue/clear), 56-cap pack = £159.82. Label: 2, counselling, see below

**Dose**

Severe pain in cancer

• By mouth

**Child 12–18 years** 4 mg every 12 hours, increased if necessary according to severity of pain

**Counselling** Swallow whole or open capsule and sprinkle contents on soft food

## METHADONE HYDROCHLORIDE

**Cautions** see notes above; also history of cardiac conduction abnormalities, family history of sudden death (ECG monitoring recommended; see also QT-interval prolongation, below)

**QT-interval prolongation** Children with the following risk factors for QT-interval prolongation should be carefully monitored while taking methadone: heart or liver disease, electrolyte abnormalities, or concomitant treatment with drugs that can prolong QT interval; children requiring more than 100 mg daily should also be monitored

**Contra-indications** see notes above; also phaeochromocytoma

**Hepatic impairment** see notes above

**Renal impairment** see notes above

**Pregnancy** see notes above

**Breast-feeding** withdrawal symptoms in infant; breast-feeding permissible during maintenance but dose should be as low as possible and infant monitored to avoid sedation

**Side-effects** see notes above; also QT-interval prolongation; torsade de pointes, hypothermia, restlessness, raised intracranial pressure, dysmenorrhoea, dry eyes, and hyperprolactinaemia

**Licensed use** not licensed for use in children

**Indications and dose**

Neonatal opioid withdrawal dose may vary, consult local guidelines

• By mouth

**Neonate** initially 100 micrograms/kg increased by 50 micrograms/kg every 6 hours until symptoms are controlled; for maintenance, total daily dose that controls symptoms given in 2 divided doses; to withdraw, reduce dose over 7–10 days

**Methadone** (Non-proprietary) [CD2]

Oral solution 1 mg/mL, methadone hydrochloride 1 mg/mL, net price 30 mL = 62p, 50 mL = £1.04, 100 mL = £1.27, 500 mL = £11.34. Label: 2

Brands include *Eptadone®*, *Metharose®* (sugar-free), *Physeptone* (also as sugar-free)

> **Safe Practice**
> This preparation is 2½ times the strength of Methadone Linctus; many preparations of this strength are licensed for opioid dependence only but some are also licensed for analgesia in severe pain

## MORPHINE SALTS

**Cautions** see notes above; also pancreatitis, cardiac arrhythmias, severe cor pulmonale

**Contra-indications** see notes above; also delayed gastric emptying, acute abdomen; heart failure secondary to chronic lung disease; phaeochromocytoma

**Hepatic impairment** see notes above

**Renal impairment** see notes above

**Pregnancy** see notes above

**Breast-feeding** therapeutic doses unlikely to affect infant

**Side-effects** see notes above; also paralytic ileus, abdominal pain, anorexia, dyspepsia, exacerbation of pancreatitis, taste disturbance, hypertension, hypothermia, syncope, bronchospasm, inhibition of cough reflex, restlessness, seizures, paraesthesia, asthenia, malaise, disorientation, excitation, agitation, delirium, raised intracranial pressure, amenorrhoea, myoclonus, muscle fasciculation, rhabdomyolysis, nystagmus

**Licensed use** *Oramorph*® solution not licensed for use in children under 1 year; *Oramorph*® unit dose vials not licensed for use in children under 6 years; *Sevredol*® tablets not licensed for use in children under 3 years; *Filnarine*® SR tablets not licensed for use in children under 6 years; *MST Continus*® preparations licensed to treat children with cancer pain (age-range not specified by manufacturer); *MXL*® capsules not licensed for use in children under 1 year; suppositories not licensed for use in children

### Indications and dose

**Pain**

- **By subcutaneous injection**

  **Neonate** initially 100 micrograms/kg every 6 hours, adjusted according to response

  **Child 1–6 months** initially 100–200 micrograms/kg every 6 hours, adjusted according to response

  **Child 6 months–2 years** initially 100–200 micrograms/kg every 4 hours, adjusted according to response

  **Child 2–12 years** initially 200 micrograms/kg every 4 hours, adjusted according to response

  **Child 12–18 years** initially 2.5–10 mg every 4 hours, adjusted according to response

- **By intravenous injection over at least 5 minutes**

  **Neonate** initially 50 micrograms/kg every 6 hours, adjusted according to response

  **Child 1–6 months** initially 100 micrograms/kg every 6 hours, adjusted according to response

  **Child 6 months–12 years** initially 100 micrograms/kg every 4 hours, adjusted according to response

  **Child 12–18 years** initially 5 mg every 4 hours, adjusted according to response

- **By intravenous administration**

  **Neonate** initially *by intravenous injection* (over at least 5 minutes) 50 micrograms/kg then *by continuous intravenous infusion* 5–20 micrograms/kg/hour adjusted according to response

  **Child 1–6 months** initially *by intravenous injection* (over at least 5 minutes) 100 micrograms/kg then *by continuous intravenous infusion* 10–30 micrograms/kg/hour adjusted according to response

  **Child 6 months–12 years** initially *by intravenous injection* (over at least 5 minutes) 100 micrograms/kg then *by continuous intravenous infusion* 20–30 micrograms/kg/hour adjusted according to response

  **Child 12–18 years** initially *by intravenous injection* (over at least 5 minutes) 5 mg then *by continuous intravenous infusion* 20–30 micrograms/kg/hour adjusted according to response

- **By mouth or by rectum**

  **Child 1–3 months** initially 50–100 micrograms/kg every 4 hours, adjusted according to response

  **Child 3–6 months** 100–150 micrograms/kg every 4 hours, adjusted according to response

  **Child 6–12 months** 200 micrograms/kg every 4 hours, adjusted according to response

  **Child 1–2 years** initially 200–300 micrograms/kg every 4 hours, adjusted according to response

  **Child 2–12 years** initially 200–300 micrograms/kg (max. 10 mg) every 4 hours, adjusted according to response

  **Child 12–18 years** initially 5–10 mg every 4 hours, adjusted according to response

- **By continuous subcutaneous infusion**

  **Child 1–3 months** 10 micrograms/kg/hour, adjusted according to response

  **Child 3 months–18 years** 20 micrograms/kg/hour, adjusted according to response

**Neonatal opioid withdrawal** under specialist supervision

- **By mouth**

  **Neonate** initially 40 micrograms/kg every 4 hours until symptoms controlled, increase dose if necessary; reduce frequency gradually over 6–10 days, and stop when 40 micrograms/kg once daily achieved; dose may vary, consult local guidelines

**Administration** for *continuous intravenous infusion*, dilute with Glucose 5% or 10% or Sodium Chloride 0.9%

*Neonatal intensive care*, dilute 2.5 mg/kg body-weight to a final volume of 50 mL with infusion fluid; an intravenous infusion rate of 0.1 mL/hour provides a dose of 5 micrograms/kg/hour

### ◢ Oral solutions

**Note** For advice on transfer from oral solutions of morphine to modified-release preparations of morphine, see Pain Management with Opioids, (p. 16)

**Morphine Oral Solutions**

PoM or CD2

Oral solutions of morphine can be prescribed by writing the formula:
Morphine hydrochloride 5 mg
Chloroform water to 5 mL

**Note** The proportion of morphine hydrochloride may be altered when specified by the prescriber; if above 13 mg per 5 mL the solution becomes CD2. For sample prescription see Controlled Drugs and Drug Dependence, p. 8. It is usual to adjust the strength so that the dose volume is 5 or 10 mL.

**Oramorph**® (Boehringer Ingelheim)
Oramorph® oral solution PoM, morphine sulfate 10 mg/5 mL, net price 100-mL pack = £1.78; 300-mL pack = £4.95; 500-mL pack = £7.47. Label: 2
Oramorph® concentrated oral solution CD2, sugar-free, morphine sulfate 100 mg/5 mL, net price 30-mL pack = £4.98; 120-mL pack = £18.59 (both with calibrated dropper). Label: 2

### ◢ Tablets

**Sevredol**® (Napp) CD2
Tablets, f/c, scored, morphine sulfate 10 mg (blue), net price 56-tab pack = £5.28; 20 mg (pink), 56-tab pack = £10.55; 50 mg (pale green), 56-tab pack = £28.02. Label: 2

### ◢ Modified-release 12-hourly oral preparations

**Filnarine**® SR (Teva UK) CD2
Tablets, m/r, f/c, morphine sulfate 10 mg (pink), net price 60-tab pack = £3.30; 30 mg (blue), 60-tab pack = £7.89; 60 mg (pink), 60-tab pack = £15.39; 100 mg (white), 60-tab pack = £24.37; 200 mg (white), 60-tab pack = £48.74. Label: 2, 25

**Dose**

- **By mouth**

  Every 12 hours, dose adjusted according to daily morphine requirements; for further advice on determining dose, see Pain Management with Opioids, (p. 16); dosage requirements should be reviewed if the brand is altered

**Note** Prescriptions must also specifiy 'tablets' (i.e. 'Filnarine SR tablets')

**4**

**Central nervous system**

**MST Continus®** (Napp) [CD2]

Tablets, m/r, f/c, morphine sulfate 5 mg (white), net price 60-tab pack = £3.29; 10 mg (brown), 60-tab pack = £5.16; 15 mg (green), 60-tab pack = £9.61; 30 mg (purple), 60-tab pack = £12.40; 60 mg (orange), 60-tab pack = £24.20; 100 mg (grey), 60-tab pack = £38.30; 200 mg (green), 60-tab pack = £76.62. Label: 2, 25

Suspension (= sachet of granules to mix with water), m/r, pink, morphine sulfate 20 mg/sachet, net price 30-sachet pack = £24.58; 30 mg/sachet, 30-sachet pack = £25.54; 60 mg/sachet, 30-sachet pack = £51.09; 100 mg/sachet, 30-sachet pack = £85.15; 200 mg/sachet pack, 30-sachet pack = £170.30. Label: 2, 13

**Dose**

- **By mouth**

  Every 12 hours, dose adjusted according to daily morphine requirements; for further advice on determining dose, see Pain Management with Opioids, (p. 16); dosage requirements should be reviewed if the brand is altered

**Note** Prescriptions must also specify 'tablets' or 'suspension' (i.e. 'MST Continus tablets' or 'MST Continus suspension')

◢ **Modified-release 24-hourly oral preparations**

**MXL®** (Napp) [CD2]

Capsules, m/r, morphine sulfate 30 mg (light blue), net price 28-cap pack = £10.91; 60 mg (brown), 28-cap pack = £14.95; 90 mg (pink), 28-cap pack = £22.04; 120 mg (green), 28-cap pack = £29.15; 150 mg (blue), 28-cap pack = £36.43; 200 mg (red-brown), 28-cap pack = £46.15. Label: 2, counselling, see below

**Dose**

- **By mouth**

  Every 24 hours, dose adjusted according to daily morphine requirements; for further advice on determining dose, see Pain Management with Opioids, (p. 16); dosage requirements should be reviewed if the brand is altered

**Counselling** Swallow whole or open capsule and sprinkle contents on soft food

**Note** Prescriptions must also specify 'capsules' (i.e. 'MXL capsules')

◢ **Suppositories**

**Morphine** (Non-proprietary) [CD2]

Suppositories, morphine sulfate 10 mg, net price 12 = £11.21; 15 mg, 12 = £8.85; 30 mg, 12 = £13.47. Label: 2

**Note** Both the strength of the suppositories and the morphine salt contained in them must be specified by the prescriber

Other strengths of morphine sulfate suppositories available from 'special-order' manufacturers or specialist importing companies, see p. 823

◢ **Injections**

**Morphine Sulfate** (Non-proprietary) [CD2]

Injection, morphine sulfate 10, 15, 20, and 30 mg/mL, net price 1- and 2-mL amp (all) = 72p–£1.40

Intravenous infusion, morphine sulfate 1 mg/mL, net price 50-mL vial = £5.00; 2 mg/mL, 50-mL vial = £5.89

**Minijet®** **Morphine Sulphate** (UCB Pharma) [CD2]

Injection, morphine sulfate 1 mg/mL, net price 10-mL disposable syringe = £15.00

◢ **Injection with antiemetic**

For prescribing information on cyclizine, see section 4.6

**Caution** **Not** recommended in palliative care, see Nausea and Vomiting, p. 18

**Cyclimorph®** (Amdipharm) [CD2]

Cyclimorph-10® Injection, morphine tartrate 10 mg, cyclizine tartrate 50 mg/mL, net price 1-mL amp = £1.75

**Dose**

**Moderate to severe pain** (short-term use only)

- **By subcutaneous, intramuscular, or intravenous injection**

  **Child 12–18 years** 1 mL, repeated not more often than every 4 hours, max. 3 doses in any 24-hour period

Cyclimorph-15® Injection, morphine tartrate 15 mg, cyclizine tartrate 50 mg/mL, net price 1-mL amp = £1.82

**Dose**

**Moderate to severe pain** (short-term use only)

- **By subcutaneous, intramuscular, or intravenous injection**

  **Child 12–18 years** 1 mL, repeated not more often than every 4 hours, max. 3 doses in any 24-hour period

## ■ OXYCODONE HYDROCHLORIDE

**Cautions** see notes above; also toxic psychosis; pancreatitis

**Contra-indications** see notes above; also acute abdomen; delayed gastric emptying; chronic constipation; cor pulmonale; acute porphyria (section 9.8.2)

**Hepatic impairment** max. initial dose 2.5 mg every 6 hours in children not currently treated with an opioid with mild impairment; avoid in moderate to severe impairment; see also notes above

**Renal impairment** max. initial dose 2.5 mg every 6 hours in children not currently treated with an opioid with mild to moderate impairment; avoid if estimated glomerular filtration rate less than 10 mL/minute/1.73m²; see also notes above

**Pregnancy** see notes above

**Breast-feeding** present in milk—avoid

**Side-effects** see notes above; also diarrhoea, abdominal pain, anorexia, dyspepsia; bronchospasm, dyspnoea, impaired cough reflex; asthenia, anxiety; chills; *less commonly* paralytic ileus, cholestasis, gastritis, flatulence, dysphagia, taste disturbance, belching, hiccups, vasodilatation, supraventricular tachycardia, syncope, amnesia, hypoaesthesia, restlessness, seizures, hypotonia, paraesthesia, disorientation, malaise, agitation, speech disorder, tremor, pyrexia, amenorrhoea, thirst, dehydration, muscle fasciculation, and dry skin

**Licensed use** not licensed for use in children

**Indications and dose**

**Moderate to severe pain in palliative care** (see also Pain Management with Opioids, (p. 16))

- **By mouth**

  **Child 1 month–12 years** initially 200 micrograms/kg (up to 5 mg) every 4–6 hours, dose increased if necessary according to severity of pain

  **Child 12–18 years** initially 5 mg every 4–6 hours, dose increased if necessary according to severity of pain

**Oxycodone** (Non-proprietary) (CD2)

Oral solution, oxycodone hydrochloride 5 mg/5 mL, net price 250-mL pack = £8.70. Label: 2

Concentrated oral solution, oxycodone hydrochloride 10 mg/mL, net price 120-mL pack = £41.80. Label: 2

**Oxynorm**® (Napp) (CD2)

Capsules, oxycodone hydrochloride 5 mg (orange/beige), net price 56-cap pack = £11.36; 10 mg (white/beige), 56-cap pack = £22.73; 20 mg (pink/beige), 56-cap pack = £45.47. Label: 2

Liquid (= oral solution), sugar-free, oxycodone hydrochloride 5 mg/5 mL, net price 250 mL = £9.66. Label: 2

Concentrate (= concentrated oral solution), sugar-free, oxycodone hydrochloride 10 mg/mL, net price 120 mL = £46.39. Label: 2

◀ **Modified release**

**OxyContin**® (Napp) (CD2)

Tablets, f/c, m/r, oxycodone hydrochloride 5 mg (blue), net price 28-tab pack = £12.46; 10 mg (white), 56-tab pack = £24.91; 15 mg (grey), 56-tab pack = £37.41; 20 mg (pink), 56-tab pack = £49.82; 30 mg (brown), 56-tab pack = £74.81; 40 mg (yellow), 56-tab pack = £99.66; 60 mg (red), 56-tab pack = £149.66; 80 mg (green), 56-tab pack = £199.33; 120 mg (purple), 56-tab pack = £299.31. Label: 2, 25

**Dose**

**Moderate to severe pain in palliative care**

● By mouth

**Child 8–12 years** initially, 5 mg every 12 hours, increased if necessary according to severity of pain

**Child 12–18 years** initially, 10 mg every 12 hours, increased if necessary according to severity of pain

■ **PAPAVERETUM** ◢

**Safe Practice**

Do **not** confuse with papaverine

A mixture of 253 parts of morphine hydrochloride, 23 parts of papaverine hydrochloride and 20 parts of codeine hydrochloride

To avoid confusion, the figures of 7.7 mg/mL or 15.4 mg/mL should be used for prescribing purposes

**Cautions**  see notes above; supraventricular tachycardia

**Contra-indications**  see notes above; heart failure secondary to chronic lung disease; phaeochromocytoma

**Hepatic impairment**  see notes above

**Renal impairment**  see notes above

**Pregnancy**  see notes above

**Breast-feeding**  therapeutic doses unlikely to affect infant

**Side-effects**  see notes above; also hypothermia

**Indications and dose**

**Premedication, postoperative analgesia, severe chronic pain**

● By subcutaneous or intramuscular injection

**Neonate** 115 micrograms/kg repeated every 4 hours if necessary

**Child 1–12 months** 154 micrograms/kg repeated every 4 hours if necessary

**Child 1–6 years** 1.93–3.85 mg repeated every 4 hours if necessary

**Child 6–12 years** 3.85–7.7 mg repeated every 4 hours if necessary

**Child 12–18 years** 7.7–15.4 mg repeated every 4 hours if necessary

● By intravenous injection

Generally 25–50% of the corresponding subcutaneous or intramuscular dose

**Papaveretum** (Non-proprietary) (CD2) ◢

Injection, papaveretum 15.4 mg/mL (providing the equivalent of 10 mg of anhydrous morphine/mL), net price 1-mL amp = £1.64

■ **PETHIDINE HYDROCHLORIDE**
  (Meperidine)

**Cautions**  see notes above; not suitable for severe continuing pain; accumulation of metabolites may result in neurotoxicity; cardiac arrhythmias, severe cor pulmonale

**Contra-indications**  see notes above; phaeochromocytoma

**Hepatic impairment**  see notes above

**Renal impairment**  see notes above

**Pregnancy**  see notes above

**Breast-feeding**  present in milk but not known to be harmful

**Side-effects**  see notes above; also restlessness, tremor, and hypothermia; convulsions reported in overdosage

**Indications and dose**

**Obstetric analgesia**

● By subcutaneous or by intramuscular injection

**Child 12–18 years** 1 mg/kg (max. 100 mg), repeated 1–3 hours later if necessary; max. 400 mg in 24 hours

**Pethidine** (Non-proprietary) (CD2)

Injection, pethidine hydrochloride 50 mg/mL, net price 1-mL amp = 48p, 2-mL amp = 51p; 10 mg/mL, 5-mL amp = £3.17, 10-mL amp = £2.18

■ **TRAMADOL HYDROCHLORIDE**

**Cautions**  see notes above; impaired consciousness; excessive bronchial secretions; not suitable as substitute in opioid-dependent patients

General anaesthesia Not recommended for analgesia during potentially light planes of general anaesthesia (possibly increased intra-operative recall reported)

**Contra-indications**  see notes above; uncontrolled epilepsy

**Hepatic impairment**  see notes above

**Renal impairment**  see notes above

**Pregnancy**  embryotoxic in *animal* studies—manufacturer advises avoid; see also notes above

**4** Central nervous system

**Breast-feeding** amount probably too small to be harmful, but manufacturer advises avoid

**Side-effects** see notes above; also diarrhoea, retching, fatigue, paraesthesia; *less commonly* gastritis, and flatulence; *rarely* anorexia, syncope, hypertension, bronchospasm, dyspnoea, wheezing, seizures, and muscle weakness; blood disorders also reported

**Licensed use** not licensed for use in children under 12 years

**Indications and dose**

Moderate to severe pain

* By mouth

  **Child 12–18 years** 50–100 mg not more often than every 4 hours; total of more than 400 mg daily not usually required

* By intravenous injection (over 2–3 minutes) or by intravenous infusion or by intramuscular injection

  **Child 12–18 years** 50–100 mg every 4–6 hours

Postoperative pain

* By intravenous injection (over 2–3 minutes)

  **Child 12–18 years** 100 mg initially then 50 mg every 10–20 minutes if necessary up to total max. 250 mg (including initial dose) in first hour, *then* 50–100 mg every 4–6 hours; max. 600 mg daily

**Administration** for *intravenous infusion*, dilute with Glucose 5% *or* Sodium Chloride 0.9%

**Tramadol Hydrochloride** (Non-proprietary) ᴾᵒᴹ

Capsules, tramadol hydrochloride 50 mg, net price 30-cap pack = £1.22, 100-cap pack = £2.07. Label: 2

Oral drops, tramadol hydrochloride 100 mg/mL (2.5 mg/drop), net price 10 mL = £3.50. Label: 2, 13

Injection, tramadol hydrochloride 50 mg/mL, net price 2-mL amp = 95p

**Zamadol®** (Meda) ᴾᵒᴹ

Capsules, tramadol hydrochloride 50 mg, net price 100-cap pack = £8.00. Label: 2

Orodispersible tablets (*Zamadol Melt®*), tramadol hydrochloride 50 mg, net price 60-tab pack = £7.12. Label: 2, counselling, administration

**Excipients** include aspartame (section 9.4.1)

**Counselling** *Zamadol Melt®* should be sucked and then swallowed. May also be dispersed in water

Injection, tramadol hydrochloride 50 mg/mL, net price 2-mL amp = £1.10

**Zydol®** (Grünenthal) ᴾᵒᴹ

Capsules, green/yellow, tramadol hydrochloride 50 mg, net price 30-cap pack = £2.29, 100-cap pack = £7.63. Label: 2

Soluble tablets, tramadol hydrochloride 50 mg, net price 20-tab pack = £2.79, 100-tab pack = £13.33. Label: 2, 13

Injection, tramadol hydrochloride 50 mg/mL, net price 2-mL amp = 80p

◢ **Modified-release 12-hourly preparations**

**Larapam® SR** (Sandoz) ᴾᵒᴹ

Tablets, m/r, tramadol hydrochloride 100 mg, net price 60-tab pack = £17.55; 150 mg, 60-tab pack = £27.35; 200 mg, 60-tab pack = £36.50. Label: 2, 25

**Dose**

Moderate to severe pain

* By mouth

  **Child 12–18 years** initially 100 mg twice daily increased if necessary; usual max. 200 mg twice daily

**Mabron®** (Morningside) ᴾᵒᴹ

Tablets, m/r, tramadol hydrochloride 100 mg, net price 60-tab pack = £18.26; 150 mg, 60-tab pack = £27.39; 200 mg, 60-tab pack = £36.52. Label: 2, 25

**Dose**

Moderate to severe pain

* By mouth

  **Child 12–18 years** 100 mg twice daily increased if necessary; usual max. 200 mg twice daily

**Marol®** (Morningside) ᴾᵒᴹ

Tablets, m/r, tramadol hydrochloride 100 mg, net price 60-tab pack = £9.12; 150 mg, 60-tab pack = £13.68; 200 mg, 60-tab pack = £18.24. Label: 2, 25

**Dose**

Moderate to severe pain

* By mouth

  **Child 12–18 years** 100 mg twice daily increased if necessary; usual max. 200 mg twice daily

**Maxitram SR®** (Chiesi) ᴾᵒᴹ

Capsules, m/r, tramadol hydrochloride 50 mg (white), net price 60-cap pack = £4.55; 100 mg (yellow), 60-cap pack = £12.14; 150 mg (yellow), 60-cap pack = £18.21; 200 mg (yellow), 60-cap pack = £24.28. Label: 2, 25

**Dose**

Moderate to severe pain

* By mouth

  **Child 12–18 years** initially 100 mg twice daily increased if necessary; usual max. 200 mg twice daily

**Tramquel SR®** (Meda) ᴾᵒᴹ

Capsules, m/r, tramadol hydrochloride 50 mg (dark green), net price 60-cap pack = £7.20; 100 mg (white), 60-cap pack = £14.39; 150 mg (dark green), 60-cap pack = £21.59; 200 mg (yellow), 60-cap pack = £28.78. Label: 2, counselling, administration

**Dose**

Moderate to severe pain

* By mouth

  **Child 12–18 years** 50–100 mg twice daily increased if necessary; usual max. 200 mg twice daily

**Administration** Swallow whole or open capsule and swallow contents immediately without chewing

**Zamadol® SR** (Meda) [PoM]

Capsules, m/r, tramadol hydrochloride 50 mg (green), net price 60-cap pack = £7.20; 100 mg, 60-cap pack = £14.39; 150 mg (dark green), 60-cap pack = £21.59; 200 mg (yellow), 60-cap pack = £28.78. Label: 2, counselling, administration

**Dose**

**Moderate to severe pain**

- By mouth

   **Child 12–18 years** 50–100 mg twice daily increased if necessary to 150–200 mg twice daily; total of more than 400 mg daily not usually required

**Administration** Swallow whole or open capsule and swallow contents immediately without chewing

**Zeridame® SR** (Actavis) [PoM]

Tablets, m/r, tramadol hydrochloride 100 mg, net price 60-tab pack = £17.21; 150 mg, 60-tab pack = £25.82; 200 mg, 60-tab pack = £34.43. Label: 2, 25

**Dose**

**Moderate to severe pain**

- By mouth

   **Child 12–18 years** 100 mg twice daily, increased if necessary; usual max. 200 mg twice daily

**Zydol SR®** (Grünenthal) [PoM]

Tablets, m/r, f/c, tramadol hydrochloride 50 mg (yellow), net price 60-tab pack = £4.60; 100 mg, 60-tab pack = £18.26; 150 mg (beige), 60-tab pack = £27.39; 200 mg (orange), 60-tab pack = £36.52. Label: 2, 25

**Dose**

**Moderate to severe pain**

- By mouth

   **Child 12–18 years** 50–100 mg twice daily increased if necessary to 150–200 mg twice daily; total of more than 400 mg daily not usually required

◢**Modified-release 24-hourly preparations**

**Tradorec XL®** (MSD) [PoM]

Tablets, m/r, tramadol hydrochloride 100 mg, net price 30-tab pack = £14.10; 200 mg, 30-tab pack = £14.98; 300 mg, 30-tab pack = £22.47. Label: 2, 25

**Dose**

**Moderate to severe pain**

- By mouth

   **Child 12–18 years** initially 100 mg once daily, increased if necessary to max. 400 mg once daily

**Zamadol® 24hr** (Meda) [PoM]

Tablets, f/c, m/r, tramadol hydrochloride 150 mg, net price 28-tab pack = £10.70; 200 mg, 28-tab pack = £14.26; 300 mg, 28-tab pack = £21.39; 400 mg, 28-tab pack = £28.51. Label: 2, 25

**Dose**

**Moderate to severe pain**

- By mouth

   **Child 12–18 years** initially 150 mg once daily increased if necessary; max. 400 mg once daily

**Zydol XL®** (Grünenthal) [PoM]

Tablets, m/r, f/c, tramadol hydrochloride 150 mg, net price 30-tab pack = £12.18; 200 mg, 30-tab pack = £17.98; 300 mg, 30-tab pack = £24.94; 400 mg, 30-tab pack = £32.47. Label: 2, 25

**Dose**

**Moderate to severe pain**

- By mouth

   **Child 12–18 years** 150 mg once daily increased if necessary; more than 400 mg once daily not usually required

◢**With paracetamol**

section 4.7.1

## 4.7.3 Neuropathic pain

Neuropathic pain, which occurs as a result of damage to neural tissue, includes *compression neuropathies, peripheral neuropathies* (e.g. due to diabetes, HIV infection, chemotherapy), *trauma, idiopathic neuropathy, central pain* (e.g. pain following spinal cord injury and syringomyelia), *postherpetic neuralgia,* and *phantom limb pain.* The pain may occur in an area of sensory deficit and may be described as burning, shooting or scalding; it may be accompanied by pain that is evoked by a non-noxious stimulus (allodynia).

Children with chronic neuropathic pain require multidisciplinary management, which may include physiotherapy and psychological support. Neuropathic pain is generally managed with a tricyclic antidepressant such as **amitriptyline** (p. 185) or antiepileptic drugs such as **carbamazepine** (p. 219). Children with localised pain may benefit from **topical local anaesthetic** preparations section 15.2, particularly while awaiting specialist review. Neuropathic pain may respond only partially to **opioid analgesics**. A corticosteroid may help to relieve pressure in compression neuropathy and thereby reduce pain.

For the management of neuropathic pain in palliative care see Pain, (p. 16).

**Chronic facial pain**   Chronic oral and facial pain including persistent idiopathic facial pain (also termed 'atypical facial pain') and temporomandibular dysfunction (previously termed temporomandibular joint pain dysfunction syndrome) may call for prolonged use of analgesics or for other drugs. Tricyclic antidepressants (section 4.3.1) may be useful for facial pain [unlicensed indication], but are not on the Dental Practitioners' List. Disorders of this type require specialist referral and psychological support to accompany drug treatment. Children on long-term therapy need to be monitored both for progress and for side-effects.

## 4.7.4 Antimigraine drugs

4.7.4.1   Treatment of acute migraine

4.7.4.2   Prophylaxis of migraine

4.7.4.3   Cluster headache and the trigeminal autonomic cephalalgias

### 4.7.4.1 Treatment of acute migraine

Treatment of a migraine attack should be guided by response to previous treatment and the severity of the attacks. A **simple analgesic** such as paracetamol (preferably in a soluble or dispersible form) or an NSAID, usually ibuprofen, is often effective; concomitant **antiemetic** treatment may be required. If treatment with an analgesic is inadequate, an attack may be treated with a specific antimigraine compound such as the $5HT_1$-receptor agonist **sumatriptan**. **Ergot alkaloids** are associated with many side-effects and should be avoided.

Excessive use of acute treatments for migraine (opioid and non-opioid analgesics, $5HT_1$-receptor agonists, and ergotamine) is associated with medication-overuse headache (analgesic-induced headache); therefore, increasing consumption of these medicines needs careful management.

**4**

**Central nervous system**

## 5HT$_1$-receptor agonists

5HT$_1$-receptor agonists are used in the treatment of acute migraine attacks; treatment of children should be initiated by a specialist. The 5HT$_1$-receptor agonists ('triptans') act on the 5HT (serotonin) 1B/1D receptors and they are therefore sometimes referred to as 5HT$_{1B/1D}$-receptor agonists. A 5HT$_1$-receptor agonist may be used during the established headache phase of an attack and is the preferred treatment in those who fail to respond to conventional analgesics. 5HT$_1$-receptor agonists are **not** indicated for the treatment of hemiplegic, basilar, or opthalmoplegic migraine.

If a child does not respond to one 5HT$_1$-receptor agonist, an alternative 5HT$_1$-receptor agonist should be tried. For children who have prolonged attacks that frequently recur despite treatment with a 5HT$_1$-receptor agonist, combination therapy with an NSAID such as naproxen can be considered. **Sumatriptan** and **zolmitriptan** are used for migraine in children. They may also be of value in cluster headache (see also section 4.7.4.3).

**Cautions** See **interactions**: Appendix 1 (5HT$_1$ agonists).

## SUMATRIPTAN

**Cautions** see under 5HT$_1$-receptor agonists above; pre-existing cardiac disease; history of seizures; sensitivity to sulfonamides; **interactions**: Appendix 1 (5HT$_1$ agonists)
**Skilled tasks** Drowsiness may affect performance of skilled tasks (e.g. driving)
**Contra-indications** vasospasm; previous cerebrovascular accident or transient ischaemic attack; peripheral vascular disease; moderate and severe hypertension
**Hepatic impairment** reduce dose of oral therapy; avoid in severe impairment
**Renal impairment** use with caution
**Pregnancy** limited experience—avoid unless potential benefit outweighs risk
**Breast-feeding** present in milk but amount probably too small to be harmful; withhold breast-feeding for 12 hours
**Side-effects** nausea, vomiting; sensations of tingling, heat, heaviness, pressure, or tightness of any part of the body (including throat and chest—discontinue if intense, may be due to coronary vasoconstriction or to anaphylaxis), transient increase in blood pressure, flushing; dyspnoea; drowsiness, dizziness, weakness; myalgia; *also reported* diarrhoea, ischaemic colitis, hypotension, bradycardia or tachycardia, palpitation, arrhythmias, myocardial infarction, Raynaud's syndrome, anxiety, seizures, tremor, dystonia, nystagmus, arthralgia, visual disturbances, sweating; epistaxis with nasal spray
**Licensed use** tablets and injection not licensed for use in children; not licensed for treating cluster headache in children; intranasal dose for migraine not licensed

### Indications and dose

Treatment of acute migraine
• By mouth
**Child 6–10 years** 25 mg as a single dose, repeated once after at least 2 hours if migraine recurs
**Child 10–12 years** 50 mg as a single dose, repeated once after at least 2 hours if migraine recurs

**Child 12–18 years** 50–100 mg as a single dose, repeated once after at least 2 hours if migraine recurs
• By subcutaneous injection (using auto-injector)
**Child 10–18 years** 6 mg as a single dose, repeated once after at least 1 hour if migraine recurs; max. 12 mg in 24 hours
• Intranasally
**Child 12–18 years** 10–20 mg as a single dose, repeated once after at least 2 hours if migraine recurs; max. 40 mg in 24 hours

Treatment of acute cluster headache (under specialist supervision)
• By subcutaneous injection (using auto-injector)
**Child 10–18 years** 6 mg as a single dose, repeated once after at least 1 hour if headache recurs; max. 12 mg in 24 hours
• Intranasally
**Child 12–18 years** 10–20 mg as a single dose, repeated once after at least 2 hours if headache recurs; max. 40 mg in 24 hours

**Note** Child not responding to initial dose should not take second dose for same attack

**[1]Sumatriptan** (Non-proprietary) ▪PoM▪
Tablets, sumatriptan (as succinate) 50 mg, net price 6-tab pack = £1.71; 100 mg, 6-tab pack = £2.43. Label: 3, 10, patient information leaflet

**Imigran**® (GSK) ▪PoM▪
Tablets, sumatriptan (as succinate) 50 mg, net price 6-tab pack = £26.54; 100 mg, 6-tab pack = £42.90. Label: 3, 10, patient information leaflet

Injection, sumatriptan (as succinate) 12 mg/mL (= 6 mg/0.5-mL syringe), net price, treatment pack (2 × 0.5-mL prefilled syringes and auto-injector) = £42.47; refill pack 2 × 0.5-mL prefilled cartridges = £40.41. Label: 3, 10, patient information leaflet

Nasal spray, sumatriptan 10 mg/0.1-mL actuation, net price 2 unit-dose spray device = £11.80; 20 mg/0.1-mL actuation, 2 unit-dose spray device = £11.80, 6 unit-dose spray device = £35.39. Label: 3, 10, patient information leaflet

**Imigran Radis**® (GSK) ▪PoM▪
Tablets, f/c, sumatriptan (as succinate) 50 mg (pink), net price 6-tab pack = £23.90; 100 mg (white), 6-tab pack = £42.90. Label: 3, 10, patient information leaflet

## ZOLMITRIPTAN

**Cautions** see under 5HT$_1$-receptor agonists above; should not be taken within 24 hours of any other 5HT$_1$-receptor agonist; **interactions**: Appendix 1 (5HT$_1$ agonists)
**Contra-indications** vasospasm; Wolff-Parkinson-White syndrome or arrhythmias associated with accessory cardiac conduction pathways; previous cerebrovascular accident or transient ischaemic attack; ischaemic heart disease; uncontrolled hypertension

1. Sumatriptan 50 mg tablets can be sold to the public to treat previously diagnosed migraine; max. daily dose 100 mg

**Hepatic impairment** max. 5 mg in 24 hours in moderate or severe impairment

**Pregnancy** limited experience—avoid unless potential benefit outweighs risk

**Breast-feeding** use with caution—present in milk in *animal* studies

**Side-effects** abdominal pain, dry mouth, nausea, vomiting; palpitation, sensations of tingling, heat, heaviness, pressure, or tightness of any part of the body (including throat and chest—discontinue if intense, may be due to coronary vasoconstriction or to anaphylaxis); dizziness, drowsiness, headache, paraesthesia, asthenia; myalgia, muscle weakness; *less commonly* tachycardia, transient increase in blood pressure, polyuria; *rarely* urticaria; *very rarely* gastrointestinal and splenic infarction, ischaemic colitis, angina pectoris, myocardial infarction; *with nasal spray*, taste disturbance, and epistaxis

**Licensed use** not licensed for use in children

**Indications and dose**

> Treatment of acute migraine
> * By mouth
>> **Child 12–18 years** 2.5 mg, repeated after not less than 2 hours if migraine recurs (if response unsatisfactory after 3 attacks consider increasing dose to 5 mg or switching to alternative treatment); max. 10 mg in 24 hours
> * Intranasally
>> **Child 12–18 years** 5 mg (1 spray) into 1 nostril, repeated after not less than 2 hours if migraine recurs; max. 10 mg in 24 hours

> Treatment of acute cluster headache
> * Intranasally
>> **Child 12–18 years** 5 mg (1 spray) into 1 nostril, repeated after not less than 2 hours if headache recurs; max. 10 mg in 24 hours

**Zomig**® (AstraZeneca) [PoM]
Tablets, f/c, yellow, zolmitriptan 2.5 mg, net price 6-tab pack = £18.00, 12-tab pack = £36.00
Orodispersible tablets (*Zomig Rapimelt*®), zolmitriptan 2.5 mg, net price 6-tab pack = £17.90; 5 mg, 6-tab pack = £22.80. Counselling, administration
Counselling *Zomig Rapimelt*® should be placed on the tongue, allowed to disperse and swallowed
Excipients include aspartame equivalent to phenylalanine 2.81 mg/tablet (section 9.4.1)
Nasal spray, zolmitriptan 5 mg/0.1-mL unit-dose spray device, net price 6 unit-dose sprays = £36.50

## Antiemetics

Antiemetics (section 4.6), including **metoclopramide**, **domperidone**, phenothiazines, and antihistamines, relieve the nausea associated with migraine attacks. Antiemetics may be given by intramuscular injection or rectally if vomiting is a problem. Metoclopramide and domperidone have the added advantage of promoting gastric emptying and normal peristalsis; a single dose should be given at the onset of symptoms (**important:** for warnings relating to extrapyramidal effects of metoclopramide see p. 192 and p. 196).

**4.7.4.2 Prophylaxis of migraine**

Where migraine attacks are frequent, possible provoking factors such as stress should be sought; combined oral contraceptives may also provoke migraine. Preventive treatment should be considered if migraine attacks interfere with school and social life, particularly for children who:

* suffer at least two attacks a month;
* suffer an increasing frequency of headaches;
* suffer significant disability despite suitable treatment for migraine attacks;
* cannot take suitable treatment for migraine attacks.

In children it is often possible to stop prophylaxis after a period of treatment.

**Propranolol** (section 2.4) may be effective in preventing migraine in children but it is contra-indicated in those with asthma. Side-effects such as depression and postural hypotension can further limit its use.

**Pizotifen**, an antihistamine and serotonin antagonist, may also be used but its efficacy in children has not been clearly established. Common side-effects include drowsiness and weight gain.

**Topiramate** (section 4.8.1) is licensed for migraine prophylaxis.

### PIZOTIFEN

**Cautions** urinary retention; susceptibility to angle-closure glaucoma; history of epilepsy; avoid abrupt withdrawal; **interactions:** Appendix 1 (pizotifen)
Skilled tasks Drowsiness may affect performance of skilled tasks (e.g. driving); effects of alcohol enhanced

**Hepatic impairment** use with caution

**Renal impairment** use with caution

**Pregnancy** avoid unless potential benefit outweighs risk

**Breast-feeding** amount probably too small to be harmful, but manufacturer advises avoid

**Side-effects** dry mouth, nausea, dizziness, drowsiness, increased appetite, weight gain; *less commonly* constipation; *rarely* anxiety, aggression, insomnia, paraesthesia, hallucination, depression, arthralgia, myalgia; *very rarely* seizures; jaundice, hepatitis, and muscle cramps also reported

**Licensed use** 1.5-mg tablets not licensed for use in children

**Indications and dose**

> Prophylaxis of migraine
> * By mouth
>> **Child 5–18 years** initially 500 micrograms at night increased gradually up to 1.5 mg daily in divided doses; max. single dose (at night) 1 mg

**Pizotifen** (Non-proprietary) [PoM]
Tablets, pizotifen (as hydrogen malate), 500 micrograms, net price 28-tab pack = £1.28; 1.5 mg, 28-tab pack = £2.17. Label: 2

**Sanomigran**® (Novartis) [PoM]
Tablets, both ivory-yellow, s/c, pizotifen (as hydrogen malate), 500 micrograms, net price 60-tab pack = £2.06; 1.5 mg, 28-tab pack = £3.42. Label: 2
Elixir, pizotifen (as hydrogen malate) 250 micrograms/5 mL, net price 300 mL = £3.61. Label: 2

4

Central nervous system

### 4.7.4.3 Cluster headache and the trigeminal autonomic cephalalgias

Cluster headache rarely responds to standard analgesics. **Sumatriptan** given by subcutaneous injection is the drug of choice for the *treatment* of cluster headache. If an injection is unsuitable, sumatriptan nasal spray or **zolmitriptan** nasal spray may be used. Treatment should be initiated by a specialist. Alternatively, 100% **oxygen** at a rate of 10–15 litres/minute for 10–20 minutes is useful in aborting an attack.

The other trigeminal autonomic cephalalgias, paroxysmal hemicrania (sensitive to indometacin), and short-lasting unilateral neuralgiform headache attacks with conjunctival injection and tearing, are seen rarely and are best managed by a specialist.

## 4.8 Antiepileptics

| 4.8.1 | Control of the epilepsies |
| 4.8.2 | Drugs used in status epilepticus |
| 4.8.3 | Febrile convulsions |

### 4.8.1 Control of the epilepsies

The decision about when to start treatment with an antiepileptic drug and the choice of medication depends on frequency and type of seizures, neurological findings, the identification of an epilepsy syndrome, and the wishes of the child and carers. For the majority of children, epilepsy is controlled with a single antiepileptic drug.

The object of treatment is to prevent the occurrence of seizures by maintaining an effective dose of one or more antiepileptic drugs. Careful adjustment of doses is necessary, starting with low doses and increasing gradually until seizures are controlled or there are significant adverse effects.

When choosing an antiepileptic drug to use, the seizure type, epilepsy syndrome, concomitant medication, co-morbidity, age, and sex should be taken into account. For women of child-bearing age, see Pregnancy, p. 217 and Breast-feeding, p. 218.

The frequency of administration is often determined by the plasma-drug half-life, and should be kept as low as possible to encourage better adherence. Most antiepileptics, when used in usual dosage, can be given twice daily. Lamotrigine, perampanel, phenobarbital and phenytoin, which have long half-lives, can be given as a daily dose at bedtime. However, with large doses, some antiepileptics may need to be given 3 times daily to avoid adverse effects associated with high peak plasma-drug concentrations. Young children metabolise some antiepileptics more rapidly than adults and therefore may require more frequent doses and a higher amount per kilogram body-weight.

**Management**   When monotherapy with a first-line antiepileptic drug has failed, monotherapy with a second drug should be tried; the diagnosis should be checked before starting an alternative drug if the first drug showed lack of efficacy. The change from one antiepileptic drug to another should be cautious, slowly withdrawing the first drug only when the new regimen

has been established. Combination therapy with two or more antiepileptic drugs may be necessary, but the concurrent use of antiepileptic drugs increases the risk of adverse effects and drug interactions (see below). If combination therapy does not bring about worthwhile benefits, revert to the regimen (monotherapy or combination therapy) that provided the best balance between tolerability and efficacy.

**Interactions**   Interactions between antiepileptics are complex and may increase toxicity without a corresponding increase in antiepileptic effect. Interactions are usually caused by hepatic enzyme induction or inhibition; displacement from protein binding sites is not usually a problem. These interactions are highly variable and unpredictable.

For interactions of antiepileptic drugs, see **Appendix 1**; for advice on hormonal contraception and enzyme-inducing drugs, see section 7.3.1 and section 7.3.2.

Significant interactions that occur **between antiepileptics** and that may affect dosing requirements are as follows:

> **Note**
> Check under each drug for possible interactions when two or more antiepileptic drugs are used

**Carbamazepine**

*often lowers* plasma concentration of clobazam, clonazepam, lamotrigine, perampanel, phenytoin (but may also raise plasma-phenytoin concentration), tiagabine, topiramate, valproate, and an active metabolite of oxcarbazepine

*sometimes lowers* plasma concentration of ethosuximide, primidone (but tendency for corresponding increase in plasma-phenobarbital concentration), and rufinamide

*sometimes raises* plasma concentration of phenobarbital and primidone-derived phenobarbital

**Ethosuximide**

*sometimes raises* plasma concentration of phenytoin

**Lamotrigine**

*sometimes raises* plasma concentration of an active metabolite of carbamazepine (but evidence is conflicting)

**Oxcarbazepine**

*often lowers* plasma concentration of perampanel

*sometimes lowers* plasma concentration of carbamazepine (but may raise plasma concentration of an active metabolite of carbamazepine)

*sometimes raises* plasma concentration of phenytoin

*often raises* plasma concentration of phenobarbital and primidone-derived phenobarbital

**Phenobarbital** *or* **Primidone**

*often lowers* plasma concentration of clonazepam, lamotrigine, phenytoin (but may also raise plasma-phenytoin concentration), tiagabine, valproate, and an active metabolite of oxcarbazepine

*sometimes lowers* plasma concentration of ethosuximide, rufinamide, and topiramate

**Phenytoin**

*often lowers* plasma concentration of clonazepam, carbamazepine, lamotrigine, perampanel, tiagabine, topiramate, valproate, and an active metabolite of oxcarbazepine

*often raises* plasma concentration of phenobarbital and primidone-derived phenobarbital

*sometimes lowers* plasma concentration of ethosuximide, primidone (by increasing conversion to phenobarbital), and rufinamide

**Rufinamide**

*sometimes lowers* plasma concentration of carbamazepine

*sometimes raises* plasma concentration of phenytoin

**Stiripentol**

*often raises* plasma concentration of carbamazepine, clobazam, phenobarbital, primidone-derived phenobarbital, and phenytoin

**Topiramate**

*often lowers* plasma concentration of perampanel

*sometimes raises* plasma concentration of phenytoin

**Valproate**

*sometimes lowers* plasma concentration of an active metabolite of oxcarbazepine

*often raises* plasma concentration of lamotrigine, phenobarbital, primidone-derived phenobarbital, phenytoin (but may also lower), and an active metabolite of carbamazepine

*sometimes raises* plasma concentration of ethosuximide and rufinamide

**Vigabatrin**

*often lowers* plasma concentration of phenytoin

**Withdrawal** Antiepileptics should be withdrawn under specialist supervision. Avoid abrupt withdrawal, particularly of barbiturates and benzodiazepines because this can precipitate severe rebound seizures. Reduction in dosage should be gradual and, in the case of barbiturates, the withdrawal process may take months.

The decision to withdraw antiepileptics from a seizure-free child, and its timing, depends on individual circumstances such as the type of epilepsy and its cause. Even in children who have been seizure-free for several years, there is a significant risk of seizure recurrence on drug withdrawal.

Drugs should be gradually withdrawn over at least 2–3 months by reducing the daily dose by 10–25% at intervals of 1–2 weeks. Benzodiazepines may need to be withdrawn over 6 months or longer.

In children receiving several antiepileptic drugs, only one drug should be withdrawn at a time.

**Monitoring** Routine measurement of plasma concentrations of antiepileptic drugs is not usually justified, because the target concentration ranges are arbitrary and often vary between individuals. However, plasma-drug concentrations may be measured in children with worsening seizures, status epilepticus, suspected non-compliance, or suspected toxicity. Similarly, haematological and biochemical monitoring should not be undertaken unless clinically indicated.

Plasma concentration of some medications may change during pregnancy and monitoring may be required (see under Pregnancy, below).

**Antiepileptic hypersensitivity syndrome** Antiepileptic hypersensitivity syndrome is a rare but potentially fatal syndrome associated with some antiepileptic drugs (**carbamazepine, lacosamide, lamotrigine, oxcarbazepine, phenobarbital, phenytoin, primidone,** and **rufinamide**); rarely cross-sensitivity occurs between some of these antiepileptic drugs. Some other antiepileptic drugs (**eslicarbazepine, stiripentol,** and **zonisamide**) have a theoretical risk. The symptoms usually start between 1 and 8 weeks of exposure; fever, rash, and lymphadenopathy are most commonly seen. Other systemic signs include liver dysfunction, haematological, renal, and pulmonary abnormalities, vasculitis, and multi-organ failure. If signs or symptoms of hypersensitivity syndrome occur, the drug should be withdrawn immediately, the child should not be re-exposed, and expert advice should be sought.

**Driving** Older children with epilepsy may drive a motor vehicle (but not a large goods or passenger carrying vehicle) provided that they have been seizure-free for one year or, if subject to attacks only while asleep, have established a 3-year period of asleep attacks without awake attacks. Those affected by drowsiness should not drive or operate machinery.

Guidance issued by the Drivers Medical Unit of the Driver and Vehicle Licensing Agency (DVLA) recommends that patients should be advised not to drive during medication changes or withdrawal of antiepileptic drugs, and for 6 months afterwards.

Patients who have had a first or single epileptic seizure must not drive for 6 months (5 years in the case of large goods or passenger carrying vehicles) after the event; driving may then be resumed, provided the patient has been assessed by a specialist as fit to drive because no abnormality was detected on investigation.

**Pregnancy** Young women of child-bearing potential should discuss with a specialist the impact of both epilepsy, and its treatment, on the outcome of pregnancy.

There is an increased risk of teratogenicity associated with the use of antiepileptic drugs (especially if used during the first trimester and particularly if the patient takes two or more antiepileptic drugs). Valproate is associated with the highest risk of major and minor congenital malformations, and with developmental delay. Valproate should not be prescribed unless there is no safer alternative and only after a careful discussion of the risks; doses greater than 1 g daily are associated with an increased risk of teratogenicity. There is also an increased risk of teratogenicity with phenytoin, primidone, phenobarbital, lamotrigine, and carbamazepine. Topiramate carries an increased risk of cleft palate if taken in the first trimester of pregnancy. There is not enough evidence to establish the risk of teratogenicity with other antiepileptic drugs.

Prescribers should also consider carefully the choice of antiepileptic therapy in pre-pubescent girls who may later become pregnant.

Young women of child-bearing potential who take antiepileptic drugs should be given contraceptive advice. Some antiepileptic drugs can reduce the efficacy of hormonal contraceptives, and the efficacy of some antiepileptics may be affected by hormonal contraceptives (see section 7.3.1 and interactions of antiepileptics, Appendix 1).

Young women who want to become pregnant should be referred to a specialist for advice in advance of conception. For some women, the severity of seizure or the seizure type may not pose a serious threat, and drug withdrawal may be considered; therapy may be resumed after the first trimester. If treatment with antiepileptic drugs must continue throughout pregnancy, then monotherapy is preferable at the lowest effective dose.

Once an unplanned pregnancy is discovered it is usually too late for changes to be made to the treatment regimen; the risk of harm to the mother and fetus from convulsive seizures outweighs the risk of continued therapy. The likelihood of a young woman who is taking antiepileptic drugs having a baby with no malformations is at least 90%, and it is important that women do not stop taking essential treatment because of concern over harm to the fetus.

To reduce the risk of neural tube defects, folate supplementation (section 9.1.2) is advised before conception and throughout the first trimester.

The concentration of antiepileptic drugs in the plasma can change during pregnancy. Doses of phenytoin p. 226, carbamazepine, and lamotrigine should be adjusted on the basis of plasma-drug concentration monitoring; the dose of other antiepileptic drugs should be monitored carefully during pregnancy and after birth, and adjustments made on a clinical basis. Plasma-drug concentration monitoring during pregnancy is also useful to check compliance. Additionally, in patients taking topiramate or levetiracetam, it is recommended that fetal growth is monitored.

Young women who have seizures in the second half of pregnancy should be assessed for eclampsia before any change is made to antiepileptic treatment. Status epilepticus should be treated according to the standard protocol, see section 4.8.2.

Routine injection of vitamin K (section 9.6.6) at birth minimises the risk of neonatal haemorrhage associated with antiepileptics.

Withdrawal effects in the newborn may occur with some antiepileptic drugs, in particular benzodiazepines and phenobarbital, and can take several days to diminish.

### Epilepsy and Pregnancy Register

All pregnant women with epilepsy, whether taking medication or not, should be encouraged to notify the UK Epilepsy and Pregnancy Register (Tel: 0800 389 1248).

**Breast-feeding**   Young women taking antiepileptic monotherapy should generally be encouraged to breast-feed; if a young woman is on combination therapy or if there are other risk factors, such as premature birth, specialist advice should be sought.All infants should be monitored for sedation, feeding difficulties, adequate weight gain, and developmental milestones. Infants should also be monitored for adverse effects associated with the antiepileptic drug particularly with newer antiepileptics, if the antiepileptic is readily transferred into breast-milk causing high infant serum-drug concentrations (e.g. ethosuximide, lamotrigine, and primidone), or if slower metabolism in the infant causes drugs to accumulate (e.g. phenobarbital and lamotrigine). Serum-drug concentration monitoring should be undertaken in breast-fed infants if suspected adverse reactions develop; if toxicity develops it may be necessary to introduce formula feeds to limit the infant's drug exposure, or to wean the infant off breast-milk altogether.

Primidone, phenobarbital, and the benzodiazepines are associated with an established risk of drowsiness in breast-fed babies and caution is required.

Withdrawal effects may occur in infants if a mother suddenly stops breast-feeding, particularly if she is taking phenobarbital, primidone, or lamotrigine.

## Focal seizures with or without secondary generalisation

**Carbamazepine** and **lamotrigine** are the drugs of choice for focal seizures; **levetiracetam**, **oxcarbazepine** and **sodium valproate** can be considered if these are unsuitable. Other drugs that may be used as adjunctive treatment include **clobazam**, **gabapentin**, and **topiramate**.

## Generalised seizures

**Tonic-clonic seizures**   The drug of choice for tonic-clonic seizures in children is **sodium valproate**, or **lamotrigine** where sodium valproate is unsuitable. **Carbamazepine** or **oxcarbazepine** can also be considered. Other drugs that may be used as adjunctive treatment include **clobazam**, **levetiracetam** and **topiramate**.

**Absence seizures**   **Ethosuximide** and sodium valproate are the drugs of choice for absence seizures; lamotrigine can be used if these are unsuitable. Sodium valproate is also highly effective in treating the generalised tonic-clonic seizures which can co-exist with absence seizures in idiopathic primary generalised epilepsy. Second-line therapy includes clobazam, **clonazepam**, levetiracetam, topiramate or **zonisamide**.

**Myoclonic seizures**   Myoclonic seizures (myoclonic jerks) occur in a variety of syndromes, and response to treatment varies considerably. Sodium valproate is the drug of choice; consider levetiracetam or topiramate if sodium valproate is unsuitable. Second-line therapy includes clobazam, clonazepam, piracetam or **zonisamide**.

**Tonic and atonic seizures**   Tonic or atonic seizures are treated with sodium valproate; lamotrigine can be considered as adjunctive treatment if sodium valproate is ineffective or not tolerated.Second-line therapy includes **rufinamide** and topiramate.

## Epilepsy syndromes

**Infantile spasms**   Vigabatrin is the drug of choice for infantile spasms associated with tuberous sclerosis. In spasms of other causes, high doses of corticosteroids, such as **prednisolone** (section 6.3.2) or **tetracosactide** (section 6.5.1), may be more effective.

**Dravet syndrome**   Sodium valproate or **topiramate** is the treatment of choice in severe myoclonic epilepsy in infancy. **Clobazam** or **stiripentol** may be considered as adjunctive treatment.

**Lennox-Gastaut syndrome**   Sodium valproate is the first-line drug for treating Lennox-Gastaut syndrome; **lamotrigine** can be used as adjunctive treatment if sodium valproate is ineffective or not tolerated. **Rufinamide** and topiramate may be considered by tertiary epilepsy specialists.

**Landau-Kleffner syndrome**  Always discuss with or refer to tertiary epilepsy specialists.

**Neonatal seizures**  Seizures can occur before delivery, but they are most common up to 24 hours after birth. Seizures in neonates occur as a result of biochemical disturbances, inborn errors of metabolism, hypoxic ischaemic encephalopathy, drug withdrawal, meningitis, stroke, cerebral haemorrhage or malformation, or severe jaundice (kernicterus).

Seizures caused by biochemical imbalance and those in neonates with inherited abnormal pyridoxine or biotin metabolism should be corrected by treating the underlying cause (section 9.6.2). Seizures caused by drug withdrawal following intra-uterine exposure are treated with a drug withdrawal regimen.

**Phenobarbital** can be used to manage neonatal seizures where there is a risk of recurrence; **phenytoin** is an alternative. Benzodiazepines (such as **clonazepam** (p. 234) and **midazolam** (p. 236)) and **rectal paraldehyde** (p. 236) may also be useful in the management of acute neonatal seizures. Lidocaine (p. 85) may be used if other treatments are unsuccessful; lidocaine should not be given to neonates who have received phenytoin infusion because of the risk of cardiac toxicity.

## Carbamazepine and oxcarbazepine

**Carbamazepine** is a drug of choice for focal seizures. It can exacerbate myoclonic and absence seizures. It is essential to initiate carbamazepine therapy at a low dose and build this up slowly in small increments every 3–7 days. Some side-effects (such as headache, ataxia, drowsiness, nausea, vomiting, blurring of vision, dizziness, unsteadiness, and allergic skin reactions) are dose-related, and may be dose-limiting. These side-effects are more common at the start of treatment. They may be reduced by altering the timing of medication or by using a modified-release preparation.

**Oxcarbazepine** is licensed as monotherapy or adjunctive therapy for the treatment of focal seizures with or without secondary generalised tonic-clonic seizures.

## ■ CARBAMAZEPINE

**Cautions**  cardiac disease (see also Contra-indications); skin reactions (see also Blood, Hepatic, or Skin disorders, below and under Side-effects); test for HLA-B*1502 allele in individuals of Han Chinese or Thai origin (avoid unless no alternative—risk of Stevens-Johnson syndrome in the presence of HLA-B*1502 allele); history of haematological reactions to other drugs; manufacturer recommends blood counts and hepatic and renal function tests (but evidence of practical value uncertain); may exacerbate absence and myoclonic seizures; consider vitamin D supplementation in patients who are immobilised for long periods or who have inadequate sun exposure or dietary intake of calcium; susceptibility to angle-closure glaucoma; cross-sensitivity reported with oxcarbazepine, and with phenytoin (see also Anti-epileptic Hypersensitivity Syndrome, p. 217); avoid abrupt withdrawal; **interactions**: see p. 216 and Appendix 1 (carbamazepine)

**Blood, hepatic, or skin disorders**  Children or their carers should be told how to recognise signs of blood, liver, or skin disorders, and advised to seek immediate medical attention if symptoms such as fever, rash, mouth ulcers, bruising, or bleeding develop. Carbamazepine should be withdrawn immediately in cases of aggravated liver dysfunction or acute liver disease. Leucopenia that is severe, progressive, or associated with clinical symptoms requires withdrawal (if necessary under cover of a suitable alternative).

**Contra-indications**  AV conduction abnormalities (unless paced); history of bone-marrow depression; acute porphyria (section 9.8.2)

**Hepatic impairment**  metabolism impaired in advanced liver disease; see also Blood, Hepatic, or Skin Disorders, above

**Renal impairment**  use with caution

**Pregnancy**  see Pregnancy, p. 217; monitor plasma-carbamazepine concentration

**Breast-feeding**  amount probably too small to be harmful but monitor infant for possible adverse reactions; see also Breast-feeding, p. 218

**Side-effects**  see notes above; also dry mouth, nausea, vomiting, oedema, ataxia, dizziness, drowsiness, fatigue, headache, hyponatraemia (leading in rare cases to water intoxication), blood disorders (including eosinophilia, leucopenia, thrombocytopenia, haemolytic anaemia, and aplastic anaemia), dermatitis, urticaria; *less commonly* diarrhoea, constipation, involuntary movements (including nystagmus), visual disturbances; *rarely* abdominal pain, anorexia, hepatitis, jaundice, vanishing bile duct syndrome, cardiac conduction disorders, hypertension, hypotension, peripheral neuropathy, dysarthria, aggression, agitation, confusion, depression, hallucinations, restlessness, paraesthesia, lymph node enlargement, muscle weakness, systemic lupus erythematosus, delayed multi-organ hypersensitivity disorder (see also Anti-epileptic Hypersensitivity Syndrome, p. 217); *very rarely* pancreatitis, stomatitis, hepatic failure, taste disturbance, exacerbation of coronary artery disease, AV block with syncope, circulatory collapse, hypercholesterolaemia, thrombophlebitis, thromboembolism, pulmonary hypersensitivity (with dyspnoea, pneumonitis, or pneumonia), psychosis, neuroleptic malignant syndrome, osteomalacia (see Cautions), osteoporosis, galactorrhoea, gynaecomastia, impaired male fertility, interstitial nephritis, renal failure, sexual dysfunction, urinary frequency, urinary retention, arthralgia, muscle pain, muscle spasm, conjunctivitis, angle-closure glaucoma, hearing disorders, acne, alterations in skin pigmentation, alopecia, hirsutism, sweating, photosensitivity, purpura, Stevens-Johnson syndrome, toxic epidermal necrolysis, aseptic meningitis; suicidal ideation

**Pharmacokinetics**  plasma concentration for optimum response 4–12 mg/litre (20–50 micromol/litre) measured after 1–2 weeks

**Licensed use**  *suppositories* not licensed for use in trigeminal neuralgia or prophylaxis of bipolar disorder

**Indications and dose**

**Focal and generalised tonic-clonic seizures, trigeminal neuralgia, prophylaxis of bipolar disorder**

- By mouth

  **Child 1 month–12 years** initially 5 mg/kg at night or 2.5 mg/kg twice daily, increased as necessary by 2.5–5 mg/kg every 3–7 days; usual maintenance dose 5 mg/kg 2–3 times daily; doses up to 20 mg/kg daily have been used

  **Child 12–18 years** initially 100–200 mg 1–2 times daily, increased slowly to usual maintenance dose 200–400 mg 2–3 times daily; in some cases doses up to 1.8 g daily may be needed

• **By rectum**
  **Child 1 month–18 years** use approx. 25% more than the oral dose (max. 250 mg) up to 4 times daily

**Note** Different preparations may vary in bioavailability; to avoid reduced effect or excessive side-effects, it may be prudent to avoid changing the formulation

**Administration** Oral liquid has been used rectally— should be retained for at least 2 hours (but may have laxative effect)

**Carbamazepine** (Non-proprietary) PoM
Tablets, carbamazepine 100 mg, net price 28 = £5.69; 200 mg, 28 = £4.99; 400 mg, 28 = £6.59. Label: 3, 8, counselling, blood, hepatic or skin disorder symptoms (see above), driving (see notes above)
**Dental prescribing on NHS** Carbamazepine Tablets may be prescribed

**Tegretol®** (Novartis) PoM
Tablets, scored, carbamazepine 100 mg, net price 84-tab pack = £2.07; 200 mg, 84-tab pack = £3.83; 400 mg, 56-tab pack = £5.02. Label: 3, 8, counselling, blood, hepatic or skin disorder symptoms (see above), driving (see notes above)

Chewtabs, orange, carbamazepine 100 mg, net price 56-tab pack = £3.16; 200 mg, 56-tab pack = £5.88. Label: 3, 8, 21, 24, counselling, blood, hepatic or skin disorder symptoms (see above), driving (see notes above)

Liquid, sugar-free, carbamazepine 100 mg/5 mL. Net price 300-mL pack = £6.12. Label: 3, 8, counselling, blood, hepatic or skin disorder symptoms (see above), driving (see notes above)

Suppositories, carbamazepine 125 mg, net price 5 = £8.03; 250 mg, 5 = £10.71. Label: 3, 8, counselling, blood, hepatic or skin disorder symptoms (see above), driving (see notes above)

**Dose**
> **Epilepsy** for short-term use (max. 7 days) when oral therapy temporarily not possible

**Note** Suppositories of 125 mg may be considered to be approximately equivalent in therapeutic effect to tablets of 100 mg but final adjustment should always depend on clinical response (plasma concentration monitoring recommended); max. dose *by rectum* 250 mg 4 times daily

◢**Modified release**
**Carbagen® SR** (Generics) PoM
Tablets, m/r, f/c, scored, carbamazepine 200 mg, net price 56-tab pack = £5.20; 400 mg, 56-tab pack = £10.24. Label: 3, 8, 25, counselling, blood, hepatic or skin disorder symptoms (see above), driving (see notes above)
**Dose**
> **Child 5–18 years** as above; total daily dose given in 1–2 divided doses

**Tegretol® Prolonged Release** (Novartis) PoM
Tablets, m/r, scored, carbamazepine 200 mg (beige-orange), net price 56-tab pack = £5.20; 400 mg (brown-orange), 56-tab pack = £10.24. Label: 3, 8, 25, counselling, blood, hepatic or skin disorder symptoms (see above), driving (see notes above)
**Dose**
> **Child 5–18 years** as above; total daily dose given in 2 divided doses

**Administration** *Tegretol® Prolonged Release* tablets can be halved but should not be chewed

## ◢ OXCARBAZEPINE

**Cautions** hypersensitivity to carbamazepine (see also Antiepileptic Hypersensitivity Syndrome, p. 217); avoid abrupt withdrawal; hyponatraemia (monitor plasma-sodium concentration in patients at risk), heart failure (monitor body-weight), cardiac conduction disorders; avoid in acute porphyria (section 9.8.2); interactions: see p. 216 and Appendix 1 (oxcarbazepine)

**Blood, hepatic, or skin disorders** Children or their carers should be told how to recognise signs of blood, liver, or skin disorders, and advised to seek immediate medical attention if symptoms such as lethargy, confusion, muscular twitching, fever, rash, blistering, mouth ulcers, bruising, or bleeding develop

**Hepatic impairment** caution in severe impairment— no information available

**Renal impairment** halve initial dose if estimated glomerular filtration rate less than 30 mL/minute/$1.73\,m^2$, increase according to response at intervals of at least 1 week

**Pregnancy** see Pregnancy, p. 217

**Breast-feeding** amount probably too small to be harmful but manufacturer advises avoid; see also Breast-feeding, p. 218

**Side-effects** nausea, vomiting, constipation, diarrhoea, abdominal pain, dizziness, headache, drowsiness, agitation, amnesia, asthenia, ataxia, confusion, impaired concentration, depression, tremor, hyponatraemia, acne, alopecia, rash, nystagmus, visual disorders including diplopia; *less commonly* urticaria, leucopenia; *very rarely* hepatitis, pancreatitis, arrhythmias, blood disorders, multi-organ hypersensitivity (see also Antiepileptic Hypersensitivity Syndrome, p. 217), systemic lupus erythematosus, Stevens-Johnson syndrome, and toxic epidermal necrolysis; hypertension and hypothyroidism also reported; suicidal ideation

**Indications and dose**

> **Monotherapy and adjunctive therapy of focal seizures with or without secondary generalised tonic-clonic seizures**
>
> • **By mouth**
>   **Child 6–18 years** initially 4–5 mg/kg (max. 300 mg) twice daily, increased according to response in steps of up to 5 mg/kg twice daily at weekly intervals (usual maintenance dose for adjunctive therapy 15 mg/kg twice daily); max. 23 mg/kg twice daily

**Note** In adjunctive therapy the dose of concomitant antiepileptics may need to be reduced when using high doses of oxcarbazepine

**Oxcarbazepine** (Non-proprietary) PoM
Tablets, oxcarbazepine 150 mg, net price 50-tab pack = £11.02; 300 mg, 50-tab pack = £22.38; 600 mg, 50-tab pack = £44.72. Label: 3, 8, counselling, blood, hepatic or skin disorders (see above), driving (see notes above)

**Trileptal®** (Novartis) PoM
Tablets, f/c, scored, oxcarbazepine 150 mg (green), net price 50-tab pack = £10.20; 300 mg (yellow), 50-tab pack = £20.40; 600 mg (pink), 50-tab pack = £40.80. Label: 3, 8, counselling, blood, hepatic or skin disorders (see above), driving (see notes above)
Oral suspension, sugar-free, oxcarbazepine 300 mg/5 mL, net price 250 mL (with oral syringe) = £40.80. Label: 3, 8, counselling, blood, hepatic or skin disorders (see above), driving (see notes above)
**Excipients** include propylene glycol (see Excipients, p. 2)

## Ethosuximide

Ethosuximide is used for absence seizures.

### ETHOSUXIMIDE

**Cautions** avoid abrupt withdrawal; avoid in acute porphyria (section 9.8.2); **interactions:** see p. 216 and Appendix 1 (ethosuximide)

**Blood disorders** Children or their carers should be told how to recognise signs of blood disorders, and advised to seek immediate medical attention if symptoms such as fever, mouth ulcers, bruising, or bleeding develop

**Hepatic impairment** use with caution

**Renal impairment** use with caution

**Pregnancy** see Pregnancy, p. 217

**Breast-feeding** present in milk; hyperexcitability and sedation reported; see also Breast-feeding, p. 218

**Side-effects** gastro-intestinal disturbances (including nausea, vomiting, diarrhoea, abdominal pain, and anorexia), weight loss; *less frequently* headache, fatigue, drowsiness, dizziness, hiccup, ataxia, euphoria, irritability, aggression, and impaired concentration; *rarely* tongue swelling, sleep disturbances, depression, psychosis, photophobia, dyskinesia, increased libido, vaginal bleeding, myopia, gingival hypertrophy, rash; *also reported* hyperactivity, increase in seizure frequency, blood disorders (including leucopenia, agranulocytosis, pancytopenia, and aplastic anaemia—blood counts required if features of infection), systemic lupus erythematosus, Stevens-Johnson syndrome; suicidal ideation

#### Indications and dose

**Absence seizures, atypical absence, myoclonic seizures**

- By mouth

    **Child 1 month–6 years** initially 5 mg/kg (max. 125 mg) twice daily, increased every 5–7 days up to maintenance dose of 10–20 mg/kg (max. 500 mg) twice daily; total daily dose may rarely be given in 3 divided doses

    **Child 6–18 years** initially 250 mg twice daily, increased by 250 mg at intervals of 5–7 days to usual dose of 500–750 mg twice daily; occasionally up to 1 g twice daily may be needed

**Ethosuximide** (Non-proprietary) [PoM]

Capsules, ethosuximide 250 mg, net price 56-cap pack = £38.23. Label: 8, counselling, blood disorders (see above), driving (see notes above)

**Emeside®** (Chemidex) [PoM]

Syrup, black currant, ethosuximide 250 mg/5 mL, net price 200-mL pack = £6.60. Label: 8, counselling, blood disorders (see above), driving (see notes above)

**Zarontin®** (Pfizer) [PoM]

Syrup, yellow, ethosuximide 250 mg/5 mL, net price 200-mL pack = £4.22. Label: 8, counselling, blood disorders (see above), driving (see notes above)

## Gabapentin

Gabapentin is used as adjunctive therapy for the treatment of focal seizures with or without secondary generalisation; it can be used as monotherapy in children over 12 years.

### GABAPENTIN

**Cautions** avoid abrupt withdrawal; diabetes mellitus; mixed seizures (including absences); false positive readings with some urinary protein tests; history of psychotic illness; high doses of oral solution in adolescents with low body-weight—see preparations below; **interactions:** Appendix 1 (gabapentin)

**Renal impairment** reduce dose if estimated glomerular filtration rate less than 80 mL/minute/1.73 m$^2$; consult product literature

**Pregnancy** see Pregnancy, p. 217

**Breast-feeding** present in milk—manufacturer advises use only if potential benefit outweighs risk; see also Breast-feeding, p. 218

**Side-effects** nausea, vomiting, gingivitis, diarrhoea, abdominal pain, dyspepsia, constipation, dry mouth or throat, flatulence, weight gain, increased appetite, anorexia, hypertension, vasodilatation, oedema, dyspnoea, cough, hostility, confusion, emotional lability, depression, vertigo, anxiety, nervousness, abnormal thoughts, drowsiness, dizziness, malaise, ataxia, convulsions, movement disorders, speech disorder, amnesia, tremor, insomnia, headache, paraesthesia, nystagmus, abnormal reflexes, fever, flu syndrome, impotence, leucopenia, arthralgia, myalgia, twitching, visual disturbances, rhinitis, rash, pruritus, acne; *less commonly* palpitation; *also reported* pancreatitis, hepatitis, hallucinations, blood glucose fluctuations in children with diabetes, breast hypertrophy, gynaecomastia, acute renal failure, incontinence, thrombocytopenia, tinnitus, Stevens-Johnson syndrome, alopecia, hypersensitivity syndrome; suicidal ideation

**Licensed use** not licensed for use in children under 6 years; not licensed at doses over 50 mg/kg daily in children under 12 years

#### Indications and dose

**Adjunctive treatment of focal seizures with or without secondary generalisation**

- By mouth

    **Child 2–6 years** 10 mg/kg once daily on day 1, then 10 mg/kg twice daily on day 2, then 10 mg/kg 3 times daily on day 3, increased according to response to usual dose of 30–70 mg/kg daily in 3 divided doses

    **Child 6–12 years** 10 mg/kg (max. 300 mg) once daily on day 1, then 10 mg/kg (max. 300 mg) twice daily on day 2, then 10 mg/kg (max. 300 mg) 3 times daily on day 3; usual dose 25–35 mg/kg daily in 3 divided doses; max. 70 mg/kg daily in 3 divided doses

    **Child 12–18 years** 300 mg once daily on day 1, then 300 mg twice daily on day 2, then 300 mg 3 times daily on day 3 *or* initially 300 mg 3 times daily on day 1; then increased according to response in steps of 300 mg (in 3 divided doses) every 2–3 days; usual dose 0.9–3.6 g daily in 3 divided doses (max. 1.6 g 3 times daily)

**Monotherapy for focal seizures with or without secondary generalisation**

- By mouth

    **Child 12–18 years** 300 mg once daily on day 1, then 300 mg twice daily on day 2, then 300 mg 3 times daily on day 3 *or* initially 300 mg 3 times daily on day 1; then increased according to

**4 Central nervous system**

response in steps of 300 mg (in 3 divided doses) every 2–3 days; usual dose 0.9–3.6 g daily in 3 divided doses (max. 1.6 g 3 times daily)

**Note** Some children may not tolerate daily increments; longer intervals (up to weekly) may be more appropriate

**Administration** capsules can be opened but the bitter taste is difficult to mask

**Gabapentin** (Non-proprietary) PoM

Capsules, gabapentin 100 mg, net price 100-cap pack = £3.57; 300 mg, 100-cap pack = £8.83; 400 mg, 100-cap pack = £5.53. Label: 3, 5, 8, counselling, driving (see notes above)

Tablets, gabapentin 600 mg, net price 100-tab pack = £24.85; 800 mg, 100-tab pack= £36.42. Label: 3, 5, 8, counselling, driving (see notes above)

Oral solution, gabapentin 50 mg/mL, net price 150-mL pack = £57.50. Label: 3, 5, 8, counselling, driving (see notes above)

**Excipients** include propylene glycol (see Excipients, p. 2)

**Important** The levels of propylene glycol, acesulfame K and saccharin sodium may exceed the recommended WHO daily intake limits if high doses of gabapentin oral solution (Rosemont brand) are given to adolescents with low body-weight (39–50 kg)—consult product literature

**Electrolytes** $Na^+$ 0.031 mmol/mL, $K^+$ 0.097 mmol/mL

**Neurontin®** (Pfizer) PoM

Capsules, gabapentin 100 mg (white), net price 100-cap pack = £18.29; 300 mg (yellow), 100-cap pack = £42.40; 400 mg (orange), 100-cap pack = £49.06. Label: 3, 5, 8, counselling, driving (see notes above)

Tablets, f/c, gabapentin 600 mg, net price 100-tab pack = £84.80; 800 mg, 100-tab pack = £98.13. Label: 3, 5, 8, counselling, driving (see notes above)

## Lacosamide

**Lacosamide** is licensed for adjunctive treatment of focal seizures with or without secondary generalisation.

The *Scottish Medicines Consortium* (p. 3) has advised (January 2009) that lacosamide (*Vimpat®*) is accepted for restricted use within NHS Scotland as adjunctive treatment for focal seizures with or without secondary generalisation in patients from 16 years. It is restricted for specialist use in refractory epilepsy.

### LACOSAMIDE

**Cautions** risk of PR-interval prolongation (including conduction problems, severe cardiac disease, and concomitant use of drugs that prolong PR interval), elderly; **interactions:** Appendix 1 (lacosamide)

**Contra-indications** second- or third-degree AV block

**Hepatic impairment** caution in severe impairment—no information available

**Renal impairment** titrate dose with caution; max. 250 mg daily if estimated glomerular filtration rate is less than 30 mL/minute/1.73 $m^2$

**Pregnancy** see Pregnancy, p. 217

**Breast-feeding** manufacturer advises avoid—present in milk in *animal* studies; see also Breast-feeding, p. 218

**Side-effects** nausea, vomiting, constipation, flatulence, dizziness, headache, impaired coordination, cognitive disorder, drowsiness, tremor, depression, fatigue, abnormal gait, blurred vision, nystagmus, pruritus; *rarely* multi-organ hypersensitivity reaction (see Antiepileptic Hypersensitivity Syndrome, p. 217); *also reported* dyspepsia, dry mouth, AV block, bradycardia, PR-interval prolongation, atrial fibrillation, atrial flutter, aggression, agitation, psychosis, euphoria, confusion, hypoesthesia, dysarthria, irritability, muscle spasm, tinnitus, rash; suicidal ideation

**Indications and dose**

**Adjunctive treatment of focal seizures with or without secondary generalisation**

- **By mouth or by intravenous infusion over 15–60 minutes (for up to 5 days)**

  **Child 16–18 years** initially 50 mg twice daily, increased in steps of 50 mg twice daily every week; max. 200 mg twice daily

**Administration** for *intravenous infusion*, give undiluted or dilute with Glucose 5% *or* Sodium Chloride 0.9%

**Vimpat®** (UCB Pharma) PoM

Tablets, f/c, lacosamide 50 mg (pink), net price 14-tab pack = £10.81; 100 mg (yellow), 14-tab pack = £21.62, 56-tab pack = £86.50; 150 mg (salmon), 14-tab pack = £32.44, 56-tab pack £129.74; 200 mg (blue), 56-tab pack = £144.16. Label: 8, counselling, driving (see notes above)

Syrup, yellow-brown, sugar-free, strawberry flavoured, lacosamide 10 mg/mL, net price 200-mL pack = £25.74. Label: 8, counselling, driving (see notes above)

**Excipients** include aspartame (section 9.4.1), propylene glycol (see Excipients)

Intravenous infusion, lacosamide 10 mg/mL net price 200-mg vial = £29.70

**Electrolytes** $Na^+$ 2.6 mmol/200-mg vial

## Lamotrigine

**Lamotrigine** is an antiepileptic for focal seizures, primary and secondary generalised tonic-clonic seizures, and for typical absence seizures; it may exacerbate myoclonic seizures. Efficacy may not be maintained in all children treated for typical absence seizures. It may be tried for atypical absence, atonic, and tonic seizures. Lamotrigine may cause serious skin reactions; dose recommendations should be adhered to closely.

Lamotrigine is used either as sole treatment or as an adjunct to treatment with other antiepileptic drugs. Valproate increases plasma-lamotrigine concentration, whereas the enzyme-inducing antiepileptics reduce it; care is therefore required in choosing the appropriate initial dose and subsequent titration. When the potential for interaction is not known, treatment should be initiated with lower doses, such as those used with valproate.

### LAMOTRIGINE

**Cautions** closely monitor and consider withdrawal if rash, fever, or signs of hypersensitivity syndrome develop; avoid abrupt withdrawal (taper off over 2 weeks or longer) unless serious skin reaction occurs; myoclonic seizures (may be exacerbated); **interactions:** see p. 216 and Appendix 1 (lamotrigine)

**Blood disorders** Children and their carers should be alert for symptoms and signs suggestive of bone-marrow failure, such as anaemia, bruising, or infection. Aplastic anaemia, bone-marrow depression, and pancytopenia have been associated rarely with lamotrigine

4 Central nervous system

**Hepatic impairment**  halve dose in moderate impairment; quarter dose in severe impairment

**Renal impairment**  caution in renal failure; metabolite may accumulate; consider reducing maintenance dose in significant impairment

**Pregnancy**  see Pregnancy, p. 217

**Breast-feeding**  present in milk, but limited data suggest no harmful effect on infant; see also Breast-feeding, p. 218

**Side-effects**  nausea, vomiting, diarrhoea, dry mouth, aggression, agitation, headache, drowsiness, dizziness, tremor, insomnia, ataxia, back pain, arthralgia, nystagmus, diplopia, blurred vision, rash (see Skin Reactions, below); *rarely* conjunctivitis; *very rarely* hepatic failure, movement disorders, unsteadiness, increase in seizure frequency, confusion, hallucination, blood disorders (including anaemia, leucopenia, thrombocytopenia, pancytopenia—see Blood Disorders, above), hypersensitivity syndrome (see Antiepileptic Hypersensitivity Syndrome, p. 217), lupus erythematosus-like reactions; *also reported* suicidal ideation, aseptic meningitis

**Skin reactions**  Serious skin reactions including Stevens-Johnson syndrome and toxic epidermal necrolysis have developed (especially in children); most rashes occur in the first 8 weeks. Rash is sometimes associated with hypersensitivity syndrome (see Side-effects, above) and is more common in patients with history of allergy or rash from other antiepileptic drugs. Consider withdrawal if rash or signs of hypersensitivity syndrome develop. Factors associated with increased risk of serious skin reactions include concomitant use of valproate, initial lamotrigine dosing higher than recommended, and more rapid dose escalation than recommended.

**Counselling**  Warn children and their carers to see their doctor immediately if rash or signs or symptoms of hypersensitivity syndrome develop (see Antiepileptic Hypersensitivity Syndrome, p. 217)

**Indications and dose**

**Monotherapy and adjunctive treatment of focal seizures and primary and secondary generalised tonic-clonic seizures; seizures associated with Lennox-Gastaut syndrome**

• **By mouth**

**Adjunctive therapy of seizures *with valproate***

**Child 2–12 years** initially 150 micrograms/kg once daily for 14 days (those weighing under 13 kg may receive 2 mg on alternate days for first 14 days) then 300 micrograms/kg once daily for further 14 days, thereafter increased by max. of 300 micrograms/kg every 7–14 days; usual maintenance 1–5 mg/kg daily in 1–2 divided doses; max. daily dose 200 mg

**Child 12–18 years** initially 25 mg on alternate days for 14 days then 25 mg daily for further 14 days, thereafter increased by max. 50 mg every 7–14 days; usual maintenance 100–200 mg daily in 1–2 divided doses

**Adjunctive therapy of seizures (with enzyme inducing drugs) *without valproate***

**Child 2–12 years** initially 300 micrograms/kg twice daily for 14 days then 600 micrograms/kg twice daily for further 14 days, thereafter increased by max. 1.2 mg/kg every 7–14 days; usual maintenance 5–15 mg/kg daily in 1–2 divided doses; max. daily dose 400 mg

**Child 12–18 years** initially 50 mg daily for 14 days then 50 mg twice daily for further 14 days, thereafter increased by max. 100 mg every 7–14 days;

usual maintenance 100–200 mg twice daily (up to 700 mg daily has been required)

**Adjunctive therapy of seizures (without enzyme inducing drugs) *without valproate***

**Child 2–12 years** initially 300 micrograms/kg daily in 1–2 divided doses for 14 days then 600 micrograms/kg in 1–2 divided doses for further 14 days, thereafter increased by max. 600 micrograms/kg every 7–14 days; usual maintenance 1–10 mg/kg daily in 1–2 divided doses; max. 200 mg daily

**Child 12–18 years** initially 25 mg daily for 14 days, increased to 50 mg daily for further 14 days, then increased by max. 100 mg every 7–14 days; usual maintenance 100–200 mg daily in 1–2 divided doses

**Monotherapy of seizures**

**Child 12–18 years** initially 25 mg daily for 14 days, increased to 50 mg daily for further 14 days, then increased by max. 100 mg every 7–14 days; usual maintenance as monotherapy, 100–200 mg daily in 1–2 divided doses (up to 500 mg daily has been required)

**Monotherapy of typical absence seizures**

• **By mouth**

**Child 2–12 years** initially 300 micrograms/kg daily in 1–2 divided doses for 14 days, then 600 micrograms/kg daily in 1–2 divided doses for further 14 days, thereafter increased by max. 600 micrograms/kg every 7–14 days; usual maintenance 1–10 mg/kg daily in 1–2 divided doses (up to 15 mg/kg daily has been required)

**Note** Dose titration should be repeated if restarting after interval of more than 5 days

---

**Safe Practice**

Do not confuse the different combinations; see also notes above

---

**Lamotrigine** (Non-proprietary) PoM

Tablets, lamotrigine 25 mg, net price 56-tab pack = £2.25; 50 mg, 56-tab pack = £3.07; 100 mg, 56-tab pack = £4.53; 200 mg, 30-tab pack = £27.53, 56-tab pack = £7.51.Label: 8, counselling, driving (see notes above), skin reactions (see above)

Dispersible tablets, lamotrigine 5 mg, net price 28-tab pack = £2.27; 25 mg, 56-tab pack = £2.91; 100 mg, 56-tab pack = £5.86. Label: 8, 13, counselling, driving (see notes above), skin reactions (see above)

**Lamictal®** (GSK) PoM

Tablets, yellow, lamotrigine 25 mg, net price 56-tab pack = £19.61; 50 mg, 56-tab pack = £33.35; 100 mg, 56-tab pack = £57.53; 200 mg, 56-tab pack = £97.79. Label: 8, counselling, driving (see notes above), skin reactions (see above)

Dispersible tablets, chewable, lamotrigine 2 mg, net price 30-tab pack = £10.45; 5 mg, 28-tab pack = £7.82; 25 mg, 56-tab pack = £19.61; 100 mg, 56-tab pack = £57.53. Label: 8, 13, counselling, driving (see notes above), skin reactions (see above)

**4**

**Central nervous system**

**Central nervous system** 4

# Levetiracetam

Levetiracetam is used for monotherapy and adjunctive treatment of focal seizures with or without secondary generalisation, and for adjunctive treatment of myoclonic seizures in children with juvenile myoclonic epilepsy, and primary generalised tonic-clonic seizures.

## ▌ LEVETIRACETAM

**Cautions** avoid abrupt withdrawal; **interactions:** Appendix 1 (levetiracetam)

**Hepatic impairment** halve dose in severe hepatic impairment if estimated glomerular filtration rate less than 60 mL/minute/1.73 m$^2$

**Renal impairment** reduce dose if estimated glomerular filtration rate less than 80 mL/minute/1.73 m$^2$ (consult product literature)

**Pregnancy** see Pregnancy, p. 217

**Breast-feeding** present in milk—manufacturer advises avoid; see also Breast-feeding, p. 218

**Side-effects** anorexia, weight changes, abdominal pain, nausea, vomiting, dyspepsia, diarrhoea, cough, drowsiness, amnesia, ataxia, convulsion, dizziness, headache, tremor, hyperkinesia, malaise, impaired attention, aggression, agitation, depression, insomnia, anxiety, irritability, personality disorder, thrombocytopenia, myalgia, diplopia, blurred vision, rash; *also reported* pancreatitis, hepatic failure, paraesthesia, confusion, hallucinations, psychosis, suicidal ideation, leucopenia, neutropenia, pancytopenia, alopecia, toxic epidermal necrolysis, Stevens-Johnson syndrome

**Licensed use** *granules* not licensed for use in children under 6 years, for initial treatment in children with body-weight less than 25 kg, or for the administration of doses below 250 mg

### Indications and dose

#### Monotherapy of focal seizures
- **By mouth or by intravenous infusion**
  **Note** If switching between oral therapy and intravenous therapy (for those temporarily unable to take oral medication), the intravenous dose should be the same as the established oral dose

  **Child 16–18 years** initially 250 mg once daily increased after 1 week to 250 mg twice daily; thereafter, increased according to response in steps of 250 mg twice daily every 2 weeks; max. 1.5 g twice daily

#### Adjunctive therapy of focal seizures
- **By mouth**
  **Child 1–6 months** initially 7 mg/kg once daily, increased by max. 7 mg/kg twice daily every 2 weeks; max. 21 mg/kg twice daily

  **Child 6 months–18 years, body-weight under 50 kg** initially 10 mg/kg once daily, increased by max. 10 mg/kg twice daily every 2 weeks; max. 30 mg/kg twice daily

  **Child 12–18 years, body-weight over 50 kg** initially 250 mg twice daily, increased by 500 mg twice daily every 2 weeks; max. 1.5 g twice daily

- **By intravenous infusion**
  **Note** If switching between oral therapy and intravenous therapy (for those temporarily unable to take oral medication), the intravenous dose should be the same as the established oral dose

  **Child 4–18 years, body-weight under 50 kg** initially 10 mg/kg once daily, increased by max. 10 mg/kg twice daily every 2 weeks; max. 30 mg/kg twice daily

  **Child 12–18 years, body-weight over 50 kg** initially 250 mg twice daily, increased by 500 mg twice daily every 2 weeks; max. 1.5 g twice daily

#### Adjunctive therapy of myoclonic seizures and tonic-clonic seizures
- **By mouth or by intravenous infusion**
  **Note** If switching between oral therapy and intravenous therapy (for those temporarily unable to take oral medication), the intravenous dose should be the same as the established oral dose

  **Child 12–18 years, body-weight under 50 kg** initially 10 mg/kg once daily, increased by max. 10 mg/kg twice daily every 2 weeks; max. 30 mg/kg twice daily

  **Child 12–18 years, body-weight over 50 kg** initially 250 mg twice daily, increased by 500 mg twice daily every 2 weeks; max. 1.5 g twice daily

**Administration** for *intravenous infusion*, dilute requisite dose with at least 100 mL Glucose 5% or Sodium Chloride 0.9%; give over 15 minutes

For administration of *oral solution*, requisite dose may be diluted in a glass of water

**Levetiracetam** (Non-proprietary) ▣PoM▣
Tablets, levetiracetam 250 mg, net price 60-tab pack = £27.50; 500mg, 60-tab pack = £48.50; 750 mg, 60-tab pack = £83.50; 1 g, 60-tab pack = £94.50. Label: 8

Oral Solution, levetiracetam 100 mg/mL, net price 300 mL = £66.95. Label: 8

Granules, levetiracetam 250 mg/sachet, net price 60-sachet pack =£22.41; 500 mg/sachet, net price 60-sachet pack =£39.46; 1 g/sachet, net price 60-sachet pack =£76.27. Label: 8
**Brands include** *Desitrend*®

**Keppra**® (UCB Pharma) ▣PoM▣
Tablets, f/c, levetiracetam 250 mg (blue), net price 60-tab pack = £29.70; 500 mg (yellow), 60-tab pack = £52.30; 750 mg (orange), 60-tab pack = £89.10; 1 g (white), 60-tab pack = £101.10. Label: 8

Oral solution, sugar-free, levetiracetam 100 mg/mL, net price 150 mL (with 1-mL or 3-mL syringe) = £42.60, 300 mL (with 10-ml syringe) = £71.00. Label: 8

Concentrate for intravenous infusion, levetiracetam 100 mg/mL, net price 5-mL vial = £13.50
**Electrolytes** Na$^+$ 0.83 mmol/vial
**Note** For dilution before use

# Perampanel

Perampanel is licensed for adjunctive treatment of partial onset seizures with or without secondary generalised seizures.

## ▌ PERAMPANEL

**Cautions** interactions: Appendix 1 (perampanel)
**Hepatic impairment** increase at intervals of at least 2 weeks, up to max. 8 mg daily in mild or moderate impairment; avoid in severe impairment

**Renal impairment** avoid in moderate or severe impairment

**Pregnancy** see Pregnancy, p. 217; manufacturer advises avoid

**Breast-feeding** avoid—present in milk in *animal* studies

**Side-effects** nausea, changes in appetite, weight increase, aggression, dizziness, drowsiness, dysarthria, gait disturbance, irritability, anxiety, confusion, suicidal ideation and behaviour, malaise, ataxia, back pain, vertigo, blurred vision, diplopia

**Indications and dose**

> Adjunctive treatment of partial onset seizures with or without secondary generalised seizures
>
> • By mouth
>
>> **Child 12-18 years** initially 2 mg once daily before bedtime, increased according to response and tolerability in 2-mg steps at intervals of at least 2 weeks; usual maintenance 4–8 mg once daily; max. 12 mg once daily
>>
>> **Note** Titrate at intervals of at least 1 week with concomitant carbamazepine, oxcarbazepine, or phenytoin (see also Appendix 1).

**Fycompa®** (Eisai) ▼ PoM
Tablets, all f/c, perampanel 2 mg (orange), net price 7-tab pack = £35.00; 4 mg (red) 28-tab pack = £140.00; 6 mg (pink) 28-tab pack = £140.00; 8 mg (purple) 28-tab pack = £140.00; 10 mg (green) 28-tab pack = £140.00; 12 mg (blue) 28-tab pack = £140.00. Label: 3, 8, 25, counselling, driving (see notes above)

---

# Phenobarbital and primidone

**Phenobarbital** is effective for tonic-clonic, focal seizures and neonatal seizures but may cause behavioural disturbances and hyperkinesia. It may be tried for atypical absence, atonic, and tonic seizures. For therapeutic purposes phenobarbital and phenobarbital sodium should be considered equivalent in effect. Rebound seizures may be a problem on withdrawal. Monitoring the plasma-drug concentration is less useful than with other drugs because tolerance occurs.

**Primidone** is largely converted to phenobarbital and this is probably responsible for its antiepileptic action. It is used rarely in children. A low initial dose of primidone is essential.

---

## ▌PHENOBARBITAL
(Phenobarbitone)

**Cautions** see also notes above; debilitated; respiratory depression (avoid if severe); avoid abrupt withdrawal (dependence with prolonged use); history of drug and alcohol abuse; consider vitamin D supplementation in patients who are immobilised for long periods or who have inadequate sun exposure or dietary intake of calcium; avoid in acute porphyria (see section 9.8.2); **interactions:** see p. 216 and Appendix 1 (phenobarbital)

**Hepatic impairment** may precipitate coma; avoid in severe impairment

**Renal impairment** use with caution

**Pregnancy** see Pregnancy, p. 217

**Breast-feeding** avoid if possible; drowsiness may occur; see also Breast-feeding, p. 218

**Side-effects** hepatitis, cholestasis; hypotension; respiratory depression; drowsiness, lethargy, depression, ataxia, behavioural disturbances, nystagmus, irritability, hallucinations, impaired memory and cognition, hyperactivity; osteomalacia (see Cautions); megaloblastic anaemia (may be treated with folic acid), agranulocytosis, thrombocytopenia; allergic skin reactions; *very rarely* Stevens-Johnson syndrome and toxic epidermal necrolysis; suicidal ideation; Antiepileptic Hypersensitivity Syndrome (see p. 217); **overdosage:** see Emergency Treatment of Poisoning, p. 24

**Pharmacokinetics** trough plasma concentration for optimum response 15–40 mg/litre (60–180 micromol/litre)

**Indications and dose**

> All forms of epilepsy except typical absence seizures
>
> • By mouth or by intravenous injection
>
>> **Neonate** initially 20 mg/kg *by slow intravenous injection* then 2.5–5 mg/kg once daily either *by slow intravenous injection* or *by mouth*; dose and frequency adjusted according to response
>
> • By mouth
>
>> **Child 1 month–12 years** initially 1–1.5 mg/kg twice daily, increased by 2 mg/kg daily as required; usual maintenance dose 2.5–4 mg/kg once or twice daily
>>
>> **Child 12–18 years** 60–180 mg once daily

> Status epilepticus section 4.8.2
>
> **Note** For therapeutic purposes phenobarbital and phenobarbital sodium may be considered equivalent in effect

**Administration** for administration *by mouth*, tablets may be crushed

For *intravenous injection*, dilute to a concentration of 20 mg/mL with Water for Injections; give over 20 minutes (no faster than 1 mg/kg/minute)

**Phenobarbital** (Non-proprietary) CD3
Tablets, phenobarbital 15 mg, net price 28-tab pack = 95p; 30 mg, 28-tab pack = 96p; 60 mg, 28-tab pack = 71p. Label: 2, 8, counselling, driving (see notes above)

Elixir, phenobarbital 15 mg/5 mL in a suitable flavoured vehicle, containing alcohol 38%, net price 100 mL = 78p. Label: 2, 8, counselling, driving (see notes above)

**Note** Some hospitals supply **alcohol-free** formulations of varying phenobarbital strengths

Injection, phenobarbital sodium 15 mg/mL, net price 1-mL amp = £1.64; 30 mg/mL, 1-mL amp = £2.04; 60 mg/mL, 1-mL amp = £2.14; 200 mg/mL, 1-mL amp = £2.00

**Excipients** include propylene glycol (see Excipients, p. 2)

**Note** Must be diluted before intravenous administration (see Administration)

---

## ▌PRIMIDONE

**Cautions** see Phenobarbital; **interactions:** see p. 216 and Appendix 1 (phenobarbital)

**Hepatic impairment** reduce dose, may precipitate coma

**Renal impairment** see Phenobarbital

**4 Central nervous system**

**Pregnancy** see Pregnancy, p. 217
**Breast-feeding** see Breast-feeding, p. 218
**Side-effects** see Phenobarbital; also nausea, visual disturbances; *less commonly* vomiting, headache, dizziness; *rarely* psychosis, lupus erythematosus, arthralgia; *also reported* Dupuytren's contracture
**Pharmacokinetics** monitor plasma concentrations of derived phenobarbital. Optimum range as for phenobarbital

**Indications and dose**

All forms of epilepsy except typical absence seizures (but see notes above)

• By mouth

**Child under 2 years** initially 125 mg daily at bedtime, increased by 125 mg every 3 days according to response; usual maintenance, 125–250 mg twice daily

**Child 2–5 years** initially 125 mg daily at bedtime, increased by 125 mg every 3 days according to response; usual maintenance, 250–375 mg twice daily

**Child 5–9 years** initially 125 mg daily at bedtime, increased by 125 mg every 3 days according to response; usual maintenance, 375–500 mg twice a day

**Child 9–18 years** initially 125 mg daily at bedtime, increased by 125 mg every 3 days to 250 mg twice daily, then increased according to response by 250 mg every 3 days to max. 750 mg twice daily

**Mysoline®** (Acorus) [PoM]
Tablets, scored, primidone 50 mg, net price 100-tab pack = £12.60; 250 mg, 100-tab pack = £12.60.
Label: 2, 8, counselling, driving (see notes above)

## Phenytoin

Phenytoin is effective for tonic-clonic, focal, and neonatal seizures but it may worsen myoclonus. It has a narrow therapeutic index and the relationship between dose and plasma-drug concentration is non-linear; small dosage increases in some children may produce large increases in plasma-drug concentration with acute toxic side-effects. Similarly, a few missed doses or a small change in drug absorption may result in a marked change in plasma-drug concentration. Monitoring of plasma-drug concentration improves dosage adjustment.

Preparations containing phenytoin sodium are **not** bioequivalent to those containing phenytoin base (such as *Epanutin Infatabs®* and *Epanutin®* suspension); 100 mg of phenytoin sodium is approximately equivalent in therapeutic effect to 92 mg phenytoin base. The dose is the same for all phenytoin products when initiating therapy, however if switching between these products the difference in phenytoin content may be clinically significant. Care is needed when making changes between formulations and plasma-phenytoin concentration monitoring is recommended.

Symptoms of phenytoin toxicity include nystagmus, diplopia, slurred speech, ataxia, confusion, and hyperglycaemia.

Phenytoin may cause coarsening of the facial appearance, acne, hirsutism, and gingival hyperplasia and so may be particularly undesirable in adolescent patients.

When only parenteral administration is possible, fosphenytoin (section 4.8.2), a pro-drug of phenytoin, may be convenient to give. Whereas phenytoin should be given intravenously only, fosphenytoin may also be given by intramuscular injection.

## PHENYTOIN

**Cautions** see notes above; cross-sensitivity reported with cabamazepine (see also Antiepileptic Hypersensitivity Syndrome, p. 217); avoid abrupt withdrawal; HLA-B* 1502 allele in individuals of Han Chinese or Thai origin – avoid unless essential (increased risk of Stevens–Johnson syndrome); manufacturer recommends blood counts (but evidence of practical value uncertain); consider vitamin D supplementation in patients that are immobilised for long periods or who have inadequate sun exposure or dietary intake of calcium; enteral feeding (interrupt feeding for 2 hours before and after dose; more frequent monitoring may be necessary); avoid in acute porphyria (section 9.8.2); **interactions:** see p. 216 and Appendix 1 (phenytoin)
**Blood or skin disorders** Children and their carers should be told how to recognise signs of blood or skin disorders, and advised to seek immediate medical attention if symptoms such as fever, rash, mouth ulcers, bruising, or bleeding develop. Leucopenia which is severe, progressive, or associated with clinical symptoms requires withdrawal (if necessary under cover of a suitable alternative)
**Hepatic impairment** reduce dose
**Pregnancy** changes in plasma-protein binding make interpretation of plasma-phenytoin concentrations difficult—monitor unbound fraction; see also Pregnancy, p. 217
**Breast-feeding** small amounts present in milk, but not known to be harmful; see also Breast-feeding, p. 218
**Side-effects** nausea, vomiting, constipation; drowsiness, insomnia, transient nervousness, tremor, paraesthesia, dizziness, headache, anorexia; gingival hypertrophy and tenderness (maintain good oral hygiene); rash (discontinue; if mild reintroduce cautiously but discontinue immediately if recurrence), acne, hirsutism, coarsening of facial appearance; *rarely* hepatoxicity (discontinue immediately and do not readminister), peripheral neuropathy, dyskinesia, lymphadenopathy, osteomalacia (see Cautions), blood disorders (including megaloblastic anaemia, leucopenia, thrombocytopenia, and aplastic anaemia), polyarteritis nodosa, lupus erythematosus, Stevens-Johnson syndrome, and toxic epidermal necrolysis; *also reported* polyarthropathy, pneumonitis, interstitial nephritis, hypersensitivity syndrome (see Antiepileptic Hypersensitivity Syndrome, p. 217), suicidal ideation
**Pharmacokinetics** therapeutic plasma-phenytoin concentrations reduced in first 3 months of life because of reduced protein binding
Trough plasma concentration for optimum response: Neonate–3 months, 6–15 mg/litre (25–60 micromol/litre)
Child 3 months–18 years, 10–20 mg/litre (40–80 micromol/litre)
**Licensed use** licensed for use in children (age range not specified by manufacturer)

#### Indications and dose

> **All forms of epilepsy except absence seizures**
> * By intravenous injection (over 20–30 minutes) and by mouth
>
>   **Neonate** *initial loading dose by slow intravenous injection* (section 4.8.2) 18 mg/kg then *by mouth* 2.5–5 mg/kg twice daily adjusted according to response and plasma-phenytoin concentration (usual max. 7.5 mg/kg twice daily)
>
> * By mouth
>
>   **Child 1 month–12 years** initially 1.5–2.5 mg/kg twice daily, then adjusted according to response and plasma-phenytoin concentration to 2.5–5 mg/kg twice daily (usual max. 7.5 mg/kg twice daily *or* 300 mg daily)
>
>   **Child 12–18 years** initially 75–150 mg twice daily then adjusted according to response and plasma-phenytoin concentration to 150–200 mg twice daily (usual max. 300 mg twice daily)

> **Status epilepticus, acute symptomatic seizures associated with head trauma or neurosurgery** section 4.8.2

**Administration** for administration *by mouth*, interrupt enteral feeds for at least 1–2 hours before and after giving phenytoin; give with water to enhance absorption

For administration by *intravenous injection* and *intravenous infusion*, see p. 237

**Phenytoin** (Non-proprietary) PoM
Tablets, coated, phenytoin sodium 100 mg, net price 28-tab pack = £30.00. Label: 8, counselling, administration, blood or skin disorder symptoms (see above), driving (see notes above)
Note On the basis of single dose tests there are no clinically relevant differences in bioavailability between available phenytoin sodium tablets and capsules but there may be a pharmacokinetic basis for maintaining the same brand of phenytoin in some patients (see notes above)

**Epanutin**® (Pfizer) PoM
Capsules, phenytoin sodium 25 mg (white/purple), net price 28-cap pack = 66p; 50 mg (white/pink), 28-cap pack = 67p; 100 mg (white/orange), 84-cap pack = £2.83; 300 mg (white/green), 28-cap pack = £2.83. Label: 8, counselling, administration, blood or skin disorder symptoms (see above), driving (see notes above)

Chewable tablets (*Infatabs*®), yellow, scored, phenytoin 50 mg, net price 200-tab pack = £13.18. Label: 8, 24, counselling, blood or skin disorder symptoms (see above), driving (see notes above)
Note Contains phenytoin base therefore care is needed when changing to capsules or tablets containing phenytoin sodium (see notes above)

Suspension, red, phenytoin 30 mg/5 mL, net price 500 mL = £4.27. Label: 8, counselling, administration, blood or skin disorder symptoms (see above), driving (see notes above)
Note Contains phenytoin base therefore care is needed when changing to capsules or tablets containing phenytoin sodium (see notes above)

◢Parenteral preparations
Section 4.8.2

## Rufinamide

**Rufinamide** is licensed for the adjunctive treatment of seizures in Lennox-Gastaut syndrome.

The *Scottish Medicines Consortium* (p. 3) has advised (October 2008) that rufinamide (*Inovelon*®) is accepted for restricted use within NHS Scotland as adjunctive therapy in the treatment of seizures associated with Lennox-Gastaut syndrome in patients 4 years and above. It is restricted for use when alternative traditional antiepileptic drugs are unsatisfactory.

### ▌RUFINAMIDE

**Cautions** closely monitor and consider withdrawal if rash, fever, or other signs of hypersensitivity syndrome develop (see also Antiepileptic Hypersensitivity Syndrome, p. 217); avoid abrupt withdrawal; **interactions:** see p. 216 and Appendix 1 (rufinamide)

**Hepatic impairment** caution and careful dose titration in mild to moderate impairment; avoid in severe impairment

**Pregnancy** see Pregnancy, p. 217

**Breast-feeding** manufacturer advises avoid—no information available; see also Breast-feeding, p. 218

**Side-effects** nausea, vomiting, constipation, diarrhoea, dyspepsia, abdominal pain; rhinitis, epistaxis; weight loss, anorexia, dizziness, headache, drowsiness, insomnia, anxiety, fatigue, increase in seizure frequency, impaired coordination, hyperactivity, tremor, gait disturbances; influenza-like symptoms; oligomenorrhoea; back pain; nystagmus, diplopia, blurred vision; rash, and acne; hypersensitivity syndrome (see Antiepileptic Hypersensitivity Syndrome, p. 217) also reported

#### Indications and dose

> **Adjunctive treatment of seizures in Lennox-Gastaut syndrome**
> * By mouth
>
>   **Child 4–18 years** body-weight less than 30 kg, initially 100 mg twice daily increased according to response in steps of 100 mg twice daily up to every 2 days; max. 500 mg twice daily (max. 300 mg twice daily if adjunctive therapy *with valproate*)
>
>   **Child 4–18 years** body-weight over 30 kg, initially 200 mg twice daily increased according to response in steps of 200 mg twice daily up to every 2 days; body-weight 30–50 kg max. 900 mg twice daily; body-weight 50–70 kg max. 1.2 g twice daily; body-weight over 70 kg max. 1.6 g twice daily

**Administration** Tablets may be crushed and given in half a glass of water

**Inovelon**® (Eisai) PoM
Tablets, pink, f/c, scored, rufinamide 100 mg, net price 10-tab pack = £5.15; 200 mg, 60-tab pack = £61.77; 400 mg, 60-tab pack = £102.96. Label: 8, 21, counselling, driving (see notes above), hypersensitivity syndrome (see notes above)
Oral suspension, white, sugar-free, rufinamide 40 mg/mL, net price 460-mL pack = £94.71. Label: 8, 21, counselling, driving (see notes above), hypersensitivity syndrome (see notes above)
Excipients include propylene glycol

## Stiripentol

Stiripentol is licensed for use in combination with clobazam and valproate as adjunctive therapy of refractory generalised tonic-clonic seizures in children with severe myoclonic epilepsy in infancy (Dravet Syndrome). It should be used under specialist supervision.

**4**

**Central nervous system**

**Central nervous system** 4

# ▌ STIRIPENTOL

**Cautions** perform full blood count and liver function tests prior to initiating treatment and every 6 months thereafter; monitor growth; **interactions:** Appendix 1 (stiripentol)

**Contra-indications** history of psychosis

**Hepatic impairment** avoid—no information available

**Renal impairment** avoid—no information available

**Pregnancy** see Pregnancy, p. 217

**Breast-feeding** present in milk in *animal* studies; see also Breast-feeding, p. 218

**Side-effects** nausea, vomiting; aggression, anorexia, ataxia, drowsiness, dystonia, hyperexcitability, hyperkinesia, hypotonia, irritability, sleep disorders, weight loss; neutropenia; *less commonly* fatigue, photosensitivity, rash, and urticaria

**Indications and dose**

**Severe myoclonic epilepsy in infancy**

- By mouth

  **Child 3-18 years** initially 10 mg/kg in 2-3 divided doses; titrate dose over minimum of 3 days to max. 50 mg/kg/day in 2-3 divided doses

**Diacomit®** (Alan Pharmaceuticals) ▼ PoM

Capsules, stiripentol 250 mg (pink), net price 60-cap pack = £284.00; 500 mg (white), 60-cap pack = £493.00. Label: 1, 8, 21, counselling, administration

Powder, stiripentol 250 mg, net price 60-sachet pack = £284.00; 500 mg, 60-sachet pack = £493.00. Label: 1, 8, 13, 21, counselling, administration

**Excipients** include aspartame (section 9.4.1)

**Counselling** Do not take with milk, dairy products, carbonated drinks, fruit juice, or with food or drink that contains caffeine

# Tiagabine

Tiagabine is used as adjunctive treatment for focal seizures with or without secondary generalisation that are not satisfactorily controlled by other antiepileptics.

# ▌ TIAGABINE

**Cautions** avoid in acute porphyria (section 9.8.2); avoid abrupt withdrawal; **interactions:** Appendix 1 (tiagabine)

**Driving** May impair performance of skilled tasks (e.g. driving)

**Hepatic impairment** in mild to moderate impairment reduce dose, prolong the dose interval, or both; avoid in severe impairment

**Pregnancy** see Pregnancy, p. 217

**Breast-feeding** see Breast-feeding, p. 218

**Side-effects** diarrhoea; dizziness, tiredness, nervousness, tremor, impaired concentration, emotional lability, speech impairment; *rarely* confusion, depression, drowsiness, psychosis, non-convulsive status epilepticus, bruising, and visual disturbances; suicidal ideation; leucopenia also reported

**Indications and dose**

**Adjunctive treatment for focal seizures with or without secondary generalisation not satisfactorily controlled by other antiepileptics**

- By mouth

  **With enzyme-inducing drugs**

  **Child 12-18 years** initially 5-10 mg daily in 1-2 divided doses, increased in steps of 5-10 mg daily at weekly intervals; usual maintenance dose 30-45 mg daily in 2-3 divided doses

  **Without enzyme-inducing drugs**

  **Child 12-18 years** initially 5-10 mg daily in 1-2 divided doses, increased in steps of 5-10 mg daily at weekly intervals; initial maintenance dose 15-30 mg daily in 2-3 divided doses

**Gabitril®** (Cephalon) PoM

Tablets, f/c, tiagabine (as hydrochloride) 5 mg, net price 100-tab pack = £40.89; 10 mg, 100-tab pack = £81.77; 15 mg, 100-tab pack = £122.66. Label: 21

# Topiramate

Topiramate can be given alone or as adjunctive treatment in generalised tonic-clonic seizures or focal seizures. Topiramate is also licensed for prophylaxis of migraine (section 4.7.4.2).

# ▌ TOPIRAMATE

**Cautions** avoid abrupt withdrawal; risk of metabolic acidosis; risk of nephrolithiasis—ensure adequate hydration (especially in strenuous activity or warm environment); avoid in acute porphyria (section 9.8.2); **interactions:** see p. 216 and Appendix 1 (topiramate)

**Important** Topiramate has been associated with acute myopia with secondary angle-closure glaucoma, typically occurring within 1 month of starting treatment. Choroidal effusions resulting in anterior displacement of the lens and iris have also been reported. If raised intra-ocular pressure occurs:

- seek specialist ophthalmological advice;

- use appropriate measures to reduce intra-ocular pressure;

- stop topiramate as rapidly as feasible

**Hepatic impairment** use with caution in moderate to severe impairment—clearance may be reduced

**Renal impairment** use with caution if estimated glomerular filtration rate less than 60 mL/minute/1.73m$^2$—reduced clearance and longer time to steady-state plasma concentration

**Pregnancy** see Pregnancy, p. 217

**Breast-feeding** manufacturer advises avoid—present in milk; see also Breast-feeding, p. 218

**Side-effects** nausea, diarrhoea, vomiting, constipation, dyspepsia, abdominal pain, dry mouth, taste disturbance, gastritis, appetite changes, dyspnoea, impaired attention, cognitive impairment, movement disorders, seizures, tremor, malaise, impaired coordination, speech disorder, drowsiness, dizziness, sleep disturbance, anxiety, confusion, paraesthesia, aggression, mood changes, depression, agitation, irritability, nephrolithiasis, urinary disorders, anaemia, arthralgia, muscle spasm, myalgia, muscular weakness, visual disturbances, nystagmus, tinnitus, epistaxis, alopecia, rash, pruritus; *less commonly* pancreatitis, flatulence, abdominal distension, gingival bleeding, salivation, halitosis, thirst, glossodynia, bradycardia, palpitation, hypotension, postural hypotension, flushing, altered sense of smell, peripheral neuropathy, suicidal ideation, psychosis, panic attack, influenza-like symptoms, sexual dysfunction, urinary calculus, haematuria, blood disorders (including leucopenia, neutropenia, and thrombocytopenia), hypokalaemia, metabolic acidosis, dry eye, photophobia, blepharospasm, increased lacrimation, mydriasis, hearing loss, reduced sweating, skin discoloration; *rarely* Raynaud's syndrome, periorbital oedema, unilateral blindness, Stevens-Johnson syndrome, abnormal skin odour, calcinosis; *very rarely* angle-closure glaucoma; *also reported* encephalopathy, hyperammonaemia, maculopathy, toxic epidermal necrolysis

**Licensed use** not licensed for use in children for migraine prophylaxis

**Indications and dose**

> **Monotherapy of generalised tonic-clonic seizures or focal seizures with or without secondary generalisation**
>
> - **By mouth**
>   **Child 6–18 years** initially 0.5–1 mg/kg (max. 25 mg) at night for 1 week then increased in steps of 250–500 micrograms/kg (max. 25 mg) twice daily at intervals of 1–2 weeks; initial target dose 50 mg twice daily; max. 7.5 mg/kg (max. 250 mg) twice daily

> **Adjunctive treatment of generalised tonic-clonic seizures or focal seizures with or without secondary generalisation, adjunctive treatment of seizures in Lennox-Gastaut syndrome**
>
> - **By mouth**
>   **Child 2–18 years** initially 1–3 mg/kg (max. 25 mg) at night for 1 week then increased in steps of 0.5–1.5 mg/kg (max. 25 mg) twice daily at intervals of 1–2 weeks; usual dose 2.5–4.5 mg/kg twice daily; max. 7.5 mg/kg (max. 200 mg) twice daily

> **Migraine prophylaxis**
>
> - **By mouth**
>   **Child 16–18 years** initially 25 mg at night for 1 week then increased in steps of 25 mg daily at weekly intervals; usual dose 50–100 mg daily in 2 divided doses; max. 200 mg daily

**Note** If child cannot tolerate titration regimens recommended above then smaller steps or longer interval between steps may be used

**Topiramate** (Non-proprietary) PoM
Tablets, topiramate 25 mg, net price 60-tab pack = £6.17; 50 mg, 60-tab pack = £10.74; 100 mg, 60-tab pack = £12.52; 200 mg, 60-tab pack = £17.21. Label: 3, 8, counselling, driving (see notes above)

Capsules, topiramate 15 mg, net price 60-cap pack = £16.61; 25 mg, 60-cap pack = £24.91; 50 mg, 60-cap pack = £40.93. Label: 3, 8, counselling, driving (see notes above)

**Topamax®** (Janssen) PoM
Tablets, f/c, topiramate 25 mg, net price 60-tab pack = £19.29; 50 mg (light yellow), 60-tab pack = £31.69; 100 mg (yellow), 60-tab pack = £56.76; 200 mg (salmon), 60-tab pack = £110.23. Label: 3, 8, counselling, driving (see notes above)

Sprinkle capsules, topiramate 15 mg, net price 60-cap pack = £14.79; 25 mg, 60-cap pack = £22.18; 50 mg, 60-cap pack = £36.45. Label: 3, 8, counselling, administration, driving (see notes above)
**Counselling** Swallow whole or sprinkle contents of capsule on soft food and swallow immediately without chewing

## Valproate

**Valproate** (as either sodium valproate or valproic acid) is effective in controlling tonic-clonic seizures, particularly in primary generalised epilepsy. It is a drug of choice in primary generalised epilepsy, generalised absences and myoclonic seizures, and can be tried in atypical absence, atonic, and tonic seizures. Valproate should generally be avoided in children under 2 years especially with other antiepileptics, but it may be required in infants with continuing epileptic tendency. Sodium valproate has widespread metabolic effects, and monitoring of liver function tests and full blood count is essential (see Cautions below). Plasma-valproate concentrations are not a useful index of efficacy, therefore routine monitoring is unhelpful.

### ■ SODIUM VALPROATE

**Cautions** see notes above; monitor liver function before therapy and during first 6 months especially in children most at risk (see also below); measure full blood count and ensure no undue potential for bleeding before starting and before surgery; systemic lupus erythematosus; false-positive urine tests for ketones; avoid sudden withdrawal; consider vitamin D supplementation in patients that are immobilised for long periods or who have inadequate sun exposure or dietary intake of calcium; **interactions:** see p. 216 and Appendix 1 (valproate)
**Liver toxicity** Liver dysfunction (including fatal hepatic failure) has occurred in association with valproate (especially in children under 3 years and in those with metabolic or degenerative disorders, organic brain disease or severe seizure disorders associated with mental retardation) usually in first 6 months and usually involving multiple antiepileptic therapy. Raised liver enzymes during valproate treatment are usually transient but children should be reassessed clinically and liver function (including prothrombin time) monitored until return to normal—discontinue if abnormally prolonged prothrombin time (particularly in association with other relevant abnormalities)
**Blood or hepatic disorders** Children and their carers should be told how to recognise signs of blood or liver disorders and advised to seek immediate medical attention if symptoms develop
**Pancreatitis** Children and their carers should be told how to recognise signs and symptoms of pancreatitis and advised to seek immediate medical attention if symptoms such as abdominal pain, nausea, or vomiting develop; discontinue if pancreatitis is diagnosed

**Contra-indications** family history of severe hepatic dysfunction; acute porphyria (section 9.8.2)

**Hepatic impairment** avoid if possible—hepatotoxicity and hepatic failure may occasionally occur (usually in first 6 months); avoid in active liver disease; see also under Cautions

**Renal impairment** reduce dose

**Pregnancy** see Pregnancy, p. 217; neonatal bleeding (related to hypofibrinaemia) and neonatal hepatotoxicity also reported

**Breast-feeding** amount too small to be harmful; see also Breast-feeding, p. 218

**4 Central nervous system**

**Side-effects** nausea, gastric irritation, diarrhoea; weight gain; hyperammonaemia, thrombocytopenia; transient hair loss (regrowth may be curly); *less frequently* increased alertness, aggression, hyperactivity, behavioural disturbances, ataxia, tremor, and vasculitis; *rarely* hepatic dysfunction (see under Cautions; withdraw treatment immediately if persistent vomiting and abdominal pain, anorexia, jaundice, oedema, malaise, drowsiness, or loss of seizure control), lethargy, drowsiness, confusion, stupor, hallucinations, blood disorders (including anaemia, leucopenia, and pancytopenia), hearing loss, and rash; *very rarely* pancreatitis (see under Cautions), peripheral oedema, increase in bleeding time, extrapyramidal symptoms, encephalopathy, coma, gynaecomastia, Fanconi's syndrome, hirsutism, enuresis, hyponatraemia, acne, toxic epidermal necrolysis, and Stevens-Johnson syndrome; suicidal ideation; reduced bone mineral density (see Cautions); *also reported* menstrual disturbances

## Indications and dose

**All forms of epilepsy**

- **By mouth or by rectum**

  **Neonate** initially 20 mg/kg once daily; usual maintenance dose 10 mg/kg twice daily

  **Child 1 month–12 years** initially 10–15 mg/kg (max. 600 mg) daily in 1–2 divided doses; usual maintenance dose 25–30 mg/kg daily in 2 divided doses (up to 60 mg/kg daily in 2 divided doses in infantile spasms; monitor clinical chemistry and haematological parameters if dose exceeds 40 mg/kg daily)

  **Child 12–18 years** initially 600 mg daily in 1–2 divided doses increased gradually (in steps of 150–300 mg) every 3 days; usual maintenance dose 1–2 g daily in 2 divided doses; max. 2.5 g daily in 2 divided doses

- **By intravenous administration**

  **Note** If switching from oral therapy to intravenous therapy give current oral daily dose by intravenous injection *or* intermittent intravenous infusion in 2–4 divided doses, *or* by continuous intravenous infusion

  **Neonate** *by intravenous injection* 10 mg/kg twice daily

  **Child 1 month–12 years** initially 10 mg/kg *by intravenous injection,* followed *by continuous intravenous infusion,* or *by intermittent intravenous infusion* or *intravenous injection* in 2–4 divided doses up to usual range 20–40 mg/kg daily (doses above 40 mg/kg daily monitor clinical chemistry and haematological parameters)

  **Child 12–18 years** initially 10 mg/kg *by intravenous injection,* followed *by continuous intravenous infusion,* or *by intermittent intravenous infusion* or *intravenous injection* in 2–4 divided doses up to max. 2.5 g daily; usual range 1–2 g daily (20–30 mg/kg daily)

**Administration** for *rectal administration,* sodium valproate oral solution may be given rectally and retained for 15 minutes (may require dilution with water to prevent rapid expulsion).

For *intravenous injection,* may be diluted in Glucose 5% *or* Sodium Chloride 0.9% and given over 3–5 minutes.

For *intravenous infusion,* dilute injection solution with Glucose 5% *or* Sodium Chloride 0.9%

◢**Oral**

**Sodium Valproate** (Non-proprietary) PoM

Tablets (crushable), scored, sodium valproate 100 mg, net price 100-tab pack = £5.60. Label: 8, 21, counselling, pancreatitis, blood, or hepatic disorder symptoms (see above), driving (see notes above)

Tablets, e/c, sodium valproate 200 mg, net price 100-tab pack = £4.83; 500 mg, 100-tab pack = £10.09. Label: 5, 8, 25, counselling, pancreatitis, blood, or hepatic disorder symptoms (see above), driving (see notes above)

Oral solution, sodium valproate 200 mg/5 mL, net price 300 mL = £5.42. Label: 8, 21, counselling, pancreatitis, blood, or hepatic disorder symptoms (see above), driving (see notes above)

**Epilim®** (Sanofi-Aventis) PoM

Tablets (crushable), scored, sodium valproate 100 mg, net price 100-tab pack = £5.60. Label: 8, 21, counselling, pancreatitis, blood, or hepatic disorder symptoms (see above), driving (see notes above)

Tablets, e/c, lilac, sodium valproate 200 mg, net price 100-tab pack = £7.70; 500 mg, 100-tab pack = £19.25. Label: 5, 8, 25, counselling, pancreatitis, blood, or hepatic disorder symptoms (see above), driving (see notes above)

Liquid, red, sugar-free, sodium valproate 200 mg/5 mL, net price 300-mL pack = £9.33. Label: 8, 21, counselling, pancreatitis, blood, or hepatic disorder symptoms (see above), driving (see notes above)

Syrup, red, sodium valproate 200 mg/5 mL, net price 300-mL pack = £7.78. Label: 8, 21, counselling, pancreatitis, blood, or hepatic disorder symptoms (see above), driving (see notes above)

**Note** May be diluted, preferably in Syrup BP; use within 14 days

◢**Modified release**

**Epilim Chrono®** (Sanofi-Aventis) PoM

Tablets, m/r, lilac, sodium valproate 200 mg (as sodium valproate and valproic acid), net price 100-tab pack = £11.65; 300 mg, 100-tab pack = £17.47; 500 mg, 100-tab pack = £29.10. Label: 8, 21, 25, counselling, pancreatitis, blood, or hepatic disorder symptoms (see above), driving (see notes above)

**Dose**

**Epilepsy**

- **By mouth**

  **Child body-weight over 20 kg** as above, total daily dose given in 1–2 divided doses

**Epilim Chronosphere®** (Sanofi-Aventis) PoM

Granules, m/r, sodium valproate 50 mg (as sodium valproate and valproic acid), net price 30-sachet pack = £30.00; 100 mg, 30-sachet pack = £30.00; 250 mg, 30-sachet pack = £30.00; 500 mg, 30-sachet pack = £30.00; 750 mg, 30-sachet pack = £30.00; 1 g, 30-sachet pack = £30.00. Label: 8, 21, 25, counselling, administration, pancreatitis, blood, or hepatic disorder symptoms (see above), driving (see notes above)

**Dose**

**Epilepsy**

- **By mouth**

  **Child** as above to the nearest whole 50-mg sachet; total daily dose given in 1–2 divided doses

**Counselling** Granules may be mixed with soft food or drink that is cold or at room temperature and swallowed immediately without chewing

**Episenta®** (Beacon) PoM

Capsules, enclosing m/r granules, sodium valproate 150 mg, net price 100-cap pack = £7.00; 300 mg, 100-cap pack = £13.00. Label: 8, 21, 25, counselling, administration, pancreatitis, blood, or hepatic disorder symptoms (see above), driving (see notes above)

**Dose**

**Epilepsy**

* By mouth

> **Child** as above, total daily dose given in 1–2 divided doses

**Counselling** Contents of capsule may be mixed with soft food or drink that is cold or at room temperature and swallowed immediately without chewing

Granules, m/r, sodium valproate 500 mg, net price 100-sachet pack = £21.00; 1 g, 100-sachet pack = £41.00. Label: 8, 21, 25, counselling, administration, pancreatitis, blood, or hepatic disorder symptoms (see above), driving (see notes above)

**Dose**

**Epilepsy**

* By mouth

> **Child** as above, total daily dose given in 1–2 divided doses

**Counselling** Granules may be mixed with soft food or drink that is cold or at room temperature and swallowed immediately without chewing

**Epival®** (Chanelle Medical) PoM

Tablets, m/r, scored, sodium valproate 300 mg, net price 100-tab pack = £12.13; 500 mg 100-tab pack = £20.21. Label: 8, 21, 25, counselling, pancreatitis, blood, or hepatic disorder symptoms (see above), driving (see notes above)

**Dose**

**Epilepsy**

* By mouth

> **Child body-weight over 20 kg** as above, total daily dose given in 1–2 divided doses

**Counselling** Tablets may be halved but not crushed or chewed

◢ **Parenteral**

**Epilim® Intravenous** (Sanofi-Aventis) PoM

Injection, powder for reconstitution, sodium valproate, net price 400-mg vial (with 4-mL amp water for injections) = £11.58

**Episenta®** (Beacon) PoM

Injection, sodium valproate 100 mg/mL, net price 3-mL amp = £7.00

◢ **Valproic acid**

**Convulex®** (Pharmacia) PoM

Capsules, e/c, valproic acid 150 mg, net price 100-cap pack = £3.68; 300 mg, 100-cap pack = £7.35; 500 mg, 100-cap pack = £12.25. Label: 8, 21, 25, counselling, pancreatitis, blood, or hepatic disorder symptoms (see above), driving (see notes above)

**Dose**

**Epilepsy**

* By mouth

> **Child** as for sodium valproate, total daily dose given in 2–4 divided doses

**Equivalence to Sodium valproate** Manufacturer advises that Convulex® has a 1:1 dose relationship with products containing sodium valproate, but nevertheless care is needed in making changes

## Vigabatrin

Vigabatrin can be prescribed in combination with other antiepileptic treatment for focal epilepsy with or without secondary generalisation. It should not be prescribed unless all other appropriate drug combinations are ineffective or have not been tolerated, and it should be initiated and supervised by an appropriate specialist. Vigabatrin can be prescribed as monotherapy in the management of infantile spasms in West's syndrome.

About one-third of those treated with vigabatrin have suffered visual field defects; counselling and **careful monitoring** for this side-effect are required (see also Visual Field Defects under Cautions below). Vigabatrin has prominent behavioural side-effects in some children.

### ■ VIGABATRIN

**Cautions** closely monitor neurological function; avoid sudden withdrawal; history of psychosis, depression, or behavioural problems; absence seizures (may be exacerbated); **interactions:** see p. 216 and Appendix 1 (vigabatrin)

**Visual field defects** Vigabatrin is associated with visual field defects. The onset of symptoms varies from 1 month to several years after starting. In most cases, visual field defects have persisted despite discontinuation, and further deterioration after discontinuation cannot be excluded. Product literature advises visual field testing before treatment and at 6-month intervals. Children and their carers should be warned to report any new visual symptoms that develop and those with symptoms should be referred for an urgent ophthalmological opinion. Gradual withdrawal of vigabatrin should be considered.

**Contra-indications** visual field defects

**Renal impairment** consider reduced dose or increased dose interval if estimated glomerular filtration rate less than 60 mL/minute/1.73 m²

**Pregnancy** see Pregnancy, p. 217

**Breast-feeding** present in milk—manufacturer advises avoid; see also Breast-feeding, p. 218

**Side-effects** nausea, abdominal pain; oedema; drowsiness (*rarely* encephalopathic symptoms including marked sedation, stupor, and confusion with non-specific slow wave EEG—reduce dose or withdraw); fatigue, excitation, agitation, dizziness, headache, nervousness, depression, aggression, irritability, paranoia, impaired concentration, impaired memory, tremor, paraesthesia, speech disorder, weight gain; visual field defects (see under Cautions), blurred vision, nystagmus, diplopia; *less commonly* ataxia, psychosis, mania, and rash; occasional increase in seizure frequency (especially if myoclonic); *rarely* suicidal ideation and retinal disorders (including peripheral retinal neuropathy); *very rarely* hepatitis, optic neuritis and optic atrophy; *also reported* movement disorders in infantile spasms

### Indications and dose

**Adjunctive treatment of focal seizures with or without secondary generalisation not satisfactorily controlled with other antiepileptics**

* By mouth

> **Neonate** initially 15–20 mg/kg twice daily increased over 2–3 weeks to usual maintenance dose 30–40 mg/kg twice daily; max. 75 mg/kg twice daily

> **Child 1 month–2 years** initially 15–20 mg/kg twice daily increased over 2–3 weeks to usual maintenance dose 30–40 mg/kg twice daily; max. 75 mg/kg twice daily

**Child 2–12 years** initially 15–20 mg/kg (max. 250 mg) twice daily increased over 2–3 weeks to usual maintenance dose 30–40 mg/kg (max. 1.5 g) twice daily

**Child 12–18 years** initially 250 mg twice daily increased over 2–3 weeks to usual maintenance dose 1–1.5 g twice daily

**Administration** Tablets may be crushed and dispersed in liquid

- **By rectum**

    **Child 1 month–18 years** dose as for oral therapy, see above

    **Administration** dissolve contents of sachet in small amount of water and administer rectally

**Infantile spasms as monotherapy**
- **By mouth**

    **Neonate** initially 15–25 mg/kg twice daily adjusted according to response over 7 days to usual maintenance dose 40–50 mg/kg twice daily; max. 75 mg/kg twice daily

    **Child 1 month–2 years** initially 15–25 mg/kg twice daily adjusted according to response over 7 days to usual maintenance dose 40–50 mg/kg twice daily; max. 75 mg/kg twice daily

**Sabril®** (Sanofi-Aventis) [PoM]

Tablets, f/c, scored, vigabatrin 500 mg, net price 100-tab pack = £30.84. Label: 3, 8, counselling, driving (see notes above)

Powder, sugar-free, vigabatrin 500 mg/sachet. Net price 50-sachet pack = £17.08. Label: 3, 8, 13, counselling, driving (see notes above)

**Note** The contents of a sachet should be dissolved in water or a soft drink immediately before taking

## Benzodiazepines

**Clobazam** may be used as adjunctive therapy in the treatment of epilepsy. **Clonazepam** is occasionally used in tonic-clonic or focal seizures, but its sedative side-effects may be prominent. The effectiveness of clobazam and clonazepam may decrease significantly after weeks or months of continuous therapy.

**Nitrazepam** is used for treating infantile spasms.

**Hepatic impairment** Benzodiazepines can precipitate coma if used in hepatic impairment. Start with smaller initial doses or reduce dose; avoid in severe impairment.

**Renal impairment** Children with renal impairment have increased cerebral sensitivity to benzodiazepines; start with small doses in severe impairment.

**Pregnancy** There is a risk of neonatal withdrawal symptoms when benzodiazepines are used during pregnancy. Avoid regular use and use only if there is a clear indication such as seizure control. High doses administered during late pregnancy or labour may cause neonatal hypothermia, hypotonia, and respiratory depression.

**Breast-feeding** Benzodiazepines are present in milk, and should be avoided if possible during breast-feeding.

## CLOBAZAM

**Cautions** see Diazepam, section 4.8.2
**Contra-indications** see Diazepam, section 4.8.2
**Hepatic impairment** see notes above
**Renal impairment** see notes above
**Pregnancy** see notes above
**Breast-feeding** see notes above
**Side-effects** see Diazepam, section 4.8.2
**Licensed use** not licensed for use in children under 3 years (licensed for use in child 6 months–3 years in exceptional cases); not licensed as monotherapy

**Indications and dose**

Adjunctive therapy for epilepsy, monotherapy under specialist supervision for catamenial (menstruation) seizures (usually for 7–10 days each month, just before and during menstruation), cluster seizures

- **By mouth**

    **Child 1 month–6 years** initially 125 micrograms/kg twice daily, increased if necessary every 5 days to usual maintenance dose of 250 micrograms/kg twice daily; max. 500 micrograms/kg twice daily, not exceeding 15 mg twice daily

    **Child 6–18 years** initially 5 mg daily, increased if necessary every 5 days to usual maintenance dose of 0.3–1 mg/kg daily; max. 60 mg daily; daily doses of up to 30 mg may be given as a single dose at bedtime, higher doses should be divided

**¹Clobazam** (Non-proprietary) [CD4-1] [NHS]

Tablets, clobazam 10 mg. Net price 30-tab pack = £4.68. Label: 2 or 19, 8, counselling, driving (see notes above)

**Brands include** *Frisium*® [NHS]

Tablets, clobazam 5 mg available on a named patient basis

## CLONAZEPAM

**Cautions** see notes above; respiratory disease; spinal or cerebellar ataxia; myasthenia gravis (avoid if unstable); history of alcohol or drug abuse, depression or suicidal ideation; debilitated patients; avoid sudden withdrawal; acute porphyria (section 9.8.2); **interactions:** see p. 216 and Appendix 1 (anxiolytics and hypnotics)

**Driving** Drowsiness may affect performance of skilled tasks (e.g. driving); effects of alcohol enhanced

**Contra-indications** respiratory depression; acute pulmonary insufficiency; sleep apnoea syndrome; marked neuromuscular respiratory weakness including unstable myasthenia gravis
**Hepatic impairment** see notes above
**Renal impairment** see notes above
**Pregnancy** see notes above
**Breast-feeding** see notes above
**Side-effects** drowsiness, fatigue, dizziness, muscle hypotonia, coordination disturbances; also poor concentration, restlessness, confusion, amnesia, dependence, and withdrawal; salivary or bronchial hypersecretion in infants and small children; *rarely* gastrointestinal symptoms, respiratory depression, headache, paradoxical effects including aggression and anxiety, sexual dysfunction, urinary incontinence, urticaria, pruritus, reversible hair loss, skin pigmentation changes; dysarthria, and visual disturbances on long-term treatment; blood disorders reported; **overdosage:** see Emergency Treatment of Poisoning, p. 29

1. [NHS] except for epilepsy and endorsed 'SLS'

**Indications and dose**

All forms of epilepsy

- By mouth

   **Child 1 month–1 year** initially 250 micrograms at night for 4 nights, increased over 2–4 weeks to usual maintenance dose of 0.5–1 mg at night (may be given in 3 divided doses if necessary)

   **Child 1–5 years** initially 250 micrograms at night for 4 nights, increased over 2–4 weeks to usual maintenance of 1–3 mg at night (may be given in 3 divided doses if necessary)

   **Child 5–12 years** initially 500 micrograms at night for 4 nights, increased over 2–4 weeks to usual maintenance dose of 3–6 mg at night (may be given in 3 divided doses if necessary)

   **Child 12–18 years** initially 1 mg at night for 4 nights, increased over 2–4 weeks to usual maintenance dose of 4–8 mg at night (may be given in 3–4 divided doses if necessary)

**Note** Clonazepam doses in BNFC may differ from those in product literature

**Administration** for administration *by mouth*, injection solution may be given orally

**Clonazepam** (Non-proprietary) CD4-1
Tablets, clonazepam 500 micrograms, net price 100-tab pack = £3.93; 2 mg, 100 tab-pack = £5.28. Label: 2, 8, counselling, driving (see notes above)

**Rivotril®** (Roche) CD4-1
Tablets, scored, clonazepam 500 micrograms (beige), net price 100-tab pack = £3.69; 2 mg (white), 100-tab pack = £4.93. Label: 2, 8, counselling, driving (see notes above)

Injection, section 4.8.2

Liquid, clonazepam 0.5 mg/5 mL; 2 mg/5 mL; 2.5 mg/mL.
Available from 'special-order' manufacturers or specialist importing companies, see p. 823

## ▌ NITRAZEPAM

**Cautions** avoid abrupt withdrawal; respiratory disease; acute porphyria (section 9.8.2); muscle weakness and myasthenia gravis; hypoalbuminaemia; **interactions:** Appendix 1 (anxiolytics and hypnotics)

**Contra-indications** respiratory depression, acute pulmonary insufficiency, sleep apnoea syndrome; marked neuromuscular respiratory weakness including myasthenia gravis

**Hepatic impairment** see notes above

**Renal impairment** see notes above

**Side-effects** drowsiness, confusion, ataxia; see also under Diazepam (section 4.8.2); **overdosage:** see Emergency Treatment of Poisoning, p. 29

**Licensed use** not licensed for use in children

**Indications and dose**

Infantile spasms

- By mouth

   **Child 1 month–2 years** initially 125 micrograms/kg twice daily, adjusted according to response over 2–3 weeks to 250 micrograms/kg twice daily; max. 500 micrograms/kg (not exceeding 5 mg) twice daily; total daily dose may alternatively be given in 3 divided doses

**Nitrazepam** (Non-proprietary) CD4-1
Oral suspension, nitrazepam 2.5 mg/5 mL, net price 150 mL = £5.09. Label: 1, 8, counselling, driving (see notes above)
**Brands include** *Somnite®* NHS

## Other drugs

**Acetazolamide** (section 11.6), a carbonic anhydrase inhibitor, has a specific role in treating epilepsy associated with menstruation. It can also be used in conjunction with other antiepileptics for refractory tonic-clonic, absence, or focal seizures. It is occasionally helpful in atypical absence, atonic, and tonic seizures.

**Piracetam** is used as adjunctive treatment for cortical myoclonus.

## 4.8.2 Drugs used in status epilepticus

**Convulsive status epilepticus** Immediate measures to manage status epilepticus include positioning the child to avoid injury, supporting respiration including the provision of oxygen, maintaining blood pressure, and the correction of any hypoglycaemia. **Pyridoxine** (section 9.6.2) should be administered if the status epilepticus is caused by pyridoxine deficiency.

Seizures lasting 5 minutes should be treated urgently with buccal **midazolam** or intravenous **lorazepam** (repeated once after 10 minutes if seizures recur or fail to respond). Intravenous **diazepam** is effective but it carries a high risk of venous thrombophlebitis (reduced by using an emulsion formulation of diazepam injection). **Clonazepam** can also be used as an alternative. Patients should be monitored for respiratory depression and hypotension.

> **Important**
>
> If, after initial treatment with benzodiazepines, seizures recur or fail to respond 25 minutes after onset, phenytoin sodium should be used, or if the child is on regular phenytoin, give phenobarbital intravenously over 5 minutes; the paediatric intensive care unit should be contacted. Paraldehyde can be given after starting phenytoin infusion.
>
> If these measures fail to control seizures 45 minutes after onset, anaesthesia with thiopental (section 15.1.1) should be instituted with full intensive care support.

**Phenytoin sodium** can be given by intravenous infusion over 20 minutes, followed by the maintenance dosage if appropriate; monitor ECG and blood pressure, and reduce rate of administration if bradycardia or hypotension occurs. Intramuscular phenytoin should not be used (absorption is slow and erratic).

**Paraldehyde** given rectally causes little respiratory depression and is therefore useful where facilities for resuscitation are poor.

For **neonatal seizures**, see p. 219.

**Non-convulsive status epilepticus** The urgency to treat non-convulsive status epilepticus depends on the severity of the child's condition. If there is incomplete loss of awareness, oral antiepileptic therapy should be restarted or continued. Children who fail to respond to oral antiepileptic therapy or have complete

**4**

**Central nervous system**

**4 Central nervous system**

lack of awareness can be treated in the same way as convulsive status epilepticus, although anaesthesia is rarely needed.

## ▌ CLONAZEPAM

**Cautions** see Clonazepam, section 4.8.1; facilities for reversing respiratory depression with mechanical ventilation must be at hand (but see also notes above) **Intravenous infusion** Intravenous infusion of clonazepam is potentially hazardous (especially if prolonged), calling for close and constant observation and best carried out in specialist centres with intensive care facilities. Prolonged infusion may lead to accumulation and delay recovery

**Contra-indications** see Clonazepam, section 4.8.1; avoid injections containing benzyl alcohol in neonates (see under preparations below)

**Hepatic impairment** see Benzodiazepines, section 4.8.1

**Renal impairment** see Benzodiazepines, section 4.8.1

**Pregnancy** see Benzodiazepines, section 4.8.1

**Breast-feeding** see Benzodiazepines, section 4.8.1

**Side-effects** see Clonazepam, section 4.8.1; hypotension and apnoea

**Indications and dose**

### Status epilepticus

• By intravenous injection over at least 2 minutes

**Neonate** 100 micrograms/kg repeated after 24 hours if necessary (avoid unless there is no safer alternative)

**Child 1 month–12 years** 50 micrograms/kg (max. 1 mg) repeated once after 10 minutes if necessary

**Child 12–18 years** 1 mg repeated once after 10 minutes if necessary

• By intravenous infusion

**Child 1 month–12 years** initially 50 micrograms/kg (max. 1 mg) *by intravenous injection* then *by intravenous infusion* 10 micrograms/kg/hour adjusted according to response; max. 60 micrograms/kg/hour

**Child 12–18 years** initially 1 mg *by intravenous injection* then *by intravenous infusion* 10 micrograms/kg/hour adjusted according to response; max. 60 micrograms/kg/hour

### Other forms of epilepsy section 4.8.1

**Administration** for *intravenous injection*, dilute to a concentration of 500 micrograms/mL with Water for Injections

For *intravenous infusion*, dilute to a concentration of 12 micrograms/mL with Glucose 5% *or* Sodium Chloride 0.9%; incompatible with bicarbonate; adsorbed on PVC—glass infusion apparatus preferred (if PVC apparatus used, complete infusion within 2 hours)

**Rivotril®** (Roche) [CD4-1]
Injection, clonazepam 1 mg/mL in solvent, net price 1-mL amp (with 1 mL water for injections) = 60p
Excipients include benzyl alcohol (avoid in neonates unless there is no safer alternative available, see Excipients, p. 2), ethanol, propylene glycol

## ▌ DIAZEPAM

**Cautions** respiratory disease, muscle weakness and myasthenia gravis, history of drug or alcohol abuse, marked personality disorder; avoid prolonged use (and abrupt withdrawal thereafter); when given par-

enterally, close observation required until full recovery from sedation; when given intravenously, facilities for reversing respiratory depression with mechanical ventilation must be immediately available (but see also notes above); porphyria (section 9.8.2); **interactions:** Appendix 1 (anxiolytics and hypnotics)
**Skilled tasks** Drowsiness may affect performance of skilled tasks (e.g. driving); effects of alcohol enhanced

**Contra-indications** respiratory depression; marked neuromuscular respiratory weakness including unstable myasthenia gravis; acute pulmonary insufficiency; sleep apnoea syndrome; phobic or obsessional states; hyperkinesis; avoid injections containing benzyl alcohol in neonates (see under preparations below)

**Hepatic impairment** see Benzodiazepines, section 4.8.1

**Renal impairment** see Benzodiazepines, section 4.8.1

**Pregnancy** see Benzodiazepines, section 4.8.1

**Breast-feeding** see Benzodiazepines, section 4.8.1

**Side-effects** drowsiness and lightheadedness the next day, confusion and ataxia, amnesia, dependence, paradoxical increase in aggression, muscle weakness; *occasionally:* dizziness, salivation changes, gynaecomastia, gastro-intestinal disturbances, visual disturbances, dysarthria, tremor, incontinence; *rarely* hypotension, apnoea, respiratory depression, headache, vertigo, changes in libido, urinary retention, blood disorders, jaundice, skin reactions; on intravenous injection, pain, thrombophlebitis; *also reported* irritability, delusions, excitement, restlessness, hallucinations, psychosis; **overdosage:** see Emergency Treatment of Poisoning, p. 29

**Licensed use** *Diazepam Desitin®*, *Diazepam Rectubes®*, and *Stesolid Rectal Tubes®* not licensed for use in children under 1 year

**Indications and dose**

### Status epilepticus, febrile convulsions (section 4.8.3), convulsions caused by poisoning

• By intravenous injection over 3–5 minutes

**Neonate** 300–400 micrograms/kg repeated once after 10 minutes if necessary

**Child 1 month–12 years** 300–400 micrograms/kg (max. 10 mg) repeated once after 10 minutes if necessary

**Child 12–18 years** 10 mg repeated once after 10 minutes if necessary

• By rectum (as rectal solution)

**Neonate** 1.25–2.5 mg repeated once after 10 minutes if necessary

**Child 1 month–2 years** 5 mg repeated once after 10 minutes if necessary

**Child 2–12 years** 5–10 mg repeated once after 10 minutes if necessary

**Child 12–18 years** 10–20 mg repeated once after 10 minutes if necessary

### Life-threatening acute drug-induced dystonic reactions (section 4.9.2)

• By intravenous injection over 3–5 minutes

**Child 1 month–12 years** 100 micrograms/kg repeat doses as necessary

**Child 12–18 years** 5–10 mg repeat doses as necessary

### Muscle spasm section 10.2.2

**Diazepam** (Non-proprietary) [CD4-1]

Injection (solution), diazepam 5 mg/mL, net price
2-mL amp = 45p

Excipients include benzyl alcohol (avoid in neonates
unless there is no safer alternative available, see
Excipients, p. 2), ethanol, propylene glycol

Injection (emulsion), diazepam 5 mg/mL (0.5%), net
price 2-mL amp = 91p

Brands include *Diazemuls*®

Rectal tubes (= rectal solution), diazepam 2 mg/mL,
net price 1.25-mL (2.5-mg) tube = 90p, 2.5-mL (5-
mg) tube = £1.41; 4 mg/mL, 2.5-mL (10-mg) tube =
£1.88

Brands include *Diazepam Desitin*®, *Diazepam Rectubes*®,
*Stesolid*®

---

## FOSPHENYTOIN SODIUM

**Note** Fosphenytoin is a pro-drug of phenytoin

**Cautions** see Phenytoin Sodium; resuscitation facilities must be available; **interactions:** see p. 216 and
Appendix 1 (phenytoin)

**Contra-indications** see Phenytoin Sodium

**Hepatic impairment** consider 10–25% reduction in
dose or infusion rate (except initial dose for status
epilepticus)

**Renal impairment** consider 10–25% reduction in
dose or infusion rate (except initial dose for status
epilepticus)

**Pregnancy** see Phenytoin (section 4.8.1) and
Pregnancy, p. 217

**Breast-feeding** see Phenytoin (section 4.8.1)

**Side-effects** see Phenytoin Sodium; also dry mouth,
taste disturbance, vasodilatation, asthenia, dysarthria,
euphoria, incoordination, chills, visual disturbances,
tinnitus, pruritus, ecchymosis; *less commonly*
hypoaesthesia, increased or decreased reflexes, stupor, muscle weakness, muscle spasm, pain, hypoa-
cusis; *also reported* extrapyramidal disorder, twitching,
confusion, hyperglycaemia

**Important** Intravenous infusion of fosphenytoin has been
associated with severe cardiovascular reactions including
asystole, ventricular fibrillation, and cardiac arrest.
Hypotension, bradycardia, and heart block have also been
reported. The following are recommended:

- monitor heart rate, blood pressure, and respiratory
  function for duration of infusion;

- observe patient for at least 30 minutes after infusion;

- if hypotension occurs, reduce infusion rate or discontinue;

- reduce dose or infusion rate in renal or hepatic impairment.

**Indications and dose**

Expressed as **phenytoin sodium equivalent** (PE);
fosphenytoin sodium 1.5 mg ≡ phenytoin sodium
1 mg

**Status epilepticus**

- By intravenous infusion (at a rate of 2–3 mg(PE)/
  kg/minute, max. 150 mg(PE)/minute)

  **Child 5–18 years** initially 20 mg(PE)/kg, then (at a
  rate of 1–2 mg(PE)/kg/minute, max. 100 mg(PE)/
  minute) 4–5 mg(PE)/kg; total daily dose may be
  given in 1–4 divided doses; adjusted according to
  response and trough plasma-phenytoin concentration

**Prophylaxis or treatment of seizures associated
with neurosurgery or head injury**

- By intravenous infusion (at a rate of 1–2 mg(PE)/
  kg/minute, max. 100 mg(PE)/minute)

  **Child 5–18 years** initially 10–15 mg(PE)/kg then
  4–5 mg(PE)/kg daily; total daily dose may be
  given in 1–4 divided doses; adjusted according to
  response and trough plasma-phenytoin concentration

**Temporary substitution for oral phenytoin**

- By intravenous infusion (at a rate of 1–2 mg(PE)/
  kg/minute, max. 100 mg (PE)/minute)

  **Child 5–18 years** same dose and dosing frequency
  as oral phenytoin therapy

**Note** Fosphenytoin sodium doses in BNFC may differ from
those in product literature

**Note**

Prescriptions for fosphenytoin sodium should state
the dose in terms of phenytoin sodium equivalent
(PE)

**Administration** for *intermittent intravenous infusion*,
dilute to a concentration of 1.5–25 mg (PE)/mL with
Glucose 5% or Sodium Chloride 0.9%

**Pro-Epanutin**® (Pfizer) [PoM]

Injection, fosphenytoin sodium 75 mg/mL (equivalent to phenytoin sodium 50 mg/mL), net price
10-mL vial = £40.00

Electrolytes phosphate 3.7 micromol/mg fosphenytoin
sodium (phosphate 5.6 micromol/mg phenytoin sodium)

---

## LORAZEPAM

**Cautions** see Diazepam; facilities for reversing respiratory depression with mechanical ventilation must
be immediately available

**Contra-indications** see Diazepam

**Hepatic impairment** see Benzodiazepines, section
4.8.1

**Renal impairment** see Benzodiazepines, section 4.8.1

**Pregnancy** see Benzodiazepines, section 4.8.1

**Breast-feeding** see Benzodiazepines, section 4.8.1

**Side-effects** see Diazepam; hypotension and apnoea

**Licensed use** not licensed for use in febrile convulsions or convulsions caused by poisoning

**Indications and dose**

**Status epilepticus, febrile convulsions (section
4.8.3), convulsions caused by poisoning**

- By slow intravenous injection

  **Neonate** 100 micrograms/kg as a single dose,
  repeated once after 10 minutes if necessary

  **Child 1 month–12 years** 100 micrograms/kg
  (max. 4 mg) as a single dose, repeated once after
  10 minutes if necessary

  **Child 12–18 years** 4 mg as a single dose, repeated
  once after 10 minutes if necessary

**Peri-operative use**

Section 15.1.4.1

**Administration** for *intravenous injection*, dilute with an
equal volume of Sodium Chloride 0.9% (for neonates,
dilute injection solution to a concentration of
100 micrograms/mL)

◀ **Preparations**

Section 15.1.4.1

4 Central nervous system

**4 Central nervous system**

## MIDAZOLAM

**Cautions** see Midazolam, section 15.1.4.1

**Contra-indications** see Midazolam, section 15.1.4.1

**Hepatic impairment** use with caution in mild to moderate impairment; avoid in severe impairment

**Renal impairment** use with caution in chronic renal failure

**Pregnancy** see Midazolam, section 15.1.4.1 and Pregnancy, p. 217

**Breast-feeding** amount probably too small to be harmful after single doses

**Side-effects** see Midazolam, section 15.1.4.1

**Licensed use** oromucosal solution not licensed for use in children under 3 months; injection not licensed for use in status epilepticus or febrile convulsions

**Indications and dose**

> **Status epilepticus, febrile convulsions (section 4.8.3)**
>
> • **By buccal administration**
>
> > **Neonate** 300 micrograms/kg, repeated once after 10 minutes if necessary
> >
> > **Child 1–3 months** 300 micrograms/kg (max. 2.5 mg), repeated once after 10 minutes if necessary
> >
> > **Child 3 months–1 year** 2.5 mg, repeated once after 10 minutes if necessary
> >
> > **Child 1–5 years** 5 mg, repeated once after 10 minutes if necessary
> >
> > **Child 5–10 years** 7.5 mg, repeated once after 10 minutes if necessary
> >
> > **Child 10–18 years** 10 mg, repeated once after 10 minutes if necessary
>
> • **By intravenous administration**
>
> > **Neonate** initially *by intravenous injection* 150–200 micrograms/kg followed *by continuous intravenous infusion* of 60 micrograms/kg/hour (increased by 60 micrograms/kg/hour every 15 minutes until seizure controlled); max. 300 micrograms/kg/hour
> >
> > **Child 1 month–18 years** initially *by intravenous injection* 150–200 micrograms/kg followed *by continuous intravenous infusion* of 60 micrograms/kg/hour (increased by 60 micrograms/kg/hour every 15 minutes until seizure controlled); max. 300 micrograms/kg/hour

**Administration** for *intravenous injection*, dilute with Glucose 5% *or* Sodium Chloride 0.9%; rapid intravenous injection (less than 2 minutes) may cause seizure-like myoclonus in preterm neonate

*Neonatal intensive care*, dilute 15 mg/kg body-weight to a final volume of 50 mL with infusion fluid; an intravenous infusion rate of 0.1 mL/hour provides a dose of 30 micrograms/kg/hour

**Buccolam** (ViroPharma) ▼ [CD3]

Oromucosal solution, midazolam (as hydrochloride) 5 mg/mL, 0.5-mL (2.5 mg) prefilled syringe = £20.50, 1-mL (5 mg) prefilled syringe = £21.38, 1.5mL (7.5 mg) prefilled syringe = £22.25, 2-mL (10 mg) prefilled syringe = £22.88. Label: 2, counselling, administration

Note Other unlicensed formulations are also available and may have different doses—refer to product literature

◢**Parenteral preparations**

Section 15.1.4

## PARALDEHYDE

**Cautions** bronchopulmonary disease; **interactions:** Appendix 1 (paraldehyde)

**Contra-indications** gastric disorders; rectal administration in colitis

**Hepatic impairment** use with caution

**Pregnancy** avoid unless essential—crosses placenta

**Breast-feeding** avoid unless essential—present in milk

**Side-effects** rash

**Licensed use** not licensed for use in children as an enema

**Indications and dose**

> **Status epilepticus**
>
> • **By rectum**
>
> See preparation

**Paraldehyde in olive oil** (Non-proprietary) [PoM]

Enema, premixed solution of paraldehyde in olive oil in equal volumes, available from 'special–order' manufacturers or specialist importing companies, p. 823

**Dose**

> **Status epilepticus**
>
> • **By rectum**
>
> > **Neonate** 0.8 mL/kg as a single dose
> >
> > **Child 1 month–18 years** 0.8 mL/kg (max. 20 mL) as a single dose

## PHENOBARBITAL SODIUM
### (Phenobarbitone sodium)

**Cautions** see Phenobarbital, section 4.8.1; **interactions:** see p. 216 and Appendix 1 (phenobarbital)

**Hepatic impairment** see Phenobarbital, section 4.8.1

**Renal impairment** see Phenobarbital, section 4.8.1

**Pregnancy** see Pregnancy, p. 217

**Breast-feeding** see Phenobarbital, section 4.8.1

**Side-effects** see Phenobarbital, section 4.8.1

**Indications and dose**

> **Status epilepticus**
>
> • **By slow intravenous injection** (no faster than 1 mg/kg/minute)
>
> > **Neonate** initially 20 mg/kg then 2.5–5 mg/kg once or twice daily
> >
> > **Child 1 month–12 years** initially 20 mg/kg then 2.5–5 mg/kg once or twice daily
> >
> > **Child 12–18 years** initially 20 mg/kg (max. 1 g) then 300 mg twice daily

> **Other forms of epilepsy** section 4.8.1

Note For therapeutic purposes phenobarbital and phenobarbital sodium may be considered equivalent in effect

**Administration** for *intravenous injection*, dilute to a concentration of 20 mg/mL with Water for Injections

**Phenobarbital** (Non-proprietary) [CD3]

Injection, phenobarbital sodium 15 mg/mL, net price 1-mL amp = £1.64; 30 mg/mL, 1-mL amp = £2.04; 60 mg/mL, 1-mL amp = £2.14; 200 mg/mL, 1-mL amp = £2.00

Excipients include propylene glycol (see Excipients, p. 2)

Note Must be diluted before intravenous administration (see Administration)

# ▲ PHENYTOIN SODIUM

**Cautions** see notes above; respiratory depression; hypotension and heart failure; resuscitation facilities must be available; injection solutions alkaline (irritant to tissues); see also p. 226; **interactions:** see p. 216 and Appendix 1 (phenytoin)

**Contra-indications** sinus bradycardia, sino-atrial block, and second- and third-degree heart block; Stokes-Adams syndrome; acute porphyria (section 9.8.2)

**Hepatic impairment** see Phenytoin, section 4.8.1

**Pregnancy** see Phenytoin, section 4.8.1 and Pregnancy, p. 217

**Breast-feeding** see Phenytoin, section 4.8.1

**Side-effects** intravenous injection may cause cardiovascular and CNS depression (particularly if injection too rapid) with arrhythmias, hypotension, and cardiovascular collapse; alterations in respiratory function (including respiratory arrest); *also reported* tonic seizures, purple glove syndrome; see also p. 226

**Indications and dose**

> **Status epilepticus, acute symptomatic seizures associated with trauma or neurosurgery**
>
> • **By slow intravenous injection or infusion (with blood-pressure and ECG monitoring)**
>
> **Neonate** initially 20 mg/kg as a loading dose then 2.5–5 mg/kg twice daily
>
> **Child 1 month–12 years** initially 20 mg/kg as a loading dose then 2.5–5 mg/kg twice daily
>
> **Child 12–18 years** initially 20 mg/kg as a loading dose then up to 100 mg 3–4 times daily

> **Other forms of epilepsy** section 4.8.1

**Note** Phenytoin sodium doses in BNFC may differ from those in product literature

**Administration** before and after administration flush intravenous line with Sodium Chloride 0.9%.

For *intravenous injection*, give into a large vein at rate not exceeding 1 mg/kg/minute (max. 50 mg/minute).

For *intravenous infusion*, dilute to a concentration not exceeding 10 mg/mL with Sodium Chloride 0.9% and give into a large vein through an in-line filter (0.22–0.50 micron) at a rate not exceeding 1 mg/kg/minute (max. 50 mg/minute); complete administration within 1 hour of preparation

**Phenytoin** (Non-proprietary) [PoM]
Injection, phenytoin sodium 50 mg/mL with propylene glycol 40% and alcohol 10% in water for injections, net price 5-mL amp = £3.40

**Epanutin® Ready-Mixed Parenteral** (Pfizer) [PoM]
Injection, phenytoin sodium 50 mg/mL with propylene glycol 40% and alcohol 10% in water for injections. Net price 5-mL amp = £4.88

## 4.8.3 Febrile convulsions

*Brief febrile convulsions* need no specific treatment; antipyretic medication (e.g. **paracetamol**, section 4.7.1) is commonly used to reduce fever and prevent further convulsions but evidence to support this practice is lacking. *Prolonged febrile convulsions* (those lasting 5 minutes or longer), or *recurrent febrile convulsions* without recovery, must be treated actively (as for convulsive status epilepticus section 4.8.2).

Long-term anticonvulsant prophylaxis for febrile convulsions is rarely indicated.

## 4.9 Drugs used in dystonias and related disorders

4.9.1 Dopaminergic drugs used in dystonias

4.9.2 Antimuscarinic drugs used in dystonias

4.9.3 Drugs used in essential tremor, chorea, tics, and related disorders

Dystonias may result from conditions such as cerebral palsy or may be related to a deficiency of the neurotransmitter dopamine as in Segawa syndrome.

## 4.9.1 Dopaminergic drugs used in dystonias

**Levodopa**, the amino-acid precursor of dopamine, acts by replenishing depleted striatal dopamine. It is given with an extracerebral **dopa-decarboxylase inhibitor**, which reduces the peripheral conversion of levodopa to dopamine, thereby limiting side-effects such as nausea, vomiting, and cardiovascular effects; additionally, effective brain-dopamine concentrations are achieved with lower doses of levodopa. The extracerebral dopa-decarboxylase inhibitor most commonly used in children is carbidopa (in **co-careldopa**).

Levodopa therapy should be initiated at a low dose and increased in small steps; the final dose should be as low as possible. Intervals between doses should be chosen to suit the needs of the individual child.

In severe dystonias related to cerebral palsy, improvement can be expected within 2 weeks. Children with Segawa syndrome are particularly sensitive to levodopa; they may even become symptom free on small doses. Levodopa also has a role in treating metabolic disorders such as defects in tetrahydrobiopterin synthesis and dihydrobiopterin reductase deficiency. For the use of tetrahydrobiopterin in metabolic disorders see section 9.4.1.

Children may experience nausea within 2 hours of taking a dose; nausea and vomiting with co-careldopa is rarely dose-limiting, but domperidone (section 4.6) can be useful in controlling these effects.

In dystonic cerebral palsy, treatment with larger doses of levodopa is associated with the development of potentially troublesome motor complications (including response fluctuations and dyskinesias). Response fluctuations are characterised by large variations in motor performance, with normal function during the 'on' period, and weakness and restricted mobility during the 'off' period.

4 Central nervous system

## Sudden onset of sleep

Excessive daytime sleepiness and sudden onset of sleep can occur with co-careldopa.

Children starting treatment with these drugs, and their carers, should be warned of the risk and of the need to exercise caution when performing skilled tasks e.g. driving or operating machinery. Children who have experienced excessive sedation or sudden onset of sleep should refrain from performing skilled tasks until these effects have stopped occurring.

Management of excessive daytime sleepiness should focus on the identification of an underlying cause, such as depression or concomitant medication. Children, and their carers, should be counselled on improving sleep behaviour.

## CO-CARELDOPA

A mixture of carbidopa and levodopa; the proportions are expressed in the form *x*/*y* where *x* and *y* are the strengths in milligrams of carbidopa and levodopa respectively

**Cautions** see also notes above; pulmonary disease, peptic ulceration, cardiovascular disease (including history of myocardial infarction with residual arrhythmia), diabetes mellitus, osteomalacia, susceptibility to angle-closure glaucoma, history of skin melanoma (risk of activation), psychiatric illness (avoid if severe and discontinue if deterioration); warn children and carers about excessive drowsiness (see notes above); in prolonged therapy, psychiatric, hepatic, haematological, renal, and cardiovascular monitoring is advisable; warn patients to resume normal activities gradually; avoid abrupt withdrawal; **interactions:** Appendix 1 (levodopa)

**Pregnancy** use with caution—toxicity in *animal* studies

**Breast-feeding** may suppress lactation; present in milk—avoid

**Side-effects** see also notes above; anorexia, nausea and vomiting, insomnia, agitation, postural hypotension (rarely labile hypertension), dizziness, tachycardia, arrhythmias, reddish discoloration of urine and other body fluids; *rarely* hypersensitivity; *very rarely* angle-closure glaucoma; abnormal involuntary movements and psychiatric symptoms which include hypomania and psychosis may be dose-limiting; depression, drowsiness, headache, flushing, sweating, gastro-intestinal bleeding, peripheral neuropathy, taste disturbance, pruritus, rash, and liver enzyme changes also reported; syndrome resembling neuroleptic malignant syndrome reported on withdrawal

**Licensed use** not licensed for use in children

**Indications and dose**

> **Dopamine-sensitive dystonias including Segawa syndrome and dystonias related to cerebral palsy**
> • By mouth, expressed as levodopa
>> **Child 3 months–18 years** initially 250 micrograms/kg 2–3 times daily of a preparation containing 1:4 carbidopa:levodopa, increased according to response every 2–3 days to max. 1 mg/kg three times daily

## Treatment of defects in tetrahydrobiopterin synthesis and dihydrobiopterin reductase deficiency

• By mouth, expressed as levodopa

> **Neonate** initially 250–500 micrograms/kg 4 times daily of a preparation containing 1:4 carbidopa: levodopa, increased according to response every 4–5 days to maintenance dose of 2.5–3 mg/kg 4 times daily; at higher doses consider preparation containing 1:10 carbidopa:levodopa; review regularly (every 3–6 months)

> **Child 1 month–18 years** initially 250–500 micrograms/kg 4 times daily of a preparation containing 1:4 carbidopa:levodopa, increased according to response every 4–5 days to maintenance dose of 2.5–3 mg/kg 4 times daily; at higher doses consider preparation containing 1:10 carbidopa:levodopa; review regularly (every 3–6 months in early childhood)

**Co-careldopa** (Non-proprietary) [PoM]

Tablets, co-careldopa 10/100 (carbidopa 10 mg (anhydrous), levodopa 100 mg), net price 100-tab pack = £7.30. Label: 14, counselling, skilled tasks, see notes above

Tablets, co-careldopa 25/100 (carbidopa 25 mg (anhydrous), levodopa 100 mg), net price 100-tab pack = £24.45. Label: 14, counselling, skilled tasks, see notes above

Tablets, co-careldopa 25/250 (carbidopa 25 mg (anhydrous), levodopa 250 mg), net price 100-tab pack = £34.58. Label: 14, counselling, skilled tasks, see notes above

**Sinemet®** (MSD) [PoM]

Sinemet® 12.5 mg/50 mg tablets, yellow, scored, co-careldopa 12.5/50 (carbidopa 12.5 mg (anhydrous), levodopa 50 mg), net price 90-tab pack = £6.28. Label: 14, counselling, skilled tasks, see notes above

Note 2 tablets *Sinemet®* 12.5 mg/50 mg ≡ 1 tablet *Sinemet®* Plus 25 mg/100 mg

Sinemet® 10 mg/100 mg tablets, blue, scored, co-careldopa 10/100 (carbidopa 10 mg (anhydrous), levodopa 100 mg), net price 90-tab pack = £6.57. Label: 14, counselling, skilled tasks, see notes above

Sinemet® Plus 25 mg/100 mg tablets, yellow, scored, co-careldopa 25/100 (carbidopa 25 mg (anhydrous), levodopa 100 mg), net price 90-tab pack = £9.66. Label: 14, counselling, skilled tasks, see notes above

Sinemet® 25 mg/250 mg tablets, blue, scored, co-careldopa 25/250 (carbidopa 25 mg (anhydrous), levodopa 250 mg), net price 90-tab pack = £13.72. Label: 14, counselling, skilled tasks, see notes above

## 4.9.2 Antimuscarinic drugs used in dystonias

The antimuscarinic drugs **procyclidine** and **trihexyphenidyl** reduce the symptoms of dystonias, including those induced by antipsychotic drugs; there is no justification for giving them routinely in the absence of dystonic symptoms. Tardive dyskinesia is not improved by antimuscarinic drugs and may be made worse.

*Central nervous system* **4**

There are no important differences between the antimuscarinic drugs, but some children tolerate one better than another.

Procyclidine can be given parenterally and is effective emergency treatment for acute drug-induced dystonic reactions.

If treatment with an antimuscarinic is ineffective, intravenous diazepam (p. 234) can be given for life-threatening acute drug-induced dystonic reactions.

**Cautions**   Antimuscarinics should be used with caution in cardiovascular disease, hypertension, psychotic disorders, pyrexia, and in those susceptible to angle-closure glaucoma. Antimuscarinics should not be withdrawn abruptly in children taking long-term treatment. Antimuscarinics are liable to abuse. **Interactions:** Appendix 1 (Antimuscarinics).

**Skilled tasks**   Antimuscarinics can affect performance of skilled tasks (e.g. driving).

**Contra-indications**   Antimuscarinics should be avoided in gastro-intestinal obstruction and myasthenia gravis.

**Hepatic and renal impairment**   Procyclidine and trihexyphenidyl should be used with caution in children with hepatic or renal impairment.

**Side-effects**   Side-effects of antimuscarinics include constipation, dry mouth, nausea, vomiting, tachycardia, dizziness, confusion, euphoria, hallucinations, impaired memory, anxiety, restlessness, urinary retention, blurred vision, and rash. Angle-closure glaucoma occurs very rarely.

## ▌ PROCYCLIDINE HYDROCHLORIDE

**Cautions**   see notes above; **interactions:** Appendix 1 (antimuscarinics)
**Contra-indications**   see notes above
**Hepatic impairment**   see notes above
**Renal impairment**   see notes above
**Pregnancy**   use only if potential benefit outweighs risk
**Breast-feeding**   no information available
**Side-effects**   see notes above; also gingivitis
**Licensed use**   not licensed for use in children
**Indications and dose**

Dystonias
● By mouth
    **Child 7–12 years** 1.25 mg 3 times daily
    **Child 12–18 years** 2.5 mg 3 times daily

Acute dystonia
● By intramuscular or intravenous injection
    **Child under 2 years** 0.5–2 mg as a single dose
    **Child 2–10 years** 2–5 mg as a single dose
    **Child 10–18 years** 5–10 mg (occasionally more than 10 mg)
    **Note** Usually effective in 5–10 minutes but may need 30 minutes for relief

**Procyclidine** (Non-proprietary) PoM
Tablets, procyclidine hydrochloride 5 mg, net price 28-tab pack = £2.77. Counselling, driving

**Arpicolin®** (Rosemont) PoM
Syrup, sugar-free, procyclidine hydrochloride 2.5 mg/5 mL, net price 150 mL = £4.22; 5 mg/5 mL, 150 mL pack = £7.54. Counselling, driving

**Kemadrin®** (Aspen) PoM
Tablets, scored, procyclidine hydrochloride 5 mg, net price 100-tab pack = £4.72. Counselling, driving

**Kemadrin®** (Auden Mckenzie) PoM
Injection, procyclidine hydrochloride 5 mg/mL, net price 2-mL amp = £1.49

## ▌ TRIHEXYPHENIDYL HYDROCHLORIDE
(Benzhexol hydrochloride)

**Cautions**   see notes above; **interactions:** Appendix 1 (antimuscarinics)
**Contra-indications**   see notes above
**Hepatic impairment**   see notes above
**Renal impairment**   see notes above
**Pregnancy**   use only if potential benefit outweighs risk
**Breast-feeding**   avoid
**Side-effects**   see notes above
**Licensed use**   not licensed for use in children
**Indications and dose**

Dystonia
● By mouth
    **Child 3 months–18 years** initially 1–2 mg daily in 1–2 divided doses, increased every 3–7 days by 1 mg daily; adjusted according to response and side-effects; max. 2 mg/kg daily

**Trihexyphenidyl** (Non-proprietary) PoM
Tablets, trihexyphenidyl hydrochloride 2 mg, net price 84-tab pack = £19.60; 5 mg, 84-tab pack = £16.79, 100-tab pack = £15.60. Counselling, before or after food, driving

**Broflex®** (Alliance) PoM
Syrup, pink, black currant, trihexyphenidyl hydrochloride 5 mg/5 mL, net price 200 mL = £7.44. Counselling, driving

## 4.9.3 Drugs used in essential tremor, chorea, tics, and related disorders

**Haloperidol** can improve motor tics and symptoms of Tourette syndrome and related choreas (see section 4.2.1). Other treatments for Tourette syndrome include **pimozide** (p. 176) [unlicensed indication] (**important:** ECG monitoring required) and **sulpiride** (p. 176) [unlicensed indication].

**Propranolol** or another beta-adrenoceptor blocking drug (section 2.4) may be useful in treating essential tremor or tremor associated with anxiety or thyrotoxicosis.

**Botulinum toxin type A** should be used under specialist supervision. Treatment with botulinum toxin type A can be considered in children with an acquired non-progressive brain injury if rapid-onset spasticity causes postural or functional difficulties, and in children with spasticity in whom focal dystonia causes postural or functional difficulties or pain.

**4 Central nervous system**

## ▌BOTULINUM TOXIN TYPE A

**Cautions** neurological disorders (can lead to increased sensitivity and exaggerated muscle weakness); excessive weakness or atrophy in target muscle; history of dysphagia or aspiration; chronic respiratory disorder

**Contra-indications** generalised disorders of muscle activity (e.g. myasthenia gravis); infection at injection site

**Pregnancy** low risk of systemic absorption but avoid unless essential

**Breast-feeding** low risk of systemic absorption but avoid unless essential

**Side-effects** increased electrophysiologic jitter in some distant muscles; misplaced injections may paralyse nearby muscle groups and excessive doses may paralyse distant muscles; influenza-like symptoms, *rarely* arrhythmias, myocardial infarction, seizures, hypersensitivity reactions including rash, pruritus and anaphylaxis, antibody formation (substantial deterioration in response); *very rarely* exaggerated muscle weakness, dysphagia, dysphonia, respiratory disorders, aspiration, (see Counselling below)
**Specific side-effects in paediatric cerebral palsy** Drowsiness, paraesthesia, urinary incontinence, myalgia

### Indications and dose

In children over 2 years for dynamic equinus foot deformity caused by spasticity in ambulant paediatric cerebral palsy for dose consult product literature (**important**: information specific to **each individual preparation** and **not interchangeable**)

**Counselling** Children and carers should be warned of the signs and symptoms of toxin spread, such as muscle weakness and breathing difficulties; they should be advised to seek immediate medical attention if swallowing, speech or breathing difficulties occur

**Botox®** (Allergan) PoM
Injection, powder for reconstitution, botulinum toxin type A complex, net price 50-unit vial = £77.50; 100-unit vial = £138.20; 200-unit vial = £276.40. Counselling, side-effects, see under Dose above

**Dysport®** (Ipsen) PoM
Injection, powder for reconstitution, botulinum type A toxin-haemagglutinin complex, net price 300-unit vial = £92.40; 500-unit vial = £154.00. Counselling, side-effects, see under Dose above

## ▌4.10 Drugs used in substance dependence

This section includes drugs used in the treatment of neonatal abstinence syndrome and cigarette smoking.

Treatment of alcohol or opioid dependence in children requires specialist management. The UK health departments have produced guidance on the treatment of drug misuse in the UK. *Drug Misuse and Dependence: UK Guidelines on Clinical Management (2007)* is available at www.nta.nhs.uk/uploads/clinical_guidelines_2007.pdf.

**Neonatal abstinence syndrome** Neonatal abstinence syndrome occurs at birth as a result of intra-uterine exposure to opioids or high-dose benzodiazepines.

Treatment is usually initiated if:

● feeding becomes a problem and tube feeding is required;

● there is profuse vomiting or watery diarrhoea;

● the baby remains very unsettled after two consecutive feeds despite gentle swaddling and the use of a pacifier.

Treatment involves weaning the baby from the drug on which it is dependent. **Morphine** or **methadone** (section 4.7.2) can be used in babies of mothers who have been taking opioids. Morphine is widely used because the dose can be easily adjusted, but methadone may provide smoother control of symptoms. Weaning babies from opioids usually takes 7–10 days.

Weaning babies from benzodiazepines that have a long half-life is difficult to manage; **chlorpromazine** (section 4.2.1) may be used in these situations but excessive sedation may occur. For babies who are dependent on barbiturates, phenobarbital (section 4.8.1) may be tried, although it does not control gastro-intestinal symptoms.

## ▌4.10.1 Alcohol dependence

Classification not used in *BNF for Children*.

## ▌4.10.2 Nicotine dependence

Smoking cessation interventions are a cost-effective way of reducing ill health and prolonging life. Smokers should be advised to stop and offered help with follow-up when appropriate. If possible, smokers should have access to smoking cessation services for behavioural support.

Therapy to aid smoking cessation is chosen according to the smoker's likely adherence, availability of counselling and support, previous experience of smoking-cessation aids, contra-indications and adverse effects of the preparations, and the smoker's preferences. Nicotine replacement therapy is an effective aid to smoking cessation. The use of nicotine replacement therapy in an individual who is already accustomed to nicotine introduces few new risks and it is widely accepted that there are no circumstances in which it is safer to smoke than to use nicotine replacement therapy.

Some individuals benefit from having more than one type of nicotine replacement therapy prescribed, such as a combination of transdermal and oral preparations.

**Concomitant medication** Cigarette smoking increases the metabolism of some medicines by stimulating the hepatic enzyme CYP1A2. When smoking is discontinued, the dose of these drugs, in particular theophylline p. 140 and some antipsychotics (including clozapine p. 178, olanzapine p. 179, chlorpromazine p. 174, and haloperidol p. 174), may need to be reduced. Regular monitoring for adverse effects is advised.

## Nicotine replacement therapy

Nicotine replacement therapy can be used in place of cigarettes after abrupt cessation of smoking, or alternatively to reduce the amount of cigarettes used in advance of making a quit attempt. Nicotine replacement therapy can also be used to minimise passive smoking, and to treat cravings and reduce compensatory smoking after enforced abstinence in smoke-free environments. Smokers who find it difficult to achieve abstinence should consult a healthcare professional for advice.

**Choice**    Nicotine patches are a prolonged-release formulation and are applied for 16 hours (with the patch removed overnight) or for 24 hours. If the individual experiences strong cravings for cigarettes on waking, a 24-hour patch may be more suitable. Immediate-release nicotine preparations (gum, lozenges, sublingual tablets, inhalator, nasal spray, and oral spray) are used whenever the urge to smoke occurs or to prevent cravings.

The choice of nicotine replacement preparation depends largely on patient preference, and should take into account what preparations, if any, have been tried before. Patients with a high level of nicotine dependence, or who have failed with nicotine replacement therapy previously, may benefit from using a combination of an immediate-release preparation and patches to achieve abstinence.

All preparations are licensed for children over 12 years (with the exception of *Nicotinell*® lozenges which are licensed for children under 18 years only when recommended by a doctor).

**Cautions**    Most warnings for nicotine replacement therapy also apply to continued cigarette smoking, but the risk of continued smoking outweighs any risks of using nicotine preparations. Nicotine replacement therapy should be used with caution in haemodynamically unstable patients hospitalised with severe arrhythmias, myocardial infarction, or cerebrovascular accident, and in patients with phaeochromocytoma or uncontrolled hyperthyroidism. Care is also needed in individuals with diabetes mellitus—blood-glucose concentration should be monitored closely when initiating treatment.

Specific cautions for individual preparations are usually related to the local effect of nicotine. *Oral preparations* should be used with caution in patients with oesophagitis, gastritis, or peptic ulcers because swallowed nicotine can aggravate these conditions. The *gum* may also stick to and damage dentures. Acidic beverages, such as coffee or fruit juice, may decrease the absorption of nicotine through the buccal mucosa and should be avoided for 15 minutes before the use of oral nicotine replacement therapy. Care should be taken with the *inhalation cartridges* in patients with obstructive lung disease, chronic throat disease, or bronchospastic disease. The *nasal spray* can cause worsening of bronchial asthma. *Patches* should not be placed on broken skin and should be used with caution in patients with skin disorders.

**Hepatic impairment**    Nicotine replacement therapy should be used with caution in moderate to severe hepatic impairment.

**Renal impairment**    Nicotine replacement therapy should be used with caution in severe renal impairment.

**Pregnancy**    The use of nicotine replacement therapy in pregnancy is preferable to the continuation of smoking, but should be used only if smoking cessation without nicotine replacement fails. Intermittent therapy is preferable to patches but avoid liquorice-flavoured nicotine products. Patches are useful however, if the young woman is experiencing pregnancy-related nausea and vomiting. If patches are used, they should be removed before bed.

**Breast-feeding**    Nicotine is present in milk; however, the amount to which the infant is exposed is small and less hazardous than second-hand smoke. Intermittent therapy is preferred.

**Side-effects**    Some systemic effects occur on initiation of therapy, particularly if the individual is using high-strength preparations; however, the individual may confuse side-effects of the nicotine-replacement preparation with nicotine withdrawal symptoms. Common symptoms of nicotine withdrawal include malaise, headache, dizziness, sleep disturbance, coughing, influenza-like symptoms, depression, irritability, increased appetite, weight gain, restlessness, anxiety, drowsiness, aphthous ulcers, decreased heart rate, and impaired concentration.

Mild topical reactions at the beginning of treatment are common because of the irritant effect of nicotine. *Oral preparations* and *inhalation cartridges* can cause irritation of the throat, *gum*, *lozenges*, and *oral spray* can cause increased salivation, and *patches* can cause minor skin irritation. The *nasal spray* commonly causes coughing, nasal irritation, epistaxis, sneezing, and watery eyes; the *oral spray* can cause watery eyes and blurred vision.

Gastro-intestinal disturbances are common and may be caused by swallowed nicotine. Nausea, vomiting, dyspepsia, and hiccup occur most frequently. Ulcerative stomatitis has also been reported. Dry mouth is a common side-effect of *lozenges*, *patches*, *oral spray*, and *sublingual tablets*. *Lozenges* cause diarrhoea, constipation, dysphagia, oesophagitis, gastritis, mouth ulcers, bloating, flatulence, and less commonly, taste disturbance, thirst, gingival bleeding, and halitosis. The *oral spray* may also cause abdominal pain, flatulence, and taste disturbance.

Palpitations may occur with nicotine replacement therapy and rarely *patches* and *oral spray* can cause arrhythmia. The *inhalator* can very rarely cause reversible atrial fibrillation. *Patches*, *lozenges*, and *oral spray* can cause chest pain.

Paraesthesia is a common side-effect of *oral spray*. Abnormal dreams can occur with *patches*; removal of the patch before bed may help. *Lozenges* and *oral spray* may cause rash and hot flushes. Sweating and myalgia can occur with *patches* and *oral spray*; the *patches* can also cause arthralgia.

**Nicotine medicated chewing gum**    Individuals who smoke fewer than 20 cigarettes each day should use 1 piece of 2-mg strength gum when the urge to smoke occurs or to prevent cravings; individuals who smoke more than 20 cigarettes each day or who require more than 15 pieces of 2-mg strength gum each day should use the 4-mg strength. Individuals should not exceed 15 pieces of 4-mg strength gum daily. If attempting smoking cessation, treatment should continue for 3 months before reducing the dose.

**Administration**    Chew the gum until the taste becomes strong, then rest it between the cheek and gum; when the taste starts to fade, repeat this process. One piece of gum lasts for approximately 30 minutes.

**4**

**Central nervous system**

**Nicotine inhalation cartridge** The cartridges can be used when the urge to smoke occurs or to prevent cravings, up to a maximum of 12 cartridges of the 10-mg strength daily, or 6 cartridges of the 15-mg strength daily.

**Administration** Insert the cartridge into the device and draw in air through the mouthpiece; each session can last for approximately 5 minutes. The amount of nicotine from 1 puff of the cartridge is less than that from a cigarette, therefore it is necessary to inhale more often than when smoking a cigarette. A single 10-mg cartridge lasts for approximately 20 minutes of intense use; a single 15-mg cartridge lasts for approximately 40 minutes of intense use.

**Nicotine lozenge** One lozenge should be used every 1–2 hours when the urge to smoke occurs. Individuals who smoke less than 20 cigarettes each day should usually use the lower-strength lozenges; individuals who smoke more than 20 cigarettes each day and those who fail to stop smoking with the low-strength lozenges should use the higher-strength lozenges. Individuals should not exceed 15 lozenges daily. If attempting smoking cessation, treatment should continue for 6–12 weeks before attempting a reduction in dose.

**Administration** Slowly allow each lozenge to dissolve in the mouth; periodically move the lozenge from one side of the mouth to the other. Lozenges last for 10–30 minutes, depending on their size.

**Nicotine sublingual tablets** Individuals who smoke fewer than 20 cigarettes each day should initially use 1 tablet each hour, increased to 2 tablets each hour if necessary; individuals who smoke more than 20 cigarettes each day should use 2 tablets each hour. Individuals should not exceed 40 tablets daily. If attempting smoking cessation, treatment should continue for up to 3 months before reducing the dose.

**Administration** Each tablet should be placed under the tongue and allowed to dissolve.

**Nicotine oral spray** Individuals can use 1–2 sprays in the mouth when the urge to smoke occurs or to prevent cravings. Individuals should not exceed 2 sprays per episode (up to 4 sprays every hour), and a maximum of 64 sprays daily.

**Administration** The oral spray should be released into the mouth, holding the spray as close to the mouth as possible and avoiding the lips. The individual should not inhale while spraying and avoid swallowing for a few seconds after use.

**Note** If using the oral spray for the first time, or if unit not used for 2 or more days, prime the unit before administration

**Nicotine nasal spray** Individuals can use 1 spray in each nostril when the urge to smoke occurs, up to twice every hour for 16 hours daily (maximum 64 sprays daily). If attempting smoking cessation, treatment should continue for 8 weeks before reducing the dose.

**Administration** Initially 1 spray should be used in both nostrils but when withdrawing from therapy, the dose can be gradually reduced to 1 spray in 1 nostril.

**Nicotine transdermal patches** As a general guide for smoking cessation, individuals who smoke more than 10 cigarettes daily should apply a high-strength patch daily for 6–8 weeks, followed by the medium strength patch for 2 weeks, and then the low-strength patch for the final 2 weeks; individuals who smoke fewer than 10 cigarettes daily can usually start with the medium-strength patch for 6–8 weeks, followed by the low-strength patch for 2–4 weeks. A slower titration schedule can be used in patients who are not ready to quit but want to reduce cigarette consumption before a quit attempt.

If abstinence is not achieved, or if withdrawal symptoms are experienced, the strength of the patch used should be maintained or increased until the patient is stabilised. Individuals using the high-strength patch who experience excessive side-effects, that do not resolve within a few days, should change to a medium-strength patch for the remainder of the initial period and then use the low strength patch for 2–4 weeks.

**Administration** Patches should be applied on waking to dry, non-hairy skin on the hip, trunk, or upper arm and held in position for 10–20 seconds to ensure adhesion; place next patch on a different area and avoid using the same site for several days.

---

## ◀ NICOTINE

**Cautions** see notes above; **interactions:** Appendix 1 (nicotine)

**Hepatic impairment** see notes above

**Renal impairment** see notes above

**Pregnancy** see notes above

**Breast-feeding** see notes above

**Side-effects** see notes above

**Indications and dose**
See notes above

**Nicorette®** (McNeil)
Tablets (sublingual) (*Nicorette Microtab®*), nicotine (as a cyclodextrin complex) 2 mg, net price starter pack of 2 × 15-tablet discs with dispenser = £4.46; pack of 100 = £12.12. Label: 26, counselling, administration, see notes above
**Note** Also available as *NicAssist®*

Chewing gum, sugar-free, nicotine (as resin) 2 mg, net price pack of 30 = £3.41, pack of 105 = £9.37, pack of 210 = £14.82; 4 mg, pack of 30 = £3.99, pack of 105 = £11.48, pack of 210 = £18.24. Counselling, administration, see notes above
**Note** Available in mint, freshfruit, freshmint, and icy white flavours (icy white flavour not available for pack size of 210 pieces). Also available as *NicAssist®*

Mint lozenge, sugar-free, nicotine (as bitartrate) 2 mg, net price pack of 24 = £2.55, pack of 96 = £8.29. Label: 24, counselling, administration, see notes above

Patches, self-adhesive, beige, nicotine, '5 mg' patch (releasing approx. 5 mg/16 hours), net price 7 = £9.07; '10 mg' patch (releasing approx. 10 mg/16 hours), 7 = £9.07; '15 mg' patch (releasing approx. 15 mg/16 hours), 2 = £2.85, 7 = £9.07. Counselling, administration, see notes above
**Note** Also available as *NicAssist®*

Invisi patches, self-adhesive, beige, nicotine, '10 mg' patch (releasing approx. 10 mg/16 hours), net price 7 = £9.97; '15 mg' patch (releasing approx. 15 mg/16 hours), 7 = £9.97; '25 mg' patch (releasing approx. 25 mg/16 hours), 7 = £9.97. Counselling, administration, see notes above
**Note** Also available as *NicAssist® Translucent* patches

*4 Central nervous system*

Oral spray (*Nicorette Quickmist® mouthspray*), nicotine 1 mg/metered dose, net price 150-dose pack = £11.48, 2 × 150-dose pack = £18.50. Counselling, administration, see notes above
**Note** Contains < 100 mg ethanol per dose

Nasal spray, nicotine 500 micrograms/metered spray, net price 200-spray unit = £13.40. Counselling, administration, see notes above
**Note** Also available as *NicAssist®*

Inhalator (nicotine-impregnated plug for use in inhalator mouthpiece), nicotine 10 mg/cartridge, net price 6-cartridge pack = £4.46, 42-cartridge pack = £14.01; 15 mg/cartridge, 4-cartridge pack = £4.14 , 20-cartridge pack = £14.03, 36-cartridge pack = £22.33. Counselling, administration, see notes above
**Note** Also available as *NicAssist®*

**Nicotinell®** (Novartis Consumer Health)
Chewing gum, sugar-free, nicotine (as polacrilin complex) 2 mg, net price pack of 12 = £1.71, pack of 24 = £3.01, pack of 72 = £6.69, pack of 96 = £8.26, pack of 204 = £14.23; 4 mg, pack of 12 = £1.70, pack of 24 = £3.30, pack of 72 = £8.29, pack of 96 = £10.26. Counselling, administration, see notes above
**Note** Also available in fruit, liquorice, icemint, and mint flavours

Mint lozenge, sugar-free, nicotine (as bitartrate) 1 mg, net price pack of 12 = £1.71, pack of 36 = £4.27, pack of 96 = £9.12; 2 mg, pack of 12 = £1.99, pack of 36 = £4.95, pack of 96 = £10.60. Label: 24, counselling, administration, see notes above
**Excipients** include aspartame (section 9.4.1)

TTS Patches, self-adhesive, all yellowish-ochre, nicotine, '*10*' patch (releasing approx. 7 mg/24 hours), net price 7 = £9.12; '*20*' patch (releasing approx. 14 mg/24 hours), 2 = £2.57, 7 = £9.40; '*30*' patch (releasing approx. 21 mg/24 hours), 2 = £2.85, 7 = £9.97, 21 = £24.51. Counselling, administration, see notes above

**NiQuitin®** (GSK Consumer Healthcare)
Chewing gum, sugar-free, mint-flavour, nicotine 2 mg (white), net price pack of 12 = £1.71, pack of 24 = £2.85, pack of 96 = £8.55; 4 mg (yellow), pack of 12 = £1.71, pack of 24 = £2.85, pack of 96 = £8.55. Counselling, administration, see notes above

Lozenges, sugar-free, nicotine (as resinate) 1.5 mg (cherry- and mint-flavoured), net price pack of 20 = £3.18, pack of 60 = £8.93; 2 mg (mint-flavoured), pack of 36 = £5.12, pack of 72 = £9.97; 4 mg (mint-flavoured), pack of 20 = £3.18, pack of 36 = £5.12, pack of 60 = £8.93, pack of 72 = £9.97. Label: 24, counselling, administration, see notes above
**Excipients** include aspartame (section 9.4.1); contains 0.65 mmol Na$^+$/lozenge
**Note** Nicotine (as resinate) also available as *Niquitin® Pre-quit* lozenges and *Niquitin® Minis* lozenges

Patches, self-adhesive, pink/beige, nicotine '*7 mg*' patch (releasing approx. 7 mg/24 hours), net price 7 = £9.97; '*14 mg*' patch (releasing approx. 14 mg/24 hours), 7 = £9.97; '*21 mg*' patch (releasing approx. 21 mg/24 hours), 7 = £9.97, 14 = £18.79. Counselling, administration, see notes above
**Note** Also available as a clear patch

## 4.10.3 Opioid dependence

Classification not used in *BNF for Children*.

## 4.11 Drugs for dementia

Classification not used in *BNF for Children*.

# 5 Infections

This chapter includes advice on the drug management of the following:

anthrax, p. 299

bacterial infections: table 1, summary of antibacterial treatment, p. 246

bacterial infections: table 2, summary of antibacterial prophylaxis, p. 256

Lyme disease, p. 262

MRSA infections, p. 261

oral infections, p. 245 and p. 253

## Notifiable diseases

Doctors must notify the Proper Officer of the local authority (usually the consultant in communicable disease control) when attending a patient suspected of suffering from any of the diseases listed below; a form is available from the Proper Officer.

| | |
|---|---|
| Anthrax | Mumps |
| Botulism | Paratyphoid fever |
| Brucellosis | Plague |
| Cholera | Poliomyelitis, acute |
| Diarrhoea (infectious bloody) | Rabies |
| Diphtheria | Rubella |
| Encephalitis, acute | SARS |
| Food poisoning | Scarlet fever |
| Haemolytic uraemic syndrome | Smallpox |
| | Streptococcal disease (Group A, invasive) |
| Haemorrhagic fever (viral) | Tetanus |
| Hepatitis, viral | Tuberculosis |
| Legionnaires' disease | Typhoid fever |
| Leprosy | Typhus |
| Malaria | Whooping cough |
| Measles | Yellow fever |
| Meningitis | |
| Meningococcal septicaemia | |

Note

It is good practice for doctors to also inform the consultant in communicable disease control of instances of other infections (e.g. psittacosis) where there could be a public health risk.

## 5.1 Antibacterial drugs

**Choice of a suitable drug** Before selecting an antibacterial the clinician must first consider two factors—the child and the known or likely causative organism. Factors related to the child which must be considered include history of allergy, renal and hepatic function, susceptibility to infection (i.e. whether immunocompromised), ability to tolerate drugs by mouth, severity of illness, ethnic origin, age and, if an adolescent female, whether pregnant, breast-feeding or taking an oral contraceptive.

The known or likely organism and its antibacterial sensitivity, in association with the above factors, will suggest one or more antibacterials, the final choice depending on the microbiological, pharmacological, and toxicological properties.

The principles involved in selection of an antibacterial must allow for a number of variables including age, changing renal and hepatic function, increasing bacterial resistance, and information on side-effects. Duration of therapy, dosage, and route of administration depend on site, type and severity of infection and response.

**Antibacterial policies** Local policies often limit the antibacterials that may be used to achieve reasonable economy consistent with adequate cover, and to reduce the development of resistant organisms. A policy may indicate a range of drugs for general use, and permit other drugs only on the advice of the microbiologist or paediatric infectious diseases specialist.

**Before starting therapy** The following principles should be considered before starting:

- Viral infections should not be treated with antibacterials. However, antibacterials may be indicated for treatment of secondary bacterial infection (e.g. bacterial pneumonia secondary to influenza);

- Samples should be taken for culture and sensitivity testing whenever possible; 'blind' antibacterial prescribing for unexplained pyrexia usually leads to further difficulty in establishing the diagnosis;

- Knowledge of **prevalent organisms** and their current **sensitivity** is of great help in choosing an antibacterial before bacteriological confirmation is available. Generally, narrow-spectrum antibacterials are preferred to broad-spectrum antibacterials unless there is a clear clinical indication (e.g. life-threatening sepsis);

- The **dose** of an antibacterial varies according to a number of factors including age, weight, hepatic function, renal function, and severity of infection. The prescribing of the so-called 'standard' dose in serious infections may result in failure of treatment or even death of the patient; therefore it is important to prescribe a dose appropriate to the condition. An inadequate dose may also increase the likelihood of antibacterial resistance. On the other hand, for an antibacterial with a narrow margin between the toxic and therapeutic dose (e.g. an aminoglycoside) it is also important to avoid an excessive dose and the concentration of the drug in the plasma may need to be monitored;

- The **route** of administration of an antibacterial often depends on the severity of the infection. Life-threatening infections often require intravenous therapy. Antibacterials that are well absorbed may be given by mouth even for some serious infections. Parenteral administration is also appropriate when the oral route cannot be used (e.g. because of vomiting) or if absorption is inadequate (e.g. in neonates and young children). Whenever possible painful intramuscular injections should be avoided in children;

- **Duration** of therapy depends on the nature of the infection and the response to treatment. Courses should not be unduly prolonged because they encourage resistance, they may lead to side-effects and they are costly. However, in certain infections such as tuberculosis or osteomyelitis it may be necessary to treat for prolonged periods. The prescription for an antibacterial should specify the duration of treatment or the date when treatment is to be reviewed.

**Oral bacterial infections** Antibacterial drugs should only be prescribed for the *treatment* of oral infections on the basis of defined need. They may be used in conjunction with (but not as an alternative to) other appropriate measures, such as providing drainage or extracting a tooth.

The 'blind' prescribing of an antibacterial for unexplained pyrexia, cervical lymphadenopathy, or facial swelling can lead to difficulty in establishing the diagnosis. A sample should always be taken for bacteriology in the case of severe oral infection.

Oral infections which may require antibacterial treatment include acute periapical or periodontal abscess, cellulitis, acutely created oral-antral communication (and acute sinusitis), severe pericoronitis, localised osteitis, acute necrotising ulcerative gingivitis, and destructive forms of chronic periodontal disease. Most of these infections are readily resolved by the early establishment of drainage and removal of the cause (typically an infected necrotic pulp). Antibacterials may be required if treatment has to be delayed, in immunocompromised patients, or in those with conditions such as diabetes; see also Table 1, section 5.1. Certain rarer infections including bacterial sialadenitis, osteomyelitis, actinomycosis, and infections involving fascial spaces such as Ludwig's angina, require antibiotics and specialist hospital care.

**5**

**Infections**

Antibacterial drugs may also be useful after dental surgery in some cases of spreading infection. Infection may spread to involve local lymph nodes, to fascial spaces (where it can cause airway obstruction), or into the bloodstream (where it can lead to cavernous sinus thrombosis and other serious complications). Extension of an infection can also lead to maxillary sinusitis; osteomyelitis is a complication, which usually arises when host resistance is reduced.

If the oral infection fails to respond to antibacterial treatment within 48 hours the antibacterial should be changed, preferably on the basis of bacteriological investigation. Failure to respond may also suggest an incorrect diagnosis, lack of essential additional measures (such as drainage), poor host resistance, or poor patient compliance.

Combination of a penicillin (or a macrolide) with metronidazole may sometimes be helpful for the treatment of severe or resistant oral infections.

See also **Penicillins** (section 5.1.1), **Cephalosporins** (section 5.1.2.1), **Tetracyclines** (section 5.1.3), **Macrolides** (section 5.1.5), **Clindamycin** (section 5.1.6), **Metronidazole** (section 5.1.11), and **Fusidic acid** (section 13.10.1.2).

**Superinfection** In general, broad-spectrum antibacterial drugs such as the cephalosporins are more likely to be associated with adverse reactions related to the selection of resistant organisms e.g. *fungal infections* or *antibiotic-associated colitis* (pseudomembranous colitis); other problems associated with superinfection include vaginitis and pruritus ani.

**Therapy** Suggested treatment is shown in Table 1. When the pathogen has been isolated treatment may be changed to a more appropriate antibacterial if necessary. If no bacterium is cultured the antibacterial can be continued or stopped on clinical grounds. Infections for which prophylaxis is useful are listed in table 2.

**Switching from parenteral to oral treatment** The ongoing parenteral administration of an antibacterial should be reviewed regularly. In older children it may be possible to switch to an oral antibacterial; in neonates and infants this should be done more cautiously because of the relatively high incidence of bacteraemia and the possibility of variable oral absorption.

**Prophylaxis** Infections for which antibacterial prophylaxis is useful are listed in Table 2. In most situations, only a short course of prophylactic antibacterial is needed. Longer-term antibacterial prophylaxis is appropriate in specific indications such as vesico-ureteric reflux

## Table 1. Summary of antibacterial therapy

> If treating a patient suspected of suffering from a notifiable disease, the consultant in communicable disease control should be informed (see p. 244)

### Gastro-intestinal system

### Gastro-enteritis
Frequently self-limiting and may not be bacterial.

Antibacterial not usually indicated

### Campylobacter enteritis
Frequently self-limiting; treat if immunocompromised or if severe infection.

Clarithromycin[1]

*Alternative*, ciprofloxacin
  Strains with decreased sensitivity to ciprofloxacin isolated frequently

### Salmonella (non-typhoid)
Treat invasive or severe infection. Do not treat less severe infection unless there is a risk of developing invasive infection (e.g. immunocompromised children, those with haemoglobinopathy, or children under 6 months of age).

Ciprofloxacin *or* cefotaxime

### Shigellosis
Antibacterial not indicated for mild cases.

Azithromycin *or* ciprofloxacin

*Alternatives if micro-organism sensitive*, amoxicillin *or* trimethoprim

1. Where clarithromycin is suggested azithromycin or erythromycin may be used

### Typhoid fever

Infections from Middle-East, South Asia, and South-East Asia may be multiple-antibacterial-resistant and sensitivity should be tested.

Cefotaxime[1]

  Azithromycin may be an alternative in mild or moderate disease caused by multiple-antibacterial-resistant micro-organisms

  *Alternative if micro-organism sensitive*, ciprofloxacin *or* chloramphenicol

### *Clostridium difficile* infection

Oral metronidazole

  *Suggested duration of treatment 10–14 days*

  *For third or subsequent episode of infection, for severe infection, for infection not responding to metronidazole, or in children intolerant of metronidazole*, oral vancomycin

  *Suggested duration of treatment 10–14 days*

  *For infection not responding to vancomycin, or for life-threatening infection, or in patients with ileus*, oral vancomycin + i/v metronidazole

  *Suggested duration of treatment 10–14 days*

### Necrotising enterocolitis in neonates

Benzylpenicillin + gentamicin + metronidazole *or* amoxicillin[2] + gentamicin + metronidazole *or* amoxicillin[2] + cefotaxime + metronidazole

### Peritonitis

A cephalosporin + metronidazole *or* amoxicillin + gentamicin + metronidazole *or* piperacillin with tazobactam alone

### Peritonitis: peritoneal dialysis-associated

Vancomycin[3] + ceftazidime added to dialysis fluid *or* vancomycin added to dialysis fluid + ciprofloxacin by mouth

  *Suggested duration of treatment 14 days or longer*

## Cardiovascular system

### Endocarditis: initial 'blind' therapy

Flucloxacillin (*or* benzylpenicillin if symptoms less severe) + gentamicin

  *If cardiac prostheses present, or if penicillin-allergic, or if meticillin-resistant Staphylococcus aureus suspected*, vancomycin + rifampicin + gentamicin

### Endocarditis caused by staphylococci

Flucloxacillin

  Add rifampicin for at least 2 weeks in prosthetic valve endocarditis.

  *Suggested duration of treatment at least 4 weeks (at least 6 weeks for prosthetic valve endocarditis)*

  *If penicillin-allergic or if meticillin-resistant Staphylococcus aureus*, vancomycin + rifampicin

  *Suggested duration of treatment at least 4 weeks (at least 6 weeks for prosthetic valve endocarditis)*

### Native-valve endocarditis caused by fully-sensitive streptococci (e.g. viridans streptococci)

Benzylpenicillin

  *Suggested duration of treatment 4 weeks*

  *Alternative if a large vegetation, intracardial abscess, or infected emboli are absent*, benzylpenicillin + gentamicin

  *Suggested duration of treatment 2 weeks*

  *If penicillin-allergic*, vancomycin

  *Suggested duration of treatment 4 weeks*

1. Where cefotaxime is suggested ceftriaxone may be used
2. Where amoxicillin is suggested ampicillin may be used
3. Where vancomycin is suggested teicoplanin may be used

### Native-valve endocarditis caused by less-sensitive streptococci

Benzylpenicillin + gentamicin
*Suggested duration of treatment* 4–6 weeks (stop gentamicin after 2 weeks for micro-organisms moderately sensitive to penicillin)

*If aminoglycoside cannot be used and if streptococci moderately sensitive to penicillin,* benzylpenicillin
*Suggested duration of treatment* 4 weeks

*If penicillin-allergic or highly penicillin-resistant,* vancomycin[1] + gentamicin
*Suggested duration of treatment* 4–6 weeks (stop gentamicin after 2 weeks for micro-organisms moderately sensitive to penicillin)

### Prosthetic valve endocarditis caused by streptococci

Benzylpenicillin + gentamicin
*Suggested duration of treatment* at least 6 weeks (stop gentamicin after 2 weeks if micro-organisms fully sensitive to penicillin)

*If penicillin-allergic or highly penicillin-resistant,* vancomycin[1] + gentamicin
*Suggested duration of treatment* at least 6 weeks (stop gentamicin after 2 weeks if micro-organisms fully sensitive to penicillin)

### Endocarditis caused by enterococci (e.g. *Enterococcus faecalis*)

Amoxicillin[2] + gentamicin
If gentamicin-resistant, substitute gentamicin with streptomycin.
*Suggested duration of treatment* at least 4 weeks (at least 6 weeks for prosthetic valve endocarditis)

*If penicillin-allergic or penicillin-resistant,* vancomycin[1] + gentamicin
If gentamicin-resistant, substitute gentamicin with streptomycin.
*Suggested duration of treatment* at least 4 weeks (at least 6 weeks for prosthetic valve endocarditis)

### Endocarditis caused by haemophilus, actinobacillus, cardiobacterium, eikenella, and kingella species ('HACEK' micro-organisms)

Amoxicillin[2] + gentamicin
*Suggested duration of treatment* 4 weeks (6 weeks for prosthetic valve endocarditis); stop gentamicin after 2 weeks

*If amoxicillin-resistant,* ceftriaxone + gentamicin
*Suggested duration of treatment* 4 weeks (6 weeks for prosthetic valve endocarditis); stop gentamicin after 2 weeks

---

## Respiratory system

### *Haemophilus influenzae* epiglottitis

Cefotaxime[3]
*If history of immediate hypersensitivity reaction to penicillin or to cephalosporins,* chloramphenicol

### Pneumonia: community-acquired

Children under 2 years with mild symptoms of lower respiratory tract infection (particularly those vaccinated with pneumococcal polysaccharide conjugate vaccine and haemophilus type b conjugate vaccine) are unlikely to have pneumonia; antibacterial treatment may be considered if symptoms persist

*Neonate,* benzylpenicillin + gentamicin

*Child 1 month–18 years,* amoxicillin[2] by mouth
Pneumococci with decreased penicillin sensitivity have been isolated in the UK, but are not common.
If no response to treatment, add clarithromycin[4]
If staphylococci suspected (e.g. in influenza or measles), give by mouth amoxicillin + flucloxacillin *or* co-amoxiclav alone
If septicaemia, complicated pneumonia, or if oral administration not possible, initiate treatment with i/v amoxicillin *or* i/v co-amoxiclav *or* i/v cefuroxime *or* i/v cefotaxime[3]
*Suggested duration of treatment* 7 days (may extend treatment to 14 days in some cases e.g. if staphylococci suspected)

*Child 1 month–18 years, if penicillin-allergic,* clarithromycin[4]
*Suggested duration of treatment* 7 days (may extend treatment to 14 days in some cases e.g if staphylococci suspected)

---

1. Where vancomycin is suggested teicoplanin may be used
2. Where amoxicillin is suggested ampicillin may be used
3. Where cefotaxime is suggested ceftriaxone may be used
4. Where clarithromycin is suggested azithromycin or erythromycin may be used

### Pneumonia possibly caused by atypical pathogens
Clarithromycin[1]
*Suggested duration of treatment* 10–14 days
*Alternative for chlamydial or mycoplasma infections in children over 12 years*, doxycycline
*Suggested duration of treatment* 10–14 days

### Pneumonia: hospital-acquired
*Early-onset infection* (less than 5 days after admission to hospital), treat as for severe community-acquired pneumonia of unknown aetiology; if life-threatening infection, or if recent history of antibacterial treatment, or if resistant organisms suspected, treat as for late-onset hospital-acquired pneumonia

*Late-onset infection* (more than 5 days after admission to hospital), an antpseudomonal penicillin (e.g. piperacillin with tazobactam) *or* another antipseudomonal beta-lactam
If meticillin-resistant *Staphylococcus aureus* suspected, add vancomycin.
If severe illness caused by *Pseudomonas aeruginosa*, add an aminoglycoside.
*Suggested duration of treatment* 7 days (longer if *Pseudomonas aeruginosa* confirmed)

## Cystic fibrosis
### Staphylococcal lung infection in cystic fibrosis
Flucloxacillin
If child already taking flucloxacillin prophylaxis or if severe exacerbation, add sodium fusidate or rifampicin; use flucloxacillin at treatment dose
*If penicillin-allergic*, clarithromycin[1] *or* clindamycin
Use clarithromycin only if micro-organism sensitive

### *Haemophilus influenzae* lung infection in cystic fibrosis
Amoxicillin *or* a broad-spectrum cephalosporin
In severe exacerbation use a third-generation cephalosporin (e.g. cefotaxime)

### Pseudomonal lung infection in cystic fibrosis
Ciprofloxacin + *nebulised* colistimethate sodium
*For severe exacerbation*, an antipseudomonal beta-lactam antibacterial + parenteral tobramycin

## Central nervous system
### Meningitis: initial empirical therapy
- Transfer patient to hospital urgently.
- If *meningococcal disease* (meningitis with non-blanching rash or meningococcal septicaemia) suspected, benzylpenicillin (see p. 260 for dose) should be given before transfer to hospital, so long as this does not delay the transfer. If a patient with suspected bacterial meningitis without non-blanching rash cannot be transferred to hospital urgently, benzylpenicillin (see p. 260 for dose) should be given before the transfer. Cefotaxime (section 5.1.2) may be an alternative in penicillin allergy; chloramphenicol (section 5.1.7) may be used if history of immediate hypersensitivity reaction to penicillins or to cephalosporins.
- In hospital, consider adjunctive treatment with dexamethasone (section 6.3.2), preferably starting before or with first dose of antibacterial, but no later than 12 hours after starting antibacterial; avoid dexamethasone in septic shock, meningococcal septicaemia, or if immunocompromised, or in meningitis following surgery.
- In hospital, if aetiology unknown

*Neonate and child 1–3 months*, cefotaxime[2] + amoxicillin[3]
Consider adding vancomycin if prolonged or multiple use of other antibacterials in the last 3 months, or if travelled, in the last 3 months, to areas outside the UK with highly penicillin- and cephalosporin-resistant pneumococci
*Suggested duration of treatment* at least 14 days

*Child 3 months–18 years*, cefotaxime[2]
Consider adding vancomycin if prolonged or multiple use of other antibacterials in the last 3 months, or if travelled, in the last 3 months, to areas outside the UK with highly penicillin- and cephalosporin-resistant pneumococci
*Suggested duration of treatment* at least 10 days

1. Where clarithromycin is suggested azithromycin or erythromycin may be used
2. Where cefotaxime is suggested ceftriaxone may be used
3. Where amoxicillin is suggested ampicillin may be used

5 Infections

**Meningitis caused by group B streptococcus**

Benzylpenicillin + gentamicin *or* cefotaxime[1] alone

*Suggested duration of treatment* at least 14 days; stop gentamicin after 5 days

**Meningitis caused by meningococci**

Benzylpenicillin *or* cefotaxime[1]

*Suggested duration of treatment* 7 days.

To eliminate nasopharyngeal carriage in patients treated with benzylpenicillin or cefotaxime see Table 2, section 5.1

*If history of immediate hypersensitivity reaction to penicillin or to cephalosporins,* chloramphenicol

*Suggested duration of treatment* 7 days.

To eliminate nasopharyngeal carriage see Table 2, section 5.1

**Meningitis caused by pneumococci**

Cefotaxime[1]

Consider adjunctive treatment with dexamethasone (section 6.3.2), preferably starting before or with first dose of antibacterial, but no later than 12 hours after starting antibacterial (may reduce penetration of vancomycin into cerebrospinal fluid).

If micro-organism penicillin-sensitive, replace cefotaxime with benzylpenicillin.

If micro-organism highly penicillin- and cephalosporin-resistant, add vancomycin and if necessary rifampicin.

*Suggested duration of antibacterial treatment* 14 days

**Meningitis caused by *Haemophilus influenzae***

Cefotaxime[1]

Consider adjunctive treatment with dexamethasone (section 6.3.2), preferably starting before or with first dose of antibacterial, but no later than 12 hours after starting antibacterial.

*Suggested duration of antibacterial treatment* 10 days.

For *H. influenzae* type b give rifampicin for 4 days before hospital discharge to those under 10 years of age or to those in contact with vulnerable household contacts (see Table 2, section 5.1)

*If history of immediate hypersensitivity reaction to penicillin or to cephalosporins, or if micro-organism resistant to cefotaxime,* chloramphenicol

Consider adjunctive treatment with dexamethasone (section 6.3.2), preferably starting before or with first dose of antibacterial, but no later than 12 hours after starting antibacterial.

*Suggested duration of antibacterial treatment* 10 days.

For *H. influenzae* type b give rifampicin for 4 days before hospital discharge to those under 10 years of age or to those in contact with vulnerable household contacts (see Table 2, section 5.1)

**Meningitis caused by Listeria**

Amoxicillin[2] + gentamicin

*Suggested duration of treatment* 21 days.

Consider stopping gentamicin after 7 days

*If history of immediate hypersensitivity reaction to penicillin,* co-trimoxazole

*Suggested duration of treatment* 21 days

## Urinary tract

**Urinary-tract infection**

*Child under 3 months of age,* i/v amoxicillin[2] + gentamicin *or* i/v cephalosporin alone

*Child over 3 months of age with uncomplicated lower urinary-tract infection,* trimethoprim *or* nitrofurantoin

*Suggested duration of treatment* 3 days.

Re-assess child if unwell 24–48 hours after initial assessment

*Child over 3 months of age, alternative for uncomplicated lower urinary-tract infection,* amoxicillin[2] *or* oral cephalosporin (e.g. cefalexin)

Use amoxicillin only if micro-organism sensitive.

*Suggested duration of treatment* 3 days.

Re-assess child if unwell 24–48 hours after initial assessment

*Child over 3 months of age with acute pyelonephritis,* a cephalosporin *or* co-amoxiclav

*Suggested duration of treatment* 7–10 days

1. Where cefotaxime is suggested ceftriaxone may be used
2. Where amoxicillin is suggested ampicillin may be used

## Genital system

### Uncomplicated genital chlamydial infection, non-gonococcal urethritis, and non-specific genital infection

Contact tracing recommended.

*Child under 12 years*, erythromycin
> *Suggested duration of treatment* 14 days

*Child 12–18 years*, azithromycin *or* doxycycline
> *Suggested duration of treatment* azithromycin as a single dose or doxycycline for 7 days

*Child 12–18 years, alternative*, erythromycin
> *Suggested duration of treatment* 14 days

### Gonorrhoea: uncomplicated

Contact tracing recommended. Consider chlamydia co-infection. Choice of antibacterial depends on locality where infection acquired.

*Child under 12 years*, ceftriaxone
> *Suggested duration of treatment* single-dose

*Child 12–18 years*, cefixime
> *Suggested duration of treatment* single-dose

*Child 12–18 years, alternative if micro-organism sensitive*, ciprofloxacin
> *Suggested duration of treatment* single-dose

*Child 12–18 years with pharyngeal infection*, ceftriaxone
> *Suggested duration of treatment* single-dose

### Pelvic inflammatory disease

Contact tracing recommended

*Child 2–12 years*, erythromycin + metronidazole + i/m ceftriaxone
> *Suggested duration of treatment* 14 days (use i/m ceftriaxone as a single dose)

*Child 12–18 years*, doxycycline + metronidazole + i/m ceftriaxone
> If severely ill, seek specialist advice.
> *Suggested duration of treatment* 14 days (use i/m ceftriaxone as a single dose)

### Neonatal congenital syphilis

Benzylpenicillin
> Also consider treating neonates with suspected congenital syphilis whose mothers were treated inadequately for syphilis, or whose mothers were treated for syphilis in the 4 weeks before delivery, or whose mothers were treated with non-penicillin antibacterials for syphilis.
> *Suggested duration of treatment* 10 days

### Syphilis

Contact tracing recommended.

*Child under 12 years*, benzylpenicillin *or* procaine benzylpenicillin [unlicensed]
> *Suggested duration of treatment* 10 days

*Child 12–18 years, early syphilis (infection of less than 2 years)*, benzathine benzylpenicillin [unlicensed]
> *Suggested duration of treatment* single-dose (repeat dose after 7 days for females in the third trimester of pregnancy)

*Child 12–18 years, alternatives for early syphilis*, doxycycline *or* erythromycin
> *Suggested duration of treatment* 14 days

*Child 12–18 years, late latent syphilis (asymptomatic infection of more than 2 years)*, benzathine benzylpenicillin [unlicensed]
> *Suggested duration of treatment* once weekly for 2 weeks

*Child 12–18 years, alternative for late latent syphilis*, doxycycline
> *Suggested duration of treatment* 28 days

*Child 12–18 years who is an asymptomatic contact of a patient with infectious syphilis*, doxycycline
> *Suggested duration of treatment* 14 days

**5**

**Infections**

███████ **Blood**

## Septicaemia

*Neonate less than 72 hours old*, benzylpenicillin + gentamicin

> If Gram-negative septicaemia suspected, use benzylpenicillin + gentamicin + cefotaxime; stop benzylpenicillin if Gram-negative infection confirmed.
>
> *Suggested duration of treatment* usually 7 days

*Neonate more than 72 hours old*, flucloxacillin + gentamicin *or* amoxicillin[1] + cefotaxime

> *Suggested duration of treatment* usually 7 days

*Child 1 month–18 years with community-acquired septicaemia*, aminoglycoside + amoxicillin[1] *or* cefotaxime[2] alone

> If pseudomonas or resistant micro-organisms suspected, use a broad-spectrum antipseudomonal beta-lactam antibacterial.
>
> If anaerobic infection suspected, add metronidazole.
>
> If Gram-positive infection suspected, add flucloxacillin *or* vancomycin[3].
>
> *Suggested duration of treatment* at least 5 days

*Child 1 month–18 years with hospital-acquired septicaemia*, a broad-spectrum antipseudomonal beta-lactam antibacterial (e.g. piperacillin with tazobactam, ticarcillin with clavulanic acid, imipenem with cilastatin, *or* meropenem)

> If pseudomonas suspected, or if multiple-resistant organisms suspected, or if severe sepsis, add aminoglycoside.
>
> If meticillin-resistant Staphylococcus aureus suspected, add vancomycin[3].
>
> If anaerobic infection suspected, add metronidazole to a broad-spectrum cephalosporin.
>
> *Suggested duration of treatment* at least 5 days

## Septicaemia related to vascular catheter

Vancomycin[3]

> If Gram-negative sepsis suspected, especially in the immunocompromised, add a broad-spectrum antipseudomonal beta-lactam.
>
> Consider removing vascular catheter, particularly if infection caused by *Staphylococcus aureus*, pseudomonas, or candida

## Meningococcal septicaemia

If meningococcal disease suspected, a single dose of benzylpenicillin (see p. 260 for dose) should be given before urgent transfer to hospital, so long as this does not delay the transfer; cefotaxime (section 5.1.2) may be an alternative in penicillin allergy; chloramphenicol may be used if history of immediate hypersensitivity reaction to penicillin or to cephalosporins.

Benzylpenicillin *or* cefotaxime[2]

> To eliminate nasopharyngeal carriage in patients treated with benzylpenicillin or cefotaxime see Table 2, section 5.1

*If history of immediate hypersensitivity reaction to penicillin or to cephalosporins*, chloramphenicol

> To eliminate nasopharyngeal carriage see Table 2, section 5.1

███████ **Musculoskeletal system**

## Osteomyelitis

Seek specialist advice if chronic infection or prostheses present.

Flucloxacillin

> Consider adding fusidic acid or rifampicin for initial 2 weeks.
>
> *Suggested duration of treatment* 6 weeks for acute infection

*If penicillin-allergic*, clindamycin

> Consider adding fusidic acid or rifampicin for initial 2 weeks.
>
> *Suggested duration of treatment* 6 weeks for acute infection

*If meticillin-resistant* Staphylococcus aureus *suspected*, vancomycin[3]

> Consider adding fusidic acid or rifampicin for initial 2 weeks.
>
> *Suggested duration of treatment* 6 weeks for acute infection

1. Where amoxicillin is suggested ampicillin may be used
2. Where cefotaxime is suggested ceftriaxone may be used
3. Where vancomycin is suggested teicoplanin may be used

## Septic arthritis
Seek specialist advice if prostheses present.

Flucloxacillin
*Suggested duration of treatment* 4–6 weeks (longer if infection complicated)

*If penicillin-allergic*, clindamycin
*Suggested duration of treatment* 4–6 weeks (longer if infection complicated)

*If meticillin-resistant* Staphylococcus aureus *suspected*, vancomycin[1]
*Suggested duration of treatment* 4–6 weeks (longer if infection complicated)

*If gonococcal arthritis or Gram-negative infection suspected*, cefotaxime[2]
*Suggested duration of treatment* 4–6 weeks (longer if infection complicated; treat gonococcal infection for 2 weeks)

## Eye

### Purulent conjunctivitis
Chloramphenicol eye drops
See also section 11.3.1

### Congenital chlamydial conjunctivitis
Erythromycin (by mouth)
*Suggested duration of treatment* 14 days

### Congenital gonococcal conjunctivitis
Cefotaxime[2]
*Suggested duration of treatment* single-dose

## Ear, nose, and oropharynx

### Pericoronitis
Antibacterial required only in presence of systemic features of infection, or of trismus, or persistent swelling despite local treatment.

Metronidazole
*Suggested duration of treatment* 3 days or until symptoms resolve

*Alternative*, amoxicillin
*Suggested duration of treatment* 3 days or until symptoms resolve

### Gingivitis: acute necrotising ulcerative
Antibacterial required only if systemic features of infection.

Metronidazole
*Suggested duration of treatment* 3 days or until symptoms resolve

*Alternative*, amoxicillin
*Suggested duration of treatment* 3 days or until symptoms resolve

### Periapical or periodontal abscess
Antibacterial required only in severe disease with cellulitis or if systemic features of infection.

Amoxicillin
*Suggested duration of treatment* 5 days

*Alternative*, metronidazole
*Suggested duration of treatment* 5 days

### Periodontitis
Antibacterial used as an adjunct to debridement in severe disease or disease unresponsive to local treatment alone.

Metronidazole

*Alternative in child over 12 years*, doxycycline

---

1. Where vancomycin is suggested teicoplanin may be used
2. Where cefotaxime is suggested ceftriaxone may be used

5
Infections

## Throat infections

Most throat infections are caused by viruses and many do not require antibacterial therapy. Consider antibacterial, if history of valvular heart disease, if marked systemic upset, if peritonsillar cellulitis or abscess, or if at increased risk from acute infection (e.g. in immunosuppression, cystic fibrosis); prescribe antibacterial for beta-haemolytic streptococcal pharyngitis.

### Phenoxymethylpenicillin

In severe infection, initial parenteral therapy with benzylpenicillin, then oral therapy with phenoxymethylpenicillin *or* amoxicillin[1]. **Avoid** amoxicillin if possibility of glandular fever, see section 5.1.1.3.

*Suggested duration of treatment* 10 days

### *If penicillin-allergic*, clarithromycin[2]

*Suggested duration of treatment* 10 days

## Sinusitis

Antibacterial should usually be used only for persistent symptoms and purulent discharge lasting at least 7 days or if severe symptoms. Also, consider antibacterial for those at high risk of serious complications (e.g. in immunosuppression, cystic fibrosis).

### Amoxicillin[1] *or* clarithromycin[2]

*Suggested duration of treatment* 7 days.

Consider oral co-amoxiclav if no improvement after 48 hours.

In severe infection, initial parenteral therapy with co-amoxiclav or cefuroxime may be required

## Otitis externa

Consider systemic antibacterial if spreading cellulitis or child systemically unwell.

For topical preparations see section 12.1.1.

### Flucloxacillin

### *If penicillin-allergic*, clarithromycin[2]

### *If pseudomonas suspected*, ciprofloxacin (*or* an aminoglycoside)

## Otitis media

Many infections caused by viruses. Most uncomplicated cases resolve without antibacterial treatment. In children without systemic features, antibacterial treatment may be started after 72 hours if no improvement. Consider earlier treatment if deterioration, if systemically unwell, if at high risk of serious complications (e.g. in immunosuppression, cystic fibrosis), if mastoiditis present, or in children under 2 years of age with bilateral otitis media.

### Amoxicillin[1]

Consider co-amoxiclav if no improvement after 48 hours.

In severe infection, initial parenteral therapy with co-amoxiclav or cefuroxime.

*Suggested duration of treatment* 5 days (longer if severely ill)

### *If penicillin-allergic*, clarithromycin[2]

*Suggested duration of treatment* 5 days (longer if severely ill)

## Skin

### Impetigo: small areas of skin infected

Seek local microbiology advice before using topical treatment in hospital.

### Topical fusidic acid

*Suggested duration of treatment* 7 days is usually adequate (max. 10 days)

### *Alternative if meticillin-resistant Staphylococcus aureus*, topical mupirocin

*Suggested duration of treatment* 7 days is usually adequate (max. 10 days)

1. Where amoxicillin is suggested ampicillin may be used
2. Where clarithromycin is suggested azithromycin or erythromycin may be used

### Impetigo: widespread infection

Oral flucloxacillin

If streptococci suspected in severe infection, add phenoxymethylpenicillin.

*Suggested duration of treatment* 7 days

*If penicillin-allergic,* oral clarithromycin[1]

*Suggested duration of treatment* 7 days

### Erysipelas

Phenoxymethylpenicillin *or* benzylpenicillin

If severe infection, replace phenoxymethylpenicillin or benzylpenicillin with high-dose flucloxacillin; if meticillin-resistant *S. aureus* suspected, see section 5.1.1.2.

*Suggested duration of treatment* at least 7 days

*If penicillin-allergic,* clindamycin *or* clarithromycin[1]

If meticillin-resistant *S.aureus* suspected in severe infection, see section 5.1.1.2.

*Suggested duration of treatment* at least 7 days

### Cellulitis

Flucloxacillin (high dose)

If streptococcal infection confirmed, replace flucloxacillin with phenoxymethylpenicillin or benzylpenicillin.

If Gram-negative bacteria or anaerobes suspected (e.g. facial infection, orbital infection, or infection caused by animal or human bites), use broad-spectrum antibacterials; if periumbilical cellulitis, use flucloxacillin + gentamicin.

If meticillin-resistant *S. aureus* suspected, see section 5.1.1.2

*If penicillin-allergic,* clindamycin *or* clarithromycin[1]

If Gram-negative bacteria suspected, use broad-spectrum antibacterials.

If meticillin-resistant *S aureus* suspected, see section 5.1.1.2

### Staphylococcal scalded skin syndrome

Flucloxacillin

*Suggested duration of treatment* 7–10 days

*If penicillin-allergic,* clarithromycin[1]

*Suggested duration of treatment* 7–10 days

### Animal and human bites

Cleanse wound thoroughly. For tetanus-prone wound, give human tetanus immunoglobulin (with a tetanus-containing vaccine if necessary, according to immunisation history and risk of infection), see under Tetanus Vaccines, section 14.4. Consider rabies prophylaxis (section 14.4) for bites from animals in endemic countries; assess risk of blood-borne viruses (including HIV, hepatitis B and C) and give appropriate prophylaxis to prevent viral spread.

Co-amoxiclav

*If penicillin-allergic,* clindamycin

### Acne

See section 13.6.

### Paronychia or 'septic spots' in neonate

Flucloxacillin

If systemically unwell, add an aminoglycoside

### Surgical wound infection

Flucloxacillin or co-amoxiclav

5

Infections

---

1. Where clarithromycin is suggested azithromycin or erythromycin may be used

## Table 2. Summary of antibacterial prophylaxis

### Prevention of recurrence of rheumatic fever
Phenoxymethylpenicillin by mouth

**Child 1 month–6 years** 125 mg twice daily

**Child 6–18 years** 250 mg twice daily

*or*

Erythromycin by mouth

**Child 1 month–2 years** 125 mg twice daily

**Child 2–18 years** 250 mg twice daily

### Prevention of secondary case of invasive group A streptococcal infection[1]
Phenoxymethylpenicillin by mouth

**Neonate** 12.5 mg/kg (max. 62.5 mg) every 6 hours for 10 days

**Child 1 month–1 year** 62.5 mg every 6 hours for 10 days

**Child 1–6 years** 125 mg every 6 hours for 10 days

**Child 6–12 years** 250 mg every 6 hours for 10 days

**Child 12–18 years** 250–500 mg every 6 hours for 10 days

If child penicillin allergic,

*either* erythromycin by mouth

**Child 1 month–2 years** 125 mg every 6 hours for 10 days

**Child 2–8 years** 250 mg every 6 hours for 10 days

**Child 8–18 years** 250–500 mg every 6 hours for 10 days

*or* azithromycin by mouth [unlicensed indication]

**Child 6 months–12 years** 12 mg/kg (max. 500 mg) once daily for 5 days

**Child 12–18 years** 500 mg once daily for 5 days

### Prevention of secondary case of meningococcal meningitis[2]
Ciprofloxacin by mouth [unlicensed indication]

**Neonate** 30 mg/kg (max. 125 mg) as a single dose

**Child 1 month–5 years** 30 mg/kg (max. 125 mg) as a single dose

**Child 5–12 years** 250 mg as a single dose

**Child 12–18 years** 500 mg as a single dose

*or*

Rifampicin by mouth

**Neonate** 5 mg/kg every 12 hours for 2 days

**Child 1 month–1 year** 5 mg/kg every 12 hours for 2 days

**Child 1–12 years** 10 mg/kg (max. 600 mg) every 12 hours for 2 days

**Child 12–18 years** 600 mg every 12 hours for 2 days

*or*

Ceftriaxone by intramuscular injection [unlicensed indication]

**Child 1 month–12 years** 125 mg as a single dose

**Child 12–18 years** 250 mg as a single dose

### Prevention of secondary case of *Haemophilus influenzae* type b disease[2]
Rifampicin by mouth

**Child 1–3 months** 10 mg/kg once daily for 4 days

**Child 3 months–12 years** 20 mg/kg (max. 600 mg) once daily for 4 days

**Child 12–18 years** 600 mg once daily for 4 days

*or (if rifampicin cannot be used)*

Ceftriaxone by intramuscular injection, or by intravenous injection, or by intravenous infusion [unlicensed indication]

**Child 1 month–12 years** 50 mg/kg (max. 1 g) once daily for 2 days; by intravenous infusion only

**Child 12–18 years** 1 g once daily for 2 days

Give antibacterial prophylaxis to all household contacts of an index case with confirmed or suspected invasive *Haemophilus influenzae* type b disease if there is a vulnerable individual in the household. Also, give antibacterial prophylaxis to the index case if they are under 10 years of age or if they are in contact with vulnerable household contacts. Vulnerable individuals include the immunocompromised, those with asplenia, or children under 10 years of age. For immunisation against *Haemophilus influenzae* type b disease, see section 14.4

### Prevention of secondary case of diphtheria in non-immune patient
Erythromycin[3] by mouth

**Child 1 month–2 years** 125 mg every 6 hours for 7 days

**Child 2–8 years** 250 mg every 6 hours for 7 days

**Child 8–18 years** 500 mg every 6 hours for 7 days

Treat for further 10 days if nasopharyngeal swabs positive after first 7 days' treatment. For immunisation against diphtheria see section 14.4

### Prevention of pertussis
Clarithromycin[4] by mouth

**Neonate** 7.5 mg/kg twice daily for 7 days

**Child 1 month–12 years**

**Body-weight under 8 kg** 7.5 mg/kg twice daily for 7 days

**Body-weight 8–11 kg** 62.5 mg twice daily for 7 days

**Body-weight 12–19 kg** 125 mg twice daily for 7 days

**Body-weight 20–29 kg** 187.5 mg twice daily for 7 days

**Body-weight 30–40 kg** 250 mg twice daily for 7 days

**Child 12–18 years** 500 mg twice daily for 7 days

Within 3 weeks of onset of cough in the index case, give antibacterial prophylaxis to vulnerable close contacts and to other close contacts who are in contact with vulnerable individuals. Vulnerable contacts include neonates, unimmunised or partially immunised children under 10 years of age, females in the last month of pregnancy, the immunocompromised, or those with chronic illness (e.g. asthma, congenital heart disease). For immunisation against pertussis see section 14.4

---

1. For details of those who should receive chemoprophylaxis contact a consultant in communicable disease control (or a consultant in infectious diseases or the local Health Protection Agency Laboratory)
2. For details of those who should receive chemoprophylaxis contact a consultant in communicable disease control (or a consultant in infectious diseases or the local Health Protection Agency laboratory). Unless there has been direct exposure of the mouth or nose to infectious droplets from a patient with meningococcal disease who has received less than 24 hours of antibacterial treatment, healthcare workers do not generally require chemoprophylaxis
3. Where erythromycin is suggested another macrolide (e.g. azithromycin or clarithromycin) may be used
4. Where clarithromycin is suggested azithromycin or erythromycin may be used

## Prevention of pneumococcal infection in asplenia or in patients with sickle-cell disease

Phenoxymethylpenicillin by mouth

**Child under 1 year** 62.5 mg twice daily

**Child 1–5 years** 125 mg twice daily

**Child 5–18 years** 250 mg twice daily

If cover also needed for *H. influenzae* in child give amoxicillin instead

**Child 1 month–5 years** 125 mg twice daily

**Child 5–12 years** 250 mg twice daily

**Child 12–18 years** 500 mg twice daily

If penicillin-allergic, erythromycin by mouth

**Child 1 month–2 years** 125 mg twice daily

**Child 2–8 years** 250 mg twice daily

**Child 8–18 years** 500 mg twice daily
**Note** Antibacterial prophylaxis is not fully reliable; for vaccines in asplenia see p. 603. Antibacterial prophylaxis may be discontinued in children over 5 years of age with sickle-cell disease who have received pneumococcal immunisation and who do not have a history of severe pneumococcal infection

## Prevention of *Staphylococcus aureus* lung infection in cystic fibrosis

*Primary prevention*, flucloxacillin by mouth

**Neonate** 125 mg twice daily

**Child 1 month–3 years** 125 mg twice daily

*Secondary prevention*, flucloxacillin by mouth

**Child 1 month–18 years** 50 mg/kg (max. 1 g) twice daily

## Prevention of tuberculosis in susceptible close contacts or those who have become tuberculin positive[1]

Isoniazid for 6 months

**Neonate** 10 mg/kg daily

**Child 1 month –12 years** 10 mg/kg daily (max. 300 mg daily)

**Child 12–18 years** 300 mg daily

*or* isoniazid + rifampicin for 3 months

**Child 1 month–12 years** isoniazid 10 mg/kg daily (max. 300 mg daily) + rifampicin 10 mg/kg daily (max. 450 mg daily if body-weight less than 50 kg; max. 600 mg daily if body-weight over 50 kg)

**Child 12–18 years** isoniazid 300 mg daily + rifampicin 600 mg daily (rifampicin 450 mg daily if body-weight less than 50 kg)

*or* (if isoniazid-resistant tuberculosis) rifampicin for 6 months

**Child 1 month–12 years** 10 mg/kg daily (max. 450 mg daily if body-weight less than 50 kg; max. 600 mg daily if body-weight over 50 kg)

**Child 12–18 years** 600 mg daily (450 mg daily if body-weight less than 50 kg)

---

1. For details of those who should receive chemoprophylaxis contact the lead clinician for local tuberculosis services (or a consultant in communicable disease control). See also section 5.1.9, for advice on immunocompromised patients and on prevention of tuberculosis

## Prevention of urinary-tract infection

Trimethoprim by mouth

**Neonate** 2 mg/kg at night

**Child 1 month–12 years** 2 mg/kg (max. 100 mg) at night

*or*

**Child 6 weeks–6 months** 12.5 mg at night

**Child 6 months–6 years** 25 mg at night

**Child 6–12 years** 50 mg at night

**Child 12–18 years** 100 mg at night

*or* nitrofurantoin by mouth

**Child 3 months–12 years** 1 mg/kg at night

**Child 12–18 years** 50–100 mg at night
Antibacterial prophylaxis can be considered for recurrent infection, significant urinary-tract anomalies, or significant kidney damage. See also section 5.1.13

## Prevention of infection from animal and human bites

Co-amoxiclav alone (*or* clindamycin if penicillin-allergic)
Cleanse wound thoroughly. For tetanus-prone wound, give human tetanus immunoglobulin (with a tetanus-containing vaccine if necessary, according to immunisation history and risk of infection), see under Tetanus vaccines, section 14.4. Consider rabies prophylaxis (section 14.4) for bites from animals in endemic countries. Assess risk of blood-borne viruses (including HIV, hepatitis B and C) and give appropriate prophylaxis to prevent viral spread. Antibacterial prophylaxis recommended for wounds less than 48–72 hours old when the risk of infection is high (e.g. bites from humans or cats; bites to the hand, foot, face, or genital area; bites involving oedema, crush or puncture injury, or other moderate to severe injury; wounds that cannot be debrided adequately; patients with diabetes mellitus, cirrhosis, asplenia, prosthetic joints or valves, or those who are immunocompromised). Give antibacterial prophylaxis for up to 5 days

## Prevention of infection in gastro-intestinal procedures

### Operations on stomach or oesophagus[2]

Single dose[3] of i/v gentamicin *or* i/v cefuroxime *or* i/v co-amoxiclav

  Add i/v teicoplanin[4] if high risk of meticillin-resistant *Staphylococcus aureus*

### Open biliary surgery[2]

Single dose[3] of i/v cefuroxime + i/v metronidazole[5] *or* i/v gentamicin + i/v metronidazole[5] *or* i/v co-amoxiclav alone

  Add i/v teicoplanin[4] if high risk of meticillin-resistant *Staphylococcus aureus*

### Resections of colon and rectum, and resections in inflammatory bowel disease, and appendicectomy[2]

Single dose[3] of i/v gentamicin + i/v metronidazole[5] *or* i/v cefuroxime + i/v metronidazole[5] *or* i/v co-amoxiclav alone

  Add i/v teicoplanin[4] if high risk of meticillin-resistant *Staphylococcus aureus*

---

2. Intravenous antibacterial prophylaxis should be given up to 30 minutes before the procedure
3. Additional intra-operative or postoperative doses of antibacterial may be given for prolonged procedures or if there is major blood loss
4. Where teicoplanin is suggested vancomycin may be used
5. Metronidazole may alternatively be given by suppository but to allow adequate absorption, it should be given 2 hours before surgery

**Endoscopic retrograde cholangiopancreatography[1]**

Single dose of i/v gentamicin *or* oral or i/v ciprofloxacin
> Prophylaxis recommended if pancreatic pseudocyst, immunocompromised, history of liver transplantation, or risk of incomplete biliary drainage. For biliary complications following liver transplantation, add i/v amoxicillin or i/v teicoplanin[2]

**Percutaneous endoscopic gastrostomy or jejunostomy[1]**

Single dose of i/v co-amoxiclav or i/v cefuroxime
> Use single dose of i/v teicoplanin[2] if history of allergy to penicillins or cephalosporins, or if high risk of meticillin-resistant *Staphylococcus aureus*

## Prevention of infection in orthopaedic surgery

### Closed fractures[1]

Single dose[3] of i/v cefuroxime *or* i/v flucloxacillin
> If history of allergy to penicillins or to cephalosporins or if high risk of meticillin-resistant *Staphylococcus aureus*, use single dose[3] of i/v teicoplanin[2]

### Open fractures

i/v co-amoxiclav alone *or* i/v cefuroxime + i/v metronidazole (*or* i/v clindamycin alone if history of allergy to penicillins or to cephalosporins)
> Add i/v teicoplanin[2] if high risk of meticillin-resistant *Staphylococcus aureus*. Start prophylaxis within 3 hours of injury and continue until soft tissue closure (max. 72 hours).
> At first debridement also use a single dose of i/v cefuroxime + i/v metronidazole + i/v gentamicin *or* i/v co-amoxiclav + i/v gentamicin (*or* i/v clindamycin + i/v gentamicin if history of allergy to penicillins or to cephalosporins).
> At time of skeletal stabilisation and definitive soft tissue closure[1] use a single dose of i/v gentamicin and i/v teicoplanin[2]

### High lower-limb amputation[1]

i/v co-amoxiclav alone *or* i/v cefuroxime + i/v metronidazole[4]
> Continue antibacterial prophylaxis for at least 2 doses after procedure (max. duration of prophylaxis 5 days). If history of allergy to penicillin or to cephalosporins, or if high risk of meticillin-resistant *Staphylococcus aureus*, use i/v teicoplanin[2] + i/v gentamicin + i/v metronidazole[4]

## Prevention of infection in obstetric surgery

### Termination of pregnancy

Single dose[3] of oral metronidazole
> If genital chlamydial infection cannot be ruled out, give doxycycline (section 5.1.3) postoperatively

## Prevention of endocarditis

> ### NICE guidance
> ### Antimicrobial prophylaxis against infective endocarditis in children and adults undergoing interventional procedures (March 2008)
>
> Antibacterial prophylaxis and chlorhexidine mouthwash are **not** recommended for the prevention of endocarditis in patients undergoing dental procedures.
>
> Antibacterial prophylaxis is **not** recommended for the prevention of endocarditis in patients undergoing procedures of the:
> * upper and lower respiratory tract (including ear, nose, and throat procedures and bronchoscopy);
> * genito-urinary tract (including urological, gynaecological, and obstetric procedures);
> * upper and lower gastro-intestinal tract.
>
> While these procedures can cause bacteraemia, there is no clear association with the development of infective endocarditis. Prophylaxis may expose patients to the adverse effects of antimicrobials when the evidence of benefit has not been proven.
>
> Any infection in patients at risk of endocarditis[5] should be investigated promptly and treated appropriately to reduce the risk of endocarditis.
>
> If patients at risk of endocarditis[5] are undergoing a gastro-intestinal or genito-urinary tract procedure at a site where infection is suspected, they should receive appropriate antibacterial therapy that includes cover against organisms that cause endocarditis.
>
> Patients at risk of endocarditis[5] should be:
> * advised to maintain good oral hygiene;
> * told how to recognise signs of infective endocarditis, and advised when to seek expert advice.

> ### Dermatological procedures
> Advice of a Working Party of the British Society for Antimicrobial Chemotherapy is that patients who undergo dermatological procedures[6] do not require antibacterial prophylaxis against endocarditis.

---

5. Patients at risk of endocarditis include those with valve replacement, acquired valvular heart disease with stenosis or regurgitation, structural congenital heart disease (including surgically corrected or palliated structural conditions, but excluding isolated atrial septal defect, fully repaired ventricular septal defect, fully repaired patent ductus arteriosus, and closure devices considered to be endothelialised), hypertrophic cardiomyopathy, or a previous episode of infective endocarditis

6. The British Association of Dermatologists Therapy Guidelines and Audit Subcommittee advise that such dermatological procedures include skin biopsies and excision of moles or of malignant lesions

---

1. Intravenous antibacterial prophylaxis should be given up to 30 minutes before the procedure
2. Where teicoplanin is suggested vancomycin may be used
3. Additional intra-operative or postoperative doses of antibacterial may be given for prolonged procedures or if there is major blood loss
4. Metronidazole may alternatively be given by suppository but to allow adequate absorption, it should be given 2 hours before surgery

## Joint prostheses and dental treatment

> **Joint prostheses and dental treatment**
>
> Advice of a Working Party of the British Society for Antimicrobial Chemotherapy is that patients with prosthetic joint implants (including total hip replacements) do not require antibacterial prophylaxis for dental treatment. The Working Party considers that it is unacceptable to expose patients to the adverse effects of antibacterials when there is no evidence that such prophylaxis is of any benefit, but that those who develop any intercurrent infection require prompt treatment with antibacterials to which the infecting organisms are sensitive.
>
> The Working Party has commented that joint infections have rarely been shown to follow dental procedures and are even more rarely caused by oral streptococci.

## Immunosuppression and indwelling intraperitoneal catheters

> **Immunosuppression and indwelling intraperitoneal catheters**
>
> Advice of a Working Party of the British Society for Antimicrobial Chemotherapy is that patients who are immunosuppressed (including transplant patients) and patients with indwelling intraperitoneal catheters do not require antibacterial prophylaxis for dental treatment provided there is no other indication for prophylaxis.
>
> The Working Party has commented that there is little evidence that dental treatment is followed by infection in immunosuppressed and immunodeficient patients nor is there evidence that dental treatment is followed by infection in patients with indwelling intraperitoneal catheters.

a penicillin. Children who are allergic to one penicillin will be allergic to all because the hypersensitivity is related to the basic penicillin structure. As patients with a history of immediate hypersensitivity to penicillins may also react to the cephalosporins and other beta-lactam antibiotics, they should not receive these antibiotics; aztreonam may be less likely to cause hypersensitivity in penicillin-sensitive patients and can be used with caution. If a penicillin (or another beta-lactam antibiotic) is essential in a child with immediate hypersensitivity to penicillin then specialist advice should be sought on hypersensitivity testing or using a beta-lactam antibiotic with a different structure to the penicillin that caused the hypersensitivity (see also p. 268).

Individuals with a history of a minor rash (i.e. non-confluent, non-pruritic rash restricted to a small area of the body) or a rash that occurs more than 72 hours after penicillin administration are probably not allergic to penicillin and in these individuals a penicillin should not be withheld unnecessarily for serious infections; the possibility of an allergic reaction should, however, be borne in mind. Other beta-lactam antibiotics (including cephalosporins) can be used in these patients.

**Other side effects**   A rare but serious toxic effect of the penicillins is encephalopathy due to cerebral irritation. This may result from excessively high doses or in patients with severe renal failure. The penicillins should **not** be given by intrathecal injection because they can cause encephalopathy which may be fatal.

Another problem relating to high doses of penicillin, or normal doses given to patients with renal failure, is the accumulation of electrolyte since most injectable penicillins contain either sodium or potassium.

Diarrhoea frequently occurs during oral penicillin therapy. It is most common with broad-spectrum penicillins, which can also cause antibiotic-associated colitis.

**5  Infections**

## 5.1.1  Penicillins

**5.1.1.1  Benzylpenicillin and phenoxymethylpenicillin**
**5.1.1.2  Penicillinase-resistant penicillins**
**5.1.1.3  Broad-spectrum penicillins**
**5.1.1.4  Antipseudomonal penicillins**
**5.1.1.5  Mecillinams**

The penicillins are bactericidal and act by interfering with bacterial cell wall synthesis. They diffuse well into body tissues and fluids, but penetration into the cerebrospinal fluid is poor except when the meninges are inflamed. They are excreted in the urine in therapeutic concentrations.

**Hypersensitivity reactions**   The most important side-effect of the penicillins is hypersensitivity which causes rashes and anaphylaxis and can be fatal. Allergic reactions to penicillins occur in 1–10% of exposed individuals; anaphylactic reactions occur in fewer than 0.05% of treated patients. Individuals with a history of anaphylaxis, urticaria, or rash immediately after penicillin administration are at risk of immediate hypersensitivity to a penicillin; these individuals should not receive

### 5.1.1.1  Benzylpenicillin and phenoxymethylpenicillin

Benzylpenicillin (Penicillin G) remains an important and useful antibiotic but is inactivated by bacterial beta-lactamases. It is effective for many streptococcal (including pneumococcal), gonococcal, and meningococcal infections and also for anthrax (section 5.1.12), diphtheria, gas-gangrene, leptospirosis, and treatment of Lyme disease (section 5.1.1.3) in children. It is also used in combination with gentamicin for the empirical treatment of sepsis in neonates less than 48 hours old. Pneumococci, meningococci, and gonococci which have decreased sensitivity to penicillin have been isolated; **benzylpenicillin is no longer the drug of first choice for pneumococcal meningitis.** Although benzylpenicillin is effective in the treatment of tetanus, metronidazole (section 5.1.11) is preferred. Benzylpenicillin is inactivated by gastric acid and absorption from the gastro-intestinal tract is low; therefore it must be given by injection.

**Benzathine benzylpenicillin** or **procaine benzylpenicillin** is used in the treatment of syphilis (see Table 1 section 5.1); both are available from 'special-order' manufacturers or specialist importing companies, see p. 823.

Phenoxymethylpenicillin (Penicillin V) has a similar antibacterial spectrum to benzylpenicillin, but is less active. It is gastric acid-stable, so is suitable for oral administration. It should not be used for serious infections because absorption can be unpredictable and plasma concentrations variable. It is indicated principally for respiratory-tract infections in children, for streptococcal tonsillitis, and for continuing treatment after one or more injections of benzylpenicillin when clinical response has begun. It should not be used for meningococcal or gonococcal infections. Phenoxymethylpenicillin is used for prophylaxis against streptococcal infections following rheumatic fever and against pneumococcal infections following splenectomy or in sickle cell disease.

**Oral infections**  Phenoxymethylpenicillin is effective for dentoalveolar abscess.

## BENZYLPENICILLIN SODIUM
(Penicillin G)

**Cautions**  history of allergy; false-positive urinary glucose (if tested for reducing substances); **interactions:** Appendix 1 (penicillins)

**Contra-indications**  penicillin hypersensitivity

**Renal impairment**  neurotoxicity—high doses may cause convulsions. Estimated glomerular filtration rate 10–50 mL/minute/1.73 m$^2$, use normal dose every 8–12 hours; estimated glomerular filtration rate less than 10 mL/minute/1.73 m$^2$ use normal dose every 12 hours

**Pregnancy**  not known to be harmful

**Breast-feeding**  trace amounts in milk, but appropriate to use

**Side-effects**  hypersensitivity reactions including urticaria, fever, joint pains, rashes, angioedema, anaphylaxis, serum sickness-like reactions; *rarely* CNS toxicity including convulsions (especially with high doses or in severe renal impairment), interstitial nephritis, haemolytic anaemia, leucopenia, thrombocytopenia and coagulation disorders; also reported diarrhoea (including antibiotic-associated colitis)

**Indications and dose**

Mild to moderate susceptible infections (including throat infections, otitis media, pneumonia, cellulitis, neonatal sepsis, Table 1, section 5.1)

• By intramuscular injection or by slow intravenous injection or infusion (intravenous route recommended in neonates and infants)

Neonate under 7 days 25 mg/kg every 12 hours; increased to 25 mg/mg every 8 hours if necessary

Neonate 7–28 days 25 mg/kg every 8 hours; dose doubled in severe infection

Child 1 month–18 years 25 mg/kg every 6 hours; increased to 50 mg/kg every 4–6 hours (max. 2.4 g every 4 hours) in severe infection

Endocarditis (combined with another antibacterial if necessary, see Table 1, section 5.1)

• By slow intravenous injection or infusion

Child 1 month–18 years 25 mg/kg every 4 hours, increased if necessary to 50 mg/kg (max. 2.4 g) every 4 hours

Meningitis, meningococcal disease

• By intravenous infusion

Neonate under 7 days 50 mg/kg every 12 hours

Neonate 7–28 days 50 mg/kg every 8 hours

Child 1 month–18 years 50 mg/kg every 4–6 hours (max. 2.4 g every 4 hours)

Important. If meningococcal disease (meningitis with non-blanching rash or meningococcal septicaemia) is suspected, a single dose of benzylpenicillin should be given before transferring the child to hospital urgently, so long as this does not delay the transfer. If a child with suspected bacterial meningitis without non-blanching rash cannot be transferred to hospital urgently, a single dose of benzylpenicillin should be given before the transfer. Suitable doses of benzylpenicillin by intravenous injection (or by intramuscular injection) are: Infant under 1 year 300 mg; Child 1–9 years 600 mg, 10 years and over 1.2 g. In penicillin allergy, cefotaxime (section 5.1.2) may be an alternative; chloramphenicol (section 5.1.7) may be used if there is a history of anaphylaxis to penicillins

**Administration**  Intravenous route recommended in neonates and infants. For *intravenous infusion*, dilute with Glucose 5% *or* Sodium Chloride 0.9%; give over 15–30 minutes. Longer administration time is particularly important when using doses of 50 mg/kg (or greater) to avoid CNS toxicity

> **Safe practice**
> Intrathecal injection of benzylpenicillin is **not** recommended

**Crystapen**® (Genus) [PoM]
Injection, powder for reconstitution, benzylpenicillin sodium (unbuffered), net price 600-mg vial = 95p, 2-vial 'GP pack' = £2.64; 1.2-g vial = £1.89
Electrolytes  Na$^+$ 1.68 mmol/600-mg vial; 3.36 mmol/1.2-g vial

## PHENOXYMETHYLPENICILLIN
(Penicillin V)

**Cautions**  see under Benzylpenicillin; **interactions:** Appendix 1 (penicillins)

**Contra-indications**  see under Benzylpenicillin

**Pregnancy**  not known to be harmful

**Breast-feeding**  trace amounts in milk, but appropriate to use

**Side-effects**  see under Benzylpenicillin

**Indications and dose**

Susceptible infections including oral infections, tonsillitis, otitis media, erysipelas, cellulitis

• By mouth

Child 1 month–1 year 62.5 mg 4 times daily (increased up to 12.5 mg/kg 4 times daily if necessary)

Child 1–6 years 125 mg 4 times daily (increased up to 12.5 mg/kg 4 times daily if necessary)

Child 6–12 years 250 mg 4 times daily (increased up to 12.5 mg/kg 4 times daily if necessary)

Child 12–18 years 500 mg 4 times daily (increased up to 1 g 4 times daily if necessary)

Prevention of pneumococcal infection in asplenia or sickle cell disease, see Table 2, section 5.1

Prevention of recurrence of rheumatic fever, see Table 2, section 5.1

Prevention of group A streptococcal infection, see Table 2, section 5.1

**Phenoxymethylpenicillin** (Non-proprietary) PoM

Tablets, phenoxymethylpenicillin (as potassium salt) 250 mg, net price 28-tab pack = £1.27. Label: 9, 23

**Dental prescribing on NHS** Phenoxymethylpenicillin Tablets may be prescribed

Oral solution, phenoxymethylpenicillin (as potassium salt) for reconstitution with water, net price 125 mg/5 mL, 100 mL = £1.90; 250 mg/5 mL, 100 mL = £2.59. Label: 9, 23

**Note** Sugar-free versions are available and can be ordered by specifying 'sugar-free' on the prescription

**Dental prescribing on NHS** Phenoxymethylpenicillin Oral Solution may be prescribed

---

**5.1.1.2  Penicillinase-resistant penicillins**

Most staphylococci are now resistant to benzylpenicillin because they produce penicillinases. **Flucloxacillin**, however, is not inactivated by these enzymes and is thus effective in infections caused by penicillin-resistant staphylococci, which is the main indication for its use. Flucloxacillin is acid-stable and can, therefore, be given by mouth as well as by injection.

Flucloxacillin is well absorbed from the gut. For a warning on hepatic disorders see under Flucloxacillin.

**MRSA**  Infection from *Staphylococcus aureus* strains resistant to meticillin [now discontinued] (meticillin-resistant *Staph. aureus*, MRSA) and to flucloxacillin can be difficult to manage. Treatment is guided by the sensitivity of the infecting strain.

**Rifampicin** (section 5.1.9) or **sodium fusidate** (section 5.1.7) should **not** be used alone because resistance may develop rapidly. **Clindamycin** alone or a combination of rifampicin and sodium fusidate can be used for *skin and soft-tissue infections* caused by MRSA; a **tetracycline** is an alternative in children over 12 years of age. A **glycopeptide** (e.g. vancomycin, section 5.1.7) can be used for severe skin and soft-tissue infections associated with MRSA. A combination of a glycopeptide and sodium fusidate *or* a glycopeptide and rifampicin can be considered for skin and soft-tissue infections that have failed to respond to a single antibacterial. **Linezolid** (section 5.1.7) should be reserved for skin and soft-tissue infections that have not responded to other antibacterials or for children who cannot tolerate other antibacterials.

A **glycopeptide** can be used for *pneumonia* associated with MRSA. **Linezolid** should be reserved for hospital-acquired pneumonia that has not responded to other antibacterials or for children who cannot tolerate other antibacterials.

**Trimethoprim** or **nitrofurantoin** can be used for *urinary-tract infections* caused by MRSA; a **tetracycline** is an alternative in children over 12 years of age. A glycopeptide can be used for urinary-tract infections that are severe or resistant to other antibacterials.

A **glycopeptide** can be used for *septicaemia* associated with MRSA.

For the management of endocarditis, osteomyelitis, or septic arthritis associated with MRSA, see Table 1, section 5.1.

Prophylaxis with vancomycin or teicoplanin (alone or in combination with another antibacterial active against other pathogens) is appropriate for patients undergoing surgery if:

● there is a history of MRSA colonisation or infection without documented eradication;

● there is a risk that the patient's MRSA carriage has recurred;

● the patient comes from an area with a high prevalence of MRSA.

It is important that hospitals have infection control guidelines to minimise MRSA transmission, including policies on isolation and treatment of MRSA carriers and on hand hygiene. For eradication of nasal carriage of MRSA, see section 12.2.3.

---

## ▌FLUCLOXACILLIN

**Cautions**  see under Benzylpenicillin (section 5.1.1.1); risk of kernicterus in jaundiced neonates when high doses given parenterally; **interactions:** Appendix 1 (penicillins)

> **Hepatic disorders**
> Cholestatic jaundice and hepatitis may occur very rarely, up to two months after treatment with flucloxacillin has been stopped. Administration for more than 2 weeks and increasing age are risk factors. Healthcare professionals are reminded that:
> ● flucloxacillin should not be used in patients with a history of hepatic dysfunction associated with flucloxacillin;
> ● flucloxacillin should be used with caution in patients with hepatic impairment;
> ● careful enquiry should be made about hypersensitivity reactions to beta-lactam antibacterials.

**Contra-indications**  see under Benzylpenicillin (section 5.1.1.1)

**Hepatic impairment**  see Cautions and Hepatic Disorders above

**Renal impairment**  use normal dose every 8 hours if estimated glomerular filtration rate less than 10 mL/minute/1.73 m$^2$

**Pregnancy**  not known to be harmful

**Breast-feeding**  trace amounts in milk, but appropriate to use

**Side-effects**  see under Benzylpenicillin (section 5.1.1.1); also gastro-intestinal disturbances; *very rarely* hepatitis and cholestatic jaundice reported (see also Hepatic Disorders above)

**Indications and dose**

> **Infections due to beta-lactamase-producing staphylococci including otitis externa; adjunct in pneumonia, impetigo, cellulitis**
> ● By mouth
>> **Neonate under 7 days** 25 mg/kg twice daily
>> **Neonate 7–21 days** 25 mg/kg 3 times daily
>> **Neonate 21–28 days** 25 mg/kg 4 times daily
>> **Child 1 month–2 years** 62.5–125 mg 4 times daily
>> **Child 2–10 years** 125–250 mg 4 times daily
>> **Child 10–18 years** 250–500 mg 4 times daily
> ● By intramuscular injection
>> **Child 1 month–18 years** 12.5–25 mg/kg every 6 hours (max. 500 mg every 6 hours)

**5** Infections

- **By slow intravenous injection or by intravenous infusion**

  **Neonate under 7 days** 25 mg/kg every 12 hours; may be doubled in severe infection

  **Neonate 7–21 days** 25 mg/kg every 8 hours; may be doubled in severe infection

  **Neonate 21–28 days** 25 mg/kg every 6 hours; may be doubled in severe infection

  **Child 1 month–18 years** 12.5–25 mg/kg every 6 hours (max. 1 g every 6 hours); may be doubled in severe infection

**Osteomyelitis (Table 1, section 5.1), cerebral abscess, staphylococcal meningitis**

- **By slow intravenous injection or by intravenous infusion**

  **Neonate under 7 days** 50–100 mg/kg every 12 hours

  **Neonate 7–21 days** 50–100 mg/kg every 8 hours

  **Neonate 21–28 days** 50–100 mg/kg every 6 hours

  **Child 1 month–18 years** 50 mg/kg (max. 2 g) every 6 hours

**Endocarditis (Table 1, section 5.1)**

- **By slow intravenous injection or by intravenous infusion**

  **Child 1 month–18 years** 50 mg/kg (max. 2 g) every 6 hours

**Prevention of staphylococcal lung infection in cystic fibrosis**

Table 2, section 5.1

**Staphylococcal lung infection in cystic fibrosis**

- **By mouth**

  **Child 1 month–18 years** 25 mg/kg (max. 1 g) 4 times daily; total daily dose may alternatively be given in 3 divided doses

- **By slow intravenous injection or by intravenous infusion**

  **Child 1 month–18 years** 50 mg/kg (max. 2 g) every 6 hours

**Administration** for *intermittent intravenous infusion*, dilute reconstituted solution in Glucose 5% *or* Sodium Chloride 0.9% and give over 30–60 minutes

**Flucloxacillin** (Non-proprietary) [PoM]

Capsules, flucloxacillin (as sodium salt) 250 mg, net price 28 = £2.07; 500 mg, 28 = £3.21. Label: 9, 23
**Brands include** *Floxapen®, Fluclomix®, Ladropen®*

Oral solution (= elixir or syrup), flucloxacillin (as sodium salt) for reconstitution with water, 125 mg/ 5 mL, net price 100 mL = £4.41; 250 mg/5 mL, 100 mL = £31.28. Label: 9, 23
**Note** Sugar-free versions are available and can be ordered by specifying 'sugar-free' on the prescription

Injection, powder for reconstitution, flucloxacillin (as sodium salt). Net price 250-mg vial = £1.23; 500-mg vial = £2.45; 1-g vial = £4.90

### 5.1.1.3   Broad-spectrum penicillins

**Ampicillin** is active against certain Gram-positive and Gram-negative organisms but is inactivated by penicillinases including those produced by *Staphylococcus*

*aureus* and by common Gram-negative bacilli such as *Escherichia coli*. Ampicillin is also active against *Listeria* spp. and enterococci. Almost all staphylococci, approx. 60% of *E. coli* strains and approx. 20% of *Haemophilus influenzae* strains are now resistant. The likelihood of resistance should therefore be considered before using ampicillin for the 'blind' treatment of infections; in particular, it should not be used for hospital patients without checking sensitivity.

Ampicillin can be given by mouth, but less than half the dose is absorbed and absorption is further decreased by the presence of food in the gut. Ampicillin is well excreted in the bile and urine.

**Amoxicillin** is a derivative of ampicillin and has a similar antibacterial spectrum. It is better absorbed than ampicillin when given by mouth, producing higher plasma and tissue concentrations; unlike ampicillin, absorption is not affected by the presence of food in the stomach.

Amoxicillin or ampicillin are principally indicated for the treatment of community-acquired pneumonia and middle ear infections, both of which may be due to *Streptococcus pneumoniae* and *H. influenzae*, and for urinary-tract infections (section 5.1.13). They are also used in the treatment of endocarditis and listerial meningitis. Amoxicillin may also be used for the treatment of Lyme disease [not licensed], see below.

Maculopapular rashes occur commonly with ampicillin (and amoxicillin) but are not usually related to true penicillin allergy. They often occur in children with glandular fever; broad-spectrum penicillins should not therefore be used for 'blind' treatment of a sore throat. The risk of rash is also increased in children with acute or chronic lymphocytic leukaemia or in cytomegalovirus infection.

**Co-amoxiclav** consists of amoxicillin with the beta-lactamase inhibitor clavulanic acid. Clavulanic acid itself has no significant antibacterial activity but, by inactivating beta-lactamases, it makes the combination active against beta-lactamase-producing bacteria that are resistant to amoxicillin. These include resistant strains of *Staph. aureus*, *E. coli*, and *H. influenzae*, as well as many *Bacteroides* and *Klebsiella* spp. Co-amoxiclav should be reserved for infections likely, or known, to be caused by amoxicillin-resistant beta-lactamase-producing strains.

A combination of ampicillin with flucloxacillin (as co-fluampicil) is available to treat infections involving either streptococci or staphylococci (e.g. cellulitis).

**Lyme disease**   Lyme disease should generally be treated by those experienced in its management. **Amoxicillin** [unlicensed indication], **cefuroxime axetil** or **doxycycline** are the antibacterials of choice for *early Lyme disease* or *Lyme arthritis* but doxycycline should only be used in children over 12 years of age. If these antibacterials are contra-indicated, a **macrolide** (e.g. clarithromycin) can be used for early Lyme disease. Intravenous administration of **ceftriaxone**, **cefotaxime** (section 5.1.2.1), or **benzylpenicillin** (p. 260) is recommended for Lyme disease associated with cardiac or neurological complications. The duration of treatment is usually 2–4 weeks; Lyme arthritis may require further treatment.

**Oral infections** Amoxicillin or ampicillin are as effective as phenoxymethylpenicillin (section 5.1.1.1) but they are better absorbed; however, they may encourage emergence of resistant organisms.

Like phenoxymethylpenicillin, amoxicillin and ampicillin are ineffective against bacteria that produce beta-lactamases. Co-amoxiclav is active against beta-lactamase-producing bacteria that are resistant to amoxicillin. Co-amoxiclav may be used for severe dental infection with spreading cellulitis or dental infection not responding to first-line antibacterial treatment.

## AMOXICILLIN
(Amoxycillin)

**Cautions** see under Ampicillin; maintain adequate hydration with high doses (particularly during parenteral therapy); **interactions:** Appendix 1 (penicillins)

**Contra-indications** see under Ampicillin

**Renal impairment** risk of crystalluria with high doses (particularly during parenteral therapy). Reduce dose in severe impairment; rashes more common

**Pregnancy** not known to be harmful

**Breast-feeding** trace amounts in milk, but appropriate to use

**Side-effects** see under Ampicillin

**Indications and dose**

Susceptible infections including urinary-tract infections, sinusitis, uncomplicated community-acquired pneumonia, oral infections (Table 1, section 5.1), Lyme disease (see notes above), salmonellosis
- By mouth

Neonate 7–28 days 30 mg/kg (max. 62.5 mg) 3 times daily; dose doubled in severe infection

Child 1 month–1 year 62.5 mg 3 times daily; dose doubled in severe infection, community-acquired pneumonia, salmonellosis, or Lyme disease

Child 1–5 years 125 mg 3 times daily; dose doubled in severe infection, community-acquired pneumonia, salmonellosis, or Lyme disease

Child 5–18 years 250 mg 3 times daily; dose doubled in severe infection, community-acquired pneumonia, salmonellosis, or Lyme disease

- By intravenous injection or infusion

Neonate under 7 days 30 mg/kg every 12 hours; dose doubled in severe infection, community-acquired pneumonia, or salmonellosis

Neonate 7–28 days 30 mg/kg every 8 hours; dose doubled in severe infection, community-acquired pneumonia, or salmonellosis

Child 1 month–18 years 20–30 mg/kg (max. 500 mg) every 8 hours; dose doubled in severe infection (max. 4 g daily)

Otitis media (but see Table 1, section 5.1)
- By mouth

Child 1 month–18 years 40 mg/kg daily in 3 divided doses (max. 1.5 g daily in 3 divided doses)

Listerial meningitis (in combination with another antibacterial, Table 1, section 5.1), group B streptococcal infection, enterococcal endocarditis (in combination with another antibiotic)
- By intravenous infusion

Neonate under 7 days 50 mg/kg every 12 hours; dose may be doubled in meningitis

Neonate 7–28 days 50 mg/kg every 8 hours; dose may be doubled in meningitis

Child 1 month–18 years 50 mg/kg every 4–6 hours (max. 2 g every 4 hours)

Cystic fibrosis (treatment of asymptomatic *H. influenzae* carriage or mild exacerbations)
- By mouth

Child 1 month–1 year 125 mg 3 times daily

Child 1–7 years 250 mg 3 times daily

Child 7–18 years 500 mg 3 times daily

*Helicobacter pylori* eradication section 1.3

**Note** Amoxicillin doses in BNFC may differ from those in product literature

**Administration** Displacement value may be significant when reconstituting injection, consult local guidelines. Dilute intravenous injection to a concentration of 50 mg/mL (100 mg/mL for neonates). May be further diluted with Glucose 5% *or* Glucose 10% *or* Sodium chloride 0.9% *or* 0.45% for intravenous infusion. Give intravenous infusion over 30 minutes when using doses over 30 mg/kg

**Amoxicillin** (Non-proprietary) PoM
Capsules, amoxicillin (as trihydrate) 250 mg, net price 21 = £1.07; 500 mg, 21 = £1.31. Label: 9
Brands include *Amix®, Amoram®, Amoxident®, Galenamox®, Rimoxallin®*
Dental prescribing on NHS Amoxicillin Capsules may be prescribed
Oral suspension, amoxicillin (as trihydrate) for reconstitution with water, 125 mg/5 mL, net price 100 mL = £1.22; 250 mg/5 mL, 100 mL = £1.39. Label: 9
Note Sugar-free versions are available and can be ordered by specifying 'sugar-free' on the prescription
Brands include *Amoram®, Galenamox®, Rimoxallin®*
Dental prescribing on NHS Amoxicillin Oral Suspension may be prescribed
Injection, powder for reconstitution, amoxicillin (as sodium salt), net price 250-mg vial = 32p; 500-mg vial = 66p; 1-g vial = £1.16

**Amoxil®** (GSK) PoM
Capsules, both maroon/gold, amoxicillin (as trihydrate), 250 mg, net price 21-cap pack = £3.45; 500 mg, 21-cap pack = £6.91. Label: 9
Paediatric suspension, amoxicillin 125 mg (as trihydrate)/1.25 mL when reconstituted with water, net price 20 mL (peach- strawberry- and lemon-flavoured) = £3.25. Label: 9, counselling, use of pipette
Excipients include sucrose 600 mg/1.25 mL
Injection, powder for reconstitution, amoxicillin (as sodium salt), net price 500-mg vial = 56p; 1-g vial = £1.12
Electrolytes Na$^+$ 3.3 mmol/g

## AMPICILLIN

**Cautions** history of allergy; erythematous rashes common in glandular fever (see notes above);

increased risk of erythematous rashes in cyto-megalovirus infection, and acute or chronic lympho-cytic leukaemia (see notes above); **interactions:** Appendix 1 (penicillins)

**Contra-indications** penicillin hypersensitivity

**Renal impairment** if estimated glomerular filtration rate less than $10 \, mL/minute/1.73 \, m^2$ reduce dose or frequency—rashes more common

**Pregnancy** not known to be harmful

**Breast-feeding** trace amounts in milk, but appropriate to use

**Side-effects** nausea, vomiting, diarrhoea; rashes (discontinue treatment); rarely, antibiotic-associated colitis; see also under Benzylpenicillin (section 5.1.1.1)

**Indications and dose**

**Susceptible infections including urinary-tract infections, otitis media, sinusitis, uncomplicated community-acquired pneumonia, oral infections (Table 1, section 5.1), salmonellosis**

• By mouth

**Neonate 7–21 days** 30 mg/kg (max. 62.5 mg) 3 times daily; dose doubled in severe infection

**Neonate 21–28 days** 30 mg/kg (max. 62.5 mg) 4 times daily; dose doubled in severe infection

**Child 1 month–1 year** 62.5 mg 4 times daily; dose doubled in severe infection, community-acquired pneumonia, or salmonellosis

**Child 1–5 years** 125 mg 4 times daily; dose doubled in severe infection, community-acquired pneumonia, or salmonellosis

**Child 5–12 years** 250 mg 4 times daily; dose doubled in severe infection, community-acquired pneumonia, or salmonellosis

**Child 12–18 years** 250–500 mg 4 times daily; dose doubled in severe infection

• By intravenous injection or infusion

**Neonate under 7 days** 30 mg/kg every 12 hours; dose doubled in severe infection, community-acquired pneumonia, or salmonellosis

**Neonate 7–21 days** 30 mg/kg every 8 hours; dose doubled in severe infection, community-acquired pneumonia, or salmonellosis

**Neonate 21–28 days** 30 mg/kg every 6 hours; dose doubled in severe infection, community-acquired pneumonia, or salmonellosis

**Child 1 month–18 years** 25 mg/kg (max. 500 mg) every 6 hours; dose doubled in severe infection

**Listerial meningitis, group B streptococcal infection, enterococcal endocarditis** (in combination with another antibacterial, see Table 1, section 5.1)

• By intravenous infusion

**Neonate under 7 days** 50 mg/kg every 12 hours; dose doubled in meningitis

**Neonate 7–21 days** 50 mg/kg every 8 hours; dose doubled in meningitis

**Neonate 21–28 days** 50 mg/kg every 6 hours; dose doubled in meningitis

**Child 1 month–18 years** 50 mg/kg every 4–6 hours (max. 2 g every 4 hours)

**Administration** *Oral*: administer at least 30 minutes before food

*Injection*: displacement value may be significant when reconstituting injection, consult local guidelines. Dilute intravenous injection to a concentration of 50–100 mg/mL. May be further diluted with glucose 5% or 10% or sodium chloride 0.9% or 0.45% for infusion. Give over 30 minutes when using doses of greater than 50 mg/kg to avoid CNS toxicity including convulsions.

**Ampicillin** (Non-proprietary) PoM

Capsules, ampicillin 250 mg, net price 28 = £7.18; 500 mg, 28 = £32.93. Label: 9, 23
**Brands include** *Rimacillin*®
**Dental prescribing on NHS** Ampicillin Capsules may be prescribed

Oral suspension, ampicillin 125 mg/5 mL when reconstituted with water, net price 100 mL = £9.23; 250 mg/5 mL, 100 mL = £14.17. Label: 9, 23
**Brands include** *Rimacillin*®
**Dental prescribing on NHS** Ampicillin Oral Suspension may be prescribed

Injection, powder for reconstitution, ampicillin (as sodium salt), net price 500-mg vial = £7.83

**Penbritin**® (Chemidex) PoM

Capsules, both grey/red, ampicillin (as trihydrate) 250 mg, net price 28-cap pack = £2.10; 500 mg, 28-cap pack = £5.28. Label: 9, 23

Syrup, apricot- caramel- and peppermint-flavoured, ampicillin (as trihydrate) for reconstitution with water, 125 mg/5 mL, net price 100 mL = £3.78; 250 mg/5 mL, 100 mL = £7.39. Label: 9, 23
**Excipients** include sucrose 3.6 g/5 mL

◢**With flucloxacillin**

**Co-fluampicil** (Non-proprietary) PoM

Capsules, co-fluampicil 250/250 (flucloxacillin 250 mg as sodium salt, ampicillin 250 mg as trihydrate), net price 28-cap pack = £14.73. Label: 9, 22
**Brands include** *Flu-Amp*®

Syrup, co-fluampicil 125/125 (flucloxacillin 125 mg as magnesium salt, ampicillin 125 mg as trihydrate)/ 5 mL when reconstituted with water, net price 100 mL = £4.99. Label: 9, 22

**Magnapen**® (Wockhardt) PoM

Injection 500 mg, powder for reconstitution, co-fluampicil 250/250 (flucloxacillin 250 mg as sodium salt, ampicillin 250 mg as sodium salt), net price per vial = £1.33
**Electrolytes** Na+ 1.3 mmol/vial

## ◢ CO-AMOXICLAV

A mixture of amoxicillin (as the trihydrate or as the sodium salt) and clavulanic acid (as potassium cla-vulanate); the proportions are expressed in the form $x/y$ where $x$ and $y$ are the strengths in milligrams of amoxicillin and clavulanic acid respectively

**Cautions** see under Ampicillin and notes above; maintain adequate hydration with high doses (particularly during parenteral therapy); **interactions:** Appendix 1 (penicillins)
**Cholestatic jaundice** Cholestatic jaundice can occur either during or shortly after the use of co-amoxiclav. An epidemiological study has shown that the risk of acute liver toxicity was about 6 times greater with co-amoxiclav than with amoxicillin; these reactions have only rarely been reported in children. Jaundice is usually self-limiting and

very rarely fatal. The duration of treatment should be appropriate to the indication and should not usually exceed 14 days

**Contra-indications** penicillin hypersensitivity, history of co-amoxiclav-associated or penicillin-associated jaundice or hepatic dysfunction

**Hepatic impairment** monitor liver function in liver disease. See also Cholestatic Jaundice above

**Renal impairment** risk of crystalluria with high doses (particularly during parenteral therapy).

*Co-amoxiclav 125/31 suspension, 250/62 suspension, 250/125 tablets, or 500/125 tablets*: use normal dose every 12 hours if estimated glomerular filtration rate 10–30 mL/minute/1.73 m². Use the normal dose recommended for mild or moderate infections every 12 hours if estimated glomerular filtration rate less than 10 mL/minute/1.73 m².

*Co-amoxiclav 400/57 suspension*: avoid if estimated glomerular filtration rate less than 30 mL/minute/1.73 m².

*Co-amoxiclav injection*: use normal initial dose and then use half normal dose every 12 hours if estimated glomerular filtration rate 10–30 mL/minute/1.73 m²; use normal initial dose and then use half normal dose every 24 hours if estimated glomerular filtration rate less than 10 mL/minute/1.73 m²

**Pregnancy** not known to be harmful

**Breast-feeding** trace amounts in milk, but appropriate to use

**Side-effects** see under Ampicillin; hepatitis, cholestatic jaundice (see above); Stevens-Johnson syndrome, toxic epidermal necrolysis, exfoliative dermatitis, vasculitis reported; rarely prolongation of bleeding time, dizziness, headache, convulsions (particularly with high doses or in renal impairment); superficial staining of teeth with suspension, phlebitis at injection site

**Indications and dose**

> Infections due to beta-lactamase-producing strains (where amoxicillin alone not appropriate) including respiratory-tract infections, bone and joint infections, genito-urinary and abdominal infections, cellulitis, animal bites
>
> • By mouth, expressed as co-amoxiclav (see also under Other Oral Preparations below)
>
> **Neonate** 0.25 mL/kg of *125/31* suspension 3 times daily
>
> **Child 1 month–1 year** 0.25 mL/kg of *125/31* suspension 3 times daily; dose doubled in severe infection
>
> **Child 1–6 years** 5 mL of *125/31* suspension 3 times daily *or* 0.25 mL/kg of *125/31* suspension 3 times daily; dose doubled in severe infection
>
> **Child 6–12 years** 5 mL of *250/62* suspension 3 times daily *or* 0.15 mL/kg of *250/62* suspension 3 times daily; dose doubled in severe infection
>
> **Child 12–18 years** one *250/125* strength tablet 3 times daily; increased in severe infections to one *500/125* strength tablet 3 times daily
>
> • By intravenous injection over 3–4 minutes or by intravenous infusion, expressed as co-amoxiclav
>
> **Neonate** 30 mg/kg every 12 hours
>
> **Child 1–3 months** 30 mg/kg every 12 hours
>
> **Child 3 months–18 years** 30 mg/kg (max. 1.2 g) every 8 hours

> Severe dental infection with spreading cellulitis or dental infection not responding to first-line antibacterial, see notes above
>
> • By mouth, expressed as co-amoxiclav
>
> **Child 12–18 years** one *250/125* strength tablet every 8 hours for 5 days

**Administration** for *intermittent intravenous infusion* dilute reconstituted solution to a concentration of 10 mg/mL with Sodium Chloride 0.9%; give over 30–40 minutes

**Co-amoxiclav** (Non-proprietary) ⓅoM

Tablets, co-amoxiclav 250/125 (amoxicillin 250 mg as trihydrate, clavulanic acid 125 mg as potassium salt), net price 21-tab pack = £2.63. Label: 9
**Dental prescribing on NHS** Co-amoxiclav 250/125 Tablets may be prescribed

Tablets, co-amoxiclav 500/125 (amoxicillin 500 mg as trihydrate, clavulanic acid 125 mg as potassium salt), net price 21-tab pack = £4.38. Label: 9

Oral suspension, co-amoxiclav 125/31 (amoxicillin 125 mg as trihydrate, clavulanic acid 31.25 mg as potassium salt)/5 mL when reconstituted with water, net price 100 mL = £2.49. Label: 9
**Note** Sugar-free versions are available and can be ordered by specifying 'sugar-free' on the prescription
**Dental prescribing on NHS** Co-amoxiclav 125/31 Suspension may be prescribed

Oral suspension, co-amoxiclav 250/62 (amoxicillin 250 mg as trihydrate, clavulanic acid 62.5 mg as potassium salt)/5 mL when reconstituted with water, net price 100 mL = £6.29. Label: 9
**Note** Sugar-free versions are available and can be ordered by specifying 'sugar-free' on the prescription
**Dental prescribing on NHS** Co-amoxiclav 250/62 Suspension may be prescribed

Injection 500/100, powder for reconstitution, co-amoxiclav 500/100 (amoxicillin 500 mg as sodium salt, clavulanic acid 100 mg as potassium salt), net price per vial = £1.21

Injection 1000/200, powder for reconstitution, co-amoxiclav 1000/200 (amoxicillin 1 g as sodium salt, clavulanic acid 200 mg as potassium salt), net price per vial = £2.63

**Augmentin®** (GSK) ⓅoM

Tablets 375 mg, f/c, co-amoxiclav 250/125 (amoxicillin 250 mg as trihydrate, clavulanic acid 125 mg as potassium salt), net price 21-tab pack = £4.19. Label: 9

Tablets 625 mg, f/c, co-amoxiclav 500/125 (amoxicillin 500 mg as trihydrate, clavulanic acid 125 mg as potassium salt). Net price 21-tab pack = £8.00. Label: 9

Suspension '125/31 SF', sugar-free, co-amoxiclav 125/31 (amoxicillin 125 mg as trihydrate, clavulanic acid 31.25 mg as potassium salt)/5 mL when reconstituted with water. Net price 100 mL (raspberry- and orange-flavoured) = £4.08. Label: 9
**Excipients** include aspartame 12.5 mg/5 mL (section 9.4.1)

Suspension '250/62 SF', sugar-free, co-amoxiclav 250/62 (amoxicillin 250 mg as trihydrate, clavulanic acid 62.5 mg as potassium salt)/5 mL when reconstituted with water. Net price 100 mL (raspberry- and orange-flavoured) = £5.74. Label: 9

**Excipients** include aspartame 12.5 mg/5 mL (section 9.4.1)

Injection 600 mg, powder for reconstitution, co-amoxiclav 500/100 (amoxicillin 500 mg as sodium salt, clavulanic acid 100 mg as potassium salt). Net price per vial = £1.31

**Electrolytes** Na$^+$ 1.35 mmol, K$^+$ 0.5 mmol/600-mg vial

Injection 1.2 g, powder for reconstitution, co-amoxiclav 1000/200 (amoxicillin 1 g as sodium salt, clavulanic acid 200 mg as potassium salt). Net price per vial = £2.61

**Electrolytes** Na$^+$ 2.7 mmol, K$^+$ 1 mmol/1.2-g vial

### ◢ Other oral preparations

**Co-amoxiclav** (Non-proprietary) PoM

Suspension '400/57', co-amoxiclav 400/57 (amoxicillin 400 mg as trihydrate, clavulanic acid 57 mg as potassium salt)/5 mL when reconstituted with water. Net price 35 mL = £4.13, 70 mL = £5.79. Label: 9

**Excipients** may include aspartame (section 9.4.1)

**Note** Sugar-free versions are available and can be ordered by specifying 'sugar-free' on the prescription

**Brands** include *Augmentin-Duo*®

**Dose**

> **Child 2 months–2 years** 0.15 mL/kg twice daily, doubled in severe infection
>
> **Child 2–6 years (13–21 kg)** 2.5 mL twice daily, doubled in severe infection
>
> **Child 7–12 years (22–40 kg)** 5 mL twice daily, doubled in severe infection
>
> **Child 12–18 years (over 40 kg)** 10 mL twice daily, increased to 10 mL three times daily in severe infection

### 5.1.1.4 Antipseudomonal penicillins

**Piperacillin**, a ureidopenicillin, is only available in combination with the beta-lactamase inhibitor tazobactam. **Ticarcillin**, a carboxypenicillin, is only available in combination with the beta-lactamase inhibitor clavulanic acid (section 5.1.1.3). Both preparations have a broad spectrum of activity against a range of Gram-positive and Gram-negative bacteria, and anaerobes. Piperacillin with tazobactam has activity against a wider range of Gram-negative organisms than ticarcillin with clavulanic acid and it is more active against *Pseudomonas aeruginosa*. These antibacterials are not active against MRSA.

These antipseudomonal penicillins are used in the treatment of septicaemia, hospital-acquired pneumonia, complicated infections involving the urinary-tract, skin and soft-tissue or intra-abdomen. They may be used for the empirical treatment of septicaemia in immunocompromised children but otherwise should generally be reserved for serious infections resistant to other antibacterials. For severe pseudomonas infections (especially in neutropenia or endocarditis) these antipseudomonal penicillins can be given with an aminoglycoside (e.g. gentamicin, section 5.1.4) since they have a synergistic effect.

Piperacillin with tazobactam is used in cystic fibrosis for the treatment of *Ps. aeruginosa* colonisation when ciprofloxacin and nebulised colistimethate sodium have been ineffective; it can also be used in infective exacerbations, when it is combined with an aminoglycoside.

Owing to the sodium content of many of these antibiotics, high doses may lead to hypernatraemia.

---

## ◢ PIPERACILLIN WITH TAZOBACTAM

**Cautions** see under Benzylpenicillin (section 5.1.1.1); interactions: Appendix 1 (penicillins)

**Contra-indications** see under Benzylpenicillin (section 5.1.1.1)

**Renal impairment** dose expressed as a combination of piperacillin and tazobactam (both as sodium salts). Child under 12 years 78.75 mg/kg (max. 4.5 g) every 8 hours if estimated glomerular filtration rate less than 50 mL/minute/1.73 m$^2$. Child 12–18 years max. 4.5 g every 8 hours if estimated glomerular filtration rate 20–40 mL/minute/1.73 m$^2$; max. 4.5 g every 12 hours if estimated glomerular filtration rate less than 20 mL/minute/1.73 m$^2$

**Pregnancy** manufacturer advises use only if potential benefit outweighs risk

**Breast-feeding** trace amounts in milk, but appropriate to use

**Side-effects** see under Benzylpenicillin (section 5.1.1.1); also nausea, vomiting, diarrhoea; *less commonly* stomatitis, dyspepsia, constipation, jaundice, hypotension, headache, insomnia, injection-site reactions; *rarely* abdominal pain, hepatitis, eosinophilia; *very rarely* hypoglycaemia, hypokalaemia, pancytopenia, Stevens-Johnson syndrome, toxic epidermal necrolysis

**Licensed use** not licensed for use in children under 12 years (except for children 2–12 years with neutropenia and complicated intra-abdominal infections)

**Indications and dose**

> Expressed as a combination of piperacillin and tazobactam (both as sodium salts) in a ratio of 8:1

> **Hospital-acquired pneumonia, septicaemia, complicated infections involving the urinary-tract or skin and soft tissues**
> - **By intravenous infusion**
>   > **Neonate** 90 mg/kg every 8 hours
>   >
>   > **Child 1 month–12 years** 90 mg/kg every 6–8 hours; (max 4.5 g every 6 hours)
>   >
>   > **Child 12–18 years** 4.5 g every 8 hours, increased to 4.5 g every 6 hours in severe infections

> **Infections in children with neutropenia**
> - **By intravenous infusion**
>   > **Child 1 month–18 years** 90 mg/kg (max. 4.5 g) every 6 hours

> **Complicated intra-abdominal infections**
> - **By intravenous infusion**
>   > **Child 2–12 years** 112.5 mg/kg (max. 4.5 g) every 8 hours
>   >
>   > **Child 12–18 years** 4.5 g every 8 hours, increased to 4.5 g every 6 hours in severe infection

**Administration** displacement value may be significant when reconstituting injection, consult local guidelines. For *intravenous infusion*, dilute reconstituted solution to a concentration of 15–90 mg/mL with Glucose 5% *or* Sodium Chloride 0.9%; give over 30 minutes

**Piperacillin with tazobactam** (Non-proprietary) PoM
Injection 2.25 g, powder for reconstitution, piperacillin 2 g (as sodium salt), tazobactam 250 mg (as sodium salt), net price 2.25-g vial = £7.16
Injection 4.5 g, powder for reconstitution, piperacillin 4 g (as sodium salt), tazobactam 500 mg (as sodium salt), net price 4.5-g vial = £14.21

**Tazocin**® (Pfizer) PoM
Injection 2.25 g, powder for reconstitution, piperacillin 2 g (as sodium salt), tazobactam 250 mg (as sodium salt), net price 2.25-g vial = £7.65
**Electrolytes**  Na+ 5.58 mmol/2.25-g vial
Injection 4.5 g, powder for reconstitution, piperacillin 4 g (as sodium salt), tazobactam 500 mg (as sodium salt), net price 4.5-g vial = £15.17
**Electrolytes**  Na+ 11.16 mmol/4.5-g vial

---

## ◼ TICARCILLIN WITH CLAVULANIC ACID

**Cautions**  see under Benzylpenicillin (section 5.1.1.1); interactions: Appendix 1 (penicillins)
**Cholestatic Jaundice**  For a warning on cholestatic jaundice possibly associated with clavulanic acid, see under Co-amoxiclav

**Contra-indications**  see under Benzylpenicillin (section 5.1.1.1)

**Hepatic impairment**  manufacturer advises caution in severe impairment; also cholestatic jaundice, see under Co-amoxiclav

**Renal impairment**  Neonate reduce dose if estimated glomerular filtration rate less than 60 mL/minute/ 1.73 m². Child 1 month–18 years use normal dose every 8 hours if estimated glomerular filtration rate 30–60 mL/minute/1.73 m²; use half normal dose every 8 hours if estimated glomerular filtration rate 10–30 mL/minute/1.73 m²; use half normal dose every 12 hours if estimated glomerular filtration rate less than 10 mL/minute/1.73 m²

**Pregnancy**  not known to be harmful

**Breast-feeding**  trace amounts in milk, but appropriate to use

**Side-effects**  see under Benzylpenicillin (section 5.1.1.1); also nausea, vomiting, coagulation disorders, haemorrhagic cystitis (more frequent in children), injection-site reactions, Stevens-Johnson syndrome, toxic epidermal necrolysis, hypokalaemia, eosinophilia

**Indications and dose**

Expressed as a combination of ticarcillin (as sodium salt) and clavulanic acid (as potassium salt) in a ratio of 15:1

**Infections due to *Pseudomonas* and *Proteus* spp.**
see notes above

● **By intravenous infusion**

**Preterm neonate body-weight under 2 kg** 80 mg/kg every 12 hours

**Preterm neonate body-weight over 2 kg and neonate** 80 mg/kg every 8 hours, increased to every 6 hours in more severe infections

**Child 1 month–18 years and body-weight under 40 kg** 80 mg/kg every 8 hours, increased to every 6 hours in more severe infections

**Child under 18 years and body-weight over 40 kg** 3.2 g every 6–8 hours, increased to every 4 hours in more severe infections

---

**Administration**  Displacement value may be important, consult local guidelines. For intermittent infusion, dilute reconstituted solution further to a concentration of 16–32 mg/mL with glucose 5%; infuse over 30–40 minutes.

**Timentin**® (GSK) PoM
Injection 3.2 g, powder for reconstitution, ticarcillin 3 g (as sodium salt), clavulanic acid 200 mg (as potassium salt). Net price per vial = £5.33
**Electrolytes**  Na+ 16 mmol, K+ 1 mmol /3.2-g vial

---

**5.1.1.5**  **Mecillinams**

Pivmecillinam has significant activity against many Gram-negative bacteria including *Escherichia coli*, klebsiella, enterobacter, and salmonellae. It is not active against *Pseudomonas aeruginosa* or enterococci. Pivmecillinam is hydrolysed to mecillinam, which is the active drug.

---

## ◼ PIVMECILLINAM HYDROCHLORIDE

**Cautions**  see under Benzylpenicillin (section 5.1.1.1); also liver and renal function tests required in long-term use; avoid in acute porphyria (section 9.8.2); interactions: Appendix 1 (penicillins)

**Contra-indications**  see under Benzylpenicillin (section 5.1.1.1); also carnitine deficiency, oesophageal strictures, gastro-intestinal obstruction, infants under 3 months

**Pregnancy**  not known to be harmful, but manufacturer advises avoid

**Breast-feeding**  trace amounts in milk, but appropriate to use

**Side-effects**  see under Benzylpenicillin (section 5.1.1.1); nausea, vomiting, abdominal pain, headache, dizziness; also reported mouth ulcers, oesophagitis, reduced serum and total body carnitine (especially with long-term or repeated use)

**Licensed use**  not licensed for use in children under 3 months

**Indications and dose**

**Acute uncomplicated cystitis**
● **By mouth**
**Child body-weight over 40 kg** initially 400 mg then 200 mg every 8 hours for 3 days

**Chronic or recurrent bacteriuria**
**Child body-weight over 40 kg** 400 mg every 6–8 hours

**Urinary-tract infections**
**Child body-weight under 40 kg** 5–10 mg/kg every 6 hours; total daily dose may alternatively be given in 3 divided doses

**Salmonellosis** not recommended therefore no dose stated

**Counselling** Tablets should be swallowed whole with plenty of fluid during meals while sitting or standing

**Selexid**® (LEO) PoM
Tablets, f/c, pivmecillinam hydrochloride 200 mg, net price 10-tab pack = £4.50. Label: 9, 21, 27, counselling, posture (see Dose above)

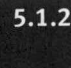

## 5.1.2 Cephalosporins, carbapenems, and other beta-lactams

### 5.1.2.1 Cephalosporins
### 5.1.2.2 Carbapenems
### 5.1.2.3 Other beta-lactam antibiotics

Antibiotics in this section include the **cephalosporins**, such as cefotaxime, ceftazidime, cefuroxime, cefalexin and cefradine, the **monobactam**, aztreonam, and the **carbapenems**, imipenem (a thienamycin derivative), meropenem, and ertapenem.

### 5.1.2.1 Cephalosporins

The cephalosporins are broad-spectrum antibacterials which are used for the treatment of septicaemia, pneumonia, meningitis, biliary-tract infections, peritonitis, and urinary-tract infections. The pharmacology of the cephalosporins is similar to that of the penicillins, excretion being principally renal. Cephalosporins penetrate the cerebrospinal fluid poorly unless the meninges are inflamed; cefotaxime and ceftriaxone are suitable cephalosporins for infections of the CNS (e.g meningitis).

The principal side-effect of the cephalosporins is hypersensitivity and about 0.5–6.5% of penicillin-sensitive patients will also be allergic to the cephalosporins. Patients with a history of immediate hypersensitivity to penicillin should not receive a cephalosporin. If a cephalosporin is essential in these patients because a suitable alternative antibacterial is not available, then cefixime, cefotaxime, ceftazidime, ceftriaxone, or cefuroxime can be used with caution; cefaclor, cefadroxil, cefalexin, and cefradine should be avoided.

Antibiotic-associated colitis may occur with the use of broad-spectrum cephalosporins, particularly second- and third-generation cephalosporins.

**Cefuroxime** is a 'second generation' cephalosporin that is less susceptible than the earlier cephalosporins to inactivation by beta-lactamases. It is, therefore, active against certain bacteria that are resistant to the other drugs and has greater activity against *Haemophilus influenzae*.

**Cefotaxime**, **ceftazidime** and **ceftriaxone** are 'third generation' cephalosporins with greater activity than the 'second generation' cephalosporins against certain Gram-negative bacteria. However, they are less active than cefuroxime against Gram-positive bacteria, most notably *Staphylococcus aureus*. Their broad antibacterial spectrum may encourage superinfection with resistant bacteria or fungi.

**Ceftazidime** has good activity against pseudomonas. It is also active against other Gram-negative bacteria.

**Ceftriaxone** has a longer half-life and therefore needs to be given only once daily. Indications include serious infections such as septicaemia, pneumonia, and meningitis. The calcium salt of ceftriaxone forms a precipitate in the gall bladder which may rarely cause symptoms but these usually resolve when the antibacterial is stopped. In neonates, ceftriaxone may displace bilirubin from plasma-albumin and should be avoided in neonates with unconjugated hyperbilirubinaemia, hypoalbuminaemia, acidosis or impaired bilirubin binding.

**Orally active cephalosporins**   The orally active 'first generation' cephalosporins, **cefalexin**, **cefradine**, and **cefadroxil** and the 'second generation' cephalosporin, **cefaclor**, have a similar antimicrobial spectrum. They are useful for urinary-tract infections which do not respond to other drugs or which occur in pregnancy, respiratory-tract infections, otitis media, sinusitis, and skin and soft-tissue infections. Cefaclor has good activity against *H. influenzae*, but it is associated with protracted skin reactions especially in children. Cefadroxil has a long duration of action and can be given twice daily; it has poor activity against *H. influenzae*. **Cefuroxime axetil**, an ester of the 'second generation' cephalosporin cefuroxime, has the same antibacterial spectrum as the parent compound; it is poorly absorbed and needs to be given with food to maximise absorption.

**Cefixime** and **cefpodoxime proxetil** are orally active 'third generation' cephalosporins. Cefixime has a longer duration of action than the other cephalosporins that are active by mouth. It is only licensed for acute infections. Cefpodoxime proxetil is more active than the other oral cephalosporins against respiratory bacterial pathogens and it is licensed for upper and lower respiratory-tract infections.

For treatment of Lyme disease, see section 5.1.1.3.

**Oral infections**   The cephalosporins offer little advantage over the penicillins in dental infections, often being less active against anaerobes. Infections due to oral streptococci (often termed viridans streptococci) which become resistant to penicillin are usually also resistant to cephalosporins. This is of importance in the case of children who have had rheumatic fever and are on long-term penicillin therapy. Cefalexin and cefradine have been used in the treatment of oral infections.

---

## CEFACLOR

**Cautions**   sensitivity to beta-lactam antibacterials (avoid if history of immediate hypersensitivity reaction, see also notes above and p. 259); false positive urinary glucose (if tested for reducing substances) and false positive Coombs' test; **interactions**: Appendix 1 (cephalosporins)

**Contra-indications**   cephalosporin hypersensitivity

**Renal impairment**   no dosage adjustment required, manufacturer advises caution

**Pregnancy**   not known to be harmful

**Breast-feeding**   present in milk in low concentration, but appropriate to use

**Side-effects**   diarrhoea (rarely antibiotic-associated colitis), nausea and vomiting, abdominal discomfort, headache; allergic reactions including rashes, pruritus, urticaria, serum sickness-like reactions with rashes, fever and arthralgia, and anaphylaxis; Stevens-Johnson syndrome, toxic epidermal necrolysis reported; disturbances in liver enzymes, transient hepatitis and cholestatic jaundice; other side-effects reported include eosinophilia and blood disorders (including thrombocytopenia, leucopenia, agranulocytosis, aplastic anaemia and haemolytic anaemia); reversible interstitial nephritis, hyperactivity, nervousness, sleep disturbances, hallucinations, confusion, hypertonia, and dizziness

5 Infections

**Indications and dose**

Infections due to sensitive Gram-positive and Gram-negative bacteria but see notes above

● By mouth

**Child 1 month–12 years** 20 mg/kg daily in 3 divided doses, doubled for severe infection (usual max. 1 g daily)

*or*

**Child 1 month–1 year** 62.5 mg 3 times daily; dose doubled for severe infections

**Child 1–5 years** 125 mg 3 times daily; dose doubled for severe infections

**Child 5–12 years** 250 mg 3 times daily; dose doubled for severe infections

**Child 12–18 years** 250 mg 3 times daily; dose doubled for severe infections (max. 4 g daily)

---

Asymptomatic carriage of *Haemophilus influenzae* or mild exacerbations in cystic fibrosis

● By mouth

**Child 1 month–1 year** 125 mg every 8 hours

**Child 1–7 years** 250 mg 3 times daily

**Child 7–18 years** 500 mg 3 times daily

**Cefaclor** (Non-proprietary) PoM

Capsules, cefaclor (as monohydrate) 250 mg, net price 21-cap pack = £5.09; 500 mg, 50-cap pack = £31.99. Label: 9
Brands include *Keftid*®

Suspension, cefaclor (as monohydrate) for reconstitution with water, 125 mg/5 mL, net price 100 mL = £8.33; 250 mg/5 mL, 100 mL = £6.97. Label: 9
Note Sugar-free versions are available and can be ordered by specifying 'sugar-free' on the prescription
Brands include *Keftid*®

**Distaclor**® (Flynn) PoM

Capsules, cefaclor (as monohydrate) 500 mg (violet/grey), net price 21-cap pack = £18.19. Label: 9

Suspension, both pink, cefaclor (as monohydrate) for reconstitution with water, 125 mg/5 mL, net price 100 mL = £4.13; 250 mg/5 mL, 100 mL = £8.26. Label: 9

**Distaclor MR**® (Flynn) PoM

Tablets, m/r, both blue, cefaclor (as monohydrate) 375 mg. Net price 14-tab pack = £8.31. Label: 9, 21, 25
**Dose**

Susceptible infections

**Child 12–18 years** 375 mg every 12 hours with food, dose doubled for pneumonia

Lower urinary-tract infections

**Child 12–18 years** 375 mg every 12 hours with food

---

■ **CEFADROXIL**

**Cautions** see under Cefaclor; **interactions**: Appendix 1 (cephalosporins)

**Contra-indications** see under Cefaclor

**Renal impairment** reduce dose if estimated glomerular filtration rate less than 50 mL/minute/1.73 m²

**Pregnancy** not known to be harmful

**Breast-feeding** present in milk in low concentration, but appropriate to use

**Side-effects** see under Cefaclor
**Indications and dose**

Infections due to sensitive Gram-positive and Gram-negative bacteria but see notes above

● By mouth

**Child 6–18 years**

**Body-weight under 40 kg** 500 mg twice daily;

**Body-weight over 40 kg** 0.5–1 g twice daily (1 g once daily for skin, soft-tissue and uncomplicated urinary-tract infections)

**Cefadroxil** (Non-proprietary) PoM

Capsules, cefadroxil (as monohydrate) 500 mg, net price 20-cap pack = £4.83. Label: 9

---

■ **CEFALEXIN**
(Cephalexin)

**Cautions** see under Cefaclor; **interactions**: Appendix 1 (cephalosporins)

**Contra-indications** see under Cefaclor

**Renal impairment** reduce dose in moderate impairment

**Pregnancy** not known to be harmful

**Breast-feeding** present in milk in low concentration, but appropriate to use

**Side-effects** see under Cefaclor
**Indications and dose**

Infections due to sensitive Gram-positive and Gram-negative bacteria but see notes above

● By mouth

**Neonate under 7 days** 25 mg/kg (max. 125 mg) twice daily

**Neonate 7–21 days** 25 mg/kg (max. 125 mg) 3 times daily

**Neonate 21–28 days** 25 mg/kg (max. 125 mg) 4 times daily

**Child 1 month–12 years** 12.5 mg/kg twice daily; dose doubled in severe infection; max. 25 mg/kg 4 times daily (max. 1 g 4 times daily)

*or*

**Child 1 month–1 year** 125 mg twice daily

**Child 1–5 years** 125 mg 3 times daily

**Child 5–12 years** 250 mg 3 times daily

**Child 12–18 years** 500 mg 2–3 times daily, increased to 1–1.5 g 3–4 times daily for severe infection

---

Prophylaxis of recurrent urinary-tract infection

● By mouth

**Child 1 month–18 years** 12.5 mg/kg at night (max. 125 mg at night)

**Cefalexin** (Non-proprietary) PoM

Capsules, cefalexin 250 mg, net price 28-cap pack = £1.66; 500 mg, 21-cap pack = £2.09. Label: 9
Dental prescribing on NHS Cefalexin Capsules may be prescribed

Tablets, cefalexin 250 mg, net price 28-tab pack = £1.94; 500 mg, 21-tab pack = £2.39. Label: 9
Dental prescribing on NHS Cefalexin Tablets may be prescribed

5 Infections

Oral suspension, cefalexin for reconstitution with water, 125 mg/5 mL, net price 100 mL = £1.75; 250 mg/5 mL, 100 mL = £2.15. Label: 9

**Dental prescribing on NHS** Cefalexin Oral Suspension may be prescribed

**Ceporex®** (Co-Pharma) [PoM]

Capsules, both caramel/grey, cefalexin 250 mg, net price 28-cap pack = £4.02; 500 mg, 28-cap pack = £7.85. Label: 9

Tablets, all pink, f/c, cefalexin 250 mg, net price 28-tab pack = £4.02; 500 mg, 28-tab pack = £7.85. Label: 9

Syrup, all orange, cefalexin for reconstitution with water, 125 mg/5 mL, net price 100 mL = £1.43; 250 mg/5 mL, 100 mL = £2.87; 500 mg/5 mL, 100 mL = £5.57. Label: 9

**Keflex®** (Flynn) [PoM]

Capsules, cefalexin 250 mg (green/white), net price 28-cap pack = £1.46; 500 mg (pale green/dark green), 21-cap pack = £1.98. Label: 9

Tablets, both peach, cefalexin 250 mg, net price 28-tab pack = £1.60; 500 mg (scored), 21-tab pack = £2.08. Label: 9

Suspension, cefalexin for reconstitution with water, 125 mg/5 mL, net price 100 mL = 84p; 250 mg/5 mL, 100 mL = £1.40. Label: 9

## CEFIXIME

**Cautions** see under Cefaclor; **interactions:** Appendix 1 (cephalosporins)

**Contra-indications** see under Cefaclor

**Renal impairment** reduce dose if estimated glomerular filtration rate less than 20 mL/minute/1.73 m$^2$

**Pregnancy** not known to be harmful

**Breast-feeding** manufacturer advises avoid unlesss essential—no information available

**Side-effects** see under Cefaclor

**Indications and dose**

Acute infections due to sensitive Gram-positive and Gram-negative bacteria, but see notes above

- By mouth

    **Child 6 months–1 year** 75 mg daily

    **Child 1–5 years** 100 mg daily

    **Child 5–10 years** 200 mg daily

    **Child 10–18 years** 200–400 mg daily or 100–200 mg twice daily

Uncomplicated gonorrhoea [unlicensed indication, see also Table 1, section 5.1]

- By mouth

    **Child 12–18 years** 400 mg as a single dose

**Suprax®** (Sanofi-Aventis) [PoM]

Tablets, f/c, scored, cefixime 200 mg. Net price 7-tab pack = £13.23. Label: 9

Paediatric oral suspension, cefixime 100 mg/5 mL when reconstituted with water, net price 100 mL (with spoon for measuring 3.75 mL or 5 mL) = £18.91. Label: 9

## CEFOTAXIME

**Cautions** see under Cefaclor; **interactions:** Appendix 1 (cephalosporins)

**Contra-indications** see under Cefaclor

**Renal impairment** usual initial dose, then use half normal dose if estimated glomerular filtration rate less than 5 mL/minute/1.73 m$^2$

**Pregnancy** not known to be harmful

**Breast-feeding** present in milk in low concentration, but appropriate to use

**Side-effects** see under Cefaclor; rarely arrhythmias following rapid injection reported

**Indications and dose**

Infections due to sensitive Gram-positive and Gram-negative bacteria, surgical prophylaxis, Haemophilus epiglottitis and meningitis (Table 1, section 5.1) see also notes above

- By intramuscular or by intravenous injection or intravenous infusion

    **Neonate under 7 days** 25 mg/kg every 12 hours; dose doubled in severe infection and meningitis

    **Neonate 7–21 days** 25 mg/kg every 8 hours; dose doubled in severe infection and meningitis

    **Neonate 21–28 days** 25 mg/kg every 6–8 hours; dose doubled in severe infection and meningitis

    **Child 1 month–18 years** 50 mg/kg every 8–12 hours; increase to every 6 hours in very severe infections and meningitis (max. 12 g daily)

    **Important.** If meningococcal disease (meningitis with non-blanching rash or meningococcal septicaemia) is suspected, and the child cannot be given benzylpenicillin (e.g. because of an allergy), a single dose of cefotaxime can be given (if available) before urgent transfer to hospital, so long as this does not delay the transfer. If a child with suspected bacterial meningitis without non-blanching rash cannot be transferred to hospital urgently and cannot be given benzylpenicillin, a single dose of cefotaxime can be given before transfer. Suitable doses of cefotaxime by intravenous injection (or by intramuscular injection) are Child under 12 years 50 mg/kg; Child over 12 years 1 g; chloramphenicol (section 5.1.7) may be used if there is a history of anaphylaxis to penicillins or cephalosporins

Congenital gonococcal conjunctivitis

- By intramuscular injection

    **Neonate** 100 mg/kg (max. 1 g) as a single dose

Uncomplicated gonorrhoea

- By intramuscular injection

    **Child 12–18 years** 500 mg as a single dose

Severe exacerbations of Haemophilus influenzae infection in cystic fibrosis

- By intravenous injection or intravenous infusion

    **Child 1 month–18 years** 50 mg/kg every 6–8 hours (max. 12 g daily)

**Administration** Displacement value may be significant, consult local guidelines. For intermittent intravenous infusion dilute in glucose 5% or sodium chloride 0.9%; administer over 20–60 minutes; incompatible with alkaline solutions

**Cefotaxime** (Non-proprietary) [PoM]

Injection, powder for reconstitution, cefotaxime (as sodium salt), net price 500-mg vial = £2.14; 1-g vial = £4.31; 2-g vial = £8.57

## CEFPODOXIME

**Cautions**  see under Cefaclor; **interactions**: Appendix 1 (cephalosporins)

**Contra-indications**  see under Cefaclor

**Renal impairment**  increase dose interval to every 24 hours if estimated glomerular filtration rate 10–40 mL/minute/1.73 m². Increase dose interval to every 48 hours if estimated glomerular filtration rate less than 10 mL/minute/1.73 m²

**Pregnancy**  not known to be harmful

**Breast-feeding**  present in milk in low concentration —manufacturer advises avoid

**Side-effects**  see under Cefaclor

**Indications and dose**

Upper respiratory-tract infections (but in pharyngitis and tonsillitis reserved for infections which are recurrent, chronic, or resistant to other antibacterials), lower respiratory-tract infections (including bronchitis and pneumonia), skin and soft tissue infections, uncomplicated urinary-tract infections

- By mouth

    **Child 15 days–6 months** 4 mg/kg twice daily

    **Child 6 months–2 years** 40 mg twice daily

    **Child 3–8 years** 80 mg twice daily

    **Child 9–12 years** 100 mg twice daily

    **Child 12–18 years** 100 mg twice daily (increased to 200 mg twice daily in sinusitis, skin and soft tissue infections, uncomplicated upper urinary tract infections and if necessary in lower respiratory tract infections)

**Orelox**® (Sanofi-Aventis) `PoM`

Tablets, f/c, cefpodoxime 100 mg (as proxetil), net price 10-tab pack = £9.78. Label: 5, 9, 21

Oral suspension, cefpodoxime (as proxetil) for reconstitution with water, 40 mg/5 mL, net price 100 mL = £11.50. Label: 5, 9, 21

Excipients  include aspartame (section 9.4.1)

## CEFRADINE
(Cephradine)

**Cautions**  see under Cefaclor; **interactions**: Appendix 1 (cephalosporins)

**Contra-indications**  see under Cefaclor

**Renal impairment**  reduce dose if estimated glomerular filtration rate less than 20 mL/minute/1.73 m²

**Pregnancy**  not known to be harmful

**Breast-feeding**  present in milk in low concentration, but appropriate to use

**Side-effects**  see under Cefaclor

**Licensed use**  not licensed for use in children for prevention of *Staphylococcus aureus* lung infection in cystic fibrosis

**Indications and dose**

Infections due to sensitive Gram-positive and Gram-negative bacteria but see notes above

- By mouth

    **Child 7–12 years** 12.5–25 mg/kg twice daily (total daily dose may alternatively be given in 3–4 divided doses)

    **Child 12–18 years** 0.5–1 g twice daily *or* 250–500 mg 4 times daily; up to 1 g 4 times daily in severe infections

Prevention of *Staphylococcus aureus* lung infection in cystic fibrosis

- By mouth

    **Child 7–18 years** 2 g twice daily

**Cefradine** (Non-proprietary) `PoM`

Capsules, cefradine 250 mg, net price 20-cap pack = £2.86; 500 mg, 20-cap pack = £4.50. Label: 9

Brands include *Nicef*®

Dental prescribing on NHS Cefradine Capsules may be prescribed

## CEFTAZIDIME

**Cautions**  see under Cefaclor; **interactions**: Appendix 1 (cephalosporins)

**Contra-indications**  see under Cefaclor

**Hepatic impairment**  manufacturer advises caution in severe impairment

**Renal impairment**  reduce dose if estimated glomerular filtration rate less than 50 mL/minute/1.73 m²—consult product literature

**Pregnancy**  not known to be harmful

**Breast-feeding**  present in milk in low concentration, but appropriate to use

**Side-effects**  see under Cefaclor; also taste disturbances, paraesthesia

**Licensed use**  nebulised route unlicensed

**Indications and dose**

Infections due to sensitive Gram-positive and Gram-negative bacteria but see notes above

- By intravenous injection or infusion

    **Neonate under 7 days** 25 mg/kg every 24 hours; dose doubled in severe infection and meningitis

    **Neonate 7–21 days** 25 mg/kg every 12 hours; dose doubled in severe infection and meningitis

    **Neonate 21–28 days** 25 mg/kg every 8 hours; dose doubled in severe infection and meningitis

    **Child 1 month–18 years** 25 mg/kg every 8 hours; dose doubled in severe infection, febrile neutropenia and meningitis (max. 6 g daily)

Pseudomonal lung infection in cystic fibrosis

- By intravenous injection or infusion (or by deep intramuscular injection if intravenous administration not possible)

    **Child 1 month–18 years** 50 mg/kg every 8 hours (max. 9 g daily); single doses over 1 g intravenous route only

Chronic *Burkholderia cepacia* infection in cystic fibrosis

- By inhalation of nebulised solution

    **Child 1 month–18 years** 1 g twice daily

**Administration**  For parenteral administration, intravenous route recommended in children. Displacement value may be significant, consult local guidelines. For intermittent intravenous infusion dilute reconstituted solution further to a concentration of not more than 40 mg/mL in Glucose 5% or Glucose 10% or Sodium chloride 0.9%; give over 20–30 minutes

**5 Infections**

For nebulisation, dissolve dose in 3 mL of water for injection

**Ceftazidime** (Non-proprietary) PoM
Injection, powder for reconstitution, ceftazidime (as pentahydrate), with sodium carbonate, net price 1-g vial = £8.50; 2-g vial = £17.90

**Fortum®** (GSK) PoM
Injection, powder for reconstitution, ceftazidime (as pentahydrate), with sodium carbonate, net price 500-mg vial = £4.40, 1-g vial = £8.79, 2-g vial = £17.59, 3-g vial = £25.76
Electrolytes  Na⁺ 2.3 mmol/g

**Kefadim®** (Flynn) PoM
Injection, powder for reconstitution, ceftazidime (as pentahydrate), with sodium carbonate, net price 1-g vial = £7.92; 2-g vial = £15.84
Electrolytes  Na⁺ 2.3 mmol/g

## CEFTRIAXONE

**Cautions** see under Cefaclor; neonates; may displace bilirubin from serum albumin, administer over 60 minutes in neonates (see also Contra-indications); treatment longer than 14 days, renal failure, dehydration—risk of ceftriaxone precipitation in gall bladder; **interactions:** Appendix 1 (cephalosporins)

**Contra-indications** see under Cefaclor; neonates less than 41 weeks postmenstrual age; neonates over 41 weeks postmenstrual age with jaundice, hypoalbuminaemia, or acidosis; concomitant treatment with intravenous calcium (including total parenteral nutrition containing calcium) in neonates over 41 weeks postmenstrual age—risk of precipitation in urine and lungs

**Hepatic impairment** if hepatic impairment is accompanied by severe renal impairment, reduce dose and monitor plasma concentration

**Renal impairment** max. 50 mg/kg daily (max. 2 g daily) in severe renal impairment; also monitor plasma concentration if hepatic impairment accompanied by severe renal impairment

**Pregnancy** not known to be harmful

**Breast-feeding** present in milk in low concentration, but appropriate to use

**Side-effects** see under Cefaclor; calcium ceftriaxone precipitates in urine (particularly in very young, dehydrated or those who are immobilised) or in gall bladder—consider discontinuation if symptomatic; rarely prolongation of prothrombin time, pancreatitis

**Licensed use** not licensed for congenital gonococcal conjunctivitis or early syphilis; not licensed for prophylaxis of meningococcal meningitis or *Haemophilus influenzae* type b disease; not licensed for use in children under 12 years of age for uncomplicated gonorrhoea or pelvic inflammatory disease

**Indications and dose**

Infections due to sensitive Gram-positive and Gram-negative bacteria
• By intravenous infusion over 60 minutes
  **Neonate** 20–50 mg/kg once daily
• By deep intramuscular injection, or by intravenous injection over 2–4 minutes, or by intravenous infusion
  **Child 1 month–12 years**
  **Body-weight under 50 kg** 50 mg/kg once daily; up to 80 mg/kg daily in severe infections and

meningitis; doses of 50 mg/kg and over by intravenous infusion only
  **Body-weight 50 kg and over** dose as for child 12–18 years
  **Child 12–18 years** 1 g daily; 2–4 g daily in severe infections and meningitis; intramuscular doses over 1 g divided between more than one site; single intravenous doses above 1 g by intravenous infusion only

Congenital gonococcal conjunctivitis
• By intravenous infusion over 60 minutes or by deep intramuscular injection
  **Neonate** 25–50 mg/kg (max.125 mg) as a single dose

Uncomplicated gonorrhoea, pelvic inflammatory disease (Table 1, section 5.1)
• By deep intramuscular injection
  **Child under 12 years**
  **Body-weight under 45 kg** 125 mg as a single dose
  **Body-weight over 45 kg** 250 mg as a single dose
  **Child 12–18 years** 250 mg as a single dose

Early syphilis
• By deep intramuscular injection
  **Child 12–18 years** 500 mg daily for 10 days

Surgical prophylaxis
• By deep intramuscular injection or by intravenous injection over at least 2–4 minutes, or (for colorectal surgery) by intravenous infusion
  **Child 12–18 years** 1 g up to 30 minutes before the procedure; colorectal surgery, 2 g up to 30 minutes before the procedure; intramuscular doses over 1 g divided between more than one site

Prophylaxis of meningococcal meningitis Table 2, section 5.1

Prophylaxis of *Haemophilus influenzae* type b disease Table 2, section 5.1

**Administration** Displacement value may be significant, consult local guidelines. For *intravenous infusion*, dilute reconstituted solution with Glucose 5% or 10% or Sodium Chloride 0.9%; give over at least 30 minutes (60 minutes in neonates). Not to be given simultaneously with parenteral nutrition or infusion fluids containing calcium, even by different infusion lines; may be infused sequentially with infusion fluids containing calcium if flush with sodium chloride 0.9% between infusions or give infusions by different infusion lines at different sites; see also Contra-indications above

For *intramuscular injection* ceftriaxone may be mixed with 1% Lidocaine Hydrochloride Injection to reduce pain at intramuscular injection site; final concentration 250–350 mg/mL.

**Ceftriaxone** (Non-proprietary) PoM
Injection, powder for reconstitution, ceftriaxone (as sodium salt), net price 1-g vial = £10.17; 2-g vial = £20.36

**Rocephin®** (Roche) [PoM]

Injection, powder for reconstitution, ceftriaxone (as sodium salt), net price 250-mg vial = £2.40; 1-g vial = £9.58; 2-g vial = £19.18

Electrolytes Na⁺ 3.6 mmol/g

## CEFUROXIME

**Cautions** see under Cefaclor; **interactions:** Appendix 1 (cephalosporins)

**Contra-indications** see under Cefaclor

**Renal impairment** reduce parenteral dose if estimated glomerular filtration rate less than 20 mL/minute/1.73 m²

**Pregnancy** not known to be harmful

**Breast-feeding** present in milk in low concentration, but appropriate to use

**Side-effects** see under Cefaclor

**Licensed use** not licensed for treatment of Lyme disease in children under 12 years

### Indications and dose

Infections due to sensitive Gram-positive and Gram-negative bacteria

• By mouth (as cefuroxime axetil)

**Child 3 months–2 years** 10 mg/kg (max. 125 mg) twice daily

**Child 2–12 years** 15 mg/kg (max. 250 mg) twice daily

**Child 12–18 years** 250 mg twice daily; dose doubled in severe lower respiratory-tract infections, or if pneumonia suspected; dose reduced to 125 mg twice daily in lower urinary-tract infection

• By intravenous injection or infusion or by intramuscular injection

**Neonate under 7 days** 25 mg/kg every 12 hours; dose doubled in severe infection, intravenous route only

**Neonate 7–21 days** 25 mg/kg every 8 hours; dose doubled in severe infection, intravenous route only

**Neonate 21–28 days** 25 mg/kg every 6 hours; dose doubled in severe infection, intravenous route only

**Child 1 month–18 years** 20 mg/kg (max. 750 mg) every 8 hours; increase to 50–60 mg/kg (max. 1.5 g) every 6–8 hours in severe infection and cystic fibrosis

Lyme disease (see also section 5.1.1.3)

• By mouth

**Child 3 months–12 years** 15 mg/kg (max. 500 mg) twice daily for 14–21 days (for 28 days in Lyme arthritis)

**Child 12–18 years** 500 mg twice daily for 14–21 days (for 28 days in Lyme arthritis)

Surgical prophylaxis

• By intravenous injection

**Child 1 month–18 years** 50 mg/kg (max. 1.5 g) up to 30 minutes before the procedure; up to 3 further doses of 30 mg/kg (max. 750 mg) may be given by *intramuscular or intravenous injection* every 8 hours for high-risk procedures

**Administration** Single doses over 750 mg should be administered by the intravenous route only.

Displacement value may be significant when reconstituting injection, consult local guidelines. For intermittent intravenous infusion, dilute reconstituted solution further in glucose 5% or sodium chloride 0.9%; give over 30 minutes.

**Cefuroxime** (Non-proprietary) [PoM]

Tablets, cefuroxime (as axetil) 250 mg, net price 14-tab pack = £10.39. Label: 9, 21, 25

Injection, powder for reconstitution, cefuroxime (as sodium salt), net price 750-mg vial = £2.52; 1.5-g vial = £5.05

**Zinacef®** (GSK) [PoM]

Injection, powder for reconstitution, cefuroxime (as sodium salt). Net price 250-mg vial = 94p; 750-mg vial = £2.34; 1.5-g vial = £4.70

Electrolytes Na⁺ 1.8 mmol/750-mg vial

**Zinnat®** (GSK) [PoM]

Tablets, both f/c, cefuroxime (as axetil) 125 mg, net price 14-tab pack = £4.56; 250 mg, 14-tab pack = £9.11. Label: 9, 21, 25

Suspension, cefuroxime (as axetil) 125 mg/5 mL when reconstituted with water, net price 70 mL (tutti-frutti-flavoured) = £5.20. Label: 9, 21

Excipients include aspartame (section 9.4.1), sucrose 3.1 g/5 mL

### 5.1.2.2 Carbapenems

The carbapenems are beta-lactam antibacterials with a broad-spectrum of activity which includes many Gram-positive and Gram-negative bacteria, and anaerobes; **imipenem** and **meropenem** have good activity against *Pseudomonas aeruginosa*. The carbapenems are not active against meticillin-resistant *Staphylococcus aureus* and *Enterococcus faecium*.

Imipenem and meropenem are used for the treatment of severe hospital-acquired infections and polymicrobial infections caused by multiple-antibacterial resistant organisms (including septicaemia, hospital-acquired pneumonia, intra-abdominal infections, skin and soft-tissue infections, and complicated urinary-tract infections).

**Ertapenem** is licensed for treating abdominal and gynaecological infections and for community-acquired pneumonia, but it is not active against atypical respiratory pathogens and it has limited activity against penicillin-resistant pneumococci. Unlike the other carbapenems, ertapenem is not active against *Pseudomonas* or against *Acinetobacter* spp.

Imipenem is partially inactivated in the kidney by enzymatic activity and is therefore administered in combination with **cilastatin**, a specific enzyme inhibitor, which blocks its renal metabolism. Meropenem and ertapenem are stable to the renal enzyme which inactivates imipenem and therefore can be given without cilastatin.

Side-effects of imipenem with cilastatin are similar to those of other beta-lactam antibiotics; neurotoxicity has been observed at very high dosage, in renal failure, or in patients with CNS disease. Meropenem has less seizure-inducing potential and can be used to treat central nervous system infection. Ertapenem has been associated with seizures uncommonly.

5 Infections

## ERTAPENEM

**Cautions** hypersensitivity to beta-lactam antibacterials (avoid if history of immediate hypersensitivity reaction, see also p. 259); renal impairment, CNS disorders—risk of seizures; **interactions:** Appendix 1 (ertapenem)

**Renal impairment** risk of seizures; avoid if estimated glomerular filtration rate less than 30 mL/minute/1.73 m$^2$

**Pregnancy** manufacturer advises avoid unless potential benefit outweighs risk

**Breast-feeding** present in milk—manufacturer advises avoid

**Side-effects** diarrhoea, nausea, vomiting, headache, injection-site reactions, rash (also reported with eosinophilia and systemic symptoms), pruritus, raised platelet count; *less commonly* dry mouth, taste disturbances, dyspepsia, abdominal pain, anorexia, constipation, melaena, antibiotic-associated colitis, bradycardia, hypotension, chest pain, oedema, pharyngeal discomfort, dyspnoea, dizziness, sleep disturbances, confusion, anxiety, depression, agitation, tremor, pelvic peritonitis, renal impairment, muscle cramp, scleral disorder, blood disorders (including neutropenia, thrombocytopenia, haemorrhage), hypoglycaemia, electrolyte disturbances; *also reported* hallucinations, dyskinesia, muscular weakness

### Indications and dose

**Abdominal infections, acute gynaecological infections, community-acquired pneumonia**

- By intravenous infusion

  **Child 3 months–13 years** 15 mg/kg every 12 hours (max. 1 g daily)

  **Child 13–18 years** 1 g once daily

**Administration** reconstitute 1 g with 10 mL Water for Injections or Sodium Chloride 0.9%; for *intravenous infusion*, dilute requisite dose in Sodium Chloride 0.9% to a final concentration not exceeding 20 mg/mL; give over 30 minutes; incompatible with glucose solutions

**Invanz®** (MSD) PoM
Intravenous infusion, powder for reconstitution, ertapenem (as sodium salt), net price 1-g vial = £31.65
Electrolytes Na$^+$ 6 mmol/1-g vial

## IMIPENEM WITH CILASTATIN

**Cautions** CNS disorders (e.g. epilepsy); hypersensitivity to beta-lactam antibacterials (avoid if history of immediate hypersensitivity reaction, see also p. 259); **interactions:** Appendix 1 (imipenem with cilastatin)

**Renal impairment** reduce dose if estimated glomerular filtration rate less than 70 mL/minute/1.73 m$^2$; risk of CNS side-effects

**Pregnancy** manufacturer advises avoid unless potential benefit outweighs risk (toxicity in *animal* studies)

**Breast-feeding** present in milk but unlikely to be absorbed

**Side-effects** nausea (may reduce rate of infusion), vomiting, diarrhoea (rarely antibiotic-associated colitis), eosinophilia, rash (rarely toxic epidermal necrolysis and Stevens-Johnson syndrome); *less commonly* hypotension, seizures, myoclonic activity, dizziness, drowsiness, hallucinations, confusion, leucopenia, thrombocytopenia, thrombocytosis, positive Coombs' test; *rarely* taste disturbances, hepatitis, encephalopathy, anaphylactic reactions, paraesthesia, tremor, acute renal failure, polyuria, tooth, tongue or urine discoloration, hearing loss; *very rarely*, abdominal pain, heartburn, glossitis, tachycardia, palpitation, flushing, cyanosis, dyspnoea, hyperventilation, headache, asthenia, haemolytic anaemia, aggravation of myasthenia gravis, polyarthralgia, tinnitus, hypersalivation, hyperhidrosis

**Licensed use** not licensed for use in children under 1 year; not licensed for use in children with renal impairment

### Indications and dose

**Aerobic and anaerobic Gram-positive and Gram-negative infections, hospital-acquired septicaemia** Table 1, section 5.1; not indicated for CNS infections

- By intravenous infusion

  expressed in terms of imipenem

  **Neonate under 7 days** 20 mg/kg every 12 hours

  **Neonate 7–21 days** 20 mg/kg every 8 hours

  **Neonate 21–28 days** 20 mg/kg every 6 hours

  **Child 1–3 months** 20 mg/kg every 6 hours

  **Child 3 months–18 years** 15 mg/kg (max. 500 mg) every 6 hours; infection caused by Pseudomonas or other less sensitive organisms, life-threatening infection, or empirical treatment of infection in febrile patients with neutropenia, 25 mg/kg (max. 1 g) every 6 hours

**Cystic fibrosis**

- By intravenous infusion

  **Child 1 month–18 years** 25 mg/kg (max. 1 g) every 6 hours

**Administration** for *intravenous infusion* dilute to a concentration of 5 mg (as imipenem)/mL in Sodium Chloride 0.9%; give up to 500 mg (as imipenem) over 20–30 minutes; give dose greater than 500 mg (as imipenem) over 40–60 minutes

**Imipenem with cilastatin** (Non-proprietary) PoM
Intravenous infusion, powder for reconstitution, imipenem (as monohydrate) 500 mg with cilastatin (as sodium salt) 500 mg, net price per vial = £12.00

**Primaxin®** (MSD) PoM
Intravenous infusion, powder for reconstitution, imipenem (as monohydrate) 500 mg with cilastatin (as sodium salt) 500 mg, net price per vial = £12.00
Electrolytes Na$^+$ 1.6 mmol/vial

## MEROPENEM

**Cautions** hypersensitivity to beta-lactam antibacterials (avoid if history of immediate hypersensitivity reaction, see also p. 259); **interactions:** Appendix 1 (meropenem)

**Hepatic impairment** monitor liver function

**Renal impairment** use normal dose every 12 hours if estimated glomerular filtration rate 26–50 mL/minute/1.73 m$^2$; use half normal dose every 12 hours if estimated glomerular filtration rate 10–25 mL/minute/1.73 m$^2$; use half normal dose every 24 hours if estimated glomerular filtration rate less than 10 mL/minute/1.73 m$^2$

**Pregnancy** use only if potential benefit outweighs risk—no information available

**Breast-feeding** unlikely to be absorbed (but manufacturer advises avoid)

**Side-effects** nausea, vomiting, diarrhoea (antibiotic-associated colitis reported), abdominal pain, disturbances in liver function tests, headache, thrombocythaemia, rash, pruritus; *less commonly* paraesthesia, eosinophilia, thrombocytopenia, leucopenia; *rarely* convulsions; also reported haemolytic anaemia, positive Coombs' test, Stevens-Johnson syndrome, toxic epidermal necrolysis

**Licensed use** not licensed for use in children under 3 months

**Indications and dose**

Aerobic and anaerobic Gram-positive and Gram-negative infections (see notes above), hospital-acquired septicaemia Table 1, section 5.1

- **By intravenous injection over 5 minutes or by intravenous infusion**

  **Neonate under 7 days** 20 mg/kg every 12 hours, dose doubled in severe infection

  **Neonate 7–28 days** 20 mg/kg every 8 hours; dose doubled in severe infection

  **Child 1 month–12 years**

  **Body-weight under 50 kg** 10–20 mg/kg every 8 hours

  **Body-weight over 50 kg** dose as for child 12–18 years

  **Child 12–18 years** 0.5–1 g every 8 hours

Meningitis

- **By intravenous infusion**

  **Neonate under 7 days** 40 mg/kg every 12 hours

  **Neonate 7–28 days** 40 mg/kg every 8 hours

  **Child 1 month–12 years**

  **Body-weight under 50 kg** 40 mg/kg every 8 hours

  **Body-weight over 50 kg** dose as for child 12–18 years

  **Child 12–18 years** 2 g every 8 hours

Exacerbations of chronic lower respiratory-tract infections in cystic fibrosis

- **By intravenous infusion**

  **Child 1 month–12 years**

  **Body-weight under 50 kg** 40 mg/kg every 8 hours

  **Body-weight over 50 kg** dose as for child 12–18 years

  **Child 12–18 years** 2 g every 8 hours

**Administration** displacement value may be significant when reconstituting injection, consult local guidelines. For *intravenous infusion*, dilute reconstituted solution further to a concentration of 1–20 mg/mL in Glucose 5% *or* Sodium Chloride 0.9%; give over 15–30 minutes

**Meropenem** (Non-proprietary) (PoM)
Injection, powder for reconstitution, meropenem (as trihydrate), net price 500-mg vial = £7.74; 1-g vial = £15.47

**Meronem**® (AstraZeneca) (PoM)
Injection, powder for reconstitution, meropenem (as trihydrate), net price 500-mg vial = £8.60; 1-g vial = £17.19
Electrolytes Na$^+$ 3.9 mmol/g

**5.1.2.3 Other beta-lactam antibiotics**

Aztreonam is a monocyclic beta-lactam ('monobactam') antibiotic with an antibacterial spectrum limited to Gram-negative aerobic bacteria including *Pseudomonas aeruginosa*, *Neisseria meningitidis*, and *Haemophilus influenzae*; it should not be used alone for 'blind' treatment since it is not active against Gram-positive organisms. Aztreonam is also effective against *Neisseria gonorrhoeae* (but not against concurrent chlamydial infection). Side-effects are similar to those of the other beta-lactams although aztreonam may be less likely to cause hypersensitivity in penicillin-sensitive patients.

Aztreonam may be administered by nebuliser for the treatment of chronic *Ps. aeruginosa* infection in cystic fibrosis.

**AZTREONAM**

**Cautions** hypersensitivity to beta-lactam antibiotics; interactions: Appendix 1 (aztreonam)
Specific cautions for inhaled treatment Other inhaled drugs should be administered before aztreonam; a bronchodilator should be administered before each dose. Measure lung function before and after initial dose of aztreonam and monitor for bronchospasm. Haemoptysis—risk of further haemorrhage

**Contra-indications** aztreonam hypersensitivity

**Hepatic impairment** use injection with caution and monitor liver function

**Renal impairment** if estimated glomerular filtration rate 10–30 mL/minute/1.73 m$^2$, usual initial dose of injection, then half normal dose; if estimated glomerular filtration rate less than 10 mL/minute/1.73 m$^2$, usual initial dose of injection, then one-quarter normal dose

**Pregnancy** no information available; manufacturer of injection advises avoid; manufacturer of powder for nebuliser solution advises avoid unless essential

**Breast-feeding** amount in milk probably too small to be harmful

**Side-effects**
Specific side-effects for parenteral treatment *Rarely* gastro-intestinal bleeding, antibiotic-associated colitis, jaundice, hepatitis, hypotension, chest pain, dyspnoea, seizures, paraesthesia, confusion, dizziness, asthenia, headache, insomnia, breast tenderness, blood disorders (including thrombocytopenia and neutropenia), myalgia, diplopia, tinnitus, halitosis; also reported nausea, vomiting, abdominal pain, diarrhoea, mouth ulcers, taste disturbances, flushing, bronchospasm, rash (including toxic epidermal necrolysis and erythema multiforme)
Specific side-effects for inhaled treatment Wheezing, bronchospasm, cough, haemoptysis, pyrexia, arthralgia, rash, rhinorrhoea, pharyngolaryngeal pain

**Licensed use** injection not licensed for use in children under 7 days

## Indications and dose

**Gram-negative infections including *Pseudomonas aeruginosa*, *Haemophilus influenzae*, and *Neisseria meningitidis***

- By intravenous injection over 3–5 minutes or by intravenous infusion

  **Neonate under 7 days** 30 mg/kg every 12 hours

  **Neonate 7–28 days** 30 mg/kg every 6–8 hours

  **Child 1 month–2 years** 30 mg/kg every 6–8 hours

  **Child 2–12 years** 30 mg/kg every 6–8 hours increased to 50 mg/kg every 6–8 hours in severe infection and cystic fibrosis (max. 2 g every 6 hours)

  **Child 12–18 years** 1 g every 8 hours or 2 g every 12 hours; 2 g every 6–8 hours for severe infections (including systemic *Ps. aeruginosa* and lung infections in cystic fibrosis)

**Chronic pulmonary *Pseudomonas aeruginosa* infection in patients with cystic fibrosis**

- By inhalation of nebulised solution

  **Child 6–18 years** 75 mg 3 times daily (at least 4 hours apart) for 28 days, subsequent courses repeated after 28-day interval without aztreonam nebuliser solution

**Administration** Displacement value of injection may be significant, consult local guidelines. For intermittent intravenous infusion, dilute reconstituted solution further in Glucose 5% *or* Sodium chloride 0.9% to a concentration of less than 20 mg/mL; to be given over 20–60 minutes

◢**Parenteral**

**Azactam®** (Squibb) [PoM]
Injection, powder for reconstitution, aztreonam. Net price 1-g vial = £9.40; 2-g vial = £18.82

◢**Inhalation**

**Cayston®** (Gilead) [PoM]
Powder for nebuliser solution, aztreonam (as lysine), net price 84 × 75 mg vials (with solvent and nebuliser handset) = £2566.50

## 5.1.3 Tetracyclines

The tetracyclines are broad-spectrum antibiotics whose value has decreased owing to increasing bacterial resistance. In children over 12 years of age they are useful for infections caused by chlamydia (trachoma, psittacosis, salpingitis, urethritis, and lymphogranuloma venereum), rickettsia (including Q-fever), brucella (doxycycline with either streptomycin or rifampicin), and the spirochaete, *Borrelia burgdorferi* (Lyme disease—see section 5.1.1.3). They are also used in respiratory and genital mycoplasma infections, in acne, in destructive (refractory) periodontal disease, in exacerbations of chronic respiratory diseases (because of their activity against *Haemophilus influenzae*), and for leptospirosis in penicillin hypersensitivity (as an alternative to erythromycin).

Microbiologically, there is little to choose between the various tetracyclines, the only exception being **minocycline** which has a broader spectrum; it is active against *Neisseria meningitidis* and has been used for meningococcal prophylaxis but is no longer recommended because of side-effects including dizziness and vertigo (see Table 2, section 5.1 for current recommendations). Compared to other tetracyclines, minocycline is associated with a greater risk of lupus-erythematosus-like syndrome. Minocycline sometimes causes irreversible pigmentation.

For the role of tetracyclines in the management of meticillin-resistant *Staphylococcus aureus* (MRSA) infections, see p. 261.

**Oral infections** In children over 12 years of age, tetracyclines can be effective against oral anaerobes but the development of resistance (especially by oral streptococci) has reduced their usefulness for the treatment of acute oral infections; they may still have a role in the treatment of destructive (refractory) forms of periodontal disease. Doxycycline has a longer duration of action than tetracycline or oxytetracycline and need only be given once daily; it is reported to be more active against anaerobes than some other tetracyclines.

For the use of doxycycline in the treatment of recurrent aphthous ulceration, oral herpes, or as an adjunct to gingival scaling and root planing for periodontitis, see section 12.3.1 and section 12.3.2.

**Cautions** Tetracyclines may increase muscle weakness in patients with myasthenia gravis, and exacerbate systemic lupus erythematosus. Antacids, and aluminium, calcium, iron, magnesium and zinc salts decrease the absorption of tetracyclines; milk also reduces the absorption of demeclocycline, oxytetracycline, and tetracycline. Other **interactions:** Appendix 1 (tetracyclines).

**Contra-indications** Deposition of tetracyclines in growing bone and teeth (by binding to calcium) causes staining and occasionally dental hypoplasia, and they should **not** be given to children under 12 years, or to pregnant or breast-feeding women. However, doxycycline may be used in children for treatment and post-exposure prophylaxis of anthrax when an alternative antibacterial cannot be given [unlicensed indication]. Tetracyclines should not be given to children with acute porphyria (section 9.8.2).

**Hepatic impairment** Tetracyclines should be avoided or used with caution in children with hepatic impairment. Tetracyclines should also be used with caution in those receiving potentially hepatotoxic drugs.

**Renal impairment** With the exception of **doxycycline** and **minocycline**, the tetracyclines may exacerbate renal failure and should **not** be given to children with renal impairment.

**Pregnancy** Tetracyclines should **not** be given to pregnant women; effects on skeletal development have been documented in the first trimester in *animal* studies. Administration during the second or third trimester may cause discoloration of the child's teeth, and maternal hepatotoxicity has been reported with large parenteral doses.

**Breast-feeding** Tetracyclines should **not** be given to women who are breast-feeding (although absorption and therefore discoloration of teeth in the infant is probably usually prevented by chelation with calcium in milk).

**Side-effects** Side-effects of the tetracyclines include nausea, vomiting, diarrhoea (antibiotic-associated colitis reported occasionally), dysphagia, and oesophageal irritation. Other rare side-effects include hepatotoxicity, pancreatitis, blood disorders, photosensitivity (particularly with demeclocycline), and hypersensitivity reactions (including rash, exfoliative dermatitis, Stevens-Johnson syndrome, urticaria, angioedema, anaphylaxis, pericarditis). Headache and visual disturbances may indicate benign intracranial hypertension (discontinue treatment); bulging fontanelles have been reported in infants.

## ■ TETRACYCLINE

**Cautions** see notes above
**Contra-indications** see notes above
**Hepatic impairment** see notes above; max. 1 g daily in divided doses
**Renal impairment** see notes above
**Pregnancy** see notes above
**Breast-feeding** see notes above
**Side-effects** see notes above; also acute renal failure, skin discoloration

**Indications and dose**

Susceptible infections see notes above

- By mouth

  **Child 12–18 years** 250 mg 4 times daily, increased in severe infections to 500 mg 3–4 times daily

Acne section 13.6.2

Non-gonococcal urethritis

- By mouth

  **Child 12–18 years** 500 mg 4 times daily for 7–14 days (21 days if failure or relapse after first course)

**Tetracycline** (Non-proprietary) PoM
Tablets, coated, tetracycline hydrochloride 250 mg, net price 28-tab pack = £13.67. Label: 7, 9, 23, counselling, posture
**Dental prescribing on NHS** Tetracycline Tablets may be prescribed

## ■ DEMECLOCYCLINE HYDROCHLORIDE

**Cautions** see notes above, but photosensitivity more common (avoid exposure to sunlight or sun lamps)
**Contra-indications** see notes above
**Hepatic impairment** see notes above; max. 1 g daily in divided doses
**Renal impairment** see notes above
**Pregnancy** see notes above
**Breast-feeding** see notes above
**Side-effects** see notes above; also reversible nephrogenic diabetes insipidus, acute renal failure

**Indications and dose**

Susceptible infections see notes above

- By mouth

  **Child 12–18 years** 150 mg 4 times daily *or* 300 mg twice daily

**Demeclocycline hydrochloride** (Non-proprietary) PoM
Capsules, demeclocycline hydrochloride 150 mg, net price 28-cap pack = £25.09. Label: 7, 9, 11, 23

## ■ DOXYCYCLINE

**Cautions** see notes above; alcohol dependence; photosensitivity reported (avoid exposure to sunlight or sun lamps)

**Contra-indications** see notes above
**Hepatic impairment** see notes above
**Renal impairment** use with caution (avoid excessive doses)
**Pregnancy** see notes above
**Breast-feeding** see notes above
**Side-effects** see notes above; also anorexia, dry mouth, flushing, anxiety, and tinnitus
**Licensed use** not licensed for use in children under 12 years

**Indications and dose**

Susceptible infections see notes above

- By mouth

  **Child 12–18 years** 200 mg on first day, then 100 mg daily; severe infections (including refractory urinary-tract infections) 200 mg daily

Early syphilis

- By mouth

  **Child 12–18 years** 100 mg twice daily for 14 days

Late latent syphilis

- By mouth

  **Child 12–18 years** 100 mg twice daily for 28 days

Uncomplicated genital chlamydia, non-gonococcal urethritis, pelvic inflammatory disease Table 1, section 5.1

- By mouth

  **Child 12–18 years** 100 mg twice daily for 7 days (14 days in pelvic inflammatory disease)

Lyme disease (see also section 5.1.1.3)

- By mouth

  **Child 12–18 years** 100 mg twice daily for 10–14 days (for 28 days in Lyme arthritis)

Anthrax (treatment or post-exposure prophylaxis) see also section 5.1.12

- By mouth

  **Child under 12 years** (only if alternative antibacterial cannot be given) 2.5 mg/kg twice daily (max. 100 mg twice daily)

  **Child 12–18 years** 100 mg twice daily

Acne section 13.6.2

Adjunct to gingival scaling and root planing for periodontitis section 12.3.1

**Counselling** Capsules should be swallowed whole with plenty of fluid during meals while sitting or standing
**Note** Doxycycline doses in BNF for Children may differ from those in product literature

**Doxycycline** (Non-proprietary) PoM
Capsules, doxycycline (as hyclate) 50 mg, net price 28-cap pack = £1.79; 100 mg, 8-cap pack = £1.16. Label: 6, 9, 11, 27, counselling, posture
**Brands include** *Doxylar*®
**Dental prescribing on NHS** Doxycycline Capsules 100 mg may be prescribed

**Vibramycin-D**® (Pfizer) PoM
Dispersible tablets, yellow, scored, doxycycline 100 mg, net price 8-tab pack = £4.91. Label: 6, 9, 11, 13
**Dental prescribing on NHS** May be prescribed as Dispersible Doxycycline Tablets

**5 Infections**

# LYMECYCLINE

**Cautions** see notes above
**Contra-indications** see notes above
**Hepatic impairment** see notes above
**Renal impairment** see notes above
**Pregnancy** see notes above
**Breast-feeding** see notes above
**Side-effects** see notes above
**Indications and dose**

> Susceptible infections see notes above
> • By mouth
>> **Child 12–18 years** 408 mg twice daily, increased to 1.224–1.632 g daily in severe infections
>
> Acne
> • By mouth
>> **Child 12–18 years** 408 mg daily for at least 8 weeks

**Lymecycline** (Non-proprietary) (PoM)
Capsules, lymecycline 408 mg(= tetracycline 300 mg), net price 28-cap pack = £7.77. Label: 6, 9

**Tetralysal 300**® (Galderma) (PoM)
Capsules, red/yellow, lymecycline 408 mg (= tetracycline 300 mg). Net price 28-cap pack = £7.77, 56-cap pack = £14.97. Label: 6, 9

# MINOCYCLINE

**Cautions** see notes above; if treatment continued for longer than 6 months, monitor every 3 months for hepatotoxicity, pigmentation and for systemic lupus erythematosus—discontinue if these develop or if pre-existing systemic lupus erythematosus worsens
**Contra-indications** see notes above
**Hepatic impairment** see notes above
**Renal impairment** use with caution (avoid excessive doses)
**Pregnancy** see notes above
**Breast-feeding** see notes above
**Side-effects** see notes above; also dizziness and vertigo (more common in women); *rarely* anorexia, tinnitus, impaired hearing, hyperaesthesia, paraesthesia, acute renal failure, pigmentation (sometimes irreversible), and alopecia; *very rarely* systemic lupus erythematosus, discoloration of conjunctiva, tears, and sweat
**Indications and dose**

> Susceptible infections see notes above
> • By mouth
>> **Child 12–18 years** 100 mg twice daily

Acne section 13.6.2

**Counselling** Tablets or capsules should be swallowed whole with plenty of fluid while sitting or standing

**Minocycline** (Non-proprietary) (PoM)
Capsules, minocycline (as hydrochloride) 50 mg, net price 56-cap pack = £15.27; 100 mg, 28-cap pack = £13.09. Label: 6, 9, counselling, posture
Brands include *Aknemin*®

Tablets, minocycline (as hydrochloride) 50 mg, net price 28-tab pack = £4.93; 100 mg, 28-tab pack = £9.52. Label: 6, 9, counselling, posture

**◢Modified release**
**Minocycline m/r preparations** (PoM)
Capsules, m/r, minocycline (as hydrochloride) 100 mg, net price 56-cap pack = £20.08. Label: 6, 25
Brands include *Acnamino*® MR, *Minocin MR*®, *Sebomin MR*®
**Dose**

> Acne
> • By mouth
>> **Child 12–18 years** 1 capsule daily

# OXYTETRACYCLINE

**Cautions** see notes above
**Contra-indications** see notes above
**Hepatic impairment** see notes above
**Renal impairment** see notes above
**Pregnancy** see notes above
**Breast-feeding** see notes above
**Side-effects** see notes above
**Indications and dose**

> Susceptible infections see notes above
> • By mouth
>> **Child 12–18 years** 250–500 mg 4 times daily

Acne section 13.6.2

**Oxytetracycline** (Non-proprietary) (PoM)
Tablets, coated, oxytetracycline dihydrate 250 mg, net price 28-tab pack = £1.28. Label: 7, 9, 23
Brands include *Oxymycin*®
**Dental prescribing on NHS** Oxtetracycline Tablets may be prescribed

# 5.1.4 Aminoglycosides

These include amikacin, gentamicin, neomycin, streptomycin, and tobramycin. All are bactericidal and active against some Gram-positive and many Gram-negative organisms. Amikacin, gentamicin, and tobramycin are also active against *Pseudomonas aeruginosa*; streptomycin is active against *Mycobacterium tuberculosis* and is now almost entirely reserved for tuberculosis (section 5.1.9).

The aminoglycosides are not absorbed from the gut (although there is a risk of absorption in inflammatory bowel disease and liver failure) and must therefore be given by injection for systemic infections.

The important side-effects of aminoglycosides are ototoxicity and nephrotoxicity; they occur most commonly in children with renal failure.

**Gentamicin** is the aminoglycoside of choice in the UK and is used widely for the treatment of serious infections. It has a broad spectrum but is inactive against anaerobes and has poor activity against haemolytic streptococci and pneumococci. When used for the 'blind' therapy of undiagnosed serious infections it is usually given in conjunction with a penicillin or metronidazole (or both). Gentamicin is used together with another antibiotic for the treatment of endocarditis (see below and Table 1, section 5.1).

Loading and maintenance doses may be calculated on the basis of the patient's weight and renal function (e.g. using a nomogram); adjustments are then made according to serum-gentamicin concentrations. High doses are occasionally indicated for serious infections, especially in the neonate, children with cystic fibrosis or the immunocompromised patient; whenever possible treatment should not exceed 7 days.

**Amikacin** is more stable than gentamicin to enzyme inactivation. Amikacin is used in the treatment of serious infections caused by gentamicin-resistant Gram-negative bacilli.

**Tobramycin** has similar activity to gentamicin. It is slightly more active against *Ps. aeruginosa* but shows less activity against certain other Gram-negative bacteria. Tobramycin can be administered by nebuliser or by inhalation of powder for the treatment of *Ps. aeruginosa* infection in cystic fibrosis (see Cystic Fibrosis, below).

**Neomycin** is too toxic for parenteral administration and can only be used for infections of the skin or mucous membranes or to reduce the bacterial population of the colon prior to bowel surgery or in hepatic failure. Oral administration may lead to malabsorption. Small amounts of neomycin may be absorbed from the gut in children with hepatic failure and, as these children may also be uraemic, cumulation may occur with resultant ototoxicity.

**Cystic fibrosis**    A higher dose of parenteral aminoglycoside is often required in children with cystic fibrosis because renal clearance of the aminoglycoside is increased. For the role of aminoglycosides in the treatment of pseudomonal lung infections in cystic fibrosis see Table 1, section 5.1. Inhaled tobramycin is used for chronic pseudomonal lung infection in cystic fibrosis; however, resistance may develop, and some children do not respond to treatment.

---

**NICE guidance**
**Tobramycin by dry powder inhalation for pseudomonal lung infection in cystic fibrosis (March 2013)**

Tobramycin dry powder for inhalation is recommended for chronic pulmonary infection caused by *Pseudomonas aeruginosa* in patients with cystic fibrosis only if there is an inadequate response to colistimethate sodium, or if colistimethate sodium cannot be used because of contra-indications or intolerance. The manufacturer must provide tobramycin dry powder for inhalation at the discount agreed as part of the patient access scheme to primary, secondary and tertiary care in the NHS.

Patients currently receiving tobramycin dry powder for inhalation can continue treatment until they, their carers, and their clinicians consider it appropriate to stop.

www.nice.org.uk/TA276

---

**Endocarditis**    **Gentamicin** is used in combination with other antibiotics for the treatment of bacterial endocarditis (Table 1, section 5.1). Serum-gentamicin concentration should be determined twice each week (more often in renal impairment). **Streptomycin** may be used as an alternative in gentamicin-resistant enterococcal endocarditis.

**Once daily dosage**    *Once daily administration* of aminoglycosides is more convenient, provides adequate serum concentrations, and has largely superseded *multiple-daily dose regimens* (given in 2–3 divided doses during the 24 hours). Local guidelines on dosage and serum concentrations should be consulted. A once-daily, high-dose regimen of an aminoglycoside should be avoided in children with endocarditis or burns of more than 20% of the total body surface area, or in children over 1 month of age with a creatinine clearance of less than 20 mL/minute/1.73m$^2$. There is insufficient evidence to recommend a once daily, high-dose regimen of an aminoglycoside in pregnancy. The *extended interval dose regimen* is used in neonates to reflect the changes in renal function that occur with increasing gestational and postnatal age (see Neonates below).

**Serum concentrations**    Serum concentration monitoring avoids both excessive and subtherapeutic concentrations thus preventing toxicity and ensuring efficacy. Serum-aminoglycoside concentration should be measured in all children receiving parenteral aminoglycosides and **must** be determined in neonates, in obesity, and in cystic fibrosis, *or* if high doses are being given, *or* if there is renal impairment.

In children with normal renal function, aminoglycoside concentration should be measured initially after 3 or 4 doses of a multiple daily dose regimen; children with renal impairment may require earlier and more frequent measurement of aminoglycoside concentration.

Blood samples should be taken just before the next dose is administered ('trough' concentration). If the pre-dose ('trough') concentration is high, the interval between doses must be increased. For multiple daily dose regimens, blood samples should also be taken approximately 1 hour after intramuscular or intravenous administration ('peak' concentration). If the post-dose ('peak') concentration is high, the dose must be decreased.

**Cautions**    The main side-effects of the aminoglycosides are dose-related, therefore, care must be taken with dosage and, whenever possible, parenteral treatment should not exceed 7 days. Renal function should be assessed before starting an aminoglycoside and during treatment. If possible, dehydration should be corrected before starting an aminoglycoside. Auditory and vestibular function should also be monitored during treatment. In order to optimise the dose and avoid toxicity, serum-aminoglycoside concentrations should be monitored in children receiving parenteral aminoglycosides (see also Serum Concentrations).

Aminoglycosides should be used with caution in those with conditions characterised by muscular weakness (avoid in myasthenia gravis). If possible, aminoglycosides should not be given with potentially ototoxic drugs (e.g. cisplatin). Administration of an aminoglycoside and of an ototoxic diuretic (e.g. furosemide) should be separated by as long a period as practicable. **Interactions**: Appendix 1 (aminoglycosides)

**Contra-indications**    Aminoglycosides may impair neuromuscular transmission and should not be given to patients with myasthenia gravis

**Renal impairment**    Excretion of aminoglycosides is principally via the kidney and accumulation occurs in renal impairment. Ototoxicity and nephrotoxicity occur commonly in patients with renal failure. If there is impairment of renal function, the interval between doses must be increased; if the renal impairment is severe, the dose itself should be reduced as well. Serum-aminoglycoside concentrations **must** be moni-

**5**

**Infections**

tored in patients with renal impairment, see Serum Concentrations above; renal, auditory, and vestibular function should also be monitored. A once-daily, high-dose regimen of an aminoglycoside should be avoided in children over 1 month of age with a creatinine clearance less than $20\,mL/minute/1.73\,m^2$.

**Pregnancy** There is a risk of auditory or vestibular nerve damage in the infant when aminoglycosides are used in the second and third trimesters of pregnancy. The risk is greatest with streptomycin (section 5.1.9). The risk is probably very small with gentamicin and tobramycin, but their use should be avoided unless essential (if given, serum-aminoglycoside concentration monitoring is essential).

**Neonates** As aminoglycosides are eliminated principally via the kidney, neonatal treatment must reflect the changes in glomerular filtration that occur with increasing gestational and postnatal age. The *extended interval dose regimen* is used in neonates, and serum-aminoglycoside concentrations **must** be measured. In patients on single daily dose regimens it may become necessary to prolong the dose interval to more than 24 hours if the trough concentration is high.

**Side-effects** The important side-effects of the aminoglycosides are nephrotoxicity and irreversible ototoxicity (including vestibular and auditory damage). Rash occurs commonly with streptomycin, but less frequently with the other aminoglycosides. Rare side-effects include nausea, vomiting, antibiotic-associated colitis, peripheral neuropathy, electrolyte disturbances (notably hypomagnesaemia on prolonged therapy, but also hypocalcaemia and hypokalaemia), and stomatitis. Side-effects reported very rarely include blood disorders and CNS effects (including headache, encephalopathy, and convulsions). Aminoglycosides may impair neuromuscular transmission; large doses given during surgery have been responsible for a transient myasthenic syndrome in patients with normal neuromuscular function.

---

### █ GENTAMICIN

**Cautions** see notes above; **interactions:** Appendix 1 (aminoglycosides)

**Contra-indications** see notes above

**Renal impairment** see notes above

**Pregnancy** see notes above

**Side-effects** see notes above

**Pharmacokinetics** *Extended interval dose regimen in neonates:* pre-dose ('trough') concentration should be less than 2 mg/litre

*Once daily dose regimen:* pre-dose ('trough') concentration should be less than 1 mg/litre

*Multiple daily dose regimen:* one hour ('peak') serum concentration should be 5–10 mg/litre (3–5 mg/litre for endocarditis, 8–12 mg/litre in cystic fibrosis); pre-dose ('trough') concentration should be less than 2 mg/litre (less than 1 mg/litre for endocarditis)

*Intrathecal/intraventricular injection:* cerebrospinal fluid concentration should not exceed 10 mg/litre

---

### Indications and dose

> To avoid excessive dosage in obese children, use ideal weight for height to calculate parenteral dose and monitor serum-gentamicin concentration closely

**Neonatal sepsis**

● Extended interval dose regimen by slow intravenous injection or intravenous infusion

Neonate less than 32 weeks postmenstrual age 4–5 mg/kg every 36 hours

Neonate 32 weeks and over postmenstrual age 4–5 mg/kg every 24 hours

● Multiple daily dose regimen by slow intravenous injection

Neonate less than 29 weeks postmenstrual age 2.5 mg/kg every 24 hours

Neonate 29–35 weeks postmenstrual age 2.5 mg/kg every 18 hours

Neonate over 35 weeks postmenstrual age 2.5 mg/kg every 12 hours

**Septicaemia, meningitis and other CNS infections, biliary-tract infection, acute pyelonephritis, endocarditis (see notes above), pneumonia in hospital patients, adjunct in listerial meningitis (Table 1, section 5.1)**

● Once daily dose regimen (not for endocarditis or meningitis) by intravenous infusion

Child 1 month–18 years initially 7 mg/kg, then adjusted according to serum-gentamicin concentration

● Multiple daily dose regimen by intramuscular or by slow intravenous injection over at least 3 minutes

Child 1 month–12 years 2.5 mg/kg every 8 hours

Child 12–18 years 2 mg/kg every 8 hours

**Pseudomonal lung infection in cystic fibrosis**

● Multiple daily dose regimen by slow intravenous injection over at least 3 minutes or by intravenous infusion

Child 1 month–18 years 3 mg/kg every 8 hours

**Bacterial ventriculitis and CNS infection (supplement to systemic therapy)**

● By intrathecal or intraventricular injection, seek specialist advice

Neonate seek specialist advice

Child 1 month–18 years 1 mg daily (increased if necessary to 5 mg daily)

Note only preservative-free, intrathecal preparation should be used

**Eye** section 11.3.1

**Ear** section 12.1.1

Note Local guidelines may vary

**Administration** for *intravenous infusion,* dilute in Glucose 5% or Sodium Chloride 0.9%; give over 30 minutes

For *nebulisation,* dilute preservative-free preparation in 3 mL sodium chloride 0.9%. Administer after physiotherapy and bronchodilators

For *intrathecal* or *intraventricular injection,* use preservative-free intrathecal preparations only

**Gentamicin** (Non-proprietary) [PoM]

Injection, gentamicin (as sulfate), net price 40 mg/mL, 1-mL amp = £1.40, 2-mL amp = £1.54, 2-mL vial = £1.48

Paediatric injection, gentamicin (as sulfate) 10 mg/mL, net price 2-mL vial = £1.80

Intrathecal injection, gentamicin (as sulfate) 5 mg/mL, net price 1-mL amp = 74p

Intravenous infusion, gentamicin (as sulfate) 1 mg/mL in sodium chloride intravenous infusion 0.9%, net price 80-mL (80 mg) bottle = £1.95; 3 mg/mL, 80-mL (240 mg) bottle = £5.95, 120-mL (360 mg) bottle = £8.45

**Cidomycin®** (Sanofi-Aventis) [PoM]

Injection, gentamicin (as sulfate) 40 mg/mL. Net price 2-mL amp or vial = £1.48

**Genticin®** (Amdipharm) [PoM]

Injection, gentamicin (as sulfate) 40 mg/mL. Net price 2-mL amp = £1.40

**Isotonic Gentamicin Injection** (Baxter) [PoM]

Intravenous infusion, gentamicin (as sulfate) 800 micrograms/mL in sodium chloride intravenous infusion 0.9%. Net price 100-mL (80-mg) *Viaflex®* bag = £1.61

Electrolytes Na⁺ 15.4 mmol/100-mL bag

---

## ▌ AMIKACIN

**Cautions** see notes above; **interactions**: Appendix 1 (aminoglycosides)

**Contra-indications** see notes above

**Renal impairment** see notes above

**Pregnancy** see notes above

**Side-effects** see notes above

**Pharmacokinetics** *Multiple dose regimen*: one-hour ('peak') serum concentration should not exceed 30 mg/litre; pre-dose ('trough') concentration should be less than 10 mg/litre

*Once daily dose regimen*: pre-dose ('trough') concentration should be less than 5 mg/litre

**Licensed use** dose for cystic fibrosis not licensed

**Indications and dose**

> To avoid excessive dosage in obese children, use ideal weight for height to calculate dose and monitor serum-amikacin concentration closely

**Neonatal sepsis**

● Extended interval dose regimen by slow intravenous injection over 3–5 minutes or by intravenous infusion

**Neonate** 15 mg/kg every 24 hours

● Multiple daily dose regimen by intramuscular or by slow intravenous injection or by infusion

**Neonate** loading dose of 10 mg/kg then 7.5 mg/kg every 12 hours

**Serious Gram-negative infections resistant to gentamicin**

● By slow intravenous injection over 3–5 minutes

**Child 1 month–12 years** 7.5 mg/kg every 12 hours

**Child 12–18 years** 7.5 mg/kg every 12 hours, increased to 7.5 mg/kg every 8 hours in severe

infections, max. 500 mg every 8 hours for up to 10 days (max. cumulative dose 15 g)

**Once daily dose regimen (not for endocarditis or meningitis)**

● By intravenous injection or infusion

**Child 1 month–18 years** initially 15 mg/kg, then adjusted according to serum-amikacin concentration

**Pseudomonal lung infection in cystic fibrosis**

● Multiple daily dose regimen by slow intravenous injection or infusion

**Child 1 month–18 years** 10 mg/kg every 8 hours (max. 500 mg every 8 hours)

Note Local dosage guidelines may vary

**Administration** for *intravenous infusion*, dilute with Glucose 5% *or* Sodium Chloride 0.9%; give over 30–60 minutes

**Amikacin** (Non-proprietary) [PoM]

Injection, amikacin (as sulfate) 250 mg/mL. Net price 2-mL vial = £10.14

Electrolytes Na⁺ 0.56 mmol/500-mg vial

**Amikin®** (Bristol-Myers Squibb) [PoM]

Injection, amikacin (as sulfate) 50 mg/mL. Net price 2-mL vial = £2.07

Electrolytes Na⁺ < 0.5 mmol/vial

---

## ▌ TOBRAMYCIN

**Cautions** see notes above; **interactions**: Appendix 1 (aminoglycosides)

**Specific cautions for inhaled treatment** Other inhaled drugs should be administered before tobramycin. Measure lung function before and after initial dose of tobramycin and monitor for bronchospasm; if bronchospasm occurs in a child not using a bronchodilator, repeat test using bronchodilator. Monitor renal function before treatment and then annually. Severe haemoptysis—risk of further haemorrhage

**Contra-indications** see notes above

**Renal impairment** see notes above

**Pregnancy** see notes above

**Side-effects** see notes above; *on inhalation*, cough (more frequent by inhalation of powder), bronchospasm (see Cautions), dysphonia, taste disturbances, pharyngitis, mouth ulcers, salivary hypersecretion, laryngitis, haemoptysis, epistaxis

**Pharmacokinetics** *Extended interval dose regimen in neonates*: pre-dose ('trough') concentration should be less than 2 mg/litre

*Once daily dose regimen*: pre-dose ('trough') concentration should be less than 1 mg/litre

*Multiple daily dose regimen*: one-hour ('peak') serum concentration should not exceed 10 mg/litre (8–12 mg/litre in cystic fibrosis); pre-dose ('trough') concentration should be less than 2 mg/litre

**5**

**Infections**

**5 Infections**

## Indications and dose

> To avoid excessive dosage in obese children, use ideal weight for height to calculate parenteral dose and monitor serum-tobramycin concentration closely

**Neonatal sepsis**
- Extended interval dose regimen by intravenous injection over 3–5 minutes or by intravenous infusion

  **Neonate less than 32 weeks postmenstrual age** 4–5 mg/kg every 36 hours

  **Neonate 32 weeks and over postmenstrual age** 4–5 mg/kg every 24 hours

- Multiple daily dose regimen by slow intravenous injection or by intravenous infusion

  **Neonate under 7 days** 2 mg/kg every 12 hours

  **Neonate 7–28 days** 2–2.5 mg/kg every 8 hours

**Septicaemia, meningitis and other CNS infections, biliary-tract infection, acute pyelonephritis, pneumonia in hospital patients**
- Multiple daily dose regimen by slow intravenous injection over 3–5 minutes

  **Child 1 month–12 years** 2–2.5 mg/kg every 8 hours

  **Child 12–18 years** 1 mg/kg every 8 hours; in severe infections up to 5 mg/kg daily in divided doses every 6–8 hours (reduced to 3 mg/kg daily as soon as clinically indicated)

- Once daily dose regimen by intravenous infusion

  **Child 1 month–18 years** initially 7 mg/kg, then adjusted according to serum-tobramycin concentration

**Pseudomonal lung infection in cystic fibrosis**
- Multiple daily dose regimen by slow intravenous injection over 3–5 minutes

  **Child 1 month–18 years** 8–10 mg/kg/daily in 3 divided doses

- Once daily dose regimen by intravenous infusion over 30 minutes

  **Child 1 month–18 years** initially 10 mg/kg (max. 660 mg), then adjusted according to serum-tobramycin concentration

**Chronic pulmonary *Pseudomonas aeruginosa* infection in patients with cystic fibrosis**
- By inhalation of nebulised solution

  **Child 6–18 years** 300 mg every 12 hours for 28 days, subsequent courses repeated after 28-day interval without tobramycin nebuliser solution

- By inhalation of powder

  **Child 6–18 years** 112 mg every 12 hours for 28 days, subsequent courses repeated after 28-day interval without tobramycin inhalation powder

**Note** Local dosage guidelines may vary

**Administration** for *intravenous infusion*, dilute with Glucose 5% *or* Sodium Chloride 0.9%; give over 20–60 minutes

◢**Parenteral**

**Tobramycin** (Non-proprietary) [PoM]

Injection, tobramycin (as sulfate) 40 mg/mL, net price 1-mL (40-mg) vial = £4.00, 2-mL (80-mg) vial = £4.16, 6-mL (240-mg) vial = £19.20

◢**Inhalation**

**Bramitob**® (Chiesi) [PoM]

Nebuliser solution, tobramycin 75 mg/mL, net price 56 x 4-mL (300-mg) unit = £1187.00

**Tobi**® (Novartis) [PoM]

Nebuliser solution, tobramycin 60 mg/mL, net price 56 × 5-mL (300-mg) unit = £1187.20

Podhaler (dry powder for inhalation), tobramycin 28 mg/capsule, net price 56-cap pack (with *Tobi*® *Podhaler* device) = £447.50, 224-cap pack (with 5 *Tobi*® *Podhaler* devices) = £1790.00. Counselling, administration

## 5.1.5 Macrolides

The macrolides have an antibacterial spectrum that is similar but not identical to that of penicillin; they are thus an alternative in penicillin-allergic patients. They are active against many-penicillin-resistant staphylococci, but some are now also resistant to the macrolides.

Indications for the macrolides include campylobacter enteritis, respiratory infections (including pneumonia, whooping cough, Legionella, chlamydia, and mycoplasma infection), and skin infections.

**Erythromycin** is also used in the treatment of early syphilis, uncomplicated genital chlamydial infection, and non-gonococcal urethritis. Erythromycin has poor activity against *Haemophilus influenzae*. Erythromycin causes nausea, vomiting, and diarrhoea in some patients; in mild to moderate infections this can be avoided by giving a lower dose or the total dose in 4 divided doses, but if a more serious infection, such as Legionella pneumonia, is suspected higher doses are needed.

**Azithromycin** is a macrolide with slightly less activity than erythromycin against Gram-positive bacteria, but enhanced activity against some Gram-negative organisms including *H. influenzae*. Plasma concentrations are very low, but tissue concentrations are much higher. It has a long tissue half-life and once daily dosage is recommended. Azithromycin is also used in the treatment of uncomplicated genital chlamydial infection, non-gonococcal urethritis, typhoid [unlicensed indication], and trachoma [unlicensed indication] (section 11.3.1).

**Clarithromycin** is an erythromycin derivative with slightly greater activity than the parent compound. Tissue concentrations are higher than with erythromycin. It is given twice daily. Clarithromycin is also used in regimens for *Helicobacter pylori* eradication (section 1.3).

For the role of erythromycin, azithromycin, and clarithromycin in the treatment of Lyme disease, see section 5.1.1.3.

**Spiramycin** is also a macrolide (section 5.4.7).

**Oral infections**  The macrolides are an alternative for oral infections in penicillin-allergic patients or where a beta-lactamase producing organism is involved. However, many organisms are now resistant to macrolides or rapidly develop resistance; their use should therefore be limited to short courses. Metronidazole (section 5.1.11) may be preferred as an alternative to a penicillin.

**Cautions**  Macrolides should be used with caution in children with a predisposition to QT interval prolongation (including electrolyte disturbances and concomitant use of drugs that prolong the QT interval). Macrolides may aggravate myasthenia gravis.

**Side-effects** Nausea, vomiting, abdominal discomfort, and diarrhoea are the most common side-effects of the macrolides, but they are mild and less frequent with azithromycin and clarithromycin than with erythromycin. Hepatotoxicity (including cholestatic jaundice) and rash occur less frequently. Other side-effects reported rarely or very rarely include pancreatitis, antibiotic-associated colitis, QT interval prolongation, arrhythmias, Stevens-Johnson syndrome, and toxic epidermal necrolysis. Generally reversible hearing loss (sometimes with tinnitus) has been reported after large doses of a macrolide; it occurs commonly after long-term therapy with azithromycin. Intravenous infusion may cause local tenderness and phlebitis.

## ■ AZITHROMYCIN

**Cautions** see notes above; **interactions:** Appendix 1 (macrolides)

**Hepatic impairment** manufacturers advise avoid in severe liver disease—no information available

**Renal impairment** use with caution if estimated glomerular filtration rate less than 10 mL/minute/1.73 m²

**Pregnancy** manufacturers advise use only if adequate alternatives not available

**Breast-feeding** present in milk; use only if no suitable alternative

**Side-effects** see notes above; also anorexia, dyspepsia, flatulence, dizziness, headache, malaise, paraesthesia, arthralgia, disturbances in taste and vision; *less commonly* constipation, gastritis, chest pain, oedema, anxiety, sleep disturbances, hypoaesthesia, leucopenia, photosensitivity; *rarely* agitation; also reported syncope, convulsions, smell disturbances, interstitial nephritis, acute renal failure, thrombocytopenia, haemolytic anaemia, tongue discoloration

**Licensed use** not licensed for typhoid fever, Lyme disease, chronic *Pseudomonas aeruginosa* infection in cystic fibrosis, or prophylaxis of group A streptococcal infection

### Indications and dose

> **Respiratory-tract infections, otitis media, skin and soft-tissue infections**
> - By mouth
>   **Child over 6 months** 10 mg/kg once daily (max. 500 mg once daily) for 3 days
>   *or*
>   **Body-weight 15–25 kg** 200 mg once daily for 3 days
>   **Body-weight 26–35 kg** 300 mg once daily for 3 days
>   **Body-weight 36–45 kg** 400 mg once daily for 3 days
>   **Body-weight over 45 kg** 500 mg once daily for 3 days

> **Infection in cystic fibrosis**
> - By mouth
>   **Child 6 months–18 years** 10 mg/kg once daily (max. 500 mg once daily) for 3 days; course repeated after 1 week, then repeat as necessary

> **Chronic *Pseudomonas aeruginosa* infection in cystic fibrosis**
> - By mouth
>   **Child 6–18 years**
>   **Body-weight 25–40 kg** 250 mg 3 times a week
>   **Body-weight over 40 kg** 500 mg 3 times a week

> **Uncomplicated genital chlamydial infections and non-gonococcal urethritis**
> - By mouth
>   **Child 12–18 years** 1 g as a single dose

> **Lyme disease (see also section 5.1.1.3), mild to moderate typhoid due to multiple-antibacterial resistant organisms**
> - By mouth
>   **Child 6 months–18 years** 10 mg/kg once daily (max. 500 mg) for 7–10 days (for 7 days in typhoid)

> **Prevention of group A streptococcal infection**
> Table 2, section 5.1

**Azithromycin** (Non-proprietary) ⓅoM
Capsules, azithromycin (as dihydrate) 250 mg, net price 4-cap pack = £9.82, 6-cap pack = £14.73. Label: 5, 9, 23
**Dental prescribing on NHS** Azithromycin Capsules may be prescribed

Tablets, azithromycin (as monohydrate hemi-ethanolate) 250 mg, net price 4-tab pack = £9.83; 500 mg, 3-tab pack = £6.75. Label: 5, 9
**Dental prescribing on NHS** Azithromycin Tablets may be prescribed
**Note** Azithromycin tablets can be sold to the public for the treatment of confirmed, asymptomatic *Chlamydia trachomatis* genital infection in those over 16 years of age, and for the epidemiological treatment of their sexual partners, subject to max. single dose of 1 g, max. daily dose 1 g, and a pack size of 1 g

Oral suspension, azithromycin (as monohydrate) 200 mg/5 mL when reconstituted with water, net price 15-mL pack = £5.81, 30-mL pack = £11.04. Label: 5, 9
**Dental prescribing on NHS** Azithromycin Oral Suspension 200 mg/5 mL may be prescribed

**Zithromax**® (Pfizer) ⓅoM
Capsules, azithromycin (as dihydrate) 250 mg, net price 4-cap pack = £7.16, 6-cap pack = £10.74. Label: 5, 9, 23

Oral suspension, cherry/banana-flavoured, azithromycin (as dihydrate) 200 mg/5 mL when reconstituted with water. Net price 15-mL pack = £4.06, 22.5-mL pack = £6.10, 30-mL pack = £11.04. Label: 5, 9

## ■ CLARITHROMYCIN

**Cautions** see notes above; **interactions:** Appendix 1 (macrolides)

**Hepatic impairment** hepatic dysfunction including jaundice reported

**Renal impairment** use half normal dose if estimated glomerular filtration rate less than 30 mL/minute/1.73 m²; avoid *Klaricid XL*® if estimated glomerular filtration rate less than 30 mL/minute/1.73 m²

**5**
**Infections**

**Pregnancy** manufacturer advises avoid unless potential benefit outweighs risk

**Breast-feeding** manufacturer advises avoid unless potential benefit outweighs risk—present in milk

**Side-effects** see notes above; also dyspepsia, tooth and tongue discoloration, smell and taste disturbances, stomatitis, glossitis, and headache; *less commonly* arthralgia and myalgia; *rarely* tinnitus; *very rarely* dizziness, insomnia, nightmares, anxiety, confusion, psychosis, paraesthesia, convulsions, hypoglycaemia, renal failure, interstitial nephritis, leucopenia, and thrombocytopenia

**Licensed use** tablets and intravenous infusion not licensed for use in children under 12 years

**Indications and dose**

> **Respiratory-tract infections, mild to moderate skin and soft-tissue infections, otitis media (see also Table 1, section 5.1)**
>
> • By mouth
>
> > **Neonate** 7.5 mg/kg twice daily
> >
> > **Child 1 month–12 years**
> > **Body-weight under 8 kg** 7.5 mg/kg twice daily
> > **Body-weight 8–11 kg** 62.5 mg twice daily
> > **Body-weight 12–19 kg** 125 mg twice daily
> > **Body-weight 20–29 kg** 187.5 mg twice daily
> > **Body-weight 30–40 kg** 250 mg twice daily
> >
> > **Child 12–18 years** 250 mg twice daily for 7 days, increased if necessary in severe infections to 500 mg every 12 hours for up to 14 days
>
> • By intravenous infusion into large proximal vein
>
> > **Child 1 month–12 years** 7.5 mg/kg every 12 hours
> > **Child 12–18 years** 500 mg every 12 hours
>
> **Lyme disease** (see also section 5.1.1.3)
>
> • By mouth
>
> > **Child 1 month–12 years** 7.5 mg/kg (max. 500 mg) twice daily for 14–21 days
> >
> > **Child 12–18 years** 500 mg twice daily for 14–21 days
>
> *Helicobacter pylori* **eradication** section 1.3
>
> **Prevention of pertussis** Table 2, section 5.1

**Administration** for intermittent intravenous infusion dilute reconstituted solution further in Glucose 5% *or* Sodium chloride 0.9% to a concentration of 2 mg/mL; give into large proximal vein over 60 minutes

**Clarithromycin** (Non-proprietary) PoM
Tablets, clarithromycin 250 mg, net price 14-tab pack = £3.17; 500 mg, 14-tab pack = £4.10. Label: 9
**Dental prescribing on NHS** Clarithromycin Tablets may be prescribed

Oral suspension, clarithromycin for reconstitution with water 125 mg/5 mL, net price 70 mL = £6.82; 250 mg/5 mL, 70 mL = £13.63. Label: 9
**Dental prescribing on NHS** Clarithromycin Oral Suspension may be prescribed

Intravenous infusion, powder for reconstitution, clarithromycin; net price 500-mg vial = £10.31

**Klaricid**® (Abbott Healthcare) PoM
Tablets, both yellow, f/c, clarithromycin 250 mg, net price 14-tab pack = £6.30; 500 mg, 14-tab pack = £10.17, 20-tab pack = £14.54. Label: 9

Paediatric suspension, clarithromycin for reconstitution with water 125 mg/5 mL, net price 70 mL = £4.73, 100 mL = £8.14; 250 mg/5 mL, 70 mL = £9.46. Label: 9

Granules, clarithromycin 250 mg/sachet, net price 14-sachet pack = £11.68. Label: 9, 13

Intravenous infusion, powder for reconstitution, clarithromycin. Net price 500-mg vial = £9.45
**Electrolytes** Na⁺< 0.5 mmol/500-mg vial

**Klaricid XL**® (Abbott Healthcare) PoM
Tablets, m/r, yellow, clarithromycin 500 mg, net price 7-tab pack = £6.46, 14-tab pack = £12.71. Label: 9, 21, 25
**Dose**

> • By mouth
>
> > **Child 12–18 years** 500 mg once daily (doubled in severe infections) for 7–14 days

## ▎ ERYTHROMYCIN

**Cautions** see notes above; neonate under 2 weeks (risk of hypertrophic pyloric stenosis); avoid in acute porphyria (section 9.8.2); **interactions:** Appendix 1 (macrolides)

**Hepatic impairment** may cause idiosyncratic hepatotoxicity

**Renal impairment** reduce dose in severe renal impairment (ototoxicity)

**Pregnancy** not known to be harmful

**Breast-feeding** only small amounts in milk—not known to be harmful

**Side-effects** see notes above

**Indications and dose**

> **Susceptible infections in patients with penicillin hypersensitivity, oral infections (see notes above), campylobacter enteritis, respiratory-tract infections (including Legionella infection), skin infections, chlamydial ophthalmia, prevention and treament of pertussis (see also Table 2, section 5.1)**
>
> • By mouth
>
> > **Neonate** 12.5 mg/kg every 6 hours
> >
> > **Child 1 month–2 years** 125 mg 4 times daily; dose doubled in severe infections
> >
> > **Child 2–8 years** 250 mg 4 times daily; dose doubled in severe infections
> >
> > **Child 8–18 years** 250–500 mg 4 times daily; dose doubled in severe infections
> >
> > **Note** Total daily dose may be given in two divided doses
>
> • By intravenous infusion
>
> > **Neonate** 10–12.5 mg/kg every 6 hours
> >
> > **Child 1 month–18 years** 12.5 mg/kg (max. 1 g) every 6 hours
>
> **Early syphilis**
>
> • By mouth
>
> > **Child 12–18 years** 500 mg 4 times daily for 14 days

**Uncomplicated genital chlamydia, non-gonococcal urethritis, pelvic inflammatory disease (see also Table 1, section 5.1)**

- By mouth

  **Child 1 month–2 years** 12.5 mg/kg 4 times daily for 14 days

  **Child 2–12 years** 250 mg twice daily for 14 days

  **Child 12–18 years** 500 mg twice daily for 14 days

**Lyme disease** (see also section 5.1.1.3)

- By mouth

  **Child 1 month–18 years** 12.5 mg/kg (max. 500 mg) 4 times daily for 14–21 days

**Prophylaxis against pneumococcal infection** Table 2, section 5.1

**Gastric stasis** section 1.2

**Acne vulgaris** section 13.6

**Diphtheria prophylaxis** Table 2, section 5.1

**Prevention of group A streptococcal infection** Table 2, section 5.1

**Administration** Dilute reconstituted solution further in glucose 5% (neutralised with Sodium bicarbonate) or sodium chloride 0.9% to a concentration of 1–5 mg/mL; give over 20–60 minutes

Concentration of up to 10 mg/mL may be used in fluid-restriction if administered via a central venous catheter

**Erythromycin** (Non-proprietary) [PoM]

Capsules, enclosing e/c microgranules, erythromycin 250 mg, net price 28-cap pack = £15.00. Label: 5, 9, 25

Brands include *Tiloryth*®

Tablets, e/c, erythromycin 250 mg, net price 28 = £1.54. Label: 5, 9, 25

Dental prescribing on NHS Erythromycin Tablets e/c may be prescribed

**Erythromycin Ethyl Succinate** (Non-proprietary) [PoM]

Oral suspension, erythromycin (as ethyl succinate) for reconstitution with water 125 mg/5 mL, net price 100 mL = £1.99; 250 mg/5 mL, 100 mL = £2.64; 500 mg/5 mL, 100 mL = £4.31. Label: 9

Note Sugar-free versions are available and can be ordered by specifying 'sugar-free' on the prescription

Brands include *Primacine*®

Dental prescribing on NHS Erythromycin Ethyl Succinate Oral Suspension may be prescribed

**Erythromycin Lactobionate** (Non-proprietary) [PoM]

Intravenous infusion, powder for reconstitution, erythromycin (as lactobionate), net price 1-g vial = £9.98

**Erymax**® (Cephalon) [PoM]

Capsules, opaque orange/clear orange, enclosing orange and white e/c pellets, erythromycin 250 mg, net price 28-cap pack = £5.61, 112-cap pack = £22.44. Label: 5, 9, 25

**Erythrocin**® (Amdipharm) [PoM]

Tablets, both f/c, erythromycin (as stearate), 250 mg, net price 100–tab pack = £18.20; 500 mg, 100–tab pack = £36.40. Label: 9

Dental prescribing on NHS May be prescribed as Erythromycin Stearate Tablets

**Erythroped**® (Amdipharm) [PoM]

Suspension SF, sugar-free, banana-flavoured, erythromycin (as ethyl succinate) for reconstitution with water, 125 mg/5 mL (*Suspension PI SF*), net price 140 mL = £3.06; 250 mg/5 mL, 140 mL = £5.95; 500 mg/5 mL (*Suspension SF Forte*), 140 mL = £10.56. Label: 9

**Erythroped A**® (Amdipharm) [PoM]

Tablets, yellow, f/c, erythromycin 500 mg (as ethyl succinate). Net price 28-tab pack = £10.78. Label: 9

Dental prescribing on NHS May be prescribed as Erythromycin Ethyl Succinate Tablets

## 5.1.6 Clindamycin

Clindamycin is active against Gram-positive cocci, including streptococci and penicillin-resistant staphylococci, and also against many anaerobes, especially *Bacteroides fragilis*. It is well concentrated in bone and excreted in bile and urine.

Clindamycin is recommended for staphylococcal joint and bone infections such as osteomyelitis, and intra-abdominal sepsis; it is an alternative to macrolides for erysipelas or cellulitis in penicillin-allergic patients. It is also used in combination with other antibacterials for cellulitis in immunocompromised children. Clindamycin can also be used for infections associated with meticillin-resistant *Staphylococcus aureus* (MRSA) in bone and joint infections, and skin and soft-tissue infections.

Clindamycin has been associated with antibiotic-associated colitis (section 1.5), which may be fatal. Although it can occur with most antibacterials, antibiotic-associated colitis occurs more frequently with clindamycin. Children should therefore discontinue treatment immediately if diarrhoea develops.

**Oral infections** Clindamycin should not be used routinely for the treatment of oral infections because it may be no more effective than penicillins against anaerobes and there may be cross-resistance with erythromycin-resistant bacteria. Clindamycin can be used for the treatment of dentoalveolar abscess that has not responded to penicillin or to metronidazole.

### CLINDAMYCIN

**Cautions** discontinue immediately if diarrhoea or colitis develops; monitor liver and renal function if treatment exceeds 10 days, and in neonates and infants; avoid rapid intravenous administration; avoid in acute porphyria (section 9.8.2); **interactions**: Appendix 1 (clindamycin)

**Contra-indications** diarrhoeal states; avoid injections containing benzyl alcohol in neonates (see under preparations below)

**Pregnancy** not known to be harmful

**Breast-feeding** amount probably too small to be harmful; bloody diarrhoea reported in 1 infant

**Side-effects** diarrhoea (discontinue treatment), abdominal discomfort, oesophagitis, oesophageal ulcers, taste disturbances, nausea, vomiting, antibio-

5 Infections

tic-associated colitis; jaundice; leucopenia, eosinophilia, and thrombocytopenia reported; polyarthritis reported; rash, pruritus, urticaria, anaphylactoid reactions, Stevens-Johnson syndrome, toxic epidermal necrolysis, exfoliative and vesiculobullous dermatitis reported; pain, induration, and abscess after intramuscular injection; thrombophlebitis after intravenous injection

**Indications and dose**

**Staphylococcal bone and joint infections, peritonitis** see notes above

- **By mouth**

  **Neonate under 14 days** 3–6 mg/kg 3 times daily

  **Neonate 14–28 days** 3–6 mg/kg 4 times daily

  **Child 1 month–12 years** 3–6 mg/kg (max. 450 mg) 4 times daily

  **Child 12–18 years** 150–300 mg 4 times daily; in severe infections 450 mg 4 times daily

- **By deep intramuscular injection or by intravenous infusion**

  **Child 1 month–12 years** 3.75–6.25 mg/kg 4 times daily; increased up to 10 mg/kg 4 times daily in severe infections; total daily dose may alternatively be given in 3 divided doses

  **Child 12–18 years** 150–675 mg 4 times daily; total daily dose may alternatively be given in 2–3 divided doses; in life-threatening infection up to 1.2 g 4 times daily; single doses above 600 mg by intravenous infusion only; single doses by intravenous infusion not to exceed 1.2 g

**Staphylococcal lung infection in cystic fibrosis**

- **By mouth**

  **Child 1 month–18 years** 5–7 mg/kg (max. 600 mg) 4 times daily

**Treatment of falciparum malaria**, see p. 332

**Administration** for *intravenous infusion*, dilute to a concentration of not more than 18 mg/mL with Glucose 5% or Sodium Chloride 0.9%; give over 10–60 minutes at a max. rate of 20 mg/kg/hour

**Clindamycin** (Non-proprietary) PoM
Capsules, clindamycin (as hydrochloride) 150 mg, net price 24-cap pack = £11.75. Label: 9, 27, counselling, see above (diarrhoea)
**Dental prescribing on NHS** Clindamycin Capsules may be prescribed

Injection, clindamycin (as phosphate) 150 mg/mL, net price 2-mL amp = £5.80, 4-mL amp = £11.65

Liquid, 75 mg/5 mL available from 'special-order' manufacturers or specialist importing companies, see p. 823

**Dalacin C®** (Pharmacia) PoM
Capsules, clindamycin (as hydrochloride) 75 mg (green/white), net price 24-cap pack = £7.45; 150 mg, (white), 24-cap pack = £13.72. Label: 9, 27, counselling, see above (diarrhoea)
**Dental prescribing on NHS** May be prescribed as Clindamycin Capsules

Injection, clindamycin (as phosphate) 150 mg/mL, net price 2-mL amp = £6.20, 4-mL amp = £12.35
**Excipients** include benzyl alcohol (avoid in neonates, see Excipients, p. 2)

---

## 5.1.7 Some other antibacterials

Antibacterials discussed in this section include chloramphenicol, fusidic acid, glycopeptide antibiotics (vancomycin and teicoplanin), linezolid, and the polymyxin, colistimethate sodium.

## Chloramphenicol

**Chloramphenicol** is a potent broad-spectrum antibiotic; however, it is associated with serious haematological side-effects when given systemically and should therefore be reserved for the treatment of life-threatening infections, particularly those caused by *Haemophilus influenzae*, and also for typhoid fever. Chloramphenicol is also used in cystic fibrosis for the treatment of respiratory *Burkholderia cepacia* infection resistant to other antibacterials.

Grey baby syndrome may follow excessive doses in neonates with immature hepatic metabolism; monitoring of plasma concentrations is recommended.

Chloramphenicol eye drops (section 11.3.1) and chloramphenicol ear drops (section 12.1.1) are also available.

### CHLORAMPHENICOL

**Cautions** avoid repeated courses and prolonged treatment; blood counts required before and periodically during treatment; monitor plasma-chloramphenicol concentration in neonates (see below); interactions: Appendix 1 (chloramphenicol)

**Contra-indications** acute porphyria (section 9.8.2)

**Hepatic impairment** avoid if possible—increased risk of bone-marrow depression; reduce dose and monitor plasma-chloramphenicol concentration

**Renal impairment** avoid in severe impairment unless no alternative; dose-related depression of haematopoiesis

**Pregnancy** manufacturer advises avoid; neonatal grey-baby syndrome if used in third trimester

**Breast-feeding** manufacturer advises avoid; use another antibiotic; may cause bone-marrow toxicity in infant; concentration in milk usually insufficient to cause 'grey-baby syndrome'

**Side-effects** blood disorders including reversible and irreversible aplastic anaemia (with reports of resulting leukaemia), peripheral neuritis, optic neuritis, headache, depression, urticaria, erythema multiforme, nausea, vomiting, diarrhoea, stomatitis, glossitis, dry mouth; nocturnal haemoglobinuria reported; grey syndrome (abdominal distension, pallid cyanosis, circulatory collapse) may follow excessive doses in neonates with immature hepatic metabolism (see Pharmacokinetics below)

**Pharmacokinetics** plasma concentration monitoring required in neonates and preferred in those under 4 years of age, and in hepatic impairment; recommended peak plasma concentration (approx. 2 hours after administration by mouth, intravenous injection or infusion) 10–25 mg/litre; pre-dose ('trough') concentration should not exceed 15 mg/litre

**Indications and dose**

See notes above

- **By intravenous injection**

  **Neonate up to 14 days** 12.5 mg/kg twice daily

  **Neonate 14–28 days** 12.5 mg/kg 2–4 times daily

  **Note** Check dosage carefully; overdosage can be fatal (see also pharmacokinetics above)

- **By mouth or by intravenous injection or infusion**

  **Child 1 month–18 years** 12.5 mg/kg every 6 hours; dose may be doubled in severe infections such as septicaemia, meningitis and epiglottitis providing plasma-chloramphenicol concentrations are measured and high doses reduced as soon as indicated

**Administration** Displacement value may be significant for injection, consult local guidelines. For intermittent intravenous infusion, dilute reconstituted solution further in glucose 5% *or* sodium chloride 0.9%

**Chloramphenicol** (Non-proprietary) PoM

Capsules, chloramphenicol 250 mg. Net price 60 = £377.00

**Kemicetine®** (Pharmacia) PoM

Injection, powder for reconstitution, chloramphenicol (as sodium succinate). Net price 1-g vial = £1.39
Electrolytes  Na+ 3.14 mmol/g

## Fusidic acid

**Fusidic acid** and its salts are narrow-spectrum antibiotics. The only indication for their use is in infections caused by penicillin-resistant staphylococci, especially osteomyelitis, as they are well concentrated in bone; they are also used for staphylococcal endocarditis. A second antistaphylococcal antibiotic is usually required to prevent emergence of resistance during treatment.

### ■ SODIUM FUSIDATE

**Cautions** monitor liver function with high doses or on prolonged therapy; elimination may be reduced in hepatic impairment or biliary disease or biliary obstruction; **interactions**: Appendix 1 (fusidic acid)

**Hepatic impairment** impaired biliary excretion, avoid or reduce dose; possibly increased risk of hepatotoxicity, monitor liver function

**Pregnancy** not known to be harmful; manufacturer advises use only if potential benefit outweighs risk

**Breast-feeding** present in milk; manufacturer advises caution

**Side-effects** nausea, vomiting, abdominal pain, dyspepsia, diarrhoea, drowsiness, dizziness; *less commonly* anorexia, headache, malaise, rash, pruritus; also reported, reversible jaundice especially after high dosage (withdraw therapy if persistent), acute renal failure (usually with jaundice), blood disorders

**Indications and dose**

Penicillin-resistant staphylococcal infection including osteomyelitis, staphylococcal endocarditis in combination with other antibacterials see under Preparations, below

**Fucidin®** (LEO) PoM

Tablets, f/c, sodium fusidate 250 mg, net price 10-tab pack = £6.02. Label: 9

**Dose**

As sodium fusidate

- **By mouth**

  **Child 12–18 years** 500 mg every 8 hours, dose doubled for severe infections

**Skin infection** as sodium fusidate

- **By mouth**

  **Child 12–18 years** 250 mg every 12 hours for 5–10 days

Suspension, off-white, banana- and orange-flavoured, fusidic acid 250 mg/5 mL, net price 50 mL = £6.73. Label: 9, 21

**Dose**

As fusidic acid

- **By mouth**

  **Neonate** 15 mg/kg 3 times daily

  **Child 1 month–1 year** 15 mg/kg 3 times daily

  **Child 1–5 years** 250 mg 3 times daily

  **Child 5–12 years** 500 mg 3 times daily

  **Child 12–18 years** 750 mg 3 times daily

  **Note** Fusidic acid is incompletely absorbed and doses recommended for suspension are proportionately higher than those for sodium fusidate tablets

## Vancomycin and teicoplanin

The glycopeptide antibiotics **vancomycin** and **teicoplanin** have bactericidal activity against aerobic and anaerobic Gram-positive bacteria including multi-resistant staphylococci. However, there are reports of *Staphylococcus aureus* with reduced susceptibility to glycopeptides. There are increasing reports of glycopeptide-resistant *Enterococci*.

They are used *parenterally* in the treatment of serious infections caused by Gram-positive cocci. Teicoplanin is similar to vancomycin, but has a significantly longer duration of action, allowing once daily administration after the loading dose. Teicoplanin is associated with a lower incidence of nephrotoxicity than vancomycin.

They are also used for surgical prophylaxis when there is a high risk of MRSA ( Table 2, section 5.1).

Penetration into cerebrospinal fluid is poor; vancomycin may be administered by the *intrathecal* or *intraventricular* route for treatment of meningitis [unlicensed].

Vancomycin (added to dialysis fluid) is also used in the treatment of peritonitis associated with peritoneal dialysis [unlicensed route] (Table 1, section 5.1).

Vancomycin given *by mouth* for 10–14 days is effective in the treatment of *Clostridium difficile* infection (see also section 1.5); low doses are considered adequate (higher dose may be considered if the infection fails to respond or if it is life-threatening). Vancomycin should **not** be given by mouth for systemic infections since it is not significantly absorbed.

### ■ VANCOMYCIN

**Cautions** avoid rapid infusion (risk of anaphylactoid reactions, see Side-effects); rotate infusion sites; avoid if history of deafness; all patients require plasma-vancomycin measurement (after 3 or 4 doses if renal function normal, earlier if renal impairment), blood counts, urinalysis, and renal function tests; monitor auditory function in renal impairment; teicoplanin sensitivity; systemic absorption may follow oral

**5 Infections**

administration especially in inflammatory bowel disorders or following multiple doses; **interactions:** Appendix 1 (vancomycin)

**Specific cautions for inhaled treatment** Administer inhaled bronchodilator before vancomycin. Measure lung function before and after initial dose of vancomycin and monitor for bronchospasm.

**Renal impairment** reduce dose—monitor plasma-vancomycin concentration and renal function regularly; see also Cautions above

**Pregnancy** manufacturer advises use only if potential benefit outweighs risk—plasma-vancomycin concentration monitoring essential to reduce risk of fetal toxicity

**Breast-feeding** present in milk—significant absorption following oral administration unlikely

**Side-effects** after parenteral administration: nephrotoxicity including renal failure and interstitial nephritis; ototoxicity (discontinue if tinnitus occurs); blood disorders including neutropenia (usually after 1 week or high cumulative dose), rarely agranulocytosis and thrombocytopenia; nausea; chills, fever; eosinophilia, anaphylaxis, rashes (including exfoliative dermatitis, Stevens-Johnson syndrome, toxic epidermal necrolysis, and vasculitis); phlebitis (irritant to tissue); on rapid infusion, severe hypotension (including shock and cardiac arrest), wheezing, dyspnoea, urticaria, pruritus, flushing of the upper body ('red man' syndrome), pain and muscle spasm of back and chest

**Pharmacokinetics** plasma concentration monitoring required; pre-dose ('trough') concentration should be 10–15 mg/litre (15–20 mg/litre for less sensitive strains of meticillin-resistant *Staphylococcus aureus*)

**Licensed use** not licensed for intraventricular use or inhalation

**Indications and dose**

Infections due to Gram-positive bacteria including osteomyelitis, septicaemia and soft-tissue infections see notes above

- **By intravenous infusion**

  **Neonate less than 29 weeks postmenstrual age** 15 mg/kg every 24 hours, adjusted according to plasma concentration

  **Neonate 29–35 weeks postmenstrual age** 15 mg/kg every 12 hours, adjusted according to plasma concentration

  **Neonate over 35 weeks postmenstrual age** 15 mg/kg every 8 hours, adjusted according to plasma concentration

  **Child 1 month–18 years** 15 mg/kg every 8 hours (maximum daily dose 2 g), adjusted according to plasma concentration

*Clostridium difficile* infection (see also notes above)

- **By mouth**

  **Child 1 month–5 years** 5 mg/kg 4 times daily for 10–14 days (increased up to 10 mg/kg 4 times daily if infection fails to respond or is life-threatening)

  **Child 5–12 years** 62.5 mg 4 times daily for 10–14 days (increased up to 250 mg 4 times daily if infection fails to respond or is life-threatening)

  **Child 12–18 years** 125 mg 4 times daily for 10–14 days (increased up to 500 mg 4 times daily if infection fails to respond or is life-threatening)

CNS infection e.g. ventriculitis

- **By intraventricular administration, seek specialist advice**

  **Neonate** 10 mg once every 24 hours

  **Child 1 month–18 years** 10 mg once every 24 hours

  **Note** for all children reduce to 5 mg daily if ventricular size reduced or increase to 15–20 mg once daily if ventricular size increased. Adjust dose according to CSF concentration after 3-4 days; aim for pre-dose ('trough') concentration less than 10 mg/litre. If CSF not draining freely reduce dose frequency to once every 2–3 days

Peritonitis associated with peritoneal dialysis
Add to each bag of dialysis fluid to achieve a concentration of 20–25 mg/litre

Eradication of meticillin-resistant *Staphylococcus aureus* from the respiratory tract in cystic fibrosis

- **By inhalation of nebulised solution**

  **Child 1 month–18 years** 4 mg/kg (max. 250 mg) 2 or 4 times daily for 5 days

**Note** Vancomycin doses in BNF for Children may differ from those in product literature

**Administration** Displacement value may be significant, consult product literature and local guidelines. For intermittent intravenous infusion, the reconstituted preparation should be further diluted in sodium chloride 0.9% *or* glucose 5% to a concentration of up to 5 mg/mL; give over at least 60 minutes (rate not to exceed 10 mg/minute for doses over 500 mg); use continuous infusion only if intermittent not available (limited evidence); 10 mg/mL can be used if infused via a central venous line over at least 1 hour

Injection may be given orally; flavouring syrups may be added to the solution at the time of administration

*For nebulisation* administer required dose in 4 mL of sodium chloride 0.9% (or water for injections).

> **Safe Practice**
> For intraventricular administration, seek specialist advice

**Vancomycin** (Non-proprietary) [PoM]

Capsules, vancomycin (as hydrochloride) 125 mg, net price 28-cap pack = £132.47; 250 mg, 28-cap pack = £132.47. Label: 9

Injection, powder for reconstitution, vancomycin (as hydrochloride), for use as an infusion, net price 500-mg vial = £7.25; 1-g vial = £14.50
**Note** Can be used to prepare solution for oral administration

**Vancocin®** (Flynn) [PoM]

Matrigel capsules, vancomycin (as hydrochloride) 125 mg, net price 28-cap pack = £88.31. Label: 9

Injection, powder for reconstitution, vancomycin (as hydrochloride), for use as an infusion, net price 500-mg vial = £8.05; 1-g vial = £16.11
**Note** Can be used to prepare solution for oral administration

# TEICOPLANIN

**Cautions** vancomycin sensitivity; blood counts and liver and kidney function tests required—monitor renal and auditory function on prolonged administration during renal impairment or if other nephrotoxic or neurotoxic drugs given; monitor plasma-teicoplanin concentration if severe sepsis or burns, deep-seated staphylococcal infection (including bone and joint infection), endocarditis, renal impairment, and in intravenous drug abusers; **interactions:** Appendix 1 (teicoplanin)

**Renal impairment** from day 4, use normal dose every 48 hours if estimated glomerular filtration rate 40–60 mL/minute/1.73 m$^2$ and use normal dose every 72 hours if estimated glomerular filtration rate less than 40 mL/minute/1.73 m$^2$; see also Cautions above

**Pregnancy** manufacturer advises use only if potential benefit outweighs risk

**Breast-feeding** no information available

**Side-effects** rash, pruritus; *less commonly* nausea, vomiting, diarrhoea, bronchospasm, dizziness, headache, fever, leucopenia, thrombocytopenia, eosinophilia, tinnitus, mild hearing loss, vestibular disorders, thrombophlebitis; *also reported* renal failure, exfoliative dermatitis, Stevens-Johnson syndrome, toxic epidermal necrolysis

**Pharmacokinetics** plasma-teicoplanin concentration is not measured routinely because there is no clear relationship between plasma-teicoplanin concentration and toxicity. However, the plasma-teicoplanin concentration can be used to optimise treatment in some patients (see Cautions). Pre-dose ('trough') concentration should be greater than 10 mg/litre (greater than 15–20 mg/litre in endocarditis) but less than 60 mg/litre

**Indications and dose**

> **Potentially serious Gram-positive infections including endocarditis, and serious infections due to Staphylococcus aureus**
>
> • **By intravenous injection or intravenous infusion over 30 minutes**
>
> **Neonate** initially 16 mg/kg for one dose followed 24 hours later by 8 mg/kg once daily (intravenous infusion only)
>
> **Child 1 month–18 years** initially 10 mg/kg (max. 400 mg) every 12 hours for 3 doses, then 6 mg/kg (max. 400 mg) once daily (after first 3 doses, subsequent doses can be given by intramuscular injection, if necessary, although intravenous route preferable; in severe infections (including burns, septicaemia, septic arthritis and osteomyelitis) initially 10 mg/kg every 12 hours for 3 doses then 10 mg/kg once daily

**Administration** For intermittent intravenous infusion, dilute reconstituted solution further in sodium chloride 0.9% *or* glucose 5%; give over 30 minutes. Intermittent intravenous infusion preferred in neonates

**Targocid**® (Sanofi-Aventis) PoM
Injection, powder for reconstitution, teicoplanin, net price 200-mg vial (with diluent) = £3.57; 400-mg vial (with diluent) = £6.10
Electrolytes Na$^+$ < 0.5 mmol/200- and 400-mg vial

---

## Linezolid

Linezolid, an oxazolidinone antibacterial, is active against Gram-positive bacteria including meticillin-resistant *Staphylococcus aureus* (MRSA), and glycopeptide-resistant enterococci. Resistance to linezolid can develop with prolonged treatment or if the dose is less than that recommended. Linezolid should be reserved for infections caused by Gram-positive bacter-

ia when the organisms are resistant to other antibacterials or when patients cannot tolerate other antibacterials. Linezolid is **not** active against common Gram-negative organisms; it must be given in combination with other antibacterials for mixed infections that also involve Gram-negative organisms. There is limited information on use in children and expert advice should be sought. A higher incidence of blood disorders and optic neuropathy have been reported in patients receiving linezolid for more than the maximum recommended duration of 28 days.

### ▌ LINEZOLID

**Cautions** monitor full blood count (including platelet count) weekly (see also Blood Disorders below); unless close observation and blood-pressure monitoring possible, avoid in uncontrolled hypertension, phaeochromocytoma, carcinoid tumour, thyrotoxicosis, bipolar depression, schizophrenia, or acute confusional states; **interactions:** Appendix 1 (MAOIs)

> **Blood disorders**
>
> Haematopoietic disorders (including thrombocytopenia, anaemia, leucopenia, and pancytopenia) have been reported in patients receiving linezolid. It is recommended that full blood counts are monitored weekly. Close monitoring is recommended in patients who:
> * receive treatment for more than 10–14 days;
> * have pre-existing myelosuppression;
> * are receiving drugs that may have adverse effects on haemoglobin, blood counts, or platelet function;
> * have severe renal impairment.
>
> If significant myelosuppression occurs, treatment should be stopped unless it is considered essential, in which case intensive monitoring of blood counts and appropriate management should be implemented.

> **CHM advice (optic neuropathy)**
>
> Severe optic neuropathy may occur rarely, particularly if linezolid is used for longer than 28 days. The CHM recommends that:
> * patients should be warned to report symptoms of visual impairment (including blurred vision, visual field defect, changes in visual acuity and colour vision) immediately;
> * patients experiencing new visual symptoms (regardless of treatment duration) should be evaluated promptly, and referred to an ophthalmologist if necessary;
> * visual function should be monitored regularly if treatment is required for longer than 28 days.

**Monoamine oxidase inhibition** Linezolid is a reversible, non-selective monoamine oxidase inhibitor (MAOI). Patients should avoid consuming large amounts of tyramine-rich foods (such as mature cheese, yeast extracts, undistilled alcoholic beverages, and fermented soya bean products). In addition, linezolid should not be given with another MAOI or within 2 weeks of stopping another MAOI. Unless close observation and blood-pressure monitoring is possible, avoid in those receiving SSRIs, 5HT$_1$ agonists ('triptans'), tricyclic antidepressants, sympathomimetics, dopaminergics, buspirone, pethidine and possibly other opioid analgesics. For other interactions see Appendix 1 (MAOIs)

**Contra-indications** see Monoamine Oxidase Inhibition above

**Hepatic impairment** no dose adjustment necessary but in severe hepatic impairment use only if potential benefit outweighs risk

**Renal impairment** no dose adjustment necessary but metabolites may accumulate if estimated glomerular filtration rate less than 30 mL/minute/1.73 m²; see also Blood Disorders above

**Pregnancy** manufacturer advises use only if potential benefit outweighs risk—no information available

**Breast-feeding** manufacturer advises avoid—present in milk in *animal* studies

**Side-effects** diarrhoea (antibiotic-associated colitis reported), nausea, vomiting, taste disturbances, headache; *less commonly* thirst, dry mouth, glossitis, stomatitis, tongue discoloration, abdominal pain, dyspepsia, gastritis, constipation, pancreatitis, hypertension, fever, fatigue, dizziness, insomnia, hypoaesthesia, paraesthesia, tinnitus, polyuria, leucopenia, thrombocytopenia, eosinophilia, electrolyte disturbances, blurred vision, rash, pruritus, diaphoresis, injection-site reactions; *rarely* tachycardia, transient ischaemic attacks, renal failure; also reported tooth discoloration, convulsions, lactic acidosis, hyponatraemia, pancytopenia, anaemia, Stevens-Johnson syndrome, toxic epidermal necrolysis; peripheral and optic neuropathy reported on prolonged therapy (see also CHM Advice above)

**Licensed use** not licensed for use in children

**Indications and dose**

> Pneumonia, complicated skin and soft-tissue infections caused by Gram-positive bacteria (initiated under expert supervision)
> - By mouth or by intravenous infusion over 30–120 minutes
>   **Neonate under 7 days** 10 mg/kg every 12 hours, increase to every 8 hours if poor response
>   **Neonate over 7 days** 10 mg/kg every 8 hours
>   **Child 1 month–12 years** 10 mg/kg (max. 600 mg) every 8 hours
>   **Child 12–18 years** 600 mg every 12 hours

**Zyvox**® (Pharmacia) [PoM]
Tablets, f/c, linezolid 600 mg, net price 10-tab pack = £445.00. Label: 9, 10, patient information leaflet

Suspension, yellow, linezolid 100 mg/5 mL when reconstituted with water, net price 150 mL (orange-flavoured) = £222.50. Label: 9, 10 patient information leaflet
Excipients include aspartame 20 mg/5 mL (section 9.4.1)

Intravenous infusion, linezolid 2 mg/mL, net price 300-mL *Excel*® bag = £44.50
Excipients include Na⁺ 5 mmol/300-mL bag, glucose 13.71 g/300-mL bag

## Polymyxins

The polymyxin antibiotic, **colistimethate sodium** (colistin sulfomethate sodium), is active against Gram-negative organisms including *Pseudomonas aeruginosa*, *Acinetobacter baumanii*, and *Klebsiella pneumoniae*. It is **not** absorbed by mouth and is given by injection for a systemic effect. Intravenous administration of colistimethate sodium should be reserved for Gram-negative infections resistant to other antibacterials; its major adverse effects are dose-related neurotoxicity and nephrotoxicity.

Colistimethate sodium is also given by inhalation of a nebulised solution as an adjunct to standard antibacterial therapy in patients with cystic fibrosis.

Both colistimethate sodium and polymyxin B are included in some preparations for topical application.

## COLISTIMETHATE SODIUM
### (Colistin sulfomethate sodium)

**Cautions** acute porphyria (section 9.8.2); **interactions:** Appendix 1 (polymyxins)
**Specific cautions for parenteral treatment** Monitor renal function
**Specific cautions for inhaled treatment** Measure lung function before and after initial dose of colistimethate sodium and monitor for bronchospasm; if bronchospasm occurs in a child not using a bronchodilator, repeat test using a bronchodilator before the dose of colistimethate sodium

**Contra-indications** myasthenia gravis

**Renal impairment** reduce dose and monitor plasma-colistimethate sodium concentration during parenteral treatment–consult product literature

**Pregnancy** clinical use suggests probably safe when used by inhalation of nebulised solution; use parenteral treatment only if potential benefit outweighs risk

**Breast-feeding** present in milk but poorly absorbed from gut; manufacturers advise avoid (or use only if potential benefit outweighs risk)

**Side-effects**
**Specific side-effects for parenteral treatment** Neurotoxicity reported especially with excessive doses (including apnoea, perioral and peripheral paraesthesia, vertigo, headache, muscle weakness; rarely vasomotor instability, slurred speech, confusion, psychosis, visual disturbances), nephrotoxicity; rash
**Specific side-effects for inhaled treatment** Sore throat, sore mouth, cough, bronchospasm

**Pharmacokinetics** plasma concentration monitoring recommended in renal impairment; recommended 'peak' plasma-colistimethate sodium concentration (approx. 1 hour after intravenous injection or infusion) 5–15 mg/litre; pre-dose ('trough') concentration 2–6 mg/litre

**Licensed use** *Promixin*® powder for nebuliser solution not licensed for use in children under 2 years

**Indications and dose**

> *Pseudomonas aeruginosa* infection in cystic fibrosis
> - By slow intravenous injection into a totally implantable venous access device, or by intravenous infusion (but see notes above)
>   **Child 1 month–18 years**
>   **Body-weight under 60 kg** 25 000 units/kg every 8 hours
>   **Body-weight over 60 kg** 2 million units every 8 hours
> - By inhalation of nebulised solution
>   **Child 1 month–2 years** 0.5–1 million units twice daily; increased to 1 million units 3 times daily for subsequent respiratory isolates of *Ps. aeruginosa*
>   **Child 2–18 years** 1–2 million units twice daily; increased to 2 million units 3 times daily for subsequent respiratory isolates of *Ps. aeruginosa*

**Administration** For *intravenous infusion*, dilute to a concentration of 40 000 units/mL with Sodium Chloride 0.9%; give over 30 minutes

For *slow intravenous injection* into a totally implantable venous access device, dilute to a concentration of 90 000 units/mL with Sodium Chloride 0.9% for child under 12 years (200 000 units/mL for child over 12 years)

For *nebulisation* administer required dose in 2–4 mL of sodium chloride 0.9% (*or* water for injections) *or* a 1:1 mixture of sodium chloride 0.9% and water for injection

**Colistimethate sodium** (Non-proprietary) ▸PoM◂
Injection, powder for reconstitution, colistimethate sodium, net price 1 million-unit vial = £1.68

**Colomycin®** (Forest) ▸PoM◂
Injection, powder for reconstitution, colistimethate sodium, net price 1 million-unit vial = £1.68; 2 million-unit vial = £3.09
**Electrolytes** (before reconstitution) Na+< 0.5 mmol/1 million-unit and 2 million-unit vial
**Note** *Colomycin®* Injection may be used for nebulisation

**Promixin®** (Profile) ▸PoM◂
Powder for nebuliser solution, colistimethate sodium, net price 1 million-unit vial = £4.60.

Injection, powder for reconstitution, colistimethate sodium, net price 1 million unit-vial = £2.30
**Electrolytes** (before reconstitution) Na+< 0.5 mmol/1 million-unit vial

## 5.1.8 Sulfonamides and trimethoprim

The importance of the sulfonamides has decreased as a result of increasing bacterial resistance and their replacement by antibacterials which are generally more active and less toxic.

Sulfamethoxazole and trimethoprim are used in combination (as **co-trimoxazole**) because of their synergistic activity. However, co-trimoxazole is associated with rare but serious side-effects e.g. Stevens-Johnson syndrome and blood dyscrasias, notably bone marrow depression and agranulocytosis (see Restrictions on the Use of Co-trimoxazole below). Co-trimoxazole should be avoided in children less than 6 weeks of age (except for treatment and prophylaxis of *pneumocystis pneumonia*) because of the risk of kernicterus. There is a risk of haemolytic anaemia if used in children with glucose-6-phosphate dehydrogenase (G6PD) deficiency (section 9.1.5).

---

**Restrictions on the use of co-trimoxazole**
Co-trimoxazole is the drug of choice in the prophylaxis and treatment of *Pneumocystis jirovecii* (*Pneumocystis carinii*) pneumonia; it is also indicated for nocardiasis, *Stenotrophomonas maltophilia* infection [unlicensed indication], and toxoplasmosis. It should only be considered for use in *infections of the urinary tract* when there is bacteriological evidence of sensitivity to co-trimoxazole and good reason to prefer this combination to a single antibacterial; similarly it should only be used in *acute otitis media in children* when there is good reason to prefer it. Co-trimoxazole is also used for the treatment of infections caused by *Burkholderia cepacia* in cystic fibrosis [unlicensed indication].

---

**Trimethoprim** can be used alone for urinary- and respiratory-tract infections and for shigellosis and invasive salmonella infections. Trimethoprim has side-effects similar to co-trimoxazole but they are less severe and occur less frequently.

For *topical preparations* of sulfonamides used in the treatment of burns see section 13.10.1.1.

## ▌ CO-TRIMOXAZOLE

A mixture of trimethoprim and sulfamethoxazole (sulphamethoxazole) in the proportions of 1 part to 5 parts

**Cautions** maintain adequate fluid intake; avoid in blood disorders (unless under specialist supervision); monitor blood counts on prolonged treatment; discontinue immediately if blood disorders or rash develop; predisposition to folate deficiency; asthma; G6PD deficiency (section 9.1.5); avoid in infants under 6 weeks (except for treatment or prophylaxis of pneumocystis pneumonia); **interactions:** Appendix 1 (trimethoprim, sulfamethoxazole)

**Contra-indications** acute porphyria (section 9.8.2)

**Hepatic impairment** manufacturer advises avoid in severe liver disease

**Renal impairment** use half normal dose if estimated glomerular filtration rate 15–30 mL/minute/1.73 m²; avoid if estimated glomerular filtration rate less than 15 mL/minute/1.73 m² and if plasma-sulfamethoxazole concentration cannot be monitored

**Pregnancy** teratogenic risk in first trimester (trimethoprim a folate antagonist). Neonatal haemolysis and methaemoglobinaemia in third trimester; fear of increased risk of kernicterus in neonates appears to be unfounded

**Breast-feeding** small risk of kernicterus in jaundiced infants and of haemolysis in G6PD-deficient infants (due to sulfamethoxazole)

**Side-effects** nausea, diarrhoea; headache, hyperkalaemia; rash (*very rarely* including Stevens-Johnson syndrome, toxic epidermal necrolysis, photosensitivity)—discontinue immediately; *less commonly* vomiting; *very rarely* glossitis, stomatitis, anorexia, liver damage (including jaundice and hepatic necrosis), pancreatitis, antibiotic-associated colitis, myocarditis, cough and shortness of breath, pulmonary infiltrates, aseptic meningitis, depression, convulsions, peripheral neuropathy, ataxia, tinnitus, vertigo, hallucinations, hypoglycaemia, blood disorders (including leucopenia, thrombocytopenia, megaloblastic anaemia, eosinophilia), hyponatraemia, renal disorders including interstitial nephritis, arthralgia, myalgia, vasculitis, systemic lupus erythematosus, and uveitis; rhabdomyolysis reported in HIV-infected patients

**Pharmacokinetics** plasma concentration monitoring may be required with high doses or during moderate to severe renal impairment; seek expert advice

**Licensed use** not licensed for use in children under 6 weeks

*(margin)* **5** Infections

**5 Infections**

## Indications and dose

**Treatment of susceptible infections (but see notes above)** dose expressed as co-trimoxazole

- **By mouth**

  **Child 6 weeks–12 years** 24 mg/kg twice daily

  *or*

  **Child 6 weeks–6 months** 120 mg twice daily

  **Child 6 months–6 years** 240 mg twice daily

  **Child 6–12 years** 480 mg twice daily

  **Child 12–18 years** 960 mg twice daily

- **By intravenous infusion**

  **Child 6 weeks–18 years** 18 mg/kg every 12 hours; increased in severe infection to 27 mg/kg (max. 1.44 g) every 12 hours

**Treatment of *Pneumocystis jirovecii* (*P. carinii*) infections (undertaken where facilities for appropriate monitoring available—consult microbiologist and product literature)**

- **By mouth or by intravenous infusion**

  **Child 1 month–18 years** 60 mg/kg every 12 hours for 14–21 days; total daily dose may alternatively be given in 3–4 divided doses

  **Note** oral route preferred

**Prophylaxis of *Pneumocystis jirovecii* (*P. carinii*) infections**

- **By mouth**

  **Child 1 month–18 years** 450 mg/m$^2$ (max. 960 mg) twice daily for three days of the week (either consecutively or on alternate days)

  **Note** dose regimens may vary, consult local guidelines

**Note** 480 mg of co-trimoxazole consists of sulfamethoxazole 400 mg and trimethoprim 80 mg

**Administration** for intermittent intravenous infusion may be further diluted in glucose 5% and 10% or sodium chloride 0.9%. Dilute contents of 1 ampoule (5 mL) to 125 mL, 2 ampoules (10 mL) to 250 mL or 3 ampoules (15 mL) to 500 mL; suggested duration of infusion 60–90 minutes (but may be adjusted according to fluid requirements); if fluid restriction necessary, 1 ampoule (5 mL) may be diluted with 75 mL glucose 5% and the required dose infused over max. 60 minutes; check container for haze or precipitant during administration. In severe fluid restriction may be given undiluted via a central venous line

**Co-trimoxazole** (Non-proprietary) [PoM]

Tablets, co-trimoxazole 480 mg, net price 28-tab pack = £18.99; 960 mg, 100 = £23.46. Label: 9
**Brands include** *Fectrim®, Fectrim® Forte*

Paediatric oral suspension, co-trimoxazole 240 mg/5 mL, net price 100 mL = £1.12. Label: 9

Oral suspension, co-trimoxazole 480 mg/5 mL. Net price 100 mL = £4.41. Label: 9

**Septrin®** (Aspen) [PoM]

Tablets, co-trimoxazole 480 mg, net price 100-tab pack = £15.52. Label: 9

Forte tablets, scored, co-trimoxazole 960 mg, net price 100-tab pack = £23.46. Label: 9

Adult suspension, co-trimoxazole 480 mg/5 mL, net price 100 mL (vanilla-flavoured) = £4.41. Label: 9

Paediatric suspension, sugar-free, co-trimoxazole 240 mg/5 mL. Net price 100 mL (banana- and vanilla-flavoured) = £2.45. Label: 9

Intravenous infusion, co-trimoxazole 96 mg/mL. To be diluted before use. Net price 5-mL amp = £1.78
**Electrolytes** Na$^+$ 1.7 mmol/5 mL
**Excipients** include alcohol 13.2%, propylene glycol, sulfites

## ▌ TRIMETHOPRIM

**Cautions** predisposition to folate deficiency; manufacturer recommends blood counts on long-term therapy (but evidence of practical value unsatisfactory); neonates (specialist supervision required); acute porphyria (section 9.8.2); **interactions:** Appendix 1 (trimethoprim)

**Blood disorders** On long-term treatment, patients and their carers should be told how to recognise signs of blood disorders and advised to seek immediate medical attention if symptoms such as fever, sore throat, rash, mouth ulcers, purpura, bruising or bleeding develop

**Contra-indications** blood dyscrasias

**Renal impairment** use half normal dose after 3 days if estimated glomerular filtration rate 15–30 mL/minute/1.73 m$^2$; use half normal dose if estimated glomerular filtration rate less than 15 mL/minute/1.73 m$^2$ (monitor plasma-trimethoprim concentration if estimated glomerular filtration rate less than 10 mL/minute/1.73 m$^2$)

**Pregnancy** teratogenic risk in first trimester (folate antagonist); manufacturers advise avoid

**Breast-feeding** present in milk—short-term use not known to be harmful

**Side-effects** gastro-intestinal disturbances including nausea and vomiting, pruritus, rashes, hyperkalaemia, depression of haematopoiesis; rarely erythema multiforme, toxic epidermal necrolysis, photosensitivity and other allergic reactions including angioedema and anaphylaxis; aseptic meningitis reported

**Licensed use** not licensed for use in children under 6 weeks

## Indications and dose

**Urinary-tract infections; respiratory-tract infections**

- **By mouth**

  **Neonate** initially 3 mg/kg as a single dose then 1–2 mg/kg twice daily

  **Child 1 month–12 years** 4 mg/kg (max. 200 mg) twice daily

  *or*

  **Child 6 weeks–6 months** 25 mg twice daily

  **Child 6 months–6 years** 50 mg twice daily

  **Child 6–12 years** 100 mg twice daily

  **Child 12–18 years** 200 mg twice daily

**Prophylaxis of urinary-tract infection**

Table 2, section 5.1

**Pneumocystis pneumonia** see p. 344

**Trimethoprim** (Non-proprietary) (PoM)
Tablets, trimethoprim 100 mg, net price 28 = 94p;
200 mg, 14-tab pack = 91p. Label: 9
Brands include *Trimopan*®

Suspension, trimethoprim 50 mg/5 mL, net price
100 mL = £2.37. Label: 9

## 5.1.9 Antituberculosis drugs

Tuberculosis is treated in two phases—an *initial phase* using 4 drugs and a *continuation phase* using two drugs in fully sensitive cases. Treatment requires specialised knowledge, particularly where the disease involves resistant organisms or non-respiratory organs.

The regimens given below are recommended for the treatment of tuberculosis in the UK; variations occur in other countries. Either the unsupervised regimen or the supervised regimen described below should be used; the two regimens should **not** be used concurrently. Compliance with therapy is a major determinant of its success. Treatment needs to be carefully monitored in families in whom concordance may be problematic.

**Initial phase** The concurrent use of 4 drugs during the initial phase is designed to reduce the bacterial population as rapidly as possible and to prevent the emergence of drug-resistant bacteria. The drugs are best given as combination preparations, provided the respective dose of each drug is appropriate, unless the child is unable to swallow the tablets or one of the components cannot be given because of resistance or intolerance. The treatment of choice for the initial phase is the daily use of isoniazid, rifampicin, pyrazinamide and ethambutol. However, care is needed in young children receiving ethambutol because of the difficulty in testing eyesight and in obtaining reports of visual symptoms (see below). Treatment should be started without waiting for culture results if clinical features or histology results are consistent with tuberculosis; treatment should be continued even if initial culture results are negative. The initial phase drugs should be continued for 2 months. Where a positive culture for *M. tuberculosis* has been obtained, but susceptibility results are not available after 2 months, treatment with rifampicin, isoniazid, pyrazinamide and ethambutol should be continued until full susceptibility is confirmed, even if this is for longer than 2 months.

Streptomycin is rarely used in the UK although it may be used in the initial phase of treatment if resistance to isoniazid has been established before therapy is commenced and ethambutol is contra-indicated.

**Continuation phase** After the initial phase, treatment is continued for a further 4 months with isoniazid and rifampicin (preferably given as a combination preparation). Longer treatment is necessary for meningitis, direct spinal cord involvement, and for resistant organisms which may also require modification of the regimen.

**Unsupervised treatment** The following regimen should be used for those who are likely to take antituberculous drugs reliably **without supervision** by a healthcare worker. Children and families who are unlikely to comply with daily administration of antituberculous drugs should be treated with the regimen described under Supervised Treatment.

### Recommended dosage for standard unsupervised 6-month treatment

| | |
|---|---|
| **Isoniazid** (for 6 months) | Child 1 month–18 years 10 mg/kg (max. 300 mg) once daily |
| **Rifampicin** (for 6 months) | Child 1 month–18 years 15 mg/kg once daily (max. 450 mg daily if body-weight under 50 kg; max. 600 mg daily if body-weight 50 kg and over) |
| **Pyrazinamide** (for 2-month initial phase only) | Child 1 month–18 years 35 mg/kg once daily (max. 1.5 g daily if body-weight under 50 kg; max. 2 g daily if body-weight 50 kg and over) |
| **Ethambutol** (for 2-month initial phase only) | Child 1 month–18 years 20 mg/kg once daily |

Note In general, doses should be rounded up to facilitate administration of suitable volumes of liquid or an appropriate strength of tablet. The exception is ethambutol due to the risk of toxicity. Doses may also need to be recalculated to allow for weight gain in younger children.
The fixed-dose combination preparations (*Rifater*®, *Rifinah*®) are unlicensed for use in children. Consideration may be given to use of these preparations in older children, provided the respective dose of each drug is appropriate for the weight of the child.

**Pregnancy** The standard regimen (above) may be used during pregnancy. Streptomycin should not be given in pregnancy.

**Breast-feeding** The standard regimen (above) may be used during breast-feeding.

**Neonates** Congenital tuberculosis is acquired from maternal extrapulmonary sites at birth, particularly the genital tract; if infection is suspected, the baby will require treatment with isoniazid 10 mg/kg once daily, rifampicin 15 mg/kg once daily, pyrazinamide 35 mg/kg once daily, and ethambutol 20 mg/kg once daily. Isoniazid, rifampicin, pyrazinamide, and ethambutol are used for 2 months during the initial phase of treatment. After the initial phase, treatment is continued for a further 4 months with isoniazid and rifampicin.

**Supervised treatment** Drug administration needs to be **fully supervised** by a healthcare worker (directly observed therapy, DOT) in children or families who cannot comply reliably with the treatment regimen. These patients are given isoniazid, rifampicin, pyrazinamide and ethambutol (or streptomycin) 3 times a week under supervision for the first 2 months followed by

**5 Infections**

isoniazid and rifampicin 3 times a week for a further 4 months.

## Recommended dosage for intermitttent supervised 6-month treatment

| | |
|---|---|
| **Isoniazid** (for 6 months) | Child 1 month–18 years 15 mg/kg (max. 900 mg) 3 times a week |
| **Rifampicin** (for 6 months) | Child 1 month–18 years 15 mg/kg (max. 900 mg) 3 times a week |
| **Pyrazinamide** (for 2-month initial phase only) | Child 1 month–18 years 50 mg/kg 3 times a week (max. 2 g 3 times a week if body-weight under 50 kg; max. 2.5 g 3 times a week if body-weight 50 kg and over) |
| **Ethambutol** (for 2-month initial phase only) | Child 1 month–18 years 30 mg/kg 3 times a week |

**Note** In general, doses should be rounded up to facilitate administration of suitable volumes of liquid or an appropriate strength of tablet. The exception is ethambutol due to the risk of toxicity. Doses may also need to be recalculated to allow for weight gain in younger children.
The fixed-dose combination preparations (*Rifater*®, *Rifinah*®) are unlicensed for use in children. Consideration may be given to use of these preparations in older children, provided the respective dose of each drug is appropriate for the weight of the child.

**Immunocompromised patients**   Multi-resistant *Mycobacterium tuberculosis* may be present in immuno-compromised children. The organism should always be cultured to confirm its type and drug sensitivity. Confirmed *M. tuberculosis* infection sensitive to first-line drugs should be treated with a standard 6-month regimen; after completing treatment, children should be closely monitored. The regimen may need to be modified if infection is caused by resistant organisms, and specialist advice is needed.

Specialist advice should be sought about tuberculosis treatment or chemoprophylaxis in a HIV-positive individual; care is required in choosing the regimen and in avoiding potentially serious interactions. Starting anti-retroviral treatment in the first 2 months of anti-tuberculosis treatment increases the risk of immune reconstitution syndrome.

Infection may also be caused by other mycobacteria e.g. *M. avium* complex in which case specialist advice on management is needed.

**Corticosteroids**   A corticosteroid should be given (in addition to antituberculosis therapy) for meningeal or pericardial tuberculosis.

**Prevention of tuberculosis**   Chemoprophylaxis may be required in children who are close contacts of a case of smear-positive pulmonary tuberculosis and who are severely immunosuppressed (including congenital immunodeficiencies, cytotoxic or immunosuppressive therapy) and in those who have evidence of latent tuberculosis and require treatment with immuno-suppressants; expert advice should be sought.

Chemoprophylaxis involves use of either isoniazid alone for 6 months or of isoniazid and rifampicin for 3 months (see Table 2, section 5.1).

For prevention of tuberculosis in susceptible close contacts or those who have become tuberculin-positive, see Table 2, section 5.1. For advice on immunisation against tuberculosis and tuberculin testing, see section 14.4.

**Monitoring**   Since isoniazid, rifampicin and pyrazinamide are associated with liver toxicity, *hepatic function* should be checked before treatment with these drugs. Those with pre-existing liver disease should have frequent checks particularly in the first 2 months. If there is no evidence of liver disease (and pre-treatment liver function is normal), further checks are only necessary if the patient develops fever, malaise, vomiting, jaundice or unexplained deterioration during treatment. In view of the need to comply fully with antituberculous treatment on the one hand and to guard against serious liver damage on the other, children and their carers should be informed carefully how to recognise signs of liver disorders and advised to discontinue treatment and seek **immediate** medical attention should symptoms of liver disease occur.

*Renal function* should be checked before treatment with antituberculous drugs and appropriate dosage adjustments made. Streptomycin or ethambutol should preferably be avoided in patients with renal impairment, but if used, the dose should be reduced and the plasma-drug concentration monitored.

*Visual acuity* should be tested before ethambutol is used (see below).

> Major causes of treatment failure are incorrect prescribing by the physician and inadequate compliance by the child or their carer. Monthly tablet counts and urine examination (rifampicin imparts an orange-red coloration) may be useful indicators of compliance with treatment. Avoid both excessive and inadequate dosage. Treatment should be supervised by a specialist paediatrician.

**Isoniazid** is cheap and highly effective. Like rifampicin it should always be included in any antituberculous regimen unless there is a specific contra-indication. Its only common side-effect is peripheral neuropathy which is more likely to occur where there are pre-existing risk factors such as diabetes, chronic renal failure, pregnancy, malnutrition and HIV infection. In these circumstances pyridoxine (section 9.6.2) should be given prophylactically from the start of treatment. Other side-effects such as hepatitis (important: see Monitoring above) and psychosis are rare.

**Rifampicin**, a rifamycin, is a key component of any antituberculous regimen. Like isoniazid it should always be included unless there is a specific contra-indication.

During the first two months ('initial phase') of rifampicin administration transient disturbance of liver function with elevated serum transaminases is common but generally does not require interruption of treatment. Occasionally more serious liver toxicity requires a change of treatment particularly in those with pre-existing liver disease (important: see Monitoring above).

On intermittent treatment six toxicity syndromes have been recognised—influenza-like, abdominal, and respiratory symptoms, shock, renal failure, and thrombocytopenic purpura—and can occur in 20 to 30% of patients.

Rifampicin induces hepatic enzymes which accelerate the metabolism of several drugs including oestrogens, corticosteroids, phenytoin, sulfonylureas, and anticoagulants; **interactions**: Appendix 1 (rifamycins). **Important**: the effectiveness of hormonal contraceptives is reduced and alternative family planning advice should be offered (section 7.3.1).

**Rifabutin** is indicated in adults for *prophylaxis* against *M. avium* complex infections in patients with a low CD4 count; it is also licensed in adults for the *treatment* of non-tuberculous mycobacterial disease and pulmonary tuberculosis. There is limited experience in children. As with rifampicin it induces hepatic enzymes and the effectiveness of hormonal contraceptives is reduced requiring alternative family planning methods.

**Pyrazinamide** is a bactericidal drug only active against intracellular dividing forms of *Mycobacterium tuberculosis*; it exerts its main effect only in the first two or three months. It is particularly useful in tuberculous meningitis because of good meningeal penetration. It is not active against *M. bovis*. Serious liver toxicity may occasionally occur (important: see Monitoring above).

**Ethambutol** is included in a treatment regimen if isoniazid resistance is suspected; it can be omitted if the risk of resistance is low.

Side-effects of ethambutol are largely confined to visual disturbances in the form of loss of acuity, colour blindness, and restriction of visual fields. These toxic effects are more common where excessive dosage is used or if the child's renal function is impaired. The earliest features of ocular toxicity are subjective and children and their carers should be advised to discontinue therapy immediately if deterioration in vision develops and promptly seek further advice. Early discontinuation of the drug is almost always followed by recovery of eyesight. Those who cannot understand warnings about visual side-effects should, if possible, be given an alternative drug. In particular, ethambutol should be used with caution in children until they are at least 5 years old and capable of reporting symptomatic visual changes accurately.

Where possible visual acuity should be tested by Snellen chart before treatment with ethambutol.

**Streptomycin** is now rarely used in the UK except for resistant organisms. Plasma-drug concentration should be measured in patients with impaired renal function in whom streptomycin must be used with great care.

Drug-resistant tuberculosis should be treated by a specialist paediatrician with experience in such cases, and where appropriate facilities for infection-control exist. Second-line drugs available for infections caused by resistant organisms, or when first-line drugs cause unacceptable side-effects, include amikacin, capreomycin, cycloserine, newer macrolides (e.g. azithromycin and clarithromycin), quinolones (e.g. moxifloxacin) and protionamide (prothionamide; no longer on UK market). Availability of suitable formulations may limit choice in children.

## CYCLOSERINE

**Cautions** monitor haematological, renal, and hepatic function; **interactions**: Appendix 1 (cycloserine)

**Contra-indications** epilepsy, depression, severe anxiety, psychotic states, alcohol dependence, acute porphyria (section 9.8.2)

**Renal impairment** increase interval between doses if creatinine clearance less than 50 mL/minute/1.73m² and monitor blood-cycloserine concentration

**Pregnancy** manufacturer advises use only if potential benefit outweighs risk—crosses the placenta

**Breast-feeding** present in milk—amount too small to be harmful

**Side-effects** mainly neurological, including headache, dizziness, vertigo, drowsiness, tremor, convulsions, confusion, psychosis, depression (discontinue or reduce dose if symptoms of CNS toxicity); rashes, allergic dermatitis (discontinue or reduce dose); megaloblastic anaemia; changes in liver function tests; heart failure at high doses reported

**Pharmacokinetics** blood concentration should not exceed a peak concentration of 30 mg/litre (measured 3–4 hours after the dose); penetrates CNS

**Licensed use** licensed for use in children (age range not specified by manufacturer)

### Indications and dose

**Tuberculosis resistant to first-line drugs, used in combination with other drugs**

• By mouth

   **Child 2–12 years** initially 5 mg/kg (max. 250 mg) twice daily, adjusted according to blood concentration and response up to 10 mg/kg (max. 500 mg) twice daily

   **Child 12–18 years** initially 250 mg twice daily for 2 weeks adjusted according to blood concentration and response to max. 500 mg twice daily

**Cycloserine** (King) [PoM]
Capsules, red/grey cycloserine 250 mg, net price 100-cap pack = £333.80. Label: 2, 8

## ETHAMBUTOL HYDROCHLORIDE

**Cautions** test visual acuity before treatment and warn patients to report visual changes—see notes above; young children (see notes above)—routine ophthalmological monitoring recommended

**Contra-indications** optic neuritis, poor vision

**Renal impairment** if creatinine clearance less than 30 mL/minute/1.73 m², use 15–25 mg/kg (max. 2.5 g) 3 times a week and monitor plasma-ethambutol concentration; risk of optic nerve damage

**Pregnancy** not known to be harmful; see also p. 293

**Breast-feeding** amount too small to be harmful; see also p. 293

**Side-effects** optic neuritis, red/green colour blindness, peripheral neuritis, rarely rash, pruritus, urticaria, thrombocytopenia

**Pharmacokinetics** 'peak' concentration (2–2.5 hours after dose) should be 2–6 mg/litre (7–22 micromol/litre); 'trough' (pre-dose) concentration should be less than 1 mg/litre (4 micromol/litre)

### Indications and dose

**Tuberculosis, used in combination with other drugs** see notes above

**Ethambutol** (Non-proprietary) [PoM]
Tablets, ethambutol hydrochloride 100 mg, net price 56-tab pack = £12.00; 400 mg, 56-tab pack = £44.18. Label: 8

## ISONIAZID

**Cautions** see Monitoring in notes above; also slow acetylator status (increased risk of side-effects); epilepsy; history of psychosis; alcohol dependence, malnutrition, diabetes mellitus, HIV infection (risk of peripheral neuritis); acute porphyria (section 9.8.2); **interactions:** Appendix 1 (isoniazid)

**Hepatic disorders** Children and their carers should be told how to recognise signs of liver disorder, and advised to discontinue treatment and seek immediate medical attention if symptoms such as persistent nausea, vomiting, malaise or jaundice develop

**Contra-indications** drug-induced liver disease

**Hepatic impairment** use with caution; monitor liver function regularly and particularly frequently in the first 2 months; see also Hepatic Disorders above

**Renal impairment** risk of ototoxicity and peripheral neuropathy; prophylactic pyridoxine recommended

**Pregnancy** not known to be harmful; prophylactic pyridoxine recommended; see also p. 293

**Breast-feeding** monitor infant for possible toxicity; theoretical risk of convulsions and neuropathy; prophylactic pyridoxine advisable in mother; see also p. 293

**Side-effects** nausea, vomiting, constipation, dry mouth; peripheral neuritis with high doses (pyridoxine prophylaxis, see notes above), optic neuritis, convulsions, psychotic episodes, vertigo; hypersensitivity reactions including fever, Stevens-Johnson syndrome, purpura; blood disorders including agranulocytosis, haemolytic anaemia, aplastic anaemia; hepatitis; pancreatitis; interstitial pneumonitis; systemic lupus erythematosus-like syndrome, pellagra, hyperreflexia, difficulty with micturition, hyperglycaemia, and gynaecomastia reported; hearing loss and tinnitus (in children with end-stage renal impairment); when used with tyramine or histamine rich foods, tachycardia, palpitation, hypotension, flushing, headache, dizziness, and sweating also reported

**Indications and dose**

> Tuberculosis, used in combination with other drugs see notes above

**Isoniazid** (Non-proprietary) [PoM]

Tablets, isoniazid 50 mg, net price 56-tab pack = £11.10; 100 mg, 28-tab pack = £11.30. Label: 8, 22

Injection, isoniazid 25 mg/mL, net price 2-mL amp = £11.04

## ▎ PYRAZINAMIDE

**Cautions** see Monitoring in notes above; also diabetes; **interactions:** Appendix 1 (pyrazinamide)

**Hepatic disorders** Children and their carers should be told how to recognise signs of liver disorder, and advised to discontinue treatment and seek immediate medical attention if symptoms such as persistent nausea, vomiting, malaise or jaundice develop

**Contra-indications** acute porphyria (section 9.8.2)

**Hepatic impairment** monitor hepatic function—idiosyncratic hepatotoxicity more common; avoid in severe hepatic impairment; see also Hepatic Disorders above

**Renal impairment** if estimated glomerular filtration rate less than 30 mL/minute/1.73 m², use 25–30 mg/kg 3 times a week

**Pregnancy** manufacturer advises use only if potential benefit outweighs risk; see also p. 293

**Breast-feeding** amount too small to be harmful; see also p. 293

**Side-effects** hepatotoxicity including fever, anorexia, hepatomegaly, splenomegaly, jaundice, liver failure; nausea, vomiting, dysuria, arthralgia, sideroblastic

anaemia, thrombocytopenia, rash and occasionally photosensitivity

**Indications and dose**

> Tuberculosis in combination with other drugs see notes above

**Zinamide®** (Genus)

Tablets, scored, pyrazinamide 500 mg, net price 30-tab pack = £31.35. Label: 8

## ▎ RIFABUTIN

**Cautions** see under Rifampicin; acute porphyria (section 9.8.2)

**Contra-indications** rifamycin hypersensitivity

**Hepatic impairment** reduce dose in severe impairment

**Renal impairment** use half normal dose if estimated glomerular filtration rate less than 30 mL/minute/1.73 m²

**Pregnancy** manufacturer advises avoid—no information available

**Breast-feeding** manufacturer advises avoid—no information available

**Side-effects** nausea, vomiting; leucopenia, thrombocytopenia, anaemia, rarely haemolysis; raised liver enzymes, jaundice, rarely hepatitis; uveitis following high doses or administration with drugs which raise plasma concentration—see also **interactions:** Appendix 1 (rifamycins); arthralgia, myalgia, influenza-like syndrome, dyspnoea; also hypersensitivity reactions including fever, rash, eosinophilia, bronchospasm, shock; skin, urine, saliva and other body secretions coloured orange-red; asymptomatic corneal opacities reported with long-term use

**Licensed use** not licensed for use in children

**Indications and dose**

> Prophylaxis of *Mycobacterium avium* complex infections in immunosuppressed patients with low CD4 count (see product literature) Also see notes above
> * **By mouth**
>   **Child 1–12 years** 5 mg/kg (max. 300 mg) once daily
>   **Child 12–18 years** 300 mg once daily

> Treatment of non-tuberculous mycobacterial disease, in combination with other drugs
> * **By mouth**
>   **Child 1month–12 years** 5 mg/kg once daily for up to 6 months after cultures negative
>   **Child 12–18 years** 450–600 mg once daily for up to 6 months after cultures negative

> Treatment of pulmonary tuberculosis, in combination with other drugs
> * **By mouth**
>   **Child 12–18 years** 150–450 mg daily for at least 6 months

**Mycobutin®** (Pharmacia) [PoM]

Capsules, red-brown, rifabutin 150 mg. Net price 30-cap pack = £90.38. Label: 8, 14, counselling, lenses, see under Rifampicin

# ■ RIFAMPICIN

**Cautions** see Monitoring in notes above; also liver function tests and blood counts in hepatic disorders, and on prolonged therapy, see also below; acute porphyria (section 9.8.2); **important:** effectiveness of hormonal contraceptives is reduced and alternative family planning advice should be offered (see also section 7.3.1); discolours soft contact lenses; see also notes above; **interactions:** Appendix 1 (rifamycins)
**Note** If treatment interrupted re-introduce with low dosage and increase gradually; discontinue permanently if serious side-effects develop
**Hepatic disorders** Children and their carers should be told how to recognise signs of liver disorder, and advised to discontinue treatment and seek immediate medical attention if symptoms such as persistent nausea, vomiting, malaise or jaundice develop

**Contra-indications** jaundice; rifamycin hypersensitivity

**Hepatic impairment** impaired elimination; monitor liver function; avoid or do not exceed 8 mg/kg daily; see also Cautions above

**Renal impairment** use with caution if dose above 10 mg/kg daily

**Pregnancy** manufacturers advise very high doses teratogenic in *animal* studies in first trimester; risk of neonatal bleeding may be increased in third trimester; see also p. 293

**Breast-feeding** amount too small to be harmful; see also p. 293

**Side-effects** gastro-intestinal symptoms including anorexia, nausea, vomiting, diarrhoea (antibiotic-associated colitis reported); headache, drowsiness; those occurring mainly on intermittent therapy include influenza-like symptoms (with chills, fever, dizziness, bone pain), respiratory symptoms (including shortness of breath), collapse and shock, haemolytic anaemia, disseminated intravascular coagulation and acute renal failure, thrombocytopenic purpura; alterations of liver function, jaundice; flushing, urticaria, and rashes; other side-effects reported include oedema, psychoses, adrenal insufficiency, muscular weakness and myopathy, exfoliative dermatitis, toxic epidermal necrolysis, Stevens-Johnson syndrome, pemphigoid reactions, leucopenia, eosinophilia, menstrual disturbances; urine, saliva, and other body secretions coloured orange-red; thrombophlebitis reported if infusion used for prolonged period

**Licensed use** not licensed for use in children for pruritus due to cholestasis

**Indications and dose**

Tuberculosis, in combination with other drugs see notes above

Prophylaxis of meningococcal meningitis and *Haemophilus influenzae* (type b) infection Table 2, section 5.1

Brucellosis, legionnaires disease, serious staphylococcal infections, in combination with other antibacterials
• By mouth or by intravenous infusion
　**Neonates** 5–10 mg/kg twice daily
　**Child 1 month–1 year** 5–10 mg/kg twice daily
　**Child 1–18 years** 10 mg/kg (max. 600 mg) twice daily

Pruritus due to cholestasis
• By mouth
　**Child 1 month–18 years** 5–10 mg/kg (max. 600 mg) once daily

**Administration** Displacement value may be significant, consult local reconstitution guidelines; reconstitute with solvent provided. May be further diluted with glucose 5% or sodium chloride 0.9% to a final concentration of 1.2 mg/mL. Infuse over 2–3 hours.

**Rifampicin** (Non-proprietary) (PoM)
Capsules, rifampicin 150 mg, net price 100 = £20.82; 300 mg, 100 = £46.21. Label: 8, 14, 22, counselling, see contact lenses above

**Rifadin®** (Sanofi-Aventis) (PoM)
Capsules, rifampicin 150 mg (blue/red), net price 100-cap pack = £18.32; 300 mg (red), 100-cap pack = £36.63. Label: 8, 14, 22, counselling, see contact lenses above
Syrup, red, rifampicin 100 mg/5 mL (raspberry-flavoured). Net price 120 mL = £3.56. Label: 8, 14, 22, counselling, see contact lenses above
**Excipients** include sucrose
Intravenous infusion, powder for reconstitution, rifampicin. Net price 600-mg vial (with solvent) = £7.67
**Electrolytes** Na$^+$< 0.5 mmol/vial

**Rimactane®** (Sandoz) (PoM)
Capsules, rifampicin 150 mg (red), net price 60-cap pack = £11.35; 300 mg (red/brown), 60-cap pack = £22.69. Label: 8, 14, 22, counselling, see contact lenses above

◀ **Combined preparations**
See notes above

**Rifater®** (Sanofi-Aventis) (PoM)
Tablets, pink, s/c, rifampicin 120 mg, isoniazid 50 mg, pyrazinamide 300 mg. Net price 100-tab pack = £21.95. Label: 8, 14, 22, counselling, see contact lenses above

**Rifinah® 150/100** (Sanofi-Aventis) (PoM)
Tablets, pink, s/c, rifampicin 150 mg, isoniazid 100 mg, net price 84-tab pack = £15.91. Label: 8, 14, 22, counselling, see contact lenses above

**Rifinah® 300/150** (Sanofi-Aventis) (PoM)
Tablets, orange, s/c, rifampicin 300 mg, isoniazid 150 mg, net price 56-tab pack = £21.02. Label: 8, 14, 22, counselling, see contact lenses above
**Note** Some stock packaged as *Rifinah 150/300*

# ■ STREPTOMYCIN

**Cautions** see under Aminoglycosides, section 5.1.4; measure plasma-concentration in renal impairment; interactions: Appendix 1 (aminoglycosides)

**Contra-indications** see under Aminoglycosides, section 5.1.4

**Renal impairment** see under Aminoglycosides, section 5.1.4

**Pregnancy** see under Aminoglycosides, section 5.1.4

**Side-effects** see under Aminoglycosides, section 5.1.4; also hypersensitivity reactions, paraesthesia of mouth

**5 Infections**

**Pharmacokinetics** one-hour ('peak') concentration should be 15–40 mg/litre; pre-dose ('trough') concentration should be less than 5 mg/litre (less than 1 mg/litre in renal impairment)

**Licensed use** not licensed for use in children

**Indications and dose**

> Tuberculosis, resistant to other treatment, in combination with other drugs
> * By deep intramuscular injection
>> **Child 1 month–18 years** 15 mg/kg (max. 1 g) once daily

> Adjunct to doxycycline in brucellosis, expert advice essential
> * By deep intramuscular injection
>> **Child 1 month–18 years** 5–10 mg/kg every 6 hours; total daily dose may alternatively be given in 2–3 divided doses

**Important** Side-effects increase after a cumulative dose of 100 g, which should only be exceeded in exceptional circumstances

**Streptomycin Sulfate** (Non-proprietary) [PoM]
Injection, powder for reconstitution, streptomycin (as sulfate), net price 1-g vial = £8.25
Available as an unlicensed preparation from UCB Pharma

## 5.1.10 Antileprotic drugs

Classification not used in *BNF for Children*.

## 5.1.11 Metronidazole

**Metronidazole** is an antimicrobial drug with high activity against anaerobic bacteria and protozoa. It is also used for surgical and gynaecological sepsis in which its activity against colonic anaerobes, especially *Bacteroides fragilis*, is important. Metronidazole by mouth is effective for the treatment of *Clostridium difficile* infection (see also section 1.5); it can be given by intravenous infusion if oral treatment is inappropriate. Metronidazole is well absorbed orally and the intravenous route is normally reserved for severe infections. Metronidazole by the rectal route is an effective alternative to the intravenous route when oral administration is not possible. Intravenous metronidazole is used for the treatment of established cases of tetanus; diazepam (section 10.2.2) and tetanus immunoglobulin (section 14.5.2) are also used.

Topical metronidazole (section 13.10.1.2) reduces the odour produced by anaerobic bacteria in fungating tumours; it is also used in the management of rosacea (section 13.6).

**Oral infections** Metronidazole is an alternative to a penicillin for the treatment of many oral infections where the patient is allergic to penicillin or the infection is due to beta-lactamase-producing anaerobes (Table 1, section 5.1). It is the drug of first choice for the treatment of acute necrotising ulcerative gingivitis (Vincent's infection) and pericoronitis; amoxicillin is a suitable alternative (section 5.1.1.3). For these purposes treatment with metronidazole for 3 days is sufficient, but the duration of treatment may need to be longer in pericoronitis. Tinidazole is licensed for the treatment of acute ulcerative gingivitis.

## ▣ METRONIDAZOLE

**Cautions** disulfiram-like reaction with alcohol, clinical and laboratory monitoring advised if treatment exceeds 10 days; **interactions:** Appendix 1 (metronidazole)

**Hepatic impairment** in severe liver disease reduce total daily dose to one-third, and give once daily; use with caution in hepatic encephalopathy

**Pregnancy** manufacturer advises avoidance of high-dose regimens; use only if potential benefit outweighs risk

**Breast-feeding** significant amount in milk; manufacturer advises avoid large single doses though otherwise compatible; may give milk a bitter taste

**Side-effects** gastro-intestinal disturbances (including nausea and vomiting), taste disturbances, furred tongue, oral mucositis, anorexia; *very rarely* hepatitis, jaundice, pancreatitis, drowsiness, dizziness, headache, ataxia, psychotic disorders, darkening of urine, thrombocytopenia, pancytopenia, myalgia, arthralgia, visual disturbances, rash, pruritus, and erythema multiforme; on prolonged or intensive therapy peripheral neuropathy, transient epileptiform seizures, and leucopenia; also reported aseptic meningitis, optic neuropathy

**Indications and dose**

> Protozoal infections section 5.4.2

> Anaerobic infections (usually treated for 7 days and for 10–14 days in *Clostridium difficile* infection)
> * By mouth
>> **Child 1–2 months** 7.5 mg/kg every 12 hours
>> **Child 2 months–12 years** 7.5 mg/kg (max. 400 mg) every 8 hours
>> **Child 12–18 years** 400 mg every 8 hours
> * By rectum
>> **Child 1 month–1 year** 125 mg 3 times daily for 3 days, then twice daily thereafter
>> **Child 1–5 years** 250 mg 3 times daily for 3 days, then twice daily thereafter
>> **Child 5–10 years** 500 mg 3 times daily, for 3 days, then twice daily thereafter
>> **Child 10–18 years** 1 g 3 times daily for 3 days, then twice daily thereafter
> * By intravenous infusion over 20–30 minutes
>> **Neonate** 7.5 mg/kg every 12 hours
>> **Child 1–2 months** 7.5 mg/kg every 12 hours
>> **Child 2 months–18 years** 7.5 mg/kg (max. 500 mg) every 8 hours

> Pelvic inflammatory disease (see also Table 1, section 5.1)
> * By mouth
>> **Child 12–18 years** 400 mg twice daily for 14 days

> Acute ulcerative gingivitis and other acute dental infections
> * By mouth
>> **Child 1–3 years** 50 mg every 8 hours
>> **Child 3–7 years** 100 mg every 12 hours
>> **Child 7–10 years** 100 mg every 8 hours
>> **Child 10–18 years** 200–250 mg every 8 hours

*Helicobacter pylori* eradication section 1.3

### Surgical prophylaxis

- By mouth

  **Child 1 month–12 years** 30 mg/kg (max. 500 mg) 2 hours before the procedure

  **Child 12–18 years** 400–500 mg 2 hours before the procedure; up to 3 further doses of 400–500 mg may be given every 8 hours for high-risk procedures

- By intravenous infusion

  **Neonate under 40 weeks postmenstrual age** 10 mg/kg up to 30 minutes before the procedure

  **Neonate over 40 weeks postmenstrual age** 20–30 mg/kg up to 30 minutes before the procedure

  **Child 1 month–12 years** 30 mg/kg (max. 500 mg) up to 30 minutes before the procedure

  **Child 12–18 years** 500 mg up to 30 minutes before the procedure; up to 3 further doses of 500 mg may be given every 8 hours for high-risk procedures

- By rectum

  **Child 5–10 years** 500 mg 2 hours before surgery; up to 3 further doses of 500 mg may be given every 8 hours for high-risk procedures

  **Child 10–18 years** 1 g 2 hours before surgery; up to 3 further doses of 1 g may be given every 8 hours for high-risk procedures

**Metronidazole** (Non-proprietary) PoM

Tablets, metronidazole 200 mg, net price 21-tab pack = £1.36; 400 mg, 21-tab pack = £1.35. Label: 4, 9, 21, 25, 27

Brands include *Vaginyl*®

**Dental prescribing on NHS** Metronidazole Tablets may be prescribed

Tablets, metronidazole 500 mg, net price 21-tab pack = £29.84. Label: 4, 9, 21, 25, 27

**Dental prescribing on NHS** Metronidazole Tablets may be prescribed

Suspension, metronidazole (as benzoate) 200 mg/ 5 mL. Net price 100 mL = £11.43. Label: 4, 9

Brands include *Norzol*®

**Dental prescribing on NHS** Metronidazole Oral Suspension may be prescribed

Intravenous infusion, metronidazole 5 mg/mL. Net price 20-mL amp = £1.56, 100-mL container = £3.41

**Flagyl**® (Winthrop) PoM

Tablets, both f/c, ivory, metronidazole 200 mg, net price 21-tab pack = £4.49; 400 mg, 14-tab pack = £6.34. Label: 4, 9, 21, 25, 27

Suppositories, metronidazole 500 mg, net price 10 = £15.18; 1 g, 10 = £23.06. Label: 4, 9

**Metrolyl**® (Sandoz) PoM

Intravenous infusion, metronidazole 5 mg/mL, net price 100-mL Steriflex® bag = £1.22

Electrolytes Na⁺ 14.53 mmol/100-mL bag

Suppositories, metronidazole 500 mg, net price 10 = £12.34; 1 g, 10 = £18.34. Label: 4, 9

## 5.1.12 Quinolones

**Ciprofloxacin** is active against both Gram-positive and Gram-negative bacteria. It is particularly active against Gram-negative bacteria, including salmonella, shigella, campylobacter, neisseria, and pseudomonas. Ciprofloxacin has only moderate activity against Gram-positive bacteria such as *Streptococcus pneumoniae* and *Enterococcus faecalis*; it should not be used for pneumococcal pneumonia. It is active against chlamydia and some mycobacteria. Most anaerobic organisms are not susceptible. Ciprofloxacin is licensed in children over 1 year of age for pseudomonal infections in cystic fibrosis, for complicated urinary-tract infections, and for treatment and prophylaxis of inhalation anthrax. When the benefits of treatment outweigh the risks, ciprofloxacin is licensed in children over 1 year of age for severe infections of the respiratory tract and of the gastro-intestinal system (including typhoid fever). It is also used in the treatment of septicaemia caused by multi-resistant organisms (usually hospital acquired) and gonorrhoea (although resistance is increasing). Ciprofloxacin is also used in the prophylaxis of meningococcal disease.

**Nalidixic acid** may be used in uncomplicated urinary-tract infections that are resistant to other antibiotics.

Many staphylococci are resistant to quinolones and their use should be avoided in MRSA infections.

**Ofloxacin** eye drops are used in ophthalmic infections (section 11.3.1).

There is much less experience of the other quinolones in children; expert advice should be sought.

**Anthrax** *Inhalation* or *gastro-intestinal anthrax* should be treated initially with either **ciprofloxacin** or, in children over 12 years, **doxycycline** [unlicensed indication] (section 5.1.3) combined with one or two other antibacterials (such as amoxicillin, benzylpenicillin, chloramphenicol, clarithromycin, clindamycin, imipenem with cilastatin, rifampicin [unlicensed indication], and vancomycin). When the condition improves and the sensitivity of the *Bacillus anthracis* strain is known, treatment may be switched to a single antibacterial. Treatment should continue for 60 days because germination may be delayed.

*Cutaneous anthrax* should be treated with either ciprofloxacin [unlicensed indication] or doxycycline [unlicensed indication] (section 5.1.3) for 7 days. Treatment may be switched to amoxicillin (section 5.1.1.3) if the infecting strain is susceptible. Treatment may need to be extended to 60 days if exposure is due to aerosol. A combination of antibacterials for 14 days is recommended for cutaneous anthrax with systemic features, extensive oedema, or lesions of the head or neck.

Ciprofloxacin or doxycycline may be given for *post-exposure prophylaxis*. If exposure is confirmed, antibacterial prophylaxis should continue for 60 days. Antibacterial prophylaxis may be switched to amoxicillin after 10–14 days if the strain of *B. anthracis* is susceptible. Vaccination against anthrax (section 14.4) may allow the duration of antibacterial prophylaxis to be shortened.

**Cautions** Quinolones should be used with caution in children with a history of epilepsy or conditions that predispose to seizures, in G6PD deficiency (section 9.1.5), myasthenia gravis (risk of exacerbation). Exposure to excessive sunlight should be avoided (discontinue if photosensitivity occurs). Quinolones can pro-long the QT interval. Ciprofloxacin and nalidixic acid should be used with caution in children with risk factors for QT interval prolongation (e.g. electrolyte distur-bances, acute myocardial infarction, heart failure with reduced left ventricular ejection fraction, bradycardia, congenital long QT syndrome, concomitant use with other drugs known to prolong the QT interval, history of symptomatic arrhythmias). The CSM has warned that quinolones may induce **convulsions** in patients with or without a history of convulsions; taking NSAIDs at the same time may also induce them. Other **interactions:** Appendix 1 (quinolones).

Quinolones cause arthropathy in the weight-bearing joints of immature *animals* and are therefore generally not recommended in children and growing adolescents. However, the significance of this effect in humans is uncertain and in some specific circumstances short-term use of a quinolone in children is justified. Nalidixic acid is used for resistant urinary-tract infections in children over 3 months of age.

---

### Tendon damage

Tendon damage (including rupture) has been reported rarely in patients receiving quinolones. Tendon rupture may occur within 48 hours of start-ing treatment; cases have also been reported several months after stopping a quinolone. Healthcare pro-fessionals are reminded that:

- quinolones are contra-indicated in patients with a history of tendon disorders related to quinolone use;
- the risk of tendon damage is increased by the con-comitant use of corticosteroids;
- if tendinitis is suspected, the quinolone should be discontinued immediately.

---

**Contra-indications** Quinolone hypersensitivity.

**Pregnancy** Quinolones should be avoided in pregnancy because they have been shown to cause arthropathy in *animal* studies; safer alternatives are available; however, a single dose of ciprofloxacin may be used for the prevention of a secondary case of meningococcal meningitis.

**Side-effects** Side-effects of the quinolones include nausea, vomiting, diarrhoea (rarely antibiotic-associated colitis), headache, and dizziness. Less frequent side-effects include dyspepsia, abdominal pain, anorexia, sleep disturbances, asthenia, confusion, anxiety, depres-sion, hallucinations, tremor, blood disorders (including eosinophilia, leucopenia, thrombocytopenia), arthralgia, myalgia, rash (very rarely Stevens-Johnson syndrome and toxic epidermal necrolysis), disturbances in vision and taste. Other side-effects reported rarely or very rarely include hepatic dysfunction (including jaundice and hepatitis), hypotension, vasculitis, dyspnoea, con-vulsions, psychoses, paraesthesia, renal failure, inter-stitial nephritis, tendon inflammation and damage (see also Tendon Damage above), photosensitivity, distur-bances in hearing and smell. The drug should be **dis-continued** if psychiatric, neurological or hypersensi-tivity reactions (including severe rash) occur.

---

### ■ CIPROFLOXACIN

**Cautions** see notes above; avoid excessive alkalinity of urine and ensure adequate fluid intake (risk of

crystalluria); **interactions:** Appendix 1 (quinolones) **Skilled tasks** May impair performance of skilled tasks (e.g. driving)

**Contra-indications** see notes above

**Renal impairment** reduce dose if estimated glom-erular filtration rate less than 30 mL/minute/ 1.73 m$^2$—consult product literature

**Pregnancy** see notes above

**Breast-feeding** amount probably too small to be harmful but manufacturer advises avoid

**Side-effects** see notes above; also flatulence, pain and phlebitis at injection site; *rarely* dysphagia, pan-creatitis, chest pain, tachycardia, syncope, oedema, hot flushes, abnormal dreams, sweating, hyperglyc-aemia, and erythema nodosum; *very rarely* movement disorders, tinnitus, vasculitis, and tenosynovitis

**Licensed use** licensed for use in children over 1 year for complicated urinary-tract infections, for pseudo-monal lower respiratory-tract infections in cystic fibrosis, for prophylaxis and treatment of inhalational anthrax; licensed for use in children over 1 year for other infections where the benefit is considered to outweigh the potential risks; not licensed for use in children for gastro-intestinal anthrax; not licensed for use in children for prophylaxis of meningococcal meningitis; not licensed for use in children under 1 year of age

### Indications and dose

**Complicated urinary-tract infections**

- **By mouth**
  **Neonate** 10 mg/kg twice daily
  **Child 1 month–18 years** 10 mg/kg twice daily; dose doubled in severe infection (max. 750 mg twice daily)

- **By intravenous infusion over 60 minutes**
  **Neonate** 6 mg/kg every 12 hours
  **Child 1 month–18 years** 6 mg/kg every 8 hours; increased to 10 mg/kg every 8 hours in severe infection (max. 400 mg every 8 hours)

**Severe respiratory-tract infections, gastro-intes-tinal infections; see notes above**

- **By mouth**
  **Neonate** 15 mg/kg twice daily
  **Child 1 month–18 years** 20 mg/kg (max. 750 mg) twice daily

- **By intravenous infusion over 60 minutes**
  **Neonate** 10 mg/kg every 12 hours
  **Child 1 month–18 years** 10 mg/kg (max. 400 mg) every 8 hours

**Pseudomonal lower respiratory-tract infection in cystic fibrosis**

- **By mouth**
  **Child 1 month–18 years** 20 mg/kg (max. 750 mg) twice daily

- **By intravenous infusion over 60 minutes**
  **Child 1 month–18 years** 10 mg/kg (max. 400 mg) every 8 hours

**Gonorrhoea**

- **By mouth**
  **Child 12–18 years** 500 mg as a single dose

**Anthrax (treatment and post-exposure prophy-laxis, see notes above)**
- **By mouth**
  **Child 1 month–18 years** 15 mg/kg (max. 500 mg) twice daily
- **By intravenous infusion over 60 minutes**
  **Child 1 month–18 years** 10 mg/kg (max. 400 mg) every 12 hours

**Eye infections** section 11.3.1

**Prophylaxis of meningococcal meningitis** Table 2, section 5.1

**Ciprofloxacin** (Non-proprietary) PoM
Tablets, ciprofloxacin (as hydrochloride) 100 mg, net price 6-tab pack = £1.42; 250 mg, 10-tab pack = 96p, 20-tab pack = £1.09; 500 mg, 10-tab pack = £1.06, 20-tab pack = £1.22; 750 mg, 10-tab pack = £6.15. Label: 7, 9, 25, counselling, driving

Intravenous infusion, ciprofloxacin (as lactate) 2 mg/mL, net price 50-mL bottle = £8.00, 100-mL bottle = £15.00, 200-mL bottle = £22.00

**Ciproxin**® (Bayer) PoM
Tablets, all f/c, ciprofloxacin (as hydrochloride) 250 mg (scored), net price 10-tab pack = £6.59; 500 mg (scored), 10-tab pack = £12.49; 750 mg, 10-tab pack = £17.78. Label: 7, 9, 25, counselling, driving

Suspension, strawberry-flavoured, ciprofloxacin for reconstitution with diluent provided, 250 mg/5 mL, net price 100 mL = £16.83. Label: 7, 9, 25, counselling, driving

Intravenous infusion, ciprofloxacin (as lactate) 2 mg/mL, in sodium chloride 0.9%, net price 50-mL bottle = £7.61, 100-mL bottle = £15.02, 200-mL bottle = £22.85
Electrolytes  Na⁺ 15.4 mmol/100-mL bottle

---

### ◼ NALIDIXIC ACID

**Cautions**  see notes above; avoid in acute porphyria (section 9.8.2); false positive urinary glucose (if tested for reducing substances); monitor blood counts, renal and liver function if treatment exceeds 2 weeks; **interactions:** Appendix 1 (quinolones)
**Contra-indications**  see notes above
**Hepatic impairment**  manufacturer advises caution in liver disease
**Renal impairment**  use with caution; avoid if estimated glomerular filtration rate less than 20 mL/minute/1.73 m²
**Pregnancy**  see notes above
**Breast-feeding**  risk to infant very small but one case of haemolytic anaemia reported
**Side-effects**  see notes above; also reported toxic psychosis, increased intracranial pressure, cranial nerve palsy, peripheral neuropathy, metabolic acidosis
**Licensed use**  not licensed for use in children under 3 months of age

**Indications and dose**
**Urinary tract infection resistant to other antibiotics**
- **By mouth**
  **Child 3 months–12 years** 12.5 mg/kg 4 times daily for 7 days, reduced to 7.5 mg/kg 4 times daily in prolonged therapy or 15 mg/kg twice daily for prophylaxis
  **Child 12–18 years** 900 mg 4 times daily for 7 days, reduced in chronic infections to 600 mg 4 times daily

**Nalidixic acid** (Rosemont) PoM
Suspension, pink, nalidixic acid 300 mg/5 mL, net price 150 mL (raspberry- and strawberry-flavoured) = £12.50. Label: 9, 11
Excipients  include sucrose 450 mg/5 mL

---

## 5.1.13  Urinary-tract infections

Urinary-tract infection is more common in adolescent girls than in boys; when it occurs in adolescent boys there is frequently an underlying abnormality of the renal tract. Recurrent episodes of infection are an indication for radiological investigation especially in children in whom untreated pyelonephritis may lead to permanent kidney damage.

*Escherichia coli* is the most common cause of urinary-tract infection; *Staphylococcus saprophyticus* is also common in sexually active young women. Less common causes include Proteus and Klebsiella spp. *Pseudomonas aeruginosa* infections usually occur in the hospital setting and may be associated with functional or anatomical abnormalities of the renal tract. *Staphylococcus epidermidis* and *Enterococcus faecalis* infection may complicate catheterisation or instrumentation.

A specimen of urine should be collected for culture and sensitivity testing before starting antibacterial therapy;
- in children under 3 years of age;
- in children with suspected upper urinary-tract infection, complicated infection, or recurrent infection;
- if resistant organisms are suspected;
- if urine dipstick testing gives a single positive result for leucocyte esterase or nitrite;
- if clinical symptoms are not consistent with results of dipstick testing;
- in pregnant women.

Treatment should not be delayed while waiting for results. The antibacterial chosen should reflect current local bacterial sensitivity to antibacterials.

Urinary-tract infections in children require prompt antibacterial treatment to minimise the risk of renal scarring. Uncomplicated 'lower' urinary-tract infections in *children over 3 months* of age can be treated with trimethoprim, nitrofurantoin, a first generation cephalosporin, or amoxicillin for 3 days; children should be reassessed if they continue to be unwell 24–48 hours after the initial assessment.

Acute pyelonephritis in children over 3 months of age can be treated with a first generation cephalosporin or co-amoxiclav for 7–10 days. If the patient is severely ill, then the infection is best treated initially by intravenous injection of a broad-spectrum antibacterial such as cefotaxime or co-amoxiclav; gentamicin is an alternative.

*Children under 3 months of age* should be transferred to hospital and treated initially with intravenous antibacterials such as ampicillin with gentamicin, or cefotaxime alone, until the infection responds; full doses of oral antibacterials are then given for a further period.

**Resistant infections** Widespread bacterial resistance to ampicillin, amoxicillin, and trimethoprim has been reported. Alternatives for resistant organisms include co-amoxiclav (amoxicillin with clavulanic acid), an oral cephalosporin, pivmecillinam, or a quinolone.

**Antibacterial prophylaxis** Recurrent episodes of infection are an indication for imaging tests. *Antibacterial prophylaxis* with low doses of trimethoprim or nitrofurantoin may be considered for children with recurrent infection, significant urinary-tract anomalies, or significant kidney damage. Nitrofurantoin is contraindicated in children under 3 months of age because of the theoretical possibility of haemolytic anaemia.

**Pregnancy** Urinary-tract infection in *pregnancy* may be asymptomatic and requires prompt treatment to prevent progression to acute pyelonephritis. Penicillins and cephalosporins are suitable for treating urinary-tract infection during pregnancy. Nitrofurantoin may also be used but it should be avoided at term. Sulfonamides, quinolones, and tetracyclines should be avoided during pregnancy; trimethoprim should also preferably be avoided particularly in the first trimester.

**Renal impairment** In *renal failure* antibacterials normally excreted by the kidney accumulate with resultant toxicity unless the dose is reduced. This applies especially to the aminoglycosides which should be used with great caution; tetracyclines, methamine, and nitrofurantoin should be avoided altogether.

---

### ▋ NITROFURANTOIN

**Cautions** anaemia; diabetes mellitus; electrolyte imbalance; vitamin B and folate deficiency; pulmonary disease; on long-term therapy, monitor liver function and monitor for pulmonary symptoms (discontinue if deterioration in lung function); susceptibility to peripheral neuropathy; false positive urinary glucose (if tested for reducing substances); urine may be coloured yellow or brown; **interactions:** Appendix 1 (nitrofurantoin)

**Contra-indications** infants less than 3 months old, G6PD deficiency (section 9.1.5), acute porphyria (section 9.8.2)

**Hepatic impairment** use with caution; cholestatic jaundice and chronic active hepatitis reported

**Renal impairment** avoid if estimated glomerular filtration rate less than 60 mL/minute/1.73 m$^2$; risk of peripheral neuropathy; ineffective because of inadequate urine concentrations

**Pregnancy** avoid at term—may produce neonatal haemolysis

**Breast-feeding** avoid; only small amounts in milk but enough to produce haemolysis in G6PD-deficient infants (section 9.1.5)

**Side-effects** anorexia, nausea, vomiting, and diarrhoea; acute and chronic pulmonary reactions (pulmonary fibrosis reported; possible association with lupus erythematosus-like syndrome); peripheral neuropathy; also reported, hypersensitivity reactions (including angioedema, anaphylaxis, sialadenitis, urticaria, rash and pruritus); rarely, cholestatic jaun-

dice, hepatitis, exfoliative dermatitis, erythema multiforme, pancreatitis, arthralgia, blood disorders (including agranulocytosis, thrombocytopenia, and aplastic anaemia), benign intracranial hypertension, and transient alopecia

**Indications and dose**

**Acute uncomplicated urinary-tract infection**

● By mouth

**Child 3 months–12 years** 750 micrograms/kg 4 times daily for 3–7 days

**Child 12–18 years** 50 mg 4 times daily for 3–7 days; increased to 100 mg 4 times daily in severe chronic recurrent infections

**Prophylaxis of urinary-tract infection** (but see Cautions above)

Table 2, section 5.1

**Nitrofurantoin** (Non-proprietary) [PoM]
Tablets, nitrofurantoin 50 mg, net price 28-tab pack = £1.84; 100 mg, 28-tab pack = £4.43 Label: 9, 14, 21

Oral suspension, nitrofurantoin 25 mg/5 mL, net price 300 mL = £99.05. Label: 9, 14, 21
Note Sugar-free versions are available and can be ordered by specifying 'sugar-free' on the prescription

**Furadantin**® (Mercury) [PoM]
Tablets, all yellow, scored, nitrofurantoin 50 mg, net price 100-tab pack = £9.79; 100 mg, 100-tab pack = £18.11. Label: 9, 14, 21

**Macrodantin**® (Mercury) [PoM]
Capsules, yellow/white, nitrofurantoin 50 mg (as macrocrystals), net price 30-cap pack = £2.49; 100 mg (yellow/white), 30-cap pack = £4.81. Label: 9, 14, 21

◢ **Modified release**

**Macrobid**® (Mercury) [PoM]
Capsules, m/r, blue/yellow, nitrofurantoin 100 mg (as nitrofurantoin macrocrystals and nitrofurantoin monohydrate). Net price 14-cap pack = £4.89. Label: 9, 14, 21, 25

**Dose**

**Uncomplicated urinary-tract infection**

**Child 12–18 years** 1 capsule twice daily with food

**Genito-urinary surgical prophylaxis**

**Child 12–18 years** 1 capsule twice daily on day of procedure and for 3 days after

---

### 5.2  Antifungal drugs

**5.2.1  Triazole antifungals**

**5.2.2  Imidazole antifungals**

**5.2.3  Polyene antifungals**

**5.2.4  Echinocandin antifungals**

**5.2.5  Other antifungals**

---

### Treatment of fungal infections

The systemic treatment of common fungal infections is outlined below; specialist treatment is required in most forms of systemic or disseminated fungal infections. For local treatment of fungal infections, see section 7.2.2 (genital), section 7.4.4 (bladder), section 11.3.2 (eye), section 12.1.1 (ear), section 12.3.2 (oropharynx), and section 13.10.2 (skin).

**Aspergillosis**  Aspergillosis most commonly affects the respiratory tract but in severely immunocompromised patients, invasive forms can affect the heart, brain, and skin. **Voriconazole** (section 5.2.1) is the treatment of choice for aspergillosis; **liposomal amphotericin** (section 5.2.3) is an alternative first-line treatment when voriconazole cannot be used. **Caspofungin** (section 5.2.4) or **itraconazole** (section 5.2.1) can be used in patients who are refractory to, or intolerant of voriconazole and liposomal amphotericin. Itraconazole is also used for the treatment of chronic pulmonary aspergillosis or as an adjunct in the treatment of allergic bronchopulmonary aspergillosis.

**Candidiasis**  Many superficial candidal infections, including infections of the skin (section 13.10.2), are treated locally. Systemic antifungal treatment is required in widespread or intractable infection. Vaginal candidiasis can be treated with locally acting antifungals (section 7.2.2); alternatively, **fluconazole** (section 5.2.1) can be given by mouth.

*Oropharyngeal candidiasis* generally responds to topical therapy (section 12.3.2). Fluconazole is given by mouth for unresponsive infections; it is reliably absorbed and is effective. **Itraconazole** (section 5.2.1) can be used for infections that do not respond to fluconazole. Topical therapy may not be adequate in immunocompromised children and an oral triazole antifungal is preferred.

For *invasive or disseminated candidiasis*, either **amphotericin** (section 5.2.3) by intravenous infusion or an **echinocandin** (section 5.2.4) can be used. **Fluconazole** (section 5.2.1) is an alternative for *Candida albicans* infection in clinically stable children who have not received an azole antifungal recently. Amphotericin should be considered for the initial treatment of CNS candidiasis. **Voriconazole** (section 5.2.1) can be used for infections caused by fluconazole-resistant *Candida* spp. when oral therapy is required, or in children intolerant of amphotericin or an echinocandin. In refractory cases, **flucytosine** (section 5.2.5) can be used with intravenous amphotericin.

**Cryptococcosis**  Cryptococcosis is uncommon but infection in the immunocompromised, especially HIV-positive children, can be life-threatening; cryptococcal meningitis is the most common form of fungal meningitis. The treatment of choice in cryptococcal meningitis is **amphotericin** (section 5.2.3) by intravenous infusion with **flucytosine** (section 5.2.5) by intravenous infusion for 2 weeks, followed by **fluconazole** (section 5.2.1) by mouth for 8 weeks or until cultures are negative. In cryptococcosis, fluconazole is sometimes given alone as an alternative in HIV-positive children with mild localised infection or in those who cannot tolerate amphotericin. Following successful treatment, fluconazole can be used for prophylaxis against relapse until immunity recovers.

**Histoplasmosis**  Histoplasmosis is rare in temperate climates; it can be life-threatening, particularly in HIV-infected children. **Itraconazole** (section 5.2.1) can be used for the treatment of immunocompetent children with indolent non-meningeal infection, including chronic pulmonary histoplasmosis. **Amphotericin** (section 5.2.3) by intravenous infusion is preferred in children with fulminant or severe infections. Following successful treatment, itraconazole can be used for prophylaxis against relapse until immunity recovers.

**Skin and nail infections**  Mild localised fungal infections of the skin (including tinea corporis, tinea cruris, and tinea pedis) respond to topical therapy (section 13.10.2). Systemic therapy is appropriate if topical therapy fails, if many areas are affected, or if the site of infection is difficult to treat such as in infections of the nails (onychomycosis) and of the scalp (tinea capitis).

Oral imidazole or triazole antifungals (particularly **itraconazole**) and **terbinafine** are used more frequently than griseofulvin because they have a broader spectrum of activity and require a shorter duration of treatment.

*Tinea capitis* is treated systemically; additional topical application of an antifungal (section 13.10.2) may reduce transmission. **Griseofulvin** (section 5.2.5) is used for tinea capitis; it is effective against infections caused by *Trichophyton tonsurans* and *Microsporum* spp. **Terbinafine** (section 5.2.5) is used for tinea capitis caused by *T. tonsurans* [unlicensed indication]; the role of terbinafine in the management of *Microsporum* infections is uncertain. **Fluconazole** (section 5.2.1) or **itraconazole** (section 5.2.1) are alternatives in the treatment of tinea capitis caused by *T. tonsurans* or *Microsporum* spp. [both unlicensed indications].

*Pityriasis versicolor* (section 13.10.2) may be treated with **itraconazole** (section 5.2.1) by mouth if topical therapy is ineffective; **fluconazole** (section 5.2.1) by mouth is an alternative. Oral **terbinafine** is **not** effective for pityriasis versicolor.

Antifungal treatment may not be necessary in asymptomatic children with tinea infection of the nails. If treatment is necessary, a systemic antifungal is more effective than topical therapy. **Terbinafine** (section 5.2.5) and **itraconazole** (section 5.2.1) have largely replaced griseofulvin for the systemic treatment of *onychomycosis*, particularly of the toenail; they should be used under specialist advice. Although terbinafine is not licensed for use in children, it is considered to be the drug of choice for onychomycosis. Itraconazole can be administered as intermittent 'pulse' therapy. For the role of topical antifungals in the treatment of onychomycosis, see section 13.10.2.

**Immunocompromised children**  Immunocompromised children are at particular risk of fungal infections and may receive antifungal drugs prophylactically; oral triazole antifungals are the drugs of choice for prophylaxis. **Fluconazole** (section 5.2.1) is more reliably absorbed than **itraconazole** (section 5.2.1), but fluconazole is not effective against *Aspergillus* spp. Itraconazole is preferred in patients at risk of invasive aspergillosis. **Micafungin** (section 5.2.4) can be used for prophylaxis of candidiasis in patients undergoing haematopoietic stem cell transplantation when fluconazole or itraconazole cannot be used.

**Amphotericin** (section 5.2.3) by intravenous infusion or **caspofungin** (section 5.2.4) is used for the empirical *treatment* of serious fungal infections in immunocompromised children; caspofungin is not effective against fungal infections of the CNS.

## 5.2.1 Triazole antifungals

For the role of triazole antifungal drugs in the prevention and systemic treatment of fungal infections, see p. 302. **Fluconazole** is very well absorbed after oral administration. It also achieves good penetration into the cerebrospinal fluid to treat fungal meningitis. Fluconazole is

**5 Infections**

excreted largely unchanged in the urine and can be used to treat candiduria.

**Itraconazole** is active against a wide range of dermatophytes. There is limited information available on use in children. Itraconazole capsules require an acid environment in the stomach for optimal absorption.

Itraconazole has been associated with liver damage and should be avoided or used with caution in children with liver disease; fluconazole is less frequently associated with hepatotoxicity.

**Voriconazole** is a broad-spectrum antifungal drug which is licensed in adults for the treatment of life-threatening infections.

## ▌ FLUCONAZOLE

**Cautions** concomitant use with hepatotoxic drugs, monitor liver function with high doses or extended courses—discontinue if signs or symptoms of hepatic disease (risk of hepatic necrosis); susceptibility to QT interval prolongation; **interactions:** Appendix 1 (antifungals, triazole)

**Contra-indications** acute porphyria (section 9.8.2)

**Hepatic impairment** toxicity with related drugs

**Renal impairment** usual initial dose then halve subsequent doses if estimated glomerular filtration rate less than 50 mL/minute/1.73m²

**Pregnancy** manufacturer advises avoid—multiple congenital abnormalities reported with long-term high doses

**Breast-feeding** present in milk but amount probably too small to be harmful

**Side-effects** nausea, abdominal discomfort, diarrhoea, flatulence, headache, rash (discontinue treatment or monitor closely if infection invasive or systemic); less frequently dyspepsia, vomiting, taste disturbance, hepatic disorders, angioedema, anaphylaxis, dizziness, seizures, alopecia, pruritus, toxic epidermal necrolysis, Stevens-Johnson syndrome (severe cutaneous reactions more likely in AIDS patients), hyperlipidaemia, leucopenia, thrombocytopenia, and hypokalaemia reported

**Licensed use** not licensed for tinea infections in children, or for vaginal candidiasis in girls under 16 years, or for prevention of relapse of cryptococcal meningitis after completion of primary therapy in children with AIDS

**Indications and dose**

> **Mucosal candidiasis (except genital)**
> * By mouth or by intravenous infusion
>
> **Neonate under 2 weeks** 3–6 mg/kg on first day then 3 mg/kg every 72 hours
>
> **Neonate 2–4 weeks** 3–6 mg/kg on first day then 3 mg/kg every 48 hours
>
> **Child 1 month–12 years** 3–6 mg/kg on first day then 3 mg/kg (max. 100 mg) daily for 7–14 days in oropharyngeal candidiasis (max. 14 days except in severely immunocompromised patients); for 14–30 days in other mucosal infections (e.g. oesophagitis, candiduria, non-invasive bronchopulmonary infections)
>
> **Child 12–18 years** 50 mg daily (100 mg daily in unusually difficult infections) given for 7–14 days in oropharyngeal candidiasis (max. 14 days except in severely immunocompromised patients); for

14–30 days in other mucosal infections (e.g. oesophagitis, candiduria, non-invasive bronchopulmonary infections)

> **Vaginal candidiasis (see also Recurrent Vulvovaginal Candidiasis, section 7.2.2)**
> * By mouth
>
> **Child under 16 years (post-puberty)** a single dose of 150 mg
>
> **Child 16–18 years** a single dose of 150 mg

> **Candidal balanitis**
> * By mouth
>
> **Child 16–18 years** a single dose of 150 mg

> **Tinea pedis, corporis, cruris, pityriasis versicolor, and dermal candidiasis**
> * By mouth
>
> **Child 1 month–18 years** 3 mg/kg (max. 50 mg) daily for 2–4 weeks (for up to 6 weeks in tinea pedis); max. duration of treatment 6 weeks

> **Tinea capitis**
> * By mouth
>
> **Child 1–18 years** 6 mg/kg (max. 300 mg) daily for 2–4 weeks

> **Invasive candidal infections (including candidaemia and disseminated candidiasis) and cryptococcal infections (including meningitis)**
> * By mouth or by intravenous infusion
>
> **Neonate under 2 weeks** 6–12 mg/kg every 72 hours, treatment continued according to response (at least 8 weeks for cryptococcal meningitis)
>
> **Neonate 2–4 weeks** 6–12 mg/kg every 48 hours, treatment continued according to response (at least 8 weeks for cryptococcal meningitis)
>
> **Child 1 month–18 years** 6–12 mg/kg (max. 800 mg) daily, treatment continued according to response (at least 8 weeks for cryptococcal meningitis)

> **Prevention of relapse of cryptococcal meningitis in HIV-infected patients after completion of primary therapy**
> * By mouth or by intravenous infusion
>
> **Child 1 month–18 years** 6 mg/kg (max. 200 mg) daily

> **Prevention of fungal infections in immunocompromised patients**
> * By mouth or by intravenous infusion
>
> **Neonate under 2 weeks** according to extent and duration of neutropenia, 3–12 mg/kg every 72 hours
>
> **Neonate 2–4 weeks** according to extent and duration of neutropenia, 3–12 mg/kg every 48 hours
>
> **Child 1 month–18 years** according to extent and duration of neutropenia, 3–12 mg/kg (max. 400 mg) daily; 12 mg/kg (max. 400 mg) daily if high risk of systemic infections e.g. following bone-marrow transplantation; commence treatment before anticipated onset of neutropenia and continue for 7 days after neutrophil count in desirable range

**Administration** for *intravenous infusion*, give over 10–30 minutes; do not exceed an infusion rate of 5–10 mL/minute

**Fluconazole** (Non-proprietary) (PoM)
[1]Capsules, fluconazole 50 mg, net price 7-cap pack = £1.14; 150 mg, single-capsule pack = 98p; 200 mg, 7-cap pack = £5.04. Label: 9, (50 and 200 mg)
**Dental prescribing on NHS** Fluconazole Capsules 50 mg may be prescribed

Intravenous infusion, fluconazole 2 mg/mL, net price 25-mL bottle = £7.31; 100-mL bottle = £29.27; 50-mL infusion bag = £2.70; 100-mL infusion bag = £3.89

**Diflucan**® (Pfizer) (PoM)
[1]Capsules, fluconazole 50 mg (blue/white), net price 7-cap pack = £16.61; 150 mg (blue), single-capsule pack = £7.12; 200 mg (purple/white), 7-cap pack = £66.42. Label: 9, (50 and 200 mg)

Oral suspension, orange-flavoured, fluconazole for reconstitution with water, 50 mg/5 mL, net price 35 mL = £16.61; 200 mg/5 mL, 35 mL = £66.42. Label: 9
**Dental prescribing on NHS** May be prescribed as Fluconazole Oral Suspension 50 mg/5 mL

Intravenous infusion, fluconazole 2 mg/mL in sodium chloride intravenous infusion 0.9%, net price 25-mL bottle = £7.32; 100-mL bottle = £29.28
**Electrolytes** Na⁺ 15 mmol/100-mL bottle

## ITRACONAZOLE

**Cautions** absorption reduced in AIDS and neutropenia (monitor plasma-itraconazole concentration and increase dose if necessary); susceptibility to congestive heart failure (see also Heart Failure, below); **interactions:** Appendix 1 (antifungals, triazole)
**Hepatotoxicity** Potentially life-threatening hepatotoxicity reported very rarely—discontinue if signs of hepatitis develop. Avoid or use with caution if history of hepatotoxicity with other drugs or in active liver disease. Monitor liver function if treatment continues for longer than one month, if receiving other hepatotoxic drugs, if history of hepatotoxicity with other drugs, or in hepatic impairment
**Counselling** Children or their carers should be told how to recognise signs of liver disorder and advised to seek prompt medical attention if symptoms such as anorexia, nausea, vomiting, fatigue, abdominal pain or dark urine develop

> **Heart failure**
> Following reports of heart failure, caution is advised when prescribing itraconazole to patients at high risk of heart failure. Those at risk include:
> * patients receiving high doses and longer treatment courses;
> * those with cardiac disease;
> * patients receiving treatment with negative inotropic drugs, e.g. calcium channel blockers.
> Itraconazole should be avoided in patients with ventricular dysfunction or a history of heart failure unless the infection is serious.

**Contra-indications** acute porphyria (section 9.8.2)
**Hepatic impairment** use only if potential benefit outweighs risk of hepatotoxicity (see Hepatotoxicity above); dose reduction may be necessary

---

1. Capsules can be sold to the public for vaginal candidiasis and associated candidal balanitis in those aged 16–18 years, in a container or packaging containing not more than 150 mg and labelled to show a max. dose of 150 mg

**Renal impairment** risk of congestive heart failure; bioavailability of oral formulations possibly reduced; use intravenous infusion with caution if estimated glomerular filtration rate 30–80 mL/minute/1.73 m$^2$ (monitor renal function); avoid intravenous infusion if estimated glomerular filtration rate less than 30 mL/minute/1.73 m$^2$

**Pregnancy** manufacturer advises use only in life-threatening situations (toxicity at high doses in *animal* studies); ensure effective contraception during treatment and until the next menstrual period following end of treatment

**Breast-feeding** small amounts present in milk—may accumulate; manufacturer advises avoid

**Side-effects** nausea, abdominal pain, rash; *less commonly* vomiting, dyspepsia, taste disturbances, flatulence, diarrhoea, constipation, oedema, headache, dizziness, paraesthesia (discontinue treatment if neuropathy), menstrual disorder, and alopecia; *rarely* pancreatitis, dyspnoea, hypoaesthesia, urinary frequency, leucopenia, visual disturbances, and tinnitus; also reported, heart failure (see Cautions above), hypertriglyceridaemia, hepatitis (see Hepatotoxicity above), erectile dysfunction, thrombocytopenia, hypokalaemia, myalgia, arthralgia, photosensitivity, toxic epidermal necrolysis, and Stevens-Johnson Syndrome; *with intravenous injection* hypertension and hyperglycaemia

**Licensed use** *Sporanox*® capsules and *Sporanox*® *Pulse* are not licensed for use in children under 12 years; *Sporanox*® liquid and *Sporanox*® infusion are not licensed for use in children (age range not specified by manufacturer)

**Indications and dose**

**Oropharyngeal candidiasis**
* By mouth
    **Child 1 month–12 years** 3–5 mg/kg once daily; max. 100 mg daily (200 mg daily in AIDS or neutropenia) for 15 days
    **Child 12–18 years** 100 mg once daily (200 mg once daily in AIDS or neutropenia) for 15 days

**Pityriasis versicolor**
* By mouth
    **Child 1 month–12 years** 3–5 mg/kg (max. 200 mg) once daily for 7 days
    **Child 12–18 years** 200 mg once daily for 7 days

**Tinea corporis and tinea cruris**
* By mouth
    **Child 1 month–12 years** 3–5 mg/kg (max. 100 mg) once daily for 15 days
    **Child 12–18 years** *either* 100 mg once daily for 15 days *or* 200 mg once daily for 7 days

**Tinea pedis and tinea manuum**
* By mouth
    **Child 1 month–12 years** 3–5 mg/kg (max. 100 mg) once daily for 30 days
    **Child 12–18 years** *either* 100 mg once daily for 30 days *or* 200 mg twice daily for 7 days

**Tinea capitis**
* By mouth
    **Child 1–18 years** 3–5 mg/kg (max. 200 mg) daily for 2–6 weeks

### Onychomycosis
- **By mouth**

  **Child 1–12 years** course ('pulse') of 5 mg/kg (max. 200 mg) daily for 7 days; subsequent courses repeated after 21 day intervals; fingernails 2 courses, toenails 3 courses

  **Child 12–18 years** *either* 200 mg once daily for 3 months *or* course ('pulse') of 200 mg twice daily for 7 days, subsequent courses repeated after 21-day intervals; fingernails 2 courses, toenails 3 courses

### Systemic aspergillosis, candidiasis and cryptococcosis including cryptococcal meningitis where other antifungal drugs inappropriate or ineffective (limited information available)
- **By mouth**

  **Child 1 month–18 years** 5 mg/kg (max. 200 mg) once daily; increased in invasive or disseminated disease and in cryptococcal meningitis to 5 mg/kg (max. 200 mg) twice daily

- **By intravenous infusion**

  **Child 1 month–18 years** 2.5 mg/kg (max. 200 mg) every 12 hours for 2 days, then 2.5 mg/kg (max. 200 mg) once daily for max. 12 days

### Histoplasmosis
- **By mouth**

  **Child 1 month–18 years** 5 mg/kg (max. 200 mg) 1–2 times daily

### Maintenance in HIV-infected patients to prevent relapse of underlying fungal infection and prophylaxis in neutropenia when standard therapy inappropriate
- **By mouth**

  **Child 1 month–18 years** 5 mg/kg (max. 200 mg) once daily, increased to 5 mg/kg (max. 200 mg) twice daily if low plasma-itraconazole concentration (see Cautions)

### Prophylaxis of deep fungal infections (when standard therapy inappropriate) in patients with haematological malignancy or undergoing bone-marrow transplantation who are expected to become neutropenic
- **By mouth (liquid preparation only)**

  **Child 1 month–18 years** 2.5 mg/kg twice daily starting before transplantation or before chemotherapy (taking care to avoid interaction with cytotoxic drugs) and continued until neutrophil count recovers

**Administration** For *intravenous infusion*, dilute 250 mg with 50 mL Sodium Chloride 0.9% and give requisite dose through an in-line filter (0.2 micron) over 60 minutes

**Itraconazole** (Non-proprietary) [PoM]
Capsules, enclosing coated beads, itraconazole 100 mg, net price 15-cap pack = £7.21. Label: 5, 9, 21, 25, counselling, hepatotoxicity

**Sporanox®** (Janssen) [PoM]
Capsules, blue/pink, enclosing coated beads, itraconazole 100 mg, net price 4-cap pack = £3.67; 15-cap pack = £13.77; 28-cap pack (*Sporanox®-Pulse*) = £25.72; 60-cap pack = £55.10. Label: 5, 9, 21, 25, counselling, hepatotoxicity

Oral liquid, sugar-free, cherry-flavoured, itraconazole 10 mg/mL, net price 150 mL (with 10-mL measuring cup) = £45.80. Label: 9, 23, counselling, administration, hepatotoxicity
**Counselling** Do not take with food; swish around mouth and swallow, do not rinse afterwards
Concentrate for intravenous infusion, itraconazole 10 mg/mL. For dilution before use. Net price 25-mL amp (with infusion bag and filter) = £62.58
**Excipients** include propylene glycol

## ◢ VORICONAZOLE

**Cautions** electrolyte disturbances, cardiomyopathy, bradycardia, symptomatic arrhythmias, history of QT interval prolongation, concomitant use with other drugs that prolong QT interval; avoid exposure to sunlight; patients at risk of pancreatitis; monitor renal function; **interactions:** Appendix 1 (antifungals, triazole)
**Hepatotoxicity** Hepatitis, cholestasis, and fulminant hepatic failure reported uncommonly usually in first 10 days; risk increased in patients with haematological malignancy. Monitor liver function before treatment and during treatment

**Contra-indications** acute porphyria (section 9.8.2)

**Hepatic impairment** Child 2–12 years no information available. Child 12–18 years in mild to moderate hepatic cirrhosis use usual initial dose then halve subsequent doses; no information available for severe hepatic cirrhosis—manufacturer advises use only if potential benefit outweighs risk. See also Hepatotoxicity above.

**Renal impairment** Child 2–12 years no information available. Child 12–18 years intravenous vehicle may accumulate if estimated glomerular filtration rate less than 50 mL/minute/1.73 m$^2$—use intravenous infusion only if potential benefit outweighs risk, and monitor renal function; alternatively, use tablets or oral suspension (no dose adjustment required)

**Pregnancy** toxicity in *animal* studies—manufacturer advises avoid unless potential benefit outweighs risk; effective contraception required during treatment

**Breast-feeding** manufacturer advises avoid—no information available

**Side-effects** nausea, vomiting, abdominal pain, diarrhoea, jaundice (see Hepatotoxicity above), oedema, hypotension, chest pain, respiratory distress syndrome, sinusitis, headache, dizziness, asthenia, anxiety, depression, confusion, agitation, hallucinations, paraesthesia, tremor, influenza-like symptoms, hypoglycaemia, haematuria, blood disorders (including anaemia, thrombocytopenia, leucopenia, pancytopenia), acute renal failure, hypokalaemia, visual disturbances, (including altered perception, blurred vision, and photophobia), rash, pruritus, photosensitivity, alopecia, cheilitis, injection-site reactions; *less commonly* dyspepsia, duodenitis, cholecystitis, pancreatitis, hepatitis (see Hepatotoxicity above), constipation, arrhythmias (including QT interval prolongation), syncope, raised serum cholesterol, hypersensitivity reactions (including flushing), ataxia, nystagmus, hypoaesthesia, adrenocortical insufficiency, arthritis, blepharitis, optic neuritis, scleritis, glossitis, gingivitis, psoriasis, Stevens-Johnson syndrome; *rarely* pseudomembranous colitis, taste disturbances (more common with oral suspension), convulsions, insomnia, tinnitus, hearing disturbances, extrapyramidal effects, hypertonia, hypothyroidism, hyperthyroidism, discoid lupus erythematosus, toxic epidermal necrolysis, pseudoporphyria, retinal haemorrhage, optic atrophy; also reported squamous cell carcinoma of skin (particularly in presence of phototoxicity or in the immunosuppressed)

**Indications and dose**

Invasive aspergillosis; serious infections caused by *Scedosporium* spp., *Fusarium* spp., or invasive fluconazole-resistant *Candida* spp. (including *C. krusei*)

- By mouth

  **Child 2–12 years** (transfer to oral suspension after initial intravenous therapy) 9 mg/kg every 12 hours (reduced in steps of 1 mg/kg if not tolerated; increased in steps of 1 mg/kg if inadequate response); max. 350 mg every 12 hours (reduced in steps of 50 mg if not tolerated; increased in steps of 50 mg if inadequate response)

  **Child 12–15 years**

  **Body-weight under 50 kg** dose as for child 2–12 years

  **Body-weight over 50 kg** dose as for child 15–18 years and body-weight over 40 kg

  **Child 15–18 years, body-weight under 40 kg** 200 mg every 12 hours for 2 doses then 100 mg every 12 hours, increased if necessary to 150 mg every 12 hours

  **Child 15–18 years, body-weight over 40 kg** 400 mg every 12 hours for 2 doses then 200 mg every 12 hours, increased if necessary to 300 mg every 12 hours

- By intravenous infusion

  **Child 2–12 years** 9 mg/kg every 12 hours for 2 doses then 8 mg/kg every 12 hours (reduced in steps of 1 mg/kg if not tolerated; increased in steps of 1 mg/kg if inadequate response) for max. 6 months

  **Child 12–15 years**

  **Body-weight under 50 kg** dose as for child 2–12 years

  **Body-weight over 50 kg** dose as for child 15–18 years

  **Child 15–18 years** 6 mg/kg every 12 hours for 2 doses then 4 mg/kg every 12 hours (reduced to 3 mg/kg every 12 hours if not tolerated) for max. 6 months

**Administration** For *intravenous infusion*, reconstitute each 200 mg with 19 mL Water for Injections to produce a 10 mg/mL solution; dilute dose to concentration of 0.5–5 mg/mL with Glucose 5% *or* Sodium Chloride 0.9% and give at a rate not exceeding 3 mg/kg/hour

**Vfend®** (Pfizer) (PoM)
Tablets, f/c, voriconazole 50 mg, net price 28-tablet pack = £275.68; 200 mg, 28-tab pack = £1102.74. Label: 9, 11, 23

Oral suspension, voriconazole 200 mg/5 mL when reconstituted with water, net price 75 mL (orange-flavoured) = £551.37. Label: 9, 11, 23

Intravenous infusion, powder for reconstitution, voriconazole, net price 200-mg vial = £77.14
**Excipients** include sulfobutylether beta cyclodextrin sodium (risk of accumulation in renal impairment)
**Electrolytes** Na$^+$ 9.47 mmol/vial

## 5.2.2 Imidazole antifungals

The imidazole antifungals include clotrimazole, econazole, ketoconazole, and tioconazole. They are used for the local treatment of vaginal candidiasis (section 7.2.2) and for dermatophyte infections (section 13.10.2).

Ketoconazole is better absorbed by mouth than other imidazoles. However, its use is restricted because it is associated with fatal hepatotoxicity (see below).

Miconazole (section 12.3.2) can be used locally for oral infections; it is also effective in intestinal infections. Systemic absorption may follow use of miconazole oral gel and may result in significant drug interactions.

### KETOCONAZOLE

**Cautions** predisposition to adrenocortical insufficiency; **interactions**: Appendix 1 (antifungals, imidazole)
**Hepatotoxicity** Potentially life-threatening hepatotoxicity reported very rarely; risk of hepatotoxicity greater if given for longer than 10 days. Monitor liver function before treatment, then on weeks 2 and 4 of treatment, then every month. Avoid or use with caution if abnormal liver function tests (avoid in active liver disease) or if history of hepatotoxicity with other drugs.
**Counselling** Children and their carers should be told how to recognise signs of liver disorder and advised to seek prompt medical attention if symptoms such as anorexia, nausea, vomiting, fatigue, abdominal pain, jaundice, or dark urine develop

**Contra-indications** acute porphyria (section 9.8.2)
**Hepatic impairment** avoid (see also Hepatotoxicity above)
**Pregnancy** manufacturer advises avoid unless potential benefit outweighs risk (teratogenicity in *animal* studies)
**Breast-feeding** manufacturer advises avoid
**Side-effects** nausea, vomiting, abdominal pain; pruritus; *less commonly* diarrhoea, headache, dizziness, drowsiness, and rash; also reported fatal liver damage (see Hepatotoxicity above), dyspepsia, raised intracranial pressure, paraesthesia, adrenocortical insufficiency, erectile dysfunction, menstrual disorders, azoospermia (with high doses), gynaecomastia, thrombocytopenia, photophobia, photosensitivity, and alopecia

**Indications and dose**

Dermatophytoses and *Malassezia* folliculitis *either* resistant to fluconazole, terbinafine, or itraconazole *or* in patients intolerant of these antifungals; chronic mucocutaneous, cutaneous, and oropharyngeal candidiasis *either* resistant to fluconazole or itraconazole *or* in patients intolerant of these antifungals

- By mouth

  **Child body-weight 15–30 kg** 100 mg once daily

  **Child body-weight over 30 kg** 200 mg once daily, increased if response inadequate to 400 mg once daily

  **Note** Treatment continued until symptoms have cleared and cultures negative, but see Cautions (max. duration of treatment 4 weeks for *Malassezia* infection)

**Nizoral®** (Janssen) (PoM)
Tablets, scored, ketoconazole 200 mg. Net price 30-tab pack = £14.02. Label: 5, 9, 21, Counselling, hepatotoxicity

**5 Infections**

## 5.2.3 Polyene antifungals

The polyene antifungals include amphotericin and nystatin; neither drug is absorbed when given by mouth. Nystatin is used for oral, oropharyngeal, and perioral infections by local application in the mouth (section 12.3.2). Nystatin is also used for *Candida albicans* infection of the skin (section 13.10.2)

**Amphotericin** by intravenous infusion is used for the treatment of systemic fungal infections and is active against most fungi and yeasts. It is highly protein bound and penetrates poorly into body fluids and tissues. When given parenterally amphotericin is toxic and side-effects are common. Lipid formulations of amphotericin (*Abelcet*® and *AmBisome*®) are significantly less toxic and are recommended when the conventional formulation of amphotericin is contra-indicated because of toxicity, especially nephrotoxicity, or when response to conventional amphotericin is inadequate; lipid formulations are more expensive. For the role of amphotericin in the systemic treatment of fungal infections, see p. 302.

## AMPHOTERICIN
### (Amphotericin B)

**Cautions** when given parenterally, toxicity common (close supervision necessary and close observation required for at least 30 minutes after test dose; see Anaphylaxis below); hepatic and renal function tests, blood counts and plasma electrolyte (including plasma-potassium and magnesium concentration) monitoring required; corticosteroids (avoid except to control reactions); avoid rapid infusion (risk of arrhythmias); **interactions:** Appendix 1 (amphotericin)

**Anaphylaxis** Anaphylaxis occurs rarely with any intravenous amphotericin product and a test dose is advisable before the first infusion in children over 1 month of age; the patient should be carefully observed for at least 30 minutes after the test dose. Prophylactic antipyretics or hydrocortisone should only be used in patients who have previously experienced acute adverse reactions (in whom continued treatment with amphotericin is essential)

**Renal impairment** use only if no alternative; nephrotoxicity may be reduced with use of lipid formulation

**Pregnancy** not known to be harmful, but manufacturers advise avoid unless potential benefit outweighs risk

**Breast-feeding** no information available

**Side-effects** anorexia, nausea and vomiting, diarrhoea, epigastric pain; febrile reactions, headache, muscle and joint pain; anaemia; disturbances in renal function (including hypokalaemia and hypomagnesaemia) and renal toxicity; also cardiovascular toxicity (including arrhythmias, blood pressure changes), blood disorders, neurological disorders (including hearing loss, diplopia, convulsions, peripheral neuropathy, encephalopathy), abnormal liver function (discontinue treatment), rash, anaphylactoid reactions (see Anaphylaxis, above); pain and thrombophlebitis at injection site

**Licensed use** intravenous conventional formulation amphotericin (*Fungizone*®) is licensed for use in children (age range not specified by manufacturer); *Ambisome*® not licensed for use in children under 1 month

### Indications and dose

**Systemic fungal infections**

- **By intravenous infusion**

See preparations

**Note** Different preparations of intravenous amphotericin vary in their pharmacodynamics, pharmacokinetics, dosage, and administration; these preparations should **not** be considered interchangeable. To avoid confusion, prescribers should specify the brand to be dispensed.

**Fungizone**® (Squibb) [PoM]

Intravenous infusion, powder for reconstitution, amphotericin (as sodium deoxycholate complex), net price 50-mg vial = £3.88
**Electrolytes** Na⁺< 0.5 mmol/vial

**Dose**

**Systemic fungal infection**

- **By intravenous infusion**

**Neonate** 1 mg/kg once daily, increased if necessary to 1.5 mg/kg daily; after 7 days, may be reduced to 1–1.5 mg/kg on alternate days

**Child 1 month–18 years** initial test dose of 100 micrograms/kg (max. 1 mg) included as part of first dose of 250 micrograms/kg daily; increased over 2–4 days, if tolerated, to 1 mg/kg daily; in severe infection max. 1.5 mg/kg daily or on alternate days

**Note** prolonged treatment usually necessary; if interrupted for longer than 7 days, recommence at 250 micrograms/kg daily and increase gradually

**Administration** For *intravenous infusion*, reconstitute each vial with 10 mL Water for Injections and shake immediately to produce a 5 mg/mL colloidal solution; dilute further in Glucose 5% to a concentration of 100 micrograms/mL (in fluid-restricted children, up to 400 micrograms/mL given via a central line); pH of glucose solution must not be below 4.2 (check each container—consult product literature for details of buffer); infuse over 4–6 hours, or if tolerated over a minimum of 2 hours (initial test dose given over 20–30 minutes); begin infusion immediately after dilution and protect from light; incompatible with Sodium Chloride solutions—flush existing intravenous line with Glucose 5% or use separate line; an in-line filter (pore size no less than 1 micron) may be used

### ◢ Lipid formulations

**Abelcet**® (Cephalon) [PoM]

Intravenous infusion, amphotericin 5 mg/mL as lipid complex with L-α-dimyristoylphosphatidylcholine and L-α-dimyristoylphosphatidylglycerol, net price 20-mL vial = £77.43 (hosp. only)
**Electrolytes** Na⁺ 3.12 mmol/vial

**Dose**

Severe invasive candidiasis; severe systemic fungal infections in children not responding to conventional amphotericin or to other antifungal drugs or where toxicity or renal impairment precludes conventional amphotericin, including invasive aspergillosis, cryptococcal meningitis and disseminated cryptococcosis in children with HIV

- **By intravenous infusion**

**Child 1 month–18 years** initial test dose of 100 micrograms/kg (max. 1 mg) then 5 mg/kg once daily

**Administration** for *intravenous infusion*, allow suspension to reach room temperature, shake gently to ensure no yellow settlement, withdraw requisite dose (using 17–19 gauge needle) into one or more 20-mL syringes; replace needle on syringe with a 5-

micron filter needle provided (fresh needle for each syringe) and dilute in Glucose 5% to a concentration of 2 mg/mL; preferably give *via* an infusion pump at a rate of 2.5 mg/kg/hour (initial test dose given over 15 minutes); an in-line filter (pore size no less than 15 micron) may be used; do not use sodium chloride or other electrolyte solutions—flush existing intravenous line with Glucose 5% or use separate line

**AmBisome®** (Gilead) PoM
Intravenous infusion, powder for reconstitution, amphotericin 50 mg encapsulated in liposomes, net price 50-mg vial = £96.69
**Electrolytes** Na$^+$< 0.5 mmol/vial
**Excipients** include sucrose 900 mg/vial
**Dose**

> **Severe systemic or deep mycoses where toxicity (particularly nephrotoxicity) precludes use of conventional amphotericin; suspected or proven infection in febrile neutropenic patients unresponsive to broad-spectrum antibacterials**
> - **By intravenous infusion**
>   **Neonate** 1 mg/kg once daily; increased if necessary to 3 mg/kg once daily; max. 5 mg/kg once daily
>   **Child 1 month–18 years** initial test dose 100 micrograms/kg (max. 1 mg) then 3 mg/kg once daily; max. 5 mg/kg once daily

> **Visceral leishmaniasis** see section 5.4.5 and product literature

**Administration** for *intravenous infusion*, reconstitute each vial with 12 mL Water for Injections and shake vigorously to produce a preparation containing 4 mg/mL; withdraw requisite dose from vial and introduce into Glucose 5% or 10% through the 5-micron filter provided, to produce a final concentration of 0.2–2 mg/mL; infuse over 30–60 minutes, or if non-anaphylactic infusion-related reactions occur infuse over 2 hours (initial test dose given over 10 minutes); an in-line filter (pore size no less than 1 micron) may be used; incompatible with sodium chloride solutions—flush existing intravenous line with Glucose 5% or 10%, or use separate line

pruritus, sweating, injection-site reactions; *less commonly* abdominal pain, dyspepsia, dysphagia, dry mouth, taste disturbances, anorexia, constipation, flatulence, cholestasis, hepatic dysfunction, ascites, palpitation, arrhythmia, chest pain, heart failure, thrombophlebitis, hypertension, bronchospasm, cough, dizziness, fatigue, paraesthesia, hypoaesthesia, sleep disturbances, tremor, anxiety, disorientation, hyperglycaemia, renal failure, hypocalcaemia, metabolic acidosis, anaemia, thrombocytopenia, leucopenia, myalgia, muscular weakness, blurred vision, and erythema multiforme; *also reported*, acute respiratory distress syndrome, anaphylaxis, and hypercalcaemia

**Indications and dose**

> **Invasive aspergillosis (see notes above); invasive candidiasis (see notes above); empirical treatment of systemic fungal infections in patients with neutropenia**
> - **By intravenous infusion**
>   **Neonate** 25 mg/m$^2$ once daily
>   **Child 1 month–3 months** 25 mg/m$^2$ once daily
>   **Child 3 months–1 year** 50 mg/m$^2$ once daily
>   **Child 1–18 years** 70 mg/m$^2$ (max. 70 mg) on first day then 50 mg/m$^2$ (max. 70 mg) once daily; increased to 70 mg/m$^2$ (max. 70 mg) daily if lower dose tolerated but inadequate response

**Administration** for *intravenous infusion*, allow vial to reach room temperature; initially reconstitute 50 mg with 10.5 mL Water for Injections to produce a 5.2 mg/mL solution, or reconstitute 70 mg with 10.5 mL Water for Injections to produce a 7.2 mg/mL solution; mix gently to dissolve; dilute requisite dose to a final concentration not exceeding 500 micrograms/mL with Sodium Chloride 0.9%; give over 60 minutes; incompatible with glucose solutions

**Cancidas®** (MSD) PoM
Intravenous infusion, powder for reconstitution, caspofungin (as acetate), net price 50-mg vial = £327.67; 70-mg vial = £416.78

## 5.2.4 Echinocandin antifungals

The echinocandin antifungals include **caspofungin** and **micafungin**. They are only active against *Aspergillus* spp. and *Candida* spp; however micafungin is not used for the treatment of aspergillosis. Echinocandins are not effective against fungal infections of the CNS. For the role of echinocandin antifungals in the prevention and systemic treatment of fungal infections, see p. 302.

## CASPOFUNGIN

**Cautions** interactions: Appendix 1 (caspofungin)
**Hepatic impairment** usual initial dose, then use 70% of normal maintenance dose in moderate impairment; no information available for severe impairment
**Pregnancy** manufacturer advises avoid unless essential—toxicity in *animal* studies
**Breast-feeding** present in milk in *animal* studies—manufacturer advises avoid
**Side-effects** nausea, diarrhoea, vomiting; tachycardia, hypotension, flushing; dyspnoea; headache; hypokalaemia, hypomagnesaemia; arthralgia; rash,

## MICAFUNGIN

**Cautions** monitor renal function; **interactions**: Appendix 1 (micafungin)
**Hepatotoxicity** Potentially life-threatening hepatotoxicity reported. Monitor liver function—discontinue if significant and persistent abnormalities in liver function tests develop. Use with caution in hepatic impairment (avoid if severe) or if receiving other hepatotoxic drugs. Risk of hepatic side-effects greater in children under 1 year of age
**Hepatic impairment** use with caution in mild to moderate impairment; avoid in severe impairment; see also Hepatotoxicity above
**Renal impairment** use with caution; deterioration in renal function
**Pregnancy** manufacturer advises avoid unless essential—toxicity in *animal* studies
**Breast-feeding** manufacturer advises use only if potential benefit outweighs risk—present in milk in *animal* studies
**Side-effects** nausea, vomiting, diarrhoea, abdominal pain, hepatomegaly; blood pressure changes, tachycardia; headache, fever; hypokalaemia, hypomagnesaemia, hypocalcaemia, leucopenia, anaemia, throm-

bocytopenia, renal failure; rash, phlebitis; *less commonly* dyspepsia, constipation, hepatitis and cholestasis (see also Hepatotoxicity above), taste disturbances, anorexia, palpitation, bradycardia, flushing, dyspnoea, sleep disturbances, anxiety, confusion, dizziness, tremor, pancytopenia, eosinophilia, hyponatraemia, hyperkalaemia, hypophosphataemia, hyperhidrosis, and pruritus; *rarely* haemolytic anaemia; also reported disseminated intravascular coagulation, Stevens-Johnson syndrome, toxic epidermal necrolysis

### Indications and dose

Invasive candidiasis

- By intravenous infusion

  **Neonate** (seek specialist advice) 2 mg/kg once daily (increased to 4 mg/kg daily if inadequate response) for at least 14 days

  **Child 1 month–18 years, body-weight under 40 kg** 2 mg/kg once daily (increased to 4 mg/kg daily if inadequate response) for at least 14 days

  **Child 1 month–18 years, body-weight over 40 kg** 100 mg once daily (increased to 200 mg daily if inadequate response) for at least 14 days

Oesophageal candidiasis

- By intravenous infusion

  **Child 16–18 years, body-weight under 40 kg** 3 mg/kg once daily

  **Child 16–18 years, body-weight over 40 kg** 150 mg once daily

Prophylaxis of candidiasis in children undergoing bone-marrow transplantation or who are expected to become neutropenic for over 10 days

- By intravenous infusion

  **Neonate** 1 mg/kg once daily; continue for at least 7 days after neutrophil count in desirable range

  **Child 1 month–18 years, body-weight under 40 kg** 1 mg/kg once daily; continue for at least 7 days after neutrophil count in desirable range

  **Child 1 month–18 years, body-weight over 40 kg** 50 mg once daily; continue for at least 7 days after neutrophil count in desirable range

**Administration** for *intravenous infusion* reconstitute each vial with 5 mL Glucose 5% *or* Sodium Chloride 0.9%; gently rotate vial, without shaking, to dissolve; dilute requisite dose to a concentration of 0.5–2 mg/mL with Glucose 5% *or* Sodium Chloride 0.9%; protect infusion from light; give over 60 minutes

**Mycamine**® (Astellas) PoM
Intravenous infusion, powder for reconstitution, micafungin (as sodium), net price 50-mg vial = £196.08; 100-mg vial = £341.00

## 5.2.5 Other antifungals

**Flucytosine** is used with amphotericin in a synergistic combination. Bone marrow depression can occur which limits its use, particularly in children with AIDS; weekly blood counts are necessary during prolonged therapy. Resistance to flucytosine can develop during therapy and sensitivity testing is essential before and during treatment. For the role of flucytosine in the treatment

of systemic candidiasis and cryptococcal meningitis, see p. 302.

**Griseofulvin** is effective for widespread or intractable dermatophyte infections but has been superseded by newer antifungals, particularly for nail infections. Griseofulvin is used in the treatment of tinea capitis. It is the drug of choice for trichophyton infections in children, see p. 303. Duration of therapy is dependent on the site of the infection and may extend to a number of months.

**Terbinafine** is the drug of choice for fungal nail infections and is also used for ringworm infections where oral treatment is considered appropriate (see p. 303).

## ◼ FLUCYTOSINE

**Cautions** blood disorders; liver- and kidney-function tests and blood counts required (weekly in blood disorders); **interactions:** Appendix 1 (flucytosine)

**Renal impairment** liver- and kidney-function tests and blood counts required weekly; use normal dose every 12 hours if creatinine clearance 20–40 mL/minute; use normal dose every 24 hours if creatinine clearance 10–20 mL/minute; use initial normal dose if creatinine clearance less than 10 mL/minute and then adjust dose according to plasma-flucytosine concentration

**Pregnancy** teratogenic in *animal* studies; manufacturer advises use only if potential benefit outweighs risk

**Breast-feeding** manufacturer advises avoid

**Side-effects** nausea, vomiting, diarrhoea, rashes; less frequently cardiotoxicity, confusion, hallucinations, convulsions, headache, sedation, vertigo, alterations in liver function tests (hepatitis and hepatic necrosis reported), and toxic epidermal necrolysis; blood disorders including thrombocytopenia, leucopenia, and aplastic anaemia reported

**Pharmacokinetics** for plasma-concentration monitoring blood should be taken shortly before starting the next infusion. Plasma concentration for optimum response 25–50 mg/litre (200–400 micromol/litre)—should not be allowed to exceed 80 mg/litre (620 micromol/litre)

**Licensed use** tablets not licensed

### Indications and dose

Systemic yeast and fungal infections, adjunct to amphotericin in severe systemic candidiasis and in other severe or long-standing infections

- By intravenous infusion or by mouth

  **Neonate** 50 mg/kg every 12 hours

  **Child 1 month–18 years** 50 mg/kg every 6 hours; extremely sensitive organisms, 25–37.5 mg/kg every 6 hours may be sufficient; treatment continued usually for not more than 7 days

Cryptococcal meningitis (adjunct to amphotericin, see Cryptococcosis, p. 303)

- By intravenous infusion or by mouth

  **Neonate** 50 mg/kg every 12 hours

  **Child 1 month–18 years** 25 mg/kg every 6 hours for 2 weeks

**Administration** for *intravenous infusion*, give over 20–40 minutes

**Ancotil®** (Meda) [PoM]
Intravenous infusion, flucytosine 10 mg/mL. Net price 250-mL infusion bottle = £30.33 (hosp. only)
Electrolytes Na⁺ 34.5 mmol/250-mL bottle
**Note** Flucytosine tablets may be available from 'special-order' manufacturers or specialist importing companies, see p. 823

## GRISEOFULVIN

**Cautions** interactions: Appendix 1 (griseofulvin)
**Skilled tasks** May impair performance of skilled tasks; effects of alcohol enhanced
**Contra-indications** systemic lupus erythematosus (risk of exacerbation); acute porphyria (section 9.8.2)
**Hepatic impairment** avoid in severe liver disease
**Pregnancy** avoid (fetotoxicity and teratogenicity in *animals*); effective contraception required during and for at least 1 month after administration to women (**important**: effectiveness of oral contraceptives may be reduced, additional contraceptive precautions e.g. barrier method, required); also males should avoid fathering a child during and for at least 6 months after treatment
**Breast-feeding** avoid—no information available
**Side-effects** nausea, vomiting, diarrhoea, headache; also reported, abdominal pain, dyspepsia, hepatotoxicity, glossitis, taste disturbances, sleep disturbances, dizziness, fatigue, confusion, agitation, depression, impaired co-ordination and hearing, peripheral neuropathy, menstrual disturbances, renal failure, leucopenia, systemic lupus erythematosus, rash (including rarely erythema multiforme, toxic epidermal necrolysis), and photosensitivity
**Licensed use** tablets and suspension licensed for use in children (age range not specified by manufacturer)

**Indications and dose**

> **Dermatophyte infections where topical therapy has failed or is inappropriate**
> * By mouth
>   **Child 1 month–12 years** 10 mg/kg (max. 500 mg) once daily or in divided doses; in severe infection dose may be doubled, reducing when response occurs
>   **Child 12–18 years** 500 mg once daily or in divided doses; in severe infection dose may be doubled, reducing when response occurs

> **Tinea capitis caused by *Trichophyton tonsurans***
> * By mouth
>   **Child 1 month–12 years** 15–20 mg/kg (max. 1 g) once daily or in divided doses
>   **Child 12–18 years** 1 g once daily or in divided doses

**Griseofulvin** (Non-proprietary) [PoM]
Tablets, griseofulvin 125 mg, net price 100 = £34.86; 500 mg, 100 = £90.34. Label: 9, 21, counselling, skilled tasks

**Fulsovin®** (Kappin) [PoM]
Oral suspension, griseofulvin 125 mg/5 mL, net price 100 mL (peppermint-flavoured) = £59.90. Label: 9, 21, counselling, skilled tasks

## TERBINAFINE

**Cautions** psoriasis (risk of exacerbation); autoimmune disease (risk of lupus-erythematosus-like effect) interactions: Appendix 1 (terbinafine)
**Hepatic impairment** manufacturer advises avoid—elimination reduced
**Renal impairment** use half normal dose if estimated glomerular filtration rate less than 50 mL/minute/1.73 m² and no suitable alternative available
**Pregnancy** manufacturer advises use only if benefit outweighs risk—no information available
**Breast-feeding** avoid—present in milk
**Side-effects** abdominal discomfort, anorexia, nausea, diarrhoea; headache; rash and urticaria occasionally with arthralgia or myalgia; *less commonly* taste disturbance; *rarely* liver toxicity (including jaundice, cholestasis and hepatitis)—discontinue treatment, angioedema, dizziness, malaise, paraesthesia, hypoaesthesia, photosensitivity; *very rarely* psychiatric disturbances, blood disorders (including leucopenia and thrombocytopenia), lupus erythematosus-like effect, exacerbation of psoriasis, serious skin reactions (including Stevens-Johnson syndrome and toxic epidermal necrolysis)—discontinue treatment if progressive skin rash; also reported, pancreatitis, vasculitis, influenza-like symptoms, rhabdomyolysis, disturbances in smell
**Licensed use** not licensed for use in children

**Indications and dose**

> **Dermatophyte infections of the nails, ringworm infections (including tinea pedis, cruris, corporis, and capitis) where oral therapy appropriate (due to site, severity or extent)**
> * By mouth
>   **Child over 1 year; body-weight 10–20 kg** 62.5 mg once daily
>   **Child body-weight 20–40 kg** 125 mg once daily
>   **Child body-weight over 40 kg** 250 mg once daily
>   **Note** treatment usually for 4 weeks in tinea capitis, 2–6 weeks in tinea pedis, 2–4 weeks in tinea cruris, 4 weeks in tinea corporis, 6 weeks–3 months in nail infections (occasionally longer in toenail infections)

**Fungal skin infections** section 13.10.2

**Terbinafine** (Non-proprietary) [PoM]
Tablets, terbinafine (as hydrochloride) 250 mg, net price 14-tab pack = £2.33, 28-tab pack = £3.02. Label: 9

**Lamisil®** (Novartis) [PoM]
Tablets, off-white, scored, terbinafine (as hydrochloride) 250 mg, net price 14-tab pack = £21.30, 28-tab pack = £41.09. Label: 9

## 5.3 Antiviral drugs

**5.3.1** HIV infection
**5.3.2** Herpesvirus infections
**5.3.3** Viral hepatitis
**5.3.4** Influenza
**5.3.5** Respiratory syncytial virus

The majority of virus infections resolve spontaneously in immunocompetent subjects. A number of specific treatments for viral infections are available, particularly

**5**
**Infections**

for the immunocompromised. This section includes notes on herpes simplex and varicella-zoster, human immunodeficiency virus, cytomegalovirus, respiratory syncytial virus, viral hepatitis and influenza.

## 5.3.1   HIV infection

There is no cure for infection caused by the human immunodeficiency virus (HIV) but a number of drugs slow or halt disease progression. Drugs for HIV infection (antiretrovirals) may be associated with serious side-effects. Although antiretrovirals increase life expectancy considerably and decrease the risk of complications associated with premature ageing, mortality and morbidity remain slightly higher than in uninfected individuals.

The natural progression of HIV disease is different in children compared to adults; drug treatment should only be undertaken by specialists within a formal paediatric HIV clinical network. Guidelines and dose regimens are under constant review and for this reason some dose recommendations have not been included in *BNF for Children*.

Further information on the management of children with HIV can be obtained from the Children's HIV Association (CHIVA) www.chiva.org.uk; and further information on antiretroviral use and toxicity can be obtained from the Paediatric European Network for Treatment of AIDS (PENTA) website www.pentatrials.org.

**Principles of treatment**   Treatment is aimed at suppressing viral replication for as long as possible; it should be started before the immune system is irreversibly damaged. The need for early drug treatment should, however, be balanced against the risk of toxicity. Commitment to treatment and strict adherence over many years are required; the regimen chosen should take into account convenience and the child's tolerance of treatment. The development of drug resistance is reduced by using a combination of drugs; such combinations should have synergistic or additive activity while ensuring that their toxicity is not additive. It is recommended that viral sensitivity to antiretroviral drugs is established before starting treatment or before switching drugs if the infection is not responding.

**Initiation of treatment**   Treatment is started in all HIV infected children under 1 year of age regardless of clinical and immunological parameters. In children over 1 year of age, treatment is based on the child's age, CD4 cell count, viral load, and symptoms. The choice of antiviral treatment for children should take into account the method and frequency of administration, risk of side-effects, compatibility of drugs with food, palatability, and the appropriateness of the formulation. Initiating treatment with a combination of drugs ('highly active antiretroviral therapy' which includes 2 nucleoside reverse transcriptase inhibitors with *either* a non-nucleoside reverse transcriptase inhibitor *or* a boosted protease inhibitor) is recommended. Abacavir and lamivudine are the nucleoside reverse transcriptase inhibitors of choice for initial therapy; however, zidovudine and lamivudine are used in children who are positive for the HLA-B*5701 allele. Nevirapine is the preferred non-nucleoside reverse transcriptase inhibitor in children under 3 years of age, but efavirenz is preferred in older children. Lopinavir with ritonavir is the preferred boosted protease inhibitor for initial therapy. The metabolism of many antiretrovirals varies in young children; it may therefore be necessary to adjust the dose according to the plasma-drug concentration. Children who require treatment for both HIV and chronic hepatitis B should receive antivirals that are active against both diseases (section 5.3.3).

**Switching therapy**   Deterioration of the condition (including clinical, virological changes, and CD4 cell changes) may require a complete change of therapy. The choice of an alternative regimen depends on factors such as the response to previous treatment, tolerance, and the possibility of cross-resistance.

**Pregnancy**   Treatment of HIV infection in pregnancy aims to reduce the risk of toxicity to the fetus (although the teratogenic potential of most antiretroviral drugs is unknown), to minimise the viral load and disease progression in the mother, and to prevent transmission of infection to the neonate. **All treatment options require careful assessment by a specialist.** Zidovudine monotherapy reduces transmission of infection to the neonate. However, combination antiretroviral therapy maximises the chance of preventing transmission and represents optimal therapy for the mother. Combination antiretroviral therapy may be associated with a greater risk of preterm delivery. Local protocols and national guidelines (www.bhiva.org) should be consulted for recommendations on treatment during pregnancy and the perinatal period.

**Breast-feeding**   Breast-feeding by HIV-positive mothers may cause HIV infection in the infant and should be avoided.

**Post-exposure prophylaxis**   Children exposed to HIV infection through needlestick injury or by another route should be sent immediately to an accident and emergency department for post-exposure prophylaxis [unlicensed indication]. Antiretrovirals for prophylaxis are chosen on the basis of efficacy and potential for toxicity. Recommendations have been developed by the Children's HIV Association, www.chiva.org.uk.

**Drugs used for HIV infection**   Zidovudine, a nucleoside reverse transcriptase inhibitor (or 'nucleoside analogue'), was the first anti-HIV drug to be introduced. Other nucleoside reverse transcriptase inhibitors include **abacavir, didanosine, emtricitabine, lamivudine, stavudine,** and **tenofovir.** There are concerns about renal toxicity and effects on bone mineralisation when tenofovir is used in prepubertal children.

The protease inhibitors include **atazanavir, darunavir, fosamprenavir** (a pro-drug of amprenavir), **indinavir, lopinavir, ritonavir, saquinavir,** and **tipranavir.** Indinavir is no longer recommended because it is associated with nephrolithiasis. Ritonavir in low doses boosts the activity of atazanavir, darunavir, fosamprenavir, lopinavir, saquinavir, and tipranavir increasing the persistence of plasma concentrations of these drugs; at such a low dose, ritonavir has no intrinsic antiviral activity. A combination of lopinavir with low-dose ritonavir is available for use in children. The protease inhibitors are metabolised by cytochrome P450 enzyme systems and therefore have a significant potential for drug interactions. Protease inhibitors are associated with lipodystrophy and metabolic effects (see below).

The non-nucleoside reverse transcriptase inhibitors **efavirenz, etravirine,** and **nevirapine** are active against the subtype HIV-1 but not HIV-2, a subtype that is rare in the UK. These drugs may interact with a number of drugs metabolised in the liver. Nevirapine is associated with a high incidence of rash (including Stevens-Johnson syndrome) and rarely fatal hepatitis. Rash is also associated with efavirenz and etravirine but it is usually milder. Psychiatric or CNS disturbances are common with efavirenz. CNS disturbances are often self-limiting and can be reduced by taking the dose at bedtime (especially in the first 2–4 weeks of treatment). Efavirenz has also been associated with an increased plasma cholesterol concentration. Etravirine is used in regimens containing a boosted protease inhibitor for HIV infection resistant to other non-nucleoside reverse transcriptase inhibitors and protease inhibitors.

**Enfuvirtide**, which inhibits the fusion of HIV to the host cell, is licensed for managing infection that has failed to respond to a regimen of other antiretroviral drugs. Enfuvirtide should be combined with other potentially active antiretroviral drugs; it is given by subcutaneous injection.

**Maraviroc** is an antagonist of the CCR5 chemokine receptor. It is used in patients exclusively infected with CCR5–tropic HIV.

**Raltegravir** is an inhibitor of HIV integrase. It is used for the treatment of HIV infection resistant to multiple antiretrovirals.

**Immune reconstitution syndrome**   Improvement in immune function as a result of antiretroviral treatment may provoke a marked inflammatory reaction against residual opportunistic organisms.

**Lipodystrophy syndrome**   Metabolic effects associated with antiretroviral treatment include *fat redistribution, insulin resistance,* and *dyslipidaemia;* collectively these have been termed *lipodystrophy syndrome.* Children should be encouraged to lead a healthy lifestyle that reduces their long-term cardiovascular risk. Plasma lipids and blood glucose should be measured before starting antiretroviral therapy, after 3–6 months of treatment, and then at least annually. Insulin resistance and hyperglycaemia occur only rarely in children.

Fat redistribution (with loss of subcutaneous fat, increased abdominal fat, 'buffalo hump' and breast enlargement) is associated with regimens containing protease inhibitors and nucleoside reverse transcriptase inhibitors. Stavudine, and to a lesser extent zidovudine, are associated with a higher risk of lipoatrophy and should be used only if alternative regimens are not suitable.

Dyslipidaemia is associated with antiretroviral treatment, particularly with protease inhibitors; in children, hypercholesterolaemia appears to be more common than hypertriglyceridaemia. Protease inhibitors and some nucleoside reverse transcriptase inhibitors are associated with insulin resistance and hyperglycaemia, but they occur rarely in children. Of the protease inhibitors, atazanavir and darunavir are less likely to cause dyslipidaemia, while saquinavir and atazanavir are less likely to impair glucose tolerance.

**Osteonecrosis**   Osteonecrosis has been reported in children with advanced HIV disease or following long-term exposure to combination antiretroviral therapy.

# Nucleoside reverse transcriptase inhibitors

## Cautions

**Lactic acidosis** Life-threatening lactic acidosis associated with hepatomegaly and hepatic steatosis has been reported with nucleoside reverse transcriptase inhibitors. They should be used with caution in children with hepatomegaly, hepatitis (especially hepatitis C treated with interferon alfa and ribavirin), liver-enzyme abnormalities and with other risk factors for liver disease and hepatic steatosis. Treatment with the nucleoside reverse transcriptase inhibitor should be **discontinued** in case of symptomatic hyperlactataemia, lactic acidosis, progressive hepatomegaly or rapid deterioration of liver function. Stavudine, especially with didanosine, is associated with a higher risk of lactic acidosis and should be used only if alternative regimens are not suitable.

**Hepatic impairment**   Nucleoside reverse transcriptase inhibitors should be used with caution in children with hepatic impairment (greater risk of hepatic side-effects, see also Lactic Acidosis above). However, some nucleoside reverse transcriptase inhibitors are used in children who also have chronic hepatitis B.

**Pregnancy**   See p. 312

**Breast-feeding**   See p. 312

**Side-effects**   Side-effects of the nucleoside reverse transcriptase inhibitors include gastro-intestinal disturbances (such as nausea, vomiting, abdominal pain, flatulence and diarrhoea), anorexia, pancreatitis, liver damage (see also Lactic Acidosis, above), dyspnoea, cough, headache, insomnia, dizziness, fatigue, blood disorders (including anaemia, neutropenia, and thrombocytopenia), myalgia, arthralgia, rash, urticaria, and fever. See notes above for Lipodystrophy Syndrome (above) and Osteonecrosis (above).

## ABACAVIR

**Cautions** see notes above; also test for HLA-B*5701 allele before treatment (or if re-starting treatment and HLA-B*5701 status not known)—increased risk of hypersensitivity reaction in presence of HLA-B*5701 allele; **interactions:** Appendix 1 (abacavir)
**Hypersensitivity reactions** Life-threatening hypersensitivity reactions reported—characterised by fever or rash and possibly nausea, vomiting, diarrhoea, abdominal pain, dyspnoea, cough, lethargy, malaise, headache, and myalgia; less frequently mouth ulceration, oedema, hypotension, sore throat, acute respiratory distress syndrome, anaphylaxis, paraesthesia, arthralgia, conjunctivitis, lymphadenopathy, lymphocytopenia and renal failure; rarely myolysis; laboratory abnormalities may include raised liver function tests (see Lactic Acidosis above) and creatine kinase; symptoms usually appear in the first 6 weeks, but may occur at any time; monitor for symptoms every 2 weeks for 2 months; discontinue immediately if any symptom of hypersensitivity develops and do not rechallenge (risk of more severe hypersensitivity reaction); discontinue if hypersensitivity cannot be ruled out, even when other diagnoses possible—if rechallenge necessary it must be carried out in hospital setting; if abacavir is stopped for any reason other than hypersensitivity, exclude hypersensitivity reaction as the cause and rechallenge only if medical assistance is readily available; care needed with concomitant use of drugs which cause skin toxicity
**Counselling** Children and carers should be told the importance of regular dosing (intermittent therapy may increase the risk of sensitisation), how to recognise signs of

Infections

5

hypersensitivity, and advised to seek immediate medical attention if symptoms develop or before re-starting treatment; children or their carers should be advised to keep Alert Card with them at all times

**Hepatic impairment** see notes above; also avoid in moderate impairment unless essential; avoid in severe impairment

**Renal impairment** manufacturer advises avoid in end-stage renal disease; avoid *Kivexa*® or *Trizivir*® if estimated glomerular filtration rate less than 50 mL/minute/1.73 m²

**Pregnancy** manufacturer advises avoid (toxicity in *animal* studies); see also Pregnancy, p. 312

**Breast-feeding** see p. 312

**Side-effects** see notes above; also hypersensitivity reactions (see above); *very rarely* Stevens-Johnson syndrome and toxic epidermal necrolysis; rash and gastro-intestinal disturbances more common in children

**Licensed use** *Trizivir*® not licensed for use in children

**Indications and dose**

> **HIV infection in combination with other antiretroviral drugs**
>
> • By mouth
>
> **Child 3 months–12 years** 8 mg/kg (max. 300 mg) twice daily *or* 16 mg/kg (max. 600 mg) once daily
>
> *or*
>
> **Body-weight 14–21 kg** 150 mg twice daily *or* 300 mg once daily
>
> **Body-weight 21–30 kg** 150 mg in the morning and 300 mg in the evening *or* 450 mg once daily
>
> **Body-weight over 30 kg** 300 mg twice daily *or* 600 mg once daily
>
> **Child 12–18 years** 300 mg twice daily *or* 600 mg once daily

**Ziagen**® (ViiV) [PoM]
Tablets, yellow, f/c, scored, abacavir (as sulfate) 300 mg, net price 60-tab pack = £208.95. Counselling, hypersensitivity reactions

Oral solution, sugar-free, banana and strawberry flavoured, abacavir (as sulfate) 20 mg/mL, net price 240-mL = £55.72. Counselling, hypersensitivity reactions
Excipients include propylene glycol

◢**With lamivudine**
For cautions, contra-indications and side-effects see under individual drugs

**Kivexa**® (ViiV) [PoM]
Tablets, orange, f/c, abacavir (as sulfate) 600 mg, lamivudine 300 mg, net price 30-tab pack = £352.25. Counselling, hypersensitivity reactions
Dose

> **HIV infection in combination with other antiretroviral drugs**
>
> • By mouth
>
> **Child 12–18 years and body-weight over 40 kg** 1 tablet once daily

◢**With lamivudine and zidovudine**
**Note** use only if child is stabilised (for 6–8 weeks) on the individual components in the same proportions. For cautions, contra-indications and side-effects see under individual drugs

**Trizivir**® (ViiV) [PoM]
Tablets, blue-green, f/c, abacavir (as sulfate) 300 mg, lamivudine 150 mg, zidovudine 300 mg, net

price 60-tab pack = £509.06. Counselling, hypersensitivity reactions
Dose

> **HIV infection**
>
> • By mouth
>
> **Child body-weight over 30 kg** 1 tablet twice daily

---

## ▌ DIDANOSINE
### (ddI, DDI)

**Cautions** see notes above; also history of pancreatitis (preferably avoid, otherwise extreme caution, see also below); peripheral neuropathy or hyperuricaemia (see under Side-effects); ophthalmological examination (including visual acuity, colour vision, and dilated fundus examination) recommended annually or if visual changes occur; **interactions:** Appendix 1 (didanosine)
**Pancreatitis** If symptoms of pancreatitis develop or if serum lipase is raised and pancreatitis is confirmed, discontinue treatment. Whenever possible avoid concomitant treatment with other drugs known to cause pancreatic toxicity (e.g. intravenous pentamidine isetionate); monitor closely if concomitant therapy unavoidable. Since significant elevations of triglycerides cause pancreatitis monitor closely if triglycerides elevated

**Hepatic impairment** see notes above

**Renal impairment** reduce dose if estimated glomerular filtration rate less than 60 mL/minute/1.73 m²; consult product literature

**Pregnancy** manufacturer advises use only if potential benefit outweighs risk

**Breast-feeding** see p. 312

**Side-effects** see notes above; also pancreatitis (less common in children, see also under Cautions); liver failure, non-cirrhotic portal hypertension, anaphylactic reactions, peripheral neuropathy (switch to another antiretroviral if peripheral neuropathy develops), diabetes mellitus, hypoglycaemia, acute renal failure, rhabdomyolysis, dry eyes, retinal and optic nerve changes, dry mouth, parotid gland enlargement, sialadenitis, alopecia, hyperuricaemia (suspend if raised significantly)

**Licensed use** tablets not licensed for use in children under 3 months; EC capsules not licensed for use in children under 6 years

**Indications and dose**

> **HIV infection in combination with other antiretroviral drugs**
>
> • By mouth
>
> **Neonate 14–28 days** 50–100 mg/m² twice daily
>
> **Child 1–8 months** 50–100 mg/m² twice daily
>
> **Child 8 months–18 years** 180–240 mg/m² once daily; usual dose 200 mg/m² once daily; max. 400 mg daily

**Videx**® (Bristol-Myers Squibb) [PoM]
Tablets, with calcium and magnesium antacids, didanosine 25 mg, net price 60-tab pack = £25.06. Label: 23, counselling, administration, see below
Excipients include aspartame equivalent to phenylalanine 36.5 mg per tablet (section 9.4.1)
**Note** Antacids in formulation may affect absorption of other drugs—see **interactions:** Appendix 1 (antacids)
**Administration** to ensure sufficient antacid, each dose to be taken as at least 2 tablets (child under 1 year 1 tablet) chewed thoroughly, crushed or dispersed in water; clear apple juice may be added for flavouring; tablets to be taken 2 hours after

lopinavir with ritonavir capsules and oral solution or atazanavir with ritonavir

Videx® EC capsules, enclosing e/c granules, didanosine 125 mg, net price 30-cap pack = £48.18; 200 mg, 30-cap pack = £77.09; 250 mg, 30-cap pack = £96.37; 400 mg, 30-cap pack = £154.19. Label: 25, counselling, administration, see below
**Administration**  capsules should be swallowed whole and taken at least 2 hours before or 2 hours after food

## ◢ EMTRICITABINE
(FTC)

**Cautions**  see notes above; also on discontinuation, monitor patients with hepatitis B (risk of exacerbation of hepatitis); **interactions:** Appendix 1 (emtricitabine)
**Hepatic impairment**  see notes above and Cautions above
**Renal impairment**  reduce dose or increase dosage interval if estimated glomerular filtration rate less than 50 mL/minute/1.73 m², consult product literature
**Pregnancy**  see p. 312
**Breast-feeding**  see p. 312
**Side-effects**  see notes above; also abnormal dreams, pruritus, and hyperpigmentation

### Indications and dose
See preparations

**Emtriva®** (Gilead) PoM
Capsules, white/blue, emtricitabine 200 mg, net price 30-cap pack = £163.50
**Dose**
> **HIV infection in combination with other anti-retroviral drugs**
> • By mouth
> **Child body-weight over 33 kg** 200 mg once daily

Oral solution, orange, emtricitabine 10 mg/mL, net price 170-mL pack (candy-flavoured) = £46.50
**Electrolytes**  Na⁺ 460 micromol/mL
**Dose**
> **HIV infection in combination with other anti-retroviral drugs**
> • By mouth
> **Child 4 months–18 years**
> **Body-weight under 33 kg** 6 mg/kg once daily
> **Body-weight over 33 kg** 240 mg once daily

**Note**  240 mg oral solution ≡ 200 mg capsule; where appropriate the capsule may be used instead of the oral solution
**Missed dose**  If a dose is more than 12 hours late, the missed dose should not be taken and the next dose should be taken at the normal time

◢ **With tenofovir**
See under Tenofovir

◢ **With efavirenz and tenofovir**
See under Tenofovir

## ◢ LAMIVUDINE
(3TC)

**Cautions**  see notes above; **interactions:** Appendix 1 (lamivudine)
**Chronic hepatitis B**  Recurrent hepatitis in patients with chronic hepatitis B may occur on discontinuation of

lamivudine. When treating chronic hepatitis B with lamivudine, monitor liver function tests every 3 months, and viral markers of hepatitis B every 3–6 months, more frequently in patients with advanced liver disease or following transplantation (monitoring to continue for at least 1 year after discontinuation)
**Hepatic impairment**  see notes above and Cautions above
**Renal impairment**  reduce dose if estimated glomerular filtration rate less than 50 mL/minute/1.73 m²; consult product literature
**Pregnancy**  see p. 312
**Breast-feeding**  can be used with caution in women infected with chronic hepatitis B alone, providing that adequate measures are taken to prevent hepatitis B infection in infants; for women infected with HIV, see p. 312
**Side-effects**  see notes above; also peripheral neuropathy, muscle disorders including rhabdomyolysis, nasal symptoms, alopecia
**Licensed use**  *Epivir®* not licensed for use in children under 3 months; *Zeffix®* not licensed for use in children

### Indications and dose
See preparations

**Epivir®** (ViiV) PoM
Tablets, f/c, lamivudine 150 mg (scored, white), net price 60-tab pack = £143.32; 300 mg (grey), 30-tab pack = £157.51

Oral solution, banana- and strawberry-flavoured, lamivudine 50 mg/5 mL, net price 240-mL pack = £39.01
**Excipients**  include sucrose 1 g/5 mL
**Dose**
> **HIV infection in combination with other anti-retroviral drugs**
> • By mouth
> **Child 1–3 months** 4 mg/kg twice daily
> **Child 3 months–12 years** 4 mg/kg (max. 150 mg) twice daily *or* 8 mg/kg (max. 300 mg) once daily
> *or*
> **Body-weight 14–21 kg** 75 mg twice daily *or* 150 mg once daily
> **Body-weight 21–30 kg** 75 mg in the morning and 150 mg in the evening *or* 225 mg once daily
> **Body-weight over 30 kg** 150 mg twice daily *or* 300 mg once daily
> **Child 12–18 years** 150 mg twice daily *or* 300 mg once daily

**Zeffix®** (ViiV) PoM
Tablets, brown, f/c, lamivudine 100 mg, net price 28-tab pack = £78.09
**Dose**
> **Chronic hepatitis B infection** *either* with compensated liver disease (with evidence of viral replication and histology of active liver inflammation or fibrosis) when first-line treatments cannot be used, *or* (in combination with another antiviral drug without cross-resistance to lamivudine) with decompensated liver disease
> • By mouth
> **Child 2–12 years** 3 mg/kg (max. 100 mg) once daily
> **Child 12–18 years** 100 mg once daily
> **Note**  Children receiving lamivudine for concomitant HIV infection should continue to receive lamivudine in a dose appropriate for HIV infection

◢ **With abacavir**
See under Abacavir

◢With zidovudine
See under Zidovudine

◢With abacavir and zidovudine
See under Abacavir

---

## ▌ STAVUDINE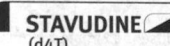
(d4T)

**Cautions** see notes above; also history of peripheral neuropathy, excessive alcohol intake, concomitant use of isoniazid—risk of peripheral neuropathy (see under Side-effects); history of pancreatitis or concomitant use with other drugs associated with pancreatitis; **interactions:** Appendix 1 (stavudine)

**Hepatic impairment** see notes above

**Renal impairment** risk of peripheral neuropathy; reduce dose to 50% if estimated glomerular filtration rate 25–50 mL/minute/1.73 m$^2$; reduce dose to 25% if estimated glomerular filtration rate less than 25 mL/minute/1.73 m$^2$

**Pregnancy** manufacturer advises use only if potential benefit outweighs risk

**Breast-feeding** see p. 312

**Side-effects** see notes above; also peripheral neuropathy (switch to another antiretroviral if peripheral neuropathy develops), abnormal dreams, cognitive dysfunction, drowsiness, depression, pruritus; *less commonly* anxiety, gynaecomastia

**Licensed use** capsules not licensed for use in children under 3 months

### Indications and dose

HIV infection in combination with other antiretroviral drugs when no suitable alternative available and when prescribed for shortest period possible

- By mouth

  Child 1 month–18 years

  **Body-weight under 30 kg** 1 mg/kg twice daily, preferably at least 1 hour before food

  **Body-weight 30–60 kg** 30 mg twice daily, preferably at least 1 hour before food

  **Body-weight over 60 kg** 40 mg twice daily, preferably at least 1 hour before food

**Zerit**® (Bristol-Myers Squibb) [PoM] ◢
Capsules, stavudine 20 mg (brown), net price 56-cap pack = £139.46; 30 mg (light orange/dark orange), 56-cap pack = £146.25; 40 mg (dark orange), 56-cap pack = £150.66 (all hosp. only)

Oral solution, cherry-flavoured, stavudine for reconstitution with water, 1 mg/mL, net price 200 mL = £22.94

---

## ▌ TENOFOVIR DISOPROXIL

**Cautions** see notes above; also test renal function and serum phosphate before treatment, then every 4 weeks (more frequently if at increased risk of renal impairment) for 1 year and then every 3 months, interrupt treatment if renal function deteriorates or serum phosphate decreases; concomitant or recent use of nephrotoxic drugs; **interactions:** Appendix 1 (tenofovir)

*Chronic hepatitis B* When treating chronic hepatitis B with tenofovir, monitor liver function tests every 3 months and viral markers for hepatitis B every 3–6 months during treatment (continue monitoring for at least 1 year after discontinuation—recurrent hepatitis may occur on discontinuation)

**Hepatic impairment** see notes above and Cautions above; manufacturer of *Atripla*® advises caution in mild impairment; avoid *Atripla*® in moderate to severe impairment

**Renal impairment** increase dose interval if estimated glomerular filtration rate less than 50 mL/minute/1.73 m$^2$; avoid *Atripla*® if estimated glomerular filtration rate less than 50 mL/minute/1.73 m$^2$; avoid *Truvada*® if estimated glomerular filtration rate less than 30 mL/minute/1.73 m$^2$

**Pregnancy** see p. 312

**Breast-feeding** see p. 312

**Side-effects** see notes above; also hypophosphataemia; *rarely* renal failure, proximal renal tubulopathy, nephrogenic diabetes insipidus; also reported reduced bone density

### Indications and dose

HIV infection in combination with other antiretroviral drugs when first-line nucleoside reverse transcriptase inhibitors cannot be used because of resistance or contra-indications

- By mouth
- **Child 2–18 years** 6.5 mg/kg (max. 245 mg) once daily

  *or*

  Child 6–18 years

  **Body-weight 17–22 kg** 123 mg once daily

  **Body-weight 22–28 kg** 163 mg once daily

  **Body-weight 28–35 kg** 204 mg once daily

  **Body-weight over 35 kg** 245 mg once daily

Chronic hepatitis B infection with compensated liver disease (with evidence of viral replication, and histology of active liver inflammation or fibrosis)

- By mouth

  Child 12–18 years, body-weight over 35 kg 245 mg once daily

**Missed dose** If a dose is more than 12 hours late, the missed dose should not be taken and the next dose should be taken at the normal time

**Viread**® (Gilead) [PoM]
Tablets, f/c, tenofovir disoproxil (as fumarate) 123 mg (white), net price 30-tab pack = £120.71; 163 mg (white), 30-tab pack = £159.98; 204 mg (white), 30-tab pack = £200.22; 245 mg (blue), 30-tab pack = £240.46. Label: 21

Granules, sugar-free, tenofovir disoproxil (as fumarate) 33 mg/g, net price 60 g (with 1-g scoop) = £64.12. Label: 21, counselling, administration

Note 7.5 scoops of granules contains approx. 245 mg tenofovir disoproxil (as fumarate)

Administration Mix 1 scoop of granules with 1 tablespoon of soft food (e.g. yoghurt, apple sauce) and take immediately without chewing. Do **not** mix granules with liquids

◢With emtricitabine
For **cautions**, **contra-indications**, and **side-effects** see under individual drugs

**Truvada**® (Gilead) [PoM]
Tablets, blue, f/c, tenofovir disoproxil (as fumarate) 245 mg, emtricitabine 200 mg, net price 30-tab pack

= £418.50. Label: 21, Counselling, administration
Children with swallowing difficulties may disperse tablet in
half a glass of water, orange juice, or grape juice (but bitter
taste)

◢With efavirenz and emtricitabine

For **cautions**, **contra-indications**, and **side-effects**
see under individual drugs

**Atripla**® (Gilead) PoM
Tablets, pink, f/c, efavirenz 600 mg, emtricitabine
200 mg, tenofovir disoproxil (as fumarate) 245 mg,
net price 30-tab pack = £626.90. Label: 23, 25

---

◢ **ZIDOVUDINE**
(Azidothymidine, AZT)

**Note** The abbreviation AZT which is sometimes used for
zidovudine has also been used for another drug

**Cautions**  see notes above; also haematological toxicity particularly with high dose and advanced disease—monitor full blood count after 4 weeks of
treatment, then every 3 months; vitamin $B_{12}$ deficiency (increased risk of neutropenia); if anaemia or
myelosuppression occur, reduce dose or interrupt
treatment according to product literature, or consider
other treatment; **interactions**: Appendix 1 (zidovudine)

**Contra-indications**  abnormally low neutrophil count
or haemoglobin concentration (consult product literature); neonates with hyperbilirubinaemia requiring
treatment other than phototherapy, or with raised
transaminase (consult product literature); acute porphyria (section 9.8.2)

**Hepatic impairment**  see notes above; also accumulation may occur

**Renal impairment**  reduce dose if estimated glomerular filtration rate less than 10 mL/minute/1.73 m²;
consult product literature

**Pregnancy**  see p. 312

**Breast-feeding**  see p. 312

**Side-effects**  see notes above; also anaemia (may
require transfusion), taste disturbance, chest pain,
influenza-like symptoms, paraesthesia, neuropathy,
convulsions, dizziness, drowsiness, anxiety, depression, loss of mental acuity, myopathy, gynaecomastia,
urinary frequency, sweating, pruritus, pigmentation of
nails, skin and oral mucosa

**Indications and dose**

HIV infection in combination with other antiretroviral drugs

• By mouth

**Child 1 month–18 years** 180 mg/m² (max.
300 mg) twice daily

or

**Body-weight 4–9 kg** 12 mg/kg twice daily
**Body-weight 9–30 kg** 9 mg/kg twice daily
**Body-weight over 30 kg** 250–300 mg twice daily

or

**Body-weight 8–14 kg** 100 mg twice daily
**Body-weight 14–21 kg** 100 mg in the morning and
200 mg in the evening
**Body-weight 21–28 kg** 200 mg twice daily
**Body-weight 28–30 kg** 200–250 mg twice daily

• By intravenous infusion over 1 hour in children
temporarily unable to take zidovudine by mouth

**Child 3 months–12 years** 60–80 mg/m² every 6
hours (approximating to 9–12 mg/kg twice daily
by mouth) usually for not more than 2 weeks

**Child 12–18 years** 0.8–1 mg/kg every 4 hours
(approximating to 1.2–1.5 mg/kg every 4 hours by
mouth) usually for not more than 2 weeks

Prevention of maternal-fetal HIV transmission
seek specialist advice (combination therapy preferred)

**Administration**  for *intermittent intravenous infusion*,
dilute to a concentration of 2 mg/mL or 4 mg/mL
with Glucose 5% and give over 1 hour.
For administration *by mouth*, *Combivir*® tablets may
be crushed and mixed with semi-solid food or liquid
just before administration

**Zidovudine** (Non-proprietary) PoM
Capsules, zidovudine 100 mg, net price 60-cap pack
= £50.17; 250 mg, 60-cap pack = £125.44

**Retrovir**® (ViiV) PoM
Capsules, zidovudine 100 mg (white), net price 100-
cap pack = £104.54; 250 mg (blue/white), 40-cap
pack = £104.54

Oral solution, sugar-free, strawberry-flavoured, zidovudine 50 mg/5 mL, net price 200-mL pack with
10-mL oral syringe = £20.91

Injection, zidovudine 10 mg/mL. For dilution and
use as an intravenous infusion. Net price 20-mL vial
= £10.50

◢With lamivudine

For **cautions**, **contra-indications**, and **side-effects**
see under individual drugs

**Combivir**® (ViiV) PoM
Tablets, f/c, zidovudine 300 mg, lamivudine 150 mg,
net price 60-tab pack = £300.12

**Dose**

HIV infection in combination with other antiretrovirals

• By mouth

**Child body-weight 14–21 kg** half a tablet twice daily
**Child body-weight 21–30 kg** half a tablet in the morning
and one tablet in the evening
**Child body-weight over 30 kg** one tablet twice daily

◢With abacavir and lamivudine

See under Abacavir

---

## Protease inhibitors

**Cautions**  Protease inhibitors should be used with
caution in diabetes (see also Lipodystrophy Syndrome,
p. 313). Caution is also needed in children with haemophilia who may be at increased risk of bleeding.

**Contra-indications**  Protease inhibitors should not
be given to patients with acute porphyria (but see
section 9.8.2).

**Hepatic impairment**  Protease inhibitors should be
used with caution in children with chronic hepatitis B or
C (increased risk of hepatic side-effects).

**Pregnancy**  See p. 312

5  Infections

**Breast-feeding**  See p. 312

**Side-effects**  Side-effects of the protease inhibitors include gastro-intestinal disturbances (including diarrhoea, nausea, vomiting, abdominal pain, flatulence), anorexia, hepatic dysfunction, pancreatitis; blood disorders including anaemia, neutropenia, and thrombocytopenia; sleep disturbances, fatigue, headache, dizziness, paraesthesia, myalgia, myositis, rhabdomyolysis; taste disturbances; rash, pruritus, Stevens-Johnson syndrome, hypersensitivity reactions including anaphylaxis; see also Lipodystrophy Syndrome (p. 313) and Osteonecrosis (p. 313).

### ATAZANAVIR

**Cautions**  see notes above; concomitant use with drugs that prolong PR interval; cardiac conduction disorders; predisposition to QT interval prolongation (including electrolyte disturbances, concomitant use of drugs that prolong QT interval); **interactions:** Appendix 1 (atazanavir)
**Rash**  Mild to moderate rash occurs commonly, usually within the first 3 weeks of therapy. Severe rash occurs less frequently and may be accompanied by systemic symptoms. Discontinue if severe rash develops

**Contra-indications**  see notes above

**Hepatic impairment**  see notes above; also use with caution in mild impairment; avoid in moderate to severe impairment

**Pregnancy**  manufacturer advises use only if potential benefit outweighs risk; theoretical risk of hyperbilirubinaemia in neonate if used at term

**Breast-feeding**  see p. 312

**Side-effects**  see notes above; also AV block; *less commonly* mouth ulcers, dry mouth, cholelithiasis, hypertension, syncope, chest pain, torsades de pointes, dyspnoea, peripheral neuropathy, abnormal dreams, amnesia, disorientation, depression, anxiety, weight changes, increased appetite, gynaecomastia, nephrolithiasis, urinary frequency, haematuria, proteinuria, arthralgia, alopecia; *rarely* cholecystitis, hepatosplenomegaly, oedema, palpitation, abnormal gait

**Indications and dose**

HIV infection in combination with other antiretroviral drugs
* By mouth
With low-dose ritonavir
**Child 6-18 years**
**Body-weight 15-20 kg** 150 mg once daily
**Body-weight 20-40 kg** 200 mg once daily
**Body-weight over 40 kg** 300 mg once daily

**Reyataz®** (Bristol-Myers Squibb) ▼ PoM
Capsules, atazanavir (as sulfate) 150 mg (dark blue/light blue), net price 60-cap pack = £303.38; 200 mg (dark blue), 60-cap pack = £303.38; 300 mg (red/blue), 30-cap pack = £303.38. Label: 5, 21

### DARUNAVIR

**Cautions**  see notes above; also sulfonamide sensitivity; monitor liver function before and during treatment; **interactions:** Appendix 1 (daruanvir)
**Rash**  Mild to moderate rash occurs commonly, usually within the first 4 weeks of therapy and resolves without

stopping treatment. Severe skin rash (including Stevens-Johnson syndrome and toxic epidermal necrolysis) occurs less frequently and may be accompanied by fever, malaise, arthralgia, myalgia, oral lesions, conjunctivitis, hepatitis, or eosinophilia; treatment should be stopped if severe rash develops

**Contra-indications**  see notes above

**Hepatic impairment**  see notes above; also manufacturer advises caution in mild to moderate impairment; avoid in severe impairment—no information available

**Pregnancy**  manufacturer advises use only if potential benefit outweighs risk—no information available

**Breast-feeding**  see p. 312

**Side-effects**  see notes above; also haematemesis, myocardial infarction, chest pain, QT interval prolongation, syncope, bradycardia, tachycardia, palpitation, hypertension, flushing, peripheral oedema, dyspnoea, cough, peripheral neuropathy, anxiety, confusion, memory impairment, depression, abnormal dreams, convulsions, increased appetite, weight changes, pyrexia, hypothyroidism, osteoporosis, gynaecomastia, erectile dysfunction, reduced libido, dysuria, polyuria, nephrolithiasis, renal failure, arthralgia, visual disturbances, dry eyes, conjunctival hyperaemia, rhinorrhoea, throat irritation, dry mouth, stomatitis, nail discoloration, acne, seborrhoeic dermatitis, eczema, increased sweating, and alopecia

**Indications and dose**

In combination with other antiretroviral drugs, for HIV infection resistant to other protease inhibitors in children previously treated with antiretrovirals
* By mouth
With low-dose ritonavir
**Child 3-18 years**
**Body-weight 15-30 kg** 375 mg twice daily
**Body-weight 30-40 kg** 450 mg twice daily
**Body-weight over 40 kg** 600 mg twice daily
**Missed dose**  If a dose is more than 6 hours late, the missed dose should not be taken and the next dose should be taken at the normal time

**Prezista®** (Janssen) PoM
Tablets, f/c, darunavir (as ethanolate) 75 mg (white), net price 480-tab pack = £446.70; 150 mg (white), 240-tab pack = £446.70; 400 mg (light orange), 60-tab pack = £297.80; 600 mg (orange), 60-tab pack = £446.70. Label: 21

Oral suspension, sugar-free, strawberry-flavoured, darunavir (as ethanolate) 100 mg/mL, net price 200-mL= £248.17. Label: 21

### FOSAMPRENAVIR

**Note**  Fosamprenavir is a pro-drug of amprenavir

**Cautions**  see notes above; **interactions:** Appendix 1 (fosamprenavir)
**Rash**  Rash may occur, usually in the second week of therapy; discontinue permanently if severe rash with systemic or allergic symptoms or, mucosal involvement; if rash mild or moderate, may continue without interruption—usually resolves within 2 weeks and may respond to antihistamines

**Contra-indications**  see notes above

**Hepatic impairment**  see notes above; also manufacturer advises caution in mild impairment; reduce dose in moderate to severe impairment

**Pregnancy** toxicity in *animal* studies; manufacturer advises use only if potential benefit outweighs risk

**Breast-feeding** see p. 312

**Side-effects** see notes above; also reported, rash including rarely Stevens-Johnson syndrome (see also Rash above)

### Indications and dose

**HIV infection in combination with other anti-retroviral drugs**

• By mouth

With low-dose ritonavir

**Child 6–18 years**

**Body-weight 25–39 kg** 18 mg/kg (max. 700 mg) twice daily

**Body-weight over 39 kg** 700 mg twice daily

Note 700 mg fosamprenavir is equivalent to approx. 600 mg amprenavir

**Telzir®** (ViiV) PoM

Tablets, f/c, pink, fosamprenavir (as calcium) 700 mg, net price 60-tab pack = £258.97

Oral suspension, fosamprenavir (as calcium) 50 mg/ mL, net price 225-mL pack (grape-bubblegum-and peppermint-flavoured) (with 10-mL oral syringe) = £69.06. Counselling, administration

Excipients include propylene glycol

Administration In children, oral suspension should be taken with food

**Kaletra®** (AbbVie) PoM

Tablets, pale yellow, f/c, lopinavir 100 mg, ritonavir 25 mg, net price 60-tab pack = £76.85. Label: 25

Dose

**HIV infection in combination with other anti-retroviral drugs**

• By mouth

**Child 2–18 years with body-weight under 40 kg**

**Body surface area 0.5–0.9 m²** 2 tablets twice daily

**Body surface area 0.9–1.4 m²** 3 tablets twice daily

Tablets, yellow, f/c, lopinavir 200 mg, ritonavir 50 mg, net price 120-tab pack = £307.39. Label: 25

Dose

**HIV infection in combination with other anti-retroviral drugs**

• By mouth

**Child 2–18 years with body surface area greater than 1.4 m² or body-weight 40 kg and over** 2 tablets twice daily

Oral solution, lopinavir 400 mg, ritonavir 100 mg/ 5 mL, net price 5 × 60-mL packs = £307.39. Label: 21

Excipients include propylene glycol 153 mg/mL (see Excipients, p. 2), alcohol 42%

Dose

**HIV infection in combination with other anti-retroviral drugs**

• By mouth

**Child 2–18 years** 2.9 mL/m² (max. 5 mL) twice daily with food

Counselling Oral solution tastes bitter

## ▌ LOPINAVIR WITH RITONAVIR

**Cautions** see notes above; concomitant use with drugs that prolong QT or PR interval; cardiac conduction disorders, structural heart disease; pancreatitis (see below); monitor liver function before and during treatment; **interactions:** Appendix 1 (lopinavir, ritonavir)

Pancreatitis Signs and symptoms suggestive of pancreatitis (including raised serum lipase) should be evaluated—discontinue if pancreatitis diagnosed

**Contra-indications** see notes above

**Hepatic impairment** see notes above; also avoid oral solution—high propylene glycol content; manufacturer advises avoid tablets in severe impairment

**Renal impairment** avoid oral solution due to high propylene glycol content

**Pregnancy** avoid oral solution due to high propylene glycol content; manufacturer advises use tablets only if potential benefit outweighs risk (toxicity in *animal* studies)

**Breast-feeding** see p. 312

**Side-effects** see notes and Cautions above; also colitis, weight changes, hypertension, anxiety, neuropathy, sexual dysfunction, amenorrhoea, menorrhagia, arthralgia, night sweats; *less commonly* gastrointestinal ulcer, rectal bleeding, dry mouth, stomatitis, artherosclerosis, AV block, cerebrovascular accident, deep vein thrombosis, abnormal dreams, convulsions, tremor, nephritis, haematuria, visual disturbances, tinnitus, alopecia

### Indications and dose

See preparations

## ▌ RITONAVIR

**Cautions** see notes above; concomitant use with drugs that prolong PR interval; cardiac conduction disorders, structural heart disease; pancreatitis (see below); **interactions:** Appendix 1 (ritonavir)

Pancreatitis Signs and symptoms suggestive of pancreatitis (including raised serum lipase) should be evaluated—discontinue if pancreatitis diagnosed

**Contra-indications** see notes above

**Hepatic impairment** see notes above; also avoid in decompensated liver disease; in severe impairment without decompensation, use 'booster' doses with caution (avoid treatment doses)

**Pregnancy** manufacturer advises use only if potential benefit outweighs risk—toxicity in *animal* studies

**Breast-feeding** see p. 312

**Side-effects** see notes and Cautions above; also diarrhoea (may impair absorption—close monitoring required), vasodilatation, cough, throat irritation, anxiety, perioral and peripheral paraesthesia, hyperaesthesia, fever, decreased blood-thyroxine concentration, electrolyte disturbances, raised uric acid, dry mouth, mouth ulcers, and sweating; *less commonly* increased prothrombin time and dehydration; *rarely* toxic epidermal necrolysis; also reported syncope, postural hypotension, seizures, menorrhagia, renal failure

**5**

**Infections**

**Infections** 5

### Indications and dose

**Low-dose ritonavir to increase the effect of atazanavir**
- By mouth

  **Child 6–18 years**
  **Body-weight 15–20 kg** 80–100 mg once daily
  **Body-weight over 20 kg** 100 mg once daily

**Low-dose ritonavir to increase the effect of darunavir**
- By mouth

  **Child 3–18 years**
  **Body-weight 15–30 kg** 50 mg twice daily
  **Body-weight 30–40 kg** 60 mg twice daily
  **Body-weight over 40 kg** 100 mg twice daily

**Low-dose ritonavir to increase the effect of fosamprenavir**
- By mouth

  **Child 6–18 years**
  **Body-weight 25–33 kg** 3 mg/kg twice daily
  **Body-weight over 33 kg** 100 mg twice daily

**Low-dose ritonavir to increase the effect of saquinavir**
- By mouth

  **Child 16–18 years** 100 mg twice daily

**Low-dose ritonavir to increase the effect of tipranavir**
- By mouth

  **Child 2–12 years** 150 mg/m$^2$ (max. 200 mg) twice daily
  **Child 12–18 years** 200 mg twice daily

**High-dose ritonavir (in combination with other antiretroviral drugs) for treatment of HIV infection, but tolerability is poor**
- By mouth

  **Child 2–18 years** initially 250 mg/m$^2$ twice daily, increased by 50 mg/m$^2$ at intervals of 2–3 days to 350 mg/m$^2$ twice daily (max. 600 mg twice daily)

**Norvir®** (AbbVie) [PoM]
Tablets, f/c, ritonavir 100 mg, net price 30-tab pack = £19.44. Label: 21, 25
Oral solution, sugar-free, ritonavir 400 mg/5 mL, net price 5 × 90-mL packs (with measuring cup) = £403.20. Label: 21, counselling, administration
**Excipients** include alcohol, propylene glycol
**Counselling** Oral solution contains 43% alcohol; bitter taste can be masked by mixing with chocolate milk; do not mix with water, measuring cup must be dry
Administration of ritonavir and didanosine should be separated by at least 2 hours

◀**With lopinavir**
See under Lopinavir with ritonavir

### SAQUINAVIR

**Cautions** see notes above; monitor ECG before starting treatment and then on day 3 or 4 of treatment—discontinue if QT interval over 480 milliseconds, if QT interval more than 20 milliseconds above baseline, or if prolongation of PR interval; concomitant use of garlic (avoid garlic capsules—reduces plasma-saqui-

navir concentration); **interactions:** Appendix 1 (saquinavir)
**Counselling** Children and their carers should be told how to recognise signs of arrhythmia and advised to seek medical attention if symptoms such as palpitation or syncope develop
**Contra-indications** see notes above; predisposition to cardiac arrhythmias (including congenital QT prolongation, bradycardia, history of symptomatic arrhythmias, heart failure with reduced left ventricular ejection fraction, electrolyte disturbances, concomitant use of drugs that prolong QT or PR interval); concomitant use of drugs that increase plasma-saquinavir concentration (avoid unless no alternative treatment available)
**Hepatic impairment** see notes above; also manufacturer advises caution in moderate impairment; avoid in decompensated liver disease
**Renal impairment** use with caution if estimated glomerular filtration rate less than 30 mL/minute/1.73 m$^2$
**Pregnancy** manufacturer advises use only if potential benefit outweighs risk
**Breast-feeding** see p. 312
**Side-effects** see notes above; also dyspnoea, increased appetite, peripheral neuropathy, convulsions, changes in libido, renal impairment, dry mouth, and alopecia

### Indications and dose

**HIV infection in combination with other antiretroviral drugs in children previously treated with antiretroviral therapy**
- By mouth

  With low-dose ritonavir

  **Child 16–18 years** 1 g twice daily

**HIV infection in combination with other antiretroviral drugs in children not previously treated with antiretroviral therapy**
- By mouth

  With low-dose ritonavir

  **Child 16–18 years** 500 mg twice daily for 7 days then 1 g twice daily

**Invirase®** (Roche) [PoM]
Tablets, orange, f/c, saquinavir (as mesilate) 500 mg, net price 120-tab pack = £251.26. Label: 21, counselling, arrhythmias

### TIPRANAVIR

**Cautions** see notes above; also patients at risk of increased bleeding from trauma, surgery, or other pathological conditions; concomitant use of drugs that increase risk of bleeding; **interactions:** Appendix 1 (tipranavir)
**Hepatotoxicity** Potentially life-threatening hepatotoxicity reported; monitor liver function before treatment then every 2 weeks for 1 month, then every 3 months. Discontinue if signs or symptoms of hepatitis develop or if liver-function abnormality develops (consult product literature)
**Contra-indications** see notes above
**Hepatic impairment** see notes above; also manufacturer advises caution in mild impairment; avoid in moderate or severe impairment—no information available
**Pregnancy** manufacturer advises use only if potential benefit outweighs risk—toxicity in *animal* studies
**Breast-feeding** see p. 312

**Side-effects** see notes above; also dyspnoea, anorexia, peripheral neuropathy, influenza-like symptoms, renal impairment, and photosensitivity; *rarely* dehydration

### Indications and dose

> **HIV infection resistant to other protease inhibitors, in combination with other antiretroviral drugs in children previously treated with antiretrovirals**
>
> For dose, see preparations

**Aptivus**® (Boehringer Ingelheim) [PoM]

Capsules, pink, tipranavir 250 mg, net price 120-cap pack = £441.00. Label: 5, 21
Excipients include ethanol 100 mg per capsule

Dose
> With low-dose ritonavir
> - **By mouth**
>   **Child 12–18 years** 500 mg twice daily

Oral solution, toffee-and mint-flavoured, tipranavir 100 mg/mL, net price 95-mL pack = £129.65. Label: 5, 21, counselling, crystallisation
Excipients include vitamin E 78 mg/mL

Dose
> With low-dose ritonavir
> - **By mouth**
>   **Child 2–12 years** 375 mg/m$^2$ (max. 500 mg) twice daily

Note The bioavailability of *Aptivus*® oral solution is higher than that of the capsules; the oral solution is **not** interchangeable with the capsules on a milligram-for-milligram basis

Counselling Children and carers should be told to observe the oral solution for crystallisation; the bottle should be replaced if more than a thin layer of crystals form (doses should continue to be taken at the normal time until the bottle is replaced)

---

## Non-nucleoside reverse transcriptase inhibitors

### ■ EFAVIRENZ

**Cautions** history of mental illness or seizures; monitor liver function if receiving other hepatotoxic drugs; **interactions:** Appendix 1 (efavirenz)
Rash Rash, usually in the first 2 weeks, is the most common side-effect; discontinue if severe rash with blistering, desquamation, mucosal involvement or fever; if rash mild or moderate, may continue without interruption—usually resolves within 1 month
Psychiatric disorders Children or their carers should be advised to seek immediate medical attention if symptoms such as severe depression, psychosis or suicidal ideation occur

**Contra-indications** acute porphyria (but see section 9.8.2)

**Hepatic impairment** in mild to moderate liver disease, monitor for dose-related side-effects (e.g. CNS effects) and liver function; avoid in severe impairment; greater risk of hepatic side-effects in chronic hepatitis B or C

**Renal impairment** manufacturer advises caution in severe renal failure—no information available

**Pregnancy** manufacturer advises avoid (effective contraception required during treatment and for 12 weeks after treatment); use efavirenz only if no alternative available

**Breast-feeding** see p. 312

**Side-effects** rash including Stevens-Johnson syndrome (see Rash above); abdominal pain, diarrhoea, nausea, vomiting; anxiety, depression, sleep disturbances, abnormal dreams, dizziness, headache, fatigue, impaired concentration (administration at bedtime especially in first 2–4 weeks reduces CNS effects); pruritus; *less commonly* pancreatitis, hepatitis, flushing, psychosis, mania, suicidal ideation, amnesia, ataxia, tremor, convulsions, gynaecomastia, blurred vision, tinnitus; *rarely* hepatic failure, photosensitivity; also reported raised serum cholesterol (see Lipodystrophy syndrome, p. 313); see also Osteonecrosis, p. 313

### Indications and dose

> See preparations

**Sustiva**® (Bristol-Myers Squibb) [PoM]

Capsules, efavirenz 50 mg (yellow/white), net price 30-cap pack = £16.73; 100 mg (white), 30-cap pack = £33.41; 200 mg (yellow), 90-cap pack = £200.27. Label: 23

Dose
> **HIV infection in combination with other antiretroviral drugs**
> - **By mouth**
>   **Child 3–18 years**
>   **Body-weight 13–15 kg** 200 mg once daily
>   **Body-weight 15–20 kg** 250 mg once daily
>   **Body-weight 20–25 kg** 300 mg once daily
>   **Body-weight 25–32.5 kg** 350 mg once daily
>   **Body-weight 32.5–40 kg** 400 mg once daily
>   **Body-weight 40 kg and over** 600 mg once daily

Administration Capsules may be opened and contents added to food (contents have a peppery taste) [unlicensed use]

Tablets, f/c, yellow, efavirenz 600 mg, net price 30-tab pack = £200.27. Label: 23

Dose
> **HIV infection in combination with other antiretroviral drugs**
> - **By mouth**
>   **Child body-weight over 40 kg** 600 mg once daily

Oral solution, sugar-free, strawberry and mint flavour, efavirenz 30 mg/mL, net price 180-mL pack = £53.84

Dose
> **HIV infection in combination with other antiretroviral drugs**
> - **By mouth**
>   **Child 3–5 years**
>   **Body-weight 13–15 kg** 360 mg once daily
>   **Body-weight 15–20 kg** 390 mg once daily
>   **Body-weight 20–25 kg** 450 mg once daily
>   **Body-weight 25–32.5 kg** 510 mg once daily
>
>   **Child 5–18 years**
>   **Body-weight 13–15 kg** 270 mg once daily
>   **Body-weight 15–20 kg** 300 mg once daily
>   **Body-weight 20–25 kg** 360 mg once daily
>   **Body-weight 25–32.5 kg** 450 mg once daily
>   **Body-weight 32.5–40 kg** 510 mg once daily
>   **Body-weight 40 kg and over** 720 mg once daily

Note The bioavailability of *Sustiva*® oral solution is lower than that of the capsules and tablets; the oral solution is **not** interchangeable with either capsules or tablets on a milligram-for-milligram basis

### ◢ With emtricitabine and tenofovir

See under Tenofovir

5 Infections

## ETRAVIRINE

**Cautions** interactions: Appendix 1 (etravirine)
**Hypersensitivity reactions** Rash, usually in the second week, is the most common side-effect and appears more frequently in females. Life-threatening hypersensitivity reactions reported usually during week 3–6 of treatment and characterised by rash, eosinophilia, and systemic symptoms (including fever, general malaise, myalgia, arthralgia, blistering, oral lesions, conjunctivitis, and hepatitis). Discontinue permanently if hypersensitivity reaction or severe rash develop. If rash mild or moderate (without signs of hypersensitivity reaction), may continue without interruption— usually resolves within 2 weeks
**Counselling** Children and carers should be told how to recognise hypersensitivity reactions and advised to seek immediate medical attention if hypersensitivity reaction or severe rash develop

**Contra-indications** acute porphyria (but see section 9.8.2)

**Hepatic impairment** use with caution in moderate impairment; avoid in severe impairment—no information available; greater risk of hepatic side-effects in chronic hepatitis B or C

**Pregnancy** manufacturer advises use only if potential benefit outweighs risk

**Breast-feeding** see p. 312

**Side-effects** rash (including Stevens-Johnson syndrome rarely and toxic epidermal necrolysis very rarely; see also Hypersensitivity Reactions above); gastro-oesophageal reflux, nausea, abdominal pain, flatulence, gastritis; hypertension; peripheral neuropathy; diabetes, hyperlipidaemia (see also Lipodystrophy Syndrome, p. 313); renal failure; anaemia; less commonly pancreatitis, haematemesis, hepatitis, chest pain, bronchospasm, drowsiness, malaise, gynaecomastia, blurred vision, dry mouth, and sweating; also reported, haemorrhagic stroke; see also Osteonecrosis, p. 313

**Licensed use** not licensed for use in children

**Indications and dose**

> **In combination with other antiretroviral drugs (including a boosted protease inhibitor) for HIV infection resistant to other non-nucleoside reverse transcriptase inhibitors and protease inhibitors**
>
> For dose, consult Guidelines (see notes above)

**Administration** for children with swallowing difficulties, tablets may be dispersed in a glass of water just before administration

**Intelence®** (Janssen) [PoM]
Tablets, etravirine 100 mg, net price 120-tab pack = £301.27; 200 mg, 60-tab pack = £301.27. Label: 21, counselling, rash, and hypersensitivity reactions
**Note** Dispense in original container (contains desiccant)

## NEVIRAPINE

**Cautions** chronic hepatitis B or C, high CD4 cell count, and females (all at greater risk of hepatic side-effects); interactions: Appendix 1 (nevirapine)
**Hepatic disease** Potentially life-threatening hepatotoxicity including fatal fulminant hepatitis reported usually in first 6 weeks; close monitoring required during first 18 weeks; monitor liver function before treatment then every 2 weeks for 2 months then after 1 month and then regularly; discontinue permanently if abnormalities in liver function tests accompanied by hypersensitivity reaction (rash, fever, arthralgia, myalgia, lymphadenopathy, hepatitis, renal impairment, eosinophilia, granulocytopenia); suspend if severe abnormalities in liver function tests but no hypersensitivity reaction—discontinue permanently if

significant liver function abnormalities recur; monitor patient closely if mild to moderate abnormalities in liver function tests with no hypersensitivity reaction
**Rash** Rash, usually in first 6 weeks, is most common side-effect; incidence reduced if introduced at low dose and dose increased gradually; monitor closely for skin reactions during first 18 weeks; discontinue permanently if severe rash or if rash accompanied by blistering, oral lesions, conjunctivitis, facial oedema, general malaise or hypersensitivity reactions; if rash mild or moderate may continue without interruption but dose should not be increased until rash resolves
**Counselling** Children and carers should be told how to recognise hypersensitivity reactions and advised to discontinue treatment and seek immediate medical attention if severe skin reaction, hypersensitivity reactions or symptoms of hepatitis develop

**Contra-indications** acute porphyria (but see section 9.8.2); post-exposure prophylaxis

**Hepatic impairment** manufacturer advises avoid modified-release preparation—no information available; use 'immediate-release' preparation with caution in moderate impairment and avoid in severe impairment; see also Hepatic Disease, above

**Renal impairment** manufacturer advises avoid modified-release preparation—no information available

**Pregnancy** although manufacturer advises caution, may be appropriate to use if clearly indicated; see also p. 312

**Breast-feeding** see p. 312

**Side-effects** rash including Stevens-Johnson syndrome and toxic epidermal necrolysis (see also Cautions above), nausea, vomiting, abdominal pain, diarrhoea, hepatitis (see also Hepatic Disease above), hypersensitivity reactions (may involve hepatic reactions and rash, see also Hepatic Disease above), headache, fatigue, fever, granulocytopenia; less commonly anaemia, myalgia, arthralgia; see also Osteonecrosis, p. 313

**Licensed use** 'immediate-release' tablets not licensed for use in children weighing less than 50 kg or with body surface area less than 1.25 m$^2$; 'immediate-release' tablets and suspension not licensed for once daily dose after the initial dose titration

**Indications and dose**

> **HIV infection in combination with other antiretroviral drugs**
> • By mouth
>
> **Neonate 14–28 days** 150–200 mg/m$^2$ once daily of 'immediate-release' preparation for first 14 days, then (if no rash present) 150–200 mg/m$^2$ twice daily of 'immediate-release' preparation
>
> **Child 1 month–3 years** 150–200 mg/m$^2$ (max. 200 mg) once daily of 'immediate-release' preparation for first 14 days, then (if no rash present) 150–200 mg/m$^2$ (max. 200 mg) twice daily or 300–400 mg/m$^2$ (max. 400 mg) once daily of 'immediate-release' preparation
>
> **Child 3–18 years** 150–200 mg/m$^2$ (max. 200 mg) once daily of 'immediate-release' preparation for first 14 days,
>
> then (if no rash present after initial dose titration) 150–200 mg/m$^2$ (max. 200 mg) twice daily of 'immediate-release' preparation
>
> or (if no rash present after initial dose titration)
> **Body surface area 0.58–0.83m$^2$** 200 mg once daily of modified-release preparation or 'immediate-release' preparation

**Body surface area 0.84–1.17m²** 300 mg once daily of modified-release preparation or 'immediate-release' preparation

**Body surface area over 1.17m²** 400 mg once daily of modified-release preparation or 'immediate-release' preparation

**Note** Initial dose titration using 'immediate-release' preparation should not exceed 28 days; if rash not resolved within 28 days, alternative treatment should be sought. If treatment interrupted for more than 7 days, restart using the lower dose of the 'immediate-release' preparation for the first 14 days as for new treatment

**Viramune®** (Boehringer Ingelheim) PoM
Tablets, nevirapine 200 mg, net price 14-tab pack = £39.67, 60-tab pack = £170.00. Counselling, hypersensitivity reactions
Suspension, nevirapine 50 mg/5 mL, net price 240-mL pack = £50.40. Counselling, hypersensitivity reactions
Prolonged-release tablets, m/r, yellow, nevirapine 50 mg, net price 180-tab pack = £127.50; 100 mg, 90-tab pack = £127.50; 400 mg, 30-tab pack = £170.00. Label: 25, counselling, hypersensitivity reactions

## Other antiretrovirals

### ENFUVIRTIDE

**Cautions**
**Hypersensitivity reactions** Hypersensitivity reactions including rash, fever, nausea, vomiting, chills, rigors, low blood pressure, respiratory distress, glomerulonephritis, and raised liver enzymes reported; discontinue immediately if any signs or symptoms of systemic hypersensitivity develop and do not rechallenge
**Counselling** Children and carers should be told how to recognise signs of hypersensitivity, and advised to discontinue treatment and seek prompt medical attention if symptoms develop
**Hepatic impairment** manufacturer advises caution—no information available; chronic hepatitis B or C (possibly greater risk of hepatic side-effects)
**Pregnancy** manufacturer advises use only if potential benefit outweighs risk
**Breast-feeding** see p. 312
**Side-effects** injection-site reactions; pancreatitis, gastro-oesophageal reflux disease, anorexia, weight loss; hypertriglyceridaemia; peripheral neuropathy, asthenia, tremor, anxiety, nightmares, irritability, impaired concentration, vertigo; pneumonia, sinusitis, influenza-like illness; diabetes mellitus; haematuria; renal calculi, lymphadenopathy; myalgia; conjunctivitis; dry skin, acne, erythema, skin papilloma; *less commonly* hypersensitivity reactions (see Cautions); see also Osteonecrosis, p. 313

**Indications and dose**
HIV infection in combination with other antiretroviral drugs for resistant infection or for children intolerant to other antiretroviral regimens
• By subcutaneous injection
**Child 6–16 years** 2 mg/kg (max. 90 mg) twice daily
**Child 16–18 years** 90 mg twice daily

**Administration** for *subcutaneous injection*, reconstitute with 1.1 mL Water for Injections and allow to stand (for up to 45 minutes) to dissolve; do **not** shake or invert vial

**Fuzeon®** (Roche) PoM
Injection, powder for reconstitution, enfuvirtide 108 mg (= enfuvirtide 90 mg/mL when reconstituted with 1.1 mL Water for Injections), net price 108-mg vial = £18.03 (with solvent, syringe, and alcohol swabs). Counselling, hypersensitivity reactions

### MARAVIROC

**Cautions** cardiovascular disease; chronic hepatitis B or C; **interactions:** Appendix 1 (maraviroc)
**Hepatic impairment** use with caution
**Renal impairment** if estimated glomerular filtration rate less than 80 mL/minute/1.73 m², consult product literature
**Pregnancy** manufacturer advises use only if potential benefit outweighs risk—toxicity in *animal* studies
**Breast-feeding** see p. 312
**Side-effects** nausea, diarrhoea, abdominal pain, flatulence, anorexia, depression, insomnia, malaise, headache, anaemia, rash; *less commonly* seizures, renal failure, proteinuria, myositis; *rarely* hepatitis, angina, pancytopenia, granulocytopenia, Stevens-Johnson syndrome; see also Osteonecrosis, p. 313
**Licensed use** not licensed for use in children

**Indications and dose**
CCR5–tropic HIV infection in combination with other antiretroviral drugs in children previously treated with antiretrovirals
For dose, consult Guidelines (see notes above)

**Celsentri®** (ViiV) PoM
Tablets, blue, f/c, maraviroc 150 mg, net price 60-tab pack = £519.14; 300 mg, 60-tab pack = £519.14

### RALTEGRAVIR

**Cautions** risk factors for myopathy or rhabdomyolysis; psychiatric illness (may exacerbate underlying illness including depression); **interactions:** Appendix 1 (raltegravir)
**Rash** Rash occurs commonly. Discontinue if severe rash or rash accompanied by fever, malaise, arthralgia, myalgia, blistering, mouth ulceration, conjunctivitis, angioedema, hepatitis, or eosinophilia
**Hepatic impairment** chronic hepatitis B or C (greater risk of hepatic side-effects); use with caution in severe impairment—no information available
**Pregnancy** manufacturer advises avoid—toxicity in *animal* studies
**Breast-feeding** see p. 312
**Side-effects** diarrhoea, nausea, vomiting, abdominal pain, flatulence, hypertriglyceridaemia, dizziness, headache, insomnia, abnormal dreams, asthenia, rash (including less commonly Stevens-Johnson syndrome, rash with eosinophilia and systemic symptoms; see also Rash above); *less commonly* gastritis, hepatitis, pancreatitis, dry mouth, gastro-oesophageal reflux, taste disturbances, pain on swallowing, peptic ulcer, constipation, rectal bleeding, lipodystrophy (see Lipodystrophy Syndrome, p. 313), palpitation, ventricular extrasystoles, bradycardia, hypertension, flushing, chest pain, oedema, dysphonia, epistaxis, nasal congestion, drowsiness, anxiety, appetite changes, confusion, impaired memory and attention, depression, suicidal ideation, pyrexia, chills, carpal tunnel syndrome, tremor, peripheral neuropathy, erectile dysfunction, gynaecomastia, menopausal symptoms, osteopenia, renal failure, nocturia,

polydipsia, anaemia, thrombocytopenia, neutropenia, arthralgia, myalgia, rhabdomyolysis, visual disturbances, tinnitus, gingivitis, glossitis, acne, pruritus, hyperhidrosis, dry skin, skin papilloma, and alopecia; see also Osteonecrosis, p. 313

**Indications and dose**

**In combination with other antiretroviral drugs for HIV infection resistant to multiple antiretrovirals**

- By mouth

    **Child 16–18 years** 400 mg twice daily

**Isentress®** (MSD) ▣PoM

Tablets, pink, f/c, raltegravir (as potassium salt) 400 mg, net price 60-tab pack = £616.22. Label: 25

### 5.3.2  Herpesvirus infections

**5.3.2.1**  Herpes simplex and varicella–zoster infection

**5.3.2.2**  Cytomegalovirus infection

### 5.3.2.1  Herpes simplex and varicella–zoster infection

The two most important herpesvirus pathogens are herpes simplex virus (herpesvirus hominis) and varicella–zoster virus.

**Herpes simplex infections**  Herpes infection of the mouth and lips and in the eye is generally associated with herpes simplex virus serotype 1 (HSV-1); other areas of the skin may also be infected, especially in immunodeficiency. Genital infection is most often associated with HSV-2 and also HSV-1. Treatment of herpes simplex infection should start as early as possible and usually within 5 days of the appearance of the infection.

In individuals with good immune function, mild infection of the eye (ocular herpes, section 11.3.3) and of the lips (herpes labialis or cold sores, section 13.10.3) is treated with a topical antiviral drug. Primary herpetic gingivostomatitis is managed by changes to diet and with analgesics (section 12.3.2). Severe infection, neonatal herpes infection or infection in immunocompromised individuals requires treatment with a systemic antiviral drug. After completing parenteral treatment of neonatal herpes simplex encephalitis, oral suppression therapy with aciclovir for 6 months can be considered on specialist advice. Primary or recurrent genital herpes simplex infection is treated with an antiviral drug given by mouth. Persistance of a lesion or recurrence in an immunocompromised child may signal the development of resistance.

Specialist advice should be sought for systemic treatment of herpes simplex infection in pregnancy.

**Varicella–zoster infections**  Regardless of immune function and the use of any immunoglobulins, neonates with *chickenpox* should be treated with a parenteral antiviral to reduce the risk of severe disease. Oral therapy is not recommended as absorption is variable.

Chickenpox in otherwise healthy children between 1 month and 12 years is usually mild and antiviral treatment is not usually required. Chickenpox is more severe in adolescents than in children; antiviral treatment started within 24 hours of the onset of rash may reduce the duration and severity of symptoms in otherwise healthy adolescents. Antiviral treatment is generally recommended in immunocompromised patients and those at special risk (e.g. because of severe cardiovascular or respiratory disease or chronic skin disorder); in such cases, an antiviral is given for 10 days with at least 7 days of parenteral treatment.

In pregnancy severe chickenpox may cause complications, especially varicella pneumonia. Specialist advice should be sought for the treatment of chickenpox during pregnancy.

Neonates and children who have been exposed to chickenpox and are at special risk of complications may require prophylaxis with varicella-zoster immunoglobulin (see under Disease-specific Immunoglobulins, section 14.5.2). Prophylactic intravenous aciclovir should be considered for neonates whose mothers develop chickenpox 4 days before to 2 days after delivery.

In *herpes zoster* (shingles) systemic antiviral treatment can reduce the severity and duration of pain, reduce complications, and reduce viral shedding. Treatment with the antiviral should be started within 72 hours of the onset of rash and is usually continued for 7–10 days. Immunocompromised patients at high risk of disseminated or severe infection should be treated with a parenteral antiviral drug. Chronic pain which persists after the rash has healed (postherpetic neuralgia) requires specific management (section 4.7.3).

**Choice**  Aciclovir is active against herpesviruses but does not eradicate them. Uses of aciclovir include systemic treatment of varicella–zoster and the systemic and topical treatment of herpes simplex infections of the skin (section 13.10.3) and mucous membranes (section 7.2.2). It is used by mouth for severe herpetic stomatitis (see also p. 547). Aciclovir eye ointment (section 11.3.3) is used for herpes simplex infections of the eye; it is combined with systemic treatment for ophthalmic zoster.

**Famciclovir**, a prodrug of penciclovir, is similar to aciclovir and is licensed in adults for use in herpes zoster and genital herpes; there is limited information available on use in children. Penciclovir itself is used as a cream for herpes simplex labialis (section 13.10.3).

**Valaciclovir** is an ester of aciclovir, licensed in adults for herpes zoster and herpes simplex infections of the skin and mucous membranes (including genital herpes); it is also licensed in children over 12 years for preventing cytomegalovirus disease following solid organ transplantation. Valaciclovir may be used for the treatment of mild herpes zoster in immunocompromised children over 12 years; treatment should be initiated under specialist supervision.

### ▶ ACICLOVIR
(Acyclovir)

**Cautions**  maintain adequate hydration (especially with infusion or high doses, or during renal impairment); interactions: Appendix 1 (aciclovir)

**Renal impairment**  see Cautions above; also risk of neurological reactions increased; use normal *intravenous* dose every 12 hours if estimated glomerular filtration rate 25–50 mL/minute/1.73 m$^2$ (every 24 hours if estimated glomerular filtration rate 10–25 mL/minute/1.73 m$^2$); consult product literature for intravenous dose if estimated glomerular filtration rate less than 10 mL/minute/1.73 m$^2$. For *herpes zoster*, use normal oral dose every 8 hours if estimated glomerular filtration rate 10–25 mL/minute/1.73 m$^2$ (every 12 hours if estimated glomerular filtration rate less than 10 mL/minute/1.73 m$^2$). For *herpes simplex*, use normal oral dose every 12 hours if estimated glomerular filtration rate less than 10 mL/minute/1.73 m$^2$

**Pregnancy** not known to be harmful—manufacturers advise use only when potential benefit outweighs risk

**Breast-feeding** significant amount in milk after systemic administration; not known to be harmful but manufacturers advise caution

**Side-effects** nausea, vomiting, abdominal pain, diarrhoea, headache, fatigue, rash, urticaria, pruritus, photosensitivity; *very rarely* hepatitis, jaundice, dyspnoea, neurological reactions (including dizziness, confusion, hallucinations, convulsions, ataxia, dysarthria, and drowsiness), acute renal failure, anaemia, thrombocytopenia, and leucopenia; on *intravenous infusion*, severe local inflammation (sometimes leading to ulceration), and *very rarely* agitation, tremors, psychosis and fever

**Licensed use** tablets and suspension not licensed for suppression of herpes simplex or for treatment of herpes zoster in children (age range not specified by manufacturer); intravenous infusion not licensed for herpes zoster in children under 18 years; tablets and suspension not licensed for attenuation of chickenpox (if varicella-zoster immunoglobulin not indicated) in children under 18 years

### Indications and dose

Herpes simplex treatment

- By mouth

  **Child 1 month–2 years** 100 mg 5 times daily, usually for 5 days (longer if new lesions appear during treatment or if healing incomplete); dose doubled if immunocompromised or if absorption impaired

  **Child 2–18 years** 200 mg 5 times daily, usually for 5 days (longer if new lesions appear during treatment or if healing incomplete); dose doubled if immunocompromised or if absorption impaired

- By intravenous infusion

  **Neonate** 20 mg/kg every 8 hours for 14 days (for at least 21 days if CNS involvement—confirm cerebrospinal fluid negative for herpes simplex virus before stopping treatment)

  **Child 1–3 months** 20 mg/kg every 8 hours for 14 days (for at least 21 days if CNS involvement—confirm cerebrospinal fluid negative for herpes simplex virus before stopping treatment)

  **Child 3 months–12 years** 250 mg/m$^2$ every 8 hours usually for 5 days, doubled to 500 mg/m$^2$ every 8 hours in the immunocompromised or in simplex encephalitis (given for at least 21 days in encephalitis—confirm cerebrospinal fluid negative for herpes simplex virus before stopping treatment)

  **Child 12–18 years** 5 mg/kg every 8 hours usually for 5 days, doubled to 10 mg/kg every 8 hours in the immunocompromised or in simplex encephalitis (given for at least 14 days in encephalitis (at least 21 days if also immunocompromised)—confirm cerebrospinal fluid negative

for herpes simplex virus before stopping treatment)

  **Note** To avoid excessive dose in obese patients parenteral dose should be calculated on the basis of ideal weight for height

Herpes simplex prophylaxis in the immunocompromised

- By mouth

  **Child 1 month–2 years** 100–200 mg 4 times daily

  **Child 2–18 years** 200–400 mg 4 times daily

Herpes simplex suppression

- By mouth

  **Child 12–18 years** 400 mg twice daily *or* 200 mg 4 times daily; increased to 400 mg 3 times daily if recurrences occur on standard suppressive therapy or for suppression of genital herpes during late pregnancy (from 36 weeks gestation); therapy interrupted every 6–12 months to reassess recurrence frequency—consider restarting after two or more recurrences

Chickenpox and herpes zoster infection

- By mouth

  **Child 1 month–2 years** 200 mg 4 times daily for 5 days (for herpes zoster in the immunocompromised continue for 2 days after crusting of lesions)

  **Child 2–6 years** 400 mg 4 times daily for 5 days (for herpes zoster in the immunocompromised continue for 2 days after crusting of lesions)

  **Child 6–12 years** 800 mg 4 times daily for 5 days (for herpes zoster in the immunocompromised continue for 2 days after crusting of lesions)

  **Child 12–18 years** 800 mg 5 times daily for 7 days (for herpes zoster in the immunocompromised continue for 2 days after crusting of lesions)

- By intravenous infusion

  **Neonate** 10–20 mg/kg every 8 hours for at least 7 days (given for 10–14 days in encephalitis, possibly longer if also immunocompromised)

  **Child 1–3 months** 10–20 mg/kg every 8 hours for at least 7 days (given for 10–14 days in encephalitis, possibly longer if also immunocompromised)

  **Child 3 months–12 years** 250 mg/m$^2$ every 8 hours usually for 5 days, doubled to 500 mg/m$^2$ every 8 hours in the immunocompromised or in encephalitis (given for 10–14 days in encephalitis, possibly longer if also immunocompromised)

  **Child 12–18 years** 5 mg/kg every 8 hours usually for 5 days, doubled to 10 mg/kg every 8 hours in the immunocompromised or in encephalitis (given for 10–14 days in encephalitis, possibly longer if also immunocompromised)

  **Note** To avoid excessive dose in obese patients parenteral dose should be calculated on the basis of ideal weight for height

Prophylaxis of chickenpox after delivery (see notes above)

- By intravenous infusion

  **Neonate** 10 mg/kg every 8 hours; continued until serological tests confirm absence of virus

**Attenuation of chickenpox if varicella–zoster immunoglobulin not indicated**

- **By mouth**

  **Child 1 month–18 years** 10 mg/kg 4 times daily for 7 days starting 1 week after exposure

**Herpesvirus skin infections** section 13.10.3

**Herpesvirus eye infections** section 11.3.3

**Administration** for *intravenous infusion*, reconstitute to 25 mg/mL with Water for Injections or Sodium Chloride 0.9% then dilute to concentration of 5 mg/mL with Sodium Chloride 0.9% *or* Sodium Chloride and Glucose and give over 1 hour; alternatively, may be administered in a concentration of 25 mg/mL using a suitable infusion pump and central venous access and given over 1 hour

**Aciclovir** (Non-proprietary) [PoM]

Tablets, aciclovir 200 mg, net price 25-tab pack = £4.45; 400 mg, 56-tab pack = £8.10; 800 mg, 35-tab pack = £10.21. Label: 9

**Dental prescribing on NHS** Aciclovir Tablets 200 mg or 800 mg may be prescribed

Dispersible tablets, aciclovir 200 mg, net price 25-tab pack = £2.05; 400 mg, 56-tab pack = £7.24; 800 mg, 35-tab pack = £7.02. Label: 9

Suspension, aciclovir 200 mg/5 mL, net price 125 mL = £38.22; 400 mg/5 mL, 100 mL = £41.55. Label: 9

**Dental prescribing on NHS** Aciclovir Oral Suspension 200 mg/5 mL may be prescribed

Intravenous infusion, powder for reconstitution, aciclovir (as sodium salt), net price 250-mg vial = £9.13; 500-mg vial = £20.22

**Electrolytes** Na⁺ 1.1 mmol/250-mg vial

Intravenous infusion, aciclovir (as sodium salt), 25 mg/mL, net price 10-mL (250-mg) vial = £10.37; 20-mL (500-mg) vial = £19.21; 40-mL (1-g) vial = £40.44

**Electrolytes** Na⁺ 1.16 mmol/250-mg vial

**Zovirax®** (GSK) [PoM]

Tablets, all dispersible, f/c, aciclovir 200 mg, net price 25-tab pack = £17.71; 800 mg (scored, *Shingles Treatment Pack*), 35-tab pack = £65.80. Label: 9

Suspension, both off-white, sugar-free, aciclovir 200 mg/5 mL (banana-flavoured), net price 125 mL = £29.53; 400 mg/5 mL (*Double Strength Suspension*, orange-flavoured), 100 mL = £33.01. Label: 9

Intravenous infusion, powder for reconstitution, aciclovir (as sodium salt), net price 250-mg vial = £9.96; 500-mg vial = £17.72

**Electrolytes** Na⁺ 1.1 mmol/250-mg vial

---

## VALACICLOVIR

**Note** Valaciclovir is a pro-drug of aciclovir

**Cautions** see under Aciclovir

**Hepatic impairment** manufacturer advises caution with high doses used for preventing cytomegalovirus disease—no information available in children

**Renal impairment** maintain adequate hydration; for *herpes zoster*, 1 g every 12 hours if estimated glomerular filtration rate 30–50 mL/minute/1.73 m² (1 g every 24 hours if estimated glomerular filtration rate

10–30 mL/minute/1.73 m²; 500 mg every 24 hours if estimated glomerular filtration rate less than 10 mL/minute/1.73 m²); for *treatment of herpes simplex*, 500 mg (1 g in immunocompromised or HIV-positive children) every 24 hours if estimated glomerular filtration rate less than 30 mL/minute/1.73 m²; for *treatment of herpes labialis*, if estimated glomerular filtration rate 30–50 mL/minute/1.73 m², initially 1 g, then 1 g 12 hours after initial dose (if estimated glomerular filtration rate 10–30 mL/minute/1.73 m², initally 500 mg, then 500 mg 12 hours after initial dose; if estimated glomerular filtration rate less than 10 mL/minute/1.73 m², 500 mg as a single dose); for *suppression of herpes simplex*, 250 mg (500 mg in immunocompromised or HIV-positive children) every 24 hours if estimated glomerular filtration rate less than 30 mL/minute/1.73 m²; reduce dose according to estimated glomerular filtration rate for *cytomegalovirus prophylaxis* following solid organ transplantation (consult product literature)

**Pregnancy** see under Aciclovir

**Breast-feeding** see under Aciclovir

**Side-effects** see under Aciclovir but neurological reactions more frequent with high doses

**Licensed use** not licensed for treatment of herpes zoster in children; not licensed for treatment or suppression of herpes simplex infection in immunocompromised or HIV-positive children

### Indications and dose

**Herpes zoster in immunocompromised**

- **By mouth**

  **Child 12–18 years** 1 g 3 times daily for at least 7 days (continue for 2 days after crusting of lesions)

**Treatment of herpes simplex**

- **By mouth**

  **Child 12–18 years** first episode, 500 mg twice daily for 5 days, longer if new lesions appear during treatment or if healing incomplete (1 g twice daily for 10 days in immunocompromised or HIV-positive children); recurrent infection, 500 mg twice daily for 3–5 days (1 g twice daily for 5–10 days in immunocompromised or HIV-positive children)

**Treatment of herpes labialis**

- **By mouth**

  **Child 12–18 years** initially 2 g, then 2 g 12 hours after initial dose

**Suppression of herpes simplex**

- **By mouth**

  **Child 12–18 years** 500 mg daily in 1–2 divided doses (in immunocompromised or HIV-positive children, 500 mg twice daily); therapy interrupted every 6–12 months to reassess recurrence frequency—consider restarting after two or more recurrences

**Prevention of cytomegalovirus disease following solid organ transplantation (preferably starting within 72 hours of transplantation)**

- **By mouth**

  **Child 12–18 years** 2 g 4 times daily usually for 90 days

**Valaciclovir** (Non-proprietary) [PoM]
Tablets, valaciclovir 500 mg, net price 10-tab pack = £19.43, 42 tab-pack = £79.04. Label: 9

**Valtrex®** (GSK) [PoM]
Tablets, f/c, valaciclovir (as hydrochloride) 250 mg, net price 60-tab pack = £123.28; 500 mg, 10-tab pack = £20.59, 42-tab pack = £86.30. Label: 9

## 5.3.2.2 Cytomegalovirus infection

Recommendations for the optimum maintenance therapy of cytomegalovirus (CMV) infections and the duration of treatment are subject to rapid change.

**Ganciclovir** is related to aciclovir but it is more active against cytomegalovirus; it is also much more toxic than aciclovir and should therefore be prescribed under specialist supervision and only when the potential benefit outweighs the risks. Ganciclovir is administered by intravenous infusion for the *initial treatment* of CMV infection. The use of ganciclovir may also be considered for symptomatic congenital CMV infection. Ganciclovir causes profound myelosuppression when given with zidovudine; the two should not normally be given together particularly during initial ganciclovir therapy. The likelihood of ganciclovir resistance increases in patients with a high viral load or in those who receive the drug over a long duration; cross-resistance to cidofovir is common.

**Valaciclovir** (section 5.3.2.1) is licensed for use in children over 12 years for prevention of cytomegalovirus disease following renal transplantation.

**Foscarnet** is also active against cytomegalovirus; it is toxic and can cause renal impairment.

**Cidofovir** is given in combination with probenecid for CMV retinitis in AIDS patients when ganciclovir and foscarnet are contra-indicated. Cidofovir is nephrotoxic. There is limited information on its use in children.

## ▌GANCICLOVIR

**Cautions** close monitoring of full blood count (severe deterioration may require correction and possibly treatment interruption); history of cytopenia; potential carcinogen and teratogen; radiotherapy; ensure adequate hydration during intravenous administration; vesicant—infuse into vein with adequate flow preferably using plastic cannula; possible risk of long-term carcinogenic or reproductive toxicity; **interactions**: Appendix 1 (ganciclovir)

**Contra-indications** hypersensitivity to valganciclovir, ganciclovir, aciclovir, or valaciclovir; abnormally low haemoglobin, neutrophil, or platelet counts (consult product literature)

**Renal impairment** reduce dose if estimated glomerular filtration rate less than 70 mL/minute/1.73 m²; consult product literature

**Pregnancy** avoid—teratogenic risk; ensure effective contraception during treatment and barrier contraception for males during and for at least 90 days after treatment

**Breast-feeding** avoid—no information available

**Side-effects** diarrhoea, nausea, vomiting, dyspepsia, abdominal pain, constipation, flatulence, dysphagia, taste disturbance, hepatic dysfunction; dyspnoea, chest pain, cough; headache, insomnia, convulsions, dizziness, peripheral neuropathy, depression, anxiety;

confusion, abnormal thinking, fatigue, weight loss, anorexia; infection, pyrexia, night sweats; anaemia, leucopenia, thrombocytopenia, pancytopenia, renal impairment; myalgia, arthralgia; macular oedema, retinal detachment, vitreous floaters, eye pain; ear pain; dermatitis, pruritus; injection-site reactions; *less commonly* mouth ulcers, pancreatitis, arrhythmias, hypotension, anaphylactic reactions, psychosis, tremor, male infertility, haematuria, disturbances in hearing and vision, and alopecia

**Licensed use** not licensed for use in children

**Indications and dose**

> **Life-threatening or sight-threatening cytomegalovirus infections in immunocompromised patients only; prevention of cytomegalovirus disease following immunosuppressive therapy following organ transplantation**
> • By intravenous infusion
>> **Child 1 month–18 years** initially (induction) 5 mg/kg every 12 hours for 14–21 days for treatment or for 7–14 days for prevention; maintenance (for patients at risk of relapse of retinitis), 6 mg/kg daily on 5 days per week *or* 5 mg/kg daily until adequate recovery of immunity; if retinitis progresses initial induction treatment may be repeated
>
> **Congenital cytomegalovirus infection of the CNS**
> • By intravenous infusion
>> **Neonate** 6 mg/kg every 12 hours for 6 weeks
>
> **Local treatment of CMV retinitis** section 11.3.3

**Administration** for *intravenous infusion*, reconstitute with Water for Injections (500 mg/10 mL) then dilute to a concentration of not more than 10 mg/mL with Glucose 5% *or* Sodium Chloride 0.9% and give over 1 hour

**Cymevene®** (Roche) [PoM]
Intravenous infusion, powder for reconstitution, ganciclovir (as sodium salt). Net price 500-mg vial = £29.77
Electrolytes Na⁺ 2 mmol/500-mg vial
Caution in handling Ganciclovir is toxic and personnel should be adequately protected during handling and administration; if solution comes into contact with skin or mucosa, wash off immediately with soap and water

## ▌FOSCARNET SODIUM

**Cautions** monitor electrolytes, particularly calcium and magnesium; monitor serum creatinine every second day during induction and every week during maintenance; ensure adequate hydration; avoid rapid infusion; **interactions**: Appendix 1 (foscarnet)

**Renal impairment** reduce dose; consult product literature

**Pregnancy** avoid

**Breast-feeding** avoid—present in milk in *animal* studies

**Side-effects** nausea, vomiting, diarrhoea (occasionally constipation and dyspepsia), abdominal pain, anorexia; changes in blood pressure and ECG; headache, fatigue, mood disturbances (including psychosis), asthenia, paraesthesia, convulsions, tremor, dizziness, and other neurological disorders; rash; impairment of renal function including acute renal failure; hypocalcaemia (sometimes symptomatic) and other electrolyte disturbances; abnormal liver function tests; decreased haemoglobin concentration, leucopenia, granulocytopenia, thrombocytopenia; thrombophlebitis if given undiluted by peripheral vein; genital irritation and ulceration (due to high concentrations excreted in urine); isolated reports of pancreatitis

**Licensed use**   not licensed for use in children

**Indications and dose**

### CMV disease

- By intravenous infusion

  **Child 1 month–18 years** induction 60 mg/kg every 8 hours for 2–3 weeks then maintenance 60 mg/kg daily, increased to 90–120 mg/kg if tolerated; if disease progresses on maintenance dose, repeat induction regimen

### Mucocutaneous herpes simplex infection

- By intravenous infusion

  **Child 1 month–18 years** 40 mg/kg every 8 hours for 2–3 weeks or until lesions heal

**Administration**   for *intravenous infusion*, give undiluted solution via a central venous catheter; alternatively dilute to a concentration of 12 mg/mL with Glucose 5% *or* Sodium Chloride 0.9% for administration via a peripheral vein; give over at least 1 hour (give doses greater than 60 mg/kg over 2 hours)

**Foscavir**® (Clinigen)  PoM
Intravenous infusion, foscarnet sodium hexahydrate 24 mg/mL, net price 250-mL bottle = £34.49

---

### 5.3.3  Viral hepatitis

Treatment for viral hepatitis should be initiated by a specialist in hepatology or infectious diseases. The management of uncomplicated acute viral hepatitis is largely symptomatic. Hepatitis B and hepatitis C viruses are major causes of chronic hepatitis. For details on immunisation against hepatitis A and B infections, see section 14.4 (active immunisation) and section 14.5 (passive immunisation).

**Chronic hepatitis B**   Interferon alfa (section 8.2.4), peginterferon alfa-2a, lamivudine (section 5.3.1), adefovir dipivoxil, entecavir, and tenofovir disoproxil have a role in the treatment of chronic hepatitis B in adults, but their role in children has not been well established. Specialist supervision is required for the management of chronic hepatitis B.

Tenofovir, or a combination of tenofovir with either emtricitabine or lamivudine, may be used with other antiretrovirals, as part of 'highly active antiretroviral therapy' (section 5.3.1) in children who require treatment for both HIV and chronic hepatitis B. If children infected with both HIV and chronic hepatitis B only require treatment for chronic hepatitis B, they should receive antivirals that are not active against HIV. Management of these children should be co-ordinated between HIV and hepatology specialists.

**Chronic hepatitis C**   Treatment should be considered for children with moderate or severe liver disease. Specialist supervision is required and the regimen is chosen according to the genotype of the infecting virus

and the viral load. A combination of **ribavirin** (section 5.3.5) with either **interferon alfa** (section 8.2.4) or **peginterferon alfa-2b** is licensed for use in children over 3 years with chronic hepatitis C. A combination of peginterferon alfa (BNF Section 8.2.4) and ribavirin is preferred.

---

### 5.3.4  Influenza

For advice on immunisation against influenza, see section 14.4.

**Oseltamivir** and **zanamivir** reduce replication of influenza A and B viruses by inhibiting viral neuraminidase. They are most effective for the treatment of influenza if started within a few hours of the onset of symptoms; oseltamivir is licensed for use within 48 hours of the first symptoms while zanamivir is licensed for use within 36 hours of the first symptoms. In otherwise healthy individuals they reduce the duration of symptoms by about 1–1.5 days. For further information on the treatment of influenza, see NICE guidance, p. 329.

Oseltamivir and zanamivir are licensed for post-exposure prophylaxis of influenza when influenza is circulating in the community. Oseltamivir should be given within 48 hours of exposure to influenza while zanamivir should be given within 36 hours of exposure to influenza (see also NICE guidance, p. 329). However, in children with severe influenza or in those who are immunocompromised, antivirals may still be effective after this time if viral shedding continues [unlicensed use]. Oseltamivir and zanamivir are also licensed for use in exceptional circumstances (e.g. when vaccination does not cover the infecting strain) to prevent influenza in an epidemic.

There is evidence that some strains of influenza A virus have reduced susceptibility to oseltamivir, but may retain susceptibility to zanamivir. Resistance to oseltamivir may be greater in severely immunocompromised children.

### Oseltamivir in children under 1 year of age

Data on the use of oseltamivir in children under 1 year of age is limited. Furthermore, oseltamivir may be ineffective in neonates because they may not be able to metabolise oseltamivir to its active form. However, oseltamivir can be used (under specialist supervision) for the treatment or post-exposure prophylaxis of influenza in children under 1 year of age. The Department of Health has advised (May 2009) that during a pandemic, treatment with oseltamivir can be overseen by healthcare professionals experienced in assessing children.

**Amantadine** is licensed for prophylaxis and treatment of influenza A in children over 10 years of age, but it is no longer recommended (see NICE guidance, p. 329).

Information on pandemic influenza, avian influenza, and swine influenza can be found at www.hpa.org.uk.

**Pregnancy and breast-feeding**   Although safety data are limited, either oseltamivir or zanamivir can be used in women who are pregnant or breast-feeding when the potential benefit outweighs the risk (e.g. during a pandemic). Oseltamivir is the preferred drug in women who are breast-feeding.

Infections

**5**

Infections

### NICE guidance

**Oseltamivir, zanamivir, and amantadine for prophylaxis and treatment of influenza (September 2008 and February 2009)**

The drugs described here are not a substitute for vaccination, which remains the most effective way of preventing illness from influenza.

- Amantadine is **not** recommended for prophylaxis or treatment of influenza.
- Oseltamivir or zanamivir are **not** recommended for seasonal prophylaxis against influenza.
- When influenza is circulating in the community[1], either oseltamivir or zanamivir is recommended (in accordance with UK licensing) for post-exposure prophylaxis in at-risk patients who are not effectively protected by influenza vaccine, and who have been in close contact with someone suffering from influenza-like illness in the same household or residential setting. Oseltamivir should be given within 48 hours of exposure to influenza while zanamivir should be given within 36 hours of exposure to influenza.
- When influenza is circulating in the community[1], oseltamivir or zanamivir is recommended (in accordance with UK licensing) for the treatment of influenza in at-risk patients who can start treatment within 48 hours (within 36 hours for zanamivir) of the onset of symptoms.
- During local outbreaks of influenza-like illness, when there is a high level of certainty that influenza is present, either oseltamivir or zanamivir may be used for post-exposure prophylaxis or treatment in at-risk patients (regardless of influenza vaccination) living in long-term residential or nursing homes.

At-risk[2] patients are those who have one or more of the following conditions:

- chronic respiratory disease (including asthma);
- chronic heart disease;
- chronic renal disease;
- chronic liver disease;
- chronic neurological disease;
- immunosuppression;
- diabetes mellitus.

This guidance does not cover the circumstances of a pandemic, an impending pandemic, or a widespread epidemic of a new strain of influenza to which there is little or no immunity in the community.

www.nice.org.uk/TA158
www.nice.org.uk/TA168

---

### ⬛ OSELTAMIVIR

**Renal impairment** for *treatment*, use 40% of normal dose twice daily if estimated glomerular filtration rate 30–60 mL/minute/1.73 m$^2$ (40% of normal dose once daily if estimated glomerular filtration rate 10–30 mL/minute/1.73 m$^2$); for *prevention*, use 40% of normal dose once daily if estimated glomerular filtration rate 30–60 mL/minute/1.73 m$^2$ (40% of normal dose every 48 hours if estimated glomerular filtration rate 10–30 mL/minute/1.73 m$^2$); avoid for *treatment* and *prevention* if estimated glomerular filtration rate less than 10 mL/minute/1.73 m$^2$

**Pregnancy** use only if potential benefit outweighs risk (e.g. during a pandemic); see also p. 328

**Breast-feeding** amount probably too small to be harmful; use only if potential benefit outweighs risk; (e.g. during a pandemic); see also p. 328

**Side-effects** nausea, vomiting, abdominal pain, dyspepsia, headache; *less commonly* arrhythmias, convulsions, altered consciousness, eczema, rash; *rarely* hepatitis, gastro-intestinal bleeding, neuropsychiatric disorders, thrombocytopenia, visual disturbances, Stevens-Johnson syndrome, toxic epidermal necrolysis

**Licensed use** not licensed for use in children under 1 year unless there is a pandemic

**Indications and dose**

**Prevention of influenza**

- **By mouth**

  **Neonate** (see notes above) 2 mg/kg once daily for 10 days for post-exposure prophylaxis

  **Child 1–3 months** (see notes above) 2.5 mg/kg once daily for 10 days for post-exposure prophylaxis

  **Child 3 months–1 year** (see notes above) 3 mg/kg once daily for 10 days for post-exposure prophylaxis

  **Child 1–13 years**

  **Body-weight 10–15 kg** 30 mg once daily for 10 days for post-exposure prophylaxis; for up to 6 weeks during an epidemic

  **Body-weight 15–23 kg** 45 mg once daily for 10 days for post-exposure prophylaxis; for up to 6 weeks during an epidemic

  **Body-weight 23–40 kg** 60 mg once daily for 10 days for post-exposure prophylaxis; for up to 6 weeks during an epidemic

  **Body-weight over 40 kg** 75 mg once daily for 10 days for post-exposure prophylaxis; for up to 6 weeks during an epidemic

  **Child 13–18 years** 75 mg once daily for 10 days for post-exposure prophylaxis; for up to 6 weeks during an epidemic

**Treatment of influenza**

- **By mouth**

  **Neonate** (see notes above) 2 mg/kg twice daily for 5 days

  **Child 1–3 months** (see notes above) 2.5 mg/kg twice daily for 5 days

  **Child 3 months–1 year** (see notes above) 3 mg/kg twice daily for 5 days

  **Child 1–13 years**

  **Body-weight 10–15 kg** 30 mg twice daily for 5 days

  **Body-weight 15–23 kg** 45 mg twice daily for 5 days

  **Body-weight 23–40 kg** 60 mg twice daily for 5 days

  **Body-weight over 40 kg** 75 mg twice daily for 5 days

  **Child 13–18 years** 75 mg twice daily for 5 days

**Administration** if suspension not available, capsules can be opened and the contents mixed with a small amount of sweetened food, such as sugar water or chocolate syrup, just before administration

---

1. National surveillance schemes, including those run by Public Health England, should be used to indicate when influenza is circulating in the community.
2. The Department of Health in England has advised (November 2010 and April 2011) that 'at risk patients' also includes children who are at risk of developing medical complications from influenza (treatment only) or females who are pregnant.

**¹Tamiflu®** (Roche) [PoM]

Capsules, oseltamivir (as phosphate) 30 mg (yellow), net price 10-cap pack = £7.71; 45 mg (grey), 10-cap pack = £15.41; 75 mg (grey-yellow), 10-cap pack = £15.41. Label: 9

Oral suspension, sugar-free, tutti-frutti-flavoured, oseltamivir (as phosphate) for reconstitution with water, 30 mg/5 mL, net price 65 mL = £10.27. Label: 9

Excipients include sorbitol 900 mg/5 mL

Note Solutions prepared by 'Special Order' manufacturers may be a different concentration

## ZANAMIVIR

**Cautions** asthma and chronic pulmonary disease (risk of bronchospasm—short-acting bronchodilator should be available; avoid in severe asthma unless close monitoring possible and appropriate facilities available to treat bronchospasm); uncontrolled chronic illness; other inhaled drugs should be administered before zanamivir

**Pregnancy** use only if potential benefit outweighs risk (e.g. during a pandemic); see also p. 328

**Breast-feeding** amount probably too small to be harmful; use only if potential benefit outweighs risk (e.g. during a pandemic); see also p. 328

**Side-effects** rash; *less commonly* bronchospasm, dyspnoea, angioedema, urticaria; *rarely* Stevens-Johnson syndrome, toxic epidermal necrolysis; also reported neuropsychiatric disorders

**Indications and dose**

Post-exposure prophylaxis of influenza

• By inhalation of powder

**Child 5–18 years** 10 mg once daily for 10 days

Prevention of influenza during an epidemic

• By inhalation of powder

**Child 5–18 years** 10 mg once daily for up to 28 days

Treatment of influenza

• By inhalation of powder

**Child 5–18 years** 10 mg twice daily for 5 days (for up to 10 days if resistance to oseltamivir suspected)

**¹Relenza®** (GSK) [PoM]

Dry powder for inhalation disks containing 4 blisters of zanamivir 5 mg/blister, net price 5 disks with *Diskhaler®* device = £16.36

## 5.3.5 Respiratory syncytial virus

**Ribavirin** inhibits a wide range of DNA and RNA viruses. It is licensed for administration by inhalation for the treatment of severe bronchiolitis caused by the respiratory syncytial virus (RSV) in infants, especially when they have other serious diseases. However, there is no evidence that ribavirin produces clinically relevant benefit in RSV bronchiolitis. Ribavirin is given by mouth with peginterferon alfa or interferon alfa for the treatment of chronic hepatitis C infection (see Viral Hepatitis, section 5.3.3). Ribavirin is also effective in Lassa

fever and has also been used parenterally in the treatment of life-threatening RSV, parainfluenza virus, and adenovirus infections in immunocompromised children [unlicensed indications].

**Palivizumab** is a monoclonal antibody licensed for preventing serious lower respiratory-tract disease caused by respiratory syncytial virus in children at high risk of the disease; it should be prescribed under specialist supervision and on the basis of the likelihood of hospitalisation.

Palivizumab is recommended for:

• children under 9 months of age with chronic lung disease (defined as requiring oxygen for at least 28 days from birth) and who were born preterm[2];

• children under 6 months of age with haemodynamically significant, acyanotic congenital heart disease who were born preterm[2].

Palivizumab should be considered for:

• children under 2 years of age with severe combined immunodeficiency syndrome;

• children under 1 year of age who require long-term ventilation;

• children 1–2 years of age who require long-term ventilation and have an additional co-morbidity (including cardiac disease or pulmonary hypertension).

## PALIVIZUMAB

**Cautions** moderate to severe acute infection or febrile illness; thrombocytopenia; serum-palivizumab concentration may be reduced after cardiac surgery; hypersensitivity to humanised monoclonal antibodies

**Side-effects** fever, injection-site reactions, nervousness; *less commonly* diarrhoea, vomiting, constipation, haemorrhage, rhinitis, cough, wheeze, pain, drowsiness, asthenia, hyperkinesia, leucopenia, and rash; also reported, apnoea, hypersensitivity reactions (including anaphylaxis), convulsions and thrombocytopenia

**Licensed use** licensed for the prevention of serious lower respiratory-tract disease caused by respiratory syncytial virus (RSV) in children under 6 months of age (at the start of the RSV season) and born at less than 35 weeks postmenstrual age, or in children under 2 years of age who have received treatment for bronchopulmonary dysplasia in the last 6 months, or in children under 2 years of age with haemodynamically significant congenital heart disease

**Indications and dose**

Prevention of serious disease caused by respiratory syncytial virus infection (see notes above)

• By intramuscular injection (preferably in antero-lateral thigh)

**Neonate** 15 mg/kg once a month during season of RSV risk

**Child 1 month–2 years** 15 mg/kg once a month during season of RSV risk (child undergoing cardiac bypass surgery, 15 mg/kg as soon as stable after surgery, then once a month during season of risk); injection volume over 1 mL should be divided between 2 or more sites

---

1. [NHS] except for the treatment and prophylaxis of influenza as indicated in the notes above and NICE guidance; endorse prescription 'SLS'

2. For details of the preterm age groups included in the recommendations, see *Immunisation against Infectious Disease* (2006), available at www.gov.uk/dh

**Synagis®** (AbbVie) [PoM]

Injection, powder for reconstitution, palivizumab, net price 50-mg vial = £360.40; 100-mg vial = £663.11

---

## ◣ RIBAVIRIN
(Tribavirin)

**Cautions**

**Specific cautions for inhaled treatment** Maintain standard supportive respiratory and fluid management therapy; monitor electrolytes closely; monitor equipment for precipitation; pregnant women (and those planning pregnancy) should avoid exposure to aerosol

**Specific cautions for systemic treatment** Exclude pregnancy before treatment in females of childbearing age; effective contraception essential during treatment and for 4 months after treatment in females and for 7 months after treatment in males of childbearing age; routine monthly pregnancy tests recommended; condoms must be used if partner of male patient is pregnant (ribavirin excreted in semen); cardiac disease (assessment including ECG recommended before and during treatment—discontinue if deterioration); determine full blood count, platelets, electrolytes, serum creatinine, liver function tests and uric acid before starting treatment and then on weeks 2 and 4 of treatment, then as indicated clinically—adjust dose if adverse reactions or laboratory abnormalities develop (consult product literature); eye examination recommended before oral treatment; eye examination also recommended during oral treatment if pre-existing ophthalmological disorder or if decrease in vision reported—discontinue treatment if ophthalmological disorder deteriorates or if new ophthalmological disorder develops; test thyroid function before treatment and then every 3 months; patients with a transplant—risk of rejection; risk of growth retardation, the reversibility of which is uncertain—if possible, consider starting treatment after pubertal growth spurt

Interactions: Appendix 1 (ribavirin)

**Contra-indications**

**Specific contra-indications for systemic treatment** Severe, uncontrolled cardiac disease in children with chronic hepatitis C; haemoglobinopathies; severe debilitating medical conditions; autoimmune disease (including autoimmune hepatitis); history of severe psychiatric condition

**Hepatic impairment** no dosage adjustment required; use oral ribavirin with caution in severe hepatic dysfunction or decompensated cirrhosis

**Renal impairment** plasma-ribavirin concentration increased; manufacturer advises avoid oral ribavirin if estimated glomerular filtration rate less than 50 mL/minute/1.73 m$^2$; manufacturer advises use intravenous preparation with caution if estimated glomerular filtration rate less than 30 mL/minute/1.73 m$^2$

**Pregnancy** avoid; teratogenicity in *animal* studies; see also Cautions above

**Breast-feeding** avoid—no information available

**Side-effects**

**Specific side-effects for inhaled treatment** Worsening respiration, bacterial pneumonia, and pneumothorax reported; rarely non-specific anaemia and haemolysis

**Specific side-effects for oral treatment** Haemolytic anaemia (anaemia may be improved by epoetin); also (in combination with peginterferon alfa or interferon alfa) nausea, vomiting, dyspepsia, abdominal pain, flatulence, constipation, diarrhoea, colitis, chest pain, palpitation, tachycardia, peripheral oedema, changes in blood pressure, syncope, flushing, pallor, cough, dyspnoea, tachypnoea, headache, dizziness, hyperkinesia, asthenia, impaired concentration and memory, sleep disturbances, abnormal dreams, anxiety, depression, suicidal ideation, psychoses, dysphagia, weight loss, dysphonia, paraesthesia, hypoaesthesia, ataxia, hypertonia, influenza-like symptoms, growth retardation (including decrease in height and weight), thyroid disorders, hyperglycaemia, menstrual disturbances, virilism, breast pain, testicular pain, sexual dysfunction, micturition disorders, leucopenia, thrombocytopenia, lymphadenopathy, dehydration, hypocalcaemia, myalgia, arthralgia, hyperuricaemia, visual disturbances, eye pain, dry eyes, hearing impairment, tinnitus, earache, dry mouth, taste disturbances, mouth ulcers, stomatitis, glossitis, tooth disorder, gingivitis, alopecia, pruritus, dry skin, skin discoloration, rash (including very rarely Stevens-Johnson syndrome and toxic epidermal necrolysis), increased sweating, psoriasis, photosensitivity, and acne; *less commonly* pancreatitis, gastro-intestinal bleeding, and hypertriglyceridaemia; *rarely* peptic ulcer, arrhythmias, cardiomyopathy, myocardial infarction, pericarditis, stroke, interstitial pneumonitis, pulmonary embolism, seizures, renal failure, vasculitis, rheumatoid arthritis, systemic lupus erythematosus, sarcoidosis, optic neuropathy, and retinal haemorrhage; *very rarely* aplastic anaemia and peripheral ischaemia

**Licensed use** inhalation licensed for use in children (age range not specified by manufacturer); intravenous preparation not licensed

### Indications and dose

**Bronchiolitis**

* **By aerosol inhalation or nebulisation (via small particle aerosol generator)**

  **Child 1 month–2 years** inhale solution containing 20 mg/mL for 12–18 hours for at least 3 days; max. 7 days

**Life-threatening RSV, parainfluenza virus, and adenovirus infection in immunocompromised children** (seek expert advice)

* **By intravenous infusion over 15 minutes**

  **Child 1 month–18 years** 33 mg/kg as a single dose, then 16 mg/kg every 6 hours for 4 days, then 8 mg/kg every 8 hours for 3 days

**Chronic hepatitis C (in combination with interferon alfa or peginterferon alfa) in previously untreated children without liver decompensation**

* **By mouth**

  **Child over 3 years; body-weight under 47 kg** 15 mg/kg daily in 2 divided doses

  **Child body-weight 47–50 kg** 200 mg in the morning and 400 mg in the evening

  **Child body-weight 50–65 kg** 400 mg twice daily

  **Child body-weight 65–81 kg** 400 mg in the morning and 600 mg in the evening

  **Child body-weight 81–105 kg** 600 mg twice daily

  **Child body-weight over 105 kg** 600 mg in the morning and 800 mg in the evening

**Rebetol®** (MSD) [PoM]

Capsules, ribavirin 200 mg, net price 84-cap pack = £160.90, 140-cap pack = £267.81, 168-cap pack = £321.38. Label: 21

Oral solution, ribavirin 200 mg/5 mL, net price 100 mL (bubble-gum-flavoured) = £67.08. Label: 21

**Virazole®** (Meda) [PoM]

Inhalation◣, ribavirin 6 g for reconstitution with 300 mL water for injections. Net price 3 × 6-g vials = £349.00

Intravenous infusion, 100 mg/mL, 10-mL amp
Available on a named-patient basis from Valeant

**5**

**Infections**

## 5.4 Antiprotozoal drugs

Advice on specific problems available from:

**Advice for healthcare professionals**

PHE (Public Health England) Malaria    (020) 7637 0248
Reference Laboratory    (Fax)
www.hpa.org.uk/infections/topics_az/    (prophylaxis only)
malaria

National Travel Health Network and    0845 602 6712
Centre

Travel Medicine Team, Health    (0141) 300 1100
Protection, Scotland    (weekdays 2–4
(registered users of Travax only)    p.m. only)
www.travax.nhs.uk

(for registered users of the NHS Travax
website only)

Birmingham    (0121) 424 0357

Liverpool    (0151) 705 3100

London    0845 155 5000
   (treatment)

Oxford    (01865) 225 430

**Advice for travellers**

Hospital for Tropical Diseases, Travel    020 7950 7799
Healthline

www.fitfortravel.nhs.uk

WHO advice on international travel and health
www.who.int/ith

National Travel Health Network and
Centre (NaTHNaC)
www.nathnac.org/travel/index.htm

## 5.4.1   Antimalarials

Recommendations on the prophylaxis and treatment of malaria reflect guidelines agreed by UK malaria specialists. Choice will depend on the age of the child (see below).

The centres listed above should be consulted for advice on special problems.

### Treatment of malaria

If the infective species is **not known**, or if the infection is **mixed**, initial treatment should be as for *falciparum malaria* with quinine, *Malarone®* (proguanil with atovaquone), or *Riamet®* (artemether with lumefantrine). Falciparum malaria can progress rapidly in unprotected children and antimalarial treatment should be considered in those with features of severe malaria and possible exposure, even if the initial blood tests for the organism are negative.

### Falciparum malaria (treatment)

Falciparum malaria (malignant malaria) is caused by *Plasmodium falciparum*. In most parts of the world *P. falciparum* is now resistant to chloroquine which should not therefore be given for treatment.

Quinine, *Malarone®* (proguanil with atovaquone), or *Riamet®* (artemether with lumefantrine) can be given *by mouth* if the child can swallow and retain tablets and there are no serious manifestations (e.g. impaired consciousness); quinine should be given *by intravenous infusion* (see below) if the child is seriously ill or unable to take tablets. **Mefloquine** is now rarely used for treatment because of concerns about resistance.

*Oral.* **Quinine** is well tolerated by children although the salts are bitter.

The dosage regimen for quinine *by mouth* is:
10 mg/kg (of quinine salt[1]; max. 600 mg) every 8 hours for 7 days
*together with or followed by*
*either* **clindamycin** 7–13 mg/kg (max. 450 mg) every 8 hours for 7 days [unlicensed indication]
*or*, in children over 12 years, **doxycycline** 200 mg once daily for 7 days

If the parasite is likely to be sensitive, **pyrimethamine** with **sulfadoxine** as a single dose [unlicensed] may be given (instead of either clindamycin or doxycycline) together with, or after, a course of quinine.

The dose regimen for pyrimethamine with sulfadoxine by mouth is:
Child up to 4 years and body-weight over 5 kg pyrimethamine 12.5 mg with sulfadoxine 250 mg as a single dose

Child 5–6 years pyrimethamine 25 mg with sulfadoxine 500 mg as a single dose

Child 7–9 years pyrimethamine 37.5 mg with sulfadoxine 750 mg as a single dose

Child 10–14 years pyrimethamine 50 mg with sulfadoxine 1 g as a single dose

Child 14–18 years pyrimethamine 75 mg with sulfadoxine 1.5 g as a single dose

Alternatively, *Malarone®*, or *Riamet®* may be given instead of quinine. It is not necessary to give clindamycin, doxycycline, or pyrimethamine with sulfadoxine after *Malarone®* or *Riamet®* treatment.

The dose regimen for *Malarone®* by mouth is:
Child body-weight 5–9 kg 2 'paediatric' tablets once daily for 3 days

Child body-weight 9–11 kg 3 'paediatric' tablets once daily for 3 days

Child body-weight 11–21 kg 1 'standard' tablet once daily for 3 days

Child body-weight 21–31 kg 2 'standard' tablets once daily for 3 days

Child body-weight 31–40 kg 3 'standard' tablets once daily for 3 days

Child body-weight over 40 kg 4 'standard' tablets once daily for 3 days

The dose regimen for *Riamet®* by mouth is:
Child body-weight 5–15 kg 1 tablet initially, followed by 5 further doses of 1 tablet each given at 8, 24, 36, 48, and 60 hours (total 6 tablets over 60 hours)

Child body-weight 15–25 kg 2 tablets initially, followed by 5 further doses of 2 tablets each given at

---

1. Valid for quinine hydrochloride, dihydrochloride, and sulfate; not valid for quinine bisulfate which contains a correspondingly smaller amount of quinine.

8, 24, 36, 48, and 60 hours (total 12 tablets over 60 hours)

Child body-weight 25–35 kg 3 tablets initially, followed by 5 further doses of 3 tablets each given at 8, 24, 36, 48, and 60 hours (total 18 tablets over 60 hours)

Child 12–18 years and body-weight over 35 kg, 4 tablets initially followed by 5 further doses of 4 tablets each given at 8, 24, 36, 48, and 60 hours (total 24 tablets over 60 hours)

*Parenteral.* If the child is seriously ill or unable to swallow tablets, or if more than 2% of red blood cells are parasitized, **quinine** should be given *by intravenous infusion.* The dose regimen for quinine *by intravenous infusion* is calculated on a mg/kg basis:

Neonates and children, loading dose[1,2] of 20 mg/kg (up to maximum 1.4 g) of quinine salt[3] infused over 4 hours *then 8 hours after the start of the loading dose,* maintenance dose of 10 mg/kg[4] (up to maximum 700 mg) of quinine salt[3] infused over 4 hours every 8 hours (until child can swallow tablets to complete the 7-day course *together with or followed by either* clindamycin or doxycycline as above).

Specialist advice should be sought in difficult cases (e.g. very high parasite count, deterioration on optimal doses of quinine, infection acquired in quinine-resistant areas of south-east Asia) because intravenous **artesunate** may be available for 'named-patient' use.

**Pregnancy**   Falciparum malaria is particularly dangerous in pregnancy, especially in the last trimester. The treatment doses of oral and intravenous quinine given above (including the loading dose) can safely be given in pregnancy. Clindamycin [unlicensed indication] should be given for 7 days with or after quinine. Doxycycline should be avoided in pregnancy (affects teeth and skeletal development in fetus); pyrimethamine with sulfadoxine, *Malarone®*, and *Riamet®* are also best avoided until more information is available. Specialist advice should be sought in difficult cases (e.g. very high parasite count, deterioration on optimal doses of quinine, infection acquired in quinine-resistant areas of south east Asia) because intravenous artesunate may be available for 'named patient' use.

---

## Benign malarias (treatment)

Benign malaria is usually caused by *Plasmodium vivax* and less commonly by *P. ovale* and *P. malariae.* **Chloroquine**[5] is the drug of choice for the treatment of benign malarias (but chloroquine-resistant *P. vivax* infection has

been reported from Indonesia, New Guinea and some adjacent islands).

Chloroquine alone is adequate for *P. malariae* infections but in the case of *P. vivax* and *P. ovale*, a *radical cure* (to destroy parasites in the liver and thus prevent relapses) is required. This is achieved with **primaquine**[6] given after the chloroquine.

The dosage regimen of chloroquine *by mouth* for benign malaria in children is:

initial dose of 10 mg/kg of base (max. 620 mg) *then*

a single dose of 5 mg/kg of base (max. 310 mg) after 6–8 hours *then*

a single dose of 5 mg/kg of base (max. 310 mg) daily for 2 days

For a *radical cure*, **primaquine**[6] [unlicensed] is then given to children over 6 months of age; specialist advice should be sought for children under 6 months of age. Primaquine is given in a dose of 250 micrograms/kg (max. 15 mg) daily for 14 days in *P. ovale* infection or 500 micrograms/kg (max. 30 mg) daily for 14 days in *P. vivax* infection.

**Parenteral**   If the child is unable to take oral therapy, quinine can be given by *intravenous infusion.* The dose is 10 mg/kg[4] (max. 700 mg) of quinine salt[3] infused over 4 hours every 8 hours, changed to oral chloroquine as soon as the child's condition permits.

**Pregnancy**   Treatment doses of chloroquine can be given for benign malaria. In the case of *P. vivax* or *P. ovale*, however, the radical cure with primaquine should be **postponed** until the pregnancy is over; instead chloroquine should be continued at a dose of 10 mg/kg (max. 310 mg) each week during the pregnancy.

---

## Prophylaxis against malaria

The recommendations on prophylaxis reflect guidelines agreed by UK malaria specialists; the advice is aimed at residents of the UK who travel to endemic areas. The choice of drug for a particular child should take into account:

- risk of exposure to malaria;

- extent of drug resistance;

- efficacy of the recommended drugs;

- side-effects of the drugs;

- patient-related factors (e.g. age, pregnancy, renal or hepatic impairment, compliance with prophylactic regimen).

Prophylactic doses are based on guidelines agreed by UK malaria experts and may differ from advice in product literature. **Weight is a better guide than age.** If in doubt obtain advice from specialist centre, see p. 332.

**Protection against bites**   Prophylaxis is **not absolute**, and breakthrough infection can occur with any of the drugs recommended. Personal protection

---

1. In intensive care units the loading dose can alternatively be given as quinine salt[3] 7 mg/kg infused over 30 minutes followed immediately by 10 mg/kg over 4 hours then (after 8 hours) maintenance dose as described.
2. **Important:** the loading dose of 20 mg/kg should **not** be used if the patient has received quinine or mefloquine during the previous 12 hours
3. Valid for quinine hydrochloride, dihydrochloride, and sulfate; not valid for quinine bisulfate which contains a correspondingly smaller amount of quinine.
4. Maintenance dose should be reduced to 5–7 mg/kg of quinine salt[3] in children with severe renal impairment, severe hepatic impairment, or if parenteral treatment is required for more than 48 hours.
5. For the treatment of chloroquine-resistant benign malaria *Malarone®* [unlicensed indication], quinine, or *Riamet®* [unlicensed indication] can be used; as with chloroquine, primaquine should be given for radical cure.
6. Before starting primaquine, blood should be tested for glucose-6-phosphate dehydrogenase (G6PD) activity since the drug can cause haemolysis in G6PD-deficient patients. Specialist advice should be obtained in G6PD deficiency. In mild G6PD deficiency, primaquine in a dose of 750 micrograms/kg (max. 45 mg) once a week for 8 weeks, has been found useful and without undue harmful effects.

5 Infections

against being bitten is very important. Mosquito nets impregnated with permethrin provide the most effective barrier protection against insects (infants should sleep with a mosquito net stretched over the cot or baby carrier); mats and vaporised insecticides are also useful. Diethyltoluamide (DEET) 20–50% in lotions, sprays, or roll-on formulations is safe and effective when applied to the skin of adults and children over 2 months of age. It can also be used during pregnancy and breast-feeding. The duration of protection varies according to the concentration of DEET and is longest for DEET 50%. Long sleeves and trousers worn after dusk also provide protection.

**Length of prophylaxis**  In order to determine tolerance and to establish habit, prophylaxis should generally be started one week (preferably 2–3 weeks in the case of mefloquine) before travel into an endemic area (or if not possible at earliest opportunity up to 1 or 2 days before travel); *Malarone®* or doxycycline prophylaxis should be started 1–2 days before travel. Prophylaxis should be continued for **4 weeks after leaving** (except for *Malarone®* prophylaxis which should be stopped 1 week after leaving).

In those requiring long-term prophylaxis, chloroquine and proguanil may be used for periods of over 5 years. Mefloquine is licensed for use up to 1 year (although it has been used for up to 3 years without undue problems). Doxycycline can be used for up to 2 years. In clinical trials *Malarone®* has been used for an average duration of 27 days, however, it can be used for up to 1 year (and possibly longer) with caution. Specialist advice should be sought for long-term prophylaxis.

**Return from malarial region**  It is important to be aware that **any illness** that occurs within 1 year and **especially within 3 months of return might be malaria** even if all recommended precautions against malaria were taken. Travellers and carers of children should be **warned** of this and told that if they develop any illness **particularly within 3 months** of their return they should go **immediately** to a doctor and specifically mention their exposure to malaria.

**Epilepsy**  Both chloroquine and mefloquine are unsuitable for malaria prophylaxis in children with a history of epilepsy. In areas *without chloroquine resistance*, proguanil alone is recommended; in areas *with chloroquine resistance*, doxycycline or *Malarone®* may be considered. The metabolism of doxycycline may be influenced by antiepileptics (see **interactions:** Appendix 1 (tetracyclines)).

**Asplenia**  Asplenic children (or those with severe splenic dysfunction) are at particular risk of severe malaria. If travel to malarious areas is unavoidable, rigorous precautions are required against contracting the disease.

**Renal impairment**  Avoidance (or dosage reduction) of proguanil is recommended since it is excreted by the kidneys. *Malarone®* should not be used for prophylaxis in children with estimated glomerular filtration rate less than 30 mL/minute/1.73 m². Chloroquine is only partially excreted by the kidneys and reduction of the dose for prophylaxis is not required except in severe impairment. Mefloquine is considered to be appropriate to use in renal impairment and does not require dosage reduction. Doxycycline is also considered to be appropriate.

**Pregnancy**  Travel to malarious areas should be avoided during pregnancy; if travel is unavoidable, effective prophylaxis must be used. Chloroquine and proguanil can be given in the usual doses during pregnancy, but these drugs are not appropriate for most areas because their effectiveness has declined, particularly in sub-saharan Africa; in the case of proguanil, folic acid 5 mg daily should be given. The centres listed on p. 332 should be consulted for advice on prophylaxis in chloroquine-resistant areas. Although the manufacturer advises that mefloquine should not be used during pregnancy, particularly in the first trimester, unless the potential benefit outweighs the risk, studies of mefloquine in pregnancy (including use in the first trimester) indicate that it can be considered for travel to chloroquine-resistant areas. Doxycycline is contra-indicated during pregnancy. *Malarone®* should be avoided during pregnancy unless there is no suitable alternative.

**Breast-feeding**  Prophylaxis is required in **breast-fed infants**; although antimalarials are present in milk, the amounts are too variable to give reliable protection.

## Specific recommendations

Where a journey requires two regimens, the regimen for the higher risk area should be used for the whole journey. Those travelling to remote or little-visited areas may require expert advice.

> Risk may vary in different parts of a country—check under all risk levels

> **Important**
> Settled immigrants and their carers (or long-term visitors) to the UK may be unaware that they will have **lost some of their immunity** and also that the areas where they previously lived **may now be malarious**

## North Africa, the Middle East, and Central Asia

**Very low risk**  Risk *very low* in Algeria, Egypt (but *low risk* in El Faiyum, see below), Georgia (south-east, July–October), rural north Iraq (May–October), Kyrgystan (but *low risk* in south-west, see below), Libya, most tourist areas of Turkey (but *low risk* in Adana and border with Syria, see below), Uzbekistan (extreme south-east only):

> chemoprophylaxis not recommended but avoid mosquito bites and consider malaria if fever presents

**Low risk**  Risk *low* in Azerbaijan (southern border areas, June–September), Egypt (El Faiyum only, June–October), Iran (northern border with Azerbaijan, May–October; *variable risk* in rural south-east provinces; see below), Kyrgystan (south-west, May–October), north border of Syria (May–October), Turkey (plain around Adana and east of there, border with Syria, March–November):

> chloroquine *or* (if chloroquine not appropriate) proguanil hydrochloride

**Variable risk** Risk *variable* and *chloroquine resistance present* in Afghanistan (below 2000 m, May–November), Iran (rural south-east provinces, March–November, see also *Low Risk* above), Oman (remote rural areas only), Saudi Arabia (south-west and rural areas of western region; no risk in Mecca, Medina, Jeddah, or high-altitude areas of Asir Province), Tajikistan (June–October), Yemen (no risk in Sana'a):

> chloroquine + proguanil hydrochloride *or* (if chloroquine + proguanil not appropriate and child over 12 years) doxycycline

## Sub-Saharan Africa

*No chemoprophylaxis recommended* for Cape Verde (some risk on São Tiago) and Mauritius (but avoid mosquito bites and consider malaria if fever presents)

**Very high risk** Risk *very high* (or *locally very high*) and *chloroquine resistance very widespread* in Angola, Benin, Botswana (northern half, November–June), Burkina Faso, Burundi, Cameroon, Central African Republic, Chad, Comoros, Congo, Democratic Republic of the Congo (formerly Zaïre), Djibouti, Equatorial Guinea, Eritrea, Ethiopia (below 2000 m; no risk in Addis Ababa), Gabon, Gambia, Ghana, Guinea, Guinea-Bissau, Ivory Coast, Kenya, Liberia, Madagascar, Malawi, Mali, Mauritania (all year in south; July–October in north), Mozambique, Namibia (all year along Kavango and Kunene rivers; November–June in northern third), Niger, Nigeria, Principe, Rwanda, São Tomé, Senegal, Sierra Leone, Somalia, South Africa (low-altitude areas of Mpumalanga and Limpopo Provinces, Kruger National Park, and north-east KwaZulu-Natal as far south as Jozini), Sudan, Swaziland, Tanzania, Togo, Uganda, Zambia, Zimbabwe (all year in Zambezi valley; November–June in other areas below 1200 m; risk negligible in Harare and Bulawayo):

> mefloquine *or* doxycycline (if child over 12) *or* *Malarone*®

**Note** In Zimbabwe and neighbouring countries, pyrimethamine with dapsone (also known as *Deltaprim*®) prophylaxis is used by local residents (sometimes with chloroquine—this regimen is not recommended).

## South Asia

**Low risk** Risk *low* in Bangladesh (but *high risk* in Chittagong Hill Tracts, see below), India (Kerala [southern states], Tamil Nadu, Karnataka, Southern Andhra Pradesh [including Hyderabad], Mumbai, Rajasthan [including Jaipur], Uttar Pradesh [including Agra], Haryana, Uttaranchal, Himachal Pradesh, Jammu, Kashmir, Punjab, Delhi; *variable risk* in other areas, see below; *high risk* in Assam), Sri Lanka (but *variable risk* north of Vavuniya, see below):

> chemoprophylaxis not recommended but avoid mosquito bites and consider malaria if fever present

**Variable risk** Risk *variable* and *chloroquine resistance usually moderate* in southern districts of Bhutan, India (*low risk* in some areas, see above; *high risk* in Assam, see below), Nepal (below 1500 m, especially Terai districts; no risk in Kathmandu), Pakistan (below 2000 m), Sri Lanka (north of Vavuniya; *low risk* in other areas, see above):

> chloroquine + proguanil hydrochloride *or* (if chloroquine + proguanil not appropriate) mefloquine *or* doxycycline *or* *Malarone*®

**High risk** Risk *high* and *chloroquine resistance high* in Bangladesh (only in Chittagong Hill Tracts; *low risk* in other areas, see above), India (Assam only; see also *Low Risk* and *Variable Risk* above):

> mefloquine *or* doxycycline (if child over 12) *or* *Malarone*® *or* (if mefloquine, doxycycline, or *Malarone*® not appropriate) chloroquine + proguanil hydrochloride

## South-East Asia

**Very low risk** Risk *very low* in Bali, Brunei, Cambodia (Angkor Wat and Siem Reap, but no risk in Phnom Penh; *substantial risk* in other areas, see below; *great risk* in western provinces, see below), main tourist areas of China (but *substantial risk* in Yunnan and Hainan, see below), Hong Kong, Korea (both North and South), Malaysia (both East and West including Cameron Highlands, but *substantial risk* in Sabah [except Kota Kinabalu], and *variable risk* in deep forests, see below), Singapore, Thailand (**important**: regional risk exists, see under *Great Risk*, below), Vietnam (cities, coast between Ho Chi Minh and Hanoi, and Mekong River until close to Cambodian border; *substantial risk* in other areas, see below):

> chemoprophylaxis not recommended but avoid mosquito bites and consider malaria if fever presents

**Variable risk** Risk *variable* and *some chloroquine resistance* in Indonesia (very low risk in Bali, and cities but *substantial risk* in Irian Jaya [West Papua] and Lombok, see below), rural Philippines below 600 m (no risk in cities, Cebu, Bohol, and Catanduanes), deep forests of peninsular Malaysia and Sarawak (but *substantial risk* in Sabah, see below):

> chloroquine + proguanil hydrochloride *or* (if chloroquine + proguanil not appropriate) mefloquine *or* doxycycline *or* *Malarone*®

**Substantial risk** Risk *substantial* and *drug resistance common* in Cambodia (no risk or *very low risk* in some areas, see above; *great risk* in western provinces, see below), China (Yunnan and Hainan; see also *Very Low Risk* above), East Timor, Irian Jaya [West Papua], Lombok, Malaysia (Sabah; see also *Very Low Risk* and *Variable Risk* above), Vietnam (*very low risk* in some areas, see above):

> mefloquine *or* doxycycline (if child over 12) *or* *Malarone*®

**5**
**Infections**

**Great risk and drug resistance present**   Risk *great and widespread chloroquine and mefloquine resistance present* in western provinces of Cambodia (see also *Very Low Risk* and *Substantial Risk* above), Laos (no risk in Vientiane), borders of Thailand with Cambodia, Laos and Myanmar (*very low risk* in Chang Rai and Kwai Bridge, see above), Myanmar (formerly Burma):

> doxycycline (if child over 12) *or Malarone*®

## Oceania

**Risk**   Risk *high* and *chloroquine resistance high* in Papua New Guinea (below 1800 m), Solomon Islands, Vanuatu:

> doxycycline (if child over 12) *or* mefloquine *or Malarone*®

## Central and South America and the Caribbean

**Very low risk**   Risk *very low* in Jamaica:

> chemoprophylaxis not recommended but avoid mosquito bites and consider malaria if fever presents

**Variable to low risk**   Risk *variable to low* in Argentina (rural areas along northern borders only; no risk in Iguacu Falls), rural Belize (except Belize district), Bolivia (below 2500 m; *high risk* in Amazon basin area, see below), Costa Rica (Limon Province except Puerto Limon and northern canton of Pococci), Dominican Republic (no risk in Santiago and Santo Domingo), El Salvador (Santa Ana province in west), Guatemala (below 1500 m), Haiti, Honduras, Mexico (states of Oaxaca and Chiapas), Nicaragua, Panama (west of Panama Canal but *variable to high risk* east of Panama Canal, see below), rural Paraguay, Peru (rural areas east of the Andes and west of the Amazon basin area below 2000 m; *high risk* in Amazon basin area, see below), Venezuela (north of Orinoco river; *high risk* south of and including Orinoco river and Amazon basin area, see below; Caracas and Margarita Island free of malaria):

> chloroquine *or* (if chloroquine not appropriate) proguanil hydrochloride

**Variable to high risk**   Risk *variable to high and chloroquine resistance present* in rural areas of Ecuador (below 1500 m; no malaria in Galapagos Islands and Guayaquil; see below for Esmeraldas Province), Panama (east of Panama Canal):

> chloroquine + proguanil hydrochloride *or* (if chloroquine + proguanil not appropriate) mefloquine *or* doxycycline (if child over 12) *or Malarone*®

**High risk**   Risk *high* and *marked chloroquine resistance* in Bolivia (Amazon basin area; see also *variable to low risk* above), Brazil (throughout 'Legal Amazon' area which includes the Amazon basin area, Mato Grosso

and Maranhao only; elsewhere *very low risk*—no chemoprophylaxis), Colombia (most areas below 800 m), Ecuador (Esmeraldas Province; *variable to high risk* in other areas, see above), French Guiana, all interior regions of Guyana, Peru (Amazon basin area; see also *variable to low risk* above), Suriname (except Paramaribo and coast), Venezuela (Amazon basin area, areas south of and including Orinoco river; see also *variable to low risk* above):

> mefloquine *or* doxycycline (if child over 12) *or Malarone*®

## Standby treatment [unlicensed]

> Children and their carers visiting remote, malarious areas for prolonged periods should carry standby treatment if they are likely to be more than 24 hours away from medical care. Self-medication should be **avoided** if medical help is accessible.
>
> In order to avoid excessive self-medication, the traveller should be provided with **written instructions** that urgent medical attention should be sought if fever (38°C or more) develops 7 days (or more) after arriving in a malarious area and that self-treatment is indicated if medical help is not available within 24 hours of fever onset.
>
> In view of the continuing emergence of resistant strains and of the different regimens required for different areas expert advice should be sought on the best treatment course for an individual traveller. A drug used for chemoprophylaxis should not be considered for standby treatment for the same traveller.

## Artemether with lumefantrine

Artemether with lumefantrine is licensed for the *treatment of acute uncomplicated falciparum malaria.*

### ▌ ARTEMETHER WITH LUMEFANTRINE

**Cautions**   electrolyte disturbances, concomitant use with other drugs known to cause QT-interval prolongation; monitor patients unable to take food (greater risk of recrudescence); avoid in acute porphyria (section 9.8.2); **interactions**: Appendix 1 (artemether with lumefantrine)
  **Skilled tasks**   Dizziness may affect performance of skilled tasks

**Contra-indications**   history of arrhythmias, of clinically relevant bradycardia, and of congestive heart failure accompanied by reduced left ventricular ejection fraction; family history of sudden death or of congenital QT interval prolongation

**Hepatic impairment**   manufacturer advises caution in severe impairment—monitor ECG and plasma potassium concentration

**Renal impairment**   manufacturer advises caution in severe impairment—monitor ECG and plasma potassium concentration

**Pregnancy**   toxicity in *animal* studies with artemether; manufacturer advises use only if potential benefit outweighs risk

**Breast-feeding** manufacturer advises avoid breast-feeding for at least 1 week after last dose; present in milk in *animal* studies

**Side-effects** abdominal pain, anorexia, diarrhoea, vomiting, nausea; palpitation, prolonged QT interval; cough; headache, dizziness, sleep disturbances, asthenia, paraesthesia; arthralgia, myalgia; pruritus, rash; *less commonly* ataxia, hypoaesthesia, clonus

### Indications and dose

Treatment of acute uncomplicated falciparum malaria see p. 332

Treatment of benign malaria see p. 333

**Administration** tablets may be crushed just before administration

**Riamet®** (Novartis) [PoM]
Tablets, yellow, artemether 20 mg, lumefantrine 120 mg, net price 24-tab pack = £22.50. Label: 21, counselling, skilled tasks

## Chloroquine

Chloroquine is used for the *prophylaxis of malaria* in areas of the world where the *risk of chloroquine-resistant falciparum malaria is still low*. It is also used with proguanil when chloroquine-resistant falciparum malaria is present but this regimen may not give optimal protection (see specific recommendations by country, p. 334).

Chloroquine is **no longer recommended** for the *treatment of falciparum malaria* owing to widespread resistance, nor is it recommended if the infective species is *not known* or if the infection is *mixed*; in these cases treatment should be with quinine, *Malarone®*, or *Riamet®* (for details, see p. 332). It is still recommended for the *treatment of benign malarias* (for details, see p. 333).

### ■ CHLOROQUINE

**Cautions** may exacerbate psoriasis, neurological disorders (avoid for prophylaxis if history of epilepsy, see notes above), may aggravate myasthenia gravis, severe gastro-intestinal disorders, G6PD deficiency (see section 9.1.5); ophthalmic examination with long-term therapy; avoid concurrent therapy with hepatotoxic drugs—other **interactions**: Appendix 1 (chloroquine and hydroxychloroquine)

**Hepatic impairment** use with caution in moderate to severe impairment

**Renal impairment** manufacturers advise caution; see also Prophylaxis Against Malaria, p. 334

**Pregnancy** benefit of prophylaxis and treatment in malaria outweighs risk; see also Benign Malarias (treatment), p. 333 and Prophylaxis Against Malaria, p. 334

**Breast-feeding** amount in milk probably too small to be harmful; see also Prophylaxis Against Malaria, p. 334

**Side-effects** gastro-intestinal disturbances, headache; also hypotension, convulsions, visual disturbances, depigmentation or loss of hair, skin reactions (rashes, pruritus); rarely, bone-marrow suppression, hypersensitivity reactions such as urticaria and angio-edema; other side-effects (not usually associated with malaria prophylaxis or treatment), see under Antimalarials, section 10.1.3; very toxic in **overdosage**—immediate advice from poisons centres essential (see also p. 28)

### Indications and dose

Prophylaxis of malaria

• By mouth

Dose (expressed as chloroquine base) preferably started 1 week before entering endemic area and continued for 4 weeks after leaving (see notes above)

**Child up to 12 weeks, body-weight under 6 kg** 37.5 mg once weekly

**Child 12 weeks–1 year, body-weight 6–10 kg** 75 mg once weekly

**Child 1–4 years, body-weight 10–16 kg** 112.5 mg once weekly

**Child 4–8 years, body-weight 16–25 kg** 150 mg once weekly (or 155 mg once weekly if tablets used)

**Child 8–13 years, body-weight 25–45 kg** 225 mg once weekly (or 232.5 mg once weekly if tablets used)

**Child over 13 years, body-weight over 45 kg** 310 mg once weekly

**Counselling** Warn travellers about **importance** of avoiding mosquito bites, **importance** of taking prophylaxis regularly, and **importance** of immediate visit to doctor if ill within 1 year and **especially** within 3 months of return. For details, see notes above

Treatment of benign malaria see p. 333

**Note** Chloroquine doses in BNFC may differ from those in product literature

**¹Avloclor®** (AstraZeneca) [PoM]
Tablets, scored, chloroquine phosphate 250 mg (≡ chloroquine base 155 mg). Net price 20-tab pack = £1.22. Label: 5, counselling, prophylaxis, see above

**¹Malarivon®** (Wallace Mfg) [PoM]
Syrup, chloroquine phosphate 80 mg/5 mL (≡ chloroquine base 50 mg/5 mL), net price 75 mL = £8.75. Label: 5, counselling, prophylaxis, see above

**¹Nivaquine®** (Sanofi-Aventis) [PoM]
Syrup, golden, chloroquine sulfate 68 mg/5 mL (≡ chloroquine base 50 mg/5 mL), net price 100 mL = £4.60. Label: 5, counselling, prophylaxis, see above

◢**With proguanil**
For cautions and side-effects of proguanil see Proguanil; for dose see Chloroquine and Proguanil

**¹Paludrine/Avloclor®** (AstraZeneca)
Tablets, travel pack of 14 tablets of chloroquine phosphate 250 mg (≡ chloroquine base 155 mg) and 98 tablets of proguanil hydrochloride 100 mg, net price 112-tab pack = £8.79. Label: 5, 21, counselling, prophylaxis, see above

## Mefloquine

Mefloquine is used for the *prophylaxis of malaria* in areas of the world where there is a *high risk of chloroquine-resistant falciparum malaria* (for details, see specific recommendations by country, p. 334).

Mefloquine is now rarely used for the *treatment of falciparum malaria* because of increased resistance. It

---

1. Can be sold to the public provided it is licensed and labelled for the prophylaxis of malaria. Drugs for malaria prophylaxis not prescribable on the NHS; health authorities may investigate circumstances under which antimalarials are prescribed

is rarely used for the treatment of benign malarias because better tolerated alternatives are available. Mefloquine should not be used for treatment if it has been used for prophylaxis.

### MEFLOQUINE

**Cautions** cardiac conduction disorders; epilepsy (avoid for prophylaxis); not recommended in infants under 3 months (5 kg); **interactions:** Appendix 1 (mefloquine)

**Skilled tasks** Dizziness or a disturbed sense of balance may affect performance of skilled tasks; effects may persist for up to 3 weeks

**Contra-indications** hypersensitivity to quinine; avoid for prophylaxis if history of psychiatric disorders (including depression) or convulsions

**Hepatic impairment** avoid for chemoprophylaxis in severe liver disease

**Pregnancy** manufacturer advises adequate contraception during prophylaxis and for 3 months after stopping (teratogenicity in *animal* studies), but see also p. 334

**Breast-feeding** present in milk but risk to infant minimal; see also, p. 334

**Side-effects** nausea, vomiting, dyspepsia, abdominal pain, diarrhoea; headache, dizziness, sleep disturbances; *less frequently* anorexia, bradycardia, fatigue, abnormal dreams, fever, tinnitus, and neuropsychiatric reactions (including sensory and motor neuropathies, tremor, ataxia, anxiety, depression, panic attacks, agitation, hallucinations, psychosis, convulsions); *rarely* suicidal ideation; *very rarely* pneumonitis; also reported, circulatory disorders (including hypotension and hypertension), chest pain, tachycardia, palpitation, cardiac conduction disorders, oedema, dyspnoea, encephalopathy, leucopenia, leucocytosis, thrombocytopenia, muscle weakness, myalgia, arthralgia, visual disturbances, vestibular disorders, rash (including Stevens-Johnson syndrome), pruritus, and alopecia

**Licensed use** not licensed for use in children under 5 kg body-weight and under 3 months

**Indications and dose**

**Prophylaxis of malaria** preferably started 2½ weeks before entering endemic area and continued for 4 weeks after leaving (see notes above)

- By mouth

    **Child body-weight 5–16 kg** 62.5 mg once weekly

    **Child body-weight 16–25 kg** 125 mg once weekly

    **Child body-weight 25–45 kg** 187.5 mg once weekly

    **Child body-weight over 45 kg** 250 mg once weekly

    **Long-term chemoprophylaxis** Mefloquine prophylaxis can be taken for up to 1 year

    **Counselling** Inform travellers and carers of children travelling about adverse reactions of mefloquine and, if they occur, to seek medical advice on alternative antimalarials before the next dose is due. Also warn travellers and carers of children travelling about **importance** of avoiding mosquito bites, **importance** of taking prophylaxis regularly, and **importance** of immediate visit to doctor if ill within 1 year and **especially** within 3 months of return. For details, see notes above

    **Note** Mefloquine doses in BNFC may differ from those in product literature

**Administration** Tablet may be crushed and mixed with food such as jam or honey just before administration

**¹Lariam®** (Roche) ▣PoM▣

Tablets, scored, mefloquine (as hydrochloride) 250 mg. Net price 8-tab pack = £14.53. Label: 21, 27, counselling, skilled tasks, prophylaxis, see above

## Primaquine

Primaquine is used to eliminate the liver stages of *P. vivax* or *P. ovale following chloroquine treatment* (for details, see p. 333).

### PRIMAQUINE

**Cautions** G6PD deficiency (test blood, see under Benign Malarias (treatment), p. 333); systemic diseases associated with granulocytopenia (e.g. juvenile idiopathic arthritis, lupus erythematosus); **interactions:** Appendix 1 (primaquine)

**Pregnancy** risk of neonatal haemolysis and methaemoglobinaemia in third trimester; see also, p. 333

**Breast-feeding** no information available; theoretical risk of haemolysis in G6PD-deficient infants

**Side-effects** nausea, vomiting, anorexia, abdominal pain; *less commonly* methaemoglobinaemia, haemolytic anaemia especially in G6PD deficiency, leucopenia

**Licensed use** not licensed

**Indications and dose**

**Adjunct in the treatment of *Plasmodium vivax* and *P. ovale* malaria (eradication of liver stages)** for dose see Benign Malarias, p. 333

**Primaquine** (Non-proprietary)

Tablets, primaquine (as phosphate) 7.5 mg or 15 mg
Available from 'special-order' manufacturers or specialist importing companies, see p. 823

## Proguanil

Proguanil is used (usually *with chloroquine*, but occasionally *alone*) for the *prophylaxis of malaria*, (for details, see specific recommendations by country, p. 334).

Proguanil used alone is not suitable for the *treatment of malaria*; however, *Malarone®* (a combination of atovaquone with proguanil) is licensed for the treatment of acute uncomplicated falciparum malaria.

*Malarone®* is also used for the *prophylaxis of falciparum malaria* in areas of *widespread mefloquine or chloroquine resistance*. *Malarone®* is also used as an alternative to mefloquine or doxycycline. *Malarone®* is particularly suitable for short trips to highly chloroquine-resistant areas because it needs to be taken only for 7 days after leaving an endemic area.

### PROGUANIL HYDROCHLORIDE

**Cautions** interactions: Appendix 1 (proguanil)

**Renal impairment** (see notes under Prophylaxis against malaria). Use half normal dose if estimated glomerular filtration rate 20–60 mL/minute/1.73 m². Use one-quarter normal dose on alternate days if

---

1. Drugs for malaria prophylaxis not prescribable on the NHS; health authorities may investigate circumstances under which antimalarials prescribed

estimated glomerular filtration rate 10–20 mL/minute/1.73 m$^2$. Use one-quarter normal dose once weekly if estimated glomerular filtration rate less than 10 mL/minute/1.73 m$^2$; increased risk of haematological toxicity.

**Pregnancy**  benefit of prophylaxis in malaria outweighs risk; adequate folate supplements should be given to mother; see also p. 334

**Breast-feeding**  amount in milk probably too small to be harmful when used for malaria prophylaxis; see also p. 334

**Side-effects**  mild gastric intolerance, diarrhoea, and constipation; occasionally mouth ulcers and stomatitis; *very rarely* cholestasis, vasculitis, skin reactions and hair loss

### Indications and dose

Prophylaxis of malaria preferably started 1 week before entering endemic area and continued for 4 weeks after leaving (see notes above)

- By mouth

  **Child up to 12 weeks, body-weight under 6 kg** 25 mg once daily

  **Child 12 weeks–1 year, body-weight 6–10 kg** 50 mg once daily

  **Child 1–4 years, body-weight 10–16 kg** 75 mg once daily

  **Child 4–8 years, body-weight 16–25 kg** 100 mg once daily

  **Child 8–13 years, body-weight 25–45 kg** 150 mg once daily

  **Child over 13 years, body-weight over 45 kg** 200 mg once daily

  **Counselling**  Warn travellers and carers of children travelling about **importance** of avoiding mosquito bites, **importance** of taking prophylaxis regularly, and **importance** of immediate visit to doctor if ill within 1 year and **especially** within 3 months of return. For details, see notes above

  **Note**  Proguanil doses in BNFC may differ from those in product literature

**Administration**  Tablets may be crushed and mixed with food such as milk, jam or honey just before administration

**[1]Paludrine®** (AstraZeneca)
Tablets, scored, proguanil hydrochloride 100 mg. Net price 98-tab pack = £7.43. Label: 21, counselling, prophylaxis, see above

◢**With chloroquine**
See under Chloroquine

## ◣ PROGUANIL HYDROCHLORIDE WITH ATOVAQUONE

**Cautions**  diarrhoea or vomiting (reduced absorption of atovaquone); efficacy not evaluated in cerebral or complicated malaria (including hyperparasitaemia, pulmonary oedema or renal failure); **interactions:** see Appendix 1 (proguanil, atovaquone)

**Renal impairment**  avoid for malaria prophylaxis and, if possible, for treatment if estimated glomerular filtration rate less than 30 mL/minute/1.73 m$^2$

**Pregnancy**  manufacturer advises avoid unless essential

**Breast-feeding**  use only if no suitable alternative available; see also Breast-feeding, p. 334

**Side-effects**  abdominal pain, nausea, vomiting, diarrhoea; cough; headache, dizziness, insomnia, abnormal dreams, depression, anorexia, fever; rash, pruritus; *less frequently* stomatitis, palpitation, anxiety, blood disorders, hyponatraemia, and hair loss; also reported hepatitis, cholestasis, tachycardia, hallucinations, seizures, vasculitis, mouth ulcers, photosensitivity, Stevens-Johnson syndrome

### Indications and dose

See preparations

**Counselling**  Warn travellers about **importance** of avoiding mosquito bites, **importance** of taking prophylaxis regularly, and **importance** of immediate visit to doctor if ill within 1 year and **especially** within 3 months of return. For details, see Prophylaxis against malaria, above

**[2]Malarone®** (GSK) [PoM]
Tablets ('standard'), pink, f/c, proguanil hydrochloride 100 mg, atovaquone 250 mg. Net price 12-tab pack = £25.21. Label: 21, counselling, prophylaxis, see above

**Dose**

Prophylaxis of malaria started 1–2 days before entering endemic area and continued for 1 week after leaving

- By mouth

  **Child body-weight over 40 kg** 1 tablet daily

Treatment of malaria

- By mouth

  **Child body-weight 11–21 kg** 1 tablet daily for 3 days

  **Child body-weight 21–31 kg** 2 tablets once daily for 3 days

  **Child body-weight 31–40 kg** 3 tablets once daily for 3 days

  **Child body-weight over 40 kg** 4 tablets once daily for 3 days

**[2]Malarone® Paediatric** (GSK) [PoM]
Paediatric tablets, pink, f/c, proguanil hydrochloride 25 mg, atovaquone 62.5 mg, net price 12-tab pack = £6.26. Label: 21, counselling, prophylaxis, see above

**Dose**

Prophylaxis of malaria started 1–2 days before entering endemic area and continued for 1 week after leaving

- By mouth

  **Child body-weight 11–21 kg** 1 tablet once daily

  **Child body-weight 21–31 kg** 2 tablets once daily

  **Child body-weight 31–40 kg** 3 tablets once daily

  **Child body-weight over 40 kg** use *Malarone®* ('standard') tablets, see above

Treatment of malaria

- By mouth

  **Child body-weight 5–9 kg** 2 tablets once daily for 3 days

  **Child body-weight 9–11 kg** 3 tablets once daily for 3 days

  **Child body-weight 11 kg and over** use *Malarone®* ('standard') tablets, see above

**Administration**  tablets may be crushed and mixed with food or milky drink just before administration

5 Infections

---

1. Can be sold to the public provided it is licensed and labelled for the prophylaxis of malaria. Drugs for malaria prophylaxis not prescribable on the NHS; health authorities may investigate circumstances under which antimalarials are prescribed

2. Drugs for malaria prophylaxis not prescribable on the NHS; health authorities may investigate circumstances under which antimalarials prescribed

## Pyrimethamine

Pyrimethamine should not be used alone, but is used with sulfadoxine.

Pyrimethamine with sulfadoxine is not recommended for the *prophylaxis of malaria*, but can be used in the treatment of *falciparum malaria* with (or following) *quinine*.

### PYRIMETHAMINE WITH SULFADOXINE

**Cautions** see under Pyrimethamine (section 5.4.7) and under Co-trimoxazole (section 5.1.8); not recommended for prophylaxis (severe side-effects on long-term use); **interactions**: Appendix 1 (pyrimethamine, sulfonamides)

**Contra-indications** see under Pyrimethamine (section 5.4.7) and under Co-trimoxazole (section 5.1.8); sulfonamide allergy

**Pregnancy** possible teratogenic risk in *first trimester* as pyrimethamine is a folate antagonist; in *third trimester*—risk of neonatal haemolysis and methaemoglobinaemia; fear of increased risk of neonatal kernicterus appears unfounded; see also p. 333

**Breast-feeding** small risk of neonatal kernicterus in jaundiced infants; risk of haemolysis in G6PD-deficient child due to sulfadoxine

**Side-effects** see under Pyrimethamine (section 5.4.7) and under Co-trimoxazole (section 5.1.8); pulmonary infiltrates (e.g. eosinophilic or allergic alveolitis) reported—discontinue if cough or shortness of breath

**Licensed use** not licensed for use in children of body-weight under 5 kg

**Indications and dose**

> **Adjunct to quinine in treatment of *Plasmodium falciparum* malaria** see p. 332

> **Prophylaxis** not recommended by UK malaria experts

**Pyrimethamine with sulfadoxine** (Non-proprietary) PoM

Tablets, scored, pyrimethamine 25 mg, sulfadoxine 500 mg, net price 3-tab pack = 74p

Note Also known as *Fansidar®*

Available from 'special-order' manufacturers or specialist importing companies, see p. 823

## Quinine

Quinine is not suitable for the *prophylaxis of malaria*.

Quinine is used for the *treatment of falciparum malaria* or if the infective species is *not known* or if the infection is *mixed* (for details see p. 332).

### QUININE

**Cautions** cardiac disease (including atrial fibrillation, conduction defects, heart block)—monitor ECG during parenteral treatment; monitor blood glucose and electrolyte concentration during parenteral treatment; G6PD deficiency (see section 9.1.5); **interactions**: Appendix 1 (quinine)

**Contra-indications** haemoglobinuria, myasthenia gravis, optic neuritis, tinnitus

**Hepatic impairment** for treatment of malaria in severe impairment, reduce parenteral maintenance dose to 5–7 mg/kg of quinine salt

**Renal impairment** for treatment of malaria in severe impairment, reduce parenteral maintenance dose to 5–7 mg/kg of quinine salt

**Pregnancy** risk of teratogenesis with high doses in *first trimester*, but in malaria benefit of treatment outweighs risk, see also p. 333

**Breast-feeding** present in milk but not known to be harmful

**Side-effects** cinchonism, including tinnitus, hearing impairment, vertigo, headache, nausea, vomiting, abdominal pain, diarrhoea, visual disturbances (including temporary blindness), confusion; cardiovascular effects (see Cautions); dyspnoea; hypersensitivity reactions including angioedema, rashes, hot and flushed skin; hypoglycaemia (especially after parenteral administration); blood disorders (including thrombocytopenia and intravascular coagulation); acute renal failure; muscle weakness; photosensitivity; very toxic in **overdosage**—immediate advice from poisons centres essential (see also p. 28)

**Licensed use** injection not licensed

**Indications and dose**

> **Treatment of malaria** see p. 332

> Note Quinine (anhydrous base) 100 mg ≡ quinine bisulfate 169 mg ≡ quinine dihydrochloride 122 mg ≡ quinine hydrochloride 122 mg ≡ quinine sulfate 121 mg. Quinine bisulfate 300-mg tablets are available but provide less quinine than 300 mg of the dihydrochloride, hydrochloride, or sulfate

**Administration** for *intravenous infusion*, dilute to a concentration of 2 mg/mL (max. 30 mg/mL in fluid restriction) with Glucose 5% *or* Sodium Chloride 0.9% and give over 4 hours

**Quinine Sulfate** (Non-proprietary) PoM

Tablets, coated, quinine sulfate 200 mg, net price 28-tab pack = £2.20; 300 mg, 28-tab pack = £2.12

**Quinine Dihydrochloride** (Non-proprietary) PoM

Injection, quinine dihydrochloride 300 mg/mL. For dilution and use as an infusion. 1- and 2-mL amps

Available from 'special-order' manufacturers or specialist importing companies, see p. 823

Note Intravenous injection of quinine is so hazardous that it has been superseded by infusion

## Tetracyclines

Doxycycline (section 5.1.3) is used in children over 12 years for the *prophylaxis of malaria* in areas of *widespread mefloquine or chloroquine resistance*. Doxycycline is also used as an alternative to mefloquine or *Malarone®* (for details, see specific recommendations by country, p. 334).

Doxycycline is also used as an *adjunct to quinine in the treatment of falciparum malaria* (for details see p. 332).

### DOXYCYCLINE

**Cautions** section 5.1.3

**Contra-indications** section 5.1.3

**Hepatic impairment** section 5.1.3

**Renal impairment** section 5.1.3

**Pregnancy** section 5.1.3

**Breast-feeding** section 5.1.3

**Side-effects** section 5.1.3

**Licensed use** not licensed for use in children under 12 years

**Indications and dose**

> **Prophylaxis of malaria** preferably started 1–2 days before entering endemic area and continued for 4 weeks after leaving (see notes above)
> * **By mouth**
>> **Child over 12 years** 100 mg once daily
>
> **Treatment of falciparum malaria** see p. 332

◢Preparations
Section 5.1.3

<hr>

## 5.4.2 Amoebicides

**Metronidazole** is the drug of choice for *acute invasive amoebic dysentery* since it is very effective against vegetative forms of *Entamoeba histolytica* which can cause ulceration of the large intestine. **Tinidazole** is also effective. Metronidazole and tinidazole are also active against amoebae which may have migrated to the liver. Treatment with metronidazole (or tinidazole) is followed by a 10-day course of diloxanide furoate.

**Diloxanide furoate** is the drug of choice for asymptomatic patients with *E. histolytica* cysts in the faeces; metronidazole and tinidazole are relatively ineffective. Diloxanide furoate is relatively free from toxic effects and the usual course is of 10 days, given alone for chronic infections or following metronidazole or tinidazole treatment.

For *amoebic abscesses* of the liver **metronidazole** is effective; tinidazole is an alternative. Aspiration of the abscess is indicated where it is suspected that it may rupture or where there is no improvement after 72 hours of metronidazole; the aspiration may need to be repeated. Aspiration aids penetration of metronidazole and, for abscesses with large volume of pus, if carried out in conjunction with drug therapy, may reduce the period of disability.

Diloxanide furoate is not effective against hepatic amoebiasis, but a 10-day course should be given at the completion of metronidazole or tinidazole treatment to destroy any amoebae in the gut.

<hr>

### ◼ DILOXANIDE FUROATE

**Pregnancy** manufacturer advises avoid—no information available

**Breast-feeding** manufacturer advises avoid

**Side-effects** flatulence, vomiting, urticaria, pruritus

**Licensed use** not licensed for use in children under 25 kg body-weight

**Indications and dose**

> **Chronic amoebiasis and as adjunct to metronidazole or tinidazole in acute amoebiasis**
> * **By mouth**
>> **Child 1 month–12 years** 6.6 mg/kg 3 times daily for 10 days
>>
>> **Child 12–18 years** 500 mg 3 times daily for 10 days

**Diloxanide** (Sovereign) [PoM]
Tablets, diloxanide furoate 500 mg, net price 30-tab pack = £93.50. Label: 9

<hr>

### ◼ METRONIDAZOLE

**Cautions** section 5.1.11

**Hepatic impairment** section 5.1.11

**Pregnancy** section 5.1.11

**Breast-feeding** section 5.1.11

**Side-effects** section 5.1.11

**Indications and dose**

> **Anaerobic infections** section 5.1.11

> **Invasive intestinal amoebiasis, extra-intestinal amoebiasis (including liver abscess)**
> * **By mouth**
>> **Child 1–3 years** 200 mg 3 times daily for 5 days in intestinal infection (for 5–10 days in extra-intestinal infection)
>>
>> **Child 3–7 years** 200 mg 4 times daily for 5 days in intestinal infection (for 5–10 days in extra-intestinal infection)
>>
>> **Child 7–10 years** 400 mg 3 times daily for 5 days in intestinal infection (for 5–10 days in extra-intestinal infection)
>>
>> **Child 10–18 years** 800 mg 3 times daily for 5 days in intestinal infection (for 5–10 days in extra-intestinal infection)

> **Urogenital trichomoniasis**
> * **By mouth**
>> **Child 1–3 years** 50 mg 3 times daily for 7 days
>>
>> **Child 3–7 years** 100 mg twice daily for 7 days
>>
>> **Child 7–10 years** 100 mg 3 times daily for 7 days
>>
>> **Child 10–18 years** 200 mg 3 times daily for 7 days or 400–500 mg twice daily for 5–7 days, or 2 g as a single dose

> **Giardiasis**
> * **By mouth**
>> **Child 1–3 years** 500 mg once daily for 3 days
>>
>> **Child 3–7 years** 600–800 mg once daily for 3 days
>>
>> **Child 7–10 years** 1 g once daily for 3 days
>>
>> **Child 10–18 years** 2 g once daily for 3 days or 400 mg 3 times daily for 5 days or 500 mg twice daily for 7–10 days

◢Preparations
Section 5.1.11

<hr>

### ◼ TINIDAZOLE

**Cautions** see under Metronidazole (section 5.1.11); avoid in acute porphyria (section 9.8.2); **interactions:** Appendix 1 (tinidazole)

**Pregnancy** manufacturer advises avoid in first trimester

**Breast-feeding** present in milk—manufacturer advises avoid breast-feeding during and for 3 days after stopping treatment

**Side-effects** see under Metronidazole (section 5.1.11)

**Licensed use** licensed for use in children (age range not specified by manufacturer)

**Indications and dose**

**Intestinal amoebiasis**
- By mouth

  **Child 1 month–12 years** 50–60 mg/kg (max. 2 g) once daily for 3 days

  **Child 12–18 years** 2 g once daily for 2–3 days

**Amoebic involvement of liver**
- By mouth

  **Child 1 month–12 years** 50–60 mg/kg (max. 2 g) once daily for 5 days

  **Child 12–18 years** 1.5–2 g once daily for 3–6 days

**Urogenital trichomoniasis and giardiasis**
- By mouth

  **Child 1 month–12 years** single dose of 50–75 mg/kg (max. 2 g) (repeated once if necessary)

  **Child 12–18 years** single dose of 2 g (repeated once if necessary)

**Fasigyn**® (Pfizer) [PoM]

Tablets, f/c, tinidazole 500 mg, net price 16-tab pack = £11.04. Label: 4, 9, 21, 25

## 5.4.3 Trichomonacides

**Metronidazole** (section 5.4.2) is the treatment of choice for *Trichomonas vaginalis* infection. Contact tracing is recommended and sexual contacts should be treated simultaneously. If metronidazole is ineffective, **tinidazole** (section 5.4.2) may be tried.

## 5.4.4 Antigiardial drugs

**Metronidazole** (section 5.4.2) is the treatment of choice for *Giardia lamblia* infections. Tinidazole (section 5.4.2) may be used as an alternative to metronidazole.

## 5.4.5 Leishmaniacides

Cutaneous leishmaniasis frequently heals spontaneously but if skin lesions are extensive or unsightly, treatment is indicated, as it is in visceral leishmaniasis (kala-azar). Leishmaniasis should be treated under specialist supervision.

**Sodium stibogluconate**, an organic pentavalent antimony compound, is the treatment of choice for visceral leishmaniasis. The dose is 20 mg/kg daily (max. 850 mg) for at least 20 days by intramuscular or intravenous injection; the dosage varies with different geographical regions and expert advice should be obtained. Skin lesions can also be treated with sodium stibogluconate.

**Amphotericin** is used with or after an antimony compound for visceral leishmaniasis unresponsive to the antimonial alone; side-effects may be reduced by using liposomal amphotericin (*AmBisome*®—section 5.2.3) at a dose of 1–3 mg/kg daily for 10–21 days to a cumulative dose of 21–30 mg/kg *or* at a dose of 3 mg/kg for 5 consecutive days followed by a single dose of 3 mg/kg 6 days later. *Abelcet*®, a lipid formulation of amphotericin is also likely to be effective but less information is available.

**Pentamidine isetionate** (pentamidine isethionate) (section 5.4.8) has been used in antimony-resistant visceral leishmaniasis, but although the initial response is often good, the relapse rate is high; it is associated with serious side-effects. Other treatments include paromomycin [unlicensed], available from 'special-order' manufacturers or specialist importing companies, see p. 823

## ▮ SODIUM STIBOGLUCONATE

**Cautions** intravenous injections must be given slowly over 5 minutes (to reduce risk of local thrombosis) and stopped if coughing or substernal pain; mucocutaneous disease (see below); treat intercurrent infection (e.g. pneumonia); monitor ECG before and during treatment; heart disease (withdraw if conduction disturbances occur); predisposition to QT interval prolongation (including concomitant use with drugs that prolong the QT interval); **interactions:** Appendix 1 (sodium stibogluconate)

**Mucocutaneous disease** Successful treatment of mucocutaneous leishmaniasis may induce severe inflammation around the lesions (may be life-threatening if pharyngeal or tracheal involvement)—may require corticosteroid

**Hepatic impairment** use with caution

**Renal impairment** avoid in significant impairment

**Pregnancy** manufacturer advises use only if potential benefit outweighs risk

**Breast-feeding** amount probably too small to be harmful

**Side-effects** anorexia, nausea, vomiting, abdominal pain; ECG changes; coughing (see Cautions); headache, lethargy, arthralgia, myalgia; *rarely* jaundice, flushing, bleeding from nose or gum, substernal pain (see Cautions), vertigo, fever, sweating, and rash; also reported pancreatitis and anaphylaxis; pain and thrombosis on intravenous administration, intramuscular injection also painful

**Licensed use** licensed for use in children (age range not specified by manufacturer)

**Indications and dose**

**Leishmaniasis** for dose, see notes above

**Administration** injection should be filtered immediately before administration using a filter of 5 microns or less; see also Cautions above

**Pentostam**® (GSK) [PoM]

Injection, sodium stibogluconate equivalent to pentavalent antimony 100 mg/mL. Net price 100-mL bottle = £66.43

# 5.4.6 Trypanocides

The prophylaxis and treatment of trypanosomiasis is difficult and differs according to the strain of organism. Expert advice should therefore be obtained.

# 5.4.7 Drugs for toxoplasmosis

Most infections caused by *Toxoplasma gondii* are self-limiting, and treatment is not necessary. Exceptions are children with eye involvement (toxoplasma choroido-retinitis), and those who are immunosuppressed. Toxoplasmic encephalitis is a common complication of AIDS. The treatment of choice is a combination of **pyrimethamine** and **sulfadiazine**, given for several weeks (expert advice **essential**). Pyrimethamine is a folate antagonist, and adverse reactions to this combination are relatively common (folinic acid supplements (see p. 417) and weekly blood counts needed). Alternative regimens use combinations of pyrimethamine with clindamycin or clarithromycin or azithromycin. Long-term secondary prophylaxis is required after treatment of toxoplasmosis in immunocompromised patients; prophylaxis should continue until immunity recovers.

If toxoplasmosis is acquired in pregnancy, transplacental infection may lead to severe disease in the fetus; specialist advice should be sought on management. Spiramycin may reduce the risk of transmission of maternal infection to the fetus. When there is evidence of placental or fetal infection, pyrimethamine may be given with sulfadiazine and folinic acid after the first trimester.

In neonates without signs of toxoplasmosis, but born to mothers known to have become infected, spiramycin is given while awaiting laboratory results. If toxoplasmosis is confirmed in the infant, pyrimethamine and sulfadiazine are given for 12 months, together with folinic acid.

## PYRIMETHAMINE

**Cautions** blood counts required with prolonged treatment; history of seizures—avoid large loading doses; **interactions:** Appendix 1 (pyrimethamine)

**Hepatic impairment** manufacturer advises caution

**Renal impairment** manufacturer advises caution

**Pregnancy** theoretical teratogenic risk in first trimester (folate antagonist); adequate folate supplement should be given to mother

**Breast-feeding** present in milk—avoid breast-feeding during toxoplasmosis treatment; avoid other folate antagonists

**Side-effects** depression of haematopoiesis with high doses, rashes, insomnia

**Licensed use** not licensed for use in children under 5 years

**Indications and dose**

> **Toxoplasmosis in pregnancy (in combination with sulfadiazine and folinic acid (section 8.1)),** see notes above
> * By mouth
>> **Child 12–18 years** 50 mg once daily until delivery

> **Congenital toxoplasmosis (in combination with sulfadiazine and folinic acid (section 8.1)),**
> * By mouth
>> **Neonate** 1 mg/kg twice daily for 2 days, *then* 1 mg/kg once daily for 6 months, *then* 1 mg/kg 3 times a week for 6 months

> **Malaria** no dose stated because not recommended alone

**Daraprim®** (GSK) (PoM) ◢
Tablets, scored, pyrimethamine 25 mg. Net price 30-tab pack = £2.60

## SPIRAMYCIN

**Cautions** cardiac disease, arrhythmias (including predisposition to QT interval prolongation)

**Contra-indications** sensitivity to other macrolides

**Hepatic impairment** use with caution

**Breast-feeding** present in breast milk

**Side-effects** gastro-intestinal disturbances including nausea, vomiting, diarrhoea; dizziness, headache; rash; hepatotoxicity; *rarely,* prolongation of QT interval, thrombocytopenia and vasculitis

**Licensed use** not licensed

**Indications and dose**

> **Toxoplasmosis in pregnancy** see notes above
> * By mouth
>> **Child 12–18 years** 1.5 g twice daily until delivery

> **Chemoprophylaxis of congenital toxoplasmosis**
> * By mouth
>> **Neonate** 50 mg/kg twice daily

**Spiramycin** (Non-proprietary)
Tablets, spiramycin 750 000 units (250 mg); 1.5 million units (500 mg); 3 million units (1 g)
Syrup, spiramycin 75 000 units/mL (25 mg/mL)
**Note** 3000 units ≡ 1 mg spiramycin
Available from 'special-order' manufacturers or specialist importing companies, see p. 823

## SULFADIAZINE
(Sulphadiazine)

**Cautions** see under Co-trimoxazole, section 5.1.8; **interactions:** Appendix 1 (sulfonamides)

**Contra-indications** see under Co-trimoxazole, section 5.1.8

**Hepatic impairment** use with caution in mild to moderate impairment; avoid in severe impairment

**Renal impairment** use with caution in mild to moderate impairment; avoid in severe impairment; high risk of crystalluria

**Pregnancy** risk of neonatal haemolysis and methaemoglobinaemia in third trimester; fear of increased risk of kernicterus in neonates appears to be unfounded

**Breast-feeding** small risk of kernicterus in jaundiced infants and of haemolysis in G6PD-deficient infants

**Side-effects** see under Co-trimoxazole, section 5.1.8; also hypothyroidism, benign intracranial hypertension, optic neuropathy

**Licensed use** not licensed for use in toxoplasmosis

**Indications and dose**

> **Toxoplasmosis in pregnancy (in combination with pyrimethamine and folinic acid (section 8.1))** , see notes above
> * By mouth
>> **Child 12–18 years** 1 g 3 times daily until delivery

> **Congenital toxoplasmosis (in combination with pyrimethamine and folinic acid (section 8.1))**
> * By mouth
>> **Neonate** 50 mg/kg twice daily for 12 months

**Sulfadiazine** (Non-proprietary) PoM
Tablets, sulfadiazine 500 mg, net price 56-tab pack = £37.50. Label: 9, 27

## 5.4.8 Drugs for pneumocystis pneumonia

Pneumonia caused by *Pneumocystis jirovecii* (*Pneumocystis carinii*) occurs in immunosuppressed children; it is a common cause of pneumonia in AIDS. Pneumocystis pneumonia should generally be treated by those experienced in its management. Blood gas measurement is used to assess disease severity.

## Treatment

The recommended duration of treatment is generally 14–21 days.

**Mild to moderate disease** Co-trimoxazole (section 5.1.8) in high dosage is the drug of choice for the treatment of mild to moderate pneumocystis pneumonia.

**Atovaquone** or a combination of **dapsone** with **trimethoprim** 5 mg/kg every 6–8 hours (section 5.1.8) is given by mouth for the treatment of mild to moderate disease [unlicensed indication] in children who cannot tolerate co-trimoxazole.

A combination of **clindamycin** (section 5.1.6) and **primaquine** (section 5.4.1) may be used in the treatment of mild to moderate disease [unlicensed indication]; this combination is associated with considerable toxicity.

**Severe disease** Co-trimoxazole (section 5.1.8) in high dosage, given by mouth or by intravenous infusion, is the drug of choice for the treatment of severe pneumocystis pneumonia. **Pentamidine isetionate** given by intravenous infusion is an alternative for children who cannot tolerate co-trimoxazole, or who have not responded to it. Pentamidine isetionate is a potentially toxic drug that can cause severe hypotension during or immediately after infusion. If there is clinical improvement after 7–10 days of intravenous therapy with pentamidine isetionate, patients can be switched to oral treatment (e.g. atovaquone) to complete 21 days treatment.

Corticosteroid treatment can be lifesaving in those with severe pneumocystis pneumonia (see Adjunctive Therapy below).

**Adjunctive therapy** In moderate to severe pneumocystis infections associated with HIV infection, prednisolone (section 6.3.2) is given by mouth in a dose of 2 mg/kg (max. 80 mg daily) for 5 days (alternatively, hydrocortisone may be given parenterally); the dose is then reduced over the next 16 days and then stopped. Corticosteroid treatment should ideally be started at the same time as the anti-pneumocystis therapy and certainly no later than 24–72 hours afterwards. The corticosteroid should be withdrawn before anti-pneumocystis treatment is complete.

## Prophylaxis

Prophylaxis against pneumocystis pneumonia should be given to all children with a history of this infection, and to all HIV-infected infants aged 1 month–1 year. Prophylaxis against pneumocystis pneumonia should also be considered for severely immunocompromised children. Prophylaxis should continue until immunity recovers sufficiently. It should not be discontinued if the child has oral candidiasis, continues to lose weight, or is receiving cytotoxic therapy or long-term immunosuppressant therapy.

**Co-trimoxazole** (section 5.1.8) by mouth is the drug of choice for prophylaxis against pneumocystis pneumonia. Co-trimoxazole may be used in infants born to mothers with a high risk of transmission of infection.

Inhaled **pentamidine isetionate** is better tolerated than parenteral pentamidine. Intermittent inhalation of pentamidine isetionate is used for prophylaxis against pneumocystis pneumonia in children unable to tolerate co-trimoxazole. It is effective but children may be prone to extrapulmonary infection. Alternatively, **dapsone** can be used.

## ATOVAQUONE

**Cautions** initial diarrhoea and difficulty in taking with food may reduce absorption (and require alternative therapy); other causes of pulmonary disease should be sought and treated; **interactions:** Appendix 1 (atovaquone)

**Hepatic impairment** manufacturer advises caution—monitor more closely

**Renal impairment** manufacturer advises caution—monitor more closely

**Pregnancy** manufacturer advises avoid unless potential benefit outweighs risk—no information available

**Breast-feeding** manufacturer advises avoid

**Side-effects** nausea, diarrhoea, vomiting, headache, insomnia, fever, anaemia, neutropenia, hyponatraemia, rash, pruritus; also reported, Stevens-Johnson syndrome

**Licensed use** not licensed for use in children

**Indications and dose**

> **Treatment of *Pneumocystis jirovecii* (*P. carinii*) pneumonia in children intolerant of co-trimoxazole**
> * By mouth
>> **Child 1–3 months** 15–20 mg/kg twice daily with food (particularly high fat) for 14–21 days
>>
>> **Child 3 months–2 years** 22.5 mg/kg twice daily with food (particularly high fat) for 14–21 days
>>
>> **Child 2–18 years** 15–20 mg/kg (max. 750 mg) twice daily with food (particularly high fat) for 14–21 days

**Wellvone®** (GSK) PoM

Suspension, sugar-free, atovaquone 750 mg/5 mL, net price 226 mL (tutti-frutti-flavoured) = £405.31. Label: 21

◢**With proguanil hydrochloride**

See section 5.4.1

## ▮ DAPSONE

**Cautions** cardiac or pulmonary disease; anaemia (treat severe anaemia before starting); susceptibility to haemolysis including G6PD deficiency (section 9.1.5); avoid in acute porphyria (section 9.8.2); **interactions:** Appendix 1 (dapsone)

**Blood disorders** On long-term treatment, children and their carers should be told how to recognise signs of blood disorders and advised to seek immediate medical attention if symptoms such as fever, sore throat, rash, mouth ulcers, purpura, bruising or bleeding develop

**Pregnancy** neonatal haemolysis and methaemo-globinaemia reported in third trimester; folic acid 5 mg daily should be given to mother throughout pregnancy

**Breast-feeding** haemolytic anaemia; although significant amount in milk, risk to infant very small unless infant is G6PD deficient

**Side-effects** haemolysis, methaemoglobinaemia, neuropathy, allergic dermatitis (rarely including toxic epidermal necrolysis and Stevens-Johnson syndrome), anorexia, nausea, vomiting, tachycardia, headache, insomnia, psychosis, hepatitis, agranulo-cytosis; dapsone syndrome (rash with fever and eosinophilia)—discontinue immediately (may progress to exfoliative dermatitis, hepatitis, hypoal-buminaemia, psychosis and death)

**Licensed use** not licensed for treatment of *P. jirovecii* pneumonia; monotherapy not licensed for children for prophylaxis of *P. jirovecii* pneumonia

**Indications and dose**

> **Treatment of *Pneumocystis jirovecii* (*P. carinii*) pneumonia (in combination with trimethoprim)**
>
> • **By mouth**
>
> **Child 1 month–12 years** 2 mg/kg (max. 100 mg) once daily
>
> **Child 13–18 years** 100 mg once daily

> **Prophylaxis of *Pneumocystis jirovecii* (*P. carinii*) pneumonia**
>
> • **By mouth**
>
> **Child 1 month–18 years** 2 mg/kg (max. 100 mg) once daily

**Dapsone** (Non-proprietary) PoM

Tablets, dapsone 50 mg, net price 28-tab pack = £32.53; 100 mg 28-tab pack = £47.44. Label: 8

## ▮ PENTAMIDINE ISETIONATE

**Cautions** risk of severe hypotension following administration (monitor blood pressure before starting treatment, during administration, and at regular intervals until treatment concluded; child should be lying down when receiving drug parenterally); hypo-kalaemia, hypomagnesaemia, coronary heart disease, bradycardia, history of ventricular arrhythmias, concomitant use with other drugs known to prolong Q-T interval; hypertension or hypotension; hyperglyc-

aemia or hypoglycaemia; leucopenia, thrombocyto-penia, or anaemia; carry out laboratory monitoring according to product literature; care required to protect personnel during handling and administration; **interactions:** Appendix 1 (pentamidine isetionate)

**Hepatic impairment** use with caution

**Renal impairment** reduce intravenous dose for pneumocystis pneumonia if creatinine clearance less than 10 mL/minute: in *life-threatening infection*, use 4 mg/kg once daily for 7–10 days, then 4 mg/kg on alternate days to complete course of at least 14 days; in *less severe infection*, use 4 mg/kg on alternate days for at least 14 doses

**Pregnancy** manufacturer advises avoid unless essential

**Breast-feeding** manufacturer advises avoid unless essential—no information available

**Side-effects** severe reactions, sometimes fatal, due to hypotension, hypoglycaemia, pancreatitis, and arrhythmias; also leucopenia, thrombocytopenia, acute renal failure, hypocalcaemia; also reported: azotaemia, abnormal liver-function tests, anaemia, hyperkalaemia, nausea and vomiting, dizziness, syncope, flushing, hyperglycaemia, rash, and taste disturbances; Stevens-Johnson syndrome reported; on inhalation, bronchoconstriction (may be prevented by prior use of bronchodilators), cough and shortness of breath; discomfort, pain, induration, abscess formation, and muscle necrosis at injection site

**Licensed use** not licensed for prevention of pneumocystis pneumonia in children

**Indications and dose**

> **Treatment of *Pneumocystis jirovecii* (*P. carinii*) pneumonia**
>
> • **By intravenous infusion**
>
> **Child 1 month–18 years** 4 mg/kg once daily

> **Prophylaxis of *Pneumocystis jirovecii* (*P. carinii*) pneumonia**
>
> • **By inhalation of nebulised solution (using suitable equipment—consult product literature)**
>
> **Child 5–18 years** 300 mg every 4 weeks *or* 150 mg every 2 weeks

> **Visceral leishmaniasis (kala-azar, section 5.4.5)**
>
> • **By deep intramuscular injection**
>
> **Child 1–18 years** 3–4 mg/kg on alternate days to max. total of 10 injections; course may be repeated if necessary

> **Cutaneous leishmaniasis**
>
> • **By deep intramuscular injection**
>
> **Child 1–18 years** 3–4 mg/kg once or twice weekly until condition resolves (but see also section 5.4.5)

> **Trypanosomiasis**
>
> • **By deep intramuscular injection or intravenous infusion**
>
> **Child 1–18 years** 4 mg/kg daily or on alternate days to total of 7–10 injections

**Administration** Direct intravenous injection should be avoided whenever possible and **never** given rapidly; intramuscular injections should be deep and preferably given into the buttock.

For *intravenous infusion*, reconstitute 300 mg with 3–5 mL Water for Injections (displacement value may be

**5**

**Infections**

significant), then dilute required dose with 50–250 mL Glucose 5% or Sodium Chloride 0.9%; give over at least 60 minutes

**Pentacarinat®** (Sanofi-Aventis) [PoM]
Injection, powder for reconstitution, pentamidine isetionate, net price 300-mg vial = £30.45
**Caution in handling** Pentamidine isetionate is toxic and personnel should be adequately protected during handling and administration—consult product literature
**Note** *Pentacarinat®* Injection (dissolved in water for injection) may be used for nebulisation

## 5.5 Anthelmintics

**5.5.1 Drugs for threadworms**
**5.5.2 Ascaricides**
**5.5.3 Drugs for tapeworm infections**
**5.5.4 Drugs for hookworms**
**5.5.5 Schistosomicides**
**5.5.6 Filaricides**
**5.5.7 Drugs for cutaneous larva migrans**
**5.5.8 Drugs for strongyloidiasis**

Advice on prophylaxis and treatment of helminth infections is available from the following specialist centres:

| | |
|---|---|
| Birmingham | (0121) 424 0357 |
| Scottish Centre for Infection and Environmental Health (registered users of Travax only) | (0141) 300 1100 (weekdays 12–5 p.m. only) |
| Liverpool | (0151) 705 3100 |
| London | (0845) 155 5000 (treatment) |

### 5.5.1 Drugs for threadworms
(pinworms, Enterobius vermicularis)

Anthelmintics are effective in threadworm infections, but their use needs to be combined with hygienic measures to break the cycle of auto-infection. All members of the family require treatment.

Adult threadworms do not live for longer than 6 weeks and for development of fresh worms, ova must be swallowed and exposed to the action of digestive juices in the upper intestinal tract. Direct multiplication of worms does not take place in the large bowel. Adult female worms lay ova on the perianal skin which causes pruritus; scratching the area then leads to ova being transmitted on fingers to the mouth, often via food eaten with unwashed hands. Washing hands and scrubbing nails before each meal and after each visit to the toilet is essential. A bath taken immediately after rising will remove ova laid during the night.

**Mebendazole** is the drug of choice for treating threadworm infection in children over 6 months. It is given as a single dose; as reinfection is very common, a second dose may be given after 2 weeks.

**Piperazine** is available in combination with sennosides.

### MEBENDAZOLE

**Cautions** interactions: Appendix 1 (mebendazole)
**Note** The patient information leaflet in the *Vermox®* pack includes the statement that it is not suitable for women known to be pregnant or for children under 2 years

**Pregnancy** manufacturer advises avoid—toxicity in *animal* studies
**Breast-feeding** amount present in milk too small to be harmful but manufacturer advises avoid
**Side-effects** abdominal pain; *less commonly* diarrhoea, flatulence; *rarely* hepatitis, convulsions, dizziness, neutropenia, urticaria, alopecia, rash (including Stevens-Johnson syndrome and toxic epidermal necrolysis)
**Licensed use** not licensed for use in children under 2 years

**Indications and dose**
Threadworms
● By mouth
**Child 6 months–18 years** 100 mg as a single dose; if reinfection occurs second dose may be needed after 2 weeks

Whipworms, hookworms (section 5.5.4)
● By mouth
**Child 1–18 years** 100 mg twice daily for 3 days

Roundworms (section 5.5.2)
● By mouth
**Child 1–2 years** 100 mg twice daily for 3 days
**Child 2–18 years** 100 mg twice daily for 3 days *or* 500 mg as a single dose

**¹Mebendazole** (Non-proprietary) [PoM]
Tablets, chewable, mebendazole 100 mg

**Vermox®** (Janssen) [PoM]
Tablets, orange, scored, chewable, mebendazole 100 mg. Net price 6-tab pack = £1.36
Oral suspension, mebendazole 100 mg/5 mL (banana-flavoured). Net price 30 mL = £1.59

### PIPERAZINE

**Cautions** epilepsy
**Note** Packs on sale to the general public carry a warning to avoid in epilepsy, liver or kidney disease, and to seek medical advice in pregnancy
**Hepatic impairment** manufacturer advises avoid
**Renal impairment** use with caution; avoid in severe renal impairment; risk of neurotoxicity
**Pregnancy** not known to be harmful but manufacturer advises avoid in first trimester
**Breast-feeding** present in milk—manufacturer advises avoid breast-feeding for 8 hours after dose (express and discard milk during this time)
**Side-effects** nausea, vomiting, colic, diarrhoea, allergic reactions including urticaria, bronchospasm, and rare reports of arthralgia, fever, Stevens-Johnson syndrome and angioedema; *rarely* dizziness, muscular inco-ordination ('worm wobble'); drowsiness, nystagmus, vertigo, blurred vision, confusion and clonic contractions in children with neurological or renal abnormalities

**Indications and dose**
See under preparation, below

1. Mebendazole tablets can be sold to the public if supplied for oral use in the treatment of enterobiasis in children over 2 years provided its container or package is labelled to show a max. single dose of 100 mg and it is supplied in a container or package containing not more than 800 mg

◢**With sennosides**

For cautions, contra-indications, side-effects of senna see section 1.6.2

**Pripsen®** (Thornton & Ross)

Oral powder, piperazine phosphate 4 g, total sennosides (calculated as sennoside B) 15.3 mg/sachet. Net price two-dose sachet pack = £1.98. Label: 13

**Dose**

(stirred into milk or water)

**Threadworms**

● By mouth

**Child 3 months–1 year** 1 level 2.5-mL spoonful as a single dose in the morning, repeated after 14 days

**Child 1–6 years** 1 level 5-mL spoonful as a single dose in the morning, repeated after 14 days

**Child 6–18 years** content of 1 sachet as a single dose (in the morning), repeated after 14 days

**Roundworms** first dose as for threadworms; repeat at monthly intervals for up to 3 months if reinfection risk

## 5.5.2 Ascaricides
(common roundworm infections)

**Mebendazole** (section 5.5.1) is effective against *Ascaris lumbricoides* and is generally considered to be the drug of choice.

**Levamisole** [unlicensed] (available from 'special-order' manufacturers or specialist importing companies, see p. 823) is an alternative when mebendazole cannot be used. It is very well tolerated; mild nausea or vomiting has been reported in about 1% of treated patients.

**Piperazine** may be given in a single dose, see Piperazine, above.

##  LEVAMISOLE

**Cautions** epilepsy; juvenile idiopathic arthritis; Sjögren's syndrome

**Contra-indications** blood disorders

**Hepatic impairment** use with caution—dose adjustment may be necessary

**Pregnancy** embryotoxic in *animal* studies, avoid if possible

**Breast-feeding** no information available

**Side-effects** nausea, vomiting, diarrhoea; dizziness, headache; on *prolonged treatment* taste disturbances, insomnia, convulsions, influenza-like syndrome, blood disorders, vasculitis, arthralgia, myalgia, rash

**Licensed use** not licensed

**Indications and dose**

**Roundworm (*Ascaris lumbricoides*)**

● By mouth

**Child 1 month–18 years** 2.5–3 mg/kg (max. 150 mg) as a single dose

**Hookworm**

● By mouth

**Child 1 month–18 years** 2.5 mg/kg (max. 150 mg) as a single dose repeated after 7 days if severe

**Nephrotic syndrome (specialist supervision section 6.3.2)**

● By mouth

**Child 1month–18 years** 2.5 mg/kg (max. 150 mg) on alternate days

**Levamisole** (Non-proprietary) PoM

Tablets, levamisole (as hydrochloride) 50 mg Label: 4

Available from 'special-order' manufacturers or specialist importing companies, see p. 823

## 5.5.3 Drugs for tapeworm infections

### Taenicides

**Niclosamide** [unlicensed] (available from 'special-order' manufacturers or specialist importing companies, see p. 823) is the most widely used drug for tapeworm infections and side-effects are limited to occasional gastro-intestinal upset, lightheadedness, and pruritus; it is not effective against larval worms. Fears of developing cysticercosis in *Taenia solium* infections have proved unfounded. All the same, an antiemetic can be given before treatment and a laxative can be given 2 hours after niclosamide.

**Praziquantel** [unlicensed] is available from Merck Serono (*Cysticide®*); it is as effective as niclosamide and is given to children over 4 years of age as a single dose of 5–10 mg/kg after a light breakfast (*or* as a single dose of 25 mg/kg for *Hymenolepis nana*).

### Hydatid disease

Cysts caused by *Echinococcus granulosus* grow slowly and asymptomatic children do not always require treatment. Surgical treatment remains the method of choice in many situations. **Albendazole** [unlicensed] (available from 'special-order' manufacturers or specialist importing companies, see p. 823 is used in conjunction with surgery to reduce the risk of recurrence or as primary treatment in inoperable cases. Albendazole is given to children over 2 years of age in a dose of 7.5 mg/kg twice daily (max. 400 mg twice daily) for 28 days followed by 14-day break and then repeated for up to 2–3 cycles. Alveolar echinococcosis due to *E. multilocularis* is usually fatal if untreated. Surgical removal with albendazole cover is the treatment of choice, but where effective surgery is impossible, repeated cycles of albendazole (for a year or more) may help. Careful monitoring of liver function is particularly important during drug treatment.

## 5.5.4 Drugs for hookworms
(ancylostomiasis, necatoriasis)

Hookworms live in the upper small intestine and draw blood from the point of their attachment to their host. An iron-deficiency anaemia may occur and, if present, effective treatment of the infection requires not only expulsion of the worms but treatment of the anaemia.

**Mebendazole** (section 5.5.1) has a useful broad-spectrum activity, and is effective against hookworms. **Albendazole** [unlicensed] (available from 'special-order' manufacturers or specialist importing companies, see p. 823) given as a single dose of 400 mg in children over 2 years, is an alternative. **Levamisole** is also effective (section 5.5.2).

**5** Infections

## 5.5.5 Schistosomicides
(bilharziasis)

Adult *Schistosoma haematobium* worms live in the genito-urinary veins and adult *S. mansoni* in those of the colon and mesentery. *S. japonicum* is more widely distributed in veins of the alimentary tract and portal system.

Praziquantel [unlicensed] is available from Merck Serono (*Cysticide®*) and is effective against all human schistosomes. In children over 4 years the dose is 20 mg/kg followed after 4–6 hours by a further dose of 20 mg/kg (20 mg/kg 3 times daily for one day for *S. japonicum* infections). No serious adverse effects have been reported. Of all the available schistosomicides, it has the most attractive combination of effectiveness, broad-spectrum activity, and low toxicity.

## 5.5.6 Filaricides

Diethylcarbamazine [unlicensed] (available from 'special-order' manufacturers or specialist importing companies, see p. 823) is effective against microfilariae and adult worms of *Loa loa, Wuchereria bancrofti*, and *Brugia malayi*. To minimise reactions, treatment in children over 1 month is commenced with a dose of diethylcarbamazine citrate 1 mg/kg in divided doses on the first day and increased gradually over 3 days to 6 mg/kg daily (3 mg/kg daily if child under 10 years) in divided doses; length of treatment varies according to infection type, and usually gives a radical cure for these infections. Close medical supervision is necessary particularly in the early phase of treatment. In heavy infections there may be a febrile reaction, and in heavy *Loa loa* infection there is a small risk of encephalopathy. In such cases specialist advice should be sought, and treatment must be given under careful in-patient supervision and stopped at the first sign of cerebral involvement.

Ivermectin [unlicensed] (available from 'special-order' manufacturers or specialist importing companies, see p. 823) is very effective in *onchocerciasis* and it is now the drug of choice. In children over 5 years, a single dose of 150 micrograms/kg by mouth produces a prolonged reduction in microfilarial levels. Retreatment at intervals of 6 to 12 months depending on symptoms must be given until the adult worms die out. Reactions are usually slight and most commonly take the form of temporary aggravation of itching and rash. Diethylcarbamazine or suramin should no longer be used for onchocerciasis because of their toxicity.

## 5.5.7 Drugs for cutaneous larva migrans
(creeping eruption)

Dog and cat hookworm larvae may enter human skin where they produce slowly extending itching tracks usually on the foot. Single tracks can be treated with topical tiabendazole (no commercial preparation available). Multiple infections respond to **ivermectin**, **albendazole** or **tiabendazole** (thiabendazole) by mouth (all unlicensed and available from 'special-order' manufacturers or specialist importing companies, see p. 823).

## 5.5.8 Drugs for strongyloidiasis

Adult forms of *Strongyloides stercoralis* live in the gut and produce larvae which penetrate the gut wall and invade the tissues, setting up a cycle of auto-infection. Ivermectin [unlicensed] in a dose of 200 micrograms/kg daily for 2 days is the treatment of choice for chronic *Strongyloides* infection in children over 5 years. Albendazole [unlicensed] is an alternative in children over 2 years given in a dose of 400 mg twice daily for 3 days, repeated after 3 weeks if necessary.

Both of these drugs are available from 'special-order' manufacturers or specialist importing companies, see p. 823.

# 6 Endocrine system

This chapter includes advice on the drug management of the following:

Adrenal suppression during illness, trauma or surgery, p. 371

Serious infections in patients taking corticosteroids, p. 372

Nephrotic syndrome, p. 371

Delayed puberty, p. 377

Precocious puberty, p. 380

Diabetes insipidus, p. 385

For hormonal contraception, see section 7.3.

## 6.1 Drugs used in diabetes

6.1.1 Insulins

6.1.2 Antidiabetic drugs

6.1.3 Diabetic ketoacidosis

6.1.4 Treatment of hypoglycaemia

6.1.5 Treatment of diabetic nephropathy and neuropathy

6.1.6 Diagnostic and monitoring devices for diabetes mellitus

Diabetes mellitus occurs because of a lack of insulin or resistance to its action. It is diagnosed by measuring fasting or random blood-glucose concentration (and occasionally by oral glucose tolerance test). Although there are many subtypes, the two principle classes of diabetes are type 1 diabetes and type 2 diabetes.

*Type 1 diabetes*, (formerly referred to as insulin-dependent diabetes mellitus (IDDM)), is due to a deficiency of insulin following autoimmune destruction of pancreatic beta cells and is the most common form of diabetes in children. Children with type 1 diabetes require administration of insulin.

*Type 2 diabetes*, (formerly referred to as non-insulin-dependent diabetes mellitus (NIDDM)), is rare in children but the incidence is increasing, particularly in adolescents, as obesity increases. It results from reduced secretion of insulin or from peripheral resistance to the action of insulin, or from a combination of both. Although children may be controlled on diet alone, many require oral antidiabetic drugs or insulin to maintain satisfactory control. There is limited information available on the use of oral anti-diabetic drugs in children (see section 6.1.2). In overweight individuals, type 2 diabetes may be prevented by losing weight and increasing physical activity.

*Genetic defects of beta-cell function* (formerly referred to as maturity-onset diabetes of the young (MODY)), describes a number of rare disease states, characterised by onset of mild hyperglycaemia, generally before 25 years of age. A sulfonylurea, such as gliclazide (p. 359), may be effective in these patients.

**Treatment of diabetes** Treatment should be aimed at alleviating symptoms and minimising the risk of long-term complications (see below).

6 Endocrine system

Diabetes is a strong risk factor for cardiovascular disease later in life. Other risk factors for cardiovascular disease (smoking, hypertension, obesity and hyperlipidaemia) should be addressed. The use of an ACE inhibitor (section 2.5.5.1) and of a lipid-regulating drug (section 2.12) can be beneficial in children with diabetes and a high cardiovascular disease risk. For reference to the use of an ACE inhibitor in the management of diabetic nephropathy, see section 6.1.5.

**Prevention of diabetic complications** Although rare, retinopathy, neuropathy and nephropathy can occur in children with diabetes. Screening for complications should begin 5 years after diagnosis of diabetes or from 12 years of age. Optimal glycaemic control in both type 1 diabetes and type 2 diabetes reduces, in the long term, the risk of microvascular complications including retinopathy, development of proteinuria and to some extent neuropathy.

A measure of the total glycosylated (or glycated) haemoglobin ($HbA_1$) or a specific fraction ($HbA_{1c}$) provides a good indication of long-term glycaemic control. Overall it is ideal to aim for an $HbA_{1c}$ concentration of 48–59 mmol/mol or less (reference range 20–42 mmol/mol), but this cannot always be achieved and for those using insulin there is a significantly increased risk of disabling hypoglycaemia.

> ### Measurement of $HbA_{1c}$
>
> $HbA_{1c}$ values are expressed in *mmol of glycosylated haemoglobin per mol of haemoglobin (mmol/mol)*, a standardised unit specific for $HbA_{1c}$ created by the International Federation of Clinical Chemistry and Laboratory Medicine (IFCC). $HbA_{1c}$ values were previously aligned to the assay used in the Diabetes Control and Complications Trial (DCCT) and expressed as a percentage.
>
> #### Equivalent values
>
> | IFCC-$HbA_{1c}$ (mmol/mol) | DCCT-$HbA_{1c}$ (%) |
> | --- | --- |
> | 42 | 6.0 |
> | 48 | 6.5 |
> | 53 | 7.0 |
> | 59 | 7.5 |
> | 64 | 8.0 |
> | 75 | 9.0 |

Laboratory measurement of serum-fructosamine concentration is technically simpler and cheaper than the measurement of $HbA_{1c}$ and can be used to assess control over short periods of time, particularly when $HbA_{1c}$ monitoring is invalid (e.g. disturbed erythrocyte turnover or abnormal haemoglobin type).

Tight control of blood pressure in hypertensive children with type 2 diabetes may reduce mortality significantly and protects visual acuity (by reducing considerably the risks of maculopathy and retinal photocoagulation) (see also section 2.5).

**Driving** Information on the requirements for driving vehicles by individuals receiving treatment for diabetes is available in the BNF (section 6.1) or from the DVLA at www.dvla.gov.uk/medical.aspx.

## 6.1.1 Insulins

### 6.1.1.1 Short-acting insulins
### 6.1.1.2 Intermediate- and long-acting insulins
### 6.1.1.3 Hypodermic equipment

Insulin is a polypeptide hormone that plays a key role in the regulation of carbohydrate, fat, and protein metabolism. There are differences in the amino-acid sequence of animal insulins, human insulins, and the human insulin analogues. Human sequence insulin may be produced semisynthetically by enzymatic modification of porcine insulin (emp) or biosynthetically by recombinant DNA technology using bacteria (crb, prb) or yeast (pyr).

Immunological resistance to insulin action is uncommon. Preparations of human sequence insulin should theoretically be less immunogenic than other insulin preparations, but no real advantage has been shown in trials.

Insulin is inactivated by gastro-intestinal enzymes, and must therefore be given by injection; the subcutaneous route is ideal in most circumstances. Insulin is usually injected into the thighs, buttocks, or abdomen; absorption from a limb site can be increased if the limb is used in strenuous exercise after the injection. Generally, subcutaneous insulin injections cause few problems; lipodystrophy may occur and is a factor in poor glycaemic control. Lipodystrophy can be minimised by using different injection sites in rotation. Local allergic reactions are rare.

Insulin should be given to all children with type 1 diabetes; it may also be needed to treat type 2 diabetes either when other methods cannot control the condition or during periods of acute illness or peri-operatively. Insulin is required in all instances of ketoacidosis (section 6.1.3), which can develop rapidly in children.

> ### NHS Diabetes guidance
> ### Safe and Effective Use of Insulin in Hospitalised Patients (March 2010)
> Available at www.diabetes.nhs.uk

**Management of diabetes with insulin** The aim of treatment is to achieve the best possible control of blood-glucose concentration without making the child or carer obsessional and to avoid disabling hypoglycaemia; close co-operation is needed between the child or carer and the medical team to achieve good control and thereby reduce the risk of complications.

Insulin preparations can be divided into 3 types:

- those of **short** duration which have a relatively rapid onset of action, namely soluble insulin and the rapid-acting insulin analogues, insulin aspart, insulin glulisine, and insulin lispro (section 6.1.1.1);
- those with an **intermediate** action, e.g. isophane insulin (section 6.1.1.2); and
- those whose action is slower in onset and lasts for **long** periods, e.g. protamine zinc insulin, insulin detemir, and insulin glargine (section 6.1.1.2).

The duration of action of a particular type of insulin can vary from one child to another, and needs to be assessed individually.

Mixtures of insulin preparations may be required and appropriate combinations have to be determined for the individual child. Treatment should be started with several doses of short-acting insulin (soluble insulin or a rapid-acting insulin analogue) given throughout the day with a longer-acting insulin given once or twice daily. Alternatively, for those who have difficulty with, or prefer not to use, multiple daily injection regimens or in whom such regimens fail to achieve adequate glycaemic control, a mixture of premixed short- and intermediate-acting insulins (most commonly in a proportion of 30% soluble insulin and 70% isophane insulin) can be given twice daily. The dose of short-acting or rapid-acting insulin (or the proportion of the short-acting soluble insulin component in premixed insulin) can be increased in those with excessive postprandial hyperglycaemia. The dose of insulin is increased gradually according to the child's individual requirements, taking care to avoid troublesome hypoglycaemia.

Initiation of insulin may be followed by a partial remission phase or 'honeymoon period' when lower doses of insulin are required than are subsequently necessary to maintain glycaemic control.

### Examples of insulin regimens

- Multiple injection regimen: short-acting insulin or rapid-acting insulin analogue, before meals
  With intermediate-acting or long-acting insulin, once or twice daily;

- Short-acting insulin or rapid-acting insulin analogue mixed with intermediate-acting insulin, twice daily (before breakfast and the main evening meal);

- Short-acting insulin or rapid-acting insulin analogue mixed with intermediate-acting insulin, before breakfast
  With short-acting or rapid-acting insulin analogue alone, before afternoon snack or the main evening meal, and intermediate-acting insulin or long-acting insulin, at bedtime;

- Continuous subcutaneous insulin infusion (see below).

**Insulin requirements** Most prepubertal children require around 0.6–0.8 units/kg/day of insulin after the initial temporary remission phase. Unless the child has a very sedentary life-style, a requirement for higher doses may indicate poor compliance, poor absorption of insulin from the injection site (e.g. because of lipohypertrophic sites), or the beginning of puberty. During puberty up to 1.5–2 units/kg/day of insulin may be required, especially during growth spurts. Around 1 year after menarche or after the growth spurt in boys, the dose may need to be adjusted to avoid excessive weight gain. Insulin requirements can be *increased* by infection, stress, and accidental or surgical trauma. Insulin requirements can be *reduced* in very active individuals, in those with certain endocrine disorders (e.g. Addison's disease, hypopituitarism), or in coeliac disease. Insulin requirements should be assessed frequently in all these circumstances.

**Hepatic impairment** Insulin requirements may be decreased in patients with hepatic impairment.

**Renal impairment** Insulin requirements may decrease in patients with renal impairment and therefore dose reduction may be necessary. The compensatory response to hypoglycaemia is impaired in renal impairment.

**Pregnancy and breast-feeding** During pregnancy and breast-feeding, insulin requirements may alter and doses should be assessed frequently by an experienced diabetes physician. The dose of insulin generally needs to be increased in the second and third trimesters of pregnancy. The short-acting insulin analogues, insulin aspart and insulin lispro, are not known to be harmful, and may be used during pregnancy and breast-feeding. Evidence of the safety of long-acting insulin analogues in pregnancy is limited, therefore isophane insulin is recommended where longer-acting insulins are needed; insulin detemir may also be considered.

**Insulin administration** Insulin is generally given by *subcutaneous injection*; the injection site should be rotated to prevent lipodystrophy. Injection devices ('pens') (section 6.1.1.3), which hold the insulin in a cartridge and meter the required dose, are convenient to use. Insulin syringes (for use with needles) are less popular with children and carers, but may be required for insulins not available in cartridge form.

For intensive insulin regimens multiple subcutaneous injections (3 or more times daily) are usually recommended.

Short-acting insulins (soluble insulin, insulin aspart, insulin glulisine, and insulin lispro) can also be given by *continuous subcutaneous infusion* using a portable infusion pump. This device delivers a continuous basal insulin infusion and patient-activated bolus doses at meal times. This technique can be useful for children who suffer recurrent hypoglycaemia or marked morning rise in blood-glucose concentration despite optimised multiple-injection regimens (see also NICE guidance below). Children on subcutaneous insulin infusion must be highly motivated, able to monitor their blood-glucose concentration or have it monitored by a carer, and have expert training, advice, and supervision from an experienced healthcare team.

> **NICE guidance**
> **Continuous subcutaneous insulin infusion for the treatment of diabetes mellitus (type 1) (July 2008)**
> Continuous subcutaneous insulin infusion is recommended as an option in children over 12 years with type 1 diabetes:
> - who suffer repeated or unpredictable hypoglycaemia, whilst attempting to achieve optimal glycaemic control with multiple-injection regimens, **or**
> - whose glycaemic control remains inadequate (HbA$_{1c}$ over 8.5% [69 mmol/mol]) despite optimised multiple-injection regimens (including the use of long-acting insulin analogues where appropriate).
>
> Continuous subcutaneous insulin infusion is also recommended as an option for children under 12 years with type 1 diabetes for whom multiple-injection regimens are considered impractical or inappropriate. Children on insulin pumps should undergo a trial of multiple-injection therapy between the ages of 12 and 18 years.
> www.nice.org.uk/TA151

Soluble insulin by the *intravenous route* is reserved for urgent treatment e.g in diabetic ketoacidosis, and for fine control in serious illness and in the peri-operative period (see under Diabetes and Surgery, below).

**6 Endocrine system**

**Monitoring** All carers and children need to be trained to monitor blood-glucose concentrations (section 6.1.6). Since blood-glucose concentration varies substantially throughout the day, 'normoglycaemia' cannot always be achieved throughout a 24-hour period without always causing damaging hypoglycaemia. It is therefore best to recommend that children should maintain a blood-glucose concentration of between 4 and 10 mmol/litre for most of the time (4–8 mmol/litre before meals and less than 10 mmol/litre after meals), while accepting that on occasions, for brief periods, it will be above these values; efforts should be made to prevent the blood-glucose concentration from falling below 4 mmol/litre. Children using multiple injection regimens should understand how to adjust their insulin dose according to their carbohydrate intake. With fixed-dose insulin regimens, the carbohydrate intake needs to be regulated, and should be distributed throughout the day to match the insulin regimen. The intake of energy and of simple and complex carbohydrates should be adequate to allow normal growth and development but obesity must be avoided.

**Hypoglycaemia** Hypoglycaemia is a potential problem for all children using insulin, and they and their carers should be given careful instruction on how to avoid it.

Very tight control of diabetes lowers the blood-glucose concentration needed to trigger hypoglycaemic symptoms; an increase in the frequency of hypoglycaemic episodes may reduce the warning symptoms experienced by the child. Loss of warning of hypoglycaemia among insulin-treated children can be a serious hazard, especially for cyclists and drivers.

To restore the warning signs, episodes of hypoglycaemia must be minimised; this involves appropriate adjustment of insulin type, dose, and frequency, together with suitable timing and quantity of meals and snacks.

**Diabetes and surgery** Children with type 1 diabetes should undergo surgery in centres with facilities for, and expertise in, the care of children with diabetes. Detailed local protocols should be available to all healthcare professionals involved in the treatment of these children.

Children with type 1 diabetes who require surgery:

- should be admitted to hospital for general anaesthesia;

- should receive insulin, even if they are fasting, to avoid ketoacidosis;

- should receive glucose infusion when fasting before an anaesthetic to prevent hypoglycaemia;

- should have careful monitoring of blood-glucose concentration because surgery may cause hyperglycaemia.

**Elective surgery** Surgery in children with diabetes is best scheduled early on the list, preferably in the morning. If glycaemic control is poor it is advisable to admit the child well in advance of surgery. On the *evening before surgery*, blood-glucose should be measured frequently, especially before meals and snacks and at bedtime; urine should be tested for ketones. The usual evening or bedtime insulin and bedtime snack should be given. Ketosis or severe hypoglycaemia require correction, preferably by overnight intravenous infusion (section 6.1.3 and

section 6.1.4), and the surgery may need to be postponed.

For *minor procedures that require fasting*, a slight modification of the usual regimen may be all that is necessary e.g. for early morning procedures delay insulin and food until immediately after the procedure.

For *other types of elective surgery*, consult local treatment protocols.

**Emergency surgery** Intravenous fluids and an insulin infusion should be started immediately (see Intravenous Fluids and Continuous Insulin Infusion, below). If ketoacidosis is present the recommendations for diabetic ketoacidosis should be followed (section 6.1.3).

**Intravenous fluids and continuous insulin infusion** Blood-glucose and plasma-electrolyte concentrations must be measured frequently in a child receiving intravenous support. Intravenous infusion should be continued until after the child starts to eat and drink. The following infusions should be used and adjusted according to the child's fluid and electrolyte requirements:

- Constant infusion of sodium chloride 0.45% and glucose 5% intravenous infusion together with potassium chloride 20 mmol/litre (provided that plasma-potassium concentration is not raised) at a rate determined by factors such as volume depletion and age; the amount of potassium chloride infused is adjusted according to plasma electrolyte measurements;

- Constant infusion of soluble insulin 1 unit/mL in sodium chloride 0.9% intravenous infusion initially at a rate of 0.025 units/kg/hour (up to 0.05 units/kg/hour if the child is unwell), then adjusted according to blood-glucose concentration (frequent monitoring necessary) in line with locally agreed protocols and the child's volume depletion and age;

- Blood-glucose concentration should be maintained between 5 and 10 mmol/litre. If the glucose concentration falls below 5 mmol/litre, glucose 10% intravenous infusion may be required; conversely, if the glucose concentration persistently exceeds 14 mmol/litre, sodium chloride 0.9% intravenous infusion should be substituted;

- The insulin infusion may be stopped temporarily for 10–15 minutes if blood-glucose concentration falls below 4 mmol/litre.

The usual subcutaneous insulin regimen should be started before the first meal (but the dose may need to be 10–20% higher than usual if the child is still bedbound or unwell) and the intravenous insulin infusion stopped 1 hour later. If glycaemic control is not adequately achieved, additional insulin can be given in the following ways:

- additional doses of soluble insulin at any of the 4 injection times (before meals or bedtime) *or*

- temporary addition of intravenous insulin infusion to subcutaneous regimen *or*

- complete reversion to intravenous insulin infusion (particularly if the child is unwell).

**Neonatal hyperglycaemia** Newborn babies are relatively intolerant of glucose, especially in the first week of life and if premature. If intravenous glucose is necessary e.g. for total parenteral nutrition, infuse at a lower rate for 6–12 hours and the glucose intolerance should resolve. Insulin is not needed for such transient glucose intolerance, but may be needed if blood-glucose concentration is persistently high.

**Neonatal diabetes**   Neonatal diabetes is a rare condition that presents with acidosis, dehydration, hyperglycaemia, and rarely ketosis; it responds to continuous insulin infusion. When the neonate is stable, treatment can be switched to subcutaneous insulin given once or twice a day. Treatment is normally required for 4–6 weeks in transient forms, but may be required permanently in some cases.

### 6.1.1.1   Short-acting insulins

**Soluble insulin** is a short-acting form of insulin. For maintenance regimens it is usual to inject it 15 to 30 minutes before meals.

Soluble insulin is the most appropriate form of insulin for use in diabetic emergencies and at the time of surgery. It can be given intravenously and intramuscularly, as well as subcutaneously.

When injected subcutaneously, soluble insulin has a rapid onset of action (30 to 60 minutes), a peak action between 2 and 4 hours, and a duration of action of up to 8 hours.

When injected intravenously, soluble insulin has a very short half-life of only about 5 minutes and its effect disappears within 30 minutes.

The rapid-acting human insulin analogues, **insulin aspart**, **insulin glulisine**, and **insulin lispro**, have a faster onset (10–20 minutes) and shorter duration of action (2–5 hours) than soluble insulin; as a result, compared with soluble insulin, fasting and preprandial blood-glucose concentrations are a little higher, postprandial blood-glucose concentration is a little lower, and hypoglycaemia occurs slightly less frequently. These rapid-acting insulins are ideal for prandial dosing in a multiple injection regimen in combination with a long-acting insulin once or twice daily. Insulin aspart, insulin glulisine, and insulin lispro can be administered by subcutaneous infusion (see Insulin Administration, above). Insulin aspart and insulin lispro can also be administered intravenously and can be used as alternatives to soluble insulin for diabetic emergencies and at the time of surgery.

### ▌ INSULIN
(Insulin Injection; Neutral Insulin; Soluble Insulin)

A sterile solution of insulin (i.e. bovine or porcine) or of human insulin; pH 6.6–8.0

**Cautions**   section 6.1.1; interactions: Appendix 1 (antidiabetics)

**Hepatic impairment**   section 6.1.1

**Renal impairment**   section 6.1.1

**Pregnancy**   section 6.1.1

**Breast-feeding**   section 6.1.1

**Side-effects**   see notes above; transient oedema; local reactions and fat hypertrophy at injection site; rarely hypersensitivity reactions including urticaria, rash; overdose causes hypoglycaemia

**Indications and dose**

**Hyperglycaemia during illness, neonatal diabetes, neonatal hyperglycaemia**
- By intravenous infusion
  **Neonate** 0.02–0.125 units/kg/hour, adjusted according to blood-glucose concentration, see also notes above
  **Child 1 month–18 years** 0.025–0.1 units/kg/hour, adjusted according to blood-glucose concentration, see also notes above

**Diabetes mellitus**
- By subcutaneous injection
  According to requirements (see notes above)
  **Note** Rotate injection site to reduce local reactions and fat hypertrophy

**Diabetic ketoacidosis** section 6.1.3

**Surgery in children with diabetes** section 6.1.1

**Administration**   For *intravenous infusion*, dilute to a concentration of 1 unit/mL with Sodium Chloride 0.9% and mix thoroughly; insulin may be adsorbed by plastics, flush giving set with 5 mL of infusion fluid containing insulin.
*Neonatal intensive care*, dilute 5 units to a final volume of 50 mL with infusion fluid; an intravenous infusion rate of 0.1 mL/kg/hour provides a dose of 0.01 units/kg/hour

◢**Highly purified animal**
**Counselling** Show container to child or carer and confirm the expected version is dispensed
**Hypurin® Bovine Neutral** (Wockhardt) (PoM)
Injection, soluble insulin (bovine, highly purified) 100 units/mL. Net price 10-mL vial = £18.48; cartridges (for *Autopen® Classic*) 5 × 3 mL = £27.72

**Hypurin® Porcine Neutral** (Wockhardt) (PoM)
Injection, soluble insulin (porcine, highly purified) 100 units/mL. Net price 10-mL vial = £16.80; cartridges (for *Autopen® Classic*) 5 × 3 mL = £25.20

◢**Human sequence**
**Counselling** Show container to child or carer and confirm the expected version is dispensed
**Actrapid®** (Novo Nordisk) (PoM)
Injection, soluble insulin (human, pyr) 100 units/mL. Net price 10-mL vial = £7.48
**Note** Not recommended for use in subcutaneous insulin infusion pumps—may precipitate in catheter or needle

**Humulin S®** (Lilly) (PoM)
Injection, soluble insulin (human, prb) 100 units/mL. Net price 10-mL vial = £15.68; 5 × 3-mL cartridge (for *Autopen® Classic* or *HumaPen®*) = £19.08

**Insuman® Rapid** (Sanofi-Aventis) (PoM)
Injection, soluble insulin (human, crb) 100 units/mL, net price 5 × 3-mL cartridge (for *ClikSTAR®* and *Autopen® 24*) = £17.50
**Note** Not recommended for use in subcutaneous insulin infusion pumps

◢**Mixed preparations**
See Biphasic Isophane Insulin (section 6.1.1.2)

**6**   **Endocrine system**

## INSULIN ASPART
### (Recombinant human insulin analogue)

**Cautions** section 6.1.1; **interactions**: Appendix 1 (antidiabetics)

**Hepatic impairment** section 6.1.1

**Renal impairment** section 6.1.1

**Pregnancy** section 6.1.1

**Breast-feeding** section 6.1.1

**Side-effects** see under Insulin

**Licensed use** not licensed for use in children under 2 years

**Indications and dose**

Diabetes mellitus

- By subcutaneous injection

  Immediately before meals or when necessary shortly after meals, according to requirements

- By subcutaneous infusion, or intravenous injection, or intravenous infusion

  According to requirements

**Administration** for *intravenous infusion*, dilute to a concentration of 0.05–1 unit/mL with Glucose 5% *or* Sodium Chloride 0.9% and mix thoroughly; insulin may be adsorbed by plastics, flush giving set with 5 mL of infusion fluid containing insulin.

**NovoRapid**® (Novo Nordisk) [PoM]

Injection, insulin aspart (recombinant human insulin analogue) 100 units/mL, net price 10-mL vial = £16.28; *Penfill*® cartridge (for *Innovo*® and *Novo-Pen*® devices) 5 × 3-mL = £28.84; 5 × 3-mL *Flex-Pen*® prefilled disposable injection devices (range 1–60 units, allowing 1-unit dosage adjustment) = £32.00; 5 × 3-mL *FlexTouch*® prefilled disposable injection devices (range 1–80 units, allowing 1-unit dosage adjustment)= £32.13

Counselling Show container to child or carer and confirm the expected version is dispensed

## INSULIN GLULISINE
### (Recombinant human insulin analogue)

**Cautions** section 6.1.1; **interactions**: Appendix 1 (antidiabetics)

**Hepatic impairment** section 6.1.1

**Renal impairment** section 6.1.1

**Pregnancy** section 6.1.1

**Breast-feeding** section 6.1.1

**Side-effects** see under Insulin

**Licensed use** not licensed for children under 6 years

**Indications and dose**

Diabetes mellitus

- By subcutaneous injection

  Immediately before meals or when necessary shortly after meals, according to requirements

- By subcutaneous infusion or intravenous infusion

  According to requirements

**Apidra**® (Sanofi-Aventis) [PoM]

Injection, insulin glulisine (recombinant human insulin analogue) 100 units/mL, net price 10-mL vial = £16.60; 5 × 3-mL cartridge (for *ClikSTAR*® and *Autopen*® 24) = £28.30; 5 × 3-mL *Apidra*® *SoloStar*® prefilled disposable injection devices (range 1–80 units, allowing 1-unit dosage adjustment) = £25.00

Counselling Show container to patient and confirm that patient is expecting the version dispensed

Note The *Scottish Medicines Consortium* (p. 3) has advised (October 2008) that *Apidra*® is accepted for restricted use within NHS Scotland for the treatment of children over 6 years with diabetes mellitus in whom the use of a short-acting insulin analogue is appropriate

## INSULIN LISPRO
### (Recombinant human insulin analogue)

**Cautions** section 6.1.1; children under 12 years (use only if benefit likely compared to soluble insulin); **interactions**: Appendix 1 (antidiabetics)

**Hepatic impairment** section 6.1.1

**Renal impairment** section 6.1.1

**Pregnancy** section 6.1.1

**Breast-feeding** section 6.1.1

**Side-effects** see under Insulin

**Licensed use** not licensed for use in children under 2 years

**Indications and dose**

Diabetes mellitus

- By subcutaneous injection

  Shortly before meals or when necessary shortly after meals, according to requirements

- By subcutaneous infusion, or intravenous injection, or intravenous infusion

  According to requirements

**Administration** For *intravenous infusion*, dilute to a concentration of 0.1–1 unit/mL with Glucose 5% *or* Sodium Chloride 0.9% and mix thoroughly; insulin may be adsorbed by plastics, flush giving set with 5 mL of infusion fluid containing insulin.

**Humalog**® (Lilly) [PoM]

Injection, insulin lispro (recombinant human insulin analogue) 100 units/mL, net price 10-mL vial = £16.61; 5 × 3-mL cartridge (for *Autopen*® *Classic* or *HumaPen*®) = £28.31; 5 × 3-mL *Humalog*® *Kwik-Pen* prefilled disposable injection devices (range 1–60 units, allowing 1-unit dosage adjustment) = £29.46

Counselling Show container to child or carer and confirm the expected version is dispensed

### 6.1.1.2 Intermediate- and long-acting insulins

When given by subcutaneous injection, intermediate- and long-acting insulins have an onset of action of approximately 1–2 hours, a maximal effect at 4–12 hours, and a duration of 16–35 hours. Some are given twice daily in conjunction with short-acting (soluble) insulin, and others are given once daily. Soluble insulin can be mixed with intermediate and long-acting insulins (except insulin detemir and insulin glargine), essentially retaining the properties of the two components, although there may be some blunting of the initial effect of the soluble insulin component (especially on mixing with protamine zinc insulin, see below).

Close monitoring of blood glucose is essential when introducing a change to the insulin regimen; the total daily dose as well as any concomitant treatment may need to be adjusted.

Isophane insulin is a suspension of insulin with prot-amine; it is of particular value for initiation of twice-daily insulin regimens. Isophane can be mixed with soluble insulin before injection but ready-mixed preparations may be more appropriate (biphasic isophane insulin, biphasic insulin aspart, or biphasic insulin lispro).

Insulin zinc suspension (30% amorphous, 70% crystalline) has a more prolonged duration of action.

Protamine zinc insulin is usually given once daily with short-acting (soluble) insulin. It has the drawback of binding with the soluble insulin when mixed in the same syringe and is now rarely used.

Insulin detemir and insulin glargine are long-acting human insulin analogues with a prolonged duration of action; insulin detemir is given once or twice daily and insulin glargine is given once daily. These long-acting insulins are ideal for once or twice daily dosing in a multiple injection regimen in combination with a short-acting insulin before meals.

NICE (May 2009) has recommended that, if insulin is required in patients with type 2 diabetes, insulin detemir or insulin glargine may be considered for those:

- who require assistance with injecting insulin *or*
- whose lifestyle is significantly restricted by recurrent symptomatic hypoglycaemia *or*
- who would otherwise need twice-daily basal insulin injections in combination with oral antidiabetic drugs *or*
- who cannot use the device needed to inject isophane insulin.

## INSULIN DETEMIR
(Recombinant human insulin analogue—long-acting)

**Cautions** section 6.1.1; **interactions**: Appendix 1 (antidiabetics)
**Hepatic impairment** section 6.1.1
**Renal impairment** section 6.1.1
**Pregnancy** section 6.1.1
**Breast-feeding** section 6.1.1
**Side-effects** see under Insulin (section 6.1.1.1)
**Indications and dose**
> Diabetes mellitus
- By subcutaneous injection
  Child over 2 years according to requirements

**Levemir®** (Novo Nordisk) (PoM)
Injection, insulin detemir (recombinant human insulin analogue) 100 units/mL, net price 5 × 3-mL cartridge (for *NovoPen®* devices) = £42.00; 5 × 3-mL *FlexPen®* prefilled disposable injection device (range 1–60 units, allowing 1-unit dosage adjustment) = £42.00; 5 × 3-mL *Levemir InnoLet®* prefilled disposable injection devices (range 1–50 units, allowing 1-unit dosage adjustment) = £44.85
**Counselling** Show container to child or carer and confirm the expected version is dispensed

## INSULIN GLARGINE
(Recombinant human insulin analogue—long acting)

**Cautions** section 6.1.1; **interactions**: Appendix 1 (antidiabetics)
**Hepatic impairment** section 6.1.1
**Renal impairment** section 6.1.1
**Pregnancy** section 6.1.1
**Breast-feeding** section 6.1.1
**Side-effects** see under Insulin (section 6.1.1.1)
**Indications and dose**
> Diabetes mellitus
- By subcutaneous injection
  Child over 2 years according to requirements

**Lantus®** (Sanofi-Aventis) (PoM)
Injection, insulin glargine (recombinant human insulin analogue) 100 units/mL, net price 10-mL vial = £26.00; 5 × 3-mL cartridge (for *ClikSTAR®* and *Autopen® 24*) = £39.00; 5 × 3-mL *Lantus® SoloStar®* prefilled disposable injection devices (range 1–80 units, allowing 1-unit dosage adjustment) = £40.36
**Note** The *Scottish Medicines Consortium* (p. 3) has advised (October 2002) that insulin glargine is accepted for restricted use within NHS Scotland for the treatment of type 1 diabetes:

- in those who are at risk of or experience unacceptable frequency or severity of nocturnal hypoglycaemia on attempting to achieve better hypoglycaemic control during treatment with other insulins
- as a once daily insulin therapy for patients who require a carer to administer their insulin.

It is **not** recommended for routine use in patients with type 2 diabetes unless they suffer from recurrent episodes of hypoglycaemia or require assistance with their insulin injections.

**Counselling** Show container to child or carer and confirm the expected version is dispensed

## INSULIN ZINC SUSPENSION
(Insulin Zinc Suspension (Mixed)—long acting)

A sterile neutral suspension of bovine insulin or of human insulin in the form of a complex obtained by the addition of a suitable zinc salt; consists of rhombohedral crystals (10–40 microns) and of particles of no uniform shape (not exceeding 2 microns)

**Cautions** section 6.1.1; **interactions**: Appendix 1 (antidiabetics)
**Hepatic impairment** section 6.1.1
**Renal impairment** section 6.1.1
**Pregnancy** section 6.1.1
**Breast-feeding** section 6.1.1
**Side-effects** see under Insulin (section 6.1.1.1)
**Indications and dose**
> Diabetes mellitus
- By subcutaneous injection
  According to requirements

◢ **Highly purified animal**

**Hypurin® Bovine Lente** (Wockhardt) (PoM)
Injection, insulin zinc suspension (bovine, highly purified) 100 units/mL. Net price 10-mL vial = £27.72
**Counselling** Show container to child or carer and confirm the expected version is dispensed

6 Endocrine system

## ISOPHANE INSULIN
(Isophane Insulin Injection; Isophane
Protamine Insulin Injection; Isophane Insulin
(NPH)—intermediate acting)

A sterile suspension of bovine or porcine insulin or of human
insulin in the form of a complex obtained by the addition of
protamine sulfate or another suitable protamine

**Cautions** section 6.1.1; **interactions:** Appendix 1
(antidiabetics)

**Hepatic impairment** section 6.1.1

**Renal impairment** section 6.1.1

**Pregnancy** section 6.1.1

**Breast-feeding** section 6.1.1

**Side-effects** see under Insulin (section 6.1.1.1); protamine may cause allergic reactions

**Indications and dose**

Diabetes mellitus

• By subcutaneous injection

According to requirements

◢Highly purified animal

**Counselling** Show container to child or carer and confirm
the expected version is dispensed

**Hypurin®  Bovine Isophane** (Wockhardt) PoM
Injection, isophane insulin (bovine, highly purified)
100 units/mL. Net price 10-mL vial = £27.72; cartridges (for *Autopen® Classic*) 5 × 3 mL = £41.58

**Hypurin® Porcine Isophane** (Wockhardt) PoM
Injection, isophane insulin (porcine, highly purified)
100 units/mL. Net price 10-mL vial = £25.20; cartridges (for *Autopen® Classic*) 5 × 3 mL = £37.80

◢Human sequence

**Counselling** Show container to child or carer and confirm
the expected version is dispensed

**Insulatard®** (Novo Nordisk) PoM
Injection, isophane insulin (human, pyr) 100 units/
mL. Net price 10-mL vial = £7.48; *Insulatard Penfill®*
cartridge (for *Innovo®*, or *Novopen®* devices) 5 ×
3 mL = £22.90; 5 × 3-mL *Insulatard InnoLet®* prefilled disposable injection devices (range 1–50 units,
allowing 1-unit dosage adjustment) = £20.40

**Humulin I®** (Lilly) PoM
Injection, isophane insulin (human, prb) 100nits/mL,
net price 10-mL vial = £15.68; 5 × 3-mL cartridge
(for *Autopen® Classic* or *HumaPen®*) = £19.08; 5 ×
3-mL *Humulin 1 KwikPen®* prefilled disposable injection devices (range 1–60 units, allowing 1-unit
dosage adjustment) = £21.70

**Insuman® Basal** (Sanofi-Aventis) PoM
Injection, isophane insulin (human, crb) 100 units/
mL, net price 5-mL vial = £5.61; 5 × 3-mL cartridge (for *ClikSTAR®* and *Autopen® 24*) = £17.50; 5
× 3-mL *Insuman® Basal Solostar®* prefilled disposable injection devices (range 1–80 units, allowing 1-
unit dosage adjustment) = £19.80

◢Mixed preparations

See Biphasic Isophane Insulin (p. 357)

## PROTAMINE ZINC INSULIN
(Protamine Zinc Insulin Injection—long acting)

A sterile suspension of insulin in the form of a complex
obtained by the addition of a suitable protamine and zinc
chloride; this preparation was included in BP 1980 but is not
included in BP 1988

**Cautions** section 6.1.1; see also notes above; **interactions:** Appendix 1 (antidiabetics)

**Hepatic impairment** section 6.1.1

**Renal impairment** section 6.1.1

**Pregnancy** section 6.1.1

**Breast-feeding** section 6.1.1

**Side-effects** see under Insulin (section 6.1.1.1); protamine may cause allergic reactions

**Indications and dose**

Diabetes mellitus

• By subcutaneous injection

According to requirements

**Hypurin® Bovine Protamine Zinc** (Wockhardt) PoM
Injection, protamine zinc insulin (bovine, highly purified) 100 units/mL. Net price 10-mL vial = £27.72
**Counselling** Show container to child or carer and confirm
the expected version is dispensed

## Biphasic insulins

Biphasic insulins are pre-mixed insulin preparations
containing various combinations of short-acting (soluble) or rapid-acting (analogue) insulin and an intermediate-acting insulin.

The percentage of short-acting insulin varies from 10%
to 50%. These preparations should be administered by
subcutaneous injection up to 15 minutes before or soon
after a meal.

## BIPHASIC INSULIN ASPART
(Intermediate-acting insulin)

**Cautions** section 6.1.1; **interactions:** Appendix 1
(antidiabetics)

**Hepatic impairment** section 6.1.1

**Renal impairment** section 6.1.1

**Pregnancy** section 6.1.1

**Breast-feeding** section 6.1.1

**Side-effects** see under Insulin (section 6.1.1.1); protamine may cause allergic reactions

**Indications and dose**

Diabetes mellitus

• By subcutaneous injection

Up to 10 minutes before or soon after a meal,
according to requirements

**NovoMix® 30** (Novo Nordisk) PoM
Injection, biphasic insulin aspart (recombinant
human insulin analogue), 30% insulin aspart, 70%
insulin aspart protamine, 100 units/mL, net price 5
× 3-mL *Penfill®* cartridges (for *Innovo®* and *Novo-
Pen®* devices) = £28.84; 5 × 3-mL *FlexPen®* prefilled disposable injection devices (range 1–60 units,
allowing 1-unit dosage adjustment) = £32.00
**Counselling** Show container to child or carer and confirm
the expected version is dispensed; the proportions of the two
components should be checked **carefully** (the order in which
the proportions are stated may not be the same in other
countries)

## BIPHASIC INSULIN LISPRO
(Intermediate-acting insulin)

**Cautions** see section 6.1.1 and Insulin Lispro; **interactions:** Appendix 1 (antidiabetics)

**Hepatic impairment** section 6.1.1

**Renal impairment** section 6.1.1

**Pregnancy**  section 6.1.1

**Breast-feeding**  section 6.1.1

**Side-effects**  see under Insulin (section 6.1.1.1); protamine may cause allergic reactions

### Indications and dose

Diabetes mellitus

- **By subcutaneous injection**

  Up to 15 minutes before or soon after a meal, according to requirements

**Humalog® Mix25** (Lilly) PoM

Injection, biphasic insulin lispro (recombinant human insulin analogue), 25% insulin lispro, 75% insulin lispro protamine, 100 units/mL, net price 10-mL vial = £16.61; 5 × 3-mL cartridge (for *Autopen® Classic* or *HumaPen®*) = £29.46; 5 × 3-mL *Humalog® Mix25 KwikPen* prefilled disposable injection devices (range 1–60 units allowing 1-unit dosage adjustment) = £30.98

Counselling Show container to child or carer and confirm the expected version is dispensed; the proportions of the two components should be checked **carefully** (the order in which the proportions are stated may not be the same in other countries)

**Humalog® Mix50** (Lilly) PoM

Injection, biphasic insulin lispro (recombinant human insulin analogue), 50% insulin lispro, 50% insulin lispro protamine, 100 units/mL, net price 5 × 3-mL cartridge (for *Autopen® Classic* or *HumaPen®*) = £29.46; 5 × 3-mL *Humalog® Mix50 KwikPen* prefilled disposable injection devices (range 1–60 units, allowing 1-unit dosage adjustment) = £30.98

Counselling Show container to child or carer and confirm the expected version is dispensed; the proportions of the two components should be checked **carefully** (the order in which the proportions are stated may not be the same in other countries)

### ▌ BIPHASIC ISOPHANE INSULIN

(Biphasic Isophane Insulin Injection—intermediate acting)

A sterile buffered suspension of either porcine or human insulin complexed with protamine sulfate (or another suitable protamine) in a solution of insulin of the same species

**Cautions**  section 6.1.1; **interactions:** Appendix 1 (antidiabetics)

**Hepatic impairment**  section 6.1.1

**Renal impairment**  section 6.1.1

**Pregnancy**  section 6.1.1

**Breast-feeding**  section 6.1.1

**Side-effects**  see under Insulin (section 6.1.1.1); protamine may cause allergic reactions

### Indications and dose

Diabetes mellitus

- **By subcutaneous injection**

  According to requirements

**◀ Highly purified animal**

Counselling Show container to child or carer and confirm the expected version is dispensed; the proportions of the two components should be checked **carefully** (the order in which the proportions are stated may not be the same in other countries)

**Hypurin® Porcine 30/70 Mix** (Wockhardt) PoM

Injection, biphasic isophane insulin (porcine, highly purified), 30% soluble, 70% isophane, 100 units/mL, net price 10-mL vial = £16.80; cartridges (for *Autopen® Classic*) 5 × 3 mL = £25.20

**◀ Human sequence**

Counselling Show container to child or carer and confirm the expected version is dispensed; the proportions of the two components should be checked **carefully** (the order in which the proportions are stated may not be the same in other countries)

**Humulin M3®** (Lilly) PoM

Injection, biphasic isophane insulin (human, prb), 30% soluble, 70% isophane, 100 units/mL, net price 10-mL vial = £15.68; 5 × 3-mL cartridge (for *Autopen® Classic* or *HumaPen®*) = £19.08; 5 × 3-mL *Humulin M3 KwikPen* prefilled disposable injection devices (range 1–60 units, allowing 1-unit dosage adjustment) = £21.70

**Insuman® Comb 15** (Sanofi-Aventis) PoM

Injection, biphasic isophane insulin (human, crb), 15% soluble, 85% isophane, 100 units/mL, net price 5 × 3-mL cartridge (for *ClikSTAR®* and *Autopen® 24*) = £17.50

**Insuman® Comb 25** (Sanofi-Aventis) PoM

Injection, biphasic isophane insulin (human, crb), 25% soluble, 75% isophane, 100 units/mL, net price 5-mL vial = £5.61; 5 × 3-mL cartridge (for *ClikSTAR®* and *Autopen® 24*) = £17.50; 5 × 3-mL *Insuman® Comb 25 SoloStar* prefilled disposable injection devices (range 1–80 units, allowing 1-unit dosage adjustment) = £19.80

**Insuman® Comb 50** (Sanofi-Aventis) PoM

Injection, biphasic isophane insulin (human, crb), 50% soluble, 50% isophane, 100 units/mL, net price; 5 × 3-mL cartridge (for *ClikSTAR®* and *Autopen® 24*) = £17.50

### 6.1.1.3  Hypodermic equipment

Carers and children should be advised on the safe disposal of lancets, single-use syringes, and needles. Suitable arrangements for the safe disposal of contaminated waste must be made before these products are prescribed for patients who are carriers of infectious diseases.

**◀ Injection devices**

**Autopen®** (Owen Mumford)

Injection device; *Autopen® 24* (for use with Sanofi-Aventis 3-mL insulin cartridges), allowing 1-unit dosage adjustment, max. 21 units (single-unit version) *or* 2 unit dosage adjustment, max. 42 units (2 unit version), net price (both) = £15.73; *Autopen® Classic* (for use with Lilly and Wockhardt 3-mL insulin cartridges), allowing 1-unit dosage adjustment, max. 21 units (single-unit version) *or* 2 unit dosage adjustment, max. 42 units (2-unit version), net price (all) = £15.97

**ClikSTAR®** (Sanofi-Aventis)

Injection device, for use with *Lantus®*, *Apidra®*, and *Insuman®* 3-mL insulin cartridges; allowing 1-unit dose adjustment, max. 80 units, net price = £25.00

**HumaPen® Luxura** (Lilly)

Injection device, for use with *Humulin®* and *Humalog®* 3-mL cartridges; allowing 1-unit dosage adjustment, max. 60 units, net price = £26.36

6

Endocrine system

**HumaPen® Luxura HD** (Lilly)

Injection device, for use with *Humulin®* and *Humalog®* 3-mL cartridges; allowing 0.5-unit dosage adjustment, max. 30 units, net price = £26.36

**HumaPen® Memoir** (Lilly)

Injection device, for use with *Humalog®* 3-mL cartridges; allowing 1-unit dosage adjustment, max. 60 units, net price = £26.82

**Injex®** (Ocon Chemicals)

Needle-free insulin delivery device, for use with any 10-mL vial of insulin, allowing 1-unit dosage adjustment, max. 30 units, net price *starter set (Injex® device, reset box, transporter, 9 x 10-mL vial adaptors, 165 ampoules) = £149.36; 4-month refill pack (6 x 10-mL vial adaptors, 100 ampoules) = £24.47; ampoule pack (50 ampoules) = £12.28; vial adaptor pack (20 x 10-mL vial adaptors) = £12.23*

**InsuJet®** (European Pharma)

Needle-free insulin delivery device, for use with any 10-mL vial or 3-mL cartridge of insulin, allowing 1-unit dosage adjustment, max. 40 units, net price *starter set (InsuJet® device, nozzle cap, nozzle and piston, 1 x 10-mL adaptor, 1 x 3-mL adaptor, 1 catridge cap removal key) = £143.60; nozzle pack (15 nozzles) = £28.40, cartridge adaptor pack (15 adaptors) = £21.70, vial adaptor pack (15 adaptors) = £21.70*

**NovoPen® 4** (Novo Nordisk)

Injection device, for use with *Penfill®* 3-mL insulin cartridges; allowing 1-unit dosage adjustment, max. 60 units, net price = £26.56

**NovoPen Echo®** (Novo Nordisk)

Injection device, for use with *Penfill®* 3-mL insulin cartridges; allowing 0.5-unit dosage adjustment, max. 30 units, net price =£26.86

◄**Lancets, needles, syringes, and accessories**

Lancets, needles, syringes, and accessories are listed under Hypodermic Equipment in Part IXA of the Drug Tariff (Part III of the Northern Ireland Drug Tariff, Part 3 of the Scottish Drug Tariff).

> The Drug Tariffs can be accessed online at:
> National Health Service Drug Tariff for England and Wales: www.ppa.org.uk/ppa/edt_intro.htm
> Health and Personal Social Services for Northern Ireland Drug Tariff: www.dhsspsni.gov.uk/pas-tariff
> Scottish Drug Tariff: www.isdscotland.org/Health-Topics/Prescribing-and-Medicines/Scottish-Drug-Tariff/

## 6.1.2 Antidiabetic drugs

6.1.2.1 **Sulfonylureas**

6.1.2.2 **Biguanides**

6.1.2.3 **Other antidiabetic drugs**

Oral antidiabetic drugs are used for the treatment of type 2 diabetes mellitus. They should be prescribed only if the child fails to respond adequately to restriction of energy and carbohydrate intake and an increase in physical activity. They should be used to augment the effect of diet and exercise, and not to replace them.

In children, type 2 diabetes does not usually occur until adolescence and information on the use of oral antidiabetic drugs in children is limited. Treatment with oral antidiabetic drugs should be initiated under specialist supervision **only**; the initial dose should be at the lower end of the adult dose range and then adjusted according to response.

Metformin (section 6.1.2.2) is the oral antidiabetic drug of choice because there is most experience with this drug in children. If dietary changes and metformin do not control the diabetes adequately, either a sulfonylurea (section 6.1.2.1) or insulin (section 6.1.1) can be added.

Alternatively, oral therapy may be substituted with insulin.

When insulin is added to oral therapy, it is generally given at bedtime as isophane or long-acting insulin, and when insulin replaces an oral regimen it may be given as twice-daily injections of a biphasic insulin (or isophane insulin mixed with soluble insulin), or a multiple injection regimen. Weight gain and hypoglycaemia may be complications of insulin therapy but weight gain can be reduced if the insulin is given in combination with metformin.

**Pregnancy and breast-feeding** During pregnancy, women with *pre-existing diabetes* can be treated with metformin [unlicensed use], either alone or in combination with insulin (section 6.1.1). Metformin can be continued, or glibenclamide resumed, during breast-feeding for those with pre-existing diabetes. Women with *gestational diabetes* may be treated, with or without concomitant insulin (section 6.1.1), with glibenclamide from 11 weeks gestation (after organogenesis) [unlicensed use] or with metformin [unlicensed use]. Women with gestational diabetes should discontinue hypoglycaemic treatment after giving birth.

Other oral hypoglycaemic drugs are contra-indicated in pregnancy and breast-feeding.

### 6.1.2.1 Sulfonylureas

The sulfonylureas are not the first choice oral antidiabetics in children. They act mainly by augmenting insulin secretion and consequently are effective only when some residual pancreatic beta-cell activity is present; during long-term administration they also have an extrapancreatic action. All can cause hypoglycaemia but this is uncommon and usually indicates excessive dosage. Sulfonylurea-induced hypoglycaemia can persist for many hours and must always be treated in hospital.

Sulfonylureas are considered for children in whom metformin is contra-indicated or not tolerated. Several sulfonylureas are available but experience in children is limited; choice is determined by side-effects and the duration of action as well as the child's age and renal function. Glibenclamide, a long-acting sulfonylurea, is associated with a greater risk of hypoglycaemia and for this reason is generally avoided in children. Shorter-acting alternatives, such as **tolbutamide**, may be preferred.

Insulin therapy should be instituted temporarily during intercurrent illness (such as coma, infection, and trauma). Sulfonylureas should be omitted on the morning of surgery; insulin is often required because of the ensuing hyperglycaemia in these circumstances.

Sulfonylureas can be useful in the management of certain forms of diabetes that result from genetic defects of beta-cell function; there is most experience with gliclazide.

**Cautions** Sulfonylureas encourage weight gain and should be prescribed only if poor control and symptoms persist despite adequate attempts at dieting; metformin (section 6.1.2.2) is considered the drug of choice in children. Caution is needed in children with G6PD deficiency (section 9.1.5).

**Contra-indications** Sulfonylureas should be avoided where possible in acute porphyria (section 9.8.2). Sulfonylureas are contra-indicated in the presence of ketoacidosis.

**Hepatic impairment** Sulfonylureas should be avoided or a reduced dose should be used in severe hepatic impairment, because there is an increased risk of hypoglycaemia. Jaundice may occur.

**Renal impairment** Sulfonylureas should be used with care in those with mild to moderate renal impairment, because of the hazard of hypoglycaemia; they should be avoided where possible in severe renal impairment. If necessary, the short-acting drug tolbutamide can be used in renal impairment, as can gliclazide which is principally metabolised in the liver, but careful monitoring of blood-glucose concentration is essential; care is required to use the lowest dose that adequately controls blood glucose.

**Pregnancy** The use of sulfonylureas in pregnancy should generally be avoided because of the risk of neonatal hypoglycaemia; however, glibenclamide can be used during the second and third trimesters of pregnancy in women with gestational diabetes, see section 6.1.2.

**Breast-feeding** The use of sulfonylureas (except glibenclamide [unlicensed use], see section 6.1.2) in breast-feeding should be avoided because there is a theoretical possibility of hypoglycaemia in the infant.

**Side-effects** Side-effects of sulfonylureas are generally mild and infrequent and include gastro-intestinal disturbances such as nausea, vomiting, diarrhoea and constipation.

Sulfonylureas can occasionally cause a disturbance in liver function, which rarely leads to cholestatic jaundice, hepatitis, and hepatic failure. Hypersensitivity reactions can occur, usually in the first 6–8 weeks of therapy. They consist mainly of allergic skin reactions which progress rarely to erythema multiforme or exfoliative dermatitis, fever, and jaundice; photosensitivity has rarely been reported with glipizide. Blood disorders are also rare but include leucopenia, thrombocytopenia, agranulocytosis, pancytopenia, haemolytic anaemia, and aplastic anaemia.

## GLIBENCLAMIDE

**Cautions** see notes above; **interactions:** Appendix 1 (antidiabetics)
**Contra-indications** see notes above
**Hepatic impairment** see notes above
**Renal impairment** see notes above
**Pregnancy** see notes above
**Breast-feeding** see notes above
**Side-effects** see notes above

**Licensed use** not licensed for use in children
**Indications and dose**

> Type 2 diabetes mellitus, maturity-onset diabetes of the young (specialist management only, see notes above)
> • By mouth
>> **Child 12–18 years** initially 2.5 mg daily with or immediately after breakfast, adjusted according to response, max. 15 mg daily

**Glibenclamide** (Non-proprietary) ᴾᵒᴹ
Tablets, glibenclamide 2.5 mg, net price 28-tab pack = 95p; 5 mg, 28-tab pack = £1.07

## GLICLAZIDE

**Cautions** see notes above; **interactions:** Appendix 1 (antidiabetics)
**Contra-indications** see notes above
**Hepatic impairment** see notes above
**Renal impairment** see notes above
**Pregnancy** see notes above
**Breast-feeding** see notes above
**Side-effects** see notes above
**Licensed use** not licensed for use in children
**Indications and dose**

> Type 2 diabetes mellitus, maturity-onset diabetes of the young (specialist management only, see notes above)
> • By mouth
>> **Child 12–18 years** initially 20 mg once daily with breakfast, adjusted according to response; up to 160 mg as a single dose; max. 160 mg twice daily

**Gliclazide** (Non-proprietary) ᴾᵒᴹ
Tablets, gliclazide 40 mg, net price 28-tab pack = £3.36; 80 mg, 28-tab pack = £1.10, 60-tab pack = £1.52
Brands include *Zicron*®

**Diamicron**® (Servier) ᴾᵒᴹ
Tablets, scored, gliclazide 80 mg, net price 60-tab pack = £4.38

## TOLBUTAMIDE

**Cautions** see notes above; **interactions:** Appendix 1 (antidiabetics)
**Contra-indications** see notes above
**Hepatic impairment** see notes above
**Renal impairment** see notes above
**Pregnancy** see notes above
**Breast-feeding** see notes above
**Side-effects** see notes above; also headache, tinnitus
**Licensed use** not licensed for use in children
**Indications and dose**

> Type 2 diabetes mellitus (see notes above), specialist management only
> • By mouth
>> **Child 12–18 years** 0.5–1.5 g (max. 2 g) daily in divided doses with or immediately after meals *or* as a single dose with or immediately after breakfast

**Tolbutamide** (Non-proprietary) ᴾᵒᴹ
Tablets, tolbutamide 500 mg. Net price 28-tab pack = £1.74

**6**

**Endocrine system**

## 6.1.2.2 Biguanides

**Metformin**, the only available biguanide, has a different mode of action from the sulfonylureas, and is not interchangeable with them. It exerts its effect mainly by decreasing gluconeogenesis and by increasing peripheral utilisation of glucose; since it acts only in the presence of endogenous insulin it is effective only if there are some residual functioning pancreatic islet cells.

Metformin is the drug of first choice in children with type 2 diabetes, in whom strict dieting has failed to control diabetes. When the combination of strict diet and metformin treatment fails, other options to be considered under specialist management only, include:

- combining with insulin (section 6.1.1) but weight gain and hypoglycaemia can be problems (weight gain minimised if insulin given at night);

- combining with a sulfonylurea (section 6.1.2.1) (reports of increased hazard with this combination remain unconfirmed).

Insulin treatment is almost always required in medical and surgical emergencies; insulin should also be substituted before elective surgery (omit metformin on the morning of surgery and give insulin if required).

Hypoglycaemia does not usually occur with metformin; other advantages are the lower incidence of weight gain and lower plasma-insulin concentration. It does not exert a hypoglycaemic action in non-diabetic subjects unless given in overdose.

Gastro-intestinal side-effects are initially common with metformin, and may persist in some children, particularly when high doses are given. A slow increase in dose may improve tolerability.

Very rarely, metformin can provoke lactic acidosis which is most likely to occur in children with renal impairment, see Lactic Acidosis below.

### METFORMIN HYDROCHLORIDE

**Cautions** see notes above; determine renal function before treatment and at least annually (at least twice a year in patients with additional risk factors for renal impairment, or if deterioration suspected); **interactions:** Appendix 1 (antidiabetics)

**Lactic acidosis** Use with caution in renal impairment—increased risk of lactic acidosis; avoid in significant renal impairment. Withdraw or interrupt treatment in those at risk of tissue hypoxia or sudden deterioration in renal function, such as those with dehydration, severe infection, shock, sepsis, acute heart failure, respiratory failure, or hepatic impairment

**Contra-indications** ketoacidosis; use of general anaesthesia (suspend metformin on the morning of surgery and restart when renal function returns to baseline)

**Iodine-containing X-ray contrast media** Intravascular administration of iodinated contrast agents can cause renal failure, which can increase the risk of lactic acidosis with metformin—see Lactic Acidosis above. Suspend metformin prior to the test; restart no earlier than 48 hours after the test if renal function has returned to baseline

**Hepatic impairment** withdraw if tissue hypoxia likely

**Renal impairment** see under Cautions

**Pregnancy** used in pregnancy for both pre-existing and gestational diabetes—see also Pregnancy and Breast-feeding, p. 358

**Breast-feeding** may be used during breast-feeding—see also Pregnancy and Breast-feeding, p. 358

**Side-effects** anorexia, nausea, vomiting, diarrhoea (usually transient), abdominal pain, taste disturbance; *rarely* lactic acidosis (withdraw treatment), decreased vitamin-$B_{12}$ absorption, erythema, pruritus and urticaria; hepatitis also reported

**Licensed use** not licensed for use in children under 10 years

### Indications and dose

**Diabetes mellitus** (see notes above) specialist supervision **only**

- **By mouth**

  **Child 8–10 years** initially 200 mg once daily adjusted according to response at intervals of at least 1 week; max. 2 g daily in 2–3 divided doses

  **Child 10–18 years** initially 500 mg once daily adjusted according to response at intervals of at least 1 week; max. 2 g daily in 2–3 divided doses

**Metformin** (Non-proprietary) PoM

Tablets, coated, metformin hydrochloride 500 mg, net price 28-tab pack = £1.07, 84-tab pack= £1.57; 850 mg, 56-tab pack = £1.67. Label: 21

Oral solution, sugar-free, metformin hydrochloride 500 mg/5 mL, net price 100 mL = £62.48. Label: 21
Brands include *Metsol*®

**Glucophage**® (Merck Serono) PoM

Tablets, f / c, metformin hydrochloride 500 mg, net price 84-tab pack = £2.88; 850 mg, 56-tab pack = £3.20. Label: 21

Oral powder, sugar-free, metformin hydrochloride 500 mg/sachet, net price 30-sachet pack = £3.29, 60-sachet pack = £6.58; 1 g/sachet, 30-sachet pack = £6.58, 60-sachet pack = £13.16. Label: 13, 21, counselling, administration

**Excipients** include aspartame (section 9.4.1)

**Counselling** The contents of each sachet should be mixed with 150 mL of water and taken immediately

The *Scottish Medicines Consortium* (p. 3) has advised (March 2010) that *Glucophage*® oral powder is accepted for restricted use within NHS Scotland for the treatment of type 2 diabetes mellitus in patients who are unable to swallow the solid dosage form.

## 6.1.2.3 Other antidiabetic drugs

There is little experience of the use of **acarbose** in children. It has been used in older children; therapy should be initiated by an appropriate expert.

The use of nateglinide in combination with a sulfonylurea is generally reserved for the management of some subtypes of diabetes resulting from genetic defects of beta-cell function or other syndromes of diabetes and requires specialist management.

## 6.1.3 Diabetic ketoacidosis

The management of diabetic ketoacidosis involves the replacement of fluid and electrolytes and the administration of insulin. Guidelines for the Management of Diabetic Ketoacidosis, published by the British Society of Paediatric Endocrinology and Diabetes[1], should be followed. Clinically well children with mild ketoacidosis

1. Available at www.bsped.org.uk

who are dehydrated up to 5% usually respond to oral rehydration and subcutaneous insulin. For those who do not respond, or are clinically unwell, or are dehydrated by more than 5%, insulin and replacement fluids are best given by intravenous infusion.

- To restore circulating volume for children in *shock*, give 10 mL/kg **sodium chloride 0.9%** as a rapid infusion, repeat as necessary up to a maximum of 30 mL/kg.

- Further fluid should be given by intravenous infusion at a rate that replaces deficit and provides maintenance over 48 hours; initially use **sodium chloride 0.9%**, changing to **sodium chloride 0.45%** and **glucose 5%** after 12 hours if response is adequate and plasma-sodium concentration is stable.

- Include **potassium chloride** in the fluids unless anuria is suspected, adjust according to plasma-potassium concentration.

- Insulin infusion is necessary to switch off ketogenesis and reverse acidosis; it should not be started until at least 1 hour after the start of intravenous rehydration fluids.

- **Soluble insulin** should be diluted (and **mixed thoroughly**) with **sodium chloride 0.9%** intravenous infusion to a concentration of 1 unit/mL and infused at a rate of 0.1 units/kg/hour.

- **Sodium bicarbonate** infusion (1.26% or 2.74%) is rarely necessary and is used only in cases of extreme acidosis (blood pH less than 6.9) and shock, since the acid-base disturbance is normally corrected by treatment with insulin.

- Once blood glucose falls to 14 mmol/litre, **glucose intravenous infusion 5%** *or* **10%** should be added to the fluids.

- The insulin infusion rate can be reduced to no less than 0.05 units/kg/hour when blood-glucose concentration has fallen to 14 mmol/litre *and* blood pH is greater than 7.3 *and* a glucose infusion has been started (see above); it is continued until the child is ready to take food by mouth. Subcutaneous insulin can then be started.

- The insulin infusion should not be stopped until 1 hour after starting subcutaneous soluble or long-acting insulin, or 10 minutes after starting subcutaneous insulin aspart, or insulin glulisine, or insulin lispro.

Hyperosmolar hyperglycaemic state or hyperosmolar hyperglycaemic nonketotic coma occurs rarely in children. Treatment is similar to that of diabetic ketoacidosis, although lower rates of insulin infusion and slower rehydration may be required.

## 6.1.4    Treatment of hypoglycaemia

Prompt treatment of hypoglycaemia in children from any cause is essential as severe hypoglycaemia may cause subsequent neurological damage. Hyperinsulinism, fatty acid oxidation disorders and glycogen storage disease are less common causes of acute hypoglycaemia in children.

Initially glucose 10–20 g is given by mouth either in liquid form or as granulated sugar or sugar lumps.

Approximately 10 g of glucose is available from non-diet versions of *Lucozade*® *Energy Original* 55 mL, *Coca-Cola*® 100 mL, and *Ribena*® *Blackcurrant* 19 mL (to be diluted), 2 teaspoons of sugar, and also from 3 sugar lumps[1]. If necessary this can be repeated in 10–15 minutes. After initial treatment, a snack providing sustained availability of carbohydrate (e.g. a sandwich, fruit, milk, or biscuits) or the next meal, if it is due, can prevent blood-glucose concentration from falling again.

Hypoglycaemia which causes unconsciousness or seizures is an emergency. **Glucagon**, a polypeptide hormone produced by the alpha cells of the islets of Langerhans, increases blood-glucose concentration by mobilising glycogen stored in the liver. In hypoglycaemia, if sugar cannot be given by mouth, glucagon can be given by injection. Carbohydrates should be given as soon as possible to restore liver glycogen; glucagon is not appropriate for chronic hypoglycaemia. Glucagon can be issued to parents or carers of insulin-treated children for emergency use in hypoglycaemic attacks. It is often advisable to prescribe it on an 'if necessary' basis for hospitalised insulin-treated children, so that it can be given rapidly by the nurses during a hypoglycaemic emergency. If not effective in 10 minutes intravenous glucose should be given.

Alternatively, 5 mL/kg of glucose intravenous infusion 10% (500 mg/kg of glucose) (section 9.2.2) can be given intravenously into a large vein through a large-gauge needle; care is required since this concentration is irritant especially if extravasation occurs. Glucose intravenous infusion 50% is **not** recommended, as it is very viscous and hypertonic. Close monitoring is necessary, particularly in the case of an overdose with a long-acting insulin because further administration of glucose may be required. Children whose hypoglycaemia is caused by an oral antidiabetic drug should be transferred to hospital because the hypoglycaemic effects of these drugs can persist for many hours.

Glucagon is not effective in the treatment of hypoglycaemia due to fatty acid oxidation or glycogen storage disorders.

**Neonatal hypoglycaemia** Neonatal hypoglycaemia at birth is treated with **glucose intravenous infusion 10%** given at a rate of 5 mL/kg/hour. An initial dose of 2.5 mL/kg over 5 minutes may be required if hypoglycaemia is severe enough to cause loss of consciousness or seizures. Mild asymptomatic persistent hypoglycaemia may respond to a single dose of **glucagon**. Glucagon has also been used in the short-term management of endogenous hyperinsulinism.

---

▌ **GLUCAGON**

**Cautions** see notes above, insulinoma, glucagonoma; ineffective in chronic hypoglycaemia, starvation, and adrenal insufficiency; delayed hypoglycaemia when used as a diagnostic test—deaths reported (ensure a meal is eaten before discharge)

**Contra-indications** phaeochromocytoma

**Side-effects** nausea, vomiting, diarrhoea, hypokalaemia, rarely hypersensitivity reactions

---

1. Proprietary products of quick-acting carbohydrate (e.g. *GlucoGel*®, *Dextrogel*®, *GSF-Syrup*®, *Rapilose*® gel) are available on prescription for the patient to keep to hand in case of hypoglycaemia

**6** Endocrine system

**Licensed use** unlicensed for growth hormone test and hyperinsulinism

**Indications and dose**

**Hypoglycaemia associated with diabetes**

- By subcutaneous, intramuscular, or intravenous injection

  **Neonate** 20 micrograms/kg

  **Child 1 month–2 years** 500 micrograms

  **Child 2–18 years, body-weight less than 25 kg** 500 micrograms; **body-weight over 25 kg** 1 mg

**Endogenous hyperinsulinism**

- By intramuscular or intravenous injection

  **Neonate** 200 micrograms/kg (max. 1 mg) as a single dose

  **Child 1 month–2 years** 1 mg as a single dose

- By continuous intravenous infusion

  **Neonate** 1–18 micrograms/kg/hour, adjusted according to response (max. 50 micrograms/kg/hour)

  **Child 1 month–2 years** 1–10 micrograms/kg/hour, increased if necessary

  **Administration** Do not add to infusion fluids containing calcium—precipitation may occur

**Diagnosis of growth hormone secretion** specialist centre only (section 6.5.1)

- By intramuscular injection

  **Child 1 month–18 years** 100 micrograms/kg (max. 1 mg) as a single dose; dose may vary, consult local guidelines

**Beta-blocker poisoning** , see p. 29

**Note** 1 unit of glucagon = 1 mg of glucagon

**¹GlucaGen® HypoKit** (Novo Nordisk) [PoM]
Injection, powder for reconstitution, glucagon (rys) as hydrochloride with lactose, net price 1-mg vial with prefilled syringe containing water for injection = £11.52

## Chronic hypoglycaemia

**Diazoxide** is useful in the management of chronic hypoglycaemia due to excessive insulin secretion, either from a tumour involving the islets of Langerhans or from persisting hyperinsulinaemic hypoglycaemia of infancy (nesidioblastosis, see also glucagon above). Diazoxide has no place in the management of acute hypoglycaemia. **Chlorothiazide** 3–5 mg/kg twice daily (section 2.2.1) reduces diazoxide-induced sodium and water retention and has the added benefit of potentiating the glycaemic effect of diazoxide.

If diazoxide and chlorothiazide fail to suppress excessive glucose requirements in chronic hypoglycaemia then **octreotide** or **nifedipine** (section 2.6.2) can be added. Octreotide suppresses secretion of growth hormone, but growth is unlikely to be affected in the long term.

## ■ DIAZOXIDE

**Cautions** ischaemic heart disease; monitor blood pressure, during prolonged use monitor white cell and platelet count, and regularly assess growth, bone, and

psychological development; avoid the intravenous route if possible; extravasation can cause tissue necrosis and single doses of 300 mg have been associated with angina and cerebral and myocardial infarction; **interactions:** Appendix 1 (diazoxide)

**Renal impairment** increased sensitivity to hypotensive and hyperglycaemic effect; dose reduction may be required

**Pregnancy** prolonged use in second or third trimesters may produce alopecia and impaired glucose tolerance in neonate; inhibits uterine activity

**Side-effects** anorexia, nausea, vomiting, hyperuricaemia, sodium and water retention, hyperglycaemia, hypotension, oedema, tachycardia, arrhythmias, extrapyramidal effects; hypertrichosis on prolonged treatment

**Indications and dose**

**Chronic intractable hypoglycaemia**

- By mouth or by intravenous injection

  **Neonate** initially 5 mg/kg twice daily to establish response, adjust dose according to response; usual maintenance dose 1.5–3 mg/kg 2–3 times daily; up to 7 mg/kg 3 times daily may be required in some cases, higher doses unlikely to be beneficial

  **Child 1 month–18 years** initially 1.7 mg/kg 3 times daily then adjusted according to response; usual maintenance dose 1.5–3 mg/kg 2–3 times daily; up to 5 mg/kg 3 times daily may be required in some cases, higher doses unlikely to be beneficial

**Hypertensive emergencies and resistant hypertension** section 2.5.1.1

**Eudemine®** (UCB Pharma) [PoM]
Tablets, diazoxide 50 mg, net price 100 = £44.64

Injection, see section 2.5.1

## ■ OCTREOTIDE

**Cautions** avoid abrupt withdrawal of short-acting octreotide—see Side-effects below; in insulinoma (risk of increased depth and duration of hypoglycaemia—monitor closely when initiating treatment and changing doses); diabetes mellitus (antidiabetic requirements may be reduced); monitor thyroid function on long-term therapy; monitor liver function; **interactions:** Appendix 1 (octreotide)

**Pregnancy** possible effect on fetal growth, avoid unless benefit outweighs risk; effective contraception required during treatment

**Breast-feeding** avoid unless essential—present in milk in *animal* studies

**Side-effects** anorexia, nausea, vomiting, abdominal pain, bloating, flatulence, diarrhoea, constipation, and steatorrhoea (administer between meals or at bedtime to reduce gastro-intestinal side-effects); bradycardia, dyspnoea, headache, dizziness; postprandial glucose tolerance may be impaired, rarely persistent hyperglycaemia with chronic administration; hypoglycaemia has also been reported; reduced gall bladder motility and bile flow; gallstones reported after long-term treatment; abrupt withdrawal of subcutaneous octreotide is associated with biliary colic and pancreatitis; rash, alopecia; pain and irritation at injection

---

1. [PoM] restriction does not apply where administration is for saving life in emergency

site—sites should be rotated; *rarely* pancreatitis shortly after administration; hepatitis also reported

**Licensed use** not licensed in children

**Indications and dose**

> **Persistent hyperinsulinaemic hypoglycaemia unresponsive to diazoxide and glucose**
> - By subcutaneous injection
>
>   **Neonate** initially 2–5 micrograms/kg every 6–8 hours, adjusted according to response; up to 7 micrograms/kg every 4 hours may rarely be required
>
>   **Child 1 month–18 years** initially 1–2 micrograms/kg every 4–6 hours, dose adjusted according to response; up to 7 micrograms/kg every 4 hours may rarely be required
>
> **Bleeding from oesophageal or gastric varices**
> - By continuous intravenous infusion
>
>   **Child 1 month–18 years** 1 microgram/kg/hour, higher doses may be required initially; when no active bleeding reduce dose over 24 hours; usual max. 50 micrograms/hour

**Administration** for *intravenous infusion*, dilute with Sodium Chloride 0.9% to a concentration of 10–50%

**Sandostatin**® (Novartis) (PoM)

Injection, octreotide (as acetate) 50 micrograms/mL, net price 1-mL amp = £2.98; 100 micrograms/mL, 1-mL amp = £5.60; 200 micrograms/mL 5-mL vial = £69.66; 500 micrograms/mL, 1-mL amp = £27.10

---

## 6.1.5 Treatment of diabetic nephropathy and neuropathy

### Diabetic nephropathy

Regular review of diabetic children over 12 years of age should include an annual test for microalbuminuria (the earliest sign of nephropathy). If reagent strip tests (*Micral-Test II*® (NHS) or *Microbumintest*® (NHS)) are used and prove positive, the result should be confirmed by laboratory analysis of a urine sample. Microalbuminuria can occur transiently during puberty; if it persists (at least 3 positive tests) treatment with an ACE inhibitor (section 2.5.5.1) or an angiotensin-II receptor antagonist (section 2.5.5.2) under specialist guidance should be considered; to minimise the risk of renal deterioration, blood pressure should be carefully controlled (section 2.5).

ACE inhibitors can potentiate the hypoglycaemic effect of insulin and oral antidiabetic drugs; this effect is more likely during the first weeks of combined treatment and in children with renal impairment.

For the treatment of hypertension in diabetes, see section 2.5.

### Diabetic neuropathy

Clinical neuropathy is rare in children whose diabetes is well controlled.

## 6.1.6 Diagnostic and monitoring devices for diabetes mellitus

### Blood monitoring

Blood **glucose** monitoring using a meter gives a direct measure of the glucose concentration at the time of the test and can detect hypoglycaemia as well as hyperglycaemia. Carers and children should be properly trained in the use of blood glucose monitoring systems and the appropriate action to take on the results obtained. Inadequate understanding of the normal fluctuations in blood glucose can lead to confusion and inappropriate action.

Children using multiple injection regimens should understand how to adjust their insulin dose according to their carbohydrate intake. With fixed-dose insulin regimens, the carbohydrate intake needs to be regulated, and should be distributed throughout the day to match the insulin regimen.

**Note** In the UK blood-glucose concentration is expressed in mmol/litre and Diabetes UK advises that these units should be used for self-monitoring of blood glucose. In other European countries units of mg/100 mL (or mg/dL) are commonly used.

It is advisable to check that the meter is pre-set in the correct units.

If the blood glucose level is high or if the child is unwell, blood **ketones** should be measured according to local guidelines in order to detect diabetic ketoacidosis (section 6.1.3). Children and their carers should be trained in the use of blood ketone monitoring systems and to take appropriate action on the results obtained, including when to seek medical attention.

### Urinalysis

Reagent strips are available for measuring glucose in the urine. It is rarely necessary for children to test themselves for ketones unless they become unwell—see also Blood Monitoring, above.

Microalbuminuria can be detected with *Micral-Test II*® (NHS) but this should be followed by confirmation in the laboratory, since false positive results are common.

◀ **Glucose**

**Diabur-Test 5000**® (Roche Diagnostics)

Reagent strips, for detection of glucose in urine. Net price 50-strip pack = £2.87

**Diastix**® (Bayer Diabetes Care)

Reagent strips, for detection of glucose in urine. Net price 50-strip pack = £2.78

**Medi-Test**® **Glucose** (BHR)

Reagent strips, for detection of glucose in urine. Net price 50-strip pack = £2.33

**Mission**® **Glucose** (Spirit)

Reagent strips, for detection of glucose in urine. Net price 50-strip pack = £2.29

◀ **Ketones**

**Ketostix**® (Bayer Diabetes Care)

Reagent strips, for detection of ketones in urine. Net price 50-strip pack = £2.95

6　Endocrine system

## Meters and test strips

| Meter (all NHS) | Type of monitoring | Compatible test strips | Test strip net price | Sensitivity range (mmol/litre) | Manufacturer |
|---|---|---|---|---|---|
| Accu-Chek® Active[1] | Blood glucose | Active® | 50-strip pack = £15.70 | 0.6–33.3 | Roche Diagnostics |
| Accu-Chek® Advantage[1] | Blood glucose | Advantage Plus® | 50-strip pack = £15.71 | 0.6–33.3 | Roche Diagnostics |
| Accu-Chek® Aviva | Blood glucose | Aviva® | 50-strip pack = £15.41 | 0.6–33.3 | Roche Diagnostics |
| Accu-Chek® Aviva Expert | Blood glucose | Aviva® | 50-strip pack = £15.41 | 0.6–33.3 | Roche Diagnostics |
| Accu-Chek® Compact Plus[1] | Blood glucose | Compact® | 3 × 17-strip pack = £15.29 | 0.6–33.3 | Roche Diagnostics |
| Accu-Chek® Mobile | Blood glucose | Mobile® | 100 tests = £31.54 | 0.3–33.3 | Roche Diagnostics |
| Accu-Chek® Aviva Nano | Blood glucose | Aviva | 50-strip pack = £15.41 | 0.6–33.3 | Roche Diagnostics |
| Accutrend®[1] | Blood glucose | BM-Accutest® | 50-strip pack = £14.31 | 1.1–33.3 | Roche Diagnostics |
| Ascensia Breeze®[1] | Blood glucose | Ascensia® Autodisc | 5 × 10-disc pack = £14.73 | 0.6–33.3 | Bayer Diabetes Care |
| Ascensia Esprit® 2[1] | Blood glucose | Ascensia® Autodisc | 5 × 10-disc pack = £14.73 | 0.6–33.3 | Bayer Diabetes Care |
| BGStar®[2] | Blood glucose | BGStar® | 50-strip pack = £14.73 | 1.1–33.3 | Sanofi |
| Breeze 2® | Blood glucose | Breeze 2® | 5 × 10-disc pack = £14.70 | 0.6–33.3 | Bayer Diabetes Care |
| CareSens N®[2] | Blood glucose | CareSens N® | 50-strip pack = £12.75 | 1.1–33.3 | Spirit Healthcare |
| Clever Chek® | Blood glucose | Clever Chek® | 50-strip pack = £16.30 | 1.1–33.3 | BBI Healthcare |
| Contour® | Blood glucose | Contour® Formerly Ascensia® Microfill | 50-strip pack = £15.11 | 0.6–33.3 | Bayer Diabetes Care |
| Contour® XT | Blood glucose | Contour® Next | 50-strip pack = £14.85 | 0.6–33.3 | Bayer Diabetes Care |
| FreeStyle®[1] | Blood glucose | FreeStyle® | 50-strip pack = £15.43 | 1.1–27.8 | Abbott |
| FreeStyle Freedom®[1] | Blood glucose | FreeStyle® | 50-strip pack = £15.43 | 1.1–27.8 | Abbott |
| FreeStyle Freedom Lite® | Blood glucose | FreeStyle Lite® | 50-strip pack = £15.42 | 1.1–27.8 | Abbott |
| FreeStyle Lite® | Blood glucose | FreeStyle Lite® | 50-strip pack = £15.42 | 1.1–27.8 | Abbott |
| FreeStyle Mini®[1] | Blood glucose | FreeStyle® | 50-strip pack = £15.43 | 1.1–27.8 | Abbott |
| GlucoDock® module (for use with iPhone®, iPod touch®, or iPad®) | Blood glucose | GlucoDock® | 50-strip pack = £14.90 | 1.1–33.3 | Medisana |
| GlucoMen® Glycó[1] | Blood glucose | GlucoMen® | 50-strip pack = £13.67 | 1.1–33.3 | Menarini Diagnostics |
| GlucoMen® GM | Blood glucose | GlucoMen® GM | 50-strip pack = £15.22 | 0.6–33.3 | Menarini Diagnostics |
| GlucoMen® LX | Blood glucose | GlucoMen® LX Sensor | 50-strip pack = £15.20 | 1.1–33.3 | Menarini Diagnostics |
| GlucoMen® LX Plus | Blood glucose | GlucoMen® LX Sensor | 50-strip pack = £15.20 | 1.1–33.3 | Menarini Diagnostics |
| | Blood ketones | GlucoMen®LX Ketone | 10-strip pack = £20.32 | 0–0.8 | Menarini Diagnostics |
| GlucoMen® PC[1] | Blood glucose | GlucoMen® | 50-strip pack = £13.67 | 1.1–33.3 | Menarini Diagnostics |

1. Meter no longer available
2. Free of charge from diabetes healthcare professionals

Endocrine system

6

| Meter (all [NHS]) | Type of monitoring | Compatible test strips | Test strip net price | Sensitivity range (mmol/litre) | Manufacturer |
|---|---|---|---|---|---|
| GlucoMen® Visio | Blood glucose | GlucoMen® Visio Sensor | 50-strip pack = £15.33 | 1.1–33.3 | Menarini Diagnostics |
| GlucoRx®2 | Blood glucose | GlucoRx® | 50-strip pack = £9.45 | 1.1–33.3 | GlucoRx |
| GlucoRx Nexus®2 | Blood glucose | GlucoRx Nexus® | 50-strip pack = £9.95 | 1.1–33.3 | GlucoRx |
| Glucotrend®1 | Blood glucose | Active® | 50-strip pack = £14.76 | 0.6–33.3 | Roche Diagnostics |
| iBGStar® | Blood glucose | BGStar® | 50-strip pack = £14.73 | 1.1–33.3 | Sanofi |
| IME-DC® | Blood glucose | IME-DC® | 50-strip pack = £14.10 | 1.1–33.3 | Arctic Medical |
| Mendor Discreet® | Blood glucose | Mendor Discreet® | 50-strip pack = £14.73 | 1.1–33.3 | Merck Serono |
| Microdot®+2 | Blood glucose | Microdot®+ | 50-strip pack = £10.00 | 1.1–29.2 | Cambridge Sensors |
| MyGlucoHealth® | Blood glucose | MyGlucoHealth® | 50-strip pack = £15.50 | 0.6–33.3 | Entra Health |
| Omnitest®3 | Blood glucose | Omnitest®3 | 50-strip pack = £12.00 | 0.6–33.3 | B. Braun |
| One Touch® II1 | Blood glucose | One Touch® | 50-strip pack = £14.59 | 1.1–33.3 | LifeScan |
| One Touch® Basic1 | Blood glucose | One Touch® | 50-strip pack = £14.59 | 1.1–33.3 | LifeScan |
| One Touch® Profile1 | Blood glucose | One Touch® | 50-strip pack = £14.59 | 1.1–33.3 | LifeScan |
| One Touch Ultra®1 | Blood glucose | One Touch Ultra® | 50-strip pack = £15.27 | 1.1–33.3 | LifeScan |
| One Touch Ultra 2®2 | Blood glucose | One Touch Ultra® | 50-strip pack = £15.27 | 1.1–33.3 | LifeScan |
| One Touch UltraEasy®2 | Blood glucose | One Touch Ultra® | 50-strip pack = £15.27 | 1.1–33.3 | LifeScan |
| One Touch UltraSmart®2 | Blood glucose | One Touch Ultra® | 50-strip pack = £15.27 | 1.1–33.3 | LifeScan |
| One Touch® VerioPro2 | Blood glucose | One Touch® Verio | 50-strip pack = £14.99 | 1.1–33.3 | LifeScan |
| One Touch® Vita2 | Blood glucose | One Touch® Vita | 50-strip pack = £15.07 | 1.1–33.3 | LifeScan |
| Optium®1 | Blood ketones | Optium® β-ketone | 10-strip pack = £20.63 | 0–8.0 | Abbott |
| Optium Xceed® | Blood glucose | FreeStyle Optium® Formerly Optium Plus | 50-strip pack = £15.33 | 1.1–27.8 | Abbott |
| | Blood ketones | FreeStyle Optium® β-ketone | 10-strip pack = £20.63 | 0–8.0 | Abbott |
| SD CodeFree® | Blood glucose | SD CodeFree® | 50-strip pack = £6.99 | 0.6–33.3 | SD Biosensor |
| Sensocard Plus®1 | Blood glucose | Sensocard® | 50-strip pack = £16.30 | 1.1–33.3 | BBI Healthcare |
| SuperCheck2®2 | Blood glucose | SuperCheck2® | 50-strip pack = £8.49 | 1.1–33.3 | Apollo Medical |
| TRUEone® | Blood glucose | All-in-one test strips and meter | 50-strip pack with meter = £14.81 | 1.1–33.3 | Nipro Diagnostics |
| TRUEresult®2 | Blood glucose | TRUEresult® | 50-strip pack = £14.81 | 1.1–33.3 | Nipro Diagnostics |
| TRUEresult twist®2 | Blood glucose | TRUEresult® | 50-strip pack = £14.81 | 1.1–33.3 | Nipro Diagnostics |
| TRUEtrack® | Blood glucose | TRUEtrack® | 50-strip pack = £14.80 | 1.1–33.3 | Nipro Diagnostics |
| WaveSense JAZZ®2 | Blood glucose | WaveSense JAZZ® | 50-strip pack = £9.87 | 1.1–33.3 | AgaMatrix |

1. Meter no longer available
2. Free of charge from diabetes healthcare professionals

6

Endocrine system

**Mission® Ketone** (Spirit)
Reagent strips, for detection of ketones in urine. Net price 50-strip pack = £2.50

◀**Protein**

**Albustix®** (Siemens)
Reagent strips, for detection of protein in urine. Net price 50-strip pack = £4.10

**Medi-Test® Protein 2** (BHR)
Reagent strips, for detection of protein in urine. Net price 50-strip pack = £3.27

◀**Other reagent strips available for urinalysis include:**

*Combur-3 Test®* 🅝🅗🅢 (glucose and protein—Roche Diagnostics),

*Clinitek Microalbumin®* 🅝🅗🅢 (albumin and creatinine—Siemens),

*Ketodiastix®* 🅝🅗🅢 (glucose and ketones—Bayer Diagnostics),

*Medi-Test Combi 2®* 🅝🅗🅢 (glucose and protein—BHR),

*Micral-Test II®* 🅝🅗🅢 (albumin—Roche Diagnostics),

*Microalbustix®* 🅝🅗🅢 (albumin and creatinine—Siemens),

*Uristix®* 🅝🅗🅢 (glucose and protein—Siemens)

## Oral glucose tolerance test

The oral glucose tolerance test is used mainly for diagnosis of impaired glucose tolerance; it is not recommended or necessary for routine diagnostic use when severe symptoms of hyperglycaemia are present. However, it is used for the investigation of insulin resistance, glycogen storage disease, and excessive growth hormone secretion. In children who have less severe symptoms and blood-glucose concentrations that do not establish or exclude diabetes (e.g. impaired fasting glycaemia), an oral glucose tolerance test may be required. A dose of 1.75 g/kg (max. 75 g) of anhydrous glucose is used. It is also used to establish the presence of gestational diabetes; this generally involves giving anhydrous glucose 75 g (equivalent to Glucose BP 82.5 g) by mouth to the fasting patient, and measuring blood-glucose concentration at intervals. The appropriate amount of glucose should be given with 200–300 mL fluid. Alternatively anhydrous glucose 75 g can be given as 113 mL *Polycal®* with extra fluid to administer a total volume of 200–300 mL, or as *Rapilose®* OGTT oral solution.

## 6.2    Thyroid and antithyroid drugs

**6.2.1**    Thyroid hormones
**6.2.2**    Antithyroid drugs

## 6.2.1    Thyroid hormones

Thyroid hormones are used in hypothyroidism (juvenile myxoedema), and also in diffuse non-toxic goitre, congenital or neonatal hypothyroidism, and Hashimoto's thyroiditis (lymphadenoid goitre). Neonatal hypothyroidism requires prompt treatment to facilitate normal development.

**Levothyroxine sodium** (thyroxine sodium) is the treatment of choice for *maintenance* therapy.

Doses for congenital hypothyroidism and juvenile myxoedema should be titrated according to clinical response, growth assessment, and measurement of plasma thyroxine and thyroid-stimulating hormone concentrations. In congenital hypothyroidism higher initial doses may normalise metabolism more quickly, with associated beneficial effects on mental development.

**Liothyronine sodium** has a similar action to levothyroxine but is more rapidly metabolised and has a more rapid effect; 20–25 micrograms is equivalent to approximately 100 micrograms of levothyroxine. Its effects develop after a few hours and disappear within 24 to 48 hours of discontinuing treatment. It may be used in *severe hypothyroid states* when a rapid response is desired.

Liothyronine by intravenous injection is the treatment of choice in *hypothyroid coma*. Adjunctive therapy includes intravenous fluids, hydrocortisone, and treatment of infection; assisted ventilation is often required.

## ▌ LEVOTHYROXINE SODIUM
(Thyroxine sodium)

**Cautions** panhypopituitarism or predisposition to adrenal insufficiency (initiate corticosteroid therapy before starting levothyroxine); cardiac disorders (monitor ECG; start at low dose and carefully titrate); long-standing hypothyroidism, diabetes insipidus, diabetes mellitus (dose of antidiabetic drugs including insulin may need to be increased); **interactions:** Appendix 1 (thyroid hormones)

**Pregnancy** monitor maternal serum-thyrotrophin concentration—levothyroxine may cross the placenta and excessive maternal concentration may be detrimental to fetus

**Breast-feeding** amount too small to affect tests for neonatal hypothyroidism

**Side-effects** usually at excessive dosage include diarrhoea, vomiting, anginal pain, arrhythmias, palpitation, tachycardia, benign intracranial hypertension; tremor, restlessness, excitability, insomnia, headache, flushing, sweating, fever, heat intolerance, weight loss, nervousness; craniosynostosis and premature closure of epiphyses; menstrual irregularities; eosinophilia, liver dysfunction; muscle cramps, muscular weakness; transient hair loss; hypersensitivity reactions including rash, pruritus and oedema also reported

**Indications and dose**

> Levothyroxine equivalent to 100 micrograms/m²/day can be used as a guide to the requirements in children

**Hypothyroidism**
• **By mouth**
**Neonate** initially 10–15 micrograms/kg once daily (max. 50 micrograms daily), adjusted in steps of 5 micrograms/kg every 2 weeks or as necessary; usual maintenance dose 20–50 micrograms daily

**Child 1 month–2 years** initially 5 micrograms/kg once daily (max. 50 micrograms daily) adjusted in steps of 10–25 micrograms daily every 2–4 weeks until metabolism normalised; usual maintenance dose 25–75 micrograms daily

**Child 2–12 years** initially 50 micrograms once daily adjusted in steps of 25 micrograms daily every 2–4 weeks until metabolism normalised; usual maintenance dose 75–100 micrograms daily

**Child 12–18 years** initially 50 micrograms once daily adjusted in steps of 25–50 micrograms daily every 3–4 weeks until metabolism normalised; usual maintenance dose 100–200 micrograms daily

**Levothyroxine** (Non-proprietary) [PoM]
Tablets, levothyroxine sodium 25 micrograms, net price 28-tab pack = £2.22; 50 micrograms, 28-tab pack = £1.09; 100 micrograms, 28-tab pack = £1.09
Brands include *Eltroxin*®

Oral solution, levothyroxine sodium 25 micrograms/ 5 mL, net price 100 mL = £42.75; 50 micrograms/ 5 mL, 100 mL = £44.90; 100 micrograms/5 mL, 100 mL = £52.75
Brands include *Evotrox*® (sugar-free)
**Note** All strengths of levothyroxine oral solution by Almus and branded as *Evotrox*®, have been reformulated (August 2010) leading to an increase in potency of approximately 10%; the manufacturer advises that the recommended dose has not changed, but recommends increased monitoring of patients on these preparations as dose adjustments may be necessary

---

### ■ LIOTHYRONINE SODIUM
(L-Tri-iodothyronine sodium)

**Cautions** severe and prolonged hypothyroidism (initiate corticosteroid therapy in adrenal insufficiency); cardiac disorders (monitor ECG; start at low dose and carefully titrate); diabetes insipidus, diabetes mellitus (dose of antidiabetic drugs including insulin may need to be increased); **interactions:** Appendix 1 (thyroid hormones)

**Pregnancy** does not cross the placenta in significant amounts; monitor maternal thyroid function tests—dosage adjustment may be necessary

**Breast-feeding** amount too small to affect tests for neonatal hypothyroidism

**Side-effects** usually at excessive dosage include diarrhoea; anginal pain, arrhythmias, palpitation, tachycardia; restlessness, excitability, headache, flushing, sweating, weight loss; muscle cramps, muscle weakness

**Indications and dose**
See also notes above

**Hypothyroidism**
● **By mouth**
  **Child 12–18 years** initially 10–20 micrograms daily gradually increased to 60 micrograms daily in 2–3 divided doses
● **By slow intravenous injection**
  (replacement for oral levothyroxine)
  Convert **daily** levothyroxine dose to liothyronine (see notes above for approximate equivalence) and give in 2–3 divided doses, adjusted according to response

**Hypothyroid coma**
● **By slow intravenous injection**
  **Child 12–18 years** 5–20 micrograms repeated every 12 hours or up to every 4 hours if necessary; *alternatively* initially 50 micrograms then 25 micrograms every 8 hours reducing to 25 micrograms twice daily

**Liothyronine sodium** (Mercury) [PoM]
Tablets, scored, liothyronine sodium 20 micrograms, net price 28-tab pack = £26.15

**Triiodothyronine** (Goldshield) [PoM]
Injection, powder for reconstitution, liothyronine sodium (with dextran). Net price 20-microgram amp = £37.92

---

### 6.2.2 Antithyroid drugs

Antithyroid drugs are used for hyperthyroidism either to prepare children for thyroidectomy or for long-term management. In the UK **carbimazole** is the most commonly used drug. **Propylthiouracil** should be reserved for children who are intolerant of, or who experience sensitivity reactions to, carbimazole (sensitivity is not necessarily displayed to both drugs), and for whom other treatments are inappropriate. Both drugs act primarily by interfering with the synthesis of thyroid hormones.

Treatment in children should be undertaken by a specialist.

> **Neutropenia and agranulocytosis**
> Doctors are reminded of the importance of recognising bone marrow suppression induced by carbimazole and the need to stop treatment promptly.
> 1.  Children and their carers should be asked to report symptoms and signs suggestive of infection, especially sore throat.
> 2.  A white blood cell count should be performed if there is any clinical evidence of infection.
> 3.  Carbimazole should be stopped promptly if there is clinical or laboratory evidence of neutropenia.

**Carbimazole** or **propylthiouracil** are initially given in large doses to block thyroid function. This dose is continued until the child becomes euthyroid, usually after 4 to 8 weeks, and is then gradually reduced to a maintenance dose of 30–60% of the initial dose. Alternatively high-dose treatment is continued in combination with levothyroxine replacement (*blocking-replacement regimen*); this is particularly useful when dose adjustment proves difficult. Treatment is usually continued for 12 to 24 months. The blocking-replacement regimen is **not** suitable during pregnancy. Hypothyroidism should be avoided particularly during pregnancy as it can cause fetal goitre.

When substituting, carbimazole 1 mg is considered equivalent to propylthiouracil 10 mg but the dose may need adjusting according to response.

Rashes and pruritus are common with carbimazole but they can be treated with antihistamines without discontinuing therapy; alternatively propylthiouracil can be substituted. If a child on carbimazole develops a sore throat it should be reported immediately because of the

**6**

**Endocrine system**

rare complication of agranulocytosis (see Neutropenia and Agranulocytosis, above).

**Iodine** has been used as an adjunct to antithyroid drugs for 10 to 14 days before partial thyroidectomy; however, there is little evidence of a beneficial effect. Iodine should not be used for long-term treatment because its antithyroid action tends to diminish.

**Radioactive sodium iodide** ($^{131}$I) solution is used increasingly for the treatment of thyrotoxicosis at all ages, particularly where medical therapy or compliance is a problem, in patients with cardiac disease, and in patients who relapse after thyroidectomy.

**Propranolol** (section 2.4) is useful for rapid relief of thyrotoxic symptoms and can be used in conjunction with antithyroid drugs or as an adjunct to radioactive iodine. Beta-blockers are also useful in neonatal thyrotoxicosis and in supraventricular arrhythmias due to hyperthyroidism. Propranolol has been used in conjunction with iodine to prepare mildly thyrotoxic patients for surgery but it is preferable to make the patient euthyroid with carbimazole. Laboratory tests of thyroid function are not altered by beta-blockers. Most experience in treating thyrotoxicosis has been gained with propranolol but **atenolol** (section 2.4) is also used.

*Thyrotoxic crisis* ('thyroid storm') requires emergency treatment with intravenous administration of fluids, propranolol and hydrocortisone as sodium succinate, as well as oral iodine solution and carbimazole or propylthiouracil which may need to be administered by nasogastric tube.

**Neonatal hyperthyroidism** is treated with carbimazole or propylthiouracil, usually for 8 to 12 weeks. In severe symptomatic disease iodine may be needed to block the thyroid and propranolol required to treat peripheral symptoms.

**Pregnancy** Radioactive iodine therapy is contraindicated during pregnancy. Propylthiouracil and carbimazole can be given but the blocking-replacement regimen (see above) is **not** suitable. Rarely, carbimazole has been associated with congenital defects, including aplasia cutis of the neonate, therefore propylthiouracil remains the drug of choice during the first trimester of pregnancy. In the second trimester, consider switching to carbimazole because of the potential risk of hepatotoxicity with propylthiouracil. Both propylthiouracil and carbimazole cross the placenta and in high doses can cause fetal goitre and hypothyroidism—the lowest dose that will control the hyperthyroid state should be used (requirements in Graves' disease tend to fall during pregnancy).

**Breast-feeding** Carbimazole and propylthiouracil are present in breast milk but this does not preclude breast-feeding as long as neonatal development is closely monitored and the lowest effective dose is used.

## CARBIMAZOLE

**Hepatic impairment** use with caution in mild to moderate impairment; avoid in severe hepatic impairment

**Pregnancy** see notes above

**Breast-feeding** amount in milk may be sufficient to affect neonatal thyroid function, therefore lowest effective dose should be used; see notes above

**Side-effects** nausea, mild gastro-intestinal disturbances, taste disturbance, hepatic disorders (including hepatitis and jaundice), headache, fever, malaise, rash, pruritus, arthralgia; *rarely* myopathy, alopecia, bone marrow suppression (including pancytopenia and agranulocytosis, see Neutropenia and Agranulocytosis above), hypersensitivity reactions

**Indications and dose**

**Hyperthyroidism (including Graves' disease)**

● **By mouth**

**Neonate** initially 750 micrograms/kg daily in single or divided doses until euthyroid then adjust as necessary (see notes above); higher initial doses (up to 1 mg/kg daily) are occasionally required, particularly in thyrotoxic crisis

**Child 1 month–12 years** initially 750 micrograms/kg (max. 30 mg) daily in single or divided doses until euthyroid then adjusted as necessary (see notes above); higher initial doses occasionally required, particularly in thyrotoxic crisis

**Child 12–18 years** initially 30 mg daily in single or divided doses until euthyroid then adjusted as necessary (see notes above); higher initial doses occasionally required, particularly in thyrotoxic crisis

**Counselling** Warn child and carers to tell doctor **immediately** if sore throat, mouth ulcers, bruising, fever, malaise, or non-specific illness develops

**Carbimazole** (Non-proprietary) [PoM]
Tablets, carbimazole 5 mg, net price 100-tab pack = £4.53; 20 mg, 100-tab pack = £16.83. Counselling, blood disorder symptoms

**Neo-Mercazole®** (Amdipharm) [PoM]
Tablets, both pink, carbimazole 5 mg, net price 100-tab pack = £3.85; 20 mg, 100-tab pack = £11.44. Counselling, blood disorder symptoms
**Administration** tablets may be crushed in water and used immediately

## IODINE AND IODIDE

**Cautions** not for long-term treatment

**Pregnancy** neonatal goitre and hypothyroidism; see also notes above

**Breast-feeding** stop breast-feeding; danger of neonatal hypothyroidism or goitre; appears to be concentrated in milk; see also notes above

**Side-effects** hypersensitivity reactions including coryza-like symptoms, headache, lacrimation, conjunctivitis, pain in salivary glands, laryngitis, bronchitis, rashes; on prolonged treatment depression, insomnia, impotence; goitre in infants of mothers taking iodides

**Indications and dose**

See under preparation

**Aqueous Iodine Oral Solution**
Oral solution, iodine 5%, potassium iodide 10% in purified water, freshly boiled and cooled, total iodine 130 mg/mL, net price 500 mL = £6.24. Label: 27

**Dose**

**Neonatal thyrotoxicosis**

● **By mouth**

**Neonate** 0.05–0.1 mL 3 times daily

**Thyrotoxicosis (pre-operative)**

● By mouth

**Neonate** 0.1–0.3 mL 3 times daily

**Child 1 month–18 years** 0.1–0.3 mL 3 times daily

**Thyrotoxic crisis**

● By mouth

**Child 1 month–1 year** 0.2–0.3 mL 3 times daily

**Administration** Dilute well with milk or water

## ▎PROPYLTHIOURACIL

**Cautions** monitor for hepatotoxicity

**Hepatotoxicity** Severe hepatic reactions have been reported, including fatal cases and cases requiring liver transplant—discontinue if significant liver-enzyme abnormalities develop

**Counselling** Patients should be told how to recognise signs of liver disorder and advised to seek prompt medical attention if symptoms such as anorexia, nausea, vomiting, fatigue, abdominal pain, jaundice, dark urine, or pruritus develop

**Hepatic impairment** reduce dose (see also Hepatotoxicity above)

**Renal impairment** estimated glomerular filtration rate 10–50 mL/minute/1.73 m$^2$, use 75% of normal dose; estimated glomerular filtration rate less than 10 mL/minute/1.73 m$^2$, use 50% of normal dose

**Pregnancy** see notes above

**Breast-feeding** monitor infant's thyroid status but amount in milk probably too small to affect infant; high doses may affect neonatal thyroid function; see also notes above

**Side-effects** see under Carbimazole; leucopenia; *rarely* cutaneous vasculitis, thrombocytopenia, aplastic anaemia, hypoprothrombinaemia, hepatic disorders (including hepatitis, hepatic failure, encephalopathy, hepatic necrosis; see also Hepatotoxicity above), nephritis, lupus erythematous-like syndromes

**Licensed use** not licensed for use in children under 6 years of age

**Indications and dose**

**Hyperthyroidism (including Graves' disease)**

● By mouth

**Neonate** initially 2.5–5 mg/kg twice daily until euthyroid then adjusted as necessary (see notes above); higher doses occasionally required, particularly in thyrotoxic crisis

**Child 1 month–1 year** initially 2.5 mg/kg 3 times daily until euthyroid then adjusted as necessary (see notes above); higher doses occasionally required, particularly in thyrotoxic crisis

**Child 1–5 years** initially 25 mg 3 times daily until euthyroid then adjusted as necessary (see notes above); higher doses occasionally required, particularly in thyrotoxic crisis

**Child 5–12 years** initially 50 mg 3 times daily until euthyroid then adjusted as necessary (see notes above); higher doses occasionally required, particularly in thyrotoxic crisis

**Child 12–18 years** initially 100 mg 3 times daily administered until euthyroid then adjusted as necessary (see notes above); higher doses occasionally required, particularly in thyrotoxic crisis

**Propylthiouracil** (Non-proprietary) PoM

Tablets, propylthiouracil 50 mg, net price 56-tab pack = £47.11, 100-tab pack = £67.38

## ▎PROPRANOLOL HYDROCHLORIDE

**Cautions** see section 2.4

**Contra-indications** see section 2.4

**Hepatic impairment** section 2.4

**Renal impairment** section 2.4

**Pregnancy** section 2.4

**Breast-feeding** section 2.4

**Side-effects** see section 2.4

**Indications and dose**

**Hyperthyroidism with autonomic symptoms, thyrotoxicosis, thyrotoxic crisis**

● By mouth

**Neonate** initially 250–500 micrograms/kg every 6–8 hours, adjusted according to response

**Child 1 month–18 years** initially 250–500 micrograms/kg every 8 hours, then adjusted according to response; doses up to 1 mg/kg every 8 hours occasionally required, max. 40 mg every 8 hours

● By intravenous injection over 10 minutes

**Neonate** initially 20–50 micrograms/kg every 6–8 hours, adjusted according to response

**Child 1 month–18 years** initially 25–50 micrograms/kg (max. 5 mg) every 6–8 hours, adjusted according to response

◀**Preparations**

See section 2.4

## 6.3 Corticosteroids

6.3.1 Replacement therapy
6.3.2 Glucocorticoid therapy

## 6.3.1 Replacement therapy

The adrenal cortex normally secretes hydrocortisone (cortisol) which has glucocorticoid activity and weak mineralocorticoid activity. It also secretes the mineralocorticoid aldosterone.

In deficiency states, physiological replacement is best achieved with a combination of **hydrocortisone** (section 6.3.2) and the mineralocorticoid **fludrocortisone**; hydrocortisone alone does not usually provide sufficient mineralocorticoid activity for complete replacement.

In *Addison's disease* or following adrenalectomy, **hydrocortisone** by mouth is usually required. This is given in 2–3 divided doses, the larger in the morning and the smaller in the evening, mimicking the normal diurnal rhythm of cortisol secretion. The optimum daily dose is determined on the basis of clinical response. Glucocorticoid therapy is supplemented by fludrocortisone.

In *acute adrenocortical insufficiency*, **hydrocortisone** is given intravenously (preferably as sodium succinate) every 6 to 8 hours in sodium chloride intravenous infusion 0.9%.

In *hypopituitarism*, glucocorticoids should be given as in adrenocortical insufficiency, but since production of aldosterone is also regulated by the renin-angiotensin system a mineralocorticoid is not usually required. Additional replacement therapy with levothyroxine

*6 Endocrine system*

(section 6.2.1) and sex hormones (section 6.4) should be given as indicated by the pattern of hormone deficiency.

In *congenital adrenal hyperplasia*, the pituitary gland increases production of corticotropin to compensate for reduced formation of cortisol; this results in excessive adrenal androgen production. Treatment is aimed at suppressing corticotropin using hydrocortisone (section 6.3.2). Careful and continual dose titration is required to avoid growth retardation and toxicity; for this reason potent, synthetic glucocorticoids such as dexamethasone are usually reserved for use in adolescents. The dose is adjusted according to clinical response and measurement of adrenal androgens and 17-hydroxyprogesterone. Salt-losing forms of congenital adrenal hyperplasia (where there is a lack of aldosterone production) also require mineralocorticoid replacement and salt supplementation (particularly in early life). The dose of mineralocorticoid is adjusted according to electrolyte concentration and plasma-renin activity.

## ▌ FLUDROCORTISONE ACETATE

**Cautions** section 6.3.2; **interactions:** Appendix 1 (corticosteroids)

**Contra-indications** section 6.3.2

**Hepatic impairment** see section 6.3.2

**Renal impairment** see section 6.3.2

**Pregnancy** see section 6.3.2

**Breast-feeding** see section 6.3.2

**Side-effects** section 6.3.2

**Indications and dose**

> Mineralocorticoid replacement in adrenocortical insufficiency
>
> • By mouth
>
> **Neonate** initially 50 micrograms once daily, adjusted according to response; usual range 50–200 micrograms daily; higher doses may be required
>
> **Child 1 month–18 years** initially 50–100 micrograms once daily; maintenance 50–300 micrograms once daily, adjusted according to response

**Note** Dose adjustment may be required if salt supplements are administered

**Florinef®** (Squibb) [PoM]
Tablets, scored, fludrocortisone acetate 100 micrograms. Net price 100-tab pack = £5.05. Label: 10, steroid card

## 6.3.2 Glucocorticoid therapy

In comparing the relative potencies of corticosteroids in terms of their anti-inflammatory (glucocorticoid) effects it should be borne in mind that high glucocorticoid activity in itself is of no advantage unless it is accompanied by relatively low mineralocorticoid activity (see Disadvantages of Corticosteroids below). The mineralocorticoid activity of **fludrocortisone** (section 6.3.1) is so high that its anti-inflammatory activity is of no clinical relevance. The table below shows equivalent anti-inflammatory doses.

### Equivalent anti-inflammatory doses of corticosteroids

This table takes no account of mineralocorticoid effects, nor does it take account of variations in duration of action

| Prednisolone 1 mg | ≡ | Betamethasone 150 micrograms |
|---|---|---|
| | ≡ | Deflazacort 1.2 mg |
| | ≡ | Dexamethasone 150 micrograms |
| | ≡ | Hydrocortisone 4 mg |
| | ≡ | Methylprednisolone 800 micrograms |
| | ≡ | Triamcinolone 800 micrograms |

The relatively high mineralocorticoid activity of **hydrocortisone**, and the resulting fluid retention, makes it unsuitable for disease suppression on a long-term basis. However, hydrocortisone can be used for adrenal replacement therapy (section 6.3.1). Hydrocortisone is used on a short-term basis by intravenous injection for the emergency management of some conditions. The relatively moderate anti-inflammatory potency of hydrocortisone also makes it a useful topical corticosteroid for the management of inflammatory skin conditions because side-effects (both topical and systemic) are less marked (section 13.4).

**Prednisolone** has predominantly glucocorticoid activity and is the corticosteroid most commonly used by mouth for long-term disease suppression.

**Betamethasone** and **dexamethasone** have very high glucocorticoid activity in conjunction with insignificant mineralocorticoid activity. This makes them particularly suitable for high-dose therapy in conditions where fluid retention would be a disadvantage.

Betamethasone and dexamethasone also have a long duration of action and this, coupled with their lack of mineralocorticoid action makes them particularly suitable for conditions which require suppression of corticotropin (corticotrophin) secretion. Some esters of betamethasone and of **beclometasone** (beclomethasone) exert a considerably more marked topical effect (e.g. on the skin or the lungs) than when given by mouth; use is made of this to obtain topical effects whilst minimising systemic side-effects (e.g. for skin applications and asthma inhalations).

**Deflazacort** has a high glucocorticoid activity; it is derived from prednisolone.

## Use of corticosteroids

Dosages of corticosteroids vary widely in different diseases and in different children. If the use of a corticosteroid can save or prolong life, as in exfoliative dermatitis, pemphigus, acute leukaemia or acute transplant rejection, high doses may need to be given, because the complications of therapy are likely to be less serious than the effects of the disease itself.

When long-term corticosteroid therapy is used in some chronic diseases, the adverse effects of treatment may become greater than the disabilities caused by the disease. To minimise side-effects the maintenance dose should be kept as low as possible.

When potentially less harmful measures are ineffective corticosteroids are used topically for the treatment of inflammatory conditions of the skin (section 13.4). Corticosteroids should be avoided or used only under specialist supervision in psoriasis (section 13.5).

Corticosteroids are used both topically (by rectum) and systemically (by mouth or intravenously) in the management of ulcerative colitis and Crohn's disease (section 1.5 and section 1.7.2).

Use can be made of the mineralocorticoid activity of fludrocortisone to treat postural hypotension in autonomic neuropathy.

High-dose corticosteroids should be avoided for the management of septic shock. However, low-dose hydrocortisone can be used in septic shock (section 2.7.1) that is resistant to volume expansion and catecholamines, and is accompanied by suspected or proven adrenal insufficiency.

The suppressive action of glucocorticoids on the hypothalamic-pituitary-adrenal axis is greatest and most prolonged when they are given at night. In most adults a single dose of 1 mg of dexamethasone at night is sufficient to inhibit corticotropin secretion for 24 hours. This is the basis of the 'overnight dexamethasone suppression test' for diagnosing Cushing's syndrome.

Betamethasone and dexamethasone are also appropriate for conditions where water retention would be a disadvantage.

A corticosteroid can be used in the management of raised intracranial pressure or cerebral oedema that occurs as a result of malignancy (see also p. 18); high doses of betamethasone or dexamethasone are generally used. However, a corticosteroid should **not** be used for the management of head injury or stroke because it is unlikely to be of benefit and may even be harmful.

In acute hypersensitivity reactions, such as angioedema of the upper respiratory tract and anaphylaxis, corticosteroids are indicated as an adjunct to emergency treatment with adrenaline (epinephrine) (section 3.4.3). In such cases hydrocortisone (as sodium succinate) by intravenous injection may be required.

In the management of asthma, corticosteroids are preferably used by inhalation (section 3.2) but systemic therapy along with bronchodilators is required for the emergency treatment of severe acute asthma (section 3.1.1).

Betamethasone is used in women at risk of preterm delivery to reduce the incidence of neonatal respiratory distress syndrome [unlicensed use].

Dexamethasone should not be used routinely for the prophylaxis and treatment of chronic lung disease in neonates because of an association with adverse neurological effects.

Corticosteroids may be useful in conditions such as auto-immune hepatitis, rheumatoid arthritis, and sarcoidosis; they may also lead to remissions of acquired haemolytic anaemia (section 9.1.3) and thrombocytopenic purpura (section 9.1.4).

High doses of a corticosteroid (usually prednisolone) are used in the treatment of *glomerular kidney disease*, including *nephrotic syndrome*. The condition frequently recurs; a corticosteroid given in high doses and for prolonged periods may delay relapse but the higher incidence of adverse effects limits the overall benefit. Those who suffer frequent relapses may be treated with prednisolone given in a low dose (daily or on alternate days) for 3–6 months; the dose should be adjusted to minimise effects on growth and development. Other drugs used in the treatment of glomerular kidney disease include levamisole (section 5.5.2), cyclophosphamide and chlorambucil (section 8.1.1), and ciclosporin (section 8.2.2). *Congenital nephrotic syndrome* may be resistant to corticosteroids and immunosuppressants; indometacin (section 10.1.1) and an ACE inhibitor such as captopril (section 2.5.5.1) have been used.

Corticosteroids can improve the prognosis of serious conditions such as systemic lupus erythematosus and polyarteritis nodosa; the effects of the disease process may be suppressed and symptoms relieved, but the underlying condition is not cured, although it may ultimately remit. It is usual to begin therapy in these conditions at fairly high dose and then to reduce the dose to the lowest commensurate with disease control.

For other references to the use of corticosteroids see Prescribing in Palliative Care (p. 17), section 8.2.2 (immunosuppression), section 10.1.2 (rheumatic diseases), section 11.4 (eye), section 12.1.1 (otitis externa), section 12.2.1 (allergic rhinitis), and section 12.3.1 (aphthous ulcers).

## Administration

Whenever possible *local treatment* with creams, intra-articular injections, inhalations, eye-drops, or enemas should be used in preference to *systemic treatment*. The suppressive action of a corticosteroid on cortisol secretion is least when it is given as a single dose in the morning. In an attempt to reduce pituitary-adrenal suppression further, the total dose for two days can sometimes be taken as a single dose on alternate days; alternate-day administration has not been very successful in the management of asthma (section 3.2). Pituitary-adrenal suppression can also be reduced by means of intermittent therapy with short courses. In some conditions it may be possible to reduce the dose of corticosteroid by adding a small dose of an immunosuppressive drug (section 8.2.1).

## Cautions and contra-indications of corticosteroids

### Adrenal suppression

During prolonged therapy with corticosteroids, adrenal atrophy develops and can persist for years after stopping. Abrupt withdrawal after a prolonged period can lead to acute adrenal insufficiency, hypotension, or death (see Withdrawal of Corticosteroids, below). Withdrawal can also be associated with fever, myalgia, arthralgia, rhinitis, conjunctivitis, painful itchy skin nodules, and weight loss.

To compensate for a diminished adrenocortical response caused by prolonged corticosteroid treatment, any significant intercurrent illness, trauma, or surgical procedure requires a temporary increase in corticosteroid dose, or if already stopped, a temporary re-introduction of corticosteroid treatment. To avoid a precipitous fall in blood pressure during anaesthesia or in the immediate postoperative period, anaesthetists **must** know whether a patient is taking or has been taking a corticosteroid. A regimen for corticosteroid replacement may be necessary before and after surgery.

Children on long-term corticosteroid treatment should carry a Steroid Treatment Card (see p. 372) which gives guidance on minimising risk and provides details of prescriber, drug, dosage and duration of treatment.

---

## STEROID TREATMENT CARD

### I am a patient on STEROID treatment which must not be stopped suddenly

- If you have been taking this medicine for more than three weeks, the dose should be reduced gradually when you stop taking steroids unless your doctor says otherwise.

- Read the patient information leaflet given with the medicine.

- Always carry this card with you and show it to anyone who treats you (for example a doctor, nurse, pharmacist or dentist). For one year after you stop the treatment, you must mention that you have taken steroids.

- If you become ill, or if you come into contact with anyone who has an infectious disease, consult your doctor promptly. If you have never had chickenpox, you should avoid close contact with people who have chickenpox or shingles. If you do come into contact with chickenpox, see your doctor urgently.

- Make sure that the information on the card is kept up to date.

---

## Infections

Prolonged courses of corticosteroids increase susceptibility to infections and severity of infections; clinical presentation of infections may also be atypical. Serious infections, e.g. *septicaemia* and *tuberculosis*, may reach an advanced stage before being recognised, and *amoebiasis* or *strongyloidiasis* may be activated or exacerbated (exclude before initiating a corticosteroid in those at risk or with suggestive symptoms). Fungal or viral *ocular infections* may also be exacerbated (see also section 11.4.1).

**Chickenpox**   Unless they have had chickenpox, children receiving oral or parenteral corticosteroids for purposes other than replacement should be regarded as being *at risk of severe chickenpox* (see Steroid Treatment Card). Manifestations of fulminant illness include pneumonia, hepatitis and disseminated intravascular coagulation; rash is not necessarily a prominent feature.

Passive immunisation with varicella–zoster immunoglobulin (section 14.5.2) is needed for exposed non-immune children receiving systemic corticosteroids or for those who have used them within the previous 3

months. Confirmed chickenpox warrants specialist care and urgent treatment (section 5.3.2.1). Corticosteroids should not be stopped and dosage may need to be increased.

Topical, inhaled or rectal corticosteroids are less likely to be associated with an increased risk of severe chickenpox.

**Measles**   Children taking corticosteroids, and their carers, should be advised to take particular care to avoid exposure to measles and to seek urgent medical advice if exposure occurs. Prophylaxis with intramuscular normal immunoglobulin (section 14.5.1) may be needed.

## Withdrawal of corticosteroids

The magnitude and speed of dose reduction in corticosteroid withdrawal should be determined on a case-by-case basis, taking into consideration the underlying condition that is being treated, and individual patient factors such as the likelihood of relapse and the duration of corticosteroid treatment. *Gradual* withdrawal of systemic corticosteroids should be considered in those whose disease is unlikely to relapse and have:

- received more than 40 mg prednisolone (or equivalent) daily for more than 1 week *or* 2 mg/kg daily for 1 week *or* 1 mg/kg daily for 1 month;

- been given repeat doses in the evening;

- received more than 3 weeks' treatment;

- recently received repeated courses (particularly if taken for longer than 3 weeks);

- taken a short course within 1 year of stopping long-term therapy;

- other possible causes of adrenal suppression.

Systemic corticosteroids may be stopped abruptly in those whose disease is unlikely to relapse *and* who have received treatment for 3 weeks or less *and* who are not included in the patient groups described above.

During corticosteroid withdrawal the dose may be reduced rapidly down to physiological doses (equivalent to prednisolone $2–2.5 \text{ mg/m}^2$ daily) and then reduced more slowly. Assessment of the disease may be needed during withdrawal to ensure that relapse does not occur.

## Psychiatric reactions

Systemic corticosteroids, particularly in high doses, are linked to psychiatric reactions including euphoria, nightmares, insomnia, irritability, mood lability, suicidal thoughts, psychotic reactions, and behavioural disturbances. A serious paranoid state or depression with risk of suicide can be induced, particularly in children with a history of mental disorder. These reactions frequently subside on reducing the dose or discontinuing the corticosteroid but they may also require specific management. Children and their carers should be advised to seek medical advice if psychiatric symptoms (especially depression and suicidal thoughts) occur and they should also be alert to the rare possibility of such reactions during withdrawal of corticosteroid treatment.

Systemic corticosteroids should be prescribed with care in those predisposed to psychiatric reactions, including those who have previously suffered corticosteroid-induced psychosis, or who have a personal or family history of psychiatric disorders.

## Advice to children and carers

A patient information leaflet should be supplied to every patient when a systemic corticosteroid is prescribed. Children and carers should especially be advised of the following (for details, see Infections, Adrenal Suppression, and Psychiatric Reactions above and Withdrawal of Corticosteroids below):

- **Immunosuppression** Prolonged courses of corticosteroids can increase susceptibility to infection and serious infections can go unrecognised. Unless already immune, children are at risk of severe **chickenpox** and should avoid close contact with people who have chickenpox or shingles. Similarly, precautions should also be taken against contracting **measles**.

- **Adrenal suppression** If the corticosteroid is given for longer than 3 weeks, treatment must not be stopped abruptly. Adrenal suppression can last for a year or more after stopping treatment and the child or carer must mention the course of corticosteroid when receiving treatment for any illness or injury;

- **Mood and behaviour changes** Corticosteroid treatment, especially with high doses, can alter mood and behaviour early in treatment—the child can become confused, irritable and suffer from delusion and suicidal thoughts. These effects can also occur when corticosteroid treatment is being withdrawn. Medical advice should be sought if worrying psychological changes occur;

- **Other serious effects** Serious gastro-intestinal, musculoskeletal, and ophthalmic effects which require medical help can also occur; for details see Side-effects of Corticosteroids, p. 373.

## Steroid treatment cards

Steroid treatment cards (see p. 372) should be issued where appropriate, and are available for purchase from:

3M Security Print and Systems Limited
Gorse Street, Chadderton
Oldham, OL9 9QH
Tel: 0845 610 1112GP practices can obtain supplies through their Primary Care Trust (PCT) or Agency stores. NHS Hospitals can order supplies from www.nhsforms.co.uk or by emailing nhsforms@mmm.com

## Other cautions and contra-indications

*Other cautions include*: growth restriction—possibly irreversible, frequent monitoring required if history of tuberculosis (or X-ray changes), hypertension, congestive heart failure, diabetes mellitus including family history, osteoporosis, susceptibility to angle-closure glaucoma (including family history), ocular herpes simplex—risk of corneal perforation, severe affective disorders (particularly if history of steroid-induced psychosis—see also Psychiatric Reactions above), epilepsy, peptic ulcer, hypothyroidism, history of steroid myopathy, ulcerative colitis, diverticulitis, recent intestinal anastomoses, thromboembolic disorders, myasthenia gravis; **interactions**: Appendix 1 (corticosteroids)

*Other contra-indications include*: systemic infection (unless specific therapy given); avoid live virus vaccines in those receiving immunosuppressive doses (serum antibody response diminished)

## Hepatic impairment

When corticosteroids are administered orally or parenterally, the plasma-drug concentration may be increased in children with hepatic impairment. Corticosteroids should be used with caution in hepatic impairment and the child should be monitored closely.

## Renal impairment

Oral and parenteral preparations of corticosteroids should be used with caution in children with renal impairment.

## Pregnancy and breast-feeding

The benefit of treatment with corticosteroids during pregnancy and breast-feeding outweighs the risk; pregnant women with fluid retention should be monitored closely. Corticosteroid cover will be required during labour.

Following a review of the data on the safety of systemic corticosteroids used in pregnancy and breast-feeding the CSM (May 1998) concluded:

- corticosteroids vary in their ability to cross the placenta; betamethasone and dexamethasone cross the placenta readily while 88% of prednisolone is inactivated as it crosses the placenta;

- there is no convincing evidence that systemic corticosteroids increase the incidence of congenital abnormalities such as cleft palate or lip;

- when administration is prolonged or repeated during pregnancy, systemic corticosteroids increase the risk of intra-uterine growth restriction; there is no evidence of intra-uterine growth restriction following short-term treatment (e.g. prophylactic treatment for neonatal respiratory distress syndrome);

- any adrenal suppression in the neonate following prenatal exposure usually resolves spontaneously after birth and is rarely clinically important;

- prednisolone appears in small amounts in breast milk but maternal doses of up to 40 mg daily are unlikely to cause systemic effects in the infant; infants should be monitored for adrenal suppression if the mothers are taking a higher dose.

## Side-effects of corticosteroids

Overdosage or prolonged use can exaggerate some of the normal physiological actions of corticosteroids leading to mineralocorticoid and glucocorticoid side-effects.

Corticosteroids suppress growth and can affect the development of puberty. It is important to use the lowest effective dose; alternate-day regimens may be appropriate and limit growth reduction. For the effect of corticosteroids given in pregnancy, see Pregnancy and Breast-feeding, above.

**Mineralocorticoid** side-effects include hypertension, sodium and water retention, and potassium and calcium loss. They are most marked with fludrocortisone, but are significant with hydrocortisone, corticotropin, and tetracosactide. Mineralocorticoid actions are negligible with the high potency glucocorticoids, betamethasone and dexamethasone, and occur only slightly with methylprednisolone, prednisolone, and triamcinolone.

**Glucocorticoid** side-effects include diabetes and osteoporosis (section 6.6); in addition high doses are asso-

6

Endocrine system

ciated with avascular necrosis of the femoral head. Muscle wasting (proximal myopathy) can also occur. Corticosteroid therapy is also weakly linked with peptic ulceration; there is no conclusive evidence that the use of enteric-coated preparations of prednisolone reduces the risk of peptic ulceration. See also Psychiatric Reactions, p. 372.

High doses of corticosteroids can cause Cushing's syndrome, with moon face, striae, and acne; it is usually reversible on withdrawal of treatment, but this must always be gradually tapered to avoid symptoms of acute adrenal insufficiency (**important:** see also Adrenal Suppression, p. 371).

Side-effects can be minimised by using the lowest effective dose for the minimum period possible.

*Other side effects include: gastro-intestinal effects:* dyspepsia, abdominal distension, acute pancreatitis, oesophageal ulceration and candidiasis; *musculoskeletal effects:* muscle weakness, vertebral and long bone fractures, tendon rupture; *endocrine effects:* menstrual irregularities and amenorrhoea, hirsutism, weight gain, negative nitrogen and calcium balance, increased appetite; increased susceptibility to and severity of infection, reactivation of dormant tuberculosis; *neuropsychiatric effects:* psychological dependence, insomnia, increased intracranial pressure with papilloedema (usually after withdrawal), aggravation of schizophrenia, aggravation of epilepsy; *ophthalmic effects:* papilloedema, posterior subcapsular cataracts, corneal or scleral thinning and exacerbation of ophthalmic viral or fungal disease, increased intra-ocular pressure, exophthalmos, *very rarely* angle-closure glaucoma; *also* impaired healing, petechiae, ecchymoses, facial erythema, suppression of skin test reactions, urticaria, hyperhidrosis, skin atrophy, bruising, telangiectasia, myocardial rupture following recent myocardial infarction, congestive heart failure, leucocytosis, hyperglycaemia, hypersensitivity reactions (including anaphylaxis), thromboembolism, nausea, malaise, hiccups, headache, vertigo.

For other references to the side-effects of corticosteroids see section 1.5 (gastro-intestinal system), section 3.2 (asthma), section 11.4 (eye) and section 13.4 (skin).

### ▌BETAMETHASONE

**Cautions** see notes above
**Contra-indications** see notes above
**Hepatic impairment** see notes above
**Renal impairment** see notes above
**Pregnancy** see notes above; transient effect on fetal movements and heart rate
**Breast-feeding** see notes above
**Side-effects** see notes above
**Licensed use** *Betnesol*® tablets not licensed for use as mouthwash
**Indications and dose**

> Suppression of inflammatory and allergic disorders; congenital adrenal hyperplasia; see also notes above

* By slow intravenous injection or by intravenous infusion

**Child 1 month–1 year** initially 1 mg repeated up to 4 times in 24 hours according to response

**Child 1–6 years** initially 2 mg repeated up to 4 times in 24 hours according to response

**Child 6–12 years** initially 4 mg repeated up to 4 times in 24 hours according to response

**Child 12–18 years** initially 4–20 mg repeated up to 4 times in 24 hours according to response

**Eye** section 11.4.1

**Ear** section 12.1.1

**Nose** section 12.2.1

**Mouth** section 12.3.1

**Administration** For *intravenous infusion*, dilute with Glucose 5% or Sodium Chloride 0.9%

**Betnesol**® (UCB Pharma) ▣PoM▣
Injection, betamethasone 4 mg (as sodium phosphate)/mL. Net price 1-mL amp = £1.17. Label: 10, steroid card

### ▌DEFLAZACORT

**Cautions** see notes above
**Contra-indications** see notes above
**Hepatic impairment** see notes above
**Renal impairment** see notes above
**Pregnancy** see notes above
**Breast-feeding** see notes above
**Side-effects** see notes above
**Indications and dose**

> Inflammatory and allergic disorders

* By mouth

**Child 1 month–12 years** 0.25–1.5 mg/kg once daily or on alternate days; up to 2.4 mg/kg (max. 120 mg) daily has been used in emergency situations

**Child 12–18 years** 3–18 mg once daily or on alternate days; up to 2.4 mg/kg (max. 120 mg) daily has been used in emergency situations

> Nephrotic syndrome

* By mouth

**Child 1 month–18 years** initially 1.5 mg/kg once daily (max. 120 mg) reduced to lowest effective dose for maintenance

**Calcort**® (Sanofi-Aventis) ▣PoM▣
Tablets, deflazacort 6 mg, net price 60-tab pack = £15.82. Label: 5, 10, steroid card

### ▌DEXAMETHASONE

**Cautions** see notes above
**Contra-indications** see notes above
**Hepatic impairment** see notes above
**Renal impairment** see notes above
**Pregnancy** see notes above
**Breast-feeding** see notes above
**Side-effects** see notes above; also perineal irritation may follow intravenous administration of the phosphate ester
**Licensed use** consult product literature; not licensed for use in bacterial meningitis

**Indications and dose**

**Inflammatory and allergic disorders**

- **By mouth**

    **Child 1 month–18 years** 10–100 micrograms/kg daily in 1–2 divided doses, adjusted according to response; up to 300 micrograms/kg daily may be required in emergency situations

- **By intramuscular injection or slow intravenous injection or infusion**

    **Child 1 month–12 years** 83–333 micrograms/kg daily in 1–2 divided doses; max. 20 mg daily

    **Child 12–18 years** initially 0.4–20 mg daily

**Life-threatening cerebral oedema**

- **By intravenous injection**

    **Child under 35 kg body-weight** initially 16.7 mg, then 3.3 mg every 3 hours for 3 days, then 3.3 mg every 6 hours for 1 day, then 1.7 mg every 6 hours for 4 days, then decrease by 0.8 mg daily

    **Child over 35 kg body-weight** initially 20.8 mg, then 3.3 mg every 2 hours for 3 days, then 3.3 mg every 4 hours for 1 day, then 3.3 mg every 6 hours for 4 days, then decrease by 1.7 mg daily

**Bacterial meningitis** (see section 5.1)

- **By slow intravenous injection**

    **Child 3 months–18 years** 150 micrograms/kg (max. 10 mg) every 6 hours for 4 days starting before or with first dose of antibacterial

**Physiological replacement**

- **By mouth or by slow intravenous injection**

    **Child 1 month–18 years** 250–500 micrograms/m² every 12 hours, adjusted according to response

**Croup** section 3.1

**Nausea and vomiting with chemotherapy** section 8.1

**Rheumatic disease** section 10.1.2

**Eye** section 11.4.1

**Administration** for administration *by mouth* tablets may be dispersed in water or injection solution given by mouth

For *intravenous infusion* dilute with Glucose 5% or Sodium Chloride 0.9%; give over 15–20 minutes

**Dexamethasone** (Non-proprietary) PoM

Tablets, dexamethasone 500 micrograms, net price 28-tab pack = £38.00; 2 mg, 50-tab pack = £7.46, 100-tab pack = £13.85. Label: 10, steroid card, 21

Oral solution, sugar-free, dexamethasone (as sodium phosphate) 2 mg/5 mL, net price 150-mL = £42.30. Label: 10, steroid card, 21
**Brands include** *Dexsol*®, *Martapan*®

Injection, dexamethasone (as sodium phosphate) 3.3 mg/mL, net price 1-mL amp = 83p. Label: 10, steroid card

Injection, dexamethasone (as sodium phosphate) 4 mg/mL, net price 1-mL amp = 83p, 2-mL vial = £1.27. Label: 10, steroid card

---

## HYDROCORTISONE

**Cautions** see notes above
**Contra-indications** see notes above
**Hepatic impairment** see notes above
**Renal impairment** see notes above
**Pregnancy** see notes above
**Breast-feeding** see notes above
**Side-effects** see notes above; also phosphate ester associated with paraesthesia and pain (particularly in the perineal region)

**Indications and dose**

**Congenital adrenal hyperplasia** see also section 6.3.1

- **By mouth**

    **Neonate** 9–15 mg/m² in 3 divided doses, adjusted according to response

    **Child 1 month–18 years** 9–15 mg/m² in 3 divided doses, adjusted according to response

**Acute adrenocortical insufficiency (***Addisonian crisis***)** see also notes above and section 6.3.1

- **By slow intravenous administration**

    **Neonate** initially 10 mg *by slow intravenous injection* then 100 mg/m² daily *by continuous intravenous infusion* or in divided doses every 6–8 hours; adjusted according to response; when stable reduce over 4–5 days to oral maintenance dose

    **Child 1 month–12 years** initially 2–4 mg/kg *by slow intravenous injection* or *infusion* then 2–4 mg/kg every 6 hours; adjusted according to response; when stable reduce over 4–5 days to oral maintenance dose

    **Child 12–18 years** 100 mg every 6 to 8 hours by *slow intravenous injection* or *infusion*

**Adrenal hypoplasia, Addison's disease, chronic maintenance or replacement therapy**

- **By mouth**

    **Neonate** 8–10 mg/m² daily in 3 divided doses; higher doses may be needed

    **Child 1 month–18 years** 8–10 mg/m² daily in 3 divided doses; higher doses may be needed
    **Note** Give larger doses in the morning and smaller doses in the evening

**Inflammatory bowel disease—induction of remission** see also section 1.5.2

- **By intravenous injection**

    **Child 2–18 years** 2.5 mg/kg (max. 100 mg) every 6 hours

- **By continuous intravenous infusion**

    **Child 2–18 years** 10 mg/kg daily (max. 400 mg daily)

**Acute hypersensitivity reactions, angioedema** see also section 3.4.3

- **By intramuscular or intravenous injection**

    **Child under 6 months** initially 25 mg 3 times daily, adjusted according to response

    **Child 6 months–6 years** initially 50 mg 3 times daily, adjusted according to response

    **Child 6–12 years** initially 100 mg 3 times daily, adjusted according to response

**6**

**Endocrine system**

**Child 12–18 years** initially 200 mg 3 times daily, adjusted according to response

**Hypotension resistant to inotropic treatment and volume replacement (limited evidence)**

• By intravenous injection

**Neonate** initially 2.5 mg/kg repeated if necessary after 4 hours, then 2.5 mg/kg every 6 hours for 48 hours or until blood pressure recovers, then dose reduced gradually over at least 48 hours

**Child 1 month–18 years** 1 mg/kg (max. 100 mg) every 6 hours

**Severe acute asthma** p. 132

**Eye** section 11.4.1

**Haemorrhoids** section 1.7.2

**Rheumatic disease** section 10.1.2

**Shock** section 2.7.1

**Skin** section 13.4

**Administration**   for *intravenous administration*, dilute with Glucose 5% or Sodium Chloride 0.9%; for *intermittent infusion* give over 20–30 minutes.
For administration *by mouth*, injection solution may be swallowed [unlicensed use] but consider phosphate content; alternatively *Corlan®* pellets (section 12.3.1) may be swallowed [unlicensed use]—pellets should not be cut as may not provide appropriate dose

**Hydrocortisone®** (Non-proprietary) ᴘᴏᴹ
Tablets, scored, hydrocortisone 10 mg, net price 30-tab pack = £44.25; 20 mg, 30-tab pack = £47.17. Label: 10, steroid card, 21

[1]**Efcortesol®** (Sovereign) ᴘᴏᴹ ◢
Injection, hydrocortisone 100 mg (as sodium phosphate)/mL, net price 1-mL amp = £1.08, 5-mL amp = £4.89. Label: 10, steroid card
**Note**  Paraesthesia and pain (particularly in the perineal region) may follow intravenous injection of the phosphate ester

[1]**Solu-Cortef®** (Pharmacia) ᴘᴏᴹ
Injection, powder for reconstitution, hydrocortisone (as sodium succinate). Net price 100-mg vial = 92p, 100-mg vial with 2-mL amp water for injections = £1.16. Label: 10, steroid card

**Indications and dose**
**Inflammatory and allergic disorders**

• By mouth, slow intravenous injection or by intravenous infusion

**Child 1 month–18 years** 0.5–1.7 mg/kg daily in 2–4 divided doses depending on condition and response

**Treatment of graft rejection reactions**

• By intravenous injection

**Child 1 month–18 years** 10–20 mg/kg or 400–600 mg/m² (max. 1 g) once daily for 3 days

**Severe erythema multiforme, lupus nephritis, systemic onset juvenile idiopathic arthritis**

• By intravenous injection

**Child 1 month–18 years** 10–30 mg/kg (max. 1 g) once daily or on alternate days for up to 3 doses

**Immunosuppression** section 8.2.2

**Rheumatic disease** section 10.1.2

**Skin** section 13.4

**Administration**   intravenous injection given over 30 minutes; for intravenous infusion may be diluted with sodium chloride intravenous infusion 0.9% or 0.45%, or glucose intravenous infusion 5% or 10%

**Medrone®** (Pfizer) ᴘᴏᴹ
Tablets, scored, methylprednisolone 2 mg (pink), net price 30-tab pack = £3.88; 4 mg, 30-tab pack = £6.19; 16 mg, 30-tab pack = £17.17; 100 mg (blue), 20-tab pack = £48.32. Label: 10, steroid card, 21

**Solu-Medrone®** (Pharmacia) ᴘᴏᴹ
Injection, powder for reconstitution, methylprednisolone (as sodium succinate) (all with solvent). Net price 40-mg vial = £1.58; 125-mg vial = £4.75; 500-mg vial = £9.60; 1-g vial = £17.30; 2-g vial = £32.86. Label: 10, steroid card

◢ **Intramuscular depot**
**Depo-Medrone®** (Pharmacia) ᴘᴏᴹ
Injection (aqueous suspension), methylprednisolone acetate 40 mg/mL. Net price 1-mL vial = £2.87; 2-mL vial = £5.15; 3-mL vial = £7.47. Label: 10, steroid card
**Dose**

• By deep intramuscular injection into gluteal muscle
seek specialist advice

## METHYLPREDNISOLONE

**Cautions**  see notes above; rapid intravenous administration of large doses associated with cardiovascular collapse

**Contra-indications**  see notes above

**Hepatic impairment**  see notes above

**Renal impairment**  see notes above

**Pregnancy**  see notes above

**Breast-feeding**  see notes above

**Side-effects**  see notes above

1.  ᴘᴏᴹ restriction does not apply where administration is for saving life in emergency

## PREDNISOLONE

**Cautions**  see notes above; also Duchenne's muscular dystrophy (possible transient rhabdomyolysis and myoglobinuria following strenuous physical activity)

**Contra-indications**  see notes above

**Hepatic impairment**  see notes above

**Renal impairment**  see notes above

**Pregnancy**  see notes above

**Breast-feeding**  see notes above

**Side-effects**  see notes above

## Indications and dose

**Autoimmune inflammatory disorders (including juvenile idiopathic arthritis, connective tissue disorders and systemic lupus erythematosus)**

- By mouth

    **Child 1 month–18 years** initially 1–2 mg/kg once daily (usual max. 60 mg daily), then reduced after a few days if appropriate

**Autoimmune hepatitis**

- By mouth

    **Child 1 month–18 years** initially 2 mg/kg once daily (max. 40 mg daily) then reduced to minimum effective dose

**Corticosteroid replacement therapy**

- By mouth

    **Child 12–18 years** 2–2.5 mg/m$^2$ daily in 1–2 divided doses adjusted according to response

**Infantile spasms**

- By mouth

    **Child 1 month–2 years** initially 10 mg 4 times daily for 14 days (if seizures not controlled after 7 days increase to 20 mg 3 times daily for 7 days); reduce dose gradually over 15 days until stopped (patients taking 40 mg daily, reduce dose in steps of 10 mg every 5 days, then stop; patients taking 60 mg daily, reduce dose to 40 mg daily for 5 days, then 20 mg daily for 5 days, then 10 mg daily for 5 days, then stop)

**Idiopathic thrombocytopenic purpura**

- By mouth

    **Child 1–10 years** 1–2 mg/kg daily for max. 14 days *or* 4 mg/kg daily for max. 4 days

**Nephrotic syndrome**

- By mouth

    **Child 1 month–18 years** initially 60 mg/m$^2$ once daily (max. 80 mg daily) for 4–6 weeks until proteinuria ceases then 40 mg/m$^2$ on alternate days for 4–6 weeks, then withdraw by reducing dose gradually; prevention of relapse 0.5–1 mg/kg once daily or on alternate days for 3–6 months

**Asthma** see p. 144

**Ear** section 12.1.1

**Eye** section 11.4.1

**Immunosuppression** section 8.2.2

**Inflammatory bowel disease** section 1.5.2

**Pneumocystis pneumonia** section 5.4.8

**Rheumatic disease** section 10.1.2

**Prednisolone** (Non-proprietary) (PoM)

Tablets, prednisolone 1 mg, net price 28-tab pack = 93p; 5 mg, 28-tab pack = £1.03; 25 mg, 56-tab pack = £30.00. Label: 10, steroid card, 21

Tablets, both e/c, prednisolone 2.5 mg, net price 28-tab pack = £4.65, 100-tab pack = £30.79; 5 mg, 28-tab pack = £4.73, 100-tab pack = £31.04. Label: 5, 10, steroid card, 25

**Brands include** *Deltacortril®*

Soluble tablets, prednisolone 5 mg (as sodium phosphate), net price 30-tab pack = £8.95. Label: 10, steroid card, 13, 21

## 6.4 Sex hormones

### 6.4.1 Female sex hormones
### 6.4.2 Male sex hormones and antagonists
### 6.4.3 Anabolic steroids

Sex hormone replacement therapy is indicated in children for the treatment of gonadotrophin deficiency, gonadal disorders, or delayed puberty that interferes with quality of life. Indications include constitutional delay in puberty, congenital or acquired hypogonadotrophic hypogonadism, hypergonadotrophic hypogonadism (Turner's syndrome, Klinefelter's syndrome), endocrine disorders (Cushing's syndrome or hyperprolactinaemia), and chronic illnesses, such as cystic fibrosis or sickle-cell disease, that may affect the onset of puberty.

Replacement therapy is generally started at the appropriate age for the development of puberty and should be managed by a paediatric endocrinologist. Patients with constitutional delay, chronic illness, or eating disorders may need only small doses of hormone supplements for 4 to 6 months to induce puberty and endogenous sex hormone production, which is then sustained. Patients with organic causes of hormone deficiency will require life-long replacement, adjusted to allow normal development.

Inadequate treatment may lead to poor bone mineralisation, resulting in fractures and osteoporosis.

### 6.4.1 Female sex hormones

#### 6.4.1.1 Oestrogens
#### 6.4.1.2 Progestogens

#### 6.4.1.1 Oestrogens

Oestrogens are necessary for the development of female secondary sexual characteristics. If onset of puberty is delayed because of organic pathology, puberty can be induced with ethinylestradiol in increasing doses, guided by breast staging and uterine scans. Cyclical progestogen replacement is added after 12–18 months of oestrogen treatment (see section 6.4.1.2). Once the adult dosage of oestrogen has been reached (20 micrograms ethinylestradiol daily), it may be more convenient to provide replacement either as a low-dose oestrogen containing oral contraceptive formulation [unlicensed indication] (see section 7.3.1) or as a combined oestrogen and progestogen hormone replacement therapy preparation [unlicensed indication] (see BNF section 6.4.1.1). There is limited experience in the use of transdermal patches or gels in children; compliance and skin irritation are sometimes a problem.

Ethinylestradiol is occasionally used, under **specialist supervision**, for the management of hereditary haemorrhagic telangiectasia (but evidence of benefit is limited), for the prevention of tall stature, and in tests of growth hormone secretion (see below). Side-effects include nausea and fluid retention.

Topical oestrogen creams are used in the treatment of labial adhesions (see section 7.2.1)

## ETHINYLESTRADIOL
(Ethinyloestradiol)

**Cautions** see Combined Hormonal Contraceptives (section 7.3.1); **interactions**: Appendix 1 (Oestrogens)

**Contra-indications** cardiovascular disease (sodium retention with oedema), personal or family history of thromboembolism, acute porphyria; see also Combined Hormonal Contraceptives (section 7.3.1)

**Hepatic impairment** avoid in liver disease including disorders of hepatic excretion (e.g. Dubin-Johnson or Rotor syndromes), infective hepatitis (until liver function returns to normal), and jaundice

**Pregnancy** avoid

**Breast-feeding** avoid

**Side-effects** nausea, vomiting, headache, breast tenderness, changes in body weight, fluid retention, depression, chorea, skin reactions, chloasma, hypertension, may irritate contact lenses, impairment of liver function, hepatic tumours, rarely photosensitivity; see also Combined Hormonal Contraceptives (section 7.3.1)

**Licensed use** unlicensed for use in children

**Indications and dose**

See notes above

### Induction of sexual maturation in girls
- By mouth

  Initially 2 micrograms daily, increasing every 6 months to 5 micrograms, then to 10 micrograms, and then to 20 micrograms daily

  **Note** after 12–18 months of treatment give progestogen for 7 days of each 28-day cycle

### Maintenance of sexual maturation in girls
- By mouth

  20 micrograms daily with cyclical progestogen for 7 days of each 28-day cycle

### Prevention of tall stature in girls
- By mouth

  **Girls 2–12 years** 20–50 micrograms daily

### Pituitary priming before growth hormone secretion test in girls
- By mouth

  **Girls with bone age above 10 years** 100 micrograms daily for 3 days before test

**Ethinylestradiol** (Non-proprietary) [PoM]
Tablets, ethinylestradiol (unlicensed) 10 micrograms, net price 21-tab pack = £29.95; 50 micrograms, 21-tab pack = £38.20; 1 mg, 28-tab pack = £49.50
**Note** 2 microgram tablets available from 'special-order' manufacturers or specialist-importing companies, see p. 823

### 6.4.1.2 Progestogens

There are two main groups of progestogen, *progesterone and its analogues* (dydrogesterone and medroxyprogesterone) and *testosterone analogues* (norethisterone and norgestrel). The newer progestogens (desogestrel, norgestimate, and gestodene) are all derivatives of nor-

gestrel; levonorgestrel is the active isomer of norgestrel and has twice its potency. Progesterone and its analogues are less androgenic than the testosterone derivatives and neither progesterone nor dydrogesterone causes virilisation.

In delayed puberty cyclical progestogen is added after 12–18 months of oestrogen therapy (section 6.4.1.1) to establish a menstrual cycle; usually levonorgestrel 30 micrograms or norethisterone 5 mg daily are used for the last 7 days of each 28 day cycle.

Norethisterone is also used to postpone menstruation during a cycle; treatment is started 3 days before the expected onset of menstruation.

## NORETHISTERONE

**Cautions** conditions that may worsen with fluid retention e.g. epilepsy, hypertension, migraine, asthma, cardiac dysfunction; susceptibility to thromboembolism (particular caution with high dose); history of depression; diabetes (monitor closely); **interactions**: Appendix 1 (progestogens)

**Contra-indications** history of liver tumours, severe liver impairment; severe arterial disease, undiagnosed vaginal bleeding; acute porphyria (section 9.8.2); history during pregnancy of idiopathic jaundice, severe pruritus, or pemphigoid gestationis

**Hepatic impairment** caution; avoid if severe

**Renal impairment** use with caution

**Pregnancy** avoid

**Breast-feeding** higher doses may suppress lactation and alter milk composition; use lowest effective dose

**Side-effects** menstrual disturbances, premenstrual-like syndrome (including bloating, fluid retention, breast tenderness), weight gain, nausea, headache, dizziness, insomnia, drowsiness, depression; skin reactions (including urticaria, pruritus, rash, and acne), hirsutism and alopecia; jaundice and anaphylactoid reactions also reported

**Licensed use** not licensed for use in children

**Indications and dose**

See notes above

### Induction and maintenance of sexual maturation in females (combined with an oestrogen after 12–24 months oestrogen therapy)
- By mouth

  5 mg once daily for the last 7 days of a 28-day cycle

### Postponement of menstruation
- By mouth

  5 mg 3 times daily, starting 3 days before expected onset of menstruation

**Norethisterone** (Non-proprietary) [PoM]
Tablets, norethisterone 5 mg, net price 30-tab pack = £2.18

**Primolut N**® (Bayer) [PoM]
Tablets, norethisterone 5 mg. Net price 30-tab pack = £1.89

**Utovlan**® (Pharmacia) [PoM]
Tablets, norethisterone 5 mg, net price 30-tab pack = £1.40, 90-tab pack = £4.21

# 6.4.2 Male sex hormones and antagonists

Androgens cause masculinisation; they are used as replacement therapy in androgen deficiency, in delayed puberty, and in those who are hypogonadal due to either pituitary or testicular disease.

When given to patients with hypopituitarism androgens can lead to normal sexual development and potency but not to fertility. If fertility is desired, the usual treatment is with gonadotrophins or pulsatile gonadotrophin-releasing hormone (section 6.5.1) which stimulates spermatogenesis as well as androgen production.

Intramuscular depot preparations of **testosterone esters** are preferred for replacement therapy. Testosterone enantate or propionate or alternatively *Sustanon®*, which consists of a mixture of testosterone esters and has a longer duration of action, can be used. For induction of puberty, depot testosterone injections are given monthly and the doses increased every 6 to 12 months according to response. Single ester testosterone injections may need to be given more frequently. Implants of testosterone can be used for hypogonadism; the implants are replaced every 4 to 5 months.

Oral **testosterone undecanoate** is used for induction of puberty. An alternative approach that promotes growth rather than sexual maturation uses oral oxandrolone (section 6.4.3).

Chorionic gonadotrophin (section 6.5.1) has also been used in delayed puberty in the male to stimulate endogenous testosterone production, but has little advantage over testosterone.

Caution should be used when androgens or chorionic gonadotrophin are used in treating boys with delayed puberty since the fusion of epiphyses is hastened and may result in short stature.

Testosterone topical gel is also available but experience of use in children under 15 years is limited. Topical testosterone is applied to the penis in the treatment of microphallus; an extemporaneously prepared cream should be used because the alcohol in proprietary gel formulations causes irritation.

---

## TESTOSTERONE AND ESTERS

**Cautions** cardiac impairment, hypertension, epilepsy, migraine, diabetes mellitus, skeletal metastases (risk of hypercalcaemia); **interactions**: Appendix 1 (testosterone)

**Contra-indications** history of primary liver tumours, hypercalcaemia, nephrosis

**Hepatic impairment** avoid if possible—fluid retention and dose-related toxicity

**Renal impairment** use with caution—potential for fluid retention

**Pregnancy** avoid; causes masculinisation of female fetus

**Breast-feeding** avoid; may cause masculinisation in the female infant or precocious development in the male infant; high doses suppress lactation

**Side-effects** headache, depression, gastro-intestinal bleeding, nausea, cholestatic jaundice, changes in libido, gynaecomastia, polycythaemia, anxiety, asthenia, paraesthesia, hypertension, electrolyte disturbances including sodium retention with oedema and hypercalcaemia, weight gain; increased bone growth; androgenic effects such as hirsutism, male-pattern baldness, seborrhoea, acne, pruritus; excessive frequency and duration of penile erection, precocious sexual development and premature closure of epiphyses in pre-pubertal males, suppression of spermatogenesis in males and virilism in females; *rarely* liver tumours; sleep apnoea also reported; *with gel*, local irritation and allergic reactions

**Licensed use** *Sustanon 250®* and testosterone enantate not licensed for use in children

**Indications and dose**

See also under preparations; specialist use only

### Induction and maintenance of sexual maturation in males

- **By mouth** (as testosterone undecanoate)

  **Child over 12 years** 40 mg on alternate days increasing according to response up to 120 mg daily

- **By deep intramuscular injection** (as testosterone enantate)

  **Child over 12 years** 25–50 mg/m² every month increasing dose every 6–12 months according to response

### Treatment of microphallus

- **Topically**

  Apply 3 times daily for 3 weeks

  **Note** Use only specially manufactured preparation (see notes above)

◢ **Oral**

**Restandol® Testocaps** (Organon) [CD4-2]
Capsules, orange, testosterone undecanoate 40 mg in oily solution, net price 30-cap pack = £8.55; 60-cap pack = £17.10. Label: 21, 25

◢ **Intramuscular**

**Testosterone Enantate** (Non-proprietary) [CD4-2]
Injection (oily), testosterone enantate 250 mg/mL, net price 1-mL amp = £13.33

**Sustanon 250®** (Organon) [CD4-2]
Injection (oily), testosterone propionate 30 mg, testosterone phenylpropionate 60 mg, testosterone isocaproate 60 mg, and testosterone decanoate 100 mg/mL, net price 1-mL amp = £6.45
**Excipients** include arachis (peanut) oil, benzyl alcohol (see Excipients p. 2)

**Virormone®** (Nordic) [CD4-2]
Injection, testosterone propionate 50 mg/mL, net price 2-mL amp = £4.50
**Dose**

### Delayed puberty in males

- **By intramuscular injection**
  50 mg once weekly

◢ **Implant**

**Testosterone** (Organon) [CD4-2]
Implant, testosterone 100 mg, net price = £7.40; 200 mg = £13.79
**Dose**

### Maintenance of sexual maturation in males

**Child over 16 years** 100–600 mg; 600 mg usually maintains plasma-testosterone concentration within the normal range for 4–5 months

◀Cream

**Testosterone** (CD4-2)

Cream, testosterone 5% (other strengths available)

Available from 'special-order' manufacturers or specialist importing companies, see p. 823

## Anti-androgens and precocious puberty

The gonadorelin stimulation test (section 6.5.1) is used to distinguish between *gonadotrophin-dependent (central) precocious puberty* and *gonadotrophin-independent precocious puberty*. Treatment requires specialist management.

Gonadorelin analogues, used in the management of gonadotrophin-dependent precocious puberty, delay development of secondary sexual characteristics and growth velocity.

**Testolactone** and **cyproterone** are used in the management of gonadotrophin-independent precocious puberty, resulting from McCune-Albright syndrome, familial male precocious puberty (testotoxicosis), hormone-secreting tumours, and ovarian and testicular disorders. Testolactone inhibits the aromatisation of testosterone, the rate limiting step in oestrogen synthesis. Cyproterone is a progestogen with anti-androgen properties.

Spironolactone (section 2.2.3) is sometimes used in combination with testolactone because it has some androgen receptor blocking properties.

High blood concentration of sex hormones may activate release of gonadotrophin releasing hormone, leading to development of secondary, central gonadotrophin-dependent precocious puberty. This may require the addition of gonadorelin analogues to prevent progression of pubertal development and skeletal maturation.

## ▌CYPROTERONE ACETATE

**Cautions**  blood counts initially and throughout treatment; monitor adrenocortical function regularly; diabetes mellitus (see also Contra-indications)

**Skilled tasks**  Fatigue and lassitude may impair performance of skilled tasks (e.g. driving)

**Contra-indications**  severe diabetes (with vascular changes), sickle-cell anaemia, liver disease including Dubin-Johnson and Rotor syndromes, previous or existing liver tumours, malignant or wasting diseases, meningioma or history of meningioma, severe depression, history of thromboembolic disorders

**Hepatic impairment**  avoid—dose-related toxicity, see Side-effects below

**Side-effects**  fatigue and lassitude, breathlessness, weight changes, reduced sebum production (may clear acne), changes in hair pattern, gynaecomastia (rarely leading to galactorrhoea and benign breast nodules); rarely hypersensitivity reactions, rash and osteoporosis; inhibition of spermatogenesis (see notes above); hepatotoxicity reported (including jaundice, hepatitis and hepatic failure)

**Hepatotoxicity**  Direct hepatic toxicity such as jaundice, hepatitis and hepatic failure, including fatal cases, have been reported (usually after several months) with cyproterone acetate dosages of 100 mg and above. Liver function tests should be performed before and regularly during treatment and whenever symptoms suggestive of hepatotoxicity occur—if confirmed cyproterone should normally be withdrawn unless the hepatotoxicity can be explained by another cause such as metastatic disease (in which case cyproterone should be continued only if the perceived benefit exceeds the risk)

**Licensed use**  unlicensed for use in children

**Indications and dose**

> Gonadotrophin-independent precocious puberty)
> (specialist use only; see also notes above)
>
> • By mouth
>
> Initially 25 mg twice daily, adjusted according to response

**Cyproterone Acetate** (Non-proprietary) (PoM)

Tablets, cyproterone acetate 50 mg, net price 56-tab pack = £31.54. Label: 21, counselling, driving

**Note** 10 mg tablets available from 'special-order' manufacturers or specialist-importing companies, see p. 823

**Androcur**® (Bayer) (PoM)

Tablets, scored, cyproterone acetate 50 mg, net price 56-tab pack = £24.41. Label: 21, counselling, driving

## ▌TESTOLACTONE

**Cautions**  interactions: Appendix 1 (testolactone)

**Pregnancy**  avoid

**Breast-feeding**  no information available

**Side-effects**  nausea, vomiting, anorexia, diarrhoea; hypertension; peripheral neuropathy; weight changes; changes in hair pattern; rarely hypersensitivity reactions, rash

**Indications and dose**

> Gonadotrophin-independent precocious puberty
> (specialist use only; see also notes above)
>
> • By mouth
>
> 5 mg/kg 3–4 times daily; up to 10 mg/kg 4 times daily may be required

**Testolactone** (PoM)

Tablets, testolactone 50 mg

Available from 'special-order' manufacturers or specialist importing companies, see p. 823

## ▌GOSERELIN

**Cautions**  monitor bone mineral density

**Contra-indications**  undiagnosed vaginal bleeding

**Pregnancy**  avoid

**Breast-feeding**  avoid

**Side-effects**  changes in blood pressure, headache, mood changes including depression, hypersensitivity reactions including urticaria, pruritus, rash, asthma and anaphylaxis; changes in scalp and body hair, weight changes, withdrawal bleeding, ovarian cysts (may require withdrawal), breast swelling and tenderness (males and females), visual disturbances, paraesthesia, local reactions at injection site

**Licensed use**  not licensed for use in children

**Indications and dose**

> Gonadotrophin-dependent precocious puberty
>
> See notes above; for doses, see under preparations below
>
> **Note** Injections may be required more frequently in some cases

**Administration**  Rotate injection site to prevent atrophy and nodule formation

6 Endocrine system

**Novgos**® (Genus) [PoM]
Implant, goserelin (as acetate) 3.6 mg in prefilled
syringe, net price = £58.50
Dose

* **Implant, by subcutaneous injection into anterior abdominal wall**
  3.6 mg every 28 days

**Zoladex**® (AstraZeneca) [PoM]
Implant, goserelin (as acetate) 3.6 mg in *Safe-System*® syringe applicator, net price each = £65.00
Dose

* **Implant, by subcutaneous injection into anterior abdominal wall**
  3.6 mg every 28 days

**Zoladex**® **LA** (AstraZeneca) [PoM]
Implant, goserelin (as acetate) 10.8 mg in *SafeSystem*® syringe applicator, net price each = £235.00
Dose

* **Implant, by subcutaneous injection into anterior abdominal wall**
  10.8 mg every 12 weeks

---

## ▌ LEUPRORELIN ACETATE

**Cautions**   see Goserelin
**Contra-indications**   see Goserelin
**Pregnancy**   avoid—teratogenic in *animal* studies
**Breast-feeding**   avoid
**Side-effects**   see Goserelin
**Licensed use**   not licensed for use in children
**Indications and dose**

> Gonadotrophin-dependent precocious puberty
>
> See notes above; for doses, see under preparations below
>
> Note   Injections may be required more frequently in some cases

**Administration**   Rotate injection site to prevent atrophy and nodule formation

**Prostap**® **SR** (Wyeth) [PoM]
Injection (microsphere powder for reconstitution),
leuprorelin acetate, net price 3.75-mg vial with
1-mL vehicle-filled syringe = £75.24
Dose

* **By subcutaneous or by intramuscular injection**
  3.75 mg every four weeks (half this dose is sometimes
  used in children with body-weight under 20 kg)

**Prostap**® **3** (Wyeth) [PoM]
Injection (microsphere powder for reconstitution),
leuprorelin acetate, net price 11.25-mg vial with
2-mL vehicle-filled syringe = £225.72
Dose

* **By subcutaneous or by intramuscular injection**
  11.25 mg every 12 weeks

---

## ▌ TRIPTORELIN

**Cautions**   see Goserelin
**Contra-indications**   see Goserelin
**Pregnancy**   avoid
**Breast-feeding**   avoid
**Side-effects**   see Goserelin; also gastro-intestinal disturbances; asthenia; arthralgia

**Indications and dose**

> Gonadotrophin-dependent precocious puberty
>
> See notes above; for doses, see under preparations below

**Administration**   rotate injection site to prevent atrophy and nodule formation

**Decapeptyl**® **SR** (Ipsen) [PoM]
Injection, (powder for suspension), m/r, triptorelin
(as acetate), net price 11.25-mg vial (with diluent) =
£207.00
Dose

* **By intramuscular injection**
  11.25 mg every 3 months
  Note   Each vial includes an overage to allow accurate
  administration of 11.25 mg dose

**Gonapeptyl**® **Depot** (Ferring) [PoM]
Injection (powder for suspension), triptorelin (as
acetate), net price 3.75-mg prefilled syringe (with
prefilled syringe of vehicle) = £81.69
Dose

* **By subcutaneous or intramuscular injection**
  **Body-weight under 20 kg** initially 1.875 mg on days 0,
  14, and 28, then 1.875 mg every 4 weeks
  **Body-weight 20–30 kg** initially 2.5 mg on days 0, 14, and
  28, then 2.5 mg every 4 weeks
  **Body-weight over 30 kg** initially 3.75 mg on days 0, 14,
  and 28, then 3.75 mg every 4 weeks; discontinue when
  bone maturation consistent with age over 12 years in
  girls and over 13 years in boys
  Note   May be given every 3 weeks if necessary

---

## 6.4.3   Anabolic steroids

Anabolic steroids have some androgenic activity but in
girls they cause less virilisation than androgens. They
are used in the treatment of some *aplastic anaemias*
(section 9.1.3). Oxandrolone is used to stimulate late
pre-pubertal growth prior to induction of sexual maturation in boys with short stature and in girls with Turner's
syndrome; specialist management is required.

---

## ▌ OXANDROLONE

**Cautions**   see Testosterone (section 6.4.2); **interactions:** Appendix 1 (oxandrolone)
**Contra-indications**   see Testosterone (section 6.4.2)
**Hepatic impairment**   see Testosterone (section 6.4.2)
**Renal impairment**   see Testosterone (section 6.4.2)
**Pregnancy**   see Testosterone (section 6.4.2)
**Breast-feeding**   see Testosterone (section 6.4.2)
**Side-effects**   see Testosterone (section 6.4.2)
**Indications and dose**

> Stimulation of late pre-pubertal growth in boys
> with short stature
>
> * By mouth
>   **Boys 10–18 years (or appropriate age)** 1.25–
>   2.5 mg daily for 3–6 months

> Stimulation of late pre-pubertal growth in girls
> with Turner's syndrome
>
> * By mouth
>   **Girls** in combination with growth hormone 0.625–
>   2.5 mg daily

6 Endocrine system

**Oxandrolone**

Tablets, oxandrolone 2.5 mg

Available from 'special-order' manufacturers or specialist importing companies, see p. 823

# 6.5 Hypothalamic and pituitary hormones

**6.5.1** Hypothalamic and anterior pituitary hormones including growth hormone

**6.5.2** Posterior pituitary hormones and antagonists

Use of preparations in these sections requires detailed prior investigation of the patient and *should be reserved for specialist centres.*

## 6.5.1 Hypothalamic and anterior pituitary hormones including growth hormone

### Anterior pituitary hormones

#### Corticotrophins

**Tetracosactide** (tetracosactrin), an analogue of corticotropin (adrenocorticotrophic hormone, ACTH), is used to test adrenocortical function; failure of plasma-cortisol concentration to rise after administration of tetracosactide indicates adrenocortical insufficiency. A low-dose test is considered by some clinicians to be more sensitive when used to confirm established, partial adrenal suppression.

Tetracosactide should be given only if no other ACTH preparations have been given previously. Tetracosactide depot injection (*Synacthen Depot®*) is also used in the treatment of infantile spasms (see Infantile spasms, section 4.8.1) but it is contra-indicated in neonates because of the presence of benzyl alcohol in the injection. Corticotropin-releasing factor, corticorelin, (also known as corticotropin-releasing hormone, CRH) is used to test anterior pituitary function and secretion of corticotropin.

### ▌ TETRACOSACTIDE
(Tetracosactrin)

**Cautions** as for corticosteroids, section 6.3.2; **important**: risk of anaphylaxis (medical supervision; consult product literature); history of atopic allergy (e.g. asthma, eczema, hayfever); history of hypersensitivity; **interactions**: Appendix 1 (corticosteroids)

**Contra-indications** as for corticosteroids, section 6.3.2; avoid injections containing benzyl alcohol in neonates (see under preparations); history of hypersensitivity to corticotrophins

**Hepatic impairment** see section 6.3.2

**Renal impairment** see section 6.3.2

**Pregnancy** avoid (but may be used diagnostically if essential)

**Breast-feeding** avoid (but may be used diagnostically if essential)

**Side-effects** as for corticosteroids, section 6.3.2

**Licensed use** not licensed for low-dose test for adrenocortical insufficiency or treatment of infantile spasms

**Indications and dose**

See notes above and under preparations below

**Synacthen®** (Alliance) (PoM)

Injection, tetracosactide 250 micrograms (as acetate)/mL. Net price 1-mL amp = £2.70

**Dose**

**Diagnosis of adrenocortical insufficiency (30-minute test)**

• By intramuscular or intravenous injection
  **Standard-dose test** 145 micrograms/m² (max. 250 micrograms) as a single dose
  **Low-dose test** 300 nanograms/m² as a single dose
  **Administration** may be diluted in sodium chloride 0.9% to 250 nanograms/mL

**Synacthen Depot®** (Alliance) (PoM)

Injection (aqueous suspension), tetracosactide acetate 1 mg/mL, with zinc phosphate complex. Net price 1-mL amp = £3.87

**Excipients** include benzyl alcohol (avoid in neonates, see Excipients p. 2)

**Dose**

**Infantile spasms**

• By intramuscular injection
  **Child 1 month–2 years** initially 500 micrograms on alternate days, adjusted according to response

### ▌ CORTICORELIN
(Corticotrophin-releasing hormone, CRH)

**Pregnancy** avoid

**Breast-feeding** avoid

**Side-effects** flushing of face, neck and upper body, hypotension, mild sensation of taste or smell

**Licensed use** not licensed

**Indications and dose**

**Test of anterior pituitary function**

• By intravenous injection over 30 seconds
  **Child 1 month–18 years** 1 microgram/kg (max. 100 micrograms) as a single dose

**CRH Ferring®** (Shire) (PoM)

Injection, corticorelin 100 micrograms

## Gonadotrophins

Gonadotrophins are occasionally used in the treatment of hypogonadotrophic hypogonadism and associated oligospermia. There is no justification for their use in primary gonadal failure.

Chorionic gonadotrophin is used in the investigation of testicular function in suspected primary hypogonadism and incomplete masculinisation. It has also been used in delayed puberty in boys to stimulate endogenous testosterone production, but it has little advantage over testosterone (section 6.4.2).

### ▌ CHORIONIC GONADOTROPHIN
(Human Chorionic Gonadotrophin; HCG)

A preparation of a glycoprotein fraction secreted by the placenta and obtained from the urine of pregnant women having the action of the pituitary luteinising hormone

**Cautions** cardiac impairment, asthma, epilepsy, migraine; prepubertal boys (risk of premature epiphyseal closure or precocious puberty)

**Contra-indications** androgen-dependent tumours

**Renal impairment** use with caution

**Side-effects** oedema (reduce dose), headache, tiredness, mood changes, gynaecomastia, local reactions

**Licensed use** unlicensed in children for test of testicular function

**Indications and dose**

> **Test of testicular function**
> • By intramuscular injection
> Short stimulation test:
> **Child 1 month–18 years** 1500–2000 units once daily for 3 days
> Prolonged stimulation test:
> **Child 1 month–18 years** 1500–2000 units twice weekly for 3 weeks

> **Hypogonadotrophic hypogonadism**
> • By intramuscular injection
> **Child 1 month–18 years** 1000–2000 units twice weekly, adjusted to response

> **Undescended testes**
> • By intramuscular injection
> **Child 7–18 years** initially 500 units 3 times weekly (1000 units twice weekly if over 17 years); adjusted to response; up to 4000 units 3 times weekly may be required; continue for 1–2 months after testicular descent

**Choragon®** (Ferring) (CD4-2)
Injection, powder for reconstitution, chorionic gonadotrophin. Net price 5000-unit amp (with solvent) = £3.26. For intramuscular injection

**Pregnyl®** (Organon) (CD4-2)
Injection, powder for reconstitution, chorionic gonadotrophin. Net price 1500-unit amp = £2.12; 5000-unit amp = £3.15 (both with solvent). For subcutaneous or intramuscular injection

# Growth hormone

Growth hormone is used to treat proven deficiency of the hormone, Prader-Willi syndrome, Turner's syndrome, growth disturbance in children born small for postmenstrual age, chronic renal insufficiency, and short stature homeobox-containing gene (SHOX) deficiency (see NICE guidance below). Growth hormone is also used in Noonan syndrome and idiopathic short stature [unlicensed indications] under specialist management. Treatment should be initiated and monitored by a paediatrician with expertise in managing growth-hormone disorders; treatment can be continued under a shared-care protocol by a general practitioner.

Growth hormone of human origin (HGH; somatotrophin) has been replaced by a growth hormone of human sequence, **somatropin**, produced using recombinant DNA technology.

---

> **NICE guidance**
> **Somatropin for the treatment of growth failure in children (May 2010)**
> Somatropin is recommended for children with growth failure who:
> • have growth-hormone deficiency;
> • have Turner's syndrome;
> • have Prader-Willi syndrome;
> • have chronic renal insufficiency;
> • are born small for postmenstrual age with subsequent growth failure at 4 years of age or later;
> • have short stature homeobox-containing gene (SHOX) deficiency.
> Treatment should be discontinued if growth velocity increases by less than 50% from baseline in the first year of treatment.
> www.nice.org.uk/TA188

**Mecasermin**, a human insulin-like growth factor-I (rhIGF-I), is licensed to treat growth failure in children with severe primary insulin-like growth factor-I deficiency (section 6.7.4).

## ▌ SOMATROPIN
(Recombinant Human Growth Hormone)

**Cautions** diabetes mellitus (adjustment of antidiabetic therapy may be necessary), papilloedema (see under Side-effects), relative deficiencies of other pituitary hormones (notably hypothyroidism—manufacturers recommend periodic thyroid function tests but limited evidence of clinical value), history of malignant disease, disorders of the epiphysis of the hip (monitor for limping), resolved intracranial hypertension (monitor closely), initiation of treatment close to puberty not recommended in child born small for postmenstrual age; Silver-Russell syndrome; rotate subcutaneous injection sites to prevent lipoatrophy; **interactions:** Appendix 1 (somatropin)

**Contra-indications** evidence of tumour activity (complete antitumour therapy and ensure intracranial lesions inactive before starting); not to be used after renal transplantation or for growth promotion in children with closed epiphyses (or near closure in Prader-Willi syndrome); severe obesity or severe respiratory syndrome in Prader-Willi syndrome

**Pregnancy** interrupt treatment if pregnancy occurs

**Breast-feeding** absorption from milk unlikely

**Side-effects** headache, funduscopy for papilloedema recommended if severe or recurrent headache, visual problems, nausea and vomiting occur—if papilloedema confirmed consider benign intracranial hypertension (rare cases reported); fluid retention (peripheral oedema), arthralgia, myalgia, carpal tunnel syndrome, paraesthesia, antibody formation, hypothyroidism, insulin resistance, hyperglycaemia, hypoglycaemia, reactions at injection site; leukaemia in children with growth hormone deficiency also reported

**Licensed use** not licensed for use in Noonan syndrome

**Indications and dose**

> **Gonadal dysgenesis (Turner's syndrome)**
> • By subcutaneous injection
> 45–50 micrograms/kg daily or 1.4 mg/m² daily

**6 Endocrine system**

**Deficiency of growth hormone**

- By subcutaneous or intramuscular injection

  23–39 micrograms/kg daily *or* 0.7–1 mg/m² daily

**Prader-Willi syndrome**

- By subcutaneous injection

  **Children with growth velocity greater than 1 cm/
  year** in combination with energy-restricted diet,
  35 micrograms/kg daily *or* 1 mg/m² daily; max.
  2.7 mg daily

**Chronic renal insufficiency (renal function
decreased to less than 50%)**

- By subcutaneous injection

  45–50 micrograms/kg daily *or* 1.4 mg/m² daily
  (higher doses may be needed) adjusted if necessary after 6 months

**Growth disturbance in children born small for
postmenstrual age whose growth has not caught
up by 4 years of age or later; Noonan syndrome**

- By subcutaneous injection

  35 micrograms/kg daily *or* 1 mg/m² daily

**SHOX deficiency**

- By subcutaneous injection

  45–50 micrograms/kg daily

**Genotropin®** (Pharmacia) CD4-2
Injection, two-compartment cartridge containing
powder for reconstitution, somatropin (rbe) and diluent, net price 5.3-mg (16-unit) cartridge = £122.87,
12-mg (36-unit) cartridge = £278.20. For use with
*Genotropin® Pen* JHS device (available free of charge
from clinics). For subcutaneous injection

GoQuick® injection, two-compartment, multi-dose
disposable, prefilled pen containing powder for
reconstitution, somatropin (rbe) and diluents, net
price 5.3-mg (16-unit) prefilled pen = £122.87; 12-
mg (36-unit) prefilled pen = £278.20. For subcutaneous injection

MiniQuick® injection, two-compartment single-dose
syringe containing powder for reconstitution, somatropin (rbe) and diluent, net price 0.2-mg (0.6-unit)
syringe = £4.64; 0.4-mg (1.2-unit) syringe = £9.27;
0.6-mg (1.8-unit) syringe = £13.91; 0.8-mg (2.4-unit)
syringe = £18.55; 1-mg (3-unit) syringe = £23.18;
1.2-mg (3.6-unit) syringe = £27.82; 1.4-mg (4.2-unit)
syringe = £32.46; 1.6-mg (4.8-unit) syringe = £37.09;
1.8-mg (5.4-unit) syringe = £41.73; 2-mg (6-unit)
syringe = £46.37. For subcutaneous injection

**Humatrope®** (Lilly) CD4-2
Injection, powder for reconstitution, somatropin
(rbe), net price 6-mg (18-unit) cartridge = £108.00;
12-mg (36-unit) cartridge = £216.00; 24-mg (72-unit)
cartridge = £432.00; all supplied with diluent. For
subcutaneous or intramuscular injection; cartridges
for subcutaneous injection

**Norditropin®** (Novo Nordisk) CD4-2
SimpleXx® injection, somatropin (epr) 3.3 mg
(10 units)/mL, net price 1.5-mL (5-mg, 15-unit) cartridge = £106.35; 6.7 mg (20 units)/mL,1.5-mL (10-
mg, 30-unit) cartridge = £212.70; 10 mg (30 units)/
mL, 1.5-mL (15-mg, 45-unit) cartridge = £319.05.
For use with appropriate *NordiPen®* JHS device

(available free of charge from clinics). For subcutaneous injection

NordiFlex® injection, multidose disposable prefilled
pen, somatropin (rbe) 10 mg (30 units)/mL, net price
1.5mL (15-mg, 45-unit) prefilled pen = £347.70. For
use with *NovoFine®* or *NovoTwist®* needles. For subcutaneous injection

**NutropinAq®** (Ipsen) CD4-2
Injection, somatropin (rbe), net price 10 mg
(30 units) 2-mL cartridge = £203.00. For use with
*NutropinAq®* Pen JHS device (available free of
charge from clinics). For subcutaneous injection

**Omnitrope®** (Sandoz) CD4-2
Injection, somatropin (rbe) 3.3 mg (10 units)/mL, net
price 1.5 mL (5-mg, 15-unit) cartridge = £86.77;
6.7 mg (20 units)/mL, 1.5 mL (10-mg, 30-unit) cartridge = £173.50. For use with *Omnitrope Pen 5®* JHS
and *Omnitrope Pen 10®* JHS devices respectively
(available free of charge from clinics). For subcutaneous injection
**Excipients** include benzyl alcohol (in 5-mg cartridge)
(avoid in neonates, see Excipients, p. 2)
**Note** Biosimilar medicine, see p. 2

**Saizen®** (Merck Serono) CD4-2
Injection, somatropin (rmc), 5.83 mg (17.5 units)/
mL, net price 1.03-mL (6-mg, 18-unit) cartridge =
£139.08; 8 mg (24 units)/mL, 1.5-mL (12-mg, 36-
unit) cartridge = £278.16, 2.5-mL (20-mg, 60-unit)
cartridge = £463.60. For use with *cool.click®* JHS
needle-free autoinjector device or *easypod®* JHS
autoinjector device (available free of charge from
clinics). For subcutaneous injection

Click.easy®, powder for reconstitution, somatropin
(rmc), net price 8-mg (24-unit) vial (in *Click.easy®*
device with diluent) = £185.44. For use with *One.
click®* JHS autoinjector device or *cool.click®* JHS
needle-free autoinjector device or *easypod®* JHS
autoinjector device (available free of charge from
clinics). For subcutaneous injection

**Zomacton®** (Ferring) CD4-2
Injection, powder for reconstitution, somatropin
(rbe), net price 4-mg (12-unit) vial (with diluent) =
£79.69. For use with *ZomaJet 2 Vision* JHS needle-
free device (available free of charge from clinics) or
with needles and syringes; 10-mg (30-unit) vial (with
diluent) = £199.23, for use with *ZomaJet Vision
X®* JHS needle-free device (available free of charge
from clinics) or with needles and syringes. For subcutaneous injection
**Excipients** include benzyl alcohol (in 4-mg vial) (avoid in
neonates, see Excipients, p. 2)

## Hypothalamic hormones

**Gonadorelin** when injected intravenously in post-pub-
ertal girls leads to a rapid rise in plasma concentrations
of both luteinising hormone (LH) and follicle-stimulating
hormone (FSH). It has not proved to be very helpful,
however, in distinguishing hypothalamic from pituitary
lesions. It is used in the assessment of delayed or
precocious puberty.

Other growth hormone stimulation tests involve the use
of insulin, glucagon, arginine, and clonidine [all unlicensed uses]. The tests should be carried out in specialist centres.

## GONADORELIN

(Gonadotrophin-releasing hormone; GnRH; LH–RH)

**Cautions**  pituitary adenoma

**Pregnancy**  avoid

**Breast-feeding**  avoid

**Side-effects**  rarely nausea, headache, abdominal pain, increased menstrual bleeding; rarely, hypersensitivity reaction on repeated administration of large doses; irritation at injection site

**Licensed use**  not licensed for use in children under 1 year

**Indications and dose**

Assessment of anterior pituitary function; assessment of delayed puberty

• By subcutaneous or intravenous injection

 **Child 1–18 years** 2.5 micrograms/kg (max. 100 micrograms) as a single dose

**Gonadorelin®** (Intrapharm) [PoM]

Injection, powder for reconstitution, gonadorelin. Net price 100-microgram vial (with diluent) = £67.00 (hosp. only)

Excipients  include benzyl alcohol (avoid in neonates, see Excipients p. 2)

---

## 6.5.2 Posterior pituitary hormones and antagonists

### Posterior pituitary hormones

**Diabetes insipidus**  Diabetes insipidus is caused by either a deficiency of anti-diuretic hormone (ADH, vasopressin) secretion (cranial, neurogenic, or pituitary diabetes insipidus) or by failure of the renal tubules to react to secreted antidiuretic hormone (nephrogenic diabetes insipidus).

**Vasopressin** (antidiuretic hormone, ADH) is used in the treatment of *pituitary diabetes insipidus* as is its analogue **desmopressin**. Dosage is tailored to produce a regular diuresis every 24 hours to avoid water intoxication. Treatment may be required permanently or for a limited period only in diabetes insipidus following trauma or pituitary surgery.

Desmopressin is more potent and has a longer duration of action than vasopressin; unlike vasopressin it has no vasoconstrictor effect. It is given by mouth or intranasally for maintenance therapy, or by injection in the postoperative period or in unconscious patients. Desmopressin is also used in the differential diagnosis of diabetes insipidus; following an intramuscular or intranasal dose, restoration of the ability to concentrate urine after water deprivation confirms a diagnosis of pituitary diabetes insipidus. Failure to respond suggests nephrogenic diabetes insipidus. Fluid input must be managed carefully to avoid hyponatraemia; this test is not usually recommended in young children.

In *nephrogenic* and *partial pituitary diabetes insipidus* benefit may be gained from the paradoxical antidiuretic effect of thiazides (section 2.2.1) e.g. chlorothiazide 10–20 mg/kg (max. 500 mg) twice daily.

---

**Other uses**  Desmopressin is also used to boost factor VIII concentration in mild to moderate haemophilia and in von Willebrand's disease; it is also used to test fibrinolytic response. For a comment on use of desmopressin in nocturnal enuresis see section 7.4.2.

Vasopressin infusion is used to control variceal bleeding in portal hypertension, before introducing more definitive treatment. **Terlipressin**, a derivative of vasopressin, and octreotide are used similarly but experience in children is limited.

---

## DESMOPRESSIN

**Cautions**  see under Vasopressin; less pressor activity, but still considerable caution in cardiovascular disease and in hypertension (not indicated for nocturnal enuresis or nocturia in these circumstances); also considerable caution in cystic fibrosis; in nocturia and nocturnal enuresis limit fluid intake from 1 hour before dose until 8 hours afterwards; in nocturia periodic blood pressure and weight checks needed to monitor for fluid overload; **interactions:** Appendix 1 (desmopressin)

For cautions specifically relating to the use of desmopressin in nocturnal enuresis see section 7.4.2

**Hyponatraemic convulsions**  Patients being treated for primary nocturnal enuresis should be warned to avoid fluid overload (including during swimming) and to stop taking desmopressin during an episode of vomiting or diarrhoea (until fluid balance normal). The risk of hyponatraemic convulsions can also be minimised by keeping to the recommended starting doses and by avoiding concomitant use of drugs which increase secretion of vasopressin (e.g. tricyclic antidepressants)

**Contra-indications**  cardiac insufficiency and other conditions treated with diuretics; psychogenic polydipsia and polydipsia in alcohol dependence

**Renal impairment**  use with caution; antidiuretic effect may be reduced

**Pregnancy**  small oxytocic effect in third trimester; increased risk of pre-eclampsia

**Breast-feeding**  amount too small to be harmful

**Side-effects**  fluid retention, and hyponatraemia (in more serious cases with convulsions) on administration without restricting fluid intake; stomach pain, headache, nausea, vomiting, allergic reactions, and emotional disturbance in children also reported; epistaxis, nasal congestion, rhinitis with nasal spray

**Licensed use**  consult product literature for individual preparations; not licensed for assessment of antidiuretic hormone secretion

**Indications and dose**

Assessment of antidiuretic hormone secretion (congenital deficiency suspected) (specialist use only)

• Intranasally

 **Child 1 month–2 years** initially 100–500 nanograms as a single dose

Assessment of antidiuretic hormone secretion (congenital deficiency not suspected) (specialist use only)

• Intranasally

 **Child 1 month–2 years** 1–5 micrograms as a single dose

6

Endocrine system

6 Endocrine system

**Test for suspected diabetes insipidus (water deprivation test)**

- **Intranasally**

  **Neonate** not recommended, use trial of treatment

  **Child 1 month–2 years** 5–10 micrograms as a single dose; not usually recommended, see notes above

  **Child 2–12 years** 10–20 micrograms as a single dose, see notes above

  **Child 12–18 years** 20 micrograms as a single dose, see notes above

- **By subcutaneous or intramuscular injection**

  **Neonate** not recommended, use trial of treatment

  **Child 1 month–2 years** 400 nanograms as a single dose; not usually recommended, see notes above

  **Child 2–12 years** 0.5–1 microgram as a single dose, see notes above

  **Child 12–18 years** 1–2 micrograms as a single dose, see notes above

**Diabetes insipidus, treatment**

- **By mouth**

  (as desmopressin acetate)

  **Neonate** initially 1–4 micrograms 2–3 times daily, adjusted according to response

  **Child 1 month–2 years** initially 10 micrograms 2–3 times daily, adjusted according to response (range 30–150 micrograms daily)

  **Child 2–12 years** initially 50 micrograms 2–3 times daily, adjusted according to response (range 100–800 micrograms daily)

  **Child 12–18 years** initially 100 micrograms 2–3 times daily, adjusted according to response (range 0.2–1.2 mg daily)

- **Sublingually**

  (as desmopressin base)

  **Child 2–18 years** initially 60 micrograms 3 times daily, adjusted according to response (range 40–240 micrograms 3 times daily)

- **Intranasally**

  (as desmopressin acetate)

  **Neonate** initially 100–500 nanograms, adjusted according to response (range 1.25–10 micrograms daily in 1–2 divided doses)

  **Child 1 month–2 years** initially 2.5–5 micrograms 1–2 times daily, adjusted according to response

  **Child 2–12 years** initially 5–20 micrograms 1–2 times daily, adjusted according to response

  **Child 12–18 years** initially 10–20 micrograms 1–2 times daily, adjusted according to response

- **By subcutaneous or intramuscular injection**

  **Neonate** initially 100 nanograms once daily, adjusted according to response (intramuscular route only)

  **Child 1 month–12 years** initially 400 nanograms once daily, adjusted according to response

  **Child 12–18 years** initially 1–4 micrograms once daily, adjusted according to response

**Primary nocturnal enuresis**

- **By mouth**

  (as desmopressin acetate)

  **Child 5–18 years** 200 micrograms at bedtime, increased to 400 micrograms at bedtime only if lower dose not effective (**important:** see also Cautions), reassess after 3 months by withdrawing treatment for at least 1 week

- **Sublingually**

  (as desmopressin base)

  **Child 5–18 years** 120 micrograms at bedtime, increased to 240 micrograms at bedtime only if lower dose not effective (**important:** see also Cautions); reassess after 3 months by withdrawing treatment for at least 1 week

**Fibrinolytic response testing**

- **By intravenous injection over 20 minutes or by subcutaneous injection**

  **Child 2–18 years** 300 nanograms/kg as a single dose; blood sampled after 20 minutes for fibrinolytic activity

**Mild to moderate haemophilia and von Willebrand's disease**

- **By intravenous infusion over 20 minutes or by subcutaneous injection**

  **Child 1 month–18 years** 300 nanograms/kg as a single dose immediately before surgery or after trauma; may be repeated at intervals of 12 hours if no tachycardia

- **Intranasally**

  **Child 1–18 years** 4 micrograms/kg as a single dose, for pre-operative use give 2 hours before procedure

**Renal function testing**

- **Intranasally**

  **Child 1 month–1 year** 10 micrograms (empty bladder at time of administration and restrict fluid intake to 50% at next 2 feeds to avoid fluid overload)

  **Child 1–15 years** 20 micrograms (empty bladder at time of administration and restrict fluid intake to 500 mL from 1 hour before until 8 hours after administration to avoid fluid overload)

  **Child 15–18 years** 40 micrograms (empty bladder at time of administration and restrict fluid intake to 500 mL from 1 hour before until 8 hours after administration to avoid fluid overload)

- **By subcutaneous or intramuscular injection**

  **Child 1 month–1 year** 400 nanograms (empty bladder at time of administration and restrict fluid intake to 50% at next 2 feeds to avoid fluid overload)

  **Child 1–18 years** 2 micrograms (empty bladder at time of administration and restrict fluid intake to 500 mL from 1 hour before until 8 hours after administration to avoid fluid overload)

**Desmopressin acetate** (Non-proprietary) PoM

Tablets, desmopressin acetate 100 micrograms, net price 90-tab pack = £50.57; 200 micrograms, 30-tab pack = £24.36, 90-tab pack = £69.82. Counselling, fluid intake, see above

Nasal spray, desmopressin acetate 10 micrograms/metered spray, net price 6-mL unit (60 metered sprays) = £18.74. Counselling, fluid intake, see above
**Brands include** *Presinex*®
**Note** Children requiring dose of less than 10 micrograms should be given *DDAVP*® intranasal solution

**DDAVP**® (Ferring) PoM
Tablets, both scored, desmopressin acetate 100 micrograms, net price 90-tab pack = £44.12; 200 micrograms, 90-tab pack = £88.23. Counselling, fluid intake, see above
**Note** Tablets may be crushed

Oral lyophilisates, (*DDAVP*® *Melt*), desmopressin (as acetate) 60 micrograms, net price 100-tab pack = £50.53; 120 micrograms, 100-tab pack = £101.07; 240 micrograms, 100-tab pack = £202.14. For sublingual administration. Label: 26, counselling, fluid intake, see notes above

Intranasal solution, desmopressin acetate 100 micrograms/mL. Net price 2.5-mL dropper bottle and catheter = £9.72. Counselling, fluid intake, see above
**Administration** May be diluted with Sodium Chloride 0.9% to a concentration of 10 micrograms/mL

Injection, desmopressin acetate 4 micrograms/mL. Net price 1-mL amp = £1.10
**Administration** May be administered orally [unlicensed]; for intravenous infusion, higher doses used in mild to moderate haemophilia and von Willebrand's disease may be diluted with 30–50 mL Sodium Chloride 0.9% intravenous infusion

**Desmomelt**® (Ferring) PoM
Oral lyophilisates, desmopressin (as acetate) 120 micrograms, net price 30-tab pack = £30.34; 240 micrograms, 30-tab pack = £60.68. For sublingual administration. Label: 26, counselling, fluid intake, see above

**Desmotabs**® (Ferring) PoM
Tablets, scored, desmopressin acetate 200 micrograms, net price 30-tab pack = £29.43. Counselling, fluid intake, see above
**Note** tablets may be crushed

**Desmospray**® (Ferring) PoM
Nasal spray, desmopressin acetate 10 micrograms/metered spray, net price 6-mL unit (60 metered sprays) = £25.02. Counselling, fluid intake, see above
**Note** Children requiring dose of less than 10 micrograms should be given *DDAVP*® intranasal solution

**Low dose Desmospray**® (Ferring) PoM
Nasal spray, desmopressin acetate 2.5 micrograms/metered spray
Available from Ferring on a named-patient basis

**Octim**® (Ferring) PoM
Nasal spray, desmopressin acetate 150 micrograms/metered spray, net price 2.5-mL unit (25 metered sprays) = £576.60. Counselling, fluid intake, see above

Injection, desmopressin acetate 15 micrograms/mL, net price 1-mL amp = £19.22
**Administration** for *intravenous infusion* dilute with 50 mL of Sodium Chloride 0.9% and give over 20 minutes

## ▌ TERLIPRESSIN ACETATE

**Cautions** see under Vasopressin
**Contra-indications** see under Vasopressin
**Pregnancy** avoid
**Breast-feeding** no information available
**Side-effects** see under Vasopressin, but effects milder
**Licensed use** unlicensed for use in children
**Indications and dose**

> Adjunct in acute massive haemorrhage of gastrointestinal tract or oesophageal varices (specialist use only)
>
> - By intravenous injection
>   **Child 12–18 years** initially 2 mg then 1–2 mg every 4–6 hours until bleeding is controlled; max. duration of treatment 72 hours

**Glypressin**® (Ferring) PoM
Injection, powder for reconstitution, terlipressin acetate, net price 1-mg vial with 5 mL diluent = £18.47
Injection, solution for injection, terlipressin acetate, 0.12 mg/mL, net price 1-mg (8.5 mL) vial = £19.39

**Variquel**® (Sinclair IS) PoM
Injection, powder for reconstitution, terlipressin acetate, net price 1-mg vial with 5 mL diluent = £17.90

## ▌ VASOPRESSIN

**Cautions** heart failure, hypertension, asthma, epilepsy, migraine or other conditions which might be aggravated by water retention; avoid fluid overload
**Contra-indications** vascular disease (especially disease of coronary arteries) unless extreme caution, chronic nephritis (until reasonable blood nitrogen concentrations attained)
**Renal impairment** see Contra-indications
**Pregnancy** oxytocic effect in third trimester
**Breast-feeding** not known to be harmful
**Side-effects** fluid retention, pallor, tremor, sweating, vertigo, headache, nausea, vomiting, belching, abdominal cramps, desire to defaecate, hypersensitivity reactions (including anaphylaxis), constriction of coronary arteries (may cause anginal attacks and myocardial ischaemia), peripheral ischaemia and rarely gangrene
**Licensed use** not licensed for use in children
**Indications and dose**

> Adjunct in acute massive haemorrhage of gastrointestinal tract or oesophageal varices (specialist use only)
>
> - By continuous intravenous infusion (may also be infused directly into the superior mesenteric artery)
>   **Child 1 month–18 years** initially 0.3 units/kg (max. 20 units) over 20–30 minutes *then* 0.3 units/kg/hour, adjusted according to response (max. 1 unit/kg/hour); if bleeding stops, continue at same dose for 12 hours, then withdraw gradually over 24–48 hours; max. duration of treatment 72 hours

**6**

**Endocrine system**

**Administration** for *intravenous infusion* dilute with Glucose 5% or Sodium Chloride 0.9% to a concentration of 0.2–1 unit/mL

◀ **Synthetic vasopressin**

**Pitressin®** (Goldshield) [PoM]
Injection, argipressin (synthetic vasopressin) 20 units/mL, net price 1-mL amp = £17.14 (hosp. only)

## 6.6 Drugs affecting bone metabolism

6.6.1  Calcitonin
6.6.2  Bisphosphonates

The two main disorders of bone metabolism that occur in children are rickets and osteoporosis. The two most common forms of rickets are Vitamin D deficiency rickets (section 9.6.4) and hypophosphataemic rickets (section 9.5.2). See also calcium (section 9.5.1.1).

## Osteoporosis

Osteoporosis in children may be primary (e.g. *osteogenesis imperfecta*, and *idiopathic juvenile osteoporosis*), or secondary (e.g. due to inflammatory disorders, immobilisation, or corticosteroids); specialist management is required.

**Corticosteroid-induced osteoporosis** To reduce the risk of osteoporosis doses of oral corticosteroids should be as low as possible and courses of treatment as short as possible.

### 6.6.1 Calcitonin

Calcitonin is involved with parathyroid hormone in the regulation of bone turnover and hence in the maintenance of calcium balance and homeostasis. **Calcitonin (salmon)** (**salcatonin**, synthetic or recombinant salmon calcitonin) is used by specialists to lower the plasma-calcium concentration in children with hypercalcaemia associated with malignancy.

### ◀ CALCITONIN (SALMON)/ SALCATONIN

**Cautions** history of allergy (skin test advised); heart failure; avoid prolonged use—risk of malignancy (use lowest effective dose for shortest possible time); monitor bone growth

**Contra-indications** hypocalcaemia

**Renal impairment** use with caution

**Pregnancy** avoid unless essential, toxicity in *animal* studies

**Breast-feeding** avoid unless essential, may inhibit lactation

**Side-effects** nausea, vomiting, diarrhoea, abdominal pain, taste disturbance, flushing, dizziness, headache, fatigue, malignancy (with long-term use) musculoskeletal pain; *less commonly* hypertension, oedema, cough, polyuria, visual disturbances, injection-site reactions, rash, hypersensitivity reactions including pruritus; *also reported* tremor

**Licensed use** not licensed in children

**Indications and dose**

**Hypercalcaemia (experience limited in children)** (specialist use only)

• **By subcutaneous or intramuscular injection**
    **Child 1 month–18 years** 2.5–5 units/kg every 12 hours, max. 400 units every 6–8 hours, adjusted according to response (no additional benefit with over 8 units/kg every 6 hours)

• **By slow intravenous infusion**
    **Child 1 month–18 years** 5–10 units/kg over at least 6 hours

**Osteoporosis** (specialist use only)
    Refer for specialist advice, experience very limited

**Administration** for *intravenous infusion*, dilute injection solution (e.g. 400 units in 500 mL) with Sodium Chloride 0.9% and give over at least 6 hours; glass or hard plastic containers should not be used; some loss of potency on dilution and administration—use diluted solution without delay

**Miacalcic®** (Novartis) [PoM]
Injection, calcitonin (salmon) 50 units/mL, net price 1-mL amp = £3.42; 100 units/mL, 1-mL amp = £6.85; 200 units/mL, 2-mL vial = £30.75

### 6.6.2 Bisphosphonates

Bisphosphonates are adsorbed on to hydroxyapatite crystals in bone, slowing both their rate of growth and dissolution, and therefore reducing the rate of bone turnover.

A bisphosphonate such as **disodium pamidronate** is used in the management of severe forms of *osteogenesis imperfecta* and other causes of osteoporosis in children to reduce the number of fractures; the long-term effects of bisphosphonates in children have not been established. Single doses of biphosphonates are also used to manage hypercalaemia (section 9.5.1.2). Treatment should be initiated under specialist advice **only**.

> **Bisphosphonates: osteonecrosis of the jaw**
>
> The risk of osteonecrosis of the jaw is substantially greater for patients receiving intravenous bisphosphonates in the treatment of cancer than for patients receiving oral bisphosphonates for osteoporosis or Paget's disease.
>
> Risk factors for developing osteonecrosis of the jaw that should be considered are: potency of bisphosphonate (highest for zoledronate), route of administration, cumulative dose, duration and type of malignant disease, concomitant treatment, smoking, comorbid conditions, and history of dental disease.
>
> All patients should have a dental check-up (and any necessary remedial work should be performed) before bisphosphonate treatment, or as soon as possible after starting treatment.
>
> During bisphosphonate treatment patients should maintain good oral hygiene, receive routine dental check-ups, and report any oral symptoms.
>
> Guidance for dentists in primary care is included in *Oral Health Management of Patients Prescribed Bisphosphonates: Dental Clinical Guidance*, Scottish Dental Clinical Effectiveness Programme, April 2011 (available at www.sdcep.org.uk).

*(left margin)* **6** Endocrine system

<table>
<tr><td>

MHRA/CHM advice
**Bisphosphonates: atypical femoral fractures (June 2011)**

Atypical femoral fractures have been reported rarely with bisphosphonate treatment, mainly in patients receiving long-term treatment for osteoporosis.

The need to continue bisphosphonate treatment for osteoporosis should be re-evaluated periodically based on an assessment of the benefits and risks of treatment for individual patients, particularly after 5 or more years of use.

Patients should be advised to report any thigh, hip, or groin pain during treatment with a bisphosphonate.

Discontinuation of bisphosphonate treatment in patients suspected to have an atypical femoral fracture should be considered after an assessment of the benefits and risks of continued treatment.

</td></tr>
</table>

## ALENDRONIC ACID

**Cautions** upper gastro-intestinal disorders (dysphagia, symptomatic oesophageal disease, gastritis, duodenitis, or ulcers—see also under Contra-indications and Side-effects); history (within 1 year) of ulcers, active gastro-intestinal bleeding, or surgery of the upper gastro-intestinal tract; correct disturbances of calcium and mineral metabolism (e.g. vitamin-D deficiency, hypocalcaemia) before starting and monitor serum-calcium concentration during treatment; consider dental check-up before initiating bisphosphonate (risk of osteonecrosis of the jaw, see Bisphosphonates: Osteonecrosis of the Jaw, p. 388); exclude other causes of osteoporosis; atypical femoral fractures, see MHRA/CHM advice, above; **interactions**: Appendix 1 (bisphosphonates)

**Contra-indications** abnormalities of oesophagus and other factors which delay emptying (e.g. stricture or achalasia), hypocalcaemia

**Renal impairment** avoid if estimated glomerular filtration rate is less than $35 \, \text{mL/minute/} 1.73 \, \text{m}^2$

**Pregnancy** avoid

**Breast-feeding** no information available

**Side-effects** oesophageal reactions (see below), abdominal pain and distension, dyspepsia, regurgitation, melaena, diarrhoea or constipation, flatulence, musculoskeletal pain, headache; *rarely* rash, pruritus, erythema, photosensitivity, uveitis, scleritis, transient decrease in serum phosphate; nausea, vomiting, gastritis, peptic ulceration, hypersensitivity reactions (including urticaria and angioedema), atypical femoral fractures with long term use, see MHRA/ CHM advice, above; myalgia, malaise, and fever at initiation of treatment; *very rarely* severe skin reactions (including Stevens-Johnson syndrome), osteonecrosis of the jaw (see Bisphosphonates: Osteonecrosis of the Jaw, p. 388)

**Oesophageal reactions** Severe oesophageal reactions (oesophagitis, oesophageal ulcers, oesophageal stricture and oesophageal erosions) have been reported; patients should be advised to stop taking the tablets and to seek medical attention if they develop symptoms of oesophageal irritation such as dysphagia, new or worsening heartburn, pain on swallowing or retrosternal pain

**Licensed use** not licensed for use in children

### Indications and dose

See notes above, specialist use only

**Counselling** Swallow the tablets whole with a full glass of water on an empty stomach at least 30 minutes before breakfast (and any other oral medication); stand or sit upright for at least 30 minutes and do not lie down until after eating breakfast. Do not take the tablets at bedtime or before rising

**Alendronic acid** (Non-proprietary) ℗ₒ𝖬

Tablets, alendronic acid (as sodium alendronate) 10 mg, net price 28-tab pack = £1.44; 70 mg, 4-tab pack = £1.10. Counselling, administration

Oral solution, sugar-free, alendronic acid (as sodium alendronate) 70 mg/100 mL, net price 4 × 100-mL single-use bottles = £22.80.Counselling, administration

**Counselling** oral solution intended for single use only; swallow required dose with plenty of water while sitting or standing; to be taken on an empty stomach at least 30 minutes before breakfast (or another oral medicine); patients should stand or sit upright for at least 30 minutes after taking the solution

**Fosamax**® (MSD) ℗ₒ𝖬

Tablets, alendronic acid (as sodium alendronate) 10 mg, 28-tab pack = £23.12. Counselling, administration

**Fosamax**® **Once Weekly** (MSD) ℗ₒ𝖬

Tablets, alendronic acid (as sodium alendronate) 70 mg, net price 4-tab pack = £22.80. Counselling, administration

## DISODIUM PAMIDRONATE

Disodium pamidronate was formerly called aminohydroxypropylidenediphosphonate disodium (APD)

**Cautions** cardiac disease; previous thyroid surgery (risk of hypocalcaemia); monitor serum electrolytes, calcium, and phosphate—possibility of convulsions due to electrolyte changes; ensure adequate hydration; avoid concurrent use with other bisphosphonates; consider dental check-up before initiating bisphosphonate (risk of osteonecrosis of the jaw, see Bisphosphonates: Osteonecrosis of the Jaw, p. 388); atypical femoral fractures, see MHRA/CHM advice, above; **interactions**: Appendix 1 (bisphosphonates)

**Skilled tasks** Patients should be warned against driving, cycling, or performing skilled tasks immediately after treatment (somnolence or dizziness can occur)

**Hepatic impairment** use with caution in severe impairment—no information available

**Renal impairment** monitor renal function in renal disease or predisposition to renal impairment (e.g. in tumour-induced hypercalcaemia)

**Pregnancy** avoid—toxicity in *animal* studies

**Breast-feeding** avoid

**Side-effects** hypophosphataemia, transient rise in body temperature, fever and influenza-like symptoms (sometimes accompanied by malaise, rigors, fatigue, and flushes); arthralgia, myalgia, bone pain, nausea, vomiting, headache, lymphocytopenia, hypomagnesaemia; *rarely* muscle cramps, atypical femoral fractures, see MHRA/CHM advice, above, anorexia, abdominal pain, diarrhoea, constipation, dyspepsia, agitation, confusion, dizziness, insomnia, somnolence, lethargy, anaemia, leucopenia, hypotension or hypertension, rash, pruritus, symptomatic hypocalcaemia (paraesthesia, tetany), hyperkalaemia or hypokalaemia, hypernatraemia; osteonecrosis of the jaw (see Bisphosphonates: Osteonecrosis of the Jaw,

**6  Endocrine system**

p. 388); isolated cases of seizures, hallucinations, thrombocytopenia, haematuria, acute renal failure, deterioration of renal disease, conjunctivitis and other ocular symptoms; atrial fibrillation, and reactivation of herpes simplex and zoster also reported; also local reactions at injection site

**Licensed use** not licensed for use in children

**Indications and dose**

See notes above, specialist use only

**Disodium pamidronate** (Non-proprietary) PoM
Concentrate for intravenous infusion, disodium pamidronate 3 mg/mL, net price 5-mL vial = £27.50, 10-mL vial = £55.00; 6 mg/mL, 10-mL vial = £95.00; 9 mg/mL, 10-mL vial = £165.00; 15 mg/mL, 1-mL vial = £29.83, 2-mL vial = £59.66, 4-mL vial = £119.32, 6-mL vial £170.46

**Aredia Dry Powder®** (Novartis) PoM
Injection, powder for reconstitution, disodium pamidronate, for use as an infusion. Net price 15-mg vial = £29.83; 30-mg vial = £59.66; 90-mg vial = £170.45 (all with diluent)

### ▌RISEDRONATE SODIUM

**Cautions** oesophageal abnormalities and other factors which delay transit or emptying (e.g. stricture or achalasia—see also under Side-effects); correct hypocalcaemia before starting, correct other disturbances of bone and mineral metabolism (e.g. Vitamin-D deficiency) at onset of treatment; consider dental check-up before initiating bisphosphonate (risk of osteonecrosis of the jaw, see Bisphosphonates: Osteonecrosis of the Jaw, p. 388); atypical femoral fractures, see MHRA/CHM advice, p. 389; **interactions**: Appendix 1 (bisphosphonates)

**Contra-indications** hypocalcaemia (see Cautions above)

**Renal impairment** avoid if estimated glomerular filtration rate is less than 30 mL/minute/1.73 m$^2$

**Pregnancy** avoid

**Breast-feeding** avoid

**Side-effects** abdominal pain, dyspepsia, nausea, diarrhoea, constipation, headache, musculoskeletal pain; *less commonly* oesophagitis, oesophageal ulcer, dysphagia, gastritis, duodenitis, uveitis; *rarely* glossitis, oesophageal stricture, atypical femoral fractures, see MHRA/CHM advice, p. 389; *also reported* gastroduodenal ulceration, hepatic disorders, Stevens-Johnson syndrome, toxic epidermal necrolysis, hair loss, cutaneous vasculitis, osteonecrosis of the jaw (see Bisphosphonates: Osteonecrosis of the Jaw, p. 388)

**Oesophageal reactions** Children and their carers should be advised to stop taking the tablets and seek medical attention if they develop symptoms of oesophageal irritation such as dysphagia, pain on swallowing, retrosternal pain, or heartburn

**Licensed use** not licensed for use in children

**Indications and dose**

See notes above, specialist use only

**Counselling** Swallow tablets whole with full glass of water; on rising, take on an empty stomach at least 30 minutes before first food or drink of the day **or**, if taking at any other time of the day, avoid food and drink for at least 2 hours before or after risedronate (particularly avoid calcium-containing products e.g. milk; also avoid iron and mineral supplements and antacids); stand or sit upright for at least 30 minutes; do not take tablets at bedtime or before rising

**Risedronate Sodium** (Non-proprietary) PoM
Tablets, risedronate sodium 5 mg, net price 28-tab pack = £17.99; 30 mg, 28-tab pack = £143.95; 35 mg, 4-tab pack = £19.12. Counselling, administration, food, and calcium (see above)

**Actonel®** (Warner Chilcott) PoM
Tablets, f/c, risedronate sodium 5 mg (yellow), net price 28-tab pack = £17.99; 30 mg (white), 28-tab pack = £143.95. Counselling, administration, food, and calcium (see above)

**Actonel Once a Week®** (Warner Chilcott) PoM
Tablets, f/c, orange, risedronate sodium 35 mg, net price 4-tab pack = £19.12. Counselling, administration, food and calcium (see above)

### ▌SODIUM CLODRONATE

**Cautions** monitor renal and hepatic function and white cell count; also monitor serum calcium and phosphate periodically; renal dysfunction reported in patients receiving concomitant NSAIDs; maintain adequate fluid intake during treatment; consider dental check-up before initiating bisphosphonate (risk of osteonecrosis of the jaw, see Bisphosphonates: Osteonecrosis of the Jaw, p. 388); atypical femoral fractures, see MHRA/CHM advice, p. 389; **interactions**: Appendix 1 (bisphosphonates)

**Contra-indications** acute gastro-intestinal inflammatory conditions

**Renal impairment** use half normal dose if estimated glomerular filtration rate 10–30 mL/minute/1.73 m$^2$; avoid if estimated glomerular filtration rate less than 10 mL/minute/1.73 m$^2$

**Pregnancy** avoid

**Breast-feeding** manufacturer advises avoid—no information available

**Side-effects** nausea, vomiting, diarrhoea, skin reactions, bronchospasm; *rarely* atypical femoral fractures, see MHRA/CHM advice, p. 389; *very rarely* osteonecrosis of the jaw (see Bisphosphonates: Osteonecrosis of the Jaw, p. 388); *also reported* renal impairment

**Licensed use** not licensed for use in children

**Indications and dose**

See notes above, specialist use only

**Counselling** Avoid food for 2 hours before and 1 hour after oral treatment, particularly calcium-containing products e.g. milk; also avoid iron and mineral supplements and antacids; maintain adequate fluid intake

**Bonefos®** (Bayer) PoM
Capsules, yellow, sodium clodronate 400 mg. Net price 120-cap pack = £139.83. Counselling, food and calcium

Tablets, f/c, scored, sodium clodronate 800 mg. Net price 60-tab pack = £146.43. Counselling, food and calcium

**Clasteon®** (Beacon) PoM
Capsules, blue/white, sodium clodronate 400 mg, net price 30-cap pack = £34.96, 120-cap pack = £139.83. Counselling, food and calcium

Tablets, f/c, sodium clodronate 800 mg, net price 60-tab pack = £146.43. Counselling, food and calcium

**Loron®** (Intrapharm) PoM
Loron 520® tablets, f/c, scored, sodium clodronate 520 mg, net price 60-tab pack = £152.59. Label: 10, patient information leaflet, counselling, food and calcium

## 6.7　Other endocrine drugs

**6.7.1**　Bromocriptine and other dopaminergic drugs
**6.7.2**　Drugs affecting gonadotrophins
**6.7.3**　Metyrapone
**6.7.4**　Somatomedins

### 6.7.1　Bromocriptine and other dopaminergic drugs

Classification not used in *BNF for Children*.

### 6.7.2　Drugs affecting gonadotrophins

Classification not used in *BNF for Children*. See section 6.4.2 for use in precocious puberty.

### 6.7.3　Metyrapone

**Metyrapone** is a competitive inhibitor of 11β-hydroxylation in the adrenal cortex; the resulting inhibition of cortisol (and to a lesser extent aldosterone) production leads to an increase in ACTH production which, in turn, leads to increased synthesis and release of cortisol precursors. It is used as a test of anterior pituitary function.

Most types of *Cushing's syndrome* are treated surgically. Metyrapone may be useful to control the symptoms of the disease or to prepare the child for surgery. The dosages used are either low, and tailored to cortisol production, or high, in which case corticosteroid replacement therapy is also needed.

**Ketoconazole** (section 5.2.2) is also used by specialists for the management of *Cushing's syndrome* [unlicensed indication].

### ▌ METYRAPONE

**Cautions** gross hypopituitarism (risk of precipitating acute adrenal failure); hypertension on long-term administration; hypothyroidism (delayed response); many drugs interfere with diagnostic estimation of steroids; avoid in acute porphyria (section 9.8.2) **Skilled tasks** Drowsiness may affect the performance of skilled tasks (e.g. driving)

**Contra-indications** adrenocortical insufficiency (see Cautions)

**Hepatic impairment** use with caution (delayed response)

**Pregnancy** avoid (may impair biosynthesis of fetal-placental steroids)

**Breast-feeding** avoid—no information available

**Side-effects** occasional nausea, vomiting, dizziness, headache, hypotension, sedation; rarely abdominal pain, allergic skin reactions, hypoadrenalism, hirsutism

**Licensed use** licensed for use in children

**Indications and dose**

> Differential diagnosis of ACTH-dependent Cushing's syndrome
> • By mouth
>> **Child 1 month–18 years** 15 mg/kg (or 300 mg/m²) every 4 hours for 6 doses; minimum dose 250 mg every 4 hours, max. 750 mg every 4 hours

> Management of Cushing's syndrome
> • By mouth
>> Range 250 mg–6 g daily, adjusted according to cortisol production; see notes above

**Metopirone®** (HRA Pharma) PoM
Capsules, ivory, metyrapone 250 mg, net price 100-cap pack = £363.66. Label: 21, counselling, driving

### 6.7.4　Somatomedins

Somatomedins are a group of polypeptide hormones structurally related to insulin and commonly known as insulin-like growth factors (IGFs). **Mecasermin**, a human insulin-like growth factor-I (rhIGF-I), is the principal mediator of the somatotropic effects of human growth hormone and is used to treat growth failure in children with severe primary insulin-like growth factor-I deficiency.

### ▌ MECASERMIN
#### (Recombinant human insulin-like growth factor-I; rhIGF-I)

**Cautions** correct hypothyroidism before initiating treatment; diabetes mellitus (adjustment of antidiabetic therapy may be necessary); monitor ECG before and on termination of treatment (and during treatment if ECG abnormal); papilloedema (see under Side-effects); monitor for disorders of the epiphysis of the hip (monitor for limping); monitor for signs of tonsillar hypertrophy (snoring, sleep apnoea, and chronic middle ear effusions)

**Contra-indications** evidence of tumour activity (discontinue treatment)

**Pregnancy** avoid unless essential; contraception advised in women of child-bearing potential

**Breast-feeding** avoid

**Side-effects** headache, funduscopy for papilloedema recommended if severe or recurrent headache, visual problems, nausea and vomiting occur—if papilloedema confirmed consider benign intracranial hypertension (rare cases reported); cardiomegaly, ventricular hypertrophy, tachycardia; convulsions, sleep apnoea, night terrors, dizziness, nervousness; tonsillar hypertrophy (see Cautions above); hypoglycaemia (especially in first month, and in younger children), hyperglycaemia, gynaecomastia; arthralgia, myalgia; visual disturbance, impaired hearing; antibody formation; injection-site reactions (rotate site)

6　Endocrine system

**Indications and dose**

Growth failure in children with severe primary
insulin-like growth factor-I deficiency

• By subcutaneous injection

Child 2–18 years initially 40 micrograms/kg twice
daily for 1 week, if tolerated increase dose in steps
of 40 micrograms/kg to max. 120 micrograms/kg
twice daily; discontinue if no response within 1
year

Counselling Dose should be administered just before or
after food; do not increase dose if a dose is missed

Note Reduce dose if hypoglycaemia occurs despite
adequate food intake; withhold injection if patient unable to
eat

**Increlex®** (Ipsen) PoM
Injection, mecasermin 10 mg/mL, net price 4-mL
vial = £605.00. Counselling, administration
Excipients include benzyl alcohol (avoid in neonates, see
Excipients, p. 2)

# 7 Obstetrics, gynaecology, and urinary-tract disorders

## 7.1 Drugs used in obstetrics

This section is not included in *BNF for Children*. See BNF for management of obstetrics.

For the management of ductus arteriosus, see section 2.14.

## 7.2 Treatment of vaginal and vulval conditions

### 7.2.1 Preparations for vaginal and vulval changes
### 7.2.2 Vaginal and vulval infections

Pre-pubertal girls may be particularly susceptible to vulvovaginitis. Barrier preparations (section 13.2.2) applied after cleansing can be useful when the symptoms are due to non-specific irritation, but systemic drugs are required in the treatment of bacterial infection (section 5.1) or threadworm infestation (section 5.5.1). Intravaginal preparations, particularly those that require the use of an applicator, are not generally suitable for young girls; topical preparations may be useful in some adolescent girls.

In older girls symptoms are often restricted to the vulva, but infections almost invariably involve the vagina, which should also be treated; treatment should be as for adults, see BNF section 7.2.2.

### 7.2.1 Preparations for vaginal and vulval changes

Topical oestrogen creams containing **estriol** 0.01% (*Gynest*®) are used in the treatment of labial adhesions (for details of preparation, see BNF section 7.2.1); treatment is usually restricted to symptomatic cases. Estriol cream should be applied to the adhesions once or twice daily for 2–6 weeks; adhesions may recur following treatment.

### 7.2.2 Vaginal and vulval infections

Effective specific treatments are available for the common vaginal infections.

#### Fungal infections

Vaginal fungal infections are not normally a problem in younger girls but can occur in adolescents. *Candidal*

7 Obstetrics, gynaecology, and urinary-tract disorders

*vulvitis* can be treated locally with cream, but is almost invariably associated with vaginal infection which should also be treated. *Vaginal candidiasis*, rare in girls before puberty, can be treated with antifungal pessaries or cream inserted high into the vagina (including during menstruation), however, these are not recommended for pre-pubertal girls and treatment with an external cream may be more appropriate. Single-dose intravaginal preparations offer an advantage when compliance is a problem. Local irritation can occur on application of vaginal antifungal products.

**Imidazole** drugs (clotrimazole, econazole, fenticonazole, and miconazole) are effective against candida in short courses of 1 to 3 days according to the preparation used; treatment can be repeated if initial course fails to control symptoms or if symptoms recur. Vaginal applications may be supplemented with antifungal cream for vulvitis and to treat other superficial sites of infection.

Oral treatment of vaginal infection with fluconazole (section 5.2.1) may be considered for girls post-puberty.

**Vulvovaginal candidiasis in pregnancy** Vulvovaginal candidiasis is common during pregnancy and can be treated with vaginal application of an imidazole (such as clotrimazole), and a topical imidazole cream for vulvitis. Pregnant women need a longer duration of treatment, usually about 7 days, to clear the infection. There is limited absorption of imidazoles from the skin and vagina. Oral antifungal treatment should be avoided during pregnancy.

**Recurrent vulvovaginal candidiasis** Recurrent vulvovaginal candidiasis is very rare in children, but can occur if there are predisposing factors such as antibacterial therapy, pregnancy, diabetes mellitus, or possibly oral contraceptive use. Reservoirs of infection can also lead to recontamination and should be treated; these include other skin sites such as the digits, nail beds, and umbilicus, as well as the gastro-intestinal tract and the bladder. The sexual partner may also be the source of re-infection and, if symptomatic, should be treated with a topical imidazole cream at the same time.

Treatment against candida may need to be extended for 6 months in recurrent vulvovaginal candidiasis. Some recommended regimens suitable for older children [all unlicensed] include:

- initially, fluconazole (section 5.2.1) 150 mg by mouth every 72 hours for 3 doses, then 150 mg once every week for 6 months;
- initially, intravaginal application of a topical imidazole for 10–14 days, then clotrimazole 500-mg pessary once every week for 6 months.

## PREPARATIONS FOR VAGINAL AND VULVAL CANDIDIASIS

**Cautions** avoid intravaginal preparations (particularly those that require use of an applicator) in young girls who are not sexually active, unless there is no alternative; **interactions**: Appendix 1 (miconazole)

**Pregnancy** see notes above

**Side-effects** occasional local irritation

**Licensed use** consult product literature for individual preparations

**Indications and dose**

See notes above and under preparations below

**Clotrimazole** (Non-proprietary)
Cream (topical), clotrimazole 1%, net price 20 g = £1.52, 50 g = £4.12
**Condoms** effect on latex condoms and diaphragms not yet known
Dose
Apply to anogenital area 2–3 times daily

Pessary, clotrimazole 500 mg, net price 1 pessary with applicator = £3.13
Dose
Insert 1 pessary at night as a single dose; can be repeated once if necessary

**Canesten®** (Bayer Consumer Care)
Cream (topical), clotrimazole 1%, net price 20 g = £2.14; 50 g = £3.50
**Excipients** include benzyl alcohol, cetostearyl alcohol, polysorbates
**Condoms** damages latex condoms and diaphragms
Dose
Apply to anogenital area 2–3 times daily

Thrush Cream (topical), clotrimazole 2%, net price 20 g = £3.99
**Excipients** include benzyl alcohol, cetostearyl alcohol, polysorbates
**Condoms** damages latex condoms and diaphragms
Dose
Apply to anogenital area 2–3 times daily

Intravaginal cream (*10% VC®*) (PoM), clotrimazole 10%, net price 5-g applicator pack = £4.50
**Excipients** include benzyl alcohol, cetostearyl alcohol, polysorbates
**Condoms** damages latex condoms and diaphragms
Dose
Insert 5 g at night as a single dose; may be repeated once if necessary

Note Brands for sale to the public include *Canesten® Internal Cream*

Cream Combi, clotrimazole 10% vaginal cream and 2% topical cream, net price 5-g vaginal cream (with applicator) and 10-g topical cream = £6.81
**Excipients** include benzyl alcohol, cetostearyl alcohol, polysorbates
**Condoms** damages latex condoms and diaphragms
Dose
See under individual components

Pessaries, clotrimazole 200 mg, 3 pessaries with applicator = £3.63
**Condoms** damages latex condoms and diaphragms
Dose
Insert 200 mg for 3 nights; course may be repeated once if necessary

Pessary, clotrimazole 500 mg, net price 1 pessary with applicator = £2.00
**Excipients** none as listed in section 13.1.3
**Condoms** damages latex condoms and diaphragms
Dose
Insert 1 pessary at night as a single dose; may be repeated once if necessary

Pessary Combi, clotrimazole 500-mg pessary and cream (topical) 2%, net price 1 pessary and 10-g cream = £5.21

**Excipients** include benzyl alcohol, cetostearyl alcohol, polysorbates

**Condoms** damages latex condoms and diaphragms
**Dose**
> See under individual components

Soft Gel Pessary, clotrimazole 500 mg, net price 1 pessary with applicator = £6.41

**Condoms** damages latex condoms and diaphragms
**Dose**
> Insert 1 pessary at night as a single dose; may be repeated once if necessary

Soft Gel Pessary Combi, clotrimazole 500-mg soft gel pessary and cream (topical) 2%, net price 1 pessary and 10-g cream = £5.73

**Excipients** include benzyl alcohol, cetostearyl alcohol, polysorbates

**Condoms** damages latex condoms and diaphragms
**Dose**
> See under individual components

**Gyno-Daktarin®** (Janssen) (PoM)

Ovule (= vaginal capsule) (*Gyno-Daktarin 1®*), miconazole nitrate 1.2 g in a fatty basis, net price 1 ovule = £2.94

**Excipients** include hydroxybenzoates (parabens)

**Condoms** damages latex condoms and diaphragms
**Dose**
> Insert 1 ovule at night as a single dose; can be repeated once if necessary

**Gyno-Pevaryl®** (Janssen) (PoM)

Pessaries, econazole nitrate 150 mg, net price 3 pessaries = £2.78

**Excipients** none as listed in section 13.1.3

**Condoms** damages latex condoms and diaphragms
**Dose**
> Insert 1 pessary for 3 nights; course can be repeated once if necessary

Pessary (*Gyno-Pevaryl 1®*), econazole nitrate 150 mg, formulated for single-dose therapy, net price 1 pessary with applicator = £2.95

**Excipients** none as listed in section 13.1.3

**Condoms** damages latex condoms and diaphragms
**Dose**
> Insert 1 pessary at night as a single dose; can be repeated once if necessary

**Gynoxin®** (Recordati) (PoM)

Intravaginal cream, fenticonazole nitrate 2%, net price 30 g with applicator = £3.74

**Excipients** include cetyl alcohol, hydrogenated wool fat, propylene glycol

**Condoms** damages latex condoms and diaphragms
**Dose**
> Insert 5-g applicatorful intravaginally twice daily for 3 days

Vaginal capsule, fenticonazole nitrate 200 mg, net price 3 vaginal capsules = £2.42

**Excipients** include hydroxybenzoates (parabens)

**Condoms** damages latex condoms and diaphragms
**Dose**
> Insert 1 vaginal capsule at night for 3 nights

Vaginal capsule, fenticonazole nitrate 600 mg, net price 1 vaginal capsule = £2.62

**Excipients** include hydroxybenzoates (parabens)

**Condoms** damages latex condoms and diaphragms
**Dose**
> Insert 1 vaginal capsule at night as a single dose

**Nizoral®** (Janssen) (PoM)

Cream (topical), ketoconazole 2%, net price 30 g = £3.40

**Excipients** include polysorbates, propylene glycol, stearyl alcohol

**Condoms** effect on latex condoms and diaphragms not yet known
**Dose**
> Apply to anogenital area once or twice daily

## Other infections

*Trichomonal infections* commonly involve the lower urinary tract as well as the genital system and need systemic treatment with metronidazole (section 5.1.11) or tinidazole (section 5.4.2).

*Bacterial infections* with Gram-negative organisms are particularly common in association with gynaecological operations and trauma. Metronidazole is effective against certain Gram-negative organisms, especially *Bacteroides* spp. and can be used prophylactically in gynaecological surgery.

Clindamycin cream and metronidazole gel are indicated for bacterial vaginosis.

The antiviral drugs aciclovir, famciclovir, and valaciclovir can be used in the treatment of genital infection due to *herpes simplex virus*, the HSV type 2 being a major cause of genital ulceration. They have a beneficial effect on virus shedding and healing, generally giving relief from pain and other symptoms. See section 5.3 for systemic preparations, and section 13.10.3 for topical preparations.

## PREPARATIONS FOR OTHER VAGINAL INFECTIONS

**Cautions** avoid intravaginal preparations (particularly those that require the use of an applicator) in young girls who are not sexually active, unless there is no alternative.

**Balance Activ Rx®** (BBI Healthcare)

Vaginal gel, lactic acid 4.9%, glycogen 0.1%, net price 7 x 5 mL-tube = £5.25

**Excipients** include propylene glycol
**Dose**
**Prevention of bacterial vaginosis**
> Insert contents of 1 tube once or twice weekly

**Dalacin®** (Pharmacia) (PoM)

Cream, clindamycin 2% (as phosphate), net price 40-g pack with 7 applicators = £10.86

**Excipients** include benzyl alcohol, cetostearyl alcohol, polysorbates, propylene glycol

**Condoms** damages latex condoms and diaphragms

**Side-effects** irritation, cervicitis and vaginitis; poorly absorbed into the blood—low risk of systemic effects, see section 5.1.6

**Licensed use** not licensed for use in children
**Dose**
**Bacterial vaginosis**
> Insert 5-g applicatorful at night for 3–7 nights

**Zidoval®** (Meda) PoM
Vaginal gel, metronidazole 0.75%, net price 40-g
pack with 5 applicators = £4.31
**Excipients** include disodium edetate, hydroxybenzoates
(parabens), propylene glycol
**Side-effects** local effects including irritation,
candidiasis, abnormal discharge, pelvic discomfort
**Licensed use** not licensed for use in children under 18
years
**Note** Not recommended during menstruation; some
absorption may occur, see section 5.1.11 for systemic effects
**Dose**

**Bacterial vaginosis**

Insert 5-g applicatorful at night for 5 nights

## 7.3 Contraceptives

7.3.1   **Combined hormonal contraceptives**
7.3.2   **Progestogen-only contraceptives**
7.3.3   **Spermicidal contraceptives**
7.3.4   **Contraceptive devices**
7.3.5   **Emergency contraception**

The Fraser Guidelines[1] should be followed when prescribing contraception for women under 16 years. The
UK Medical Eligibility Criteria for Contraceptive Use
(available at www.fsrh.org) is published by the Faculty
of Sexual and Reproductive Healthcare; it categorises
the risks of using contraceptive methods with pre-existing medical conditions.

**Hormonal contraception** is the most effective method
of fertility control, but can have major and minor side-
effects, especially for certain groups of women. Hormonal contraception should only be used by adolescents
after menarche.

**Intra-uterine devices** are a highly effective method of
contraception but may produce undesirable local side-
effects. They may be used in women of all ages irrespective of parity but are less appropriate for those with
an increased risk of pelvic inflammatory disease.

**Barrier methods** alone (condoms, diaphragms, and
caps) are less effective but can be reliable for well-
motivated couples if used in conjunction with a **spermicide**. Occasionally sensitivity reactions occur. A
female condom (*Femidom®*) is also available; it is pre-
lubricated but does not contain a spermicide.

## 7.3.1 Combined hormonal contraceptives

Oral contraceptives containing an oestrogen and a
progestogen ('combined oral contraceptives') are effective preparations for general use. Advantages of combined oral contraceptives include:

- reliable and reversible;
- reduced dysmenorrhoea and menorrhagia;
- reduced incidence of premenstrual tension;
- reduced risk of symptomatic fibroids and functional
  ovarian cysts;
- less benign breast disease;

---

1. See Department of Health Guidance (July 2004): Best
   practice guidance for doctors and other health professionals on the provision of advice and treatment to young
   people under 16 on contraception, sexual and reproductive health. Available at www.dh.gov.uk

- reduced risk of ovarian and endometrial cancer;
- reduced risk of pelvic inflammatory disease.

Combined oral contraceptives containing a fixed
amount of an oestrogen and a progestogen in each
active tablet are termed 'monophasic'; those with varying amounts of the two hormones are termed 'phasic'. A
transdermal patch and a vaginal ring, both containing an
oestrogen with a progestogen, are also available.

**Choice** The majority of combined oral contraceptives contain ethinylestradiol as the oestrogen component; mestranol and estradiol valerate are also used.
The ethinylestradiol content of combined oral contraceptives ranges from 20 to 40 micrograms. Generally a
preparation with the lowest oestrogen and progestogen
content which gives good cycle control and minimal
side-effects in the individual woman is chosen.

- *Low strength preparations* (containing ethinylestradiol 20 micrograms) are particularly appropriate for
  women with risk factors for circulatory disease,
  provided a combined oral contraceptive is otherwise suitable.

- *Standard strength preparations* (containing ethinylestradiol 30 or 35 micrograms or in 30–40 microgram
  *phased* preparations) are appropriate for standard
  use—but see Risk of Venous Thromboembolism
  below. Phased preparations are generally reserved
  for women who *either* do not have withdrawal
  bleeding *or* who have breakthrough bleeding with
  monophasic products.

The progestogens desogestrel, drospirenone, and gestodene (in combination with ethinylestradiol) may be
considered for women who have side-effects (such as
acne, headache, depression, breast symptoms, and
breakthrough bleeding) with other progestogens. However, women should be advised that these progestogens
have also been associated with an increased risk of
*venous thromboembolism*. Drospirenone, a derivative of
spironolactone, has anti-androgenic and anti-mineralo-
corticoid activity; it should be used with care if an
increased plasma-potassium concentration might be
hazardous.

The progestogen norelgestromin is combined with ethinylestradiol in a transdermal patch (*Evra®*).

The vaginal contraceptive ring contains the progestogen etonogestrel combined with ethinylestradiol
(*NuvaRing®*).

**Risk of venous thromboembolism** There is an
increased risk of venous thromboembolic disease (particularly during the first year) in users of oral contraceptives, but this risk is considerably smaller than that
associated with pregnancy (about 60 cases of venous
thromboembolic disease per 100 000 pregnancies). In
all cases the risk of venous thromboembolism increases
with age and in the presence of other risk factors for
venous thromboembolism, such as obesity.

The incidence of venous thromboembolism in healthy,
non-pregnant women who are not taking an oral contraceptive is about 5–10 cases per 100 000 women per
year. For those using combined oral contraceptives
containing second-generation progestogens, such as
levonorgestrel, this incidence is about 20 per 100 000
women per year of use. The risk of venous thromboembolism with transdermal patches may be slightly
increased compared with combined oral contraceptives
that contain levonorgestrel. Some studies have reported

a greater risk of venous thromboembolism in women using combined oral contraceptives containing the third-generation progestogens desogestrel and gestodene; the incidence in these women is about 40 per 100 000 women per year of use. The absolute risk of venous thromboembolism in women using combined oral contraceptives containing these third-generation progestogens is very small and well below the risk associated with pregnancy. The risk of venous thromboembolism in women using a combined oral contraceptive containing drospirenone may be similar to that associated with combined oral contraceptives containing third-generation progestogens. The risk of venous thromboembolism associated with vaginal ring use compared to the risk with other combined hormonal contraceptives is unknown.

Provided that women are informed of the relative risks of venous thromboembolism and accept them, the choice of oral contraceptive is for the woman together with the prescriber jointly to make in light of her individual medical history and any contra-indications.

**Travel** Women taking oral contraceptives or using the patch or vaginal ring are at an increased risk of deep-vein thrombosis during travel involving long periods of immobility (over 3 hours). The risk may be reduced by appropriate exercise during the journey and possibly by wearing graduated compression hosiery.

**Missed pill** The critical time for loss of contraceptive protection is when a pill is omitted at the *beginning* or *end* of a cycle (which lengthens the pill-free interval).

If a woman forgets to take a pill, it should be taken as soon as she remembers, and the next one taken at the normal time (even if this means taking 2 pills together). A missed pill is one that is 24 or more hours late; for women taking *Qlaira*®, see below. If a woman misses only one pill, she should take an active pill as soon as she remembers and then resume normal pill-taking. No additional precautions are necessary.

If a woman misses 2 or more pills (especially from the first 7 in a packet), she may not be protected. She should take an active pill as soon as she remembers and then resume normal pill-taking. In addition, she must either abstain from sex or use an additional method of contraception such as a condom for the next 7 days. If these 7 days run beyond the end of the packet, the next packet should be started at once, omitting the pill-free interval (or, in the case of *everyday* (ED) pills, omitting the 7 inactive tablets).

A missed pill for a woman taking *Qlaira*® is one that is 12 hours or more late; for information on how to manage missed pills in women taking *Qlaira*®, refer to product literature.

Emergency contraception (section 7.3.5) is recommended if 2 or more combined oral contraceptive tablets are missed from the first 7 tablets in a packet and unprotected intercourse has occurred since finishing the last packet.

**Delayed application or detached patch** If a patch is partly detached for less than 24 hours, reapply to the same site or replace with a new patch immediately; no additional contraception is needed and the next patch should be applied on the usual 'change day'. If a patch remains detached for more than 24 hours or if the user is not aware when the patch became detached, then stop the current contraceptive cycle and start a new cycle by applying a new patch, giving a new

'Day 1'; an additional non-hormonal contraceptive must be used concurrently for the first 7 days of the new cycle.

If application of a new patch at the start of a new cycle is delayed, contraceptive protection is lost. A new patch should be applied as soon as remembered giving a new 'Day 1'; additional non-hormonal methods of contraception should be used for the first 7 days of the new cycle. If application of a patch in the middle of the cycle is delayed (i.e. the patch is not changed on day 8 or day 15):

- for up to 48 hours, apply a new patch immediately; next patch 'change day' remains the same and no additional contraception is required;

- for more than 48 hours, contraceptive protection may have been lost. Stop the current cycle and start a new 4-week cycle immediately by applying a new patch giving a new 'Day 1'; additional non-hormonal contraception should be used for the first 7 days of the new cycle.

If the patch is not removed at the end of the cycle (day 22), remove it as soon as possible and start the next cycle on the usual 'change day', the day after day 28; no additional contraception is required.

**Expulsion, delayed insertion or removal, or broken vaginal ring** If the vaginal ring is expelled for *less than 3 hours*, rinse the ring with cool water and reinsert immediately; no additional contraception is needed.

If the ring remains outside the vagina for *more than 3 hours* or if the user does not know when the ring was expelled, contraceptive protection may be reduced:

- if ring expelled during week 1 or 2 of cycle, rinse ring with cool water and reinsert; use additional precautions (barrier methods) for next 7 days;

- if ring expelled during week 3 of cycle, either insert a new ring to start a new cycle *or* allow a withdrawal bleed and insert a new ring no later than 7 days after ring was expelled; latter option only available if ring was used continuously for at least 7 days before expulsion.

If insertion of a new ring at the start of a new cycle is delayed, contraceptive protection is lost. A new ring should be inserted as soon as possible; additional precautions (barrier methods) should be used for the first 7 days of the new cycle. If intercourse occurred during the extended ring-free interval, pregnancy should be considered.

No additional contraception is required if the removal of the ring is delayed by up to 1 week (4 weeks of continuous use). The 7-day ring-free interval should be observed and subsequently a new ring should be inserted. Contraceptive protection may be reduced with continuous use of the ring for more than 4 weeks—pregnancy should be ruled out before inserting a new ring.

If the ring breaks during use, remove it and insert a new ring immediately; additional precautions (barrier methods) should be used for the first 7 days of the new cycle.

**Diarrhoea and vomiting** Vomiting and persistent, severe diarrhoea can interfere with the absorption of combined oral contraceptives. If vomiting occurs within 2 hours of taking a combined oral contraceptive another pill should be taken as soon as possible. In cases of persistent vomiting or severe diarrhoea lasting more

**7**

**Obstetrics, gynaecology, and urinary-tract disorders**

than 24 hours, additional precautions should be used during and for 7 days (9 days for *Qlaira*®) after recovery (see also under Missed pill, above). If the vomiting and diarrhoea occurs during the last 7 tablets, the next pill-free interval should be omitted (in the case of ED tablets the inactive ones should be omitted).

**Interactions**  The effectiveness of *combined* oral contraceptives, *progestogen-only* oral contraceptives (section 7.3.2.1), contraceptive patches, and vaginal rings can be considerably reduced by interaction with drugs that induce hepatic enzyme activity (e.g. **carbamazepine, nevirapine, oxcarbazepine, phenytoin, phenobarbital, primidone, ritonavir, St John's Wort, topiramate,** and, above all, **rifabutin** and **rifampicin**). A condom together with a long-acting method, such as an injectable contraceptive, may be more suitable for patients with HIV infection or at risk of HIV infection; advice on the possibility of interaction with anti-retroviral drugs should be sought from HIV specialists.

Women taking combined hormonal contraceptives who require enzyme-inducing drugs should be advised to change to a contraceptive method that is unaffected by enzyme-inducers (e.g. some parenteral progestogen-only contraceptives (p. 404), intra-uterine devices) for the duration of treatment and for 4 weeks after stopping. If a change in contraceptive method is undesirable or inappropriate the following options should be discussed:

- For a *short course (2 months or less) of an enzyme-inducing drug* (except rifampicin or rifabutin—see below), continue with a combined oral contraceptive providing ethinylestradiol 30 micrograms or more daily and use a 'tricycling' regimen (i.e. taking 3 packets of monophasic tablets without a break followed by a shortened tablet-free interval of 4 days [unlicensed use]). Additional contraceptive precautions should also be used whilst taking the enzyme-inducing drug and for 4 weeks after stopping. Another option is to follow the advice for long-term courses, below.

  For women using combined hormonal contraceptive patches or vaginal rings, additional contraceptive precautions are also required whilst taking the enzyme-inducing drug and for 4 weeks after stopping. If concomitant administration runs beyond the 3 weeks of patch or vaginal ring use, a new treatment cycle should be started immediately, without a patch-free or ring-free break.

- For a *long-term course (over 2 months) of an enzyme-inducing drug* (except rifampicin or rifabutin—see below), adjust the dose of combined oral contraceptive to provide ethinylestradiol 50 micrograms or more daily [unlicensed use] and use a 'tricycling' regimen (as above); continue for the duration of treatment with the enzyme-inducing drug and for 4 weeks after stopping.

  If breakthrough bleeding occurs (and all other causes are ruled out) it is recommended that the dose of ethinylestradiol is increased by increments of 10 micrograms up to a maximum of 70 micrograms daily [unlicensed use], or to use additional precautions, or to change to a method unaffected by enzyme-inducing drugs.

  Contraceptive patches and vaginal rings are not recommended for women taking enzyme-inducing drugs over a long period.

- For any course of **rifampicin** or **rifabutin**, an alternative method of contraception (such as an

IUD) is **always** recommended because they are such potent enzyme-inducing drugs; the alternative method of contraception should be continued for 4 weeks after stopping the enzyme-inducing drug.

For information on interactions of oral progestogen-only contraceptives, see also p. 403; for information on interactions of parenteral progestogen-only contraceptives, see also p. 404; for information on interactions of the intra-uterine progestogen-only device, see also p. 405; for information on interactions of hormonal emergency contraception, see also p. 409

### Antibacterials that do not induce liver enzymes

Latest recommendations are that no additional contraceptive precautions are required when *combined* oral contraceptives are used with antibacterials that do not induce liver enzymes (e.g. ampicillin, doxycycline), unless diarrhoea or vomiting occur (see above). These recommendations should be discussed with the woman, who should also be advised that guidance in patient information leaflets may differ. It is also currently recommended that no additional contraceptive precautions are required when contraceptive patches or vaginal rings are used with antibacterials that do not induce liver enzymes. There have been concerns that some antibacterials that do not induce liver enzymes reduce the efficacy of *combined* oral contraceptives by impairing the bacterial flora responsible for recycling ethinylestradiol from the large bowel; however, there is a lack of evidence to support this interaction.

**Surgery**  Oestrogen-containing contraceptives should preferably be discontinued (and adequate alternative contraceptive arrangements made) 4 weeks before major elective surgery and all surgery to the legs or surgery which involves prolonged immobilisation of a lower limb; they should normally be recommenced at the first menses occurring at least 2 weeks after full mobilisation. A progestogen-only contraceptive may be offered as an alternative and the oestrogen-containing contraceptive restarted after mobilisation, as above. When discontinuation of an oestrogen-containing contraceptive is not possible, e.g. after trauma or if a patient admitted for an elective procedure is still on an oestrogen-containing contraceptive, thromboprophylaxis (with unfractionated or low molecular weight heparin and graduated compression hosiery) is advised. These recommendations do not apply to minor surgery with short duration of anaesthesia, e.g. laparoscopic sterilisation or tooth extraction, or to women using oestrogen-free hormonal contraceptives.

**Reason to stop immediately**  Combined hormonal contraceptives should be stopped (pending investigation and treatment), if any of the following occur:

- sudden severe chest pain (even if not radiating to left arm);
- sudden breathlessness (or cough with blood-stained sputum);
- unexplained swelling or severe pain in calf of one leg;
- severe stomach pain;
- serious neurological effects including unusual severe, prolonged headache especially if first time or getting progressively worse *or* sudden partial or complete loss of vision *or* sudden disturbance of hearing or other perceptual disorders *or* dysphasia *or* bad fainting attack or collapse *or* first unexplained epileptic seizure *or* weakness, motor disturbances, very marked numbness suddenly affecting one side or one part of body;
- hepatitis, jaundice, liver enlargement;

- very high blood pressure;
- prolonged immobility after surgery or leg injury;
- detection of a risk factor which contra-indicates treatment (see Cautions and Contra-indications under Combined Hormonal Contraceptives below).

## COMBINED HORMONAL CONTRACEPTIVES

**Cautions** see notes above; also risk factors for venous thromboembolism (see below and also notes above), arterial disease and migraine, see below; personal or family history of hypertriglyceridaemia (increased risk of pancreatitis); hyperprolactinaemia (seek specialist advice); history of severe depression especially if induced by hormonal contraceptive; undiagnosed breast mass; gene mutations associated with breast cancer (e.g. BRCA 1); sickle-cell disease; inflammatory bowel disease including Crohn's disease; reduced efficacy of contraceptive patch in women with body-weight ≥ 90 kg; active trophoblastic disease (until return to normal of urine- and plasma-gonadotrophin concentration) —seek specialist advice; **interactions**: see above and Appendix 1 (oestrogens, progestogens)

**Risk factors for venous thromboembolism** See also notes above. Use with **caution** if any of following factors present but **avoid** if two or more factors present:

- *family history of venous thromboembolism* in first-degree relative aged under 45 years (avoid contraceptive containing desogestrel or gestodene, *or* avoid if known prothrombotic coagulation abnormality e.g. factor V Leiden or antiphospholipid antibodies (including lupus anticoagulant));
- *obesity*—caution if obese according to BMI (adjusted for age and gender); in those who are markedly obese, avoid unless no suitable alternative;
- *long-term immobilisation* e.g. in a wheelchair (avoid if confined to bed or leg in plaster cast);
- *history of superficial thrombophlebitis*;
- *smoking*.

**Risk factors for arterial disease** Use with **caution** if any one of following factors present but **avoid** if two or more factors present:

- *family history of arterial disease* in first degree relative aged under 45 years (avoid if atherogenic lipid profile);
- *diabetes mellitus* (avoid if diabetes complications present);
- *hypertension* (avoid if blood pressure very high);
- *smoking* (avoid if smoking 40 or more cigarettes daily);
- *obesity*—caution if obese according to BMI (adjusted for age and gender); in those who are markedly obese, avoid unless no suitable alternative;
- *migraine without aura* (avoid if *migraine with aura* (focal symptoms), *or* severe migraine frequently lasting over 72 hours despite treatment, *or* migraine treated with ergot derivatives).

**Migraine** Women should report any increase in headache frequency or onset of focal symptoms (discontinue immediately and refer urgently to neurology expert if focal neurological symptoms not typical of aura persist for more than 1 hour—see also Reason to stop immediately in notes above)

**Contra-indications** see notes above; also personal history of venous or arterial thrombosis, severe or multiple risk factors for arterial disease or for venous thromboembolism (see above), heart disease associated with pulmonary hypertension or risk of embolus; sclerosing treatment for varicose veins; migraine with aura (see also above); transient cerebral ischaemic attacks without headaches; systemic lupus erythematosus; acute porphyria (section 9.8.2); gall-

stones; history of haemolytic uraemic syndrome or history during pregnancy of pruritus, cholestatic jaundice, chorea, pemphigoid gestationis; history of breast cancer but can be used after 5 years if no evidence of disease and non-hormonal methods unacceptable; undiagnosed vaginal bleeding

**Hepatic impairment** avoid in active liver disease including disorders of hepatic excretion (e.g. Dubin-Johnson or Rotor syndromes), infective hepatitis (until liver function returns to normal), and liver tumours

**Pregnancy** not known to be harmful

**Breast-feeding** avoid until weaning or for 6 months after birth (adverse effects on lactation)

**Side-effects** see notes above; also nausea, vomiting, abdominal cramps, liver impairment, hepatic tumours; fluid retention, thrombosis (more common when factor V Leiden present or in blood groups A, B, and AB; see also notes above), hypertension, changes in lipid metabolism; headache, depression, chorea, nervousness, irritability; changes in libido, breast tenderness, enlargement, and secretion; reduced menstrual loss, 'spotting' in early cycles, absence of withdrawal bleeding, amenorrhoea after discontinuation, changes in vaginal discharge, cervical erosion; contact lenses may irritate, visual disturbances; leg cramps; skin reactions, chloasma, photosensitivity; rarely gallstones and systemic lupus erythematosus

**Breast cancer** There is a small increase in the risk of having breast cancer diagnosed in women taking the combined oral contraceptive pill; this relative risk may be due to an earlier diagnosis. In users of combined oral contraceptive pills the cancers are more likely to be localised to the breast. The most important factor for diagnosing breast cancer appears to be the age at which the contraceptive is stopped rather than the duration of use; any increase in the rate of diagnosis diminishes gradually during the 10 years after stopping and disappears by 10 years

**Cervical cancer** Use of combined oral contraceptives for 5 years or longer is associated with a small increased risk of cervical cancer; the risk diminishes after stopping and disappears by about 10 years. The risk of cervical cancer with transdermal patches and vaginal rings is not yet known

**Note** The possible small increase in the risk of breast cancer and cervical cancer should be weighed against the protective effect against cancers of the ovary and endometrium

**Licensed use** consult product literature for the licensing status of individual preparations

### Indications and dose

**Contraception, menstrual symptoms** (section 6.4.1.2)

- **By mouth**

  Each tablet should be taken at approximately same time each day; if delayed, contraceptive protection may be lost (see Missed Pill, above)

  *21-day combined (monophasic) preparations,* 1 tablet daily for 21 days; subsequent courses repeated after a 7-day interval (during which withdrawal bleeding occurs); if reasonably certain woman is not pregnant, first course can be started on any day of cycle—if starting on day 6 of cycle or later, additional precautions (barrier methods) necessary during first 7 days

  *Every day (ED) combined (monophasic) preparations,* 1 *active* tablet daily for 21 days, followed by 1 *inactive* tablet daily for 7 days (see also Combined Oral Contraceptives table, below); subsequent courses repeated without interval (withdrawal bleeding occurs when *inactive* tablets being taken); if reasonably certain woman is not pregnant, first

**7** Obstetrics, gynaecology, and urinary-tract disorders

course can be started on any day of cycle—if starting on day 6 of cycle or later, additional precautions (barrier methods) necessary during first 7 days

*Phasic preparations*, see Combined Oral Contraceptives table, below

**Changing to combined preparation containing different progestogen** If previous contraceptive used correctly, or pregnancy can reasonably be excluded, start the first *active* tablet of new brand immediately *Changing to Qlaira®*: start the first *active* Qlaira® tablet on the day after taking the last *active* tablet of the previous brand

*Changing from Qlaira®*: start the new brand after taking the last *active* Qlaira® tablet; if the *inactive* tablets are taken before starting new brand, additional precautions (barrier methods) should be used during first 7 days of taking the new brand

**Changing from progestogen-only tablet** If previous contraceptive used correctly, or pregnancy can reasonably be excluded, start new brand immediately, additional precautions (barrier methods) necessary for first 7 days

*Changing to Qlaira®*: start any day, additional precautions (barrier methods) necessary for first 9 days

**Secondary amenorrhoea (exclude pregnancy)** Start any day, additional precautions (barrier methods) necessary during first 7 days (9 days for Qlaira®)

**After childbirth (not breast-feeding)** Start 3 weeks after birth (increased risk of thrombosis if started earlier); later than 3 weeks postpartum additional precautions (barrier methods) necessary for first 7 days (9 days for Qlaira®)

**After abortion or miscarriage** Start same day

- **By transdermal application**

Apply first patch on day 1 of cycle, change patch on days 8 and 15; remove third patch on day 22 and apply new patch after 7-day patch-free interval to start subsequent contraceptive cycle

**Note** If first patch applied later than day 1, additional precautions (barrier methods) should be used for the next 7 days

**Changing from combined oral contraception** Apply patch on the first day of withdrawal bleeding; if no withdrawal bleeding within 5 days of taking last *active* tablet, rule out pregnancy before applying first patch. Unless patch is applied on first day of withdrawal bleeding, additional precautions (barrier methods) should be used concurrently for first 7 days

**Changing from progestogen-only method** From an implant, apply first patch on the day implant removed; from an injection, apply first patch when next injection due; from oral progestogen, first patch may be applied on any day after stopping pill. For all methods additional precautions (barrier methods) should be used concurrently for first 7 days

**After childbirth (not breast-feeding)** Start 4 weeks after birth; if started later than 4 weeks after birth additional precautions (barrier methods) should be used for first 7 days

**After abortion or miscarriage** Before 20 weeks' gestation start immediately; no additional contraception required if started immediately. After 20 weeks' gestation start on day 21 after abortion or on the first day of first spontaneous menstruation; additional precautions (barrier methods) should be used for first 7 days after applying the patch

- **By vagina**

Insert ring into vagina on day 1 of cycle and leave in for 3 weeks; remove ring on day 22; subsequent courses repeated after 7-day ring-free interval (during which withdrawal bleeding occurs)

**Note** If first ring inserted later than day 1, additional precautions (barrier methods) should be used for the next 7 days

**Changing from combined hormonal contraception** Insert ring at the latest on the day after the usual tablet-free, patch-free, or inactive-tablet interval. If previous contraceptive used correctly, or pregnancy can reasonably be excluded, can switch to ring on any day of cycle

**Changing from progestogen-only method** From an implant or intra-uterine progestogen-only device, insert ring on the day implant or intra-uterine progestogen-only device removed; from an injection, insert ring when injection next due; from oral preparation, first ring may be inserted on any day after stopping pill. For all methods additional precautions (barrier methods) should be used concurrently for first 7 days

**After first trimester abortion** Start immediately

**After childbirth (not breast-feeding) or second trimester abortion** Start 4 weeks after birth or abortion; if started later than 4 weeks after birth or abortion additional precautions (barrier methods) should be used for first 7 days

---

## Oral (low and standard strength)

For information on these preparations, see Combined Oral Contraceptives table, p. 401

---

## Transdermal (standard strength)

◢**Ethinylestradiol with Norelgestromin**

See Risk of Venous Thromboembolism (in notes above) before prescribing

**Evra®** (Janssen) [PoM]
Patches, self-adhesive (releasing ethinylestradiol approx. 33.9 micrograms/24 hours and norelgestromin approx. 203 micrograms/24 hours); net price 9-patch pack = £16.70. Counselling, administration

**Dose**

> 1 patch to be applied once weekly for three weeks, followed by a 7-day patch-free interval; subsequent courses repeated after 7-day patch-free interval (during which withdrawal bleeding occurs); for starting routines see under Dose above

**Note** Adhesives or bandages should not be used to hold patch in place. If patch no longer sticky do not reapply but use a new patch.

The *Scottish Medicines Consortium* has advised (September 2003) that *Evra®* patches should be restricted for use in women who are likely to comply poorly with combined oral contraceptives

---

## Vaginal (low strength)

◢**Ethinylestradiol with Etonogestrel**

See Risk of Venous Thromboembolism (in notes above) before prescribing

**NuvaRing®** (Organon) ▼ [PoM]
Vaginal ring, releasing ethinylestradiol approx. 15 micrograms/24 hours and etonogestrel approx. 120 micrograms/24 hours, net price 3-ring pack = £27.00. Counselling, administration

**Dose**

> 1 ring to be inserted into the vagina for 3 weeks, removed on day 22; subsequent courses repeated after 7-day ring-free interval (during which withdrawal bleeding occurs); for starting routines see under Dose above

**Counselling** The presence of the ring should be checked regularly. In case of expulsion see Expulsion, Delayed Insertion or Removal, or Broken Vaginal Ring, p. 397

## Combined Oral Contraceptives

See Risk of Venous Thromboembolism (in notes above) before prescribing

| Type of preparation | Oestrogen content | Progestogen content | Tablets per cycle | Brand | Price, 3-cycle pack (unless stated) | Manufacturer |
|---|---|---|---|---|---|---|
| [1]Monophasic low strength (21-day preparations) | Ethinylestradiol 20 micrograms | Desogestrel 150 micrograms | 21 | Gedarel® 20/150 | £5.98 | Consilient |
| | | | | Mercilon® | £7.97 | Organon |
| | | Gestodene 75 micrograms | 21 | Femodette® | £8.85 | Bayer |
| | | | | Millinette® 20/75 | £6.37 | Consilient |
| | | | | Sunya 20/75® | £6.62 | Stragen |
| | | Norethisterone acetate 1 mg | 21 | Loestrin 20® | £2.75 | Galen |
| [1]Monophasic standard strength (21-day preparations) | Ethinylestradiol 30 micrograms | Desogestrel 150 micrograms | 21 | Gedarel® 30/150 | £4.93 | Consilient |
| | | | | Marvelon® | £6.45 | Organon |
| | | Drospirenone 3 mg | 21 | [2]Yasmin® | £14.70 | Bayer |
| | | Gestodene 75 micrograms | 21 | Femodene® | £6.73 | Bayer |
| | | | | Katya 30/75® | £5.03 | Stragen |
| | | | | Millinette® 30/75 | £4.85 | Consilient |
| | | Levonorgestrel 150 micrograms | 21 | Levest® | £2.55 | Morningside |
| | | | | Microgynon 30® | £2.82 | Bayer |
| | | | | Ovranette® | £2.20 | Pfizer |
| | | | | Rigevidon® | £1.89 | Consilient |
| | | Norethisterone acetate 1.5 mg | 21 | Loestrin 30® | £3.95 | Galen |
| | Ethinylestradiol 35 micrograms | Norgestimate 250 micrograms | 21 | Cilest® | 3-cycle pack = £2.87; 6-cycle pack = £5.74 | Janssen |
| | | Norethisterone 500 micrograms | 21 | Brevinor® | £1.99 | Pharmacia |
| | | | | Ovysmen® | £1.49 | Janssen |
| | | Norethisterone 1 mg | 21 | Norimin® | £2.28 | Pharmacia |
| | Mestranol 50 micrograms | Norethisterone 1 mg | 21 | Norinyl-1® | £2.19 | Pharmacia |
| [3]Monophasic standard strength (28-day 'Every day' preparations) | Ethinylestradiol 30 micrograms | Gestodene 75 micrograms | 21 active 7 inactive | Femodene® ED | £6.73 | Bayer |
| | Ethinylestradiol 30 micrograms | Levonorgestrel 150 micrograms | 21 active 7 inactive | Microgynon 30 ED® | £2.54 | Bayer |

**7 Obstetrics, gynaecology, and urinary-tract disorders**

1. *Dose* 1 tablet daily for 21 days starting on day 1–5 of cycle (if reasonably certain woman is not pregnant, first course can be started on any day of cycle); subsequent courses repeated after 7-day tablet-free interval (during which withdrawal bleeding occurs); for starting and changing routines see under Indications and Dose above
2. *Caution* use with care if increased plasma-potassium concentration might be hazardous; *renal impairment* avoid if eGFR less than 30 mL/minute/1.73 m$^2$
3. *Dose* 1 tablet daily for 28 days starting on day 1–5 of cycle with first active tablet (withdrawal bleeding occurs when inactive tablets being taken) (if reasonably certain woman is not pregnant, first course can be started on any day of cycle); subsequent courses repeated without interval; for starting and changing routines see under Indications and Dose above

**Obstetrics, gynaecology, and urinary-tract disorders** · 7

## Combined Oral Contraceptives (*continued*)

See Risk of Venous Thromboembolism (in notes above) before prescribing

| Type of preparation | Oestrogen content | Progestogen content | Tablets per cycle | Brand | Price, 3-cycle pack (unless stated) | Manufacturer |
|---|---|---|---|---|---|---|
| [1]Phasic standard strength (21-day preparations) | Ethinylestradiol 30 micrograms | Gestodene 50 micrograms | 6 | Triadene® | £8.99 | Bayer |
| | Ethinylestradiol 40 micrograms | Gestodene 70 micrograms | 5 | | | |
| | Ethinylestradiol 30 micrograms | Gestodene 100 micrograms | 10 | | | |
| | Ethinylestradiol 30 micrograms | Levonorgestrel 50 micrograms | 6 | Logynon® | £3.96 | Bayer |
| | Ethinylestradiol 40 micrograms | Levonorgestrel 75 micrograms | 5 | TriRegol® | £2.87 | Consilient |
| | Ethinylestradiol 30 micrograms | Levonorgestrel 125 micrograms | 10 | | | |
| | Ethinylestradiol 35 micrograms | Norethisterone 500 micrograms | 7 | BiNovum® | £1.96 | Janssen |
| | Ethinylestradiol 35 micrograms | Norethisterone 1 mg | 14 | | | |
| | Ethinylestradiol 35 micrograms | Norethisterone 500 micrograms | 7 | Synphase® | 1-cycle pack = £1.20 | Pharmacia |
| | Ethinylestradiol 35 micrograms | Norethisterone 1 mg | 9 | | | |
| | Ethinylestradiol 35 micrograms | Norethisterone 500 micrograms | 5 | | | |
| | Ethinylestradiol 35 micrograms | Norethisterone 500 micrograms | 7 | TriNovum® | £2.72 | Janssen |
| | Ethinylestradiol 35 micrograms | Norethisterone 750 micrograms | 7 | | | |
| | Ethinylestradiol 35 micrograms | Norethisterone 1 mg | 7 | | | |
| [2]Phasic standard strength (28-day 'Every day' preparation) | Ethinylestradiol 30 micrograms | Levonorgestrel 50 micrograms | 6 active | Logynon ED® | £3.82 | Bayer |
| | Ethinylestradiol 40 micrograms | Levonorgestrel 75 micrograms | 5 active | | | |
| | Ethinylestradiol 30 micrograms | Levonorgestrel 125 micrograms | 10 active | | | |
| | | | 7 inactive | | | |
| [3]Phasic (28-day 'Every day' preparation) | Estradiol valerate 3 mg | | 2 active | Qlaira® | £25.18 | Bayer |
| | Estradiol valerate 2 mg | Dienogest 2 mg | 5 active | | | |
| | Estradiol valerate 2 mg | Dienogest 3 mg | 17 active | | | |
| | Estradiol valerate 1 mg | | 2 active | | | |
| | | | 2 inactive | | | |

1. *Dose* 1 tablet daily for 21 days starting on day 1–5 of cycle (if reasonably certain woman is not pregnant, first course can be started on any day of cycle); subsequent courses repeated after 7-day tablet-free interval (during which withdrawal bleeding occurs); for starting and changing routines see under Indications and Dose above
2. *Dose* 1 tablet daily for 28 days starting on day 1–5 of cycle with first active tablet (withdrawal bleeding occurs when inactive tablets being taken) (if reasonably certain woman is not pregnant, first course can be started on any day of cycle); subsequent courses repeated without interval; for starting and changing routines see under Indications and Dose above
3. *Dose* 1 tablet daily for 28 days starting on day 1 of cycle with first active tablet (withdrawal bleeding occurs when inactive tablets being taken); subsequent courses repeated without interval; for starting and changing routines see under Indications and Dose above

## 7.3.2 Progestogen-only contraceptives

| 7.3.2.1 | Oral progestogen-only contraceptives |
| 7.3.2.2 | Parenteral progestogen-only contraceptives |
| 7.3.2.3 | Intra-uterine progestogen-only device |

### 7.3.2.1 Oral progestogen-only contraceptives

Oral progestogen-only preparations may offer a suitable alternative when oestrogens are contra-indicated (including those patients with venous thrombosis or a past history or predisposition to venous thrombosis), but have a higher failure rate than combined preparations. They are suitable for heavy smokers, and for those with hypertension, valvular heart disease, diabetes mellitus, and migraine. Menstrual irregularities (oligomenorrhoea, menorrhagia) are more common but tend to resolve on long-term treatment.

**Interactions**  Effectiveness of oral progestogen-only preparations is not affected by antibacterials that do not induce liver enzymes. The efficacy of oral progestogen-only preparations is, however, reduced by enzyme-inducing drugs and an alternative contraceptive method, unaffected by the interacting drug, is recommended during treatment with an enzyme-inducing drug and for at least 4 weeks afterwards—see p. 398 and Appendix 1 (progestogens). For a short course of an enzyme-inducing drug, if a change in contraceptive method is undesirable or inappropriate, the progestogen-only oral method may be continued in combination with additional contraceptive precautions (e.g. barrier methods) for the duration of treatment with the enzyme-inducing drug and for 4 weeks after stopping.

**Surgery**  All progestogen-only contraceptives (including those given by injection) are suitable for use as an alternative to combined oral contraceptives before major elective surgery, before all surgery to the legs, or before surgery which involves prolonged immobilisation of a lower limb.

**Starting routine**  One tablet daily, on a continuous basis, starting on day 1 of cycle and taken at the same time each day (if delayed by longer than 3 hours (12 hours for *Cerazette*®) contraceptive protection may be lost). Additional contraceptive precautions are not necessary when initiating treatment.

**Changing from a combined oral contraceptive**  Start on the day following completion of the combined oral contraceptive course without a break (or in the case of ED tablets omitting the inactive ones).

**After childbirth**  Oral progestogen-only contraceptives can be started up to and including day 21 postpartum without the need for additional contraceptive precautions. If started more than 21 days postpartum, additional contraceptive precautions are required for 2 days.

**Missed pill**  The following advice is now recommended by family planning organisations:

'If you forget a pill, take it as soon as you remember and carry on with the next pill at the right time. If the pill was more than 3 hours (12 hours for *Cerazette*®) overdue you are not protected. Continue normal pill-taking but you must also use another method, such as the condom, for the next 2 days.'

The Faculty of Sexual and Reproductive Healthcare recommends emergency contraception (see p. 408) if one or more progestogen-only contraceptive tablets are missed or taken more than 3 hours (12 hours for *Cerazette*®) late and unprotected intercourse has occurred before 2 further tablets have been correctly taken.

**Diarrhoea and vomiting**  Vomiting and persistent, severe diarrhoea can interfere with the absorption of oral progestogen-only contraceptives. If vomiting occurs within 2 hours of taking an oral progestogen-only contraceptive, another pill should be taken as soon as possible. If a replacement pill is not taken within 3 hours (12 hours for *Cerazette*®) of the normal time for taking the progestogen-only pill, or in cases of persistent vomiting or very severe diarrhoea, additional precautions should be used during illness and for 2 days after recovery (see also under Missed pill above).

### ORAL PROGESTOGEN-ONLY CONTRACEPTIVES
(Progestogen-only pill, 'POP')

**Cautions**  arterial disease; sex-steroid dependent cancer; past ectopic pregnancy; malabsorption syndromes; active trophoblastic disease (until return to normal of urine- and plasma-gonadotrophin concentration)—seek specialist advice; systemic lupus erythematosus with positive (or unknown) antiphospholipid antibodies; functional ovarian cysts; history of jaundice in pregnancy; **interactions:** see notes above and Appendix 1 (progestogens)

Other conditions  The product literature advises caution in patients with history of thromboembolism, hypertension, diabetes mellitus and migraine; evidence for caution in these conditions is unsatisfactory

**Contra-indications**  undiagnosed vaginal bleeding; severe arterial disease; acute porphyria (section 9.8.2); history of breast cancer but can be used after 5 years if no evidence of disease and non-hormonal contraceptive methods unacceptable

**Hepatic impairment**  caution in active liver disease; and recurrent cholestatic jaundice, avoid in liver tumour

**Pregnancy**  not known to be harmful

**Breast-feeding**  progestogen-only contraceptives do not affect lactation; see also After Childbirth above

**Side-effects**  menstrual irregularities (see also notes above); nausea, vomiting, headache, dizziness, breast discomfort, depression, skin disorders, disturbance of appetite, changes in libido

Breast cancer  There is a small increase in the risk of having breast cancer diagnosed in women using, or who have recently used, a progestogen-only contraceptive pill; this relative risk may be due to an earlier diagnosis. The most important risk factor appears to be the age at which the contraceptive is stopped rather than the duration of use; the risk disappears gradually during the 10 years after stopping and there is no excess risk by 10 years. A possible small increase in the risk of breast cancer should be weighed against the benefits

**Licensed use**  consult product literature for the licensing status of individual preparations

### Indications and dose

**Contraception**

- By mouth

  1 tablet daily at same time each day, starting on day 1 of cycle then continuously; if administration delayed for 3 hours (12 hours for *Cerazette*®) or more it should be regarded as a 'missed pill', see notes above

**7  Obstetrics, gynaecology, and urinary-tract disorders**

**Cerazette®** (Organon) PoM

Tablets, f/c, desogestrel 75 micrograms, net price 3 × 28-tab pack = £8.68

The *Scottish Medicines Consortium* (p. 3) has advised (September 2003) that *Cerazette®* should be restricted for use in women who cannot tolerate oestrogen-containing contraceptives or in whom such preparations are contra-indicated

**Femulen®** (Pfizer) PoM

Tablets, etynodiol diacetate 500 micrograms, net price 3 × 28-tab pack = £3.31

**Micronor®** (Janssen) PoM

Tablets, norethisterone 350 micrograms, net price 3 × 28-tab pack = £1.66

**Norgeston®** (Bayer) PoM

Tablets, s/c, levonorgestrel 30 micrograms, net price 35-tab pack = 92p

**Noriday®** (Pharmacia) PoM

Tablets, norethisterone 350 micrograms, net price 3 × 28-tab pack = £2.10

### 7.3.2.2 Parenteral progestogen-only contraceptives

**Medroxyprogesterone acetate** (*Depo-Provera®*) is a long-acting progestogen given by intramuscular injection; it is as effective as the combined oral preparations but because of its prolonged action it should never be given without *full counselling backed by the patient information leaflet*. It may be used as a short-term or long-term contraceptive for women who have been counselled about the likelihood of menstrual disturbance and the potential for a delay in return to full fertility. Delayed return of fertility and irregular cycles may occur after discontinuation of treatment but there is no evidence of permanent infertility. Troublesome bleeding has been reported in patients given medroxyprogesterone acetate in the immediate puerperium; delaying the first injection until 6 weeks after the birth may minimise bleeding problems. If the woman is not breast-feeding, the first injection may be given within 5 days postpartum (she should be warned that the risk of heavy or prolonged bleeding may be increased). The manufacturer advises that in women who are breast-feeding, the first dose should be delayed until 6 weeks after the birth; however, evidence suggests no harmful effect to infant if given earlier. The benefits of using medroxyprogesterone acetate in breast-feeding women outweigh any risks.

Reduction in bone mineral density and, rarely, osteoporosis and osteoporotic fractures have also been reported with medroxyprogesterone acetate. The reduction in bone mineral density occurs in the first 2–3 years of use and then stabilises. See also below.

- In adolescents, medroxyprogesterone acetate (*Depo-Provera®*) should be used only when other methods of contraception are inappropriate;
- in all women, the benefits of using medroxyprogesterone acetate beyond 2 years should be evaluated against the risks;
- in women with risk factors for osteoporosis, a method of contraception other than medroxyprogesterone acetate should be considered.

**Norethisterone enantate** (*Noristerat®*) is a long-acting progestogen given as an oily injection which provides contraception for 8 weeks; it is used as short-term

interim contraception e.g. before vasectomy becomes effective.

An **etonogestrel-releasing implant** (*Nexplanon®*) is also available. It is a highly effective long-acting contraceptive, consisting of a single flexible rod that is inserted subdermally into the lower surface of the upper arm and provides contraception for up to 3 years. The manufacturer advises that in heavier women, blood-etonogestrel concentrations are lower and therefore the implant may not provide effective contraception during the third year; they advise that earlier replacement may be considered in such patients, however, evidence to support this recommendation is lacking. Local reactions such as bruising and itching can occur at the insertion site. The contraceptive effect of etonogestrel is rapidly reversed on removal of the implant. *The doctor or nurse administering (or removing) the system should be fully trained in the technique and should provide full counselling reinforced by the patient information leaflet.*

*Implanon®*, also an etonogestrel-releasing implant, has been discontinued (October 2010), but some women may have the implant in place until 2013.

**Cautions, contra-indications, and side-effects** The cautions, contra-indications, and side-effects of oral progestogen-only contraceptives apply to parenteral progestogen-only contraceptives, except that parenteral preparations reliably inhibit ovulation and therefore protect against ectopic pregnancy and functional ovarian cysts.

**Interactions** Effectiveness of parenteral progestogen-only contraceptives is not affected by antibacterials that do not induce liver enzymes. The effectiveness of norethisterone and medroxyprogesterone acetate intramuscular injections is not affected by enzyme-inducing drugs and they may be continued as normal during courses of these drugs. However, effectiveness of the etonogestrel-releasing implant may be reduced by enzyme-inducing drugs and an alternative contraceptive method, unaffected by the interacting drug, is recommended during treatment with the enzyme-inducing drug and for at least 4 weeks after stopping. For a short course of an enzyme-inducing drug, if a change in contraceptive method is undesirable or inappropriate, the implant may be continued in combination with additional contraceptive precautions (e.g. condom) for the duration of treatment with the enzyme-inducing drug and for 4 weeks after stopping it.

### PARENTERAL PROGESTOGEN-ONLY CONTRACEPTIVES

**Cautions** see notes above and under preparations; possible risk of breast cancer, see oral progestogen-only contraceptives (section 7.3.2.1); history during pregnancy of pruritus or of deterioration of otosclerosis, disturbances of lipid metabolism; **interactions:** see notes above and Appendix 1 (progestogens)

**Counselling** Full counselling backed by *patient information leaflet* required before administration

**Contra-indications** see notes above; history of breast cancer but can be used after 5 years if no evidence of disease and non-hormonal contraceptive methods unacceptable

**Hepatic impairment** see Oral Progestogen-only Contraceptives, section 7.3.2.1

**Pregnancy** not known to be harmful; for *Implanon®* or *Nexplanon®* if pregnancy occurs remove implant

**Breast-feeding**   progestogen-only contraceptives do not affect lactation; see also notes above

**Side-effects**   see notes above; injection-site reactions; *with medroxyprogesterone acetate injection,* weight gain also reported

    **Cervical cancer** Use of injectable progestogen-only contraceptives is associated with a small increased risk of cervical cancer; this increased risk may be similar to that seen with combined oral contraceptives, see p. 399. The risk of cervical cancer with other progestogen-only contraceptives is not yet known.

**Licensed use**   consult product literature for the licensing status of individual preparations

### Indications and dose

    **Contraception** see also notes above and under preparations (roles vary according to preparation)

        For dose see under preparations

### ◢Injectable preparations

**Depo-Provera®** (Pfizer) [PoM]

    Injection (aqueous suspension), medroxyprogesterone acetate 150 mg/mL, net price 1-mL prefilled syringe = £6.01, 1-mL vial = £6.01. Counselling, see patient information leaflet

**Dose**

- **By deep intramuscular injection**

    150 mg within first 5 days of cycle or within first 5 days after parturition (delay until 6 weeks after parturition if breast-feeding); for long-term contraception, repeated every 12 weeks (if interval greater than 12 weeks and 5 days, rule out pregnancy before next injection and advise patient to use additional contraceptive measures (e.g. barrier) for 14 days after the injection)

**Noristerat®** (Bayer) [PoM]

    Injection (oily), norethisterone enantate 200 mg/mL, net price 1-mL amp = £3.38. Counselling, see patient information leaflet

**Dose**

- **By deep intramuscular injection**

    Given very slowly *into gluteal muscle,* short-term contraception, 200 mg within first 5 days of cycle or immediately after parturition (duration 8 weeks); may be repeated once after 8 weeks (withhold breast-feeding for neonates with severe or persistent jaundice requiring medical treatment)

### ◢Implants

**Nexplanon®** (Organon) ▼ [PoM]

    Implant, containing etonogestrel 68 mg in radiopaque flexible rod, net price = £79.46. Counselling, see patient information leaflet

**Dose**

- **By subdermal implantation**

    No hormonal contraceptive use in previous month, 1 implant inserted during first 5 days of cycle; postpartum, 1 implant inserted 21–28 days after delivery; in breast-feeding mothers, 1 implant inserted after 28 days postpartum; abortion or miscarriage in the second trimester, 1 implant inserted 21–28 days after abortion or miscarriage; abortion or miscarriage in first trimester, 1 implant inserted within 5 days; changing from other hormonal contraceptive, consult product literature; remove implant within 3 years of insertion

---

**7.3.2.3**   **Intra-uterine progestogen-only device**

The progestogen-only intra-uterine system, *Mirena®,* releases **levonorgestrel** directly into the uterine cavity.

It is used as a contraceptive, for the treatment of primary menorrhagia and for the prevention of endometrial hyperplasia during oestrogen replacement therapy. This may therefore be a contraceptive method of choice for women who have excessively heavy menses.

The effects of the progestogen-only intra-uterine system are mainly local and hormonal including prevention of endometrial proliferation, thickening of cervical mucus, and suppression of ovulation in some women (in some cycles). In addition to the progestogenic activity, the intra-uterine system itself may contribute slightly to the contraceptive effect. Return of fertility after removal is rapid and appears to be complete. *The doctor or nurse administering (or removing) the system should be fully trained in the technique and should provide full counselling reinforced by the patient information leaflet.*

Advantages of the progestogen-only intra-uterine system over copper intra-uterine devices are that there may be an improvement in any dysmenorrhoea and a reduction in blood loss; there is also evidence that the frequency of pelvic inflammatory disease may be reduced (particularly in the youngest age groups who are most at risk).

In primary menorrhagia, menstrual bleeding is reduced significantly within 3–6 months of inserting the progestogen-only intra-uterine system, probably because it prevents endometrial proliferation. Another treatment should be considered if menorrhagia does not improve within this time (section 6.4.1.2).

**Cautions and contra-indications**   Generally the cautions and contra-indications for the progestogen-only intra-uterine system are as for standard intra-uterine devices (section 7.3.4). Although the progestogen-only intra-uterine system produces little systemic progestogenic activity, it is usually avoided for 5 years after any evidence of breast cancer. However, the system can be considered for a woman in long-term remission from breast cancer who has menorrhagia and requires effective contraception. Since levonorgestrel is released close to the site of the main contraceptive action (on cervical mucus and endometrium) progestogenic side-effects and interactions are less likely; in particular, enzyme-inducing drugs are unlikely to significantly reduce the contraceptive effect of the progestogen-only intra-uterine system and additional contraceptive precautions are not required.

**Side-effects**   Initially, changes in the pattern and duration of menstrual bleeding (spotting or prolonged bleeding) are common; endometrial disorders should be ruled out before insertion and the patient should be fully counselled (and provided with a patient information leaflet). Improvement in progestogenic side-effects, such as mastalgia and in the bleeding pattern usually occurs a few months after insertion and bleeding may often become very light or absent. Functional ovarian cysts (usually asymptomatic) can occur and usually resolve spontaneously (ultrasound monitoring recommended).

---

■   **INTRA-UTERINE PROGESTOGEN-ONLY SYSTEM**

**Cautions**   see notes above; history of depression; advanced uterine atrophy; systemic lupus erythematosus with positive (or unknown) antiphospholipid antibodies; **interactions:** see notes above and Appendix 1 (progestogens)

**Contra-indications** see notes above; not suitable for emergency contraception

**Hepatic impairment** see Oral Progestogen-only Contraceptives, section 7.3.2.1

**Pregnancy** avoid; if pregnancy occurs remove system

**Breast-feeding** progestogen-only contraceptives do not affect lactation

**Side-effects** see notes above; also abdominal pain, expulsion, peripheral oedema, depression (sometimes severe), nervousness, salpingitis, pelvic inflammatory disease, pelvic pain, back pain; *rarely* uterine perforation, hirsutism, hair loss, pruritus, migraine, rash

**Licensed use** not licensed for use in women under 18 years

**Indications and dose**

See under preparation

**Mirena**® (Bayer) [PoM]

Intra-uterine system, T-shaped plastic frame (impregnated with barium sulfate and with threads attached to base) with polydimethylsiloxane reservoir releasing levonorgestrel 20 micrograms/24 hours, net price = £85.66. Counselling, see patient information leaflet

**Dose**

**Contraception and menorrhagia**

Insert into uterine cavity within 7 days of onset of menstruation, or any time if replacement, or any time if reasonably certain the woman is not pregnant and there is no risk of conception (additional precautions (e.g. barrier methods) necessary for next 7 days), or immediately after first-trimester termination by curettage; postpartum insertions should be delayed until at least 4 weeks after delivery; effective for 5 years

**Note** When system is removed (and not immediately replaced) and pregnancy is not desired, remove during first few days of menstruation, otherwise additional precautions (e.g. barrier methods) should be used for at least 7 days before removal

**Prevention of endometrial hyperplasia during oestrogen replacement therapy**

Insert during last days of menstruation or withdrawal bleeding or anytime if amenorrhoeic; effective for 4 years

**7.3.3 Spermicidal contraceptives**

Spermicidal contraceptives are useful additional safeguards but do **not** give adequate protection if used alone unless fertility is already significantly diminished. They have two components: a spermicide and a vehicle which itself may have some inhibiting effect on sperm activity. They are suitable for use with barrier methods, such as diaphragms or caps; however, spermicidal contraceptives are not generally recommended for use with condoms, as there is no evidence of any additional protection compared with non-spermicidal lubricants.

Spermicidal contraceptives are not suitable for use in those with or at high risk of sexually transmitted infections (including HIV); high frequency use of the spermicide nonoxinol '9' has been associated with genital lesions, which may increase the risk of acquiring these infections.

---

Products such as petroleum jelly (*Vaseline*®), baby oil and oil-based vaginal and rectal preparations are likely to damage condoms and contraceptive diaphragms made from latex rubber, and may render them less effective as a barrier method of contraception and as a protection from sexually transmitted infections (including HIV).

**Gygel**® (Marlborough)

Gel, nonoxinol '9' 2%, net price 30 g = £4.25

**Excipients** include hydroxybenzoates (parabens), propylene glycol, sorbic acid

**Condoms** No evidence of harm to latex condoms and diaphragms

**Pregnancy** toxicity in *animal* studies

**Breast-feeding** present in milk in *animal* studies

**7.3.4 Contraceptive devices**

## Intra-uterine devices

The intra-uterine device (IUD) is a suitable contraceptive for women of all ages irrespective of parity; however, it is less appropriate for those with an increased risk of pelvic inflammatory disease e.g. women under 25 years (see below).

The most effective intra-uterine devices have at least 380 mm$^2$ of copper and have banded copper on the arms. Smaller devices have been introduced to minimise side-effects; these consist of a plastic carrier wound with copper wire or fitted with copper bands; some also have a central core of silver to prevent fragmentation of the copper.

A frameless, copper-bearing intra-uterine device (*Gyne-Fix*®) is also available. It consists of a knotted, polypropylene thread with 6 copper sleeves; the device is anchored in the uterus by inserting the knot into the uterine fundus.

The timing and technique of fitting an intra-uterine device are critical for its subsequent performance. *The healthcare professional inserting (or removing) the device should be fully trained in the technique and should provide full counselling, backed, where available, by the patient information leaflet.* Devices should not be fitted during the heavy days of the period; they are best fitted after the end of menstruation and before the calculated time of implantation.

The main excess risk of infection occurs in the first 20 days after insertion and is believed to be related to existing carriage of a sexually transmitted infection. Women under 25 years are at a higher risk of sexually transmitted infections, and pre-insertion screening (for chlamydia, and depending on sexual history and local prevalence of disease, *Neisseria gonorrhoeae*) should be performed. If results are unavailable at the time of fitting an intra-uterine device for emergency contraception, appropriate prophylactic antibacterial cover should be given. The woman should be advised to attend *as an emergency* if she experiences sustained pain during the next 20 days.

An intra-uterine device should not be removed in mid-cycle unless an additional contraceptive was used for the previous 7 days. If removal is essential post-coital contraception should be considered.

If an intra-uterine device fails and the woman wishes to continue to full-term the device should be removed in the first trimester if possible.

## ■ INTRA-UTERINE CONTRACEPTIVE DEVICES

**Cautions** see notes above; also anaemia, menorrhagia (progestogen intra-uterine system might be preferable, section 7.3.2.3), endometriosis, severe primary dysmenorrhoea, history of pelvic inflammatory disease, diabetes, fertility problems, nulliparity and young age, severely scarred uterus (including after endometrial resection) or severe cervical stenosis; drug- or disease-induced immunosuppression (risk of infection—avoid if marked immunosuppression); epilepsy (risk of seizure at time of insertion); increased risk of expulsion if inserted before uterine involution; gynaecological examination before insertion, 6–8 weeks after then annually but counsel women to seek medical attention promptly in case of significant symptoms, especially pain; anticoagulant therapy (avoid if possible)

**Contra-indications** severe anaemia, recent sexually transmitted infection (if not fully investigated and treated), unexplained uterine bleeding, distorted or small uterine cavity, genital malignancy, active trophoblastic disease (until return to normal of urine- and plasma-gonadotrophin concentration), pelvic inflammatory disease, established or marked immunosuppression; *copper devices:* copper allergy, Wilson's disease, medical diathermy

**Pregnancy** remove device; if pregnancy occurs, increased likelihood that it may be ectopic

**Breast-feeding** not known to be harmful

**Side-effects** uterine or cervical perforation, displacement, expulsion; pelvic infection may be exacerbated, menorrhagia, dysmenorrhoea, allergy; *on insertion*: pain (alleviated by NSAID such as ibuprofen 30 minutes before insertion) and bleeding, occasionally epileptic seizure and vasovagal attack

**Indications and dose**
See notes above

**Ancora® 375 Ag** (RF Medical)
Intra-uterine device, copper wire with silver core, wound on vertical stem of U-shaped plastic carrier, surface area approx. 375 mm$^2$, impregnated with barium sulfate for radio-opacity, threads attached to base of vertical stem; preloaded in inserter, net price = £9.95
For uterine length over 6.5 cm; replacement every 5 years (see also notes above)

**Ancora® 375 Cu** (RF Medical)
Intra-uterine device, copper wire, wound on vertical stem of U-shaped plastic carrier, surface area approx. 375 mm$^2$, impregnated with barium sulfate for radio-opacity, threads attached to base of vertical stem; preloaded in inserter, net price = £7.95
For uterine length over 6.5 cm; replacement every 5 years (see also notes above)

**Copper T 380A®** (RF Medical)
Intra-uterine device, copper wire, wound on vertical stem of T-shaped plastic carrier with copper sleeve on each arm, total surface area approx. 380 mm$^2$, impregnated with barium sulfate for radio-opacity, threads attached to base of vertical stem; with loading capsule, net price = £8.95
For uterine length 6.5–9 cm; replacement every 10 years (see also notes above)

**Cu-Safe® T300** (Williams) ⦿🅷🆂
Intra-uterine device, copper wire, wound on vertical stem of T-shaped plastic carrier, surface area approx. 300 mm$^2$, impregnated with barium sulfate for radio-opacity, monofilament thread attached to base of vertical stem; preloaded in inserter, net price = £9.11
For uterine length over 5 cm; replacement every 5 years (see also notes above)

**Flexi-T 300®** (Durbin)
Intra-uterine device, copper wire, wound on vertical stem of T-shaped plastic carrier, surface area approx. 300 mm$^2$, impregnated with barium sulfate for radio-opacity, monofilament thread attached to base of vertical stem; preloaded in inserter, net price = £9.47
For uterine length over 5 cm; replacement every 5 years (see also notes above)

**Flexi-T® + 380** (Durbin)
Intra-uterine device, copper wire, wound on vertical stem of T-shaped plastic carrier with copper sleeve on each arm, total surface area approx. 380 mm$^2$, impregnated with barium sulfate for radio-opacity, monofilament thread attached to base of vertical stem; preloaded in inserter, net price = £10.06
For uterine length over 6 cm; replacement every 5 years (see also notes above)

**GyneFix®** (Williams)
Intra-uterine device, 6 copper sleeves with surface area of 330 mm$^2$ on polypropylene thread, net price = £26.64
Suitable for all uterine sizes; replacement every 5 years

**Load® 375** (Durbin)
Intra-uterine device, copper wire, wound on vertical stem of U-shaped plastic carrier, surface area approx. 375 mm$^2$, impregnated with barium sulfate for radio-opacity, monofilament thread attached to base of vertical stem; preloaded in inserter, net price = £8.52
For uterine length over 7 cm; replacement every 5 years (see also notes above)

**Mini TT 380® Slimline** (Durbin)
Intra-uterine device, copper wire, wound on vertical stem of T-shaped plastic carrier with copper sleeves fitted flush on to distal portion of each horizontal arm, total surface area approx. 380 mm$^2$, impregnated with barium sulfate for radio-opacity, thread attached to base of vertical stem; easy-loading system, no capsule, net price = £12.46
For minimum uterine length 5 cm; replacement every 5 years (see also notes above)

**Multiload® Cu375** (Organon)
Intra-uterine device, as *Load® 375*, with copper surface area approx. 375 mm$^2$ and vertical stem length 3.5 cm, net price = £9.24
For uterine length 6–9 cm; replacement every 5 years (see also notes above)

**Multi-Safe® 375** (Williams)
Intra-uterine device, copper wire, wound on vertical stem of U-shaped plastic carrier, surface area approx. 375 mm$^2$, impregnated with barium sulfate for radio-opacity, monofilament thread attached to base of vertical stem; preloaded in inserter, net price = £8.80
For uterine length 6–9cm; replacement every 5 years (see also notes above)

**7 Obstetrics, gynaecology, and urinary-tract disorders**

**MultiSafe® 375 Short Stem** (Williams) [JHS]
Intra-uterine device, copper wire, wound on vertical stem of U-shaped plastic carrier, surface area approx. 375 mm², impregnated with barium sulfate for radio-opacity, monofilament thread attached to base of vertical stem; preloaded in inserter, net price = £8.80
  For uterine length 5–7cm; replacement every 5 years (see also notes above)

**Neo-Safe® T380** (Williams)
Intra-uterine device, copper wire, wound on vertical stem of T-shaped plastic carrier, surface area approx. 380 mm², impregnated with barium sulfate for radio-opacity, threads attached to base of vertical stem, net price = £13.80
  For uterine length 6.5–9 cm; replacement every 5 years (see also notes above)

**Novaplus T 380® Ag** (RF Medical)
Intra-uterine device, copper wire with silver core, wound on vertical stem of T-shaped plastic carrier, surface area approx. 380 mm², impregnated with barium sulfate for radio-opacity, threads attached to base of vertical stem, net price = £12.50
  'Mini' size for minimum uterine length 5 cm; 'Normal' size for uterine length 6.5–9 cm; replacement every 5 years (see also notes above)

**Novaplus T 380® Cu** (RF Medical)
Intra-uterine device, copper wire, wound on vertical stem of T-shaped plastic carrier, surface area approx. 380 mm², impregnated with barium sulfate for radio-opacity, threads attached to base of vertical stem, net price = £10.95
  'Mini' size for minimum uterine length 5 cm; 'Normal' size for uterine length 6.5–9 cm; replacement every 5 years (see also notes above)

**Nova-T® 380** (Bayer)
Intra-uterine device, copper wire with silver core, wound on vertical stem of T-shaped plastic carrier, surface area approx. 380 mm², impregnated with barium sulfate for radio-opacity, threads attached to base of vertical stem, net price = £12.97
  For uterine length 6.5–9 cm; replacement every 5 years (see also notes above)

**T-Safe® 380A Quickload** (Williams)
Intra-uterine device, copper wire, wound on vertical stem of T-shaped plastic carrier with copper collar on the distal portion of each arm, total surface area approx. 380 mm², impregnated with barium sulfate for radio-opacity, threads attached to base of vertical stem, net price = £10.29; available with a capsule loading device (T-Safe® CU 380A [JHS]), net price £10.29
  For uterine length 6.5–9 cm; replacement every 10 years (see also notes above)

**TT 380® Slimline** (Durbin)
Intra-uterine device, copper wire, wound on vertical stem of T-shaped plastic carrier, with copper sleeves fitted flush on to distal portion of each horizontal arm, total surface area approx. 380 mm², impregnated with barium sulfate for radio-opacity, thread attached to base of vertical stem; easy-loading system, no capsule, net price = £12.46
  For uterine length 6.5–9 cm; replacement every 10 years (see also notes above)

**UT 380 Short®** (Durbin)
Intra-uterine device, copper wire, wound on vertical stem of T-shaped plastic carrier, surface area approx. 380 mm², impregnated with barium sulfate for radio-opacity, thread attached to base of vertical stem; net price = £11.22
  For uterine length 5–7 cm; replacement every 5 years (see also notes above)

**UT 380 Standard®** (Durbin)
Intra-uterine device, copper wire, wound on vertical stem of T-shaped plastic carrier, surface area approx. 380 mm², impregnated with barium sulfate for radio-opacity, thread attached to base of vertical stem; net price = £11.22
  For uterine length 6.5–9 cm; replacement every 5 years (see also notes above)

## Other contraceptive devices

◢**Silicone contraceptive caps**
**Silicone Contraceptive Pessary**
Silicone, sizes 22, 26, and 30 mm, net price = £15.00
  **Brands include** *FemCap®*

◢**Rubber contraceptive diaphragms**
**Type A Diaphragm with Flat Metal Spring**
Transparent rubber with flat metal spring, sizes 55–95 mm (rising in steps of 5 mm), net price = £5.78
  **Brands include** *Reflexions®*

◢**Silicone contraceptive diaphragms**
**Type B Diaphragm with Coiled Metal Spring**
Silicone with coiled metal spring, sizes 60–90 mm (rising in steps of 5 mm), net price = £8.35
  **Brands include** *Milex Omniflex®*

**Type C Arcing Spring diaphragm**
Silicone with arcing spring, sizes 60–90 mm (rising in steps of 5 mm), net price = £8.35
  **Brands include** *Milex Arcing Style®, Ortho All-Flex®*

## 7.3.5 Emergency contraception

## Hormonal methods

Hormonal emergency contraceptives include **levonorgestrel** and **ulipristal**; either drug should be taken as soon as possible after unprotected intercourse to increase efficacy.

Levonorgestrel is effective if taken within 72 hours (3 days) of unprotected intercourse and may also be used between 72 and 96 hours after unprotected intercourse [unlicensed use], but efficacy decreases with time. Ulipristal, a progesterone receptor modulator, is effective if taken within 120 hours (5 days) of unprotected intercourse.

Levonorgestrel is less effective than insertion of an intra-uterine device (see below). Ulipristal is as effective as levonorgestrel but it's efficacy compared to an intra-uterine device is not yet known.

If vomiting occurs within 2 hours of taking levonorgestrel or within 3 hours of taking ulipristal, a replacement dose should be given. If an anti-emetic is required domperidone is preferred.

When prescribing or supplying hormonal emergency contraception, women should be advised:

- that their next period may be early or late;
- that a barrier method of contraception needs to be used until the next period;
- to seek medical attention promptly if any lower abdominal pain occurs because this could signify an ectopic pregnancy;
- to return in 3 to 4 weeks if the subsequent menstrual bleed is abnormally light, heavy or brief, or is absent, or if she is otherwise concerned (if there is any doubt as to whether menstruation has occurred, a pregnancy test should be performed at least 3 weeks after unprotected intercourse).

**Interactions**   The effectiveness of levonorgestrel, and possibly ulipristal is reduced in women taking enzyme-inducing drugs (and possibly for 4 weeks after stopping); a copper intra-uterine device can be offered instead. If the copper intra-uterine device is undesirable or inappropriate, the dose of levonorgestrel should be increased to a total of 3 mg taken as a single dose [unlicensed dose—advise women accordingly]. There is no need to increase the dose for emergency contraception if the patient is taking antibacterials that are not enzyme inducers.

### ■ LEVONORGESTREL

**Cautions**   see notes above; past ectopic pregnancy; severe malabsorption syndromes; active trophoblastic disease (until return to normal of urine- and plasma-gonadotrophin concentration)—seek specialist advice; **interactions:** see notes above and Appendix 1 (progestogens)

**Contra-indications**   acute porphyria (section 9.8.2)

**Pregnancy**   not known to be harmful

**Breast-feeding**   progestogen-only contraceptives do not affect lactation

**Side-effects**   menstrual irregularities (see also notes above), nausea, low abdominal pain, fatigue, headache, dizziness, breast tenderness, vomiting

**Licensed use**   consult product literature

**Indications and dose**

Emergency contraception

- By mouth

  1.5 mg as a single dose as soon as possible after coitus, preferably within 12 hours but no later than after 72 hours (but see also notes above)

[1]**Levonelle® One Step** (Bayer)
Tablets, levonorgestrel 1.5 mg, net price 1-tab pack = £13.83

**Levonelle® 1500** (Bayer) [PoM]
Tablets, levonorgestrel 1.5 mg, net price 1-tab pack = £5.20

### ■ ULIPRISTAL ACETATE

**Cautions**   see notes above; uncontrolled severe asthma; effectiveness of combined hormonal and progestogen-only contraceptives may be reduced—additional precautions (barrier methods) required for 14 days for combined and parenteral progestogen-

only hormonal contraceptives (16 days for *Qlaira*®) and 9 days for oral progestogen-only contraceptives; **interactions:** see notes above and Appendix 1 (ulipristal)

**Contra-indications**   repeated use within a menstrual cycle

**Hepatic impairment**   manufacturer advises avoid in severe impairment—no information available

**Pregnancy**   limited information available

**Breast-feeding**   manufacturer advises avoid for 1 week after administration—present in milk

**Side-effects**   gastro-intestinal disturbances (including nausea, vomiting, diarrhoea, and abdominal pain); dizziness, fatigue, headache, menstrual irregularities (see notes above); back pain, muscle spasms; *less commonly* tremor, hot flushes, uterine spasm, breast tenderness, dry mouth, blurred vision, pruritus, and rash

**Indications and dose**

Emergency contraception

- By mouth

  30 mg as a single dose as soon as possible after coitus, but no later than after 120 hours

**ellaOne**® (HRA Pharma) [PoM]
Tablets, ulipristal acetate 30 mg, net price 1-tab pack = £16.95

## Intra-uterine device

Insertion of an intra-uterine device is more effective than oral levonorgestrel for emergency contraception, see also notes above. A copper intra-uterine contraceptive device (section 7.3.4) can be inserted up to 120 hours (5 days) after unprotected intercourse; sexually transmitted infections should be tested for and insertion of the device should usually be covered by antibacterial prophylaxis (e.g. azithromycin 1 g as a single dose). If intercourse has occurred more than 5 days previously, the device can still be inserted up to 5 days after the earliest likely calculated ovulation (i.e. within the minimum period before implantation), regardless of the number of episodes of unprotected intercourse earlier in the cycle.

## 7.4  Drugs for genito-urinary disorders

7.4.1   Drugs for urinary retention

7.4.2   Drugs for urinary frequency, enuresis, and incontinence

7.4.3   Drugs used in urological pain

7.4.4   Bladder instillations and urological surgery

7.4.5   Drugs for erectile dysfunction

For drugs used in the treatment of urinary-tract infections see section 5.1.13.

## 7.4.1  Drugs for urinary retention

*Acute retention* is painful and is treated by catheterisation.

*Chronic retention* is painless and often long-standing. Clean intermittent catheterisation may be considered.

*7 Obstetrics, gynaecology, and urinary-tract disorders*

---

1. Can be sold to women over 16 years; when supplying emergency contraception to the public, pharmacists should refer to guidance issued by the Royal Pharmaceutical Society

After the cause has been established and treated, drugs may be required to increase detrusor muscle tone.

Alpha-blockers such as doxazosin and tamsulosin can be used in some cases of dysfunctional voiding.

## Alpha-blockers

The selective alpha-blockers **doxazosin** and **tamsulosin** can be used to improve bladder emptying in children with dysfunctional voiding where the post-void residual urine volume is significant; treatment should be under specialist advice only. Alpha-blockers can reduce blood pressure rapidly after the first dose and should be introduced with caution.

### DOXAZOSIN

**Cautions** see under Doxazosin (section 2.5.4)

**Contra-indications** see under Doxazosin (section 2.5.4)

**Hepatic impairment** see under Doxazosin (section 2.5.4)

**Pregnancy** see under Doxazosin (section 2.5.4)

**Breast-feeding** see under Doxazosin (section 2.5.4)

**Side-effects** see under Doxazosin (section 2.5.4)

**Licensed use** not licensed for use in children

**Indications and dose**

**Dysfunctional voiding** (see notes above)
* By mouth

**Child 4–12 years** initially 0.5 mg daily increased at monthly intervals according to response; maximum 2 mg daily

**Child 12–18 years** initially 1 mg daily, dose may be doubled at intervals of 1 month according to response; usual maintenance 2–4 mg daily; max. 8 mg daily

**Hypertension** section 2.5.4

◀**Preparations**
Section 2.5.4

### TAMSULOSIN HYDROCHLORIDE

**Cautions** care with initial dose (postural hypotension); cataract surgery (risk of intra-operative floppy iris syndrome); **interactions:** Appendix 1 (alpha-blockers)

**Driving** May affect performance of skilled tasks e.g. driving

**Contra-indications** history of postural hypotension

**Hepatic impairment** avoid in severe impairment

**Renal impairment** use with caution if estimated glomerular filtration rate less than 10 mL/minute/1.73 m²

**Side-effects** dizziness, headache, asthenia; abnormal ejaculation; *less commonly* nausea, vomiting, constipation, diarrhoea, palpitation, postural hypotension, syncope, rhinitis, rash, pruritus, and urticaria; *very rarely* angioedema and priapism; also drowsiness, blurred vision, dry mouth, and oedema; *also reported* intra-operative floppy iris syndrome

**Licensed use** not licensed for use in children

**Indications and dose**

**Dysfunctional voiding** (see notes above)
* By mouth

**Child 12–18 years** 400 micrograms once daily

**Tamsulosin hydrochloride** (Non-proprietary) ⓅoM

Capsules, m/r, tamsulosin hydrochloride 400 micrograms, net price 30-cap pack = £4.62. Label: 25, counselling, driving

**Brands include** *Bazetham®* MR, *Contiflo®* XL, *Diffundox®* XL, *Losinate®* MR, *Pinexel®* PR, *Prosurin®* XL, *Stronazon®* MR, *Tabphyn®* MR

**Flomaxtra® XL** (Astellas) ⓅoM

Tablets, m/r, tamsulosin hydrochloride 400 micrograms, net price 30-tab pack = £10.47. Label: 25, counselling, driving

### 7.4.2 Drugs for urinary frequency, enuresis, and incontinence

## Urinary incontinence

Antimuscarinic drugs reduce symptoms of urgency and urge incontinence and increase bladder capacity; **oxybutynin** also has a direct relaxant effect on urinary smooth muscle. Oxybutynin can be considered first for children under 12 years. Side-effects limit the use of oxybutynin, but they may be reduced by starting at a lower dose and then slowly titrating upwards; alternatively oxybutynin can be given by intravesicular instillation. **Tolterodine** is also effective for urinary incontinence; it can be considered for children over 12 years, or for younger children who have failed to respond to oxybutynin. Modified-release preparations of oxybutynin and tolterodine are available; they may have fewer side-effects. Antimuscarinic treatment should be reviewed soon after it is commenced, and then at regular intervals; a response generally occurs within 6 months but occasionally may take longer. Children with nocturnal enuresis may require specific additional measures if night-time symptoms also need to be controlled (see p. 411).

**Cautions** Antimuscarinic drugs should be used with caution in autonomic neuropathy and in children susceptible to angle-closure glaucoma. Antimuscarinics can worsen hyperthyroidism, congestive heart failure, arrhythmias, and tachycardia. For **interactions,** see Appendix 1 (antimuscarinics).

**Contra-indications** Antimuscarinic drugs should be avoided in myasthenia gravis, significant bladder outflow obstruction or urinary retention, severe ulcerative colitis, toxic megacolon, and in gastro-intestinal obstruction or intestinal atony.

**Side-effects** Side-effects of antimuscarinic drugs include dry mouth, gastro-intestinal disturbances including constipation, blurred vision, dry eyes, drowsiness, difficulty in micturition (less commonly urinary retention), palpitation, and skin reactions (including dry skin, rash, and photosensitivity); also headache, diarrhoea, angioedema, arrhythmias, and tachycardia. Central nervous system stimulation, such as restlessness, disorientation, hallucination, and convulsions may occur. Antimuscarinic drugs may reduce sweating leading to heat sensations and fainting in hot environments or in patients with fever, and *very rarely* may precipitate angle-closure glaucoma.

### OXYBUTYNIN HYDROCHLORIDE

**Cautions** see notes above; acute porphyria (section 9.8.2)

**Contra-indications** see notes above

**Hepatic impairment** manufacturer advises caution

**Renal impairment** manufacturer advises caution

**Pregnancy** manufacturer advises avoid unless essential—toxicity in *animal* studies

**Breast-feeding** manufacturer advises avoid—present in milk in *animal* studies

**Side-effects** see notes above; also dizziness; *less commonly* anorexia, facial flushing; *rarely* night terrors

**Licensed use** not licensed for use in children under 5 years; intravesical instillation not licensed for use in children

**Indications and dose**

> Urinary frequency, urgency and incontinence, neurogenic bladder instability
> - By mouth
>   - **Child 2–5 years** 1.25–2.5 mg 2–3 times daily;
>   - **Child 5–12 years** 2.5–3 mg twice daily, increased to 5 mg 2–3 times daily
>   - **Child 12–18 years** 5 mg 2–3 times daily, increased if necessary to max. 5 mg 4 times daily
> - By intravesical instillation
>   - **Child 2–18 years** 5 mg 2–3 times daily

> Nocturnal enuresis associated with overactive bladder
> - By mouth
>   - **Child 5–18 years** 2.5–3 mg twice daily increased to 5 mg 2–3 times daily (last dose before bedtime)

**Oxybutynin Hydrochloride** (Non-proprietary) [PoM]
Tablets, oxybutynin hydrochloride 2.5 mg, net price 56-tab pack = £6.58; 3 mg, 56-tab pack = £9.15; 5 mg, 56-tab pack = £5.53, 84-tab pack = £12.50. Label: 3

Intravesical instillation, oxybutynin (as hydrochloride) 5 mg/30 mL.
Available from 'special-order' manufacturers or specialist importing companies, see p. 823

**Cystrin®** (Winthrop) [PoM]
Tablets, oxybutynin hydrochloride 5 mg (scored), net price 84-tab pack = £21.99. Label: 3

**Ditropan®** (Sanofi-Aventis) [PoM]
Tablets, both blue, scored, oxybutynin hydrochloride 2.5 mg, net price 84-tab pack = £6.59; 5 mg, 84-tab pack = £12.82. Label: 3

◄**Modified release**

**Lyrinel® XL** (Janssen) [PoM]
Tablets, m/r, oxybutynin hydrochloride 5 mg (yellow), net price 30-tab pack = £10.81; 10 mg (pink), 30-tab pack = £21.62. Label: 3, 25

**Dose**

> Urinary frequency, urgency, and incontinence associated with idiopathic overactive bladder or neurogenic bladder instability; nocturnal enuresis associated with overactive bladder (see also Nocturnal Enuresis, below)
> - By mouth
>   - **Child 5–18 years** initially 5 mg once daily adjusted according to response in steps of 5 mg at weekly intervals; max. 15 mg once daily

Note Children taking immediate-release oxybutynin may be transferred to the nearest equivalent daily dose of *Lyrinel® XL*

## ■ TOLTERODINE TARTRATE

**Cautions** see notes above; history of QT-interval prolongation; concomitant use with other drugs known to prolong QT interval

**Contra-indications** see notes above

**Hepatic impairment** reduce dose; avoid modified-release preparations

**Renal impairment** reduce dose and avoid modified-release preparations if estimated glomerular filtration rate less than $30 \, mL/minute/1.73 \, m^2$

**Pregnancy** manufacturer advises avoid—toxicity in *animal* studies

**Breast-feeding** manufacturer advises avoid—no information available

**Side-effects** see notes above; also chest pain, peripheral oedema; sinusitis, bronchitis; paraesthesia, fatigue, dizziness, vertigo, weight gain; *less commonly* memory impairment; *also reported* flushing

**Licensed use** not licensed for use in children

**Indications and dose**

> Urinary frequency, urgency, incontinence
> - By mouth
>   - **Child 2–18 years** 1 mg once daily, increased according to response; max. 2 mg twice daily

> Nocturnal enuresis associated with overactive bladder
> - By mouth
>   - **Child 5–18 years** 1 mg once daily at bedtime, increased according to response; max. 2 mg twice daily

**Tolterodine Tartrate** (Non-proprietary) [PoM]
Tablets, tolterodine tartrate 1 mg, net price 56-tab pack = £4.35; 2 mg, 56-tab pack = £4.58. Label: 3

**Detrusitol®** (Pfizer) [PoM]
Tablets, f/c, tolterodine tartrate 1 mg, net price 56-tab pack = £29.03; 2 mg, 56-tab pack = £30.56

◄**Modified release**

**Tolterodine Tartrate** (Non-proprietary) [PoM]
Capsules, m/r, tolterodine tartrate 4 mg, net price 28-cap pack = £20.62. Label: 3, 25
**Brands include** *Santizor XL®*
Note Children stabilised on immediate-release tolterodine tartrate 2 mg twice daily may be transferred to modified-release tolterodine tartrate 4 mg once daily

**Detrusitol® XL** (Pfizer) [PoM]
Capsules, blue, m/r, tolterodine tartrate 4 mg, net price 28-cap pack = £25.78. Label: 25
Note Children stabilised on immediate-release tolterodine tartrate 2 mg twice daily may be transferred to *Detrusitol® XL* 4 mg once daily

## Nocturnal enuresis in children

*Nocturnal enuresis* is common in young children, but persists in a small proportion by 10 years of age. For children under 5 years, reassurance and advice on the management of nocturnal enuresis can be useful for some families. Treatment may be considered in children over 5 years depending on their maturity and motivation, the frequency of nocturnal enuresis, and the needs of the child and their family.

Initially, advice should be given on fluid intake, diet, toileting behaviour, and reward systems; for children who do not respond to this advice, further treatment may be necessary. An **enuresis alarm** should be first-line treatment for motivated, well supported children; alarms have a lower relapse rate than drug treatment when discontinued. Treatment should be reviewed after 4 weeks, and, if there are early signs of response, continued until a minimum of 2 weeks' uninterrupted dry nights have been achieved. If complete dryness is not achieved after 3 months, only continue if the condition is still improving and the child remains motivated to use the alarm. If initial alarm treatment is unsuccessful, consider combination treatment with **desmopressin** (see below), or desmopressin alone if the alarm is no longer appropriate or desirable.

**Desmopressin** (section 6.5.2), an analogue of vasopressin, is given by oral or by sublingual administration; it should not be given intranasally for nocturnal enuresis due to an increased incidence of side-effects. Desmopressin alone can be offered to children over 5 years of age if an alarm is inappropriate or undesirable, or when rapid or short-term results are the priority (for example to cover periods away from home); desmopressin alone can also be used if there has been a partial response to a combination of desmopressin and an alarm following initial treatment with an alarm. Treatment should be assessed after 4 weeks and continued for 3 months if there are signs of response. Desmopressin should be withdrawn at regular intervals (for 1 week every 3 months) for full reassessment. Particular care is needed to avoid fluid overload by restricting fluid intake from 1 hour before taking desmopressin until 8 hours after. When stopping treatment with desmopressin, gradual withdrawal should be considered.

Nocturnal enuresis associated with daytime symptoms (overactive bladder) can be managed with antimuscarinic drugs (see Urinary incontinence, p. 410) in combination with desmopressin. Treatment should be prescribed only after specialist assessment and should be continued for 3 months; the course can be repeated if necessary.

The tricyclic antidepressant **imipramine** (section 4.3.1) may be considered for children who have not responded to all other treatments and have undergone specialist assessment, however, behavioural disturbances can occur and relapse is common after withdrawal. Treatment should not normally exceed 3 months unless a physical examination is made and the child is fully reassessed; toxicity following overdosage with tricyclics is of particular concern.

## 7.4.3 Drugs used in urological pain

**Lidocaine gel** is a useful topical application in *urethral pain* or to relieve the discomfort of catheterisation (section 15.2).

## Alkalinisation of urine

*Alkalinisation* of urine can be undertaken with **potassium citrate**. The alkalinising action may relieve the discomfort of *cystitis* caused by lower urinary tract infections.

## ◼ POTASSIUM CITRATE

**Cautions**  cardiac disease; **interactions:** Appendix 1 (potassium salts)

**Renal impairment**  close monitoring required—high risk of hyperkalaemia; avoid in severe impairment

**Side-effects**  hyperkalaemia on prolonged high dosage, mild diuresis

**Indications and dose**

> Relief of discomfort in mild urinary-tract infections, alkalinisation of urine for dose see preparations below

**Potassium Citrate Mixture BP**
(Potassium Citrate Oral Solution)
Oral solution, potassium citrate 30%, citric acid monohydrate 5% in a suitable vehicle with a lemon flavour. Extemporaneous preparations should be recently prepared according to the following formula: potassium citrate 3 g, citric acid monohydrate 500 mg, syrup 2.5 mL, quillaia tincture 0.1 mL, lemon spirit 0.05 mL, double-strength chloroform water 3 mL, water to 10 mL. Contains about 28 mmol $K^+$/10 mL. Label: 27

**Dose**

- By mouth
  **Child 1–6 years** 5 mL 3 times daily well diluted with water
  **Child 6–18 years** 10 mL 3 times daily well diluted with water

**Note** Proprietary brands of potassium citrate are on sale to the public for the relief of discomfort in mild urinary-tract infections

## 7.4.4 Bladder instillations and urological surgery

**Bladder infection**  Various solutions are available as irrigations or washouts.

Aqueous **chlorhexidine** (section 13.11.2) can be used in the management of common infections of the bladder but it is ineffective against most *Pseudomonas* spp. Solutions containing chlorhexidine 1 in 5000 (0.02%) are used, but they may irritate the mucosa and cause burning and haematuria (in which case they should be discontinued); sterile **sodium chloride solution 0.9%** (physiological saline) is usually adequate and is preferred as a mechanical irrigant.

**Dissolution of blood clots**  Clot retention is usually treated by irrigation with sterile **sodium chloride solution 0.9%** but sterile **sodium citrate solution for bladder irrigation 3%** may also be helpful.

## Maintenance of indwelling urinary catheters

The deposition which occurs in catheterised patients is usually chiefly composed of phosphate and to minimise this the catheter (if latex) should be changed at least as often as every 6 weeks. If the catheter is to be left for longer periods a silicone catheter should be used together with the appropriate use of catheter maintenance solutions. Repeated blockage usually indicates that the catheter needs to be changed.

## CATHETER PATENCY SOLUTIONS

**Chlorhexidine 0.02%**
Brands include *Uro-Tainer Chlorhexidine*®, 100-mL sachet = £2.60

**Sodium chloride 0.9%**
Brands include *OptiFlo S*®, 50- and 100-mL sachets = £3.20; *Uriflex S*®, 100-mL sachet = £2.40; *Uriflex SP*®, with integral drug additive port, 100-mL sachet = £2.40; *Uro-Tainer Sodium Chloride*®, 50- and 100-mL sachets = £3.25; *Uro-Tainer M*®, with integral drug additive port, 50- and 100-mL sachets = £2.90

**Solution G**
Citric acid 3.23%, magnesium oxide 0.38%, sodium bicarbonate 0.7%, disodium edetate 0.01%. Brands include *OptiFlo G*®, 50- and 100-mL sachets = £3.40; *Uriflex G*®, 100-mL sachet = £2.40; *Uro-Tainer*® Twin Suby G, 2 × 30-mL = £4.46

**Solution R**
Citric acid 6%, gluconolactone 0.6%, magnesium carbonate 2.8%, disodium edetate 0.01%. Brands include *OptiFlo R*®, 50- and 100-mL sachets = £3.40; *Uriflex R*®, 100-mL sachet = £2.40; *Uro-Tainer*® Twin Solutio R, 2 × 30-mL = £4.46

## Diluents for bladder instillation

 ## SODIUM CHLORIDE

**Indications and dose**

**Diluent for instillation of drugs to the bladder**
consult product literature

**Sodium Chloride 0.9% Solution for Intravesical Use** (Non-proprietary)
Intravesical instillation, sodium chloride 0.9%, net price 50-mL bag = £9.66

## 7.4.5 Drugs for erectile dysfunction

This section is not included in *BNF for Children*. Adolescents presenting with erectile dysfunction should be referred to a specialist.

# 8 Malignant disease and immunosuppression

The management of childhood cancer is complex and is generally confined to specialist regional centres and some associated shared-care units.

Cytotoxic drugs have both anti-cancer activity and the potential for damage to normal tissue. In children, chemotherapy is almost always started with curative intent, but may be continued as palliation if the disease is refractory.

Chemotherapy with a combination of two or more cytotoxic drugs aims to reduce the development of resistance and to improve cytotoxic effect. Treatment protocols generally incorporate a series of treatment courses at defined intervals with clear criteria for starting each course, such as adequate bone-marrow recovery and renal or cardiac function. The principal component of treatment for leukaemias in children is cytotoxic therapy, whereas solid tumours may be managed with surgery or radiotherapy in addition to chemotherapy.

---

**Guidelines for handling cytotoxic drugs**

- Trained personnel should reconstitute cytotoxics;
- Reconstitution should be carried out in designated pharmacy areas;
- Protective clothing (including gloves, gowns, and masks) should be worn;
- The eyes should be protected and means of first aid should be specified;
- Pregnant staff should avoid exposure to cytotoxic drugs (all females of child-bearing age should be informed of the reproductive hazard);
- Use local procedures for dealing with spillages and safe disposal of waste material, including syringes, containers, and absorbent material;
- Staff exposure to cytotoxic drugs should be monitored.

---

Only medical or nursing staff who have received appropriate training should administer parenteral cytotoxics. In most instances central venous access will be required for the intravenous administration of cytotoxics to children; care is required to avoid the risk of extravasation (see Side-effects of Cytotoxic Drugs and their Management).

Safe system requirements for cytotoxic medicines:

- Cytotoxic drugs for the treatment of cancer should be given as part of a wider pathway of care that is co-ordinated by a multi-disciplinary team;

- Cytotoxic drugs should be prescribed, dispensed and administered only in the context of a written protocol or treatment plan;

- Injectable cytotoxic drugs should only be dispensed if they are prepared for administration;

- Oral cytotoxic medicines should be dispensed with clear directions for use.

### Risks of incorrect dosing of oral anti-cancer medicines

The National Patient Safety Agency has advised (January 2008) that the prescribing and use of oral cytotoxic medicines should be carried out to the same standard as parenteral cytotoxic therapy. Standards to be followed to achieve this include:

- non-specialists who prescribe or administer oral cytotoxic medication should have access to written protocols and treatment plans, including guidance on the monitoring and treatment of toxicity

- staff dispensing oral cytotoxic medicines should confirm that the prescribed dose is appropriate for the patient. Patients and their carers should have written information that includes details of the intended oral anti-cancer regimen, the treatment plan, and arrangements for monitoring, taken from the original protocol from the initiating hospital. Staff dispensing oral cytotoxic medicines should also have access to this information, and to advice from an experienced cancer pharmacist in the initiating hospital

### Doses

Doses of cytotoxic drugs are determined using a variety of different methods including age, body-surface area, or body-weight. Alternatively, doses may be fixed. Doses may be further adjusted following consideration of a patient's neutrophil count, renal and hepatic function, and history of previous adverse effects to the cytotoxic drug. Doses may also differ depending on whether a drug is used alone or in combination.

Because of the complexity of dosage regimens in the treatment of malignant disease, dose statements have been omitted from many of the drug entries in this chapter.

## Side-effects of cytotoxic drugs and their management

Side-effects common to most cytotoxic drugs are discussed below whilst side-effects characteristic of a particular drug or class of drugs (e.g. neurotoxicity with vinca alkaloids) are mentioned in the appropriate sections. Manufacturers' product literature, hospital-trust protocols, and treatment protocols should be consulted for full details of side-effects of individual drugs.

Side-effects of cytotoxic drugs often do not occur at the time of administration, but days or weeks later. It is therefore important that children, their carers, and healthcare professionals can identify symptoms that cause concern and can contact an expert for advice. Toxicities should be accurately recorded using a recognised scoring system such as the Common Toxicity Criteria for Adverse Events (CTCAE) developed by the National Cancer institute.

**Extravasation of intravenous drugs**  A number of cytotoxic drugs will cause severe local tissue irritation and necrosis if leakage into the extravascular compartment occurs. For information on the prevention and management of extravasation injury, see section 10.3.

**Gastro-intestinal effects**  Management of gastro-intestinal effects of cytotoxic drugs includes the use of antacids, $H_2$-receptor antagonists, and proton pump inhibitors to protect the gastric mucosa, laxatives to treat constipation, and enteral and parenteral nutritional support.

**Oral mucositis**  Good oral hygiene keeps the mouth clean and moist and helps to prevent mucositis; prevention is more effective than treatment of the complication. Good oral hygiene measures for children over 6 months include brushing teeth with a soft small brush with fluoride toothpaste 2–3 times daily, and rinsing the mouth frequently. Daily fluoride supplements (section 9.5.3) can be used on the advice of the child's dental team. For children under 6 months or when it is not possible to brush teeth, carers should be instructed how to clean the mouth using an oral sponge moistened with water or with an antimicrobial solution such as diluted chlorhexidine. Mucositis related to chemotherapy can be extremely painful and may, in some circumstances, require opioid analgesia (section 4.7.2). Secondary infection with candida is frequent; treatment with a systemically absorbed antifungal, such as fluconazole (section 5.2), is effective.

**Nausea and vomiting**  Nausea and vomiting cause considerable distress to many children who receive chemotherapy, and to a lesser extent abdominal radiotherapy, and may lead to refusal of further treatment; prophylaxis of nausea and vomiting is therefore extremely important. Symptoms may be acute (occurring within 24 hours of treatment), delayed (first occurring more than 24 hours after treatment), or anticipatory (occurring prior to subsequent doses). Delayed and anticipatory symptoms are more difficult to control than acute symptoms and require different management.

Susceptibility to nausea and vomiting may increase with repeated exposure to the cytotoxic drug.

Drugs may be divided according to their emetogenic potential and some examples are given below, but the symptoms vary according to the dose, to other drugs administered, and to the individual's susceptibility to emetogenic stimuli.

**8**

**Malignant disease and immunosuppression**

*Mildly emetogenic treatment*—fluorouracil, etoposide, low doses of methotrexate, the vinca alkaloids, and abdominal radiotherapy.

*Moderately emetogenic treatment*—carboplatin, doxorubicin, intermediate and low doses of cyclophosphamide, mitoxantrone, and high doses of methotrexate.

*Highly emetogenic treatment*—cisplatin, dacarbazine, and high doses of alkylating drugs.

Anti-emetic drugs, when given regularly, help prevent or ameliorate emesis associated with chemotherapy in children.

**Prevention of acute symptoms** For patients at *low risk of emesis*, pretreatment with metoclopramide (or less commonly domperidone) continued for up to 24 hours after chemotherapy, is often effective (section 4.6); a $5HT_3$-receptor antagonist (section 4.6) may also be of benefit.

For patients at *high risk of emesis* or when other treatment is inadequate, a $5HT_3$-receptor antagonist (section 4.6) is often highly effective. The addition of dexamethasone and other anti-emetics may also be required.

**Prevention of delayed symptoms** Dexamethasone, given by mouth, is the drug of choice for preventing delayed symptoms; it is used alone or with metoclopramide. The $5HT_3$-receptor antagonists may have a role in preventing uncontrolled symptoms.

**Prevention of anticipatory symptoms** Good symptom control is the best way to prevent anticipatory symptoms. Lorazepam can be helpful for its amnesiac, sedative, and anxiolytic effects.

**Bone-marrow suppression** All cytotoxic drugs except vincristine and bleomycin cause bone-marrow suppression. This commonly occurs 7 to 10 days after administration, but is delayed for certain drugs, such as melphalan. Peripheral blood counts must be checked before each treatment. The duration and severity of neutropenia can be reduced by the use of granulocyte-colony stimulating factors (section 9.1.6); their use should be reserved for children who have previously experienced severe neutropenia.

Cytotoxic drugs may be contra-indicated in children with acute infection; any infection should be treated before, or when starting, cytotoxic drugs.

Infection in a child with neutropenia requires immediate broad-spectrum antibacterial treatment that covers all likely pathogens (Table 1, section 5.1). Appropriate bacteriological investigations should be conducted as soon as possible. Children taking cytotoxic drugs who have signs or symptoms of infection (or their carers) should be advised to seek prompt medical attention. All children should be investigated and treated under the supervision of an appropriate oncology or haematology specialist. Antifungal treatment (section 5.2) may be required in a child with prolonged neutropenia or fever lasting longer than 4–5 days. Chickenpox and measles can be particularly hazardous in immunocompromised children. Varicella–zoster immunoglobulin (section 14.5.2) is indicated if the child does not have immunity against varicella and has had close contact with infectious chickenpox or herpes zoster. Antiviral prophylaxis (section 5.3.2.1) can be considered in addition to varicella–zoster immunoglobulin or as an alternative if varicella–zoster immunoglobulin is inappropriate. If an immunocompromised child has come into close contact with an infectious individual with measles,

normal immunoglobulin (section 14.5.1) should be given.

For advice on the use of live vaccines in individuals with impaired immune response, see section 14.1.

**Alopecia** Reversible hair loss is a common complication, although it varies in degree between drugs and individual patients.

**Pregnancy and reproductive function** Most cytotoxic drugs are teratogenic and should not be administered during pregnancy, especially during the first trimester. Exclude pregnancy before treatment with cytotoxic drugs. Considerable caution is necessary if a pregnant woman presents with cancer requiring chemotherapy, and specialist advice should always be sought.

Contraceptive advice should be given to men and women before cytotoxic therapy begins (and should cover the duration of contraception required after therapy has ended).

Regimens that do not contain an alkylating drug or procarbazine may have less effect on fertility, but those with an alkylating drug or procarbazine carry the risk of causing permanent male sterility (there is no effect on potency). Pretreatment counselling and consideration of sperm storage may be appropriate. Women are less severely affected, though the span of reproductive life may be shortened by the onset of a premature menopause. No increase in fetal abnormalities or abortion rate has been recorded in patients who remain fertile after cytotoxic chemotherapy.

**Long-term and delayed toxicity** Cytotoxic drugs may produce specific organ-related toxicity in children (e.g. cardiotoxicity with doxorubicin or nephrotoxicity with cisplatin and ifosfamide). Manifestations of such toxicity may not appear for several months or even years after cancer treatment. Careful follow-up of survivors of childhood cancer is therefore vital; national and local guidelines have been developed to facilitate this.

**Thromboembolism** Venous thromboembolism can be a complication of cancer itself, but chemotherapy increases the risk.

**Tumour lysis syndrome** Tumour lysis syndrome occurs secondary to spontaneous or treatment related rapid destruction of malignant cells. Patients at risk of tumour lysis syndrome include those with non-Hodgkin's lymphoma (especially if high grade and bulky disease), Burkitt's lymphoma, acute lymphoblastic leukaemia and acute myeloid leukaemia (particularly if high white blood cell counts or bulky disease), and occasionally those with solid tumours. Pre-existing hyperuricaemia, dehydration and renal impairment are also predisposing factors. Features, include hyperkalaemia, hyperuricaemia, and hyperphosphataemia with hypocalcaemia; renal damage and arrhythmias can follow. Early recognition of patients at risk, and initiation of prophylaxis or therapy for tumour lysis syndrome, is essential.

## Drugs for cytotoxic-induced side-effects

### Hyperuricaemia

Hyperuricaemia, which may be present in high-grade lymphoma and leukaemia, can be markedly worsened by chemotherapy and is associated with acute renal failure.

Allopurinol is used routinely in children at low to moderate risk of hyperuricaemia. It should be started 24 hours before treatment; patients should be adequately hydrated (consideration should be given to omitting phosphate and potassium from hydration fluids). The dose of mercaptopurine or azathioprine should be reduced if allopurinol is given concomitantly (see Appendix 1).

Rasburicase is a recombinant urate oxidase used in children who are at high-risk of developing hyperuricaemia. It rapidly reduces plasma-uric acid concentration and may be of particular value in preventing complications following treatment of leukaemias or bulky lymphomas.

## ■ ALLOPURINOL

**Cautions** ensure adequate fluid intake; for hyperuricaemia associated with cancer therapy, allopurinol treatment should be started before cancer therapy; **interactions:** Appendix 1 (allopurinol)

**Hepatic impairment** reduce dose, monitor hepatic function

**Renal impairment** manufacturer advises reduce dose or increase dose interval in severe impairment; adjust dose to maintain plasma-oxipurinol concentration below 100 micromol/litre

**Pregnancy** toxicity not reported; manufacturer advises use only if no safer alternative and disease carries risk for mother or child

**Breast-feeding** present in milk—not known to be harmful

**Side-effects** rashes (**withdraw** therapy; if rash mild re-introduce cautiously but **discontinue** immediately if recurrence—hypersensitivity reactions occur rarely and include exfoliation, fever, lymphadenopathy, arthralgia, and eosinophilia resembling Stevens-Johnson or toxic epidermal necrolysis, vasculitis, hepatitis, renal impairment, and *very rarely* seizures); gastro-intestinal disorders; *rarely* malaise, headache, vertigo, drowsiness, visual and taste disturbances, hypertension, alopecia, hepatotoxicity, paraesthesia and neuropathy, blood disorders (including leucopenia, thrombocytopenia, haemolytic anaemia and aplastic anaemia)

**Indications and dose**

Prophylaxis of hyperuricaemia associated with cancer chemotherapy, prophylaxis of hyperuricaemic nephropathy, enzyme disorders causing increased serum urate e.g. Lesch-Nyhan syndrome

• By mouth

**Child 1 month–15 years** 10–20 mg/kg daily (max. 400 mg daily), preferably after food

**Child 15–18 years** initially 100 mg daily, increased according to response; max. 900 mg daily (doses over 300 mg daily given in divided doses); preferably after food

**Allopurinol** (Non-proprietary) PoM
Tablets, allopurinol 100 mg, net price 28-tab pack = £1.18; 300 mg, 28-tab pack = £1.32. Label: 8, 21, 27
Brands include *Caplenal*®, *Cosuric*®, *Rimapurinol*®

**Zyloric**® (Aspen) PoM
Tablets, allopurinol 100 mg, net price 100-tab pack = £10.19; 300 mg, 28-tab pack = £7.31. Label: 8, 21, 27

## ■ RASBURICASE

**Cautions** monitor closely for hypersensitivity; atopic allergies; may interfere with test for uric acid—consult product literature

**Contra-indications** G6PD deficiency (section 9.1.5)

**Pregnancy** manufacturer advises avoid—no information available

**Breast-feeding** manufacturer advises avoid—no information available

**Side-effects** fever; nausea, vomiting; less frequently diarrhoea, headache, hypersensitivity reactions (including rash, bronchospasm and anaphylaxis); haemolytic anaemia, methaemoglobinaemia

**Licensed use** not licensed for use in children

**Indications and dose**

Prophylaxis and treatment of acute hyperuricaemia with initial chemotherapy for haematological malignancy

• By intravenous infusion

Consult local treatment protocol for details

**Fasturtec**® (Sanofi-Aventis) PoM
Intravenous infusion, powder for reconstitution, rasburicase, net price 1.5-mg vial (with solvent) = £57.88; 7.5-mg vial (with solvent) = £241.20

## Methotrexate-induced mucositis and myelosuppression

Folinic acid (given as calcium folinate) is used to counteract the folate-antagonist action of methotrexate and thus speed recovery from methotrexate-induced mucositis or myelosuppression ('folinic acid rescue').

The calcium salt of **levofolinic acid**, a single isomer of folinic acid, is also used following methotrexate administration. The dose of calcium levofolinate is generally half that of calcium folinate.

The disodium salts of folinic acid and levofolinic acid are also used for rescue therapy following methotrexate administration.

The efficacy of high dose methotrexate is enhanced by delaying initiation of folinic acid for at least 24 hours, local protocols define the correct time. Folinic acid is normally continued until the plasma-methotrexate concentration falls to 45–90 nanograms/mL (100–200 nanomol/litre).

In the treatment of methotrexate overdose, folinate should be administered immediately; other measures to enhance the elimination of methotrexate are also necessary.

## ■ FOLINIC ACID

**Cautions** avoid simultaneous administration of methotrexate; **not** indicated for pernicious anaemia or other megaloblastic anaemias due to vitamin $B_{12}$ deficiency; **interactions:** Appendix 1 (folates)

**Contra-indications**

Safe Practice
Intrathecal injection **contra-indicated**

**Pregnancy** not known to be harmful; benefit outweighs risk

**Breast-feeding** presence in milk unknown but benefit outweighs risk

8 Malignant disease and immunosuppression

8   Malignant disease and immunosuppression

**Side-effects** *rarely* pyrexia after parenteral use; gastro-intestinal disturbances, insomnia, agitation, and depression after high doses

**Licensed use** consult product literature for licensing status of individual preparations

**Indications and dose**

> See under preparation

◢Calcium folinate

(Calcium leucovorin)

**Calcium Folinate** (Non-proprietary) PoM
Tablets, scored, folinic acid (as calcium salt) 15 mg, net price 10-tab pack = £39.20, 30-tab pack = £85.74
Brands include *Refolinon*®
Note Not all strengths and pack sizes are available from all manufacturers

Injection, folinic acid (as calcium salt) 3 mg/mL, net price 1-mL amp = £4.00, 10-mL amp = £4.62; 7.5 mg/mL, net price 2-mL amp = £7.80; 10 mg/mL, net price 5-mL vial = £19.41, 10-mL vial = £35.09, 30-mL vial = £94.69, 35-mL vial = £90.98
Brands include *Refolinon*®
Note Not all strengths and pack sizes are available from all manufacturers

Injection, powder for reconstitution, folinic acid (as calcium salt), net price 15-mg vial = £4.46; 30-mg vial = £8.36

**Dose**

**Reduction of methotrexate-induced toxicity**

- By mouth, by intravenous injection or by intravenous infusion
  See notes above. Consult local treatment protocol for details

**Methotrexate overdose**

- By intravenous injection or by intravenous infusion
  See notes above. Consult local treatment protocol for details

**Megaloblastic anaemia due to folate deficiency**

- By mouth
  **Child up to 12 years** 250 microgram/kg once daily
  **Child 12–18 years** 15 mg once daily

**Metabolic disorders leading to folate deficiency**

- By mouth or by intravenous infusion
  **Child up to 18 years** 15 mg once daily; larger doses may be required in older children

**Prevention of megaloblastic anaemia associated with pyrimethamine and sulfadiazine treatment of congenital toxoplasmosis**

- By mouth
  **Neonate** 5 mg 3 times a week (increased up to 20 mg 3 times a week if neutropenic)
  **Child 1 month–1 year** 10 mg 3 times a week

◢Disodium folinate

**Sodiofolin**® (Medac) PoM
Injection, folinic acid (as disodium salt) 50 mg/mL, net price 2-mL vial = £35.09, 8-mL vial = £126.25

**Dose**

**Antidote to methotrexate**

- By intravenous injection or by intravenous infusion
  Consult local treatment protocols for details

## LEVOFOLINIC ACID

Note Levofolinic acid is an isomer of folinic acid

**Cautions** see Folinic acid

**Contra-indications**

> **Safe Practice**
> Intrathecal injection **contra-indicated**

**Pregnancy** see Folinic acid

**Breast-feeding** see Folinic acid

**Side-effects** see Folinic acid

**Indications and dose**

**Reduction of methotrexate-induced toxicity**

- By intramuscular injection or by intravenous injection or by intravenous infusion
  See notes above. Consult local treatment protocol for details

**Methotrexate overdose**

- By intramuscular injection or by intravenous injection or by intravenous infusion
  See notes above. Consult local treatment protocol for details

◢Calcium levofolinate

(Calcium levoleucovorin)

**Calcium Levofolinate** (Non-proprietary)
Injection, levofolinic acid (as calcium salt) 10 mg/mL, net price 17.5-mL vial = £84.63

**Isovorin**® (Pfizer) PoM
Injection, levofolinic acid (as calcium salt) 10 mg/mL, net price 2.5-mL vial = £11.62, 17.5-mL vial = £81.33

◢Disodium levofolinate

**Levofolinic Acid** (Non-proprietary) PoM
Injection, levofolinic acid (as disodium salt) 50 mg/mL, net price 1-mL vial = £24.70, 4-mL vial = £80.40

## Urothelial toxicity

Haemorrhagic cystitis is a common manifestation of urothelial toxicity which occurs with the oxazaphosphorines, cyclophosphamide and ifosfamide; it is caused by the metabolite acrolein. Adequate hydration is essential to reduce the risk of urothelial toxicity. **Mesna** reacts specifically with acrolein in the urinary tract, preventing toxicity. Mesna is given for the same duration as cyclophosphamide or ifosfamide. It is generally given intravenously; the dose of mesna is equal to or greater than that of the oxazaphosphorine. For the role of nebulised mesna as a mucolytic in cystic fibrosis, see section 3.7.

## MESNA

**Contra-indications** hypersensitivity to thiol-containing compounds

**Pregnancy** not known to be harmful

**Side-effects** nausea, vomiting, colic, diarrhoea, fatigue, headache, limb and joint pains, depression, irritability, rash, hypotension and tachycardia; rarely hypersensitivity reactions (more common in patients with auto-immune disorders)

**Licensed use** not licensed for use in children

## Indications and dose

**Urothelial toxicity following oxazaphosphorine therapy**

- By intravenous injection or by continuous intravenous infusion

  See notes above. Consult local treatment protocol for details

**Mucolytic in cystic fibrosis** section 3.7

**Mesna** (Non-proprietary) PoM

Tablets, f/c, mesna 400 mg, net price 10-tab pack = £42.90; 600 mg, 10-tab pack = £61.10

Injection, mesna 100 mg/mL, net price 4-mL amp = £3.95; 10-mL amp = £9.77

**Note** For oral administration contents of ampoule are taken in a flavoured drink such as orange juice or cola which may be stored in a refrigerator for up to 24 hours in a sealed container

## 8.1.1　Alkylating drugs

Extensive experience is available with these drugs, which are among the most widely used in cancer chemotherapy. They act by damaging DNA, thus interfering with cell replication. In addition to the side-effects common to many cytotoxic drugs (section 8.1), problems associated specifically with alkylating drugs include:

- an adverse effect on gametogenesis which may be reversible, particularly in females; amenorrhoea may also occur, which also may be reversible;

- a marked increase in the incidence of secondary tumours and leukaemia, particularly when alkylating drugs are combined with extensive irradiation;

- fluid retention with oedema and dilutional hyponatraemia in younger children; the risk of this complication is higher in the first 2 days and also when given with concomitant vinca alkaloids;

- urothelial toxicity with intravenous use; adequate hydration may reduce this risk; mesna (section 8.1) provides further protection against urotoxic effects of cyclophosphamide and ifosfamide.

## BUSULFAN
(Busulphan)

**Cautions** see section 8.1 and notes above; monitor full blood count regularly throughout treatment; monitor liver function; previous mediastinal or pulmonary radiation therapy; avoid in acute porphyria (but see section 9.8.2); **interactions:** Appendix 1 (busulfan)

**Hepatic impairment** manufacturer advises monitor hepatic function—no information available

**Pregnancy** avoid (teratogenic in *animals*); manufacturers advise effective contraception during and for 6 months after treatment in men or women; see also Pregnancy and Reproductive Function, p. 416

**Breast-feeding** discontinue breast-feeding

**Side-effects** see section 8.1 and notes above; also hepatotoxicity (including hepatic veno-occlusive disease, hyperbilirubinaemia, jaundice, and fibrosis); cardiac tamponade in thalassaemia; pneumonia, skin hyperpigmentation; *rarely* progressive pulmonary

fibrosis, seizures, aplastic anaemia, visual disturbances, hypersensitivity reactions (including urticaria, erythema); *very rarely* myasthenia gravis, gynaecomastia

## Indications and dose

**Conditioning treatment before haematopoietic stem-cell transplantation**

- By mouth or by intravenous infusion

  Consult local treatment protocol for details

**Myleran®** (Alkopharma) PoM

Tablets, f/c, busulfan 2 mg, net price 25-tab pack = £5.20

**Busilvex®** (Fabre) PoM

Concentrate for intravenous infusion, busulfan 6 mg/mL, net price 10-mL vial = £201.25

**Busulfan**

Capsules, busulfan 25 mg

Available from 'special-order' manufacturers or specialist importing companies, p. 823

## CHLORAMBUCIL

**Cautions** see section 8.1 and notes above; monitor full blood count regularly throughout treatment; increased seizure risk in children with nephrotic syndrome or history of epilepsy; avoid in acute porphyria (but see section 9.8.2)

**Hepatic impairment** manufacturer advises consider dose reduction in severe impairment—limited information available

**Pregnancy** avoid; manufacturer advises effective contraception during treatment in men or women; see also Pregnancy and Reproductive Function, p. 416

**Breast-feeding** discontinue breast-feeding

**Side-effects** see section 8.1 and notes above; also *less commonly* skin rash (possible progression to Stevens-Johnson syndrome and toxic epidermal necrolysis); *rarely* seizures, hepatotoxicity and jaundice; *very rarely* irreversible bone-marrow suppression, pulmonary fibrosis, tremor, peripheral neuropathy, sterile cystitis, sterility in prepubertal and pubertal males

**Licensed use** not licensed for use in nephrotic syndrome

## Indications and dose

**Hodgkin's disease**

- By mouth

  Consult local treatment protocol for details

**Non-Hodgkin's lymphoma**

- By mouth

  Consult local treatment protocol for details

**Relapsing steroid-sensitive nephrotic syndrome; initiated in specialist centres** (see also section 6.3.2, p. 371)

- By mouth

  **Child 3 months–18 years** 200 micrograms/kg once daily for 8 weeks

**Leukeran®** (Alkopharma) PoM

Tablets, f/c, brown, chlorambucil 2 mg, net price 25-tab pack = £8.36

8　Malignant disease and immunosuppression

## CYCLOPHOSPHAMIDE

**Cautions** see section 8.1 and notes above; previous or concurrent mediastinal irradiation—risk of cardiotoxicity; diabetes mellitus; avoid in acute porphyria (but see section 9.8.2); **interactions:** Appendix 1 (cyclophosphamide)

**Contra-indications** haemorrhagic cystitis

**Hepatic impairment** reduce dose—consult local treatment protocol for details

**Renal impairment** reduce dose—consult local treatment protocol for details

**Pregnancy** avoid; manufacturer advises effective contraception during and for at least 3 months after treatment in men or women; see also Pregnancy and Reproductive Function, p. 416

**Breast-feeding** discontinue breast-feeding during and for 36 hours after stopping treatment

**Side-effects** see section 8.1 and notes above; *also* anorexia; pancreatitis; cardiotoxicity at high doses; interstitial pulmonary fibrosis; inappropriate secretion of anti-diuretic hormone, disturbances of carbohydrate metabolism; urothelial toxicity; pigmentation of palms, nails and soles; *rarely* hepatotoxicity and renal dysfunction

**Licensed use** not licensed for use in children

**Indications and dose**

> Acute lymphoblastic leukaemia, non-Hodgkin's lymphoma, retinoblastoma, neuroblastoma, rhabdomyosarcoma, soft-tissue sarcomas, Ewing tumour, neuroectodermal tumours (including medulloblastoma), infant brain tumours, ependymona, high-dose conditioning for bone marrow transplantation, lupus nephritis
> * By mouth or by intravenous infusion
>   Consult local treatment protocol for details

> Steroid-sensitive nephrotic syndrome see also section 6.3.2, p. 371
> * By mouth
>   **Child 3 months–18 years** 2–3 mg/kg once daily for 8 weeks
> * By intravenous infusion
>   **Child 3 months–18 years** 500 mg/m$^2$ once a month for 6 months

**Administration** Consult local treatment protocol for details

**Cyclophosphamide** (Non-proprietary) PoM
Tablets, s/c, cyclophosphamide (anhydrous) 50 mg, net price 100 = £20.20. Label: 25, 27

Injection, powder for reconstitution, cyclophosphamide, net price 500-mg vial = £5.66; 1-g vial = £10.66

## IFOSFAMIDE

**Cautions** see section 8.1 and notes above; ensure satisfactory electrolyte balance, and renal function before each course (risk of tubular dysfunction, Fanconi's syndrome, or diabetes insipidus if renal toxicity not treated promptly); avoid in acute porphyria (but see section 9.8.2); **interactions:** Appendix 1 (ifosfamide)

**Contra-indications** urinary tract obstruction; acute infection (including urinary-tract infection); urothelial damage

**Hepatic impairment** avoid
**Renal impairment** avoid

**Pregnancy** avoid (teratogenic and carcinogenic in *animals*); manufacturer advises adequate contraception during and for at least 6 months after treatment in men or women; see also Pregnancy and Reproductive Function, p. 416

**Breast-feeding** discontinue breast-feeding

**Side-effects** see section 8.1 and notes above; *also* drowsiness, confusion, disorientation, restlessness, psychosis; urothelial toxicity causing haemorrhagic cystitis and dysuria, renal toxicity (see Cautions above); *less commonly* severe encephalopathy; *rarely* diarrhoea, constipation, convulsions, anorexia; *very rarely* jaundice, thrombophlebitis, syndrome of inappropriate antidiuretic hormone secretion

**Indications and dose**

> Rhabdomyosarcoma, soft-tissue sarcomas, Ewing tumour, germ cell tumour, osteogenic sarcoma
> * By intravenous infusion
>   Consult local treatment protocol for details

**Ifosfamide** (Non-proprietary) PoM
Injection, powder for reconstitution, ifosfamide, net price 1-g vial = £43.53; 2-g vial = £88.62 (hosp. only)

## MELPHALAN

**Cautions** see section 8.1 and notes above; monitor full blood count before and throughout treatment; for high-dose intravenous administration establish adequate hydration (see notes above), consider use of prophylactic anti-infective agents; haematopoietic stem cell transplantation essential for high dose treatment (consult local treatment protocol for details); avoid in acute porphyria (but see section 9.8.2); **interactions:** Appendix 1 (melphalan)

**Renal impairment** reduce dose initially—consult product literature

**Pregnancy** avoid; manufacturer advises adequate contraception during treatment in men or women; see also Pregnancy and Reproductive Function, p. 416

**Breast-feeding** discontinue breast-feeding

**Side-effects** see section 8.1 and notes above

**Licensed use** childhood neuroblastoma

**Indications and dose**

> High intravenous dose with haematopoietic stem cell transplantation in the treatment of childhood neuroblastoma and some other advanced embryonal tumours
> * Intravenous infusion
>   Consult local treatment protocol for details

**Alkeran**® (Genopharm) PoM
Injection, powder for reconstitution, melphalan 50 mg (as hydrochloride). Net price 50-mg vial (with solvent-diluent) = £33.13

## THIOTEPA

**Cautions** see section 8.1; avoid in acute porphyria (but see section 9.8.2); **interactions:** Appendix 1 (thiotepa)

**Pregnancy** avoid (teratogenic and embryotoxic in *animals*); see also Pregnancy and Reproductive Function, p. 416

**Breast-feeding** discontinue breast-feeding

**Side-effects** see section 8.1

**Indications and dose**

> Conditioning treatment before haematopoietic stem cell transplantation in the treatment of haematological disease or solid tumours, in combination with other chemotherapy
> * By intravenous infusion
>   Consult local treatment protocol for details

**Tepadina®** (Adienne) [PoM]

Injection, powder for reconstitution, thiotepa, net price 15-mg vial £123.00; 100-mg vial = £736.00

Note The *Scottish Medicines Consortium* (p. 3) has advised (June 2012) that thiotepa (*Tepadina®*) is not recommended for use within NHS Scotland in combination with other chemotherapy as conditioning treatment in children or adults with haematological disease, or solid tumours prior to haematopoietic stem cell transplantation.

## 8.1.2 Cytotoxic antibiotics

Cytotoxic antibiotics are widely used. Many act as radiomimetics and simultaneous use of radiotherapy should be **avoided** because it may markedly increase toxicity.

**Daunorubicin**, **doxorubicin**, and **epirubicin** are anthracycline antibiotics. **Mitoxantrone** (mitozantrone) is an anthracycline derivative.

All anthracycline antibiotics have been associated with varying degrees of cardiac toxicity—this may be idiosyncratic and reversible, but is commonly related to total cumulative dose and is irreversible. Cardiac function should be monitored before and at regular intervals throughout treatment and afterwards. Caution is necessary with concomitant use of cardiotoxic drugs, or drugs that reduce cardiac contractility. Anthracycline antibiotics should not normally be used in children with left ventricular dysfunction. Epirubicin and mitoxantrone are considered less toxic, and may be suitable for children who have received high cumulative doses of other anthracyclines.

### BLEOMYCIN

**Cautions** see section 8.1; ensure monitoring of pulmonary function—investigate any shortness of breath before initiation; caution in handling—irritant to tissues

**Contra-indications** acute pulmonary infection or significantly reduced lung function

**Renal impairment** reduce dose—consult local treatment protocol for details

**Pregnancy** avoid (teratogenic and carcinogenic in *animal* studies); see also Pregnancy and Reproductive Function, p. 416

**Breast-feeding** discontinue breast-feeding

**Side-effects** see section 8.1, less bone marrow suppression; anorexia; pulmonary toxicity e.g. pulmonary fibrosis (usually dose-related and delayed); fever (directly following administration), fatigue; dermatological and mucous membrane toxicity, localised skin hyperpigmentation; rarely cardiorespiratory collapse and hyperpyrexia

**Licensed use** not licensed for use in children

**Indications and dose**

> Some germ cell tumours, Hodgkin's lymphoma
> * By intravenous infusion
>   Consult local treatment protocol for details

**Bleomycin** (Non-proprietary) [PoM]

Injection, powder for reconstitution, bleomycin (as sulfate), net price 15 000-unit vial = £15.56

Note To conform to the European Pharmacopoeia vials previously labelled as containing '15 units' of bleomycin are now labelled as containing 15 000 units. The amount of bleomycin in the vial has not changed.

Brands include *Bleo-Kyowa®*

### DACTINOMYCIN
(Actinomycin D)

**Cautions** see section 8.1 and notes above; caution in handling—irritant to tissues

**Hepatic impairment** consider dose reduction if raised serum bilirubin or biliary obstruction; consult local treatment protocols

**Pregnancy** avoid (teratogenic in *animal* studies); see also Pregnancy and Reproductive Function, p. 416

**Breast-feeding** discontinue breast-feeding

**Side-effects** see section 8.1 and notes above; *less commonly* cheilitis, dysphagia; fever, malaise, lethargy; anaemia, hypoglycaemia; myalgia; acne; *rarely* hepatotoxicity (possibly dose-related)

**Licensed use** not licensed for use in children under 12 years

**Indications and dose**

> Wilms' tumour, childhood rhabdomyosarcoma and other soft tissue sarcomas, Ewing's sarcoma
> * By intravenous injection
>   Consult local treatment protocol for details

**Dactinomycin** (Non-proprietary) [PoM]

Injection, powder for reconstitution, dactinomycin Available from 'special-order' manufacturers or specialist importing companies, see p. 823

### DAUNORUBICIN

**Cautions** see section 8.1 and notes above; caution in handling—irritant to tissues

**Contra-indications** myocardial insufficiency, recent myocardial infarction, severe arrhythmia; previous treatment with maximum cumulative doses of daunorubicin or other anthracycline

**Hepatic impairment** reduce dose according to serum bilirubin concentration—consult local treatment protocol for details; avoid in severe impairment

**Renal impairment** reduce dose—consult local treatment protocol for details; avoid in severe impairment

**Pregnancy** avoid (teratogenic and carcinogenic in *animal* studies), see also Pregnancy and Reproductive Function, p. 416

**Breast-feeding** discontinue breast-feeding

**Side-effects** see section 8.1 and notes above, leucopenia, less commonly mucositis; cardiac toxicity (usually 1–6 months after initiation of therapy); fever; red urine discolouration

**Licensed use** *DaunoXome®* not licensed for use in children

8   Malignant disease and immunosuppression

## Indications and dose

**Acute myelogenous leukaemia, acute lymphocytic leukaemia**
- By intravenous infusion

Consult local treatment protocol for details

**Daunorubicin** (Non-proprietary) [PoM]
Injection, powder for reconstitution, daunorubicin (as hydrochloride), net price 20-mg vial = £55.00

◣ Lipid formulation
**DaunoXome®** (Gilead) [PoM]
Concentrate for intravenous infusion, daunorubicin encapsulated in liposomes. For dilution before use, net price 50-mg vial = £137.67

## ▮ DOXORUBICIN HYDROCHLORIDE

**Cautions** see section 8.1 and notes above; caution in handling—irritant to tissues; **interactions:** Appendix 1 (doxorubicin)

**Contra-indications** severe myocardial insufficiency, recent myocardial infarction, severe arrhythmia; previous treatment with maximum cumulative doses of doxorubicin or other anthracycline

**Hepatic impairment** reduce dose according to bilirubin concentration—consult local treatment protocol for details; avoid in severe impairment

**Pregnancy** avoid (teratogenic and toxic in *animal* studies); manufacturer of liposomal product advises effective contraception during and for at least 6 months after treatment in men or women; see also Pregnancy and Reproductive Function, p. 416

**Breast-feeding** discontinue breast-feeding

**Side-effects** see section 8.1 and notes above; red urine discoloration; thrombophlebitis over injection site; less commonly bronchospasm, fever, amenorrhoea, and skin rash

**Licensed use** not licensed for use in children

## Indications and dose

**Paediatric malignancies including Ewing's sarcoma, osteogenic sarcoma, Wilms' tumour, neuroblastoma, retinoblastoma, some liver tumours, acute lymphoblastic leukaemia, Hodgkin's lymphoma, non-Hodgkin's lymphoma**
- By intravenous infusion

Consult local treatment protocol for details

**Doxorubicin** (Non-proprietary) [PoM]
Injection, powder for reconstitution, doxorubicin hydrochloride, net price 10-mg vial = £18.72; 50-mg vial = £96.86

Injection, doxorubicin hydrochloride 2 mg/mL, net price 5-mL vial = £20.60, 25-mL vial = £103.00, 100-mL vial = £275.00

## ▮ EPIRUBICIN HYDROCHLORIDE

**Cautions** see section 8.1 and notes above; caution in handling—irritant to tissues

**Contra-indications** severe myocardial insufficiency, recent myocardial infarction, severe arrhythmia, unstable angina, myocardiopathy; previous treatment with maximum cumulative doses of epirubicin or other anthracycline

**Hepatic impairment** reduce dose according to bilirubin concentration—consult local treatment protocol for details; avoid in severe impairment

**Renal impairment** dose reduction may be necessary in severe impairment

**Pregnancy** avoid (carcinogenic in *animal* studies); see also Pregnancy and Reproductive Function, p. 416

**Breast-feeding** discontinue breast-feeding

**Side-effects** see section 8.1 and notes above; red urine discoloration; anaphylaxis

**Licensed use** not licensed for use in children

## Indications and dose

**Recurrent acute lymphoblastic leukaemia, rhabdomyosarcoma, other soft tissue tumours of childhood**
- Intravenous infusion

Consult local treatment protocol for details

**Epirubicin hydrochloride** (Non-proprietary) [PoM]
Injection, epirubicin hydrochloride 2 mg/mL, net price 5-mL vial = £18.31, 25-mL vial = £92.13, 50-mL vial = £95.54, 100-mL vial = £306.20

Injection, powder for reconstitution, epirubicin hydrochloride, net price 50-mg vial = £91.54

**Pharmorubicin® Solution for Injection** (Pharmacia) [PoM]
Injection, epirubicin hydrochloride 2 mg/mL, net price 5-mL vial = £19.31, 25-mL vial = £96.54, 100-mL vial = £386.16

## ▮ MITOXANTRONE
(Mitozantrone)

**Cautions** see section 8.1 and notes above

**Hepatic impairment** use with caution—consult local treatment protocol

**Pregnancy** avoid; effective contraception during and for at least 6 months after treatment in men or women; see also Pregnancy and Reproductive Function, p. 416

**Breast-feeding** discontinue breast-feeding

**Side-effects** see section 8.1 and notes above; transient blue-green discoloration of urine; less commonly gastro-intestinal bleeding, anorexia, allergic reactions, dyspnoea, fatigue, fever, amenorrhoea, and transient blue discoloration of skin and nails

**Licensed use** not licensed for use in children

## Indications and dose

**Acute myeloid leukaemia, recurrent acute lymphoblastic leukaemia**
- By intravenous infusion

Consult local treatment protocol for details

**Mitoxantrone** (Non-proprietary) [PoM]
Concentrate for intravenous infusion, mitoxantrone (as hydrochloride) 2 mg/mL, net price 10-mL vial = £100.00

**Onkotrone®** (Baxter) [PoM]
Concentrate for intravenous infusion, mitoxantrone (as hydrochloride) 2 mg/mL, net price 10-mL vial = £121.85, 12.5-mL vial = £152.33, 15-mL vial = £203.04

## 8.1.3 Antimetabolites

Antimetabolites are incorporated into new nuclear material or they combine irreversibly with cellular enzymes and prevent normal cellular division. **Cytarabine, fludarabine, mercaptopurine, methotrexate**, and **tioguanine** are commonly used in paediatric chemotherapy.

**Methotrexate** inhibits the enzyme dihydrofolate reductase, essential for the synthesis of purines and pyrimidines. It is given by mouth, intravenously, intramuscularly, or intrathecally. Methotrexate causes myelosuppression, mucositis, and rarely pneumonitis. It is **contra-indicated** in significant renal impairment because it is excreted primarily by the kidney. It is also contra-indicated in patients with severe hepatic impairment. It should also be **avoided** in the presence of significant pleural effusion or ascites because it can accumulate in these fluids, and its subsequent return to the circulation may cause myelosuppression. Systemic toxicity may follow intrathecal administration and blood counts should be carefully monitored. Folinic acid (section 8.1) following methotrexate administration helps to prevent methotrexate-induced mucositis and myelosuppression.

**Cytarabine** acts by interfering with pyrimidine synthesis. It is given subcutaneously, intravenously, or intrathecally. It is a potent myelosuppressant and requires careful haematological monitoring. A liposomal formulation of cytarabine for intrathecal use is available for lymphomatous meningitis.

**Fludarabine** is generally well tolerated but does cause myelosuppression, which may be cumulative.

> **Fludarabine** has a potent and prolonged immunosuppressive effect. Children treated with fludarabine are more prone to serious bacterial, opportunistic fungal, and viral infections, and prophylactic therapy is recommended in children at risk. To prevent potentially fatal transfusion-related graft-versus-host reaction, only irradiated blood products should be administered. Prescribers should consult specialist literature when using highly immunosuppressive drugs.

**Clofarabine** is licensed for the treatment of acute lymphoblastic leukaemia in children who have relapsed or are refractory after receiving at least two previous regimens. It is given by intravenous infusion.

**Nelarabine** is licensed for the treatment of T-cell acute lymphoblastic leukaemia and T-cell lymphoblastic lymphoma in children who have relapsed or who are refractory after receiving at least two previous regimens. It is given by intravenous infusion. Neurotoxicity is common with nelarabine, and close monitoring for neurological events is strongly recommended—discontinue treatment if neurotoxicity occurs.

**Mercaptopurine** is used as maintenance therapy for acute lymphoblastic leukaemia and in the management of ulcerative colitis and Crohn's disease (section 1.5). Azathioprine, which is metabolised to mercaptopurine, is generally used as an immunosuppressant (section 8.2.1 and section 10.1.3). The dose of both drugs should be reduced if the child is receiving allopurinol since it interferes with their metabolism. For the role of thio-

purine methyltransferase (TPMT) in the metabolism of azathioprine see section 8.2.1.

**Tioguanine** (thioguanine) is given by mouth for the treatment of acute lymphoblastic leukaemia; it is given at various stages of treatment in short-term cycles. Tioguanine has a lower incidence of gastro-intestinal side-effects than mercaptopurine. Long-term therapy with tioguanine is no longer recommended because of the high risk of liver toxicity.

## ▌CLOFARABINE

**Cautions** see section 8.1; cardiac disease

**Hepatic impairment** manufacturer advises caution in mild to moderate impairment; avoid in severe impairment

**Renal impairment** manufacturer advises caution in mild to moderate impairment; avoid in severe impairment

**Pregnancy** manufacturer advises avoid (teratogenic in *animal* studies); see also Pregnancy and Reproductive Function, p. 416

**Breast-feeding** discontinue breast-feeding

**Side-effects** see section 8.1; also diarrhoea, abdominal pain, jaundice; tachycardia, flushing, hypotension, pericardial effusion, oedema, haematoma; dyspnoea, cough; anxiety, agitation, dizziness, drowsiness, restlessness; headache, paraesthesia, peripheral neuropathy, restlessness; haematuria; arthralgia, myalgia; rash, pruritus, hand-foot (desquamative) syndrome, increased sweating; pancreatitis also reported

**Licensed use** not licensed for use in children under 1 year

**Indications and dose**

> **Relapsed or refractory acute lymphoblastic leukaemia**
> - By intravenous infusion
>   Consult local treatment protocol for details

**Evoltra**® (Sanofi-Aventis) ▼ PoM
Concentrate for intravenous infusion, clofarabine 1 mg/mL, net price 20-mL vial = £1153.20
Electrolytes Na$^+$ 3.08 mmol/vial

## ▌CYTARABINE

**Cautions** see section 8.1 and notes above; **interactions**: Appendix 1 (cytarabine)

**Hepatic impairment** reduce dose—consult product literature

**Renal impairment** consult local treatment protocols

**Pregnancy** avoid (teratogenic in *animal* studies); see also Pregnancy and Reproductive Function, p. 416

**Breast-feeding** discontinue breast-feeding

**Side-effects** see section 8.1 and notes above; 'cytarabine syndrome'—6–12 hours after intravenous administration—characterised by fever and malaise, myalgia, bone pain, maculopapular rash, and occasionally chest pain; *less commonly* conjunctivitis (consider prophylactic corticosteroid eye drops), neurotoxicity, renal and hepatic dysfunction, jaundice; *rarely* severe spinal cord toxicity following intrathecal administration

**Licensed use** *Depocyte*® intrathecal injection not licensed for use in children

**Malignant disease and immunosuppression** 8

**Indications and dose**

**Acute lymphoblastic leukaemia, acute myeloid leukaemia, non-Hodgkin's lymphoma**

- By intravenous injection, by intravenous infusion, or by subcutaneous injection

Consult local treatment protocol for details

**Meningeal leukaemia, meningeal neoplasms**

- By intrathecal injection

Consult local treatment protocol for details

**Note**
Based on weight or body-surface area, children may tolerate higher doses of cytarabine than adults

**Cytarabine** (Non-proprietary) PoM

Injection (for intravenous, subcutaneous or intrathecal use), cytarabine 20 mg/mL, net price 5-mL vial = £4.00

Injection (for intravenous or subcutaneous use), cytarabine 20 mg/mL, net price 5-mL vial = £3.90, 25-mL vial = £19.50

Injection (for intravenous or subcutaneous use), cytarabine 100 mg/mL, net price 1-mL vial = £4.00; 5-mL vial = £20.00; 10-mL vial = £39.00; 20-mL vial = £77.50

◢ **Lipid formulation for intrathecal use**

**DepoCyte®** (Napp) PoM

Intrathecal injection, cytarabine encapsulated in liposomes, net price 50-mg vial = £1223.75

◼ **FLUDARABINE PHOSPHATE**

**Cautions** see section 8.1 and notes above; monitor for signs of haemolysis; monitor for neurological toxicity; worsening of existing and increased susceptibility to skin cancer; **interactions:** Appendix 1 (fludarabine)

**Contra-indications** haemolytic anaemia

**Renal impairment** reduce dose by up to 50% if creatinine clearance 30–70 mL/minute/1.73 m²; avoid if creatinine clearance less than 30 mL/minute/1.73 m²

**Pregnancy** avoid (embryotoxic and teratogenic in *animal* studies); manufacturer advises effective contraception during and for at least 6 months after treatment in men or women; see also Pregnancy and Reproductive Function, p. 416

**Breast-feeding** discontinue breast-feeding

**Side-effects** see section 8.1 and notes above; also diarrhoea, anorexia; oedema; pneumonia, cough; peripheral neuropathy, visual disturbances; chills, fever, malaise, weakness; rash; *less commonly* gastro-intestinal haemorrhage, pulmonary toxicity (including pulmonary infiltrates, pneumonitis, and fibrosis), and confusion; *rarely* heart failure, arrhythmia, coma, seizures, agitation, myelodysplastic syndrome, acute myeloid leukaemia, optic neuropathy, blindness, Stevens-Johnson syndrome, toxic epidermal necrolysis, skin cancer, and haemorrhagic cystitis

**Licensed use** not licensed for use in children

**Indications and dose**

**Poor prognosis or relapsed acute myeloid leukaemia, relapsed acute lymphoblastic leukaemia, conditioning before bone marrow transplantation**

- By mouth, by intravenous injection, or by intravenous infusion

Consult local treatment protocol for details

**Fludarabine phosphate** (Non-proprietary) PoM

Injection, powder for reconstitution, fludarabine phosphate, net price 50-mg vial = £140.40

**Fludara®** (Sanofi-Aventis) PoM

Tablets, f/c, pink, fludarabine phosphate 10 mg, net price 15-tab pack = £268.12, 20-tab pack = £350.70

Injection, powder for reconstitution, fludarabine phosphate, net price 50-mg vial = £147.07

◼ **MERCAPTOPURINE**
(6-Mercaptopurine)

**Cautions** see section 8.1 and notes above; thiopurine methyltransferase status (see section 8.2.1); monitor liver function—discontinue if jaundice develops; **interactions:** Appendix 1 (mercaptopurine)

**Hepatic impairment** may need dose reduction

**Renal impairment** manufacturer advises consider reducing dose

**Pregnancy** avoid (teratogenic); see also Pregnancy and Reproductive Function, p. 416

**Breast-feeding** discontinue breast-feeding

**Side-effects** see section 8.1 and notes above; gastro-intestinal effects less common; hepatotoxicity (more frequent at higher doses); *rarely* intestinal ulceration, pancreatitis, fever, crystalluria with haematuria, rash, and hyperpigmentation; *very rarely* lymphoma

**Licensed use** not licensed for use in children for acute lymphoblastic lymphoma or T-cell non-Hodgkins lymphoma

**Indications and dose**

**Acute lymphoblastic leukaemia, lymphoblastic lymphomas**

- By mouth

Consult local treatment protocol for details

**Severe ulcerative colitis and Crohn's disease** section 1.5.3

**Important** *Puri-Nethol®* tablets and *Xaluprine®* oral suspension are **not** bioequivalent; haematological monitoring is advised when switching formulations

**Puri-Nethol®** (Alkopharma) PoM

Tablets, yellow, scored, mercaptopurine 50 mg, net price 25-tab pack = £22.54

**Xaluprine®** (Nova) PoM

Oral Suspension, mercaptopurine, 20 mg/mL, net price 100 mL (raspberry-flavoured) = £170.00
Excipients include aspartame (section 9.4.1)

**Mercaptopurine**

Capsules, mercaptopurine 10 mg
Available from 'special-order' manufacturers or specialist importing companies, p. 823

# METHOTREXATE

**Cautions** see section 8.1 and section 10.1.3; monitor renal and hepatic function; peptic ulceration, ulcerative colitis, diarrhoea, and ulcerative stomatitis; porphyria (section 9.8.2); **interactions:** Appendix 1 (methotrexate)

**Hepatic impairment** avoid in severe impairment—consult local treatment protocol for details

**Renal impairment** reduce dose—risk of nephrotoxicity at high doses; avoid in severe impairment

**Pregnancy** avoid (teratogenic; fertility may be reduced during therapy but this may be reversible); manufacturer advises effective contraception during and for at least 3 months after treatment in men or women; see also Pregnancy and Reproductive Function, p. 416

**Breast-feeding** discontinue breast-feeding—present in milk

**Side-effects** see section 8.1; also anorexia, abdominal discomfort, dyspepsia, gastro-intestinal ulceration and bleeding, diarrhoea, toxic megacolon, hepatotoxicity (see Cautions above); hypotension, pericarditis, pericardial tamponade, thrombosis; pulmonary oedema, pleuritic pain, pulmonary fibrosis, interstitial pneumonitis (see also Pulmonary Toxicity, p. 510); anaphylactic reactions, urticaria; dizziness, chills, fever, drowsiness, insomnia, malaise, headache, mood changes, abnormal cranial sensations, neurotoxicity, confusion, psychosis, paraesthesia, cerebral oedema; precipitation of diabetes; menstrual disturbances, vaginitis, cystitis, reduced libido, impotence; haematuria, dysuria, renal failure; osteoporosis, arthralgia, myalgia, vasculitis; conjunctivitis, blepharitis, visual disturbances; rash, pruritus, Stevens-Johnson syndrome, toxic epidermal necrolysis, photosensitivity, changes in nail and skin pigmentation, telangiectasia, acne, furunculosis, ecchymosis; injection-site reactions

## Indications and dose

**Maintenance and remission of acute lympho-blastic leukaemia, lymphoblastic lymphoma**

- By mouth
  - Consult local treatment protocol for details

**Treatment of early stage Burkitt's lymphoma, non-Hodgkin's lymphoma, osteogenic sarcoma, some CNS tumours including infant brain tumours, acute lymphoblastic leukaemia**

- By intravenous injection or infusion
  - Consult local treatment protocol for details

**Meningeal leukaemia, treatment and prevention of CNS involvement of leukaemia**

- By intrathecal injection
  - Consult local treatment protocol for details

**Severe Crohn's disease** section 1.5.3

**Rheumatic disease** section 10.1.3

**Psoriasis** section 13.5.3

**Methotrexate** (Non-proprietary) PoM
Injection, methotrexate (as sodium salt) 2.5 mg/mL, net price 2-mL vial = £1.68

Injection, methotrexate (as sodium salt) 25 mg/mL, net price 2-mL vial = £3.00, 20-mL vial = £30.00

Injection, methotrexate 100 mg/mL (not for intrathecal use), net price 10-mL vial = £78.33, 50-mL vial = £380.07

◢ **Oral preparations**
Section 10.1.3

# NELARABINE

**Cautions** see section 8.1 and notes above; previous or concurrent intrathecal chemotherapy or craniospinal irradiation (increased risk of neurotoxicity)
**Skilled tasks** Drowsiness may affect performance of skilled tasks (e.g. cycling or driving)

**Pregnancy** avoid (teratogenic in *animal* studies); manufacturer advises effective contraception during and for at least 3 months after treatment in men and women; see also Pregnancy and Reproductive Function, p. 416

**Breast-feeding** discontinue breast-feeding

**Side-effects** see section 8.1 and notes above; also constipation, diarrhoea; confusion, seizures, drowsiness, peripheral neurological disorders, demyelination, hypoesthesia, paraesthesia, ataxia, tremor, headache, asthenia, fatigue; pyrexia; hypoglycaemia, electrolyte disturbances; arthralgia; benign and malignant tumours also reported

## Indications and dose

**T-cell acute lymphoblastic leukaemia, T-cell lymphoblastic lymphoma**

- By intravenous infusion
  - Consult local treatment protocol for details

**Atriance**® (GSK) ▼ PoM
Intravenous infusion, nelarabine 5 mg/mL, net price 50-mL vial = £222.00
**Electrolytes** Na⁺ 3.75 mmol/vial

# TIOGUANINE
(Thioguanine)

**Cautions** see section 8.1 and notes above; thiopurine methyltransferase status (see section 8.2.1); monitor liver function weekly—discontinue if liver toxicity develops; **interactions:** Appendix 1 (tioguanine)

**Hepatic impairment** reduce dose

**Renal impairment** reduce dose

**Pregnancy** avoid (teratogenicity reported when men receiving tioguanine have fathered children); ensure effective contraception during treatment in men or women; see also Pregnancy and Reproductive Function, p. 416

**Breast-feeding** discontinue breast-feeding

**Side-effects** see section 8.1; also stomatitis and hepatotoxicity; *rarely* intestinal necrosis and perforation

## Indications and dose

**Infant acute lymphoblastic leukaemia**

- By mouth
  - Consult local treatment protocol for details

**Lanvis**® (Alkopharma) PoM
Tablets, yellow, scored, tioguanine 40 mg, net price 25-tab pack = £54.49

## 8.1.4 Vinca alkaloids and etoposide

The vinca alkaloids, **vinblastine** and **vincristine** are used to treat a variety of cancers including leukaemias, lymphomas, and some solid tumours.

Neurotoxicity, usually as peripheral or autonomic neuropathy, occurs with all vinca alkaloids and is a limiting side-effect of vincristine; it occurs less often with vinblastine. Children with neurotoxicity commonly have peripheral paraesthesia, loss of deep tendon reflexes, abdominal pain, and constipation; ototoxicity has been reported. If symptoms of neurotoxicity are severe, doses should be reduced, but children generally tolerate vincristine better than adults. Motor weakness can also occur and dose reduction or discontinuation of therapy may be appropriate if motor weakness increases. Recovery from neurotoxic effects is usually slow but complete.

Myelosuppression is the dose-limiting side-effect of vinblastine; vincristine causes negligible myelosuppression. The vinca alkaloids may cause reversible alopecia. They cause severe local irritation and care must be taken to avoid extravasation. Constipation is common with vinblastine and vincristine; prophylactic use of laxatives may be considered.

### Safe Practice
Vinblastine and vincristine are for **intravenous administration only**. Inadvertent intrathecal administration can cause severe neurotoxicity, which is usually fatal.

The National Patient Safety Agency has advised (August 2008) that teenage patients treated in an adolescent unit should receive their vinca alkaloid dose in a 50 mL minibag. Teenagers and children treated in a child unit may receive their vinca alkaloid dose in a syringe.

**Etoposide**, usually given by slow intravenous infusion, is used to treat acute leukaemias, lymphomas, and some solid tumours. Etoposide may also be given by mouth but it is unpredictably absorbed.

### ◾ ETOPOSIDE

**Cautions** see section 8.1 and notes above; **interactions**: Appendix 1 (etoposide)

**Hepatic impairment** avoid in severe impairment

**Renal impairment** consider dose reduction—consult local treatment protocol for details

**Pregnancy** avoid (teratogenic in *animal* studies); see also Pregnancy and Reproductive Function, p. 416

**Breast-feeding** discontinue breast-feeding

**Side-effects** see section 8.1, dose limiting myelosuppression, mucositis more common if given with doxorubicin; anaphylaxis associated with concentrated infusions; hypotension associated with rapid infusion; irritant to tissues if extravasated

**Licensed use** not licensed for use in children

### Indications and dose
Stage 4 neuroblastoma, germ-cell tumours, intracranial germ-cell tumours, rhabdomyosarcoma, soft-tissue sarcomas, neuroectodermal tumours (including medulloblastoma), relapsed Hodgkin's disease, non-Hodgkin's lymphoma, Ewing tumour, acute lymphoblastic leukaemia, acute myeloid leukaemia
- By mouth or by intravenous infusion
  Consult local treatment protocol for details

**Etoposide** (Non-proprietary) PoM
Concentrate for intravenous infusion, etoposide 20 mg/mL, net price 5-mL vial = £12.15, 10-mL vial = £29.00, 25-mL vial = £60.75
**Brands include** *Eposin*®

**Etopophos**® (Bristol-Myers Squibb) PoM
Injection, powder for reconstitution, etoposide (as phosphate), net price 100-mg vial = £26.17 (hosp. only)

**Vepesid**® (Bristol-Myers Squibb) PoM
Capsules, both pink, etoposide 50 mg, net price 20 = £99.82; 100 mg, 10-cap pack = £87.23 (hosp. only). Label: 23

### ◾ VINBLASTINE SULFATE

**Cautions** see section 8.1 and notes above; caution in handling; **interactions**: Appendix 1 (vinblastine)

**Contra-indications** see notes above

### Safe Practice
Intrathecal injection **contra-indicated**

**Hepatic impairment** dose reduction may be necessary—consult local treatment protocol for details

**Pregnancy** avoid (limited experience suggests fetal harm; teratogenic in *animal* studies); see also Pregnancy and Reproductive Function, p. 416

**Breast-feeding** discontinue breast-feeding

**Side-effects** see section 8.1 and notes above; abdominal pain, constipation, leucopenia, muscle pain; less commonly peripheral neuropathy; rarely paralytic ileus; irritant to tissues if extravasated

**Licensed use** licensed for use in children (age range not specified by manufacturer)

### Indications and dose
Hodgkin's disease and other lymphomas
- By intravenous injection
  Consult local treatment protocol for details

**Vinblastine** (Non-proprietary) PoM
Injection, vinblastine sulfate 1 mg/mL, net price 10-mL vial = £13.09

**Velbe**® (Genus) PoM
Injection, powder for reconstitution, vinblastine sulfate, net price 10-mg amp = £14.15

### ◾ VINCRISTINE SULFATE

**Cautions** see section 8.1 and notes above; neuromuscular disease; ileus; caution in handling; **interactions**: Appendix 1 (vincristine)

**Contra-indications** see notes above

### Safe Practice
Intrathecal injection **contra-indicated**

**Hepatic impairment** dose reduction may be necessary—consult local treatment protocol for details

**Pregnancy** avoid (teratogenicity and fetal loss in *animal* studies); see also Pregnancy and Reproductive Function, p. 416

**Breast-feeding** discontinue breast-feeding

**Side-effects** see section 8.1 and notes above; constipation (see notes above), diarrhoea, intestinal necrosis, paralytic ileus may occur in young children; dose-limiting neuromuscular effects (see notes above); urinary retention, rarely convulsions followed by coma; inappropriate secretion of antidiuretic hormone; irritant to tissues if extravasated

**Licensed use** licensed for use in children (age range not specified by manufacturer)

**Indications and dose**

Acute leukaemias, lymphomas, paediatric solid tumours

- By intravenous injection

  Consult local treatment protocol for details

**Vincristine** (Non-proprietary) PoM

Injection, vincristine sulfate 1 mg/mL, net price 1-mL vial = £13.47; 2-mL vial = £26.66; 5-mL vial = £44.16

**Oncovin®** (Genus) PoM

Injection, vincristine sulfate 1 mg/mL, net price 1-mL vial = £14.18; 2-mL vial = £28.05

---

## 8.1.5 Other antineoplastic drugs

### Amsacrine

**Amsacrine** has an action and toxic effects similar to those of doxorubicin (section 8.1.2) and is given *intravenously*. It is occasionally used in acute myeloid leukaemia.

### ▌AMSACRINE

**Cautions** see section 8.1 and notes above; consider monitoring cardiac function; monitor electrolytes (fatal arrhythmias possible if hypokalaemia); previous treatment with anthracyclines; also caution in handling—irritant to skin and tissues

**Hepatic impairment** manufacturer advises reduce initial dose by 20–30%

**Renal impairment** manufacturer advises reduce initial dose by 20–30%

**Pregnancy** avoid (teratogenic and toxic in *animal* studies); may reduce fertility; see also Pregnancy and Reproductive Function, p. 416

**Breast-feeding** discontinue breast-feeding

**Side-effects** see section 8.1; mucositis; phlebitis; *less commonly* diarrhoea, cardiotoxicity, haematuria, renal impairment, hepatotoxicity, skin rash; *rarely* acute renal failure, grand mal seizures

**Licensed use** not licensed for use in children

**Indications and dose**

Acute myeloid leukaemia

- By intravenous infusion

  Consult local treatment protocol for details

**Amsidine®** (Goldshield) PoM

Concentrate for intravenous infusion, amsacrine 5 mg (as lactate)/mL, when reconstituted by mixing two solutions. Net price 1.5-mL (75-mg) amp with 13.5-mL diluent vial = £54.08 (hosp. only)

---

### Asparaginase

**Asparaginase** is used almost exclusively in the treatment of acute lymphoblastic leukaemia. Hypersensitivity reactions may occur and facilities for the management of anaphylaxis should be available. A number of different preparations of asparaginase exist and only the product specified in the treatment protocol should be used.

**Crisantaspase** is the enzyme asparaginase produced by *Erwinia chrysanthemi*. Preparations of asparaginase derived from *Escherichia coli* are also available. Children who are hypersensitive to asparaginase derived from one organism may tolerate asparaginase derived from another organism but cross-sensitivity occurs in about 20–30% of individuals.

---

### ▌CRISANTASPASE

**Cautions** see section 8.1 and notes above

**Contra-indications** history of pancreatitis related to asparaginase therapy

**Pregnancy** avoid; see also Pregnancy and Reproductive Function, p. 416

**Breast-feeding** discontinue breast-feeding

**Side-effects** see section 8.1; also liver dysfunction, pancreatitis, diarrhoea; coagulation disorders; lethargy, drowsiness, confusion, dizziness, neurotoxicity, convulsions, headache; *less commonly* changes in blood lipids, anaphylaxis, hyperglycaemia; *rarely* CNS depression; *very rarely* myalgia; abdominal pain and hypertension also reported

**Indications and dose**

Acute lymphoblastic leukaemia, acute myeloid leukaemia, non-Hodgkin's lymphoma

- By intravenous, intramuscular or subcutaneous injection

  Consult local treatment protocol for details

**Erwinase®** (EUSA Pharma) PoM

Injection, powder for reconstitution, crisantaspase, net price 10 000-unit vial = £301.70

◢**Preparations**

Preparations of asparaginase derived from *Escherichia coli* are available but they are not licensed, they include: *Medac®* asparaginase, *Elspar®* asparaginase, and *Oncaspar®* pegaspargase.

---

### Dacarbazine and temozolomide

**Dacarbazine** is a component of a commonly used combination for Hodgkin's disease (ABVD—doxorubicin [previously *Adriamycin®*], bleomycin, vinblastine, and dacarbazine). It is given *intravenously*.

**Temozolomide** is structurally related to dacarbazine and is used in children for second-line treatment of malignant glioma.

**8** Malignant disease and immunosuppression

## DACARBAZINE

**Cautions**   see section 8.1; caution in handling

**Hepatic impairment**   dose reduction may be required in combined hepatic and renal impairment; avoid in severe impairment

**Renal impairment**   dose reduction may be required in combined renal and hepatic impairment; avoid in severe impairment

**Pregnancy**   avoid (carcinogenic and teratogenic in *animal* studies); ensure effective contraception during and for at least 6 months after treatment in men or women; see also Pregnancy and Reproductive Function, p. 416

**Breast-feeding**   discontinue breast-feeding

**Side-effects**   see section 8.1; *also* anorexia; *less commonly* facial flushing, confusion, headache, seizures, facial paraesthesia, influenza-like symptoms, blurred vision, renal impairment, rash; *rarely* diarrhoea, hepatotoxicity including liver necrosis and hepatic vein thrombosis, photosensitivity, irritant to skin and tissues, injection-site reactions

**Indications and dose**

Hodgkin's disease, paediatric solid tumours

- By intravenous injection or by intravenous infusion

  Consult local treatment protocol for details

**Dacarbazine** (Non-proprietary) PoM
Injection, powder for reconstitution, dacarbazine (as citrate), net price 100-mg vial = £5.05; 200-mg vial = £7.16; 500-mg vial = £16.50; 600-mg vial = £22.50; 1-g vial = £31.80

## TEMOZOLOMIDE

**Cautions**   see section 8.1; **interactions**: Appendix 1 (temozolomide)

**Hepatic impairment**   use with caution in severe impairment—no information available

**Renal impairment**   manufacturer advises caution—no information available

**Pregnancy**   avoid (teratogenic and embryotoxic in *animal* studies); manufacturer advises adequate contraception during treatment; men should avoid fathering a child during and for at least 6 months after treatment; see also Pregnancy and Reproductive Function, p. 416

**Breast-feeding**   discontinue breast-feeding

**Side-effects**   see section 8.1

**Indications and dose**

Treatment of malignant glioma

- By mouth

  Consult local treatment protocol for details

**Temozolomide** (Non-proprietary) PoM
Capsules, temozolomide 5 mg, net price 5-cap pack = £13.58; 20 mg, 5-cap pack = £54.30; 100 mg, 5-cap pack = £271.52; 140 mg, 5-cap pack = £380.18; 180 mg, 5-cap pack = £488.74; 250 mg, 5-cap pack = £678.80. Label: 23, 25
Brands include *Temomedac*®

**Temodal**® (MSD) PoM
Capsules, temozolomide 5 mg (green/white), net price 5-cap pack = £16.29; 20 mg (yellow/white), 5-cap pack = £65.16; 100 mg (pink/white), 5-cap pack = £325.80; 140 mg (blue/white), 5-cap pack = £456.12; 180 mg (orange/white), 5-cap pack = £586.44; 250 mg (white), 5-cap pack = £814.50. Label: 23, 25

## Mitotane

**Mitotane** is used in children for the symptomatic treatment of advanced or inoperable adrenocortical carcinoma. It selectively inhibits the activity of the adrenal cortex, necessitating corticosteroid replacement therapy (section 6.3.1); the dose of glucocorticoid should be increased in case of shock, trauma, or infection. Neuropsychological impairment can occur, possibly secondary to hypothyroidism, and growth retardation has also been reported in children treated with mitotane.

## MITOTANE

**Cautions**   see notes above; risk of accumulation in overweight patients; monitor plasma-mitotane concentration—consult product literature; avoid in acute porphyria (section 9.8.2); **interactions**: Appendix 1 (mitotane)

**Skilled tasks** Central nervous system toxicity may affect performance of skilled tasks

**Counselling** Children and their carers should be warned to contact doctor immediately if injury, infection, or illness occurs (because of the risk of acute adrenal insufficiency)

**Hepatic impairment**   manufacturer advises caution in mild to moderate impairment—monitoring of plasma-mitotane concentration recommended; avoid in severe impairment

**Renal impairment**   manufacturer advises caution in mild to moderate renal impairment—monitoring of plasma-mitotane concentration recommended; avoid in severe impairment

**Pregnancy**   manufacturer advises avoid—women of child-bearing age should use effective contraception during and after treatment; see also Pregnancy and Reproductive Function, p. 416

**Breast-feeding**   discontinue breast-feeding

**Side-effects**   see section 8.1 and notes above; *also* gastro-intestinal disturbances (including nausea, vomiting, diarrhoea, epigastric discomfort), anorexia, liver disorders; hypercholesterolaemia, hypertriglyceridaemia; ataxia, confusion, asthenia, myasthenia, paraesthesia, drowsiness, neuropathy, cognitive impairment, movement disorder, dizziness, headache; gynaecomastia; prolonged bleeding time, leucopenia, thrombocytopenia, anaemia; rash; *rarely* hypersalivation, hypertension, postural hypotension, flushing, pyrexia, haematuria, proteinuria, haemorrhagic cystitis, hypouricaemia, visual disturbances and ocular disorders

**Licensed use**   not licensed for use in children

**Indications and dose**

Symptomatic treatment of advanced or inoperable adrenocortical carcinoma

- By mouth

  Consult local treatment protocol for details

**Lysodren**® (HRA Pharma) PoM
Tablets, scored, mitotane 500 mg, net price 100-tab pack = £590.97. Label: 2, 10, 21, counselling, skilled tasks, adrenal suppression

## Platinum compounds

**Carboplatin** is used in the treatment of a variety of paediatric malignancies; it is given by intravenous infusion. Carboplatin can be given in an outpatient setting and is better tolerated than cisplatin; nausea and vomiting are less severe and nephrotoxicity, neurotoxicity, and ototoxicity are much less of a problem. Carboplatin is, however, more myelosuppressive than cisplatin.

**Cisplatin** is of value in children with a variety of malignancies; it is given by intravenous infusion. Cisplatin requires intensive intravenous hydration; routine use of intravenous fluids containing potassium or magnesium may also be required to help control hypokalaemia and hypomagnesaemia. Treatment may be complicated by severe nausea and vomiting; delayed vomiting may occur and is difficult to control. Cisplatin has dose-related and potentially cumulative side-effects including nephrotoxicity, neurotoxicity, and ototoxicity. Baseline testing of renal function and hearing is required; for children with pre-existing renal or hearing impairment or marked bone-marrow suppression, consideration should be given to withholding treatment or using another drug.

### ■ CARBOPLATIN

**Cautions** see section 8.1 and notes above; consider therapeutic drug monitoring; **interactions:** Appendix 1 (platinum compounds)

**Renal impairment** reduce dose and monitor haematological parameters and renal function; avoid if creatinine clearance less than $20 \, mL/minute/1.73 \, m^2$

**Pregnancy** avoid (teratogenic and embryotoxic in *animal* studies); see also Pregnancy and Reproductive Function, p. 416

**Breast-feeding** discontinue breast-feeding

**Side-effects** see section 8.1 and notes above

**Licensed use** not licensed for use in children

**Indications and dose**

> Stage 4 neuroblastoma, germ cell tumours, low-grade gliomas (including astrocytomas), neuroectodermal tumours (including medulloblastoma), rhabdomyosarcoma (metastatic and non-metastatic disease), soft-tissue sarcomas, retinoblastoma, high risk Wilms' tumour, some liver tumours
> - By intravenous infusion
>   Consult local treatment protocol for details

**Carboplatin** (Non-proprietary) (PoM)
Injection, carboplatin 10 mg/mL, net price 5-mL vial = £22.04, 15-mL vial = £56.92, 45-mL vial = £168.85, 60-mL vial = £260.00

### ■ CISPLATIN

**Cautions** see section 8.1 and notes above; monitor full blood count, renal function, audiology, and plasma electrolytes; **interactions:** Appendix 1 (platinum compounds)

**Renal impairment** avoid if possible—nephrotoxic

**Pregnancy** avoid (teratogenic and toxic in *animal* studies); manufacturer advises effective contraception during and for at least 3 months after treatment in men or women; see also Pregnancy and Reproductive Function, p. 416

**Breast-feeding** discontinue breast-feeding

**Side-effects** see section 8.1 and notes above; also peripheral neuropathy; hypophosphataemia, hypocalcaemia, hyperuricaemia also reported

**Licensed use** not licensed for use in children

**Indications and dose**

> Osteogenic sarcoma, stage 4 neuroblastoma, some liver tumours, infant brain tumours, intracranial germ-cell tumours
> - By intravenous infusion
>   Consult local treatment protocol for details

**Cisplatin** (Non-proprietary) (PoM)
Injection, cisplatin 1 mg/mL, net price 10-mL vial = £5.85, 50-mL vial = £24.50, 100-mL vial = £50.22

Injection, powder for reconstitution, cisplatin, net price 50-mg vial = £17.00

## Procarbazine

**Procarbazine** is most often used in Hodgkin's disease. It is given *by mouth*. It is a weak monoamine-oxidase inhibitor and dietary restriction is rarely considered necessary. Alcohol ingestion may cause a disulfiram-like reaction.

### ■ PROCARBAZINE

**Cautions** see section 8.1 and notes above; **interactions:** Appendix 1 (procarbazine)

**Hepatic impairment** caution in mild to moderate impairment; avoid in severe impairment

**Renal impairment** caution in mild to moderate impairment; avoid in severe impairment

**Pregnancy** avoid (teratogenic in *animal* studies and isolated reports in humans); see also Pregnancy and Reproductive Function, p. 416

**Breast-feeding** discontinue breast-feeding

**Side-effects** see section 8.1 and notes above; hypersensitivity rash (discontinue treatment)

**Indications and dose**

> Hodgkin's lymphoma, gliomas
> - By mouth
>   Consult local treatment protocol for details

**Procarbazine** (Non-proprietary) (PoM)
Capsules, ivory, procarbazine (as hydrochloride) 50 mg, net price 50-cap pack = £199.60. Label: 4

## Protein kinase inhibitors

**Everolimus,** a protein kinase inhibitor, is licensed in children from the age of 3 years for the treatment of subependymal giant cell astrocytoma associated with tuberous sclerosis complex who require therapeutic intervention but are not amenable to surgery.

**Imatinib,** a tyrosine kinase inhibitor, is licensed in children for the treatment of newly diagnosed Philadelphia-chromosome-positive chronic myeloid leukaemia when bone marrow transplantation is not considered first line treatment, and for Philadelphia-chromosome-positive chronic myeloid leukaemia in chronic phase after failure of interferon alfa, or in accelerated phase, or in blast crisis.

**8** Malignant disease and immunosuppression

**8 Malignant disease and immunosuppression**

## EVEROLIMUS

**Cautions** see section 8.1; monitor blood-glucose concentration, serum-triglycerides and serum-cholesterol before treatment and periodically thereafter; concomitant use of drugs that increase risk of bleeding; history of bleeding disorders; monitor renal function before treatment and periodically thereafter; reduce dose or discontinue if severe side-effects occur—consult product literature; **interactions**: Appendix 1 (everolimus)

**Pneumonitis** Non-infectious pneumonitis reported. Children and their carers should be advised to seek urgent medical advice if new or worsening respiratory symptoms occur

**Hepatic impairment** consult product literature

**Pregnancy** manufacturer advises avoid (toxicity in *animal* studies); effective contraception must be used during and for up to 8 weeks after treatment; see also Pregnancy and Reproductive Function, p. 416

**Breast-feeding** manufacturer advises avoid

**Side-effects** see section 8.1; also diarrhoea, dry mouth, abdominal pain, dysphagia, anorexia, taste disturbance, chest pain, hypertension, hyperlipidaemia, hypercholesterolaemia, peripheral oedema, pneumonitis (including interstitial lung disease), asthenia, fatigue, headache, insomnia, convulsions, irritability, increased susceptibility to infections (including pneumonia, aspergillosis, and candidiasis), hyperglycaemia, hypoglycaemia, dehydration, renal failure, electrolyte disturbance, arthralgia, eyelid oedema, epistaxis, skin and nail disorders (including hand-foot syndrome); *less commonly* congestive heart failure, myalgia, agitation, aggression, rhabdomyolysis and impaired wound healing; hepatitis B reactivation and haemorrhage also reported

**Indications and dose**

**Subependymal giant cell astrocytoma associated with tuberous sclerosis complex**

- By mouth

Consult product literature

**Votubia**® (Novartis) ▼ PoM
Tablets, white-yellow, everolimus, 2.5 mg, net price 30-tab pack = £1200.00; 5 mg, 30-tab pack = £2250.00; 10 mg, 30-tab pack = £2970.00. Label: 25, counselling, pneumonitis

**Note** *Votubia*® tablets may be dispersed in approximately 30 mL of water by gently stirring, immediately before drinking. After solution has been swallowed, any residue must be re-dispersed in the same volume of water and swallowed

## IMATINIB

**Cautions** see section 8.1; cardiac disease; risk factors for heart failure; history of renal failure; monitor for fluid retention; monitor liver function (see also Hepatic Impairment, below); monitor growth in children (may cause growth retardation); **interactions**: Appendix 1 (imatinib)

**Hepatic impairment** start with minimum recommended dose; reduce dose further if not tolerated; consult local treatment protocol

**Renal impairment** start with minimum recommended dose; reduce dose further if not tolerated; consult local treatment protocol

**Pregnancy** manufacturer advises avoid unless potential benefit outweighs risk; effective contraception required during treatment; see also Pregnancy and Reproductive Function, p. 416

**Breast-feeding** discontinue breast-feeding

**Side-effects** see section 8.1; also abdominal pain, appetite changes, constipation, diarrhoea, flatulence, gastro-oesophageal reflux, taste disturbance, weight changes, dry mouth; oedema (including pulmonary oedema, pleural effusion, and ascites), flushing, haemorrhage; cough, dyspnoea; dizziness, headache, insomnia, hypoaesthesia, paraesthesia; influenza-like symptoms; cramps, arthralgia; visual disturbances, lacrimation, conjunctivitis, dry eyes; epistaxis; dry skin, sweating, rash, pruritus, photosensitivity; *less commonly* gastric ulceration, pancreatitis, hepatic dysfunction (rarely hepatic failure, hepatic necrosis), dysphagia, heart failure, tachycardia, palpitation, syncope, hypertension, hypotension, cold extremities, cough, acute respiratory failure, depression, drowsiness, anxiety, peripheral neuropathy, tremor, migraine, impaired memory, vertigo, gynaecomastia, menorrhagia, irregular menstruation, sexual dysfunction, electrolyte disturbances, renal failure, urinary frequency, gout, tinnitus, hearing loss; skin hyperpigmentation; *rarely* intestinal obstruction, gastro-intestinal perforation, inflammatory bowel disease, arrhythmia, atrial fibrillation, myocardial infarction, angina, pulmonary fibrosis, pulmonary hypertension, increased intracranial pressure, convulsions, confusion, haemolytic anaemia, rhabdomyolysis, myopathy, aseptic necrosis of bone, cataract, glaucoma, angioedema, exfoliative dermatitis, and Stevens-Johnson syndrome; *also reported* growth retardation in children

**Indications and dose**

**Chronic phase and advanced phase chronic myeloid leukaemia**

- By mouth

Consult local treatment protocol for details

**Glivec**® (Novartis) PoM
Tablets, f/c, imatinib (as mesilate) 100 mg (yellow-brown, scored), net price 60-tab pack = £802.04; 400 mg (yellow), 30-tab pack = £1604.08. Label: 21, 27

**Counselling** Tablets may be dispersed in water or apple juice

# Tretinoin

**Tretinoin** is licensed for the induction of remission in acute promyelocytic leukaemia. It is used in previously untreated children as well as in those who have relapsed after standard chemotherapy or who are refractory to it.

## TRETINOIN

**Note** Tretinoin is the acid form of vitamin A

**Cautions** exclude pregnancy before starting treatment, see also Pregnancy below; monitor full blood count and coagulation profile, liver function, serum calcium and plasma lipids before and during treatment; increased risk of thrombo-embolism during first month of treatment; **interactions**: Appendix 1 (retinoids)

**Hepatic impairment** reduce dose—consult local treatment protocol for details

**Renal impairment** reduce dose—consult local treatment protocol for details

**Pregnancy** teratogenic; effective contraception must be used for at least 1 month before oral treatment, during treatment and for at least 1 month after stopping (oral progestogen-only contraceptives **not** considered effective); see also Pregnancy and Reproductive Function, p. 416

**Breast-feeding** discontinue breast-feeding

**Side-effects** retinoic acid syndrome (fever, dyspnoea, acute respiratory distress, pulmonary infiltrates, pleural effusion, hyperleukocytosis, hypotension, oedema, weight gain, hepatic, renal and multi-organ failure) requires immediate treatment—consult product literature; gastro-intestinal disturbances, pancreatitis; arrhythmias, flushing, oedema; headache, benign intracranial hypertension (children particularly susceptible—consider dose reduction if intractable headache), shivering, dizziness, confusion, anxiety, depression, insomnia, paraesthesia, visual and hearing disturbances (children particularly susceptible to nervous system effects); raised liver enzymes, serum creatinine and lipids; bone and chest pain, alopecia, erythema, rash, pruritus, sweating, dry skin and mucous membranes, cheilitis; thromboembolism, hypercalcaemia, and genital ulceration reported

**Indications and dose**

**Acute promyelocytic leukaemia**

● By mouth

　Consult treatment protocol for details

**Vesanoid**® (Roche) ▼PoM▼

　Capsules, yellow/brown, tretinoin 10 mg, net price 100-cap pack = £160.63. Label: 21, 25

---

## 8.2　Drugs affecting the immune response

**8.2.1　Antiproliferative immunosuppressants**

**8.2.2　Corticosteroids and other immunosuppressants**

**8.2.3　Anti-lymphocyte monoclonal antibodies**

**8.2.4　Other immunomodulating drugs**

---

### Immunosuppressant therapy

Immunosuppressants are used to suppress rejection in organ transplant recipients and to treat a variety of chronic inflammatory and autoimmune diseases. Solid organ transplant patients are maintained on drug regimens, which may include antiproliferative drugs (azathioprine or mycophenolate mofetil), calcineurin inhibitors (ciclosporin or tacrolimus), corticosteroids, or sirolimus. Choice is dependent on the type of organ, time after transplant, and clinical condition of the patient. Specialist management is required and other immunomodulators may be used to initiate treatment or to treat rejection.

> **Bioavailability**
>
> Different formulations of the same immunosuppressant may vary in bioavailability and to avoid reduced effect or excessive side-effects, it is important not to change formulation except on the advice of a transplant specialist.

**Impaired immune responsiveness** Infections in the immunocompromised child can be severe and show atypical features. Specific local protocols should be followed for the management of infection. Corticosteroids may suppress clinical signs of infection and allow diseases such as septicaemia or tuberculosis to reach an advanced stage before being recognised. Children should be up-to-date with their childhood vaccinations before initiation of immunosuppressant therapy (e.g. before transplantation); vaccination with varicella-zoster vaccine (section 14.4) is also necessary during this period—**important**: for advice on measles exposure, see section 14.5.1, and chickenpox (varicella) exposure, see section 14.5.2. For advice on the use of live vaccines in individuals with impaired immune response, see section 14.1. For general comments and warnings relating to corticosteroids and immunosuppressants, see section 6.3.2.

**Pregnancy** Transplant patients immunosuppressed with azathioprine should not discontinue it on becoming pregnant. However, there have been reports of premature birth and low birth-weight following exposure to azathioprine, particularly in combination with corticosteroids. Spontaneous abortion has been reported following maternal or paternal exposure. Azathioprine is teratogenic in *animal* studies.

There is less experience of ciclosporin in pregnancy but it does not appear to be any more harmful than azathioprine. The use of these drugs during pregnancy needs to be supervised in specialist units.

## 8.2.1　Antiproliferative immunosuppressants

**Azathioprine** is widely used for transplant recipients and it is also used to treat a number of auto-immune conditions (see section 10.1.3), usually when corticosteroid therapy alone provides inadequate control. It is metabolised to mercaptopurine, and doses should be reduced to one quarter of the original dose when allopurinol is given concurrently. Blood tests and monitoring for signs of myelosuppression are essential in long-term treatment with azathioprine.

> **Thiopurine methyltransferase**
>
> The enzyme thiopurine methyltransferase (TPMT) metabolises thiopurine drugs (azathioprine, mercaptopurine, tioguanine); the risk of myelosuppression is increased in patients with reduced activity of the enzyme, particularly for the few individuals in whom TPMT activity is undetectable. Consider measuring TPMT activity before starting azathioprine, mercaptopurine, or tioguanine therapy. Patients with absent TPMT activity should not receive thiopurine drugs; those with reduced TPMT activity may be treated under specialist supervision.

**Mycophenolate mofetil** is metabolised to mycophenolic acid which has a more selective mode of action than azathioprine. It is used in combination with a corticosteroid and either ciclosporin or tacrolimus for the prophylaxis of acute rejection in transplant recipients. Compared with similar regimens incorporating azathioprine, mycophenolate mofetil may reduce the risk of acute rejection episodes; the risk of opportunistic infections (particularly due to tissue-invasive cytomegalovirus) and the occurrence of blood disorders such as leucopenia may be higher. Children may suffer a high incidence of side-effects, particularly gastro-intestinal effects, calling for temporary reduction in dose or interruption of treatment.

Cases of pure red cell aplasia have been reported with azathioprine and with mycophenolate mofetil; dose reduction or discontinuation should be considered under specialist supervision.

> **NICE guidance (immunosuppressive therapy for renal transplantation in children and adolescents)**
> See p. 433

Cyclophosphamide (section 8.1.1) is less commonly prescribed as an immunosuppressant.

## ◢ AZATHIOPRINE

**Cautions** see Bioavailability, p. 431; thiopurine methyltransferase status (see notes above); monitor for toxicity throughout treatment; monitor full blood count weekly (more frequently with higher doses or if severe hepatic or renal impairment) for first 4 weeks (manufacturer advises weekly monitoring for 8 weeks but evidence of practical value unsatisfactory), thereafter reduce frequency of monitoring to at least every 3 months; **interactions**: Appendix 1 (azathioprine)

**Bone marrow suppression** Children and their carers should be warned to report immediately any signs or symptoms of bone marrow suppression e.g. inexplicable bruising or bleeding, infection

**Contra-indications** hypersensitivity to mercaptopurine

**Hepatic impairment** reduce dose; monitor liver function; see also Cautions

**Renal impairment** reduce dose; see also Cautions

**Pregnancy** see section 8.2; treatment should not normally be initiated during pregnancy

**Breast-feeding** present in milk in low concentration; no evidence of harm in small studies—use if potential benefit outweighs risk

**Side-effects** hypersensitivity reactions (including malaise, dizziness, vomiting, diarrhoea, fever, rigors, myalgia, arthralgia, rash, hypotension and interstitial nephritis—calling for immediate withdrawal); dose-related bone marrow suppression (see also Cautions); liver impairment, cholestatic jaundice, hair loss and increased susceptibility to infections and colitis in patients also receiving corticosteroids; nausea; *rarely* pancreatitis, pneumonitis, hepatic veno-occlusive disease, lymphoma, red cell aplasia—see notes above

### Indications and dose

**Suppression of transplant rejection**

- By mouth, or (if oral route not possible) by intravenous infusion (see also note below)
  Consult local treatment protocol for details

  **Child 1 month–18 years** maintenance, 1–3 mg/kg once daily, adjusted according to response; total daily dose may alternatively be given in 2 divided doses

**Severe ulcerative colitis and Crohn's disease** section 1.5.3

**Systemic lupus erythematosus, vasculitis, autoimmune conditions when corticosteroid therapy alone has proved inadequate** section 10.1.3

**Administration** Consult local treatment protocol for details

For *intravenous injection*, reconstitute 50 mg with 5–15 mL Water for Injections; give over at least 1 minute

For *intravenous infusion*, reconstitute 50 mg with 5–15 mL Water for Injections; dilute requisite dose to a concentration of 0.25–2.5 mg/mL in Glucose 5% *or* Sodium Chloride 0.9%

**Note** Intravenous injection is alkaline and very irritant. Intravenous route should therefore be used **only** if oral route not feasible and discontinued as soon as oral route can be tolerated. To reduce irritation flush line with infusion fluid

**Azathioprine** (Non-proprietary) [PoM]
Tablets, azathioprine 25 mg, net price 28-tab pack = £6.67; 50 mg, 56-tab pack = £5.56. Label: 21
**Brands include** *Azamune*®

**Imuran**® (Aspen) [PoM]
Tablets, both f/c, azathioprine 25 mg (orange), net price 100-tab pack = £10.99; 50 mg (yellow), 100-tab pack = £7.99. Label: 21

Injection, powder for reconstitution, azathioprine (as sodium salt), net price 50-mg vial = £15.38

## ◢ MYCOPHENOLATE MOFETIL

**Cautions** see Bioavailability, p. 431; full blood counts every week for 4 weeks then twice a month for 2 months then every month in the first year (consider interrupting treatment if neutropenia develops); active gastro-intestinal disease (risk of haemorrhage, ulceration and perforation); delayed graft function; increased susceptibility to skin cancer (avoid exposure to strong sunlight); possible decreased effectiveness of vaccination—avoid live vaccines; **interactions**: Appendix 1 (mycophenolate mofetil)

**Bone marrow suppression** Children and their carers should be warned to report immediately any signs or symptoms of bone marrow suppression e.g. infection or inexplicable bruising or bleeding

**Renal impairment** manufacturer advises consider dose reduction if estimated glomerular filtration rate less than 25 mL/minute/1.73 m²

**Pregnancy** manufacturer advises avoid—congenital malformations reported; effective contraception required before treatment, during treatment, and for 6 weeks after discontinuation of treatment

**Breast-feeding** manufacturer advises avoid—present in milk in *animal* studies

**Side-effects** taste disturbance, gingival hyperplasia, nausea, constipation, flatulence, anorexia, weight loss, diarrhoea, vomiting, abdominal pain, gastro-intestinal inflammation, ulceration, and bleeding, hepatitis, jaundice, pancreatitis, stomatitis, ileus, pleural effusion, oedema, tachycardia, hypertension, hypotension, vasodilatation, cough, dyspnoea, insomnia, agitation, confusion, depression, anxiety, convulsions, paraesthesia, myasthenic syndrome, tremor, dizziness, headache, influenza-like syndrome, infections, hyperglycaemia, renal impairment, malignancy (particularly of the skin), blood disorders (including leucopenia, anaemia, thrombocytopenia, pancytopenia, and red cell aplasia—see notes above), disturbances of electrolytes and blood lipids, arthralgia, alopecia, acne, skin hypertrophy, and rash; *also reported* intestinal villous atrophy, progressive multifocal leucoencephalopathy, interstitial lung disease, pulmonary fibrosis

**Licensed use** not licensed for use in children under 2 years for the prophylaxis of acute rejection in renal transplantation; not licensed for use in children for the prophylaxis of acute rejection in hepatic transplantation

### Indications and dose

**Prophylaxis of acute rejection in renal transplantation in combination with a corticosteroid and ciclosporin**

* **By mouth**

  Consult local treatment protocol for details

  **Child 1 month–18 years** 600 mg/m$^2$ twice daily (max. 2 g daily)

**Prophylaxis of acute rejection in renal transplantation in combination with a corticosteroid and tacrolimus**

* **By mouth**

  Consult local treatment protocol for details

  **Child 1 month–18 years** 300 mg/m$^2$ twice daily (max. 2 g daily)

**Prophylaxis of acute rejection in hepatic transplantation in combination with a corticosteroid and ciclosporin or tacrolimus**

* **By mouth**

  Consult local treatment protocol for details

  **Child 1 month–18 years** 10 mg/kg twice daily, increased to 20 mg/kg twice daily (max. 2 g daily)

**Note** Tablets and capsules not appropriate for dose titration in children with body surface area less than 1.25 m$^2$

**Mycophenolate Mofetil** (Non-proprietary) PoM

Capsules, mycophenolate mofetil 250 mg, net price 100-cap pack = £35.00

Tablets, mycophenolate mofetil 500 mg, net price 50-tab pack = £31.50

Brands include *Arzip*®

**CellCept**® (Roche) PoM

Capsules, blue/brown, mycophenolate mofetil 250 mg, net price 100-cap pack = £82.26

Tablets, lavender, mycophenolate mofetil 500 mg, net price 50-tab pack = £82.26

Oral suspension, mycophenolate mofetil 1 g/5 mL when reconstituted with water, net price 175 mL = £115.16

Excipients include aspartame (section 9.4.1)

## 8.2.2 Corticosteroids and other immunosuppressants

The corticosteroids prednisolone and dexamethasone are widely used in paediatric oncology; they have a marked antitumour effect. Dexamethasone is preferred for acute lymphoblastic leukaemia whilst prednisolone may be used for Hodgkin's disease, non-Hodgkin's lymphoma, and B-cell lymphoma and leukaemia.

Dexamethasone is the corticosteroid of choice in paediatric supportive and palliative care. For children who are not receiving a corticosteroid as a component of their chemotherapy, dexamethasone may be used to reduce raised intracranial pressure (see p. 19), or to help control emesis when combined with an appropriate anti-emetic (see p. 18). For more information on gluco-

corticoid therapy, including the disadvantages of treatment, see section 6.3.2.

The corticosteroids are also powerful immunosuppressants. They are used to prevent organ transplant rejection, and in high dose to treat rejection episodes.

**Ciclosporin** (cyclosporin), a calcineurin inhibitor, is a potent immunosuppressant which is virtually non-myelotoxic but markedly nephrotoxic. It may be used in organ and tissue transplantation, for prevention of graft rejection following bone marrow, kidney, liver, pancreas, heart, lung, and heart-lung transplantation, and for prophylaxis and treatment of graft-versus-host disease. Ciclosporin also has a role in steroid-sensitive and steroid-resistant nephrotic syndrome; in corticosteroid-sensitive nephrotic syndrome it may be given with prednisolone (section 6.3).

**Tacrolimus** is also a calcineurin inhibitor. Although not chemically related to ciclosporin it has a similar mode of action and side-effects.

**Sirolimus** is a non-calcineurin inhibiting immunosuppressant.

**Basiliximab** is a monoclonal antibody that prevents T-lymphocyte proliferation; it is used for prophylaxis of acute rejection in allogeneic renal transplantation. It is given with ciclosporin and corticosteroid immunosuppression regimens; its use should be confined to specialist centres.

**Antithymocyte immunoglobulin** (rabbit) is used for the prophylaxis of organ rejection in renal and heart allograft recipients and for the treatment of corticosteroid-resistant allograft rejection in renal transplantation. Tolerability is increased by pretreatment with an intravenous corticosteroid and antihistamine; an antipyretic drug such as paracetamol may also be beneficial.

> **NICE guidance**
> **Immunosuppressive therapy for renal transplantation in children and adolescents (April 2006)**
> NICE has recommended that for induction therapy in the prophylaxis of organ rejection, either basiliximab or daclizumab [discontinued] are options for combining with a calcineurin inhibitor. For each individual, ciclosporin or tacrolimus is chosen as the calcineurin inhibitor on the basis of side-effects. Mycophenolate mofetil is recommended as part of an immunosuppressive regimen **only if:**
> * the calcineurin inhibitor is not tolerated, particularly if nephrotoxicity endangers the transplanted kidney; *or*
> * there is very high risk of nephrotoxicity from the calcineurin inhibitor, requiring a reduction in the dose of the calcineurin inhibitor or its avoidance.
>
> Mycophenolic acid is not recommended as part of an immunosuppressive regimen for renal transplantation in children or adolescents.
> Sirolimus [not licensed for use in children] is recommended as a component of immunosuppressive regimen **only if** intolerance necessitates the withdrawal of a calcineurin inhibitor.
> These recommendations may not be consistent with the marketing authorisation of some of the products.
> www.nice.org.uk/TA99

**8 Malignant disease and immunosuppression**

## ANTITHYMOCYTE IMMUNOGLOBULIN (RABBIT)

**Cautions** see notes above; monitor blood count

**Contra-indications** infection

**Pregnancy** manufacturer advises use only if potential benefit outweighs risk—no information available

**Breast-feeding** manufacturer advises avoid—no information available

**Side-effects** nausea, vomiting, dysphagia, diarrhoea; hypotension; infusion-related reactions (including cytokine release syndrome and anaphylaxis, see notes above), serum sickness; fever, shivering, increased susceptibility to infection; increased susceptibility to malignancy; lymphopenia, neutropenia, thrombocytopenia; myalgia; pruritus, rash

### Indications and dose

Heart transplantation

• **By intravenous infusion over at least 6 hours**

**Child 1 month–18 years** 1–2.5 mg/kg daily for 3–5 days starting the day of transplantation

**Note** To avoid excessive dosage in obese patients, calculate dose on the basis of ideal body weight

Renal transplantation

• **By intravenous infusion over at least 6 hours**

**Child 1–18 years** 1–1.5 mg/kg daily for 3–9 days starting the day of transplantation

**Note** To avoid excessive dosage in obese patients, calculate dose on the basis of ideal body weight

Corticosteroid-resistant renal graft rejection

• **By intravenous infusion over at least 6 hours**

**Child 1–18 years** 1.5 mg/kg daily for 7–14 days

**Note** To avoid excessive dosage in obese patients, calculate dose on the basis of ideal body weight

**Administration** For *continuous intravenous infusion* reconstitute each vial with 5 mL water for injections to produce a solution of 5 mg/mL; gently rotate to dissolve. Dilute requisite dose with Glucose 5% or Sodium Chloride 0.9% to an approx. concentration of 0.5 mg/mL; begin infusion immediately after dilution; give through an in-line filter (pore size 0.22 micron); incompatible with unfractionated heparin and hydrocortisone in glucose infusion—precipitation reported

**Thymoglobuline®** (Sanofi Aventis) [PoM]
Intravenous infusion, powder for reconstitution, rabbit anti-human thymocyte immunoglobulin, net price 25-mg vial = £158.77

## BASILIXIMAB

**Pregnancy** manufacturer advises avoid—no information available; adequate contraception must be used during treatment and for 16 weeks after last dose

**Breast-feeding** manufacturer advises avoid—no information available

**Side-effects** severe hypersensitivity reactions and cytokine release syndrome reported

### Indications and dose

Prophylaxis of acute rejection in allogeneic renal transplantation used in combination with ciclosporin and corticosteroid-containing immunosuppression regimens

• **By intravenous injection or by intravenous infusion**

Consult local treatment protocol for details

**Child over 1 year, body-weight under 35 kg** 10 mg within 2 hours before transplant surgery and 10 mg 4 days after surgery

**Child body-weight over 35 kg** 20 mg within 2 hours before transplant surgery and 20 mg 4 days after surgery

**Note** Withhold second dose if severe hypersensitivity or graft loss occurs

**Administration** For *intravenous infusion*, dilute reconstituted solution to a concentration not exceeding 400 micrograms/mL, with Glucose 5% or Sodium Chloride 0.9%; give over 20–30 minutes

**Simulect®** (Novartis) [PoM]
Injection, powder for reconstitution, basiliximab, net price 10-mg vial = £758.69, 20-mg vial = £842.38 (both with water for injections). For intravenous infusion

## CICLOSPORIN
(Cyclosporin)

**Cautions** monitor kidney function—dose dependent increase in serum creatinine and urea during first few weeks may necessitate discontinuation (exclude rejection of kidney transplant); monitor liver function (see also Hepatic Impairment below); monitor blood pressure—discontinue if hypertension develops that cannot be controlled by antihypertensives; hyperuricaemia; monitor serum potassium especially in renal dysfunction (risk of hyperkalaemia); monitor serum magnesium; measure blood lipids before treatment and after the first month of treatment; monitor whole blood ciclosporin concentration (trough level dependent on indication—consult local treatment protocol for details); use with tacrolimus specifically contra-indicated; for patients other than transplant recipients, preferably avoid other immunosuppressants (increased risk of infection and malignancies, including lymphoma and skin cancer); avoid excessive exposure to UV light, including sunlight; **interactions:** Appendix 1 (ciclosporin)

**Additional cautions in nephrotic syndrome** *Contra-indicated* in uncontrolled hypertension, uncontrolled infections, and malignancy; in long-term management, perform renal biopsies every 1–2 years

**Additional cautions** Atopic Dermatitis and Psoriasis, section 13.5.3; Rheumatoid Arthritis, section 10.1.3

**Hepatic impairment** dosage adjustment based on bilirubin and liver enzymes may be needed

**Renal impairment** dose as in normal renal function but see Cautions above; in *nephrotic syndrome* reduce dose by 25–50% if serum creatinine more than 30% above baseline on more than one measurement

**Pregnancy** crosses placenta; see Immunosuppressant Therapy, p. 431

**Breast-feeding** present in milk—manufacturer advises avoid

**Side-effects** anorexia, nausea, vomiting, abdominal pain, diarrhoea, gingival hyperplasia, hepatic dysfunction, hypertension, tremor, headache, paraesthesia, fatigue, renal dysfunction (renal structural changes on long-term administration; see also under Cautions), hyperuricaemia, hyperkalaemia, hypomagnesaemia, hyperlipidaemia, hypercholesterolaemia, muscle cramps, myalgia, hypertrichosis; *less commonly* oedema, weight gain, signs of encephalopathy, anaemia, thrombocytopenia; *rarely* pancreatitis, motor polyneuropathy, menstrual disturbances, gynaecomastia, micro-angiopathic haemolytic anaemia, haemolytic uraemic syndrome, hyperglycaemia, muscle weakness, myopathy, visual disturbances secondary to benign intracranial hypertension (discontinue); *also reported with infusion* anaphylaxis

**Licensed use** not licensed for use in children under 3 months

### Indications and dose

Prevention of graft rejection following bone-marrow, kidney, liver, pancreas, heart, lung, and heart-lung transplantation, prophylaxis and treatment of graft-versus-host disease
- By mouth or by intravenous infusion
  Consult local treatment protocols for details

Nephrotic syndrome see also section 6.3.2, p. 371
- By mouth
  Child 1 month–18 years 3 mg/kg twice daily, increase if necessary in corticosteroid-resistant disease; for maintenance reduce to lowest effective dose according to whole blood-ciclosporin concentrations, proteinuria, and renal function

Refractory ulcerative colitis section 1.5.3

Severe psoriasis, severe eczema section 13.5.3

> **Important**
>
> Patients should be stabilised on a particular brand of oral ciclosporin because switching between formulations without close monitoring may lead to clinically important changes in blood-ciclosporin concentration. Prescribing and dispensing of ciclosporin should be by brand name to avoid inadvertent switching. If it is necessary to switch a patient to a different brand of ciclosporin, the patient should be monitored closely for changes in blood-ciclosporin concentration, serum-creatinine, blood pressure, and transplant function.

**Capimune®** (Mylan) [PoM]
Capsules, ciclosporin 25 mg (grey), net price 30-cap pack = £13.80; 50 mg (white), 30-cap pack = £27.00; 100 mg (grey), 30-cap pack = £51.50. Counselling, administration
**Excipients** include propylene glycol (see Excipients, p. 2)
**Note** Contains ethanol
**Counselling** Total daily dose should be taken in 2 divided doses

**Capsorin®** (Morningside) [PoM]
Capsules, ciclosporin 25 mg (grey), net price 30-cap pack = £13.11; 50 mg (white), 30-cap pack = £25.65; 100 mg (grey), 30-cap pack = £48.93. Counselling, administration
**Note** Contains ethanol
**Counselling** Total daily dose should be taken in 2 divided doses

**Deximune®** (Dexcel) [PoM]
Capsules, grey, ciclosporin 25 mg, net price 30-cap pack = £13.94; 50 mg 30-cap pack = £27.31; 100 mg 30-cap pack = £51.83. Counselling, administration
**Note** Contains ethyl lactate which is metabolised to ethanol
**Counselling** Total daily dose should be taken in 2 divided doses

**Neoral®** (Novartis) [PoM]
Capsules, ciclosporin 10 mg (yellow/white), net price 60-cap pack = £18.48; 25 mg (blue/grey), 30-cap pack = £18.59; 50 mg (yellow/white), 30-cap pack = £36.41; 100 mg (blue/grey), 30-cap pack = £69.11. Counselling, administration
**Excipients** include propylene glycol (see Excipients, p. 2)
**Note** Contains ethanol

Oral solution, yellow, sugar-free, ciclosporin 100 mg/mL, net price 50 mL = £103.55. Counselling, administration
**Excipients** include propylene glycol (see Excipients, p. 2)
**Note** Contains ethanol
**Counselling** Total daily dose should be taken in 2 divided doses
Mix solution with orange juice (or squash) or apple juice (to improve taste) or with water immediately before taking (and rinse with more to ensure total dose). Do not mix with grapefruit juice. Keep medicine measure away from other liquids (including water)

**Sandimmun®** (Novartis) [PoM]
Concentrate for intravenous infusion (oily), ciclosporin 50 mg/mL. To be diluted before use, net price 1-mL amp = £1.94; 5-mL amp = £9.17
**Excipients** include polyoxyl castor oil (risk of anaphylaxis, see Excipients, p. 2)
**Note** Contains ethanol
**Administration** For *intravenous infusion*, dilute to a concentration of 0.5–2.5 mg/mL with Glucose 5% *or* Sodium Chloride 0.9%; give over 2–6 hours; not to be used with PVC equipment; observe patient for signs of anaphylaxis for at least 30 minutes after starting infusion and at frequent intervals thereafter
**Note** Capsules and oral solution available direct from Novartis for children who cannot be transferred to a different oral preparation

## SIROLIMUS

**Cautions** monitor renal function when given with ciclosporin; monitor whole blood-sirolimus trough concentration (Afro-Caribbean patients may require higher doses); hyperlipidaemia (monitor lipids); monitor urine proteins; increased susceptibility to infection (especially urinary-tract infection); increased susceptibility to lymphoma and other malignancies, particularly of the skin (limit exposure to UV light); **interactions**: Appendix 1 (sirolimus)

**Hepatic impairment** monitor blood-sirolimus trough concentration; dose reduction may be necessary, consult local treatment protocol for details

**Pregnancy** avoid unless essential—toxicity in *animal* studies; effective contraception must be used during treatment and for 12 weeks after stopping

**Breast-feeding** discontinue breast-feeding

**Side-effects** abdominal pain, constipation, nausea, diarrhoea, ascites, stomatitis, oedema, tachycardia, hypertension, hypercholesterolaemia, hypertriglyceridaemia, venous thromboembolism, pleural effusion, pneumonitis, headache, pyrexia, proteinuria, haemolytic uraemic syndrome, anaemia, thrombocytopenia, thrombotic thrombocytopenic purpura, leucopenia,

8

Malignant disease and immunosuppression

neutropenia, hypokalaemia, hypophosphataemia, hyperglycaemia, lymphocele, arthralgia, osteonecrosis, epistaxis, acne, rash, impaired healing; *less commonly* pancreatitis, pulmonary embolism, pulmonary haemorrhage, pericardial effusion, nephrotic syndrome, pancytopenia; *rarely* interstitial lung disease, alveolar proteinosis, hepatic necrosis, lymphoedema, hypersensitivity reactions (including anaphylactic reactions, angiodema, exfoliative dermatitis, hypersensitivity vasculitis); *also reported* focal segmental glomerulosclerosis, reversible impairment of male fertility

**Licensed use**   not licensed for use in children

**Indications and dose**

> See NICE guidance, p. 433
>
> • **By mouth**
>
>> Consult local treatment protocols for details

**Rapamune®** (Pfizer) [PoM]
Tablets, coated, sirolimus 0.5 mg (tan), net price 30-tab pack = £69.00; 1 mg (white), 30-tab pack = £86.49; 2 mg (yellow), 30-tab pack = £172.98. Counselling, administration
**Important** The 0.5-mg tablet is not bioequivalent to the 1-mg, 2-mg, and 5-mg tablets. Multiples of 0.5-mg tablets should **not** be used as a substitute for other tablet strengths
Oral solution, sirolimus 1 mg/mL, net price 60 mL = £162.41. Counselling, administration
**Note** Contains ethanol
**Administration**   food may affect absorption (give at the same time with respect to food). Mix solution with at least 60 mL water or orange juice in a glass or plastic container immediately before taking; refill container with at least 120 mL of water or orange juice and drink immediately (to ensure total dose). Do not mix with any other liquids

## TACROLIMUS

**Cautions**   monitor blood pressure, ECG (**important:** see cardiomyopathy below), fasting blood-glucose concentration, haematological and neurological (including visual) parameters, electrolytes, hepatic and renal function; monitor whole blood-tacrolimus trough concentration (especially during episodes of diarrhoea)—consult local treatment protocol for details; QT-interval prolongation; neurotoxicity; increased risk of infections, malignancies, and lymphoproliferative disorders; avoid excessive exposure to UV light (including sunlight); **interactions:** Appendix 1 (tacrolimus)
**Skilled tasks** May affect performance of skilled tasks (e.g. driving)

**Contra-indications**   hypersensitivity to macrolides; avoid concurrent administration with ciclosporin (care if patient has previously received ciclosporin)

**Hepatic impairment**   dose reduction may be necessary in severe impairment

**Pregnancy**   exclude before treatment; avoid unless potential benefit outweighs risk—risk of premature delivery, intra-uterine growth restriction, and hyperkalaemia; toxicity in *animal* studies

**Breast-feeding**   avoid—present in breast milk

**Side-effects**   nausea, vomiting, diarrhoea, constipation, dyspepsia, flatulence, bloating, weight changes, anorexia, gastro-intestinal inflammation, ulceration, and perforation, hepatic dysfunction, jaundice, cholestasis, ascites, bile-duct abnormalities, oedema, tachycardia, hypertension, haemorrhage, thromboembolic and ischaemic events, dyspnoea, pleural effusion, parenchymal lung disorders, sleep disturbances, tremor, headache, peripheral neuropathy, mood changes, depression, confusion, anxiety, psychosis, seizures, paraesthesia, dizziness, renal impairment, renal failure, renal tubular necrosis, urinary abnormalities, hyperglycaemia, electrolyte disturbances (including hyperkalaemia, hypokalaemia, and hyperuricaemia), blood disorders (including anaemia, leucopenia, pancytopenia, and thrombocytopenia), arthralgia, muscle cramp, visual disturbances, photophobia, tinnitus, impaired hearing, alopecia, sweating, acne; *less commonly* paralytic ileus, gastro-intestinal reflux disease, peritonitis, pancreatitis, heart failure, arrhythmia, cardiac arrest, cerebrovascular accident, cardiomyopathy (**important:** see Cardiomyopathy below), palpitation, respiratory failure, coma, speech disorder, amnesia, paralysis, influenza-like symptoms, encephalopathy, coagulation disorders, cataract, photosensitivity, hypoglycaemia, dysmenorrhoea, hypertonia, dermatitis; *rarely* pericardial effusion, respiratory distress syndrome, posterior reversible encephalopathy syndrome, dehydration, thrombotic thrombocytopenic purpura, blindness, toxic epidermal necrolysis, hirsutism; *very rarely* myasthenia, haemorrhagic cystitis, Stevens Johnson syndrome; *also reported* pure red cell aplasia, agranulocytosis, haemolytic anaemia
**Cardiomyopathy** Cardiomyopathy has been reported in children. Children should be monitored by echocardiography for hypertrophic changes—consider dose reduction or discontinuation if these occur

**Licensed use**   *Advagraf®* not licensed for use in children

**Indications and dose**

> See under preparations and consult local treatment protocols

> Atopic eczema (topical use) section 13.5.3

> ---
>
> **MHRA/CHM advice**
> **Oral tacrolimus products: prescribe and dispense by brand name only, to minimise the risk of inadvertent switching between products, which has been associated with reports of toxicity and graft rejection (June 2012)**
> Inadvertent switching between oral tacrolimus products has been associated with reports of toxicity and graft rejection. To ensure maintenance of therapeutic response when a patient is stabilised on a particular brand, oral tacrolimus products should be prescribed and dispensed by brand name only.
> • *Adoport®, Prograf®, Capexion®, Tacni®,* and *Vivadex®* are immediate-release capsules taken twice daily, once in the morning and once in the evening;
> • *Modigraf®* granules are used to prepare an immediate-release oral suspension which is taken twice daily, once in the morning and once in the evening;
> • *Advagraf®* is a prolonged-release capsule that is taken once daily in the morning.
> Switching between tacrolimus brands requires careful supervision and therapeutic monitoring by an appropriate specialist.

**Administration**   For *continuous intravenous infusion* over 24 hours, dilute to a concentration of 4–100 micrograms/mL with Glucose 5% *or* Sodium Chloride 0.9%, to a total volume between 20–500 mL. Tacrolimus is incompatible with PVC

**Adoport**® (Sandoz) PoM

Capsules, tacrolimus (as monohydrate) 500 micrograms (white/ivory), net price 50-cap pack = £50.50; 1 mg (white/brown), 50-cap pack = £65.52, 100-cap pack = £131.02; 5 mg (white/orange), 50-cap pack = £242.05. Label: 23, counselling, skilled tasks

**Dose**

**Prophylaxis of graft rejection following liver transplantation, starting 12 hours after transplantation**

- By mouth

  **Neonate** initially 150 micrograms/kg twice daily, adjusted according to whole-blood concentration

  **Child 1 month–18 years** initially 150 micrograms/kg twice daily, adjusted according to whole-blood concentration

**Prophylaxis of graft rejection following kidney transplantation, starting within 24 hours of transplantation**

- By mouth

  **Neonate** initially 150 micrograms/kg twice daily, adjusted according to whole-blood concentration

  **Child 1 month–18 years** initially 150 micrograms/kg twice daily, adjusted according to whole-blood concentration

  **Note** A lower initial dose of 100 micrograms/kg twice daily has been used in adolescents to prevent very high 'trough' concentrations

**Prophylaxis of graft rejection following heart transplantation** *without antibody induction*, **starting within 12 hours of transplantation**

- By mouth

  **Neonate** initially 150 micrograms/kg twice daily as soon as clinically possible (8–12 hours after discontinuation of intravenous infusion), adjusted according to whole-blood concentration

  **Child 1 month–18 years** initially 150 micrograms/kg twice daily as soon as clinically possible (8–12 hours after discontinuation of intravenous infusion), adjusted according to whole-blood concentration

**Prophylaxis of graft rejection following heart transplantation** *following antibody induction*, **starting within 5 days of transplantation**

- By mouth

  **Neonate** initially 50–150 micrograms/kg twice daily, adjusted according to whole-blood concentration

  **Child 1 month–18 years** initially 50–150 micrograms/kg twice daily, adjusted according to whole-blood concentration

**Allograft rejection resistant to conventional immunosuppressive therapy** Consult local treatment protocol

**Capexion**® (Generics) PoM

Capsules, tacrolimus 500 micrograms, (ivory), net price 50-cap pack = £52.50; 1 mg (white), 50-cap pack = £68.20, 100-cap pack = £136.20; 5 mg (red), 50-cap pack = £252.00. Label: 23, counselling, skilled tasks

**Dose**

**Prophylaxis of graft rejection following liver transplantation, starting 12 hours after transplantation**

- By mouth

  **Neonate** initially 150 micrograms/kg twice daily, adjusted according to whole-blood concentration

  **Child 1 month–18 years** initially 150 micrograms/kg twice daily, adjusted according to whole-blood concentration

**Prophylaxis of graft rejection following kidney transplantation, starting within 24 hours of transplantation**

- By mouth

  **Neonate** initially 150 micrograms/kg twice daily, adjusted according to whole-blood concentration

  **Child 1 month–18 years** initially 150 micrograms/kg twice daily, adjusted according to whole-blood concentration

  **Note** A lower initial dose of 100 micrograms/kg twice daily has been used in adolescents to prevent very high 'trough' concentrations

**Prophylaxis of graft rejection following heart transplantation** *without antibody induction*, **starting within 12 hours of transplantation**

- By mouth

  **Neonate** initially 150 micrograms/kg twice daily, as soon as clinically possible (8–12 hours after discontinuation of intravenous infusion), adjusted according to whole-blood concentration

  **Child 1 month–18 years** initially 150 micrograms/kg twice daily, as soon as clinically possible (8–12 hours after discontinuation of intravenous infusion), adjusted according to whole-blood concentration

**Prophylaxis of graft rejection following heart transplantation** *following antibody induction*, **starting within 5 days of transplantation**

- By mouth

  **Neonate** initially 50–150 micrograms/kg twice daily, adjusted according to whole-blood concentration

  **Child 1 month–18 years** initially 50–150 micrograms/kg twice daily, adjusted according to whole-blood concentration

**Allograft rejection resistant to conventional immunosuppressive therapy** Consult local treatment protocol

**Modigraf**® (Astellas) ▼ PoM

Granules, tacrolimus (as monohydrate), 200 micrograms, net price 50-sachet pack = £71.30; 1 mg, 50-sachet pack = £356.65. Label: 13, 23, counselling, skilled tasks

**Dose**

**Prophylaxis of graft rejection following liver transplantation, starting 12 hours after transplantation**

- By mouth

  **Neonate** initially 150 micrograms/kg twice daily, adjusted according to whole-blood concentration

  **Child 1 month–18 years** initially 150 micrograms/kg twice daily, adjusted according to whole-blood concentration

**Prophylaxis of graft rejection following kidney transplantation, starting within 24 hours of transplantation**

- By mouth

  **Neonate** initially 150 micrograms/kg twice daily, adjusted according to whole-blood concentration

  **Child 1 month–18 years** initially 150 micrograms/kg twice daily, adjusted according to whole-blood concentration

  **Note** A lower initial dose of 100 micrograms/kg twice daily has been used in adolescents to prevent very high 'trough' concentrations

**8**

**Malignant disease and immunosuppression**

**Prophylaxis of graft rejection following heart transplantation** *without antibody induction* **starting within 12 hours of transplantation**

• By mouth

  **Neonate** initially 150 micrograms/kg twice daily as soon as clinically possible (8–12 hours after discontinuing intravenous infusion), adjusted according to whole-blood concentration

  **Child 1 month–18 years** initially 150 micrograms/kg twice daily as soon as clinically possible (8–12 hours after discontinuing intravenous infusion), adjusted according to whole-blood concentration

**Prophylaxis of graft rejection following heart transplantation** *following antibody induction* **starting within 5 days of transplantation**

• By mouth

  **Neonate** initially 50–150 micrograms/kg twice daily, adjusted according to whole-blood concentration

  **Child 1 month–18 years** initially 50–150 micrograms/kg twice daily, adjusted according to whole-blood concentration

**Allograft rejection resistant to conventional immunosuppressive therapy** Consult local treatment protocol

**Note** The *Scottish Medicines Consortium* (p. 3) has advised (November 2010) that tacrolimus granules for oral suspension (*Modigraf*®) are accepted for restricted use within NHS Scotland in patients for whom tacrolimus is an appropriate choice of immunosuppressive therapy and where small changes (less than 500 micrograms) in dosing increments are required (such as, in paediatric patients) or in seriously ill patients who are unable to swallow tacrolimus capsules.

**Prograf**® (Astellas) PoM

Capsules, tacrolimus (as monohydrate) 500 micrograms (yellow), net price 50-cap pack = £61.88; 1 mg (white), 50-cap pack = £80.28, 100-cap pack = £160.54; 5 mg (greyish-red), 50-cap pack = £296.58. Label: 23, counselling, skilled tasks

Concentrate for intravenous infusion, tacrolimus 5 mg/mL. To be diluted before use. Net price 1-mL amp = £58.46

**Excipients** include polyoxyl castor oil (risk of anaphylaxis, see Excipients, p. 2)

**Dose**

**Prophylaxis of graft rejection following liver transplantation, starting 12 hours after transplantation**

• By mouth

  **Neonate** initially 150 micrograms/kg twice daily, adjusted according to whole-blood concentration

  **Child 1 month–18 years** initially 150 micrograms/kg twice daily, adjusted according to whole-blood concentration

• By continuous intravenous infusion (only if oral route inappropriate)

  **Neonate** 50 micrograms/kg over 24 hours for up to 7 days (then transfer to oral therapy), adjusted according to whole-blood concentration

  **Child 1 month–18 years** 50 micrograms/kg over 24 hours for up to 7 days (then transfer to oral therapy), adjusted according to whole-blood concentration

**Prophylaxis of graft rejection following kidney transplantation, starting within 24 hours of transplantation**

• By mouth

  **Neonate** initially 150 micrograms/kg twice daily, adjusted according to whole-blood concentration

  **Child 1 month–18 years** initially 150 micrograms/kg twice daily, adjusted according to whole-blood concentration

  **Note** A lower initial dose of 100 micrograms/kg twice daily has been used in adolescents to prevent very high 'trough' concentrations

• By continuous intravenous infusion (only if oral route inappropriate)

  **Neonate** 75–100 micrograms/kg over 24 hours for up to 7 days (then transfer to oral therapy), adjusted according to whole-blood concentration

  **Child 1 month–18 years** 75–100 micrograms/kg over 24 hours for up to 7 days (then transfer to oral therapy), adjusted according to whole-blood concentration

**Prophylaxis of graft rejection following heart transplantation** *without antibody induction,* **starting within 12 hours of transplantation**

• By mouth

  **Neonate** initially 150 micrograms/kg twice daily as soon as clinically possible (8–12 hours after discontinuation of intravenous infusion), adjusted according to whole-blood concentration

  **Child 1 month–18 years** initially 150 micrograms/kg twice daily as soon as clinically possible (8–12 hours after discontinuation of intravenous infusion), adjusted according to whole-blood concentration

• By continuous intravenous infusion

  **Neonate** 30–50 micrograms/kg over 24 hours for up to 7 days (then transfer to oral therapy), adjusted according to whole-blood concentration

  **Child 1 month–18 years** 30–50 micrograms/kg over 24 hours for up to 7 days (then transfer to oral therapy), adjusted according to whole-blood concentration

**Prophylaxis of graft rejection following heart transplantation** *following antibody induction,* **starting within 5 days of transplantation**

• By mouth

  **Neonate** initially 50–150 micrograms/kg twice daily, adjusted according to whole-blood concentration

  **Child 1 month–18 years** initially 50–150 micrograms/kg twice daily, adjusted according to whole-blood concentration

**Allograft rejection resistant to conventional immunosuppressive therapy** Consult local treatment protocol

**Tacni**® (TEVA UK) PoM

Capsules, tacrolimus 500 micrograms (ivory), net price 50-cap pack = £50.48; 1 mg (white), 50-cap pack = £65.49, 100-cap pack = £130.99; 5 mg (red), 50-cap pack = £242.01. Label: 23, counselling, skilled tasks

**Dose**

**Prophylaxis of graft rejection following liver transplantation, starting 12 hours after transplantation**

• By mouth

  **Neonate** initially 150 micrograms/kg twice daily, adjusted according to whole-blood concentration

  **Child 1 month–18 years** initially 150 micrograms/kg twice daily, adjusted according to whole-blood concentration

**Prophylaxis of graft rejection following kidney transplantation, starting within 24 hours of transplantation**

• By mouth

  **Neonate** initially 150 micrograms/kg twice daily, adjusted according to whole-blood concentration

  **Child 1 month–18 years** initially 150 micrograms/kg twice daily, adjusted according to whole-blood concentration

  **Note** A lower initial dose of 100 micrograms/kg twice daily has been used in adolescents to prevent very high 'trough' concentrations

**Prophylaxis of graft rejection following heart transplantation *without antibody induction*, starting within 12 hours of transplantation**

- By mouth

  **Neonate** initially 150 micrograms/kg twice daily, as soon as clinically possible (8–12 hours after discontinuation of intravenous infusion), adjusted according to whole-blood concentration

  **Child 1 month–18 years** initially 150 micrograms/kg twice daily, as soon as clinically possible (8–12 hours after discontinuation of intravenous infusion), adjusted according to whole-blood concentration

**Prophylaxis of graft rejection following heart transplantation *following antibody induction*, starting within 5 days of transplantation**

- By mouth

  **Neonate** initially 50–150 micrograms/kg twice daily, adjusted according to whole-blood concentration

  **Child 1 month–18 years** initially 50–150 micrograms/kg twice daily, adjusted according to whole-blood concentration

**Allograft rejection resistant to conventional immunosuppressive therapy** Consult local treatment protocol

---

**Vivadex®** (Dexcel) PoM

Capsules, tacrolimus 500 micrograms (ivory), net price 50-cap pack = £46.41; 1 mg (white), 50-cap pack = £60.21, 100-cap pack = £120.41; 5 mg (red), 50-cap pack = £222.44. Label: 23, counselling, skilled tasks

**Dose**

**Prophylaxis of graft rejection following liver transplantation, starting 12 hours after transplantation**

- By mouth

  **Neonate** initially 150 micrograms/kg twice daily, adjusted according to whole-blood concentration

  **Child 1 month–18 years** initially 150 micrograms/kg twice daily, adjusted according to whole-blood concentration

**Prophylaxis of graft rejection following kidney transplantation, starting within 24 hours of transplantation**

- By mouth

  **Neonate** initially 150 micrograms/kg twice daily, adjusted according to whole-blood concentration

  **Child 1 month–18 years** initially 150 micrograms/kg twice daily, adjusted according to whole-blood concentration

  **Note** A lower initial dose of 100 micrograms/kg twice daily has been used in adolescents to prevent very high 'trough' concentrations

**Prophylaxis of graft rejection following heart transplantation *without antibody induction*, starting within 12 hours of transplantation**

- By mouth

  **Neonate** initially 150 micrograms/kg twice daily as soon as clinically possible (8–12 hours after discontinuation of intravenous infusion), adjusted according to whole-blood concentration

  **Child 1 month–18 years** initially 150 micrograms/kg twice daily as soon as clinically possible (8–12 hours after discontinuation of intravenous infusion), adjusted according to whole-blood concentration

**Prophylaxis of graft rejection following heart transplantation *following antibody induction*, starting within 5 days of transplantation**

- By mouth

  **Neonate** initially 50–150 micrograms/kg twice daily, adjusted according to whole-blood concentration

  **Child 1 month–18 years** initially 50–150 micrograms/kg twice daily, adjusted according to whole-blood concentration

**Allograft rejection resistant to conventional immunosuppressive therapy** Consult local treatment protocol

◢**Modified release**

*Advagraf®* is not licensed for use in children

**Advagraf®** (Astellas) PoM

Capsules, m/r, tacrolimus (as monohydrate) 500 micrograms (yellow/orange), net price 50-cap pack = £35.79; 1 mg (white/orange), 50-cap pack = £71.59, 100-cap pack = £143.17; 3 mg (red/orange), 50-cap pack = £214.76; 5 mg (red/orange), 50-cap pack = £266.92. Label: 23, 25, counselling, skilled tasks

## 8.2.3 Anti-lymphocyte monoclonal antibodies

**Rituximab**, a monoclonal antibody which causes lysis of B lymphocytes, has been used as a component of the treatment of post-transplantation lymphoproliferative disease, non-Hodgkin's lymphoma, Hodgkin's lymphoma, and severe cases of resistant immune modulated disease including idiopathic thrombocytopenia purpura, haemolytic anaemia, and systemic lupus erythematosus. Full resuscitation facilities should be at hand and as with other cytotoxics, treatment should be undertaken under the close supervision of a specialist.

Rituximab should be used with caution in children receiving cardiotoxic chemotherapy or with a history of cardiovascular disease; in adults exacerbation of angina, arrhythmia, and heart failure have been reported. Transient hypotension occurs frequently during infusion and antihypertensives may need to be withheld for 12 hours before infusion. Progressive multifocal leucoencephalopathy (which is usually fatal or causes severe disability) has been reported in association with rituximab; children treated with rituximab should be monitored for cognitive, neurological, or psychiatric signs and symptoms. If progressive multifocal leucoencephalopathy is suspected, suspend treatment until it has been excluded.

Infusion-related side-effects (including cytokine release syndrome) are reported commonly with rituximab and occur predominantly during the first infusion; they include fever and chills, nausea and vomiting, allergic reactions (such as rash, pruritus, angioedema, bronchospasm and dyspnoea), flushing and tumour pain. Children should be given paracetamol and an antihistamine before each dose of rituximab to reduce these effects. Premedication with a corticosteroid should also be considered. The infusion may have to be stopped temporarily and the infusion-related effects treated—consult product literature or local treatment protocol for appropriate management. Evidence of pulmonary infiltration and features of tumour lysis syndrome should be sought if infusion-related effects occur.

**8 Malignant disease and immunosuppression**

Fatalities following **severe** cytokine release syndrome (characterised by severe dyspnoea) and associated with features of tumour lysis syndrome have occurred 1–2 hours after infusion of rituximab. Children with a high tumour burden as well as those with pulmonary insufficiency or infiltration are at increased risk and should be monitored **very closely** (and a slower rate of infusion considered).

**Alemtuzumab** is no longer licensed but is available through a patient access programme for oncological and transplant indications.

### RITUXIMAB

**Cautions** see notes above—but for full details (including monitoring) consult product literature or local treatment protocol

**Pregnancy** avoid unless potential benefit to mother outweighs risk of B-lymphocyte depletion in fetus—effective contraception (in both sexes) required during and for 12 months after treatment

**Breast-feeding** avoid breast-feeding during and for 12 months after treatment

**Side-effects** see notes above—but for full details (including monitoring and management of side-effects) consult product literature

**Licensed use** not licensed for use in children

**Indications and dose**

  See notes above

- By intravenous infusion

    Consult local treatment protocol for details

**MabThera**® (Roche) ℗ℴ𝔐
Concentrate for intravenous infusion, rituximab 10 mg/mL, net price 10-mL vial = £174.63, 50-mL vial = £873.15

## 8.2.4 Other immunomodulating drugs

## Interferon alfa

**Interferon alfa** has shown some antitumour effect and may have a role in inducing early regression of life-threatening corticosteroid-resistant haemangiomas of infancy. Interferon alfa preparations are also used in the treatment of chronic hepatitis B, and chronic hepatitis C ideally in combination with ribavirin (section 5.3.3). Interferon alfa should always be used under the close supervision of a specialist. Side-effects are dose-related, but commonly include anorexia, nausea, influenza-like symptoms, and lethargy. Ocular side-effects and depression (including suicidal behaviour) have also been reported. Myelosuppression may occur, particularly affecting granulocyte counts. Cardiovascular problems (hypotension, hypertension, and arrhythmias), nephrotoxicity and hepatotoxicity have been reported and monitoring of hepatic function is recommended. Hypertriglyceridaemia, sometimes severe, has been observed; monitoring of lipid concentration is recommended. Other side-effects include hypersensitivity reactions, thyroid abnormalities, hyperglycaemia, alopecia, psoriasiform rash, confusion, coma and seizures, and reversible motor problems in young children. Rarely pulmonary infiltrates, pneumonitis, and pneumonia have occurred; respiratory symptoms should be

investigated and if pulmonary infiltrates are suspected or lung function is impaired the discontinuation of interferon alfa should be considered.

### INTERFERON ALFA

**Cautions** consult product literature and local treatment protocol for details; **interactions:** Appendix 1 (interferons)

**Contra-indications** consult product literature and local treatment protocol for details; avoid injections containing benzyl alcohol in neonates (see under preparations below)

**Hepatic impairment** close monitoring in mild to moderate impairment; avoid if severe

**Renal impairment** close monitoring required in mild to moderate impairment; avoid in severe impairment

**Pregnancy** avoid unless potential benefit outweighs risk (toxicity in *animal* studies); effective contraception required during treatment—consult product literature

**Breast-feeding** unlikely to be harmful

**Side-effects** see notes above, consult product literature and local treatment protocols for details

**Licensed use** not licensed for use in children for chronic active hepatitis B; *Roferon-A*® not licensed for use in children

**Indications and dose**

  **Induction of early regression of life-threatening corticosteroid resistant haemangiomata of infancy**

- By subcutaneous injection

    Consult local treatment protocol for details

  **Chronic active hepatitis B infection** see under preparations below

  **Chronic active hepatitis C infection** see under preparations below

**IntronA**® (MSD) ℗ℴ𝔐
Injection, interferon alfa-2b (rbe) 10 million units/mL, net price 1-mL vial = £42.35, 2.5-mL vial = £105.95. For subcutaneous injection or intravenous infusion

Injection pen, interferon alfa-2b (rbe), net price 15 million units/mL, 1.5-mL cartridge = £76.28; 25 million units/mL, 1.5-mL cartridge = £127.14; 50 million units/mL, 1.5-mL cartridge = £254.28. For subcutaneous injection
Note Each 1.5-mL multidose cartridge delivers 6 doses of 0.2 mL i.e. a total of 1.2 mL

**Dose**

  **Chronic active hepatitis B**

- By subcutaneous injection

    **Child 2–18 years** 5–10 million units/m$^2$ 3 times weekly

  **Chronic active hepatitis C** (in combination with oral ribavirin, see p. 331)

- By subcutaneous injection

    **Child 3–18 years** 3 million units/m$^2$ 3 times weekly

**Roferon-A**® (Roche) ℗ℴ𝔐
Injection, interferon alfa-2a (rbe). Net price 6 million units/mL, 0.5-mL (3 million-unit) prefilled syringe = £14.20; 9 million units/mL, 0.5-mL (4.5 million-unit) prefilled syringe = £21.29; 12 million units/mL, 0.5-mL (6 million-unit) prefilled syringe = £28.37; 18 million units/mL, 0.5-mL (9 million-unit) prefilled

syringe = £42.57; 30 million units/mL, 0.6-mL (18 million-unit) cartridge = £85.15, for use with *Roferon* pen device. For subcutaneous injection (cartridges, vials, and prefilled syringes) and intramuscular injection (cartridges and vials)

**Excipients** include benzyl alcohol (avoid in neonates, see Excipients, p. 2)

**Dose**

> **Chronic active hepatitis B**
>
> • By subcutaneous injection
>
> **Child 2–18 years** 2.5–5 million units/m² 3 times weekly; up to 10 million units/m² has been used 3 times weekly

## Interferon gamma

**Interferon gamma-1b** is used to reduce the frequency of serious infection in chronic granulomatous disease and in severe malignant osteopetrosis.

### ■ INTERFERON GAMMA-1b
(Immune interferon)

**Cautions** seizure disorders (including seizures associated with fever); cardiac disease (including ischaemia, congestive heart failure, and arrhythmias); monitor before and during treatment: haematological tests (including full blood count, differential white cell count, and platelet count), blood chemistry tests (including renal and liver function tests) and urinalysis; avoid simultaneous administration of foreign proteins including immunological products (risk of exaggerated immune response); **interactions:** Appendix 1 (interferons)

**Hepatic impairment** manufacturer advises caution in severe impairment—risk of accumulation

**Renal impairment** manufacturer advises caution in severe impairment—risk of accumulation

**Pregnancy** manufacturers advise avoid unless potential benefit outweighs risk (toxicity in *animal* studies); effective contraception required during treatment—consult product literature

**Breast-feeding** manufacturer advises avoid—no information available

**Side-effects** nausea, vomiting, diarrhoea, abdominal pain; headache, fatigue, fever, chills, depression; myalgia, arthralgia; rash, injection-site reactions; *rarely* confusion and systemic lupus erythematosus; also reported, neutropenia, thrombocytopenia, proteinuria and raised liver enzymes

**Indications and dose**

> See notes above and under Preparations below

**Immukin**® (Boehringer Ingelheim) [PoM]
Injection, recombinant human interferon gamma-1b 200 micrograms/mL, net price 0.5-mL vial = £66.67

**Dose**

> • By subcutaneous injection
>
> **Body surface area 0.5 m² or less** 1.5 micrograms/kg 3 times a week
>
> **Body surface area greater than 0.5 m²** 50 micrograms/m² 3 times a week
>
> Not recommended for infant under 6 months with chronic granulomatous disease

## Canakinumab

**Canakinumab** is a recombinant human monoclonal antibody that selectively inhibits interleukin-1beta receptor binding. It is licensed for the treatment of

cryopyrin-associated periodic syndromes, including severe forms of familial cold auto-inflammatory syndrome (or familial cold urticaria), Muckle-Wells syndrome, and neonatal-onset multisystem inflammatory disease (also known as chronic infantile neurological cutaneous and articular syndrome). These are rare inherited auto-inflammatory disorders.

### ■ CANAKINUMAB

**Cautions** history of recurrent infection or predisposition to infection; monitor neutrophil count before starting treatment, 1–2 months after starting treatment, and periodically thereafter; children should receive all recommended vaccinations (including pneumococcal and inactivated influenza vaccine) before starting treatment; avoid live vaccines unless potential benefit outweighs risk—consult product literature and section 14.1, p. 600 for further information

**Tuberculosis** Children should be evaluated for latent and active tuberculosis before starting treatment and monitored for signs and symptoms of tuberculosis during and after treatment

**Contra-indications** severe active infection (see also Cautions); neutropenia; concomitant use with tumour necrosis factor inhibitors (possible increased risk of infections)

**Hepatic impairment** no information available

**Renal impairment** limited information available but manufacturer advises no dose adjustment required

**Pregnancy** manufacturer advises avoid unless potential benefit outweighs risk; effective contraception required during treatment and for up to 3 months after last dose

**Breast-feeding** consider if benefit outweighs risk—not known if present in human milk

**Side-effects** vertigo, increased susceptibility to infection, injection-site reactions

**Indications and dose**

> **Cryopyrin-associated periodic syndromes**
>
> • By subcutaneous injection
>
> **Child 4–18 years**
>
> **Body-weight 15–40 kg** 2 mg/kg every 8 weeks; if response inadequate 7 days after starting treatment, consider a second dose of 2 mg/kg; if a full response is then achieved, subsequent dosing should be 4 mg/kg every 8 weeks
>
> **Body-weight over 40 kg** 150 mg every 8 weeks; if response inadequate 7 days after starting treatment, consider a second dose of 150 mg; if a full response is then achieved, subsequent dosing should be 300 mg every 8 weeks

**Ilaris**® (Novartis) ▼ [PoM]
Injection, powder for reconstitution, canakinumab, net price 150-mg vial = £9927.80

## Mifamurtide

**Mifamurtide** is licensed in children and adolescents for the treatment of high-grade, resectable, non-metastatic osteosarcoma after complete surgical resection. It is used in combination with chemotherapy.

NICE guidance
Mifamurtide for the treatment of
osteosarcoma (October 2011)

Mifamurtide in combination with postoperative
multi-agent chemotherapy is recommended (within
its licensed indication), as an option for the treatment of high-grade resectable non-metastatic osteosarcoma after macroscopically complete surgical
resection in children, adolescents and young adults
and when mifamurtide is made available at a
reduced cost to the NHS under the patient access
scheme.
www.nice.org.uk/TA235

# MIFAMURTIDE

**Cautions** asthma and chronic obstructive pulmonary
disease—consider prophylactic bronchodilator therapy; history of autoimmune, inflammatory, or collagen disease; monitor renal function, hepatic function and clotting parameters; monitor patients with
history of venous thrombosis, vasculitis, or unstable
cardiovascular disorders for persistent or worsening
symptoms during administration—consult product
literature **interactions**: Appendix 1 (mifamurtide)

**Hepatic impairment** use with caution—no information available

**Renal impairment** use with caution—no information
available

**Pregnancy** avoid; effective contraception required

**Breast-feeding** avoid—no information available

**Side-effects** gastro-intestinal disturbances (including
anorexia, nausea, vomiting, diarrhoea, constipation,
abdominal pain, dyspepsia); tachycardia, hypertension, palpitations, hypotension, phlebitis; oedema,
respiratory disorders (including dyspnoea, epistaxis,
cough, tachypnoea, haemoptysis, pleural effusion);
confusion, depression, insomnia, headache, dizziness,
paraesthesia, hypoaesthesia, tremor, drowsiness,
anxiety; hypokalaemia, anaemia, leucopenia, thrombocytopenia, granulocytopenia; haematuria, dysuria,
pollakiuria; musculoskeletal pain; blurred vision;
vertigo, tinnitus, hearing loss; sweating, alopecia,
rash, dry skin, flushing

**Indications and dose**

- See notes above
- By intravenous infusion (over 1 hour)
  Consult local treatment protocols for details

**Mepact**® (Takeda) ▼ PoM
Intravenous infusion, powder for reconstitution,
mifamurtide, net price 4-mg vial = £2375.00

# 8.3 Sex hormones and hormone antagonists in malignant disease

Classification not used in *BNF for Children*.

# 9 Nutrition and blood

## 9.1 Anaemias and some other blood disorders

9.1.1 Iron-deficiency anaemias
9.1.2 Drugs used in megaloblastic anaemias
9.1.3 Drugs used in hypoplastic, haemolytic, and renal anaemias
9.1.4 Drugs used in platelet disorders
9.1.5 G6PD deficiency
9.1.6 Drugs used in neutropenia

Before initiating treatment for anaemia it is essential to determine which type is present. Iron salts may be harmful and result in iron overload if given alone to patients with anaemias other than those due to iron deficiency.

### 9.1.1 Iron-deficiency anaemias

9.1.1.1 Oral iron
9.1.1.2 Parenteral iron

*Treatment* with an iron preparation is justified only in the presence of a demonstrable iron-deficiency state. Before starting treatment, it is important to exclude any serious underlying cause of the anaemia (e.g. gastro-intestinal bleeding). The possibility of thalassaemia should be considered in children of Mediterranean or Indian sub-continent descent.

*Prophylaxis* with an iron preparation may be appropriate in those with a poor diet, malabsorption, menorrhagia, pregnancy, in haemodialysis patients, and in the management of low birth-weight infants such as preterm neonates.

### 9.1.1.1 Oral iron

Iron salts should be given by mouth unless there are good reasons for using another route.

Ferrous salts show only marginal differences between one another in efficiency of absorption of iron. Haemoglobin regeneration rate is little affected by the type of salt used provided sufficient iron is given, and in most patients the speed of response is not critical. Choice of preparation is thus usually decided by formulation, palatability, incidence of side-effects, and cost.

9 Nutrition and blood

**Treatment of iron-deficiency anaemia** The oral dose of **elemental iron** to treat deficiency is 3–6 mg/kg (max. 200 mg) daily given in 2–3 divided doses. Iron supplementation may also be required to produce an optimum response to erythropoietins in iron-deficient children with chronic renal failure or in preterm neonates. (See also Prophylaxis of iron deficiency, below.)
**Prescribing** Express the dose in terms of elemental iron and iron salt and select the most appropriate preparation; specify both the iron salt and formulation on the prescription. The iron content of artificial formula feeds should also be considered.

### Iron content of different iron salts

| Iron salt | Amount | Content of ferrous iron |
|---|---|---|
| Ferrous fumarate | 200 mg | 65 mg |
| Ferrous gluconate | 300 mg | 35 mg |
| Ferrous sulfate | 300 mg | 60 mg |
| Ferrous sulfate, dried | 200 mg | 65 mg |
| Sodium feredetate | 190 mg | 27.5 mg |

**Therapeutic response** The haemoglobin concentration should rise by about 100–200 mg/100 mL (1–2 g/litre) per day or 2 g/100 mL (20 g/litre) over 3–4 weeks. When the haemoglobin is in the normal range, treatment should be continued for a further 3 months to replenish the iron stores. Epithelial tissue changes such as atrophic glossitis and koilonychia are usually improved, but the response is often slow. The most common reason for lack of response in children is poor compliance; poor absorption is rare in children.

**Prophylaxis of iron deficiency** In neonates, haemoglobin and haematocrit concentrations change rapidly. These changes are not due to iron deficiency and cannot be corrected by iron supplementation. Similarly, neonatal anaemia resulting from repeated blood sampling does not respond to iron therapy.

All babies, including preterm neonates, are born with substantial iron stores but these stores can become depleted unless dietary intake is adequate. All babies require an iron intake of 400–700 nanograms daily to maintain body stores. Iron in breast milk is well absorbed but that in artificial feeds or in cow's milk is less so. Most artificial formula feeds are sufficiently fortified with iron to prevent deficiency and their iron content should be taken into account when considering further iron supplementation.

**Dose** Prophylactic iron supplementation (elemental iron 5 mg daily) may be required in babies of low birth-weight who are solely breast-fed; supplementation is started 4–6 weeks after birth and continued until mixed feeding is established.

Infants with a poor diet may become anaemic in the second year of life, particularly if cow's milk, rather than fortified formula feed, is a major part of the diet.

**Compound preparations** Some oral preparations contain **ascorbic acid** to aid absorption of the iron, but the therapeutic advantage of such preparations is minimal and cost may be increased.

There is no justification for the inclusion of other ingredients, such as the **B group of vitamins**, except **folic acid** for pregnant women, see p. 447.

**Side-effects** Gastro-intestinal irritation can occur with iron salts. Nausea and epigastric pain are dose-related, but the relationship between dose and altered bowel habit (constipation or diarrhoea) is less clear. Oral iron can exacerbate diarrhoea in patients with inflammatory bowel disease.

Iron preparations taken orally can be constipating and occasionally lead to faecal impaction.

If side-effects occur, the dose may be reduced; alternatively, another iron salt may be used, but an improvement in tolerance may simply be a result of a lower content of elemental iron. The incidence of side-effects due to ferrous sulfate is no greater than with other iron salts when compared on the basis of equivalent amounts of elemental iron.

Iron preparations are an important cause of accidental overdose in children and as little as 20 mg/kg of elemental iron can lead to symptoms of toxicity. For the treatment of **iron overdose**, see Emergency Treatment of Poisoning, p. 29.

**Counselling** Although iron preparations are best absorbed on an empty stomach, they can be taken after food to reduce gastro-intestinal side-effects; they may discolour stools.

## FERROUS SULFATE

**Cautions** interactions: Appendix 1 (iron)
**Side-effects** see notes above
**Indications and dose**
> Iron-deficiency anaemia, prophylaxis of iron deficiency see notes above and preparations

**Ferrous Sulfate** (Non-proprietary)
Tablets, coated, dried ferrous sulfate 200 mg (65 mg iron), net price 28-tab pack = £1.15
Dose
> **Child 6–18 years** prophylactic, 1 tablet daily; therapeutic, 1 tablet 2–3 times daily, see notes above

**Ironorm® Drops** (Wallace Mfg)
Oral drops, ferrous sulfate 125 mg (25 mg iron)/mL, net price 15 mL = £4.95
Dose
> **Child 1 month–6 years** prophylactic 0.3 mL daily, but see notes above
> **Child 6–18 years** prophylactic 0.6 mL daily

## FERROUS FUMARATE

**Cautions** interactions: Appendix 1 (iron)
**Side-effects** see notes above
**Indications and dose**
> Iron-deficiency anaemia, prophylaxis of iron deficiency see notes above and preparations

**Fersaday®** (Mercury)
Tablets, brown, f/c, ferrous fumarate 322 mg (100 mg iron). Net price 28-tab pack = 79p
Dose
> **Child 12–18 years** prophylactic, 1 tablet daily; therapeutic, 1 tablet twice daily

**Ferrous Fumarate** (Non-proprietary)
Tablets, ferrous fumarate 210 mg (68 mg iron), net price 84 = £1.44
Dose
> **Child 12–18 years**, prophylactic, 1 tablet 1–2 times daily; therapeutic, 1 tablet 2–3 times daily

Syrup, ferrous fumarate approx. 140 mg (45 mg iron)/5 mL, net price 200 mL = £3.73

**9 Nutrition and blood**

### Dose

> **Preterm neonate** see notes above
>
> **Neonate** see notes above
>
> **Child 1 month–12 years** see notes above
>
> **Child 12–18 years** prophylactic, 5 mL twice daily; therapeutic, 10 mL twice daily

**Fersamal®** (Mercury)

Syrup, ferrous fumarate approx. 140 mg (45 mg iron)/5 mL. Net price 200 mL = £3.73

### Dose

> **Preterm neonate** see notes above
>
> **Neonate** see notes above
>
> **Child 1 month–12 years** see notes above
>
> **Child 12–18 years** prophylactic, 5 mL twice daily; therapeutic, 10 mL twice daily

**Galfer®** (Thornton & Ross)

Capsules, red/green, ferrous fumarate 305 mg (100 mg iron), net price 100 = £2.00

### Dose

> **Child 12–18 years** prophylactic, 1 capsule daily; therapeutic, 1 capsule twice daily

Syrup, brown, sugar-free ferrous fumarate 140 mg (45 mg iron)/5 mL. Net price 300 mL = £5.33

### Dose

> **Preterm neonate and body-weight up to 3 kg** prophylactic, 0.5 mL daily, see notes above
>
> **Neonate** prophylactic and therapeutic, 0.25 mL/kg twice daily (total daily dose may alternatively be given in 3 divided doses), see notes above
>
> **Child 1 month–12 years** prophylactic and therapeutic, 0.25 mL/kg twice daily (total daily dose may alternatively be given in 3 divided doses); max 20 mL daily, see notes above
>
> **Child 12–18 years** prophylactic, 10 mL once daily; therapeutic, 10 mL 1–2 times daily

## ▌ FERROUS GLUCONATE

**Cautions** interactions: Appendix 1 (iron)

**Side-effects** see notes above

### Indications and dose

> Iron-deficiency anaemia see notes above and preparation

**Ferrous Gluconate** (Non-proprietary)

Tablets, red, coated, ferrous gluconate 300 mg (35 mg iron), net price 28 = £2.95

### Dose

> **Child 6–12 years** prophylactic and therapeutic, 1–3 tablets daily
>
> **Child 12–18 years** prophylactic, 2 tablets daily; therapeutic, 4–6 tablets daily in divided doses

## ▌ POLYSACCHARIDE-IRON COMPLEX

**Cautions** interactions: Appendix 1 (iron)

**Side-effects** see notes above

### Indications and dose

> Iron-deficiency anaemia, prophylaxis of iron deficiency see notes above and preparation

**Niferex®** (Tillomed)

Elixir, brown, sugar-free, polysaccharide-iron complex equivalent to 100 mg of iron/5 mL. Net price 240-mL pack = £6.06; ⒮ℍⓈ[1] 30-mL dropper bottle for paediatric use = £2.16. Counselling, use of dropper

### Dose

> **Neonate** (from dropper bottle) 1 drop (approx. 500 micrograms iron) per 450 g body-weight 3 times daily, see notes above
>
> **Child 1 month–2 years** (from dropper bottle) 1 drop (approx. 500 micrograms iron) per 450 g body-weight 3 times daily, see notes above
>
> **Child 2–6 years** therapeutic, 2.5 mL daily
>
> **Child 6–12 years** therapeutic, 5 mL daily
>
> **Child 12–18 years** prophylactic, 2.5 mL daily; therapeutic, 5 mL 1–2 times daily (5 mL once daily if required during second and third trimester of pregnancy)

## ▌ SODIUM FEREDETATE
(Sodium ironedetate)

**Cautions** interactions: Appendix 1 (iron)

**Side-effects** see notes above

**Licensed use** not licensed for prophylaxis of iron deficiency

### Indications and dose

> Iron-deficiency anaemia, prophylaxis of iron deficiency see notes above and preparation

**Sytron®** (Archimedes)

Elixir, sugar-free, sodium feredetate 190 mg equivalent to 27.5 mg of iron/5 mL. Net price 100 mL = £1.07

### Dose

> **Neonate** prophylactic, 1 mL daily, see notes above; therapeutic, up to 2.5 mL twice daily (smaller doses should be used initially), see notes above
>
> **Child 1 month–1 year** prophylactic, 1 mL daily, see notes above; therapeutic, up to 2.5 mL twice daily (smaller doses should be used initially), see notes above
>
> **Child 1–5 years** therapeutic, 2.5 mL 3 times daily
>
> **Child 5–12 years** therapeutic, 5 mL 3 times daily
>
> **Child 12–18 years** therapeutic, 5 mL increasing gradually to 10 mL 3 times daily

### 9.1.1.2 Parenteral iron

Iron can be administered parenterally as **iron dextran**, **iron sucrose**, or **ferric carboxymaltose**. Parenteral iron is generally reserved for use when oral therapy is unsuccessful because the child cannot tolerate oral iron, or does not take it reliably, or if there is continuing blood loss, or in malabsorption.

Many children with chronic renal failure who are receiving haemodialysis (and some who are receiving peritoneal dialysis) also require iron by the intravenous route on a regular basis (see also Erythropoietins, section 9.1.3).

With the exception of children with severe renal failure receiving haemodialysis, parenteral iron does not produce a faster haemoglobin response than oral iron provided that the oral iron preparation is taken reliably and is absorbed adequately.

Anaphylactic reactions can occur with parenteral iron complexes; facilities for cardiopulmonary resuscitation

1. ⒮ℍⓈ except 30-mL paediatric dropper bottle for prophylaxis and treatment of iron deficiency in infants born prematurely; endorse prescription 'SLS'

must be available. Depending on the preparation, a small test dose may be required. If children complain of acute symptoms particularly nausea, back pain, breathlessness, or develop hypotension, the infusion should be stopped.

## FERRIC CARBOXYMALTOSE

A ferric carboxymaltose complex containing 5% (50 mg/mL) of iron

**Cautions** hypersensitivity can occur with parenteral iron and facilities for cardiopulmonary resuscitation must be available; oral iron should not be given until 5 days after last injection; allergic disorders including asthma and eczema; infection (discontinue if ongoing bacteraemia)

**Hepatic impairment** use with caution; avoid in conditions where iron overload increases risk of impairment

**Pregnancy** avoid in first trimester; crosses the placenta in *animal* studies; may influence skeletal development

**Side-effects** gastro-intestinal disturbances; headache, dizziness; rash; injection-site reactions; *less commonly* hypertension, hypotension, flushing, chest pain, peripheral oedema, hypersensitivity reactions (including anaphylaxis), fatigue, paraesthesia, malaise, pyrexia, rigors, myalgia, arthralgia, back pain, pruritus, and urticaria; *rarely* dyspnoea

**Licensed use** not licensed for use in children under 14 years

**Indications and dose**

Iron-deficiency anaemia see notes above

- By slow intravenous injection or by intravenous infusion

    Calculated according to body-weight and iron deficit, consult product literature

**Ferinject®** (Vifor) ▼ (PoM)
Injection, iron (as ferric carboxymaltose) 50 mg/mL, net price 2-mL vial = £21.75, 10-mL vial = £108.75
**Electrolytes** Na⁺ 0.24 mmol/mL

## IRON DEXTRAN

A complex of ferric hydroxide with sucrose containing 5% (50 mg/mL) of iron

**Cautions** oral iron should not be given until 5 days after last injection
**Anaphylaxis** Anaphylactic reactions can occur with parenteral iron and a test dose is recommended before *each* dose; the patient should be carefully observed for 60 minutes after the first test dose and for 15 minutes after subsequent test doses. Facilities for cardiopulmonary resuscitation must be available; risk of allergic reactions increased in immune or inflammatory conditions

**Contra-indications** history of allergic disorders including asthma, and eczema; infection; active rheumatoid arthritis

**Hepatic impairment** avoid in severe impairment
**Renal impairment** avoid in acute renal failure
**Pregnancy** avoid in first trimester
**Side-effects** *less commonly* nausea, vomiting, abdominal pain, flushing, dyspnoea, anaphylactic reactions (see Anaphylaxis above), and rash; *rarely* diarrhoea, chest pain, hypotension, angioedema, arrhythmias, tachycardia, dizziness, restlessness, fatigue, seizures, tremor,

impaired consciousness, myalgia, arthralgia, sweating, and injection-site reactions; *very rarely* hypertension, palpitation, headache, paraesthesia, haemolysis, and transient deafness

**Licensed use** not licensed for use in children under 14 years

**Indications and dose**

Iron-deficiency anaemia see notes above

- By slow intravenous injection or by intravenous infusion

    Calculated according to body-weight and iron deficit, consult product literature

**CosmoFer®** (Pharmacosmos) (PoM)
Injection, iron (as iron dextran) 50 mg/mL, net price 2-mL amp = £7.97; 10-mL amp = £39.85

## IRON SUCROSE

A complex of ferric hydroxide with sucrose containing 2% (20 mg/mL) of iron

**Cautions** oral iron should not be given until 5 days after last injection; infection (discontinue if ongoing bacteraemia)
**Anaphylaxis** Anaphylactic reactions can occur with parenteral iron and a test dose is recommended before the first dose; the patient should be carefully observed for 15 minutes. Facilities for cardiopulmonary resuscitation must be available

**Contra-indications** history of allergic disorders including asthma, eczema, and anaphylaxis

**Hepatic impairment** use with caution; avoid in conditions where iron overload increases risk of impairment

**Pregnancy** avoid in first trimester
**Side-effects** taste disturbances; *less commonly* nausea, vomiting, abdominal pain, diarrhoea, hypotension, tachycardia, flushing, palpitation, chest pain, bronchospasm, dyspnoea, headache, dizziness, fever, myalgia, pruritus, rash, and injection-site reactions; *rarely* peripheral oedema, hypertension, anaphylactic reactions (see Anaphylaxis above), fatigue, asthenia, and paraesthesia; bradycardia, confusion, arthralgia, and increased sweating also reported

**Licensed use** not licensed for use in children
**Indications and dose**

Iron-deficiency anaemia see notes above

- By slow intravenous injection or by intravenous infusion

    Calculated according to body-weight and iron deficit, consult product literature

**Venofer®** (Vifor) (PoM)
Injection, iron (as iron sucrose) 20 mg/mL, net price 5-mL vial = £9.35

## 9.1.2 Drugs used in megaloblastic anaemias

Megaloblastic anaemias are rare in children; they may result from a lack of either vitamin B₁₂ or folate, and it is essential to establish in every case which deficiency is present and the underlying cause. In emergencies, when delay might be dangerous, it is sometimes necessary to administer both substances after the bone marrow test while plasma assay results are awaited. Normally, however, appropriate treatment should not be instituted until the results of tests are available.

Vitamin $B_{12}$ is used in the treatment of megaloblastosis caused by *prolonged nitrous oxide anaesthesia*, which inactivates the vitamin, and in the rare disorders of *congenital transcobalamin II deficiency, methylmalonic acidaemia* and *homocystinuria* (see section 9.8.1).

Vitamin $B_{12}$ should be given prophylactically after *total ileal resection*.

Apart from dietary deficiency, all other causes of vitamin $B_{12}$ deficiency are attributable to malabsorption. There is little place for the use of low-dose vitamin $B_{12}$ orally and none for vitamin $B_{12}$ intrinsic factor complexes given by mouth. Vitamin $B_{12}$ in large oral doses [unlicensed] may be effective.

**Hydroxocobalamin** has completely replaced cyanocobalamin as the form of vitamin $B_{12}$ of choice for therapy; it is retained in the body longer than cyanocobalamin and thus for maintenance therapy can be given at intervals of up to 3 months. Treatment is generally initiated with frequent administration of intramuscular injections to replenish the depleted body stores. Thereafter, maintenance treatment, which is usually for life, can be instituted. There is no evidence that doses larger than those recommended provide any additional benefit in vitamin $B_{12}$ neuropathy.

**Folic acid** has few indications for long-term therapy since most causes of folate deficiency are self-limiting or will yield to a short course of treatment. It should not be used in undiagnosed megaloblastic anaemia unless vitamin $B_{12}$ is administered concurrently otherwise neuropathy may be precipitated (see above).

In *folate-deficient megaloblastic anaemia* (e.g. because of poor nutrition, pregnancy, or treatment with antiepileptics), daily folic acid supplementation for 4 months brings about haematological remission and replenishes body stores; higher doses may be necessary in malabsorption states. In pregnancy, folic acid 5 mg daily is continued to term.

For prophylaxis in *chronic haemolytic states, malabsorption* or *in renal dialysis*, folic acid is given daily or sometimes weekly, depending on the diet and the rate of haemolysis.

Folic acid is also used for the prevention of methotrexate-induced side-effects in juvenile idiopathic arthritis (see also section 10.1.3, p. 509), severe Crohn's disease (see section 1.5.3, p. 53), and severe psoriasis (see section 13.5.3, p. 574).

For *prophylaxis in pregnancy*, see Prevention of Neural Tube Defects below.

Folic acid is actively excreted in breast milk and is well absorbed by the infant. It is also present in cow's milk and artificial formula feeds but is heat labile. Serum and red cell folate concentrations fall after delivery and urinary losses are high, particularly in low birth-weight neonates. Although symptomatic deficiency is rare in the absence of malabsorption or prolonged diarrhoea, it is common for neonatal units to give supplements of folic acid to all preterm neonates from 2 weeks of age until full-term corrected age is reached, particularly if heated breast milk is used without an artificial formula fortifier.

**Folinic acid** is also effective in the treatment of folate-deficient megaloblastic anaemia but it is normally only used in association with cytotoxic drugs (see section 8.1); it is given as calcium folinate.

**Prevention of neural tube defects**  Folic acid supplements taken before and during pregnancy can reduce the occurrence of neural tube defects. The risk of a neural tube defect occurring in a child should be assessed and folic acid given as follows:

Women at a low risk of conceiving a child with a neural tube defect should be advised to take folic acid as a medicinal or food supplement at a dose of 400 micrograms daily before conception and until week 12 of pregnancy. Women who have not been taking folic acid and who suspect they are pregnant should start at once and continue until week 12 of pregnancy.

Couples are at a high risk of conceiving a child with a neural tube defect if either partner has a neural tube defect (or either partner has a family history of neural tube defects), if they have had a previous pregnancy affected by a neural tube defect, or if the woman has coeliac disease (or other malabsorption state), diabetes mellitus, sickle-cell anaemia, or is taking antiepileptic medicines (see also section 4.8.1).

Women in the high-risk group who wish to become pregnant (or who are at risk of becoming pregnant) should be advised to take folic acid 5 mg daily and continue until week 12 of pregnancy (women with sickle-cell disease should continue taking their normal dose of folic acid 5 mg daily (or increase the dose to 5 mg daily) and continue this throughout pregnancy).

> There is **no** justification for prescribing multiple-ingredient vitamin preparations containing vitamin $B_{12}$ or folic acid.

## HYDROXOCOBALAMIN

**Cautions**  should not be given before diagnosis fully established but see also notes above; **interactions** Appendix 1 (hydroxocobalamin)

**Breast-feeding**  present in milk but not known to be harmful

**Side-effects**  nausea, headache, dizziness; fever, hypersensitivity reactions (including rash and pruritus); injection-site reactions; hypokalaemia and thrombocytosis during initial treatment; chromaturia

**Licensed use**  licensed for use in children (age not specified by manufacturers); not licensed for use in inborn errors of metabolism

### Indications and dose

**Macrocytic anaemia without neurological involvement**

● By intramuscular injection

**Child 1 month–18 years** initially 250 micrograms–1 mg 3 times a week for 2 weeks then 250 micrograms once weekly until blood count normal, then 1 mg every 3 months

**Macrocytic anaemia with neurological involvement**

- By intramuscular injection

  **Child 1 month–18 years** initially 1 mg on alternate days until no further improvement, then 1 mg every 2 months

**Prophylaxis of macrocytic anaemias associated with vitamin B$_{12}$ deficiency**

- By intramuscular injection

  **Child 1 month–18 years** 1 mg every 2–3 months

**Leber's optic atrophy**

- By intramuscular injection

  Initially 1 mg daily for 2 weeks, then 1 mg twice weekly until no further improvement, thereafter 1 mg every 1–3 months

**Congenital transcobalamin II deficiency**

- By intramuscular injection

  **Neonate** 1 mg 3 times a week, reduce after 1 year to 1 mg once weekly or as appropriate

  **Child 1 month–18 years** 1 mg 3 times a week, reduce after 1 year to 1 mg once weekly or as appropriate

**Methylmalonic acidaemia and homocystinuria**

- By intramuscular injection

  **Child 1 month–18 years** initially 1 mg daily for 5–7 days, reduce according to response to maintenance dose of up to 1 mg once or twice weekly

**Methylmalonic acidaemia, maintenance once intramuscular response established**

- By mouth

  **Child 1 month–18 years** 5–10 mg once or twice weekly

  **Note** Some children do not respond to the oral route

**Cyanide poisoning**

  See Emergency Treatment of Poisoning, p. 31

**Hydroxocobalamin** (Non-proprietary) [PoM]

  Injection, hydroxocobalamin 1 mg/mL. Net price 1-mL amp = 74p

  **Brands include** *Cobalin-H*® (JHS), *Neo-Cytamen*® (JHS)

  Injection, hydroxocobalamin 2.5 mg/mL, 2 mL

  Available from 'special-order' manufacturers or specialist importing companies, see p. 823

  **Administration** For administration *by mouth*, injection solution may be given orally; it will not have prolonged effect via this route

  **Note** The BP directs that when Vitamin B$_{12}$ injection is prescribed or demanded hydroxocobalamin injection shall be dispensed or supplied

  Powder available from specialist importing companies

---

## FOLIC ACID

**Cautions** should never be given alone for vitamin B$_{12}$ deficiency states (may precipitate subacute combined degeneration of the spinal cord); **interactions:** Appendix 1 (folates)

**Side-effects** rarely gastro-intestinal disturbances

**Licensed use** unlicensed for limiting methotrexate toxicity

### Indications and dose

**Folate supplementation in neonates** (see notes above)

- By mouth

  **Neonate** 50 micrograms once daily *or* 500 micrograms once weekly

**Megaloblastic anaemia due to folate deficiency** (see notes above)

- By mouth

  **Neonate** initially 500 micrograms/kg once daily for up to 4 months

  **Child 1 month–1 year** initially 500 micrograms/kg once daily (max. 5 mg) for up to 4 months; up to 10 mg daily may be required in malabsorption states

  **Child 1–18 years** 5 mg daily for 4 months (until term in pregnant women); up to 15 mg daily may be required in malabsorption states

**Haemolytic anaemia; metabolic disorders**

- By mouth

  **Child 1 month–12 years** 2.5–5 mg once daily

  **Child 12–18 years** 5–10 mg once daily

**Prophylaxis of folate deficiency in dialysis**

- By mouth

  **Child 1 month–12 years** 250 microgram/kg (max. 10 mg) once daily

  **Child 12–18 years** 5–10 mg once daily

**Prevention of methotrexate side-effects in juvenile idiopathic arthritis**

- By mouth

  **Child 2–18 years** 1 mg daily *or* 5 mg once weekly, adjusted according to local guidelines

**Prevention of methotrexate side-effects in severe Crohn's disease or severe psoriasis**

- By mouth

  See section 1.5.3 and section 13.5.3

**Prevention of neural tube defects**

- By mouth

  See notes above

[1]**Folic Acid** (Non-proprietary) [PoM]

  Tablets, folic acid 400 micrograms, net price 90-tab pack = £2.37; 5 mg, 28-tab pack = £1.00

  Syrup, folic acid 2.5 mg/5 mL, net price 150 mL = £9.16

  **Brands include** *Lexpec*® (sugar-free)

---

### 9.1.3 Drugs used in hypoplastic, haemolytic, and renal anaemias

Anabolic steroids (see BNF, section 6.4.3), pyridoxine, antilymphocyte immunoglobulin, and various corticosteroids are used in hypoplastic and haemolytic anaemias.

---

1. Can be sold to the public provided daily doses do not exceed 500 micrograms

**Antilymphocyte immunoglobulin** given intravenously through a central line over 12–18 hours each day for 5 days produces a response in about 50% of cases of acquired *aplastic anaemia*; the response rate may be increased when ciclosporin is given as well. Severe reactions are common in the first 2 days and profound immunosuppression can occur; antilymphocyte immunoglobulin should be given under specialist supervision with appropriate resuscitation facilities. Alternatively, oxymetholone tablets (available from 'special-order' manufacturers or specialist importing companies, see p. 823) may be used in aplastic anaemia at a dose of 1–5 mg/kg daily for 3 to 6 months.

It is unlikely that dietary deficit of **pyridoxine** (section 9.6.2) produces clinically relevant haematological effects. However, certain forms of *sideroblastic anaemia* respond to pharmacological doses, possibly reflecting its role as a co-enzyme during haemoglobin synthesis. Pyridoxine is indicated in both *idiopathic acquired* and *hereditary sideroblastic anaemias*. Although complete cures have not been reported, some increase in haemoglobin can occur with high doses. *Reversible sideroblastic anaemias* respond to treatment of the underlying cause but pyridoxine is indicated in pregnancy, haemolytic anaemias, or during isoniazid treatment.

**Corticosteroids** (section 6.3) have an important place in the management of haematological disorders including *autoimmune haemolytic anaemia, idiopathic thrombocytopenias* (section 9.1.4) and *neutropenias*, and *major transfusion reactions*. They are also used in chemotherapy schedules for many types of *lymphoma, lymphoid leukaemias*, and *paraproteinaemias*, including *multiple myeloma*.

## Erythropoietins

**Epoetins** (recombinant human erythropoietins) are used to treat the anaemia associated with erythropoietin deficiency in chronic renal failure, see below.

**Epoetin beta** is also used for the prevention of anaemia in preterm neonates of low birth-weight; a therapeutic response may take several weeks. Only unpreserved formulations should be used as other preparations may contain benzyl alcohol (see Excipients, p. 2).

There is insufficient information to support the use of erythropoietins in children with leukaemia or in those receiving cancer chemotherapy.

**Darbepoetin** is a glycosylated derivative of epoetin; it persists longer in the body and can be administered less frequently than epoetin.

Other factors, such as iron or folate deficiency, that contribute to the anaemia of chronic renal failure should be corrected before treatment and monitored during therapy. Supplemental iron may improve the response in resistant patients and in preterm neonates (see section 9.1.1.1). Aluminium toxicity, concurrent infection, or other inflammatory disease can impair the response to erythropoietins.

### Erythropoietins—haemoglobin concentration

In chronic kidney disease, the use of erythropoietins can be considered in a child with anaemia. The aim of treatment is to relieve symptoms of anaemia and to avoid the need for blood transfusion. The optimum haemoglobin concentration is dependent on the child's age and factors such as symptoms, co-morbidities, and patient preferences. The haemoglobin concentration should not be increased beyond that which provides adequate control of symptoms of anaemia. In *adults*, overcorrection of haemoglobin concentration with erythropoietins in those with chronic kidney disease may increase the risk of serious cardiovascular events and death; haemoglobin concentrations higher than 12 g/100 mL should be avoided in children.

For MHRA/CHM advice relating to adults, see BNF section 9.1.3.

### Pure red cell aplasia

There have been very rare reports of pure red cell aplasia in patients treated with erythropoietins. In patients who develop a lack of efficacy with erythropoietin therapy and with a diagnosis of pure red cell aplasia, treatment with erythropoietins must be discontinued and testing for erythropoietin antibodies considered. Patients who develop pure red cell aplasia should **not** be switched to another form of erythropoietin.

## DARBEPOETIN ALFA

**Cautions**  see Epoetin
**Contra-indications**  see Epoetin
**Hepatic impairment**  manufacturer advises caution
**Pregnancy**  no evidence of harm in *animal* studies—manufacturer advises caution
**Breast-feeding**  manufacturer advises avoid—no information available
**Side-effects**  see Epoetin; also, oedema, injection-site pain; isolated reports of pure red cell aplasia particularly following subcutaneous administration in patients with chronic renal failure (discontinue therapy)—see also notes above

### Indications and dose

**Symptomatic anaemia associated with chronic renal failure in children on dialysis (see also notes above)**
- By intravenous or subcutaneous injection
  **Child 11–18 years** initially 450 nanograms/kg once weekly adjusted according to response by approx. 25% at intervals of at least 4 weeks; maintenance dose, given once weekly *or* once every 2 weeks

**Symptomatic anaemia associated with chronic renal failure in children not on dialysis (see also notes above)**
- By intravenous or subcutaneous injection
  **Child 11–18 years** *by subcutaneous or intravenous injection*, initially 450 nanograms/kg once weekly *or by subcutaneous injection*, initially 750 nanograms/kg once every 2 weeks; adjusted according to response by approx. 25% at intervals of at

**9 Nutrition and blood**

least 4 weeks; maintenance dose, given *subcutaneously* or *intravenously* once weekly or *subcutaneously* once every 2 weeks or *subcutaneously* once every month

Note Subcutaneous route preferred in patients not on haemodialysis. Reduce dose by approximately 25% if rise in haemoglobin concentration exceeds 2 g/100 mL over 4 weeks or if haemoglobin concentration exceeds 12 g/100 mL; if haemoglobin concentration continues to rise, despite dose reduction, suspend treatment until haemoglobin concentration decreases and then restart at a dose approximately 25% lower than the previous dose. When changing route give same dose then adjust according to weekly or fortnightly haemoglobin measurements. Adjust doses not more frequently than every 2 weeks during maintenance treatment.

### Aranesp® (Amgen) [PoM]

Injection, prefilled syringe, darbepoetin alfa, 25 micrograms/mL, net price 0.4 mL (10 micrograms) = £14.68; 40 micrograms/mL, 0.375 mL (15 micrograms) = £22.03, 0.5 mL (20 micrograms) = £29.37; 100 micrograms/mL, 0.3 mL (30 micrograms) = £44.05, 0.4 mL (40 micrograms) = £58.73, 0.5 mL (50 micrograms) = £73.41; 200 micrograms/mL, 0.3 mL (60 micrograms) = £88.09, 0.4 mL (80 micrograms) = £117.45, 0.5 mL (100 micrograms) = £146.81, 0.65 mL (130 micrograms) = £190.86; 500 micrograms/mL, 0.3 mL (150 micrograms) = £220.22, 0.6 mL (300 micrograms) = £440.43, 1 mL (500 micrograms) = £734.05

Injection (*Aranesp® SureClick*), prefilled disposable injection device, darbepoetin alfa, 40 micrograms/mL, net price 0.5 mL (20 micrograms) = £29.36; 100 micrograms/mL, net price 0.4 mL (40 micrograms) = £58.72; 200 micrograms/mL, net price 0.3 mL (60 micrograms) = £88.09, 0.4 mL (80 micrograms) = £117.45, 0.5 mL (100 micrograms) = £146.81; 500 micrograms/mL, net price 0.3 mL (150 micrograms) = £220.22, 0.6 mL (300 micrograms) = £440.43, 1 mL (500 micrograms) = £734.05

### EPOETIN ALFA, BETA, and ZETA
(Recombinant human erythropoietins)

Note The prescriber must specify which epoetin is required, see also Biosimilar medicines, p. 2

**Cautions** see notes above; also inadequately treated or poorly controlled blood pressure (monitor closely blood pressure, reticulocyte counts, haemoglobin, and electrolytes), interrupt treatment if blood pressure uncontrolled; sudden stabbing migraine-like pain is warning of hypertensive crisis; sickle-cell disease (lower target haemoglobin concentration may be appropriate); ischaemic vascular disease; thrombocytosis (monitor platelet count for first 8 weeks); epilepsy; malignant disease; increase in unfractionated or low molecular weight heparin dose may be needed during dialysis

**Contra-indications** pure red cell aplasia following erythropoietin therapy (see also notes above); uncontrolled hypertension; avoid injections containing benzyl alcohol in neonates (see under preparations, below)

**Hepatic impairment** manufacturers advise caution in chronic hepatic failure

**Pregnancy** no evidence of harm; benefits probably outweigh risks of anaemia and blood transfusion

**Breast-feeding** unlikely to be present in milk; effect on infant minimal

**Side-effects** diarrhoea, nausea, vomiting; dose-dependent increase in blood pressure or aggravation of hypertension; in isolated patients with normal or low blood pressure, hypertensive crisis with encephalopathy-like symptoms and generalised tonic-clonic seizures requiring immediate medical attention; dose-dependent increase in platelet count (but thrombocytosis rare) regressing during treatment; influenza-like symptoms (may be reduced if intravenous injection given over 5 minutes); cardiovascular events; shunt thrombosis especially if tendency to hypotension or arteriovenous shunt complications; *very rarely* sudden loss of efficacy because of pure red cell aplasia, particularly following subcutaneous administration in patients with chronic renal failure (discontinue erythropoietin therapy)—see also notes above, hyperkalaemia, hypersensitivity reactions (including anaphylaxis and angioedema), skin reactions, injection-site reactions, and peripheral oedema also reported

**Licensed use** *Eprex®* 20 000-unit, 30 000-unit, and 40 000-unit prefilled syringes not licensed for use in children

### Indications and dose

See under preparations, below

### ◀Epoetin alfa

**Binocrit® (Sandoz) [PoM]**

Injection, prefilled syringe, epoetin alfa, net price 1000 units = £5.09; 2000 units = £10.18; 3000 units = £15.27; 4000 units = £20.36; 5000 units = £25.46; 6000 units = £30.55; 8000 units = £40.73; 10 000 units = £50.91

Note Biosimilar Medicine, p. 2

**Dose**

**Symptomatic anaemia associated with chronic renal failure in children on haemodialysis (see also notes above)**

• By intravenous injection over 1–5 minutes

**Child 1 month–18 years** initially 50 units/kg 3 times weekly adjusted according to response in steps of 25 units/kg 3 times weekly at intervals of at least 4 weeks; maintenance dose, body-weight under 10 kg usually 75–150 units/kg 3 times weekly, body-weight 10–30 kg usually 60–150 units/kg 3 times weekly, body-weight over 30 kg usually 30–100 units/kg 3 times weekly

Note Reduce dose by approximately 25% if rise in haemoglobin concentration exceeds 2 g/100 mL over 4 weeks or if haemoglobin concentration exceeds 12 g/100 mL; if haemoglobin concentration continues to rise, despite dose reduction, suspend treatment until haemoglobin concentration decreases and then restart at a dose approximately 25% lower than the previous dose

**Eprex® (Janssen) [PoM]**

Injection, prefilled syringe, epoetin alfa, net price 1000 units = £5.53; 2000 units = £11.07; 3000 units = £16.60; 4000 units = £22.13; 5000 units = £27.66; 6000 units = £33.19; 8000 units = £44.25; 10 000 units = £55.31; 20 000 units = £110.62; 30 000 units = £199.11; 40 000 units = £265.48. An auto-injector device is available for use with prefilled syringes

**9** **Nutrition and blood**

Dose

### Symptomatic anaemia associated with chronic renal failure in children on haemodialysis (see also notes above)

- By intravenous injection over 1–5 minutes

  **Child 1 month–18 years** initially 50 units/kg 3 times weekly adjusted according to response in steps of 25 units/kg 3 times weekly at intervals of at least 4 weeks; maintenance dose, body-weight under 10 kg usually 75–150 units/kg 3 times weekly, body-weight 10–30 kg usually 60–150 units/kg 3 times weekly, body-weight 30–60 kg usually 30–100 units/kg 3 times weekly, body-weight over 60 kg usually 75–300 units/kg weekly (as a single dose or in divided doses)

**Note** Reduce dose by approximately 25% if rise in haemoglobin concentration exceeds 2 g/100 mL over 4 weeks or if haemoglobin concentration exceeds 12 g/100 mL; if haemoglobin concentration continues to rise, despite dose reduction, suspend treatment until haemoglobin concentration decreases and then restart at a dose approximately 25% lower than the previous dose

◀**Epoetin beta**

**NeoRecormon®** (Roche) [PoM]

Injection, prefilled syringe, epoetin beta, net price 500 units = £3.75; 2000 units = £14.98; 3000 units = £22.47; 4000 units = £29.96; 5000 units = £37.47; 6000 units = £44.94; 10 000 units = £70.14; 20 000 units = £140.28; 30 000 units = £224.69

**Excipients** include phenylalanine up to 300 micrograms/syringe (section 9.4.1)

Dose

### Symptomatic anaemia associated with chronic renal failure (see also notes above)

- By subcutaneous injection

  **Neonate** initially 20 units/kg 3 times weekly for 4 weeks, increased according to response at intervals of 4 weeks in steps of 20 units/kg 3 times weekly; total weekly dose may be given in daily doses; maintenance dose, initially reduce dose by half then adjust according to response at intervals of 1–2 weeks; total weekly maintenance dose may be given as a single dose or in 3 or 7 divided doses; max. 720 units/kg weekly

  **Child 1 month–18 years** initially 20 units/kg 3 times weekly for 4 weeks, increased according to response at intervals of 4 weeks in steps of 20 units/kg 3 times weekly; total weekly dose may be divided into daily doses; maintenance dose, initially reduce dose by half then adjust according to response at intervals of 1–2 weeks; total weekly maintenance dose may be given as a single dose or in 3 or 7 divided doses; max. 720 units/kg weekly

- By intravenous injection over 2 minutes

  **Neonate** initially 40 units/kg 3 times weekly for 4 weeks, increased according to response to 80 units/kg 3 times weekly after 4 weeks, with further increases if needed at intervals of 4 weeks in steps of 20 units/kg 3 times weekly; maintenance dose, initially reduce dose by half then adjust according to response at intervals of 1–2 weeks; max. 720 units/kg weekly

  **Child 1 month–18 years** initially 40 units/kg 3 times weekly for 4 weeks, increased according to response to 80 units/kg 3 times weekly after 4 weeks, with further increases if needed at intervals of 4 weeks in steps of 20 units/kg 3 times weekly; maintenance dose, initially reduce dose by half then adjust according to response at intervals of 1–2 weeks; max. 720 units/kg weekly

**Note** Subcutaneous route preferred in patients not on haemodialysis. Reduce dose by approximately 25% if rise in haemoglobin concentration exceeds 2 g/100 mL over 4 weeks or if haemoglobin concentration approaches or exceeds 12 g/100 mL; if haemoglobin concentration continues to rise, despite dose reduction, suspend treatment until haemoglobin concentration decreases and then restart at a dose approximately 25% lower than the previous dose.

### Prevention of anaemias of prematurity in neonates with birth-weight of 0.75–1.5 kg and post-menstrual age under 34 weeks

- By subcutaneous injection (of single-dose, unpreserved injection)

  **Neonate** 250 units/kg 3 times weekly preferably starting within 3 days of birth and continued for 6 weeks

Multidose injection, powder for reconstitution, epoetin beta, net price 50 000-unit vial = £374.48 (with solvent)

**Excipients** include phenylalanine up to 5 mg/vial (section 9.4.1), benzyl alcohol (avoid in neonates, see Excipients p. 2)

**Note** Avoid contact of reconstituted injection with glass; use only plastic materials

Dose

### Symptomatic anaemia associated with chronic renal failure (see also notes above)

- By subcutaneous injection

  **Child 3–18 years** initially 20 units/kg 3 times weekly for 4 weeks, increased according to response at intervals of 4 weeks in steps of 20 units/kg 3 times weekly; total weekly dose may be divided into daily doses; maintenance dose, initially reduce dose by half then adjust according to response at intervals of 1–2 weeks; total weekly maintenance dose may be given as a single dose or in 3 or 7 divided doses; max. 720 units/kg weekly

- By intravenous injection over 2 minutes

  **Child 3–18 years** initially 40 units/kg 3 times weekly for 4 weeks, increased according to response to 80 units/kg 3 times weekly after 4 weeks, with further increases if needed at intervals of 4 weeks in steps of 20 units/kg 3 times weekly; maintenance dose, initially reduce dose by half then adjust according to response at intervals of 1–2 weeks; max. 720 units/kg weekly

**Note** Subcutaneous route preferred in patients not on haemodialysis. Reduce dose by approximately 25% if rise in haemoglobin concentration exceeds 2 g/100 mL over 4 weeks or if haemoglobin concentration approaches or exceeds 12 g/100 mL; if haemoglobin concentration continues to rise, despite dose reduction, suspend treatment until haemoglobin concentration decreases and then restart at a dose approximately 25% lower than the previous dose.

◀**Epoetin zeta**

**Retacrit®** (Hospira) [PoM]

Injection, prefilled syringe, epoetin zeta, net price 1000 units = £5.66; 2000 units = £11.31; 3000 units = £16.97; 4000 units = £22.63; 5000 units = £28.28; 6000 units = £33.94; 8000 units = £45.25; 10 000 units = £56.57; 20 000 units = £203.64; 30 000 units = £305.46; 40 000 units = £407.27

**Excipients** include phenylalanine up to 500 micrograms/syringe (section 9.4.1)

**Note** Biosimilar Medicine, p. 2

Dose

### Symptomatic anaemia associated with chronic renal failure in children on haemodialysis (see also notes above)

- By intravenous injection over 1–5 minutes

  **Child 1 month–18 years** initially 50 units/kg 3 times weekly adjusted according to response in steps of 25 units/kg 3 times weekly at intervals of at least 4 weeks; maintenance dose, body-weight under 10 kg usually 75–150 units/kg 3 times weekly, body-weight 10–30 kg usually 60–150 units/kg 3 times weekly, body-weight over 30 kg usually 30–100 units/kg 3 times weekly

**Note** Avoid increasing haemoglobin concentration at a rate exceeding 2 g/100 mL over 4 weeks

## Sickle-cell disease

Sickle-cell disease is caused by a structural abnormality of haemoglobin resulting in deformed, less flexible red blood cells. Acute complications in the more severe forms include *sickle-cell crisis*, where infarction of the microvasculature and blood supply to organs results in severe pain. Sickle-cell crisis requires hospitalisation, intravenous fluids, analgesia (section 4.7), and treatment of any concurrent infection. Chronic complications include skin ulceration, renal failure, and increased susceptibility to infection. Pneumococcal vaccine (section 14.4), haemophilus influenzae type b vaccine (section 14.4), an annual influenza vaccine (section 14.4), and prophylactic penicillin (Table 2, section 5.1) reduce the risk of infection. Hepatitis B vaccine (section 14.4) should be considered if the child is not immune.

In most forms of sickle-cell disease, varying degrees of haemolytic anaemia are present accompanied by increased erythropoiesis; this may increase folate requirements and folate supplementation may be necessary (section 9.1.2).

**Hydroxycarbamide** can reduce the frequency of crises and the need for blood transfusions. Hydroxycarbamide should be considered, in consultation with a specialist centre, for children who have recurrent episodes of acute pain (more than 3 admissions in the previous 12 months, or who are very symptomatic in the community) or who have had 2 or more episodes of acute sickle chest syndrome in the last 2 years (or 1 episode requiring ventilatory support). Beneficial effects of hydroxycarbamide may not become evident for several months. Myelosuppression, and skin reactions are the most common side-effects.

## HYDROXYCARBAMIDE
(Hydroxyurea)

**Cautions** see section 8.1 and notes above; also monitor renal and hepatic function before and during treatment; monitor full blood count before treatment, then every 2 weeks for the first 2 months and then every 2 months thereafter (or every 2 weeks if on max. dose); leg ulcers (review treatment if cutaneous vasculitic ulcerations develop); **interactions:** Appendix 1 (hydroxycarbamide)

**Hepatic impairment** manufacturer advises caution in mild to moderate impairment; avoid in severe impairment

**Renal impairment** reduce initial dose by 50% if estimated glomerular filtration rate less than 60 mL/minute/1.73 m$^2$; avoid if estimated glomerular filtration rate less than 30 mL/minute/1.73 m$^2$

**Pregnancy** avoid (teratogenic in *animal* studies); manufacturer advises effective contraception before and during treatment; see also section 8.1

**Breast-feeding** discontinue breast-feeding

**Side-effects** see section 8.1 and notes above; also headache; *less commonly* dizziness, and rash; *rarely* reduced sperm count and activity; fever, amenorrhoea, bleeding, and hypomagnesaemia also reported

**Indications and dose**

#### Sickle-cell disease (see notes above)
- By mouth
  **Child 2–18 years** initially 10–15 mg/kg once daily, increased every 12 weeks in steps of 2.5–5 mg/kg daily according to response; usual dose 15–30 mg/kg daily (max. 35 mg/kg daily)

**Siklos®** (Nordic) [PoM]
Tablets, scored, f/c, hydroxycarbamide 100 mg, net price 60-tab pack = £100.00; 1 g, 30-tab pack = £500.00

## Iron overload

Severe tissue iron overload can occur in aplastic and other refractory anaemias, mainly as the result of repeated blood transfusions. It is a particular problem in refractory anaemias with hyperplastic bone marrow, especially *thalassaemia major*, where excessive iron absorption from the gut and inappropriate iron therapy can add to the tissue siderosis.

Iron overload associated with haemochromatosis can be treated with repeated venesection. Venesection may also be used for patients who have received multiple transfusions and whose bone marrow has recovered. Where venesection is contra-indicated, and in thalassaemia, the long-term administration of the iron chelating compound **desferrioxamine mesilate** is useful. Subcutaneous infusions of desferrioxamine are given over 8–12 hours, 3–7 times a week; the dose should reflect the degree of iron overload. The initial dose should not exceed 30 mg/kg. For established overload the dose is usually between 20 and 50 mg/kg daily. Desferrioxamine (up to 2 g per unit of blood) may also be given at the time of blood transfusion, provided that the desferrioxamine is **not** added to the blood and is **not** given through the same line as the blood (but the two may be given through the same cannula).

Iron excretion induced by desferrioxamine is enhanced by ascorbic acid (vitamin C, section 9.6.3) 100–200 mg daily by mouth; it should be given separately from food since it also enhances iron absorption. Ascorbic acid should not be given to children with cardiac dysfunction; in children with normal cardiac function ascorbic acid should be introduced 1 month after starting desferrioxamine.

Desferrioxamine infusion can be used to treat *aluminium overload* in dialysis patients; theoretically 100 mg of desferrioxamine binds with 4.1 mg of aluminium.

**Deferasirox,** an oral iron chelator, is licensed for the treatment of chronic iron overload in children over 6 years with thalassaemia major who receive frequent blood transfusions (more than 7 mL/kg/month of packed red blood cells). It is also licensed for transfusion-related chronic iron overload when desferrioxamine is contra-indicated or inadequate in children aged 2–5 years with thalassaemia major who receive frequent blood transfusions, children over 2 years with thalassaemia major who receive infrequent blood transfusions (less than 7 mL/kg/month of packed red blood cells), and in children over 2 years with other anaemias. Deferasirox is also licensed for the treatment of chronic iron overload when desferrioxamine is contra-indicated or inadequate in children over 10 years with non-transfusion-dependent thalassaemia syndromes.

The *Scottish Medicines Consortium* (p. 3) has advised (January 2007) that deferasirox is accepted for restricted use within NHS Scotland for the treatment of chronic iron overload associated with the treatment of rare acquired or inherited anaemias requiring recurrent blood transfusions. It is not recommended for patients with myelodysplastic syndromes.

**Deferiprone,** an oral iron chelator, is licensed for the treatment of iron overload in children over 6 years of age with thalassaemia major in whom desferrioxamine is contra-indicated or is inadequate. Blood dyscrasias, particularly agranulocytosis, have been reported with deferiprone.

## DEFERASIROX

**Cautions** eye and ear examinations required before treatment and annually during treatment; monitor body-weight, height and sexual development annually; monitor serum-ferritin concentration monthly; risk of gastro-intestinal ulceration and haemorrhage; platelet count less than $50 \times 10^9$/litre; consider treatment interruption if unexplained cytopenia occurs; not recommended in conditions which may reduce life expectancy (e.g. high-risk myelodysplastic syndromes); history of liver cirrhosis; test liver function before treatment, then every 2 weeks during the first month, and then monthly; measure baseline serum-creatinine and monitor renal function weekly during the first month of treatment and monthly thereafter; test for proteinuria monthly; monitor liver-iron concentration every three months in children with non-transfusion-dependent thalassaemia syndromes when serum ferritin is $\leq 800$ micrograms/litre; **interactions**: Appendix 1 (deferasirox)

**Hepatic impairment** use with caution in moderate impairment, reduce dose considerably then gradually increase to max. 50% of normal dose; avoid in severe impairment

**Renal impairment** reduce dose by 10 mg/kg if serum-creatinine increased above age-appropriate limits *or* estimated glomerular filtration rate less than 90 mL/minute/1.73 m$^2$ on 2 consecutive occasions—interrupt treatment if deterioration in renal function persists after dose reduction; avoid if estimated glomerular filtration rate less than 60 mL/minute/1.73 m$^2$

**Pregnancy** manufacturer advises avoid unless essential—toxicity in *animal* studies

**Breast-feeding** manufacturer advises avoid—present in milk in *animal* studies

**Side-effects** gastro-intestinal disturbances (including ulceration and fatal haemorrhage); headache; proteinuria; pruritus, rash; *less commonly* oedema, hepatitis, cholelithiasis, fatigue, anxiety, sleep disorder, dizziness, pyrexia, pharyngitis, glucosuria, renal tubulopathy, disturbances of hearing and vision (including lens opacity and maculopathy), and skin pigmentation; hepatic failure, acute renal failure, tubulointerstitial nephritis, blood disorders (including anaemia, agranulocytosis, neutropenia, pancytopenia, and thrombocytopenia), hypersensitivity reactions (including anaphylaxis and angioedema), and alopecia also reported

**Licensed use** see notes above

**Indications and dose**

Transfusion-related chronic iron overload
- **By mouth**
  **Child 2–18 years** initially 10–30 mg/kg once daily according to serum-ferritin concentration and amount of transfused blood (consult product literature); maintenance, adjust dose every 3–6 months in steps of 5–10 mg/kg according to serum-ferritin concentration; usual max. 30 mg/kg daily, but may be increased to max. 40 mg/kg daily and reduced in steps of 5–10 mg/kg once control achieved

Chronic iron overload in non-transfusion-dependent thalassaemia syndromes
- **By mouth**
  **Child 10–18 years** initially 10 mg/kg once daily; adjust dose according to serum-ferritin concentration and liver-iron concentration (consult product literature); max. 10 mg/kg daily

**Exjade®** (Novartis) ▼ PoM
Dispersible tablets, deferasirox 125 mg, net price 28-tab pack = £117.60; 250 mg, 28-tab pack = £235.20; 500 mg, 28-tab pack = £470.40. Label: 13, 22, counselling, administration
**Counselling** Tablets should be dispersed in water, orange juice, or apple juice; if necessary, resuspend residue and swallow

## DEFERIPRONE

**Cautions** monitor neutrophil count weekly and discontinue treatment if neutropenia develops
**Blood disorders** Patients or their carers should be told how to recognise signs of neutropenia and advised to seek immediate medical attention if symptoms such as fever or sore throat develop

**Contra-indications** history of agranulocytosis or recurrent neutropenia

**Hepatic impairment** manufacturer advises monitor liver function—interrupt treatment if persistent elevation in serum alanine aminotransferase

**Renal impairment** manufacturer advises caution—no information available

**Pregnancy** manufacturer advises avoid before intended conception and during pregnancy—teratogenic and embryotoxic in *animal* studies; contraception advised in girls of child-bearing potential

**Breast-feeding** manufacturer advises avoid—no information available

**Side-effects** gastro-intestinal disturbances (reducing dose and increasing gradually may improve tolerance), increased appetite; headache; red-brown urine discoloration; neutropenia, agranulocytosis; zinc deficiency; arthropathy

**Licensed use** see notes above

**Indications and dose**

Iron overload in thalassaemia major
- **By mouth**
  **Child 6–18 years** 25 mg/kg 3 times daily (max. 100 mg/kg daily)

**Ferriprox®** (Swedish Orphan) PoM
Tablets, f/c, scored, deferiprone 500 mg, net price 100-tab pack = £152.39; 1 g, 50-tab pack = £175.25. Label: 14, counselling, blood disorders
Oral solution, red, deferiprone 100 mg/mL, net price 500 mL = £152.39. Label: 14, counselling, blood disorders

## DESFERRIOXAMINE MESILATE
(Deferoxamine Mesilate)

**Cautions** eye and ear examinations before treatment and at 3-month intervals during treatment; monitor body-weight and height in children at 3-month intervals—risk of growth restriction with excessive doses; aluminium-related encephalopathy (may exacerbate neurological dysfunction); **interactions**: Appendix 1 (desferrioxamine)

**Renal impairment** use with caution

**Pregnancy** teratogenic in *animal* studies, manufacturer advises use only if potential benefit outweighs risk

**Breast-feeding** manufacturer advises use only if potential benefit outweighs risk—no information available

**Side-effects** nausea, vomiting, abdominal pain, headache, pyrexia, growth retardation and bone disorders (see Cautions), arthralgia, myalgia, hearing disturbances, injection-site reactions; *rarely* diarrhoea, hepatic impairment, hypotension (especially when given too rapidly by intravenous injection), anaphylaxis, Yersinia and mucormycosis infections, blood dyscrasias (including thrombocytopenia and leucopenia), leg cramps, bone pain, visual disturbances (including lens opacity and retinopathy), rash; *very rarely* acute respiratory distress, neurological disturbances (including dizziness, neuropathy, convulsions, and paraesthesia), renal impairment; muscle spasms also reported

**Indications and dose**

Chronic iron overload see notes above

Aluminium overload in dialysis patients
● By intravenous infusion
    **Child 1 month–18 years** 5 mg/kg once weekly

Iron poisoning
    See Emergency Treatment of Poisoning, p. 29

**Administration** For *intravenous* or *subcutaneous infusion*, reconstitute powder with Water for Injection to a concentration of 100 mg/mL; dilute with Glucose 5% or Sodium Chloride 0.9%. In *haemodialysis* or *haemofiltration* administer over the last hour of dialysis (may be given via the dialysis fistula). *Intraperitoneal*: may be added to dialysis fluid. In CAPD give prior to the last exchange of the day.
**Note** For full details and warnings relating to administration, consult product literature

**Desferrioxamine mesilate** (Non-proprietary) [PoM]
Injection, powder for reconstitution, desferrioxamine mesilate, net price 500-mg vial = £4.26; 2-g vial = £17.05

**Desferal**® (Novartis) [PoM]
Injection, powder for reconstitution, desferrioxamine mesilate, net price 500-mg vial = £4.67, 2-g vial = £18.66

---

## Atypical haemolytic uraemic syndrome and paroxysmal nocturnal haemoglobinuria

**Eculizumab**, a recombinant monoclonal antibody, inhibits terminal complement activation at the C5 protein and thereby reduces haemolysis and thrombotic microangiopathy. Eculizumab is used to reduce thrombotic microangiopathy in atypical haemolytic uraemic syndrome (aHUS). Eculizumab is also used in adults to reduce haemolysis in paroxysmal nocturnal haemoglobinuria (PNH), a severe and disabling form of haemolytic anaemia [unlicensed indication in children].

---

## ECULIZUMAB

**Cautions** active systemic infection; monitor child for 1 hour after infusion; for *atypical haemolytic uraemic syndrome*, monitor for thrombotic microangiopathy (measure platelet count, serum-lactate dehydrogenase concentration, and serum creatinine) during treatment and for at least 12 weeks after discontinuation; for *paroxysmal nocturnal haemoglobinuria*, monitor for intravascular haemolysis (including serum-lactate dehydrogenase concentration) during treatment and for at least 8 weeks after discontinuation

**Meningococcal infection** Vaccinate against *Neisseria meningitidis* at least 2 weeks before treatment (tetravalent vaccine against serotypes A, C, W135 and Y recommended); revaccinate according to current medical guidelines. Patients receiving eculizumab less than 2 weeks after receiving meningococcal vaccine must be given prophylactic antibiotics until 2 weeks after vaccination. Advise child and carers to report promptly any signs of meningococcal infection. Other immunisations should also be up to date (section 14.1)

**Contra-indications** unresolved *Neisseria meningitidis* infection; patients unvaccinated against *Neisseria meningitidis* (see also Cautions above)

**Pregnancy** no information available—use only if potential benefit outweighs risk; human IgG antibodies known to cross placenta; manufacturer advises effective contraception during and for 5 months after treatment

**Breast-feeding** no information available—manufacturer advises avoid breast-feeding during and for 5 months after treatment

**Side-effects** gastro-intestinal disturbances; oedema; cough, nasopharyngitis; headache, dizziness, vertigo, fatigue, dysgeusia, paraesthesia; infection (including meningococcal infection); spontaneous erection, dysuria; arthralgia, myalgia; blood disorders (including thrombocytopenia, leucopenia); alopecia, pruritus, rash; influenza-like symptoms; infusion-related reactions; *less commonly* anorexia, gingival pain, jaundice, palpitation, haematoma, hypotension, chest pain, syncope, tremor, hot flushing, epistaxis, anxiety, depression, mood changes, sleep disturbances, Graves' disease, menstrual disorders, renal impairment, malignant melanoma, muscle spasms, myelodysplastic syndrome, visual disturbances, tinnitus, hyperhidrosis, petechiae, and skin depigmentation

**Licensed use** not licensed for use in children for paroxysmal nocturnal haemoglobinuria

**Indications and dose**

Atypical haemolytic uraemic syndrome (specialist use only)
● By intravenous infusion
    **Child 2 months–18 years**
    **Body-weight 5–10 kg** initially 300 mg once a week for 2 weeks, then 300 mg once every 3 weeks
    **Body-weight 10–20 kg** initially 600 mg on week 1, then 300 mg on week 2, then 300 mg once every 2 weeks
    **Body-weight 20–30 kg** initially 600 mg once a week for 3 weeks, then 600 mg once every 2 weeks
    **Body-weight 30–40 kg** initially 600 mg once a week for 2 weeks, then 900 mg on week 3, then 900 mg once every 2 weeks

**Body-weight over 40 kg** initially 900 mg once a week for 4 weeks, then 1.2 g on week 5, then 1.2 g once every 2 weeks

**Note** Consult product literature for details of supplemental doses with concomitant plasmapheresis, plasma exchange, or plasma infusion

**Paroxysmal nocturnal haemoglobinuria** (specialist use only)

• By intravenous infusion

Refer for specialist advice, experience very limited

**Administration** dilute requisite dose to a concentration of 5 mg/mL with Glucose 5% or Sodium Chloride 0.9% and mix gently; give over 25–45 minutes; if infusion-related reactions occur, infusion time may be increased to 4 hours in child under 12 years or 2 hours in child over 12 years

**Soliris**® (Alexion) ▼ PoM
Concentrate for intravenous infusion, eculizumab 10 mg/mL, net price 30-mL vial = £3150.00. Counselling, meningococcal infection, patient information card
**Electrolytes** Na⁺ 5 mmol/vial

## 9.1.4 Drugs used in platelet disorders

**Idiopathic thrombocytopenic purpura** Acute idiopathic thrombocytopenic purpura is usually self-limiting in children. A **corticosteroid**, such as prednisolone (p. 376), is sometimes used if idiopathic thrombocytopenic purpura does not resolve spontaneously or if it is associated with severe cutaneous symptoms or mucous membrane bleeding; corticosteroid treatment should not be continued longer than 14 days regardless of the response.

**Immunoglobulin** preparations (section 14.5) may be used in idiopathic thrombocytopenic purpura or where a temporary rapid rise in platelets is needed, as in pregnancy or pre-operatively; they are often used in preference to a corticosteroid. Anti-D immunoglobulin is licensed for the management of idiopathic thrombocytopenic purpura.

Other therapy that has been tried under specialist supervision in refractory idiopathic thrombocytopenic purpura includes azathioprine (section 8.2.1), cyclophosphamide (section 8.1.1), vincristine (section 8.1.4), and ciclosporin (section 8.2.2). Rituximab is also used in specialist centres but experience of its use in children is limited. For patients with chronic severe thrombocytopenia refractory to other therapy, tranexamic acid (section 2.11) may be given to reduce the severity of haemorrhage.

Splenectomy is considered in chronic thrombocytopenic purpura if a satisfactory platelet count is not achieved with regular immunoglobulin infusions, if there is a relapse on withdrawing or reducing the dose of corticosteroid, and if other therapies are considered inappropriate.

**Essential thrombocythaemia** Anagrelide reduces platelets in essential thrombocythaemia in patients at risk of thrombo-haemorrhagic events who have not responded adequately to other drugs or who cannot tolerate other drugs.

## ■ ANAGRELIDE

**Cautions** cardiovascular disease—assess cardiac function before and during treatment; concomitant aspirin in patients at risk of haemorrhage; monitor full blood count (monitor platelet count every 2 days for 1 week, then weekly until maintenance dose established), liver function, serum creatinine, and urea; **interactions**: Appendix 1 (anagrelide)
**Skilled tasks** Dizziness may affect performance of skilled tasks (e.g. driving)

**Hepatic impairment** manufacturer advises caution in mild impairment; avoid in moderate to severe impairment

**Renal impairment** manufacturer advises avoid if estimated glomerular filtration rate less than 50 mL/minute/1.73 m²

**Pregnancy** manufacturer advises avoid (toxicity in *animal* studies)

**Breast-feeding** manufacturer advises avoid—no information available

**Side-effects** gastro-intestinal disturbances; palpitation, tachycardia, fluid retention; headache, dizziness, fatigue; anaemia; rash; *less commonly* pancreatitis, gastro-intestinal haemorrhage, congestive heart failure, hypertension, arrhythmias, syncope, chest pain, dyspnoea, sleep disturbances, paraesthesia, hypoaesthesia, depression, nervousness, confusion, amnesia, fever, weight changes, impotence, blood disorders, myalgia, arthralgia, epistaxis, dry mouth, alopecia, skin discoloration, and pruritus; *rarely* gastritis, colitis, postural hypotension, angina, myocardial infarction, vasodilatation, pulmonary infiltrates, migraine, drowsiness, impaired coordination, dysarthria, asthenia, tinnitus, renal failure, nocturia, visual disturbances, and gingival bleeding; allergic alveolitis and hepatitis also reported

**Licensed use** not licensed for use in children

**Indications and dose**

**Essential thrombocythaemia in at-risk children who have not responded adequately to other therapy or who are intolerant of it** (initiated under specialist supervision)

• By mouth

**Child 7–18 years** initially 500 micrograms daily adjusted according to response in steps of 500 micrograms daily at weekly intervals to max. 10 mg daily (max. single dose 2.5 mg); usual dose range 1–3 mg daily in divided doses

**Xagrid**® (Shire) ▼ PoM
Capsules, anagrelide (as hydrochloride), 500 micrograms, net price 100-cap pack= £337.14. Counselling, skilled tasks, see above

## 9.1.5 G6PD deficiency

Glucose 6-phosphate dehydrogenase (G6PD) deficiency is highly prevalent in individuals originating from most parts of Africa, from most parts of Asia, from Oceania, and from Southern Europe; it can also occur, rarely, in any other individuals. G6PD deficiency is more common in males than it is in females.

Individuals with G6PD deficiency are susceptible to developing acute haemolytic anaemia when they take a number of common drugs. They are also susceptible to developing acute haemolytic anaemia when they eat fava beans (broad beans, *Vicia faba*); this is termed *favism* and can be more severe in children or when the fresh fava beans are eaten raw.

When prescribing drugs for children with G6PD deficiency, the following three points should be kept in mind:

- G6PD deficiency is genetically heterogeneous; susceptibility to the haemolytic risk from drugs varies; thus, a drug found to be safe in some G6PD-deficient individuals may not be equally safe in others;

- manufacturers do not routinely test drugs for their effects in G6PD-deficient individuals;

- the risk and severity of haemolysis is almost always dose-related.

The lists below should be read with these points in mind. Ideally, information about G6PD deficiency should be available before prescribing a drug listed below. However, in the absence of this information, the possibility of haemolysis should be considered, especially if the child belongs to a group in which G6PD deficiency is common.

A very few G6PD-deficient individuals with chronic non-spherocytic haemolytic anaemia have haemolysis even in the absence of an exogenous trigger. These children must be regarded as being at high risk of severe exacerbation of haemolysis following administration of any of the drugs listed below.

---

**Drugs with *definite* risk of haemolysis in most G6PD-deficient individuals**

**Dapsone** and other sulfones (higher doses for dermatitis herpetiformis more likely to cause problems)

**Methylthioninium chloride**

**Niridazole** [not on UK market]

**Nitrofurantoin**

**Pamaquin** [not on UK market]

**Primaquine** (30 mg weekly for 8 weeks has been found to be without undue harmful effects in African and Asian people, see section 5.4.1)

**Quinolones** (including ciprofloxacin, moxifloxacin, nalidixic acid, norfloxacin, and ofloxacin)

**Rasburicase**

**Sulfonamides** (including co-trimoxazole; some sulfonamides, e.g. sulfadiazine, have been tested and found not to be haemolytic in many G6PD-deficient individuals)

---

**Drugs with *possible* risk of haemolysis in some G6PD-deficient individuals**

**Aspirin** (acceptable up to a dose of at least 1 g daily in most G6PD-deficient individuals)

**Chloroquine** (acceptable in acute malaria and malaria chemoprophylaxis)

**Menadione**, water-soluble derivatives (e.g. menadiol sodium phosphate)

**Probenecid** [not on UK market]

**Quinidine** (acceptable in acute malaria) [not on UK market]

**Quinine** (acceptable in acute malaria)

**Sulfonylureas**

---

**Note** Naphthalene in mothballs also causes haemolysis in individuals with G6PD-deficiency.

---

## 9.1.6 Drugs used in neutropenia

Recombinant human granulocyte-colony stimulating factor (rhG-CSF) stimulates the production of neutrophils and may reduce the duration of chemotherapy-induced neutropenia and thereby reduce the incidence of associated sepsis; there is as yet no evidence that it improves overall survival. **Filgrastim** (unglycosylated rhG-CSF) and **lenograstim** (glycosylated rhG-CSF) have similar effects; both have been used in a variety of clinical settings, including cytotoxic-induced neutropenia, and neutropenia following bone marrow transplantation, but they do not have any clear-cut routine indications. In congenital neutropenia filgrastim usually increases the neutrophil count with an appropriate clinical response. Prolonged use may be associated with an increased risk of myeloid malignancy.

Treatment with granulocyte-colony stimulating factors should only be prescribed by those experienced in their use.

**Neonatal neutropenia** Filgrastim has been used to treat sepsis-induced neutropenia in preterm neonates. There is no clear evidence that granulocyte-colony stimulating factors improve survival or long-term outcomes.

**Cautions** Granulocyte-colony stimulating factors should be used with caution in patients with pre-malignant or malignant myeloid conditions. Full blood counts (including differential white cell count and platelet count) should be monitored. Treatment should be withdrawn in patients who develop signs of pulmonary infiltration. There have been reports of pulmonary infiltrates leading to acute respiratory distress syndrome—patients with a history of pulmonary infiltrates or pneumonia may be at higher risk. Granulocyte-colony stimulating factors should be used with caution in children with sickle-cell disease. Spleen size should be monitored during treatment as there is a risk of splenomegaly and rupture.

**Pregnancy** There have been reports of toxicity in *animal* studies and manufacturers advise not to use granulocyte-colony stimulating factors during pregnancy unless the potential benefit outweighs the risk.

**Breast-feeding** There is no evidence for the use of granulocyte-colony stimulating factors during breast-feeding and manufacturers advise avoiding use.

**Side-effects** Side-effects of granulocyte-colony stimulating factors include gastro-intestinal disturbances, anorexia, headache, asthenia, fever, musculoskeletal pain, bone pain, rash, alopecia, injection-site reactions, thrombocytopenia, and leucocytosis. *Less commonly* chest pain can occur. Pulmonary side-effects, particularly interstitial pneumonia (see Cautions above), cutaneous vasculitis, and acute febrile neutrophilic dermatosis have *rarely* been reported.

---

### FILGRASTIM
**(Recombinant human granulocyte-colony stimulating factor, G-CSF)**

**Cautions** see notes above; also regular morphological and cytogenetic bone-marrow examinations recommended in severe congenital neutropenia (possible risk of myelodysplastic syndromes or leukaemia); secondary acute myeloid leukaemia; osteoporotic bone disease (monitor bone density if given for more than 6 months); **interactions**: Appendix 1 (filgrastim)

**Contra-indications**  severe congenital neutropenia (Kostman's syndrome) with abnormal cytogenetics

**Pregnancy**  see notes above

**Breast-feeding**  see notes above

**Side-effects**  see notes above; also mucositis, splenic enlargement, hepatomegaly, transient hypotension, epistaxis, urinary abnormalities (including dysuria, proteinuria, and haematuria), osteoporosis, exacerbation of rheumatoid arthritis, anaemia, transient decrease in blood glucose, pseudogout, and raised uric acid; *very rarely* splenic rupture

**Licensed use**  not licensed for treatment of glycogen storage disease or neonatal neutropenia

### Indications and dose

Cytotoxic-induced neutropenia

- Preferably by subcutaneous injection or by intravenous infusion (over 30 minutes)

  **Child 1 month–18 years** 5 micrograms/kg daily started not less than 24 hours after cytotoxic chemotherapy, continued until neutrophil count in normal range, usually for up to 14 days (up to 38 days in acute myeloid leukaemia)

Myeloablative therapy followed by bone-marrow transplantation

- By intravenous infusion over 30 minutes or over 24 hours or by subcutaneous infusion over 24 hours

  **Child 1 month–18 years** 10 micrograms/kg daily, started not less than 24 hours following cytotoxic chemotherapy (and within 24 hours of bone-marrow infusion), then adjusted according to absolute neutrophil count (consult product literature and local protocol)

Mobilisation of peripheral blood progenitor cells for autologous infusion, used alone

- By subcutaneous injection or by subcutaneous infusion over 24 hours

  **Child 1 month–18 years** 10 micrograms/kg daily for 5–7 days

Mobilisation of peripheral blood progenitor cells for autologous infusion following adjunctive myelosuppressive chemotherapy (to improve yield)

- By subcutaneous injection

  **Child 1 month–18 years** 5 micrograms/kg daily, started the day after completion of chemotherapy and continued until neutrophil count in normal range; for timing of leucopheresis consult product literature

Mobilisation of peripheral blood progenitor cells in normal donors for allogeneic infusion

- By subcutaneous injection

  **Child over 16 years** 10 micrograms/kg daily for 4–5 days; for timing of leucopheresis consult product literature

Severe chronic neutropenia

- By subcutaneous injection

  **Child 1 month–18 years** in severe congenital neutropenia, initially 12 micrograms/kg daily in single or divided doses (initially 5 micrograms/kg daily in idiopathic or cyclic neutropenia), adjusted according to response (consult product literature and local protocol)

Persistent neutropenia in HIV infection

- By subcutaneous injection

  **Child 1 month–18 years** initially 1 microgram/kg daily, increased as necessary until absolute neutrophil count in normal range (usual max. 4 micrograms/kg daily), then adjusted to maintain absolute neutrophil count in normal range (consult product literature)

Neonatal neutropenia

- By subcutaneous injection

  **Neonate** 10 micrograms/kg daily, discontinue if white cell count exceeds 50 × 10⁹/litre

Glycogen storage disease type 1b

- By subcutaneous injection

  5 micrograms/kg daily, adjusted as necessary

**Administration**  For *subcutaneous* or *intravenous infusion*, dilute with Glucose 5% to a concentration of not less than 15 micrograms/mL; to dilute to a concentration of 2–15 micrograms/mL, add albumin solution (human albumin solution) to produce a final albumin solution of 2 mg/mL; not compatible with Sodium Chloride solutions

**Neupogen®** (Amgen) (PoM)
Injection, filgrastim 30 million units (300 micrograms)/mL; net price 1-mL vial = £58.56
Injection (Singleject®), filgrastim 60 million units (600 micrograms)/mL, net price 0.5-mL prefilled syringe = £58.56; 96 million units (960 micrograms)/mL, 0.5-mL prefilled syringe = £93.40

**Nivestim®** (Hospira) ▼ (PoM)
Injection, prefilled syringe, filgrastim, net price 12 million-units (120 micrograms)/0.2 mL = £36.00; 30 million-units (300 micrograms)/0.5 mL = £58.00; 48 million-units (480 micrograms)/0.5 mL = £93.00
**Note** Biosimilar medicine, p. 2

**Ratiograstim®** (Ratiopharm UK) ▼ (PoM)
Injection, prefilled syringe, filgrastim, net price 30 million-units (300 micrograms)/0.5 mL = £62.26; 48 million-units (480 micrograms)/0.8 mL = £99.29
**Note** Biosimilar medicine, p. 2

**Tevagrastim®** (TEVA UK) (PoM)
Injection, prefilled syringe, filgrastim, net price 30 million-units (300 micrograms)/0.5 mL = £62.25; 48 million-units (480 micrograms)/0.8 mL = £99.29
**Note** Biosimilar medicine, p. 2

**Zarzio®** (Sandoz) (PoM)
Injection, prefilled syringe, filgrastim, net price 30 million-units (300 micrograms)/0.5 mL = £59.00; 48 million-units (480 micrograms)/0.5 mL = £94.00
**Note** Biosimilar medicine, p. 2

**9**

**Nutrition and blood**

## LENOGRASTIM
(Recombinant human granulocyte-colony stimulating factor, rHuG-CSF)

**Cautions**  see notes above

**Pregnancy**  see notes above

**Breast-feeding**  see notes above

**Side-effects**  see notes above; also splenic rupture and toxic epidermal necrolysis

**Licensed use**  not licensed for use in children for cytotoxic-induced neutropenia, mobilisation of peripheral blood progenitor cells (monotherapy or adjunctive therapy), or following peripheral stem cells transplantation

**Indications and dose**

Following peripheral stem cells or bone-marrow transplantation

- By intravenous infusion over 30 minutes or by subcutaneous injection

  **Child 2–18 years** 150 micrograms/$m^2$ daily started the day after transplantation, continued until neutrophil count stable in acceptable range (max. 28 days)

Cytotoxic-induced neutropenia

- By subcutaneous injection

  **Child 2–18 years** 150 micrograms/$m^2$ daily started the day after completion of chemotherapy, continued until neutrophil count stable in acceptable range (max. 28 days)

Mobilisation of peripheral blood progenitor cells, used alone

- By subcutaneous injection

  **Child 2–18 years** 10 micrograms/kg daily for 4–6 days (5–6 days in healthy donors)

Mobilisation of peripheral blood progenitor cells following adjunctive myelosuppressive chemotherapy (to improve yield)

- By subcutaneous injection

  **Child 2–18 years** 150 micrograms/$m^2$ daily, started 1–5 days after completion of chemotherapy and continued until neutrophil count in acceptable range; for timing of leucopheresis consult product literature

**Administration**  for *intravenous infusion*, dilute reconstituted solution to a concentration of not less than 2 micrograms/mL (*Granocyte-13*) or 2.5 micrograms/mL (*Granocyte-34*) with Sodium Chloride 0.9%

**Granocyte**® (Chugai) [PoM]
Injection, powder for reconstitution, lenograstim, net price 13.4 million-unit (105-microgram) vial = £40.11; 33.6 million-unit (263-microgram) vial = £62.54 (both with 1-mL prefilled syringe water for injections)
**Excipients**  include phenylalanine (section 9.4.1)

## 9.2  Fluids and electrolytes

| | |
|---|---|
| 9.2.1 | Oral preparations for fluid and electrolyte imbalance |
| 9.2.2 | Parenteral preparations for fluid and electrolyte imbalance |

The following tables give a selection of useful electrolyte values:

### Electrolyte concentrations—intravenous fluids

| Intravenous infusion | Millimoles per litre | | | | |
|---|---|---|---|---|---|
| | Na$^+$ | K$^+$ | HCO$_3^-$ | Cl$^-$ | Ca$^{2+}$ |
| *Normal plasma values* | 142 | 4.5 | 26 | 103 | 2.5 |
| Sodium Chloride 0.9% | 150 | — | — | 150 | — |
| Compound Sodium Lactate (Hartmann's) | 131 | 5 | 29 | 111 | 2 |
| Sodium Chloride 0.45% and Glucose 5% | 75 | — | — | 75 | — |
| Potassium Chloride 0.15% and Glucose 5% | — | 20 | — | 20 | — |
| Potassium Chloride 0.15% and Sodium Chloride 0.9% | 150 | 20 | — | 170 | — |
| Potassium Chloride 0.3% and Glucose 5% | — | 40 | — | 40 | — |
| Potassium Chloride 0.3% and Sodium Chloride 0.9% | 150 | 40 | — | 190 | — |
| *To correct metabolic acidosis* | | | | | |
| Sodium Bicarbonate 1.26% | 150 | — | 150 | — | — |
| Sodium Bicarbonate 8.4% for cardiac arrest | 1000 | — | 1000 | — | — |
| Sodium Lactate (m/6) | 167 | — | 167 | — | — |

### Electrolyte content—gastro-intestinal secretions

| Type of fluid | Millimoles per litre | | | | |
|---|---|---|---|---|---|
| | H$^+$ | Na$^+$ | K$^+$ | HCO$_3^-$ | Cl$^-$ |
| Gastric | 40–60 | 20–80 | 5–20 | — | 100–150 |
| Biliary | — | 120–140 | 5–15 | 30–50 | 80–120 |
| Pancreatic | — | 120–140 | 5–15 | 70–110 | 40–80 |
| Small bowel | — | 120–140 | 5–15 | 20–40 | 90–130 |

Faeces, vomit, or aspiration should be saved and analysed where possible if abnormal losses are suspected; where this is impracticable the approximations above may be helpful in planning replacement therapy

## 9.2.1  Oral preparations for fluid and electrolyte imbalance

| | |
|---|---|
| 9.2.1.1 | Oral potassium |
| 9.2.1.2 | Oral sodium and water |
| 9.2.1.3 | Oral bicarbonate |

Sodium and potassium salts, which may be given by mouth to prevent deficiencies or to treat established deficiencies of mild or moderate degree, are discussed in this section. Oral preparations for removing excess potassium and preparations for oral rehydration therapy are also included here. Oral bicarbonate, for metabolic acidosis, is also described in this section.

For reference to calcium, magnesium, and phosphate, see section 9.5.

## 9.2.1.1  Oral potassium

Compensation for potassium loss is especially necessary:

- in children in whom secondary hyperaldosteronism occurs, e.g. renal artery stenosis, renal tubule disorder, the nephrotic syndrome, and severe heart failure;
- in children with excessive losses of potassium in the faeces. chronic diarrhoea associated with intestinal malabsorption or laxative abuse;
- in those taking digoxin or anti-arrhythmic drugs, where potassium depletion may induce arrhythmias.

Measures to compensate for potassium loss may be required during long-term administration of drugs known to induce potassium loss (e.g. corticosteroids). Potassium supplements are **seldom required** with the small doses of diuretics given to treat hypertension; **potassium-sparing diuretics** (rather than potassium supplements) are recommended for prevention of hypokalaemia due to diuretics such as furosemide and the thiazides when these are given to eliminate oedema.

**Dosage**  If potassium salts are used for the *prevention of hypokalaemia*, then doses of potassium chloride 1–2 mmol/kg (usual max. 50 mmol potassium) daily by mouth are suitable in patients taking a normal diet. *Smaller doses* must be used if there is *renal insufficiency* to reduce the **risk** of **hyperkalaemia**. Potassium salts cause nausea and vomiting and poor compliance is a major limitation to their effectiveness (small divided doses may minimise gastric irritation); when appropriate, potassium-sparing diuretics are preferable (see also above). Regular monitoring of plasma-potassium concentration is essential in those taking potassium supplements. When there is *established potassium depletion* larger doses may be necessary, the quantity depending on the severity of any continuing potassium loss (monitoring of plasma-potassium concentration and specialist advice would be required). Potassium depletion is frequently associated with chloride depletion and with metabolic alkalosis, and these disorders require correction.

**Administration**  Potassium salts are preferably given as a liquid (or effervescent) preparation, rather than modified-release tablets; they should be given as the chloride (the use of effervescent potassium tablets BPC 1968 should be restricted to *hyperchloraemic states*, section 9.2.1.3). Potassium chloride solutions suitable for use by mouth in neonates are available from 'special-order' manufacturers or specialist importing companies, see p. 823; they should be used with care because they are hypertonic and can damage the gastric mucosa.
**Salt substitutes** A number of salt substitutes which contain significant amounts of potassium chloride are readily available as health food products (e.g. *LoSalt*® and *Ruthmol*®). These should not be used by patients with renal failure as potassium intoxication may result.

## ▌POTASSIUM CHLORIDE

**Cautions**  see notes above; cardiac disease; *with modified-release preparations*, intestinal stricture, history of peptic ulcer, hiatus hernia; **interactions:** Appendix 1 (potassium salts)

**Contra-indications**  plasma-potassium concentration above 5 mmol/litre
**Renal impairment**  close monitoring required—risk of hyperkalaemia; avoid in severe impairment
**Side-effects**  nausea, vomiting, abdominal pain, diarrhoea, flatulence; *with modified-release preparations*, gastro-intestinal obstruction, ulceration, and bleeding also reported
**Indications and dose**

### Potassium depletion

- By mouth

   **Neonate** 0.5–1 mmol/kg K⁺ twice daily (total daily dose may alternatively be given in 3 divided doses), adjusted according to plasma-potassium concentration

   **Child 1 month–18 years** 0.5–1 mmol/kg K⁺ twice daily (total daily dose may alternatively be given in 3 divided doses), adjusted according to plasma-potassium concentration

**Note**  Do not confuse Effervescent Potassium Tablets BPC 1968 (section 9.2.1.3) with effervescent potassium chloride tablets. Effervescent Potassium Tablets BPC 1968 do not contain chloride ions and their use should be restricted to hyperchloraemic states (section 9.2.1.3).

**Kay-Cee-L**® (Geistlich)
Syrup, sugar-free, red, potassium chloride 7.5% (1 mmol/mL each of K⁺ and Cl⁻), net price 500 mL = £4.07. Label: 21

**Sando-K**® (HK Pharma)
Tablets, effervescent, potassium bicarbonate and chloride equivalent to potassium 470 mg (12 mmol of K⁺) and chloride 285 mg (8 mmol of Cl⁻), net price 20 = £1.53. Label: 13, 21

### ▌Modified-release preparations

Avoid unless effervescent tablets or liquid preparations inappropriate

**Slow-K**® (Alliance)  ▄
Tablets, m/r, orange, s/c, potassium chloride 600 mg (8 mmol each of K⁺ and Cl⁻), net price 100 = £2.14. Label: 25, 27, counselling, swallow whole with fluid during meals while sitting or standing
**Note**  May be difficult to obtain

## Management of hyperkalaemia

*Acute severe hyperkalaemia* calls for urgent treatment with intravenous infusion of **soluble insulin** (0.3–0.6 units/kg/hour in neonates and 0.05–0.2 units/kg/hour in children over 1 month) with **glucose** (0.5–1 g/kg/hour (5–10 mL/kg of glucose 10%; 2.5–5 mL/kg of glucose 20% via a central venous catheter may also be considered). If insulin cannot be used, **salbutamol** (section 3.1.1.1) can be given by intravenous injection, but it has a slower onset of action and may be less effective for reducing plasma-potassium concentration.

**Calcium gluconate** (section 9.5.1.1) is given by slow intravenous injection to manage cardiac excitability caused by hyperkalaemia.

The correction of causal or compounding acidosis with **sodium bicarbonate** infusion (section 9.2.2.1) should be considered (**important**: preparations of sodium bicarbonate and calcium salts should not be administered in the same line— risk of precipitation). Intravenous **furosemide** can also be given but is less effective in children with renal impairment. Drugs exacerbating hyperkalaemia should be reviewed and stopped as appropriate; dialysis may occasionally be required.

**Ion-exchange resins** may be used to remove excess potassium in *mild hyperkalaemia* or in *moderate hyperkalaemia* when there are no ECG changes. Calcium polystyrene sulfonate is preferred unless plasma-calcium concentrations are high.

## POLYSTYRENE SULFONATE RESINS

**Cautions**   impaction of resin with excessive dosage or inadequate dilution; monitor for electrolyte disturbances (stop if plasma-potassium concentration below 5 mmol/litre); *sodium-containing resin* in congestive heart failure, hypertension, and oedema; **interactions:** Appendix 1 (polystyrene sulfonate resins)

**Contra-indications**   obstructive bowel disease; neonates with reduced gut motility; *calcium-containing resin* in hyperparathyroidism, multiple myeloma, sarcoidosis, or metastatic carcinoma

**Renal impairment**   use *sodium-containing resin* with caution

**Pregnancy**   manufacturers advise use only if potential benefit outweighs risk—no information available

**Breast-feeding**   manufacturers advise use only if potential benefit outweighs risk—no information available

**Side-effects**   faecal impaction following rectal administration, gastro-intestinal concretions following oral administration, intestinal necrosis reported with concomitant use of sorbitol, gastric irritation, anorexia, nausea, vomiting, constipation (discontinue treatment—avoid magnesium-containing laxatives), diarrhoea, hypomagnesaemia; gastro-intestinal obstruction, ulceration, necrosis, and ischaemic colitis also reported; with *calcium-containing resin*, hypercalcaemia (including in dialysed patients and occasionally those with renal impairment); with *sodium containing resin*, sodium retention, hypocalcaemia

**Indications and dose**
See under preparations

**Calcium Resonium®** (Sanofi-Aventis)
Powder, buff, calcium polystyrene sulfonate, net price 300 g = £68.47. Label: 13
**Dose**

**Hyperkalaemia associated with anuria or severe oliguria, and in dialysis patients**
* By mouth
  **Child 1 month–18 years** 0.5–1 g/kg (max. 60 g) daily in divided doses
  **Administration** Administer in a small amount of water or honey—do not give with fruit juice or squash, which have a high potassium content
* By rectum
  **Neonate** 0.5–1 g/kg daily. Irrigate colon to remove resin after 8–12 hours
  **Child 1 month–18 years** 0.5–1 g/kg (max. 30 g) daily. Irrigate colon to remove resin after 8–12 hours
  **Administration** Mix each 1 g of resin with 5 mL of water or 10% glucose

**Resonium A®** (Sanofi-Aventis)
Powder, buff, sodium polystyrene sulfonate, net price 454 g = £67.50. Label: 13
**Dose**

**Hyperkalaemia associated with anuria or severe oliguria, and in dialysis patients**
* By mouth
  **Child 1 month–18 years** 0.5–1 g/kg (max. 60 g) daily in divided doses
  **Administration** Administer in a small amount of water or honey—do not give with fruit juice or squash, which have a high potassium content
* By rectum
  **Neonate** 0.5–1 g/kg daily. Irrigate colon to remove resin after 8–12 hours
  **Child 1 month–18 years** 0.5–1 g/kg (max. 30 g) daily. Irrigate colon to remove resin after 8–12 hours
  **Administration** Mix each 1 g of resin with 5 mL of water or 10% glucose

**Sorbisterit®** (Stanningley) [PoM]
Powder, buff, calcium polystyrene sulfonate 759–949 mg/g, net price 500 g= £49.95. Label: 13, 21
**Excipients** include sucrose 51–241 mg per 1 g of powder
**Dose**

**Hyperkalaemia associated with anuria or severe oliguria, and in dialysis patients**
* By mouth
  **Child 1 month–18 years** 0.5–1 g/kg (max. 60 g) daily in at least 3 divided doses
  **Administration** Administer in a small amount of water or soft drink—do not give with fruit juice or squash, which have a high potassium content
* By rectum
  **Neonate** 0.5–1 g/kg daily. Irrigate colon to remove resin after 6 hours
  **Child 1 month–18 years** 0.5–1 g/kg (max. 40 g) daily. Irrigate colon to remove resin after 6 hours
  **Administration** Mix each 1 g of resin with 4 mL of 5% glucose

### 9.2.1.2 Oral sodium and water

Sodium chloride is indicated in states of sodium depletion. In preterm neonates in the first few weeks of life and in chronic conditions associated with mild or moderate degrees of sodium depletion, e.g. in salt-losing bowel or renal disease, oral supplements of sodium chloride (section 9.2.1.3) may be sufficient. Sodium chloride solutions suitable for use by mouth in neonates are available from 'special-order' manufacturers or specialist importing companies, see p. 823; they should be used with care because they are hypertonic. Supplementation with sodium chloride may be required to replace losses in children with cystic fibrosis particularly in warm weather.

## SODIUM CHLORIDE

**Indications and dose**
See also section 9.2.2

**Sodium supplementation in neonates**
* By mouth
  **Preterm neonate** 2 mmol/100 mL of formula feed or 3–4 mmol/100 mL of breast milk, consult dietician

### Sodium replacement

- By mouth

  **Child 1 month–18 years** according to requirements, generally 1–2 mmol/kg daily in divided doses, higher doses may be needed in severe depletion

### Chronic renal loss

- By mouth

  **Child 1 month–18 years** 1–2 mmol/kg daily in divided doses, adjusted according to requirements

**Slow Sodium®** (HK Pharma)

Tablets, m/r, sodium chloride 600 mg (approx. 10 mmol each of Na$^+$ and Cl$^-$). Net price 100-tab pack = £6.05. Label: 25

Capsules available from 'special-order' manufacturers or specialist importing companies, see p. 823

---

## Oral rehydration therapy (ORT)

Diarrhoea in children is usually self-limiting, however, in children under 6 months of age, and more particularly in those under 3 months, symptoms of dehydration may be less obvious and there is a risk of rapid and severe deterioration. Intestinal absorption of sodium and water is enhanced by glucose (and other carbohydrates). Replacement of fluid and electrolytes lost through diarrhoea can therefore be achieved by giving solutions containing sodium, potassium, and glucose or another carbohydrate such as rice starch.

Oral rehydration solutions should:

- enhance the absorption of water and electrolytes;
- replace the electrolyte deficit adequately and safely;
- contain an alkalinising agent to counter acidosis;
- be slightly hypo-osmolar (about 250 mmol/litre) to prevent the possible induction of osmotic diarrhoea;
- be simple to use in hospital and at home;
- be palatable and acceptable, especially to children;
- be readily available.

It is the policy of the World Health Organization (WHO) to promote a single oral rehydration solution but to use it flexibly (e.g. by giving extra water between drinks of oral rehydration solution to moderately dehydrated infants).

Oral rehydration solutions used in the UK are lower in sodium (50–60 mmol/litre) than the WHO formulation since, in general, patients suffer less severe sodium loss.

Rehydration should be rapid over 3 to 4 hours (except in hypernatraemic dehydration in which case rehydration should occur more slowly over 12 hours). The patient should be reassessed after initial rehydration and if still dehydrated rapid fluid replacement should continue.

Once rehydration is complete further dehydration is prevented by encouraging the patient to drink normal volumes of an appropriate fluid and by replacing continuing losses with an oral rehydration solution; in infants, breast-feeding or formula feeds should be offered between oral rehydration drinks.

For intravenous rehydration see section 9.2.2.

## ■ ORAL REHYDRATION SALTS (ORS)

**Licensed use** *Dioralyte® Relief* not licensed for use in children under 3 months

**Indications and dose**

**Fluid and electrolyte loss in diarrhoea** see notes above

- By mouth

  **Child 1 month–1 year** 1–1½ times usual feed volume

  **Child 1–12 years** 200 mL after every loose motion

  **Child 12–18 years** 200–400 mL after every loose motion

### ◢ UK formulations

**Note** After reconstitution any unused solution should be discarded no later than 1 hour after preparation unless stored in a refrigerator when it may be kept for up to 24 hours.

**Dioralyte®** (Sanofi-Aventis)

Oral powder, sodium chloride 470 mg, potassium chloride 300 mg, disodium hydrogen citrate 530 mg, glucose 3.56 g/sachet, net price 6-sachet pack = £2.25, 20-sachet pack (black currant- or citrus-flavoured or natural) = £6.72

**Note** Reconstitute 1 sachet with 200 mL of water (freshly boiled and cooled for infants); 5 sachets reconstituted with 1 litre of water provide Na$^+$ 60 mmol, K$^+$ 20 mmol, Cl$^-$ 60 mmol, citrate 10 mmol, and glucose 90 mmol

**Dioralyte® Relief** (Sanofi-Aventis)

Oral powder, sodium chloride 350 mg, potassium chloride 300 mg, sodium citrate 580 mg, cooked rice powder 6 g/sachet, net price 6-sachet pack (apricot-, black currant- or raspberry-flavoured) = £2.50, 20-sachet pack (apricot-flavoured) = £7.13

**Note** Reconstitute 1 sachet with 200 mL of water (freshly boiled and cooled for infants); 5 sachets when reconstituted with 1 litre of water provide Na$^+$ 60 mmol, K$^+$ 20 mmol, Cl$^-$ 50 mmol and citrate 10 mmol; contains aspartame (section 9.4.1)

**Electrolade®** (Actavis)

Oral powder, sodium chloride 236 mg, potassium chloride 300 mg, sodium bicarbonate 500 mg, anhydrous glucose 4 g/sachet (banana-, black currant-, lemon and lime-, or orange-flavoured). Net price 6-sachet (plain or multiflavoured) pack = £1.33, 20-sachet (single- or multiflavoured) pack = £4.99

**Note** Reconstitute 1 sachet with 200 mL of water (freshly boiled and cooled for infants); 5 sachets when reconstituted with 1 litre of water provide Na$^+$ 50 mmol, K$^+$ 20 mmol, Cl$^-$ 40 mmol, HCO$_3^-$ 30 mmol, and glucose 111 mmol

### ◢ WHO formulation

**Oral Rehydration Salts** (Non-proprietary)

Oral powder, sodium chloride 2.6 g, potassium chloride 1.5 g, sodium citrate 2.9 g, anhydrous glucose 13.5 g. To be dissolved in sufficient water to produce 1 litre (providing Na$^+$ 75 mmol, K$^+$ 20 mmol, Cl$^-$ 65 mmol, citrate 10 mmol, glucose 75 mmol/litre)

**Note** Recommended by the WHO and the United Nations Children's Fund but not commonly used in the UK

---

### 9.2.1.3 Oral bicarbonate

**Sodium bicarbonate** is given by mouth for *chronic acidotic states* such as uraemic acidosis or renal tubular acidosis. The dose for correction of metabolic acidosis is not predictable and the response must be assessed. For severe *metabolic acidosis*, sodium bicarbonate can be given intravenously (section 9.2.2).

Sodium supplements may increase blood pressure or cause fluid retention and pulmonary oedema in those at risk; hypokalaemia may be exacerbated.

Sodium bicarbonate may affect the stability or absorption of other drugs if administered at the same time. If possible, allow 1–2 hours before administering other drugs orally.

Where *hyperchloraemic acidosis* is associated with potassium deficiency, as in some renal tubular and gastrointestinal disorders it may be appropriate to give oral **potassium bicarbonate**, although acute or severe deficiency should be managed by intravenous therapy.

## █ SODIUM BICARBONATE

**Cautions** see notes above; respiratory acidosis; **interactions:** Appendix 1 (antacids)
**Indications and dose**

**Renal acidosis** (see also notes above)
- By mouth
  **Neonate** initially 1–2 mmol/kg daily in divided doses, adjusted according to response

  **Child 1 month–18 years** initially 1–2 mmol/kg daily in divided doses, adjusted according to response

**Metabolic acidosis** section 9.2.2.1

**Renal hyperkalaemia** section 9.2.2.1

**Sodium Bicarbonate** (Non-proprietary)
Capsules, sodium bicarbonate 500 mg (approx. 6 mmol each of $Na^+$ and $HCO_3^-$), net price 56-cap pack = £5.16
Tablets, sodium bicarbonate 600 mg, net price 100-tab pack = £2.48
**Important** Oral solutions of sodium bicarbonate are required occasionally; these need to be obtained from 'special-order' manufacturers or specialist importing companies, see p. 823, and the strength of sodium bicarbonate should be stated on the prescription

## █ POTASSIUM BICARBONATE

**Cautions** cardiac disease, **interactions:** Appendix 1 (potassium salts)
**Contra-indications** hypochloraemia; plasma-potassium concentration above 5 mmol/litre
**Renal impairment** close monitoring required—high risk of hyperkalaemia; avoid in severe impairment
**Side-effects** nausea, vomiting, abdominal pain, diarrhoea, and flatulence

**Potassium Tablets, Effervescent** (Non-proprietary)
Effervescent tablets, potassium bicarbonate 500 mg, potassium acid tartrate 300 mg, each tablet providing 6.5 mmol of $K^+$. To be dissolved in water before administration. Net price 56 = £33.38. Label: 13, 21
**Note** These tablets do not contain chloride; for effervescent tablets containing potassium and chloride, see under Potassium Chloride, section 9.2.1.1

## 9.2.2 Parenteral preparations for fluid and electrolyte imbalance

9.2.2.1 Electrolytes and water
9.2.2.2 Plasma and plasma substitutes

### 9.2.2.1 Electrolytes and water

Solutions of electrolytes are given intravenously, to meet normal fluid and electrolyte requirements or to replenish substantial deficits or continuing losses when it is not possible or desirable to use the oral route. When intravenous administration is not possible, fluid (as sodium chloride 0.9% or glucose 5%) can also be given subcutaneously by hypodermoclysis.

In an individual patient the nature and severity of the electrolyte imbalance must be assessed from the history and clinical and biochemical examination. Sodium, potassium, chloride, magnesium, phosphate, and water depletion can occur singly and in combination with or without disturbances of acid-base balance; for reference to the use of magnesium and phosphates, see section 9.5.

Isotonic solutions may be infused safely into a peripheral vein. Solutions more concentrated than plasma, for example 15% glucose, are best given through an indwelling catheter positioned in a large vein.

**Maintenance fluid requirements** in children are usually derived from the relationship that exists between body-weight and metabolic rate; the figures in the table below may be used as a guide outside the neonatal period. The glucose requirement is that needed to minimise gluconeogenesis from amino acids obtained as substrate from muscle breakdown. Maintenance fluids are intended only to provide hydration for a short period until enteral or parenteral nutrition can be established.

| Fluid requirements for children over 1 month: | |
|---|---|
| Body-weight | 24-hour fluid requirement |
| Under 10 kg | 100 mL/kg |
| 10–20 kg | 100 mL/kg for the first 10 kg + 50 mL/kg for each 1 kg body-weight over 10 kg |
| Over 20 kg | 100 mL/kg for the first 10 kg + 50 mL/kg for each 1 kg body-weight between 10–20 kg + 20 mL/kg for each 1 kg body-weight over 20 kg (max. 2 litres in females, 2.5 litres in males) |

**Important** The baseline fluid requirements shown in the table above should be adjusted to take account of factors that reduce water loss (e.g. increased antidiuretic hormone, renal failure, hypothermia, and high ambient humidity) or increase water loss (e.g. pyrexia or burns).

It is usual to meet these requirements by using a standard solution of sodium chloride and glucose. Solutions containing 20 mmol/litre of potassium chloride meet usual potassium requirements when given in the suggested volumes; adjustments may be needed if there is an inability to excrete fluids or electrolytes, excessive renal loss or continuing extra-renal losses. The exact requirements depend upon the nature of the clinical situation and types of losses incurred; see Caution on dilutional hyponatraemia below.

**Caution**   During parenteral hydration, fluids and electrolytes should be monitored closely and any disturbance corrected by slow infusion of an appropriate solution. The volume of fluid infused should take into account the possibility of reduced fluid loss owing to increased antidiuretic hormone and factors such as renal failure, hypothermia, and high humidity.

*Dilutional hyponatraemia* is a rare but potentially fatal risk of parenteral hydration. It may be caused by inappropriate use of hypotonic fluids such as sodium chloride 0.18% and glucose 4% intravenous infusion, especially in the postoperative period when antidiuretic hormone secretion is increased. Dilutional hyponatraemia is characterized by a rapid fall in plasma-sodium concentration leading to cerebral oedema and seizures; any child with severe hyponatraemia or rapidly changing plasma-sodium concentration should be referred urgently to a paediatric high dependency facility.

> **Safe practice**
>
> Sodium chloride 0.18% and glucose 4% intravenous infusion fluid should not be used for fluid replacement in children aged 16 years or less because of the risk of hyponatraemia; availability of this infusion should be restricted to high dependency and intensive care units, and specialist wards, such as renal, liver, and cardiac units. Local guidelines on intravenous fluids should be consulted.

**Replacement therapy**: initial intravenous replacement fluid is generally required if the child is over 10% dehydrated, or if 5–10% dehydrated and oral or enteral rehydration is not tolerated or possible. Oral rehydration is adequate, if tolerated, in the majority of those less than 10% dehydrated. Subsequent fluid and electrolyte requirements are determined by clinical assessment of fluid balance.

**Neonates**   Neonates lose water through the skin and nose, particularly if preterm or if the skin is damaged. The basic fluid requirement for a term baby in average ambient humidity is 40–60 mL/kg/day plus urinary losses. Preterm babies have very high transepidermal losses particularly in the first few days of life; they may need more fluid replacement than full term babies and up to 180 mL/kg/day may be required. Local guidelines for fluid management in the neonatal period should be consulted.

## Intravenous sodium

**Intravenous sodium chloride** in isotonic (0.9%) solution provides the most important extracellular ions in near physiological concentrations and is indicated in *sodium depletion*. It may be given for initial treatment of acute fluid loss and to replace ongoing gastro-intestinal losses from the upper gastro-intestinal tract. Intra-

venous sodium chloride is commonly given as a component of maintenance and replacement therapy, usually in combination with other electrolytes and glucose, see notes above. Sodium chloride solutions should be used cautiously in renal insufficiency, cardiac failure, cardio-respiratory diseases, hepatic cirrhosis and in children receiving glucocorticoids. Hyponatraemia with serious consequences may occur if maintenance and replacement fluids do not meet sodium requirements (see Caution, dilutional hyponatraemia, above).

*Chronic hyponatraemia* should ideally be corrected by fluid restriction. However, if sodium chloride is required, the deficit should be corrected slowly to avoid the risk of osmotic demyelination syndrome; the rise in plasma-sodium concentration should be no more than 10 mmol/litre in 24 hours.

**Sodium chloride and glucose** solutions are indicated when there is combined *water and sodium depletion*. A 1:1 mixture of isotonic sodium chloride and 5% glucose allows some of the water (free of sodium) to enter body cells which suffer most from dehydration while the sodium salt with a volume of water determined by the normal plasma $Na^+$ remains extracellular. Maintenance fluid should accurately reflect daily requirements and close monitoring is required to avoid fluid and electrolyte imbalance. Illness or injury increase the secretion of anti-diuretic hormone and therefore the ability to excrete excess water may be impaired. Inappropriate use of hypotonic solutions such as sodium chloride 0.18% and glucose 4% may also cause dilutional hyponatraemia especially in children (see Caution on dilutional hyponatraemia, above); if necessary, guidance should be sought from a clinician experienced in the management of fluid and electrolytes.

Combined sodium, potassium, chloride, and water depletion may occur, for example, with severe diarrhoea or persistent vomiting; replacement is carried out with sodium chloride intravenous infusion 0.9% and glucose intravenous infusion 5% with potassium as appropriate.

**Compound sodium lactate** (Hartmann's solution) can be used instead of isotonic sodium chloride solution during or after surgery, or in the initial management of the injured or wounded.

**Neonates**   The sodium requirement for most healthy neonates is 3 mmol/kg daily. Preterm neonates, particularly below 30 weeks gestation, may require up to 6 mmol/kg daily. *Hyponatraemia* may be caused by excessive renal loss of sodium; it may also be dilutional and restriction of fluid intake may be appropriate. Sodium supplementation is likely to be required if the serum sodium concentration is significantly reduced.

*Hypernatraemia* may also occur, most often due to dehydration (e.g. breast milk insufficiency). Severe hypernatraemia and hyponatraemia can cause fits and rarely brain damage. Sodium in drug preparations, delivered via continuous infusions, or in infusions to maintain the patency of intravascular or umbilical lines, can result in significant amounts of sodium being delivered, (e.g. 1 mL/hour of 0.9% sodium chloride infused over 24 hours is equivalent to 3.6 mmol/day of sodium).

## ▌SODIUM CHLORIDE

**Cautions**   restrict intake in impaired renal function, cardiac failure, hypertension, peripheral and pulmonary oedema, toxaemia of pregnancy; see also notes above

**9**

**Nutrition and blood**

**Side-effects** administration of large doses may give rise to sodium accumulation and oedema

**Indications and dose**

Electrolyte imbalance see notes above, also section 9.2.1.2

**Sodium Chloride** (Non-proprietary) PoM

Intravenous infusion, usual strength sodium chloride 0.9% (9 g, 150 mmol each of $Na^+$ and $Cl^-$/litre), this strength being supplied when normal saline for injection is requested. Net price 2-mL amp = 32p; 5-mL amp = 38p; 10-mL amp = 52p; 20-mL amp = £1.04; 50-mL amp = £3.63

In hospitals, 500- and 1000-mL packs, and sometimes other sizes, are available

**Note** The term 'normal saline' should **not** be used to describe sodium chloride intravenous infusion 0.9%; the term 'physiological saline' is acceptable but it is preferable to give the composition (i.e. sodium chloride intravenous infusion 0.9%).

**◢With other ingredients**
**Note** See above for warning on hyponatraemia

**Sodium Chloride and Glucose** (Non-proprietary) PoM

Intravenous infusion, sodium chloride 0.18% ($Na^+$ and $Cl^-$ each 30 mmol/litre), glucose 4%

In hospitals, usually 500-mL packs and sometimes other sizes are available

Intravenous infusion, sodium chloride 0.45% ($Na^+$ and $Cl^-$ each 75 mmol/litre), glucose 5%

In hospitals, usually 500-mL packs and sometimes other sizes are available

Intravenous infusion, sodium chloride 0.9% ($Na^+$ and $Cl^-$ each 150 mmol/litre), glucose 5%

In hospitals, usually 500-mL packs and sometimes other sizes are available

**Ringer's Solution** (Non-proprietary) PoM

Calcium chloride (dihydrate) 322 micrograms, potassium chloride 300 micrograms, sodium chloride 8.6 mg/mL, providing the following ions (in mmol/litre), $Ca^{2+}$ 2.2, $K^+$ 4, $Na^+$ 147, $Cl^-$ 156

In hospitals, 500- and 1000-mL packs, and sometimes other sizes, are available

**Sodium Lactate, Compound** (Non-proprietary) PoM

(Hartmann's Solution; Ringer-Lactate Solution)

Intravenous infusion, sodium chloride 0.6%, sodium lactate 0.32%, potassium chloride 0.04%, calcium chloride 0.027% (containing $Na^+$ 131 mmol, $K^+$ 5 mmol, $Ca^{2+}$ 2 mmol, $HCO_3^-$ (as lactate) 29 mmol, $Cl^-$ 111 mmol/litre)

In hospitals, 500- and 1000-mL packs, and sometimes other sizes, are available

## Intravenous glucose

Glucose solutions are used mainly to replace water deficit and should not be given alone except when there is no significant loss of electrolytes; prolonged administration of glucose solutions without electrolytes can lead to hyponatraemia and other electrolyte disturbances. Water depletion (dehydration) tends to occur when losses are not matched by a comparable intake, as may occur in coma or dysphagia.

Water loss rarely exceeds electrolyte losses but this can occur in fevers, hyperthyroidism, and in uncommon water-losing renal states such as diabetes insipidus or hypercalcaemia. The volume of glucose solution needed to replace deficits varies with the severity of the disorder; the rate of infusion should be adjusted to return the plasma-sodium concentration to normal over 48 hours.

Glucose solutions are also used to correct and prevent hypoglycaemia and to provide a source of energy in those too ill to be fed adequately by mouth; glucose solutions are a key component of parenteral nutrition (section 9.3).

Glucose solutions are given with insulin for the emergency management of *hyperkalaemia* (see p. 459). They are also given, after correction of hyperglycaemia, during treatment of diabetic ketoacidosis, when they must be accompanied by continuous insulin infusion (section 6.1.3).

Injections containing more than 10% glucose can be irritant and should be given into a central venous line; however, solutions containing up to 12.5% can be administered for a short period into a peripheral line.

## ◢ GLUCOSE
### (Dextrose Monohydrate)

**Note** Glucose BP is the monohydrate but Glucose Intravenous Infusion BP is a sterile solution of anhydrous glucose or glucose monohydrate, potency being expressed in terms of anhydrous glucose

**Side-effects** glucose injections especially if hypertonic may have a low pH and may cause venous irritation and thrombophlebitis

**Indications and dose**

Fluid replacement see notes above

Provision of energy section 9.3

Hypoglycaemia section 6.1.4

**Glucose** (Non-proprietary) PoM

Intravenous infusion, glucose or anhydrous glucose (potency expressed in terms of anhydrous glucose), usual strengths 5% (50 mg/mL), 10% (100 mg/mL), and 20% (200 mg/mL); 20% solution, net price 20-mL amp = £2.04; 50% solution[1], 20-mL amp = 95 p, 50-mL vial = £2.13

In hospitals, 500- and 1000-mL packs, and sometimes other sizes and strengths, are available; also available *Minijet®* *Glucose*, 50% in 50-mL disposable syringe[1]

## Intravenous potassium

**Potassium chloride and sodium chloride** intravenous infusion is the initial treatment for the correction of *severe hypokalaemia* and when sufficient potassium cannot be taken by mouth. Ready-mixed infusion solutions should be used when possible (see under Safe Practice below); for peripheral intravenous infusion, the concentration of potassium should not usually exceed 40 mmol/litre. Potassium infusions should be given slowly over at least 2–3 hours and at a rate not exceeding 0.2 mmol/kg/hour with specialist advice and ECG monitoring in difficult cases. Higher concentrations of potassium chloride or faster infusion rates may be given in very severe depletion, but require specialist advice.

Repeated measurements of plasma-potassium concentration are necessary to determine whether further infusions are required and to avoid the development of hyperkalaemia, which is especially likely in renal impairment.

---

1. PoM restriction does not apply where administration is for saving life in emergency

Initial potassium replacement therapy should **not** involve glucose infusions, because glucose may cause a further decrease in the plasma-potassium concentration.

> **Safe Practice**
>
> Potassium overdose can be fatal. Ready-mixed infusion solutions containing potassium should be used. Exceptionally, if potassium chloride concentrate is used for preparing an infusion, the infusion solution should be **thoroughly mixed**. Local policies on avoiding inadvertent use of potassium chloride concentrate should be followed.

## ▮ POTASSIUM CHLORIDE

**Cautions**   for peripheral intravenous infusion the concentration of solution should not usually exceed 3 g (40 mmol)/litre; specialist advice and ECG monitoring (see notes above); **interactions:** Appendix 1 (potassium salts)

**Contra-indications**   plasma-potassium concentration above 5 mmol/litre

**Renal impairment**   close monitoring required—high risk of hyperkalaemia; avoid in severe impairment

**Side-effects**   rapid infusion toxic to heart

**Indications and dose**

> **Electrolyte imbalance** see also oral potassium supplements, section 9.2.1.1
> - **By slow intravenous infusion**
>
>   Depending on the deficit or the daily maintenance requirements, see also notes above
>
>   **Neonate** 1–2 mmol/kg daily
>
>   **Child 1 month–18 years** 1–2 mmol/kg daily

**Administration**   see notes above

**Potassium Chloride and Glucose** (Non-proprietary) (PoM)

Intravenous infusion, usual strengths potassium chloride 0.3% (3 g, 40 mmol each of $K^+$ and $Cl^-$/litre) or 0.15% (1.5 g, 20 mmol each of $K^+$ and $Cl^-$/litre) with 5% of anhydrous glucose

In hospitals, 500- and 1000-mL packs, and sometimes other sizes, are available

**Potassium Chloride and Sodium Chloride** (Non-proprietary) (PoM)

Intravenous infusion, usual strength potassium chloride 0.15% (1.5 g/litre) with sodium chloride 0.9% (9 g/litre), containing $K^+$ 20 mmol, $Na^+$ 150 mmol, and $Cl^-$ 170 mmol/litre

In hospitals, 500- and 1000-mL packs, and sometimes other sizes, are available

**Potassium Chloride, Sodium Chloride, and Glucose** (Non-proprietary) (PoM)

Intravenous infusion, sodium chloride 0.45% (4.5 g, $Na^+$ 75 mmol/litre) with 5% of anhydrous glucose and usually sufficient potassium chloride to provide $K^+$ 10–40 mmol/litre (to be specified by the prescriber)

In hospitals, 500- and 1000-mL packs, and sometimes other sizes are available

**Potassium Chloride** (Non-proprietary) (PoM)

Sterile concentrate, potassium chloride 15% (150 mg, approximately 2 mmol each of $K^+$ and $Cl^-$/mL). Net price 10-mL amp = 48p

Solutions containing 10 and 20% of potassium chloride are also available in both 5- and 10-mL ampoules

**Important** Must be diluted with **not less** than 50 times its volume of Sodium Chloride 0.9% or other suitable diluent and **mixed well;** see Safe Practice, above

## Bicarbonate and trometamol

**Sodium bicarbonate** is used to control severe *metabolic acidosis* (pH < 7.1) particularly that caused by loss of bicarbonate (as in renal tubular acidosis or from excessive gastro-intestinal losses). Mild metabolic acidosis associated with volume depletion should first be managed by appropriate fluid replacement because acidosis usually resolves as tissue and renal perfusion are restored. In more severe metabolic acidosis or when the acidosis remains unresponsive to correction of anoxia or hypovolaemia, sodium bicarbonate (1.26%) can be infused over 3–4 hours with plasma-pH and electrolyte monitoring. In severe shock (section 2.7.1), for example in cardiac arrest, metabolic acidosis can develop without sodium depletion; in these circumstances sodium bicarbonate is best given intravenously as a small volume of hypertonic solution, such as 8.4%; plasma pH and electrolytes should be monitored. For *chronic acidotic states*, sodium bicarbonate can be given by mouth (section 9.2.1.3).

**Trometamol**   (tris(hydroxymethyl)aminomethane, THAM), an organic buffer, corrects metabolic acidosis by causing an increase in urinary pH and an osmotic diuresis. It is indicated when sodium bicarbonate is unsuitable as in carbon dioxide retention, hypernatraemia, or renal impairment. Respiratory support may be required because trometamol induces respiratory depression. It is also used during cardiac bypass surgery and, very rarely, in cardiac arrest.

## ▮ SODIUM BICARBONATE

**Indications and dose**

> **Metabolic acidosis** see also notes above
> - **By slow intravenous injection of a strong solution (up to 8.4%), or by continuous intravenous infusion of a weaker solution (usually 1.26%)**
>
>   An amount appropriate to the body base deficit

> **Renal hyperkalaemia**
> - **By slow intravenous injection**
>
>   **Neonate** 1 mmol/kg daily
>
>   **Child 1 month–18 years** 1 mmol/kg daily

> **Renal acidosis** section 9.2.1.3

**Sodium Bicarbonate** (PoM)

Intravenous infusion, usual strength sodium bicarbonate 1.26% (12.6 g, 150 mmol each of $Na^+$ and $HCO_3^-$/litre); various other strengths available

In hospitals, 500- and 1000-mL packs, and sometimes other sizes, are available

**Administration** For *peripheral infusion* dilute 8.4% solution at least 1 in 10; for *central line infusion* dilute 1 in 5 with Glucose 5% or 10% *or* Sodium Chloride 0.9%. Extravasation can cause severe tissue damage

**9**

**Nutrition and blood**

**Minijet® Sodium Bicarbonate** (UCB Pharma) [PoM]
Intravenous injection, sodium bicarbonate in disposable syringe, net price 4.2%, 10 mL = £11.03; 8.4%, 10 mL = £11.10, 50 mL = £12.15

Plasma and plasma substitutes are often used in very ill children whose condition is unstable. Therefore, close monitoring is required and fluid and electrolyte therapy should be adjusted according to the child's condition at all times.

## TROMETAMOL
(Tris(hydroxymethyl)aminomethane, THAM)

**Cautions** see notes above; extravasation can cause severe tissue damage

**Contra-indications** anuria; chronic respiratory acidosis

**Renal impairment** use with caution, may cause hyperkalaemia

**Pregnancy** limited information available, hypoglycaemia may harm fetus

**Breast-feeding** no information available

**Side-effects** respiratory depression; hypoglycaemia; hyperkalaemia in renal impairment; liver necrosis reported following administration via umbilical vein in neonates

**Licensed use** unlicensed preparation

**Indications and dose**

> Metabolic acidosis
> • By intravenous infusion
> > An amount appropriate to the body base deficit

◢ Preparations
Available from 'special-order' manufacturers or specialist importing companies, see p. 823

## Water

**Water for Injections** [PoM]
Net price 1-mL amp = £0.18; 2-mL amp = £0.20; 5-mL amp = £0.36; 10-mL amp = £0.37, 10-mL vial = £1.40; 20-mL amp = £0.92; 50-mL amp = £1.91; 100-mL vial = £2.01
**Note** Water for Injections can be sold or supplied by a pharmacist for a purpose other than parenteral administration, or when dry powder for parenteral administration has been prescribed without the Water for Injections that is needed as a diluent

## 9.2.2.2 Plasma and plasma substitutes

**Albumin solutions**, prepared from whole blood, contain soluble proteins and electrolytes but no clotting factors, blood group antibodies, or plasma cholinesterases; they may be given without regard to the recipient's blood group.

Albumin is usually used after the acute phase of illness to correct a plasma-volume deficit; hypoalbuminaemia itself is not an appropriate indication. The use of albumin solutions in acute plasma or blood loss may be wasteful; plasma substitutes are more appropriate. Concentrated albumin solutions may also be used to obtain a diuresis in hypoalbuminaemic patients (e.g. in nephrotic syndrome).

Recent evidence does not support the previous view that the use of albumin increases mortality.

## ALBUMIN SOLUTION
(Human Albumin Solution)

A solution containing protein derived from plasma, serum, or normal placentas; at least 95% of the protein is albumin. The solution may be isotonic (containing 3.5–5% protein) or concentrated (containing 15–25% protein).

**Cautions** history of cardiac or circulatory disease (administer slowly to avoid rapid rise in blood pressure and cardiac failure, and monitor cardiovascular and respiratory function); increased capillary permeability; correct dehydration when administering concentrated solution

**Contra-indications** cardiac failure; severe anaemia

**Side-effects** hypersensitivity reactions (including anaphylaxis) with nausea, vomiting, increased salivation, fever, tachycardia, hypotension and chills reported

**Indications and dose**
See notes above and under preparations, below

◢ Isotonic solutions
*Indications:* acute or sub-acute loss of plasma volume e.g. in burns, pancreatitis, trauma, and complications of surgery; plasma exchange

Available as: *Human Albumin Solution 4.5%* (50-, 100-, 250- and 400-mL bottles—Baxter); *Human Albumin Solution 5%* (250- and 500-mL bottles—Baxter); *Albunorm®* 5% (100-, 250-, and 500-mL bottles—Octapharma); *Zenalb®* 4.5% (50-, 100-, 250-, and 500-mL bottles—BPL)

◢ Concentrated solutions (20%)
*Indications:* severe hypoalbuminaemia associated with low plasma volume and generalised oedema where salt and water restriction with plasma volume expansion are required; adjunct in the treatment of hyperbilirubinaemia by exchange transfusion in the newborn; paracentesis of large volume ascites associated with portal hypertension

Available as: *Human Albumin Solution 20%* (50- and 100-mL vials—Baxter); *Albunorm®* 20% (50- and 100-mL bottles—Octapharma); *Flexbumin®* 20% (50- and 100-mL bags—Baxter); *Zenalb®* 20% (50- and 100-mL bottles—BPL)

## Plasma substitutes

**Gelatin** and the **etherified starches** (**pentastarch** and **tetrastarch**) are macromolecular substances which are metabolised slowly; they may be used at the outset to expand and maintain blood volume in shock arising from conditions such as burns or septicaemia. Plasma substitutes may be used as an immediate short-term measure to treat haemorrhage until blood is available. They are rarely needed when shock is due to sodium and water depletion because, in these circumstances, the shock responds to water and electrolyte repletion; see also section 2.7.1 for the management of shock.

Plasma substitutes should **not** be used to maintain plasma volume in conditions such as burns or peritonitis where there is loss of plasma protein, water, and electrolytes over periods of several days or weeks. In these situations, plasma or plasma protein fractions containing large amounts of albumin should be given.

Large volumes of *some* plasma substitutes can increase the risk of bleeding through depletion of coagulation factors.

> Plasma and plasma substitutes are often used in very ill children whose condition is unstable. Therefore, close monitoring is required and fluid and electrolyte therapy should be adjusted according to the child's condition at all times.
>
> The use of plasma substitutes in children requires specialist supervision due to the risk of fluid overload; use is best restricted to an intensive care setting.

**Cautions**  Plasma substitutes should be used with caution in cardiac disease, liver disease, or renal impairment; urine output should be monitored. Care should be taken to avoid haematocrit concentration from falling below 25–30% and the child should be monitored for hypersensitivity reactions.

**Side-effects**  Hypersensitivity reactions may occur including, rarely, severe anaphylactic reactions. Transient increase in bleeding time may occur.

## GELATIN

**Note**  The gelatin is partially degraded

**Cautions**  see notes above

**Pregnancy**  manufacturer of *Geloplasma*® advises avoid at the end of pregnancy

**Side-effects**  see notes above

**Indications and dose**

> Low blood volume in hypovolaemic shock, burns and cardiopulmonary bypass
> • By intravenous infusion
>   Initially 10–20 mL/kg of a 3.5–4% solution (see notes above)

**Gelofusine**® (B. Braun) PoM
Intravenous infusion, succinylated gelatin (modified fluid gelatin, average molecular weight 30 000) 40 g (4%), Na⁺ 154 mmol, Cl⁻ 124 mmol/litre, net price 500-mL *Ecobag*® = £5.15; 1-litre *Ecobag*® = £9.67
Contains traces of calcium

**Geloplasma**® (Fresenius Kabi) PoM
Intravenous infusion, partially hydrolysed and succinylated gelatin (modified liquid gelatin) (as anhydrous gelatin) 30 g (3%), Na⁺ 150 mmol, K⁺ 5 mmol, Mg²⁺ 1.5 mmol, Cl⁻ 100 mmol, lactate 30 mmol/litre, net price 500-mL bag = £5.05

**Isoplex**® (Beacon) PoM
Intravenous infusion, succinylated gelatin (modified fluid gelatin, average molecular weight 30 000) 40 g (4%), Na⁺ 145 mmol, K⁺ 4 mmol, Mg²⁺ 0.9 mmol, Cl⁻ 105 mmol, lactate 25 mmol/litre, net price 500-mL bag = £7.53; 1-litre bag = £14.54

**Volplex**® (Beacon) PoM
Intravenous infusion, succinylated gelatin (modified fluid gelatin, average molecular weight 30 000) 40 g (4%), Na⁺ 154 mmol, Cl⁻ 125 mmol/litre, net price 500-mL bag = £4.70; 1-litre bag = £9.09

## ETHERIFIED STARCH

A starch composed of more than 90% of amylopectin that has been etherified with hydroxyethyl groups; the terms tetrastarch and pentastarch reflect the degree of etherification

**Cautions**  see notes above

**Renal impairment**  use with caution in mild to moderate impairment; avoid in severe impairment

**Side-effects**  see notes above; also pruritus, raised serum amylase

**Indications and dose**

> Low blood volume
> • By intravenous infusion
>   According to the child's condition (see notes above)

◢Pentastarch

**HAES-steril**® (Fresenius Kabi) PoM
Intravenous infusion, pentastarch (weight average molecular weight 200 000) 10% in sodium chloride intravenous infusion 0.9%, net price, 500 mL = £16.50

**Hemohes**® (B. Braun) PoM
Intravenous infusion, pentastarch (weight average molecular weight 200 000), net price (both in sodium chloride intravenous infusion 0.9%) 6%, 500 mL = £12.50; 10%, 500 mL = £16.50

◢Tetrastarch

**Tetraspan**® (B. Braun) PoM
Intravenous infusion, hydroxyethyl starch (weight average molecular weight 130 000) 6% in sodium chloride 0.625%, containing Na⁺ 140 mmol, K⁺ 4 mmol, Mg²⁺ 1 mmol, Cl⁻ 118 mmol, Ca²⁺ 2.5 mmol, acetate 24 mmol, malate 5 mmol/litre, net price 500-mL bag = £13.50

**Volulyte**® (Fresenius Kabi) PoM
Intravenous infusion, hydroxyethyl starch (weight average molecular weight 130 000) 6% in sodium chloride intravenous infusion 0.6%, containing Na⁺ 137 mmol, K⁺ 4 mmol, Mg²⁺ 1.5 mmol, Cl⁻ 110 mmol, acetate 34 mmol/litre, net price 500-mL bag = £13.50

**Voluven**® (Fresenius Kabi) PoM
Intravenous infusion, hydroxyethyl starch (weight average molecular weight 130 000) 6% in sodium chloride intravenous infusion 0.9%, net price 500-mL bag = £12.50

◢Hypertonic solution

**HyperHAES**® (Fresenius Kabi) PoM
Intravenous infusion, hydroxyethyl starch (weight average molecular weight 200 000) 6% in sodium chloride intravenous infusion 7.2%, net price 250-mL bag = £28.00
**Cautions**  see notes above; also diabetes

9

Nutrition and blood

# 9.3   Intravenous nutrition

When adequate feeding through the alimentary tract is not possible, nutrients may be given by intravenous infusion. This may be in addition to oral or enteral tube feeding—**supplemental parenteral nutrition**, or may be the sole source of nutrition—**total parenteral nutrition** (TPN). Complete enteral starvation is undesirable and total parenteral nutrition is a last resort.

Indications for parenteral nutrition include prematurity; severe or prolonged disorders of the gastro-intestinal tract; preparation of undernourished patients for surgery, chemotherapy, or radiation therapy; major surgery, trauma, or burns; prolonged coma or inability to eat; and some patients with renal or hepatic failure. The composition of proprietary preparations used in children is given in the table Proprietary Infusion Fluids for Parenteral Feeding, p. 469

Parenteral nutrition requires the use of a solution containing amino acids, glucose, lipids, electrolytes, trace elements, and vitamins. This is now commonly provided by the pharmacy in the form of an amino-acid, glucose, electrolyte bag, and a separate lipid infusion or, in older children a single 'all-in-one' bag. If the patient is able to take small amounts by mouth, vitamins may be given orally.

The nutrition solution is infused through a central venous catheter inserted under full surgical precautions. Alternatively, infusion through a peripheral vein may be used for supplementary as well as total parenteral nutrition, depending on the availability of peripheral veins; factors prolonging cannula life and preventing thrombophlebitis include the use of soft polyurethane paediatric cannulas and use of nutritional solutions of low osmolality and neutral pH. Nutritional fluids should be given by a dedicated intravenous line; if not possible, compatibility with any drugs or fluids should be checked as precipitation of components may occur. Extravasation of parenteral nutrition solution can cause severe tissue damage and injury; the infusion site should be regularly monitored.

Before starting intravenous nutrition the patient should be clinically stable and renal function and acid-base status should be assessed. Appropriate biochemical tests should have been carried out beforehand and serious deficits corrected. Nutritional and electrolyte status must be monitored throughout treatment. The nutritional components of parenteral nutrition regimens are usually increased gradually over a number of days to prevent metabolic complications and to allow metabolic adaptation to the infused nutrients. The solutions are usually infused over 24 hours but this may be gradually reduced if long-term nutrition is required. Home parenteral nutrition is usually infused over 12 hours overnight.

Complications of long-term parenteral nutrition include gall bladder sludging, gall stones, cholestasis and abnormal liver function tests. For details of the prevention and management of parenteral nutrition complications, specialist literature should be consulted.

**Protein** (nitrogen) is given as mixtures of essential and non-essential synthetic L-amino acids. Ideally, all essential amino acids should be included with a wide variety of non-essential ones to provide sufficient nitrogen together with electrolytes (see also section 9.2.2). Solutions vary in their composition of amino acids; they often contain an energy source (usually glucose) and electrolytes. Solutions for use in neonates and children under 1 year of age are based on the amino acid profile of umbilical cord blood (*Primene®*) or breast milk (*Vaminolact®*) and contain amino acids that are essential in this age group; these amino acids may not be present in sufficient quantities in preparations designed for older children and adults.

**Energy** requirements must be met if amino acids are to be utilised for tissue maintenance. An appropriate energy to protein ratio is essential and requirements will vary depending on the child's age and condition. A mixture of carbohydrate and fat energy sources (usually 30–50% as fat) gives better utilisation of amino acids than glucose alone.

**Glucose** is the preferred source of carbohydrate, but frequent monitoring of blood glucose is required particularly during initiation and build-up of the regimen; insulin may be necessary. Glucose above a concentration of 12.5% must be infused through a central venous catheter to avoid thrombosis; the maximum concentration of glucose that should normally be infused in fluid restricted children is 20–25%.

In parenteral nutrition regimens, it is necessary to provide adequate **phosphate** in order to allow phosphorylation of glucose and to prevent hypophosphataemia. Neonates, particularly preterm neonates, and young children also require phosphorus and calcium to ensure adequate bone mineralisation. The compatibility and solubility of calcium and phosphorus salts is complex and unpredictable; precipitation is a risk and specialist pharmacy advice should be sought.

**Fat** (lipid) emulsions have the advantages of a high energy to fluid volume ratio, neutral pH, and iso-osmolarity with plasma, and provide essential fatty acids. Several days of adaptation may be required to attain maximal utilisation. Reactions include occasional febrile episodes (usually only with 20% emulsions) and rare anaphylactic responses. Interference with biochemical measurements such as those for blood gases and calcium may occur if samples are taken before fat has been cleared. Regular monitoring of plasma cholesterol and triglyceride is necessary to ensure clearance from the plasma, particularly in conditions where fat metabolism may be disturbed e.g. infection. Emulsions containing 20% or 30% fat should be used in neonates as they are cleared more efficiently. **Additives should not be mixed with fat emulsions unless compatibility is known.**

**Electrolytes** are usually provided as the chloride salts of potassium and sodium. Acetate salts can be used to reduce the amount of chloride infused; hyperchloraemic acidosis or hypochloraemic alkalosis can occur in preterm neonates or children with renal impairment.

> **Administration.** Because of the complex requirements relating to parenteral nutrition full details relating to administration have been omitted. In all cases *specialist pharmacy advice, product literature and other specialist literature should be consulted.*

## Proprietary Infusion Fluids for Parenteral Feeding

| Preparation | Nitrogen g/litre | [1,2]Energy kJ/litre | Electrolytes mmol/litre | | | | | Other components/litre |
|---|---|---|---|---|---|---|---|---|
| | | | K$^+$ | Mg$^{2+}$ | Na$^+$ | Acet$^-$ | Cl$^-$ | |
| ClinOleic 20% (Baxter) Net price 100 mL = £6.28; 250 mL = £10.08; 500 mL = £13.88 | — | 8360 | — | — | — | — | — | purified olive and soya oil 200 g, glycerol 22.5 g, egg phosphatides 12 g |
| Glamin (Fresenius Kabi) Net price 250 mL = £14.58; 500 mL = £27.20 | 22.4 | — | — | — | — | 62 | — | |
| Intralipid 10% (Fresenius Kabi) Net price 100 mL = £4.70; 500 mL = £10.30 | — | 4600 | — | — | — | — | — | soya oil 100 g, glycerol 22 g, purified egg phospholipids 12 g, phosphate 15 mmol |
| Intralipid 20% (Fresenius Kabi) Net price 100 mL = £7.05; 250 mL = £11.60; 500 mL = £15.45 | — | 8400 | — | — | — | — | — | soya oil 200 g, glycerol 22 g, purified egg phospholipids 12 g, phosphate 15 mmol |
| Intralipid 30% (Fresenius Kabi) Net price 333 mL = £17.30 | — | 12600 | — | — | — | — | — | soya oil 300 g, glycerol 16.7 g, purified egg phospholipids 12 g, phosphate 15 mmol |
| Lipofundin MCT/LCT 10% (B. Braun) Net price 100 mL = £7.70; 500 mL = £12.90 | — | 4430 | — | — | — | — | — | soya oil 50 g, medium chain triglycerides 50 g |
| Lipofundin MCT/LCT 20% (B. Braun) Net price 100 mL = £12.51; 250 mL = £11.30; 500 mL = £19.18 | — | 8000 | — | — | — | — | — | soya oil 100 g, medium chain triglycerides 100 g |
| [3]Primene 10% (Baxter) Net price 100 mL = £5.78, 250 mL = £7.92 | 15 | — | — | — | — | — | 19 | |
| Synthamin 9 (Baxter) Net price 500 mL = £6.66; 1000 mL = £12.34 | 9.1 | — | 60 | 5 | 70 | 100 | 70 | acid phosphate 30 mmol |
| Synthamin 9 EF (electrolyte-free) (Baxter) Net price 500 mL = £6.66; 1000 mL = £12.34 | 9.1 | — | — | — | — | 44 | 22 | — |
| Vamin 9 Glucose (Fresenius Kabi) Net price 100 mL = £3.80; 500 mL = £7.70; 1000 mL = £13.40 | 9.4 | 1700 | 20 | 1.5 | 50 | — | 50 | Ca$^{2+}$ 2.5 mmol, anhydrous glucose 100 g |
| [3]Vaminolact (Fresenius Kabi) Net price 100 mL = £4.35; 500 mL = £10.00 | 9.3 | — | — | — | — | — | — | |

1. *Note*. 1000 kcal = 4200 kJ; 1000 kJ = 238.8 kcal. All entries are PoM
2. Excludes protein- or amino acid-derived energy
3. For use in neonates and children only

## Supplementary preparations

> Compatibility with the infusion solution must be ascertained before adding supplementary preparations.

**Addiphos**® (Fresenius Kabi) PoM
Solution, sterile, phosphate 40 mmol, K$^+$ 30 mmol, Na$^+$ 30 mmol/20 mL. For addition to *Vamin*® solutions and glucose intravenous infusions. Net price 20-mL vial = £1.53

**Additrace**® (Fresenius Kabi) PoM
Solution, trace elements for addition to *Vamin*® solutions and glucose intravenous infusions, traces of Fe$^{3+}$, Zn$^{2+}$, Mn$^{2+}$, Cu$^{2+}$, Cr$^{3+}$, Se$^{4+}$, Mo$^{6+}$, F$^-$, I$^-$. For children over 40 kg. Net price 10-mL amp = £2.31

**Cernevit**® (Baxter) PoM
Solution, *dl*-alpha tocopherol 11.2 units, ascorbic acid 125 mg, biotin 69 micrograms, colecalciferol 220 units, cyanocobalamin 6 micrograms, folic acid 414 micrograms, glycine 250 mg, nicotinamide 46 mg, pantothenic acid (as dexpanthenol) 17.25 mg, pyridoxine hydrochloride 5.5 mg, retinol (as palmitate) 3500 units, riboflavin (as dihydrated sodium phosphate) 4.14 mg, thiamine (as cocarboxylase tetrahydrate) 3.51 mg. Dissolve in 5 mL water for injections. Net price per vial = £4.64

**Decan**® (Baxter) PoM
Solution, trace elements for addition to infusion solutions, Fe$^{2+}$, Zn$^{2+}$, Cu$^{2+}$, Mn$^{2+}$, F$^-$, Co$^{2+}$ I$^-$, Se$^{4+}$, Mo$^{6+}$, Cr$^{3+}$. For children over 40 kg. Net price 40-mL vial = £2.00

**Dipeptiven®** (Fresenius Kabi) [PoM]
Solution, N(2)-L-alanyl-L-glutamine 200 mg/mL (providing L-alanine 82 mg, L-glutamine 134.6 mg). For addition to infusion solutions containing amino acids. Net price 50 mL = £16.40, 100 mL = £30.50
**Dose**
Amino acid supplement for hypercatabolic or hypermetabolic states
300–400 mg/kg daily; max. 400 mg/kg daily, dose not to exceed 20% of total amino acid intake

**Glycophos® Sterile Concentrate** (Fresenius Kabi) [PoM]
Solution, sterile, phosphate 20 mmol, Na+ 40 mmol/ 20 mL. For addition to *Vamin®* and *Vaminolact®* solutions, and glucose intravenous infusions. Net price 20-mL vial = £4.60

**Peditrace®** (Fresenius Kabi) [PoM]
Solution, trace elements for addition to *Vaminolact®*, *Vamin® 14 Electrolyte-Free* solutions and glucose intravenous infusions, traces of $Zn^{2+}$, $Cu^{2+}$, $Mn^{2+}$, $Se^{4+}$, $F^-$, $I^-$. For use in neonates (when kidney function established, usually second day of life), infants, and children. Net price 10-mL vial = £4.18
**Cautions** reduced biliary excretion especially in cholestatic liver disease or in markedly reduced urinary excretion (careful biochemical monitoring required); total parenteral nutrition exceeding 1 month (measure serum manganese concentration and check liver function before commencing treatment and regularly during treatment)—discontinue if manganese concentration raised or if cholestasis develops

**Solivito N®** (Fresenius Kabi) [PoM]
Solution, powder for reconstitution, biotin 60 micrograms, cyanocobalamin 5 micrograms, folic acid 400 micrograms, glycine 300 mg, nicotinamide 40 mg, pyridoxine hydrochloride 4.9 mg, riboflavin sodium phosphate 4.9 mg, sodium ascorbate 113 mg, sodium pantothenate 16.5 mg, thiamine mononitrate 3.1 mg. Dissolve in water for injections or glucose intravenous infusion for adding to glucose intravenous infusion or *Intralipid®*, dissolve in *Vitlipid N®* or *Intralipid®* for adding to *Intralipid®* only. Net price per vial = £2.32

**Vitlipid N®** (Fresenius Kabi) [PoM]
Emulsion, adult, vitamin A 330 units, ergocalciferol 20 units, dl-alpha tocopherol 1 unit, phytomenadione 15 micrograms/mL. For addition to *Intralipid®*. For adults and children over 11 years. Net price 10-mL amp = £2.32
Emulsion, infant, vitamin A 230 units, ergocalciferol 40 units, dl-alpha tocopherol 0.7 unit, phytomenadione 20 micrograms/mL. For addition to *Intralipid®*. Net price 10-mL amp = £2.32

## 9.4 Oral nutrition

9.4.1 Foods for special diets
9.4.2 Enteral nutrition

### 9.4.1 Foods for special diets

These are preparations that have been modified to eliminate a particular constituent from a food or that are nutrient mixtures formulated as food substitutes for children who either cannot tolerate or cannot metabolise certain common constituents of food.

**Coeliac disease** Intolerance to gluten in coeliac disease is managed by completely eliminating gluten from the diet. A range of gluten-free products is available for prescription—see Appendix 2 (p. 791).

**Phenylketonuria** Phenylketonuria (hyperphenylalaninaemia, PKU), which results from the inability to metabolise phenylalanine, is managed by restricting dietary intake of phenylalanine to a small amount sufficient for tissue building and repair.

**Aspartame** (used as a sweetener in some foods and medicines) contributes to the phenylalanine intake and may affect control of phenylketonuria. If alternatives are unavailable, children with phenylketonuria should not be denied access to appropriate medication; the amount of aspartame consumed can be taken in to account in the management of the condition. Where the presence of aspartame in a preparation is specified in the product literature, aspartame is listed as an excipient in the relevant product entry in *BNF for Children*; the child or carer should be informed of this.

For further information on special dietary products used in the management of metabolic diseases, see Appendix 2.

Some rare forms of phenylketonuria are caused by a deficiency of tetrahydrobiopterin. Treatment involves oral supplementation of **tetrahydrobiopterin**; in some severe cases, the addition of the neurotransmitter precursors, levodopa (section 4.9.1) and 5-hydroxytryptophan, is also necessary.

**Sapropterin**, a synthetic form of tetrahydrobiopterin, is licensed as an adjunct to dietary restriction of phenylalanine in the management of patients with phenylketonuria and tetrahydrobiopterin deficiency.

## TETRAHYDROBIOPTERIN

**Renal impairment** use with caution—accumulation of metabolites
**Pregnancy** crosses the placenta; use only if benefit outweighs risk
**Breast-feeding** present in milk, effects unknown
**Side-effects** diarrhoea, urinary frequency, disturbed sleep
**Licensed use** not licensed
**Indications and dose**
Monotherapy in tetrahydrobiopterin-sensitive phenylketonuria (specialist use only)
• By mouth
**Child 1 month–18 years** 10 mg/kg twice daily (total daily dose may alternatively be given in 3 divided doses), adjusted according to response

In combination with neurotransmitter precursors for tetrahydrobiopterin-sensitive phenylketonuria (specialist use only)
• By mouth
**Child 1 month–2 years** initially 250–750 micrograms/kg 4 times daily (total daily dose may alternatively be given in 3 divided doses), adjusted according to response; max. 7 mg/kg daily
**Child 2–18 years** initially 250–750 micrograms/kg 4 times daily (total daily dose may alternatively be given in 3 divided doses), adjusted according to response; usual max. 10 mg/kg daily

**Tetrahydrobiopterin** (Non-proprietary)
Tablets, tetrahydrobiopterin 10 mg and 50 mg
Available from 'special-order' manufacturers or specialist importing companies, see p. 823

---

# ▌ SAPROPTERIN DIHYDROCHLORIDE

**Note** Sapropterin is a synthetic form of tetrahydrobiopterin

**Cautions** monitor blood-phenylalanine concentration before and after first week of treatment—if unsatisfactory response increase dose at weekly intervals to max. dose and monitor blood-phenylalanine concentration weekly; discontinue treatment if unsatisfactory response after 1 month; monitor blood-phenylalanine and tyrosine concentrations 1–2 weeks after dose adjustment and during treatment; history of convulsions

**Hepatic impairment** manufacturer advises caution—no information available

**Renal impairment** manufacturer advises caution—no information available

**Pregnancy** manufacturer advises caution—consider only if strict dietary management inadequate

**Breast-feeding** manufacturer advises avoid—no information available

**Side-effects** diarrhoea, vomiting, abdominal pain, nasal congestion, cough, pharyngolaryngeal pain, headache; *also reported* hypersensitivity reactions

## Indications and dose

Phenylketonuria (specialist use only)

• **By mouth**

**Child 4–18 years** initially 10 mg/kg once daily, preferably in the morning, adjusted according to response; usual dose 5–20 mg/kg daily

Tetrahydrobiopterin deficiency (specialist use only)

• **By mouth**

**Neonate** initially 2–5 mg/kg once daily, preferably in the morning, adjusted according to response; max. 20 mg/kg daily; total daily dose may alternatively be given in 2–3 divided doses

**Child 1 month–18 years** initially 2–5 mg/kg once daily, preferably in the morning, adjusted according to response; max. 20 mg/kg daily; total daily dose may alternatively be given in 2–3 divided doses

**Kuvan®** (Merck Serono) [PoM]
Dispersible tablets, sapropterin dihydrochloride 100 mg, net price 30-tab pack = £597.22, 120-tab pack = £2388.88. Label: 13, 21, counselling, tablets should be dissolved in water and taken within 20 minutes

## 9.4.2 Enteral nutrition

Children have higher nutrient requirements per kg body-weight, different metabolic rates, and physiological responses compared to adults. They have low nutritional stores and are particularly vulnerable to growth and nutritional problems during critical periods of development. Major illness, operations, or trauma impose increased metabolic demands and can rapidly exhaust nutritional reserves.

Every effort should be made to optimise oral food intake before beginning enteral tube feeding; this may include change of posture, special seating, feeding equipment,

oral desensitisation, food texture changes, thickening of liquids, increasing energy density of food, treatment of reflux or oesophagitis, as well as using age-specific nutritional supplements.

Enteral tube feeding has a role in both short-term rehabilitation and long-term nutritional management in paediatrics. It can be used as supportive therapy, in which the enteral feed supplies a proportion of the required nutrients, or as primary therapy, in which the enteral feed delivers all the necessary nutrients. Most children receiving tube feeds should also be encouraged to take oral food and drink. Tube feeding should be considered in the following situations:

• unsafe swallowing and risk of aspiration;

• inability to consume at least 60% of energy needs by mouth;

• total feeding time of more than 4 hours per day;

• weight loss or no weight gain for a period of 3 months (less for younger children and infants);

• weight for height (or length) less than 2nd percentile for age and sex.

Most feeds for enteral use (Appendix 2) contain protein derived from cows' milk or soya. Elemental feeds containing protein hydrolysates or free amino acids can be used for children who have diminished ability to break down protein, for example in inflammatory bowel disease or pancreatic insufficiency.

Even when nutritionally complete feeds are given, water and electrolyte balance should be monitored. Haematological and biochemical parameters should also be monitored, particularly in the clinically unstable child. Extra minerals (e.g. magnesium and zinc) may be needed in patients where gastro-intestinal secretions are being lost. Additional vitamins may also be needed. Feeds containing vitamin K may affect the INR in children receiving warfarin—see **interactions**: Appendix 1 (vitamins).

Choosing the best formula for children depends on several factors including: nutritional requirements, gastro-intestinal function, underlying disease, nutrient restrictions, age, and feed characteristics (nutritional composition, viscosity, osmolality, availability and cost). Children have specific dietary requirements and in many situations liquid feeds prepared for adults are totally unsuitable and should not be given. Expert advice from a dietician should be sought before prescribing enteral feeds for a child.

**Infant formula feeds** Child 0–12 months. Term infants with normal gastro-intestinal function are given either breast milk or normal infant formula during the first year of life. The average intake is between 150 mL and 200 mL/kg/day. Infant milk formulas are based on whey- or casein-dominant protein, lactose with or without maltodextrin, amylose, vegetable oil and milk fat. The composition of all normal and soya infant formulas have to meet The Infant Formula and Follow-on Formula Regulations (England and Wales) 2007, which enact the European Community Regulations 2006/141/EC; the composition of other enteral and specialist feeds has to meet the Commission Directive (1999/21/EC) on Dietary Foods for Special Medical Purposes.

A high-energy feed (Appendix 2, p. 764), which contains 9–11% of energy derived from protein can be used for infants who fail to grow adequately. Alternatively,

9

Nutrition and blood

energy supplements (Appendix 2, p. 785) may be added to normal infant formula to achieve a higher energy content (but this will reduce the protein to energy ratio) or the normal infant formula concentration may be increased slightly. Care should be taken not to present an osmotic load of more than 500 milliosmols/kg water to the normal functioning gut, otherwise osmotic diarrhoea will result. Concentrating or supplementing feeds should not be attempted without the advice of a paediatric dietician.

### Enteral feeds

**Child 1–6 years (body–weight 8–20 kg).** Ready-to-use feeds (Appendix 2, p. 764) based on caseinates, maltodextrin and vegetable oils (with or without added medium chain triglyceride (MCT) oil or fibre) are well tolerated and effective in improving nutritional status in this age group. Although originally designed for children 1–6 years (body–weight 8–20 kg), some products have ACBS approval for use in children weighing up to 30 kg (approx. 10 years of age). Enteral feeds formulated for children 1–6 years are low in sodium and potassium; electrolyte intake and biochemical status should be monitored. Older children in this age range taking small feed volumes may need to be given additional micronutrients. Fibre-enriched feeds may be helpful for children with chronic constipation or diarrhoea.

**Child 7–12 years (body-weight 21–45 kg).** Depending on age, weight, clinical condition and nutritional requirements, ready-to-use feeds (Appendix 2, p. 764) formulated for 7–12 year olds may be given at appropriate rates.

**Child over 12 years (body-weight over 45 kg).** As there are no standard enteral feeds formulated for this age group, adult formulations are used. The intake of protein, electrolytes, vitamins, and trace minerals should be carefully assessed and monitored.

**Note** Adult feeds containing more than 6 g/100 mL protein or 2 g/100 mL fibre should be used with caution and expert advice.

### Specialised formula

It is essential that any infant who is intolerant of breast milk or normal infant formula, or whose condition requires nutrient-specific adaptation, is prescribed an adequate volume of a nutritionally complete replacement formula (see Appendix 2, p. 776). In the first 4 months of life, a volume of 150–200 mL/kg/day is recommended. After 6 months, should the formula still be required, a volume of 600 mL/day should be maintained, in addition to solid food.

**Products for cow's milk protein intolerance or lactose intolerance.** There are a number of infant formulas formulated for cow's milk protein intolerance or lactose intolerance; these feeds may contain a residual amount of lactose (less than 1 g/100 mL formula)—sometimes described as clinically lactose-free or 'lactose-free' by manufacturers. If the total daily intake of these formulas is low, it may be necessary to supplement with calcium, and a vitamin and mineral supplement.

**Soya-based** infant formulas have a high phytoestrogen content and this may be a long-term reproductive health risk. The Chief Medical Officer has advised that soya-based infant formulas should not be used as the first choice for the management of infants with proven cow's milk sensitivity, lactose intolerance, galactokinase deficiency and galactosaemia. Most UK paediatricians with expertise in inherited metabolic disease still advocate soya-based formulations for infants with galactosaemia as there are concerns about the residual lactose content of low lactose formulas and protein hydrolysates based on cow's milk protein.

**Low lactose** infant formulations, based on whole cow's milk protein, are unsuitable for children with cow's milk protein intolerance. Liquid soya milks purchased from supermarkets and health food stores are not nutritionally complete and should never be used for infants under 1 year of age.

**Protein hydrolysate formulas.** Non-milk, peptide-based feeds containing hydrolysates of casein, whey, meat and soya protein, are suitable for infants with disaccharide or whole protein intolerance. The total daily intake of electrolytes, vitamins and minerals should be carefully assessed and modified to meet the child's nutritional requirements; these feeds have a high osmolality when given at recommended dilution and need gradual and careful introduction.

**Elemental (amino acid based formula).** Specially formulated elemental feeds containing essential and non-essential amino acids are available for use in infants and children under 6 years with proven whole protein intolerance. Adult elemental formula may be used for children over 6 years; the intake of electrolytes, vitamins and minerals should be carefully assessed and modified to meet nutritional requirements. These feeds have a high osmolality when given at the recommended concentration and therefore need gradual and careful introduction.

**Modular feeds.** Modular feeds (see Specialised Formulas for Specific Clinical Conditions, p. 781) are based on individual protein, fat, carbohydrate, vitamin and mineral components or modules which can be combined to meet the specific needs of a child. Modular feeds are used when nutritionally complete specialised formula are not tolerated, or if the fluid and nutrient requirements change e.g. in gastro-intestinal, renal or liver disease. The main advantage of modular feeds is their flexibility; disadvantages include their complexity and preparation difficulties. Modular feeds should not be used without the supervision of a paediatric dietician.

**Specialised formula.** Highly specialised formulas are designed to meet the specific requirements in various clinical conditions such as renal and liver diseases. When using these formulas, both the biochemical status of the child and their growth parameters need to be monitored.

### Feed thickeners

**Carob based thickeners** (Appendix 2, p. 791) may be used to thicken feeds for infants under 1 year with significant gastro-oesophageal reflux. Breast-fed infants can be given the thickener mixed to a paste with water or breast-milk prior to feeds.

**Pre-thickened formula** Milk-protein- or casein-dominant infant formula, which contains small quantities of pre-gelatinized starch, is recommended primarily for infants with mild gastro-oesophageal reflux. Pre-thickened formula is prepared in the same way as normal infant formula and flows through a standard teat. The feeds do not thicken on standing but thicken in the stomach when exposed to acid pH.

**Starched based thickeners** can be used to thicken liquids and feeds for children over 1 year of age with dysphagia.

### Dietary supplements for oral use

(Appendix 2, p. 769) Three types of prescribable fortified dietary supplements are available: fortified milk and non-milk tasting (juice-style) drinks, and fortified milk-based semi-solid preparations. The recommended daily quantity is age-dependent. The following is a useful guide: 1–2 years, 200 kcal (840 kJ); 3–5 years, 400 kcal (1680 kJ); 6–11 years, 600 kcal (2520 kJ); and over 12 years, 800 kcal (3360 kJ). Supplements containing 1.5 kcal/mL are high in protein and should not be used for children under 3 years of age. Many supplements are high in sugar or maltodextrin; care should be taken to prevent prolonged contact with teeth. Ideally supplements should be administered after meals or at bedtime so as not to affect appetite.

**Products for metabolic diseases**　There is a large range of disease-specific infant formulas and amino acid-based supplements available for use in children with metabolic diseases (see under specific metabolic diseases, Appendix 2, p. 795). Some of these formulas are nutritionally incomplete and supplementation with vitamins and other nutrients may be necessary. Many of the product names are similar; to prevent metabolic complications in children who cannot tolerate specific amino acids it is important to ensure the correct supplement is supplied.

**Preparations (Borderline substances)**　See Appendix 2.

# 9.5　Minerals

### 9.5.1　Calcium and magnesium
### 9.5.2　Phosphorus
### 9.5.3　Fluoride
### 9.5.4　Zinc

See section 9.1.1 for iron salts.

## 9.5.1　Calcium and magnesium

### 9.5.1.1　Calcium supplements
### 9.5.1.2　Hypercalcaemia and hypercalciuria
### 9.5.1.3　Magnesium

### 9.5.1.1　Calcium supplements

Calcium supplements are usually only required where dietary calcium intake is deficient. This dietary requirement varies with age and is relatively greater in childhood, pregnancy, and lactation, due to an increased demand. Hypocalcaemia may be caused by vitamin D deficiency (section 9.6.4), impaired metabolism, a failure of secretion (hypoparathyroidism), or resistance to parathyroid hormone (pseudohypoparathyroidism).

*Mild asymptomatic hypocalcaemia* may be managed with oral calcium supplements. *Severe symptomatic hypocalcaemia* requires an intravenous infusion of calcium gluconate 10% over 5 to 10 minutes, repeating the dose if symptoms persist; in exceptional cases it may be necessary to maintain a continuous calcium infusion over a day or more. Calcium chloride injection is also available, but is more irritant; care should be taken to prevent extravasation.

For the role of calcium gluconate in temporarily reducing the toxic effects of *hyperkalaemia*, see p. 459.

Persistent hypocalcaemia requires oral calcium supplements and either a vitamin D analogue (alfacalcidol or

calcitriol) for hypoparathyroidism and pseudohypoparathyroidism or natural vitamin D (calciferol) if due to vitamin D deficiency (section 9.6.4). It is important to monitor plasma and urinary calcium during long-term maintenance therapy.

**Neonates**　Hypocalcaemia is common in the first few days of life, particularly following birth asphyxia or respiratory distress. Late onset at 4–10 days after birth may be secondary to vitamin D deficiency, hypoparathyroidism or hypomagnesaemia and may be associated with seizures.

## ▌CALCIUM SALTS

**Cautions**　see notes above; sarcoidosis; history of nephrolithiasis; avoid calcium chloride in respiratory acidosis or respiratory failure; **interactions**: Appendix 1 (antacids, calcium salts)

**Contra-indications**　conditions associated with hypercalcaemia and hypercalciuria (e.g. some forms of malignant disease); see also Calcium Gluconate injection, p. 474

**Renal impairment**　use with caution; risk of hypercalcaemia and renal calculi

**Side-effects**　*rarely* gastro-intestinal disturbances; *with injection*, bradycardia, arrhythmias, peripheral vasodilatation, fall in blood pressure, sweating, injection-site reactions, severe tissue damage with extravasation

**Indications and dose**

See notes above; calcium deficiency
- By mouth

**Neonate** 0.25 mmol/kg 4 times a day, adjusted to response

**Child 1 month–4 years** 0.25 mmol/kg 4 times a day, adjusted to response

**Child 5–12 years** 0.2 mmol/kg 4 times a day, adjusted to response

**Child 12–18 years** 10 mmol 4 times a day, adjusted to response

Acute hypocalcaemia, urgent correction; hyperkalaemia (prevention of arrhythmias)
- By slow intravenous injection over 5–10 minutes

**Neonate** 0.11 mmol/kg (0.5 mL/kg of calcium gluconate 10%) as a single dose. [Some units use a dose of 0.46 mmol/kg (2 mL/kg calcium gluconate 10%) for hypocalcaemia in line with US practice]

**Child 1 month–18 years** 0.11 mmol/kg (0.5 mL/kg calcium gluconate 10%), max 4.5 mmol (20 mL calcium gluconate 10%)

Acute hypocalcaemia, maintenance
- By continuous intravenous infusion

**Neonate** 0.5 mmol/kg daily over 24 hours, adjusted to response, use oral route as soon as possible due to risk of extravasation

**Child 1 month–2 years** 1 mmol/kg daily (usual max 8.8 mmol) over 24 hours, use oral route as soon as possible due to risk of extravasation

**Child 2–18 years** 8.8 mmol over 24 hours, use oral route as soon as possible due to risk of extravasation

◢Oral preparations

**Calcium Gluconate** (Non-proprietary)

Effervescent tablets, calcium gluconate 1 g (calcium 89 mg or Ca²⁺ 2.23 mmol), net price 28-tab pack = £14.83. Label: 13

Note Each tablet usually contains 4.46 mmol Na⁺

**Calcium Lactate** (Non-proprietary)

Tablets, calcium lactate 300 mg (calcium 39 mg or Ca²⁺ 1 mmol), net price 84 = £2.92

**Adcal**® (ProStrakan)

Chewable tablets, fruit flavour, calcium carbonate 1.5 g (calcium 600 mg or Ca²⁺ 15 mmol), net price 100-tab pack = £7.25. Label: 24

**Cacit**® (Warner Chilcott)

Tablets, effervescent, pink, calcium carbonate 1.25 g, providing calcium citrate when dispersed in water (calcium 500 mg or Ca²⁺ 12.5 mmol), net price 76-tab pack = £11.81. Label: 13

**Calcichew**® (Shire)

Tablets (chewable), orange flavour, calcium carbonate 1.25 g (calcium 500 mg or Ca²⁺ 12.5 mmol), net price 100-tab pack = £9.33. Label: 24

Forte tablets (chewable), orange flavour, scored, calcium carbonate 2.5 g (calcium 1 g or Ca²⁺ 25 mmol), net price 60-tab pack = £13.16. Label: 24

Excipients include aspartame (section 9.4.1)

**Calcium-500** (Martindale)

Tablets, pink, f/c, calcium carbonate 1.25 g (calcium 500 mg or Ca²⁺ 12.5 mmol), net price 100-tab pack = £9.46. Label: 25

**Calcium-Sandoz**® (Alliance)

Syrup, orange flavour, calcium glubionate 1.09 g, calcium lactobionate 727 mg (calcium 108.3 mg or Ca²⁺ 2.7 mmol)/5 mL, net price 300 mL = £4.07

**Sandocal**® (Novartis Consumer Health)

Sandocal 1000 tablets, effervescent, orange flavour, calcium lactate gluconate 2.263 g, calcium carbonate 1.75 g, providing 1 g calcium (Ca²⁺ 25 mmol), net price 3 × 10-tab pack = £6.17. Label: 13

Excipients include aspartame (section 9.4.1)

◢Parenteral preparations

**Calcium Gluconate** (Non-proprietary) [PoM]

Injection, calcium gluconate 10% (Ca²⁺ approx. 225 micromol/mL). Net price 10-mL amp = 60p

Administration For *intravenous infusion* dilute to at least 45 micromol/mL with Glucose 5% *or* Sodium Chloride 0.9%. Maximum administration rate 45 micromol/kg/hour (or in neonates max. 22 micromol/kg/hour). May be given more concentrated via a central venous catheter. May be used undiluted (10% calcium gluconate) in emergencies. Avoid extravasation; should not be given by intramuscular injection. Incompatible with sodium bicarbonate and phosphate solutions.

Note The MHRA has advised that repeated or prolonged administration of calcium gluconate injection packaged in 10 mL *glass* containers is contra-indicated in children under 18 years and in patients with renal impairment owing to the risk of aluminium accumulation; in these patients the use of calcium gluconate injection packaged in *plastic* containers is recommended

**Calcium Chloride** (Non-proprietary) [PoM]

Injection, calcium chloride dihydrate 10% (calcium 27.3 mg or Ca²⁺ 680 micromol/mL), net price 10-mL disposable syringe = £5.10

Brands include *Minijet*® *Calcium Chloride 10%*

Injection, calcium chloride dihydrate 13.4% (calcium 36 mg or Ca²⁺ 910 micromol/mL), net price 10–mL amp = £14.94

◢With vitamin D

Section 9.6.4

### 9.5.1.2 Hypercalcaemia and hypercalciuria

**Severe hypercalcaemia** Severe hypercalcaemia calls for urgent treatment before detailed investigation of the cause. Dehydration should be corrected first with intravenous infusion of **sodium chloride 0.9%**. Drugs (such as thiazides and vitamin D compounds) which promote hypercalcaemia, should be discontinued and dietary calcium should be restricted.

If *severe hypercalcaemia persists* drugs which inhibit mobilisation of calcium from the skeleton may be required. The bisphosphonates are useful and disodium pamidronate (section 6.6.2) is probably the most effective.

**Corticosteroids** (section 6.3) are widely given, but may only be useful where hypercalcaemia is due to sarcoidosis or vitamin D intoxication; they often take several days to achieve the desired effect.

**Calcitonin** (section 6.6.1) can be used by specialists for the treatment of hypercalcaemia associated with malignancy; it is rarely effective where bisphosphonates have failed to reduce serum calcium adequately.

After treatment of severe hypercalcaemia the underlying cause must be established. *Further treatment* is governed by the same principles as for initial therapy. Salt and water depletion and drugs promoting hypercalcaemia should be avoided; oral administration of a bisphosphonate may be useful. Parathyroidectomy may be indicated for hyperparathyroidism.

**Hypercalciuria** Hypercalciuria should be investigated for an underlying cause, which should be treated. Reducing dietary calcium intake may be beneficial but severe restriction of calcium intake has not proved beneficial and may even be harmful.

### 9.5.1.3 Magnesium

Magnesium is an essential constituent of many enzyme systems, particularly those involved in energy generation; the largest stores are in the skeleton.

Magnesium salts are not well absorbed from the gastro-intestinal tract, which explains the use of magnesium sulfate (section 1.6.4) as an osmotic laxative.

Magnesium is excreted mainly by the kidneys and is therefore retained in renal failure, but significant *hypermagnesaemia* (causing muscle weakness and arrhythmias) is rare.

**Hypomagnesaemia** Since magnesium is secreted in large amounts in the gastro-intestinal fluid, excessive losses in diarrhoea, stoma or fistula are the most common causes of *hypomagnesaemia*; deficiency may also occur as a result of treatment with certain drugs. Hypomagnesaemia often causes secondary hypocalcaemia (with which it may be confused), particularly in neonates, and also hypokalaemia and hyponatraemia.

Symptomatic *hypomagnesaemia* is associated with a deficit of 0.5–1 mmol/kg. Magnesium is given initially by intravenous infusion or by intramuscular injection of **magnesium sulfate**; the intramuscular injection is painful. Plasma magnesium concentration should be measured to determine the rate and duration of infusion and the dose should be reduced in renal impairment. To prevent *recurrence of the deficit*, magnesium may be given by mouth in divided doses, but there is limited evidence of benefit. For maintenance (e.g. in intravenous nutrition), parenteral doses of magnesium are of the order of 0.2–0.4 mmol/kg (usual max. 20 mmol) $Mg^{2+}$ daily.

**Arrhythmias** Magnesium sulfate injection has also been recommended for the emergency treatment of *serious arrhythmias*, especially in the presence of hypokalaemia (when hypomagnesaemia may also be present) and when salvos of rapid ventricular tachycardia show the characteristic twisting wave front known as *torsade de pointes* (see also section 2.3.1).

## MAGNESIUM SULFATE

**Note** Magnesium Sulfate Injection BP is a sterile solution of Magnesium Sulfate Heptahydrate

**Cautions** see notes above; in severe hypomagnesaemia administer initially via controlled infusion device (preferably syringe pump); monitor blood pressure, respiratory rate, urinary output and for signs of overdosage (loss of patellar reflexes, weakness, nausea, sensation of warmth, flushing, drowsiness, double vision, and slurred speech); **interactions:** Appendix 1 (magnesium, parenteral)

**Hepatic impairment** avoid in hepatic coma if risk of renal failure

**Renal impairment** avoid or reduce dose; increased risk of toxicity

**Pregnancy** sufficient may cross the placenta in mothers treated with high doses e.g. in pre-eclampsia, causing hypotonia and respiratory depression in newborns

**Side-effects** generally associated with hypermagnesaemia, nausea, vomiting, thirst, flushing of skin, hypotension, arrhythmias, coma, respiratory depression, drowsiness, confusion, loss of tendon reflexes, muscle weakness

**Indications and dose**

Neonatal hypocalcaemia

• By deep intramuscular injection or intravenous infusion

    **Neonate** 0.4 mmol/kg $Mg^{2+}$ (100 mg/kg magnesium sulfate heptahydrate) 12 hourly for 2–3 doses

Hypomagnesaemia

• By intravenous injection over at least 10 minutes

    **Neonate** 0.4 mmol/kg $Mg^{2+}$ (100 mg/kg magnesium sulfate heptahydrate) 6–12 hourly as necessary

    **Child 1 month–12 years** 0.2 mmol/kg $Mg^{2+}$ (50 mg/kg magnesium sulfate heptahydrate) 12 hourly as necessary

    **Child 12–18 years** 4 mmol $Mg^{2+}$ (1 g magnesium sulfate heptahydrate) 12 hourly as necessary

Torsade de pointes (consult local guidelines)

• By intravenous injection over 10–15 minutes

    **Child 1 month–18 years** 0.1–0.2 mmol/kg (25–50 mg/kg magnesium sulfate heptahydrate); max. 8 mmol (2 g magnesium sulfate heptahydrate); dose repeated once if necessary

Persistent pulmonary hypertension section 2.5.1

Severe acute asthma section 3.1

**Administration** Dilute to 10% (100 mg magnesium sulfate heptahydrate in 1 mL) with Glucose 5 *or* 10%, Sodium Chloride 0.45 *or* 0.9% *or* Glucose and Sodium Chloride combinations. Up to 20% solution may be given in fluid restriction. Rate of administration should not exceed 10 mg/kg/minute of magnesium sulfate heptahydrate

**Note** Magnesium sulfate heptahydrate 1 g equivalent to $Mg^{2+}$ approx. 4 mmol

**Magnesium Sulfate Injection, BP** (Non-proprietary) [PoM]

Injection, magnesium sulfate heptahydrate 20% ($Mg^{2+}$ approx. 0.8 mmol/mL), net price 20-mL (4-g) amp = £2.75; 50% ($Mg^{2+}$ approx. 2 mmol/mL), 2-mL (1-g) amp = £2.39, 4-mL (2-g) prefilled syringe = £7.39; 5-mL (2.5-g) amp = £3.00, 10-mL (5-g) amp = 69p; 10-mL (5-g) prefilled syringe = £4.95

**Brands include** Minijet® Magnesium Sulfate Injection BP 50%

**Note** The BP directs that the label states the strength as the % w/v of magnesium sulfate heptahydrate and the approximate concentration of magnesium ions ($Mg^{2+}$) in mmol/mL

## MAGNESIUM-L-ASPARTATE

**Cautions** see under Magnesium Sulfate

**Renal impairment** avoid or reduce dose; increased risk of toxicity

**Side-effects** see under Magnesium Sulfate; also diarrhoea

**Licensed use** classified as a Food for Special Medical Purposes for use in children over 2 years

**Indications and dose**

Hypomagnesaemia (but see notes above)

• By mouth

    **Child 1 month–2 years** initially 0.2 mmol/kg of $Mg^{2+}$ 3 times daily dissolved in water, dose adjusted as required

    **Child 2–10 years** half a sachet (5 mmol $Mg^{2+}$) daily dissolved in 100 mL of water, dose adjusted as required

    **Child 10–18 years** one sachet (10 mmol $Mg^{2+}$) daily dissolved in 200 mL of water, dose adjusted as required

**Magnaspartate®** (KoRa)

Oral powder, magnesium-L-aspartate 6.5 g (10 mmol $Mg^{2+}$)/sachet, net price 10-sachet pack = £7.95

**Excipients** include sucrose

## MAGNESIUM GLYCEROPHOSPHATE

**Cautions** see under Magnesium Sulfate

**Renal impairment** avoid or reduce dose; increased risk of toxicity

**Side-effects**   see under Magnesium Sulfate; also diarrhoea

**Licensed use**   not licensed

**Indications and dose**

> Hypomagnesaemia (but see notes above)
>
> • By mouth
>
>> **Child 1 month–12 years** initially 0.2 mmol/kg $Mg^{2+}$ 3 times daily, dose adjusted as required
>>
>> **Child 12–18 years** initially 4–8 mmol $Mg^{2+}$ 3 times daily, dose adjusted as required

**Administration**   tablets may be dispersed in water

**Magnesium Glycerophosphate** (Non-proprietary)

Tablets, magnesium glycerophosphate 1 g (approximately magnesium 97 mg or $Mg^{2+}$ 4 mmol)
Available from 'special-order' manufacturers or specialist importing companies, see p. 823

Liquid, magnesium glycerophosphate 250 mg/mL (approximately magnesium 24.25 mg or $Mg^{2+}$ 1 mmol/mL)
Available from 'special-order' manufacturers or specialist importing companies, see p. 823

## 9.5.2  Phosphorus

### 9.5.2.1  Phosphate supplements
### 9.5.2.2  Phosphate-binding agents

### 9.5.2.1  Phosphate supplements

Oral phosphate supplements may be required in addition to vitamin D in children with hypophosphataemic vitamin D-resistant rickets (section 9.6.4). Diarrhoea is a common side-effect and should prompt a reduction in dosage.

Phosphate infusion is occasionally needed in phosphate deficiency arising from use of parenteral nutrition deficient in phosphate supplements; phosphate depletion also occurs in severe diabetic ketoacidosis. It is difficult to provide detailed guidelines for the treatment of *severe hypophosphatemia* because the extent of total body deficits and response to therapy are difficult to predict. High doses of phosphate may result in a transient serum elevation followed by redistribution into intracellular compartments or bone tissue; excessive doses may cause hypocalcaemia and metastatic calcification. It is essential to monitor plasma concentrations of calcium, phosphate, potassium and other electrolytes. It is recommended that severe hypophosphataemia be treated intravenously as large doses of oral phosphate may cause diarrhoea; intestinal absorption may be unreliable and dose adjustment may be necessary.

Phosphate is not the first choice for the treatment of hypercalcaemia because of the risk of precipitation of calcium phosphate in the kidney and other tissues. If used, the child should be well hydrated and electrolytes monitored.

**Neonates**   Phosphate deficiency may occur in very low-birthweight infants and may compromise bone growth if not corrected. Parenterally fed infants may be at risk of phosphate deficiency due to the limited solubility of phosphate. Some units routinely supplement expressed breast milk with phosphate, although the effect on the osmolality of the milk should be considered.

## ▮ PHOSPHATE

**Cautions**   see notes above, also cardiac disease, diabetes mellitus, dehydration; avoid extravasation with parenteral forms, severe tissue necrosis; sodium and potassium concentrations of preparations

**Renal impairment**   reduce dose; monitor closely

**Side-effects**   nausea, diarrhoea; hypotension, oedema; hypocalcaemia; acute renal failure; phlebitis; tissue necrosis on extravasation

**Indications and dose**

> Hypophosphataemia, including hypophosphataemic rickets and osteomalacia (see notes above)
>
> • By mouth
>
>> **Neonate** 1 mmol/kg daily in 1–2 divided doses, or as a supplement in breast milk
>>
>> **Child 1 month–5 years** 2–3 mmol/kg (max. 48 mmol) phosphate daily in 2–4 divided doses, adjusted as necessary
>>
>> **Child 5–18 years** 2–3 mmol/kg (max. 97 mmol) phosphate daily in 2–4 divided doses, adjusted as necessary
>>
>> Administration Caution, solubility in breast milk is limited to 1.2 mmol in 100 mL if calcium also added, contact pharmacy department for details
>
> • By intravenous infusion (see notes above, administration below, and seek specialist advice)
>
>> **Neonate** 1 mmol/kg phosphate daily, adjusted as necessary
>>
>> **Child 1 month–2 years** 0.7 mmol/kg phosphate daily, adjusted as necessary
>>
>> **Child 2–18 years** 0.4 mmol/kg phosphate daily, adjusted as necessary
>>
>> Administration (see also Important, below) Dilute injection with Sodium Chloride 0.9% or 0.45% *or* Glucose 5% or 10%. Administration rate of phosphate should not exceed 0.05 mmol/kg/hour. In emergencies in intensive care faster rates may be used—seek specialist advice

---

**Important**

Some phosphate injection preparations also contain potassium. For peripheral intravenous administration the *concentration* of potassium should not usually exceed 40 mmol/litre. The infusion solution should be **thoroughly mixed**. Local policies on avoiding inadvertent use of potassium concentrate should be followed. The potassium content of some phosphate preparations may also limit the *rate* at which they may be administered, see section 9.2.2.1.

---

**◢ Oral**

**Phosphate-Sandoz®** (HK Pharma)

Tablets, effervescent, anhydrous sodium acid phosphate 1.936 g, sodium bicarbonate 350 mg, potassium bicarbonate 315 mg, equivalent to phosphorus 500 mg (phosphate 16.1 mmol), sodium 468.8 mg ($Na^+$ 20.4 mmol), potassium 123 mg ($K^+$ 3.1 mmol). Net price 20 = £3.29. Label: 13

**◢ Injection**

**Phosphates** (Fresenius Kabi) [PoM]

Intravenous infusion, phosphates (providing phosphate 100 mmol/litre, potassium 19 mmol/litre, sodium 162 mmol/litre), net price 500 mL (*Polyfusor®*) = £3.75.

**Potassium acid phosphate** (Non-proprietary) PoM
Injection, 13.6% (1 mmol/mL phosphate, 1 mmol/mL potassium) 10 mL ampoule
Note See also Important, p. 476

**Dipotassium hydrogen phosphate** (Non-proprietary) PoM
Injection, 17.42% (1 mmol/mL phosphate and 2 mmol/mL potassium) 10 mL ampoule
Note See also Important, p. 476

**Disodium hydrogen phosphate** (Non-proprietary) PoM
Injection, 17.42% (0.6 mmol/mL phosphate and 1.2 mmol/mL sodium) 10 mL ampoule

### 9.5.2.2 Phosphate-binding agents

Calcium-containing preparations are used as phosphate-binding agents in the management of hyperphosphataemia complicating renal failure. Aluminium-containing preparations are rarely used as phosphate-binding agents and can cause aluminium accumulation.

**Sevelamer hydrochloride** is licensed for the treatment of hyperphosphataemia in adults on haemodialysis or peritoneal dialysis. Although experience is limited in children sevelamer may be useful when hypercalcaemia prevents the use of calcium carbonate.

### ALUMINIUM HYDROXIDE

**Cautions** see notes above; **interactions**: Appendix 1 (antacids)

**Side-effects** constipation; hyperaluminaemia

**Alu-Cap®** (Meda)
Capsules, green/red, dried aluminium hydroxide 475 mg (low Na+), net price 120-cap pack = £3.75
Dose

Hyperphosphataemia

• By mouth

Child 5–12 years 1–2 capsules 3–4 times daily, adjusted as necessary

Child 12–18 years 1–5 capsules 3–4 times daily, adjusted as necessary

### CALCIUM SALTS

**Cautions** interactions: Appendix 1 (antacids, calcium salts)

**Contra-indications** hypercalcaemia, hypercalciuria

**Side-effects** hypercalcaemia

**Indications and dose**

Phosphate binding in renal failure and hyperphosphataemia

• By mouth

Child 1 month–1 year 120 mg calcium carbonate 3–4 times daily with feeds, adjusted as necessary

Child 1–6 years 300 mg calcium carbonate 3–4 times daily prior to or with meals, adjusted as necessary

Child 6–12 years 600 mg calcium carbonate 3–4 times daily prior to or with meals, adjusted as necessary

Child 12–18 years 1.25 g calcium carbonate 3–4 times daily prior to or with meals, adjusted as necessary

**Adcal®**
Section 9.5.1.1

**Calcichew®**
Section 9.5.1.1

**Calcium-500**
Section 9.5.1.1

**Phosex®** (Pharmacosmos)
Tablets, yellow, scored, calcium acetate 1 g (calcium 250 mg or Ca²⁺ 6.2 mmol), net price 180-tab pack = £19.79. Counselling, tablets can be broken to aid swallowing but not chewed (bitter taste), take with meals
Dose

Phosphate-binding agent (with meals) in renal failure, according to the requirements of the patient

### SEVELAMER HYDROCHLORIDE

**Cautions** gastro-intestinal disorders; **interactions**: Appendix 1 (sevelamer)

**Contra-indications** bowel obstruction

**Pregnancy** manufacturer advises use only if potential benefit outweighs risk

**Breast-feeding** manufacturer advises use only if potential benefit outweighs risk

**Side-effects** nausea, vomiting, abdominal pain, constipation, diarrhoea, dyspepsia, flatulence; *very rarely* intestinal obstruction; *also reported* intestinal perforation, ileus, diverticulitis, pruritus, and rash

**Licensed use** not licensed for use in children under 18 years

**Indications and dose**

Hyperphosphataemia in patients on haemodialysis or peritoneal dialysis

• By mouth

Child 12–18 years initially 0.8–1.6 g 3 times daily with meals, then adjusted according to plasma-phosphate concentration

**Renagel®** (Sanofi-Aventis) PoM
Tablets, f/c, sevelamer hydrochloride 800 mg, net price 180-tab pack = £117.97. Label: 25, counselling, with meals
Excipients include propylene glycol (see Excipients, p. 2)

### 9.5.3 Fluoride

Availability of adequate fluoride confers significant resistance to dental caries. It is now considered that the topical action of fluoride on enamel and plaque is more important than the systemic effect.

When the fluoride content of drinking water is less than 700 micrograms per litre (0.7 parts per million), daily administration of fluoride tablets or drops provide suitable supplementation. Systemic fluoride supplements should not be prescribed without reference to the fluoride content of the local water supply. Infants need not receive fluoride supplements until the age of 6 months.

Dentifrices which incorporate sodium fluoride or monofluorophosphate are also a convenient source of fluoride.

Individuals who are either particularly caries prone or medically compromised may be given additional protection by use of fluoride rinses or by application of fluoride gels. Rinses may be used daily or weekly; daily use of a less concentrated rinse is more effective than weekly use of a more concentrated one. High-strength gels must be applied regularly under professional supervision; extreme caution is necessary to prevent the child from swallowing any excess. Less concentrated gels are available for home use. Varnishes are also available and are particularly valuable for young or disabled children since they adhere to the teeth and set in the presence of moisture.

Fluoride mouthwash, oral drops, tablets, and toothpaste are prescribable on form FP10D (GP14 in Scotland, WP10D in Wales; for details see preparations below).

There are also arrangements for health authorities to supply fluoride tablets in the course of pre-school dental schemes, and they may also be supplied in school dental schemes.

Fluoride gels are not prescribable on form FP10D (GP14 in Scotland, WP10D in Wales).

## FLUORIDES

**Note** Sodium fluoride 2.2 mg provides approx. 1 mg fluoride ion

**Contra-indications** not for areas where drinking water is fluoridated

**Side-effects** occasional white flecks on teeth with recommended doses; *rarely* yellowish-brown discoloration if recommended doses are exceeded

**Indications and dose**

Dose expressed as fluoride ion ($F^-$)

**Prophylaxis of dental caries—see notes above**

Water content less than $F^-$ 300 micrograms/litre (0.3 parts per million)

- **By mouth**
  **Child 6 months–3 years** $F^-$ 250 micrograms daily
  **Child 3–6 years** $F^-$ 500 micrograms daily
  **Child 6 years and over** $F^-$ 1 mg daily
  Water content between $F^-$ 300 and 700 micrograms/litre (0.3–0.7 parts per million)
  **Child 3–6 years** $F^-$ 250 micrograms daily
  **Child 6 years and over** $F^-$ 500 micrograms daily
  Water content above $F^-$ 700 micrograms/litre (0.7 parts per million), supplements not advised

**Note** These doses reflect the recommendations of the British Dental Association, the British Society of Paediatric Dentistry and the British Association for the Study of Community Dentistry (*Br Dent J* 1997; **182**: 6–7)

### ◢Tablets

**Counselling** Tablets should be sucked or dissolved in the mouth and taken preferably in the evening
There are arrangements for health authorities to supply fluoride tablets in the course of pre-school dental schemes, and they may also be supplied in school dental schemes.

**En-De-Kay®** (Manx)
Fluotabs 3–6 years, orange-flavoured, scored, sodium fluoride 1.1 mg ($F^-$ 500 micrograms), net price 200-tab pack = £2.38
**Dental prescribing on NHS** May be prescribed as Sodium Fluoride Tablets
Fluotabs 6+ years, orange-flavoured, scored, sodium fluoride 2.2 mg ($F^-$ 1 mg), net price 200-tab pack = £2.38
**Dental prescribing on NHS** May be prescribed as Sodium Fluoride Tablets

**Fluor-a-day®** (Dental Health)
Tablets, buff, sodium fluoride 1.1 mg ($F^-$ 500 micrograms), net price 200-tab pack = £2.54; 2.2 mg ($F^-$ 1 mg), 200-tab pack = £2.54
**Dental prescribing on NHS** May be prescribed as Sodium Fluoride Tablets

### ◢Oral drops

**Note** Fluoride supplements not considered necessary below 6 months of age (see notes above)

**En-De-Kay®** (Manx)
Fluodrops® (= paediatric drops), sugar-free, sodium fluoride 550 micrograms ($F^-$ 250 micrograms)/0.15 mL. Net price 60 mL = £2.38
**Dental prescribing on NHS** May be prescribed as Sodium Fluoride Oral Drops

### ◢Mouthwashes

Rinse mouth for 1 minute and spit out

**Counselling** Avoid eating, drinking, or rinsing mouth for 15 minutes after use

**Duraphat®** (Colgate-Palmolive)
Weekly dental rinse (= mouthwash), blue, sodium fluoride 0.2%. Net price 150 mL = £2.13. Counselling, see above
**Dose**

| Child 6 years and over for *weekly* use, rinse with 10 mL |

**Dental prescribing on NHS** May be prescribed as Sodium Fluoride Mouthwash 0.2%

**En-De-Kay®** (Manx)
Daily fluoride mouthrinse (= mouthwash), blue, sodium fluoride 0.05%. Net price 250 mL = £1.51
**Dose**

| Child 6 years and over for *daily* use, rinse with 10 mL |

**Dental prescribing on NHS** May be prescribed as Sodium Fluoride Mouthwash 0.05%

Fluorinse (= mouthwash), red, sodium fluoride 2%. Net price 100 mL = £4.97. Counselling, see above
**Dose**

| Child 8 years and over for *daily* use, dilute 5 drops to 10 mL of water; for *weekly* use, dilute 20 drops to 10 mL |

**Dental prescribing on NHS** May be prescribed as Sodium Fluoride Mouthwash 2%

**FluoriGard®** (Colgate-Palmolive)
Daily dental rinse (= mouthwash), blue, sodium fluoride 0.05%. Net price 500 mL = £2.61. Counselling, see above
**Dose**

| Child 6 years and over for *daily* use, rinse with 10 mL |

**Dental prescribing on NHS** May be prescribed as Sodium Fluoride Mouthwash 0.05%

### ◢Toothpastes

**Duraphat®** (Colgate-Palmolive) PoM
Duraphat® '2800 ppm' toothpaste, sodium fluoride 0.619%. Net price 75 mL = £3.26. Counselling, see below
**Dose**

| Child over 10 years apply 1 cm twice daily using a toothbrush |
| **Counselling** Brush teeth for 1 minute before spitting out. Avoid drinking or rinsing mouth for 30 minutes after use |

**Dental prescribing on NHS** May be prescribed as Sodium Fluoride Toothpaste 0.619%

Duraphat® '5000 ppm' toothpaste, sodium fluoride 1.1%. Net price 51 g = £6.50. Counselling, see below

**Dose**

> **Child over 16 years** apply 2 cm 3 times daily after meals using a toothbrush
>
> **Counselling** Brush teeth for 3 minutes before spitting out

**Dental prescribing on NHS** May be prescribed as Sodium Fluoride Toothpaste 1.1%

## 9.5.4 Zinc

Zinc supplements should not be given unless there is good evidence of deficiency (hypoproteinaemia spuriously lowers plasma-zinc concentration) or in zinc-losing conditions. Zinc deficiency can occur as a result of inadequate diet or malabsorption; excessive loss of zinc can occur in trauma, burns, and protein-losing conditions. A zinc supplement is given until clinical improvement occurs, but it may need to be continued in severe malabsorption, metabolic disease, or in zinc-losing states. Zinc is used in the treatment of Wilson's disease (section 9.8.1) and acrodermatitis enteropathica, a rare inherited abnormality of zinc absorption.

Parenteral nutrition regimens usually include trace amounts of zinc (section 9.3). If necessary, further zinc can be added to some intravenous feeding regimens.

### ZINC SULFATE

**Cautions** interactions: Appendix 1 (zinc)

**Renal impairment** accumulation may occur in acute renal failure

**Pregnancy** crosses placenta; risk theoretically minimal, but no information available

**Breast-feeding** present in milk; risk theoretically minimal, but no information available

**Side-effects** abdominal pain, dyspepsia, nausea, vomiting, diarrhoea, gastric irritation, gastritis; irritability, headache, lethargy

**Licensed use** *Solvazinc*® not licensed for use in acrodermatitis enteropathica

**Solvazinc**® (Galen)

Effervescent tablets, zinc sulfate monohydrate 125 mg (45 mg zinc), net price 30 = £4.32. Label: 13, 21

**Dose**

> **Zinc deficiency** (see notes above)
>
> ● By mouth
>
> **Neonate** 1 mg/kg elemental zinc daily
>
> **Child under 10 kg** half a tablet daily in water after food, adjusted as necessary
>
> **Child 10–30 kg** half a tablet 1–3 times daily in water after food, adjusted as necessary
>
> **Child over 30 kg** 1 tablet 1–3 times daily in water after food, adjusted as necessary
>
> **Acrodermatitis enteropathica**
>
> ● By mouth
>
> **Neonate** 0.5–1 mg/kg elemental zinc twice daily (total daily dose may alternatively be given in 3 divided doses), adjusted as necessary
>
> **Child 1 month–18 years** 0.5–1 mg/kg elemental zinc twice daily (total daily dose may alternatively be given in 3 divided doses), adjusted as necessary

## 9.6 Vitamins

| 9.6.1 | Vitamin A |
|---|---|
| 9.6.2 | Vitamin B group |
| 9.6.3 | Vitamin C |
| 9.6.4 | Vitamin D |
| 9.6.5 | Vitamin E |
| 9.6.6 | Vitamin K |
| 9.6.7 | Multivitamin preparations |

Vitamins are used for the prevention and treatment of specific deficiency states or where the diet is known to be inadequate; they may be prescribed in the NHS to prevent or treat deficiency but not as dietary supplements. Except for iron-deficiency anaemia, a primary vitamin or mineral deficiency due to simple dietary inadequacy is rare in the developed world. Some children may be at risk of developing deficiencies because of an inadequate intake, impaired vitamin synthesis or malabsorption in disease states such as cystic fibrosis and Crohn's disease.

The use of vitamins as general 'pick-me-ups' is of unproven value and the 'fad' for mega-vitamin therapy with water-soluble vitamins, such as ascorbic acid and pyridoxine, is unscientific and can be harmful. Many vitamin supplements are described as 'multivitamin' but few contain the whole range of essential vitamins and many contain relatively high amounts of vitamins A and D. Care should be taken to ensure the correct dose is not exceeded.

Dietary reference values for vitamins are available in the Department of Health publication:

> Dietary Reference Values for Food Energy and Nutrients for the United Kingdom: Report of the Panel on Dietary Reference Values of the Committee on Medical Aspects of Food Policy. *Report on Health and Social Subjects 41.* London: HMSO, 1991

**Dental patients** It is unjustifiable to treat stomatitis or glossitis with mixtures of vitamin preparations; this delays diagnosis and correct treatment.

Most patients who develop a nutritional deficiency despite an adequate intake of vitamins have malabsorption and if this is suspected the patient should be referred to a medical practitioner.

## 9.6.1 Vitamin A

Deficiency of vitamin A (retinol) is associated with ocular defects (particularly xerophthalmia) and an increased susceptibility to infections, but deficiency is rare in the UK (even in disorders of fat absorption).

Vitamin A supplementation may be required in children with liver disease, particularly cholestatic liver disease, due to the malabsorption of fat soluble vitamins. In those with complete biliary obstruction an intramuscular dose once a month may be appropriate.

Treatment is sometimes initiated with very high doses of vitamin A and the child should be monitored closely; very high doses are associated with acute toxicity.

Preterm neonates have low plasma concentrations of vitamin A and are usually given vitamin A supplements, often as part of an oral multivitamin preparation (section 9.6.7) once enteral feeding has been established.

9

Nutrition and blood

Massive overdose can cause rough skin, dry hair, an enlarged liver, and a raised erythrocyte sedimentation rate and raised serum calcium and serum alkaline phosphatase concentrations.

**Pregnancy**　In view of evidence suggesting that high levels of vitamin A may cause birth defects, women who are (or may become) pregnant are advised not to take vitamin A supplements (including tablets and fish-liver oil drops), except on the advice of a doctor or an antenatal clinic; nor should they eat liver or products such as liver paté or liver sausage.

## VITAMIN A
### (Retinol)

**Cautions**　see notes above; **interactions:** Appendix 1 (vitamins)

**Pregnancy**　excessive doses can be teratogenic; see also notes above

**Breast-feeding**　toxicity likely if mother taking high doses

**Side-effects**　see notes above

**Licensed use**　preparations containing only vitamin A are not licensed

### Indications and dose

See also notes above

### Vitamin A deficiency
- By mouth
  **Neonate** 5000 units daily
  **Child 1 month–1 year** 5000 units daily with or after food
  **Child 1–18 years** 10 000 units daily with or after food

  **Note** Higher doses may be used initially for treatment of severe deficiency

### Prevention of deficiency in complete biliary obstruction
- By intramuscular injection
  **Neonate** 50 000 units once a month
  **Child 1 month–1 year** 50 000 units once a month

**Arovit®** (Non-proprietary)
Oral solution, vitamin A 150 000 units/mL (1 drop contains approx. 5000 units)
Available from 'special-order' manufacturers or specialist importing companies, see p. 823

**Aquasol-A®** (Non-proprietary)
Injection, vitamin A (as palmitate) 50 000 units/mL, 2-mL amp
Available from 'special-order' manufacturers or specialist importing companies, see p. 823

## VITAMINS A and D

**Cautions**　see notes above and section 9.6.4; prolonged excessive ingestion of vitamins A and D can lead to hypervitaminosis; **interactions:** Appendix 1 (vitamins)

**Pregnancy**　see notes above

**Side-effects**　see notes above and section 9.6.4

**Licensed use**　not licensed in children under 6 months of age

### Indications and dose

See notes above and section 9.6.4

**Prevention of vitamin A and D deficiency** see individual preparations for dose information

### ◢Vitamins A and D
**Vitamins A and D** (Non-proprietary)
Capsules, vitamin A 4000 units, vitamin D 400 units (10 micrograms). Net price 84 = £3.44
**Note** May be difficult to obtain
Dose
　**Child 1–18 years** 1 capsule daily

### ◢Vitamins A, C and D
**Healthy Start Children's Vitamin Drops** (Non-proprietary)
Oral drops, vitamin A 5000 units, vitamin D 2000 units (50 micrograms), ascorbic acid 150 mg/mL
Available free of charge to children under 4 years in families on the Healthy Start Scheme, or alternatively may be available direct to the public—further information for healthcare professionals can be accessed at www.healthystart.nhs.uk. Beneficiaries can contact their midwife or health visitor for further information on where to obtain supplies.
Dose
**Prevention of vitamin deficiency**
- By mouth
  **Child 1 month–5 years** 5 drops daily (5 drops contain vitamin A approx. 700 units, vitamin D approx. 300 units (7.5 micrograms), ascorbic acid approx. 20 mg)

**Note** *Healthy Start Vitamins for women* (containing ascorbic acid, vitamin D, and folic acid) are also available free of charge to women on the Healthy Start Scheme during pregnancy and until their baby is one year old, or alternatively may be available direct to the public—further information for healthcare professionals can be accessed at www.healthystart.nhs.uk. Beneficiaries can contact their midwife or health visitor for further information on where to obtain supplies.

## 9.6.2　Vitamin B group

Deficiency of the B vitamins, other than vitamin $B_{12}$ (section 9.1.2), is rare in the UK and is usually treated by preparations containing thiamine ($B_1$), and riboflavin ($B_2$). Other members (or substances traditionally classified as members) of the vitamin B complex such as aminobenzoic acid, biotin, choline, inositol, and pantothenic acid or panthenol may be included in vitamin B preparations, but there is no evidence of their value as supplements; however, they can be used in the management of certain metabolic disorders (section 9.8.1). Anaphylaxis has been reported with parenteral B vitamins (see MHRA/CHM advice, below).

As with other vitamins of the B group, pyridoxine ($B_6$) deficiency is rare, but it may occur during isoniazid therapy (section 5.1.9) or penicillamine treatment in Wilson's disease (section 9.8.1) and is characterised by peripheral neuritis. High doses of **pyridoxine** are given in some metabolic disorders, such as hyperoxaluria, cystathioninuria and homocystinuria; folic acid supplementation may also be beneficial in these disorders (section 9.1.2). Pyridoxine is also used in sideroblastic anaemia (section 1.3). Rarely, seizures in the neonatal period or during infancy respond to pyridoxine treatment; pyridoxine should be tried in all cases of early-onset intractable seizures and status epilepticus.

9　Nutrition and blood

Pyridoxine has been tried for a wide variety of other disorders, but there is little sound evidence to support the claims of efficacy, and overdosage induces toxic effects.

A number of mitochondrial disorders may respond to treatment with certain B vitamins but these disorders require specialist management. **Thiamine** is used in the treatment of maple syrup urine disease, mitochondrial respiratory chain defects and, together with riboflavin, in the treatment of congenital lactic acidosis; riboflavin is also used in glutaric acidaemias and cytochrome oxidase deficiencies; biotin (section 9.8.1) is used in carboxylase defects.

Folic acid and vitamin $B_{12}$ are used in the treatment of megaloblastic anaemia (section 9.1.2). Folinic acid (available as calcium folinate) is used in association with cytotoxic therapy (section 8.1).

## ■ RIBOFLAVIN
(Riboflavine, vitamin $B_2$)

**Cautions**  see notes above

**Pregnancy**  crosses the placenta but no adverse effects reported, information at high doses limited

**Breast-feeding**  present in breast milk but no adverse effects reported, information at high doses limited

**Side-effects**  bright yellow urine

**Licensed use**  not licensed in children

**Indications and dose**

See also notes above

### Metabolic diseases
• **By mouth**

> **Neonate** 50 mg 1–2 times daily, adjusted according to response

> **Child 1 month–18 years** 50–100 mg 1–2 times daily, adjusted according to response, up to 400 mg daily has been used

**Riboflavin** (Non-proprietary)
Tablets, 10 mg, 50 mg and 100 mg
Available from 'special-order' manufacturers or specialist importing companies, see p. 823

◄Oral vitamin B complex preparations
See below

## ■ THIAMINE
(Vitamin $B_1$)

**Cautions**  anaphylactic shock may occasionally follow injection (see MHRA/CHM advice below)

---

**MHRA/CHM advice (September 2007)**

Although potentially serious allergic adverse reactions may rarely occur during, or shortly after, parenteral administration, the CHM has recommended that:
1. This should not preclude the use of parenteral thiamine in patients where this route of administration is required, particularly in patients at risk of Wernicke-Korsakoff syndrome where treatment with thiamine is essential;
2. Intravenous administration should be by infusion over 30 minutes;
3. Facilities for treating anaphylaxis (including resuscitation facilities) should be available when parenteral thiamine is administered.

---

**Breast-feeding**  severely thiamine-deficient mothers should avoid breast-feeding as toxic methyl-glyoxal present in milk

**Side-effects**  hypersensitivity reactions to injection

**Licensed use**  not licensed in children

**Indications and dose**

See also notes above

### Maple syrup urine disease
• **By mouth**

> **Neonate** 5 mg/kg daily, adjusted as necessary

> **Child 1 month–18 years** 5 mg/kg daily, adjusted as necessary

### Metabolic disorders including congenital lactic acidosis
• **By mouth or by intravenous infusion over 30 minutes**

> **Neonate** 50–200 mg once daily (total dose may alternatively be given in 2–3 divided doses), adjusted as necessary

> **Child 1 month–18 years** 100–300 mg once daily (total dose may alternatively be given in 2–3 divided doses), adjusted as necessary; up to 2 g daily may be necessary

**Thiamine** (Non-proprietary)
Tablets, thiamine hydrochloride 50 mg, net price 100 = £5.19; 100 mg, 100 = £8.04
**Brands include** *Benerva* ® [JHS]
Injection, 50 mg/mL, 2-mL vial; 100 mg/mL, 2-mL vial
Injection (intramuscular), 100 mg/mL, 5-mL vial
Available from 'special-order' manufacturers or specialist importing companies, see p. 823
**Note** Some preparations may contain phenol as a preservative

◄Oral vitamin B complex preparations
See below

## ■ PYRIDOXINE HYDROCHLORIDE
(Vitamin $B_6$)

**Cautions**  see notes above; risk of cardiovascular collapse with intravenous injection—resuscitation facilities must be available, monitor closely; **interactions:** Appendix 1 (vitamins)

**Side-effects**  sensory neuropathy reported with high doses given for extended periods

**Licensed use**  not licensed for use in children

**Indications and dose**

See also notes above

### Metabolic diseases including cystathioninuria and homocystinuria
• **By mouth**

> **Neonate** 50–100 mg 1–2 times daily

> **Child 1 month–18 years** 50–250 mg 1–2 times daily

### Treatment of isoniazid-induced neuropathy
• **By mouth**

> **Neonate** 5–10 mg daily

> **Child 1 month–12 years** 10–20 mg 2–3 times daily

> **Child 12–18 years** 30–50 mg 2–3 times daily

**9**

**Nutrition and blood**

**Prevention of isoniazid-induced neuropathy**
- **By mouth**

  **Neonate** 5 mg daily

  **Child 1 month–12 years** 5–10 mg daily

  **Child 12–18 years** 10 mg daily

**Prevention of penicillamine-induced neuropathy in Wilson's disease (see notes above)**
- **By mouth**

  **Child 1–12 years** 5–10 mg daily

  **Child 12–18 years** 10 mg daily

**Pyridoxine-dependent seizures**
- **By intravenous injection or by mouth**

  **Neonate** initial test dose 50–100 mg by intravenous injection, may be repeated; if responsive followed by an oral maintenance dose of 50–100 mg once daily, adjusted as necessary

  **Child 1 month–12 years** initial test dose 50–100 mg daily; if responsive followed by an oral dose of 20–50 mg 1–2 times daily, adjusted as necessary; doses up to 30 mg/kg or 1 g daily have been used

**Pyridoxine** (Non-proprietary)
Tablets, pyridoxine hydrochloride 10 mg, net price 500 = £8.53; 20 mg, 500 = £8.53; 50 mg, 28 = £1.52

Injection, 25 mg/mL, 2 mL vial
Available from 'special-order' manufacturers or specialist importing companies, see p. 823

---

## Oral vitamin B complex preparations
**Note** Other multivitamin preparations are in section 9.6.7.

**Vitamin B Tablets, Compound** ⊿
Tablets, nicotinamide 15 mg, riboflavin 1 mg, thiamine hydrochloride 1 mg, net price 28 = £1.00

**Vitamin B Tablets, Compound, Strong** ⊿
Tablets, brown, f/c or s/c, nicotinamide 20 mg, pyridoxine hydrochloride 2 mg, riboflavin 2 mg, thiamine hydrochloride 5 mg. Net price 28-tab pack = £2.30

**Vigranon B**® (Wallace Mfg) ⟨NHS⟩ ⊿
Syrup, thiamine hydrochloride 5 mg, riboflavin 2 mg, nicotinamide 20 mg, pyridoxine hydrochloride 2 mg, panthenol 3 mg/5 mL. Net price 150 mL = £2.41
**Dose**

**Treatment of deficiency**
- **By mouth**

  **Child 1 month–1 year** 5 mL 3 times daily

  **Child 1–12 years** 10 mL 3 times daily

  **Child 12–18 years** 10–15mL 3 times daily

**Prophylaxis of deficiency**
- **By mouth**

  **Child 1 month–1 year** 5 mL once daily

  **Child 1–12 years** 5 mL twice daily

  **Child 12–18 years** 5 mL 3 times daily

---

## 9.6.3 Vitamin C
### (Ascorbic acid)

Vitamin C therapy is essential in scurvy, but less florid manifestations of vitamin C deficiency have been reported. Vitamin C is used to enhance the excretion of iron one month after starting desferrioxamine therapy (section 9.1.3); it is given separately from food as it also enhances iron absorption. Vitamin C is also used in the treatment of some inherited metabolic disorders, particularly mitochondrial disorders; specialist management of these conditions is required.

Severe scurvy causes gingival swelling and bleeding margins as well as petechiae on the skin. This is, however, exceedingly rare and a child with these signs is more likely to have leukaemia. Investigation should not be delayed by a trial period of vitamin treatment.

Claims that vitamin C ameliorates colds or promotes wound healing have not been proved.

---

### ASCORBIC ACID
### (Vitamin C)

**Cautions** interactions: Appendix 1 (vitamins)
**Contra-indications** hyperoxaluria
**Side-effects** nausea, diarrhoea; headache, fatigue; hyperoxaluria
**Licensed use** not licensed for metabolic disorders
**Indications and dose**

**Treatment of scurvy**
- **By mouth**

  **Child 1 month–4 years** 125–250 mg daily in 1–2 divided doses

  **Child 4–12 years** 250–500 mg daily in 1–2 divided doses

  **Child 12–18 years** 500 mg–1 g daily in 1–2 divided doses

**Adjunct to desferrioxamine (see notes above)**
- **By mouth**

  **Child 1 month–18 years** 100–200 mg daily 1 hour before food

**Metabolic disorders** (tyrosinaemia type III; transient tyrosinaemia of the newborn; glutathione synthase deficiency; Hawkinsinuria)
- **By mouth**

  **Neonate** 50–200 mg daily, adjusted as necessary

  **Child 1 month–18 years** 200–400 mg daily in 1–2 divided doses, adjusted as necessary; up to 1 g daily may be required

**Ascorbic Acid** (Non-proprietary)
Tablets, ascorbic acid 50 mg, net price 28 = £1.79; 100 mg, 28 = £1.42; 200 mg, 28 = £1.42; 500 mg (label: 24), 28 = £2.34
**Excipients** may include aspartame
**Brands include** *Redoxon*® ⟨NHS⟩

Injection, ascorbic acid 100 mg/mL, net price 5-mL amp = £4.39
**Excipients** include metabisulfite

9. **Nutrition and blood**

## 9.6.4 Vitamin D

**Note** The term Vitamin D is used for a range of compounds including ergocalciferol (calciferol, vitamin $D_2$), colecalciferol (vitamin $D_3$), dihydrotachysterol, alfacalcidol ($1\alpha$-hydroxycholecalciferol), and calcitriol (1,25-dihydroxycholecalciferol).

Asymptomatic vitamin D deficiency is common in the United Kingdom; symptomatic deficiency may occur in certain ethnic groups, particularly as rickets or hypocalcaemia, and rarely in association with malabsorption. The amount of vitamin D required in infancy is related to the stores built up *in-utero* and subsequent exposure to sunlight. The amount of vitamin D in breast milk varies and some breast-fed babies, particularly if preterm or born to vitamin D deficient mothers, may become deficient. Most formula milk and supplement feeds contain adequate vitamin D to prevent deficiency.

Simple, nutritional vitamin D deficiency can be prevented by oral supplementation of 10 micrograms (400 units) of **ergocalciferol** (calciferol, vitamin $D_2$) or **colecalciferol** (vitamin $D_3$) daily, using multi-vitamin drops (section 9.6.7), preparations of vitamins A and D (section 9.6.1), manufactured 'special' solutions, or as calcium and ergocalciferol tablets (although the calcium and other vitamins in supplements are unnecessary); excessive supplementation may cause hypercalcaemia.

Inadequate bone mineralisation can be caused by a deficiency, or a lack of action of vitamin D or its active metabolite. In childhood this causes bowing and distortion of bones (rickets). In nutritional vitamin D deficiency rickets, initial high doses of ergocalciferol or colecalciferol should be reduced to supplemental doses after 8–12 weeks, as there is a significant risk of hypercalcaemia (see caution below). However, calcium supplements are recommended if there is hypocalcaemia or evidence of a poor dietary calcium intake. A single large dose of ergocalciferol or colecalciferol can also be effective for the treatment of nutritional vitamin D deficiency rickets.

Poor bone mineralisation in neonates and young children may also be due to inadequate intake of phosphate or calcium particularly during long-term parenteral nutrition—supplementation with phosphate (section 9.5.2.1) or calcium (section 9.5.1.1) may be required.

*Hypophosphataemic rickets* occurs due to abnormal phosphate excretion; treatment with high doses of oral phosphate (section 9.5.2.1), and hydroxylated (activated) forms of vitamin D allow bone mineralisation and optimise growth.

Nutritional deficiency of vitamin D is best treated with colecalciferol or ergocalciferol. Preparations containing calcium and colecalciferol are also occasionally used in children where there is evidence of combined calcium and vitamin D deficiency. Vitamin D deficiency caused by *intestinal malabsorption* or *chronic liver disease* usually requires vitamin D in pharmacological doses, such as **ergocalciferol** in doses of up to 40 000 units daily; the hypocalcaemia of *hypoparathyroidism* often requires higher doses in order to achieve normocalcaemia and alfacalcidol is generally preferred.

Vitamin D supplementation is often given in combination with calcium supplements for persistent hypocalcaemia in neonates, and in chronic renal disease.

Vitamin D requires hydroxylation, by the kidney and liver, to its active form therefore the hydroxylated derivatives **alfacalcidol** or **calcitriol** should be prescribed if patients with *severe liver or renal impairment* require vitamin D therapy. Alfacalcidol is generally preferred in children as there is more experience of its use and appropriate formulations are available. Calcitriol is unlicensed for use in children and is generally reserved for those with severe liver disease.

**Important.** All patients receiving pharmacological doses of vitamin D or its analogues should have their plasma-calcium concentration checked at intervals (initially once or twice weekly) and whenever nausea or vomiting occur.

## ERGOCALCIFEROL
### (Calciferol, Vitamin $D_2$)

**Cautions** see notes above; monitor plasma-calcium concentration in patients receiving high doses and in renal impairment; **interactions**: Appendix 1 (vitamins)

**Contra-indications** hypercalcaemia; metastatic calcification

**Pregnancy** high doses teratogenic in *animals* but therapeutic doses unlikely to be harmful

**Breast-feeding** caution with high doses as may cause hypercalcaemia in infant—monitor serum-calcium concentration

**Side-effects** symptoms of overdosage include anorexia, lassitude, nausea and vomiting, diarrhoea, constipation, weight loss, polyuria, sweating, headache, thirst, vertigo, and raised concentrations of calcium and phosphate in plasma and urine

**Licensed use** Calcium and Ergocalciferol tablets not licensed for use in children under 6 years

### Indications and dose

See also notes above

**Nutritional vitamin-D deficiency rickets**

- By mouth

  **Child 1–6 months** 3000 units daily, adjusted as necessary

  **Child 6 months–12 years** 6000 units daily, adjusted as necessary

  **Child 12–18 years** 10 000 units daily, adjusted as necessary

**Nutritional or physiological supplement; prevention of rickets**

- By mouth

  **Neonate** 400 units daily

  **Child 1 month–18 years** 400–600 units daily

**Vitamin D deficiency in intestinal malabsorption or in chronic liver disease**

- By mouth or by intramuscular injection

  **Child 1–12 years** 10 000–25 000 units daily, adjusted as necessary

  **Child 12–18 years** 10 000–40 000 units daily, adjusted as necessary

9

Nutrition and blood

**◢Pharmacological strengths**

(see notes above)

The BP directs that when calciferol is prescribed or demanded, colecalciferol or ergocalciferol should be dispensed or supplied

**Ergocalciferol** (Non-proprietary)

Tablets, ergocalciferol 250 micrograms (10 000 units), net price 100 = £21.99; 1.25 mg (50 000 units), 100 = £30.34

**Note** May be difficult to obtain

**Important** When the strength of the tablets ordered or prescribed is not clear, the intention of the prescriber or purchaser with respect to the strength (expressed in micrograms or milligrams per tablet) should be ascertained.

Injection, ergocalciferol, 7.5 mg (300 000 units)/mL in oil, net price 1-mL amp = £8.50, 2-mL amp = £9.85

**Note** Other formulations of ergocalciferol are available from 'special-order' manufacturers or specialist importing companies, see p. 823

**◢Daily supplements**

**Note** There is no plain vitamin D tablet available for treating simple deficiency (see notes above). Alternatives include vitamins capsules (section 9.6.7), preparations of vitamins A and D (section 9.6.1), and calcium and ergocalciferol tablets (see below).

For prescribing information on calcium, see section 9.5.1

**Calcium and Ergocalciferol** (Non-proprietary) (Calcium and Vitamin D)

Tablets, calcium lactate 300 mg, calcium phosphate 150 mg (calcium 97 mg or $Ca^{2+}$ 2.4 mmol), ergo-calciferol 10 micrograms (400 units). Net price 28-tab pack = £7.10. Counselling, crush before adminis-tration or may be chewed

## ■ ALFACALCIDOL
(1α-Hydroxycholecalciferol)

**Cautions** see under Ergocalciferol; also nephrolithiasis

**Contra-indications** see under Ergocalciferol

**Pregnancy** see under Ergocalciferol

**Breast-feeding** see under Ergocalciferol

**Side-effects** see under Ergocalciferol; also *rarely* nephrocalcinosis, pruritus, rash, and urticaria

**Indications and dose**

See also notes above

**Hypophosphataemic rickets; persistent hypo-calcaemia due to hypoparathyroidism or pseu-dohypoparathyroidism**

● By mouth or by intravenous injection

**Child 1 month–12 years** 25–50 nanograms/kg (max. 1 microgram) once daily, adjusted as necessary

**Child 12–18 years** 1 microgram once daily, adjusted as necessary

**Persistent neonatal hypocalcaemia**

● By mouth or by intravenous injection

**Neonate** 50–100 nanograms/kg once daily, adjusted as necessary (up to 2 micrograms/kg daily may be needed in resistant cases)

**Prevention of vitamin D deficiency in renal or cholestatic liver disease**

● By mouth or by intravenous injection

**Neonate** 20 nanograms/kg once daily, adjusted as necessary

**Child 1 month–12 years, body-weight under 20 kg** 15–30 nanograms/kg (max. 500 nanograms)

once daily; **body-weight over 20 kg** 250–500 nanograms once daily, adjusted as necessary

**Child 12–18 years** 250–500 nanograms once daily, adjusted as necessary

**Alfacalcidol** (Non-proprietary) [PoM]

Capsules, alfacalcidol 250 nanograms, net price 30-cap pack = £5.94; 500 nanograms 30-cap pack = £11.64; 1 microgram 30-cap pack = £15.91

**One-Alpha®** (LEO) [PoM]

Capsules, alfacalcidol 250 nanograms (white), net price 30-cap pack = £3.37; 500 nanograms (red), 30-cap pack = £6.27; 1 microgram (brown), 30-cap pack = £8.75

**Excipients** include sesame oil

Oral drops, sugar-free, alfacalcidol 2 micrograms/mL (1 drop contains approx. 100 nanograms), net price 10 mL = £22.49

**Excipients** include alcohol

**Note** The concentration of alfacalcidol in *One-Alpha®* drops is **10 times greater** than that of the former preparation *One-Alpha®* solution.

Injection, alfacalcidol 2 micrograms/mL, net price 0.5-mL amp = £2.16, 1-mL amp = £4.11

**Excipients** include alcohol, propylene glycol (caution in neonates, see, p. 2)

**Note** Shake ampoule for at least 5 seconds before use

## ■ CALCITRIOL
(1,25-Dihydroxycholecalciferol)

**Cautions** see under Ergocalciferol; monitor plasma calcium, phosphate, and creatinine during dosage titration

**Contra-indications** see under Ergocalciferol

**Pregnancy** see under Ergocalciferol

**Breast-feeding** see under Ergocalciferol

**Side-effects** see under Ergocalciferol

**Licensed use** not licensed for use in children

**Indications and dose**

See also notes above

**Vitamin D dependent rickets; hypophosphat-aemic rickets; persistent hypocalcaemia due to hypoparathyroidism or pseudo-hypoparathyroid-ism** (limited experience)

● By mouth

**Child 1 month–12 years** initially 15 nanograms/kg (max. 250 nanograms) once daily, increased if necessary in steps of 5 nanograms/kg (max. 250 nanograms) every 2–4 weeks

**Child 12–18 years** initially 250 nanograms once daily increased if necessary in steps of 5 nan-ograms/kg daily (max. 250 nanograms step) every 2–4 weeks; usual dose 0.5–1 microgram daily

**Administration** Contents of capsule may be admi-nistered by oral syringe

**Calcitriol** (Non-proprietary) [PoM]

Capsules, calcitriol 250 nanograms, net price 30-cap pack = £18.04, 100-cap pack = £19.15; 500 nan-ograms, 30-cap pack =£32.25, 100-cap pack = £25.76

**Rocaltrol®** (Roche) [PoM]

Capsules, calcitriol 250 nanograms (red/white), net price 100 = £18.04; 500 nanograms (red), 100 = £32.25

## COLECALCIFEROL
(Cholecalciferol, vitamin D₃)

**Cautions**  see under Ergocalciferol
**Contra-indications**  see under Ergocalciferol
**Pregnancy**  see under Ergocalciferol
**Breast-feeding**  see under Ergocalciferol
**Side-effects**  see under Ergocalciferol
**Licensed use**  *Adcal-D3®*, *Calceos®*, and *Fultium-D₃®* not licensed for use in children under 12 years; *Cacit®D3*, *Calcichew-D₃®* Forte, *Calcichew-D₃® 500 mg/400 unit*, and *Kalcipos-D®* not licensed for use in children (age range not specified by manufacturers); *Accrete D3®*, *Calfovit D3®*, and *Natecal D3®* not licensed for use in children under 18 years

**Indications and dose**

See under Ergocalciferol and notes above—alternative to Ergocalciferol, see also Pharmacological Strengths

**Fultium-D₃®** (Internis) PoM
Capsules, colecalciferol 20 micrograms (800 units), net price 30-cap pack= £3.60. Label: 25
Excipients  include arachis (peanut) oil

**Colecalciferol**
Various formulations available from 'special-order' manufacturers or specialist importing companies, see p. 823

◀**With calcium**
For prescribing information on calcium, see section 9.5.1

**Accrete D3®** (Internis)
Tablets, f/c, calcium carbonate 1.5 g (calcium 600 mg or Ca²⁺ 15 mmol), colecalciferol 10 micrograms (400 units), net price 60-tab pack = £3.60

**Adcal-D₃®** (ProStrakan)
Tablets (chewable), lemon or tutti-frutti flavour, calcium carbonate 1.5 g (calcium 600 mg or Ca²⁺ 15 mmol), colecalciferol 10 micrograms (400 units), net price 56-tab pack = £3.89, 112-tab pack = £7.78. Label: 24

Dissolve (effervescent tablets), lemon flavour, calcium carbonate 1.5 g (calcium 600 mg or Ca²⁺ 15 mmol), colecalciferol 10 micrograms (400 units), net price 56-tab pack = £4.99. Label: 13

Caplets (=tablets), f/c, calcium carbonate 750 mg (calcium 300 mg or Ca²⁺ 7.5 mmol), colecalciferol 5 micrograms (200 units), net price 112-tab pack = £3.65

**Cacit® D3** (Warner Chilcott)
Granules, effervescent, lemon flavour, calcium carbonate 1.25 g (calcium 500 mg or Ca²⁺ 12.5 mmol), colecalciferol 11 micrograms (440 units)/sachet, net price 30-sachet pack = £4.06. Label: 13

**Calceos®** (Galen)
Tablets (chewable), lemon flavour, calcium carbonate 1.25 g (calcium 500 mg or Ca²⁺ 12.5 mmol), colecalciferol 10 micrograms (400 units), net price 60-tab pack = £3.62. Label: 24

**Calcichew-D₃®** (Shire)
Calcichew-D₃® tablets (chewable), orange flavour, calcium carbonate 1.25 g (calcium 500 mg or Ca²⁺ 12.5 mmol), colecalciferol 5 micrograms (200 units), net price 100-tab pack = £7.68. Label: 24
Excipients  include aspartame (section 9.4.1)

Calcichew-D₃® Forte tablets (chewable), lemon flavour, calcium carbonate 1.25 g (calcium 500 mg or Ca²⁺ 12.5 mmol), colecalciferol 10 micrograms (400 units), net price 100-tab pack = £7.21. Label: 24
Excipients  include aspartame (section 9.4.1)

Calcichew-D₃® 500 mg/400 unit caplets, f/c, lemon flavour, calcium carbonate providing calcium 500 mg (Ca²⁺ 12.5 mmol), colecalciferol 10 micrograms (400 units), net price 100-tab pack = £7.57
Excipients  include propylene glycol (see Excipients ,p. 2)

**Calfovit D3®** (Menarini)
Powder, lemon flavour, calcium phosphate 3.1 g (calcium 1.2 g or Ca²⁺ 30 mmol), colecalciferol 20 micrograms (800 units), net price 30-sachet pack = £4.32. Label: 13, 21

**Kalcipos-D®** (Meda) PoM
Tablets (chewable), calcium carbonate providing calcium 500 mg (Ca²⁺ 12.5 mmol), colecalciferol 20 micrograms (800 units), net price 30-tab pack = £4.21. Label: 24

**Natecal D3®** (Chiesi)
Tablets (chewable), (aniseed, peppermint, and molasses flavour), calcium carbonate 1.5 g (calcium 600 mg or Ca²⁺ 15 mmol), colecalciferol 10 micrograms (400 units), net price 60-tab pack = £3.63. Label: 24
Excipients  include aspartame (section 9.4.1)

## 9.6.5  Vitamin E
(Tocopherols)

The daily requirement of vitamin E has not been well defined. Vitamin E supplements are given to children with fat malabsorption such as in cystic fibrosis and cholestatic liver disease. In children with abetalipoproteinaemia abnormally low vitamin E concentrations may occur in association with neuromuscular problems; this usually responds to high doses of vitamin E. Some neonatal units still administer a single intramuscular dose of vitamin E at birth to preterm neonates to reduce the risk of complications; no trials of long-term outcome have been carried out. The intramuscular route should also be considered in children with severe liver disease when response to oral therapy is inadequate.

Vitamin E has been tried for various other conditions but there is little scientific evidence of its value.

## ALPHA TOCOPHERYL ACETATE

**Cautions**  predisposition to thrombosis; increased risk of necrotising enterocolitis in preterm neonates (see administration); **interactions:** Appendix 1 (vitamins)
**Pregnancy**  no evidence of safety of high doses
**Breast-feeding**  excreted in milk, minimal risk although caution with large doses
**Side-effects**  diarrhoea and abdominal pain, particularly with high doses

Nutrition and blood

9

**Indications and dose**

**Vitamin E deficiency**

- **By mouth**

  **Neonate** 10 mg/kg once daily

  **Child 1 month–18 years** 2–10 mg/kg daily, up to 20 mg/kg has been used

**Malabsorption in cystic fibrosis**

- **By mouth (with food and pancreatic enzymes)**

  **Child 1 month–1 year** 50 mg once daily, adjusted as necessary

  **Child 1–12 years** 100 mg once daily, adjusted as necessary

  **Child 12–18 years** 100–200 mg once daily, adjusted as necessary

**Vitamin E deficiency in cholestasis and severe liver disease**

- **By mouth**

  **Neonate** 10 mg/kg daily

  **Child 1 month–12 years** initially 100 mg daily, adjusted according to response; up to 200 mg/kg daily may be required

  **Child 12–18 years** initially 200 mg daily, adjusted according to response; up to 200 mg/kg daily may be required

- **By intramuscular injection**

  **Neonate** 10 mg/kg once a month

  **Child 1 month–18 years** 10 mg/kg (max. 100 mg) once a month

**Malabsorption in abetalipoproteinaemia**

- **By mouth**

  **Neonate** 100 mg/kg once daily

  **Child 1 month–18 years** 50–100 mg/kg once daily

**Vitamin E Suspension** (Non-proprietary)

Suspension, alpha tocopheryl acetate 100 mg/mL. Net price 100 mL = £30.35

**Excipients** include sucrose

**Administration** consider dilution in neonates due to high osmolality (see Cautions)

**Note** Tablets containing tocopheryl acetate are available from 'special-order' manufacturers or specialist importing companies, see p. 823

**Vitamin E Injection**

Injection tocopheryl acetate 50 mg/mL, 2-mL ampoule

Available from 'special-order' manufacturers or specialist importing companies, see p. 823

## ALPHA TOCOPHEROL

**Cautions** predisposition to thrombosis; **interactions**: Appendix 1 (vitamins)

**Contra-indications** preterm neonates

**Hepatic impairment** manufacturer advises caution and monitor closely—no information available

**Renal impairment** manufacturer advises caution and monitor closely; risk of renal toxicity due to polyethylene glycol content

**Pregnancy** manufacturer advises caution; no evidence of harm in *animal* studies

**Breast-feeding** manufacturer advises use only if potential benefit outweighs risk—no information available

**Side-effects** diarrhoea; *less commonly* asthenia, headache, pruritus, disturbances in serum-potassium and serum-sodium concentrations, alopecia, and rash

**Vedrop®** (Orphan Europe) ▼ PoM

Oral solution, yellow, D-alpha tocopherol (as tocofersolan) 50 mg/mL, net price 20 mL = £54.55, 60 mL = £163.65 (all with oral syringe)

**Note** Tocofersolan is a water-soluble form of D-alpha tocopherol

**Dose**

**Vitamin E deficiency because of malabsorption in congenital or hereditary chronic cholestasis**

- **By mouth**

  **Neonate** 17 mg/kg daily, adjusted as necessary

  **Child 1 month–18 years** 17 mg/kg daily, adjusted as necessary

## 9.6.6   Vitamin K

Vitamin K is necessary for the production of blood clotting factors and proteins necessary for the normal calcification of bone.

Because vitamin K is fat soluble, children with fat malabsorption, especially in biliary obstruction or hepatic disease, may become deficient. For oral administration to prevent vitamin K deficiency in malabsorption syndromes, a water-soluble synthetic vitamin K derivative, **menadiol sodium phosphate** (see Contra-indications below) can be used if supplementation with phytomenadione by mouth has been insufficient.

Oral coumarin anticoagulants act by interfering with vitamin K metabolism in the hepatic cells and their effects can be antagonised by giving vitamin K; for advice on the use of vitamin K in haemorrhage, see section 2.8.2.

**Vitamin K deficiency bleeding** Neonates are relatively deficient in vitamin K and those who do not receive supplements are at risk of serious bleeding, including intracranial bleeding. The Chief Medical Officer and the Chief Nursing Officer have recommended that all newborn babies should receive vitamin K to prevent vitamin K deficiency bleeding (previously termed haemorrhagic disease of the newborn). Local protocols may vary and an appropriate regimen should be selected after discussion with parents in the antenatal period.

Vitamin K (as phytomenadione) 1 mg may be given by a single intramuscular injection at birth; this prevents vitamin K deficiency bleeding in virtually all babies; preterm neonates may be given 400 micrograms/kg (max. 1 mg). The intravenous route may be used in preterm neonates of very low birth-weight if intramuscular injection is not possible; however, it may not provide the prolonged protection of the intramuscular injection; any babies receiving intravenous vitamin K should be given subsequent oral doses.

Alternatively, in healthy babies who are not at particular risk of bleeding disorders, vitamin K may be given by mouth, and arrangements must be in place to ensure the appropriate regimen is followed. Two doses of a colloidal (mixed micelle) preparation of phytomenadione 2 mg should be given in the first week, the first dose being given at birth and the second at 4–7 days. For exclusively breast-fed babies, a third dose of phytomenadione 2 mg is given at 1 month of age; the third dose is omitted in formula-fed babies because formula feeds contain adequate vitamin K. An alternative regimen is to give one dose of phytomenadione 1 mg by mouth at birth (using the contents of a phytomenadione capsule, see preparation below) to protect from the risk of vitamin K deficiency bleeding in the first week; for exclusively breast-fed babies, further doses of phytomenadione 1 mg are given by mouth (using the contents of a phytomenadione capsule) at weekly intervals for 12 weeks.

For the *treatment* of vitamin K deficiency bleeding, intravenous phytomenadione is used, see Phytomenadione below.

## ■ MENADIOL SODIUM PHOSPHATE

**Cautions** G6PD deficiency (section 9.1.5) and vitamin E deficiency (risk of haemolysis); **interactions:** Appendix 1 (vitamins)

**Contra-indications** neonates and infants

**Pregnancy** avoid in late pregnancy and labour unless benefit outweighs risk of neonatal haemolytic anaemia, hyperbilirubinaemia, and kernicterus in neonate

**Indications and dose**

See notes above

> **Supplementation in vitamin K malabsorption**
> • **By mouth**
>> **Child 1–12 years** 5–10 mg daily, adjusted as necessary
>> **Child 12–18 years** 10–20 mg daily, adjusted as necessary

**Menadiol Phosphate** (Non-proprietary)
Tablets, menadiol sodium phosphate equivalent to 10 mg of menadiol phosphate, net price 100-tab pack = £58.39

## ■ PHYTOMENADIONE
(Vitamin K$_1$)

**Cautions** intravenous injections should be given very slowly—risk of vascular collapse (see also below); **interactions:** Appendix 1 (vitamins)

**Pregnancy** use if potential benefit outweighs risk

**Breast-feeding** present in milk, but see notes above

**Indications and dose**

> **Neonatal prophylaxis of vitamin-K deficiency bleeding** see notes above

> **Neonatal hypoprothrombinaemia or vitamin-K deficiency bleeding**
> • **By intravenous injection**
>> **Neonate** 1 mg repeated 8 hourly if necessary

> **Neonatal biliary atresia and liver disease**
> • **By mouth**
>> **Neonate** 1 mg daily

> **Reversal of coumarin anticoagulation when continued anticoagulation required or if no significant bleeding** (see also section 2.8.2)—seek specialist advice
> • **By intravenous injection**
>> **Child 1 month–18 years** 15–30 micrograms/kg (max. 1 mg) as a single dose, repeated as necessary

> **Reversal of coumarin anticoagulation when anticoagulation not required or if significant bleeding; treatment of haemorrhage associated with vitamin-K deficiency** (see also section 2.8.2)—seek specialist advice
> • **By intravenous injection**
>> **Child 1 month–18 years** 250–300 micrograms/kg (max. 10 mg) as a single dose

**Neokay**® (Neoceuticals) PoM
Capsules, brown, phytomenadione 1 mg in an oily basis, net price 12-cap pack = £3.95; 100-cap pack = £34.00

**Note** The contents of one capsule should be administered by cutting the narrow tubular tip off and squeezing the liquid contents into the mouth; if the baby spits out the dose or is sick within three hours of administration a replacement dose should be given

**Dose**
> **Neonatal prophylaxis of vitamin-K deficiency bleeding** see notes above

◀**Colloidal formulation**

**Konakion**® **MM** (Roche) PoM
Injection, phytomenadione 10 mg/mL in a mixed micelles vehicle. Net price 1-mL amp = 38p
**Excipients** include glycocholic acid 54.6 mg/amp, lecithin
**Cautions** reduce dose in liver impairment (glycocholic acid may displace bilirubin); reports of anaphylactoid reactions
**Administration** *Konakion® MM* may be administered by slow intravenous injection or by intravenous infusion in glucose 5%; **not** for intramuscular injection

**Konakion**® **MM Paediatric** (Roche) ▼ PoM
Injection, phytomenadione 10 mg/mL in a mixed micelles vehicle, net price 0.2-mL amp = 95p
**Excipients** include glycocholic acid 10.9 mg/amp, lecithin
**Cautions** parenteral administration in premature infants body-weight less than 2.5 kg (increased risk of kernicterus)
**Administration** *Konakion® MM Paediatric* may be administered *by mouth* or *by intramuscular injection* or *by intravenous injection*. For *intravenous injection*, may be diluted with Glucose 5% if necessary

## 9.6.7 Multivitamin preparations

Multivitamin supplements are used in children with vitamin deficiencies and also in malabsorption conditions such as cystic fibrosis or liver disease. To avoid potential toxicity, the content of all vitamin preparations, particularly vitamin A, should be considered when used together with other supplements. Supplementation is not required if nutrient enriched feeds are used; consult a dietician for further advice.

## ■ MULTIVITAMIN PREPARATIONS

**Cautions** see individual vitamins; vitamin A concentration of preparations varies

**Contra-indications** see individual vitamins

**Side-effects** see individual vitamins

**Licensed use** *Dalivit*® not licensed for use in children under 6 weeks

**Indications and dose**

See under preparations below

**9**

**Nutrition and blood**

### Vitamins

Capsules, ascorbic acid 15 mg, nicotinamide 7.5 mg, riboflavin 500 micrograms, thiamine hydrochloride 1 mg, vitamin A 2500 units, vitamin D 300 units, net price 28-cap pack = £1.50

**Dose**

##### Prevention of deficiency

- By mouth
  - **Child 1–12 years** 1 capsule daily
  - **Child 12–18 years** 2 capsules daily

##### Cystic fibrosis: prevention of deficiency

- By mouth
  - **Child 1–18 years** 2–3 capsules daily

### Abidec® (Chefaro UK)

Drops, vitamins A, B group, C, and D. Net price 25 mL (with dropper) = £2.20

**Note** Contains 1333 units of vitamin A (as palmitate) per 0.6 mL dose

**Excipients** include arachis (peanut) oil and sucrose

**Dose**

##### Prevention of deficiency

- By mouth
  - **Preterm neonate** 0.6 mL daily
  - **Neonate** 0.3 mL daily
  - **Child 1 month–1 year** 0.3 mL daily
  - **Child 1–18 years** 0.6 mL daily

##### Cystic fibrosis: prevention of deficiency

- By mouth
  - **Child 1 month–1 year** 0.6 mL daily
  - **Child 1–18 years** 1.2 mL daily

### Dalivit® (LPC)

Oral drops, vitamins A, B group, C, and D, net price 25 mL = £2.98, 50 mL = £4.85

**Note** Contains 5000 units of vitamin A (as palmitate) per 0.6 mL dose

**Excipients** include sucrose

**Dose**

##### Prevention of deficiency

- By mouth
  - **Neonate (including preterm)** 0.3 mL daily
  - **Child 1 month–1 year** 0.3 mL daily
  - **Child 1–18 years** 0.6 mL daily

##### Cystic fibrosis: prevention of deficiency

- By mouth
  - **Child 1 month–1 year** 0.6 mL daily
  - **Child 1–18 years** 1 mL daily

## Vitamin and mineral supplements and adjuncts to synthetic diets

### Forceval® (Alliance)

Capsules, brown/red, vitamins (ascorbic acid 60 mg, biotin 100 micrograms, cyanocobalamin 3 micrograms, folic acid 400 micrograms, nicotinamide 18 mg, pantothenic acid 4 mg, pyridoxine 2 mg, riboflavin 1.6 mg, thiamine 1.2 mg, vitamin A 2500 units, vitamin $D_2$ 400 units, vitamin E 10 mg, minerals and trace elements (calcium 100 mg, chromium 200 micrograms, copper 2 mg, iodine 140 micrograms, iron 12 mg, magnesium 30 mg, manganese 3 mg, molybdenum 250 micrograms, phosphorus 77 mg, potassium 4 mg, selenium 50 micrograms,

zinc 15 mg), net price 15-cap pack = £2.83, 30-cap pack = £5.19, 90-cap pack = £12.53. Label: 25

**Dose**

##### Vitamin and mineral deficiency and as adjunct in synthetic diets

**Child 12–18 years** 1 capsule daily one hour after a meal

Junior capsules, brown, vitamins (ascorbic acid 25 mg, biotin 50 micrograms, cyanocobalamin 2 micrograms, folic acid 100 micrograms, nicotinamide 7.5 mg, pantothenic acid 2 mg, pyridoxine 1 mg, riboflavin 1 mg, thiamine 1.5 mg, vitamin A 1250 units, vitamin $D_2$ 200 units, vitamin E 5 mg, vitamin $K_1$ 25 micrograms), minerals and trace elements (chromium 50 micrograms, copper 1 mg, iodine 75 micrograms, iron 5 mg, magnesium 1 mg, manganese 1.25 mg, molybdenum 50 micrograms, selenium 25 micrograms, zinc 5 mg), net price 30-cap pack = £3.52, 60-cap pack = £6.69

**Dose**

##### Vitamin and mineral deficiency and as adjunct in synthetic diets

**Child 5–12 years** 2 junior capsules daily

### Ketovite® (Essential)

Tablets [PoM], yellow, ascorbic acid 16.6 mg, riboflavin 1 mg, thiamine hydrochloride 1 mg, pyridoxine hydrochloride 330 micrograms, nicotinamide 3.3 mg, calcium pantothenate 1.16 mg, alpha tocopheryl acetate 5 mg, inositol 50 mg, biotin 170 micrograms, folic acid 250 micrograms, acetomenaphthone 500 micrograms, net price 100-tab pack = £4.17

**Dose**

##### Prevention of vitamin deficiency in disorders of carbohydrate or amino-acid metabolism and adjunct in restricted, specialised, or synthetic diets

**Child 1 month–18 years** 1 tablet 3 times daily; dose adjusted according to condition, diet, or age; use with *Ketovite® Liquid* for complete vitamin supplementation

**Administration** may be crushed immediately before use

Liquid, pink, sugar-free, vitamin A 2500 units, ergocalciferol 400 units, choline chloride 150 mg, cyanocobalamin 12.5 micrograms/5 mL, net price 150-mL pack = £2.70

**Dose**

##### Prevention of vitamin deficiency in disorders of carbohydrate or amino-acid metabolism and adjunct in restricted, specialised, or synthetic diets

**Child 1 month–18 years** 5 mL daily; dose adjusted according to condition, diet, or age; use with *Ketovite® Tablets* for complete vitamin supplementation

**Administration** may be mixed with milk, cereal, or fruit juice

## 9.7  Bitters and tonics

Classification not included in *BNF for Children*.

## 9.8  Metabolic disorders

### 9.8.1  Drugs used in metabolic disorders
### 9.8.2  Acute porphyrias

This section covers drugs used in metabolic disorders and not readily classified elsewhere.

## 9.8.1 Drugs used in metabolic disorders

Metabolic disorders should be managed under the guidance of a specialist. As many preparations are unlicensed and may be difficult to obtain, arrangements for continued prescribing and supply should be made in primary care.

General advice on the use of medicines in metabolic disorders can be obtained from:

Alder Hey Children's Hospital
Medicines Information Centre
Tel: (0151) 252 5381

and

Great Ormond Street Hospital for Children
Pharmacy
Tel: (020) 7405 9200

---

## Wilson's disease

**Penicillamine** is used in Wilson's disease (hepatolenticular degeneration) to aid the elimination of copper ions; it is also used for cystinuria. Children who are hypersensitive to penicillin may react rarely to penicillamine.

**Trientine** is used for the treatment of Wilson's disease only, in patients intolerant of penicillamine; it is **not** an alternative to penicillamine in other diseases such as cystinuria. Penicillamine-induced systemic lupus erythematosus may not resolve on transfer to trientine.

**Zinc** prevents the absorption of copper in Wilson's disease. Symptomatic patients should be treated initially with a chelating agent because zinc has a slow onset of action. When transferring from chelating treatment to zinc maintenance therapy, chelating treatment should be co-administered for 2–3 weeks until zinc produces its maximal effect.

## ▌ PENICILLAMINE

**Cautions** concomitant nephrotoxic drugs (increased risk of toxicity); monitor urine for proteinuria; monitor blood and platelet count regularly (see below); neurological involvement in Wilson's disease; **interactions**: Appendix 1 (penicillamine)

**Blood counts and urine tests** Consider withdrawal if platelet count falls below 120 000/mm$^3$ or white blood cells below 2500/mm$^3$ or if 3 successive falls within reference range (can restart at reduced dose when counts return to within reference range but permanent withdrawal necessary if recurrence of leucopenia or thrombocytopenia)

**Counselling** Warn child and carer to tell doctor immediately if sore throat, fever, infection, non-specific illness, unexplained bleeding and bruising, purpura, mouth ulcers, or rashes develop

**Contra-indications** lupus erythematosus

**Renal impairment** reduce dose and monitor renal function or avoid—consult product literature

**Pregnancy** fetal abnormalities reported rarely; avoid if possible

**Breast-feeding** manufacturer advises avoid unless potential outweighs risk—no information available

**Side-effects** initially nausea, anorexia, fever, rash; proteinuria, thrombocytopenia; *rarely* mouth ulceration, stomatitis, male and female breast enlargement, haematuria (withdraw immediately if cause

unknown), alopecia, pseudoxanthoma elasticum, elastosis perforans, skin laxity; *also reported* pancreatitis, vomiting, cholestatic jaundice, pulmonary haemorrhage, bronchiolitis, pneumonitis, neuropathy (especially if neurological involvement in Wilson's disease—prophylactic pyridoxine recommended, see section 9.6.2), taste loss (mineral supplements not recommended), blood disorders including neutropenia, agranulocytosis, aplastic anaemia, haemolytic anaemia and leucopenia, nephrotic syndrome, glomerulonephritis, Goodpasture's syndrome, lupus erythematosus, myasthenia gravis, polymyositis, rheumatoid arthritis, urticaria, dermatomyositis, pemphigus, Stevens-Johnson syndrome, late rashes (consider dose reduction)

### Indications and dose

**Wilson's disease**

• **By mouth**

**Child 1 month–18 years** 20 mg/kg (max. 2 g) daily in 2–3 divided doses 1 hour before food; usual maintenance dose for child over 12 years 0.75–1 g daily

**Cystinuria**

• **By mouth**

**Child 1 month–18 years** 20–30 mg/kg (max. 3 g) daily in 2–3 divided doses 1 hour before food (lower doses may be used initially and increased gradually), adjusted to maintain 24-hour urinary cystine below 1 mmol/litre; maintain adequate fluid intake

**Penicillamine** (Non-proprietary) [PoM]
Tablets, penicillamine 125 mg, net price 56-tab pack = £16.66; 250 mg, 56-tab pack = £25.00. Label: 6, 22, counselling, blood disorder symptoms (see above)

**Distamine**® (Alliance) [PoM]
Tablets, all f/c, penicillamine 125 mg, net price 100 = £10.34; 250 mg, 100 = £17.78. Label: 6, 22, counselling, blood disorder symptoms (see above)

## ▌ TRIENTINE DIHYDROCHLORIDE

**Cautions** see notes above; **interactions**: Appendix 1 (trientine)

**Pregnancy** teratogenic in *animal* studies—use only if benefit outweighs risk; monitor maternal and neonatal serum-copper concentrations

**Side-effects** nausea, rash; *very rarely* anaemia; duodenitis and colitis also reported

### Indications and dose

**Wilson's disease in patients intolerant of penicillamine**

• **By mouth**

**Child 2–12 years** 0.6–1.5 g daily in 2–4 divided doses before food, adjusted according to response

**Child 12–18 years** 1.2–2.4 g daily in 2–4 divided doses before food, adjusted according to response

**Trientine Dihydrochloride** (Univar) [PoM]
Capsules, trientine dihydrochloride 300 mg. Label: 6, 22

**9**

**Nutrition and blood**

## ZINC ACETATE

**Cautions**   portal hypertension (risk of hepatic decompensation when switching from chelating agent); monitor full blood count and serum cholesterol; **interactions:** Appendix 1 (zinc)

**Pregnancy**   usual dose 25 mg 3 times daily adjusted according to plasma-copper concentration and urinary copper excretion

**Breast-feeding**   manufacturer advises avoid; present in milk—may cause zinc-induced copper deficiency in infant

**Side-effects**   gastric irritation (usually transient; may be reduced if first dose taken mid-morning or with a little protein); *less commonly* sideroblastic anaemia and leucopenia

**Indications and dose**

> Dose expressed as elemental zinc

> **Wilson's disease**
> • By mouth
> **Child 1–6 years** 25 mg twice daily
> **Child 6–16 years** body-weight under 57 kg, 25 mg 3 times daily; body-weight 57 kg or over, 50 mg 3 times daily
> **Child 16–18 years** 50 mg 3 times daily

**Wilzin®** (Orphan Europe) [PoM]
Capsules, zinc (as acetate) 25 mg (blue), net price 250-cap pack = £132.00; 50 mg (orange), 250-cap pack = £242.00. Label: 23
**Administration**   capsules may be opened and the contents mixed with water

---

## Carnitine deficiency

**Carnitine** is available for the management of primary carnitine deficiency due to inborn errors of metabolism, or of secondary deficiency in haemodialysis patients.

Carnitine is also used in the treatment of some organic acidaemias; however, use in fatty acid oxidation is controversial.

## CARNITINE

**Cautions**   diabetes mellitus; monitoring of free and acyl carnitine in blood and urine recommended

**Renal impairment**   accumulation of metabolites may occur with chronic oral administration in severe impairment

**Pregnancy**   appropriate to use; no evidence of teratogenicity in *animal* studies

**Side-effects**   nausea, vomiting, abdominal pain, diarrhoea, fishy body odour; side-effects may be dose-related—monitor tolerance during first week and after any dose increase

**Licensed use**   not licensed for use by intravenous infusion; tablets, chewable tablets, and oral liquid (10%) not licensed in children under 12 years; paediatric oral solution (30%) not licensed in children over 12 years; not licensed for use in organic acidaemias

**Indications and dose**

> **Primary deficiency and organic acidaemias**
> • By mouth
> **Neonate** up to 200 mg/kg daily in 2–4 divided doses
> **Child 1 month–18 years** up to 200 mg/kg daily in 2–4 divided doses; usual max. 3 g daily
> • By intravenous infusion
> **Neonate** initially 100 mg/kg over 30 minutes followed by a continuous infusion of 4 mg/kg/hour
> **Child 1 month–18 years** initially 100 mg/kg over 30 minutes followed by a continuous infusion of 4 mg/kg/hour
> • By slow intravenous injection over 2–3 minutes
> **Neonate** up to 100 mg/kg/daily in 2–4 divided doses
> **Child 1 month–18 years** up to 100 mg/kg/daily in 2–4 divided doses

> **Secondary deficiency in dialysis patients**
> • By slow intravenous injection over 2–3 minutes
> **Child 1 month–18 years** 20 mg/kg after each dialysis session, adjusted according to plasma-carnitine concentration
> • By mouth
> (maintenance therapy if benefit gained from first intravenous course)
> **Child 1 month–18 years** 1 g daily

**Administration**   for *intravenous infusion*, dilute injection with Sodium Chloride 0.9% *or* Glucose 5% or 10%

**Carnitor®** (Sigma-Tau) [PoM]
Tablets, L-carnitine 330 mg, net price 90-tab pack = £103.95

Chewable tablets, L-carnitine 1 g, net price 10-tab pack = £35.00

Oral liquid, L-carnitine 100 mg/mL (10%), net price 10 × 10-mL (1-g) single-dose bottle = £35.00

Paediatric oral solution, L-carnitine 300 mg/mL (30%), net price 20 mL (cherry flavour) = £21.00

Injection, L-carnitine 200 mg/mL, net price 5-mL amp = £11.90

---

## Fabry's disease

**Agalsidase alfa** and **agalsidase beta**, enzymes produced by recombinant DNA technology, are licensed for long-term enzyme replacement therapy in Fabry's disease (a lysosomal storage disorder caused by deficiency of alpha-galactosidase A).

## AGALSIDASE ALFA and BETA

**Cautions**   interactions: Appendix 1 (agalsidase alfa and beta)
**Infusion-related reactions**   Infusion-related reactions very common; manage by slowing the infusion rate or interrupting the infusion, or minimise by pre-treatment with an antihistamine, antipyretic, or corticosteroid—consult product literature

**Pregnancy**   use with caution

**Breast-feeding**   use with caution—no information available

**Side-effects** gastro-intestinal disturbances, taste disturbances; tachycardia, bradycardia, palpitation, hypertension, hypotension, chest pain, oedema, flushing; dyspnoea, cough, rhinorrhoea; headache, fatigue, dizziness, asthenia, paraesthesia, syncope, neuropathic pain, tremor, sleep disturbances; influenza-like symptoms, nasopharyngitis; muscle spasms, myalgia, arthralgia; eye irritation; tinnitus; hypersensitivity reactions, angioedema, pruritus, urticaria, rash, acne; *less commonly* cold extremities, parosmia, ear pain and swelling, skin discoloration, and injection-site reactions

**Indications and dose**

Fabry's disease (specialist use only)
see under preparations

**Fabrazyme®** (Genzyme) PoM
Intravenous infusion, powder for reconstitution, agalsidase beta, net price 5-mg vial = £315.08; 35-mg vial = £2196.59
Dose
Fabry's disease (specialist use only)
• By intravenous infusion
Child 8–18 years 1 mg/kg every 2 weeks
Administration for *intravenous infusion*, reconstitute initially with Water for Injections (5 mg in 1.1 mL, 35 mg in 7.2 mL) to produce a solution containing 5 mg/mL; dilute with Sodium Chloride 0.9% (for doses less than 35 mg dilute with at least 50 mL; doses 35–70 mg dilute with at least 100 mL; doses 70–100 mg dilute with at least 250 mL; doses greater than 100 mg dilute with 500 mL) and give through an in-line low protein-binding 0.2 micron filter at an initial rate of no more than 15 mg/hour; for subsequent infusions, infusion rate may be increased gradually once tolerance has been established

**Replagal®** (Shire HGT) PoM
Concentrate for intravenous infusion, agalsidase alfa 1 mg/mL, net price 1-mL vial = £356.85; 3.5-mL vial = £1068.64
Dose
Fabry's disease (specialist use only)
• By intravenous infusion
Child 7–18 years 200 micrograms/kg every 2 weeks
Administration for *intravenous infusion*, dilute requisite dose with 100 mL Sodium Chloride 0.9% and give over 40 minutes using an in-line filter; use within 3 hours of dilution

## Gaucher's disease

**Imiglucerase**, an enzyme produced by recombinant DNA technology, is administered as enzyme replacement therapy in Gaucher's disease, a familial disorder affecting principally the liver, spleen, bone marrow, and lymph nodes.

**Velaglucerase alfa**, an enzyme produced by recombinant DNA technology, is administered as enzyme replacement therapy for the treatment of type I Gaucher's disease.

**Miglustat**, an inhibitor of glucosylceramide synthase, is licensed in adults for the treatment of mild to moderate type I Gaucher's disease in patients for whom imiglucerase is unsuitable; it is given by mouth.

## IMIGLUCERASE

**Cautions** monitor for imiglucerase antibodies; when stabilised, monitor all parameters and response to treatment at intervals of 6–12 months
**Pregnancy** manufacturer advises use with caution—limited information available
**Breast-feeding** no information available
**Side-effects** hypersensitivity reactions (including urticaria, angioedema, cyanosis, hypotension, flushing, tachycardia, paraesthesia, backache); *less commonly* nausea, vomiting, diarrhoea, abdominal cramps, fatigue, headache, dizziness, fever, arthralgia, injection-site reactions

**Indications and dose**

Gaucher's disease type I (specialist use only)
• By intravenous infusion
Neonate initially 60 units/kg once every 2 weeks, adjusted according to response; doses as low as 30 units/kg once every 2 weeks may be appropriate

Child 1 month–18 years initially 60 units/kg once every 2 weeks, adjusted according to response; doses as low as 30 units/kg once every 2 weeks may be appropriate

Gaucher's disease type III (specialist use only)
• By intravenous infusion
Neonate 60–120 units/kg once every 2 weeks, adjusted according to response

Child 1 month–18 years 60–120 units/kg once every 2 weeks, adjusted according to response

**Administration** For *intravenous infusion*, initially reconstitute with Water for Injections (200 units in 5.1 mL, 400 units in 10.2 mL) to a concentration of 40 units/mL; dilute requisite dose with Sodium Chloride 0.9% to a final volume of 100–200 mL; give initial dose at a rate not exceeding 0.5 units/kg/minute, subsequent doses to be given at a rate not exceeding 1 unit/kg/minute; administer within 3 hours of reconstitution

**Cerezyme®** (Genzyme) PoM
Intravenous infusion, powder for reconstitution, imiglucerase, net price 200-unit vial = £535.65; 400-unit vial = £1071.29
Electrolytes Na⁺ 0.62 mmol/200-unit vial, 1.24 mmol/400-unit vial

## VELAGLUCERASE ALFA

**Cautions** monitor immunoglobulin G (IgG) antibody concentration in severe infusion-related reactions or if there is a lack or loss of effect with velaglucerase alfa
**Infusion-related reactions** Infusion-related reactions very common; manage by slowing the infusion rate, or interrupting the infusion, or minimise by pre-treatment with an antihistamine, antipyretic, or corticosteroid—consult product literature
**Pregnancy** manufacturer advises use with caution—limited information available
**Breast-feeding** manufacturer advises use with caution—no information available
**Side-effects** nausea, abdominal pain, tachycardia, hypertension, hypotension, flushing, headache, dizziness, malaise, pyrexia, arthralgia, bone pain, back pain, hypersensitivity reactions, rash, urticaria

9 Nutrition and blood

## Indications and dose

**Gaucher's disease type I** (specialist use only)

- By intravenous infusion

  **Child 4–18 years** 60 units/kg once every 2 weeks; adjusted according to response to 15–60 units/kg once every 2 weeks

**Administration** for *intravenous infusion*, reconstitute each 400-unit vial with 4.3 mL water for injections; dilute requisite dose in 100 mL Sodium Chloride 0.9% and give over 60 minutes through a 0.22 micron filter; start infusion within 24 hours of reconstitution

**VPRIV®** (Shire HGT) ▼ PoM

Intravenous infusion, powder for reconstitution, velaglucerase alfa, net price 400-unit vial = £1410.20

**Electrolytes** Na⁺ 0.53 mmol/400-unit vial

## Mucopolysaccharidosis

**Laronidase**, an enzyme produced by recombinant DNA technology, is licensed for long-term replacement therapy in the treatment of non-neurological manifestations of mucopolysaccharidosis I, a lysosomal storage disorder caused by deficiency of alpha-L-iduronidase.

**Idursulfase**, an enzyme produced by recombinant DNA technology, is licensed for long-term replacement therapy in mucopolysaccharidosis II (Hunter syndrome), a lysosomal storage disorder caused by deficiency of iduronate-2-sulfatase.

**Galsulfase**, a recombinant form of human N-acetylgalactosamine-4-sulfatase, is licensed for long-term replacement therapy in mucopolysaccharidosis VI (Maroteaux-Lamy syndrome).

**Infusion-related reactions** Infusion-related reactions often occur with administration of laronidase, idursulfase, and galsulfase; they can be managed by slowing the infusion rate or interrupting the infusion, and can be minimised by pre-treatment with an antihistamine and an antipyretic. Recurrent infusion-related reactions may require pre-treatment with a corticosteroid—consult product literature for details.

## GALSULFASE

**Cautions** respiratory disease; acute febrile or respiratory illness (consider delaying treatment)
**Infusion-related reactions** See notes above

**Pregnancy** manufacturer advises avoid unless essential

**Breast-feeding** manufacturer advises avoid—no information available

**Side-effects** abdominal pain, umbilical hernia, gastroenteritis; chest pain, hypertension; dyspnoea, apnoea, nasal congestion; rigors, malaise, areflexia; pharyngitis; conjunctivitis, corneal opacity; ear pain; facial oedema

## Indications and dose

**Mucopolysaccharidosis VI** (specialist use only)

- By intravenous infusion

  **Child 5–18 years** 1 mg/kg once weekly

**Administration** for *intravenous infusion*, dilute requisite dose with Sodium Chloride 0.9% to a final volume of 250 mL and mix gently; infuse through a 0.2 micron in-line filter; give approx. 2.5% of the total volume over 1 hour, then infuse remaining volume over next 3 hours; if body-weight under 20 kg and at risk of fluid overload, dilute requisite dose in 100 mL Sodium Chloride 0.9% and give over at least 4 hours

**Naglazyme®** (BioMarin) PoM

Concentrate for intravenous infusion, galsulfase 1 mg/mL, net price 5-mL vial = £982.00

## IDURSULFASE

**Cautions** severe respiratory disease; acute febrile respiratory illness (consider delaying treatment)
**Infusion-related reactions** See notes above

**Contra-indications** women of child-bearing potential

**Pregnancy** manufacturer advises avoid

**Breast-feeding** manufacturer advises avoid—present in milk in *animal* studies

**Side-effects** gastro-intestinal disturbances, swollen tongue; arrhythmia, tachycardia, chest pain, cyanosis, peripheral oedema, hypertension, hypotension, flushing; bronchospasm, hypoxia, cough, wheezing, tachypnoea, dyspnoea; headache, dizziness, tremor; pyrexia; arthralgia; facial oedema, urticaria, pruritus, rash, infusion-site swelling, erythema; pulmonary embolism and anaphylaxis also reported

## Indications and dose

**Mucopolysaccharidosis II** (specialist use only)

- By intravenous infusion

  **Child 5–18 years** 500 micrograms/kg once weekly

**Administration** for *intravenous infusion*, dilute requisite dose in 100 mL Sodium Chloride 0.9% and mix gently (do not shake); give over 3 hours (gradually reduced to 1 hour if no infusion-related reactions)

**Elaprase®** (Shire HGT) ▼ PoM

Concentrate for intravenous infusion, idursulfase 2 mg/mL, net price 3-mL vial = £1985.00

## LARONIDASE

**Cautions** monitor immunoglobulin G (IgG) antibody concentration; **interactions:** Appendix 1 (laronidase)
**Infusion-related reactions** See notes above

**Pregnancy** manufacturer advises avoid unless essential—no information available

**Breast-feeding** manufacturer advises avoid—no information available

**Side-effects** nausea, vomiting, diarrhoea, abdominal pain; cold extremities, pallor, flushing, tachycardia, blood pressure changes; dyspnoea, cough, angioedema, anaphylaxis; headache, paraesthesia, dizziness, fatigue, restlessness; influenza-like symptoms; musculoskeletal pain, pain in extremities; rash, pruritus, urticaria, alopecia, infusion-site reactions; bronchospasm and respiratory arrest also reported

## Indications and dose

**Non-neurological manifestations of mucopolysaccharidosis I** (specialist use only)

- By intravenous infusion

  **Child 1 month–18 years** 100 units/kg once weekly

**Administration** for *intravenous infusion*, dilute with Sodium Chloride 0.9%; body-weight under 20 kg, dilute to 100 mL, body-weight over 20 kg dilute to 250 mL; give through in-line filter (0.22 micron) initially at a rate of 2 units/kg/hour then increase gradually every 15 minutes to max. 43 units/kg/hour

**Aldurazyme** (Genzyme) PoM
Concentrate for intravenous infusion, laronidase 100 units/mL, net price 5-mL vial = £444.70
Electrolytes Na⁺ 1.29 mmol/5-mL vial

## Nephropathic cystinosis

**Mercaptamine** is available for the treatment of nephropathic cystinosis. The oral dose is increased over several weeks to avoid intolerance. Mercaptamine has a very unpleasant taste and smell, which can affect compliance.

All patients receiving mercaptamine should be registered (contact local specialist centre for details).

Mercaptamine eye drops are used in the management of ocular symptoms arising from the deposition of cystine crystals in the eye.

> **Safe Practice**
> Mercaptamine has been confused with mercaptopurine; care must be taken to ensure the correct drug is prescribed and dispensed.

### ■ MERCAPTAMINE
(Cysteamine)

**Cautions** leucocyte-cystine concentration and haematological monitoring required—consult product literature; dose of phosphate supplement may need to be adjusted if transferring from phosphocysteamine to mercaptamine

**Contra-indications** hypersensitivity to penicillamine

**Pregnancy** avoid—teratogenic and toxic in *animal* studies

**Breast-feeding** avoid

**Side-effects** breath and body odour, nausea, vomiting, diarrhoea, anorexia, abdominal pain, gastroenteritis, dyspepsia, encephalopathy, headache, malaise, fever, rash; *less commonly* gastro-intestinal ulcer, seizures, hallucinations, drowsiness, nervousness, leucopenia, nephrotic syndrome

**Licensed use** eye drops not licensed

**Indications and dose**

Nephropathic cystinosis (specialist use only)
• By mouth

> **Neonate** initially one-sixth to one-quarter of the expected maintenance dose, increased gradually over 4–6 weeks; maintenance, 1.3 g/m² (approx. 50 mg/kg) daily in 4 divided doses
>
> **Child 1 month–12 years or under 50 kg** initially one-sixth to one-quarter of the expected maintenance dose, increased gradually over 4–6 weeks; maintenance, 1.3 g/m² (approx. 50 mg/kg) daily in 4 divided doses
>
> **Child 12–18 years or over 50 kg** initially one-sixth to one-quarter of the expected maintenance dose, increased gradually over 4–6 weeks; maintenance, 2 g daily in 4 divided doses

**Cystagon**® (Orphan Europe) PoM
Capsules, mercaptamine (as bitartrate) 50 mg, net price 100-cap pack = £70.00; 150 mg, 100-cap pack = £190.00. Label: 21
**Note** For child under 6 years at risk of aspiration, capsules can be opened and contents sprinkled on food (at a temperature suitable for eating); avoid adding to acidic drinks (e.g. orange juice)

◀**Eye drops**
**Mercaptamine** (Non-proprietary)
Eye drops, mercaptamine 0.11%, 10 mL
Available from 'special-order' manufacturers or specialist importing companies, see p. 823

## Pompe disease

**Alglucosidase alfa**, an enzyme produced by recombinant DNA technology, is licensed for long-term replacement therapy in Pompe disease, a lysosomal storage disorder caused by deficiency of acid alpha-glucosidase.

### ■ ALGLUCOSIDASE ALFA

**Cautions** cardiac and respiratory dysfunction—monitor closely; monitor immunoglobulin G (IgG) antibody concentration
**Infusion-related reactions** Infusion-related reactions very common, calling for use of antihistamine, antipyretic, or corticosteroid; consult product literature for details

**Pregnancy** toxicity in *animal* studies, but treatment should not be withheld

**Breast-feeding** manufacturer advises avoid—no information available

**Side-effects** nausea, vomiting, diarrhoea; flushing, tachycardia, blood pressure changes, cold extremities, cyanosis, facial oedema, chest discomfort; cough, tachypnoea, bronchospasm; headache, agitation, tremor, irritability, restlessness, paraesthesia, dizziness, fatigue; pyrexia; antibody formation; myalgia, muscle spasms; sweating, rash, pruritus, urticaria, injection-site reactions; hypersensitivity reactions (including anaphylaxis); severe skin reactions (including ulcerative and necrotising skin lesions) also reported

**Indications and dose**

Pompe disease (specialist use only)
• By intravenous infusion

> **Neonate** 20 mg/kg every 2 weeks
>
> **Child 1 month –18 years** 20 mg/kg every 2 weeks

**Administration** For *intravenous infusion*, reconstitute 50 mg with 10.3 mL Water for Injections to produce 5 mg/mL solution; gently rotate vial without shaking; dilute requisite dose with Sodium Chloride 0.9% to give a final concentration of 0.5–4 mg/mL; give through a low protein-binding in-line filter (0.2 micron) at an initial rate of 1 mg/kg/hour increased by 2 mg/kg/hour every 30 minutes to max. 7 mg/kg/hour

**Myozyme**® (Genzyme) PoM
Intravenous infusion, powder for reconstitution, alglucosidase alfa, net price 50-mg vial = £356.06

## Urea cycle disorders

**Sodium benzoate** and **sodium phenylbutyrate** are used in the management of urea cycle disorders. Both, either singly or in combination, are indicated as adjunctive therapy in all patients with neonatal-onset disease and in those with late-onset disease who have a history of hyperammonaemic encephalopathy. Sodium benzoate is also used in non-ketotic hyperglycinaemia.

Gastro-intestinal side-effects of sodium benzoate or sodium phenylbutyrate may be reduced by giving smaller doses more frequently. The preparations contain significant amounts of sodium; therefore, they should be used with caution in children with congestive heart

**9**

**Nutrition and blood**

failure, renal insufficiency and clinical conditions involving sodium retention with oedema.

The long-term management of urea cycle disorders includes oral maintenance treatment with sodium benzoate and sodium phenylbutyrate combined with a low protein diet and other drugs such as **arginine** or **citrulline**, depending on the specific disorder.

**Carglumic acid** is licensed for the treatment of hyperammonaemia due to *N*-acetylglutamate synthase deficiency and organic acidaemia.

## ARGININE

**Cautions**   monitor plasma pH and chloride

**Contra-indications**   not to be used in the treatment of arginase deficiency

**Pregnancy**   no information available

**Breast-feeding**   no information available

**Side-effects**   intravenous injection only: nausea, vomiting; flushing, hypotension; headache, numbness; hyperchloraemic metabolic acidosis; irritation at injection-site

**Licensed use**   injection and tablets not licensed in children; powder licensed for urea cycle disorders in children

**Indications and dose**

**Acute hyperammonaemia in carbamylphosphate synthetase deficiency, ornithine carbamyl transferase deficiency** (specialist use only)
- **By intravenous infusion**

  **Neonate** initially 200 mg/kg over 90 minutes followed by 8 mg/kg/hour

  **Child 1 month–18 years** initially 200 mg/kg over 90 minutes followed by 8 mg/kg/hour

**Maintenance treatment of hyperammonaemia in carbamylphosphate synthetase deficiency, ornithine carbamyl transferase deficiency** (specialist use only)
- **By mouth**

  **Neonate** 100 mg/kg daily in 3–4 divided doses

  **Child 1 month–18 years** 100 mg/kg daily in 3–4 divided doses

**Acute hyperammonaemia in citrullinaemia, arginosuccinic aciduria** (specialist use only)
- **By intravenous infusion**

  **Neonate** initially 600 mg/kg over 90 minutes followed by 25 mg/kg/hour

  **Child 1 month–18 years** initially 600 mg/kg over 90 minutes followed by 25 mg/kg/hour

**Maintenance treatment of hyperammonaemia in citrullinaemia, arginosuccinic aciduria** (specialist use only)
- **By mouth**

  **Neonate** 100–175 mg/kg 3–4 times daily, with food, adjusted according to response

  **Child 1 month–18 years** 100–175 mg/kg 3–4 times daily, with food, adjusted according to response

**L-Arginine** (Non-proprietary)

Tablets, L-arginine (as hydrochloride) 500 mg,

Oral solution, L-arginine 100 mg/mL
Available from 'special-order' manufacturers or specialist importing companies, see p. 823

Powder, L-arginine (as hydrochloride), net price 100 g = £12.27
Prescribe as a borderline substance (ACBS). For use as a supplement in urea cycle disorders other than arginase deficiency, such as hyperammonaemia types I and II, citrullinaemia, arginosuccinic aciduria, and deficiency of N-acetyl glutamate synthetase

Injection, L-arginine (as hydrochloride) 500 mg/mL, 10-mL ampoules; 100 mg/mL, 200-mL amp
Available from 'special-order' manufacturers or specialist importing companies, see p. 823
**Note** Other strengths may be available from 'special-order' manufacturers or specialist importing companies, see p. 823
**Administration** dilute to a concentration of 20 mg/mL with Sodium Chloride 0.9% or 0.45%, *or* Glucose 5% or 10%; max. concentration 100 mg/mL; may be given orally

## CARGLUMIC ACID

**Pregnancy**   manufacturer advises avoid unless essential—no information available

**Breast-feeding**   manufacturer advises avoid—present in milk in *animal* studies

**Side-effects**   sweating; *less commonly* diarrhoea, vomiting, bradycardia, pyrexia

**Indications and dose**

**Hyperammonaemia due to *N*-acetyl glutamate synthase deficiency** (under specialist supervision)
- **By mouth**

  **Neonate** initially 50–125 mg/kg twice daily immediately before feeds, adjusted according to plasma-ammonia concentration; maintenance 5–50 mg/kg twice daily; total daily dose may alternatively be given in 3–4 divided doses

  **Child 1 month–18 years** initially 50–125 mg/kg twice daily immediately before food, adjusted according to plasma-ammonia concentration; maintenance 5–50 mg/kg twice daily; total daily dose may alternatively be given in 3–4 divided doses

**Hyperammonaemia due to organic acidaemia** (under specialist supervision)
- **By mouth**

  **Neonate** initially 50–125 mg/kg twice daily immediately before feeds, adjusted according to plasma-ammonia concentration; total daily dose may alternatively be given in 3–4 divided doses

  **Child 1 month–18 years** initially 50–125 mg/kg twice daily immediately before food, adjusted according to plasma-ammonia concentration; total daily dose may alternatively be given in 3–4 divided doses

**Carbaglu®** (Orphan Europe) PoM
Dispersible tablets, carglumic acid 200 mg, net price 5-tab pack = £299.00, 60-tab pack = £3499.00.
Label: 13

**9 Nutrition and blood**

## ▌ CITRULLINE

**Pregnancy** no information available
**Breast-feeding** no information available
**Indications and dose**

> Carbamyl phosphate synthase deficiency, ornithine carbamyl transferase deficiency
>
> • **By mouth**
>
>> **Neonate** 150 mg/kg daily in 3–4 divided doses, adjusted according to response
>>
>> **Child 1 month–18 years** 150 mg/kg daily in 3–4 divided doses, adjusted according to response

**Citrulline Powder** (Non-proprietary)
Powder, L-citrulline 100 g
Available from 'special-order' manufacturers or specialist importing companies, see p. 823
Administration May be mixed with drinks or taken as a paste

## ▌ SODIUM BENZOATE

**Cautions** see notes above; neonates (risk of kernicterus and increased side-effects); **interactions:** Appendix 1 (sodium benzoate)
**Renal impairment** see notes above
**Pregnancy** no information available
**Breast-feeding** no information available
**Side-effects** nausea, vomiting, anorexia; irritability, lethargy, coma
**Licensed use** not licensed for use in children
**Indications and dose**

> Acute hyperammonaemia due to urea cycle disorders (specialist use only)
>
> • **By intravenous infusion**
>
>> **Neonate** initially 250 mg/kg over 90 minutes followed by 20 mg/kg/hour, adjusted according to response
>>
>> **Child 1 month–18 years** initially 250 mg/kg over 90 minutes followed by 20 mg/kg/hour, adjusted according to response

> Maintenance treatment of hyperammonaemia due to urea cycle disorders; non-ketotic hyperglycinaemia (specialist use only)
>
> • **By mouth**
>
>> **Neonate** 50–150 mg/kg 3–4 times daily, with food, adjusted according to response
>>
>> **Child 1 month–18 years** 50–150 mg/kg 3–4 times daily, with food, adjusted according to response

**Administration** for administration *by mouth*, oral solution or powder may be administered in fruit drinks; less soluble in acidic drinks

**Sodium Benzoate** (Non-proprietary) [PoM]
Tablets, sodium benzoate 500 mg
Available from 'special-order' manufacturers or specialist importing companies, see p. 823

Capsules, sodium benzoate 50 mg; 250 mg; 400 mg; 500 mg
Available from 'special-order' manufacturers or specialist importing companies, see p. 823

Oral solution, sodium benzoate 100 mg/mL; 200 mg/mL; 300 mg/mL
Available from 'special-order' manufacturers or specialist importing companies, see p. 823

Powder, Available from 'special-order' manufacturers or specialist importing companies, see p. 823

Injection, sodium benzoate 200 mg/mL, 5-mL amp
Note Contains Na$^+$ 1.4 mmol /mL
Available from 'special-order' manufacturers or specialist importing companies, see p. 823
Administration for *intravenous infusion*, dilute to a concentration of 20 mg/mL with Sodium Chloride 0.9% or 0.45%, *or* Glucose 5% or 10%; max. concentration 50 mg/mL

## ▌ SODIUM PHENYLBUTYRATE

**Cautions** see notes above; congestive heart failure; **interactions:** Appendix 1 (sodium phenylbutyrate)
**Hepatic impairment** manufacturer advises use with caution
**Renal impairment** manufacturer advises use with caution; see also notes above
**Pregnancy** avoid—toxicity in *animal* studies; manufacturer advises adequate contraception in women of child-bearing potential
**Breast-feeding** manufacturer advises avoid—no information available
**Side-effects** amenorrhoea and irregular menstrual cycles, decreased appetite, body odour, taste disturbances; less commonly nausea, vomiting, abdominal pain, peptic ulcer, pancreatitis, rectal bleeding, arrhythmia, oedema, syncope, depression, headache, rash, weight gain, renal tubular acidosis, aplastic anaemia, ecchymoses
**Licensed use** injection not licensed for use in children
**Indications and dose**

> Acute hyperammonaemia due to urea cycle disorders (specialist use only)
>
> • **By continuous intravenous infusion**
>
>> **Neonate** initially 250 mg/kg over 90 minutes followed by 20 mg/kg/hour adjusted according to response
>>
>> **Child 1 month–18 years** initially 250 mg/kg over 90 minutes followed by 20 mg/kg/hour adjusted according to response

> Maintenance treatment of hyperammonaemia due to urea cycle disorders (specialist use only)
>
> • **By mouth**
>
>> **Neonate** 75–150 mg/kg 3–4 times daily, with food
>>
>> **Child 1 month–18 years** 75–150 mg/kg 3–4 times daily, with food (max. 20 g daily)
>>
>> Administration Oral dose may be mixed with fruit drinks, milk, or feeds

**Sodium Phenylbutyrate** (Non-proprietary) [PoM]
Injection, sodium phenylbutyrate 200 mg/mL, 5-mL amp
Note Contains Na$^+$ 1.1 mmol /mL
Available from 'special-order' manufacturers or specialist importing companies, see p. 823
Administration for *intravenous infusion*, dilute to a concentration of 20 mg/mL (max. 50 mg/mL) with Glucose 5% or 10%

**Ammonaps®** (Swedish Orphan) [PoM]
Tablets, sodium phenylbutyrate 500 mg. Contains Na$^+$ 2.7 mmol/tablet. Net price 250-tab pack = £493.00
Granules, sodium phenylbutyrate 940 mg/g. Contains Na$^+$ 5.4 mmol/g. Net price 266-g pack = £860.00
Note Granules should be mixed with food before taking

## Other metabolic disorders

Other metabolic disorders and the drugs used in their management include:

**Amino acid disorders:** maple syrup urine disease (thiamine section 9.6.2); tyrosinaemia type III, hawkinsinuria (Vitamin C, section 9.6.3); tyrosinaemia type I (nitisinone).

**Mitochondrial disorders:** isolated carboxylase defects, defects of biotin metabolism (biotin, see below); mitochondrial myopathies (ubidecarenone); congenital lactic acidosis (riboflavin and thiamine, section 9.6.3); respiratory chain defects (thiamine, section 9.6.2); pyruvate dehydrogenase defects (sodium dichloroacetate)

**Neimann-Pick type C disease:** miglustat is available for the treatment of progressive neurological manifestations of Neimann-Pick type C disease, a neurodegenerative disorder characterised by impaired intracellular lipid trafficking.

**Homocystinuria and defects in cobalamin metabolism:** betaine, pyridoxine (section 9.6.2), hydroxocobalamin (section 9.1.2)

**Tetrahydrofolate reductase deficiency:** betaine, folic acid (section 9.1.2)

The *Scottish Medicines Consortium* (p. 3) has advised (July 2010) that betaine anhydrous (Cystadane®) is accepted for restricted use within NHS Scotland for the adjunctive treatment of homocystinuria involving deficiencies or defects in cystathionine beta-synthase, 5,10-methylene-tetrahydrofolate reductase, or cobalamin cofactor metabolism in patients who are not responsive to pyridoxine treatment.

### ▌ BETAINE

**Cautions**   monitor plasma-methionine concentration before and during treatment—interrupt treatment if symptoms of cerebral oedema occur

**Pregnancy**   manufacturer advises avoid unless essential—limited information available

**Breast-feeding**   manufacturer advises caution—no information available

**Side-effects**   *less commonly* gastro-intestinal disorders, anorexia, reversible cerebral oedema (see Cautions), agitation, depression, personality disorder, sleep disturbances, urinary incontinence, alopecia, and urticaria

**Indications and dose**

> **Adjunctive treatment of homocystinuria** (specialist use only)
> - By mouth
>
> **Neonate** 50 mg/kg twice daily, dose and frequency adjusted according to response; max. 75 mg/kg twice daily
>
> **Child 1 month–10 years** 50 mg/kg twice daily, dose and frequency adjusted according to response; max. 75 mg/kg twice daily
>
> **Child 10–18 years** 3 g twice daily, adjusted according to response; max. 10 g twice daily

**Administration**   Powder should be mixed with water, juice, milk, formula, or food until completely dissolved and taken immediately; measuring spoons are provided to measure 1 g, 150 mg, and 100 mg of *Cystadane®* powder

**Betaine** (Non-proprietary) [PoM]
Powder (for oral solution), betaine anhydrous 500 mg/mL when reconstituted.
Available from 'special-order' manufacturers or specialist importing companies, see p. 823

Tablets, betaine anhydrous 500 mg
Available from 'special-order' manufacturers or specialist importing companies, see p. 823

**Cystadane®** (Orphan Europe) [PoM]
Powder, betaine (anhydrous), net price 180 g = £347.00

### ▌ BIOTIN
(Vitamin H)

**Pregnancy**   no information available

**Breast-feeding**   no information available

**Indications and dose**

> **Isolated carboxylase defects**
> - By mouth or by slow intravenous injection
>
> **Neonate** 5 mg once daily, adjusted according to response; usual maintenance 10–50 mg daily, higher doses may be required
>
> **Child 1 month–18 years** 10 mg once daily, adjusted according to response; usual maintenance 10–50 mg daily but up to 100 mg daily may be required

> **Defects of biotin metabolism**
> - By mouth or by slow intravenous injection
>
> **Neonate** 10 mg once daily adjusted according to response; usual maintenance 5–20 mg daily but higher doses may be required
>
> **Child 1 month–18 years** 10 mg once daily adjusted according to response; usual maintenance 5–20 mg daily but higher doses may be required

**Biotin** (Non-proprietary) [PoM]
Tablets, biotin 5 mg, 20-tab pack

Injection, biotin 5 mg/mL
Available from 'special order' manufacturers or specialist importing companies, see p. 823
**Administration**   For administration *by mouth*, tablets may be crushed and mixed with food or drink

### ▌ MIGLUSTAT

**Cautions**   monitor cognitive and neurological function, growth, and platelet count

**Hepatic impairment**   manufacturer advises caution—no information available

**Renal impairment**   child 12–18 years, initially 200 mg twice daily if estimated glomerular filtration rate 50–70 mL/minute/1.73 m$^2$; child 12–18 years, initially 100 mg twice daily if estimated glomerular filtration rate 30–50 mL/minute/1.73 m$^2$; avoid if estimated glomerular filtration rate less than 30 mL/minute/1.73 m$^2$; child under 12 years—consult product literature

**Pregnancy**   manufacturer advises avoid (toxicity in *animal* studies)—effective contraception must be used during treatment; also men should avoid fathering a child during and for 3 months after treatment

**Breast-feeding**   manufacturer advises avoid—no information available

**Side-effects**   diarrhoea, flatulence, abdominal pain, dyspepsia, constipation, nausea, vomiting, anorexia, weight changes, tremor, dizziness, headache, peripheral neuropathy, ataxia, amnesia, hypoaesthesia, paraesthesia, insomnia, depression, chills, malaise, decreased libido, thrombocytopenia, muscle spasm and weakness

**Indications and dose**

Neimann-Pick type C disease  (specialist supervision only)

• By mouth

Child 4–12 years

**Body surface area less than 0.47 m²** 100 mg once daily

**Body surface area 0.47–0.73 m²** 100 mg twice daily

**Body surface area 0.73–0.88 m²** 100 mg three times daily

**Body surface area 0.88–1.25 m²** 200 mg twice daily

**Body surface area greater than 1.25 m²** 200 mg three times daily

**Child 12–18 years** 200 mg three times daily

**Zavesca®** (Actelion) PoM
Capsules, miglustat 100 mg, net price 84-cap pack = £3934.17 (hospital only)

## ▌ NITISINONE
(NTBC)

**Cautions**   slit-lamp examination of eyes recommended before treatment; monitor liver function regularly; monitor platelet and white blood cell count every 6 months

**Pregnancy**   manufacturer advises avoid unless potential benefit outweighs risk—toxicity in *animal* studies

**Breast-feeding**   manufacturer advises avoid—adverse effect in *animal* studies

**Side-effects**   thrombocytopenia, leucopenia, granulocytopenia; conjunctivitis, photophobia, corneal opacity, keratitis, eye pain; *less commonly* leucocytosis, blepharitis, pruritus, exfoliative dermatitis, and erythematous rash

**Indications and dose**

Hereditary tyrosinaemia type I (in combination with dietary restriction of tyrosine and phenylalanine)

• By mouth

**Neonate** initially 500 micrograms/kg twice daily, adjusted according to response; max. 2 mg/kg daily

**Child 1 month–18 years** initially 500 micrograms/kg twice daily, adjusted according to response; max. 2 mg/kg daily

**Administration**   capsules can be opened and the contents suspended in a small amount of water or formula diet and taken immediately

**Orfadin®** (Swedish Orphan) PoM
Capsules, nitisinone 2 mg, net price 60-cap pack = £564.00; 5 mg, 60-cap pack = £1127.00; 10 mg, 60-cap pack = £2062.00

## ▌ SODIUM DICHLOROACETATE

**Pregnancy**   no information available

**Breast-feeding**   no information available

**Side-effects**   polyneuropathy on prolonged use; abnormal oxalate metabolism; metabolic acidosis

**Indications and dose**

Pyruvate dehydrogenase defects

• By mouth

**Neonate** initially 12.5 mg/kg 4 times daily, adjusted according to response; up to 200 mg/kg daily may be required

**Child 1 month–18 years** initially 12.5 mg/kg 4 times daily, adjusted according to response; up to 200 mg/kg daily may be required

**Sodium dichloroacetate** (Non-proprietary) PoM
Powder (for oral solution), sodium dichloroacetate 50 mg/mL when reconstituted with water
Available from 'special-order' manufacturers or specialist importing companies, see p. 823

## ▌ UBIDECARENONE
(Ubiquinone, Co-enzyme Q10)

**Cautions**   may reduce insulin requirement in diabetes mellitus; **interactions**: Appendix 1 (ubidecarenone)

**Hepatic impairment**   reduce dose in moderate and severe impairment

**Side-effects**   nausea, diarrhoea, heartburn; *rarely* headache, irritability, agitation, dizziness

**Licensed use**   not licensed

**Indications and dose**

Mitochondrial disorders

• By mouth

**Neonate** initially 5 mg once or twice daily with food, adjusted according to response, up to 200 mg daily may be required

**Child 1 month–18 years** initially 5 mg once or twice daily with food, adjusted according to response, up to 300 mg daily may be required

**Ubidecarenone** (Non-proprietary) PoM
Oral solution, ubidecarenone 50 mg/10 mL

Tablets, ubidecarenone 10 mg

Capsules, ubidecarenone 10 mg, 30 mg
Available from 'special-order' manufacturers or specialist importing companies, see p. 823

## 9.8.2 Acute porphyrias

The acute porphyrias (acute intermittent porphyria, variegate porphyria, hereditary coproporphyria, and 5-aminolaevulinic acid dehydratase deficiency porphyria) are hereditary disorders of haem biosynthesis; they have a prevalence of about 1 in 10 000 of the population.

Great care must be taken when prescribing for patients with acute porphyria, since certain drugs can induce acute porphyric crises. Since acute porphyrias are hereditary, relatives of affected individuals should be screened and advised about the potential danger of certain drugs. Acute attacks of porphyria are exceptionally rare before puberty. When acute porphyria is suspected in a child, support from an expert porphyria service should be sought.

Treatment of serious or life-threatening conditions should not be withheld from patients with acute porphyria. When there is no safe alternative, treatment should be started and urinary porphobilinogen excretion should be measured regularly; if it increases or symptoms occur, the drug can be withdrawn and the acute attack treated. If an acute attack of porphyria occurs during pregnancy, contact an expert porphyria service for further advice.

**Haem arginate** is administered by short intravenous infusion as haem replacement in moderate, severe, or unremitting acute porphyria crises.

The National Acute Porphyria Service (NAPS) provides clinical support and treatment with haem arginate from three centres (University Hospital of Wales, Addenbrooke's Hospital, and King's College Hospital). To access the service telephone (029) 2074 7747 and ask for the Acute Porphyria Service.

## Drugs unsafe for use in acute porphyrias

The following list contains drugs on the UK market that have been classified as 'unsafe' in porphyria because they have been shown to be porphyrinogenic in animals or *in vitro*, or have been associated with acute attacks in patients. Absence of a drug from the following lists does not necessarily imply that the drug is safe. For many drugs no information about porphyria is available.

An up-to-date list of drugs considered **safe** in acute porphyrias is available at www.wmic.wales.nhs.uk/porphyria_info.php.

Further information may be obtained from www.porphyria-europe.org and also from:

Welsh Medicines Information Centre
University Hospital of Wales
Cardiff, CF14 4XW
Tel: (029) 2074 2979/3877
**Note** Quite modest changes in chemical structure can lead to changes in porphyrinogenicity but where possible general statements have been made about groups of drugs; these should be checked first.

---

### ▌ HAEM ARGINATE
(Human hemin)

**Pregnancy** manufacturer advises avoid unless essential

**Breast-feeding** manufacturer advises avoid unless essential—no information available

**Side-effects** pain and thrombophlebitis at injection site; *rarely* hypersensitivity reactions and fever; *also reported* headache

**Indications and dose**

Acute porphyrias (acute intermittent porphyria, porphyria variegata, hereditary coproporphyria)

• By intravenous infusion

Child 1 month–18 years 3 mg/kg once daily (max. 250 mg daily) for 4 days; if response inadequate, repeat 4-day course with close biochemical monitoring

**Normosang**® (Orphan Europe) ▼ PoM
Concentrate for intravenous infusion, haem arginate 25 mg/mL, net price 10-mL amp = £434.25
**Administration** administer over at least 30 minutes through a filter via large antebrachial or central vein; dilute requisite dose in 100 mL Sodium Chloride 0.9% in glass bottle; administer within 1 hour after dilution; max. concentration 2.5 mg/mL

## Unsafe drug groups (check first)

| | | | |
|---|---|---|---|
| Alkylating drugs[1] | Calcium channel blockers[5] | Imidazole antifungals[8] | Sulfonamides[10] |
| Amfetamines | Contraceptives, hormonal[6] | Non-nucleoside reverse | Sulfonylureas[11] |
| Anabolic steroids | Ergot derivatives[7] | transcriptase inhibitors[1] | Taxanes[1] |
| Antidepressants[2] | Gold salts | Progestogens[6] | Tetracyclines |
| Antihistamines[3] | Hormone replacement | Protease inhibitors[1] | Thiazolidinediones[1] |
| Barbiturates[4] | therapy[6] | Statins[9] | Triazole antifungals[8] |

## Unsafe drugs (check groups above first)

| | | | |
|---|---|---|---|
| Aceclofenac | Diclofenac | Metolazone | Rifabutin [19] |
| Alcohol | Disopyramide | Metronidazole[16] | Rifampicin [19] |
| Aminophylline | Disulfiram | Metyrapone | Risperidone |
| Amiodarone | Erythromycin | Mifepristone | Selegiline |
| Artemether with | Etamsylate | Minoxidil [16] | Spironolactone |
| lumefantrine | Ethosuximide | Mitotane | Sulfinpyrazone |
| Bexarotene | Etomidate | Nalidixic acid | Tamoxifen |
| Bosentan | Fenfluramine | Nitrazepam | Telithromycin |
| Bromocriptine | Flupentixol | Nitrofurantoin | Temoporfin |
| Buspirone | Flutamide | Orphenadrine | Theophylline |
| Cabergoline | Fosphenytoin | Oxcarbazepine | Tiagabine |
| Carbamazepine | Griseofulvin | Oxybutynin | Tinidazole |
| Chloral hydrate [12] | Hydralazine | Oxycodone[17] | Topiramate |
| Chloramphenicol | Indapamide | Pentazocine[17] | Toremifene |
| Chloroform[13] | Isometheptene mucate | Pentoxifylline | Trimethoprim |
| Clindamycin | Isoniazid | Phenoxybenzamine | Valproate[14] |
| Cocaine | Ketamine | Phenytoin | Xipamide |
| Colistimethate sodium | Ketorolac | Pivmecillinam | Zidovudine[1] |
| Cycloserine | Lidocaine [15] | Porfimer | Zuclopenthixol |
| Danazol | Mefenamic acid[16] | Potassium canrenoate[18] | |
| Dapsone | Meprobamate | Probenecid | |
| Dexfenfluramine | Methyldopa | Pyrazinamide | |
| Diazepam[14] | Metoclopramide[16] | Raloxifene | |

1. Contact Welsh Medicines Information Centre for further advice.
2. Includes tricyclic (and related) antidepressants and MAOIs; fluoxetine, mianserin, and venlafaxine thought to be safe.
3. Alimemazine, chlorphenamine, desloratadine, fexofenadine, ketotifen, loratadine, and promethazine thought to be safe.
4. Includes primidone and thiopental.
5. Amlodipine, felodipine, and nifedipine may be used with caution.
6. Progestogens are more porphyrinogenic than oestrogens; oestrogens may be safe at least in replacement doses. Progestogens should be avoided whenever possible by all young women susceptible to acute porphyria; however, when non-hormonal contraception is inappropriate, progestogens may be used with extreme caution if the potential benefit outweighs risk. The risk of an acute attack is greatest in young women who have had a previous attack. Long-acting progestogen preparations should never be used in those at risk of acute porphyria.
7. Includes ergometrine (oxytocin probably safe) and pergolide.
8. Applies to oral and intravenous use; topical antifungals are thought to be safe due to low systemic exposure.
9. Rosuvastatin thought to be safe.
10. Includes co-trimoxazole and sulfasalazine.
11. Glipizide is thought to be safe.
12. Although evidence of hazard is uncertain, manufacturer advises avoid.
13. Small amounts in medicines probably safe.
14. Status epilepticus has been treated successfully with intravenous diazepam.
15. When used for local anaesthesia, articaine, bupivacaine, lidocaine, prilocaine, and tetracaine are thought to be safe.
16. May be used with caution if safer alternative not available.
17. Buprenorphine, codeine, diamorphine, dihydrocodeine, fentanyl, methadone, morphine, pethidine, and tramadol are thought to be safe.
18. Evidence of hazard uncertain—contact Welsh Medicines Information Centre for further advice.
19. Rifamycins have been used in a few patients without evidence of harm—use with caution if safer alternative not available.

# 10 Musculoskeletal and joint diseases

This chapter also includes advice on the drug management of the following:

dental and orofacial pain, p. 501

extravasation, p. 518

myasthenia gravis, p. 514

soft-tissue and other musculoskeletal disorders, below

juvenile idiopathic arthritis and other inflammatory disorders, below

For treatment of septic arthritis see Table 1, section 5.1.

## 10.1 Drugs used in rheumatic diseases

### Juvenile idiopathic arthritis and other inflammatory disorders

Rheumatic diseases require symptomatic treatment to relieve pain, swelling, and stiffness, together with treatment to control and suppress disease activity. Treatment of juvenile idiopathic arthritis may involve non-steroidal anti-inflammatory drugs (NSAIDs) (section 10.1.1), a disease modifying antirheumatic drug (DMARD) (section 10.1.3) such as methotrexate or a cytokine modulator, and intra-articular, intravenous, or oral corticosteroids (section 10.1.2).

### Soft-tissue and musculoskeletal disorders

The management of children with soft-tissue injuries and strains, and musculoskeletal disorders, may include temporary rest together with the local application of heat or cold, local massage and physiotherapy. For pain relief, **paracetamol** (section 4.7.1) is often adequate and should be used first. Alternatively, the lowest effective dose of a **NSAID** (e.g. ibuprofen) can be used. If pain relief with either drug is inadequate, both paracetamol (in a full dose appropriate for the child) and a low dose of a NSAID may be required.

### 10.1.1 Non-steroidal anti-inflammatory drugs

In *single doses* non-steroidal anti-inflammatory drugs (NSAIDs) have analgesic activity comparable to that of paracetamol (section 4.7.1), but paracetamol is preferred.

In regular *full dosage* NSAIDs have both a lasting analgesic and an anti-inflammatory effect which makes them particularly useful for the treatment of continuous or regular pain associated with inflammation.

**Choice** Differences in anti-inflammatory activity between NSAIDs are small, but there is considerable variation in individual response and tolerance of these drugs. A large proportion of children will respond to any NSAID; of the others, those who do not respond to one may well respond to another. Pain relief starts soon after taking the first dose and a full analgesic effect should normally be obtained within a week, whereas an anti-inflammatory effect may not be achieved (or may not be clinically assessable) for up to 3 weeks. However, in juvenile idiopathic arthritis NSAIDs may take 4–12 weeks to be effective. If appropriate responses are not obtained within these times, another NSAID should be tried. The availability of appropriate formulations needs to be considered when prescribing NSAIDs for children.

NSAIDs reduce the production of prostaglandins by inhibiting the enzyme cyclo-oxygenase. They vary in their selectivity for inhibiting different types of cyclo-oxygenase; selective inhibition of cyclo-oxygenase-2 is associated with less gastro-intestinal intolerance. However, in children gastro-intestinal symptoms are rare in those taking NSAIDs for short periods. The role of selective inhibitors of cyclo-oxygenase-2 is undetermined in children.

**Ibuprofen** and **naproxen** are propionic acid derivatives used in children:

**Ibuprofen** combines anti-inflammatory, analgesic, and antipyretic properties. It has fewer side-effects than other NSAIDs but its anti-inflammatory properties are weaker.

**Naproxen** combines good efficacy with a low incidence of side-effects.

**Diclofenac**, **indometacin**, **mefenamic acid**, and **piroxicam** have properties similar to those of propionic acid derivatives:

**Diclofenac** is similar in efficacy to naproxen.

**Indometacin** has an action equal to or superior to that of naproxen, but with a high incidence of side-effects including headache, dizziness, and gastro-intestinal disturbances. It is rarely used in children and should be reserved for when other NSAIDs have been unsuccessful.

**Mefenamic acid** has minor anti-inflammatory properties. It has occasionally been associated with diarrhoea and haemolytic anaemia which require discontinuation of treatment.

**Piroxicam** is as effective as naproxen and has a long duration of action which permits once-daily administration. However, it has more gastro-intestinal side-effects than most other NSAIDs, and is associated with more frequent serious skin reactions (**important**: see CHMP advice, p. 506).

**Meloxicam** is a selective inhibitor of cyclo-oxygenase-2. Its use may be considered in adolescents intolerant to other NSAIDs.

**Ketorolac** can be used for the short-term management of postoperative pain (section 15.1.4.2).

**Etoricoxib**, a selective inhibitor of cyclo-oxygenase-2, is licensed for the relief of pain in osteoarthritis, rheumatoid arthritis, ankylosing spondylitis, and acute gout in children aged 16 years and over.

For the role of **aspirin** in children, see section 2.9.

**Dental and orofacial pain**   Most mild to moderate dental pain and inflammation is effectively relieved by **ibuprofen** or **diclofenac**. For information on the risks of serious gastro-intestinal side-effects see below.

For further information on the management of dental and orofacial pain, see p. 199.

**Cautions and contra-indications**   NSAIDs should be used with caution in children with a history of hypersensitivity to any NSAID—which includes those in whom attacks of asthma, angioedema, urticaria or rhinitis have been precipitated by any NSAID. NSAIDs should also be used with caution in coagulation defects. Caution may also be required in children with allergic disorders, and also in children with connective-tissue disorders, see Side-effects below.

In children with cardiac impairment, caution is required since NSAIDs may impair renal function (see also Side-effects below). All NSAIDs are contra-indicated in severe heart failure. Non-selective NSAIDs should be used with caution in uncontrolled hypertension, heart failure, ischaemic heart disease, peripheral arterial disease, cerebrovascular disease, and when used long term in children with risk factors for cardiovascular events. The selective inhibitor of cyclo-oxygenase-2, etoricoxib, is contra-indicated in ischaemic heart disease, cerebrovascular disease, peripheral arterial disease, and mild to severe heart failure. Etoricoxib should be used with caution in children with a history of cardiac failure, left ventricular dysfunction, hypertension, in children with oedema for any other reason, and in children with risk factors for cardiovascular events.

---

### NSAIDs and cardiovascular events

The risk of cardiovascular events secondary to NSAID use is undetermined in children. In adults, all NSAID use (including cyclo-oxygenase-2 selective inhibitors) can, to varying degrees, be associated with a small increased risk of thrombotic events (e.g. myocardial infarction and stroke) independent of baseline cardiovascular risk factors or duration of NSAID use; however, the greatest risk may be in those patients receiving high doses long term. A small increased thrombotic risk cannot be excluded in children.

In adults, **cyclo-oxygenase-2 selective inhibitors**, **diclofenac** (150 mg daily) and **ibuprofen** (2.4 g daily) are associated with an increased risk of thrombotic events. The increased risk for diclofenac is similar to that of **etoricoxib**. **Naproxen** (in adults, 1 g daily) is associated with a lower thrombotic risk, and lower doses of ibuprofen (in adults, 1.2 g daily or less) have not been associated with an increased risk of myocardial infarction.

The lowest effective dose of NSAID should be prescribed for the shortest period of time to control symptoms, and the need for long-term treatment should be reviewed periodically.

---

All NSAIDs (including cyclo-oxygenase-2 selective inhibitors) are contra-indicated in children with active gastro-intestinal ulceration or bleeding. Piroxicam and ketorolac are contra-indicated in children with a history of gastro-intestinal bleeding, ulceration, or perforation. Other non-selective NSAIDs are contra-indicated in children with a history of recurrent gastro-intestinal ulceration or haemorrhage (two or more distinct episodes), and in children with a history of gastro-intestinal bleeding or perforation related to previous NSAID therapy, see also NSAIDs and gastro-intestinal events below. For advice on the prophylaxis and treatment of NSAID-associated gastro-intestinal ulcers, see section 1.3. NSAIDs should also be used with caution in Crohn's disease or ulcerative colitis, as these conditions may be exacerbated.

For **interactions** of NSAIDs, see Appendix 1 (NSAIDs).

**Hepatic impairment**   NSAIDs should be used with caution in children with hepatic impairment; there is an increased risk of gastro-intestinal bleeding and fluid retention. NSAIDs should be avoided in severe liver disease; see also individual drugs.

**Renal impairment**    NSAIDs should be avoided if possible or used with caution in children with renal impairment; the **lowest effective dose** should be used for the **shortest possible duration**, and renal function should be **monitored**. Sodium and water retention may occur and renal function may deteriorate, possibly leading to renal failure; deterioration in renal function has also been reported after topical use; see also individual drugs.

**Pregnancy**    Most manufacturers advise avoiding NSAIDs during pregnancy or avoiding them unless the potential benefit outweighs risk. NSAIDs should be avoided during the third trimester because use is associated with a risk of closure of fetal ductus arteriosus *in utero* and possibly persistent pulmonary hypertension of the newborn. In addition, the onset of labour may be delayed and the duration may be increased.

See also individual monograph for etoricoxib.

**Breast-feeding**    NSAIDs should be used with caution during breast-feeding; see also individual drugs.

**Side-effects**    The side-effects of NSAIDs vary in severity and frequency. Gastro-intestinal disturbances including discomfort, nausea, diarrhoea, and occasionally bleeding and ulceration may occur (see also notes below and Cautions above).

---

### NSAIDs and gastro-intestinal events

All NSAIDs are associated with gastro-intestinal toxicity. In adults, evidence on the relative safety of NSAIDs indicates differences in the risks of serious upper gastro-intestinal side-effects—piroxicam (see also CHMP advice, p. 506) and ketorolac are associated with the highest risk; indometacin, diclofenac, and naproxen are associated with intermediate risk, and ibuprofen with the lowest risk (although high doses of ibuprofen have been associated with intermediate risk). **Selective inhibitors of cyclooxygenase-2** associated with a *lower risk* of serious upper gastro-intestinal side-effects than non-selective NSAIDs.

Children appear to tolerate NSAIDs better than adults and gastro-intestinal side-effects are less common although they do still occur and can be significant; use of gastro-protective drugs may be necessary (see also section 1.3).

---

Other side-effects include hypersensitivity reactions (particularly rashes, angioedema, and bronchospasm), headache, dizziness, nervousness, depression, drowsiness, insomnia, vertigo, hearing disturbances such as tinnitus, photosensitivity, and haematuria. Blood disorders have also occurred. Fluid retention may occur (rarely precipitating congestive heart failure); blood pressure may be raised.

---

### Asthma

All NSAIDs have the potential to worsen asthma, either acutely or as a gradual worsening of symptoms; consider both prescribed NSAIDs and those that are purchased over the counter.

---

Renal failure may be provoked by NSAIDs, especially in patients with pre-existing renal impairment (**important**, see Renal impairment above). Rarely, papillary necrosis

or interstitial fibrosis associated with NSAIDs can lead to renal failure. Hepatic damage, alveolitis, pulmonary eosinophilia, pancreatitis, visual disturbances, Stevens-Johnson syndrome, and toxic epidermal necrolysis are other rare side-effects. Induction of or exacerbation of colitis or Crohn's disease has been reported. Aseptic meningitis has been reported rarely with NSAIDs—children with connective tissue disorders such as systemic lupus erythematosus may be especially susceptible.

**Overdosage:** see Emergency Treatment of Poisoning, p. 25 .

---

### ■ DICLOFENAC POTASSIUM

**Cautions**    see notes above; avoid in acute porphyria (section 9.8.2)

**Contra-indications**    see notes above

**Hepatic impairment**    see notes above

**Renal impairment**    avoid in severe impairment; see also notes above

**Pregnancy**    see notes above

**Breast-feeding**    amount in milk too small to be harmful; see also notes above

**Side-effects**    see notes above

**Licensed use**    *Voltarol® Rapid* not licensed for use in children under 14 years or in fever

#### Indications and dose

> **Rheumatic disease and musculoskeletal disorders**
>
> ● **By mouth**
>
>   **Child 14–18 years** 75–100 mg daily in 2–3 divided doses

> **Postoperative pain**
>
> ● **By mouth**
>
>   **Child 9–14 years and body-weight over 35 kg** up to 2 mg/kg (max. 100 mg) daily in 3 divided doses
>
>   **Child 14–18 years** 75–100 mg daily in 2–3 divided doses

> **Fever in ear, nose, or throat infection**
>
> ● **By mouth**
>
>   **Child 9–18 years and body-weight over 35 kg** up to 2 mg/kg (max. 100 mg) daily in 3 divided doses

**Diclofenac Potassium** (Non-proprietary) PoM
Tablets, diclofenac potassium 25 mg, net price 28-tab pack = 81p; 50 mg, 28-tab pack = £1.55. Label: 21

[1]**Voltarol® Rapid** (Novartis) PoM
Tablets, s/c, diclofenac potassium 25 mg (red), net price 30-tab pack = £3.46; 50 mg (brown), 30-tab pack = £6.62. Label: 21

---

### ■ DICLOFENAC SODIUM

**Cautions**    see notes above; avoid in acute porphyria (section 9.8.2)

---

1.  12.5 mg tablets can be sold to the public for the treatment of headache, dental pain, period pain, rheumatic and muscular pain, backache and the symptoms of cold and flu (including fever), in patients aged over 14 years subject to max. single dose of 25 mg, max. daily dose of 75 mg for max. 3 days, and max. pack size of 18 × 12.5 mg

**Contra-indications**  see notes above; avoid suppositories in proctitis; avoid injections containing benzyl
alcohol in neonates (see preparations below)
**Intravenous use**  Additional contra-indications include
concomitant NSAID or anticoagulant use (including low-
dose heparins), history of haemorrhagic diathesis, history of
confirmed or suspected cerebrovascular bleeding,
operations with high risk of haemorrhage, history of asthma,
moderate or severe renal impairment, hypovolaemia,
dehydration

**Hepatic impairment**  see notes above

**Renal impairment**  avoid in severe impairment; see
also Intravenous Use and notes above

**Pregnancy**  see notes above

**Breast-feeding**  amount in milk too small to be
harmful; see also notes above

**Side-effects**  see notes above; suppositories may
cause rectal irritation; injection site reactions

**Licensed use**  not licensed for use in children under 1
year; *suppositories* not licensed for use in children
under 6 years except for use in children over 1 year
for juvenile idiopathic arthritis; solid dose forms
containing more than 25 mg not licensed for use in
children; *injection* not licensed for use in children

**Indications and dose**

**Inflammation and mild to moderate pain**

● By mouth or by rectum
   **Child 6 months–18 years** 0.3–1 mg/kg (max.
   50 mg) 3 times daily

**Postoperative pain**

● By rectum
   **Child 6 months–18 years**
   **Body-weight 8–12 kg** 12.5 mg twice daily for max.
   4 days
   **Body-weight over 12 kg** 1 mg/kg (max. 50 mg) 3
   times daily for max. 4 days
● By intravenous infusion or deep intramuscular
   injection into gluteal muscle
   **Child 2–18 years** 0.3–1 mg/kg once or twice daily
   for max. 2 days (max. 150 mg daily)

**Pain and inflammation in rheumatic disease
including juvenile idiopathic arthritis**

● By mouth
   **Child 6 months–18 years** 1.5–2.5 mg/kg (max.
   75 mg) twice daily; total daily dose may alternatively be given in 3 divided doses

**Administration**  for *intravenous infusion*, dilute 75 mg
with 100–500 mL Glucose 5% *or* Sodium Chloride
0.9% (previously buffered with 0.5 mL Sodium
Bicarbonate 8.4% solution *or* with 1 mL Sodium
Bicarbonate 4.2% solution); give over 30–120 minutes

**Diclofenac Sodium** (Non-proprietary) PoM
Tablets, both e/c, diclofenac sodium 25 mg, net
price 84-tab pack = £1.14; 50 mg, 84-tab pack =
£1.31. Label: 5, 25
**Brands include** *Defenac*®, *Dicloflex*®, *Diclozip*®, *Fenactol*®,
*Flamrase*®
Dispersible tablets, sugar-free, diclofenac sodium
10 mg
Available from 'special-order' manufacturers or specialist
importing companies, see p. 823
Suppositories, diclofenac sodium 100 mg, net price
10 = £3.97
**Brands include** *Econac*®

**Voltarol**® (Novartis) PoM
Tablets, e/c, diclofenac sodium 25 mg (yellow), net
price 84-tab pack = £2.94; 50 mg (brown), 84-tab
pack = £4.57. Label: 5, 25

Dispersible tablets, sugar-free, pink, diclofenac,
equivalent to diclofenac sodium 50 mg, net price
21-tab pack = £6.19. Label: 13, 21

Injection, diclofenac sodium 25 mg/mL, net price
3-mL amp = 83p
**Excipients**  include benzyl alcohol (avoid in neonates, see
Excipients, p. 2), propylene glycol

Suppositories, diclofenac sodium 12.5 mg, net price
10 = 58p; 25 mg, 10 = £1.03; 50 mg, 10 = £1.70;
100 mg, 10 = £3.03

◢**Modified release**

**Diclomax SR**® (Galen) PoM
Capsules, m/r, yellow, diclofenac sodium 75 mg,
net price 56-cap pack = £11.40. Label: 21, 25
**Dose**

**Pain and inflammation**

● By mouth
   **Child 12–18 years** 1 capsule 1–2 times daily

**Diclomax Retard**® (Galen) PoM
Capsules, m/r, diclofenac sodium 100 mg, net price
28-cap pack = £8.20. Label: 21, 25
**Dose**

**Pain and inflammation**

● By mouth
   **Child 12–18 years** 1 capsule once daily

**Motifene**® **75 mg** (Daiichi Sankyo) PoM
Capsules, e/c, m/r, diclofenac sodium 75 mg
(enclosing e/c pellets containing diclofenac sodium
25 mg and m/r pellets containing diclofenac sodium
50 mg), net price 56-cap pack = £8.00. Label: 25
**Excipients**  include propylene glycol (see Excipients, p. 2)
**Dose**

**Pain and inflammation**

● By mouth
   **Child 12–18 years** 1 capsule 1–2 times daily

**Voltarol**® **75 mg SR** (Novartis) PoM
Tablets, m/r, pink, diclofenac sodium 75 mg, net
price 28-tab pack = £6.46; 56-tab pack = £12.92.
Label: 21, 25
**Dose**

**Pain and inflammation**

● By mouth
   **Child 12–18 years** 1 tablet 1–2 times daily

**Note** Other brands of modified-release tablets containing
diclofenac sodium 75 mg include *Defenac*® SR, *Dexomon*® 75
SR, *Dicloflex*® 75 SR, *Fenactol*® 75 mg SR, *Flamatak*® 75 MR,
*Flamrase*® SR, *Flexotard*® MR 75, *Rheumatac*® Retard 75,
*Rhumalgan*® CR, *Slofenac*® SR, *Volsaid*® Retard 75

**Voltarol**® **Retard** (Novartis) PoM
Tablets, m/r, red, diclofenac sodium 100 mg, net
price 28-tab pack = £9.47. Label: 21, 25
**Dose**

**Pain and inflammation**

● By mouth
   **Child 12–18 years** 1 tablet once daily

**Note** Other brands of modified-release tablets containing
diclofenac sodium 100 mg include *Defenac*® Retard,
*Dexomon*® Retard 100, *Dicloflex*® Retard, *Fenactol*® Retard
100 mg, *Flamatak*® 100 MR, *Slofenac*® SR, *Volsaid*® Retard
100

**10 Musculoskeletal and joint diseases**

## ETORICOXIB

**Cautions** see notes above; also dehydration; monitor blood pressure before treatment, 2 weeks after initiation and periodically during treatment

**Contra-indications** see notes above; inflammatory bowel disease; uncontrolled hypertension (persistently above 140/90 mmHg)

**Hepatic impairment** max. 60 mg daily in mild impairment; max. 60 mg on alternate days or 30 mg once daily in moderate impairment; see also notes above

**Renal impairment** avoid if estimated glomerular filtration rate less than 30 mL/minute/1.73 m$^2$; see also notes above

**Pregnancy** manufacturer advises avoid (teratogenic in *animal* studies); see also notes above

**Breast-feeding** manufacturer advises avoid—present in milk in *animal* studies; see also notes above

**Side-effects** see notes above; also palpitation, fatigue, influenza-like symptoms, ecchymosis; *less commonly* dry mouth, taste disturbance, mouth ulcer, appetite and weight change, atrial fibrillation, transient ischaemic attack, chest pain, flushing, cough, dyspnoea, epistaxis, anxiety, mental acuity impaired, paraesthesia, electrolyte disturbance, myalgia and arthralgia; *very rarely* confusion and hallucinations

### Indications and dose

**Osteoarthritis**
- **By mouth**

    **Child 16–18 years** 30 mg once daily, increased if necessary to 60 mg once daily

**Rheumatoid arthritis and ankylosing spondylitis**
- **By mouth**

    **Child 16–18 years** 90 mg once daily

**Acute gout**
- **By mouth**

    **Child 16–18 years** 120 mg once daily for max. 8 days

**Arcoxia**® (MSD) [PoM]
Tablets, f/c, etoricoxib 30 mg (blue-green), net price 28-tab pack = £13.99; 60 mg (dark green), 28-tab pack = £20.11; 90 mg (white), 28-tab pack = £22.96; 120 mg (pale green), 7-tab pack = £6.03, 28-tab pack = £24.11

## IBUPROFEN

**Cautions** see notes above

**Contra-indications** see notes above

**Hepatic impairment** see notes above

**Renal impairment** avoid in severe impairment; see also notes above

**Pregnancy** see notes above

**Breast-feeding** amount too small to be harmful, but some manufacturers advise avoid; see also notes above

**Side-effects** see notes above

**Licensed use** not licensed for use in children under 3 months or body-weight under 5 kg

### Indications and dose

**Mild to moderate pain, pain and inflammation of soft-tissue injuries, pyrexia with discomfort**
- **By mouth**

    **Child 1–3 months** 5 mg/kg 3–4 times daily

    **Child 3–6 months** 50 mg 3 times daily; max. 30 mg/kg daily in 3–4 divided doses

    **Child 6 months–1 year** 50 mg 3–4 times daily; max. 30 mg/kg daily in 3–4 divided doses

    **Child 1–4 years** 100 mg 3 times daily; max. 30 mg/kg daily in 3–4 divided doses

    **Child 4–7 years** 150 mg 3 times daily; max. 30 mg/kg daily in 3–4 divided doses

    **Child 7–10 years** 200 mg 3 times daily; max. 30 mg/kg (max. 2.4 g) daily in 3–4 divided doses

    **Child 10–12 years** 300 mg 3 times daily; max. 30 mg/kg (max. 2.4 g) daily in 3–4 divided doses

    **Child 12–18 years** initially 300–400 mg 3–4 times daily; increased if necessary to max. 600 mg 4 times daily; maintenance dose of 200–400 mg 3 times daily may be adequate

**Pain and inflammation in rheumatic disease including juvenile idiopathic arthritis**
- **By mouth**

    **Child 3 months–18 years** 30–40 mg/kg (max. 2.4 g) daily in 3–4 divided doses; in systemic juvenile idiopathic arthritis up to 60 mg/kg (max. 2.4 g) daily [unlicensed] in 4–6 divided doses

**Post-immunisation pyrexia in infants** (see also p. 601)
- **By mouth**

    **Child 2–3 months** 50 mg as a single dose repeated once after 6 hours if necessary

**Closure of patent ductus arteriosus in neonates** see section 2.14

[1]**Ibuprofen** (Non-proprietary) [PoM]
Tablets, coated, ibuprofen 200 mg, net price 84-tab pack = £1.62; 400 mg, 84-tab pack = £1.72; 600 mg, 84-tab pack = £4.06. Label: 21
**Brands include** *Arthrofen*®, *Ebufac*®, *Rimafen*®
**Dental prescribing on NHS** Ibuprofen Tablets may be prescribed

Oral suspension, ibuprofen 100 mg/5 mL, net price 100 mL = £1.48, 150 mL = £2.71, 500 mL = £8.88. Label: 21
**Note** Sugar-free versions are available and can be ordered by specifying 'sugar-free' on the prescription
**Brands include** *Calprofen*®, *Feverfen*®, *Nurofen*® for Children, *Orbifen*® for Children
**Dental prescribing on NHS** Ibuprofen Oral Suspension Sugar-free may be prescribed

**Brufen**® (Abbott Healthcare) [PoM]
Tablets, f/c, ibuprofen 200 mg, net price 100-tab pack = £3.92; 400 mg, 100-tab pack = £8.16; 600 mg, 100-tab pack = £12.24. Label: 21

Syrup, orange, ibuprofen 100 mg/5 mL, net price 500 mL (orange-flavoured) = £8.88. Label: 21

Granules, effervescent, ibuprofen 600 mg/sachet, net price 20–sachet pack = £6.53. Label: 13, 21
Contains sodium approx. 6.5 mmol/sachet

1. Can be sold to the public under certain circumstances

◢Modified release

**Brufen Retard**® (Abbott Healthcare) [PoM]
Tablets, m/r, ibuprofen 800 mg, net price 56-tab pack = £6.48. Label: 25, 27

**Dose**

> **Pain and inflammation**
>
> - By mouth
>
>   **Child 12–18 years** 2 tablets daily as a single dose, preferably in the early evening, increased in severe cases to 3 tablets daily in 2 divided doses

**Fenbid**® (Mercury) [PoM]
Spansule® (= capsule m/r), maroon/pink, enclosing off-white pellets, ibuprofen 300 mg, net price 120-cap pack = £9.64. Label: 25

**Dose**

> **Pain and inflammation**
>
> - By mouth
>
>   **Child 12–18 years** initially 2 capsules twice daily, increased in severe cases to 3 capsules twice daily; then 1–2 capsules twice daily

## INDOMETACIN
(Indomethacin)

**Cautions** see notes above; also epilepsy, psychiatric disturbances; during prolonged therapy ophthalmic and blood examinations particularly advisable; avoid rectal administration in proctitis and haemorrhoids
**Skilled tasks** Dizziness may affect performance of skilled tasks (e.g. driving)

**Contra-indications** see notes above

**Hepatic impairment** see notes above

**Renal impairment** avoid in severe impairment; see also notes above

**Pregnancy** see notes above

**Breast-feeding** amount probably too small to be harmful—manufacturer advises avoid; see also notes above

**Side-effects** see notes above; *rarely* confusion, convulsions, psychiatric disturbances, syncope, blood disorders (particularly thrombocytopenia), hyperglycaemia, peripheral neuropathy, intestinal strictures; *also reported* hyperkalaemia; suppositories may cause rectal irritation and occasional bleeding

**Licensed use** not licensed for use in children

**Indications and dose**

> **Relief of pain and inflammation in rheumatic diseases including juvenile idiopathic arthritis** (but see p. 500)
>
> - By mouth
>
>   **Child 1 month–18 years** 0.5–1 mg/kg twice daily; higher doses may be used under specialist supervision

> **Closure of patent ductus arteriosus in premature babies** section 2.14

**Indometacin** (Non-proprietary) [PoM]
Capsules, indometacin 25 mg, net price 28-cap pack = £2.33; 50 mg, 28-cap pack = £2.29. Label: 21, counselling, driving, see above

Suppositories, indometacin 100 mg, net price 10 = £20.07. Counselling, driving, see above

Suspension, indometacin 5 mg/mL
Available from 'special-order' manufacturers or specialist importing companies, see p. 823

◢Modified release

**Indometacin m/r preparations** [PoM]
Capsules, m/r, indometacin 75 mg. Label: 21, 25, counselling, driving, see above
Brands include *Indolar SR*®, *Pardelprin*®

## MEFENAMIC ACID

**Cautions** see notes above; epilepsy; acute porphyria (section 9.8.2)

**Contra-indications** see notes above; inflammatory bowel disease

**Hepatic impairment** see notes above

**Renal impairment** avoid in severe impairment; see also notes above

**Pregnancy** see notes above

**Breast-feeding** amount too small to be harmful but manufacturer advises avoid; see also notes above

**Side-effects** see notes above; also diarrhoea or rashes (withdraw treatment), stomatitis; *less commonly* paraesthesia and fatigue; *rarely* hypotension, palpitation, glucose intolerance, thrombocytopenia, haemolytic anaemia (positive Coombs' test), and aplastic anaemia

**Indications and dose**

> **Acute pain including dysmenorrhoea, menorrhagia**
>
> - By mouth
>
>   **Child 12–18 years** 500 mg 3 times daily

**Mefenamic Acid** (Non-proprietary) [PoM]
Capsules, mefenamic acid 250 mg, net price 100 = £2.83. Label: 21

Tablets, mefenamic acid 500 mg, net price 28-tab pack = £2.20. Label: 21

Suspension, mefenamic acid 50 mg/5 mL, net price 125 mL = £79.98. Label: 21
**Excipients** include ethanol

**Ponstan**® (Chemidex) [PoM]
Capsules, blue/ivory, mefenamic acid 250 mg, net price 100-cap pack = £8.17. Label: 21

Forte tablets, yellow, mefenamic acid 500 mg, net price 100-tab pack = £15.72. Label: 21

## MELOXICAM

**Cautions** see notes above

**Contra-indications** see notes above

**Hepatic impairment** see notes above

**Renal impairment** avoid if estimated glomerular filtration rate less than 25 mL/minute/1.73 m$^2$; see also notes above

**Pregnancy** see notes above

**Breast-feeding** present in milk in *animal* studies—manufacturer advises avoid; see also notes above

**Side-effects** see notes above

**Licensed use** not licensed for use in children under 16 years

**10 Musculoskeletal and joint diseases**

### Indications and dose

**Relief of pain and inflammation in juvenile idiopathic arthritis and other musculoskeletal disorders in children intolerant to other NSAIDs**

- **By mouth**

  **Child 12–18 years and body-weight under 50 kg**
  7.5 mg once daily

  **Child 12–18 years and body-weight over 50 kg**
  15 mg once daily

**Meloxicam** (Non-proprietary) [PoM]

Tablets, meloxicam 7.5 mg, net price 30-tab pack = £1.36; 15 mg, 30-tab pack = £1.62

## ▌ NAPROXEN

**Cautions** see notes above; **interactions:** Appendix 1 (NSAIDs)

**Contra-indications** see notes above

**Hepatic impairment** see notes above

**Renal impairment** avoid if estimated glomerular filtration rate less than 30 mL/minute/1.73 m$^2$; see also notes above

**Pregnancy** see notes above

**Breast-feeding** amount too small to be harmful but manufacturer advises avoid; see also notes above

**Side-effects** see notes above

**Licensed use** not licensed for use in children under 5 years for juvenile idiopathic arthritis; not licensed for use in children under 16 years for musculoskeletal disorders or dysmenorrhoea

### Indications and dose

**Pain and inflammation in musculoskeletal disorders, dysmenorrhoea**

- **By mouth**

  **Child 1 month–18 years** 5 mg/kg twice daily (max. 1 g daily)

**Juvenile idiopathic arthritis**

- **By mouth**

  **Child 2–18 years** 5–7.5 mg/kg twice daily (max. 1 g daily)

[1]**Naproxen** (Non-proprietary) [PoM]

Tablets, naproxen 250 mg, net price 28-tab pack = £1.35; 500 mg, 28-tab pack = £1.72. Label: 21
**Brands include** *Arthroxen*®

Tablets, e/c, naproxen 250 mg, net price 56-tab pack = £3.18; 375 mg, 56-tab pack = £26.82; 500 mg, 56-tab pack = £4.83. Label: 5, 25

Suspension, naproxen 25 mg/mL
Available from 'special-order' manufacturers or specialist importing companies, see p. 823

1. Can be sold to the public for the treatment of primary dysmenorrhoea in women aged 15–50 years subject to max. single dose of 500 mg, max. daily dose of 750 mg for max. 3 days, and a max. pack size of 9 × 250 mg tablets

**Naprosyn**® (Roche) [PoM]

Tablets, yellow, scored, naproxen 250 mg, net price 56-tab pack = £4.29; 500 mg, 56-tab pack = £8.56. Label: 21

Tablets, e/c, (*Naprosyn EC*®), naproxen 250 mg, net price 56-tab pack = £4.29; 375 mg, 56-tab pack = £6.42; 500 mg, 56-tab pack = £8.56. Label: 5, 25

## ▌ PIROXICAM ◢

**Cautions** see notes above and CHMP advice below

**Contra-indications** inflammatory bowel disease; see also notes above

**Hepatic impairment** see notes above

**Renal impairment** see notes above

**Pregnancy** see notes above

**Breast-feeding** amount too small to be harmful; see also notes above

**Side-effects** see notes above

**Licensed use** not licensed for use in children

### Indications and dose

**Relief of pain and inflammation in juvenile idiopathic arthritis**

- **By mouth**

  **Child 6–18 years and body-weight under 15 kg**
  5 mg daily

  **Child 6–18 years and body-weight 16–25 kg**
  10 mg daily

  **Child 6–18 years and body-weight 26–45 kg**
  15 mg daily

  **Child 6–18 years and body-weight over 46 kg**
  20 mg daily

---

**CHMP advice**
**Piroxicam (June 2007)**

The CHMP has recommended restrictions on the use of piroxicam because of the increased risk of gastro-intestinal side effects and serious skin reactions. The CHMP has advised that:

- piroxicam should be initiated only by physicians experienced in treating inflammatory or degenerative rheumatic diseases
- piroxicam should not be used as first-line treatment
- in adults, use of piroxicam should be limited to the symptomatic relief of osteoarthritis, rheumatoid arthritis, and ankylosing spondylitis
- piroxicam dose should not exceed 20 mg daily
- piroxicam should no longer be used for the treatment of acute painful and inflammatory conditions
- treatment should be reviewed 2 weeks after initiating piroxicam, and periodically thereafter
- concomitant administration of a gastro-protective agent (section 1.3) should be considered

**Note**

Topical preparations containing piroxicam are not affected by these restrictions

---

**Piroxicam** (Non-proprietary) [PoM] ◢

Capsules, piroxicam 10 mg, net price 56-cap pack = £16.62; 20 mg, 28-cap pack = £22.45. Label: 21

Dispersible tablets, piroxicam 10 mg, net price 56-tab pack = £9.96; 20 mg, 28-tab pack = £32.41. Label: 13, 21

**Brexidol**® (Chiesi) [PoM] ◢

Tablets, yellow, scored, piroxicam (as betadex) 20 mg, net price 30-tab pack = £13.82. Label: 21

**Feldene®** (Pfizer) (PoM) ▨

Capsules, piroxicam 10 mg (red/blue), net price 30-cap pack = £3.86; 20 mg (white), 30-cap pack = £7.71. Label: 21

Tablets, (*Feldene Melt®*), piroxicam 20 mg, net price 30-tab pack = £10.53. Label: 10, patient information leaflet, 21

Excipients  include aspartame equivalent to phenylalanine 140 micrograms/tablet (section 9.4.1)

Note  Tablets may be halved [unlicensed] to give 10-mg dose; tablet placed on tongue and allowed to dissolve or may be swallowed

## 10.1.2  Corticosteroids

10.1.2.1  Systemic corticosteroids
10.1.2.2  Local corticosteroid injections

## 10.1.2.1  Systemic corticosteroids

The general actions, uses, and cautions of corticosteroids are described in section 6.3. In children with rheumatic diseases corticosteroids should be reserved for specific indications (e.g. when other therapies are unsuccessful or while waiting for DMARDs to take effect) and should be used only under the supervision of a specialist.

Systemic corticosteroids may be considered for the management of juvenile idiopathic arthritis in systemic disease or when several joints are affected. Systemic corticosteroids may also be considered in severe, possibly life-threatening conditions such as systemic lupus erythematosus, systemic vasculitis, juvenile dermatomyositis, Behçet's disease, and polyarticular joint disease.

In severe conditions, short courses ('pulses') of high-dose intravenous methylprednisolone or a pulsed oral corticosteroid may be particularly effective for providing rapid relief, and has fewer long-term adverse effects than continuous treatment.

Corticosteroid doses should be reduced with care because of the possibility of relapse if the reduction is too rapid. If complete discontinuation of corticosteroids is not possible, consideration should be given to alternate-day (or alternate high-dose, low-dose) administration; on days when no corticosteroid is given, or a lower dose is given, an additional dose of a NSAID may be helpful. In some conditions, alternative treatment using an antimalarial or concomitant use of an immunosuppressant drug, such as azathioprine, methotrexate or cyclophosphamide may prove useful; in less severe conditions treatment with a NSAID alone may be adequate.

Administration of corticosteroids may result in suppression of growth and may affect the development of puberty. The risk of corticosteroid-induced osteoporosis should be considered for those on long-term corticosteroid treatment (section 6.6); corticosteroids may also increase the risk of osteopenia in those unable to exercise. For the disadvantages of corticosteroid treatment see section 6.3.2.

## 10.1.2.2  Local corticosteroid injections

Corticosteroids are injected locally for an anti-inflammatory effect. In inflammatory conditions of the joints, including juvenile idiopathic arthritis, they are given by *intra-articular injection* as monotherapy, or as an adjunct to long-term therapy to reduce swelling and deformity in one or a few joints. Aseptic precautions (e.g. a no-touch technique) are essential, as is a clinician skilled in the technique; infected areas should be avoided and general anaesthesia, or local anaesthesia, or conscious sedation should be used. Occasionally an acute inflammatory reaction develops after an intra-articular or soft-tissue injection of a corticosteroid. This may be a reaction to the microcrystalline suspension of the corticosteroid used, but must be distinguished from sepsis introduced into the injection site.

Triamcinolone hexacetonide [unlicensed] is preferred for intra-articular injection because it is almost insoluble and has a long-acting (depot) effect. Triamcinolone acetonide and methylprednisolone may also be considered for intra-articular injection into larger joints, whilst hydrocortisone acetate should be reserved for smaller joints or for soft-tissue injections. Intra-articular corticosteroid injections can cause flushing and, in adults, may affect the hyaline cartilage. Each joint should usually be treated no more than 3–4 times in one year.

A smaller amount of corticosteroid may also be injected directly into soft tissues for the relief of inflammation in conditions such as *tennis* or *golfer's elbow* or *compression neuropathies*, which occur rarely in children. In *tendinitis*, injections should be made into the tendon sheath and not directly into the tendon (due to the absence of a true tendon sheath and a high risk of rupture, the Achilles tendon should not be injected).

Corticosteroid injections are also injected into soft tissues for the treatment of skin lesions (see section 13.4).

## LOCAL CORTICOSTEROID INJECTIONS

**Cautions**  see notes above and consult product literature; see also section 6.3.2

**Contra-indications**  see notes above and consult product literature; avoid injections containing benzyl alcohol in neonates (see preparation below)

**Side-effects**  see notes above and consult product literature

**Licensed use**  triamcinolone acetonide not licensed for use in children under 6 years

**Indications and dose**

See under preparations

◢Hydrocortisone acetate

**Hydrocortistab®** (Sovereign) (PoM)

Injection (aqueous suspension), hydrocortisone acetate 25 mg/mL, net price 1-mL amp = £5.72

Dose

• **By intra-articular injection**

(for details consult product literature)

**Child 1 month–12 years** 5–30 mg according to size of child and joint

**Child 12–18 years** 5–50 mg according to size of child and joint

Note  Where appropriate may be repeated at intervals of 21 days; not more than 3 joints should be treated on any one day

**10**

**Musculoskeletal and joint diseases**

◢ **Methylprednisolone acetate**

**Depo-Medrone**® (Pharmacia) [PoM]
Injection (aqueous suspension), methylprednisolone acetate 40 mg/mL, net price 1-mL vial = £2.87; 2-mL vial = £5.15; 3-mL vial = £7.47

**Depo-Medrone**® **with Lidocaine** (Pharmacia) [PoM]
Injection (aqueous suspension), methylprednisolone acetate 40 mg, lidocaine hydrochloride 10 mg/mL, net price 1-mL vial = £3.28; 2-mL vial = £5.88

◢ **Triamcinolone hexacetonide**

**Triamcinolone hexacetonide** (Non-proprietary) [PoM]
Injection, various strengths available from 'special order' manufacturers or specialist importing companies, see, p. 823

**Dose**
- **By intra-articular injection**
  (for details consult product literature)
  **Child 1–18 years** for larger joints 1 mg/kg (usual max. 20 mg, but higher doses have been used); if appropriate repeat treatment for relapse

◢ **Triamcinolone acetonide**

**Adcortyl**® **Intra-articular/Intradermal** (Squibb) [PoM]
Injection (aqueous suspension), triamcinolone acetonide 10 mg/mL, net price 1-mL amp = 90p; 5-mL vial = £3.63
**Excipients** include benzyl alcohol (avoid in neonates, see Excipients, p. 2)

**Dose**
- **By intra-articular injection**
  (for details consult product literature)
  **Child 1–18 years** for larger joints 2 mg/kg (max. 15 mg); for doses above 15 mg use *Kenalog*® *Intra-articular/Intramuscular*; if appropriate repeat treatment for relapse

**Kenalog**® **Intra-articular/Intramuscular** (Squibb) [PoM]
Injection (aqueous suspension), triamcinolone acetonide 40 mg/mL, net price 1-mL vial = £1.49

**Dose**
- **By intra-articular injection**
  (for details consult product literature)
  **Child 1–18 years** for larger joints 2 mg/kg (usual max. 40 mg, but higher doses have been used); if appropriate repeat treatment for relapse

## 10.1.3 Drugs that suppress the rheumatic disease process

Certain drugs, such as methotrexate, cytokine modulators, and sulfasalazine, are used to suppress the disease process in *juvenile idiopathic arthritis* (juvenile chronic arthritis); these drugs are known as disease-modifying antirheumatic drugs (DMARDs). In children, disease-modifying antirheumatic drugs should be used under specialist supervision.

Some children with juvenile idiopathic arthritis do not require disease-modifying antirheumatic drugs. Methotrexate is effective in juvenile idiopathic arthritis; sulfasalazine is an alternative but should be avoided in *systemic-onset juvenile idiopathic arthritis*. Gold and penicillamine are no longer used. For the role of cytokine modulators in *polyarticular juvenile idiopathic arthritis*, see p. 510.

Unlike NSAIDs, disease-modifying antirheumatic drugs can affect the progression of disease but they may require 3–6 months of treatment for a full therapeutic

response. Response to a disease-modifying antirheumatic drug may allow the dose of the NSAID to be reduced.

Disease-modifying antirheumatic drugs can improve not only the symptoms of inflammatory joint disease but also extra-articular manifestations. They reduce the erythrocyte sedimentation rate and C-reactive protein.

## Antimalarials

The antimalarial **hydroxychloroquine** is rarely used to treat juvenile idiopathic arthritis. Hydroxychloroquine can also be useful for systemic or discoid lupus erythematosus, particularly involving the skin and joints, and in sarcoidosis.

Retinopathy (see below) rarely occurs provided that the recommended doses are not exceeded.

**Mepacrine** is used on rare occasions to treat discoid lupus erythematosus [unlicensed].

**Cautions**    Hydroxychloroquine should be used with caution in neurological disorders (especially in those with a history of epilepsy), in severe gastro-intestinal disorders, in G6PD deficiency (section 9.1.5), and in acute porphyria. Hydroxychloroquine may exacerbate psoriasis and aggravate myasthenia gravis. Concurrent use of hepatotoxic drugs should be avoided; other **interactions**: Appendix 1 (chloroquine and hydroxychloroquine).

**Pregnancy**    It is not necessary to withdraw an antimalarial drug during pregnancy if the rheumatic disease is well controlled; however, the manufacturer of hydroxychloroquine advises avoiding use.

**Breast-feeding**    Hydroxychloroquine is present in breast milk leading to a risk of toxicity in infants—breast-feeding should be avoided when it is used to treat rheumatic disease.

> **Screening for ocular toxicity**
> Hydroxychloroquine is rarely associated with ocular toxicity. The British Society for Paediatric and Adolescent Rheumatology recommends that children should have their vision tested before long-term treatment with hydroxychloroquine and have an annual review of visual acuity. Children should be referred to an ophthalmologist if there is visual impairment, changes in visual acuity, or blurred vision. The Royal College of Ophthalmologists has recommended that a locally agreed protocol between the prescribing doctor and ophthalmologist be established to monitor the vision of these children.

> **Important**
> To avoid excessive dosage in obese children, the dose of hydroxychloroquine should be calculated on the basis of ideal body-weight; ocular toxicity is unlikely with doses under 5–6.5 mg/kg or max. 400 mg daily.

**Side-effects**    The side-effects of hydroxychloroquine include gastro-intestinal disturbances, headache, and skin reactions (rashes, pruritus); those occurring less frequently include ECG changes, convulsions, visual changes, retinal damage (see above), keratopathy, ototoxicity, hair depigmentation, hair loss, and discoloration of skin, nails, and mucous membranes.

10 Musculoskeletal and joint diseases

Side-effects that occur rarely include blood disorders (including thrombocytopenia, agranulocytosis, and aplastic anaemia), mental changes (including emotional disturbances and psychosis), myopathy (including cardiomyopathy and neuromyopathy), acute generalised exanthematous pustulosis, exfoliative dermatitis, Stevens-Johnson syndrome, photosensitivity, and hepatic damage; angioedema and bronchospasm have also been reported. **Important**: very toxic in overdosage—immediate advice from poisons centres essential (see also p. 28).

---

### ▌ HYDROXYCHLOROQUINE SULFATE

**Cautions**   see notes above

**Hepatic impairment**   use with caution in moderate to severe impairment

**Renal impairment**   manufacturer advises caution and monitoring of plasma-hydroxychloroquine concentration in severe impairment

**Pregnancy**   see notes above

**Breast-feeding**   see notes above

**Side-effects**   see notes above

**Licensed use**   *Plaquenil*® not licensed for use in children for dermatological conditions caused or aggravated by sunlight

**Indications and dose**

> Juvenile idiopathic arthritis, systemic and discoid lupus erythematosus, dermatological conditions caused or aggravated by sunlight
>
> • By mouth
>
> **Child 1 month–18 years** based on ideal body-weight, 5–6.5 mg/kg (max. 400 mg) once daily

**Hydroxychloroquine** (Non-proprietary) PoM
Tablets, hydroxychloroquine sulfate 200 mg, net price 60-tab pack = £5.10. Label: 21, counselling, antacids (see below)
Brands include *Quinoric*®
**Counselling** Do not take antacids for at least 4 hours before or after hydroxychloroquine to reduce possible interference with hydroxychloroquine absorption

**Plaquenil**® (Sanofi-Aventis) PoM
Tablets, f/c, hydroxychloroquine sulfate 200 mg, net price 60-tab pack = £5.25. Label: 21, counselling, antacids (see below)
**Counselling** Do not take antacids for at least 4 hours before or after hydroxychloroquine to reduce possible interference with hydroxychloroquine absorption

---

## Drugs affecting the immune response

**Methotrexate**, given as a once weekly dose, is the disease-modifying antirheumatic drug of choice in the treatment of juvenile idiopathic arthritis and also has a role in juvenile dermatomyositis, vasculitis, uveitis, systemic lupus erythematosus, localised scleroderma, and sarcoidosis; for these indications it is given by the subcutaneous, oral, or rarely, the intramuscular route. Absorption from intramuscular or subcutaneous routes may be more predictable than from the oral route; if the oral route is ineffective subcutaneous administration is generally preferred. Regular full blood counts (including differential white cell count and platelet count), renal and liver function tests are required. Folic acid may reduce mucosal or gastro-intestinal side-effects of methotrexate. The dosage regimen for folic acid has not been established—in children over 2 years a dose of 5 mg weekly [unlicensed indication], may be given on a different day from the methotrexate.

**Azathioprine** may be used in children for vasculitis which has failed to respond to other treatments, for the management of severe cases of *systemic lupus erythematosus* and other connective tissue disorders, in conjunction with corticosteroids for patients with severe or progressive renal disease, and in cases of *polymyositis* which are resistant to corticosteroids. Azathioprine has a corticosteroid-sparing effect in patients whose corticosteroid requirements are excessive.

**Ciclosporin** is rarely used in juvenile idiopathic arthritis, connective tissue diseases, vasculitis, and uveitis; it may be considered if the condition has failed to respond to other treatments.

---

### ▌ AZATHIOPRINE

**Cautions**   section 8.2.1

**Contra-indications**   section 8.2.1

**Hepatic impairment**   section 8.2.1

**Renal impairment**   section 8.2.1

**Pregnancy**   section 8.2.1

**Breast-feeding**   section 8.2.1

**Side-effects**   section 8.2.1

**Indications and dose**

> Systemic lupus erythematosus, vasculitis, autoimmune conditions usually when corticosteroid therapy alone has proved inadequate see also notes above
>
> • By mouth
>
> **Child 1 month–18 years** initially 1 mg/kg daily, adjusted according to response to max. 3 mg/kg daily (consider withdrawal if no improvement within 3 months)

> Inflammatory bowel disease section 1.5.3

> Transplantation rejection section 8.2.1

◢**Preparations**
Section 8.2.1

---

### ▌ METHOTREXATE

**Cautions**   section 8.1.3; see advice below (blood count, gastro-intestinal, liver, and pulmonary toxicity); extreme caution in blood disorders (avoid if severe); risk of accumulation in pleural effusion or ascites—drain before treatment; full blood count and liver function tests before starting treatment repeated fortnightly for at least the first 4 weeks and at this frequency after any change in dose until therapy stabilised, thereafter monthly; renal function tests before starting treatment and then regularly during treatment; children or their carers should report all symptoms and signs suggestive of infection, especially sore throat; treatment with folinic acid (as calcium folinate, section 8.1) may be required in acute toxicity; check immunity to varicella-zoster and con-

**10**

**Musculoskeletal and joint diseases**

sider vaccination (section 14.4) before initiating therapy; acute porphyria (section 9.8.2); **interactions:** see below and Appendix 1 (methotrexate)

**Blood count** Bone marrow suppression can occur abruptly; factors likely to increase toxicity include renal impairment and concomitant use with another anti-folate drug (e.g. trimethoprim). A clinically significant drop in white cell count or platelet count calls for immediate withdrawal of methotrexate and introduction of supportive therapy

**Gastro-intestinal toxicity** Withdraw treatment if stomatitis develops—may be first sign of gastro-intestinal toxicity

**Liver toxicity** Persistent 2–fold rise in liver transaminases may necessitate dose reduction or rarely discontinuation; abrupt withdrawal should be avoided as this can lead to disease flare

**Pulmonary toxicity** Acute pulmonary toxicity is rare in children treated for juvenile idiopathic arthritis, but children and carers should seek medical attention if dyspnoea, cough or fever develops; discontinue if pneumonitis suspected.

**NSAIDs** Children and carers should be advised to avoid self-medication with over-the-counter ibuprofen

**Contra-indications** see Cautions above; also active infection and immunodeficiency syndromes

**Hepatic impairment** avoid—dose-related toxicity; see also Cautions above

**Renal impairment** section 8.1.3

**Pregnancy** section 8.1.3

**Breast-feeding** section 8.1.3

**Side-effects** section 8.1.3; chronic pulmonary fibrosis; blood dyscrasias (including fatalities); liver cirrhosis

**Licensed use** *Metoject*® and *Ebetrex*® are licensed for use in children over 3 years for polyarticular forms of juvenile idiopathic arthritis; other preparations not licensed for use in children for non-malignant conditions

**Indications and dose**

Juvenile idiopathic arthritis, juvenile dermatomyositis, vasculitis, uveitis, systemic lupus erythematosus, localised scleroderma, sarcoidosis

- By mouth, subcutaneous injection, or intramuscular injection

   **Child 1 month–18 years** $10–15 \, mg/m^2$ once weekly initially, increased if necessary to max. $25 \, mg/m^2$ once weekly

> ### Safe Practice
> Note that the above dose is a **weekly** dose. To avoid error with low-dose methotrexate, it is recommended that:
> - the child or their carer is carefully advised of the **dose** and **frequency** and the reason for taking methotrexate and any other prescribed medicine (e.g. folic acid);
> - only one strength of methotrexate tablet (usually 2.5 mg) is prescribed and dispensed;
> - the prescription and the dispensing label clearly show the dose and frequency of methotrexate administration;
> - the child or their carer is warned to report immediately the onset of any feature of blood disorders (e.g. sore throat, bruising, and mouth ulcers), liver toxicity (e.g. nausea, vomiting, abdominal discomfort, and dark urine), and respiratory effects (e.g. shortness of breath).

Severe Crohn's disease section 1.5.3

Malignant disease section 8.1.3

Psoriasis section 13.5.3

**Methotrexate** (Non-proprietary) PoM

Tablets, yellow, methotrexate 2.5 mg, net price 24-tab pack = £2.39, 28-tab pack = £3.27. Counselling, dose, NSAIDs

Brands include *Maxtrex*®

Tablets, yellow, methotrexate 10 mg, net price 100-tab pack = £56.49. Counselling, dose, NSAIDs

Suspension, various strengths available from 'special-order' manufacturers or specialist importing companies, see p. 823

◀**Parenteral preparations**

See also section 8.1.3

**Ebetrex**® (Sandoz) PoM

Injection, prefilled syringe, methotrexate (as disodium salt) 10 mg/mL, net price 0.75 mL (7.5 mg) = £14.78, 1 mL (10 mg) = £15.21, 1.5 mL (15 mg) = £16.49; 20 mg/mL, 1 mL (20 mg) = £17.75, 1.25 mL (25 mg) = £18.39, 1.5 mL (30 mg) = £20.70

**Metoject**® (Medac) PoM

Injection, prefilled syringe, methotrexate (as disodium salt) 50 mg/mL, net price 0.15 mL (7.5 mg) = £14.85, 0.2 mL (10 mg) = £15.29, 0.3 mL (15 mg) = £16.57, 0.4 mL (20 mg) = £17.84, 0.5 mL (25 mg) = £18.48, 0.6 mL (30 mg) = £18.95

# Cytokine modulators

Cytokine modulators should be used under specialist supervision.

**Adalimumab, etanercept,** and **infliximab** inhibit the activity of tumour necrosis factor alpha (TNF-α). Adalimumab can be used for the management of active polyarticular juvenile idiopathic arthritis. Etanercept is licensed for the treatment of the following subtypes of juvenile idiopathic arthritis: polyarticular juvenile idiopathic arthritis in children who have had an inadequate response to methotrexate or who cannot tolerate it, oligoarthritis in chidren who have had an inadequate response to methotrexate or who cannot tolerate it, psoriatic arthritis in children over 12 years who have had an inadequate reponse to methotrexate or cannot tolerate it, and enthesitis-related arthritis in children over 12 years who have had an inadequate response to conventional therapy or cannot tolerate it. Infliximab has been used in refractory polyarticular juvenile idiopathic arthritis [unlicensed indication] when other treatments, such as etanercept, have failed.

The *Scottish Medicines Consortium* (p. 3) has advised (January 2013) that etanercept (*Enbrel*®) is accepted for restricted use within NHS Scotland for the treatment of polyarthritis (rheumatoid factor positive or negative) and extended oligoarthritis in children and adolescents from the age of 2 years who have had an inadequate response to or are intolerant of methotrexate, psoriatic arthritis in adolescents from the age of 12 years who have had an inadequate response to or are intolerant of methotrexate, and enthesitis-related arthritis in adolescents from the age of 12 years who have had an inadequate response to or are intolerant of conventional therapy. It is further restricted to use within specialist rheumatology services (including those working within the network for paediatric rheumatology).

---

**NICE guidance**
**Etanercept for the treatment of juvenile idiopathic arthritis (March 2002)**

Etanercept is recommended in children aged 4–17 years with active polyarticular-course juvenile idiopathic arthritis who have not responded adequately to methotrexate or who are intolerant of it. Etanercept should be used under specialist supervision according to the guidelines of the British Society for Paediatric and Adolescent Rheumatology [previously the British Paediatric Rheumatology Group].

Etanercept should be withdrawn if severe side-effects develop or if there is no response after 6 months or if the initial response is not maintained. A decision to continue therapy beyond 2 years should be based on disease activity and clinical effectiveness in individual cases.

Prescribers of etanercept should register consenting patients with the Biologics Registry of the British Society for Paediatric and Adolescent Rheumatology.
www.nice.org.uk/TA35

---

**Side-effects** Adalimumab, etanercept, and infliximab have been associated with infections, sometimes severe, including tuberculosis, septicaemia, and hepatitis B reactivation. Other side-effects include nausea, abdominal pain, worsening heart failure, hypersensitivity reactions, fever, headache, depression, antibody formation (including lupus erythematosus-like syndrome), pruritus, injection-site reactions, and blood disorders (including anaemia, leucopenia, thrombocytopenia, pancytopenia, aplastic anaemia).

**Abatacept** prevents the full activation of T-lymphocytes; it can be used for the management of active polyarticular juvenile idiopathic arthritis. Abatacept is not recommended for use in combination with TNF inhibitors.

The *Scottish Medicines Consortium* (p. 3) has advised (October 2011) that abatacept (*Orencia*®) is accepted for restricted use within NHS Scotland for the treatment of moderate to severe active polyarticular juvenile idiopathic arthritis in accordance with the licensed indications, when used within specialist rheumatology services (including those working within the network for paediatric rheumatology).

**Tocilizumab** antagonises the actions of interleukin-6; it can be used for the management of active systemic juvenile idiopathic arthritis when there has been an inadequate response to NSAIDs and systemic corticosteroids. Tocilizumab can be used in combination with methotrexate, or as monotherapy if methotrexate is not tolerated or is contra-indicated (see also NICE guidance below). Tocilizumab is not recommended for use with other cytokine modulators.

---

**NICE guidance**
**Tocilizumab for the treatment of systemic juvenile idiopathic arthritis (December 2011)**

Tocilizumab is recommended for the treatment of systemic juvenile idiopathic arthritis in children aged over 2 years who have not responded adequately to NSAIDs, systemic corticosteroids and methotrexate, if the manufacturer makes tocilizumab available with the discount agreed as part of the patient access scheme.

Tocilizumab is not recommended for the treatment of systemic juvenile idiopathic arthritis in children whose disease continues to respond to methotrexate or who have not been treated with methotrexate.

Children currently receiving tocilizumab for systemic juvenile idiopathic arthritis who do not meet these criteria should have the option to continue treatment until it is considered appropriate to stop.
www.nice.org.uk/TA238

---

## ▎ABATACEPT

**Cautions** predisposition to infection (screen for latent tuberculosis and viral hepatitis); do not initiate until active infections are controlled; children should be brought up to date with current immunisation schedule (section 14.1) before initiating therapy; progressive multifocal leucoencephalopathy—discontinue treatment if neurological symptoms present; **interactions:** Appendix 1 (abatacept)

**Contra-indications** severe infection (see also Cautions)

**Pregnancy** manufacturer advises avoid unless essential—effective contraception required during treatment and for 14 weeks after last dose

**Breast-feeding** present in milk in *animal* studies—manufacturer advises avoid breast-feeding during treatment and for 14 weeks after last dose

**Side-effects** abdominal pain, diarrhoea, dyspepsia, nausea, vomiting, stomatitis, flushing, hypertension, cough, dizziness, fatigue, headache, paraesthesia, infection, leucopenia, pain in extremities, conjunctivitis, rhinitis; *less commonly* gastritis, tachycardia, bradycardia, palpitation, hypotension, dyspnoea, weight gain, depression, anxiety, sleep disorder, menstrual disturbances, basal cell carcinoma, skin papilloma, thrombocytopenia, arthralgia, visual disturbance, dry eye, bruising, alopecia, dry skin, psoriasis; *also reported* lymphoma, lung cancer

**Indications and dose**

Moderate to severe active polyarticular juvenile idiopathic arthritis (in combination with methotrexate) in children who have not responded adequately to other disease-modifying anti-rheumatic drugs (including at least one tumour necrosis factor (TNF) inhibitor)

- **By intravenous infusion**

  **Child 6–17 years**

  **Body-weight less than 75 kg** 10 mg/kg, repeated 2 weeks and 4 weeks after initial infusion, then every 4 weeks

  **Body-weight 75–100 kg** 750 mg, repeated 2 weeks and 4 weeks after initial infusion, then every 4 weeks

**10**

**Musculoskeletal and joint diseases**

**Body-weight over 100 kg** 1 g, repeated 2 weeks and 4 weeks after initial infusion, then every 4 weeks

**Note** Review treatment if no response within 6 months

**Administration** for *intravenous infusion*, reconstitute each vial with 10 mL water for injections using the silicone-free syringe provided; dilute requisite dose in Sodium Chloride 0.9% to 100 mL (using the same silicone-free syringe); give over 30 minutes through a low protein-binding filter (pore size 0.2–1.2 micron)

**Orencia®** (Bristol-Myers Squibb) PoM
Intravenous infusion, powder for reconstitution, abatacept, net price 250-mg vial = £242.17
**Electrolytes** Na⁺<0.5 mmol/vial

## ADALIMUMAB

**Cautions** predisposition to infection; monitor for infection before, during, and for 4 months after treatment (see also Tuberculosis below); do not initiate until active infections are controlled; discontinue if new serious infection develops; hepatitis B virus—monitor for active infection; children should be brought up to date with current immunisation schedule (section 14.1) before initiating therapy; mild heart failure (discontinue if symptoms develop or worsen—avoid in moderate or severe heart failure); demyelinating disorders (risk of exacerbation); history or development of malignancy; monitor for non-melanoma skin cancer before and during treatment, especially in children with history of PUVA treatment for psoriasis or extensive immunosuppressant therapy; **interactions**: Appendix 1 (adalimumab)

**Tuberculosis** Children should be evaluated for tuberculosis before treatment. Active tuberculosis should be treated with standard treatment (section 5.1.9) for at least 2 months before starting adalimumab. Children who have previously received adequate treatment for tuberculosis can start adalimumab but should be monitored every 3 months for possible recurrence. In those without active tuberculosis but who were previously not treated adequately, chemoprophylaxis should ideally be completed before starting adalimumab. In children at high risk of tuberculosis who cannot be assessed by tuberculin skin test, chemoprophylaxis can be given concurrently with adalimumab. Children and their carers should be advised to seek medical attention if symptoms suggestive of tuberculosis (e.g. persistent cough, weight loss, and fever) develop

**Blood disorders** Children and their carers should be advised to seek medical attention if symptoms suggestive of blood disorders (such as fever, sore throat, bruising, or bleeding) develop

**Contra-indications** severe infection (see also Cautions)

**Pregnancy** avoid; manufacturer advises effective contraception required during treatment and for at least 5 months after last dose

**Breast-feeding** avoid; manufacturer advises avoid for at least 5 months after last dose

**Side-effects** see under Cytokine Modulators, p. 511 and Cautions above; also vomiting, dyspepsia, gastrointestinal haemorrhage, dizziness, hyperlipidaemia, hypertension, oedema, flushing, chest pain, tachycardia, cough, dyspnoea, mood changes, sleep disturbances, anxiety, paraesthesia, haematuria, renal impairment, benign tumours, skin cancer, electrolyte disturbances, hyperuricaemia, dehydration, musculoskeletal pain, eye disorders, rash, dermatitis, onycholysis, impaired healing; *less commonly* dysphagia, pancreatitis, cholelithiasis, hepatic steatosis, chole-

cystitis, arrhythmias, vascular occlusion, aortic aneurysm, interstitial lung disease, pneumonitis, tremor, erectile dysfunction, nocturia, malignancy (including solid tumours and lymphoma), rhabdomyolysis, hearing loss, tinnitus; *rarely* autoimmune hepatitis, myocardial infarction, demyelinating disorders; *also reported* pulmonary embolism, pleural effusion, sarcoidosis, Stevens-Johnson syndrome, cutaneous vasculitis, new onset or worsening psoriasis

**Indications and dose**

**Active polyarticular juvenile idiopathic arthritis (in combination with methotrexate or alone if methotrexate inappropriate) in children who have not responded adequately to one or more disease-modifying antirheumatic drug**

- By subcutaneous injection

  **Child 2–4 years** 24 mg/m² (max. 20 mg) on alternate weeks; review treatment if no response within 12 weeks

  **Child 4–13 years** 24 mg/m² (max. 40 mg) on alternate weeks; review treatment if no response within 12 weeks

  **Child 13–18 years** 40 mg on alternate weeks; review treatment if no response within 12 weeks

**Humira®** (AbbVie) PoM
Injection, adalimumab, net price 40-mg prefilled pen or prefilled syringe = £357.50; 40 mg/0.8-mL vial = £352.14. Label: 10, alert card, counselling, tuberculosis and blood disorders

## ETANERCEPT

**Cautions** predisposition to infection (avoid if predisposition to septicaemia); significant exposure to herpes zoster virus—interrupt treatment and consider varicella–zoster immunoglobulin; hepatitis B virus—monitor for active infection; monitor for worsening hepatitis C infection; children should be brought up to date with current immunisation schedule (section 14.1) before initiating therapy; heart failure (risk of exacerbation); history or increased risk of demyelinating disorders; history or development of malignancy; monitor for skin cancer before and during treatment particularly in those at risk (including children with psoriasis or a history of PUVA treatment); history of blood disorders; diabetes mellitus; **interactions**: Appendix 1 (etanercept)

**Tuberculosis** Children should be evaluated for tuberculosis before treatment. Active tuberculosis should be treated with standard treatment (section 5.1.9) for at least 2 months before starting etanercept. Children who have previously received adequate treatment for tuberculosis can start etanercept but should be monitored every 3 months for possible recurrence. In those without active tuberculosis but who were previously not treated adequately, chemoprophylaxis should ideally be completed before starting etanercept. In children at high risk of tuberculosis who cannot be assessed by tuberculin skin test, chemoprophylaxis can be given concurrently with etanercept. Children and their carers should be advised to seek medical attention if symptoms suggestive of tuberculosis (e.g. persistent cough, weight loss, and fever) develop

**Blood disorders** Children and their carers should be advised to seek medical attention if symptoms suggestive of blood disorders (such as fever, sore throat, bruising, or bleeding) develop

**Contra-indications** active infection; avoid injections containing benzyl alcohol in neonates (see preparations below)

**Hepatic impairment**  use with caution in moderate to severe alcoholic hepatitis

**Pregnancy**  avoid—limited information available; manufacturer advises effective contraception required during treatment and for 3 weeks after last dose

**Breast-feeding**  manufacturer advises avoid—present in milk in *animal* studies

**Side-effects**  see under Cytokine Modulators, p. 511; also *less commonly* interstitial lung disease, skin cancer, uveitis, rash, new onset or worsening psoriasis; *rarely* demyelinating disorders, seizures, lymphoma, Stevens-Johnson syndrome, vasculitis; *very rarely* toxic epidermal necrolysis; *also reported* appendicitis, gastritis, oesophagitis, inflammatory bowel disease, vomiting, diabetes mellitus, malignancy (including solid tumours and leukaemia), macrophage activation syndrome, and cutaneous ulcer

**Indications and dose**

**Juvenile idiopathic arthritis (see also notes above)**

- **By subcutaneous injection**

  **Child 2–17 years** 400 micrograms/kg (max. 25 mg) twice weekly, with an interval of 3–4 days between doses *or* 800 micrograms/kg (max. 50 mg) once weekly; consider discontinuation if no response after 4 months

**Severe plaque psoriasis** section 13.5.3

**Enbrel®** (Pfizer) (PoM)

Injection, powder for reconstitution, etanercept, net price 25-mg vial (with solvent) = £89.38. Label: 10, alert card, counselling, tuberculosis and blood disorders

Paediatric injection, powder for reconstitution, etanercept, net price 10-mg vial (with solvent) = £35.75; 25-mg vial (with solvent) = £89.38. Label: 10, alert card, counselling, tuberculosis and blood disorders

Excipients  include benzyl alcohol (avoid in neonates, see Excipients, p. 2)

Injection, etanercept, net price 25-mg prefilled syringe = £89.38; 50-mg prefilled pen or prefilled syringe = £178.75. Label: 10, alert card, counselling, tuberculosis and blood disorders

## TOCILIZUMAB

**Cautions**  predisposition to infection or history of recurrent or chronic infection; interrupt treatment if serious infection occurs; history of intestinal ulceration or diverticulitis; monitor hepatic transaminases; monitor neutrophil and platelet counts; low platelet or absolute neutrophil count (discontinue if absolute neutrophil count less than $0.5 \times 10^9$/litre or platelet count less than $50 \times 10^3$/microlitre); monitor lipid profile 4–8 weeks after starting treatment and then as indicated; monitor for demyelinating disorders; **interactions**: Appendix 1 (tocilizumab)

Tuberculosis  Children should be evaluated for tuberculosis before treatment. Children with latent tuberculosis should be treated with standard therapy (section 5.1.9) before starting tocilizumab

Counselling  Children and their carers should be advised to seek immediate medical attention if symptoms of infection occur, or if symptoms of diverticular perforation such as abdominal pain, haemorrhage, or fever accompanying change in bowel habits occur

**Contra-indications**  severe active infection (see also Cautions) do not initiate if absolute neutrophil count less than $2 \times 10^9$/litre (see also Cautions)

**Hepatic impairment**  manufacturer advises caution, consult product literature

**Renal impairment**  manufacturer advises monitor renal function closely in moderate or severe impairment

**Pregnancy**  manufacturer advises avoid unless essential (toxicity in *animal* studies); effective contraception required during and for 3 months after treatment

**Breast-feeding**  manufacturer advises use only if potential benefit outweighs risk —no information available

**Side-effects**  abdominal pain, mouth ulceration, gastritis, raised hepatic transaminases; peripheral oedema, hypertension, hypercholesterolaemia; headache; infection (including upper respiratory-tract infection); antibody formation, leucopenia, neutropenia; rash, pruritus; *less commonly* gastric ulcer, gastro-intestinal perforation, hypertriglyceridaemia, hypothyroidism, nephrolithiasis, infusion-related reactions, anaphylaxis, and thrombocytopenia also reported

**Indications and dose**

**Active systemic juvenile idiopathic arthritis (in combination with methotrexate or alone if methotrexate inappropriate) in children who have had an inadequate response to NSAIDs and systemic corticosteroids**

- **By intravenous infusion**

  **Child 2–18 years**

  **Body-weight less than 30 kg** 12 mg/kg once every 2 weeks; review treatment if no improvement within 6 weeks

  **Body-weight over 30 kg** 8 mg/kg once every 2 weeks; review treatment if no improvement within 6 weeks

**Administration**  for *intravenous infusion*; body-weight less than 30 kg, dilute requisite dose to a volume of 50 mL with Sodium chloride 0.9% and give over 1 hour; body-weight over 30 kg, dilute requisite dose to a volume of 100 mL with Sodium chloride 0.9% and give over 1 hour

**RoActemra®** (Roche) (PoM)

Concentrate for intravenous injection, tocilizumab 20 mg/mL, net price 4 mL (80-mg vial) = £102.40, 10 mL (200-mg) vial = £256.00, 20 mL (400-mg vial) = £512.00. Alert card, counselling, see above

## Sulfasalazine

**Sulfasalazine** has a beneficial effect in suppressing the inflammatory activity associated with some forms of juvenile idiopathic arthritis; it is generally not used in systemic-onset disease. Sulfasalazine may cause haematological abnormalities including leucopenia, neutropenia, and thrombocytopenia and close monitoring of full blood counts (including differential white cell count and platelet count) is necessary initially, and at monthly intervals during the first 3 months (liver-function tests also being performed at monthly intervals for the first 3 months). Although the manufacturer recommends renal function tests, evidence of practical value is unsatisfactory. For use of sulfasalazine also see section 1.5.1, aminosalicylates.

## SULFASALAZINE
(Sulphasalazine)

**Cautions**   see section 1.5.1 and notes above
**Contra-indications**   see section 1.5.1
**Hepatic impairment**   section 1.5.1
**Renal impairment**   section 1.5.1
**Pregnancy**   section 1.5.1
**Breast-feeding**   section 1.5.1
**Side-effects**   see section 1.5.1 and notes above
**Licensed use**   not licensed for use in children for juvenile idiopathic arthritis

**Indications and dose**

> Juvenile idiopathic arthritis (see also notes above)
> * By mouth
> **Child 2–18 years** initially 5 mg/kg twice daily for 1 week, then 10 mg/kg twice daily for 1 week, then 20 mg/kg twice daily for 1 week, maintenance dose 20–25 mg/kg twice daily; **Child 2–12 years** max. 2 g daily, **Child 12–18 years** max. 3 g daily

◢**Preparations**
Section 1.5.1

## 10.1.4   Gout and cytotoxic-induced hyperuricaemia

This section is not included in *BNF for Children*. For the role of allopurinol and rasburicase in the prophylaxis of hyperuricaemia associated with cancer chemotherapy and in enzyme disorders causing increased serum urate, see section 8.1. The management of gout in adolescents requires specialist supervision.

## 10.1.5   Other drugs for rheumatic diseases

Classification not used in *BNF for Children*.

## 10.2   Drugs used in neuromuscular disorders

**10.2.1   Drugs that enhance neuromuscular transmission**
**10.2.2   Skeletal muscle relaxants**

## 10.2.1   Drugs that enhance neuromuscular transmission

Anticholinesterases are used as first-line treatment in *ocular myasthenia gravis* and as an adjunct to immuno-suppressant therapy for *generalised myasthenia gravis*.

Corticosteroids are used when anticholinesterases do not control symptoms completely. A second-line immuno-suppressant such as azathioprine is frequently used to reduce the dose of corticosteroid.

Plasmapheresis or infusion of intravenous immuno-globulin [unlicensed indication] may induce temporary remission in severe relapses, particularly where bulbar or respiratory function is compromised or before thymectomy.

### Anticholinesterases

Anticholinesterase drugs enhance neuromuscular transmission in voluntary and involuntary muscle in myasthenia gravis. They prolong the action of acetylcholine by inhibiting the action of the enzyme acetylcholinesterase. Excessive dosage of these drugs can impair neuromuscular transmission and precipitate cholinergic crises by causing a depolarising block. This may be difficult to distinguish from a worsening myasthenic state.

Muscarinic side-effects of anticholinesterases include increased sweating, increased salivary and gastric secretions, increased gastro-intestinal and uterine motility, and bradycardia. These parasympathomimetic effects are antagonised by atropine.

**Edrophonium** has a very brief action and it is therefore used mainly for the diagnosis of myasthenia gravis. However, such testing should be performed only by those experienced in its use; other means of establishing the diagnosis are available. A single test-dose usually causes substantial improvement in muscle power (lasting about 5 minutes) in patients with the disease (if respiration already impaired, *only* in conjunction with someone skilled at intubation).

Edrophonium can also be used to determine whether a patient with myasthenia is receiving inadequate or excessive treatment with cholinergic drugs. If treatment is excessive an injection of edrophonium will either have no effect or will intensify symptoms (if respiration already impaired, give *only* in conjunction with someone skilled at intubation). Conversely, transient improvement may be seen if the patient is being inadequately treated. The test is best performed just before the next dose of anticholinesterase.

**Neostigmine** produces a therapeutic effect for up to 4 hours. Its pronounced muscarinic action is a disadvantage, and simultaneous administration of an antimuscarinic drug such as atropine or propantheline may be required to prevent colic, excessive salivation, or diarrhoea. In severe disease neostigmine can be given every 2 hours. In infants, neostigmine by either subcutaneous or intramuscular injection is preferred for the short-term management of myasthenia.

**Pyridostigmine** is less powerful and slower in action than neostigmine but it has a longer duration of action. It is preferable to neostigmine because of its smoother action and the need for less frequent dosage. It is particularly preferred in patients whose muscles are weak on waking. It has a comparatively mild gastro-intestinal effect but an antimuscarinic drug may still be required. It is inadvisable to use excessive doses because acetylcholine receptor down regulation may occur. Immunosuppressant therapy may be considered if high doses of pyridostigmine are needed. Neostigmine and pyridostigmine should be given to neonates 30 minutes before feeds to improve suckling.

Neostigmine and edrophonium are also used to reverse the actions of the non-depolarising neuromuscular blocking drugs (section 15.1.6).

## ◢ NEOSTIGMINE

**Cautions**   asthma (*extreme* caution), bradycardia, arrhythmias, recent myocardial infarction, epilepsy, hypotension, parkinsonism, vagotonia, peptic ulceration, hyperthyroidism; atropine or other antidote to

*(side text, left margin)* **10** Musculoskeletal and joint diseases

muscarinic effects may be necessary (particularly when neostigmine is given by injection), but not given routinely because it may mask signs of overdosage; **interactions:** Appendix 1 (parasympathomimetics)

**Contra-indications**  intestinal or urinary obstruction

**Renal impairment**  may need dose reduction

**Pregnancy**  manufacturer advises use only if potential benefit outweighs risk

**Breast-feeding**  amount probably too small to be harmful

**Side-effects**  nausea, vomiting, increased salivation, diarrhoea, abdominal cramps (more marked with higher doses); signs of overdosage include broncho-constriction, increased bronchial secretions, lacrimation, excessive sweating, involuntary defaecation and micturition, miosis, nystagmus, bradycardia, heart block, arrhythmias, hypotension, agitation, excessive dreaming, and weakness eventually leading to fasciculation and paralysis

**Indications and dose**

Treatment of myasthenia gravis

• By mouth (as neostigmine bromide)

**Neonate** initially 1–2 mg, then 1–5 mg every 4 hours, give 30 minutes before feeds

**Child up to 6 years** initially 7.5 mg repeated at suitable intervals throughout the day, total daily dose 15–90 mg

**Child 6–12 years** initially 15 mg repeated at suitable intervals throughout the day, total daily dose 15–90 mg

**Child 12–18 years** initially 15–30 mg repeated at suitable intervals throughout the day, total daily dose 75–300 mg (but max. most can tolerate is 180 mg daily)

• By subcutaneous or intramuscular injection (as neostigmine metilsulfate)

**Neonate** 150 micrograms/kg every 6–8 hours, 30 minutes before feeds, increased to max. 300 micrograms/kg every 4 hours, if necessary [unlicensed]

**Child 1 month–12 years** 200–500 micrograms repeated at suitable intervals throughout the day

**Child 12–18 years** 1–2.5 mg repeated at suitable intervals throughout the day

**Neostigmine** (Non-proprietary) PoM
Tablets, scored, neostigmine bromide 15 mg, net price 140 = £56.10

◀**Injection**
Section 15.1.6

## EDROPHONIUM CHLORIDE

**Cautions**  see under Neostigmine; have resuscitation facilities; *extreme* caution in respiratory distress (see notes above) and in asthma

Note  Severe cholinergic reactions can be counteracted by injection of atropine sulfate (which should always be available)

**Contra-indications**  see under Neostigmine

**Pregnancy**  see under Neostigmine

**Breast-feeding**  see under Neostigmine

**Side-effects**  see under Neostigmine

**Indications and dose**

Diagnostic test for myasthenia gravis

• By intravenous injection

**Child 1 month–12 years** 20 micrograms/kg followed after 30 seconds (if no adverse reaction has occurred) by 80 micrograms/kg

**Child 12–18 years** 2 mg followed after 30 seconds (if no adverse reaction has occurred) by 8 mg

Detection of overdosage or underdosage of cholinergic drugs

• By intravenous injection

**Child 1 month–12 years** 20 micrograms/kg (preferably just before next dose of anticholinesterase, see notes above)

**Child 12–18 years** 2 mg (preferably just before next dose of anticholinesterase, see notes above)

**Edrophonium** (Non-proprietary) PoM
Injection, edrophonium chloride 10 mg/mL, net price 1-mL amp = £19.50

## PYRIDOSTIGMINE BROMIDE

**Cautions**  see under Neostigmine; weaker muscarinic action

**Contra-indications**  see under Neostigmine

**Renal impairment**  reduce dose; excreted by kidney

**Pregnancy**  see under Neostigmine

**Breast-feeding**  see under Neostigmine

**Side-effects**  see under Neostigmine

**Indications and dose**

Treatment of myasthenia gravis

• By mouth

**Neonate** initially 1–1.5 mg/kg, increased gradually to max. 10 mg, repeated throughout the day, give 30–60 minutes before feeds

**Child 1 month–12 years** initially 1–1.5 mg/kg/day, increased gradually to 7 mg/kg/day in 6 divided doses; usual total daily dose 30–360 mg

**Child 12–18 years** 30–120 mg, repeated throughout the day; usual total daily dose 300–600 mg (but consider immunosuppressant therapy if total daily dose exceeds 360 mg, down-regulation of acetylcholine receptors possible if total daily dose exceeds 450 mg; see notes above)

**Mestinon®** (Meda) PoM
Tablets, scored, pyridostigmine bromide 60 mg, net price 200 = £45.33

## Immunosuppressant therapy

A course of **corticosteroids** (section 6.3) is an established treatment in severe cases of myasthenia gravis and may be particularly useful when antibodies to the acetylcholine receptor are present in high titre. Short courses of high-dose ('pulsed') methylprednisolone followed by maintenance therapy with oral corticosteroids may also be useful.

Corticosteroid treatment is usually initiated under specialist supervision. For disadvantages of corticosteroid treatment, see section 6.3.2. Transient but very serious worsening of symptoms can occur in the first 2–3 weeks, especially if the corticosteroid is started at a high dose. Once remission has occurred (usually after 2–6 months), the dose of prednisolone should be reduced slowly to the minimum effective dose.

**10**

**Musculoskeletal and joint diseases**

## 10.2.2 Skeletal muscle relaxants

The drugs described below are used for the relief of chronic muscle spasm or spasticity associated with neurological damage; they are not indicated for spasm associated with minor injuries. They act principally on the central nervous system with the exception of dantrolene, which has a peripheral site of action. They differ in action from the muscle relaxants used in anaesthesia (section 15.1.5), which block transmission at the neuromuscular junction.

The underlying cause of spasticity should be treated and any aggravating factors (e.g. pressure sores, infection) remedied. Skeletal muscle relaxants are effective in most forms of spasticity except the rare alpha variety. The major disadvantage of treatment with these drugs is that reduction in muscle tone can cause a loss of splinting action of the spastic leg and trunk muscles and sometimes lead to an increase in disability.

**Dantrolene** acts directly on skeletal muscle and produces fewer central adverse effects. It is generally used in resistant cases. The dose should be increased slowly.

**Baclofen** inhibits transmission at spinal level and also depresses the central nervous system. The dose should be increased slowly to avoid the major side-effects of sedation and muscular hypotonia (other adverse events are uncommon).

**Diazepam** has undoubted efficacy in some children. Sedation and occasionally extensor hypotonus are disadvantages. Other benzodiazepines also have muscle-relaxant properties.

## ■ BACLOFEN

**Cautions** psychiatric illness; respiratory impairment; epilepsy; history of peptic ulcer (avoid oral route in active peptic ulceration); diabetes; hypertonic bladder sphincter; avoid abrupt withdrawal (risk of hyperactive state, may exacerbate spasticity, and precipitate autonomic dysfunction including hyperthermia, psychiatric reactions and convulsions, see also under Withdrawal below); **interactions**: Appendix 1 (muscle relaxants)

Withdrawal Serious side-effects can occur on abrupt withdrawal; to minimise risk, discontinue by gradual dose reduction over at least 1–2 weeks (longer if symptoms occur)

Skilled tasks Drowsiness may affect performance of skilled tasks (e.g. driving); effects of alcohol enhanced

Specific cautions for intrathecal treatment coagulation disorders; previous spinal fusion procedure; malnutrition (increased risk of post-surgical complications)

**Contra-indications** Specific contra-indications for intrathecal treatment local or systemic infection

**Hepatic impairment** manufacturer advises use by mouth with caution

**Renal impairment** risk of toxicity—use smaller oral doses and if necessary increase dosage interval; if estimated glomerular filtration rate less than 15 mL/minute/1.73m$^2$ use by mouth only if potential benefit outweighs risk; excreted by kidney

**Pregnancy** manufacturer advises use only if potential benefit outweighs risk (toxicity in *animal* studies)

**Breast-feeding** present in milk—amount probably too small to be harmful

**Side-effects** gastro-intestinal disturbances, dry mouth; hypotension, respiratory or cardiovascular depression; sedation, drowsiness, confusion, dizziness, ataxia, hallucinations, nightmares, headache, euphoria, insomnia, depression, anxiety, agitation, tremor; seizure; urinary disturbances; myalgia; visual disorders; rash, hyperhidrosis; *rarely* taste disturbances, abdominal pain, changes in hepatic function, paraesthesia, erectile dysfunction, dysarthria; *very rarely* hypothermia

**Indications and dose**

Chronic severe spasticity of voluntary muscle

• By mouth

**Child under 18 years** initially 300 micrograms/kg daily in 4 divided doses, increased gradually at weekly intervals until satisfactory response; usual maintenance dose of 0.75–2 mg/kg daily in divided doses; **Child up to 8 years** max. total daily dose 40 mg/day, **Child 8–18 years** max. total daily dose 60 mg/day; review treatment if no benefit within 6 weeks of achieving maximum dose

Severe chronic spasticity of cerebral or spinal origin unresponsive to oral antispastic drugs (or oral therapy not tolerated)—specialist use only

• By intrathecal injection

**Child 4–18 years** initial *test dose* 25–50 micrograms over at least 1 minute via catheter or lumbar puncture, increased in 25-microgram steps (not more often than every 24 hours) to max. 100 micrograms to determine initial maintenance dose *then dose-titration phase*, most often using infusion pump (implanted into chest wall or abdominal wall tissues) to establish maintenance dose retaining some spasticity to avoid sensation of paralysis; initial *maintenance dose* 25–200 micrograms daily, adjusted according to response

### Safe Practice

Consult intrathecal injection product literature for details on dose testing and titration—important to monitor patients closely in appropriately equipped and staffed environment during screening and immediately after pump implantation. Resuscitation equipment must be available for immediate use. Treatment with continuous pump-administered intrathecal baclofen should be initiated within 3 months of a satisfactory response to intrathecal baclofen testing.

**Baclofen** (Non-proprietary) (PoM)

Tablets, baclofen 10 mg, net price 84-tab pack = £1.58. Label: 2, 8, 21

Oral solution, baclofen 5 mg/5 mL, net price 300 mL = £9.26. Label: 2, 8, 21

Brands include *Lyflex*® (sugar-free)

Intrathecal injection, baclofen 50 micrograms/mL, net price 1-mL amp (for test dose) = £2.19; 500 micrograms/mL, 20-mL amp (for use with implantable pump) = £48.62; 2 mg/mL, 5-mL amp (for use with implantable pump) = £48.62

**Lioresal**® (Novartis) (PoM)

Tablets, scored, baclofen 10 mg, net price 84-tab pack = £8.67. Label: 2, 8, 21

Excipients include gluten

Liquid, sugar-free, raspberry–flavoured, baclofen 5 mg/5 mL, net price 300 mL = £7.16. Label: 2, 8, 21

Intrathecal injection, baclofen 50 micrograms/mL, net price 1-mL amp (for test dose) = £2.19; 500 micrograms/mL, 20-mL amp (for use with implantable pump) = £48.62; 2 mg/mL, 5-mL amp (for use with implantable pump) = £48.62

## DANTROLENE SODIUM

**Cautions** impaired cardiac and pulmonary function; therapeutic effect may take a few weeks to develop—discontinue if no response within 6–8 weeks; **interactions:** Appendix 1 (muscle relaxants)

**Hepatotoxicity** Potentially life-threatening hepatotoxicity reported, usually if doses greater than 400 mg daily used, in females, if history of liver disorders, or concomitant use of hepatotoxic drugs; test liver function before and at intervals during therapy—discontinue if abnormal liver function tests or symptoms of liver disorder (counselling, see below); re-introduce only if complete reversal of hepatotoxicity

**Counselling** Children and their carers should be told how to recognise signs of liver disorder and advised to seek prompt medical attention if symptoms such as anorexia, nausea, vomiting, fatigue, abdominal pain, dark urine, or pruritus develop

**Skilled tasks** Drowsiness may affect performance of skilled tasks (eg. driving); effects of alcohol enhanced

**Contra-indications** acute muscle spasm; avoid when spasticity is useful, for example, locomotion

**Hepatic impairment** avoid—may cause severe liver damage; injection may be used in an emergency for malignant hyperthermia

**Pregnancy** avoid use in chronic spasticity—embryotoxic in *animal* studies

**Breast-feeding** present in milk—manufacturer advises avoid use in chronic spasticity

**Side-effects** diarrhoea (withdraw if severe, discontinue treatment if recurs on re-introduction), nausea, vomiting, anorexia, hepatotoxicity (see above), abdominal pain; pericarditis; pleural effusion, respiratory depression; headache, drowsiness, dizziness, asthenia, fatigue, seizures, fever, chills; speech and visual disturbances; rash; *less commonly* dysphagia, constipation, exacerbation of cardiac insufficiency, tachycardia, erratic blood pressure, dyspnoea, depression, confusion, nervousness, insomnia, increased urinary frequency, urinary incontinence or retention, haematuria, crystalluria, and increased sweating

**Licensed use** not licensed for use in children

**Indications and dose**

> Chronic severe spasticity of voluntary muscle
> * By mouth
>
> **Child 5–12 years** initially 500 micrograms/kg once daily; after 7 days increase to 500 micrograms/kg/dose 3 times daily; every 7 days increase by further 500 micrograms/kg/dose until satisfactory response; max. 2 mg/kg 3–4 times daily (max. total daily dose 400 mg)
>
> **Child 12–18 years** initially 25 mg once daily; increase to 3 times daily after 7 days; every 7 days increase by further 500 micrograms/kg/dose until satisfactory response; max. 2 mg/kg 3–4 times daily (max. total daily dose 400 mg)

> Malignant hyperthermia section 15.1.8

**Dantrium®** (SpePharm) [PoM]
Capsules, orange/brown, dantrolene sodium 25 mg, net price 100 = £16.87; 100 mg, 100 = £43.07. Label: 2, counselling, driving, hepatotoxicity

## DIAZEPAM

**Cautions** section 4.8.2
**Contra-indications** section 4.8.2
**Hepatic impairment** section 4.8.2
**Renal impairment** section 4.8.2
**Pregnancy** section 4.8.2
**Breast-feeding** section 4.8.2
**Side-effects** section 4.8.2; also hypotonia

**Indications and dose**

> Muscle spasm in cerebral spasticity or in post-operative skeletal muscle spasm
> * By mouth
>
> **Child 1–12 months** initially 250 microgram/kg twice daily
>
> **Child 1–5 years** initially 2.5 mg twice daily
>
> **Child 5–12 years** initially 5 mg twice daily
>
> **Child 12–18 years** initially 10 mg twice daily; max. total daily dose 40 mg

> Tetanus
> * By intravenous injection
>
> **Child 1 month–18 years** 100–300 micrograms/kg repeated every 1–4 hours
>
> * By intravenous infusion (or by nasoduodenal tube)
>
> **Child 1 month–18 years** 3–10 mg/kg over 24 hours, adjusted according to response

> Status epilepticus section 4.8.2

> Febrile convulsions section 4.8.3

**Administration** for *continuous intravenous infusion* of diazepam emulsion, dilute to a concentration of max. 400 micrograms/mL with Glucose 5% or 10%; max. 6 hours between addition and completion of infusion; diazepam absorbed by plastics of infusion bags and giving sets

For *continuous intravenous infusion* of diazepam solution, dilute to a concentration of max. 50 micrograms/mL with Glucose 5% or Sodium Chloride 0.9%; diazepam absorbed by plastics of infusion bags and giving sets

**Diazepam** (Non-proprietary) [CD4-1]
Tablets, diazepam 2 mg, net price 28 = 89p; 5 mg, 28 = 90p; 10 mg, 28 = 92p. Label: 2 or 19
Brands include *Rimapam*®[NHS], *Tensium*®[NHS]
**Dental prescribing on NHS** Diazepam Tablets may be prescribed

Oral solution, diazepam 2 mg/5 mL, net price 100 mL = £6.08. Label: 2 or 19
Brands include *Dialar*®[NHS]
**Dental prescribing on NHS** Diazepam Oral Solution 2 mg/5 mL may be prescribed

Strong oral solution, diazepam 5 mg/5 mL, net price 100-mL pack = £6.38. [NHS]Label: 2 or 19
Brands include *Dialar*®[NHS]

◀ **Parenteral preparations**
Section 4.8.2

**10 Musculoskeletal and joint diseases**

## 10.3   Drugs for the treatment of soft-tissue disorders and topical pain relief

**10.3.1**   Enzymes

**10.3.2**   Rubefacients, topical NSAIDs, capsaicin, and poultices

## Extravasation

> Local guidelines for the management of extravasation should be followed where they exist or specialist advice sought.

Extravasation injury follows leakage of drugs or intravenous fluids from the veins or inadvertent administration into the subcutaneous or subdermal tissue. It must be dealt with **promptly** to prevent tissue necrosis.

Acidic or alkaline preparations and those with an osmolarity greater than that of plasma can cause extravasation injury; excipients including alcohol and polyethylene glycol have also been implicated. Cytotoxic drugs commonly cause extravasation injury. Very young children are at increased risk. Those receiving anticoagulants are more likely to lose blood into surrounding tissues if extravasation occurs, while those receiving sedatives or analgesics may not notice the early signs or symptoms of extravasation.

**Prevention of extravasation**   Precautions should be taken to avoid extravasation; ideally, drugs likely to cause extravasation injury should be given through a central line and children receiving repeated doses of hazardous drugs peripherally should have the cannula resited at regular intervals. Attention should be paid to the manufacturers' recommendations for administration. Placing a glyceryl trinitrate patch or using glyceryl trinitrate ointment distal to the cannula may improve the patency of the vessel in children with small veins or in those whose veins are prone to collapse.

Children or their carers should be asked to report any pain or burning at the site of injection immediately.

**Management of extravasation**   If extravasation is suspected the infusion should be stopped immediately but the cannula should not be removed until after an attempt has been made to aspirate the area (through the cannula) in order to remove as much of the drug as possible. Aspiration is sometimes successful if the extravasation presents with a raised bleb or blister at the injection site and is surrounded by hardened tissue, but it is often unsuccessful if the tissue is soft or soggy. **Corticosteroids** are usually given to treat inflammation, although there is little evidence to support their use in extravasation. Hydrocortisone or dexamethasone (section 6.3.2) can be given either locally by subcutaneous injection or intravenously at a site distant from the injury. **Antihistamines** (section 3.4.1) and **analgesics** (section 4.7) may be required for symptom relief.

The management of extravasation beyond these measures is not well standardised and calls for specialist advice. Treatment depends on the nature of the offending substance; one approach is to localise and neutralise the substance whereas another is to spread and dilute it. The first method may be appropriate following extravasation of vesicant drugs and involves administration of an antidote (if available) and the application of cold compresses 3–4 times a day (consult specialist literature for details of specific antidotes). Spreading and diluting the offending substance involves infiltrating the area with physiological saline, applying warm compresses, elevating the affected limb, and administering hyaluronidase (section 10.3.1). A saline flush-out technique (involving flushing the subcutaneous tissue with physiological saline) may be effective but requires specialist advice. Hyaluronidase should **not** be administered following extravasation of vesicant drugs (unless it is either specifically indicated or used in the saline flush-out technique).

## 10.3.1   Enzymes

Hyaluronidase is used for the management of extravasation For preparations, see *BNF section 10.3.1*.

## 10.3.2   Rubefacients, topical NSAIDs, capsaicin, and poultices

Classification not used in *BNF for Children*.

# 11 Eye

## 11.1 Administration of drugs to the eye

Drugs are most commonly administered to the eye by topical application as eye drops or eye ointments. When a higher drug concentration is required within the eye, a local injection may be necessary, see Other Preparations, below.

Eye-drop dispenser devices are available to aid the instillation of eye drops from plastic bottles and some are prescribable on the NHS (consult Drug Tariff—see Appliances and Reagents, p. 813 for links to online Drug Tariffs). Product-specific devices may be supplied by manufacturers—contact individual manufacturers for further information. They are particularly useful for children in whom normal application is difficult, for the visually impaired, or otherwise physically limited patients.

**Eye drops and eye ointments**   Eye drops are generally instilled into the pocket formed by gently pulling down the lower eyelid and keeping the eye closed for as long as possible after application; in neonates and infants it may be more appropriate to administer the drop in the inner angle of the open eye. One drop is all that is needed; instillation of more than one drop at a time should be discouraged because it may increase systemic side-effects. A small amount of eye ointment is applied similarly; the ointment melts rapidly and blinking helps to spread it.

When two different eye-drop preparations are used at the same time of day, dilution and overflow can occur when one immediately follows the other. The carer or child should therefore leave an interval of at least 5 minutes between the two; the interval should be extended when eye drops with a prolonged contact time, such as gels and suspensions, are used. Eye ointment should be applied after drops. Both drops and ointment can cause transient blurred vision; children should be warned, where appropriate, not to perform skilled tasks (e.g. cycling or driving) until vision is clear.

Systemic effects may arise from absorption of drugs into the general circulation from conjunctival vessels or from the nasal mucosa after the excess preparation has drained down through the tear ducts. The extent of systemic absorption following ocular administration is highly variable; nasal drainage of drugs is associated with eye drops much more often than with eye ointments. Pressure on the lacrimal punctum for at least a minute after applying eye drops reduces nasolacrimal drainage and therefore decreases systemic absorption from the nasal mucosa.

For warnings relating to eye drops and contact lenses, see section 11.9.

11 Eye

**Eye lotions** These are solutions for the irrigation of the conjunctival sac. They act mechanically to flush out irritants or foreign bodies as a first-aid treatment. Sterile sodium chloride 0.9% solution (section 11.8.1) is usually used. Clean water will suffice in an emergency.

**Other preparations** Subconjunctival injection may be used to administer anti-infective drugs, mydriatics, or corticosteroids for conditions not responding to topical therapy; intracameral and intravitreal routes can also be used to administer certain drugs. These injections should only be used under specialist supervision.

Drugs such as antimicrobials and corticosteroids may be administered systemically to treat an eye condition.

**Preservatives and sensitisers** Information on preservatives and substances identified as skin sensitisers (section 13.1.3) is provided under Excipients statements in preparation entries.

## 11.2 Control of microbial contamination

Preparations for the eye should be sterile when issued. Eye drops in multiple-application containers may include a preservative but care should nevertheless be taken to avoid contamination of the contents during use.

Eye drops in multiple-application containers for *home use* should not be used for more than 4 weeks after first opening (unless otherwise stated by the manufacturer).

Multiple application eye drops for use in *hospital wards* are normally discarded 1 week after first opening (24 hours if preservative-free). Individual containers should be provided for each child, and for each eye if there are special concerns about contamination. Containers used before an operation should be discarded at the time of the operation and fresh containers supplied. A fresh supply should also be provided upon discharge from hospital; in specialist ophthalmology units it may be acceptable to issue containers that have been dispensed to the patient on the day of discharge.

In *out-patient departments* single-application containers should preferably be used; if multiple-application containers are used, they should be discarded at the end of each day. In clinics for occular surface disease and in accident and emergency departments, where the dangers of cross-infection are high, single-application containers should be used; if a multiple-application container is used, it should be discarded after single use.

Diagnostic dyes (section 11.8.2) should be used only from single-application containers.

In *eye surgery* single-application containers should be used if possible; if a multiple-application container is used, it should be discarded after single use. Preparations used during intra-ocular procedures and others that may penetrate into the anterior chamber must be isotonic and without preservatives and buffered if necessary to a neutral pH. Specially formulated fluids should be used for intra-ocular surgery; large volume intravenous infusion preparations are not suitable for this purpose. For all surgical procedures, a previously unopened container is used for each patient.

## 11.3 Anti-infective eye preparations

11.3.1　Antibacterials
11.3.2　Antifungals
11.3.3　Antivirals

**Eye infections** Most acute superficial eye infections can be treated topically. Blepharitis and conjunctivitis are often caused by staphylococci; keratitis and endophthalmitis may be bacterial, viral, or fungal.

Bacterial *blepharitis* is treated by lid hygiene and application of antibacterial eye drops to the conjunctival sac or to the lid margins. Systemic treatment may be required and may be necessary for 3 months or longer.

Most cases of acute bacterial conjunctivitis are self-limiting; where treatment is appropriate, antibacterial eye drops or an eye ointment are used. A poor response might indicate viral or allergic conjunctivitis or antibiotic resistance.

*Corneal ulcer* and *keratitis* require specialist treatment, usually under inpatient care, and may call for intensive topical, subconjunctival, or systemic administration of antimicrobials.

*Endophthalmitis* is a medical emergency which also calls for specialist management and requires intravitreal administration of antimicrobials; concomitant systemic treatment is required in some cases. Surgical intervention, such as vitrectomy, is sometimes indicated.

For reference to the treatment of *crab lice of the eyelashes*, see section 13.10.4

## 11.3.1 Antibacterials

Bacterial eye infections are generally treated topically with eye drops and eye ointments; systemic treatment is sometimes appropriate in blepharitis.

**Chloramphenicol** has a broad spectrum of activity and is the drug of choice for *superficial eye infections*. Chloramphenicol eye drops are well tolerated and the recommendation that chloramphenicol eye drops should be avoided because of an increased risk of aplastic anaemia is not well founded.

Other antibacterials with a broad spectrum of activity include the quinolones, **ciprofloxacin**, **levofloxacin**, **moxifloxacin**, and **ofloxacin**; the aminoglycosides, **gentamicin** and **tobramycin** are also active against a wide variety of bacteria. Gentamicin, tobramycin, quinolones (except moxifloxacin), and **polymyxin B** are effective for infections caused by *Pseudomonas aeruginosa*.

**Ciprofloxacin** eye drops are licensed for *corneal ulcers*; intensive application (especially in the first 2 days) is required throughout the day and night.

**Azithromycin** eye drops are licensed for trachomatous conjunctivitis caused by *Chlamydia trachomatis* and for purulent bacterial conjunctivitis. *Trachoma*, which results from chronic infection with *Chlamydia trachomatis*, can be treated with azithromycin by mouth [unlicensed indication].

**Fusidic acid** is useful for staphylococcal infections.

**Propamidine isetionate** is of little value in bacterial infections but is used by specialists to treat the rare, but potentially sight-threatening, condition of *acanthamoeba keratitis* (see also section 11.9).

Other antibacterial eye drops may be prepared aseptically in a specialist manufacturing unit from material supplied for injection, see section 11.8.

**Neonates**    Antibacterial eye drops are used to treat acute bacterial conjunctivitis in neonates (ophthalmia neonatorum); where possible the causative microorganism should be identified. **Chloramphenicol** eye drops are used to treat mild conjunctivitis; more serious infections also require a systemic antibacterial. Failure to respond to initial treatment requires further investigation; chlamydial infection is one of the most frequent causes of neonatal conjunctivitis and should be considered.

Azithromycin eye drops are licensed to treat trachomatous conjunctivitis caused by *Chlamydia trachomatis* and purulent bacterial conjunctivitis in neonates. Systemic infection due to *Chlamydia trachomatis* may accompany conjunctivitis in neonates and children under 3 months. Systemic treatment is required.

*Gonococcal eye infections* are treated with a single-dose of parenteral **cefotaxime** or **ceftriaxone**. *Chlamydial eye infections* should be managed with oral **erythromycin**. **Gentamicin** eye drops together with appropriate systemic antibacterials are used in the treatment of *pseudomonal eye infections*; high-strength gentamicin eye drops (1.5%) [unlicensed] are available for severe infections.

**With corticosteroids**    Many antibacterial preparations also incorporate a corticosteroid but such mixtures should **not** be used unless a patient is under close specialist supervision. In particular they should not be prescribed for undiagnosed 'red eye' which is sometimes caused by the herpes simplex virus and may be difficult to diagnose (section 11.4).

**Administration**    Frequency of application depends on the severity of the infection and the potential for irreversible ocular damage; antibacterial eye preparations are usually administered as follows:

- *Eye drops*, apply 1 drop at least every 2 hours in severe infection then reduce frequency as infection is controlled and continue for 48 hours after healing. For less severe infection 3–4 times daily is generally sufficient.

- *Eye ointment*, apply *either* at night (if eye drops used during the day) *or* 3–4 times daily (if eye ointment used alone).

## AZITHROMYCIN DIHYDRATE

**Side-effects**    ocular discomfort (including pruritus and burning), blurred vision; *less commonly* eyelid eczema, eyelid erythema, eyelid oedema, conjunctival hyperaemia, keratitis

**Indications and dose**

> **Purulent bacterial conjunctivitis**
>
> Apply twice daily for 3 days; review if no improvement after 3 days

> **Trachomatous conjunctivitis (see also Neonates above)**
>
> Apply twice daily for 3 days; review if no improvement after 3 days

### ◢ Single use

**Azyter®** (Spectrum Thea) ‾PoM‾
Eye drops, azithromycin dihydrate 1.5%, net price 6 × 0.25 g = £6.99

## CHLORAMPHENICOL

**Pregnancy**    avoid unless essential—no information on *topical* use but risk of neonatal 'grey-baby syndrome' with *oral* use in third trimester

**Breast-feeding**    avoid unless essential—*theoretical* risk of bone-marrow toxicity

**Side-effects**    transient stinging; see also notes above

**Indications and dose**

> See notes above

**Chloramphenicol** (Non-proprietary) ‾PoM‾
Eye drops, chloramphenicol 0.5%, net price 10 mL = £2.05

Eye ointment, chloramphenicol 1%, net price 4 g = £2.04

**Note**  Chloramphenicol 0.5% eye drops (max. pack size 10 mL) and 1% eye ointment (max. pack size 4 g) can be sold to the public for treatment of acute bacterial conjunctivitis in children over 2 years; max. duration of treatment 5 days

**Chloromycetin®** (Mercury) ‾PoM‾
Redidrops (= eye drops), chloramphenicol 0.5%, net price 5 mL = £1.65; 10 mL = 90p
**Excipients**  include phenylmercuric acetate

Ophthalmic ointment (= eye ointment), chloramphenicol 1%, net price 4 g = £1.08

### ◢ Single use

**Minims® Chloramphenicol** (Bausch & Lomb) ‾PoM‾
Eye drops, chloramphenicol 0.5%, net price 20 × 0.5 mL = £9.17

## CIPROFLOXACIN

**Pregnancy**    manufacturer advises use only if potential benefit outweighs risk

**Breast-feeding**    manufacturer advises caution

**Side-effects**    taste disturbance, ocular discomfort, ocular hyperaemia, corneal deposits (reversible after completion of treatment); *less commonly* nausea, headache, keratopathy, corneal infiltrates, corneal staining, photophobia, blurred vision, eyelid disorders (including oedema, exfoliation, erythema), eye irritation (including pain, swelling, pruritus, dryness), increased lacrimation, conjunctival hyperaemia; *rarely* diarrhoea, abdominal pain, dizziness, keratitis, corneal disorders including corneal epithelium defect, eye hypoaesthesia, asthenopia, diplopia, ear pain, paranasal sinus hypersecretion, rhinitis, dermatitis

**Licensed use**    eye ointment not licensed for use in children under 1 year

**Indications and dose**

> **Superficial bacterial infections**
>
> Apply eye drops 4 times daily; in severe infection apply every 2 hours during waking hours for 2 days, then 4 times daily; max. duration of treatment 21 days
>
> Apply 1.25 cm eye ointment 3 times daily for 2 days, then twice daily for 5 days

**11 Eye**

### Corneal ulcer

Apply eye drops throughout day and night, day 1 apply every 15 minutes for 6 hours then every 30 minutes, day 2 apply every hour, days 3–14 apply every 4 hours; max. duration of treatment 21 days

Apply eye ointment throughout day and night; apply 1.25 cm ointment every 1–2 hours for 2 days then every 4 hours for next 12 days

**Ciloxan®** (Alcon) [PoM]

Ophthalmic solution (= eye drops), ciprofloxacin (as hydrochloride) 0.3%, net price 5 mL = £4.70
Excipients include benzalkonium chloride

Eye ointment, ciprofloxacin (as hydrochloride) 0.3%, net price 3.5 g = £5.22

## FUSIDIC ACID

### Indications and dose

See notes above and under preparation below

**Fucithalmic®** (LEO) [PoM]

Eye drops, m/r, fusidic acid 1% in gel basis (liquifies on contact with eye), net price 5 g = £1.96
Excipients include benzalkonium chloride, disodium edetate

Dose

Apply twice daily

## GENTAMICIN

### Indications and dose

See notes above

**Genticin®** (Amdipharm) [PoM]

Drops (for ear or eye), gentamicin (as sulfate) 0.3%, net price 10 mL = £2.13
Excipients include benzalkonium chloride

**Gentamicin** (Non-proprietary) [PoM]

Eye drops, gentamicin 1.5%, 10 mL, available as a manufactured special from Moorfields Eye Hospital, see also 'special-order' manufacturers or specialist importing companies, p. 823

## LEVOFLOXACIN

**Pregnancy** manufacturer advises use only if potential benefit outweighs risk

**Breast-feeding** manufacturer advises use only if potential benefit outweighs risk

**Side-effects** ocular burning, visual disturbances; *less commonly* headache, ocular discomfort (including itching, pain, and dryness), conjunctival follicles, lid oedema, lid erythema, photophobia, rhinitis

### Indications and dose

Local treatment of infections (see also notes above)

Child 1–18 years apply every 2 hours (max. 8 times daily) for the first 2 days, then 4 times daily for 3 days

**Oftaquix®** (Kestrel Ophthalmics) [PoM]

Eye drops, levofloxacin 0.5%, net price 5 mL = £6.95
Excipients include benzalkonium chloride

Unit dose eye drops, levofloxacin 0.5%, net price 30 × 0.5-mL single use units = £17.95

## MOXIFLOXACIN

**Cautions** not recommended for neonates

**Side-effects** taste disturbances, ocular discomfort (including pain, irritation, and dryness), hyperaemia; *less commonly* vomiting, headache, paraesthesia, corneal disorders (including keratitis, erosion, and staining), conjunctival haemorrhage, eyelid erythema, visual disturbances, nasal discomfort, pharyngolaryngeal pain; *also reported* nausea, palpitation, dyspnoea, dizziness, raised intra-ocular pressure, photophobia, rash, pruritus

### Indications and dose

Local treatment of infections (see also notes above)

Child 1 month–18 years apply 3 times daily (continue treatment for 2–3 days after infection improves; review if no improvement within 5 days)

**Moxivig®** (Alcon) ▼ [PoM]

Eye drops, moxifloxacin (as hydrochloride) 0.5%, net price 5 mL = £9.80

## OFLOXACIN

**Cautions** corneal ulcer or epithelial defect (risk of corneal perforation)

**Pregnancy** manufacturer advises use only if benefit outweighs risk; systemic quinolones have caused arthropathy in *animal* studies

**Breast-feeding** manufacturer advises avoid

**Side-effects** ocular discomfort and irritation; *also reported* facial oedema, keratitis, visual disturbances, photophobia, increased lacrimation, ocular oedema, dry eyes, ocular hyperaemia

### Indications and dose

Local treatment of infections (see also notes above)

Child 1 month–18 years apply every 2–4 hours for the first 2 days, then reduce frequency to 4 times daily (max. 10 days treatment)

**Exocin®** (Allergan) [PoM]

Ophthalmic solution (= eye drops), ofloxacin 0.3%, net price 5 mL = £2.17
Excipients include benzalkonium chloride

## PROPAMIDINE ISETIONATE

**Pregnancy** manufacturer advises avoid unless essential—no information available

**Breast-feeding** manufacturer advises avoid unless essential—no information available

**Side-effects** eye pain and irritation

### Indications and dose

See under preparations below

**Brolene®** (Sanofi-Aventis)

Eye drops, propamidine isetionate 0.1%, net price 10 mL = £2.80
Excipients include benzalkonium chloride

Dose

Local treatment of infections (but see notes above)

Apply up to 4 times daily

Eye ointment, dibrompropamidine isetionate 0.15%, net price 5 g = £2.92

**Dose**

**Local treatment of infections (but see notes above)**

Apply 1–2 times daily

**Golden Eye**® (Typharm)

Eye drops, propamidine isetionate 0.1%, net price 10 mL = £2.70

Excipients  include benzalkonium chloride

**Dose**

**Local treatment of infections (but see section 11.3.1)**

Apply up to 4 times daily

Eye ointment, dibrompropamidine isetionate 0.15%, net price 5 g = £2.83

**Dose**

**Local treatment of infections (but see section 11.3.1)**

Apply 1–2 times daily

## ■ TOBRAMYCIN

**Indications and dose**

**Local treatment of infections (see also notes above)**

**Child 1–18 years** apply twice daily for 6–8 days; in severe infections, apply 4 times daily on the first day, then twice daily for 5–7 days

**Tobravisc**® (Alcon) [PoM]

Eye drops, tobramycin 0.3%, net price 5 mL = £4.74

Excipients  include benzododecinium bromide

## 11.3.2 Antifungals

Fungal infections of the cornea are rare. Orbital mycosis is rarer, and when it occurs it is usually because of direct spread of infection from the paranasal sinuses. Debility or immunosuppression can encourage fungal proliferation. The spread of infection through blood occasionally produces metastatic endophthalmitis.

Many different fungi are capable of producing ocular infection; they can be identified by appropriate laboratory procedures.

Antifungal preparations for the eye are not generally available. Treatment is normally carried out at specialist centres, but requests for information about supplies of preparations not available commercially should be addressed to the Strategic Health Authority (or equivalent in Scotland or Northern Ireland), or to the nearest hospital ophthalmology unit, or to Moorfields Eye Hospital, 162 City Road, London EC1V 2PD (tel. (020) 7253 3411) or www.moorfields.nhs.uk

## 11.3.3 Antivirals

Herpes simplex infections producing, for example, dendritic corneal ulcers, can be treated with **aciclovir**. Aciclovir eye ointment is used in combination with systemic treatment for ophthalmic zoster (section 5.3.2.1).

For systemic treatment of CMV retinitis, see section 5.3.2.2.

## ■ ACICLOVIR
(Acyclovir)

**Side-effects**  local irritation and inflammation, superficial punctate keratopathy; *rarely* blepharitis; *very rarely* hypersensitivity reactions including angioedema

**Indications and dose**

**Local treatment of herpes simplex infections**

Apply 1 cm ointment 5 times daily (continue for at least 3 days after complete healing)

**Herpes simplex skin infections** section 13.10.3

**Herpes simplex and varicella–zoster infections** section 5.3.2.1

**Zovirax**® (GSK) [PoM]

Eye ointment, aciclovir 3%, net price 4.5 g = £9.34

## 11.4 Corticosteroids and other anti-inflammatory preparations

**11.4.1**  Corticosteroids

**11.4.2**  Other anti-inflammatory preparations

## 11.4.1 Corticosteroids

Corticosteroids administered locally to the eye or given by mouth are effective for treating anterior segment inflammation in uveitis (section 11.5) and following surgery.

*Topical corticosteroids*  should normally only be used under expert supervision; three main dangers are associated with their use:

- a 'red eye', when the diagnosis is unconfirmed, may be due to herpes simplex virus, and a corticosteroid may aggravate the condition, leading to corneal ulceration, with possible damage to vision and even loss of the eye. Bacterial, fungal, and amoebic infections pose a similar hazard;

- 'steroid glaucoma' may follow the use of corticosteroid eye preparations in susceptible individuals;

- a 'steroid cataract' may follow prolonged use.

Other side-effects of ocular corticosteroids include thinning of the cornea and sclera. Prolonged use in neonates and infants can cause adrenal suppression.

Products combining a corticosteroid with an antimicrobial are used after ocular surgery to reduce inflammation and prevent infection: use of combination products is otherwise rarely justified.

*Systemic corticosteroids* (section 6.3.2) may be useful for ocular conditions. The risk of producing a 'steroid cataract' increases with the dose and duration of corticosteroid use.

## ■ BETAMETHASONE

**Cautions**  see notes above

**Side-effects**  see notes above

**11** Eye

**Indications and dose**

> **Local treatment of inflammation (short-term)**
>
> Apply eye drops every 1–2 hours until controlled then reduce frequency; eye ointment 2–4 times daily or at night when used with eye drops

**Betnesol®** (UCB Pharma) [PoM]
Drops (for ear, eye, or nose), betamethasone sodium phosphate 0.1%, net price 10 mL = £2.23
Excipients   include benzalkonium chloride, disodium edetate

Eye ointment, betamethasone sodium phosphate 0.1%, net price 3 g = £1.36

**Vistamethasone®** (Martindale) [PoM]
Drops (for ear, eye, or nose), betamethasone sodium phosphate 0.1%, net price 5 mL = £1.02; 10 mL = £1.16
Excipients   include benzalkonium chloride

◢**With neomycin**
**Betnesol-N®** (UCB Pharma) [PoM]◢
Drops (for ear, eye, or nose), see section 12.1.1

## ▌DEXAMETHASONE

**Cautions**   see notes above
**Side-effects**   see notes above
**Licensed use**   *Maxidex®* not licensed for use in children under 2 years
**Indications and dose**

> **Local treatment of inflammation (short-term)**
>
> Apply eye drops 4–6 times daily; severe conditions every 30–60 minutes until controlled then reduce frequency

**Maxidex®** (Alcon) [PoM]
Eye drops, dexamethasone 0.1%, net price 5 mL = £1.42; 10 mL = £2.80
Excipients   include benzalkonium chloride, disodium edetate, polysorbate 80

◢**Single use**
**Minims® Dexamethasone** (Bausch & Lomb) [PoM]
Eye drops, dexamethasone sodium phosphate 0.1%, net price 20 × 0.5 mL = £9.38
Excipients   include disodium edetate

◢**With antibacterials**
**Maxitrol®** (Alcon) [PoM]◢
Eye drops, dexamethasone 0.1%, neomycin 0.35% (as sulfate), polymyxin B sulfate 6000 units/mL, net price 5 mL = £1.68
Excipients   include benzalkonium chloride, polysorbate 20

Eye ointment, dexamethasone 0.1%, neomycin 0.35% (as sulfate), polymyxin B sulfate 6000 units/g, net price 3.5 g = £1.44
Excipients   include hydroxybenzoates (parabens), wool fat

**Sofradex®** (Sanofi-Aventis) [PoM]◢
Drops (for ear or eye), see section 12.1.1

## ▌FLUOROMETHOLONE

**Cautions**   see notes above
**Side-effects**   see notes above
**Licensed use**   not licensed for use in children under 2 years

**Indications and dose**

> **Local treatment of inflammation (short-term)**
>
> Apply 2–4 times daily (initially every hour for 24–48 hours then reduce frequency)

**FML®** (Allergan) [PoM]
Ophthalmic suspension (= eye drops), fluorometholone 0.1%, polyvinyl alcohol (*Liquifilm®*) 1.4%, net price 5 mL = £1.71; 10 mL = £2.95
Excipients   include benzalkonium chloride, disodium edetate, polysorbate 80

## ▌HYDROCORTISONE ACETATE

**Cautions**   see notes above
**Side-effects**   see notes above
**Indications and dose**

> **Local treatment of inflammation (short-term)**
>
> Apply twice daily or at night

**Hydrocortisone** (Non-proprietary) [PoM]
Eye ointment, hydrocortisone acetate 1%, net price 3 g = £6.71

## ▌PREDNISOLONE

**Cautions**   see notes above
**Side-effects**   see notes above
**Licensed use**   *Pred Forte®* not licensed for use in children (age range not specified by manufacturer)
**Indications and dose**

> **Local treatment of inflammation (short-term)**
>
> Apply every 1–2 hours until controlled then reduce frequency

**Pred Forte®** (Allergan) [PoM]
Eye drops, prednisolone acetate 1%, net price 5 mL = £1.52; 10 mL = £3.05
Excipients   include benzalkonium chloride, disodium edetate, polysorbate 80

**Predsol®** (UCB Pharma) [PoM]
Drops (for ear or eye), prednisolone sodium phosphate 0.5%, net price 10 mL = £1.92
Excipients   include benzalkonium chloride, disodium edetate

◢**Single use**
**Minims® Prednisolone Sodium Phosphate** (Bausch & Lomb) [PoM]
Eye drops, prednisolone sodium phosphate 0.5%, net price 20 × 0.5 mL = £10.08
Excipients   include disodium edetate

## ▌11.4.2   Other anti-inflammatory preparations

Eye drops containing **antihistamines**, such as **antazoline** (with xylometazoline as *Otrivine-Antistin®*), **azelastine**, **epinastine**, **ketotifen**, and **olopatadine**, can be used for allergic conjunctivitis.

**Sodium cromoglicate** and **nedocromil sodium** eye drops may be useful for vernal keratoconjunctivitis and other allergic forms of conjunctivitis.

**Lodoxamide** eye drops are used for allergic conjunctival conditions including seasonal allergic conjunctivitis.

**Emedastine** eye drops are licensed for seasonal allergic conjunctivitis.

**11 Eye**

## ANTAZOLINE SULFATE

**Side-effects**  transient stinging; *also reported* blurred vision, mydriasis, eye irritation

**Indications and dose**

Allergic conjunctivitis

See preparation below

**Otrivine-Antistin**® (Spectrum Thea)

Eye drops, antazoline sulfate 0.5%, xylometazoline hydrochloride 0.05%, net price 10 mL = £2.35

Excipients  include benzalkonium chloride, disodium edetate

Cautions  hypertension; hyperthyroidism; diabetes mellitus; angle-closure glaucoma; phaeochromocytoma; cardiovascular disease; urinary retention; **interactions:** Appendix 1 (antihistamines and sympathomimetics)

Dose

Child 12–18 years apply 2–3 times daily (max. duration 7 days)

Note  Xylometazoline is a sympathomimetic; absorption of antazoline and xylometazoline may result in systemic side-effects and the possibility of interaction with other drugs

## AZELASTINE HYDROCHLORIDE

**Side-effects**  mild transient irritation; bitter taste reported

**Indications and dose**

Allergic conjunctivitis, seasonal allergic conjunctivitis

Child 4–18 years apply twice daily, increased if necessary to 4 times daily

Perennial conjunctivitis

Child 12–18 years apply twice daily, increased if necessary to 4 times daily; max. duration of treatment 6 weeks

**Optilast**® (Meda) [PoM]

Eye drops, azelastine hydrochloride 0.05%, net price 8 mL = £6.40

Excipients  include benzalkonium chloride, disodium edetate

## EMEDASTINE

**Side-effects**  transient burning or stinging; blurred vision, local oedema, keratitis, irritation, dry eye, lacrimation, corneal infiltrates (discontinue) and staining; photophobia; headache, and rhinitis occasionally reported

**Indications and dose**

Seasonal allergic conjunctivitis

Child 3–18 years apply twice daily

**Emadine**® (Alcon) [PoM]

Eye drops, emedastine 0.05% (as difumarate), net price 5 mL = £7.31

Excipients  include benzalkonium chloride

## EPINASTINE HYDROCHLORIDE

**Side-effects**  burning; *less commonly* taste disturbance, headache, conjunctival hyperaemia, dry eye, eye pruritus, visual disturbance, increased lacrimation, eye pain, nasal irritation, rhinitis

**Indications and dose**

Seasonal allergic conjunctivitis

Child 12–18 years apply twice daily; max. duration of treatment 8 weeks

**Relestat**® (Allergan) [PoM]

Eye drops, epinastine hydrochloride 500 micrograms/mL, net price 5 mL = £9.90

Excipients  include benzalkonium chloride, disodium edetate

## KETOTIFEN

**Side-effects**  transient burning or stinging, punctate corneal epithelial erosion; *less commonly* dry eye, subconjunctival haemorrhage, photophobia; headache, drowsiness, skin reactions, and dry mouth also reported

**Indications and dose**

Seasonal allergic conjunctivitis

Child 3–18 years apply twice daily

**Zaditen**® (Spectrum Thea) [PoM]

Eye drops, ketotifen (as fumarate) 250 micrograms/mL, net price 5 mL = £7.80

Excipients  include benzalkonium chloride

## LODOXAMIDE

**Side-effects**  burning, stinging, itching, blurred vision, tear production disturbance, and ocular discomfort; *less commonly*, flushing, nasal dryness, dizziness, drowsiness, headache, blepharitis, and keratitis

**Indications and dose**

Allergic conjunctivitis

Child 4–18 years apply 4 times daily

Note  Improvement of symptoms may sometimes require treatment for up to 4 weeks

**Alomide**® (Alcon) [PoM]

Ophthalmic solution (= eye drops), lodoxamide (as trometamol) 0.1%, net price 10 mL = £5.21

Excipients  include benzalkonium chloride, disodium edetate

Note  Lodoxamide 0.1% eye drops can be sold to the public for treatment of allergic conjunctivitis in children over 4 years

## NEDOCROMIL SODIUM

**Side-effects**  transient burning and stinging; distinctive taste reported

**Indications and dose**

Seasonal and perennial allergic conjunctivitis

Child 6–18 years apply twice daily increased if necessary to 4 times daily; max. 12 weeks treatment for seasonal allergic conjunctivitis

Vernal keratoconjunctivitis

Child 6–18 years apply 4 times daily

**Rapitil**® (Sanofi-Aventis) [PoM]

Eye drops, nedocromil sodium 2%, net price 5 mL = £4.92

Excipients  include benzalkonium chloride, disodium edetate

11 Eye

## OLOPATADINE

**Side-effects**   local irritation; less commonly keratitis, dry eye, local oedema, photophobia; headache, asthenia, dizziness; dry nose also reported

**Indications and dose**

> **Seasonal allergic conjunctivitis**
>
> > **Child 3–18 years** apply twice daily; max. duration of treatment 4 months

**Opatanol®** (Alcon) [PoM]

Eye drops, olopatadine (as hydrochloride) 1 mg/mL, net price 5 mL = £3.91

**Excipients** include benzalkonium chloride

## SODIUM CROMOGLICATE
### (Sodium cromoglycate)

**Side-effects**   transient burning and stinging

**Indications and dose**

> **Allergic conjunctivitis, vernal keratoconjunctivitis**
>
> > Apply eye drops 4 times daily

**Sodium Cromoglicate** (Non-proprietary) [PoM]

Eye drops, sodium cromoglicate 2%, net price 13.5 mL = £1.79

**Brands include** *Hay-Crom® Aqueous, Opticrom® Aqueous, Vividrin®*

**Note** Sodium cromoglicate 2% eye drops can be sold to the public (in max. pack size of 10 mL) for treatment of acute seasonal and perennial allergic conjunctivitis

◢ **Single use**

**Catacrom®** (Moorfields)

Eye drops, sodium cromoglicate 2%, net price 30 x 0.3 mL = £8.99

## 11.5   Mydriatics and cycloplegics

Antimuscarinics dilate the pupil and paralyse the ciliary muscle; they vary in potency and duration of action.

Short-acting, relatively weak mydriatics, such as **tropicamide** 0.5% (action lasts for 4–6 hours), facilitate the examination of the fundus of the eye. **Cyclopentolate** 1% (action up to 24 hours) or **atropine** (action up to 7 days) are preferable for producing cycloplegia for refraction in young children; tropicamide may be preferred in neonates. **Phenylephrine** 2.5% is used for mydriasis in diagnostic or therapeutic procedures; mydriasis occurs within 60–90 minutes and lasts up to 5–7 hours.

Mydriatics and cycloplegics are used in the treatment of anterior uveitis, usually as an adjunct to corticosteriods (section 11.4.1). Atropine is used in anterior uveitis mainly to prevent posterior synechiae and to relieve ciliary spasm; cyclopentolate or **homatropine** (action up to 3 days) can also be used and may be preferred because they have a shorter duration of action.

**Cautions and contra-indications**   Darkly pigmented irides are more resistant to pupillary dilatation and caution should be exercised to avoid overdosage. Mydriasis can precipitate acute angle-closure glaucoma in the very few children who are predisposed to the condition because of a shallow anterior chamber. Atropine, cyclopentolate, and homatropine should be used with caution in children under 3 months owing to the possible association between cycloplegia and the development of amblyopia; also, neonates are at increased risk of systemic toxicity.

**Skilled tasks**   Children may not be able to undertake skilled tasks until vision clears after mydriasis.

**Side-effects**   Ocular side-effects of mydriatics and cycloplegics include transient stinging and raised intraocular pressure; on prolonged administration, local irritation, hyperaemia, oedema, and conjunctivitis can occur. Contact dermatitis can occur with the antimuscarinic mydriatic drugs, especially atropine.

Toxic systemic reactions to atropine and cyclopentolate can occur in neonates and children; see section 1.2 for systemic side-effects of antimuscarinic drugs.

## Antimuscarinics

## ATROPINE SULFATE

**Cautions**   see notes above

**Side-effects**   see notes above

**Licensed use**   not licensed for use in children for uveitis

**Indications and dose**

> **Cycloplegia**
>
> > **Child 3 months–18 years** apply drops or ointment twice daily for 3 days before procedure

> **Anterior uveitis**
>
> > **Child 2–18 years** 1 drop up to 4 times daily

**Atropine** (Non-proprietary) [PoM]

Eye drops, atropine sulfate 0.5%, net price 10 mL = £2.78; 1%, 10 mL = £9.50

◢ **Single use**

**Minims® Atropine Sulphate** (Bausch & Lomb) [PoM]

Eye drops, atropine sulfate 1%, net price 20 × 0.5 mL = £12.71

## CYCLOPENTOLATE HYDROCHLORIDE

**Cautions**   see notes above

**Side-effects**   see notes above

**Indications and dose**

> See notes above

> **Cycloplegia**
>
> > **Child 3 months–12 years** 1 drop of 1% eye drops 30–60 minutes before examination
> >
> > **Child 12–18 years** 1 drop of 0.5% eye drops 30–60 minutes before examination

> **Uveitis**
>
> > **Child 3 months–18 years** 1 drop of 0.5% eye drops (1% for deeply pigmented eyes) 2–4 times daily

**Mydrilate®** (Intrapharm) [PoM]

Eye drops, cyclopentolate hydrochloride 0.5%, net price 5 mL = £6.73; 1%, 5 mL = £6.73

**Excipients** include benzalkonium chloride

◢Single use

**Minims® Cyclopentolate Hydrochloride** (Bausch & Lomb) ᴾᵒᴹ

Eye drops, cyclopentolate hydrochloride 0.5% and 1%, net price 20 × 0.5 mL (both) = £9.64

## ■ HOMATROPINE HYDROBROMIDE

**Cautions**  see notes above

**Side-effects**  see notes above

**Licensed use**  not licensed for use in children under 3 months

**Indications and dose**

See notes above

**Child 3 months–2 years** (0.5% only) 1 drop daily or on alternate days adjusted according to response

**Child 2–18 years** 1 drop twice daily adjusted according to response

**Homatropine** (Non-proprietary) ᴾᵒᴹ

Eye drops, homatropine hydrobromide 1%, 10 mL, available without preservatives as a manufactured special from Moorfields Eye Hospital

Eye drops, homatropine 0.125% and 0.5%, 10 mL, available as a manufactured special from Moorfields Eye Hospital, see also 'special-order' manufacturers or specialist importing companies, p. 823

## ■ TROPICAMIDE

**Cautions**  see notes above

**Side-effects**  see notes above

**Indications and dose**

See notes above

**Funduscopy**

**Neonate and child** apply 0.5% eye drops 20 minutes before examination

**Mydriacyl®** (Alcon) ᴾᵒᴹ

Eye drops, tropicamide 0.5%, net price 5 mL = £1.29; 1%, 5 mL = £1.60

Excipients  include benzalkonium chloride, disodium edetate

◢Single use

**Minims® Tropicamide** (Bausch & Lomb) ᴾᵒᴹ

Eye drops, tropicamide 0.5% and 1%, net price 20 × 0.5 mL (both) = £9.01

## Sympathomimetics

## ■ PHENYLEPHRINE HYDROCHLORIDE

**Cautions**  see notes above; also corneal epithelial damage; ocular hyperaemia; susceptibility to angle-closure glaucoma; diabetes (avoid in long-standing diabetes); asthma; **interactions**: Appendix 1 (sympathomimetics)

**Contra-indications**  10% drops in neonates and children; cardiovascular disease; hypertension; aneurysms; thyrotoxicosis

**Pregnancy**  use only if potential benefit outweighs risk

**Breast-feeding**  use only if potential benefit outweighs risk—no information available

**Side-effects**  see notes above; also blurred vision, photophobia; systemic effects include palpitations,

tachycardia, extrasystoles, arrhythmias, hypertension; *also reported* coronary artery spasm, myocardial infarction (usually after use of 10% strength in patients with pre-existing cardiovascular disease)

**Indications and dose**

**Mydriasis**

Apply 1 drop before procedure; see also notes above

Note  A drop of proxymetacaine topical anaesthetic may be applied to the eye a few minutes before using phenylephrine to prevent stinging

◢Single use

**Minims® Phenylephrine Hydrochloride** (Bausch & Lomb)

Eye drops, phenylephrine hydrochloride 2.5%, net price 20 × 0.5 mL = £9.53

Excipients  include disodium edetate, sodium metabisulfite

## 11.6 Treatment of glaucoma

Glaucoma describes a group of disorders characterised by a loss of visual field associated with cupping of the optic disc and optic nerve damage and is generally associated with raised intra-ocular pressure.

Glaucoma is rare in children and should always be managed by a specialist. *Primary congenital glaucoma* is the most common form of glaucoma in children, followed by *secondary glaucomas*, such as following hereditary anterior segment malformations; *juvenile open-angle glaucoma* is less common and usually occurs in older children. *Primary angle closure glaucoma* (acute closed-angle glaucoma) is very rare in children; it is a medical emergency that requires urgent reduction of intra-ocular pressure, see below. Outflow of aqueous humour from the eye is restricted by bowing of the iris against the trabecular meshwork.

Treatment of glaucoma is determined by the pathophysiology and usually involves controlling raised intra-ocular pressure with surgery. Drug therapy is generally supportive, and can be used temporarily, pre-or post-operatively, or both, to reduce intra-ocular pressure. In secondary glaucomas, drug therapy is often used first-line, and long-term treatment may be required. Drugs that reduce intra-ocular pressure by different mechanisms are available for managing glaucoma. A topical beta-blocker or a prostaglandin analogue can be used. It may be necessary to combine these drugs or add others, such as carbonic anhydrase inhibitors, or miotics to control intra-ocular pressure.

**Acetazolamide** by intravenous injection can be used for the emergency management of raised intra-ocular pressure. Rarely, **mannitol**  can be given by slow intravenous infusion to reduce intra-ocular pressure (see section 2.2.5).

### Beta-blockers

Topical application of a beta-blocker to the eye reduces intra-ocular pressure effectively in primary and secondary glaucomas, probably by reducing the rate of production of aqueous humour.

**Cautions, contra-indications, and side-effects**  Systemic absorption can follow topical application to the eye; therefore, eye drops containing a beta-blocker are contra-indicated in bradycardia, heart block,

11 Eye

or uncontrolled heart failure. **Important:** for a warning to avoid in asthma, see below. Cough, rather than wheeze, may occur in children using topical beta-blockers. Consider also other cautions, contra-indications, and side-effects of beta-blockers (p. 87). Beta-blocker eye drops should be used with caution in children with corneal diseases. Local side-effects of eye drops include ocular stinging, burning, pain, itching, erythema, dry eyes and allergic reactions including anaphylaxis and blepharoconjunctivitis; occasionally corneal disorders have been reported.

**Important** Beta-blockers, even those with apparent cardioselectivity, should not be used in patients with asthma or a history of bronchospasm, unless no alternative treatment is available. In such cases the risk of inducing bronchospasm should be appreciated and appropriate precautions taken.

**Interactions**   Since systemic absorption may follow topical application the possibility of interactions, in particular with drugs such as verapamil, should be borne in mind. See also Appendix 1 (beta-blockers).

## ▮ BETAXOLOL

**Cautions**   see notes above
**Contra-indications**   see notes above
**Side-effects**   see notes above
**Licensed use**   not licensed for use in children
**Indications and dose**

See notes above

Apply twice daily

**Betaxolol** (Non-proprietary) ⓅoM
Eye drops, solution, betaxolol (as hydrochloride) 0.5%, net price 5 mL = £1.90
**Excipients**   may include benzalkonium chloride, disodium edetate

**Betoptic®** (Alcon) ⓅoM
Ophthalmic solution (= eye drops), betaxolol (as hydrochloride) 0.5%, net price 5 mL = £1.90
**Excipients**   include benzalkonium chloride, disodium edetate
Ophthalmic suspension (= eye drops), betaxolol (as hydrochloride) 0.25%, net price 5 mL = £2.66
**Excipients**   include benzalkonium chloride, disodium edetate
Unit dose eye drop suspension, betaxolol (as hydrochloride) 0.25%, net price 50 × 0.25 mL = £13.77

## ▮ CARTEOLOL HYDROCHLORIDE

**Cautions**   see notes above
**Contra-indications**   see notes above
**Side-effects**   see notes above
**Licensed use**   not licensed for use in children
**Indications and dose**

See notes above

Apply twice daily

**Teoptic®** (Spectrum Thea) ⓅoM
Eye drops, carteolol hydrochloride 1%, net price 5 mL = £7.60; 2%, 5 mL = £8.40
**Excipients**   include benzalkonium chloride

## ▮ LEVOBUNOLOL HYDROCHLORIDE

**Cautions**   see notes above
**Contra-indications**   see notes above

**Side-effects**   see notes above; anterior uveitis occasionally reported
**Licensed use**   not licensed for use in children
**Indications and dose**

See notes above

Apply once or twice daily

**Levobunolol** (Non-proprietary) ⓅoM
Eye drops, levobunolol hydrochloride 0.5%, net price 5 mL = £3.05
**Excipients**   may include benzalkonium chloride, disodium edetate, sodium metabisulfite

**Betagan®** (Allergan) ⓅoM
Eye drops, levobunolol hydrochloride 0.5%, polyvinyl alcohol (*Liquifilm®*) 1.4%, net price 5-mL = £1.85
**Excipients**   include benzalkonium chloride, disodium edetate, sodium metabisulfite
Unit dose eye drops, levobunolol hydrochloride 0.5%, polyvinyl alcohol (*Liquifilm®*) 1.4%, net price 30 × 0.4 mL = £9.98
**Excipients**   include disodium edetate

## ▮ TIMOLOL

**Cautions**   see notes above
**Contra-indications**   see notes above
**Side-effects**   see notes above
**Licensed use**   not licensed for use in children
**Indications and dose**

See notes above

Apply twice daily; long-acting preparations, see under preparations below

**Timolol** (Non-proprietary) ⓅoM
Eye drops, timolol (as maleate) 0.25%, net price 5 mL = £1.56; 0.5%, 5 mL = £1.56

**Timoptol®** (MSD) ⓅoM
Eye drops, in *Ocumeter®* metered-dose unit, timolol (as maleate) 0.25%, net price 5 mL = £3.12; 0.5%, 5 mL = £3.12
**Excipients**   include benzalkonium chloride
Unit dose eye drops, timolol (as maleate) 0.25%, net price 30 × 0.2 mL = £8.45; 0.5%, 30 × 0.2 mL = £9.65

◀**Once-daily preparations**
**Timoptol®-LA** (MSD) ⓅoM
Ophthalmic gel-forming solution (= eye drops), timolol (as maleate) 0.25%, net price 2.5 mL = £3.12; 0.5%, 2.5 mL = £3.12
**Excipients**   include benzododecinium bromide
**Dose**

Apply eye drops once daily

**Tiopex®** (Spectrum Thea) ⓅoM
Unit dose eye gel (= eye drops), timolol (as maleate) 0.1%, net price 30 × 0.4 g = £7.49
**Dose**

Apply once daily in the morning

◀**With dorzolamide**
See under Dorzolamide

## Prostaglandin analogues

The prostaglandin analogues **latanoprost**, and **travoprost**, and the synthetic prostamide, **bimatoprost**, increase uveoscleral outflow and subsequently reduce intra-ocular pressure. They are used to reduce intra-ocular pressure. Only latanoprost (*Xalatan*® and certain non-proprietary preparations of latanoprost) is licensed for use in children; for prescribing information, see BNF section 11.6. Children receiving prostaglandin analogues should be managed by a specialist and monitored for any changes to eye coloration since an increase in the brown pigment in the iris can occur; particular care is required in those with mixed coloured irides and those receiving treatment to one eye only.

## Sympathomimetics

**Apraclonidine** (section 11.8.2) is an alpha₂-adrenoceptor agonist that lowers intra-ocular pressure by reducing aqueous humour formation. Eye drops containing apraclonidine 0.5% are used for a short period to delay laser treatment or surgery for glaucoma in patients not adequately controlled by another drug; eye drops containing 1% are used for control of intraocular pressure after anterior segment laser surgery.

**Brimonidine**, an alpha₂-adrenoceptor agonist, is thought to lower intra-ocular pressure by reducing aqueous humour formation and increasing uveoscleral outflow; it is contra-indicated in neonates and children under 2 years (risk of severe systemic side-effects), and should be used with caution in children 2–12 years (increased risk of drowsiness).

## Carbonic anhydrase inhibitors and systemic drugs

The **carbonic anhydrase inhibitors**, acetazolamide, brinzolamide, and dorzolamide, reduce intra-ocular pressure by reducing aqueous humour production. Systemic use of acetazolamide also produces weak diuresis.

**Acetazolamide** is given by mouth or, rarely in children, by intravenous injection (intramuscular injections are painful because of the alkaline pH of the solution). It is used as an adjunct to other treatment for reducing intra-ocular pressure. Acetazolamide is a sulfonamide derivative; blood disorders, rashes, and other sulfonamide-related side-effects occur occasionally—children and their carers should be told to report any unusual skin rash. It is not generally recommended for long-term use; if electrolyte disturbances and metabolic acidosis occur, they can be corrected by administering potassium bicarbonate (as effervescent potassium tablets, section 9.2.1.3).

**Dorzolamide** and **brinzolamide** are topical carbonic anhydrase inhibitors. They are unlicensed in children but are used in those resistant to beta-blockers or those in whom beta-blockers are contra-indicated. They are used alone or as an adjunct to a topical beta-blocker. Brinzolamide can also be used as an adjunct to a prostaglandin analogue. Systemic absorption can rarely cause sulfonamide-like side-effects and may require discontinuation if severe.

Metabolic acidosis can occur in children using topical carbonic anhydrase inhibitors; symptoms may include poor feeding and lack of weight gain.

## ▮ ACETAZOLAMIDE

**Cautions** not generally recommended for prolonged use, but if given, monitor blood count and plasma electrolyte concentrations; pulmonary obstruction and impaired alveolar ventilation (risk of acidosis); diabetes mellitus; renal calculi; avoid extravasation at injection site (risk of necrosis); **interactions:** Appendix 1 (diuretics)

**Contra-indications** hypokalaemia, hyponatraemia, hyperchloraemic acidosis; adrenocortical insufficiency; long-term administration in chronic angle-closure glaucoma; sulfonamide hypersensitivity

**Hepatic impairment** manufacturer advises avoid

**Renal impairment** avoid; metabolic acidosis

**Pregnancy** manufacturer advises avoid, especially in first trimester (toxicity in *animal* studies)

**Breast-feeding** amount too small to be harmful

**Side-effects** see notes above; also nausea, vomiting, diarrhoea, taste disturbance, loss of appetite, paraesthesia, flushing, headache, dizziness, fatigue, irritability, excitement, ataxia, depression, thirst, polyuria; *less commonly* melaena, drowsiness, confusion, hearing disturbances, fever, glycosuria, metabolic acidosis and electrolyte disturbances on long-term therapy, haematuria, crystalluria, renal and ureteral colic, renal lesions or calculi, renal failure, blood disorders, bone marrow suppression, rash (including Stevens-Johnson syndrome and toxic epidermal necrosis); *rarely* fulminant hepatic necrosis, hepatitis, cholestatic jaundice, flaccid paralysis, convulsions, photosensitivity; *also reported* transient myopia

**Licensed use** not licensed for use in children for treatment of glaucoma

**Indications and dose**

> **Reduction of intra-ocular pressure in primary and secondary glaucoma**
> - By mouth or by intravenous injection
>   **Child 1 month–12 years** 5 mg/kg 2–4 times daily, adjusted according to response, max. 750 mg daily
>   **Child 12–18 years** 250 mg 2–4 times daily

> **Epilepsy**
> - By mouth or slow intravenous injection
>   **Neonate** initially 2.5 mg/kg 2–3 times daily, followed by 5–7 mg/kg 2–3 times daily (maintenance dose)
>   **Child 1 month–12 years** initially 2.5 mg/kg 2–3 times daily, followed by 5–7 mg/kg 2–3 times daily, max. 750 mg daily (maintenance dose)
>   **Child 12–18 years** 250 mg 2–4 times daily

> **Raised intracranial pressure**
> - By mouth or slow intravenous injection
>   **Child 1 month–12 years** initially 8 mg/kg 3 times daily, increased as necessary to max. 100 mg/kg daily

**Diamox**® (Mercury) ᴾᵒᴹ
Tablets, acetazolamide 250 mg, net price 112-tab pack = £12.68. Label: 3

Injection, powder for reconstitution, acetazolamide (as sodium salt), net price 500-mg vial = £14.76

◢**Modified release**
**Diamox® SR** (Mercury) ᴾᵒᴹ
Capsules, m/r, orange, enclosing orange f/c pellets, acetazolamide 250 mg, net price 30-cap pack = £13.88. Label: 3, 25
**Dose**
> **Child 12–18 years** glaucoma, 1–2 capsules daily

**11 Eye**

# ▉ BRINZOLAMIDE

**Cautions** systemic absorption follows topical application; renal tubular immaturity or abnormality—risk of metabolic acidosis; **interactions**: Appendix 1 (brinzolamide)

**Contra-indications** hyperchloraemic acidosis; sulfonamide hypersensitivity

**Hepatic impairment** manufacturer advises avoid

**Renal impairment** see Cautions above; also avoid if estimated glomerular filtration rate less than 30 mL/minute/1.73 m$^2$

**Pregnancy** avoid—toxicity in *animal* studies

**Breast-feeding** use only if benefit outweighs risk

**Side-effects** see notes above; also taste disturbances, dry mouth, headache, ocular disturbances (including corneal erosion, corneal oedema, photophobia, and reduced visual acuity); *less commonly* nausea, vomiting, diarrhoea, dyspepsia, oesophagitis, flatulence, oral hypoaesthesia and paraesthesia, chest pain, bradycardia, palpitation, dyspnoea, cough, upper respiratory tract congestion, pharyngitis, depression, sleep disturbances, nervousness, malaise, drowsiness, amnesia, dizziness, paraesthesia, sinusitis, decreased libido, erectile dysfunction, renal pain, epistaxis, nasal dryness, throat irritation, tinnitus, alopecia; *also reported* arrhythmia, tachycardia, hypertension, peripheral oedema, asthma, tremor, vertigo, pollakiuria, rhinitis, dermatitis, erythema

**Licensed use** not licensed for use in children

**Indications and dose**

> Reduction of intra-ocular pressure in primary and secondary glaucoma *either* as adjunct to beta-blockers or prostaglandin analogues *or* used alone if unresponsive to beta-blockers or if beta-blockers contra-indicated
>
> > Apply twice daily, increased to max. 3 times daily if necessary

**Azopt®** (Alcon) ⟨PoM⟩
Eye drops, brinzolamide 10 mg/mL, net price 5 mL = £6.56
**Excipients** include benzalkonium chloride, disodium edetate

# ▉ DORZOLAMIDE

**Cautions** systemic absorption follows topical application; history of renal calculi; neonates and infants with immature renal tubules—risk of metabolic acidosis; chronic corneal defects, low endothelial cell count, history of intra-ocular surgery; **interactions**: Appendix 1 (dorzolamide)

**Contra-indications** hyperchloraemic acidosis

**Hepatic impairment** manufacturer advises caution—no information available

**Renal impairment** see Cautions above; also avoid if estimated glomerular filtration rate less than 30 mL/minute/1.73 m$^2$

**Pregnancy** manufacturer advises avoid—toxicity in *animal* studies

**Breast-feeding** manufacturer advises avoid—no information available

**Side-effects** see notes above; also nausea, bitter taste, headache, asthenia, ocular irritation, blurred vision, lacrimation, conjunctivitis, superficial punctuate keratitis, eyelid inflammation; *less commonly* iridocyclitis; *rarely* dry mouth, dizziness, paraesthesia,

urolithiasis, eyelid crusting, transient myopia, corneal oedema, epistaxis, throat irritation, contact dermatitis, Stevens-Johnson syndrome, toxic epidermal necrolysis; *also reported* metabolic acidosis

**Licensed use** not licensed for use in children

**Indications and dose**

> Raised intra-ocular pressure in primary and secondary glaucoma *either* as adjunct to beta-blocker *or* used alone in patients unresponsive to beta-blockers or if beta-blockers contra-indicated
>
> > Used alone, apply 3 times daily; with topical beta-blocker, apply twice daily

**Dorzolamide** (Non-proprietary) ⟨PoM⟩
Eye drops, dorzolamide (as hydrochloride) 2%, net price 5 mL = £5.61
**Excipients** may include benzalkonium chloride
**Brands include** *Dorzant®*

**Trusopt®** (MSD) ⟨PoM⟩
Ophthalmic solution (= eye drops), in *Ocumeter® Plus* metered-dose unit, dorzolamide (as hydrochloride) 2%, net price 5 mL = £6.33
**Excipients** include benzalkonium chloride

Unit dose eye drops, dorzolamide (as hydrochloride) 2%, net price 60 × 0.2 mL = £24.18

◢**With timolol**
For prescribing information on timolol, see section 11.6, Beta-blockers

**Dorzolamide with Timolol** (Non-proprietary) ⟨PoM⟩
Eye drops, dorzolamide (as hydrochloride) 2%, timolol (as maleate) 0.5%, net price 5 mL = £10.05
**Excipients** may include benzalkonium chloride

**Cosopt®** (MSD) ⟨PoM⟩
Ophthalmic solution (= eye drops), in *Ocumeter® Plus* metered-dose unit, dorzolamide (as hydrochloride) 2%, timolol (as maleate) 0.5%, net price 5 mL = £10.05
**Excipients** include benzalkonium chloride

Unit dose eye drops, dorzolamide (as hydrochloride) 2%, timolol (as maleate) 0.5%, net price 60 × 0.2 mL = £28.59
**Dose**

> Raised intra-ocular pressure in open-angle glaucoma, or pseudoexfoliative glaucoma when beta-blockers alone not adequate
>
> > Apply twice daily

## Miotics

Miotics act by opening up the inefficient drainage channels in the trabecular meshwork. **Pilocarpine** is a miotic used pre- and postoperatively in goniotomy and trabeculotomy; it is used occasionally for aphakic glaucoma.

**Cautions** A darkly pigmented iris may require a higher concentration of the miotic or more frequent administration and care should be taken to avoid overdosage. Retinal detachment has occurred in susceptible individuals and those with retinal disease; therefore fundus examination is advised before starting treatment with a miotic. Care is also required in conjunctival or corneal damage. Intra-ocular pressure and visual fields should be monitored in those with chronic simple glaucoma and those receiving long-term treatment with a miotic. Miotics should be used with caution in patients with peptic ulceration, gastro-intestinal spasm, cardiac disease, hypertension, hypotension, asthma, epilepsy, hyperthyroidism, and urinary-tract obstruction.

**Counselling** Blurred vision may affect performance of skilled tasks (e.g. driving) particularly at night or in reduced lighting

**Contra-indications** Miotics are contra-indicated in conditions where pupillary constriction is undesirable such as acute iritis, anterior uveitis and some forms of secondary glaucoma. They should be avoided in acute inflammatory disease of the anterior segment.

**Pregnancy** Miotics should be avoided unless the potential benefit outweighs the risk—limited information available.

**Breast-feeding** Miotics should be avoided unless the potential benefit outweighs the risk—no information available.

**Side-effects** Ciliary spasm leads to headache and browache which may be more severe in the initial 2–4 weeks of treatment. Ocular side-effects include burning, itching, smarting, blurred vision, conjunctival vascular congestion, myopia, lens changes with chronic use, vitreous haemorrhage, and pupillary block. Systemic side-effects are rare following application to the eye.

## ■ PILOCARPINE

**Cautions** see notes above
**Contra-indications** see notes above
**Side-effects** see notes above
**Licensed use** not licensed for use in children
**Indications and dose**

See also notes above

Raised intra-ocular pressure
- **Child 1 month–2 years** 1 drop of 0.5% or 1% solution 3 times daily
- **Child 2–18 years** 1 drop 4 times daily

Pre- and postoperatively in goniotomy and trabeculotomy
   **Child 1 month–18 years** apply 1% or 2% solution once daily

**Pilocarpine Hydrochloride** (Non-proprietary) PoM
   Eye drops, pilocarpine hydrochloride 1%, 10 mL = £3.00; 2%, 10 mL = £2.87; 4%, 10 mL = £3.83
   Excipients may include benzalkonium chloride

◀Single use
**Minims® Pilocarpine Nitrate** (Bausch & Lomb) PoM
   Eye drops, pilocarpine nitrate 2%, net price 20 × 0.5 mL = £10.04

## 11.7 Local anaesthetics

**Oxybuprocaine** and **tetracaine** are widely used topical local anaesthetics. **Proxymetacaine** causes less initial stinging and is particularly useful for children. Oxybuprocaine or a combined preparation of lidocaine and fluorescein is used for tonometry. Tetracaine produces more profound anaesthesia and is suitable for use before minor surgical procedures, such as the removal of corneal sutures. It has a temporary disruptive effect on the corneal epithelium. **Lidocaine**, with or without adrenaline (epinephrine), is injected into the eyelids for minor surgery, see section 15.2, p. 649. Local anaes-

thetics should never be used for the management of ocular symptoms.

**Caution** Local anaesthetic eye drops should be avoided in preterm neonates because of the immaturity of the metabolising enzyme system.

## ■ LIDOCAINE HYDROCHLORIDE
(Lignocaine hydrochloride)

**Contra-indications** avoid in preterm neonates
**Indications and dose**

Local anaesthetic
   Use as required

**Minims® Lidocaine and Fluorescein** (Bausch & Lomb) PoM
   Eye drops, lidocaine hydrochloride 4%, fluorescein sodium 0.25%, net price 20 × 0.5 mL = £10.61

## ■ OXYBUPROCAINE HYDROCHLORIDE
(Benoxinate hydrochloride)

**Contra-indications** avoid in preterm neonates
**Indications and dose**

Local anaesthetic
   Use as required

**Minims® Oxybuprocaine Hydrochloride** (Bausch & Lomb) PoM
   Eye drops, oxybuprocaine hydrochloride 0.4%, net price 20 × 0.5 mL = £8.92

## ■ PROXYMETACAINE HYDROCHLORIDE

**Contra-indications** avoid in preterm neonates
**Indications and dose**

Local anaesthetic
   Use as required

**Minims® Proxymetacaine** (Bausch & Lomb) PoM
   Eye drops, proxymetacaine hydrochloride 0.5%, net price 20 × 0.5 mL = £9.51

◀With fluorescein
**Minims® Proxymetacaine and Fluorescein** (Bausch & Lomb) PoM
   Eye drops, proxymetacaine hydrochloride 0.5%, fluorescein sodium 0.25%, net price 20 × 0.5 mL = £10.59

## ■ TETRACAINE HYDROCHLORIDE
(Amethocaine hydrochloride)

**Contra-indications** avoid in preterm neonates
**Indications and dose**

Local anaesthetic
   Use as required

**Minims® Tetracaine Hydrochloride** (Bausch & Lomb) PoM
   Eye drops, tetracaine hydrochloride 0.5% and 1%, net price 20 × 0.5 mL (both) = £8.93

11 Eye

# 11.8 Miscellaneous ophthalmic preparations

### 11.8.1 Tear deficiency, ocular lubricants, and astringents
### 11.8.2 Ocular diagnostic and peri-operative preparations

Certain eye drops, e.g. amphotericin, ceftazidime, cefuroxime, colistimethate sodium, desferrioxamine, dexamethasone, gentamicin, and vancomycin, can be prepared aseptically in a specialist manufacturing unit from material supplied for injection.

Preparations may also be available from Moorfields Eye Hospital as manufactured specials, see also 'special-order' manufacturers or specialist importing companies, p. 823.

## 11.8.1 Tear deficiency, ocular lubricants, and astringents

Chronic soreness of the eyes associated with reduced or abnormal tear secretion often responds to tear replacement therapy. The severity of the condition and the child's preference will often guide the choice of preparation.

**Hypromellose** is the traditional choice of treatment for tear deficiency. It may need to be instilled frequently (e.g. hourly) for adequate relief. Ocular surface mucin is often abnormal in tear deficiency and the combination of hypromellose with a mucolytic such as **acetylcysteine** can be helpful.

The ability of **carbomers** to cling to the eye surface may help reduce frequency of application to 4 times daily.

**Polyvinyl alcohol** increases the persistence of the tear film and is useful when the ocular surface mucin is reduced.

**Sodium hyaluronate** eye drops are also used in the management of tear deficiency.

**Sodium chloride 0.9%** drops are sometimes useful in tear deficiency, and can be used as 'comfort drops' by contact lens wearers, and to facilitate lens removal. Special presentations of sodium chloride 0.9% and other irrigation solutions are used routinely for intra-ocular surgery and in first-aid for removal of harmful substances.

Eye ointments containing a **paraffin** can be used to lubricate the eye surface, especially in cases of recurrent corneal epithelial erosion. They may cause temporary visual disturbance and are best suited for application before sleep. Ointments should not be used during contact lens wear.

## ACETYLCYSTEINE

### Indications and dose

> **Tear deficiency, impaired or abnormal mucus production**
> Apply 3–4 times daily

**Ilube®** (Moorfields) PoM
Eye drops, acetylcysteine 5%, hypromellose 0.35%, net price 10 mL = £10.09
Excipients include benzalkonium chloride, disodium edetate

## CARBOMERS
(Polyacrylic acid)

Synthetic high molecular weight polymers of acrylic acid cross-linked with either allyl ethers of sucrose or allyl ethers of pentaerithrityl

**Licensed use** some preparations not licensed for use in children

### Indications and dose

> **Dry eyes including keratoconjunctivitis sicca, unstable tear film**
> Apply 3–4 times daily or as required

**GelTears®** (Bausch & Lomb)
Gel (= eye drops), carbomer 980 (polyacrylic acid) 0.2%, net price 10 g = £2.80
Excipients include benzalkonium chloride

**Liposic®** (Bausch & Lomb)
Gel (= eye drops), carbomer 980 (polyacrylic acid) 0.2%, net price 10 g = £2.96
Excipients include cetrimide

**Lumecare® Long Lasting Tear Gel** (Medicom)
Gel (= eye drops), carbomer 980 (polyacrylic acid) 0.2%, net price 10 g = £2.10
Excipients include cetrimide

**Viscotears®** (Alcon)
Liquid gel (= eye drops), carbomer 980 (polyacrylic acid) 0.2%, net price 10 g = £2.94
Excipients include cetrimide

◢ **Single use**
**Viscotears®** (Alcon)
Liquid gel (= eye drops), carbomer 980 (polyacrylic acid) 0.2%, net price 30 × 0.6-mL = £5.42

## CARMELLOSE SODIUM

### Indications and dose

> **Dry eye conditions**
> Apply as required

**Carmize®** (Aspire)
Eye drops, carmellose sodium 0.5%, net price 10 mL = £7.49

**Optive®** (Allergan)
Eye drops, carmellose sodium 0.5%, glycerol, net price 10 mL = £7.49

◢ **Single use**
**Carmellose** (Non-proprietary)
Eye drops, carmellose sodium 0.5%, net price 30 × 0.4 mL = £5.75
Note Each unit is resealable for up to 12 hours

**Carmize®** (Aspire)
Eye drops, carmellose sodium 0.5%, net price 30 × 0.4 mL = £5.75, 90 × 0.4 mL = £15.53; 1%, 30 × 0.4 mL = £3.00, 60 × 0.4 mL = £6.00

**Celluvisc®** (Allergan)
Eye drops, carmellose sodium 0.5%, net price 30 × 0.4 mL = £5.75, 90 × 0.4 mL = £15.53; 1%, 30 × 0.4 mL = £3.00, 60 × 0.4 mL = £10.99

## HYDROXYETHYLCELLULOSE

**Indications and dose**

Tear deficiency

Apply as required

**Minims® Artificial Tears** (Bausch & Lomb)
Eye drops, hydroxyethylcellulose 0.44%, sodium chloride 0.35%, net price 20 × 0.5 mL = £8.21

## HYPROMELLOSE

**Indications and dose**

Tear deficiency

Apply as required

Note The Royal Pharmaceutical Society has stated that where it is not possible to ascertain the strength of hypromellose prescribed, the prescriber should be contacted to clarify the strength intended.

**Hypromellose** (Non-proprietary)
Eye drops, hypromellose 0.3%, net price 10 mL = £1.61
Excipients may include benzalkonium chloride
Brands include *Lumecare*® Hypromellose

**Artelac®** (Bausch & Lomb)
Eye drops, hypromellose 0.32%, net price 10 mL = £4.99
Excipients include cetrimide, disodium edetate

**Isopto Alkaline®** (Alcon)
Eye drops, hypromellose 1%, net price 10 mL = 94p
Excipients include benzalkonium chloride

**Isopto Plain®** (Alcon)
Eye drops, hypromellose 0.5%, net price 10 mL = 81p
Excipients include benzalkonium chloride

**Tear-Lac®** (Scope Ophthalmics)
Eye drops, hypromellose 0.3%, net price 10 mL = £5.75

**Tears Naturale®** (Alcon)
Eye drops, hypromellose 0.3%, dextran '70' 0.1%, net price 15 mL = £1.60
Excipients include benzalkonium chloride, disodium edetate

◀Single use
**Artelac® SDU** (Bausch & Lomb)
Eye drops, hypromellose 0.32%, net price 30 × 0.5 mL = £16.95

**Hydromoor®** (Moorfields)
Eye drops, hypromellose 0.3%, net price 30 × 0.4 mL = £5.75

**Lumecare® Preservative Free Tear Drops** (Medicom)
Eye drops, hypromellose 0.3%, net price 30 × 0.5 mL = £5.72

**Tears Naturale® Single Dose** (Alcon)
Eye drops, hypromellose 0.3%, dextran '70' 0.1%, net price 28 × 0.4 mL = £13.26

## LIQUID PARAFFIN

**Indications and dose**

Dry eye conditions

Apply as required

**Lacri-Lube®** (Allergan)
Eye ointment, white soft paraffin 57.3%, liquid paraffin 42.5%, wool alcohols 0.2%, net price 3.5 g = £2.51, 5 g = £3.32

**VitA-POS®** (Scope Ophthalmics)
Eye ointment, retinol palmitate 250 units/g, white soft paraffin, light liquid paraffin, liquid paraffin, wool fat, net price 5 g = £2.75

## MACROGOLS
(Polyethylene glycols)

**Indications and dose**

Dry eye conditions

Apply as required

**Systane®** (Alcon)
Eye drops, polyethylene glycol 400 0.4%, propylene glycol 0.3%, hydroxypropyl guar, net price 10 mL = £4.66

**Systane® Ultra** (Alcon)
Eye drops, polyethylene glycol 400 0.4%, propylene glycol 0.3%, hydroxypropyl guar, sorbitol, net price 10 mL = £6.69

◀Single use
**Systane®** (Alcon)
Eye drops, polyethylene glycol 400 0.4%, propylene glycol 0.3%, hydroxypropyl guar, net price 28 × 0.8 mL = £4.66

**Systane® Ultra** (Alcon)
Eye drops, polyethylene glycol 400 0.4%, propylene glycol 0.3%, hydroxypropyl guar, sorbitol, net price 30 × 0.7 ml = £6.69

## PARAFFIN, YELLOW, SOFT

**Indications and dose**

See notes above

Apply 2 hourly as required

**Simple Eye Ointment**
Ointment, liquid paraffin 10%, wool fat 10%, in yellow soft paraffin, net price 4 g = £3.06

## POLYVINYL ALCOHOL

**Indications and dose**

Tear deficiency

Apply as required

**Liquifilm Tears®** (Allergan)
Ophthalmic solution (= eye drops), polyvinyl alcohol 1.4%, net price 15 mL = £1.93
Excipients include benzalkonium chloride, disodium edetate

Ophthalmic solution (= eye drops), polyvinyl alcohol 1.4%, povidone 0.6%, net price 30 × 0.4 mL = £5.35

11 Eye

**Sno Tears®** (Bausch & Lomb)
Eye drops, polyvinyl alcohol 1.4%, net price 10 mL = £1.06
Excipients include benzalkonium chloride, disodium edetate

## SODIUM CHLORIDE

### Indications and dose

Irrigation, including first-aid removal of harmful substances

Use as required

**Sodium Chloride 0.9% Solutions**
See section 13.11.1

**Balanced Salt Solution**
Solution (sterile), sodium chloride 0.64%, sodium acetate 0.39%, sodium citrate 0.17%, calcium chloride 0.048%, magnesium chloride 0.03%, potassium chloride 0.075%
For intra-ocular or topical irrigation during surgical procedures
Brands include *Iocare*®

◢ Single use
**Minims® Saline** (Bausch & Lomb)
Eye drops, sodium chloride 0.9%, net price 20 × 0.5 mL = £6.59

## SODIUM HYALURONATE

### Indications and dose

Dry eye conditions

Apply as required

**Hyabak®** (Spectrum Thea)
Eye drops, sodium hyaluronate 0.15%, net price 10 mL = £7.99

**Hylo-Care®** (Scope Ophthalmics)
Eye drops, sodium hyaluronate 0.1%, dexpanthenol 2%, net price 10 mL = £10.30

**Hylo-Forte®** (Scope Opthalmics)
Eye drops, sodium hyaluronate 0.2%, net price 10 mL = £10.80

**Hylo-Tear®** (Scope Opthalmics)
Eye drops, sodium hyaluronate 0.1%, net price 10 mL = £9.80

**Lumecare® Sodium Hyaluronate** (Medicom)
Eye drops, sodium hyaluronate 0.15%, net price 10 mL = £3.97

**Oxyal®** (Kestrel Ophthalmics)
Eye drops, sodium hyaluronate 0.15%, net price 10 ml = £4.15

**Vismed® Multi** (TRB Chemedica)
Eye drops, sodium hyaluronate 0.18%, net price 10 mL = £6.81

◢ Single use
**Clinitas®** (Altacor)
Eye drops, sodium hyaluronate 0.4%, net price 30 × 0.5 mL = £5.70
Note Each unit is resealable and may be used for up to 12 hours after first opening

**Lubristil®** (Moorfields)
Eye drops, sodium hyaluronate 0.15%, net price 20 × 0.3 mL = £4.99

**Ocusan®** (Agepha)
Eye drops, sodium hyaluronate 0.2%, net price 20 × 0.5 mL = £5.25

**Vismed®** (TRB Chemedica)
Eye drops, sodium hyaluronate 0.18%, net price 20 × 0.3 mL = £5.10

**Vismed® Gel** (TRB Chemedica)
Eye drops, sodium hyaluronate 0.3%, net price 20 × 0.45 mL = £5.98

## 11.8.2 Ocular diagnostic and peri-operative preparations

### Ocular diagnostic preparations

**Fluorescein sodium** is used in diagnostic procedures and for locating damaged areas of the cornea due to injury or disease.

## FLUORESCEIN SODIUM

### Indications and dose

Detection of lesions and foreign bodies

Sufficient to stain damaged areas

**Minims® Fluorescein Sodium** (Bausch & Lomb)
Eye drops, fluorescein sodium 1% or 2%, net price 20 × 0.5 mL (both) = £7.53

◢ With local anaesthetic
Section 11.7

### Ocular peri-operative drugs

Drugs used to prepare the eye for surgery and drugs that are injected into the anterior chamber at the time of surgery are included here.

Sodium hyaluronate is used during surgical procedures on the eye.

**Apraclonidine**, an alpha$_2$-adrenoceptor agonist, reduces intra-ocular pressure possibly by reducing the production of aqueous humour. It is used for short-term treatment only.

**Balanced Salt Solution** is used routinely in intra-ocular surgery (section 11.8.1).

## ACETYLCHOLINE CHLORIDE

**Cautions** gastro-intestinal spasm, peptic ulcer; heart failure; asthma; hyperthyroidism; urinary-tract obstruction

**Pregnancy** avoid unless potential benefit outweighs risk—no information available

**Breast-feeding** avoid unless potential benefit outweighs risk—no information available

**Licensed use** not licensed for use in children

### Indications and dose

Cataract surgery, penetrating keratoplasty, iridectomy, other anterior segment surgery requiring rapid complete miosis

Consult product literature

**Miochol-E**® (Bausch & Lomb) PoM

Intra-ocular irrigation, powder for reconstitution, acetylcholine chloride 10 mg/mL (1%) when reconstituted, net price 20-mg vial (with solvent) = £7.28

**Miphtel**® (SD Healthcare) PoM

Intra-ocular irrigation, powder for reconstitution, acetylcholine chloride 10 mg/mL (1%) when reconstituted, net price 20-mg vial (with solvent) = £7.28

## APRACLONIDINE

**Note** Apraclonidine is a derivative of clonidine

**Cautions** history of angina, severe coronary insufficiency, recent myocardial infarction, heart failure, cerebrovascular disease, vasovagal attack, hypertension; Raynaud's syndrome; thromboangiitis obliterans; depression; monitor intra-ocular pressure and visual fields; loss of effect may occur over time; suspend treatment if reduction in vision occurs in end-stage glaucoma; monitor for excessive reduction in intra-ocular pressure following peri-operative use; **interactions:** Appendix 1 (alpha$_2$-adrenoceptor stimulants)

**Skilled tasks** Drowsiness may affect performance of skilled tasks (e.g. driving)

**Contra-indications** history of severe or unstable and uncontrolled cardiovascular disease

**Hepatic impairment** manufacturer advises caution

**Renal impairment** use with caution in chronic renal failure

**Pregnancy** manufacturer advises avoid—no information available

**Breast-feeding** manufacturer advises avoid—no information available

**Side-effects** taste disturbance, conjunctivitis, dry eye, ocular intolerance (withdraw if eye pruritus, ocular hyperaemia, increased lacrimation, or oedema of the eyelids and conjunctiva occur), rhinitis; *less commonly* chest pain, asthma, dyspnoea, throat irritation, nervousness, irritability, impaired co-ordination, myalgia, mydriasis, keratitis, keratopathy, photophobia, visual impairment, corneal erosion and infiltrates, blepharospasm, blepharitis, eyelid ptosis or retraction, conjunctival vascular disorders, rhinorrhoea, parosmia; since absorption may follow topical application, systemic effects (see Clonidine, section 2.5.2) may occur

**Licensed use** 0.5% drops not licensed for use in children under 12 years; 1% drops not licensed for use in children

**Indications and dose**

See preparations below

**Iopidine**® (Alcon) PoM

Ophthalmic solution (= eye drops), apraclonidine 1% (as hydrochloride), net price 12 × 2 single use 0.25-mL units = £77.81

**Dose**

Control or prevention of postoperative elevation of intra-ocular pressure after anterior segment laser surgery

Apply 1 drop 1 hour before laser procedure then 1 drop immediately after completion of procedure

Ophthalmic solution (= eye drops), apraclonidine 0.5% (as hydrochloride), net price 5 mL = £10.88

**Excipients** include benzalkonium chloride

**Dose**

Short-term adjunctive treatment of chronic glaucoma in patients not adequately controlled by another drug (see note below)

**Child 12–18 years** apply 1 drop 3 times daily usually for max. 1 month

**Note** May not provide additional benefit if patient already using two drugs that suppress the production of aqueous humour

## DICLOFENAC SODIUM

**Licensed use** not licensed for use in children

**Indications and dose**

Inhibition of intra-operative miosis during cataract surgery (but does not possess intrinsic mydriatic properties), postoperative inflammation in cataract surgery, strabismus surgery, argon laser trabeculoplasty

Consult product literature

**Voltarol**® **Ophtha Multidose** (Spectrum Thea) PoM

Eye drops, diclofenac sodium 0.1%, net price 5 mL = £6.68

**Excipients** include benzalkonium chloride, disodium edetate, propylene glycol

◀ Single use

**Voltarol**® **Ophtha** (Spectrum Thea) PoM

Eye drops, diclofenac sodium 0.1%, net price pack of 5 single-dose units = £4.00, 40 single-dose units = £32.00

## FLURBIPROFEN SODIUM

**Licensed use** not licensed for use in children

**Indications and dose**

Inhibition of intra-operative miosis (but does not possess intrinsic mydriatic properties), control of postoperative and post-laser trabeculoplasty inflammation (if corticosteroids contra-indicated)

Consult product literature

**Ocufen**® (Allergan) PoM

Ophthalmic solution (= eye drops), flurbiprofen sodium 0.03%, polyvinyl alcohol (*Liquifilm*®) 1.4%, net price 40 × 0.4 mL = £37.15

## KETOROLAC TROMETAMOL

**Licensed use** not licensed for use in children

**Indications and dose**

Prophylaxis and reduction of inflammation and associated symptoms following ocular surgery

Consult product literature

**Acular**® (Allergan) PoM

Eye drops, ketorolac trometamol 0.5%, net price 5 mL = £3.00

**Excipients** include benzalkonium chloride, disodium edetate

## 11.9 Contact lenses

Some children and adolescents prefer to wear contact lenses rather than spectacles for both cosmetic and

**11 Eye**

medical reasons. Visual defects are corrected by either rigid ('hard' or gas permeable) lenses or soft (hydrogel) lenses; soft lenses are the most popular type, because they are initially the most comfortable, but they may not give the best vision. Lenses should usually be worn for a specified number of hours each day and removed for sleeping. The risk of infectious and non-infectious keratitis is increased by extended continuous contact lens wear in children, which is not recommended, except when medically indicated.

Contact lenses require meticulous care. Poor compliance with directions for use, and with daily cleaning and disinfection, can result in complications including ulcerative keratitis or conjunctivitis. One-day disposable lenses, which are worn only once and therefore require no disinfection or cleaning, are becoming increasingly popular.

*Acanthamoeba keratitis*, a painful and sight-threatening condition, is associated with ineffective lens cleaning and disinfection, the use of contaminated lens cases, or tap water coming into contact with the lenses. The condition is especially associated with the use of soft lenses (including frequently replaced lenses) and should be treated by specialists.

**Contact lenses and drug treatment**   Special care is required in prescribing eye preparations for contact lens users. Some drugs and preservatives in eye preparations can accumulate in hydrogel lenses and can cause adverse reactions. Therefore, unless medically indicated, the lenses should be removed before instillation of the eye preparation and not worn during the period of treatment. Alternatively, unpreserved drops can be used. Eye drops may, however, be instilled while patients are wearing rigid corneal contact lenses. Ointment preparations should never be used in conjunction with contact lens wear; oily eye drops should also be avoided.

Many drugs given systemically can also have adverse effects on contact lens wear. These include oral contraceptives (particularly those with a higher oestrogen content), drugs which reduce blink rate (e.g. anxiolytics, hypnotics, antihistamines, and muscle relaxants), drugs which reduce lacrimation (e.g. antihistamines, antimuscarinics, phenothiazines and related drugs, some beta-blockers, diuretics, and tricyclic antidepressants), and drugs which increase lacrimation (including ephedrine and hydralazine). Other drugs that can affect contact lens wear are isotretinoin (can cause conjunctival inflammation), aspirin (salicylic acid appears in tears and can be absorbed by contact lenses—leading to irritation), and rifampicin and sulfasalazine (can discolour lenses).

11 Eye

# 12 Ear, nose, and oropharynx

This chapter also includes advice on the drug management of the following:
  allergic rhinitis, p. 541
  nasal polyps, p. 541
  oropharyngeal infections, p. 547
  periodontitis, p. 546

## 12.1 Drugs acting on the ear

12.1.1  Otitis externa
12.1.2  Otitis media
12.1.3  Removal of ear wax

## 12.1.1 Otitis externa

Otitis externa is an inflammatory reaction of the lining of the ear canal usually associated with an underlying seborrhoeic dermatitis or eczema; it is important to exclude an underlying chronic otitis media before treatment is commenced. Many cases recover after thorough cleansing of the external ear canal by suction or dry mopping.

A frequent problem in resistant cases is the difficulty in applying lotions and ointments satisfactorily to the relatively inaccessible affected skin. The most effective method is to introduce a ribbon gauze dressing or sponge wick soaked with **corticosteroid** ear drops or with an astringent such as **aluminium acetate** solution. When this is not practical, the ear should be gently cleansed with a probe covered in cotton wool and the patient encouraged to lie with the affected ear uppermost for ten minutes after the canal has been filled with a liberal quantity of the appropriate solution.

Secondary infection in otitis externa may be of bacterial, fungal, or viral origin. If infection is present, a topical anti-infective which is not used systemically (such as **neomycin** or **clioquinol**) may be used, but for only about a week because excessive use may result in fungal infections that are difficult to treat. Sensitivity to the anti-infective or solvent may occur and resistance to antibacterials is a possibility with prolonged use. **Aluminium acetate** ear drops are also effective against bacterial infection and inflammation of the ear. **Chloramphenicol** may be used, but the ear drops contain propylene glycol and cause hypersensitivity reactions in about 10% of patients. Solutions containing an anti-infective and a corticosteroid (such as *Locorten-Vioform®*) are used for treating children when infection is present with inflammation and eczema. **Clotrimazole** 1% solution is used topically to treat fungal infection in otitis externa.

In view of reports of ototoxicity in patients with a perforated tympanic membrane (eardrum), manufacturers contra-indicate treatment with a topical aminoglycoside antibiotic in those with a tympanic perforation. However, many specialists do use these drops cautiously in the presence of a perforation in children with otitis media (section 12.1.2) and when other measures have failed for otitis externa.

A solution of **acetic acid** 2% acts as an antifungal and antibacterial in the external ear canal and may be used to treat mild otitis externa. More severe cases require treatment with an anti-inflammatory preparation with or without an anti-infective drug. A proprietary preparation containing acetic acid 2% (*EarCalm*® spray) is on sale to the public for children over 12 years.

For severe pain associated with otitis externa, a simple analgesic, such as **paracetamol** (section 4.7.1) or **ibuprofen** (section 10.1.1), can be used. A systemic antibacterial (Table 1, section 5.1) can be used if there is spreading cellulitis or if the child is systemically unwell. When a resistant staphylococcal infection (a boil) is present in the external auditory canal, oral **flucloxacillin** (section 5.1.1.2) is the drug of choice; oral **ciprofloxacin** (section 5.1.12) or a systemic aminoglycoside may be needed for pseudomonal infections, particularly in children with diabetes or compromised immunity.

The skin of the pinna adjacent to the ear canal is often affected by eczema. A topical corticosteroid (section 13.4) cream or ointment is then required, but prolonged use should be avoided.

**Administration**   To administer ear drops, lay the child down with the head turned to one side; for an infant pull the earlobe back and down, for an older child pull the earlobe back and up.

## Astringent preparations

### ◢ ALUMINIUM ACETATE

**Licensed use**   not licensed
**Indications and dose**

> Inflammation in otitis externa (see notes above)
>> Insert into meatus or apply on a ribbon gauze dressing or sponge wick which should be kept saturated with the ear drops

**Aluminium Acetate** (Non-proprietary)
Ear drops 13%, aluminium sulfate 2.25 g, calcium carbonate 1 g, tartaric acid 450 mg, acetic acid (33%) 2.5 mL, purified water 7.5 mL
Available as manufactured special

Ear drops 8%, dilute 8 parts aluminium acetate ear drops (13%) with 5 parts purified water. Must be freshly prepared

## Anti-inflammatory preparations

### Corticosteroids

Topical corticosteroids are used to treat inflammation and eczema in otitis externa.

**Cautions**   Prolonged use of topical corticosteroid ear preparations should be avoided.

**Contra-indications**   Corticosteroid ear preparations should be avoided in the presence of an untreated ear infection. If infection is present, the corticosteroid should be used in combination with a suitable anti-infective (see notes above).

**Side-effects**   Local sensitivity reactions may occur.

### ◢ BETAMETHASONE SODIUM PHOSPHATE

**Cautions**   see notes above
**Contra-indications**   see notes above
**Side-effects**   see notes above

**Licensed use**   licensed for use in children (age range not specified by manufacturers)
**Indications and dose**

> Eczematous inflammation in otitis externa (see notes above); for dose, see under preparations

> Eye section 11.4.1

> Nose section 12.2.1 and section 12.2.3

**Betnesol**® (UCB Pharma) [PoM]
Drops (for ear, eye, or nose), betamethasone sodium phosphate 0.1%. Net price 10 mL = £2.23
Excipients include benzalkonium chloride, disodium edetate
**Dose**
> *ear*, instil 2–3 drops every 2–3 hours; reduce frequency when relief obtained

**Vistamethasone**® (Martindale) [PoM]
Drops (for ear, eye, or nose), betamethasone sodium phosphate 0.1%. Net price 5 mL = £1.02; 10 mL = £1.16
Excipients include benzalkonium chloride, disodium edetate
**Dose**
> *ear*, instil 2–3 drops every 3–4 hours; reduce frequency when relief obtained

◢With antibacterial
**Betnesol-N**® (UCB Pharma) [PoM]
Drops (for ear, eye, or nose), betamethasone sodium phosphate 0.1%, neomycin sulfate 0.5%. Net price 10 mL = £2.30
Excipients include benzalkonium chloride, disodium edetate
**Dose**
> *ear*, instil 2–3 drops 3–4 times daily

### ◢ DEXAMETHASONE

**Cautions**   see notes above
**Contra-indications**   see notes above
**Side-effects**   see notes above
**Licensed use**   *Sofradex*® licensed for use in children (age range not specified by manufacturers)
**Indications and dose**

> Eczematous inflammation in otitis externa (see notes above); for dose, see under preparations

◢With antibacterial
**Otomize**® (Forest) [PoM]
Ear spray, dexamethasone 0.1%, neomycin sulfate 3250 units/mL, glacial acetic acid 2%. Net price 5-mL pump-action aerosol unit = £3.71
Excipients include hydroxybenzoates (parabens)
**Dose**
> **Child 2–18 years** *ear*, apply 1 metered spray 3 times daily

**Sofradex**® (Sanofi-Aventis) [PoM] ◢
Drops (for ear or eye), dexamethasone (as sodium metasulfobenzoate) 0.05%, framycetin sulfate 0.5%, gramicidin 0.005%. Net price 10 mL = £6.25
Excipients include polysorbate 80
**Dose**
> *ear*, instil 2–3 drops 3–4 times daily; *eye*, section 11.4.1

## FLUMETASONE PIVALATE
(Flumethasone Pivalate)

**Cautions** see notes above
**Contra-indications** see notes above
**Side-effects** see notes above

**Indications and dose**

> Eczematous inflammation in otitis externa (see notes above); for dose, see under preparation

◢**With antibacterial**

**Locorten-Vioform®** (Amdipharm) [PoM]
Ear drops, flumetasone pivalate 0.02%, clioquinol 1%. Net price 7.5 mL = £1.76
**Contra-indications** iodine sensitivity
Dose

> **Child 2–18 years** instil 2–3 drops into the ear twice daily for 7–10 days

> **Note** Clioquinol stains skin and clothing

## HYDROCORTISONE

**Cautions** see notes above
**Contra-indications** see notes above
**Side-effects** see notes above
**Licensed use** *Otosporin®* not licensed for use in children under 3 years; *other preparations* licensed for use in children (age range not specified by manufacturers)

**Indications and dose**

> Eczematous inflammation in otitis externa (see notes above); for dose, see under preparations

◢**With antibacterial**

**Gentisone® HC** (Amdipharm) [PoM]
Ear drops, hydrocortisone acetate 1%, gentamicin 0.3% (as sulfate). Net price 10 mL = £3.92
**Excipients** include benzalkonium chloride, disodium edetate
Dose

> *ear,* instil 2–4 drops 3–4 times daily and at night

**Otosporin®** (GSK) [PoM] ◢
Ear drops, hydrocortisone 1%, neomycin sulfate 3400 units, polymyxin B sulfate 10 000 units/mL. Net price 5 mL = £2.00; 10 mL = £4.00
**Excipients** include cetostearyl alcohol, hydroxybenzoates (parabens), polysorbate 20
Dose

> **Child 3–18 years** instil 3 drops into the ear 3–4 times daily

## PREDNISOLONE SODIUM PHOSPHATE

**Cautions** see notes above
**Contra-indications** see notes above
**Side-effects** see notes above
**Licensed use** licensed for use in children (age range not specified by manufacturers)

**Indications and dose**

> Eczematous inflammation in otitis externa (see notes above); for dose, see under preparations

Eye section 11.4.1

**Predsol®** (UCB Pharma) [PoM]
Drops (for ear or eye), prednisolone sodium phosphate 0.5%. Net price 10 mL = £1.92
**Excipients** include benzalkonium chloride, disodium edetate
Dose

> *ear,* instil 2–3 drops every 2–3 hours; reduce frequency when relief obtained

## Anti-infective preparations

## CHLORAMPHENICOL ◢

**Cautions** avoid prolonged use (see notes above)
**Side-effects** high incidence of sensitivity reactions to vehicle
**Licensed use** licensed for use in children (age range not specified by manufacturers)

**Indications and dose**

> Bacterial infection in otitis externa (but see notes above); for dose, see under preparation

**Chloramphenicol** (Non-proprietary) [PoM] ◢
Ear drops, chloramphenicol in propylene glycol, net price 5%, 10 mL = £6.22; 10%, 10 mL = £5.62
**Excipients** include propylene glycol
Dose

> *ear,* instil 2–3 drops 2–3 times daily

## CLOTRIMAZOLE

**Side-effects** occasional local irritation or sensitivity
**Licensed use** licensed for use in children (age range not specified by manufacturer)

**Indications and dose**

> Fungal infection in otitis externa (see notes above); for dose, see under preparation

**Canesten®** (Bayer Consumer Care)
Solution, clotrimazole 1% in polyethylene glycol 400 (macrogol 400). Net price 20 mL = £2.43
Dose

> *ear,* apply 2–3 times daily continuing for at least 14 days after disappearance of infection

## FRAMYCETIN SULFATE

**Cautions** avoid prolonged use (see notes above)
**Contra-indications** perforated tympanic membrane (see p. 537)
**Side-effects** local sensitivity
**Indications and dose**

> Bacterial infection in otitis externa (see notes above)

Eye section 11.3.1

◢**With corticosteroid**
**Sofradex®** see Dexamethasone, p. 538

## GENTAMICIN

**Cautions** avoid prolonged use (see notes above)
**Contra-indications** perforated tympanic membrane (but see p. 537 and section 12.1.2)
**Side-effects** local sensitivity
**Licensed use** licensed for use in children (age range not specified by manufacturer)

**12 Ear, nose, and oropharynx**

**Indications and dose**

> Bacterial infection in otitis externa (see notes above); for dose, see under preparations

**Genticin®** (Amdipharm) PoM
> Drops (for ear or eye), gentamicin 0.3% (as sulfate). Net price 10 mL = £2.13
> Excipients include benzalkonium chloride
> **Dose**
>> *ear*, instil 2–3 drops 3–4 times daily and at night; *eye*, section 11.3.1

◢**With corticosteroid**

**Gentisone® HC** see Hydrocortisone, p. 539

## ▌ NEOMYCIN SULFATE

**Cautions** avoid prolonged use (see notes above)
**Contra-indications** perforated tympanic membrane (see p. 537)
**Side-effects** local sensitivity
**Indications and dose**

> Bacterial infection in otitis externa (see notes above)

◢**With corticosteroid**

**Betnesol-N®** PoM see Betamethasone, p. 538

**Otomize®** see Dexamethasone, p. 538

**Otosporin®** see Hydrocortisone, p. 539

## 12.1.2 Otitis media

**Acute otitis media**   Acute otitis media is the commonest cause of severe aural pain in young children and may occur with even minor upper respiratory tract infections. Children diagnosed with acute otitis media should not be prescribed antibacterials routinely as many infections, especially those accompanying coryza, are caused by viruses. Most uncomplicated cases resolve without antibacterial treatment and a **simple analgesic**, such as paracetamol, may be sufficient. In children without systemic features, a **systemic antibacterial** (Table 1, section 5.1) may be started after 72 hours if there is no improvement, or earlier if there is deterioration, if the child is systemically unwell, if the child is at high risk of serious complications (e.g. in immunosuppression, cystic fibrosis), if mastoiditis is present, or in children under 2 years of age with bilateral otitis media. Perforation of the tympanic membrane in children with *acute otitis media* usually heals spontaneously without treatment; if there is no improvement, e.g. pain or discharge persists, a systemic antibacterial (Table 1, section 5.1) can be given. Topical antibacterial treatment of acute otitis media is ineffective and there is no place for ear drops containing a local anaesthetic.

**Otitis media with effusion**   Otitis media with effusion ('glue ear') occurs in about 10% of children and in 90% of children with cleft palates. Antimicrobials, corticosteroids, decongestants, and antihistamines have little place in the routine management of otitis media with effusion. If 'glue ear' persists for more than a month or two, the child should be referred for assessment and follow up because of the risk of long-term hearing impairment which can delay language development.

Untreated or resistant glue ear may be responsible for some types of *chronic otitis media*.

**Chronic otitis media**   Opportunistic organisms are often present in the debris, keratin, and necrotic bone of the middle ear and mastoid in children with chronic otitis media. The mainstay of treatment is thorough cleansing with aural microsuction, which may completely resolve long-standing infection. Cleansing may be followed by topical treatment as for otitis externa (section 12.1.1); this is particularly beneficial for discharging ears or infections of the mastoid cavity. Acute exacerbations of chronic infection may require treatment with an oral antibacterial (Table 1, section 5.1); a swab should be taken to identify infecting organisms and antibacterial sensitivity. Parenteral antibacterial treatment is required if *Pseudomonas aeruginosa* or *Proteus spp.* are present.

Manufacturers contra-indicate topical treatment with ototoxic antibacterials in the presence of a perforation (section 12.1.1). However, many specialists use ear drops containing **aminoglycosides** (e.g. neomycin) or **polymyxins** if the otitis media has failed to settle with systemic antibacterials; it is considered that the pus in the middle ear associated with otitis media carries a higher risk of ototoxicity than the drops themselves. Ciprofloxacin or ofloxacin ear drops [both unlicensed; available from 'special-order' manufacturers or specialist importing companies, see p. 823] or eye drops used in the ear [unlicensed indication] are an effective alternative to aminoglycoside ear drops for chronic otitis media in patients with perforation of the tympanic membrane.

## 12.1.3 Removal of ear wax

Ear wax (cerumen) is a normal bodily secretion which provides a protective film on the meatal skin and need only be removed if it causes hearing loss or interferes with a proper view of the ear drum.

Ear wax causing discomfort or impaired hearing may be softened with simple remedies such as **olive oil** ear drops or **almond oil** ear drops; **sodium bicarbonate** ear drops are also effective, but may cause dryness of the ear canal. If the wax is hard and impacted, the drops can be used twice daily for several days and this may reduce the need for mechanical removal of the wax. The child should lie with the affected ear uppermost for 5 to 10 minutes after a generous amount of the softening remedy has been introduced into the ear. Proprietary preparations containing organic solvents can irritate the meatal skin, and in most cases the simple remedies indicated above are just as effective and less likely to cause irritation. Docusate sodium or urea hydrogen peroxide are ingredients in a number of proprietary preparations for softening ear wax.

If necessary, wax may be removed by irrigation with water (warmed to body temperature). Ear irrigation is generally best avoided in young children, in children unable to co-operate with the procedure, in children who have had otitis media in the last 6 weeks, in otitis externa, in children with cleft palate, a history of ear drum perforation, or previous ear surgery. A child who has hearing in one ear only should not have that ear irrigated because even a very slight risk of damage is unacceptable in this situation.

For administration of ear drops, see p. 538.

**Almond Oil** (Non-proprietary)
Ear drops, almond oil in a suitable container
Allow to warm to room temperature before use

**Olive Oil** (Non-proprietary)
Ear drops, olive oil in a suitable container
Allow to warm to room temperature before use

**Sodium Bicarbonate** (Non-proprietary)
Ear drops, sodium bicarbonate 5%, net price 10 mL
= £1.25

**Cerumol**® (Thornton & Ross) ◢
Ear drops, chlorobutanol 5%, arachis (peanut) oil
57.3%. Net price 11 mL = £1.76

**Exterol**® (Dermal) ◢
Ear drops, urea–hydrogen peroxide complex 5% in
glycerol. Net price 8 mL = £1.75

**Molcer**® (Wallace Mfg) ◢
Ear drops, docusate sodium 5%. Net price 15 mL =
£5.60
Excipients include propylene glycol

**Otex**® (DDD) ◢
Ear drops, urea–hydrogen peroxide 5%. Net price
8 mL = £2.64

**Waxsol**® (Meda) ◢
Ear drops, docusate sodium 0.5%. Net price 10 mL
= £1.21

## 12.2 Drugs acting on the nose

| | |
|---|---|
| 12.2.1 | Drugs used in nasal allergy |
| 12.2.2 | Topical nasal decongestants |
| 12.2.3 | Nasal preparations for infection |

Rhinitis is often self-limiting but bacterial sinusitis may require treatment with antibacterials (Table 1, section 5.1). Many nasal preparations contain sympathomimetic drugs (section 12.2.2) which can give rise to rebound congestion (*rhinitis medicamentosa*) and may damage the nasal cilia. **Sodium chloride 0.9%** solution may be used as a douche or 'sniff' following endonasal surgery.

**Administration**   To administer nasal drops, lay the child face-upward with the neck extended, instil the drops, then sit the child up and tilt the head forward.

**Nasal polyps**   Short-term use of corticosteroid nasal drops helps to shrink nasal polyps; to be effective, the drops must be administered with the child in the 'head down' position. A short course of a systemic corticosteroid (section 6.3.2) may be required initially to shrink large polyps. A corticosteroid nasal spray can be used to maintain the reduction in swelling and also for the initial treatment of small polyps.

## 12.2.1 Drugs used in nasal allergy

Mild allergic rhinitis is controlled by **antihistamines** (see also section 3.4.1) or topical **nasal corticosteroids**; systemic nasal decongestants (section 3.10) are not recommended for use in children. Topical nasal decongestants can be used for a short period to relieve congestion and allow penetration of a topical nasal corticosteroid.

More persistent symptoms can be relieved by topical nasal **corticosteroids**; **sodium cromoglicate** is an alternative, but may be less effective. The topical antihistamine, **azelastine**, is useful for controlling breakthrough symptoms in allergic rhinitis. Azelastine is less effective than nasal corticosteroids, but probably more effective than sodium cromoglicate. In seasonal allergic rhinitis (e.g. hay fever), treatment should begin 2 to 3 weeks before the season commences and may have to be continued for several months; continuous long-term treatment may be required in perennial rhinitis.

**Montelukast** (section 3.3.2) is less effective than topical nasal corticosteroids; montelukast can be used in children with seasonal allergic rhinitis (unresponsive to other treatments) and concomitant asthma.

Children with disabling symptoms of seasonal rhinitis (e.g. students taking important examinations), may be treated with oral **corticosteroids** (section 6.3.2) for short periods. Oral corticosteroids may also be used at the beginning of a course of treatment with a corticosteroid spray to relieve severe mucosal oedema and allow the spray to penetrate the nasal mucosa.

Sometimes allergic rhinitis is accompanied by vasomotor rhinitis. In this situation, the addition of topical nasal **ipratropium bromide** (section 12.2.2) can reduce watery rhinorrhoea.

**Pregnancy**   If a pregnant woman cannot tolerate the symptoms of allergic rhinitis, treatment with nasal beclometasone, budesonide, fluticasone propionate, or sodium cromoglicate may be considered.

## Antihistamines

### ▮ AZELASTINE HYDROCHLORIDE

**Side-effects**   irritation of nasal mucosa; bitter taste (if applied incorrectly)
**Indications and dose**
**Treatment of allergic rhinitis** for dose, see under preparation

**Rhinolast**® (Meda) [PoM]
Nasal spray, azelastine hydrochloride 140 micrograms (0.14 mL)/metered spray. Net price 22 mL (157-spray unit with metered pump) = £10.45
Excipients include sodium edetate
Dose

> **Child 5–18 years** apply 140 micrograms (1 spray) into each nostril twice daily

**Note**  Preparations of azelastine hydrochloride can be sold to the public for nasal administration in aqueous form (other than by aerosol) for the treatment of seasonal allergic rhinitis or perennial allergic rhinitis in children over 5 years, subject to max. single dose of 140 micrograms per nostril, max. daily dose of 280 micrograms per nostril, and a pack size limit of 36 doses

## Corticosteroids

Nasal preparations containing corticosteroids have a useful role in the prophylaxis and treatment of allergic rhinitis (see notes above). They are also used for the symptomatic treatment of adenoidal hypertrophy.

**Cautions**   Corticosteroid nasal preparations should be avoided in the presence of untreated nasal infections, and also after nasal surgery (until healing has occurred); they should also be avoided in pulmonary tuberculosis. Systemic absorption may follow nasal administration particularly if high doses are used or if treatment is prolonged; for cautions and side-effects of systemic

**12**

**Ear, nose, and oropharynx**

corticosteroids, see section 6.3.2. The risk of systemic effects may be greater with nasal drops than with nasal sprays; drops are administered incorrectly more often than sprays. The height of children receiving prolonged treatment with nasal corticosteroids should be monitored; if growth is slowed, referral to a paediatrician should be considered.

**Side-effects** Local side-effects include dryness, irritation of nose and throat, and epistaxis. Nasal ulceration has been reported, and occurs commonly with nasal preparations containing fluticasone furoate or mometasone furoate. Nasal septal perforation (usually following nasal surgery) occurs very rarely. Raised intra-ocular pressure or glaucoma may occur rarely. Headache, smell and taste disturbances may also occur. Hyperactivity, sleep disturbances, anxiety, depression, and aggression have been reported. Hypersensitivity reactions, including bronchospasm, have also been reported.

### ▇ BECLOMETASONE DIPROPIONATE
(Beclomethasone Dipropionate)

**Cautions** see notes above

**Side-effects** see notes above

**Indications and dose**

> **Prophylaxis and treatment of allergic and vasomotor rhinitis**
>
> > **Child 6–18 years** apply 100 micrograms (2 sprays) into each nostril twice daily; max. total 400 micrograms (8 sprays) daily; when symptoms controlled, dose reduced to 50 micrograms (1 spray) into each nostril twice daily

**Beclometasone** (Non-proprietary) [PoM]
Nasal spray, beclometasone dipropionate 50 micrograms/metered spray. Net price 200-spray unit = £2.52
**Brands include** *Nasobec Aqueous®*

**Beconase®** (A&H) [PoM]
Nasal spray (aqueous suspension), beclometasone dipropionate 50 micrograms/metered spray. Net price 200-spray unit with applicator = £2.19
**Excipients** include benzalkonium chloride, polysorbate 80

### ▇ BETAMETHASONE SODIUM PHOSPHATE

**Cautions** see notes above

**Side-effects** see notes above

**Licensed use** licensed for use in children (age range not specified by manufacturer)

**Indications and dose**

> **Non-infected inflammatory conditions of nose** for dose, see under preparations

> **Eye** section 11.4.1

> **Ear** section 12.1.1

**Betnesol®** (UCB Pharma) [PoM]
Drops (for ear, eye, or nose), betamethasone sodium phosphate 0.1%, net price 10 mL = £2.23
**Excipients** include benzalkonium chloride, disodium edetate
**Dose**

> *nose*, instil 2–3 drops into each nostril 2–3 times daily

**Vistamethasone®** (Martindale) [PoM]
Drops (for ear, eye, or nose), betamethasone sodium phosphate 0.1%. Net price 5 mL = £1.02, 10 mL = £1.16
**Excipients** include benzalkonium chloride, disodium edetate
**Dose**

> *nose*, instil 2–3 drops into each nostril twice daily

### ▇ BUDESONIDE

**Cautions** see notes above; **interactions:** Appendix 1 (corticosteroids)

**Side-effects** see notes above

**Indications and dose**

> See under preparations

**Budesonide** (Non-proprietary) [PoM]
Nasal spray, budesonide 100 micrograms/metered spray, net price 100-spray unit = £5.90
**Dose**

> **Prophylaxis and treatment of allergic and vasomotor rhinitis**
>
> > **Child 12–18 years** apply 200 micrograms (2 sprays) into each nostril once daily in the morning *or* 100 micrograms (1 spray) into each nostril twice daily; when control achieved reduce to 100 micrograms (1 spray) into each nostril once daily

> **Nasal polyps**
>
> > **Child 12–18 years** apply 100 micrograms (1 spray) into each nostril twice daily for up to 3 months

**Rhinocort Aqua®** (AstraZeneca) [PoM]
Nasal spray, budesonide 64 micrograms/metered spray. Net price 120-spray unit = £2.49
**Excipients** include disodium edetate, polysorbate 80, potassium sorbate
**Dose**

> **Rhinitis**
>
> > **Child 12–18 years** 128 micrograms (2 sprays) into each nostril once daily in the morning *or* 64 micrograms (1 spray) into each nostril twice daily; when control achieved reduce to 64 micrograms (1 spray) into each nostril once daily; max. duration of treatment 3 months

> **Nasal polyps**
>
> > **Child 12–18 years** 64 micrograms (1 spray) into each nostril twice daily for up to 3 months

### ▇ FLUNISOLIDE

**Cautions** see notes above

**Side-effects** see notes above

**Indications and dose**

> **Prophylaxis and treatment of allergic rhinitis**
>
> > **Child 5–14 years** initially 25 micrograms (1 spray) into each nostril up to 3 times daily then reduced for maintenance
> >
> > **Child 14–18 years** 50 micrograms (2 sprays) into each nostril twice daily, increased if necessary to max. 3 times daily then reduced for maintenance

**Syntaris®** (IVAX) [PoM]
Aqueous nasal spray, flunisolide 25 micrograms/metered spray. Net price 240-spray unit with pump and applicator = £5.05
**Excipients** include benzalkonium chloride, butylated hydroxytoluene, disodium edetate, polysorbate 20, propylene glycol

**12 Ear, nose, and oropharynx**

## ■ FLUTICASONE PROPIONATE

**Cautions**　see notes above; **interactions:** Appendix 1 (corticosteroids)

**Side-effects**　see notes above

**Indications and dose**

> **Prophylaxis and treatment of allergic rhinitis**
>
> **Child 4–12 years** 50 micrograms (1 spray) into each nostril once daily, preferably in the morning, increased to max. twice daily if required
>
> **Child 12–18 years** 100 micrograms (2 sprays) into each nostril once daily, preferably in the morning, increased to max. twice daily if required; when control achieved reduce to 50 micrograms (1 spray) into each nostril once daily

**Nasal polyps** see *Flixonase Nasule*® below

**Flixonase**® (A&H) [PoM]
Aqueous nasal spray, fluticasone propionate 50 micrograms/metered spray. Net price 150-spray unit with applicator = £11.01
Excipients　include benzalkonium chloride, polysorbate 80

**Flixonase Nasule**® (A&H) [PoM]
Nasal drops, fluticasone propionate 400 micrograms/unit dose, net price 28 × 0.4-mL units = £12.99
Excipients　include polysorbate 20
**Dose**

> **Nasal polyps**
>
> **Child 16–18 years** instil 200 micrograms (approx. 6 drops) into each nostril once or twice daily; consider alternative treatment if no improvement after 4–6 weeks

**Nasofan**® (IVAX) [PoM]
Aqueous nasal spray, fluticasone propionate 50 micrograms/metered spray. Net price 150–spray unit = £8.41
Excipients　include benzalkonium chloride, polysorbate 80

**◢With azelastine hydrochloride**

**Dymista**® (Meda) [PoM]
Nasal spray, fluticasone propionate 50 micrograms, azelastine hydrochloride 137 micrograms/metered spray, net price 120-spray unit = £18.91
Excipients　include benzalkonium chloride, polysorbate 80
**Dose**

> **Moderate to severe seasonal and perennial allergic rhinitis, if monotherapy with antihistamine or corticosteroid is inadequate**
>
> **Child 12–18 years** 1 spray into each nostril twice daily

**◢Fluticasone furoate**

**Avamys**® (GSK) [PoM]
Nasal spray, fluticasone furoate 27.5 micrograms/metered spray, net price 120-spray unit = £6.44
Excipients　include benzalkonium chloride, disodium edetate, polysorbate 80
**Dose**

> **Prophylaxis and treatment of allergic rhinitis**
>
> **Child 6–12 years** 27.5 micrograms (1 spray) into each nostril once daily, increased if necessary to 55 micrograms (2 sprays) into each nostril once daily; when control achieved reduce to 27.5 micrograms (1 spray) into each nostril once daily
>
> **Child 12–18 years** 55 micrograms (2 sprays) into each nostril once daily; when control achieved reduce to minimum effective dose, 27.5 micrograms (1 spray) into each nostril once daily may be sufficient

## ■ MOMETASONE FUROATE

**Cautions**　see notes above
**Side-effects**　see notes above
**Indications and dose**

> See under preparation

**Nasonex**® (Schering-Plough) [PoM]
Nasal spray, mometasone furoate 50 micrograms/metered spray. Net price 140-spray unit = £7.68
Excipients　include benzalkonium chloride, polysorbate 80
**Dose**

> **Prophylaxis and treatment of allergic rhinitis**
>
> **Child 6–12 years** 50 micrograms (1 spray) into each nostril once daily
>
> **Child 12–18 years** 100 micrograms (2 sprays) into each nostril once daily, increased if necessary to max. 200 micrograms (4 sprays) into each nostril once daily; when control achieved reduce to 50 micrograms (1 spray) into each nostril once daily

## ■ TRIAMCINOLONE ACETONIDE

**Cautions**　see notes above
**Side-effects**　see notes above
**Licensed use**　not licensed for use in children under 6 years
**Indications and dose**

> **Treatment of allergic rhinitis**
>
> **Child 2–6 years** 55 micrograms (1 spray) into each nostril once daily; max. duration of treatment 3 months
>
> **Child 6–12 years** 55 micrograms (1 spray) into each nostril once daily, increased if necessary to 110 micrograms (2 sprays) into each nostril once daily; when control achieved, reduce to 55 micrograms (1 spray) into each nostril once daily; max. duration of treatment 3 months
>
> **Child 12–18 years** 110 micrograms (2 sprays) into each nostril once daily; when control achieved, reduce to 55 micrograms (1 spray) into each nostril once daily

**Nasacort**® (Sanofi-Aventis) [PoM]
Aqueous nasal spray, triamcinolone acetonide 55 micrograms/metered spray. Net price 120-spray unit = £7.39
Excipients　include benzalkonium chloride, disodium edetate, polysorbate 80

# Cromoglicate

## ■ SODIUM CROMOGLICATE
(Sodium Cromoglycate)

**Side-effects**　local irritation; *rarely* transient bronchospasm
**Licensed use**　licensed for use in children (age range not specified by manufacturers)
**Indications and dose**

> **Prophylaxis of allergic rhinitis** for dose, see under preparations

**12**

**Ear, nose, and oropharynx**

**Rynacrom®** (Sanofi-Aventis)

4% aqueous nasal spray, sodium cromoglicate 4% (5.2 mg/spray). Net price 22 mL (150-spray unit with pump) = £17.07

Excipients   include benzalkonium chloride, disodium edetate

Dose

*nose*, 1 spray into each nostril 2–4 times daily

**Vividrin®** (Bausch & Lomb)

Nasal spray, sodium cromoglicate 2%. Net price 15 mL (approx. 110-spray unit) = £11.60

Excipients   include benzalkonium chloride, edetic acid, polysorbate 80

Dose

*nose*, 1 spray into each nostril 4–6 times daily

## 12.2.2   Topical nasal decongestants

**Sodium chloride** 0.9% given as nasal drops or spray may relieve nasal congestion by helping to liquefy mucous secretions in children with rhinitis. In infants, 1–2 drops of sodium chloride 0.9% solution in each nostril before feeds will help relieve congestion and allow more effective suckling.

Inhalation of **warm moist air** is useful in the treatment of symptoms of acute nasal congestion in infants and children, but the use of boiling water for steam inhalation is dangerous for children and should **not** be recommended. Volatile substances (section 3.8) such as menthol and eucalyptus may encourage inhalation of warm moist air.

Topical nasal decongestants containing sympathomimetics can cause rebound congestion (*rhinitis medicamentosa*) following prolonged use (more than 7 days), and are therefore of limited value in the treatment of nasal congestion.

**Ephedrine nasal drops** is the least likely of the sympathomimetic nasal decongestants to cause rebound congestion and can provide relief for several hours. The more potent sympathomimetic drugs **oxymetazoline** and **xylometazoline** are more likely to cause a rebound effect.

The CHM/MHRA has stated that non-prescription cough and cold medicines containing ephedrine, oxymetazoline, or xylometazoline can be considered for up to 5 days' treatment in children aged 6–12 years after basic principles of best care have been tried; these medicines should not be used in children under 6 years of age (section 3.9.1).

Non-allergic watery rhinorrhoea often responds well to treatment with the antimuscarinic **ipratropium bromide**.

Recurrent, persistent bleeding may respond to the use of a sympathomimetic nasal spray; if infection is present, chlorhexidine and neomycin (*Naseptin®*) cream (section 12.2.3) may be effective.

Systemic nasal decongestants—see section 3.10.

**Sinusitis and oral pain**   Sinusitis affecting the maxillary antrum can cause pain in the upper jaw. Where this is associated with blockage of the opening from the sinus into the nasal cavity, it may be helpful to relieve the congestion with inhalation of warm moist air (section 3.8) or with **ephedrine nasal drops** (see above). For antibacterial treatment of sinusitis, see Table 1, section 5.1.

## Sympathomimetics

### ▌ EPHEDRINE HYDROCHLORIDE

**Cautions**   see notes above; also avoid excessive or prolonged use; hyperthyroidism; diabetes mellitus; cardiovascular disease (including hypertension); **interactions:** Appendix 1 (sympathomimetics)

**Pregnancy**   avoid

**Breast-feeding**   avoid

**Side-effects**   local irritation, nausea, headache; after excessive use tolerance with diminished effect, rebound congestion; cardiovascular effects also reported

**Licensed use**   not licensed for use in children under 12 years

**Indications and dose**

Nasal congestion (see notes above)

Child 12–18 years instil 1–2 drops (0.5% strength) into each nostril up to 4 times daily when required; max. duration 7 days

[1]**Ephedrine** (Non-proprietary)

Nasal drops, ephedrine hydrochloride 0.5%, net price 10 mL = £1.39; 1%, 10 mL = £1.63

Note   The BP directs that if no strength is specified 0.5% drops should be supplied

Dental prescribing on NHS   Ephedrine nasal drops may be prescribed

### ▌ XYLOMETAZOLINE HYDROCHLORIDE

**Cautions**   see under Ephedrine Hydrochloride and notes above; also angle-closure glaucoma; avoid excessive or prolonged use

**Pregnancy**   avoid

**Breast-feeding**   manufacturer advises caution—no information available

**Side-effects**   see under Ephedrine Hydrochloride and notes above; also reported transient visual disturbances; in small children, also restlessness, sleep disturbances, and hallucinations (discontinue treatment)

**Indications and dose**

Nasal congestion for dose, see under preparations

**Xylometazoline** (Non-proprietary)

Nasal drops, xylometazoline hydrochloride 0.1%, net price 10 mL = £1.91

Dose

Child 12–18 years instil 2–3 drops into each nostril 2–3 times daily when required; max. duration 7 days

Brands include   *Otradrops®*, *Otrivine®*[NHS]

Paediatric nasal drops, xylometazoline hydrochloride 0.05%, net price 10 mL = £1.59

Dose

Child 6–12 years instil 1–2 drops into each nostril 1–2 times daily when required; max. duration 5 days

Brands include   *Otradrops®*, *Otrivine®*[NHS]

---

1. Can be sold to the public provided no more than 180 mg of ephedrine base (or salts) are supplied at one time, and pseudoephedrine salts are not supplied at the same time; for conditions that apply to supplies made at the request of a patient, see *Medicines, Ethics and Practice*, London, Pharmaceutical Press (always consult latest edition)

Nasal spray, xylometazoline hydrochloride 0.1%, net price 10 mL = £1.91

**Dose**

> **Child 12–18 years** apply 1 spray into each nostril 1–3 times daily when required; max. duration 7 days

**Brands include** *Otrivine*® , *Otrivine*® Allergy Relief

## Antimuscarinic

### ■ IPRATROPIUM BROMIDE

**Cautions** see section 3.1.2; avoid spraying near eyes

**Side-effects** epistaxis, nasal dryness, and irritation; less frequently nausea, headache, and pharyngitis; *very rarely* antimuscarinic effects such as gastro-intestinal motility disturbances, palpitations, and urinary retention

**Indications and dose**

> **Rhinorrhoea associated with allergic and non-allergic rhinitis**
>
> > **Child 12–18 years** apply 42 micrograms (2 sprays) into each nostril 2–3 times daily

> **Asthma and reversible airways obstruction** section 3.1.2

**Rinatec**® (Boehringer Ingelheim) [PoM]

Nasal spray, ipratropium bromide 21 micrograms/metered spray. Net price 180-dose unit = £3.99

**Excipients** include benzalkonium chloride, disodium edetate

### 12.2.3 Nasal preparations for infection

There is **no** evidence that topical anti-infective nasal preparations have any therapeutic value in rhinitis or sinusitis; for elimination of nasal staphylococci, see below. Acute complications such as periorbital cellulitis require hospital treatment. For systemic treatment of sinusitis, see Table 1, section 5.1.

**Betnesol-N**® (UCB Pharma) [PoM]

Drops (for ear, eye, or nose), betamethasone sodium phosphate 0.1%, neomycin sulfate 0.5%. Net price 10 mL = £2.30

**Excipients** include benzalkonium chloride, disodium edetate

**Dose**

> *nose*, instil 2–3 drops into each nostril 2–3 times daily

**Note** *Betnesol-N*® licensed for use in children (age range not specified by manufacturer)

### Nasal staphylococci

Elimination of organisms such as staphylococci from the nasal vestibule can be achieved by the use of a cream containing **chlorhexidine** and **neomycin** (*Naseptin*®), but re-colonisation frequently occurs. Coagulase-positive staphylococci are present in the noses of 40% of the population. A nasal ointment containing **mupirocin** is also available; it should probably be held in reserve for resistant infections. In hospitals or in care establishments, mupirocin nasal ointment should be reserved for the *eradication* (in both patients and staff) of nasal carriage of meticillin-resistant *Staphylococcus aureus* (MRSA). The ointment should be applied 3 times daily for 5 days and a sample taken 2 days after treatment to

confirm eradication. The course may be repeated if the sample is positive (and the throat is not colonised). To avoid the development of resistance, the treatment course should not exceed 7 days and the course should not be repeated on more than one occasion. If the MRSA strain is mupirocin-resistant or does not respond after 2 courses, consider alternative products such as chlorhexidine and neomycin cream. For eradication of MRSA also consult local infection control policy. See section 13.10.1 for treatment of MRSA-infected open wounds. See section 5.1.1.2 for *treatment* of children with MRSA-positive throat swabs or systemic MRSA infection.

**Bactroban Nasal**® (GSK) [PoM]

Nasal ointment, mupirocin 2% (as calcium salt) in white soft paraffin basis. Net price 3 g = £5.80

**Dose**

> **For eradication of nasal carriage of staphylococci, including meticillin-resistant** *Staphylococcus aureus* **(MRSA)**
>
> Apply 2–3 times daily to the inner surface of each nostril (see notes above)

**Naseptin**® (Alliance) [PoM]

Cream, chlorhexidine hydrochloride 0.1%, neomycin sulfate 0.5%, net price 15 g = £1.90

**Excipients** include arachis (peanut) oil, cetostearyl alcohol

**Dose**

> **For eradication of nasal carriage of staphylococci**
>
> Apply to nostrils 4 times daily for 10 days

> **For preventing nasal carriage of staphylococci**
>
> Apply to nostrils twice daily

### 12.3 Drugs acting on the oropharynx

| | |
|---|---|
| 12.3.1 | Drugs for oral ulceration and inflammation |
| 12.3.2 | Oropharyngeal anti-infective drugs |
| 12.3.3 | Lozenges and sprays |
| 12.3.4 | Mouthwashes and gargles |
| 12.3.5 | Treatment of dry mouth |

### 12.3.1 Drugs for oral ulceration and inflammation

Ulceration of the oral mucosa may be caused by trauma (physical or chemical), recurrent aphthous ulcers, infections, carcinoma, dermatological disorders, nutritional deficiencies, gastro-intestinal disease, haematopoietic disorders, and drug therapy. It is important to establish the diagnosis in each case as the majority of these lesions require specific management in addition to local treatment. Local treatment aims to protect the ulcerated area, to relieve pain, to reduce inflammation, or to control secondary infection. Children with an unexplained mouth ulcer of more than 3 weeks' duration require urgent referral to hospital to exclude secondary causes such as leukaemia.

**Simple mouthwashes** A saline mouthwash (section 12.3.4) may relieve the pain of traumatic ulceration. The mouthwash is made up with warm water and used

**12 Ear, nose, and oropharynx**

at frequent intervals until the discomfort and swelling subsides.

**Antiseptic mouthwashes** Secondary bacterial infection may be a feature of any mucosal ulceration; it can increase discomfort and delay healing. Use of **chlorhexidine** mouthwash (section 12.3.4) is often beneficial and may accelerate healing of recurrent aphthous ulcers.

**Corticosteroids** Topical corticosteroid therapy may be used for some forms of oral ulceration; for aphthous ulcers it is most effective if applied in the 'prodromal' phase. Thrush or other types of candidiasis are recognised complications of corticosteroid treatment.

**Hydrocortisone oromucosal tablets** are useful in recurrent aphthous ulcers and erosive lichenoid lesions.

**Beclometasone dipropionate** inhaler (p. 146) 50–100 micrograms sprayed twice daily on the oral mucosa is used to manage oral ulceration [unlicensed indication]. Alternatively, **betamethasone** soluble tablets dissolved in water, can be used as a mouthwash to treat oral ulceration.

Systemic corticosteroid therapy (section 6.3.2) is reserved for severe conditions such as pemphigus vulgaris.

**Local analgesics** Local analgesics have a limited role in the management of oral ulceration. When applied topically their action is of a relatively short duration and analgesia cannot be maintained continuously throughout the day. When local anaesthetics are used in the mouth, care must be taken not to produce anaesthesia of the pharynx before meals as this might lead to choking.

**Benzydamine** and **Flurbiprofen** are non-steroidal anti-inflammatory drugs (NSAIDs). Benzydamine mouthwash or spray may be useful in reducing the discomfort associated with a variety of ulcerative conditions. It has also been found to be effective in reducing the discomfort of tonsillectomy and post-irradiation mucositis. Some children find the full-strength mouthwash causes some stinging and, for them, it should be diluted with an equal volume of water. Flurbiprofen lozenges are licensed for the relief of sore throat in adolescents.

**Choline salicylate** is a derivative of salicylic acid and has some analgesic action. The dental gel may provide relief for recurrent aphthous ulcers in children over 16 years of age.

**Periodontitis** Low-dose **doxycycline** (*Periostat*®) is licensed as an adjunct to scaling and root planing for the treatment of periodontitis in children over 12 years; a low dose of doxycycline reduces collagenase activity without inhibiting bacteria associated with periodontitis. For anti-infectives used in the treatment of destructive (refractory) forms of periodontal disease, see section 12.3.2 and Table 1, section 5.1. For mouthwashes used for oral hygiene and plaque inhibition, see section 12.3.4.

### ▌ BENZYDAMINE HYDROCHLORIDE

**Side-effects** occasional numbness or stinging; rarely hypersensitivity reactions

**Indications and dose**

**Painful inflammatory conditions of oropharynx**

- As a mouthwash (benzydamine hydrochloride 0.15%)

  **Child 13–18 years** rinse or gargle using 15 mL (dilute with an equal volume of water if stinging occurs) every 1½–3 hours as required, usually for not more than 7 days

- As an oromucosal spray (benzydamine hydrochloride 0.15%)

  **Child under 6 years** 1 spray per 4 kg body-weight (max. 4 sprays) onto affected area every 1½–3 hours

  **Child 6–12 years** 4 sprays onto affected area every 1½–3 hours

  **Child 12–18 years** 4–8 sprays onto affected area every 1½–3 hours

**Benzydamine hydrochloride** (Non-proprietary)
Mouthwash, benzydamine hydrochloride 0.15%, net price 300 mL = £6.50
Brands include *Oroeze*®
Oromucosal spray, benzydamine hydrochloride 0.15%, net price 30 mL = £4.24
Brands include *Oroeze*®
**Dental prescribing on NHS** Benzydamine Oromucosal Spray 0.15% may be prescribed

**Difflam**® (Meda)
Mouthwash (oral rinse), green, benzydamine hydrochloride 0.15%, net price 200 mL (*Difflam*® Sore Throat Rinse) = £2.50; 300 mL = £4.01
**Dental prescribing on NHS** May be prescribed as Benzydamine Mouthwash 0.15%

Oromucosal spray, benzydamine hydrochloride 0.15%, net price 30-mL unit = £3.17

### ▌ CORTICOSTEROIDS

**Contra-indications** untreated oral infection
**Side-effects** occasional exacerbation of local infection; thrush or other candidal infections
**Licensed use** *Hydrocortisone mucoadhesive buccal tablets* licensed for use in children (under 12 years—on medical advice only); *betamethasone soluble tablets* not licensed for use in oral ulceration

**Indications and dose**

**Oral and perioral lesions** for dose, see under preparations

**Betamethasone** (Non-proprietary) [PoM]
Soluble tablets, betamethasone 500 micrograms (as sodium phosphate), net price 100-tab pack = £8.20. Label: 10, 13, counselling, administration
**Dose**

**Oral ulceration**

**Child 12–18 years** 500 micrograms dissolved in 20 mL water and rinsed around the mouth 4 times daily; not to be swallowed

**Dental prescribing on NHS** Betamethasone Soluble Tablets 500 micrograms may be prescribed

**Hydrocortisone** (Non-proprietary)
Mucoadhesive buccal tablets (= oromucosal tablets), hydrocortisone 2.5 mg (as sodium succinate). Net price 20 = £2.03
**Dose**

1 lozenge 4 times daily, allowed to dissolve slowly in the mouth in contact with the ulcer

**Dental prescribing on NHS** May be prescribed as Hydrocortisone Oromucosal Tablets

**12 Ear, nose, and oropharynx**

## DOXYCYCLINE

**Cautions** section 5.1.3; monitor for superficial fungal infection, particularly if predisposition to oral candidiasis

**Contra-indications** section 5.1.3
**Hepatic impairment** section 5.1.3
**Renal impairment** section 5.1.3
**Pregnancy** section 5.1.3
**Breast-feeding** section 5.1.3
**Side-effects** section 5.1.3; fungal superinfection

**Indications and dose**

See under preparations

Oral herpes section 12.3.2

Other indications section 5.1.3

**Periostat®** (Alliance) [PoM]
Tablets, f/c, doxycycline (as hyclate) 20 mg, net price 56-tab pack = £16.50. Label: 6, 11, 27, counselling, posture

**Dose**

**Periodontitis (as an adjunct to gingival scaling and root planing)**

**Child 12–18 years** 20 mg twice daily for 3 months

**Counselling** Tablets should be swallowed whole with plenty of fluid, while sitting or standing
**Dental prescribing on NHS** May be prescribed as Doxycycline Tablets 20 mg

### ◢ Local application

For severe recurrent aphthous ulceration, a 100 mg doxycycline dispersible tablet can be stirred into a small amount of water then rinsed around the mouth for 2–3 minutes 4 times daily usually for 3 days; it should preferably not be swallowed [unlicensed indication].

**Note** Doxycycline stains teeth; avoid in children under 12 years of age

## FLURBIPROFEN

**Cautions** section 10.1.1
**Contra-indications** section 10.1.1
**Hepatic impairment** section 10.1.1
**Renal impairment** section 10.1.1
**Pregnancy** section 10.1.1
**Breast-feeding** section 10.1.1
**Side-effects** taste disturbance, mouth ulcers (move lozenge around mouth); see also section 10.1.1

**Indications and dose**

Relief of sore throat for dose, see under preparation

**Strefen®** (Reckitt Benckiser)
Lozenges, flurbiprofen 8.75 mg, net price 16 = £2.24

**Dose**

**Child 12–18 years** allow 1 lozenge to dissolve slowly in the mouth every 3–6 hours, max. 5 lozenges in 24 hours, for max. 3 days

## SALICYLATES

**Cautions** frequent application, especially in children, may give rise to salicylate poisoning
**Contra-indications** children under 16 years
**Reye's syndrome** The CHM has advised that topical oral pain relief products containing salicylate salts should not be used in children under 16 years, as a cautionary measure due to the theoretical risk of Reye's syndrome

**Side-effects** transient local burning sensation
**Indications and dose**

Mild oral and perioral lesions for dose, see under preparations

### ◢ Choline salicylate

**Choline Salicylate Dental Gel, BP**
Oral gel, choline salicylate 8.7% in a flavoured gel basis, net price 15 g = £1.89
**Brands include** *Bonjela®* (sugar-free)

**Dose**

**Child 16–18 years** apply ½-inch of gel with gentle massage not more often than every 3 hours

**Dental prescribing on NHS** Choline Salicylate Dental Gel may be prescribed

### ◢ Salicylic acid

**Pyralvex®** (Meda)
Oral paint, brown, rhubarb extract (anthraquinone glycosides 0.5%), salicylic acid 1%. Net price 10 mL with brush = £3.25
**Excipients** include ethanol

**Dose**

**Child 16–18 years** apply 3–4 times daily; max. duration 7 days

**Note** May cause temporary discolouration of teeth and oral mucosa

## 12.3.2 Oropharyngeal anti-infective drugs

Sore throat is usually a self-limiting condition often caused by viral infection which does not benefit from anti-infective treatment. Adequate analgesia may be all that is required. Systemic **antibacterials** (Table 1, section 5.1) should only be used in severe cases where there is concern for the child's overall clinical condition. Acute ulcerative gingivitis (Vincent's infection) requires treatment with oral **metronidazole** (section 5.1.11).

**Benzydamine** (section 12.3.1) may be beneficial in relieving pain and dysphagia in children, especially after tonsillectomy or the use of a nasogastric tube.

## Oropharyngeal viral infections

Children with varicella–zoster infection often develop painful lesions in the mouth and throat. **Benzydamine** (section 12.3.1) may be used to provide local analgesia. **Chlorhexidine** mouthwash or gel (section 12.3.4) will control plaque accumulation if toothbrushing is painful and will also help to control secondary infection in general.

In severe herpetic stomatitis systemic **aciclovir** or **valaciclovir** (section 5.3.2.1) may be used for oral lesions associated with herpes zoster. Aciclovir and valaciclovir are also used to prevent frequently recurring herpes simplex lesions of the mouth particularly when associated with the initiation of erythema multiforme. For the treatment of labial herpes simplex infections, see section 13.10.3.

Herpes infections of the mouth in children aged over 12 years may also respond to rinsing the mouth with **doxycycline** (section 12.3.1).

**12** Ear, nose, and oropharynx

# Oropharyngeal fungal infections

Fungal infections of the mouth are usually caused by *Candida* spp. (candidiasis or candidosis). Different types of oropharyngeal candidiasis are managed as follows:

**Thrush**    Acute    pseudomembranous    candidiasis (thrush), is usually an acute infection but it may persist for months in patients receiving inhaled corticosteroids, cytotoxics, or broad-spectrum antibacterials. Thrush also occurs in patients with serious systemic disease associated with reduced immunity such as leukaemia, other malignancies, and HIV infection. Any predisposing condition should be managed appropriately. When thrush is associated with corticosteroid inhalers, rinsing the mouth with water (or cleaning a child's teeth) immediately after using the inhaler may avoid the problem. Treatment with **nystatin** or **miconazole** may be needed. **Fluconazole** (section 5.2.1) is effective for unresponsive infections or if a topical antifungal drug cannot be used. Topical therapy may not be adequate in immunocompromised children and an oral triazole antifungal is preferred (section 5.2.1).

**Acute erythematous candidiasis**    Acute erythematous (atrophic) candidiasis is a relatively uncommon condition associated with corticosteroid and broad-spectrum antibacterial use and with HIV disease. It is usually treated with **fluconazole** (section 5.2.1).

**Angular cheilitis**    Angular cheilitis (angular stomatitis) is characterised by soreness, erythema and fissuring at the angles of the mouth. It may represent a nutritional deficiency or it may be related to orofacial granulomatosis or HIV infection. Both yeasts (*Candida* spp.) and bacteria (*Staphylococcus aureus* and beta-haemolytic streptococci) are commonly involved as interacting, infective factors. While the underlying cause is being identified and treated, it is often helpful to apply **miconazole** cream (p. 590) or **sodium fusidate** ointment (p. 589); if the angular cheilitis is unresponsive to treatment, **miconazole** and **hydrocortisone** cream or ointment (p. 561) can be used.

**Immunocompromised patients**    For advice on prevention of fungal infections in immunocompromised children see p. 303 .

For the role of antiseptic mouthwashes in the prevention of oral candidiasis in immunocompromised children, see section 12.3.4.

## Drugs used in oropharyngeal candidiasis

**Nystatin** is not absorbed from the gastro-intestinal tract and is applied locally (as a suspension) to the mouth for treating local fungal infections. **Miconazole** is used by local application (as an oral gel) in the mouth but it is also absorbed to the extent that potential interactions need to be considered. Miconazole also has some activity against Gram-positive bacteria including streptococci and staphylococci. In neonates, nystatin oral suspension or miconazole oral gel is used for the treatment of oropharyngeal candidiasis; to prevent re-infection it is important to ensure that the mother's breast nipples and the teats of feeding bottles are cleaned adequately.

**Fluconazole** (section 5.2.1) given by mouth is reliably absorbed; it is used for infections that do not respond to topical therapy or when topical therapy cannot be used. **Itraconazole** (section 5.2.1) can be used for fluconazole-resistant infections.

If candidal infection fails to respond after 1 to 2 weeks of treatment with antifungal drugs the child should be sent for investigation to eliminate the possibility of underlying disease. Persistent infection may also be caused by re-infection from the genito-urinary or gastro-intestinal tract.

## ▌ MICONAZOLE

**Cautions**    avoid in acute porphyria (section 9.8.2); **interactions:** Appendix 1 (antifungals, imidazole)

**Contra-indications**    impaired swallowing reflex in infants

**Hepatic impairment**    avoid

**Pregnancy**    manufacturer advises avoid if possible—toxicity at high doses in *animal* studies

**Breast-feeding**    manufacturer advises caution—no information available

**Side-effects**    nausea and vomiting, *very rarely* diarrhoea (usually on long-term treatment), hepatitis, rash, toxic epidermal necrolysis, and Stevens-Johnson syndrome

**Licensed use**    not licensed for use in children under 4 months of age or during first 5–6 months of life of an infant born pre-term

**Indications and dose**

**Prevention and treatment of oral and intestinal fungal infections**

- **By mouth**

**Neonate** (oral fungal infections only) 1 mL 2–4 times daily smeared around the inside of the mouth after feeds

**Child 1 month–2 years** 2.5 mL twice daily smeared around the inside of the mouth after food

**Child 2–6 years** 5 mL twice daily after food; retain near lesions before swallowing

**Child 6–12 years** 5 mL 4 times daily after food; retain near lesions before swallowing

**Child 12–18 years** 5–10 mL 4 times daily after food; retain near lesions before swallowing

**Note** Treatment should be continued for 48 hours after lesions have healed

**Localised lesions**

**Child 2–18 years** smear small amount on affected area with clean finger 4 times daily for 5–7 days (orthodontic appliances should be removed at night and brushed with gel); continue treatment for 48 hours after lesions have healed

**[1]Daktarin®** (Janssen) ▢PoM
Oral gel, sugar-free, orange-flavoured, miconazole 24 mg/mL (20 mg/g). Net price 15-g tube = £2.85, 80-g tube = £4.38. Label: 9, counselling, hold in mouth, after food
**Excipients** include ethanol
**Dental prescribing on NHS** May be prescribed as Miconazole Oromucosal Gel

## ▌ NYSTATIN

**Side-effects**    oral irritation and sensitisation, nausea reported

**Licensed use**    *suspension* not licensed for use in neonates for the treatment of candidiasis

---

1. 15-g tube can be sold to the public

**Indications and dose**

**Oral and perioral fungal infections**

**Neonate** 100 000 units 4 times daily after feeds

**Child 1 month–18 years** 100 000 units 4 times daily after food

**Note** Treatment is usually given for 7 days, and continued for 48 hours after lesions have healed.

**Skin infections** section 13.10.2

**Nystatin** (Non-proprietary) PoM
Oral suspension, nystatin 100 000 units/mL, net price 30 mL = £15.44. Label: 9, counselling, use of pipette, hold in mouth, after food
**Dental prescribing on NHS** Nystatin Oral Suspension may be prescribed

**Nystan**® (Squibb) PoM
Oral suspension, yellow, nystatin 100 000 units/mL. Net price 30 mL with pipette = £1.91. Label: 9, counselling, use of pipette, hold in mouth, after food

## 12.3.3 Lozenges and sprays

There is no convincing evidence that antiseptic lozenges and sprays have a beneficial action and they sometimes irritate and cause sore tongue and sore lips. Some preparations also contain local anaesthetics which relieve pain but may cause sensitisation.

## 12.3.4 Mouthwashes and gargles

Superficial infections of the mouth are often helped by warm mouthwashes which have a mechanical cleansing effect and cause some local hyperaemia. However, to be effective, they must be used frequently and vigorously. Mouthwashes may not be suitable for children under 7 years (risk of the solution being swallowed); the mouthwash or dental gel may be applied using a cotton bud.

A warm saline mouthwash is ideal for its cleansing effect and can be prepared either by dissolving half a teaspoonful of salt in a glassful of warm water or by diluting **compound sodium chloride mouthwash** with an equal volume of warm water. **Mouthwash solution-tablets** containing thymol are used to remove unpleasant tastes.

Mouthwashes containing an oxidising agent, such as **hydrogen peroxide**, may be useful in the treatment of acute ulcerative gingivitis (Vincent's infection). Hydrogen peroxide solution has also a mechanical cleansing effect arising from frothing when in contact with oral debris, but in concentrations greater than 1.5% may cause ulceration and tissue damage.

**Chlorhexidine** is an effective antiseptic which has the advantage of inhibiting plaque formation on the teeth. It does not, however, completely control plaque deposition and is not a substitute for effective toothbrushing. Moreover, chlorhexidine preparations do not penetrate significantly into stagnation areas and are therefore of little value in the control of dental caries or of periodontal disease once pocketing has developed. Chlorhexidine preparations are of little value in the control of acute necrotising ulcerative gingivitis. With prolonged use, chlorhexidine causes reversible brown staining of teeth and tongue. Chlorhexidine may be incompatible with some ingredients in toothpaste, causing an unplea-

sant taste in the mouth; rinse the mouth thoroughly with water between using toothpaste and chlorhexidine-containing products.

Chlorhexidine can be used as a mouthwash, spray or gel for secondary infection in mucosal ulceration and for controlling gingivitis, as an adjunct to other oral hygiene measures. These preparations may also be used instead of toothbrushing where there is a painful periodontal condition (e.g. primary herpetic stomatitis) or if the child has a haemorrhagic disorder, or is disabled. Chlorhexidine mouthwash is used in the prevention of oral candidiasis in immunocompromised patients. Chlorhexidine mouthwash reduces the incidence of alveolar osteitis following tooth extraction. Chlorhexidine mouthwash should not be used for the prevention of endocarditis in children undergoing dental procedures.

## CHLORHEXIDINE GLUCONATE

**Side-effects** mucosal irritation (if desquamation occurs, discontinue treatment or dilute mouthwash with an equal volume of water); taste disturbance; reversible brown staining of teeth, and of silicate or composite restorations; tongue discoloration; parotid gland swelling and hypersensitivity (including anaphylaxis) reported
**Note** Chlorhexidine gluconate may be incompatible with some ingredients in toothpaste; rinse the mouth thoroughly with water between using toothpaste and chlorhexidine-containing product

**Licensed use** licensed for use in children (age range not specified by manufacturer); *Corsodyl*® not licensed for use in children under 12 years (unless on the advice of a healthcare professional)

**Indications and dose**

See under preparations below

**Chlorhexidine** (Non-proprietary)
Mouthwash, chlorhexidine gluconate 0.2%, net price 300 mL = £2.51
**Dose**

**Oral hygiene and plaque inhibition, oral candidiasis, gingivitis, and management of aphthous ulcers**

Rinse mouth with 10 mL for about 1 minute twice daily

**Corsodyl**® (GSK Consumer Healthcare)
Dental gel, chlorhexidine gluconate 1%. Net price 50 g = £1.21
**Dose**

**Oral hygiene and plaque inhibition and gingivitis**

Brush on the teeth once or twice daily

**Oral candidiasis and management of aphthous ulcers**

Apply to affected areas once or twice daily

**Dental prescribing on NHS** May be prescribed as Chlorhexidine Gluconate Gel

Mouthwash, chlorhexidine gluconate 0.2%, net price 300 mL (original or mint) = £2.18, 600 mL (mint) = £3.85; alcohol-free, 300 mL (mint) = £2.28
**Dose**

**Oral hygiene and plaque inhibition, oral candidiasis, gingivitis, and management of aphthous ulcers**

Rinse mouth with 10 mL for about 1 minute twice daily

**Dental prescribing on NHS** May be prescribed as Chlorhexidine Mouthwash

**12 Ear, nose, and oropharynx**

Oral spray, chlorhexidine gluconate 0.2% (mint-flavoured). Net price 60 mL = £4.10

**Dose**

> **Oral hygiene and plaque inhibition, oral candidiasis, gingivitis, and management of aphthous ulcers**
>
> Apply as required to tooth, gingival, or ulcer surfaces using up to 12 actuations (approx. 0.14 mL/actuation) twice daily

**Dental prescribing on NHS** May be prescribed as Chlorhexidine Oral Spray

◢**With chlorobutanol**

**Eludril®** (Fabre)

Mouthwash or gargle, chlorhexidine gluconate 0.1%, chlorobutanol 0.5% (mint-flavoured), net price 90 mL = £1.36, 250 mL = £2.83, 500 mL = £5.06

**Dose**

> **Oral hygiene and plaque inhibition**
>
> **Child 6–18 years** use 10–15 mL (diluted with lukewarm water in measuring cup provided) 2–3 times daily

## ◢ HEXETIDINE

**Side-effects** local irritation; *very rarely* taste disturbance and transient anaesthesia

**Indications and dose**

> **Oral hygiene** for dose, see preparation below

**Oraldene®** (McNeil)

Mouthwash or gargle, red or blue-green (mint-flavoured), hexetidine 0.1%. Net price 100 mL = £1.31; 200 mL = £2.02

**Dose**

> **Child 6–18 years** use 15 mL (undiluted) 2–3 times daily

## ◢ HYDROGEN PEROXIDE

**Side-effects** hypertrophy of papillae of tongue on prolonged use

**Indications and dose**

> **Oral hygiene** (see notes above); for dose, see under preparations

**Hydrogen Peroxide Mouthwash, BP**

Mouthwash, consists of Hydrogen Peroxide Solution 6% (= approx. 20 volume) BP

**Dose**

> Rinse the mouth for 2–3 minutes with 15 mL diluted in half a tumblerful of warm water 2–3 times daily (see notes above)

**Dental prescribing on NHS** Hydrogen Peroxide Mouthwash may be prescribed

**Peroxyl®** (Colgate-Palmolive)

Mouthwash, hydrogen peroxide 1.5%, net price 300 mL = £2.54

**Dose**

> **Child 6–18 years**, rinse the mouth with 10 mL for about 1 minute 3 times daily (after meals and at bedtime) for max. 7 days

## ◢ SODIUM CHLORIDE

**Indications and dose**

> **Oral hygiene** (see notes above); for dose, see under preparation

**Sodium Chloride Mouthwash, Compound, BP**

Mouthwash, sodium bicarbonate 1%, sodium chloride 1.5% in a suitable vehicle with a peppermint flavour

**Dose**

> Extemporaneous preparations should be prepared according to the following formula: sodium chloride 1.5 g, sodium bicarbonate 1 g, concentrated peppermint emulsion 2.5 mL, double-strength chloroform water 50 mL, water to 100 mL
>
> To be diluted with an equal volume of warm water

**Dental prescribing on NHS** Compound Sodium Chloride Mouthwash may be prescribed

## ◢ THYMOL

**Indications and dose**

> **Oral hygiene** (see notes above); for dose, see under preparation

**Mouthwash Solution-tablets**

Consist of tablets which may contain antimicrobial, colouring, and flavouring agents in a suitable soluble effervescent basis to make a mouthwash suitable for dental purposes. Net price 100-tab pack = £15.09

**Dose**

> Dissolve 1 tablet in a tumblerful of warm water

**Note** Mouthwash Solution-tablets may contain ingredients such as thymol

**Dental prescribing on NHS** Mouthwash Solution-tablets may be prescribed

## 12.3.5 Treatment of dry mouth

Dry mouth (xerostomia) may be caused by drugs with antimuscarinic (anticholinergic) side-effects (e.g. antispasmodics and sedating antihistamines), by irradiation of the head and neck region or by damage to or disease of the salivary glands. Children with a persistently dry mouth may develop a burning or scalded sensation and have poor oral hygiene; they may develop dental caries, periodontal disease, and oral infections (particularly candidiasis). Dry mouth may be relieved in many patients by simple measures such as frequent sips of cool drinks or sucking pieces of ice or sugar-free fruit pastilles. Sugar-free chewing gum stimulates salivation in patients with residual salivary function.

**Artificial saliva** can provide useful relief of dry mouth. A properly balanced artificial saliva should be of a neutral pH and contain electrolytes (including fluoride) to correspond approximately to the composition of saliva. The acidic pH of some artificial saliva products may be inappropriate.

### Local treatment

Artificial saliva products with **ACBS approval** may be prescribed for children with dry mouth as a result of having (or having undergone) radiotherapy, or sicca syndrome. SST tablets may also be prescribed on the NHS.

**12 Ear, nose, and oropharynx**

## AS Saliva Orthana® (AS Pharma)

Oral spray, gastric mucin (porcine) 3.5%, xylitol 2%, sodium fluoride 4.2 mg/litre, with preservatives and flavouring agents, pH neutral, net price 50-mL bottle = £4.92; 500-mL refill = £34.27

**Dose**

> (ACBS) spray 2–3 times onto oral and pharyngeal mucosa, when required

**Dental prescribing on NHS** *AS Saliva Orthana*® Oral Spray may be prescribed

Lozenges, mucin 65 mg, xylitol 59 mg, in a sorbitol basis, pH neutral, net price 30-lozenge pack = £3.50

**Dose**

> (ACBS) allow 1 lozenge to dissolve slowly in the mouth when required

**Note** *AS Saliva Orthana*® lozenges do not contain fluoride
**Dental prescribing on NHS** *AS Saliva Orthana*® Lozenges may be prescribed

## Biotène Oralbalance® (GSK)

Saliva replacement gel, lactoperoxidase, lactoferrin, lysozyme, glucose oxidase, xylitol in a gel basis, net price 50-g tube = £4.10

**Dose**

> **Symptomatic treatment of dry mouth**
>
> Apply to gums and tongue as required

**Note** Avoid use with toothpastes containing detergents (including foaming agents)
**Dental prescribing on NHS** *Biotène Oralbalance*® Saliva Replacement Gel may be prescribed as Artificial Saliva Gel

## BioXtra® (RIS Products)

Gel, lactoperoxidase, lactoferrin, lysozyme, whey colostrum, xylitol and other ingredients, net price 40-mL tube = £3.94, 50-mL spray = £3.94

**Dose**

> (ACBS) apply to oral mucosa as required

**Dental prescribing on NHS** *BioXtra*® Gel may be prescribed

## Glandosane® (Fresenius Kabi)

Aerosol spray, carmellose sodium 500 mg, sorbitol 1.5 g, potassium chloride 60 mg, sodium chloride 42.2 mg, magnesium chloride 2.6 mg, calcium chloride 7.3 mg, and dipotassium hydrogen phosphate 17.1 mg/50 g, pH 5.75, net price 50-mL unit (neutral, lemon or peppermint flavoured) = £4.82

**Dose**

> (ACBS) spray onto oral and pharyngeal mucosa as required

**Dental prescribing on NHS** *Glandosane*® Aerosol Spray may be prescribed

## Saliveze® (Wyvern)

Oral spray, carmellose sodium (sodium carboxymethylcellulose), calcium chloride, magnesium chloride, potassium chloride, sodium chloride, and dibasic sodium phosphate, pH neutral, net price 50-mL bottle (mint-flavoured) = £3.50

**Dose**

> (ACBS) 1 spray onto oral mucosa as required

**Dental prescribing on NHS** *Saliveze*® Oral Spray may be prescribed

## Salivix® (Galen)

Pastilles, sugar-free, reddish-amber, acacia, malic acid and other ingredients. Net price 50-pastille pack = £3.50

**Dose**

> (ACBS) suck 1 pastille when required

**Dental prescribing on NHS** *Salivix*® Pastilles may be prescribed

## SST (Medac)

Tablets, sugar-free, citric acid, malic acid and other ingredients in a sorbitol base, net price 100-tab pack = £4.86

**Dose**

> **Symptomatic treatment of dry mouth in patients with impaired salivary gland function and patent salivary ducts**
>
> Allow 1 tablet to dissolve slowly in the mouth when required

**Dental prescribing on NHS** May be prescribed as Saliva Stimulating Tablets

## Xerotin® (SpePharm)

Oral spray, sugar-free, water, sorbitol, carmellose (carboxymethylcellulose), potassium chloride, sodium chloride, potassium phosphate, magnesium chloride, calcium chloride and other ingredients, pH neutral. Net price 100-mL unit = £6.86

**Dose**

> **Symptomatic treatment of dry mouth**
>
> Spray as required

**Dental prescribing on NHS** *Xerotin*® Oral Spray may be prescribed as Artificial Saliva Oral Spray

# 13 Skin

This chapter also includes advice on the management of the following:
> candidiasis, p. 590
> dermatophytoses, p. 590
> head lice, p. 594
> nappy rash, p. 559
> pityriasis versicolor, p. 590
> scabies, p. 593

For information on wound management products and elasticated garments, see BNF Appendix 5.

The British Association of Dermatologists' list of preferred unlicensed dermatological preparations (specials) is available at www.bad.org.uk.

# 13.1 Management of skin conditions

**13.1.1** Vehicles
**13.1.2** Suitable quantities for prescribing
**13.1.3** Excipients and sensitisation

When prescribing topical preparations for the treatment of skin conditions in children, the site of application, the condition being treated, and the child's (and carer's) preference for a particular vehicle all need to be taken into consideration.

**Neonates** Caution is required when prescribing topical preparations for neonates—their large body surface area in relation to body mass increases susceptibility to toxicity from systemic absorption of substances applied to the skin. Topical preparations containing potentially sensitising substances such as corticosteroids, aminoglycosides, iodine, and parasiticidal drugs should be avoided. Preparations containing alcohol should be avoided because they can dehydrate the skin, cause pain if applied to raw areas, and the alcohol can cause necrosis.

In *preterm neonates*, the skin is more fragile and offers a poor barrier, especially in the first fortnight after birth. Preterm infants, especially if below 32 weeks postmenstrual age, may also require special measures to maintain skin hydration.

## 13.1.1 Vehicles

The vehicle in topical preparations for the skin affects the degree of hydration, has a mild anti-inflammatory effect, and aids the penetration of the active drug. Therefore, the vehicle, as well as the active drug, should be chosen on the basis of their suitability for the child's skin condition.

**Applications** are usually viscous solutions, emulsions, or suspensions for application to the skin (including the scalp) or nails.

**Collodions** are painted on the skin and allowed to dry to leave a flexible film over the site of application.

**Creams** are emulsions of oil and water and are generally well absorbed into the skin. They may contain an antimicrobial preservative unless the active ingredient or basis is intrinsically bactericidal and fungicidal. Generally, creams are cosmetically more acceptable than ointments because they are less greasy and easier to apply.

**Gels** consist of active ingredients in suitable hydrophilic or hydrophobic bases; they generally have a high water content. Gels are particularly suitable for application to the face and scalp.

**Lotions** have a cooling effect and may be preferred to ointments or creams for application over a hairy area. Lotions in alcoholic basis can sting if used on broken skin. *Shake lotions* (such as calamine lotion) contain insoluble powders which leave a deposit on the skin surface.

**Ointments** are greasy preparations which are normally anhydrous and insoluble in water, and are more occlusive than creams. They are particularly suitable for chronic, dry lesions. The most commonly used ointment bases consist of soft paraffin or a combination of soft, liquid, and hard paraffin. Some ointment bases have both *hydrophilic* and *lipophilic* properties; they may have occlusive properties on the skin surface, encourage hydration, and also be miscible with water; they often have a mild anti-inflammatory effect. *Water-soluble ointments* contain macrogols which are freely soluble in water and are therefore readily washed off; they have a limited but useful role where ready removal is desirable.

**Pastes** are stiff preparations containing a high proportion of finely powdered solids such as zinc oxide and starch suspended in an ointment. They are used for circumscribed lesions such as those which occur in lichen simplex, chronic eczema, or psoriasis. They are less occlusive than ointments and can be used to protect inflamed, lichenified, or excoriated skin.

**Dusting powders** are used only rarely. They reduce friction between opposing skin surfaces. Dusting powders should not be applied to moist areas because they can cake and abrade the skin. Talc is a lubricant but it does not absorb moisture; it can cause respiratory irritation. Starch is less lubricant but absorbs water.

**Dilution**   The BP directs that creams and ointments should **not** normally be diluted but that should dilution be necessary care should be taken, in particular, to prevent microbial contamination. The appropriate diluent should be used and heating should be avoided during mixing; excessive dilution may affect the stability of some creams. Diluted creams should normally be used within 2 weeks of their preparation.

## 13.1.2 Suitable quantities for prescribing

**Suitable quantities of dermatological preparations to be prescribed for specific areas of the body**

| Area of the body | Creams and Ointments | Lotions |
|---|---|---|
| Face | 15–30 g | 100 mL |
| Both hands | 25–50 g | 200 mL |
| Scalp | 50–100 g | 200 mL |
| Both arms or both legs | 100–200 g | 200 mL |
| Trunk | 400 g | 500 mL |
| Groins and genitalia | 15–25 g | 100 mL |

The amounts shown above are usually suitable for children 12–18 years for twice daily application for 1 week; smaller quantities will be required for children under 12 years. These recommendations **do not apply** to corticosteroid preparations.

## 13.1.3 Excipients and sensitisation

Excipients in topical products rarely cause problems. If a patch test indicates allergy to an excipient, then products containing the substance should be avoided (see also Anaphylaxis, p. 157). The following excipients in topical preparations are associated, rarely, with sensitisation; the presence of these excipients is indicated in the entries for topical products. See also Excipients, under General Guidance, p. 2.

| | |
|---|---|
| Beeswax | Imidurea |
| Benzyl alcohol | Isopropyl palmitate |
| Butylated hydroxyanisole | *N*-(3-Chloroallyl)hexami- |
| Butylated hydroxytoluene | nium chloride (quater- |
| Cetostearyl alcohol | nium 15) |
| (including cetyl and | Polysorbates |
| stearyl alcohol) | Propylene glycol |
| Chlorocresol | Sodium metabisulfite |
| Edetic acid (EDTA) | Sorbic acid |
| Ethylenediamine | Wool fat and related sub- |
| Fragrances | stances including |
| Hydroxybenzoates (para- | lanolin[1] |
| bens) | |

## 13.2 Emollient and barrier preparations

| | |
|---|---|
| 13.2.1 | Emollients |
| 13.2.2 | Barrier preparations |

**Borderline substances**   The preparations marked 'ACBS' are regarded as drugs when prescribed in accordance with the advice of the Advisory Committee on Borderline Substances for the clinical conditions listed. Prescriptions issued in accordance with this advice and endorsed 'ACBS' will normally not be investigated. See Appendix 2 for listing by clinical condition.

13

Skin

---

1. Purified versions of wool fat have reduced the problem

## 13.2.1   Emollients

### 13.2.1.1   Emollient bath and shower preparations

**Emollients** hydrate the skin, soften the skin, act as barrier to water and external irritants, and are indicated for all dry or scaling disorders. Their effects are short-lived and they should be applied frequently even after improvement occurs. They are useful in dry and ecze-matous disorders, and to a lesser extent in psoriasis (section 13.5.2); they should be applied immediately after washing or bathing to maximise the effect of skin hydration. The choice of an appropriate emollient will depend on the severity of the condition, the child's (or carer's) preference, and the site of application. Emoll-ient preparations contained within tubs should be removed with a clean spoon or spatula to reduce bac-terial contamination of the emollient. Emollients should be applied in the direction of hair growth to reduce the risk of folliculitis. Ointments may exacerbate acne and folliculitis. Some ingredients rarely cause sensitisation (section 13.1.3) and this should be suspected if an eczematous reaction occurs. The use of aqueous cream as a leave-on emollient may increase the risk of skin reactions, particularly in eczema.

> **Fire hazard with paraffin-based emollients**
> Emulsifying ointment *or* 50% Liquid Paraffin and 50% White Soft Paraffin Ointment in contact with dressings and clothing is easily ignited by a naked flame. The risk is greater when these preparations are applied to large areas of the body, and clothing or dressings become soaked with the ointment. Chil-dren and their carers should be told to keep away from fire or flames and not to smoke when using these preparations. The risk of fire should be con-sidered when using large quantities of any paraffin-based emollient.

Preparations such as **aqueous cream** (section 13.2.1.1) and **emulsifying ointment** can be used as soap sub-stitutes; the preparation is rubbed on the skin before rinsing off completely. The addition of a bath oil (section 13.2.1.1) may also be helpful.

In the *neonate*, a preservative-free paraffin-based emoll-ient hydrates the skin without affecting the normal skin flora; substances such as olive oil are also used. The development of blisters (epidermolysis bullosa) or ichthyosis may be alleviated by applying liquid and white soft paraffin ointment while awaiting dermato-logical investigation.

Preparations containing an antibacterial (section 13.10.1) should be avoided unless infection is present or is a frequent complication of the dry skin condition.

**Urea** is a keratin softener and hydrating agent used in the treatment of dry, scaling conditions (including ichthyosis). It is occasionally used with other topical agents such as corticosteroids to enhance penetration of the skin.

#### ◢Non-proprietary emollient preparations

**Emulsifying Ointment, BP**
Ointment, emulsifying wax 30%, white soft paraffin 50%, liquid paraffin 20%, net price 500 g = £2.22
Excipients include cetostearyl alcohol

**Hydrous Ointment, BP**
Ointment, (oily cream), dried magnesium sulfate 0.5%, phenoxyethanol 1%, wool alcohols ointment 50%, in freshly boiled and cooled purified water, net price 500 g = £2.92

**Liquid and White Soft Paraffin Ointment, NPF**
Ointment, liquid paraffin 50%, white soft paraffin 50%, net price 500 g = £6.09

**Paraffin, White Soft, BP**
White petroleum jelly, net price 100 g = 51p

**Paraffin, Yellow Soft, BP**
Yellow petroleum jelly, net price 100 g = 49p

#### ◢Proprietary emollient preparations

**Aquamax®** (Dermato Logical)
Cream, light liquid paraffin 8%, white soft paraffin 20%, phenoxyethanol 1%, net price 30 g = £0.99, 100 g = £1.89, 500 g = £3.99
Excipients include cetostearyl alcohol, polysorbate 60

**Aquamol®** (Thornton & Ross)
Cream, containing liquid paraffin, white soft paraffin, net price 50 g = £1.22, 500-g pump pack = £6.40
Excipients include cetostearyl alcohol, chlorocresol

**Aveeno®** (J&J)
Cream, colloidal oatmeal in emollient basis, net price 100 mL = £3.97, 300-mL pump pack = £6.80
Excipients include benzyl alcohol, cetyl alcohol, isopropyl palmitate
ACBS: For endogenous and exogenous eczema, xeroderma, and ichthyosis

Lotion, colloidal oatmeal in emollient basis, net price 500 mL = £6.66
Excipients include benzyl alcohol, cetyl alcohol, isopropyl palmitate, stearyl alcohol
ACBS: as for *Aveeno®* Cream

**Cetraben®** (Genus)
Emollient cream, white soft paraffin 13.2%, light liq-uid paraffin 10.5%, net price 50-g pump pack = £1.40, 150-g pump pack = £3.98, 500-g pump pack = £5.99, 1.05-kg pump pack = £11.62
Excipients include cetostearyl alcohol, hydroxybenzoates (parabens)

**Dermamist®** (Alliance)
Spray application, white soft paraffin 10% in a basis containing liquid paraffin, fractionated coconut oil, net price 250-mL pressurised aerosol unit = £5.97
Excipients none as listed in section 13.1.3
Note Flammable

**Diprobase®** (Schering-Plough)
Cream, cetomacrogol 2.25%, cetostearyl alcohol 7.2%, liquid paraffin 6%, white soft paraffin 15%, water-miscible basis used for *Diprosone®* cream, net price 50 g = £1.28; 500-g pump pack= £6.32
Excipients include cetostearyl alcohol, chlorocresol

Ointment, liquid paraffin 5%, white soft paraffin 95%, basis used for *Diprosone®* ointment, net price 50 g = £1.28, 500 g = £5.99
Excipients none as listed in section 13.1.3

**13 Skin**

**Doublebase**® (Dermal)

Gel, isopropyl myristate 15%, liquid paraffin 15%, net price 100 g = £2.65, 500 g = £5.83
Excipients none as listed in section 13.1.3

Daylong Gel, isopropyl myristate 15%, liquid paraffin 15%, net price 100 g = £2.65, 500-g pump pack = £6.29
Excipients none as listed in section 13.1.3

**E45**® (Reckitt Benckiser)

Cream, light liquid paraffin 12.6%, white soft paraffin 14.5%, hypoallergenic anhydrous wool fat (hypoallergenic lanolin) 1% in self-emulsifying monostearin, net price 50 g = £1.61, 125 g = £2.90, 350 g = £4.85, 500-g pump pack = £5.62
Excipients include cetyl alcohol, hydroxybenzoates (parabens)

Lotion, light liquid paraffin 4%, cetomacrogol, white soft paraffin 10%, hypoallergenic anhydrous wool fat (hypoallergenic lanolin) 1% in glyceryl monostearate, net price 200 mL = £2.40, 500-mL pump pack = £4.50
Excipients include isopropyl palmitate, hydroxybenzoates (parabens), benzyl alcohol
ACBS: for symptomatic relief of dry skin conditions, such as those associated with atopic eczema and contact dermatitis

**Emollin**® (C D Medical)

Spray, liquid paraffin 50%, white soft paraffin 50% in aerosol basis, net price 150 mL = £3.92, 240 mL = £6.26
Excipients none as listed in section 13.1.3

**Epaderm**® (Mölnlycke)

Cream, yellow soft paraffin 15%, liquid paraffin 10%, emulsifying wax 5%, net price 50-g pump pack = £1.68, 500-g pump pack = £6.86
Excipients include cetostearyl alcohol, chlorocresol

Ointment, emulsifying wax 30%, yellow soft paraffin 30%, liquid paraffin 40%, net price 125 g = £3.85, 500 g = £6.53, 1 kg = £12.02
Excipients include cetostearyl alcohol

**Hydromol**® (Alliance)

Cream, sodium pidolate 2.5%, liquid paraffin 13.8%, net price 50 g = £2.04, 100 g = £3.80, 500 g = £11.09
Excipients include cetostearyl alcohol, hydroxybenzoates (parabens)

Ointment, yellow soft paraffin 30%, emulsifying wax 30%, liquid paraffin 40%, net price 125 g = £2.84, 500 g = £4.82, 1 kg = £8.96
Excipients include cetostearyl alcohol

**Lipobase**® (Astellas)

Cream, fatty cream basis used for *Locoid Lipo-cream*®, net price 50 g = £1.46
Excipients include cetostearyl alcohol, hydroxybenzoates (parabens)
For dry skin conditions, also for use during treatment with topical corticosteroid and as diluent for *Locoid Lipocream*®

**Oilatum**® (Stiefel)

Cream, light liquid paraffin 6%, white soft paraffin 15%, net price 40 g = £1.30, 150 g = £2.46, 500-mL pump pack = £4.99, 1.05-litre pump pack = £9.98
Excipients include benzyl alcohol, cetostearyl alcohol

*Oilatum*® Junior Cream, light liquid paraffin 6%, white soft paraffin 15%, 150 g = £3.38, 350-mL pump pack = £4.65, 500-mL pump pack = £4.99, 1.05-litre pump pack = £9.98
Excipients include benzyl alcohol, cetostearyl alcohol

**QV**® (Sound Opinion)

Cream, glycerol 10%, light liquid paraffin 10%, white soft paraffin 5%, net price 100 g = £2.02, 500 g = £5.80, 1.05-kg pump pack = £11.80
Excipients include cetostearyl alcohol, hydroxybenzoates (parabens)

Intensive ointment, light liquid paraffin 50.5%, white soft paraffin 20%, net price 450 g = £5.59
Excipients include cetostearyl alcohol

Lotion, white soft paraffin 5%, net price 250 mL = £3.11, 500-mL pump pack = £5.18
Excipients include cetostearyl alcohol, hydroxybenzoates (parabens)

**Ultrabase**® (Derma UK)

Cream, water-miscible, containing liquid paraffin and white soft paraffin, net price 50 g = £1.40, 500-g pump pack = £4.80
Excipients include fragrance, hydroxybenzoates (parabens), disodium edetate, stearyl alcohol

**Unguentum M**® (Almirall)

Cream, containing saturated neutral oil, liquid paraffin, white soft paraffin, net price 50 g = £1.41, 100 g = £2.78, 200-mL pump pack = £5.50, 500 g = £8.48
Excipients include cetostearyl alcohol, polysorbate 40, propylene glycol, sorbic acid

**ZeroAQS**® (Thornton & Ross)

Cream, macrogol cetostearyl ether 1.8%, liquid paraffin 6%, white soft paraffin 15%, net price 100 g = £1.65, 500 g = £3.29
Excipients include cetostearyl alcohol, chlorocresol

**Zerobase**® (Thornton & Ross)

Cream, liquid paraffin 11%, net price 50 g = £1.04, 500-g pump pack = £5.26
Excipients include cetostearyl alcohol, chlorocresol

**Zerocream**® (Thornton & Ross)

Cream, liquid paraffin 12.6%, white soft paraffin 14.5%, net price 50 g = £1.17, 500-g pump pack = £4.08
Excipients include cetyl alcohol, hydroxybenzoates (parabens), lanolin anhydrous

**Zeroguent**® (Thornton & Ross)

Cream, light liquid paraffin 8%, white soft paraffin 4%, refined soya bean oil 5%, net price 100 g = £2.33, 500 g = £6.99
Excipients include cetostearyl alcohol, polysorbate 40, propylene glycol, sorbic acid

◢**Preparations containing urea**

**Aquadrate**® (Alliance)

Cream, urea 10%, net price 100 g = £4.37
Excipients none as listed in section 13.1.3
Dose
Apply thinly twice daily

13
Skin

**Balneum®** (Almirall)
Cream, urea 5%, ceramide 0.1%, net price 50-g pump pack = £2.80, 500-g pump pack = £9.80
**Excipients** include cetostearyl alcohol, polysorbates, propylene glycol
**Dose**

> Apply twice daily

Balneum® Plus Cream, urea 5%, lauromacrogols 3%, net price 100 g = £3.29, 500-g pump pack = £16.42
**Excipients** include benzyl alcohol, polysorbates
**Dose**

> Apply twice daily

**Calmurid®** (Galderma)
Cream, urea 10%, lactic acid 5%, net price 100 g = £5.70, 500-g pump pack = £27.42
**Excipients** none as listed in section 13.1.3
**Dose**

> Apply a thick layer for 3–5 minutes, massage into area, and remove excess, usually twice daily. Use half-strength cream for 1 week if stinging occurs
>
> **Note** Can be diluted with aqueous cream (life of diluted cream 14 days)

**Dermatonics Heel Balm®** (Dermatonics)
Cream, urea 25%, net price 75 mL = £4.00, 200 mL = £9.50
**Excipients** include beeswax, lanolin
**Dose**

> **Child 12–18 years** apply once daily to dry skin on soles of feet

**E45® Itch Relief Cream** (Reckitt Benckiser)
Cream, urea 5%, macrogol lauryl ether 3%, net price 50 g = £2.55, 100 g = £3.47, 500-g pump pack = £14.99
**Excipients** include benzyl alcohol, polysorbates
**Dose**

> Apply twice daily

**Eucerin® Intensive** (Beiersdorf)
Cream, urea 10%, net price 100 mL = £7.59
**Excipients** include benzyl alcohol, isopropyl palmitate, wool fat
**Dose**

> Apply thinly and rub into area twice daily

Lotion, urea 10%, net price 250 mL = £7.93
**Excipients** include benzyl alcohol, isopropyl palmitate
**Dose**

> Apply sparingly and rub into area twice daily

**Flexitol®** (LaCorium)
Heel balm, urea 25%, net price 75 g = £3.80, 200 g = £9.40, 500 g = £14.75
**Excipients** include benzyl alcohol, cetostearyl alcohol, fragrance, lanolin
**Dose**

> **Child 12–18 years** apply 1–2 times daily to dry skin on soles of feet and heels

**Hydromol® Intensive** (Alliance)
Cream, urea 10%, net price 30 g = £1.64, 100 g = £4.37
**Excipients** none as listed in section 13.1.3
**Dose**

> Apply thinly twice daily

**Nutraplus®** (Galderma)
Cream, urea 10%, net price 100 g = £4.37
**Excipients** include hydroxybenzoates (parabens), propylene glycol
**Dose**

> Apply 2–3 times daily

◀**With antimicrobials**

**Dermol®** (Dermal)
Cream, benzalkonium chloride 0.1%, chlorhexidine hydrochloride 0.1%, isopropyl myristate 10%, liquid paraffin 10%, net price 100-g tube = £2.86, 500-g pump pack = £6.63
**Excipients** include cetostearyl alcohol
**Dose**

> Apply to skin or use as soap substitute

Dermol® 500 Lotion, benzalkonium chloride 0.1%, chlorhexidine hydrochloride 0.1%, liquid paraffin 2.5%, isopropyl myristate 2.5%, net price 500-mL pump pack = £6.03
**Excipients** include cetostearyl alcohol
**Dose**

> Apply to skin or use as soap substitute

**Eczmol®** (Genus)
Cream, chlorhexidine gluconate 1% in emollient basis, net price 250 mL = £3.70
**Excipients** include cetostearyl alcohol
**Dose**

> Apply to skin or use as soap substitute

### 13.2.1.1 Emollient bath and shower preparations

Emollient bath additives should be added to bath water; some can be applied to wet skin undiluted and rinsed off. Hydration can be improved by soaking in the bath for 10–20 minutes. In dry skin conditions soap should be avoided (see section 13.2.1 for soap substitutes).

The quantities of bath additives recommended for older children are suitable for an adult-size bath. Proportionately less should be used for a child-size bath or a washbasin; recommended bath additive quantities for younger children reflect this.

> These preparations make skin and surfaces slippery—particular care is needed when bathing a child.

**Aqueous Cream, BP**
Cream, emulsifying ointment 30%, [1]phenoxyethanol 1% in freshly boiled and cooled purified water, net price 100 g = £1.12, 500 g = £5.60
**Excipients** include cetostearyl alcohol

---

1. The BP permits use of alternative antimicrobials provided their identity and concentration are stated on the label

**Aquamax®** (Dermato Logical)

Cream wash, light liquid paraffin 8%, white soft paraffin 20%, pheonxyethanol 1%, net price 30 g = £0.99, 250 g = £2.99

Excipients   include cetostearyl alcohol, polysorbate 60

Dose

> Apply to wet or dry skin and rinse

**Aveeno®** (J&J)

Bath oil, colloidal oatmeal, white oat fraction in emollient basis, net price 250 mL = £4.49

Excipients   include beeswax, fragrance

ACBS: for endogenous and exogenous eczema, xeroderma, and ichthyosis

Dose

> Child 2–18 years add 20–30 mL to bath water or apply to wet skin and rinse

**Balneum®** (Almirall)

Balneum® bath oil, soya oil 84.75%, net price 200 mL = £2.48, 500 mL = £5.38, 1 litre = £10.39

Excipients   include butylated hydroxytoluene, propylene glycol, fragrance

Dose

> Neonate add 5–15 mL to bath water; do not use undiluted
>
> Child 1 month–2 years add 5–15 mL to bath water; do not use undiluted
>
> Child 2–18 years add 20–60 mL to bath water; do not use undiluted

Balneum Plus® bath oil, soya oil 82.95%, mixed lauromacrogols 15%, net price 500 mL = £6.66

Excipients   include butylated hydroxytoluene, propylene glycol, fragrance

Dose

> Neonate add 5 mL to bath water or apply to wet skin and rinse
>
> Child 1 month–2 years add 5 mL to bath water or apply to wet skin and rinse
>
> Child 2–18 years add 10–20 mL to bath water or apply to wet skin and rinse

**Cetraben®** (Genus)

Emollient bath additive, light liquid paraffin 82.8%, net price 500 mL = £5.75

Excipients   none as listed in section 13.1.3

Dose

> Neonate add ½ capful to bath water or apply to wet skin and rinse
>
> Child 1 month–12 years add ½–1 capful to bath water or apply to wet skin and rinse
>
> Child 12–18 years add 1–2 capfuls to bath water or apply to wet skin and rinse

**Dermalo®** (Dermal)

Bath emollient, acetylated wool alcohols 5%, liquid paraffin 65%, net price 500 mL = £3.44

Excipients   none as listed in section 13.1.3

Dose

> Neonate add 5 mL to bath water or apply to wet skin and rinse
>
> Child 1 month–12 years add 5–10 mL to bath water or apply to wet skin and rinse
>
> Child 12–18 years add 15–20 mL to bath water or apply to wet skin and rinse

**Diprobath®** (MSD)

Bath additive, isopropyl myristate 39%, light liquid paraffin 46%, net price 500 mL = £6.71

Excipients   none as listed in section 13.1.3

Dose

> Neonate add 5 mL to bath water; do not use undiluted
>
> Child 1 month–12 years add 10 mL to bath water; do not use undiluted
>
> Child 12–18 years add 25–50 mL to bath water; do not use undiluted

**Doublebase®** (Dermal)

Emollient bath additive, liquid paraffin 65%, net price 500 mL = £5.45

Excipients   include cetostearyl alcohol

Dose

> Neonate add 5–10 mL to bath water
>
> Child 1 month–12 years add 5–10 mL to bath water
>
> Child 12–18 years add 15–20 mL to bath water

Emollient shower gel, isopropyl myristate 15%, liquid paraffin 15%, net price 200 g = £5.21

Excipients   none as listed in section 13.1.3

Note   Also available as Doublebase® Emollient Wash Gel

Dose

> Apply to wet or dry skin and rinse, or apply to dry skin after showering

**E45®** (Reckitt Benckiser)

Emollient bath oil, cetyl dimeticone 5%, liquid paraffin 91%, net price 250 mL = £3.19, 500 mL = £5.11

Excipients   none as listed in section 13.1.3

ACBS: for endogenous and exogenous eczema, xeroderma, and ichthyosis

Dose

> Neonate add 5 mL to bath water or apply to wet skin and rinse
>
> Child 1 month–12 years add 5–10 mL to bath water or apply to wet skin and rinse
>
> Child 12–18 years add 15 mL to bath water or apply to wet skin and rinse

Emollient wash cream, zinc oxide 5% in an emollient basis, net price 250-mL pump pack = £3.19

Excipients   none as listed in section 13.1.3

ACBS: for endogenous and exogenous eczema, xeroderma, and ichthyosis

Dose

> Use as a soap substitute

**Hydromol®** (Alliance)

Bath and Shower Emollient, isopropyl myristate 13%, light liquid paraffin 37.8%, net price 350 mL = £3.61, 500 mL = £4.11, 1 litre = £8.19

Excipients   none as listed in section 13.1.3

Dose

> Neonate add ½ capful to bath water or apply to wet skin and rinse
>
> Child 1 month–12 years add ½–2 capfuls to bath water or apply to wet skin and rinse
>
> Child 12–18 years add 1–3 capfuls to bath water or apply to wet skin and rinse

**13**

**Skin**

**Oilatum®** (Stiefel)

Emollient bath additive (emulsion), light liquid paraffin 63.4%, net price 250 mL = £2.75, 500 mL = £4.57

Excipients   include acetylated lanolin alcohols, isopropyl palmitate, fragrance

**Dose**

> **Neonate** add ½ capful to bath water or apply to wet skin and rinse
>
> **Child 1 month–12 years** add ½–2 capfuls to bath water or apply to wet skin and rinse
>
> **Child 12–18 years** add 1–3 capfuls to bath water or apply to wet skin and rinse

Junior bath additive, light liquid paraffin 63.4%, net price 150 mL = £2.82, 250 mL = £3.25, 300 mL = £5.10, 600 mL = £5.89

Excipients   include acetylated lanolin alcohols, isopropyl palmitate

**Dose**

> **Neonate** add ½ capful to bath water or apply to wet skin and rinse
>
> **Child 1 month–12 years** add ½–2 capfuls to bath water or apply to wet skin and rinse
>
> **Child 12–18 years** add 1–3 capfuls to bath water or apply to wet skin and rinse

Shower emollient (gel), light liquid paraffin 70%, net price (with fragrance or fragrance-free) 150 g = £5.15

Excipients   none as listed in section 13.1.3

**Dose**

> Apply to wet skin and rinse

**QV®** (Sound Opinion)

Bath oil, light liquid paraffin 85.13%, net price 200 mL = £2.20, 500 mL = £4.66

Excipients   none as listed in section 13.1.3

**Dose**

> **Neonate** add 5 mL to bath water or apply to wet skin and rinse
>
> **Child 1 month–1 year** add 5 mL to bath water or apply to wet skin and rinse
>
> **Child 1–18 years** add 10 mL to bath water or apply to wet skin and rinse

Gentle wash, glycerol 15%, net price 250 mL = £3.11, 500-mL pump pack = £5.18

Excipients   include hydroxybenzoates (parabens)

**Dose**

> Use as a soap substitute

**Zerolatum®** (Thornton & Ross)

Emollient medicinal bath oil, liquid paraffin 65%, net price 500 mL = £4.79

Excipients   include acetylated wool alcohols

**Dose**

> **Child 1 month–12 years** add 5–10 mL to bath water
>
> **Child 12–18 years** add 15–20 mL to bath water

**Zeroneum®** (Thornton & Ross)

Bath oil, refined soya bean oil 83.35%, net price 500 mL = £4.48

Excipients   include butylated hydroxytoluene, fragrance, propylene glycol

**Dose**

> **Child 1 month–12 years** add 5 mL to bath water
>
> **Child 12–18 years** add 20 mL to bath water

◀**With antimicrobials**

**Dermol®** (Dermal)

Dermol® 600 Bath Emollient, benzalkonium chloride 0.5%, liquid paraffin 25%, isopropyl myristate 25%, net price 600 mL = £7.55

Excipients   include polysorbate 60

**Dose**

> **Child 1 month–2 years** add 5–15 mL to bath water; do not use undiluted
>
> **Child 2–18 years** add 15–30 mL to bath water; do not use undiluted

Dermol® 200 Shower Emollient, benzalkonium chloride 0.1%, chlorhexidine hydrochloride 0.1%, liquid paraffin 2.5%, isopropyl myristate 2.5%, net price 200 mL = £3.55

Excipients   include cetostearyl alcohol

**Dose**

> Apply to skin or use as soap substitute

Dermol® Wash Emulsion, benzalkonium chloride 0.1%, chlorhexidine hydrochloride 0.1%, liquid paraffin 2.5%, isopropyl myristate 2.5%, net price 200-mL pump pack = £3.55

Excipients   include cetostearyl alcohol

**Dose**

> Apply to skin or use as soap substitute

**Emulsiderm®** (Dermal)

Liquid emulsion, benzalkonium chloride 0.5%, liquid paraffin 25%, isopropyl myristate 25%, net price 300 mL (with 15-mL measure) = £3.85, 1 litre (with 30-mL measure) = £12.00

Excipients   include polysorbate 60

**Dose**

> **Child 1 month–2 years** add 5–10 mL to bath water or rub into dry skin until absorbed
>
> **Child 2–18 years** add 10–30 mL to bath water or rub into dry skin until absorbed

**Oilatum® Plus** (Stiefel)

Bath additive, benzalkonium chloride 6%, triclosan 2%, light liquid paraffin 52.5%, net price 500 mL = £6.98

Excipients   include acetylated lanolin alcohols, isopropyl palmitate

**Dose**

> **Child 6 months–1 year** add 1 mL to bath water; do not use undiluted
>
> **Child 1–18 years** add 1–2 capfuls to bath water; do not use undiluted

**Zerolatum® Plus** (Thornton & Ross)

Bath additive, benzalkonium chloride 6%, triclosan 2%, light liquid paraffin 51.66%, net price 500 mL = £5.82

Excipients   include acetylated lanolin alcohols, isopropyl palmitate, polysorbate 80

**Dose**

> **Child 6 months–1 year** add 1 mL to bath water; do not use undiluted
>
> **Child 1–18 years** add 1–2 capfuls to bath water; do not use undiluted

◀**With tar**

Section 13.5.2

**13 Skin**

## 13.2.2 Barrier preparations

Barrier preparations often contain water-repellent substances such as **dimeticone**, natural oils, and paraffins, to help protect the skin from abrasion and irritation; they are used to protect intact skin around stomas and pressure sores, and as a barrier against nappy rash. In neonates, barrier preparations which do not contain potentially sensitising excipients (section 13.1.3) are preferred. Where the skin has broken down, barrier preparations have a limited role in protecting adjacent skin. Barrier preparations with zinc oxide or titanium salts are used to aid healing of uninfected, excoriated skin.

**Nappy rash (Dermatitis)**  The first line of treatment is to ensure that nappies are changed frequently and that tightly fitting water-proof pants are avoided. The rash may clear when left exposed to the air and a barrier preparation, applied with each nappy change, can be helpful. A mild corticosteroid such as hydrocortisone 0.5% or 1% (section 13.4) can be used if inflammation is causing discomfort, but it should be avoided in neonates. The barrier preparation should be applied after the corticosteroid preparation to prevent further damage. Preparations containing hydrocortisone should be applied for no more than a week; the hydrocortisone should be discontinued as soon as the inflammation subsides. The occlusive effect of nappies and water-proof pants may increase absorption of corticosteroids (for cautions, see section 13.4). If the rash is associated with candidal infection, a topical antifungal such as clotrimazole cream (section 13.10.2) can be used. Topical antibacterial preparations (section 13.10.1) can be used if bacterial infection is present; treatment with an oral antibacterial may occasionally be required in severe or recurrent infection. Hydrocortisone may be used in combination with antimicrobial preparations if there is considerable inflammation, erosion, and infection.

◂ **Non-proprietary barrier preparations**
**Zinc and Castor Oil Ointment, BP**
Ointment, zinc oxide 7.5%, castor oil 50%, arachis (peanut) oil 30.5%, white beeswax 10%, cetostearyl alcohol 2%, net price 500 g = £2.93

◂ **Proprietary barrier preparations**
**Conotrane®** (Astellas)
Cream, benzalkonium chloride 0.1%, dimeticone 22%, net price 100 g = 88p, 500 g = £3.51
Excipients  include cetostearyl alcohol, fragrance

**Drapolene®** (Omega Pharma)
Cream, benzalkonium chloride 0.01%, cetrimide 0.2% in a basis containing white soft paraffin, cetyl alcohol and wool fat, net price 100 g = £1.54, 200 g = £2.50, 350 g = £3.75
Excipients  include cetyl alcohol, chlorocresol, wool fat

**Medicaid®** (LPC)
Cream, cetrimide 0.5% in a basis containing light liquid paraffin, white soft paraffin, cetostearyl alcohol, glyceryl monostearate, net price 50 g = £1.69
Excipients  include cetostearyl alcohol, fragrance, hydroxybenzoates (parabens), wool fat

**Metanium®** (Thornton & Ross)
Ointment, titanium dioxide 20%, titanium peroxide 5%, titanium salicylate 3% in a basis containing dimeticone, light liquid paraffin, white soft paraffin, and benzoin tincture, net price 30 g = £2.06
Excipients  none as listed in section 13.1.3

**Morhulin®** (Actavis)
Ointment, cod-liver oil 11.4%, zinc oxide 38%, in a basis containing liquid paraffin and yellow soft paraffin, net price 50 g = £1.91
Excipients  include wool fat derivative

**Siopel®** (Derma UK)
Barrier cream, dimeticone '1000' 10%, cetrimide 0.3%, arachis (peanut) oil, net price 50 g = £2.15
Excipients  include butylated hydroxytoluene, cetostearyl alcohol, hydroxybenzoates (parabens)

**Sprilon®** (Ayrton Saunders)
Spray application, dimeticone 1.04%, zinc oxide 12.5%, in a basis containing wool alcohols, cetostearyl alcohol, dextran, white soft paraffin, liquid paraffin, propellants, net price 115-g pressurised aerosol unit = £8.90
Excipients  include cetostearyl alcohol, hydroxybenzoates (parabens), wool fat
Note  Flammable

**Sudocrem®** (Forest)
Cream, benzyl alcohol 0.39%, benzyl benzoate 1.01%, benzyl cinnamate 0.15%, hydrous wool fat (hypoallergenic lanolin) 4%, zinc oxide 15.25%, net price 60 g = £1.38, 125 g = £2.00, 250 g = £3.35, 400 g = £4.71
Excipients  include beeswax (synthetic), propylene glycol, butylated hydroxyanisole, fragrance

## 13.3  Topical antipruritics

*Pruritus* may be caused by systemic disease (such as obstructive jaundice, endocrine disease, chronic renal disease, iron deficiency, and certain malignant diseases), skin disease (such as eczema, psoriasis, urticaria, and scabies), drug hypersensitivity, or as a side-effect of opioid analgesics. Where possible, the underlying cause should be treated. For the treatment of pruritus in palliative care, see Prescribing in Palliative Care, p. 19. Pruritus caused by cholestasis generally requires a bile acid sequestrant (section 1.9.2).

An **emollient** (section 13.2.1) may be of value where pruritus is associated with dry skin. Preparations containing **calamine** or **crotamiton** are sometimes used but are of uncertain value.

A topical preparation containing **doxepin 5%** is licensed for the relief of pruritus in eczema in children over 12 years; it can cause drowsiness and there may be a risk of sensitisation.

Topical antihistamines and local anaesthetics (section 15.2) are only marginally effective and occasionally cause sensitisation. For *insect stings* and *insect bites*, a short course of a topical corticosteroid is appropriate. Short-term treatment with a **sedating antihistamine** (section 3.4.1) may help in insect stings and in intractable pruritus where sedation is desirable. Calamine preparations are of little value for the treatment of insect stings or bites.

In *pruritus ani*, the underlying cause such as faecal soiling, eczema, psoriasis, or helminth infection should

**13**

**Skin**

be treated; for preparations used to relieve pruritus ani, see section 1.7.

## CALAMINE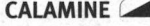

**Contra-indications**   avoid application of preparations containing zinc oxide prior to x-ray (zinc oxide may affect outcome of x-ray)

**Indications and dose**

Pruritus but see notes above

**Calamine** (Non-proprietary)
Aqueous cream, calamine 4%, zinc oxide 3%, liquid paraffin 20%, self-emulsifying glyceryl monostearate 5%, cetomacrogol emulsifying wax 5%, phenoxyethanol 0.5%, freshly boiled and cooled purified water 62.5%, net price 100 mL = 84p

Lotion (= cutaneous suspension), calamine 15%, zinc oxide 5%, glycerol 5%, bentonite 3%, sodium citrate 0.5%, liquefied phenol 0.5%, in freshly boiled and cooled purified water, net price 200 mL = 63p

Oily lotion (BP 1980), calamine 5%, arachis (peanut) oil 50%, oleic acid 0.5%, wool fat 1%, in calcium hydroxide solution, net price 200 mL = £1.57

## CROTAMITON

**Cautions**   avoid use near eyes, in buccal mucosa, or on broken or very inflamed skin; use on doctor's advice for children under 3 years

**Contra-indications**   acute exudative dermatoses

**Indications and dose**

Pruritus (including pruritus after scabies—section 13.10.4) see notes above
 Apply 2–3 times daily (for pruritus after scabies in children under 3 years apply once daily only)

**Eurax®** (Novartis Consumer Health)
Cream, crotamiton 10%, net price 30 g = £2.38, 100 g = £4.15
Excipients   include beeswax, fragrance, hydroxybenzoates (parabens), stearyl alcohol

Lotion, crotamiton 10%, net price 100 mL = £3.14
Excipients   include cetyl alcohol, fragrance, propylene glycol, sorbic acid, stearyl alcohol

## DOXEPIN HYDROCHLORIDE

**Cautions**   susceptibility to angle-closure glaucoma; urinary retention; mania; cardiac arrhythmias; severe heart disease; avoid application to large areas; **interactions:** Appendix 1 (antidepressants, tricyclic)
Skilled tasks   Drowsiness may affect performance of skilled tasks (e.g. driving); effects of alcohol enhanced

**Hepatic impairment**   manufacturer advises caution in severe liver disease

**Pregnancy**   manufacturer advises use only if potential benefit outweighs risk

**Breast-feeding**   manufacturer advises use only if potential benefit outweighs risk

**Side-effects**   drowsiness; local burning, stinging, irritation, tingling and rash; systemic side-effects such as antimuscarinic effects, headache, fever, dizziness, gastro-intestinal disturbances also reported

**Indications and dose**

Pruritus in eczema

Child 12–18 years apply thinly 3–4 times daily; usual max. 3 g per application; usual total max. 12 g daily; coverage should be less than 10% of body surface area

Depressive illness section 4.3.1

**Xepin®** (CHS) PoM
Cream, doxepin hydrochloride 5%, net price 30 g = £11.70. Label: 2, 10, patient information leaflet
Excipients   include benzyl alcohol

## 13.4 Topical corticosteroids

Topical corticosteroids are used for the treatment of inflammatory conditions of the skin (other than those arising from an infection), particularly eczema (section 13.5.1), contact dermatitis, insect stings (p. 33), and eczema of scabies (section 13.10.4). Corticosteroids suppress the inflammatory reaction during use; they are not curative and on discontinuation a rebound exacerbation of the condition may occur. They are generally used to relieve symptoms and suppress signs of the disorder when other measures such as emollients are ineffective.

Children, especially infants, are particularly susceptible to side-effects. However, concern about the safety of topical corticosteroids in children should not result in the child being undertreated. The aim is to control the condition as well as possible; inadequate treatment will perpetuate the condition. Carers of young children should be advised that treatment should **not** necessarily be reserved to 'treat only the worst areas' and they may need to be advised that patient information leaflets may contain inappropriate advice for the child's condition.

In an acute flare-up of atopic eczema, it may be appropriate to use more potent formulations of topical corticosteroids for a short period to regain control of the condition. Continuous daily application of a mild corticosteroid such as hydrocortisone 1% is equivalent to a potent corticosteroid such as betamethasone 0.1% applied intermittently.

Topical corticosteroids are of no value in the treatment of *urticaria*. They may worsen ulcerated or secondarily infected lesions. They should not be used indiscriminately in *pruritus* (where they will only benefit if inflammation is causing the itch) and are **not** recommended for *acne vulgaris*.

Systemic or very potent topical corticosteroids should be avoided or given only under specialist supervision in *psoriasis* because, although they may suppress the psoriasis in the short term, relapse or vigorous rebound occurs on withdrawal (sometimes precipitating severe pustular psoriasis). Topical use of potent corticosteroids on widespread psoriasis can lead to systemic as well as to local side-effects. It is reasonable, however, to prescribe a mild topical corticosteroid for a short period (2–4 weeks) for *flexural* and *facial psoriasis*, and to use a more potent corticosteroid such as betamethasone or fluocinonide for *psoriasis* of the *scalp, palms,* or *soles* (see below for cautions in psoriasis).

In general, the most potent topical corticosteroids should be reserved for recalcitrant dermatoses such as *chronic discoid lupus erythematosus, lichen simplex chronicus, hypertrophic lichen planus,* and *palmoplantar pustu-*

*losis*. Potent corticosteroids should generally be avoided on the face and skin flexures, but specialists occasionally prescribe them for use on these areas in certain circumstances.

When topical treatment has failed, intralesional corticosteroid injections (section 10.1.2.2) may be used. These are more effective than the very potent topical corticosteroid preparations and should be reserved for severe cases where there are localised lesions such as *keloid scars, hypertrophic lichen planus,* or *localised alopecia areata*.

**Choice** Water-miscible corticosteroid *creams* are suitable for moist or weeping lesions whereas *ointments* are generally chosen for dry, lichenified or scaly lesions or where a more occlusive effect is required. *Lotions* may be useful when minimal application to a large or hair-bearing area is required or for the treatment of exudative lesions. *Occlusive polythene or hydrocolloid dressings* increase absorption, but also increase the risk of side-effects; they are therefore used only under supervision on a short-term basis for areas of very thick skin (such as the palms and soles). Disposable nappies and tight fitting pants also increase the risk of side-effects by increasing absorption of the corticosteroid. The inclusion of urea or salicylic acid also increases the penetration of the corticosteroid.

'Wet-wrap bandaging' (section 13.5.1) increases absorption into the skin, but should be initiated only by a dermatologist and application supervised by a health-care professional trained in the technique.

In the *BNF for Children*, topical corticosteroids for the skin are categorised as 'mild', 'moderately potent', 'potent' or 'very potent' (see p. 562); the **least potent** preparation which is effective should be chosen but dilution should be avoided whenever possible.

Topical hydrocortisone is usually used in children under 1 year of age. Moderately potent and potent topical corticosteroids should be used with great care in children and for short periods (1–2 weeks) only. A very potent corticosteroid should be initiated under the supervision of a specialist.

Appropriate topical corticosteroids for specific conditions are:

- *insect bites and stings*—mild corticosteroid such as hydrocortisone 1% cream;
- *inflamed nappy rash causing discomfort* in infant over 1 month (section 13.2.2)—mild corticosteroid such as hydrocortisone 0.5% or 1% for up to 7 days (combined with antimicrobial if infected);
- *mild to moderate eczema, flexural and facial eczema or psoriasis*—mild corticosteroid such as hydrocortisone 1%;
- *severe eczema of the face and neck*—moderately potent corticosteroid for 3–5 days only, if not controlled by a mild corticosteroid;
- *severe eczema on the trunk and limbs*—moderately potent or potent corticosteroid for 1–2 weeks only, switching to a less potent preparation as the condition improves;
- *eczema affecting area with thickened skin* (e.g. soles of feet)—potent topical corticosteroid in combination with urea or salicylic acid (to increase penetration of corticosteroid).

**Perioral lesions** Hydrocortisone cream 1% can be used for up to 7 days to treat uninfected inflammatory lesions on the lips. **Hydrocortisone and miconazole**

cream or ointment is useful where infection by susceptible organisms and inflammation co-exist, particularly for initial treatment (up to 7 days) e.g. in angular cheilitis (see also p. 548). Organisms susceptible to miconazole include *Candida* spp. and many Gram-positive bacteria including streptococci and staphylococci.

**Cautions** Avoid prolonged use of a topical corticosteroid particularly on the face (and keep away from eyes). Use potent or very potent corticosteroids under specialist supervision; extreme caution is required in dermatoses of infancy including nappy rash—treatment should be limited to 5–7 days.

**Psoriasis** The use of potent or very potent corticosteroids in psoriasis can result in rebound relapse, development of generalised pustular psoriasis, and local and systemic toxicity, see notes above.

**Contra-indications** Topical corticosteroids are contra-indicated in untreated bacterial, fungal, or viral skin lesions, in acne, and in perioral dermatitis; potent corticosteroids are contra-indicated in widespread plaque psoriasis (see notes above).

**Side-effects** *Mild* and *moderately potent* topical corticosteroids are associated with few side-effects but particular care is required when treating neonates and infants, and in the use of *potent* and *very potent* corticosteroids. Absorption through the skin can rarely cause adrenal suppression and even Cushing's syndrome (section 6.3.2), depending on the area of the body being treated and the duration of treatment. Absorption of corticosteroid is greatest from severely inflamed skin, thin skin (especially on the face or genital area), from flexural sites (e.g. axillae, groin), and in infants where skin surface area is higher in relation to body-weight; absorption is increased by occlusion. Local side-effects include:

- spread and worsening of untreated infection;
- thinning of the skin which may be restored over a period after stopping treatment but the original structure may never return;
- irreversible striae atrophicae and telangiectasia;
- contact dermatitis;
- perioral dermatitis;
- acne, or worsening of acne or rosacea;
- mild depigmentation which may be reversible;
- hypertrichosis also reported.

Children and their carers should be reassured that side effects such as skin thinning and systemic effects rarely occur when topical corticosteroids are used appropriately.

> **Safe Practice**
>
> In order to minimise the side-effects of a topical corticosteroid, it is important to apply it **thinly** to affected areas **only**, no more frequently than **twice daily**, and to use the least potent formulation which is fully effective.

**Application** Topical corticosteroid preparations should be applied no more frequently than twice daily; once daily is often sufficient.

Topical corticosteroids should be spread thinly on the skin but in sufficient quantity to cover the affected areas. The length of cream or ointment expelled from a tube may be used to specify the quantity to be applied to a given area of skin. This length can be measured in terms of a *fingertip unit* (the distance from the tip of the adult index finger to the first crease). One fingertip unit (approximately 500 mg from a tube with a standard 5-mm diameter nozzle) is sufficient to cover an area that is twice that of the flat adult handprint (palm and fingers).

If a child is using topical corticosteroids of different potencies, the child and their carers should be told when to use each corticosteroid. The potency of each topical corticosteroid (see Topical Corticosteroid Preparation Potencies, below) should be included on the label with the directions for use. The label should be attached to the container (for example, the tube) rather than the outer packaging.

Mixing topical preparations on the skin should be avoided where possible; several minutes should elapse between application of different preparations.

**Compound preparations** The advantages of including other substances (such as antibacterials or antifungals) with corticosteroids in topical preparations are uncertain, but such combinations may have a place where inflammatory skin conditions are associated with bacterial or fungal infection, such as infected eczema. In these cases the antimicrobial drug should be chosen according to the sensitivity of the infecting organism and used regularly for a short period (typically twice daily for 1 week). Longer use increases the likelihood of resistance and of sensitisation.

The keratolytic effect of salicylic acid facilitates the absorption of topical corticosteroids; however, excessive and prolonged use of topical preparations containing salicylic acid may cause salicylism.

## Topical corticosteroid potencies

Potency of a topical corticosteroid preparation depends upon the formulation as well as the corticosteroid. Therefore, proprietary names are shown below.

**Mild**

> Hydrocortisone 0.1–2.5%, *Dioderm, Mildison, Synalar 1 in 10 Dilution*
>
> **Mild with antimicrobials** *Canesten HC, Daktacort, Econacort, Fucidin H, Nystaform-HC, Timodine*
>
> **Mild with crotamiton** *Eurax-Hydrocortisone*

**Moderate**

> *Betnovate-RD, Eumovate, Haelan, Modrasone, Synalar 1 in 4 Dilution, Ultralanum Plain*
>
> **Moderate with antimicrobials** *Trimovate*
>
> **Moderate with urea** *Alphaderm, Calmurid HC, Hydromol HC Intensive*

**Potent**

> Beclometasone dipropionate 0.025%, Betamethasone valerate 0.1%, *Betacap, Bettamousse, Betnovate, Cutivate, Diprosone, Elocon,* Hydrocortisone butyrate, *Locoid, Locoid Crelo, Metosyn*, Mometasone furoate 0.1%, *Nerisone, Synalar*
>
> **Potent with antimicrobials** *Aureocort,* Betamethasone and clioquinol, Betamethasone and neomycin, *Fucibet, Lotriderm, Synalar C, Synalar N*
>
> **Potent with salicylic acid** *Diprosalic*

**Very potent**

> *Dermovate, Nerisone Forte*
>
> **Very potent with antimicrobials** Clobetasol propionate 0.05% with neomycin and nystatin

---

## ▌HYDROCORTISONE

**Cautions**   see notes above
**Contra-indications**   see notes above
**Side-effects**   see notes above
**Indications and dose**

> **Mild inflammatory skin disorders such as eczemas (but for over-the-counter preparations, see below); nappy rash** (see also section 13.2.2)
>
> Apply thinly 1–2 times daily

**Hydrocortisone** (Non-proprietary) PoM
Cream, hydrocortisone 0.5%, net price, 15 g = £1.45, 30 g = £2.90; 1%, 15 g = £1.16, 30 g = £2.32, 50 g = £3.87; 2.5%, 15 g = £19.74. Label: 28, counselling, application, see p. 561. Potency: mild
**Dental prescribing on NHS**  Hydrocortisone Cream 1% 15 g may be prescribed

Ointment, hydrocortisone 0.5%, net price 15 g = £2.83, 30 g = £4.90; 1%, 15 g = £1.29, 30 g = £2.58, 50 g = £4.30; 2.5%, 15 g = £21.25. Label: 28, counselling, application, see p. 561. Potency: mild
When hydrocortisone cream or ointment is prescribed and no strength is stated, the 1% strength should be supplied

◢**Over-the-counter hydrocortisone preparations**
Skin creams and ointments containing hydrocortisone (alone or with other ingredients) can be sold to the public for the treatment of allergic contact dermatitis, irritant dermatitis, insect bite reactions and mild to moderate eczema in children over 10 years, to be applied sparingly over the affected area 1–2 times daily for max. 1 week. Over-the-counter hydrocortisone preparations should not be sold without medical advice for children under 10 years or for pregnant women; they should **not** be sold for application to the face, anogenital region, broken or infected skin (including cold sores, acne, and athlete's foot); over-the-counter hydrocortisone preparations containing clotrimazole or miconazole nitrate can be sold to the public for treatment of athlete's foot and candidal intertrigo

◢**Proprietary hydrocortisone preparations**
**Dioderm®** (Dermal) PoM
Cream, hydrocortisone 0.1%, net price 30 g = £2.39. Label: 28, counselling, application, see p. 561. Potency: mild
**Excipients**  include cetostearyl alcohol, propylene glycol
**Note**  Although this contains only 0.1% hydrocortisone, the formulation is designed to provide a clinical activity comparable to that of Hydrocortisone Cream 1% BP

**Mildison®** (Astellas) PoM
Lipocream, hydrocortisone 1%, net price 30 g = £1.71. Label: 28, counselling, application, see p. 561. Potency: mild
**Excipients**  include benzyl alcohol, cetostearyl alcohol, hydroxybenzoates (parabens)

◀ **Compound preparations**

Compound preparations with coal tar, see section 13.5.2

**Alphaderm®** (Alliance) [PoM]
Cream, hydrocortisone 1%, urea 10%, net price 30 g = £2.38; 100 g = £7.03. Label: 28, counselling, application, see p. 561. Potency: moderate
Excipients none as listed in section 13.1.3

**Calmurid HC®** (Galderma) [PoM]
Cream, hydrocortisone 1%, urea 10%, lactic acid 5%, net price 100 g = £10.51. Label: 28, counselling, application, see p. 561. Potency: moderate
Excipients none as listed in section 13.1.3
Note If stinging occurs, manufacturer advises dilute to half-strength with aqueous cream for 1 week then transfer to undiluted preparation (but see section 13.1.1 for advice to avoid dilution where possible)

**Hydromol HC Intensive®** (Alliance) [PoM]
Cream, hydrocortisone 1%, urea 10%, net price 30 g = £2.38, 100 g = £7.03. Label: 28, counselling, application, see p. 561. Potency: moderate
Excipients none as listed in section 13.1.3

◀ **With antimicrobials**
See notes above for comment on compound preparations

**Canesten HC®** (Bayer Consumer Care) [PoM]
Cream, hydrocortisone 1%, clotrimazole 1%, net price 30 g = £2.42. Label: 28, counselling, application, see p. 561. Potency: mild
Excipients include benzyl alcohol, cetostearyl alcohol
Note A 15-g tube is on sale to the public for the treatment of athlete's foot and fungal infection of skin folds with associated inflammation in children 10–18 years

**Daktacort®** (Janssen) [PoM]
Cream, hydrocortisone 1%, miconazole nitrate 2%, net price 30 g = £2.49. Label: 28, counselling, application, see p. 561. Potency: mild
Excipients include butylated hydroxyanisole, disodium edetate
Cautions interactions: Appendix 1 (antifungals, imidazole)
Dental prescribing on NHS May be prescribed as Miconazole and Hydrocortisone Cream for max. 7 days
Note A 15-g tube is on sale to the public for the treatment of athlete's foot and candidal intertrigo in children 10–18 years
Ointment, hydrocortisone 1%, miconazole nitrate 2%, net price 30 g = £2.50. Label: 28, counselling, application, see p. 561. Potency: mild
Excipients none as listed in section 13.1.3
Cautions interactions: Appendix 1 (antifungals, imidazole)
Dental prescribing on NHS May be prescribed as Miconazole and Hydrocortisone Ointment for max. 7 days

**Fucidin H®** (LEO) [PoM]
Cream, hydrocortisone acetate 1%, fusidic acid 2%, net price 30 g = £5.02, 60 g = £10.04. Label: 28, counselling, application, see p. 561. Potency: mild
Excipients include butylated hydroxyanisole, cetyl alcohol, polysorbate 60, potassium sorbate

**Nystaform-HC®** (Typharm) [PoM]
Cream, hydrocortisone 0.5%, nystatin 100 000 units/g, chlorhexidine hydrochloride 1%, net price 30 g = £2.66. Label: 28, counselling, application, see p. 561. Potency: mild
Excipients include benzyl alcohol, cetostearyl alcohol, polysorbate '60'

Ointment, hydrocortisone 1%, nystatin 100 000 units/g, chlorhexidine acetate 1%, net price 30 g = £2.66. Label: 28, counselling, application, see p. 561. Potency: mild
Excipients none as listed in section 13.1.3

**Timodine®** (Alliance) [PoM]
Cream, hydrocortisone 0.5%, nystatin 100 000 units/g, benzalkonium chloride solution 0.2%, dimeticone '350' 10%, net price 30 g = £2.80. Label: 28, counselling, application, see p. 561. Potency: mild
Excipients include butylated hydroxyanisole, cetostearyl alcohol, hydroxybenzoates (parabens), sodium metabisulfite, sorbic acid

▌ **HYDROCORTISONE BUTYRATE**

**Cautions** see notes above
**Contra-indications** see notes above
**Side-effects** see notes above
**Indications and dose**

**Severe inflammatory skin disorders such as eczemas unresponsive to less potent corticosteroids, psoriasis** see notes above
    Child 1–18 years apply thinly 1–2 times daily

**Locoid®** (Astellas) [PoM]
Cream, hydrocortisone butyrate 0.1%, net price 30 g = £1.60, 100 g = £4.93. Label: 28, counselling, application, see p. 561. Potency: potent
Excipients include cetostearyl alcohol, hydroxybenzoates (parabens)

Lipocream, hydrocortisone butyrate 0.1%, net price 30 g = £1.69, 100 g = £5.17. Label: 28, counselling, application, see p. 561. Potency: potent
Excipients include benzyl alcohol, cetostearyl alcohol, hydroxybenzoates (parabens)
Note For bland cream basis see *Lipobase®*, section 13.2.1

Ointment, hydrocortisone butyrate 0.1%, net price 30 g = £1.60, 100 g = £4.93. Label: 28, counselling, application, see p. 561. Potency: potent
Excipients none as listed in section 13.1.3

Scalp lotion, hydrocortisone butyrate 0.1%, in an aqueous isopropyl alcohol basis, net price 100 mL = £6.83. Label: 15, 28, counselling, application, see p. 561. Potency: potent
Excipients none as listed in section 13.1.3

**Locoid Crelo®** (Astellas) [PoM]
Lotion (topical emulsion), hydrocortisone butyrate 0.1% in a water-miscible basis, net price 100 g (with applicator nozzle) = £5.91. Label: 28, counselling, application, see p. 561. Potency: potent
Excipients include butylated hydroxytoluene, cetostearyl alcohol, hydroxybenzoates (parabens), propylene glycol

**13**
**Skin**

# ALCLOMETASONE DIPROPIONATE

**Cautions** see notes above
**Contra-indications** see notes above
**Side-effects** see notes above
**Licensed use** licensed for use in children (age range not specified by manufacturer)
**Indications and dose**

Inflammatory skin disorders such as eczemas
Apply thinly 1–2 times daily

**Modrasone®** (TEVA UK) [PoM]
Cream, alclometasone dipropionate 0.05%, net price 50 g = £2.68. Label: 28, counselling, application, see p. 561. Potency: moderate
Excipients include cetostearyl alcohol, chlorocresol, propylene glycol

# BECLOMETASONE DIPROPIONATE
(Beclometasone dipropionate)

**Cautions** see notes above
**Contra-indications** see notes above
**Side-effects** see notes above
**Licensed use** not licensed for use in children under 1 year
**Indications and dose**

Severe inflammatory skin disorders such as eczemas unresponsive to less potent corticosteroids, psoriasis see notes above
Apply thinly 1–2 times daily

**Beclometasone** (Non-proprietary) [PoM]
Cream, beclometasone dipropionate 0.025%, net price 30 g = £68.00. Label: 28, counselling, application, see p. 561. Potency: potent

Ointment, beclometasone dipropionate 0.025%, net price 30 g = £68.00. Label: 28, counselling, application, see p. 561. Potency: potent

# BETAMETHASONE ESTERS

**Cautions** see notes above; use of more than 100 g per week of 0.1% preparation likely to cause adrenal suppression
**Contra-indications** see notes above
**Side-effects** see notes above
**Licensed use** *Betacap®*, Betamethasone and clioquinol preparations, *Betnovate®*, and *Betnovate-RD®* not licensed for use in children under 1 year; *Bettamousse®* and *Fucibet® Lipid Cream* not licensed for use in children under 6 years; Betamethasone and neomycin preparations not licensed for use in children under 2 years; *Lotriderm®* not licensed for use in children under 12 years; *all other preparations* licensed for use in children (age range not specified by manufacturer)
**Indications and dose**

Severe inflammatory skin disorders such as eczemas unresponsive to less potent corticosteroids, psoriasis see notes above
Apply thinly 1–2 times daily

**Betamethasone Valerate** (Non-proprietary) [PoM]
Cream, betamethasone (as valerate) 0.1%, net price 30 g = £2.54, 100 g = £8.47. Label: 28, counselling, application, see p. 561. Potency: potent

Ointment, betamethasone (as valerate) 0.1%, net price 30 g = £2.80, 100 g = £9.33. Label: 28, counselling, application, see p. 561. Potency: potent

**Betacap®** (Dermal) [PoM]
Scalp application, betamethasone (as valerate) 0.1% in a water-miscible basis containing coconut oil derivative, net price 100 mL = £3.75. Label: 15, 28, counselling, application, see p. 561. Potency: potent
Excipients none as listed in section 13.1.3

**Betnovate®** (GSK) [PoM]
Cream, betamethasone (as valerate) 0.1% in a water-miscible basis, net price 30 g = £1.43, 100 g = £4.05. Label: 28, counselling, application, see p. 561. Potency: potent
Excipients include cetostearyl alcohol, chlorocresol

Ointment, betamethasone (as valerate) 0.1% in an anhydrous paraffin basis, net price 30 g = £1.43, 100 g = £4.05. Label: 28, counselling, application, see p. 561. Potency: potent
Excipients none as listed in section 13.1.3

Lotion, betamethasone (as valerate) 0.1%, net price 100 mL = £4.58. Label: 28, counselling, application, see p. 561. Potency: potent
Excipients include cetostearyl alcohol, hydroxybenzoates (parabens)

Scalp application, betamethasone (as valerate) 0.1% in a water-miscible basis, net price 100 mL = £4.99. Label: 15, 28, counselling, application, see p. 561. Potency: potent
Excipients none as listed in section 13.1.3

**Betnovate-RD®** (GSK) [PoM]
Cream, betamethasone (as valerate) 0.025% in a water-miscible basis (1 in 4 dilution of *Betnovate®* cream), net price 100 g = £3.15. Label: 28, counselling, application, see p. 561. Potency: moderate
Excipients include cetostearyl alcohol, chlorocresol

Ointment, betamethasone (as valerate) 0.025% in an anhydrous paraffin basis (1 in 4 dilution of *Betnovate®* ointment), net price 100 g = £3.15. Label: 28, counselling, application, see p. 561. Potency: moderate
Excipients none as listed in section 13.1.3

**Bettamousse®** (UCB Pharma) [PoM]
Foam (= scalp application), betamethasone valerate 0.12% (≡ betamethasone 0.1%), net price 100 g = £9.75. Label: 28, counselling, application, see p. 561. Potency: potent
Excipients include cetyl alcohol, polysorbate 60, propylene glycol, stearyl alcohol
Note Flammable

**13 Skin**

**Diprosone®** (Schering-Plough) [PoM]

Cream, betamethasone (as dipropionate) 0.05%, net price 30 g = £2.16, 100 g = £6.12. Label: 28, counselling, application, see p. 561. Potency: potent
Excipients include cetostearyl alcohol, chlorocresol

Ointment, betamethasone (as dipropionate) 0.05%, net price 30 g = £2.16, 100 g = £6.12. Label: 28, counselling, application, see p. 561. Potency: potent
Excipients none as listed in section 13.1.3

Lotion, betamethasone (as dipropionate) 0.05%, net price 30 mL = £2.73, 100 mL = £7.80. Label: 28, counselling, application, see p. 561. Potency: potent
Excipients none as listed in section 13.1.3

◀**With salicylic acid**
See notes above for comment on compound preparations
For prescribing information on salicylic acid, see p. 573

**Diprosalic®** (Schering-Plough) [PoM]

Ointment, betamethasone (as dipropionate) 0.05%, salicylic acid 3%, net price 30 g = £3.18, 100 g = £9.14. Label: 28, counselling, application, see p. 561. Potency: potent
Excipients none as listed in section 13.1.3
Dose

> Apply thinly 1–2 times daily

Scalp application, betamethasone (as dipropionate) 0.05%, salicylic acid 2%, in an alcoholic basis, net price 100 mL = £10.10. Label: 28, counselling, application, see p. 561. Potency: potent
Excipients include disodium edetate
Dose

> Apply a few drops 1–2 times daily

◀**With antimicrobials**
See notes above for comment on compound preparations

**Betamethasone and clioquinol** (Non-proprietary) [PoM]

Cream, betamethasone (as valerate) 0.1%, clioquinol 3%, net price 30 g = £9.48. Label: 28, counselling, application, see p. 561. Potency: potent
Excipients may include cetostearyl alcohol, chlorocresol
Note Stains clothing

Ointment, betamethasone (as valerate) 0.1%, clioquinol 3%, net price 30 g = £9.48. Label: 28, counselling, application, see p. 561. Potency: potent
Note Stains clothing

**Betamethasone and neomycin** (Non-proprietary) [PoM]

Cream, betamethasone (as valerate) 0.1%, neomycin sulfate 0.5%, net price 30 g = £9.48, 100 g = £28.01. Label: 28, counselling, application, see p. 561. Potency: potent
Excipients may include cetostearyl alcohol, chlorocresol

Ointment, betamethasone (as valerate) 0.1%, neomycin sulfate 0.5%, net price 30 g = £9.48, 100 g = £28.01. Label: 28, counselling, application, see p. 561. Potency: potent

**Fucibet®** (LEO) [PoM]

Cream, betamethasone (as valerate) 0.1%, fusidic acid 2%, net price 30 g = £5.32, 60 g = £10.63. Label: 28, counselling, application, see p. 561. Potency: potent
Excipients include cetostearyl alcohol, chlorocresol

Lipid cream, betamethasone (as valerate) 0.1%, fusidic acid 2%, net price 30 g = £5.62. Label: 28, counselling, application, see p. 561. Potency: potent
Excipients include cetostearyl alcohol, hydroxybenzoates (parabens)

**Lotriderm®** (TEVA UK) [PoM]

Cream, betamethasone dipropionate 0.064% (≡ betamethasone 0.05%), clotrimazole 1%, net price 30 g = £6.34. Label: 28, counselling, application, see p. 561. Potency: potent
Excipients include benzyl alcohol, cetostearyl alcohol, propylene glycol

## ■ CLOBETASOL PROPIONATE

**Cautions** see notes above

**Contra-indications** see notes above

**Side-effects** see notes above

**Licensed use** *Dermovate®* not licensed for use in children under 1 year; Clobetasol with neomycin and nystatin preparations not licensed for use in children under 2 years

**Indications and dose**

> Short-term treatment only of severe resistant inflammatory skin disorders such as recalcitrant eczemas unresponsive to less potent corticosteroids, psoriasis see notes above
>
> > Apply thinly 1–2 times daily for up to 4 weeks

**Dermovate®** (GSK) [PoM]

Cream, clobetasol propionate 0.05%, net price 30 g = £2.69, 100 g = £7.90. Label: 28, counselling, application, see p. 561. Potency: very potent
Excipients include beeswax (or beeswax substitute), cetostearyl alcohol, chlorocresol, propylene glycol

Ointment, clobetasol propionate 0.05%, net price 30 g = £2.69, 100 g = £7.90. Label: 28, counselling, application, see p. 561. Potency: very potent
Excipients include propylene glycol

Scalp application, clobetasol propionate 0.05%, in a thickened alcoholic basis, net price 30 mL = £3.07, 100 mL = £10.42. Label: 15, 28, counselling, application, see p. 561. Potency: very potent
Excipients none as listed in section 13.1.3

◀**With antimicrobials**
See notes above for comment on compound preparations

**Clobetasol with neomycin and nystatin** (Non-proprietary) [PoM]

Cream, clobetasol propionate 0.05%, neomycin sulfate 0.5%, nystatin 100 000 units/g, net price 30 g = £64.00. Label: 28, counselling, application, see p. 561. Potency: very potent

Ointment, clobetasol propionate 0.05%, neomycin sulfate 0.5%, nystatin 100 000 units/g, in a paraffin basis, net price 30 g = £64.00. Label: 28, counselling, application, see p. 561. Potency: very potent

**13**

**Skin**

## CLOBETASONE BUTYRATE

**Cautions**  see notes above
**Contra-indications**  see notes above
**Side-effects**  see notes above
**Licensed use**  licensed for use in children (age range not specified by manufacturer)
**Indications and dose**

> Eczemas and dermatitis of all types; maintenance between courses of more potent corticosteroids
>> Apply thinly 1–2 times daily

[1]**Eumovate**® (GSK) PoM
Cream, clobetasone butyrate 0.05%, net price 30 g = £1.86, 100 g = £5.44. Label: 28, counselling, application, see p. 561. Potency: moderate
Excipients  include beeswax substitute, cetostearyl alcohol, chlorocresol

Ointment, clobetasone butyrate 0.05%, net price 30 g = £1.86, 100 g = £5.44. Label: 28, counselling, application, see p. 561. Potency: moderate
Excipients  none as listed in section 13.1.3

◢With antimicrobials
See notes above for comment on compound preparations

**Trimovate**® (GSK) PoM
Cream, clobetasone butyrate 0.05%, oxytetracycline 3% (as calcium salt), nystatin 100 000 units/g, net price 30 g = £3.29. Label: 28, counselling, application, see p. 561. Potency: moderate
Excipients  include cetostearyl alcohol, chlorocresol, sodium metabisulfite
Note  Stains clothing

## DIFLUCORTOLONE VALERATE

**Cautions**  see notes above
**Contra-indications**  see notes above
**Side-effects**  see notes above
**Licensed use**  *Nerisone*® licensed for use in children (age range not specified by manufacturer); *Nerisone Forte*® not licensed for use in children under 4 years
**Indications and dose**

> Severe inflammatory skin disorders such as eczemas unresponsive to less potent corticosteroids; high strength (0.3%), short-term treatment of severe exacerbations, psoriasis see notes above
>> Apply thinly 1–2 times daily for up to 4 weeks (0.1% preparations) or 2 weeks (0.3% preparations), reducing strength as condition responds

**Nerisone**® (Meadow) PoM
Cream, diflucortolone valerate 0.1%, net price 30 g = £1.59. Label: 28, counselling, application, see p. 561. Potency: potent
Excipients  include disodium edetate, hydroxybenzoates (parabens), stearyl alcohol

Oily cream, diflucortolone valerate 0.1%, net price 30 g = £2.56. Label: 28, counselling, application, see p. 561. Potency: potent
Excipients  include beeswax

Ointment, diflucortolone valerate 0.1%, net price 30 g = £1.59. Label: 28, counselling, application, see p. 561. Potency: potent
Excipients  none as listed in section 13.1.3

**Nerisone Forte**® (Meadow) PoM
Oily cream, diflucortolone valerate 0.3%, net price 15 g = £2.09. Label: 28, counselling, application, see p. 561. Potency: very potent
Excipients  include beeswax

Ointment, diflucortolone valerate 0.3%, net price 15 g = £2.09. Label: 28, counselling, application, see p. 561. Potency: very potent
Excipients  none as listed in section 13.1.3

## FLUDROXYCORTIDE
(Flurandrenolone)

**Cautions**  see notes above
**Contra-indications**  see notes above
**Side-effects**  see notes above
**Licensed use**  licensed for use in children (age range not specified by manufacturer)
**Indications and dose**

> Inflammatory skin disorders such as eczemas
>> Apply thinly 1–2 times daily

**Haelan**® (Typharm) PoM
Cream, fludroxycortide 0.0125%, net price 60 g = £3.26. Label: 28, counselling, application, see p. 561. Potency: moderate
Excipients  include cetyl alcohol, propylene glycol

Ointment, fludroxycortide 0.0125%, net price 60 g = £3.26. Label: 28, counselling, application, see p. 561. Potency: moderate
Excipients  include beeswax, cetyl alcohol, polysorbate

Tape, polythene adhesive film impregnated with fludroxycortide 4 micrograms /cm$^2$, net price 7.5 cm × 50 cm = £9.27, 7.5 cm × 200 cm = £24.95
Dose
> Chronic localised recalcitrant dermatoses (but not acute or weeping)
>> Cut tape to fit lesion, apply to clean, dry skin shorn of hair, usually for 12 hours daily

## FLUOCINOLONE ACETONIDE

**Cautions**  see notes above
**Contra-indications**  see notes above
**Side-effects**  see notes above
**Licensed use**  not licensed for use in children under 1 year
**Indications and dose**

> Severe inflammatory skin disorders such as eczemas, psoriasis see notes above
>> Apply thinly 1–2 times daily, reducing strength as condition responds

**Synalar**® (GP Pharma) PoM
Cream, fluocinolone acetonide 0.025%, net price 30 g = £4.14, 100 g = £11.75. Label: 28, counselling, application, see p. 561. Potency: potent
Excipients  include benzyl alcohol, cetostearyl alcohol, polysorbates, propylene glycol

1. Cream can be sold to the public for short-term symptomatic treatment and control of patches of eczema and dermatitis (but not seborrhoeic dermatitis) in children over 12 years provided pack does not contain more than 15 g

13 Skin

Gel, fluocinolone acetonide 0.025%, net price 30 g = £5.56. For use on scalp and other hairy areas. Label: 28, counselling, application, see p. 561. Potency: potent
**Excipients** include hydroxybenzoates (parabens), propylene glycol

Ointment, fluocinolone acetonide 0.025%, net price 30 g = £4.14, 100 g = £11.75. Label: 28, counselling, application, see p. 561. Potency: potent
**Excipients** include propylene glycol, wool fat

**Synalar 1 in 4 Dilution**® (GP Pharma) ℗ₒₘ
Cream, fluocinolone acetonide 0.00625%, net price 50 g = £4.84. Label: 28, counselling, application, see p. 561. Potency: moderate
**Excipients** include benzyl alcohol, cetostearyl alcohol, polysorbates, propylene glycol

Ointment, fluocinolone acetonide 0.00625%, net price 50 g = £4.84. Label: 28, counselling, application, see p. 561. Potency: moderate
**Excipients** include propylene glycol, wool fat

**Synalar 1 in 10 Dilution**® (GP Pharma) ℗ₒₘ
Cream, fluocinolone acetonide 0.0025%, net price 50 g = £4.58. Label: 28, counselling, application, see p. 561. Potency: mild
**Excipients** include benzyl alcohol, cetostearyl alcohol, polysorbates, propylene glycol

◀**With antibacterials**
See notes above for comment on compound preparations

**Synalar C**® (GP Pharma) ℗ₒₘ
Cream, fluocinolone acetonide 0.025%, clioquinol 3%, net price 15 g = £2.66. Label: 28, counselling, application, see p. 561. Potency: potent
**Excipients** include cetostearyl alcohol, disodium edetate, hydroxybenzoates (parabens), polysorbates, propylene glycol

Ointment, fluocinolone acetonide 0.025%, clioquinol 3%, net price 15 g = £2.66. Label: 28, counselling, application, see p. 561. Potency: potent.
**Note** stains clothing
**Excipients** include propylene glycol, wool fat

**Synalar N**® (GP Pharma) ℗ₒₘ
Cream, fluocinolone acetonide 0.025%, neomycin sulfate 0.5%, net price 30 g = £4.36. Label: 28, counselling, application, see p. 561. Potency: potent
**Excipients** include cetostearyl alcohol, hydroxybenzoates (parabens), polysorbates, propylene glycol

Ointment, fluocinolone acetonide 0.025%, neomycin sulfate 0.5%, in a greasy basis, net price 30 g = £4.36. Label: 28, counselling, application, see p. 561. Potency: potent
**Excipients** include propylene glycol, wool fat

## ▌FLUOCINONIDE

**Cautions** see notes above
**Contra-indications** see notes above
**Side-effects** see notes above
**Licensed use** not licensed for use in children under 1 year
**Indications and dose**

Severe inflammatory skin disorders such as eczemas unresponsive to less potent corticosteroids, psoriasis see notes above

Apply thinly 1–2 times daily

**Metosyn**® (GP Pharma) ℗ₒₘ
FAPG cream, fluocinonide 0.05%, net price 25 g = £3.96, 100 g = £13.34. Label: 28, counselling, application, see p. 561. Potency: potent
**Excipients** include propylene glycol

Ointment, fluocinonide 0.05%, net price 25 g = £3.50, 100 g = £13.15. Label: 28, counselling, application, see p. 561. Potency: potent
**Excipients** include propylene glycol, wool fat

## ▌FLUOCORTOLONE

**Cautions** see notes above
**Contra-indications** see notes above
**Side-effects** see notes above
**Licensed use** licensed for use in children (age range not specified by manufacturer)
**Indications and dose**

Severe inflammatory skin disorders such as eczemas unresponsive to less potent corticosteroids, psoriasis see notes above

Apply thinly 1–2 times daily

**Ultralanum Plain**® (Meadow) ℗ₒₘ
Cream, fluocortolone caproate 0.25%, fluocortolone pivalate 0.25%, net price 50 g = £2.95. Label: 28, counselling, application, see p. 561. Potency: moderate
**Excipients** include disodium edetate, fragrance, hydroxybenzoates (parabens), stearyl alcohol

Ointment, fluocortolone 0.25%, fluocortolone caproate 0.25%, net price 50 g = £2.95. Label: 28, counselling, application, see p. 561. Potency: moderate
**Excipients** include wool fat, fragrance

## ▌FLUTICASONE PROPIONATE

**Cautions** see notes above
**Contra-indications** see notes above
**Side-effects** see notes above
**Licensed use** not licensed for use in children under 3 months
**Indications and dose**

Inflammatory skin disorders such as dermatitis and eczemas unresponsive to less potent corticosteroids, psoriasis see notes above

Apply thinly 1–2 times daily

**Cutivate**® (GSK) ℗ₒₘ
Cream, fluticasone propionate 0.05%, net price 15 g = £2.27, 30 g = £4.24. Label: 28, counselling, application, see p. 561. Potency: potent
**Excipients** include cetostearyl alcohol, imidurea, propylene glycol

Ointment, fluticasone propionate 0.005%, net price 15 g = £2.27, 30 g = £4.24. Label: 28, counselling, application, see p. 561. Potency: potent
**Excipients** include propylene glycol

## ▌MOMETASONE FUROATE

**Cautions** see notes above
**Contra-indications** see notes above
**Side-effects** see notes above
**Licensed use** not licensed for use in children under 2 years

**13**

**Skin**

### Indications and dose

> Severe inflammatory skin disorders such as eczemas unresponsive to less potent corticosteroids, psoriasis see notes above
>
> Apply thinly once daily (to scalp in case of lotion)

**Mometasone** (Non-proprietary) `PoM`

Ointment, mometasone furoate 0.1%, net price 30 g = £4.45, 100 g = £12.28. Label: 28, counselling, application, see p. 561. Potency: potent

**Elocon®** (Schering-Plough) `PoM`

Cream, mometasone furoate 0.1%, net price 30 g = £4.36, 100 g = £12.58. Label: 28, counselling, application, see p. 561. Potency: potent

Excipients  include beeswax, propylene glycol, stearyl alcohol

Ointment, mometasone furoate 0.1%, net price 30 g = £4.32, 100 g = £12.44. Label: 28, counselling, application, see p. 561. Potency: potent

Excipients  include beeswax, propylene glycol

Scalp lotion, mometasone furoate 0.1% in an aqueous isopropyl alcohol basis, net price 30 mL = £4.36. Label: 28, counselling, application, see p. 561. Potency: potent

Excipients  include propylene glycol

### ▐ TRIAMCINOLONE ACETONIDE

**Cautions**  see notes above

**Contra-indications**  see notes above

**Side-effects**  see notes above

**Licensed use**  *Aureocort®* not licensed for use in children under 8 years

### Indications and dose

> Severe inflammatory skin disorders such as eczemas unresponsive to less potent corticosteroids, psoriasis see notes above
>
> Apply thinly 1–2 times daily

◀**With antimicrobials**

See notes above for comment on compound preparations

**Aureocort®** (Mercury) `PoM`

Ointment, triamcinolone acetonide 0.1%, chlortetracycline hydrochloride 3%, in an anhydrous greasy basis containing wool fat and white soft paraffin, net price 15 g = £3.51. Label: 28, counselling, application, see p. 561. Potency: potent

Excipients  include wool fat

Note  Stains clothing

## 13.5  Preparations for eczema and psoriasis

13.5.1  **Preparations for eczema**

13.5.2  **Preparations for psoriasis**

13.5.3  **Drugs affecting the immune response**

## 13.5.1  Preparations for eczema

The main types of eczema (dermatitis) in children are atopic, irritant and allergic contact; different types may co-exist. *Atopic eczema* is the most common type and it usually involves dry skin as well as infection and lichenification caused by scratching and rubbing. *Seborrhoeic dermatitis* (see below) is also common in infants.

Management of eczema involves the removal or treatment of contributory factors; known or suspected irritants and contact allergens should be avoided. Rarely, ingredients in topical medicinal products may sensitise the skin (section 13.1.3); *BNF for Children* lists active ingredients together with excipients that have been associated with skin sensitisation.

Skin dryness and the consequent irritant eczema requires **emollients** (section 13.2.1) applied regularly (at least twice daily) and liberally to the affected area; this can be supplemented with bath or shower emollients. The use of emollients should continue even if the eczema improves or if other treatment is being used.

**Topical corticosteroids** (section 13.4) are also required in the management of eczema; the potency of the corticosteroid should be appropriate to the severity and site of the condition, and the age of the child. Mild corticosteroids are generally used on the face and on flexures; the more potent corticosteroids are generally required for use on lichenified areas of eczema or for severe eczema on the scalp, limbs, and trunk. Treatment should be reviewed regularly, especially if a potent corticosteroid is required. In children with frequent flares (2–3 per month), a topical corticosteroid can be applied on 2 consecutive days each week to prevent further flares.

Bandages (including those containing **zinc** and **ichthammol**) are sometimes applied over topical corticosteroids or emollients to treat eczema of the limbs. Dry-wrap dressings can be used to provide a physical barrier to help prevent scratching and improve retention of emollients. Wet elasticated viscose stockinette is used for 'wet-wrap' bandaging over topical corticosteroids or emollients to cool the skin and relieve itching, but there is an increased risk of infection and excessive absorption of the corticosteroid; 'wet-wrap' bandaging should be used under specialist supervision.

For details of elasticated viscose stockinette tubular bandages and garments, and silk clothing, see BNF section A5.8.3

For the role of topical **pimecrolimus** and **tacrolimus** in atopic eczema, see section 13.5.3.

**Infection**  Bacterial infection (commonly with *Staphylococcus aureus* and occasionally with *Streptococcus pyogenes*) can exacerbate eczema. A topical antibacterial (section 13.10.1) may be used for small areas of mild infection; treatment should be limited to a short course (typically 1 week) to reduce the risk of drug resistance or skin sensitisation. Associated eczema is treated simultaneously with a topical corticosteroid which can be combined with a topical antimicrobial.

Eczema involving moderate to severe, widespread, or recurrent infection requires the use of a systemic antibacterial (section 5.1, table 1) that is active against the infecting organism. Preparations that combine an antiseptic with an emollient application (section 13.2.1) and with a bath emollient (section 13.2.1.1) can also be used; antiseptic shampoos (section 13.9) can be used on the scalp.

*Intertriginous eczema* commonly involves candida and bacteria; it is best treated with a mild or moderately potent topical corticosteroid combined with a suitable antimicrobial drug. For the treatment of nappy rash, see section 13.2.2.

Widespread *herpes simplex infection* may complicate atopic eczema (eczema herpeticum) and treatment

*13 Skin*

under specialist supervision with a systemic antiviral drug (section 5.3.2.1) is indicated. Secondary bacterial infection often exacerbates eczema herpeticum.

The management of *seborrhoeic dermatitis* is described below.

**Management of other features of eczema**  *Lichenification*, which results from repeated scratching, is treated initially with a potent corticosteroid. Bandages containing **ichthammol** (to reduce pruritus) and other substances such as **zinc oxide** can be applied over the corticosteroid or emollient. **Coal tar** (section 13.5.2) and ichthammol can be useful in some cases of *chronic eczema*. *Discoid eczema*, with thickened plaques in chronic atopic eczema, is usually treated with a topical antiseptic preparation, a potent topical corticosteroid, and paste bandages containing zinc oxide and ichthammol.

A *non-sedating* antihistamine (section 3.4.1) may be of some value in relieving severe itching or urticaria associated with eczema. A *sedating* antihistamine (section 3.4.1) can be used at night if itching causes sleep disturbance, but a large dose may be needed and drowsiness may persist on the following day.

*Exudative ('weeping') eczema* requires a potent corticosteroid initially; infection may also be present and require specific treatment (see above). **Potassium permanganate** solution (1 in 10 000) can be used as a soak in exudating eczema for its antiseptic and astringent effects; treatment should be stopped when exudation stops.

*Severe refractory eczema* is best managed under specialist supervision; it may require phototherapy or drugs that act on the immune system (section 13.5.3).

**Seborrhoeic dermatitis**  *Seborrhoeic dermatitis* (*seborrhoeic eczema*) is associated with species of the yeast *Malassezia*. *Infantile seborrhoeic dermatitis* affects particularly the body folds, nappy area and scalp; it is treated with emollients and mild topical corticosteroids with suitable antimicrobials. Infantile seborrhoeic dermatitis affecting the scalp (*cradle cap*) is treated by hydrating the scalp using natural oils and the use of mild shampoo (section 13.9).

In older children, seborrhoeic dermatitis affects the scalp, paranasal areas, and eyebrows. Shampoos active against the yeast (including those containing ketoconazole and coal tar, section 13.9) and combinations of mild topical corticosteroids with suitable antimicrobials (section 13.4) are used to treat older children.

## ICHTHAMMOL

**Side-effects**  skin irritation

**Licensed use**  no information available

**Indications and dose**

> **Chronic lichenified eczema**
>
> > **Child 1–18 years** apply 1–3 times daily

**Ichthammol Ointment, BP 1980**
Ointment, ichthammol 10%, yellow soft paraffin 45%, wool fat 45%

**Zinc and Ichthammol Cream, BP**
Cream, ichthammol 5%, cetostearyl alcohol 3%, wool fat 10%, in zinc cream
Available from 'special-order' manufacturers or specialist importing companies, see p. 823

## Medicated bandages

Zinc paste bandages are used with **coal tar** or **ichthammol** in chronic lichenified skin conditions such as chronic eczema (ichthammol often being preferred since its action is considered to be milder). They are also used with **calamine** in milder eczematous skin conditions.

For information on available medicated bandages and stockings, see BNF Appendix 5.

## 13.5.2 Preparations for psoriasis

Psoriasis is characterised by epidermal thickening and scaling. It commonly affects extensor surfaces and the scalp. For mild psoriasis, reassurance and treatment with an emollient may be all that is necessary. *Guttate psoriasis* is a distinctive form of psoriasis that characteristically occurs in children and young adults, often following a streptococcal throat infection or tonsillitis.

Occasionally psoriasis is provoked or exacerbated by drugs such as lithium, chloroquine and hydroxychloroquine, beta-blockers, non-steroidal anti-inflammatory drugs, and ACE inhibitors. Psoriasis may not occur until the drug has been taken for weeks or months.

**Emollients** (section 13.2.1), in addition to their effects on dryness, scaling and cracking, may have an antiproliferative effect in psoriasis. They are particularly useful in *inflammatory psoriasis* and in *chronic stable plaque psoriasis*.

For *chronic stable plaque psoriasis* on extensor surfaces of trunk and limbs preparations containing **coal tar** are moderately effective, but the smell is unacceptable to some children. **Vitamin D** and its analogues are effective and cosmetically acceptable alternatives to preparations containing coal tar or dithranol. **Dithranol** is an effective topical antipsoriatic agent but it irritates and stains the skin and it should be used only under specialist supervision. Adverse effects of dithranol are minimised by using a 'short-contact technique' (see below) and by starting with low concentration preparations. **Tazarotene**, a topical retinoid for the treatment of mild to moderate plaque psoriasis, is not recommended for use in children under 18 years. These medications can irritate the skin particularly in the flexures and they are not suitable for the more inflammatory forms of psoriasis; their use should be suspended during an inflammatory phase of psoriasis. The efficacy and the irritancy of each substance varies between patients. If a substance irritates significantly, it should be stopped or the concentration reduced; if it is tolerated, its effects should be assessed after 4 to 6 weeks and treatment continued if it is effective.

Widespread *unstable psoriasis* of erythrodermic or generalised pustular type requires urgent specialist assessment. Initial topical treatment should be limited to using emollients frequently and generously. More localised acute or subacute *inflammatory psoriasis* with hot, spreading or itchy lesions, should be treated topically with emollients or with a corticosteroid of moderate potency.

*Scalp psoriasis* is usually scaly, and the scale may be thick and adherent. This requires softening with an emollient ointment, cream, or oil and usually combined with **salicylic acid** as a keratolytic.

Some preparations for psoriasis affecting the scalp combine salicylic acid with coal tar or **sulfur**. The preparation should be applied generously and left on for at least an hour, often more conveniently overnight, before washing it off. If a corticosteroid lotion or gel is required (e.g. for itch), it can be used in the morning.

*Flexural psoriasis* can be managed with short-term use of a mild potency topical corticosteroid. **Calcitriol** or **tacalcitol** can be used in the longer term; **calcipotriol** is more likely to cause irritation in flexures and should be avoided. Low-strength tar preparations can also be used.

*Facial psoriasis* can be treated with short-term use of a mild topical corticosteroid; if this is ineffective, calcitriol, tacalcitol, or a low-strength tar preparation can be used.

**Calcipotriol** and **tacalcitol** are analogues of vitamin D that affect cell division and differentiation. **Calcitriol** is an active form of vitamin D. Vitamin D and its analogues are used as first-line treatment for plaque psoriasis; they do not smell or stain and they may be more acceptable than tar or dithranol products. Of the vitamin D analogues, tacalcitol and calcitriol are less likely to irritate.

**Coal tar** has anti-inflammatory properties that are useful in chronic plaque psoriasis; it also has antiscaling properties. Contact of coal tar products with normal skin is not normally harmful and preparations containing coal tar can be used for widespread small lesions; however, irritation, contact allergy, and sterile folliculitis can occur. Leave-on preparations that remain in contact with the skin, such as creams or ointments, containing up to 6% coal tar may be used on children 1 month to 2 years; leave-on preparations containing coal tar 10% may be used on children over 2 years with more severe psoriasis. Tar baths and tar shampoos (see section 13.9) may also be helpful.

**Dithranol** is effective for chronic plaque psoriasis. Its major disadvantages are irritation (for which individual susceptibility varies) and staining of skin and of clothing. It should be applied to chronic extensor plaques only, carefully avoiding normal skin. Dithranol is not generally suitable for widespread small lesions nor should it be used in the flexures or on the face. Treatment should be started with a low concentration such as dithranol 0.1%, and the strength increased gradually every few days up to 3%, according to tolerance. Proprietary preparations are more suitable for home use; they are usually washed off after 20–30 minutes ('short contact' technique). Specialist nurses may apply intensive treatment with dithranol paste which is covered by stockinette dressings and usually retained overnight. Dithranol should be discontinued if even a low concentration causes acute inflammation; continued use can result in the psoriasis becoming unstable. When applying dithranol, hands should be protected by gloves or they should be washed thoroughly afterwards.

A topical **corticosteroid** (section 13.4) is not generally suitable for long-term use or as the sole treatment of extensive chronic plaque psoriasis; any early improvement is not usually maintained and there is a risk of the condition deteriorating or of precipitating an unstable form of psoriasis e.g. erythrodermic psoriasis or generalised pustular psoriasis on withdrawal. Topical use of potent corticosteroids on widespread psoriasis can also lead to systemic as well as local side-effects. However, topical corticosteroids used short-term may be appropriate to treat psoriasis in specific sites such as the face

or flexures with a mild corticosteroid, and psoriasis of the scalp, palms, and soles with a potent corticosteroid. Very potent topical corticosteroids should only be used under specialist supervision.

Combining the use of a corticosteroid with another specific topical treatment may be beneficial in chronic plaque psoriasis; the drugs may be used separately at different times of the day or used together in a single formulation. *Eczema* co-existing with psoriasis may be treated with a corticosteroid, or coal tar, or both.

**Phototherapy**   Phototherapy is available in specialist centres under the supervision of a dermatologist. Narrow band ultraviolet B (UVB) radiation is usually effective for *chronic stable psoriasis* and for *guttate psoriasis*. It can be considered for children with moderately severe psoriasis in whom topical treatment has failed, but it may irritate inflammatory psoriasis. The use of phototherapy and photochemotherapy in children is limited by concerns over carcinogenicity and premature ageing.

**Photochemotherapy** combining long-wave ultraviolet A radiation with a psoralen (PUVA) is available in specialist centres under the supervision of a dermatologist. The psoralen, which enhances the effect of irradiation, is administered either by mouth or topically. PUVA is effective in most forms of psoriasis, including the *localised palmoplantar pustular psoriasis*. Early adverse effects include phototoxicity and pruritus. Higher cumulative doses exaggerate skin ageing, increase the risk of dysplastic and neoplastic skin lesions especially squamous cancer, and pose a theoretical risk of cataracts.

Phototherapy combined with coal tar, dithranol, topical vitamin D or vitamin D analogues, or oral acitretin, allows reduction of the cumulative dose of phototherapy required to treat psoriasis.

**Systemic treatment**   Systemic treatment is required for severe, resistant, unstable or complicated forms of psoriasis, and it should be initiated only under specialist supervision. Systemic drugs for psoriasis include acitretin and drugs that affect the immune response (section 13.5.3).

**Acitretin**, a metabolite of etretinate, is a retinoid (vitamin A derivative); it is prescribed by specialists. The main indication of acitretin is severe psoriasis resistant to other forms of therapy. It is also used in disorders of keratinisation such as severe *Darier's disease* (keratosis follicularis), and some forms of *ichthyosis*. Although a minority of cases of psoriasis respond well to acitretin alone, it is only moderately effective in many cases; adverse effects are a limiting factor. A therapeutic effect occurs after 2 to 4 weeks and the maximum benefit after 4 to 6 weeks or longer. Continuous treatment for longer than 6 months is not usually necessary in psoriasis. However, some patients, particularly those with severe ichthyosis, may benefit from longer treatment, provided that the lowest effective dose is used, patients are monitored carefully for adverse effects, and the need for treatment is reviewed regularly. Topical preparations containing keratolytics should normally be stopped before administration of acitretin. Liberal use of emollients should be encouraged and topical corticosteroids can be continued if necessary.

Acitretin is teratogenic; in females of child-bearing age, the possibility of pregnancy must be excluded before treatment and effective contraception must be used during treatment and for at least 3 years afterwards (oral progestogen-only contraceptives not considered effective).

---

## Topical preparations for psoriasis

### Vitamin D and analogues

Calcipotriol, calcitriol, and tacalcitol are used for the management of *plaque psoriasis*. They should be avoided by those with calcium metabolism disorders, and used with caution in *generalised pustular* or *erythrodermic exfoliative psoriasis* (enhanced risk of hypercalcaemia). Local skin reactions (itching, erythema, burning, paraesthesia, dermatitis) are common. Hands should be washed thoroughly after application to avoid inadvertent transfer to other body areas. Aggravation of psoriasis has also been reported.

### ▲ CALCIPOTRIOL

**Cautions** see notes above; avoid use on face; avoid excessive exposure to sunlight and sunlamps

**Contra-indications** see notes above

**Hepatic impairment** manufacturers advise avoid in severe impairment

**Renal impairment** manufacturers advise avoid in severe impairment

**Pregnancy** manufacturers advise avoid unless essential

**Breast-feeding** no information available

**Side-effects** see notes above; also photosensitivity, dry skin; *rarely* facial or perioral dermatitis

**Licensed use** Calcipotriol ointment and scalp solution, and *Dovobet*® not licensed for use in children

**Indications and dose**

> **Plaque psoriasis**
>
> **Child 6–18 years** apply ointment twice daily; 6–12 years max. 50 g weekly, over 12 years max. 75 g weekly (less with scalp solution, see below)
>
> **Note** Patient information leaflet for *Dovonex*® ointment advises liberal application (but note max. recommended weekly dose, above)

> **Scalp psoriasis (specialist use only)**
>
> **Child 6–12 years** apply scalp solution twice daily; max. 30 mL weekly (less when used with ointment, see below)
>
> **Child 12–18 years** apply scalp solution twice daily; max. 45 mL weekly (less when used with ointment, see below)

**Note** When preparations used together max. total calcipotriol 2.5 mg in any one week for child 6–12 years (e.g. scalp solution 20 mL with ointment 30 g); max. 3.75 mg in any one week for child 12–18 years (e.g. scalp solution 30 mL with ointment 45 g)

**Calcipotriol** (Non-proprietary) (PoM)

Ointment, calcipotriol 50 micrograms/g, net price 120 g = £24.04

Scalp solution, calcipotriol 50 micrograms/mL, net price 60 mL = £12.53, 120 mL = £26.07

**Dovonex**® (LEO) (PoM)

Ointment, calcipotriol 50 micrograms/g, net price 30 g = £5.78

**Excipients** include disodium edetate, propylene glycol

### ◢ With betamethasone

For prescribing information, and for comment on the limited role of corticosteroids in psoriasis, see section 13.4.

**Dovobet**® (LEO) (PoM)

Ointment, betamethasone (as dipropionate) 0.05%, calcipotriol (as monohydrate) 50 micrograms/g, net price 120 g = £61.27. Label: 28

**Excipients** include butylated hydroxytoluene

**Dose**

> **Stable plaque psoriasis (specialist use only)**
>
> **Child 12–18 years** apply once daily to max. 30% of body surface for up to 4 weeks; max. 75 g weekly; if necessary, treatment should be continued beyond 4 weeks, or repeated, only on the advice of a specialist
>
> **Note** When different preparations containing calcipotriol used together, max. total calcipotriol 3.75 mg in any one week for child 12–18 years

Gel, betamethasone (as dipropionate) 0.05%, calcipotriol (as monohydrate) 50 micrograms/g, net price 60 g = £36.50, 2 × 60 g = £67.79. Label: 28

**Excipients** include butylated hydroxytoluene

**Dose**

> **Scalp psoriasis (specialist use only)**
>
> **Child 12–18 years** apply 1–4 g to scalp once daily, shampoo off after leaving on scalp overnight or during the day; usual duration of therapy 4 weeks; if necessary, treatment should be continued beyond 4 weeks, or repeated, only on the advice of a specialist

> **Mild to moderate plaque psoriasis (specialist use only)**
>
> **Child 12–18 years** apply once daily to max. 30% of body surface for up to 4 weeks; max. 75 g weekly; if necessary, treatment should be continued beyond 4 weeks, or repeated, only on the advice of a specialist
>
> **Note** When different preparations containing calcipotriol used together, max. total calcipotriol 3.75 mg in any one week for child 12–18 years

### ▲ CALCITRIOL

(1,25-Dihydroxycholecalciferol)

**Cautions** see notes above

**Contra-indications** see notes above; do not apply under occlusion

**Hepatic impairment** manufacturer advises avoid—no information available

**Renal impairment** manufacturer advises avoid—no information available

**Pregnancy** manufacturer advises use in restricted amounts only if clearly necessary and to monitor urine- and serum-calcium concentration

**Breast-feeding** manufacturer advises avoid

**Side-effects** see notes above

**Indications and dose**

> **Mild to moderate plaque psoriasis**
>
> **Child 12–18 years** apply twice daily; not more than 35% of body surface to be treated daily, max. 30 g daily

**Silkis**® (Galderma) (PoM)

Ointment, calcitriol 3 micrograms/g, net price 100 g = £13.87

**Excipients** none as listed in section 13.1.3

### ▲ TACALCITOL

**Cautions** see notes above; avoid eyes; monitor serum-calcium concentration if risk of hypercalcaemia; if used in conjunction with UV treatment, UV radiation should be given in the morning and tacalcitol applied at bedtime

**13**

**Skin**

**Contra-indications**   see notes above

**Renal impairment**   monitor serum-calcium concentration

**Pregnancy**   manufacturer advises avoid unless no safer alternative—no information available

**Breast-feeding**   manufacturer advises avoid application to breast area; no information available on presence in milk

**Side-effects**   see notes above

**Indications and dose**

> **Plaque psoriasis**
>
> **Child 12–18 years** apply once daily preferably at bedtime; max. 10 g *ointment* or 10 mL *lotion* daily
>
> **Note** When lotion and ointment used together, max. total tacalcitol 280 micrograms in any one week (e.g. lotion 30 mL with ointment 40 g)

**Curatoderm®** (Almirall) [PoM]
Lotion, tacalcitol (as monohydrate) 4 micrograms/g, net price 30 mL = £12.73
**Excipients** include disodium edetate, propylene glycol

Ointment, tacalcitol (as monohydrate) 4 micrograms/g, net price 30 g = £13.40, 60 g = £23.14, 100 g = £30.86
**Excipients** none as listed in section 13.1.3

## Tars

### ▌ TARS

**Cautions**   application to face and skin flexures; use suitable chemical protection gloves for extemporaneous preparation

**Contra-indications**   not for use in sore, acute, or pustular psoriasis or in presence of infection; avoid eyes, mucosa, genital or rectal areas; broken or inflamed skin

**Side-effects**   skin irritation and acne-like eruptions, photosensitivity; stains skin, hair, and fabric

**Indications and dose**

> **Psoriasis and occasionally chronic atopic eczema**
>
> Apply 1–3 times daily starting with low-strength preparations; proprietary preparations, see individual entries below
>
> **Note** For shampoo preparations see section 13.9

**◢Non-proprietary preparations**
May be difficult to obtain. Patients may find newer proprietary preparations more acceptable

**Coal Tar Paste, BP**
Paste, strong coal tar solution 7.5%, in compound zinc paste

**Zinc and Coal Tar Paste, BP**
Paste, zinc oxide 6%, coal tar 6%, emulsifying wax 5%, starch 38%, yellow soft paraffin 45%
**Excipients** include cetostearyl alcohol

**◢Proprietary preparations**

**Carbo-Dome®** (Sandoz)
Cream, coal tar solution 10%, in a water-miscible basis, net price 30 g = £4.77, 100 g = £16.38
**Excipients** include beeswax, hydroxybenzoates (parabens)
**Dose**
> **Psoriasis**
>
> Apply to skin 2–3 times daily; product can be diluted with a few drops of freshly boiled and cooled water before applying

**Cocois®** (UCB Pharma)
Scalp ointment, coal tar solution 12%, salicylic acid 2%, precipitated sulfur 4%, in a coconut oil emollient basis, net price 40 g (with applicator nozzle) = £6.22, 100 g = £11.69
**Excipients** include cetostearyl alcohol
**Dose**
> **Scaly scalp disorders including psoriasis, eczema, seborrhoeic dermatitis and dandruff**
>
> **Child 6–12 years** medical supervision required
>
> **Child 12–18 years** apply to scalp once weekly as necessary (if severe use daily for first 3–7 days), shampoo off after 1 hour

**Exorex®** (Forest)
Lotion, coal tar solution 5% in an emollient basis, net price 100 mL = £8.11, 250 mL = £16.24
**Excipients** include hydroxybenzoates (parabens)
**Dose**
> **Psoriasis**
>
> Apply to skin or scalp 2–3 times daily; product can be diluted with a few drops of water before applying

**Psoriderm®** (Dermal)
Cream, coal tar 6%, lecithin 0.4%, net price 225 mL = £9.42
**Excipients** include isopropyl palmitate, propylene glycol
**Dose**
> **Psoriasis**
>
> Apply to skin or scalp 1–2 times daily

Scalp lotion—section 13.9

**Sebco®** (Derma UK)
Scalp ointment, coal tar solution 12%, salicylic acid 2%, precipitated sulfur 4%, in a coconut oil emollient basis, net price 40 g = £4.54, 100 g = £8.52
**Excipients** include cetostearyl alcohol
**Dose**
> **Scaly scalp disorders including psoriasis, eczema, seborrhoeic dermatitis and dandruff**
>
> **Child 6–12 years** medical supervision required
>
> **Child 12–18 years** apply to scalp as necessary (if severe use daily for first 3–7 days), shampoo off after 1 hour

**◢Bath preparations**

**Coal Tar Solution, BP**
Solution, coal tar 20%, polysorbate '80' 5%, in alcohol (96%), net price 500 mL = £8.16. Label: 15
**Excipients** include polysorbates
**Dose**
> Use 100 mL in an adult-size bath, and proportionally less for a child's bath
>
> **Note** Strong Coal Tar Solution BP contains coal tar 40%

**Polytar Emollient®** (Stiefel)
Bath additive, coal tar solution 2.5%, arachis (peanut) oil extract of coal tar 7.5%, tar 7.5%, cade oil 7.5%, light liquid paraffin 35%, net price 500 mL = £5.78
**Excipients** include isopropyl palmitate
**Dose**
> **Psoriasis, eczema, atopic and pruritic dermatoses**
>
> Use 2–4 capfuls (15–30 mL) in adult-size bath and proportionally less for a child's bath; soak for 20 minutes

**Psoriderm®** (Dermal)
Bath emulsion, coal tar 40%, net price 200 mL = £2.74
**Excipients** include polysorbate 20

Skin

**Dose**

> **Psoriasis**
>
> Use 30 mL in adult-size bath, and proportionally less for a child's bath; soak for 5 minutes

# Dithranol

 **DITHRANOL**
(Anthralin)

**Cautions** avoid use near eyes and sensitive areas of skin; see also notes above

**Contra-indications** hypersensitivity; acute and pustular psoriasis

**Pregnancy** no adverse effects reported

**Breast-feeding** no adverse effects reported

**Side-effects** local burning sensation and irritation; stains skin, hair, and fabrics

**Licensed use** *Dithrocream*® and *Psorin*® licensed for use in children (age range not specified by manufacturer); *Micanol*® licensed for use in children, but not recommended for infants or young children (age range not specified by manufacturer)

**Indications and dose**

> **Subacute and chronic psoriasis**
>
> See notes above and under preparations
>
> **Note** Some of these dithranol preparations also contain coal tar or salicylic acid—for prescribing information see under Tars or under Salicylic Acid

◢Non-proprietary preparations

¹**Dithranol Ointment, BP** [PoM]

Ointment, dithranol, in yellow soft paraffin; usual strengths 0.1–2%. Part of basis may be replaced by hard paraffin if a stiffer preparation is required. Label: 28

**Dithranol Paste, BP**

Paste, dithranol in zinc and salicylic acid (Lassar's) paste. Usual strengths 0.1–1% of dithranol. Label: 28

◢Proprietary preparations

**Dithrocream**® (Dermal)

Cream, dithranol 0.1%, net price 50 g = £3.77; 0.25%, 50 g = £4.04; 0.5%, 50 g = £4.66; 1%, 50 g = £5.42; [PoM] 2%, 50 g = £6.79. Label: 28

**Excipients** include cetostearyl alcohol, chlorocresol

**Dose**

> For application to skin or scalp; 0.1–0.5% cream suitable for overnight treatment, 1–2% cream for max. 1 hour

**Micanol**® (GP Pharma)

Cream, dithranol 1% in a lipid-stabilised basis, net price 50 g = £16.18; [PoM] 3%, 50 g = £20.15. Label: 28

**Excipients** none as listed in section 13.1.3

**Dose**

> For application to skin or scalp, apply 1% cream for up to 30 minutes once daily, if necessary 3% cream can be used under medical supervision

**Note** At the end of contact time, use plenty of lukewarm (not hot) water to rinse off cream; soap may be used *after* the cream has been rinsed off; use shampoo before applying cream to scalp and if necessary after cream has been rinsed off

1. [PoM] if dithranol content more than 1%, otherwise may be sold to the public

**Psorin**® (LPC)

Ointment, dithranol 0.11%, coal tar 1%, salicylic acid 1.6%, net price 50 g = £9.22, 100 g = £18.44. Label: 28

**Excipients** include beeswax, wool fat

**Dose**

> For application to skin up to twice daily

Scalp gel, dithranol 0.25%, salicylic acid 1.6% in gel basis containing methyl salicylate, net price 50 g = £7.03. Label: 28

**Excipients** none as listed in section 13.1.3

**Dose**

> For application to scalp, initially apply on alternate days for 10–20 minutes; may be increased to daily application for max. 1 hour and then wash off

# Salicylic acid

 **SALICYLIC ACID**

For coal tar preparations containing salicylic acid, see under Tars p. 572; for dithranol preparations containing salicylic acid see under Dithranol, above

**Cautions** see notes above; avoid broken or inflamed skin

**Salicylate toxicity** Salicylate toxicity may occur particularly if applied on large areas of skin or on neonatal skin

**Side-effects** sensitivity, excessive drying, irritation, systemic effects after widespread use (see under Cautions)

**Indications and dose**

> **Hyperkeratotic skin disorders** see under preparation

> **Warts and calluses** section 13.7

> **Scalp conditions** section 13.9

> **Fungal nail infections** section 13.10.2

**Zinc and Salicylic Acid Paste, BP**

Paste, (Lassar's Paste), zinc oxide 24%, salicylic acid 2%, starch 24%, white soft paraffin 50%

Available from 'special-order' manufacturers or specialist importing companies, see p. 823

**Dose**

> **Child 1 month–18 years** apply twice daily

# Oral retinoids for psoriasis

 **ACITRETIN**

**Note** Acitretin is a metabolite of etretinate

**Cautions** in children use only in exceptional circumstances (premature epiphyseal closure reported); in females of childbearing age exclude pregnancy before starting (test for pregnancy within 2 weeks before treatment and monthly thereafter; start treatment on day 2 or 3 of menstrual cycle)—females of childbearing age (including those with history of infertility) should avoid pregnancy and use effective contraception (ideally 2 methods of contraception, one of which is a combined hormonal contraceptive or an intra-uterine device) for at least 1 month before, during, and for at least 3 years after treatment (oral progestogen-only contraceptives not considered effective); avoid concomitant use of keratolytics; do not donate blood during and for 2 years after stopping therapy (teratogenic risk); check liver function at start, at least every 4 weeks for first 2 months and then every 3 months; monitor serum-triglyceride and serum-cholesterol concentrations before treatment, 1 month after starting, then every 3 months; diabetes (can alter glucose tolerance—initial frequent blood glucose checks); monitor growth parameters and bone development; investigate atypical musculoskeletal symptoms; avoid excessive exposure to sunlight and unsupervised use of sunlamps; **interactions:** Appendix 1 (retinoids)

**Contra-indications** hyperlipidaemia

**Hepatic impairment** avoid in severe impairment—risk of further impairment

**Renal impairment** avoid in severe impairment; increased risk of toxicity

**Pregnancy** avoid—teratogenic; effective contraception must be used—see Cautions above

**Breast-feeding** avoid

**Side-effects** abdominal pain, diarrhoea, nausea, vomiting, dryness and inflammation of mucous membranes, peripheral oedema, reversible increase in serum-cholesterol and serum-triglyceride concentrations (with high doses), headache, arthralgia, myalgia, dryness of conjunctiva (causing conjunctivitis and decreased tolerance to contact lenses), alopecia (reversible on withdrawal), abnormal hair texture, skin exfoliation, pruritus, epidermal fragility, sticky skin, dermatitis, erythema, brittle nails, paronychia; *less commonly* hepatitis, dizziness, visual disturbances, photosensitivity; *rarely* peripheral neuropathy; *very rarely* benign intracranial hypertension (discontinue if severe headache, nausea, vomiting, or visual disturbances occur), bone pain, exostosis (skeletal hyperostosis and extra-osseous calcification reported following long-term treatment with etretinate, and premature epiphyseal closure in children, see Cautions above), night blindness, ulcerative keratitis; *also reported* taste disturbance, rectal haemorrhage, flushing, malaise, drowsiness, granulomatous lesions, impaired hearing, tinnitus, initial worsening of psoriasis, dry skin, sweating

**Indications and dose**

> **Harlequin ichthyosis** (under expert supervision only)
> * By mouth
>> **Neonate** 500 micrograms/kg once daily with food or milk (occasionally up to 1 mg/kg daily) with careful monitoring of musculoskeletal development

> **Severe extensive psoriasis resistant to other forms of therapy, palmoplantar pustular psoriasis, severe congenital ichthyosis, severe Darier's disease (keratosis follicularis)** (all under expert supervision only)
> * By mouth
>> **Child 1 month–12 years** 500 micrograms/kg once daily with food or milk (occasionally up to 1 mg/kg daily) to max. 35 mg daily with careful monitoring of musculoskeletal development (see also p. 570)
>>
>> **Child 12–18 years** initially 25–30 mg daily (Darier's disease 10 mg daily) for 2–4 weeks, then adjusted according to response, usual range 25–50 mg daily; up to 75 mg daily for short periods in psoriasis and ichthyosis (see also p. 570)

**Neotigason®** (Actavis) PoM

Capsules, acitretin 10 mg (brown/white), net price 60-cap pack = £23.80; 25 mg (brown/yellow), 60-cap pack = £55.24. Label: 10, patient information leaflet, 11, 21

### 13.5.3 Drugs affecting the immune response

Drugs affecting the immune response are used for eczema or psoriasis.

**Pimecrolimus** by topical application is licensed for *mild to moderate atopic eczema*. **Tacrolimus** is licensed for topical use in *moderate to severe atopic eczema*. Both are drugs whose long-term safety is still being evaluated and they should not usually be considered first-line treatment unless there is a specific reason to avoid or reduce the use of topical corticosteroids. Treatment with topical pimecrolimus or topical tacrolimus should be initiated only by prescribers experienced in treating atopic eczema.

> **NICE guidance**
> **Tacrolimus and pimecrolimus for atopic eczema (August 2004)**
> Topical pimecrolimus and tacrolimus are options for atopic eczema not controlled by maximal topical corticosteroid treatment or if there is a risk of important corticosteroid side-effects (particularly skin atrophy).
> Topical pimecrolimus is recommended for moderate atopic eczema on the face and neck of children aged 2–16 years and topical tacrolimus is recommended for moderate to severe atopic eczema in children over 2 years. Pimecrolimus and tacrolimus should be used within their licensed indications.
> www.nice.org.uk/TA82

The *Scottish Medicines Consortium* (p. 3) has advised (March 2010) that tacrolimus ointment (*Protopic®*) is accepted for restricted use within NHS Scotland for the prevention of flares in children aged over 2 years with moderate to severe atopic eczema in accordance with the licensed indication; initiation of treatment is restricted to doctors (including general practitioners) with a specialist interest and experience in treating atopic eczema with immunomodulatory therapy.

For the role of topical corticosteroids in eczema, see section 13.5.1, and for comment on their limited role in psoriasis, see section 13.4. A systemic corticosteroid (section 6.3.2) such as prednisolone may be used in *severe* refractory eczema.

Systemic drugs acting on the immune system are generally used by **specialists** in a hospital setting.

**Ciclosporin** by mouth can be used for *severe psoriasis* and for *severe eczema*. **Azathioprine** (section 8.2.1) or **mycophenolate mofetil** (section 8.2.1) are also used for severe refractory eczema in children.

**Methotrexate** can be used for *severe resistant psoriasis*; the dose is given **once weekly** and adjusted according to severity of the condition and haematological and biochemical measurements. Folic acid (section 9.1.2) should be given to reduce the possibility of methotrexate toxicity [unlicensed indication]. Folic acid can

**13 Skin**

be given at a dose of 5 mg once weekly on a different day to the methotrexate; alternative regimens may be used in some settings.

**Etanercept** (a cytokine modulator) is licensed in children over 6 years of age for the treatment of *severe plaque psoriasis* that is inadequately controlled by other systemic treatments and photochemotherapy, or when these other treatments cannot be used because of intolerance or contra-indications.

## CICLOSPORIN
(Cyclosporin)

**Cautions** section 8.2.2

**Additional cautions in atopic dermatitis and psoriasis** *Contra-indicated* in abnormal renal function, uncontrolled hypertension (see also below), infections not under control, and malignancy (see also below). Dermatological and physical examination, including blood pressure and renal function measurements required at least twice before starting. During treatment, monitor serum creatinine every 2 weeks for first 3 months then every month; reduce dose by 25–50% if serum creatinine increases more than 30% above baseline (even if within normal range) and discontinue if reduction not successful within one month. Discontinue if hypertension develops that cannot be controlled by dose reduction or antihypertensive therapy. Avoid excessive exposure to sunlight and avoid use of UVB or PUVA. *In atopic dermatitis*, also allow herpes simplex infections to clear before starting (if they occur during treatment withdraw if severe); *Staphylococcus aureus* skin infections not absolute contra-indication providing controlled (but avoid erythromycin unless no other alternative—see also **interactions**: Appendix 1 (ciclosporin)); investigate lymphadenopathy that persists despite improvement in atopic dermatitis. *In psoriasis*, also exclude malignancies (including those of skin and cervix) before starting (biopsy any lesions not typical of psoriasis) and treat patients with malignant or pre-malignant conditions of skin only after appropriate treatment (and if no other option); discontinue if lymphoproliferative disorder develops

**Hepatic impairment** section 8.2.2

**Renal impairment** see Cautions above

**Pregnancy** section 8.2.2

**Breast-feeding** section 8.2.2

**Side-effects** section 8.2.2

**Licensed use** not licensed for use in children under 16 years for atopic eczema (dermatitis) or psoriasis

**Indications and dose**

> **Short-term treatment (usually max. 8 weeks but may be used for longer under specialist supervision) of severe atopic dermatitis where conventional therapy ineffective or inappropriate**
>
> • **By mouth, administered in accordance with expert advice**
>
>   **Child 1 month–18 years** initially 1.25 mg/kg twice daily, if good initial response not achieved within 2 weeks, increase rapidly to max. 2.5 mg/kg twice daily; initial dose of 2.5 mg/kg twice daily if very severe
>
>   **Important** For preparations and counselling and for advice on conversion between the preparations, see section 8.2.2

> **Severe psoriasis where conventional therapy ineffective or inappropriate**
>
> • **By mouth, administered in accordance with expert advice**
>
>   **Child 1 month–18 years** initially 1.25 mg/kg twice daily, increased gradually to max. 2.5 mg/kg twice daily if no improvement within 1 month (discon-

tinue if response still insufficient after 6 weeks); initial dose of 2.5 mg/kg twice daily justified if condition requires rapid improvement

**Important** For preparations and counselling and for advice on conversion between the preparations, see section 8.2.2

**Refractory ulcerative colitis** section 1.5.3

**Transplantation and graft-versus-host disease** section 8.2.2

◢**Preparations**
Section 8.2.2

## METHOTREXATE

**Cautions** see section 8.1.3; also photosensitivity—psoriasis lesions aggravated by UV radiation (skin ulceration reported)

**Contra-indications** section 8.1.3

**Hepatic impairment** avoid—dose-related toxicity

**Renal impairment** section 8.1.3

**Pregnancy** section 8.1.3

**Breast-feeding** section 8.1.3

**Side-effects** section 8.1.3

**Licensed use** not licensed for use in children with psoriasis

**Indications and dose**

> **Severe uncontrolled psoriasis unresponsive to conventional therapy (specialist use only)**
>
> • **By mouth**
>
>   **Child 2–18 years** initially 200 micrograms/kg (max. 10 mg) once **weekly** increased according to response to 400 micrograms/kg (max. 25 mg) once **weekly**

### Safe Practice

Note that the above dose is a **weekly** dose. To avoid error with low-dose methotrexate, it is recommended that:

• the child or their carer is carefully advised of the **dose** and **frequency** and the reason for taking methotrexate and any other prescribed medicine (e.g. folic acid);

• only one strength of methotrexate tablet (usually 2.5 mg) is prescribed and dispensed;

• the prescription and the dispensing label clearly show the dose and frequency of methotrexate administration;

• the child or their carer is warned to report immediately the onset of any feature of blood disorders (e.g. sore throat, bruising, and mouth ulcers), liver toxicity (e.g. nausea, vomiting, abdominal discomfort, and dark urine), and respiratory effects (e.g. shortness of breath).

**Malignant disease** section 8.1.3

**Rheumatoid arthritis** section 10.1.3

**Severe Crohn's disease** section 1.5.3

◢**Preparations**
Section 10.1.3

## PIMECROLIMUS

**Cautions** UV light (avoid excessive exposure to sunlight and sunlamps), avoid other topical treatments except emollients at treatment site; alcohol consumption (risk of facial flushing and skin irritation)

**Contra-indications** contact with eyes and mucous membranes, application under occlusion, infection at treatment site; congenital epidermal barrier defects; generalised erythroderma; immunodeficiency; concomitant use with drugs that cause immunosuppression (may be prescribed in exceptional circumstances by specialists); application to malignant or potentially malignant skin lesions

**Side-effects** burning sensation, pruritus, erythema, skin infections (including folliculitis and *less commonly* impetigo, herpes simplex and zoster, molluscum contagiosum); *rarely* papilloma, skin discoloration, local reactions including pain, paraesthesia, peeling, dryness, oedema, and worsening of eczema; skin malignancy reported

### Indications and dose

> Short-term treatment of mild to moderate atopic eczema (including flares) when topical corticosteroids cannot be used; see also notes above
>
> > **Child 2–18 years** apply twice daily until symptoms resolve (stop treatment if eczema worsens or no response after 6 weeks)

**Elidel**® (Meda) [PoM]
Cream, pimecrolimus 1%, net price 30 g = £19.69, 60 g = £37.41, 100 g = £59.07. Label: 4, 11, 28
**Excipients** include benzyl alcohol, cetyl alcohol, propylene glycol, stearyl alcohol

## TACROLIMUS

**Cautions** UV light (avoid excessive exposure to sunlight and sunlamps); alcohol consumption (risk of facial flushing and skin irritation)

**Contra-indications** infection at treatment site; congenital epidermal barrier defects; generalised erythroderma; immunodeficiency; concomitant use with drugs that cause immunosuppression (may be prescribed in exceptional circumstances by specialists); application to malignant or potentially malignant skin lesions; application under occlusion; avoid contact with eyes and mucous membranes

**Pregnancy** manufacturer advises avoid unless essential; toxicity in *animal* studies following systemic administration

**Breast-feeding** manufacturer advises avoid—present in milk following systemic administration

**Side-effects** application-site reactions including rash, irritation, pain, and paraesthesia; herpes simplex infection, Kaposi's varicelliform eruption; application-site infections; *less commonly* acne; *also reported* rosacea, malignancies (including skin malignancy, cutaneous lymphoma, and other types of lymphomas)

### Indications and dose

> Short-term treatment of moderate to severe atopic eczema (including flares) either unresponsive to, or in children intolerant of conventional therapy; see also notes above
>
> > **Child 2–16 years** initially apply 0.03% ointment thinly twice daily for up to 3 weeks (consider other treatment if eczema worsens or if no improvement after 2 weeks) then reduce to once daily until lesion clears
> >
> > **Child 16–18 years** initially apply 0.1% ointment thinly twice daily until lesion clears (consider other treatment if eczema worsens or if no improvement after 2 weeks); reduce to once daily or switch to 0.03% ointment if clinical condition allows

> Prevention of flares in children with moderate to severe atopic eczema and 4 or more flares a year, who have responded to initial treatment with topical tacrolimus
>
> > **Child 2–16 years** apply 0.03% ointment thinly twice weekly (with an interval of 2–3 days between applications); use short-term treatment regimen during an acute flare; interrupt preventative therapy after 1 year to reassess condition
> >
> > **Child 16–18 years** apply 0.1% ointment thinly twice weekly (with an interval of 2–3 days between applications); use short-term treatment regimen during an acute flare; review need for preventative therapy after 1 year

> Other indications section 8.2.2

**Protopic**® (Astellas) [PoM]
Ointment, tacrolimus (as monohydrate) 0.03%, net price 30 g = £19.44, 60 g = £35.46; 0.1%, 30 g = £21.60, 60 g = £39.40. Label: 4, 11, 28
**Excipients** include beeswax

# Cytokine modulators

## ETANERCEPT

**Cautions** section 10.1.3
**Contra-indications** section 10.1.3
**Hepatic impairment** section 10.1.3
**Pregnancy** section 10.1.3
**Breast-feeding** section 10.1.3
**Side-effects** section 10.1.3

### Indications and dose

> Severe plaque psoriasis
> - **By subcutaneous injection**
>
> > **Child 6–18 years** 800 micrograms/kg (max. 50 mg) once weekly for up to 24 weeks; discontinue if no response after 12 weeks

> Polyarticular-course juvenile idiopathic arthritis section 10.1.3

◢**Preparations**
Section 10.1.3

# 13.6  Acne and rosacea

| | |
|---|---|
| **13.6.1** | Topical preparations for acne |
| **13.6.2** | Oral preparations for acne |

**Acne vulgaris**    Acne vulgaris commonly affects children around puberty and occasionally affects infants. Treatment of acne should be commenced early to prevent scarring; lesions may worsen before improving. The choice of treatment depends on age, severity, and whether the acne is predominantly inflammatory or comedonal.

*Mild to moderate acne* is generally treated with topical preparations, such as benzoyl peroxide, azelaic acid, and retinoids (section 13.6.1).

For *moderate to severe inflammatory acne* or where topical preparations are not tolerated or are ineffective or where application to the site is difficult, systemic treatment (section 13.6.2) with oral antibacterials may be effective. **Co-cyprindiol** (cyproterone acetate with ethinylestradiol) has anti-androgenic properties and may be useful in young women with acne refractory to other treatments.

*Severe acne*, acne unresponsive to prolonged courses of oral antibacterials, acne with scarring, or acne associated with psychological problems calls for early referral to a consultant dermatologist who may prescribe oral **isotretinoin** (section 13.6.2).

**Neonatal and infantile acne**    Inflammatory papules, pustules, and occasionally comedones may develop at birth or within the first month; most neonates with acne do not require treatment. Acne developing at 3–6 months of age may be more severe and persistent; lesions are usually confined to the face. Topical preparations containing benzoyl peroxide (at the lowest strength possible to avoid irritation), adapalene, or tretinoin may be used if treatment for infantile acne is necessary. In infants with inflammatory acne, oral **erythromycin** (section 5.1.5) is used because topical preparations for acne are not well tolerated. In cases of erythromycin-resistant acne, oral isotretinoin (section 13.6.2) can be given on the advice of a consultant dermatologist.

**Rosacea**    The adult form of rosacea rarely occurs in children. Persistent or repeated use of potent topical corticosteroids may cause periorificial rosacea (steroid acne). The pustules and papules of rosacea may be treated for at least 6 weeks with a topical **metronidazole** preparation (section 13.10.1.2), or a systemic antibacterial such as **erythromycin** (section 5.1.5), or for a child over 12 years, **oxytetracycline** (section 5.1.3). Tetracyclines are **contra-indicated** in children under 12 years of age.

## 13.6.1  Topical preparations for acne

In mild to moderate acne, comedones and inflamed lesions respond well to benzoyl peroxide (see below) or topical retinoids (see p. 579). Alternatively, topical application of an antibacterial such as erythromycin or clindamycin may be effective for inflammatory acne. However, topical antibacterials are probably no more effective than benzoyl peroxide and may promote the emergence of resistant organisms. If topical prepara-

tions prove inadequate, oral preparations may be needed (section 13.6.2). The choice of product and formulation (gel, solution, lotion, or cream) is largely determined by skin type, patient preference, and previous usage of acne products.

## Benzoyl peroxide and azelaic acid

**Benzoyl peroxide** is effective in mild to moderate acne. Both comedones and inflamed lesions respond well to benzoyl peroxide. The lower concentrations seem to be as effective as higher concentrations in reducing inflammation. It is usual to start with a lower strength and to increase the concentration of benzoyl peroxide gradually. The usefulness of benzoyl peroxide washes is limited by the short time the products are in contact with the skin. Adverse effects include local skin irritation, particularly when therapy is initiated, but the scaling and redness often subside with a reduction in benzoyl peroxide concentration, frequency, and area of application. If the acne does not respond after 2 months then use of a topical antibacterial should be considered.

**Azelaic acid** has antimicrobial and anticomedonal properties. It may be used as an alternative to benzoyl peroxide or to a topical retinoid for treating mild to moderate comedonal acne, particularly of the face; azelaic acid is less likely to cause local irritation than benzoyl peroxide.

### BENZOYL PEROXIDE

**Cautions**    avoid contact with eyes, mouth, and mucous membranes; may bleach fabrics and hair; avoid excessive exposure to sunlight

**Side-effects**    skin irritation (reduce frequency or suspend use until irritation subsides and re-introduce at reduced frequency)

**Licensed use**    *Quinoderm*® is licensed for use in children; *all other preparations*, not licensed for use in treatment of infantile acne

#### Indications and dose

**Acne vulgaris**

**Child 12–18 years** apply 1–2 times daily preferably after washing with soap and water, start treatment with lower-strength preparations

Note  May bleach clothing

**Infantile acne**

**Child 1 month–2 years** apply 1–2 times daily; start treatment with lower-strength preparations

**Acnecide**® (Galderma)
Gel, benzoyl peroxide 5% in an aqueous gel basis, net price 30 g = £5.44, 60 g = £10.88
Excipients  include propylene glycol

**Brevoxyl**® (GSK)
Cream, benzoyl peroxide 4% in an aqueous basis, net price 40 g = £3.30
Excipients  include cetyl alcohol, fragrance, stearyl alcohol

**PanOxyl**® (GSK)
Aquagel (= aqueous gel), benzoyl peroxide 2.5%, net price 40 g = £1.76; 5%, 40 g = £1.92; 10%, 40 g = £2.13
Excipients  include propylene glycol

Cream, benzoyl peroxide 5% in a non-greasy basis, net price 40 g = £1.89
Excipients  include isopropyl palmitate, propylene glycol

**13**

**Skin**

Gel, benzoyl peroxide 10% in an aqueous alcoholic basis, net price 40 g = £1.69
Excipients include fragrance

◀ **With antimicrobials**

**Duac® Once Daily** (GSK) PoM
Gel, benzoyl peroxide 5%, clindamycin 1% (as phosphate) in an aqueous basis, net price 25 g = £9.95, 50 g = £19.90
Excipients include disodium edetate
Dose

> **Acne vulgaris**
>
> **Child 12–18 years** apply once daily in the evening

**Quinoderm®** (Alliance)
Cream, benzoyl peroxide 5%, potassium hydroxy-quinoline sulfate 0.5%, in an astringent vanishing-cream basis, net price 50 g = £2.21
Excipients include cetostearyl alcohol, edetic acid (EDTA)
Cream, benzoyl peroxide 10%, potassium hydroxy-quinoline sulfate 0.5%, in an astringent vanishing-cream basis, net price 25 g = £1.30, 50 g = £2.49
Excipients include cetostearyl alcohol, edetic acid (EDTA)
Dose

> **Acne vulgaris, acneform eruptions, folliculitis**
>
> Apply 2–3 times daily

## ◤ AZELAIC ACID

**Cautions** avoid contact with eyes, mouth, and mucous membranes

**Side-effects** local irritation (reduce frequency or discontinue temporarily); *less commonly* skin discoloration; *also reported* worsening of asthma

**Indications and dose**

> See under preparations

**Finacea®** (Bayer) PoM
Gel, azelaic acid 15%, net price 30 g = £7.48
Excipients include disodium edetate, polysorbate 80, propylene glycol
Dose

> **Facial acne vulgaris**
>
> **Child 12–18 years** apply twice daily; discontinue if no improvement after 1 month

**Skinoren®** (Bayer) PoM
Cream, azelaic acid 20%, net price 30 g = £3.74
Excipients include propylene glycol
Dose

> **Acne vulgaris**
>
> **Child 12–18 years** apply twice daily (sensitive skin, once daily for first week)

## Topical antibacterials for acne

In the treatment of mild to moderate inflammatory acne, topical antibacterials may be no more effective than topical benzoyl peroxide or tretinoin. Topical antibacterials are probably best reserved for children who wish to avoid oral antibacterials or who cannot tolerate them.

Topical preparations of **erythromycin** and **clindamycin** may be used to treat *inflamed lesions* in mild to moderate acne when topical benzoyl peroxide or tretinoin is ineffective or poorly tolerated. Topical benzoyl peroxide, azelaic acid, or retinoids used in combination with an antibacterial (topical or systemic) may be more effective than an antibacterial used alone. Topical anti-bacterials can produce mild irritation of the skin, and on rare occasions cause sensitisation; gastro-intestinal disturbances have been reported with topical clindamycin.

Antibacterial resistance of *Propionibacterium acnes* is increasing; there is cross-resistance between erythromycin and clindamycin. To avoid development of resistance:

- when possible use non-antibiotic antimicrobials (such as benzoyl peroxide or azelaic acid);

- avoid concomitant treatment with different oral and topical antibacterials;

- if a particular antibacterial is effective, use it for repeat courses if needed (short intervening courses of benzoyl peroxide or azelaic acid may eliminate any resistant propionibacteria);

- do not continue treatment for longer than necessary (but treatment with a topical preparation should be continued for at least 6 months).

## ◤ ANTIBACTERIALS

**Cautions** some manufacturers advise preparations containing alcohol are not suitable for use with benzoyl peroxide; discontinue clindamycin preparations immediately if diarrhoea or colitis occur

**Indications and dose**

> **Acne vulgaris** for dose, see under preparations

**Dalacin T®** (Pharmacia) PoM
Topical solution, clindamycin 1% (as phosphate), in an aqueous alcoholic basis, net price (both with applicator) 30 mL = £4.34, 50 mL = £7.23
Excipients include propylene glycol
Dose

> Apply thinly twice daily

Lotion, clindamycin 1% (as phosphate) in an aqueous basis, net price 30 mL = £5.08, 60 mL = £10.16
Excipients include cetostearyl alcohol, hydroxybenzoates (parabens)
Dose

> Apply thinly twice daily

**Stiemycin®** (Stiefel) PoM
Solution, erythromycin 2% in an alcoholic basis, net price 50 mL = £7.69
Excipients include propylene glycol
Dose

> **Child 12–18 years** apply thinly twice daily

**Zindaclin®** (Crawford) PoM
Gel, clindamycin 1% (as phosphate), net price 30 g = £8.66
Excipients include propylene glycol
Dose

> **Child 12–18 years** apply thinly once daily

**Zineryt®** (Astellas) PoM
Topical solution, powder for reconstitution, erythromycin 40 mg, zinc acetate 12 mg/mL when reconstituted with solvent containing ethanol, net price per pack of powder and solvent to provide 30 mL = £7.71, 90 mL = £16.68
Excipients none as listed in section 13.1.3
Dose

> Apply twice daily

## Topical retinoids and related preparations for acne

Topical **tretinoin**, its isomer **isotretinoin**, and **adapalene** (a retinoid-like drug), are useful for treating comedones and inflammatory lesions in mild to moderate acne. Patients should be warned that some redness and skin peeling can occur initially but settles with time. If undue irritation occurs, the frequency of application should be reduced or treatment suspended until the reaction subsides; if irritation persists, discontinue treatment. Several months of treatment may be needed to achieve an optimal response and the treatment should be continued until no new lesions develop.

Tretinoin can be used under specialist supervision to treat infantile acne; adapalene can also be used. See also Neonatal and Infantile Acne, p. 577.

**Cautions**    Topical retinoids should be avoided in severe acne involving large areas. Contact with eyes, nostrils, mouth and mucous membranes, eczematous, broken or sunburned skin should be avoided. Topical retinoids should be used with caution on sensitive areas such as the neck, and accumulation in angles of the nose should be avoided. Exposure to UV light (including sunlight, solariums) should be avoided; if sun exposure is unavoidable, an appropriate sunscreen (section 13.8.1) or protective clothing should be used. Use of retinoids with abrasive cleaners, comedogenic or astringent cosmetics should be avoided. Allow peeling (resulting from other irritant treatments) to subside before using a topical retinoid; alternating a preparation that causes peeling with a topical retinoid may give rise to contact dermatitis (reduce frequency of retinoid application).

**Pregnancy**    Topical retinoids are contra-indicated in pregnancy; females of child-bearing age must use effective contraception (oral progestogen-only contraceptives not considered effective).

**Side-effects**    Local reactions include burning, erythema, stinging, pruritus, dry or peeling skin (discontinue if severe). Increased sensitivity to UVB light or sunlight occurs. Temporary changes of skin pigmentation with tretinoin have been reported. Eye irritation and oedema, and blistering or crusting of skin have been reported rarely.

### ■ ADAPALENE

**Cautions**    see notes above
**Pregnancy**    see notes above
**Breast-feeding**    amount of drug in milk probably too small to be harmful; ensure infant does not come in contact with treated areas
**Side-effects**    see notes above
**Licensed use**    not licensed for use in infantile acne
**Indications and dose**

> Infantile acne
>> **Child 1 month–2 years** apply thinly once daily in the evening

> Mild to moderate acne vulgaris
>> **Child 12–18 years** apply thinly once daily in the evening

**Differin**® (Galderma) ℗ₒₘ
Cream, adapalene 0.1%, net price 45 g = £11.40. Label: 11
Excipients    include disodium edetate, hydroxybenzoates (parabens)

Gel, adapalene 0.1%, net price 45 g = £11.40. Label: 11
Excipients    include disodium edetate, hydroxybenzoates (parabens), propylene glycol

**◢With benzoyl peroxide**
**Epiduo**® (Galderma) ℗ₒₘ
Gel, adapalene 0.1%, benzoyl peroxide 2.5%, net price 45 g = £17.91. Label: 11
Excipients    include disodium edetate, polysorbate 80, propylene glycol
**Dose**

> Acne vulgaris
>> **Child 9–18 years** apply thinly once daily in the evening
> **Note**  May bleach clothing and hair

### ■ ISOTRETINOIN

**Note**  Isotretinoin is an isomer of tretinoin
**Important**  For prescribing information on isotretinoin **when given by mouth**, see p. 581
**Cautions**    (*topical application* only) see notes above; also personal or familial history of non-melanoma skin cancer
**Contra-indications**    (*topical application* only) rosacea; perioral dermatitis
**Pregnancy**    (*topical application* only) see notes above
**Breast-feeding**    avoid
**Side-effects**    (*topical application* only) see notes above
**Indications and dose**

> Acne vulgaris
>> Apply thinly 1–2 times daily

**Isotrex**® (Stiefel) ℗ₒₘ
Gel, isotretinoin 0.05%, net price 30 g = £5.94. Label: 11
Excipients    include butylated hydroxytoluene

**◢With antibacterial**
**Isotrexin**® (Stiefel) ℗ₒₘ
Gel, isotretinoin 0.05%, erythromycin 2% in ethanolic basis, net price 30 g = £7.47. Label: 11
Excipients    include butylated hydroxytoluene

### ■ TRETINOIN

**Note**  Tretinoin is the acid form of vitamin A
**Cautions**    see notes above
**Contra-indications**    personal or familial history of non-melanoma skin cancer; rosacea; perioral dermatitis
**Pregnancy**    see notes above
**Breast-feeding**    amount of drug in milk after topical application probably too small to be harmful; ensure infant does not come into contact with treated areas
**Side-effects**    see notes above
**Indications and dose**

> See under preparations

> Malignant disease section 8.1.5

◢With antibacterial

**Aknemycin Plus®** (Almirall) [PoM]

Solution, tretinoin 0.025%, erythromycin 4% in an alcoholic basis, net price 25 mL = £7.05. Label: 11

Excipients none as listed in section 13.1.3

**Dose**

> **Acne (all forms), particularly that associated with oily skin**
>
> Apply thinly 1–2 times daily

## Other topical preparations for acne

A topical preparation of **nicotinamide** is available for inflammatory acne.

### ▮ NICOTINAMIDE

**Cautions** avoid contact with eyes and mucous membranes (including nose and mouth); reduce frequency of application if excessive dryness, irritation, or peeling

**Side-effects** dry skin, pruritus, erythema, burning, irritation

**Licensed use** licensed for use in children (age range not specified by manufacturer)

**Indications and dose**

> **Inflammatory acne vulgaris** see under preparations below

**Nicam®** (Dermal)

Gel, nicotinamide 4%, net price 60 g = £7.10

Excipients none as listed in section 13.1.3

**Dose**

> Apply twice daily; reduce to once daily or on alternate days if irritation occurs

## 13.6.2 Oral preparations for acne

## Oral antibacterials for acne

Oral antibacterials may be used in *moderate to severe inflammatory acne* when topical treatment is not adequately effective or is inappropriate. Concomitant anti-comedonal treatment with topical benzoyl peroxide or azelaic acid may also be required (section 13.6.1).

Tetracyclines should not be given to children under 12 years. In children over 12 years, either **oxytetracycline** or **tetracycline** (section 5.1.3) is usually given for acne in a dose of 500 mg twice daily. If there is no improvement after the first 3 months another oral antibacterial should be used. Maximum improvement usually occurs after 4 to 6 months but in more severe cases treatment may need to be continued for 2 years or longer.

**Doxycycline** and **lymecycline** (section 5.1.3) are alternatives to tetracycline in children over 12 years. Doxycycline can be used in a dose of 100 mg daily. Lymecycline is given in a dose of 408 mg daily.

Although **minocycline** is as effective as other tetracyclines for acne, it is associated with a greater risk of lupus erythematosus-like syndrome. Minocycline sometimes causes irreversible pigmentation; it is given in a dose of 100 mg once daily or 50 mg twice daily.

**Erythromycin** (section 5.1.5) in a dose of 500 mg twice daily for children over 12 years is an alternative for the management of moderate to severe acne with inflamed lesions, but propionibacteria strains resistant to erythromycin are becoming widespread and this may explain

poor response. Infants with acne requiring oral treatment with erythromycin should be given 250 mg once daily *or* 125 mg twice daily; in cases of erythromycin-resistant *P. acnes* in infants, oral isotretinoin may be used on the advice of a consultant dermatologist.

Concomitant use of different topical and systemic antibacterials is undesirable owing to the increased likelihood of the development of bacterial resistance.

## Hormone treatment for acne

**Co-cyprindiol** (cyproterone acetate with ethinylestradiol) contains an anti-androgen. It is no more effective than an oral broad-spectrum antibacterial but is useful in females of childbearing age who also wish to receive oral contraception.

Improvement of acne with co-cyprindiol probably occurs because of decreased sebum secretion which is under androgen control. Some females with moderately severe hirsutism may also benefit because hair growth is also androgen-dependent. Contra-indications of co-cyprindiol include pregnancy and a predisposition to thrombosis.

> Venous thromboembolism occurs more frequently in women taking co-cyprindiol than those taking a low-dose combined oral contraceptive. Co-cyprindiol is licensed for use in women with severe acne that has not responded to oral antibacterials and for moderately severe hirsutism; it should not be used solely for contraception. It is contra-indicated in those with a personal or close family history of venous thromboembolism. Women with severe acne or hirsutism may have an inherently increased risk of cardiovascular disease.

### ▮ CO-CYPRINDIOL

A mixture of cyproterone acetate and ethinylestradiol in the mass proportions 2000 parts to 35 parts, respectively

**Cautions** see under Combined Hormonal Contraceptives, section 7.3.1

**Contra-indications** see under Combined Hormonal Contraceptives, section 7.3.1

**Hepatic impairment** see under Combined Hormonal Contraceptives, section 7.3.1

**Pregnancy** avoid—risk of feminisation of male fetus with cyproterone

**Breast-feeding** manufacturer advises avoid; possibility of anti-androgen effects in neonate with cyproterone

**Side-effects** see under Combined Hormonal Contraceptives, section 7.3.1

**Licensed use** licensed for use in females of childbearing age

**Indications and dose**

> **Severe acne in females of childbearing age refractory to prolonged oral antibacterial therapy (but see notes above), moderately severe hirsutism**
>
> • By mouth
>
> 1 tablet daily for 21 days starting on day 1 of menstrual cycle and repeated after a 7-day interval, usually for several months; withdraw 3–4 months after acne or hirsutism completely resolved (repeat courses may be given if recurrence); long-term treatment may be necessary for severe symptoms

13 Skin

**Co-cyprindiol** (Non-proprietary) PoM

Tablets, co-cyprindiol 2000/35 (cyproterone acetate 2 mg, ethinylestradiol 35 micrograms), net price 63-tab pack = £4.70

Brands include *Acnocin®*, *Cicafem®*, *Clairette®*

**Dianette®** (Bayer) PoM

Tablets, beige, s/c, co-cyprindiol 2000/35 (cyproterone acetate 2 mg, ethinylestradiol 35 micrograms), net price 63-tab pack = £7.71

## Oral retinoid for acne

The retinoid **isotretinoin** reduces sebum secretion. It is used for the systemic treatment of nodulo-cystic and conglobate acne, severe acne, acne with scarring, or for acne which has not responded to an adequate course of a systemic antibacterial. Isotretinoin is used for the treatment of severe infantile acne resistant to erythromycin.

Isotretinoin is a toxic drug that should be prescribed **only** by, or under the supervision of, a consultant dermatologist. It is given for at least 16 weeks; repeat courses are not normally required.

Side-effects of isotretinoin include severe dryness of the skin and mucous membranes, nose bleeds, and joint pains. The drug is **teratogenic** and must **not** be given to females of child-bearing age unless they practise effective contraception (oral progestogen-only contraceptives not considered effective) and then only after detailed assessment and explanation by the physician. They must also be registered with a pregnancy prevention programme (see under Cautions below).

Although a causal link between isotretinoin use and psychiatric changes (including suicidal ideation) has not been established, the possibility should be considered before initiating treatment; if psychiatric changes occur during treatment, isotretinoin should be stopped, the prescriber informed, and specialist psychiatric advice should be sought.

### ■ ISOTRETINOIN

**Note** Isotretinoin is an isomer of tretinoin

**Cautions** see notes above; also avoid blood donation during treatment and for at least 1 month after treatment; history of depression; monitor all patients for depression; measure hepatic function and serum lipids before treatment, 1 month after starting and then every 3 months (reduce dose or discontinue if transaminase or serum lipids persistently raised); discontinue if uncontrolled hypertriglyceridaemia or pancreatitis; diabetes; dry eye syndrome (associated with risk of keratitis); avoid keratolytics; **interactions:** Appendix 1 (retinoids)

**Pregnancy prevention** In women of child-bearing potential, exclude pregnancy up to 3 days before treatment (start treatment on day 2 or 3 of menstrual cycle), every month during treatment (unless there are compelling reasons to indicate that there is no risk of pregnancy), and 5 weeks after stopping treatment—perform pregnancy test in the first 3 days of the menstrual cycle. Women must practise effective contraception for at least 1 month before starting treatment, during treatment, and for at least 1 month after stopping treatment. Women should be advised to use at least 1 method of contraception, but ideally they should use 2 methods of contraception. Oral progestogen-only contraceptives are not considered effective. Barrier methods should not be used alone, but can be used in conjunction with other contraceptive methods. Each prescription for isotretinoin should be limited to a supply of up to 30 days' treatment and dispensed within 7 days of the date stated on the prescription; repeat prescriptions or faxed prescriptions

are not acceptable. Women should be advised to discontinue treatment and to seek prompt medical attention if they become pregnant during treatment or within 1 month of stopping treatment.

**Counselling** Warn patient to avoid wax epilation (risk of epidermal stripping), dermabrasion, and laser skin treatments (risk of scarring) during treatment and for at least 6 months after stopping; patient should avoid exposure to UV light (including sunlight) and use sunscreen and emollient (including lip balm) preparations from the start of treatment

**Contra-indications** hypervitaminosis A, hyperlipidaemia

**Hepatic impairment** avoid—further impairment may occur

**Renal impairment** in severe impairment, reduce initial dose and increase gradually, if necessary, up to 1 mg/kg daily as tolerated

**Pregnancy** avoid—teratogenic; effective contraception must be used—see Pregnancy Prevention above

**Breast-feeding** avoid

**Side-effects** dryness of skin (with dermatitis, scaling, thinning, erythema, pruritus), epidermal fragility (trauma may cause blistering), dryness of lips (sometimes cheilitis), dryness of eyes (with blepharitis and conjunctivitis), dryness of pharyngeal mucosa (with hoarseness), dryness of nasal mucosa (with epistaxis), headache, myalgia and arthralgia, raised plasma-triglyceride concentration (risk of pancreatitis if triglycerides above 9 mmol/litre), raised serum-cholesterol concentration (with reduced high-density lipoprotein concentration), raised blood-glucose concentration, raised serum-transaminase concentration, haematuria and proteinuria, thrombocytopenia, thrombocytosis, neutropenia and anaemia; *rarely* mood changes (depression, aggressive behaviour, anxiety, and very rarely psychosis and suicidal ideation)—expert referral required, skin reactions (including reports of Stevens-Johnson syndrome and toxic epidermal necrolysis), alopecia; *very rarely* nausea, hepatitis, inflammatory bowel disease, gastrointestinal haemorrhage, haemorrhagic diarrhoea (discontinue treatment), benign intracranial hypertension (avoid concomitant tetracyclines), convulsions, malaise, drowsiness, dizziness, diabetes mellitus, lymphadenopathy, hyperuricaemia, glomerulonephritis, tendinitis, arthritis, raised serum-creatine kinase concentration, bone changes (including reduced bone density, early epiphyseal closure, and skeletal hyperstosis) and calcification of tendons and ligaments following long-term administration, visual disturbances (papilloedema, corneal opacities, cataracts, decreased night vision, photophobia, blurred vision, colour blindness)—expert referral required and consider withdrawal, decreased tolerance to contact lenses, keratitis, impaired hearing, Gram-positive infections of skin and mucous membranes, exacerbation of acne, acne fulminans, allergic vasculitis and granulomatous lesions, paronychia, hirsutism, nail dystrophy, skin hyperpigmentation, photosensitivity, increased sweating

**Licensed use** not licensed for use in infantile acne

### Indications and dose

**Acne vulgaris** under supervision of consultant dermatologist, see notes above

• By mouth

**Child 12–18 years** 500 micrograms/kg daily (in 1–2 divided doses), increased if necessary to 1 mg/kg daily, for 16–24 weeks (repeat treatment course after a period of at least 8 weeks if relapse after

**13**

**Skin**

first course); max. cumulative dose 150 mg/kg per course

**Severe infantile acne** under supervision of a consultant dermatologist, see p. 577

● By mouth

**Child 1 month–2 years** 200 micrograms/kg daily (in 1–2 divided doses), increased if necessary to 1 mg/kg daily, for 16–24 weeks; max. cumulative dose 150 mg/kg per course

**Isotretinoin** (Non-proprietary) PoM

Capsules, isotretinoin 5 mg, net price 56-cap pack = £14.99; 20 mg, 56-cap pack = £39.99. Label: 10, patient information leaflet, 11, 21

**Roaccutane®** (Roche) PoM

Capsules, isotretinoin 10 mg (brown-red), net price 30-cap pack = £14.54; 20 mg (brown-red/white), 30-cap pack = £20.02. Label: 10, patient information card, 11, 21

## 13.7   Preparations for warts and calluses

Warts (verruca vulgaris) are common, benign, self-limiting, and usually asymptomatic. They are caused by a human papillomavirus, which most frequently affects the hands, feet (plantar warts), and the anogenital region (see below); treatment usually relies on local tissue destruction and is required only if the warts are painful, unsightly, persistent, or cause distress. In immunocompromised children, warts may be more difficult to eradicate.

Preparations of **salicylic acid, formaldehyde, gluteraldehyde** or **silver nitrate** are used for the removal of warts on hands and feet. **Salicylic acid** is a useful keratolytic which may be considered first-line in the treatment of warts; it is also suitable for the removal of *corns and calluses*. Preparations of salicylic acid in a collodion basis are available but some children may develop an allergy to colophony in the formulation; collodion should be avoided in children allergic to elastic adhesive plaster. Cryotherapy causes pain, swelling, and blistering, and may be no more effective than topical salicylic acid in the treatment of warts.

### ▌ SALICYLIC ACID

**Cautions** significant peripheral neuropathy, patients with diabetes at risk of neuropathic ulcers; impaired peripheral circulation; protect surrounding skin and avoid broken skin; not suitable for application to face, anogenital region, or large areas

**Side-effects** skin irritation, skin ulceration (with high concentrations)

**Licensed use** not licensed for use in children under 2 years

**Indications and dose**

**Warts on hands and feet (plantar)**

For dose see preparations; apply carefully to wart and protect surrounding skin (e.g. with soft paraffin or specially designed plaster); rub wart surface gently with file or pumice stone once weekly; treatment may need to be continued for up to 3 months

**Psoriasis** section 13.5.2

**Fungal nail infections** section 13.10.2

**Cuplex®** (Crawford)

Gel, salicylic acid 11%, lactic acid 4%, in a collodion basis, net price 5 g = £2.23. Label: 15

**Dose**

Apply twice daily

**Note** Contains colophony (see notes above)

**Duofilm®** (GSK)

Paint, salicylic acid 16.7%, lactic acid 16.7%, in flexible collodion, net price 15 mL (with applicator) = £2.25. Label: 15

**Dose**

Apply daily

**Occlusal®** (Alliance)

Cutaneous solution, salicylic acid 26% in polyacrylic solution, net price 10 mL (with applicator) = £3.56. Label: 15

**Dose**

Apply daily

**Salactol®** (Dermal)

Paint, salicylic acid 16.7%, lactic acid 16.7%, in flexible collodion, net price 10 mL (with applicator) = £1.71. Label: 15

**Dose**

Apply daily

**Note** Contains colophony (see notes above)

**Salatac®** (Dermal)

Gel, salicylic acid 12%, lactic acid 4% in a collodion basis, net price 8 g (with applicator) = £2.98. Label: 15

**Dose**

Apply daily

**Verrugon®** (Ransom)

Ointment, salicylic acid 50% in a paraffin basis, net price 6 g = £3.12

**Dose**

Apply daily

### ▌ FORMALDEHYDE

**Cautions** see under Salicylic Acid

**Side-effects** see under Salicylic Acid

**Licensed use** licensed for use in children (age range not specified by manufacturer)

**Indications and dose**

**Warts, particularly plantar warts** for dose see preparation below

**Veracur®** (Typharm)

Gel, formaldehyde 0.75% in a water-miscible gel basis, net price 15 g = £2.41

**Dose**

Apply twice daily

## ◼ GLUTARALDEHYDE

**Cautions**  protect surrounding skin; not for application to face, mucosa, or anogenital areas

**Side-effects**  rashes, skin irritation (discontinue if severe); stains skin brown

**Licensed use**  licensed for use in children (age range not specified by manufacturer)

**Indications and dose**

**Warts, particularly plantar warts**

Apply twice daily

**Glutarol®** (Dermal)

Solution (= application), glutaraldehyde 10%, net price 10 mL (with applicator) = £2.07

## ◼ SILVER NITRATE

**Cautions**  protect surrounding skin and avoid broken skin; not suitable for application to face, ano-genital region, or large areas

**Side-effects**  chemical burns on surrounding skin; stains skin and fabric

**Licensed use**  no age range specified by manufacturer

**Indications and dose**

**Common warts and verrucas**

Apply moistened caustic pencil tip for 1–2 minutes; repeat after 24 hours up to max. 3 applications for warts *or* max. 6 applications for verrucas

Instructions in proprietary packs generally incorporate advice to remove dead skin before use by gentle filing and to cover with adhesive dressing after application

**Umbilical granulomas**

Apply moistened caustic pencil tip (usually containing silver nitrate 40%) for 1–2 minutes while protecting surrounding skin with soft paraffin

**AVOCA®** (Bray)

Caustic pencil, tip containing silver nitrate 40%, potassium nitrate 60%, net price = £0.94; silver nitrate 95%, potassium nitrate 5%, treatment pack (including emery file, 6 adhesive dressings and protector pads) = £1.94

## Anogenital warts

Anogenital warts (condylomata acuminata) in children are often asymptomatic and require only a simple barrier preparation. If treatment is required it should be supervised by a hospital specialist. Persistent warts on genital skin may require treatment with cryotherapy or other forms of physical ablation under general anaesthesia.

**Podophyllotoxin** (the major active ingredient of podophyllum), or **imiquimod** are used to treat external anogenital warts; these preparations can cause considerable irritation of the treated area and are therefore suitable only for children who are able to cooperate with the treatment.

## ◼ IMIQUIMOD

**Cautions**  avoid normal or broken skin and open wounds; not suitable for internal genital warts; uncircumcised males (risk of phimosis or stricture of foreskin); autoimmune disease; immunosuppressed patients

**Pregnancy**  no evidence of teratogenicity or toxicity in *animal* studies; manufacturer advises caution

**Breast-feeding**  no information available

**Side-effects**  local reactions (including itching, burning sensation, erythema, erosion, oedema, excoriation, and scabbing); headache; influenza-like symptoms; myalgia; *less commonly* local ulceration and alopecia; *rarely* Stevens-Johnson syndrome and cutaneous lupus erythematosus-like effect; *very rarely* dysuria in females; permanent hypopigmentation or hyperpigmentation reported

**Licensed use**  not licensed for use in children

**Indications and dose**

**External genital and perianal warts** (for use under specialist supervision only)

Apply thinly 3 times a week at night until lesions resolve (max. 16 weeks)

**Important**  Should be rubbed in and allowed to stay on the treated area for 6–10 hours then washed off with mild soap and water (uncircumcised males treating warts under foreskin should wash the area daily). The cream should be washed off before sexual contact

**Aldara®** (Meda) ⃞PoM⃞

Cream, imiquimod 5%, net price 12-sachet pack = £48.34. Label: 10, patient information leaflet

**Excipients**  include benzyl alcohol, cetyl alcohol, hydroxybenzoates (parabens), polysorbate 60, stearyl alcohol

**Condoms**  may damage latex condoms and diaphragms

## ◼ PODOPHYLLOTOXIN

**Cautions**  see notes above; avoid normal skin and open wounds; keep away from face; very irritant to eyes

**Pregnancy**  avoid

**Breast-feeding**  avoid

**Side-effects**  local irritation

**Licensed use**  not licensed for use in children

**Indications and dose**

See under preparations (for use under specialist supervision only)

**Condyline®** (Takeda) ⃞PoM⃞

Solution, podophyllotoxin 0.5% in alcoholic basis, net price 3.5 mL (with applicators) = £14.49. Label: 15

**Dose**

**Condylomata acuminata affecting the penis or the female external genitalia**

**Child 2–18 years** (see notes above) apply twice daily for 3 consecutive days; treatment may be repeated at weekly intervals if necessary for a total of five 3-day treatment courses; direct medical supervision for lesions in the female and for lesions greater than 4 cm$^2$ in the male; max. 50 single applications ('loops') per session (consult product literature)

**Warticon®** (GSK) ⃞PoM⃞

Cream, podophyllotoxin 0.15%, net price 5 g (with mirror) = £14.86

**Excipients**  include butylated hydroxyanisole, cetyl alcohol, hydroxybenzoates (parabens), sorbic acid, stearyl alcohol

**Dose**

**Condylomata acuminata affecting the penis or the female external genitalia**

**Child 2–18 years** (see notes above) apply twice daily for 3 consecutive days; treatment may be repeated at weekly intervals if necessary for a total of four 3-day treatment courses; direct medical supervision for lesions greater than 4 cm$^2$

**13**

**Skin**

Solution, blue, podophyllotoxin 0.5% in alcoholic basis, net price 3 mL (with applicators) = £12.38. Label: 15

**Dose**

> **Condylomata acuminata affecting the penis or the female external genitalia**
>
> **Child 2–18 years** (see notes above) apply twice daily for 3 consecutive days; treatment may be repeated at weekly intervals if necessary for a total of four 3-day treatment courses; direct medical supervision for lesions greater than 4 cm²; max. 50 single applications ('loops') per session (consult product literature)

# 13.8 Sunscreens and camouflagers

### 13.8.1 Sunscreen preparations
### 13.8.2 Camouflagers

# 13.8.1 Sunscreen preparations

Solar ultraviolet irradiation can be harmful to the skin. It is responsible for disorders such as *polymorphic light eruption, solar urticaria*, and it provokes the various *cutaneous porphyrias*. It also provokes (or at least aggravates) skin lesions of *lupus erythematosus* and may aggravate some other *dermatoses*. Certain drugs, such as demeclocycline, phenothiazines, or amiodarone, can cause photosensitivity. All these conditions (as well as *sunburn*) may occur after relatively short periods of exposure to the sun. Solar ultraviolet irradiation may provoke attacks of recurrent herpes labialis (but it is not known whether the effect of sunlight exposure is local or systemic).

The effects of exposure over longer periods include *ageing changes* and more importantly the initiation of *skin cancer*.

Solar ultraviolet radiation is approximately 200–400 nm in wavelength. The medium wavelengths (290–320 nm, known as UVB) cause *sunburn*. The long wavelengths (320–400 nm, known as UVA) are responsible for many *photosensitivity reactions* and *photodermatoses*. Both UVA and UVB contribute to long-term *photodamage* and to the changes responsible for *skin cancer* and ageing.

Sunscreen preparations contain substances that protect the skin against UVA and UVB radiation, but they are no substitute for covering the skin and avoiding sunlight. Protective clothing and sun avoidance (rather than the use of sunscreen preparations) are recommended for children under 6 months of age.

The sun protection factor (SPF, usually indicated in the preparation title) provides guidance on the degree of protection offered against UVB; it indicates the multiples of protection provided against burning, compared with unprotected skin; for example, an SPF of 8 should enable a child to remain 8 times longer in the sun without burning. However, in practice users do not apply sufficient sunscreen product and the protection is lower than that found in experimental studies. Some manufacturers use a star rating system to indicate the protection against UVA relative to protection against UVB for sunscreen products. However, the usefulness of the star rating system remains controversial. The EU Commission (September 2006) has recommended that the UVA protection factor for a sunscreen should be at least one-third of the sun protection factor (SPF); products that achieve this requirement will be labelled with a UVA logo alongside the SPF classification. Preparations that also contain reflective substances, such as titanium dioxide, provide the most effective protection against UVA.

Sunscreen preparations may rarely cause allergic reactions.

> For optimum photoprotection, sunscreen preparations should be applied **thickly** and **frequently** (approximately 2 hourly). In photodermatoses, they should be used from spring to autumn. As maximum protection from sunlight is desirable, preparations with the highest SPF should be prescribed.

## Ingredient nomenclature in sunscreen preparations

| rINN | INCI |
| --- | --- |
| amiloxate | isoamyl *p*-methoxycinnamate |
| avobenzone | butyl methoxydibenzoylmethane |
| bemotrizinol | bis-ethylhexyloxyphenol methoxyphenyl triazine |
| bisoctrizole | methylene bis-benzotriazolyl tetramethylbutylphenol |
| ecamsule | terephthalylidene dicamphor sulfonic acid |
| ensulizole | phenylbenzimidazole sulfonic acid |
| enzacamene | 4-methylbenzylidene camphor |
| octinoxate | octyl (*or* ethylhexyl) methoxycinnamate |
| octocrilene | octocrylene |
| oxybenzone | benzophenone-3 |

The European Commission Cosmetic Products Regulation (EC) 1223/2009 requires the use of INCI (International Nomenclature of Cosmetic Ingredients) for cosmetics and sunscreens. This table includes the rINN and the INCI synonym for the active ingredients of sunscreen preparations in BNFC

**Borderline substances**    The preparations marked 'ACBS' cannot be prescribed on the NHS except for skin protection against ultraviolet radiation in abnormal cutaneous photosensitivity resulting from genetic disorders or photodermatoses, including vitiligo and those resulting from radiotherapy; chronic or recurrent herpes simplex labialis. Preparations with SPF less than 30 should not normally be prescribed. See also Appendix 2.

**Anthelios®** (L'Oréal Active)

XL SPF 50+ Melt-in cream (UVA and UVB protection; UVB-SPF 50+), avobenzone 3.5%, bemotrizinol 3%, drometrizole trisiloxane 0.5%, ecamsule 1%, octocrilene 2.5%, titanium dioxide 4.2%, net price 50 mL = £3.63. ACBS

**Excipients** include disodium edetate, stearyl alcohol

**Note** For INCI synonyms, see table above

**Sunsense® Ultra** (Crawford)

Lotion (UVA and UVB protection; UVB-SPF 50+), avobenzone 2%, ensulizole 2%, enzacamene 4%, octinoxate 6%, oxybenzone 2%, titanium dioxide 3%, net price 50-mL bottle with roll-on applicator = £4.11, 125 mL = £6.86, 500-mL pump pack = £15.54. ACBS

Excipients  include butylated hydroxytoluene, cetyl alcohol, fragrance, hydroxybenzoates (parabens), propylene glycol

Note  For INCI synonyms, see table above

**Uvistat®** (LPC)

Cream (UVA and UVB protection; UVB-SPF 30), avobenzone 5%, bisotrizole 1.5%, octinoxate 7.5%, octocrilene 4%, titanium dioxide 5.2%, net price 125 mL = £7.45. ACBS

Excipients  include disodium edetate, hydroxybenzoates (parabens), propylene glycol

Note  For INCI synonyms, see table above

Cream (UVA and UVB protection; UVB-SPF 50), amiloxate 2%, avobenzone 5%, bisotrizole 6%, octinoxate 10%, octocrilene 4%, titanium dioxide 4.8%, net price 125 mL = £8.45. ACBS

Excipients  include disodium edetate, polysorbate 60, propylene glycol

Note  For INCI synonyms, see table above

Lipscreen (UVA and UVB protection; UVB-SPF 50), avobenzone 5%, bemotrizinol 3%, octinoxate 10%, octocrilene 4%, titanium dioxide 3%, net price 5 g = £2.99. ACBS

Excipients  include butylated hydroxytoluene, hydroxybenzoates (parabens)

Note  For INCI synonyms, see table above

## Photodamage

*Actinic keratoses* occur very rarely in healthy children; *actinic cheilitis* may occur on the lips of adolescents following excessive sun exposure.

**Diclofenac** gel (*Solaraze®*) and topical preparations of **fluorouracil** are licensed for the treatment of actinic keratoses but they are not licensed for use in children.

In children with photosensitivity disorders, such as erythropoietic protoporphyria, specialists may use **beta-carotene**, **mepacrine**, **chloroquine** or **hydroxychloroquine** (section 10.1.3) to reduce skin reactions.

### ▌ BETACAROTENE

Note  Betacarotene is a precursor to vitamin A

**Cautions**  monitor vitamin A intake; **interactions:** Appendix 1 (vitamins)

**Hepatic impairment**  avoid

**Renal impairment**  use with caution

**Pregnancy**  partially converted to vitamin A, but does not give rise to abnormally high serum concentration; manufacturer advises use only if potential benefit outweighs risk

**Breast-feeding**  use with caution—present in milk

**Side-effects**  loose stools; yellow discoloration of skin; *rarely*, bruising, arthralgia

**Licensed use**  not licensed for use in UK

**Indications and dose**

> **Management of photosensitivity reactions in erythropoietic protoporphyria** (specialist use only)
>
> • **By mouth**
>
>  **Child 1–5 years** 60–90 mg daily in single or divided doses

**Child 5–9 years** 90–120 mg daily in single or divided doses

**Child 9–12 years** 120–150 mg daily in single or divided doses

**Child 12–16 years** 150–180 mg daily in single or divided doses

**Child 16–18 years** 180–300 mg daily in single or divided doses

Note  Protection not total—avoid strong sunlight and use sunscreen preparations; generally 2–6 weeks of treatment (resulting in yellow coloration of palms and soles) necessary before increasing exposure to sunlight; dose should be adjusted according to level of exposure to sunlight

**Betacarotene** (Non-proprietary)

Capsules, 15 mg, 25 mg are available from 'special-order' manufacturers or specialist importing companies, see p. 823. Label: 21

## █ 13.8.2 █ Camouflagers

Disfigurement of the skin can be very distressing and may have a marked psychological effect, especially in children. Cosmetic preparations may be used to camouflage unsightly scars, skin deformities, and pigment abnormalities, such as vitiligo and birthmarks.

Opaque cover foundation or cream is used to mask skin pigment abnormalities; careful application using a combination of dark- and light-coloured cover creams set with powder helps to minimise the appearance of skin deformities.

**Borderline substances**  The preparations marked 'ACBS' cannot be prescribed on the NHS for postoperative scars and other deformities except as adjunctive therapy in the relief of emotional disturbances due to disfiguring skin disease, such as vitiligo.

**Covermark®** (Derma UK)

Classic foundation (masking cream), net price 15 mL (10 shades) = £11.86. ACBS

Excipients  include beeswax, hydroxybenzoates (parabens), fragrance

Finishing powder, net price 25 g = £11.86. ACBS

Excipients  include beeswax, hydroxybenzoates (parabens), fragrance

**Dermablend®** (L'Oréal Active)

Ultra corrective foundation, (7 shades), net price 12 g = £5.60. ACBS

Excipients  include beeswax, isopropyl palmitate

**Dermacolor®** (Fox)

Camouflage creme, (100 shades), net price 25 mL = £10.37. ACBS

Excipients  include beeswax, butylated hydroxytoluene, fragrance, propylene glycol, stearyl alcohol, wool fat

Fixing powder, (7 shades), net price 60 g = £8.77. ACBS

Excipients  include fragrance

**Keromask®** (Lornamead)

Masking cream, (24 shades), net price 15 mL = £5.68. ACBS

Excipients  include butylated hydroxyanisole, hydroxybenzoates (parabens), wool fat, propylene glycol

Finishing powder, (4 shades) net price 20 g = £5.68. ACBS

Excipients  include butylated hydroxytoluene, hydroxybenzoates (parabens)

**Veil**® (Thomas Blake)

Cover cream (40 shades), net price 19 g = £21.66, 44 g = £32.22, 70 g = £40.68. ACBS

Excipients   include hydroxybenzoates (parabens), wool fat derivative

Finishing powder, translucent, net price 35 g = £23.75. ACBS

Excipients   include butylated hydroxyanisole, hydroxybenzoates (parabens)

## 13.9  Shampoos and other preparations for scalp conditions

The detergent action of shampoo removes grease (sebum) from hair. Prepubertal children produce very little grease and require shampoo less frequently than adults. Shampoos can be used as vehicles for medicinal products, but their usefulness is limited by the short time the product is in contact with the scalp and by their irritant nature.

Oils and ointments are very useful for scaly, dry scalp conditions; if a greasy appearance is cosmetically unacceptable, the preparation may be applied at night and washed out in the morning. Alcohol-based lotions are rarely used in children; alcohol causes painful stinging on broken skin and the fumes may exacerbate asthma.

Itchy, inflammatory, eczematous scalp conditions may be relieved by a simple emollient oil such as **olive oil** or **coconut oil** (arachis oil (ground nut oil, peanut oil) is best avoided in children under 5 years). In more severe cases a topical **corticosteroid** (section 13.4) may be required. Preparations containing **coal tar** are used for the common scaly scalp conditions of childhood including seborrhoeic dermatitis, dandruff (a mild form of seborrhoeic dermatitis), and psoriasis (section 13.5.2); **salicylic acid** is used as a keratolytic in some scalp preparations.

Shampoos containing antimicrobials such as **selenium sulfide** or **ketoconazole** are used for seborrhoeic dermatitis and dandruff in which yeast infection has been implicated, and for tinea capitis (ringworm of the scalp, section 13.10.2). Bacterial infection affecting the scalp (usually secondary to eczema, head lice, or ringworm) may be treated with shampoos containing antimicrobials such as **pyrithione zinc**, **cetrimide**, or **povidone-iodine**.

In neonates and infants, *cradle cap* (which is also a form of seborrhoeic eczema) can be treated by massaging **coconut oil** or **olive oil** into the scalp; a bland emollient such as **emulsifying ointment** can be rubbed onto the affected area once or twice daily before bathing and a mild shampoo used.

◀ **Shampoos**

[1]**Ketoconazole** (Non-proprietary) PoM

Cream—section 13.10.2

1. Can be sold to the public for the prevention and treatment of dandruff and seborrhoeic dermatitis of the scalp as a shampoo formulation containing ketoconazole max. 2%, in a pack containing max. 120 mL and labelled to show a max. frequency of application of once every 3 days

Shampoo, ketoconazole 2%, net price 120 mL = £3.53

Excipients   include imidurea

Brands include   *Dandrazol*® *2% Shampoo, Nizoral*®

**Dose**

**Seborrhoeic dermatitis and dandruff**

Treatment, apply twice weekly for 2–4 weeks; prophylaxis, apply once every 1–2 weeks; leave preparation on for 3–5 minutes before rinsing

**Pityriasis versicolor**

Treatment, apply once daily for max. 5 days; prophylaxis, apply once daily for up to 3 days before sun exposure; leave preparation on for 3–5 minutes before rinsing

**Alphosyl 2 in 1**® (GSK Consumer Healthcare)

Shampoo, alcoholic coal tar extract 5%, net price 125 mL = £1.81, 250 mL = £3.43

Excipients   include hydroxybenzoates (parabens), fragrance

**Dose**

**Dandruff**

Use once or twice weekly as necessary

**Psoriasis, seborrhoeic dermatitis, scaling and itching**

Use every 2–3 days

**Capasal**® (Dermal)

Shampoo, coal tar 1%, coconut oil 1%, salicylic acid 0.5%, net price 250 mL = £4.69

Excipients   none as listed in section 13.1.3

**Dose**

**Scaly scalp disorders including psoriasis, seborrhoeic dermatitis, dandruff, and cradle cap**

Apply daily as necessary

**Ceanel Concentrate**® (Alliance)

Shampoo, cetrimide 10%, undecenoic acid 1%, net price 150 mL = £3.40, 500 mL = £9.80

Excipients   none as listed in section 13.1.3

**Dose**

**Scalp psoriasis, seborrhoeic dermatitis, dandruff**

Apply 3 times in first week then twice weekly

**Dermax**® (Dermal)

Shampoo, benzalkonium chloride 0.5%, net price 250 mL = £5.69

Excipients   none as listed in section 13.1.3

**Dose**

**Seborrhoeic scalp conditions associated with dandruff and scaling**

Apply as necessary

**Psoriderm**® (Dermal)

Scalp lotion (= shampoo), coal tar 2.5%, lecithin 0.3%, net price 250 mL = £4.74

Excipients   include disodium edetate

**Dose**

**Scalp psoriasis**

Use as necessary

**Selsun**® (Chattem UK)

Shampoo, selenium sulfide 2.5%, net price 50 mL = £1.44, 100 mL = £1.96, 150 mL = £2.75

Excipients   include fragrance

Cautions   avoid using 48 hours before or after applying hair colouring, straightening or waving preparations

**13 Skin**

Dose

**Seborrhoeic dermatitis and dandruff**

**Child 5–18 years** apply twice weekly for 2 weeks then once weekly for 2 weeks and then as necessary

**Pityriasis versicolor [unlicensed indication]**

**Child 5–18 years** apply to affected area and leave on for 10 minutes before rinsing off; apply once daily for 7 days; repeat course if necessary

**Note** diluting with a small amount of water prior to application can reduce irritation

### T/Gel® (J&J)

Shampoo, coal tar extract 2%, net price 125 mL = £3.18, 250 mL = £4.78

**Excipients** include fragrance, hydroxybenzoates (parabens), imidurea, tetrasodium edetate

Dose

**Scalp psoriasis, seborrhoeic dermatitis, dandruff**

Apply 2–3 times weekly

◀**Other scalp preparations**

### Cocois®

Section 13.5.2

### Polytar® (GSK)

Liquid, tar blend 1%, net price 250 mL = £2.23

**Excipients** include arachis (peanut) oil, fragrance, imidurea, polysorbate 80

Dose

**Scalp disorders including psoriasis, seborrhoea, eczema, pruritus, and dandruff**

Apply 1–2 times weekly

### Polytar Plus® (GSK)

Liquid, tar blend 1%, net price 500 mL = £3.91

**Excipients** include arachis (peanut) oil, fragrance, imidurea, polysorbate 80

Dose

**Scalp disorders including psoriasis, seborrhoea, pruritus, and dandruff**

Apply 1–2 times weekly

## 13.10 Anti-infective skin preparations

| | |
|---|---|
| 13.10.1 | Antibacterial preparations |
| 13.10.2 | Antifungal preparations |
| 13.10.3 | Antiviral preparations |
| 13.10.4 | Parasiticidal preparations |
| 13.10.5 | Preparations for minor cuts and abrasions |

## 13.10.1 Antibacterial preparations

| | |
|---|---|
| 13.10.1.1 | Antibacterial preparations only used topically |
| 13.10.1.2 | Antibacterial preparations also used systemically |

Topical antibacterial preparations are used to treat localised bacterial skin infections caused by Gram-positive organisms (particularly by staphylococci or streptococci). Systemic antibacterial treatment (Table 1, section 5.1) is more appropriate for deep-seated skin infections.

Problems associated with the use of topical antibacterials include bacterial resistance, contact sensitisation, and superinfection. In order to minimise the development of resistance, antibacterials used systemically (e.g. fusidic acid) should not generally be chosen for topical use. *Resistant organisms* are more common in hospitals, and whenever possible swabs should be taken for bacteriological examination before beginning treatment.

**Neomycin** applied topically may cause sensitisation and cross-sensitivity with other aminoglycoside antibacterials such as gentamicin may occur. Topical antibacterials applied over large areas can cause systemic toxicity; ototoxicity with neomycin and with **polymyxins** is a particular risk for neonates and children with renal impairment.

Superficial bacterial infection of the skin may be treated with a topical antiseptic such as **povidine–iodine** (section 13.11.4) which also softens crusts, or **hydrogen peroxide** 1% cream (section 13.11.6).

Bacterial infections such as *impetigo* and *folliculitis* can be treated with a short course of topical **fusidic acid**; **mupirocin** should be used only to treat meticillin-resistant *Staphylococcus aureus*.

For extensive or long-standing impetigo, an oral antibacterial such as **flucloxacillin** (or **clarithromycin** in children with penicillin-allergy), Table 1, section 5.1, should be used. A mild antiseptic may help to soften crusts. Mild antiseptics may be useful in reducing the spread of infection, but there is little evidence to support the use of topical antiseptics alone in the treatment of impetigo.

*Cellulitis*, a rapidly spreading deeply seated inflammation of the skin and subcutaneous tissue, requires systemic antibacterial treatment (see Table 1, section 5.1). Lower leg infections or infections spreading around wounds are almost always cellulitis. *Erysipelas*, a superficial infection with clearly defined edges (and often affecting the face), is also treated with a systemic antibacterial (see Table 1, section 5.1).

*Staphylococcal scalded-skin syndrome* requires urgent treatment with a systemic antibacterial, such as flucloxacillin (see Table 1, section 5.1).

**Mupirocin** is not related to any other antibacterial in use; it is effective for skin infections, particularly those due to Gram-positive organisms but it is not indicated for pseudomonal infection. Although *Staphylococcus aureus* strains with low-level resistance to mupirocin are emerging, it is generally useful in infections resistant to other antibacterials. To avoid the development of resistance, mupirocin or fusidic acid should not be used for longer than 10 days and local microbiology advice should be sought before using it in hospital. In the presence of mupirocin-resistant MRSA infection, a topical antiseptic, such as povidone–iodine, chlorhexidine, or alcohol, can be used (section 13.11); their use should be discussed with the local microbiologist.

Mupirocin ointment contains macrogols; extensive absorption of macrogols through the mucous membranes or through application to thin or damaged skin may result in renal toxicity, especially in neonates. Mupirocin nasal ointment is formulated in a paraffin base and may be more suitable for the treatment of MRSA-infected open wound in neonates.

**Metronidazole** gel is used topically in children to reduce the odour associated with anaerobic infections and for the treatment of periorificial rosacea (section 13.6); oral metronidazole (section 5.1.11) is used to treat wounds infected with anaerobic bacteria.

**13**

**Skin**

Retapamulin can be used for impetigo and other super-ficial bacterial skin infections caused by *Staphylococcus aureus* and *Streptococcus pyogenes* that are resistant to first-line topical antibacterials. However, it is not effec-tive against MRSA. The *Scottish Medicines Consortium* (p. 3) has advised (March 2008) that retapamulin (*Altar-go*®) is **not** recommended for use within NHS Scotland for the treatment of superficial skin infections.

Silver sulfadiazine is licensed for the prevention and treatment of infection in burns but the use of appro-priate dressings may be more effective. Systemic effects may occur following extensive application of silver sulfadiazine; its use is not recommended in neonates.

### 13.10.1.1  Antibacterial preparations only used topically

## MUPIROCIN

**Renal impairment** manufacturer advises caution when *Bactroban*® ointment used in moderate or severe impairment because it contains macrogols (polyethylene glycols)

**Pregnancy** manufacturer advises avoid unless poten-tial benefit outweighs risk—no information available

**Breast-feeding** no information available

**Side-effects** local reactions including urticaria, pru-ritus, burning sensation, rash

**Licensed use** *Bactroban*® ointment licensed for use in children (age range not specified by manufacturer); *Bactroban*® cream not recommended for use in chil-dren under 1 year

**Indications and dose**

> **Bacterial skin infections** (see also notes above)
>
> > **Child 1 month–18 years** apply up to 3 times daily for up to 10 days

**Bactroban**® (GSK) [PoM]

Cream, mupirocin (as mupirocin calcium) 2%, net price 15 g = £4.38

Excipients include benzyl alcohol, cetyl alcohol, stearyl alcohol

Ointment, mupirocin 2%, net price 15 g = £4.38

Excipients none as listed in section 13.1.3

Nasal ointment—section 12.2.3

## NEOMYCIN SULFATE

**Cautions** large areas—if large areas of skin are being treated ototoxicity may be a hazard in children, particularly in those with renal impairment

**Contra-indications** neonates

**Renal impairment** see Cautions above

**Side-effects** sensitisation (see also notes above)

**Licensed use** *Neomycin Cream BPC*—no information available

**Indications and dose**

> **Bacterial skin infections** see under preparation

**Neomycin Cream BPC** [PoM] ▨

Cream, neomycin sulfate 0.5%, cetomacrogol emulsifying ointment 30%, chlorocresol 0.1%, disodium edetate 0.01%, in freshly boiled and cooled purified water, net price 15 g = £2.17

Excipients include cetostearyl alcohol, edetic acid (EDTA)

Dose

> Apply up to 3 times daily (short-term use)

## POLYMYXINS

**Cautions** large areas—if large areas of skin are being treated nephrotoxicity and neurotoxicity may be a hazard, particularly in children with renal impairment

**Renal impairment** see Cautions above

**Side-effects** sensitisation (see also notes above)

**Licensed use** licensed for use in children (age range not specified by manufacturer)

**Indications and dose**

> **Bacterial skin infections** see under preparation

**Polyfax**® (TEVA UK) [PoM]

Ointment, polymyxin B sulfate 10 000 units, bacitra-cin zinc 500 units/g, net price 4 g = £3.26, 20 g = £4.62

Excipients none as listed in section 13.1.3

Dose

> Apply twice daily or more frequently if required

## RETAPAMULIN

**Contra-indications** contact with eyes and mucous membranes

**Side-effects** local reactions including irritation, erythema, pain, contact dermatitis, and pruritus

**Indications and dose**

> **Superficial bacterial skin infections** (but see also notes above)
>
> > **Child 9 months–18 years** apply thinly twice daily for 5 days; max. area of skin treated 2% of body surface area; review treatment if no response within 2–3 days

**Altargo**® (GSK) [PoM]

Ointment, retapamulin 1%, net price 5 g = £7.89.

Label: 28

Excipients include butylated hydroxytoluene

## SILVER SULFADIAZINE

**Cautions** G6PD deficiency; may inactivate enzymatic debriding agents—concomitant use may be inap-propriate; **interactions:** Appendix 1 (sulfonamides)

Large areas Plasma-sulfadiazine concentrations may approach therapeutic levels with *side-effects* and *interactions* as for sulfonamides (see section 5.1.8) if large areas of skin are treated. Owing to the association of sulfonamides with severe blood and skin disorders, treatment should be stopped immediately if blood disorders or rashes develop—but leucopenia developing 2–3 days after starting treatment of burns patients is reported usually to be self-limiting and silver sulfadiazine need not usually be discontinued provided blood counts are monitored carefully to ensure return to baseline within a few days. Argyria may also occur if large areas of skin are treated (or if application is prolonged).

**Contra-indications** sensitivity to sulfonamides; not recommended for neonates

**Hepatic impairment** manufacturer advises caution if significant impairment; see also Large areas, above

**Renal impairment** manufacturer advises caution if significant impairment; see also Large areas, above

**Pregnancy** risk of neonatal haemolysis and methaemoglobinaemia in third trimester

**Breast-feeding** small risk of kernicterus in jaundiced infants and of haemolysis in G6PD deficient infants

**Side-effects** allergic reactions including burning, itching and rashes; argyria reported following pro-longed use; leucopenia reported (monitor blood count)

13 Skin

**Licensed use** no age range specified by manufacturer but see contra-indications, above

**Indications and dose**

> **Prophylaxis and treatment of infection in burn wounds, for conservative management of finger-tip injuries** see under preparation below

> **Adjunct to short-term treatment of infection in pressure sores, adjunct to prophylaxis of infection in skin graft donor sites and extensive abrasions** consult product literature for details

**Flamazine**® (S&N Hlth.) PoM

Cream, silver sulfadiazine 1%, net price 20 g = £2.91, 50 g = £3.85, 250 g = £10.32, 500 g = £18.27
**Excipients** include cetyl alcohol, polysorbates, propylene glycol

**Dose**

> **Burns**

>> **Child 1 month–18 years** apply daily or more frequently if very exudative

> **Finger-tip injuries**

>> **Child 1 month–18 years** apply every 2–3 days

**Note** apply with sterile applicator

## 13.10.1.2 Antibacterial preparations also used systemically

**Sodium fusidate** is a narrow-spectrum antibacterial used for staphylococcal infections. For the role of sodium fusidate in the treatment of impetigo see p. 587.

**Metronidazole** is used topically to treat rosacea and to reduce the odour associated with anaerobic infections; oral metronidazole (section 5.1.11) is used to treat wounds infected with anaerobic bacteria.

**Angular cheilitis** An ointment containing sodium fusidate is used in the fissures of angular cheilitis when associated with staphylococcal infection. For further information on angular cheilitis, see p. 548.

## FUSIDIC ACID

**Cautions** see notes above; avoid contact with eyes

**Side-effects** rarely hypersensitivity reactions

**Licensed use** licensed for use in children (age range not specified by manufacturer)

**Indications and dose**

> **Staphylococcal skin infections**

>> Apply 3–4 times daily, usually for 7 days

> **Penicillin-resistant staphylococcal infections**

>> section 5.1.7

> **Staphylococcal eye infections**

>> section 11.3.1

**Fucidin**® (LEO) PoM

Cream, fusidic acid 2%, net price 15 g = £1.92, 30 g = £3.64
**Excipients** include butylated hydroxyanisole, cetyl alcohol

Ointment, sodium fusidate 2%, net price 15 g = £2.23, 30 g = £3.79
**Excipients** include cetyl alcohol, wool fat

**Dental prescribing on NHS** May be prescribed as Sodium Fusidate ointment

## METRONIDAZOLE

**Cautions** avoid exposure to strong sunlight or UV light

**Side-effects** skin irritation

**Licensed use** *Acea*® and *Anabact*® not licensed for use in children under 12 years; *Noritate*® not licensed for use in children under 16 years; *Metrogel*®, *Metrosa*®, *Rosiced*®, *Rozex*®, and *Zyomet*® not licensed for use in children

**Indications and dose**

> **Malodorous tumours and wounds**

>> For dose see preparations

> **Rosacea** (see also section 13.6)

>> For dose see preparations

> ***Helicobacter pylori* eradication**

>> section 1.3

> **Anaerobic infections**

>> section 5.1.11 and section 7.2.2

> **Protozoal infections**

>> section 5.4.2

**Acea**® (Ferndale) PoM

Gel, metronidazole 0.75%, net price 40 g = £9.95
**Excipients** include disodium edetate, hydroxybenzoates (parabens)

**Dose**

> **Acute inflammatory exacerbations of rosacea**

>> **Child 1–18 years** apply thinly twice daily

**Anabact**® (CHS) PoM

Gel, metronidazole 0.75%, net price 15 g = £4.47, 30 g = £7.89
**Excipients** include hydroxybenzoates (parabens), propylene glycol

**Dose**

> **Malodorous fungating tumours and skin ulcers**

>> Apply to clean wound 1–2 times daily and cover with non-adherent dressing

**Metrogel**® (Galderma) PoM

Gel, metronidazole 0.75%, net price 40 g = £6.86
**Excipients** include hydroxybenzoates (parabens), propylene glycol

**Dose**

> **Acute inflammatory exacerbations of rosacea**

>> **Child 1–18 years** apply thinly twice daily

> **Malodorous fungating tumours**

>> Apply to clean wound 1–2 times daily and cover with non-adherent dressing

**Metrosa**® (Linderma) PoM

Gel, metronidazole 0.75%, net price 40 g = £19.90
**Excipients** include propylene glycol

**Dose**

> **Acute exacerbation of rosacea**

>> **Child 1–18 years** apply thinly twice daily

**Rosiced**® (Fabre) PoM

Cream, metronidazole 0.75%, net price 30 g = £7.50
**Excipients** include propylene glycol

**Dose**

> **Inflammatory papules and pustules of rosacea**

>> **Child 1–18 years** apply twice daily for 6 weeks (longer if necessary)

**13**

**Skin**

**Rozex®** (Galderma) PoM

Cream, metronidazole 0.75%, net price 30 g = £4.11, 40 g = £6.86
**Excipients** include benzyl alcohol, isopropyl palmitate

Gel, metronidazole 0.75%, net price 30 g = £4.11, 40 g = £6.86
**Excipients** include disodium edetate, hydroxybenzoates (parabens), propylene glycol

**Dose**

> **Inflammatory papules, pustules and erythema of rosacea**
>
> **Child 1–18 years** apply twice daily

**Zyomet®** (Mercury) PoM

Gel, metronidazole 0.75%, net price 30 g = £12.00
**Excipients** include benzyl alcohol, disodium edetate, propylene glycol

**Dose**

> **Acute inflammatory exacerbations of rosacea**
>
> **Child 1–18 years** apply thinly twice daily

## 13.10.2 Antifungal preparations

Most localised fungal infections are treated with topical preparations. To prevent relapse, local antifungal treatment should be continued for 1–2 weeks after the disappearance of all signs of infection. Systemic therapy (section 5.2) is necessary for nail or scalp infection or if the skin infection is widespread, disseminated or intractable. Specimens of scale, nail or hair should be sent for mycological examination before starting treatment, unless the diagnosis is certain.

**Dermatophytoses**    Ringworm infection can affect the scalp (tinea capitis), body (tinea corporis), groin (tinea cruris), hand (tinea manuum), foot (tinea pedis, athlete's foot), or nail (tinea unguium, onychomycosis). Tinea capitis is a common childhood infection that requires systemic treatment with an oral antifungal (section 5.2); additional application of a topical antifungal, during the early stages of treatment, may reduce the risk of transmission. A topical antifungal can also be used to treat asymptomatic carriers of scalp ringworm.

Tinea corporis and tinea pedis infections in children respond to treatment with a topical **imidazole** (clotrimazole, econazole, ketoconazole, or miconazole) or **terbinafine** cream. Nystatin is less effective against tinea.

**Compound benzoic acid ointment** (Whitfield's ointment) has been used for ringworm infections but it is cosmetically less acceptable than proprietary preparations. Antifungal dusting powders are of little therapeutic value in the treatment of fungal skin infections and may cause skin irritation; they may have some role in preventing re-infection.

Antifungal treatment may not be necessary in asymptomatic children with tinea infection of the nails. If treatment is necessary, a systemic antifungal (section 5.2) is more effective than topical therapy. However, topical application of **tioconazole** may be useful for treating early onychomycosis when involvement is limited to mild distal disease, or for superficial white onychomycosis, or where there are contra-indications to systemic therapy. Chronic paronychia on the fingers (usually due to a candidal infection) should be treated with topical clotrimazole or nystatin, but these preparations should be used with caution in children who suck their fingers. Chronic paronychia of the toes (usually due to

dermatophyte infection) can be treated with topical terbinafine.

**Pityriasis versicolor**    Pityriasis (tinea) versicolor can be treated with **ketoconazole** shampoo or **selenium sulfide** shampoo (section 13.9). Topical imidazole antifungals such as **clotrimazole, econazole, ketoconazole,** and **miconazole,** or topical **terbinafine** are alternatives, but large quantities may be required.

If topical therapy fails, or if the infection is widespread, pityriasis versicolor is treated systemically with an azole antifungal (section 5.2). Relapse is common, especially in the immunocompromised.

**Candidiasis**    Candidal skin infections can be treated with topical imidazole antifungals **clotrimazole, econazole, ketoconazole,** or **miconazole;** topical terbinafine is an alternative. Topical application of **nystatin** is also effective for candidiasis but it is ineffective against dermatophytosis. Refractory candidiasis requires systemic treatment (section 5.2.1) generally with a triazole such as fluconazole; systemic treatment with griseofulvin or terbinafine is **not appropriate** for refractory candidiasis. For the treatment of oral candiasis see section 12.3.2 and for the management of nappy rash see section 13.2.2.

**Angular cheilitis**    Miconazole cream is used in the fissures of angular cheilitis when associated with *Candida*. For further information on angular cheilitis, see p. 548.

**Cautions**    Contact with eyes and mucous membranes should be avoided.

**Side-effects**    Occasional local irritation and hypersensitivity reactions include mild burning sensation, erythema, and itching. Treatment should be discontinued if symptoms are severe.

**Compound topical preparations**    Combination of an imidazole and a mild corticosteroid (such as hydrocortisone 1%) (section 13.4) may be of value in the treatment of eczematous intertrigo and, in the first few days only, of a severely inflamed patch of ringworm. Combination of a mild corticosteroid with either an imidazole or nystatin may be of use in the treatment of *intertriginous eczema* associated with candida.

### ▌ AMOROLFINE

**Cautions**    see notes above; also avoid contact with ears; use with caution in child likely to suck affected digits

**Side-effects**    see notes above

**Licensed use**    not licensed for use in children under 12 years

**Indications and dose**

> **Fungal nail infections**
>
> Apply to infected nails 1–2 times weekly after filing and cleansing; allow to dry (approx. 3 minutes); treat finger nails for 6 months, toe nails for 9–12 months (review at intervals of 3 months); avoid nail varnish or artificial nails during treatment

**Amorolfine** (Non-proprietary) PoM

Nail lacquer, amorolfine (as hydrochloride) 5%, net price 5-mL pack = £11.35, 2 × 2.5-mL pack = £19.53. Label: 10, patient information leaflet
**Brands include** *Omicur®*

**Loceryl®** (Galderma) [PoM]
Nail lacquer, amorolfine (as hydrochloride) 5%, net price 5-mL pack (with nail files, spatulas, and cleansing swabs) = £18.17. Label: 10, patient information leaflet
Excipients   none as listed in section 13.1.3

## ◼ BENZOIC ACID

**Licensed use**   licensed for use in children (age range not specified by manufacturer)
**Indications and dose**
> Ringworm (tinea) but see notes above; dose under preparation

◢With salicylic acid
For prescribing information on salicylic acid, see p. 573

**Benzoic Acid Ointment, Compound, BP**
(Whitfield's ointment)
Ointment, benzoic acid 6%, salicylic acid 3%, in emulsifying ointment
Excipients   include cetostearyl alcohol
Dose
> **Child 1 month–18 years** apply twice daily

## ◼ CLOTRIMAZOLE

**Cautions**   see notes above
**Pregnancy**   minimal absorption from skin; not known to be harmful
**Side-effects**   see notes above
**Licensed use**   licensed for use in children (age range not specified by manufacturer)
**Indications and dose**
> Fungal skin infections
>> Apply 2–3 times daily

> Vaginal candidiasis section 7.2.2

> Otitis externa section 12.1.1

**Clotrimazole** (Non-proprietary)
Cream, clotrimazole 1%, net price 20 g = £1.52

**Canesten®** (Bayer Consumer Care)
Cream, clotrimazole 1%, net price 20 g = £2.14, 50 g = £3.50
Excipients   include benzyl alcohol, cetostearyl alcohol, polysorbate 60

Solution, clotrimazole 1% in macrogol 400 (polyethylene glycol 400), net price 20 mL = £2.43. For hairy areas
Excipients   none as listed in section 13.1.3

Spray, clotrimazole 1%, in 30% isopropyl alcohol, net price 40-mL atomiser = £4.99. Label: 15. For large or hairy areas
Excipients   include propylene glycol

## ◼ ECONAZOLE NITRATE

**Cautions**   see notes above
**Pregnancy**   minimal absorption from skin; not known to be harmful
**Side-effects**   see notes above
**Licensed use**   *Pevaryl®*, no age range specified by manufacturer

**Indications and dose**
> Fungal skin infections
>> Apply twice daily

> Fungal nail infections
>> Apply once daily under occlusive dressing

> Vaginal candidiasis section 7.2.2

**Pevaryl®** (Janssen)
Cream, econazole nitrate 1%, net price 30 g = £2.65
Excipients   include butylated hydroxyanisole, fragrance

## ◼ KETOCONAZOLE

**Cautions**   see notes above
**Side-effects**   see notes above
**Indications and dose**
> Tinea pedis
>> Apply twice daily

> Other fungal infections
>> Apply 1–2 times daily

> Systemic or resistant fungal infections section 5.2.2

> Vulval candidiasis section 7.2.2

**Nizoral®** (Janssen) [PoM]
[1]Cream, ketoconazole 2%, net price 30 g = £3.40
Excipients   include cetyl alcohol, polysorbates, propylene glycol, stearyl alcohol
Note   A 15-g tube is available for sale to the public for the treatment of tinea pedis, tinea cruris, and candidal intertrigo
Shampoo—section 13.9

## ◼ MICONAZOLE NITRATE

**Cautions**   see notes above; **interactions**: Appendix 1 (antifungals, imidazole)
**Pregnancy**   absorbed from skin in small amounts; manufacturer advises caution
**Side-effects**   see notes above
**Licensed use**   licensed for use in children (age range not specified by manufacturer)
**Indications and dose**
> Fungal skin infections
>> **Neonate** apply twice daily continuing for 10 days after lesions have healed
>>> **Child 1 month–18 years** apply twice daily continuing for 10 days after lesions have healed

> Fungal nail infections
>> Apply 1–2 times daily

> Oral and intestinal fungal infections section 12.3.2

> Vaginal candidiasis section 7.2.2

**Miconazole** (Non-proprietary)
Cream, miconazole nitrate 2%, net price 20 g = £2.05, 45 g = £1.97
Dental prescribing on NHS   Miconazole cream may be prescribed

1.  [NHS] except for seborrhoeic dermatitis and pityriasis versicolor and endorsed 'SLS'

**Daktarin**® (Janssen)
Cream, miconazole nitrate 2%, net price 30 g = £1.82
Excipients   include butylated hydroxyanisole

## NYSTATIN

**Cautions**   see notes above
**Side-effects**   see notes above
**Licensed use**   licensed for use in children (age range not specified by manufacturer)
**Indications and dose**

Skin infections due to *Candida* spp. for dose, see preparation

Oral fungal infections section 12.3.2

**Nystaform**® (Typharm) [PoM]
Cream, nystatin 100 000 units/g, chlorhexidine hydrochloride 1%, net price 30 g = £2.62
Excipients   include benzyl alcohol, cetostearyl alcohol, polysorbate 60
Dose

Apply 2–3 times daily continuing for 7 days after lesions have healed.

## SALICYLIC ACID

**Cautions**   avoid broken or inflamed skin
Salicylate toxicity   Salicylate toxicity can occur particularly if applied on large areas of skin
**Side-effects**   see notes above
**Indications and dose**

Fungal nail infections, particularly tinea

Child 5–18 years apply twice daily and after washing
Note   Use with caution in child likely to suck affected digits

Hyperkeratotic skin disorders section 13.5.2

Warts and calluses section 13.7

**Phytex**® (Wynlit) ◢
Paint, salicylic acid 1.46% (total combined), tannic acid 4.89% and boric acid 3.12% (as borotannic complex), in a vehicle containing alcohol and ethyl acetate, net price 25 mL (with brush) = £2.81
Excipients   none as listed in section 13.1.3
Note   Flammable

## TERBINAFINE

**Cautions**   avoid contact with eyes
**Pregnancy**   manufacturer advises use only if potential benefit outweighs risk—*animal* studies suggest no adverse effects
**Breast-feeding**   manufacturer advises avoid—present in milk, but less than 5% of the dose is absorbed after topical application of terbinafine; avoid application to mother's chest
**Side-effects**   see notes above
**Licensed use**   not licensed for use in children

**Indications and dose**
Fungal skin infections

Apply thinly 1–2 times daily for up to 1 week in tinea pedis, 1–2 weeks in tinea corporis and tinea cruris, 2 weeks in cutaneous candidiasis and pityriasis versicolor; review after 2 weeks

Systemic therapy section 5.2.5

[1]**Terbinafine** (Non-proprietary) [PoM]
Cream, terbinafine hydrochloride 1%, net price 15 g = £5.10, 30 g = £2.69

**Lamisil**® (Novartis Consumer Health) [PoM]
Cream, terbinafine hydrochloride 1%, net price 15 g = £4.86, 30 g = £8.76
Excipients   include benzyl alcohol, cetyl alcohol, polysorbate 60, stearyl alcohol

## TIOCONAZOLE

**Cautions**   see notes above; also use with caution if child likely to suck affected digits
**Pregnancy**   manufacturer advises avoid
**Side-effects**   see notes above; also local oedema, dry skin, nail discoloration, periungual inflammation, nail pain, rash, exfoliation
**Licensed use**   licensed for use in children (age range not specified by manufacturer)
**Indications and dose**
Fungal nail infections

Apply to nails and surrounding skin twice daily for up to 6 months (may be extended to 12 months)

**Trosyl**® (Pfizer) [PoM]
Cutaneous solution, tioconazole 28%, net price 12 mL (with applicator brush) = £27.38
Excipients   none as listed in section 13.1.3

## UNDECENOATES

**Side-effects**   see notes above
**Licensed use**   *Monphytol*® not licensed for use in children under 12 years; *Mycota*® licensed for use in children (age range not specified by manufacturer)
**Indications and dose**
See under preparations

**Mycota**® (Thornton & Ross)
Cream, zinc undecenoate 20%, undecenoic acid 5%, net price 25 g = £1.64
Excipients   include fragrance
Dose
Treatment of athlete's foot

Apply twice daily continuing for 7 days after lesions have healed

Prevention of athlete's foot

Apply once daily

1. Can be sold to the public for external use in children over 16 years for the treatment of tinea pedis and tinea cruris as a cream containing terbinafine hydrochloride max. 1% in a pack containing max. 15 g; also for the treatment of tinea pedis, tinea cruris, and tinea corporis as a spray containing terbinafine hydrochloride max. 1% in a pack containing max. 30 mL or as a gel containing terbinafine hydrochloride max. 1% in a pack containing max. 30 g

13 Skin

Powder, zinc undecenoate 20%, undecenoic acid 2%, net price 70 g = £2.22
**Excipients** include fragrance
**Dose**

### Treatment of athlete's foot

Apply twice daily continuing for 7 days after lesions have healed

### Prevention of athlete's foot

Apply once daily

Spray application, undecenoic acid 3.9%, dichlorophen 0.4% (pressurised aerosol pack), net price 100 mL = £2.46
**Excipients** include fragrance
**Dose**

### Treatment of athlete's foot

Apply twice daily continuing for 7 days after lesions have healed

### Prevention of athlete's foot

Apply once daily

## 13.10.3 Antiviral preparations

See section 12.3.2 for drugs used in *herpetic stomatitis*, section 13.5.1 for *eczema herpeticum*, and section 11.3.3 for viral infections of the *eye*.

**Aciclovir** cream is used for the treatment of initial and recurrent labial, cutaneous, and genital *herpes simplex infections* in children; treatment should begin as early as possible. Systemic treatment is necessary for buccal or vaginal infections or if cold sores recur frequently (for details of systemic use see section 5.3.2.1).

**Herpes labialis** Aciclovir cream can be used for the treatment of initial and recurrent labial herpes simplex infections (cold sores). It is best applied at the earliest possible stage, usually when prodromal changes of sensation are felt in the lip and before vesicles appear.

**Penciclovir** cream is also licensed for the treatment of herpes labialis; it needs to be applied more frequently than aciclovir cream.

### ▌ ACICLOVIR
(Acyclovir)

**Cautions** avoid contact with eyes and mucous membranes
**Pregnancy** not known to be harmful—manufacturers advise use only when potential benefit outweighs risk; limited absorption from topical aciclovir preparations
**Side-effects** transient stinging or burning; occasionally erythema, itching or drying of the skin
**Licensed use** licensed for use in children (age range not specified by manufacturer)
**Indications and dose**

### Herpes simplex infections

Apply to lesions every 4 hours (5 times daily) for 5–10 days, starting at first sign of attack

### Herpes simplex and varicella–zoster infections
section 5.3.2.1

### Eye infections section 11.3.3

**Aciclovir** (Non-proprietary) (PoM)
Cream, aciclovir 5%, net price 2 g = £1.10, 10 g = £1.81
**Dental prescribing on NHS** Aciclovir Cream may be prescribed
**Note** A 2-g tube and a pump pack are on sale to the public for the treatment of cold sores

**Zovirax**® (GSK) (PoM)
Cream, aciclovir 5%, net price 2 g = £4.63, 10 g = £13.96
**Excipients** include cetostearyl alcohol, propylene glycol

### ▌ PENCICLOVIR

**Cautions** avoid contact with eyes and mucous membranes
**Side-effects** transient stinging, burning, numbness; hypersensitivity reactions also reported
**Licensed use** not licensed for use in children under 12 years

**Vectavir**® (Novartis Consumer Health) (PoM)
Cream, penciclovir 1%, net price 2 g = £4.20
**Excipients** include cetostearyl alcohol, propylene glycol
**Dose**

### Herpes labialis

Apply to lesions every 2 hours during waking hours for 4 days, starting at first sign of attack

**Dental prescribing on NHS** May be prescribed as Penciclovir Cream

## 13.10.4 Parasiticidal preparations

### Suitable quantities of parasiticidal preparations

| Area of body | Skin creams | Lotions | Cream rinses |
|---|---|---|---|
| Scalp (head lice) | — | 50–100 mL | 50–100 mL |
| Body (scabies) | 30–60 g | 100 mL | — |
| Body (crab lice) | 30–60 g | 100 mL | — |

These amounts are usually suitable for a child 12–18 years for single application

### Scabies

**Permethrin** is used for the treatment of *scabies* (*Sarcoptes scabiei*); **malathion** can be used if permethrin is inappropriate.

**Benzyl benzoate** is an irritant and should be avoided in children; it is less effective than malathion and permethrin.

**Ivermectin** (available from 'special-order' manufacturers or specialist importing companies, see p. 823), is used in combination with topical drugs, for the treatment of hyperkeratotic (crusted or 'Norwegian') scabies that does not respond to topical treatment alone.

**Application** Although acaricides have traditionally been applied after a hot bath, this is **not** necessary and there is even evidence that a hot bath may increase absorption into the blood, removing them from their site of action on the skin.

All members of the affected household should be treated simultaneously. Treatment should be applied to the

**13**

**Skin**

whole body including the scalp, neck, face, and ears. Particular attention should be paid to the webs of the fingers and toes and lotion brushed under the ends of nails. Malathion and permethrin should be applied twice, one week apart. It is important to warn users to reapply treatment to the hands if they are washed. Children with hyperkeratotic scabies may require 2 or 3 applications of acaricide on consecutive days to ensure that enough penetrates the skin crusts to kill all the mites.

**Itching**  The *itch* and *eczema* of scabies persists for some weeks after the infestation has been eliminated and treatment for pruritus and eczema (section 13.5.1) may be required. Application of **crotamiton** can be used to control itching after treatment with more effective acaricides. A topical **corticosteroid** (section 13.4) may help to reduce itch and inflammation after scabies has been treated successfully; however, persistent symptoms suggest failure of scabies eradication. Oral administration of a **sedating antihistamine** (section 3.4.1) at night may also be useful.

## Head lice

**Dimeticone** is effective against head lice (*Pediculus humanus capitis*) and acts on the surface of the organism. **Malathion**, an organophosphorous insecticide, is an alternative but resistance has been reported. Benzyl benzoate is licensed for the treatment of head lice but it is not recommended for use in children.

Head lice infestation (pediculosis) should be treated using lotion or liquid formulations only if live lice are present. Shampoos are diluted too much in use to be effective. A contact time of 8–12 hours or overnight treatment is recommended for lotions and liquids; a 2-hour treatment is not sufficient to kill eggs.

In general, a course of treatment for head lice should be 2 applications of a parasiticidal product 7 days apart to kill lice emerging from any eggs that survive the first application. All affected individuals in a household should be treated at the same time.

**Wet combing methods**  Head lice can be mechanically removed by combing wet hair meticulously with a plastic detection comb (probably for at least 30 minutes each time) over the whole scalp at 4-day intervals for a minimum of 2 weeks and continued until no lice are found on 3 consecutive sessions; hair conditioner or vegetable oil can be used to facilitate the process.

Several devices for the removal of head lice, such as combs and topical solutions, are available and some are prescribable on the NHS (consult Drug Tariff—see Appliances and Reagents, p. 813 for links to online Drug Tariffs).

## Crab lice

**Permethrin** and **malathion** are used to eliminate *crab lice* (*Pthirus pubis*); permethrin is not licensed for treatment of crab lice in children under 18 years. An aqueous preparation should be applied, allowed to dry naturally and washed off after 12 hours; a second treatment is needed after 7 days to kill lice emerging from surviving eggs. All surfaces of the body should be treated, including the scalp, neck, and face (paying particular attention to the eyebrows and other facial hair). A different insecticide should be used if a course of treatment fails.

## Parasiticidal preparations

**Dimeticone** coats head lice and interferes with water balance in lice by preventing excretion of water; it is less active against eggs and treatment should be repeated after 7 days.

**Malathion** is recommended for *scabies*, *head lice* and *crab lice* (see notes above). The risk of systemic effects associated with 1–2 applications of malathion is considered to be very low; however, except in the treatment of hyperkeratotic scabies (see notes above), applications of malathion liquid repeated at intervals of less than 1 week *or* application for more than 3 consecutive weeks should be **avoided** since the likelihood of eradication of lice is not increased.

**Permethrin** is effective for *scabies*. It is active against *head lice* but the formulation and licensed methods of application of the current products make them unsuitable for the treatment of head lice. Permethrin is also effective against *crab lice* but it is not licensed for this purpose in children under 18 years.

### ▌DIMETICONE

**Cautions**  avoid contact with eyes
**Side-effects**  skin irritation
**Licensed use**  not licensed for use in children under 6 months except under medical supervision
**Indications and dose**

> **Head lice**
>
> Rub into dry hair and scalp, allow to dry naturally, shampoo after 8 hours (or overnight); repeat application after 7 days

**Hedrin®** (Thornton & Ross)
Lotion, dimeticone 4%, net price 50 mL = £2.98, 120-mL spray pack = £7.13, 150 mL = £6.92
**Note** Patients should be told to keep their hair away from fire and flames during treatment

### ▌MALATHION

**Cautions**  avoid contact with eyes; do not use on broken or secondarily infected skin; do not use lotion more than once a week for 3 consecutive weeks; alcoholic lotions **not** recommended for head lice in children with severe eczema or asthma, or for scabies or crab lice (see notes above)
**Side-effects**  skin irritation and hypersensitivity reactions; chemical burns also reported
**Licensed use**  not licensed for use in children under 6 months except under medical supervision
**Indications and dose**

> See notes above and under preparations

> **Head lice**
>
> Rub into dry hair and scalp, allow to dry naturally, remove by washing after 12 hours; repeat application after 7 days (see also notes above)

> **Crab lice**
>
> Apply over whole body, allow to dry naturally, wash off after 12 hours or overnight; repeat application after 7 days

**13** Skin

**Scabies**

Apply over whole body, and wash off after 24 hours; if hands are washed with soap within 24 hours, they should be retreated; see also notes above; repeat application after 7 days

**Note** For scabies, manufacturer recommends application to the body but not necessarily to the head and neck. However, application should be extended to the scalp, neck, face, and ears

**Derbac-M®** (SSL)
Liquid, malathion 0.5% in an aqueous basis, net price 50 mL = £2.37, 200 mL = £5.93
**Excipients** include cetostearyl alcohol, fragrance, hydroxybenzoates (parabens)
For crab lice, head lice, and scabies

### PERMETHRIN

**Cautions** avoid contact with eyes; do not use on broken or secondarily infected skin

**Side-effects** pruritus, erythema, and stinging; rarely rashes and oedema

**Licensed use** *Dermal Cream* (scabies), not licensed for use in children under 2 months; children aged 2 months–2 years, medical supervison required; not licensed for treatment of crab lice in children under 18 years; *Creme Rinse* (head lice) not licensed for use in children under 6 months except under medical supervision

**Indications and dose**

See notes above

**Scabies**

Apply 5% preparation over whole body including face, neck, scalp and ears; wash off after 8–12 hours; if hands washed with soap within 8 hours of application, they should be treated again with cream (see notes above); repeat application after 7 days

**Note** Manufacturer recommends application to the body but to exclude head and neck. However, application should be extended to the scalp, neck, face, and ears

**Permethrin** (Non-proprietary)
Cream, permethrin 5%, net price 30 g = £5.43

**Lyclear® Creme Rinse** (Omega Pharma)
Cream rinse, permethrin 1% in basis containing isopropyl alcohol 20%, net price 59 mL = £2.38, 2 × 59-mL pack = £4.32
**Excipients** include cetyl alcohol
**Note** Use not recommended, therefore no dose stated (product too diluted in use and insufficient contact time)

**Lyclear® Dermal Cream** (Omega Pharma)
Dermal cream, permethrin 5%, net price 30 g = £5.71. Label: 10, patient information leaflet
**Excipients** include butylated hydroxytoluene, wool fat derivative

## 13.10.5 Preparations for minor cuts and abrasions

**Cetrimide** cream is used to treat minor cuts and abrasions. **Proflavine** cream may be used to treat infected wounds or burns, but has now been largely superseded by other antiseptics or suitable antibacterials.

**Cetrimide Cream, BP**
Cream, cetrimide 0.5% in a suitable water-miscible basis such as cetostearyl alcohol 5%, liquid paraffin 50% in freshly boiled and cooled purified water, net price 50 g = £1.11

**Proflavine Cream, BPC**
Cream, proflavine hemisulfate 0.1%, yellow beeswax 2.5%, chlorocresol 0.1%, liquid paraffin 67.3%, freshly boiled and cooled purified water 25%, wool fat 5%, net price 100 mL = £1.59
**Excipients** include beeswax, wool fat
**Note** Stains clothing

### Collodion

**Flexible collodion** may be used to seal minor cuts and wounds that have partially healed.

**Collodion, Flexible, BP**
Collodion, castor oil 2.5%, colophony 2.5% in a collodion basis, prepared by dissolving pyroxylin (10%) in a mixture of 3 volumes of ether and 1 volume of alcohol (90%), net price 10 mL = 38p. Label: 15
**Contra-indications** allergy to colophony in elastic adhesive plasters and tape

### Skin tissue adhesive

Tissue adhesives are used for closure of minor skin wounds and for additional suture support. They should be applied by an appropriately trained healthcare professional. Skin tissue adhesives may cause skin sensitisation.

**Dermabond ProPen®** (Ethicon)
Topical skin adhesive, sterile, octyl 2-cyanoacrylate, net price 0.5 mL = £18.38

**Epiglu®** (Schuco)
Tissue adhesive, sterile, ethyl-2-cyanoacrylate 954.5 mg/g, polymethylmethacrylate, net price 4 × 3-g vials = £149.50 (with dispensing pipettes and pallete)

**Histoacryl®** (B. Braun)
Tissue adhesive, sterile, enbucrilate, net price 5 × 200-mg unit (blue) = £32.00, 10 × 200-mg unit (blue) = £67.20, 5 × 500-mg unit (clear or blue) = £34.65, 10 × 500-mg unit (blue) = £69.30

**LiquiBand®** (MedLogic)
Tissue adhesive, sterile, enbucrilate, net price 0.5-g amp = £5.50

## 13.11 Skin cleansers, antiseptics, and desloughing agents

**13.11.1** Alcohols and saline
**13.11.2** Chlorhexidine salts
**13.11.3** Cationic surfactants and soaps
**13.11.4** Iodine
**13.11.5** Phenolics
**13.11.6** Oxidisers and dyes
**13.11.7** Desloughing agents

Soap or detergent is used with water to cleanse intact skin but they can irritate infantile skin; emollient preparations such as aqueous cream (section 13.2.1.1) or

emulsifying ointment (section 13.2.1) can be used in place of soap or detergent for cleansing dry or irritated skin.

An antiseptic is used for skin that is infected or that is susceptible to recurrent infection. Detergent preparations containing **chlorhexidine** or **povidone–iodine**, which should be thoroughly rinsed off, are used. Emollients may also contain antiseptics (section 13.2.1).

Antiseptics such as **chlorhexidine** or **povidone–iodine** are used on intact skin before surgical procedures; their antiseptic effect is enhanced by an alcoholic solvent. Antiseptic solutions containing **cetrimide** can be used if a detergent effect is also required.

Preparations containing alcohol, and regular use of povidone-iodine, should be avoided on neonatal skin (see section 13.1).

**Hydrogen peroxide**, an oxidising agent, is available as a cream and can be used for superficial bacterial skin infections.

For irrigating ulcers or wounds, lukewarm sterile **sodium chloride 0.9% solution** is used but tap water is often appropriate.

**Potassium permanganate** solution 1 in 10 000, a mild antiseptic with astringent properties, can be used as a soak for exudative eczematous areas (section 13.5.1); treatment should be stopped when the skin becomes dry. Potassium permanganate can stain skin and nails especially with prolonged use.

## 13.11.1 Alcohols and saline

### ALCOHOL

**Cautions** flammable; avoid broken skin; patients have suffered severe burns when diathermy has been preceded by application of alcoholic skin disinfectants
**Contra-indications** neonates, see section 13.1
**Indications and dose**

> Skin preparation before injection
> Apply to skin as necessary

**Industrial Methylated Spirit, BP**
Solution, 19 volumes of ethanol and 1 volume approved wood naphtha, net price '66 OP' (containing 95% by volume alcohol) 100 mL = 39p; '74 OP' (containing 99% by volume alcohol) 100 mL = 39p. Label: 15

**Surgical Spirit, BP**
Spirit, methyl salicylate 0.5 mL, diethyl phthalate 2%, castor oil 2.5%, in industrial methylated spirit, net price 100 mL = 20p. Label: 15

### SODIUM CHLORIDE

**Indications and dose**

> See notes above

**Nebuliser diluent** section 3.1.5

**Sodium depletion** section 9.2.1.2

**Electrolyte imbalance** section 9.2.2.1

**Eye** section 11.8.1

**Oral hygiene** section 12.3.4

**Sodium Chloride** (Non-proprietary)
Solution (sterile), sodium chloride 0.9%, net price 25 × 20-mL unit = £5.50, 200–mL can = £2.65, 1 litre = 97p

**Flowfusor®** (Fresenius Kabi)
Solution (sterile), sodium chloride 0.9%, net price 120-mL Bellows Pack = £1.53

**Irriclens®** (ConvaTec)
Solution in aerosol can (sterile), sodium chloride 0.9%, net price 240-mL can = £3.30

**Irripod®** (C D Medical)
Solution (sterile), sodium chloride 0.9%, net price 25 × 20-mL sachet = £5.50

**Miniversol®** (Aguettant)
Solution (sterile), sodium chloride 0.9%, net price 30 × 45-mL unit = £13.20; 30 × 100-mL unit = £19.50

**Normasol®** (Mölnlycke)
Solution (sterile), sodium chloride 0.9%, net price 25 × 25-mL sachet = £6.14; 10 × 100-mL sachet = £7.47

**Stericlens®** (C D Medical)
Solution in aerosol can (sterile), sodium chloride 0.9%, net price 100-mL can = £1.94, 240-mL can = £2.95

**Steripod® Sodium Chloride** (Medlock)
Solution (sterile), sodium chloride 0.9%, net price 25 × 20-mL sachet = £7.57

## 13.11.2 Chlorhexidine salts

### CHLORHEXIDINE

**Cautions** avoid contact with eyes, brain, meninges and middle ear; not for use in body cavities; alcoholic solutions not suitable before diathermy or for use on neonatal skin
**Side-effects** occasional sensitivity
**Indications and dose**

> See under preparations

> **Bladder irrigation and catheter patency solutions** section 7.4.4

**Chlorhexidine 0.05%** (Baxter)
2000 Solution (sterile), pink, chlorhexidine acetate 0.05%, net price 1000 mL = £0.77
For cleansing and disinfecting wounds and burns

**Cepton®** (LPC)
Skin wash (= solution), red, chlorhexidine gluconate 1%, net price 150 mL = £2.89
For use as skin wash in acne

Lotion, blue, chlorhexidine gluconate 0.1%, net price 150 mL = £2.48
For skin disinfection in acne

**13 Skin**

**ChloraPrep®** (CareFusion)

Cutaneous solution, sterile, chlorhexidine gluconate 2% in isopropyl alcohol 70%, net price (all with single applicator) 0.67 mL (with *SEPP®* applicator) = 30p, 1.5 mL (with *FREPP®* applicator) = 55p, 1.5 mL = 78p, 3 mL = 85p, 10.5 mL = £2.92, 26 mL = £6.50; (all with single applicator, with tint) 3 mL = 90p, 10.5 mL = £3.07, 26 mL = £6.83

For skin disinfection before invasive procedures; Child under 2 months not recommended

**Note** Flammable

**CX Antiseptic Dusting Powder®** (Ecolab)

Dusting powder, sterile, chlorhexidine acetate 1%, net price 15 g = £3.93

For skin disinfection

**Hibiscrub®** (Mölnlycke)

Cleansing solution, red, chlorhexidine gluconate 4%, perfumed, in a surfactant solution, net price 250 mL = £4.25, 500 mL = £5.25, 5 litres = £24.00

**Excipients** include fragrance

Use instead of soap for pre-operative hand and skin preparation and for general hand and skin disinfection

**Hibi® Liquid Hand Rub+** (Mölnlycke)

Solution, chlorhexidine gluconate 0.5%, in isopropyl alcohol 70% with emollients, net price 500 mL = £5.25

To be used undiluted for hand and skin disinfection

**Hibitane Obstetric®** (Derma UK)

Cream, chlorhexidine gluconate solution 5% (≡ 1% chlorhexidine gluconate), in a pourable water-miscible basis, net price 250 mL = £9.00

For use in obstetrics and gynaecology as an antiseptic and lubricant (for application to skin around vulva and perineum and to hands of midwife or doctor)

**Hydrex®** (Ecolab)

Solution, chlorhexidine gluconate solution 2.5% (≡ chlorhexidine gluconate 0.5%), in denatured ethanol 70%, net price 600 mL (clear) = £3.49; 600 mL (pink) = £3.49, 200-mL spray = £1.77, 500-mL spray = £3.01

**Note** Flammable

For pre-operative skin disinfection

Surgical scrub, chlorhexidine gluconate 4% in a surfactant solution, net price 250 mL = £3.39, 500 mL = £3.59

**Excipients** include fragrance

For pre-operative hand and skin preparation and for general hand disinfection

**Unisept®** (Medlock)

Solution (sterile), pink, chlorhexidine gluconate 0.05%, net price 25 × 25-mL sachet = £5.40; 10 × 100-mL sachet = £6.67

For cleansing and disinfecting wounds and burns and swabbing in obstetrics

◀**With cetrimide**

**Tisept®** (Medlock)

Solution (sterile), yellow, chlorhexidine gluconate 0.015%, cetrimide 0.15%, net price 25 × 25-mL sachet = £5.20; 10 × 100-mL sachet = £6.68

To be used undiluted for general skin disinfection and wound cleansing

**Travasept 100®** (Baxter)

Solution (sterile), yellow, chlorhexidine acetate 0.015%, cetrimide 0.15%, net price 500 mL = 72p, 1 litre = 77p

To be used undiluted in skin disinfection such as wound cleansing and obstetrics

## Concentrates

**Hibitane® Plus 5% Concentrate** (Mölnlycke)

Solution, red, chlorhexidine gluconate 5%, in a perfumed aqueous solution, net price 5 litres = £14.50

**Dose**

| Pre-operative skin preparation |
| --- |
| Dilute 1 in 10 (0.5%) with alcohol 70% |

| General skin disinfection |
| --- |
| Dilute 1 in 100 (0.05%) with water |

**Note** Alcoholic solutions not suitable for use before diathermy (see Alcohol, p. 596) or on neonatal skin

## 13.11.3  Cationic surfactants and soaps

### ▎ CETRIMIDE

**Cautions**  avoid contact with eyes; avoid use in body cavities

**Side-effects**  skin irritation and occasionally sensitisation

**Indications and dose**

| Skin disinfection |
| --- |

◀**Preparations**

Ingredient of *Tisept®* and *Travasept® 100*, see above

## 13.11.4  Iodine

### ▎ POVIDONE–IODINE

**Cautions**  broken skin (see below)

**Large open wounds**  The application of povidone–iodine to large wounds or severe burns may produce systemic adverse effects such as metabolic acidosis, hypernatraemia, and impairment of renal function

**Contra-indications**  postmenstrual age under 32 weeks; infants body-weight under 1.5 kg; regular use in neonates; thyroid disorders; concomitant lithium treatment

**Renal impairment**  avoid regular application to inflamed or broken skin or mucosa

**Pregnancy**  sufficient iodine may be absorbed to affect the fetal thyroid in the second and third trimester

**Breast-feeding**  avoid regular or excessive use

**Side-effects**  rarely sensitivity; may interfere with thyroid function tests

**Indications and dose**

| Skin disinfection see preparations |
| --- |

**Betadine®** (Ayrton Saunders)

Dry powder spray, povidone–iodine 2.5% in a pressurised aerosol unit, net price 150-g unit = £2.63

For skin disinfection, particularly minor wounds and infections; Child under 2 years not recommended

**Note** Not for use in serous cavities

**Savlon® Dry** (Novartis Consumer Health)

Powder spray, povidone–iodine 1.14% in a pressurised aerosol unit, net price 50-mL unit = £2.39

For minor wounds

**Videne®** (Ecolab)

Alcoholic tincture, povidone–iodine 10%, net price 500 mL = £3.46

**Dose**

> Apply undiluted in pre-operative skin disinfection

> **Note** Flammable—caution in procedures involving hot wire cautery and diathermy; avoid use in neonates

Antiseptic solution, povidone–iodine 10% in aqueous solution, net price 500 mL = £3.46

**Dose**

> Apply undiluted in pre-operative skin disinfection and general antisepsis

Surgical scrub, povidone–iodine 7.5% in aqueous solution, net price 500 mL = £3.46

**Dose**

> Use as a pre-operative scrub for hand and skin disinfection

## 13.11.5 Phenolics

Triclosan has been used for disinfection of the hands and wounds, and for disinfection of the skin before surgery.

## 13.11.6 Oxidisers and dyes

### ▎ HYDROGEN PEROXIDE

**Cautions** large or deep wounds; avoid on healthy skin and eyes; bleaches fabric; incompatible with products containing iodine or potassium permanganate

**Licensed use** licensed for use in children (age range not specified by manufacturer)

**Indications and dose**

> **Superficial bacterial skin infection** see under preparation below

**Crystacide®** (Derma UK)

Cream, hydrogen peroxide 1%, net price 25 g = £8.07, 40 g = £11.62

**Excipients** include edetic acid (EDTA), propylene glycol

**Dose**

> **Superficial bacterial skin infection**

> Apply 2–3 times daily for up to 3 weeks

### ▎ POTASSIUM PERMANGANATE

**Cautions** irritant to mucous membranes

**Indications and dose**

> **Cleansing and deodorising suppurating eczematous reactions (section 13.5.1) and wounds**

> For wet dressings or baths, use approx. 0.01% (1 in 10 000) solution

> **Note** Stains skin and clothing

**Potassium Permanganate Solution**

Solution, potassium permanganate 0.1% (1 in 1000) in water

**Note** to be diluted 1 in 10 to provide a 0.01% (1 in 10 000) solution

**Permitabs®** (Alliance)

Solution tablets, for preparation of topical solution, potassium permanganate 400 mg, net price 30-tab pack = £12.97

**Note** 1 tablet dissolved in 4 litres of water provides a 0.01% (1 in 10 000) solution

## 13.11.7 Desloughing agents

Alginate, hydrogel, and hydrocolloid dressings (see BNF Appendix 5) are effective in wound debridement. Sterile larvae (maggots) (available from BioMonde) are also used for managing sloughing wounds and are prescribable on the NHS.

Desloughing solutions and creams are of little clinical value. Substances applied to an open area are easily absorbed and perilesional skin is easily sensitised.

For further information on wound management products and elastic hosiery, see BNF Appendix 5.

## 13.12 Antiperspirants

**Aluminium chloride** is a potent antiperspirant used in the treatment of axillary, palmar, and plantar hyperhidrosis. Aluminium salts are also incorporated in preparations used for minor fungal skin infections associated with hyperhidrosis.

In more severe cases specialists use tap water or **glycopyrronium bromide** (as a 0.05% solution) in the iontophoretic treatment of hyperhidrosis of palms and soles. *Botox®* contains botulinum toxin type A complex (section 4.9.3) and is available for use intradermally for severe hyperhidrosis of the axillae unresponsive to topical antiperspirant or other antihidrotic treatment; intradermal treatment is unlikely to be tolerated by most children and should be administered under hospital specialist supervision.

### ▎ ALUMINIUM SALTS

**Cautions** avoid contact with eyes or mucous membranes; avoid use on broken or irritated skin; do not shave axillae or use depilatories within 12 hours of application; avoid contact with clothing

**Side-effects** skin irritation

**Licensed use** licensed for use in children (age range not specified by manufacturer)

**Indications and dose**

> **Hyperhidrosis affecting axillae, hands or feet**

> Apply liquid formulation at night to dry skin, wash off the following morning, initially apply daily then reduce frequency as condition improves—do not bathe immediately before use

> **Hyperhidrosis, bromidrosis, intertrigo, and prevention of tinea pedis and related conditions**

> Apply powder to dry skin

**Anhydrol® Forte** (Dermal)

Solution (= application), aluminium chloride hexahydrate 20% in an alcoholic basis, net price 60-mL bottle with roll-on applicator = £2.51. Label: 15

**Excipients** none as listed in section 13.1.3

**Driclor®** (Stiefel)

Application, aluminium chloride hexahydrate 20% in an alcoholic basis, net price 75-mL bottle with roll-on applicator = £3.01. Label: 15

Excipients none as listed in section 13.1.3

Note A 30-mL pack is on sale to the public

**ZeaSORB®** (Stiefel)

Dusting powder, aldioxa 0.22%, chloroxylenol 0.5%, net price 50 g = £2.61

Excipients include fragrance

## ▌GLYCOPYRRONIUM BROMIDE

**Cautions** see notes (Antimuscarinics) in section 1.2 (but poorly absorbed and systemic effects unlikely)

**Contra-indications** see notes (Antimuscarinics) in section 1.2 (but poorly absorbed and systemic effects unlikely); also infections affecting the treatment site

**Side-effects** see notes (Antimuscarinics) in section 1.2 (but poorly absorbed and systemic effects unlikely); also tingling at administration site

**Licensed use** licensed for use in children (age range not specified by manufacturer)

**Indications and dose**

**Iontophoretic treatment of hyperhidrosis**

Consult product literature; only 1 site to be treated at a time, max. 2 sites treated in any 24 hours, treatment not to be repeated within 7 days

**Other indications** section 15.1.3

**Robinul®** (Mercury) PoM

Powder, glycopyrronium bromide, net price 3 g = £175.00

## 13.13 Topical circulatory preparations

These preparations are used to improve circulation in conditions such as bruising and superficial thrombophlebitis but are of little value. First aid measures such as rest, ice, compression, and elevation should be used. Topical preparations containing heparinoids should not be used on large areas of skin, broken or sensitive skin, or mucous membranes. Chilblains are best managed by avoidance of exposure to cold; neither systemic nor topical vasodilator therapy is established as being effective.

**Hirudoid®** (Genus)

Cream, heparinoid 0.3% in a vanishing-cream basis, net price 50 g = £3.99

Excipients include cetostearyl alcohol, hydroxybenzoates (parabens)

**Dose**

**Superficial thrombophlebitis, bruising, and haematoma**

Child 5–18 years apply up to 4 times daily

Gel, heparinoid 0.3%, net price 50 g = £3.99

Excipients include propylene glycol, fragrance

**Dose**

**Superficial thrombophlebitis, bruising, and haematoma**

Child 5–18 years apply up to 4 times daily

**13 Skin**

# 14 Immunological products and vaccines

## 14.1 Active immunity

Active immunity can be acquired by natural disease or by vaccination. **Vaccines** stimulate production of antibodies and other components of the immune mechanism; they consist of either:

1. a *live attenuated* form of a virus (e.g. measles, mumps, and rubella vaccine) or bacteria (e.g. BCG vaccine), or

2. *inactivated* preparations of a virus (e.g. influenza vaccine) or bacteria, or

3. *detoxified* exotoxins produced by a micro-organism (e.g. tetanus vaccine), or

4. *extracts of* a micro-organism, which may be derived from the organism (e.g. pneumococcal vaccine) or produced by recombinant DNA technology (e.g. hepatitis B vaccine).

**Live attenuated vaccines** usually produce durable immunity but not always as long-lasting as that resulting from natural infection.

**Inactivated** vaccines may require a primary series of injections of vaccine to produce an adequate antibody response, and in most cases booster (reinforcing) injections are required; the duration of immunity varies from months to many years. Some inactivated vaccines are adsorbed onto an adjuvant (such as aluminium hydroxide) to enhance the antibody response.

> Advice in this chapter reflects that in the handbook *Immunisation against Infectious Disease* (2006), which in turn reflects the guidance of the Joint Committee on Vaccination and Immunisation (JCVI).
>
> Chapters from the handbook are available at www.immunisation.dh.gov.uk
>
> The advice in this chapter also incorporates changes announced by the Chief Medical Officer and Health Department Updates.

**Cautions** Most children can safely receive the majority of vaccines. Vaccination may be postponed if the child is suffering from an acute illness; however, it is not necessary to postpone immunisation in children with minor illnesses without fever or systemic upset. See also Predisposition to Neurological Problems, below. For individuals with bleeding disorders, see Route of Administration, below. If alcohol or disinfectant is used for cleansing the skin it should be allowed to evaporate before vaccination to prevent possible inactivation of live vaccines.

When 2 or more vaccines are required (and are not available as a combined preparation), they should be given simultaneously at different sites, preferably in a different limb; if more than one injection is to be given in the same limb, they should be administered at least 2.5 cm apart (but see also BCG Vaccines, p. 604). When 2 live vaccines cannot be given at the same time, they should be separated by an interval of at least 4 weeks. For **interactions** see Appendix I (vaccines).

*See also* Cautions under individual vaccines.

**Contra-indications** Vaccines are contra-indicated in children who have a confirmed anaphylactic reaction to a preceding dose of a vaccine containing the same antigens or vaccine component (such as antibacterials in viral vaccines). The presence of the following excipients in vaccines and immunological products has been noted under the relevant entries:

| | |
|---|---|
| Gelatin | Polymyxin B |
| Gentamicin | Streptomycin |
| Kanamycin | Thiomersal |
| Neomycin | |
| Penicillins | |

*Hypersensitivity to egg* Children with evidence of previous anaphylactic reaction to egg should not be given tick-borne encephalitis vaccine, and yellow fever vaccine should only be considered under the guidance of a specialist. Children with a history of egg allergy can be immunised with either an egg-free influenza vaccine, if available, or an influenza vaccine with an ovalbumin content less than 120 nanograms/mL (facilities should be available to treat anaphylaxis). If an influenza vaccine containing ovalbumin is being considered in those with a history of anaphylaxis to egg or egg allergy with uncontrolled asthma, these children should be referred to a specialist in hospital. See also Cautions under MMR vaccine.

See also Vaccines and HIV infection, below.

Live vaccines may be contra-indicated temporarily in children who are:

- immunosuppressed (see Impaired Immune Response, below);

- pregnant (see Pregnancy and Breast-feeding, below).

*See also* Contra-indications under individual vaccines.

**Impaired immune response** Immune response to vaccines may be reduced in immunosuppressed children and there is also a risk of generalised infection with live vaccines. Severely immunosuppressed children should not be given live vaccines (including those with severe primary immunodeficiency). Specialist advice should be sought for children being treated with high doses of corticosteroids (dose equivalents of prednisolone: **children**, 2 mg/kg (or more than 40 mg) daily for at least 1 week or 1 mg/kg daily for 1 month), or other immunosuppressive drugs[1], and for children with malignant conditions undergoing chemotherapy or generalised radiotherapy[1,2]. For special reference to *HIV infection*, see below.

The Royal College of Paediatrics and Child Health has produced a statement, *Immunisation of the Immunocompromised Child (2002)* (available at www.rcpch.ac.uk).

**Pregnancy** Live vaccines should not be administered routinely during pregnancy because of the theoretical risk of fetal infection but where there is a significant risk of exposure to disease (e.g. to yellow fever), the need for vaccination usually outweighs any possible risk to the fetus. Termination of pregnancy following inadvertent immunisation is not recommended. There is no evidence of risk from vaccinating pregnant women with inactivated viral or bacterial vaccines or toxoids. For use of specific vaccines during pregnancy, see under individual vaccines.

**Breast-feeding** Although there is a theoretical risk of live vaccine being present in breast milk, vaccination is not contra-indicated for women who are breast-feeding when there is significant risk of exposure to disease. There is no evidence of risk from vaccinating women who are breast-feeding, with inactivated viral or bacterial vaccines or toxoids. For use of specific vaccines during breast-feeding, see under individual vaccines.

**Side-effects** Injection of a vaccine may be followed by local reactions such as pain, inflammation, redness, and lymphangitis. An induration or sterile abscess may develop at the injection site. Gastro-intestinal disturbances, fever, headache, irritability, loss of appetite, fatigue, myalgia, and malaise are among the most commonly reported side-effects. Other side-effects include influenza-like symptoms, dizziness, paraesthesia, asthenia, drowsiness, arthralgia, rash, and lymphadenopathy. Hypersensitivity reactions, such as bronchospasm, angioedema, urticaria, and anaphylaxis, are very rare but can be fatal (see section 3.4.3 for management of allergic emergencies).

**Oral** vaccines, such as cholera, live poliomyelitis, rotavirus, and live typhoid, can also cause gastro-intestinal disturbances such as nausea, vomiting, abdominal pain and cramps, and diarrhoea.

See also Predisposition to Neurological Problems, below.

---

1. Live vaccines should be postponed until at least 3 months after stopping high-dose systemic corticosteroids and at least 6 months after stopping other immunosuppressive drugs or generalised radiotherapy (at least 12 months after discontinuing immunosuppressants following bone-marrow transplantation).
2. Use of normal immunoglobulin should be considered after exposure to measles (see p. 624) and varicella–zoster immunoglobulin considered after exposure to chickenpox or herpes zoster (see p. 626).

Some vaccines (e.g. poliomyelitis) produce very few reactions, while others (e.g. measles, mumps and rubella) may cause a very mild form of the disease. Occasionally more serious adverse reactions can occur—these should always be reported to the CHM (see Adverse Reactions to Drugs, p. 11).

See also Preterm Birth, p. 602.

---

### Predisposition to neurological problems

When there is a personal or family history of *febrile* convulsions, there is an increased risk of these occurring during fever from any cause including immunisation, but this is not a contra-indication to immunisation. In children who have had a seizure associated with fever without neurological deterioration, immunisation is *recommended*; advice on the *management of fever* (see Post-immunisation Pyrexia in Infants, below) should be given before immunisation. When a child has had a convulsion not associated with fever, and the neurological condition is not deteriorating, immunisation is *recommended*.

Children with stable neurological disorders (e.g. spina bifida, congenital brain abnormality, and peri-natal hypoxic-ischaemic encephalopathy) should be immunised according to the recommended schedule.

When there is a *still evolving neurological problem*, including poorly controlled epilepsy, immunisation should be deferred and the child referred to a specialist. Immunisation is recommended if a cause for the neurological disorder is identified. If a cause is not identified, immunisation should be deferred until the condition is stable.

---

### Post-immunisation pyrexia in infants

The parent should be advised that if pyrexia develops after childhood immunisation and the infant seems distressed, a dose of paracetamol can be given and, if necessary, a second dose can be given 4–6 hours later. Ibuprofen can be used if paracetamol is unsuitable, but if a second dose of ibuprofen is required, it is given 6 hours after the first dose. The parent should be warned to seek medical advice if the pyrexia persists.

For post-immunisation pyrexia in an infant aged 2–3 months, the dose of paracetamol is 60 mg; the dose of ibuprofen is 50 mg (on a doctor's advice). An oral syringe can be obtained from any pharmacy to give the small volume required.

---

Further information on adverse effects associated with specific vaccines can be found under individual vaccines.

**Vaccines and HIV infection** HIV-positive children with or without symptoms can receive the following live vaccines:

MMR (but avoid if immunity significantly impaired), varicella-zoster (but avoid if immunity significantly impaired—consult product literature);[2]

and the following inactivated vaccines:

anthrax, cholera (oral), diphtheria, haemophilus influenzae type b, hepatitis A, hepatitis B, human papillomavirus, influenza (injection), meningo-

**14**

Immunological products and vaccines

## Immunisation schedule

Vaccines for the childhood immunisation schedule should be obtained from **local health organisations** or from ImmForm (www.immform.dh.gov.uk)—not to be prescribed on FP10 (HS21 in Northern Ireland; GP10 in Scotland; WP10 in Wales).

---

### Preterm birth

Babies born preterm should receive all routine immunisations based on their actual date of birth. The risk of apnoea following vaccination is increased in preterm babies, particularly in those born at or before 28 weeks postmenstrual age. If babies at risk of apnoea are in hospital at the time of their first immunisation, they should be monitored for 48 hours after immunisation. If a baby develops apnoea, bradycardia, or desaturation after the first immunisation, the second immunisation should also be given in hospital with similar monitoring. Seroconversion may be unreliable in babies born earlier than 28 weeks' gestation or in babies treated with corticosteroids for chronic lung disease; consideration should be given to testing for antibodies against *Haemophilus influenzae* type b, meningococcal C, and hepatitis B after primary immunisation.

---

| When to immunise (for preterm infants—see note above) | Vaccine given and dose schedule (for details of dose, see under individual vaccines) |
|---|---|
| Neonates at risk only | • **BCG Vaccine** <br> See section 14.4, BCG Vaccines <br> • **Hepatitis B Vaccine** <br> See section 14.4, Hepatitis B Vaccine |
| 2 months | • **Diphtheria, Tetanus, Pertussis (Acellular, Component), Poliomyelitis (Inactivated), and Haemophilus Type b Conjugate Vaccine (Adsorbed)** <br> First dose <br> • **Pneumococcal Polysaccharide Conjugate Vaccine (Adsorbed)** <br> First dose |
| 3 months | • **Diphtheria, Tetanus, Pertussis (Acellular, Component), Poliomyelitis (Inactivated), and Haemophilus Type b Conjugate Vaccine (Adsorbed)** <br> Second dose <br> • **Meningococcal Group C Conjugate Vaccine** <br> First dose |
| 4 months | • **Diphtheria, Tetanus, Pertussis (Acellular, Component), Poliomyelitis (Inactivated), and Haemophilus Type b Conjugate Vaccine (Adsorbed)** <br> Third dose <br> • **Meningococcal Group C Conjugate Vaccine** <br> Second dose <br> • **Pneumococcal Polysaccharide Conjugate Vaccine (Adsorbed)** <br> Second dose |
| 12 –13 months | • **Measles, Mumps and Rubella Vaccine, Live (MMR)** <br> First dose <br> • **Pneumococcal Polysaccharide Conjugate Vaccine (Adsorbed)** <br> Single booster dose <br> • **Haemophilus Type b Conjugate Vaccine and Meningococcal Group C Conjugate Vaccine** <br> Single booster dose |
| Between 3 years and 4 months, and 5 years | • **Adsorbed Diphtheria [low dose], Tetanus, Pertussis (Acellular, Component) and Poliomyelitis (Inactivated) Vaccine** <br> *or* <br> **Adsorbed Diphtheria, Tetanus, Pertussis (Acellular, Component) and Poliomyelitis (Inactivated) Vaccine** <br> Single booster dose <br> **Note:** Preferably allow interval of at least 3 years after completing primary course <br> • **Measles, Mumps and Rubella Vaccine, Live (MMR)** <br> Second dose |
| 12–13 years (females only) | • **Human Papillomavirus Vaccine** <br> 3 doses; second dose 1 month, and third dose 4–6 months after first dose[1] |
| 13–18 years | • **Adsorbed Diphtheria [low dose], Tetanus, and Poliomyelitis (Inactivated) Vaccine** <br> Single booster dose |
| During adult life, women of child-bearing age susceptible to rubella | • **Measles, Mumps and Rubella Vaccine, Live (MMR)** <br> Women of child-bearing age who have not received 2 doses of a rubella-containing vaccine or who do not have a positive antibody test for rubella should be offered rubella immunisation (using the MMR vaccine)—exclude pregnancy before immunisation, but see also section 14.4, Measles, Mumps and Rubella Vaccine |

---

1. The two human papillomavirus vaccines are not interchangeable and one vaccine product should be used for the entire course.

coccal, pertussis, pneumococcal, poliomyelitis[1], rabies, tetanus, tick-borne encephalitis, typhoid (injection).

HIV-positive children should **not** receive:

> BCG, influenza (nasal spray), typhoid (oral), yellow fever[2]

**Note** The above advice differs from that for other immunocompromised children; Immunisation of HIV-infected Children issued by Children's HIV Association (CHIVA) are available at www.chiva.org.uk

**Vaccines and asplenia**    The following vaccines are recommended for asplenic children or those with splenic dysfunction:

> haemophilus influenzae type b; influenza; meningococcal A, C, W135, and Y conjugate; pneumococcal.

For antibiotic prophylaxis in asplenia see p. 257.

**Route of administration**    Vaccines should not be given intravenously. Most vaccines are given by the intramuscular route; some vaccines are given by other routes—the intradermal route for BCG vaccine, deep subcutaneous route for Japanese encephalitis and varicella vaccines, and the oral route for cholera, live poliomyelitis, rotavirus, and live typhoid vaccines. The intramuscular route should not be used in children with **bleeding disorders** such as haemophilia or thrombocytopenia; vaccines usually given by the intramuscular route should be given by deep subcutaneous injection instead.

**Note** The Department of Health has advised *against the use of jet guns* for vaccination owing to the risk of transmitting blood-borne infections, such as HIV.

## High-risk groups

For information on high-risk groups, see section 14.4 under individual vaccines

   **BCG Vaccines**, p. 604

   **Hepatitis A Vaccine**, p. 608

   **Hepatitis B Vaccine**, p. 610

   **Influenza Vaccine**, p. 612

   **Pneumococcal Vaccines**, p. 617

   **Tetanus Vaccines**, p. 620

## Children with unknown or incomplete immunisation history

For children born in the UK who present with an inadequate or unknown immunisation history, investigation into immunisations received should be carried out. Outstanding doses should be administered where the routine childhood immunisation schedule has not been completed.

> For advice on the immunisation of children coming to the UK, consult the handbook *Immunisation against Infectious Disease* (2006) (available at www.dh.gov.uk)

## 14.2 Passive immunity

Immunity with immediate protection against certain infective organisms can be obtained by injecting preparations made from the plasma of immune individuals

with adequate levels of antibody to the disease for which protection is sought (see under Immunoglobulins, section 14.5). The duration of this passive immunity varies according to the dose and the type of immunoglobulin. Passive immunity may last only a few weeks; when necessary, passive immunisation can be repeated.

Antibodies of human origin are usually termed *immunoglobulins*. The term *antiserum* is applied to material prepared in animals. Because of serum sickness and other allergic-type reactions that may follow injections of antisera, this therapy has been replaced whenever possible by the use of immunoglobulins. Reactions are theoretically possible after injection of human immunoglobulins, but reports of such reactions are very rare.

## 14.3 Storage and use

Care must be taken to store all vaccines and other immunological products under the conditions recommended in the product literature, otherwise the preparation may become ineffective. **Refrigerated storage** is usually necessary; many vaccines and immunoglobulins need to be stored at 2–8°C and not allowed to freeze. Vaccines and immunoglobulins should be protected from light. Reconstituted vaccines and opened multidose vials must be used within the period recommended in the product literature. Unused vaccines should be disposed of by incineration at a registered disposal contractor.

Particular attention must be paid to instructions on the use of diluents. Vaccines which are liquid suspensions or are reconstituted before use should be adequately mixed to ensure uniformity of the material to be injected.

## 14.4 Vaccines and antisera

**Availability**    Anthrax and yellow fever vaccines, botulism antitoxin, diphtheria antitoxin, and snake and spider venom antitoxins are available from local designated holding centres.

For antivenom, see Emergency Treatment of Poisoning, p. 33.

Enquiries for vaccines not available commercially can also be made to:

Immunisation and Countermeasures Response, Finance and Accounting
Department of Health
Wellington House
133–155 Waterloo Road
London, SE1 8UG
vaccinesupply@PHE.gov.uk

In Scotland information about availability of vaccines can be obtained from a Specialist in Pharmaceutical Public Health.

In Wales enquiries for vaccines not commercially available should be directed to:

Welsh Medicines Information Centre
University Hospital of Wales
Cardiff, CF14 4XW
Tel: (029) 2074 2979

---

1. Inactivated poliomyelitis vaccine is now used instead of oral poliomyelitis vaccine for routine immunisation of children.
2. If yellow fever risk is unavoidable, specialist advice should be sought.

**14**   Immunological products and vaccines

In Northern Ireland:

Pharmacy and Medicines Management Centre
Beech House
Antrim Hospital Site
Northern Health and Social Care Trust
Bush Road
Antrim, BT41 2RL
rphps.admin@northerntrust.hscni.net

For further details of availability, see under individual vaccines.

---

## Anthrax vaccine

Anthrax vaccine is rarely required for children. For further information see BNF section 14.4.

---

## BCG vaccines

BCG (Bacillus Calmette-Guérin) is a live attenuated strain derived from *Mycobacterium bovis* which stimulates the development of hypersensitivity to *M. tuberculosis*. BCG vaccine should be given intradermally by operators skilled in the technique (see below).

The expected reaction to successful BCG vaccination is induration at the site of injection followed by a local lesion which starts as a papule 2 or more weeks after vaccination; the lesion may ulcerate then subside over several weeks or months, leaving a small flat scar. A dry dressing may be used if the ulcer discharges, but air should **not** be excluded.

All children of 6 years and over being considered for BCG immunisation must first be given a skin test for hypersensitivity to tuberculoprotein (see under Diagnostic agents, below). A skin test is not necessary for a child under 6 years, provided that the child has not stayed for longer than 3 months in a country with an incidence[1] of tuberculosis greater than 40 per 100 000, the child has not had contact with a person with tuberculosis, and there is no family history of tuberculosis within the last 5 years.

BCG is recommended for the following groups of children if BCG immunisation has not previously been carried out and they are negative for tuberculoprotein hypersensitivity:

- neonates with a family history of tuberculosis in the last 5 years;

- all neonates and infants (0–12 months) born in areas where the incidence[1] of tuberculosis is greater than 40 per 100 000;

- neonates, infants, and children under 16 years with a parent or grandparent born in a country with an incidence[1] of tuberculosis greater than 40 per 100 000;

- new immigrants aged under 16 years who were born in, or lived for more than 3 months in a country with an incidence[1] of tuberculosis greater than 40 per 100 000;

- new immigrants aged 16–18 years from Sub-Saharan Africa or a country[1] with an incidence of tuberculosis greater than 500 per 100 000;

- contacts of those with active respiratory tuberculosis;

---

1. List of countries or primary care trusts where the incidence of tuberculosis is greater than 40 cases per 100 000 is available at www.hpa.org.uk

- children under 16 years intending to live with local people for more than 3 months in a country with an incidence[1] of tuberculosis greater than 40 per 100 000 (section 14.6).

BCG vaccine can be given simultaneously with another live vaccine (see also section 14.1), but if they are not given at the same time, an interval of 4 weeks should normally be allowed between them. When BCG is given to infants, there is no need to delay routine primary immunisations. No further vaccination should be given in the arm used for BCG vaccination for at least 3 months because of the risk of regional lymphadenitis.

For advice on chemoprophylaxis against tuberculosis, see section 5.1.9; for treatment of infection following vaccination, seek expert advice.

### ◢ BACILLUS CALMETTE-GUÉRIN VACCINE

**BCG vaccine**

**Cautions**   see section 14.1; **interactions:** Appendix 1 (vaccines)

**Contra-indications**   see section 14.1; also neonate in household contact with known or suspected case of active tuberculosis; generalised septic skin conditions (for children with eczema, lesion-free site should be used)

**Pregnancy**   see p. 601

**Breast-feeding**   see p. 601

**Side-effects**   see section 14.1 and notes above; *also* at the injection-site, subcutaneous abscess, prolonged ulceration; *rarely* disseminated complications such as osteitis or osteomyelitis

**Indications and dose**

**Immunisation against tuberculosis**

- By intradermal injection

  **Neonate** 0.05 mL

  **Child 1 month–1 year** 0.05 mL

  **Child 1–18 years** 0.1 mL

**Intradermal injection technique**  Skin is stretched between thumb and forefinger and needle (size 25G or 26G) inserted (bevel upwards) for about 3 mm into superficial layers of dermis (almost parallel with surface). Needle should be short with short bevel (can usually be seen through epidermis during insertion). Tense raised blanched bleb showing tips of hair follicles is sign of correct injection; 7 mm bleb ≡ 0.1 mL injection, 3 mm bleb ≡ 0.05 mL injection; if considerable resistance not felt, needle is too deep and should be removed and reinserted before giving more vaccine.

To be injected at insertion of deltoid muscle onto humerus (keloid formation more likely with sites higher on arm); tip of shoulder should be **avoided**.

◢Intradermal

**Bacillus Calmette-Guérin Vaccine**  [PoM]
BCG Vaccine, Dried/Tub/BCG
Injection, (powder for suspension), freeze-dried preparation of live bacteria of a strain derived from the bacillus of Calmette and Guérin
Available from health organisations or from ImmForm (SSI brand, multidose vial with diluent)

---

## Diagnostic agents

The *Mantoux test* is recommended for tuberculin skin testing, but no licensed preparation is currently available. Guidance for healthcare professionals is available at www.dh.gov.uk/immunisation.

In the Mantoux test, the diagnostic dose is administered by intradermal injection of Tuberculin Purified Protein Derivative (PPD).

The *Heaf test* (involving the use of multiple-puncture apparatus) is no longer available.

**Note** Response to tuberculin may be suppressed by live viral vaccines, viral infection, sarcoidosis, corticosteroid therapy, or immunosuppression due to disease or treatment.
Tuberculin testing should not be carried out within 4 weeks of receiving a live viral vaccine.

Two interferon gamma release assay (IGRA) tests are also available as an aid in the diagnosis of tuberculosis infection: *QuantiFERON®-TB Gold* and *T-SPOT®.TB*. Both tests measure T-cell mediated immune response to synthetic antigens. For further information on the use of interferon gamma release assay tests for tuberculosis, see www.hpa.org.uk.

### Tuberculin Purified Protein Derivative [PoM] (Tuberculin PPD)

Injection, heat-treated products of growth and lysis of appropriate *Mycobacterium* spp. 20 units/mL (2 units/0.1-mL dose) (for routine use), 1.5-mL vial; 100 units/mL (10 units/0.1-mL dose), 1.5-mL vial

**Dose**

> **Mantoux test**
>
> • **By intradermal injection**
>
>   2 units (0.1 mL of 20 units/mL strength) for routine Mantoux test; if first test is negative and a further test is considered appropriate 10 units (0.1 mL of 100 units/mL strength)

Available from ImmForm (SSI brand)

**Important** The strength of tuberculin PPD in this product may be different to the strengths of products used previously for the Mantoux test; care is required to select the correct strength

---

## Botulism antitoxin

A polyvalent botulism antitoxin is available for the post-exposure prophylaxis of botulism and for the treatment of children thought to be suffering from botulism. It specifically neutralises the toxins produced by *Clostridium botulinum* types A, B, and E. It is not effective against infantile botulism as the toxin (type A) is seldom, if ever, found in the blood in this type of infection.

Hypersensitivity reactions are a problem. It is essential to read the contra-indications, warnings, and details of sensitivity tests on the package insert. Prior to treatment checks should be made regarding previous administration of any antitoxin and history of any allergic condition, e.g. asthma, hay fever, etc. All children should be tested for sensitivity (diluting the antitoxin if history of allergy).

### Botulism Antitoxin [PoM]

A preparation containing the specific antitoxic globulins that have the power of neutralising the toxins formed by types A, B, and E of *Clostridium botulinum*.

**Note** The BP title Botulinum Antitoxin is not used because the preparation currently in use may have a different specification

**Dose**

> **Prophylaxis**
>
>   Consult product literature

Available from local designated centres, for details see TOXBASE (requires registration) www.toxbase.org. For supplies outside working hours apply to other designated centres or to the Public Health England Colindale duty doctor (Tel (020) 8200 6868). For major incidents, obtain supplies from the local blood bank

---

## Cholera vaccine

**Cholera vaccine** (oral) contains inactivated Inaba (including El-Tor biotype) and Ogawa strains of *Vibrio cholerae*, serotype O1 together with recombinant B-subunit of the cholera toxin produced in Inaba strains of *V.cholerae*, serotype O1.

Oral cholera vaccine is licensed for travellers to endemic or epidemic areas on the basis of current recommendations (see also section 14.6). Immunisation should be completed at least 1 week before potential exposure. However, there is no requirement for cholera vaccination for international travel.

Immunisation with cholera vaccine does not provide complete protection and all travellers to a country where cholera exists should be warned that scrupulous attention to food, water, and personal hygiene is **essential**.

*Injectable cholera vaccine* provides unreliable protection and is no longer available in the UK.

### ■ CHOLERA VACCINE

**Cautions** see section 14.1 and notes above
**Contra-indications** see section 14.1; also acute gastro-intestinal illness
**Pregnancy** see p. 601
**Breast-feeding** see p. 601
**Side-effects** see section 14.1; also *rarely* respiratory symptoms such as rhinitis and cough; *very rarely* sore throat, insomnia
**Indications and dose**

> See notes above
>
> • **By mouth**
>
>   **Child 2–6 years** 3 doses each separated by an interval of 1–6 weeks
>
>   **Child 6–18 years** 2 doses separated by an interval of 1–6 weeks
>
>   **Note** If more than 6 weeks have elapsed between doses, the primary course should be restarted
>
> A single booster dose can be given 2 years after primary course for children 6–18 years, and 6 months after primary course for children 2–6 years. If more than 2 years have elapsed since the last vaccination, the primary course should be repeated

**Administration** Dissolve effervescent sodium bicarbonate granules in a glassful of water (approximately 150 mL). For child over 6 years, add vaccine suspension to make one dose. For child 2–6 years, discard half (approximately 75 mL) of the solution, then add vaccine suspension to make one dose. Drink within 2 hours. Food, drink and other oral medicines should be avoided for 1 hour before and after vaccination

**Dukoral®** (Crucell) [PoM]
Oral suspension, for dilution with solution of effervescent sodium bicarbonate granules, heat- and formaldehyde-inactivated Inaba (including El-Tor biotype) and Ogawa strains of *Vibrio cholerae* bacteria and recombinant cholera toxin B-subunit produced in *V. cholerae*, net price 2-dose pack = £23.42. Counselling, administration

## Diphtheria Vaccines

Diphtheria vaccines are prepared from the toxin of *Corynebacterium diphtheriae* and adsorption on aluminium hydroxide or aluminium phosphate improves anti-

14  Immunological products and vaccines

genicity. The vaccine stimulates the production of the protective antitoxin. The quantity of diphtheria toxoid in a preparation determines whether the vaccine is defined as 'high dose' or 'low dose'. Vaccines containing the higher dose of diphtheria toxoid are used for primary immunisation of children under 10 years of age. Vaccines containing the lower dose of diphtheria toxoid are used for primary immunisation in children over 10 years. Single-antigen diphtheria vaccine is not available and adsorbed diphtheria vaccine is given as a combination product containing other vaccines.

For primary immunisation *of children aged between 2 months and 10 years* vaccination is recommended usually in the form of 3 doses (separated by 1-month intervals) of **diphtheria, tetanus, pertussis (acellular, component), poliomyelitis (inactivated) and haemophilus type b conjugate vaccine (adsorbed)** (see Immunisation schedule, section 14.1). In unimmunised children aged *over 10 years* the primary course comprises of 3 doses of **adsorbed diphtheria** [low dose], **tetanus and poliomyelitis (inactivated) vaccine**.

A booster dose should be given 3 years after the primary course (this interval can be reduced to a minimum of 1 year if the primary course was delayed). Children *under 10 years* should receive *either* **adsorbed diphtheria, tetanus, pertussis (acellular, component) and poliomyelitis (inactivated) vaccine** *or* **adsorbed diphtheria** [low dose], **tetanus, pertussis (acellular, component) and poliomyelitis (inactivated) vaccine**. Children aged *over 10 years* should receive **adsorbed diphtheria** [low dose], **tetanus, and poliomyelitis (inactivated) vaccine**.

A second booster dose, of adsorbed diphtheria [low dose], tetanus and poliomyelitis (inactivated) vaccine, should be given 10 years after the previous booster dose (this interval can be reduced to a minimum of 5 years if previous doses were delayed). For children who have been vaccinated following a tetanus-prone wound, see Tetanus vaccines, p. 620.

**Travel**   Children travelling to areas with a risk of diphtheria infection should be fully immunised according to the UK schedule (see also section 14.6). If more than 10 years have lapsed since completion of the UK schedule, a dose of **adsorbed diphtheria** [low dose], **tetanus and poliomyelitis (inactivated) vaccine** should be administered.

**Contacts**   Advice on the management of cases of diphtheria, carriers, contacts and outbreaks must be sought from health protection units. The immunisation history of infected children and their contacts should be determined; those who have been incompletely immunised should complete their immunisation and fully immunised individuals should receive a reinforcing dose. For advice on antibacterial treatment to prevent a secondary case of diphtheria in a non-immune child, see Table 2, section 5.1.

---

## ◢ DIPHTHERIA-CONTAINING VACCINES

**Cautions**   see section 14.1; see also individual components of vaccines

**Contra-indications**   see section 14.1; see also individual components of vaccines

**Pregnancy**   see p. 601

**Breast-feeding**   see p. 601

**Side-effects**   see section 14.1; also restlessness, sleep disturbances, and unusual crying in infants;

**Licensed use**   *Infanrix-IPV + Hib*® not licensed for use in children over 36 months; *Pediacel*® not licensed in children over 4 years but Department of Health recommends that these be used for children up to 10 years

### Indications and dose
See notes above and under preparations

◢**Diphtheria-containing vaccines for children under 10 years**
**Important**   For children aged 10 years or over see Diphtheria-containing Vaccines for Children Over 10 Years, p. 607, and see Diphtheria-containing Vaccines for Immunisation of Pregnant Women Against Pertussis, p. 607

### Diphtheria, Tetanus, Pertussis (Acellular, Component), Poliomyelitis (Inactivated) and Haemophilus Type b Conjugate Vaccine (Adsorbed) PoM
Injection, suspension of diphtheria toxoid, tetanus toxoid, acellular pertussis, inactivated poliomyelitis and *Haemophilus influenzae* type b (conjugated to tetanus protein), net price 0.5-mL prefilled syringe = £32.00
**Excipients**   may include neomycin, polymyxin B and streptomycin
**Dose**
### Primary immunisation
● **By intramuscular injection**
  **Child 2 months–10 years** 3 doses each of 0.5 mL separated by intervals of 1 month; *see also* notes on booster doses, above

Available as part of childhood immunisation schedule, from health organisations or ImmForm
**Brands include** *Pediacel*®

### Adsorbed Diphtheria, Tetanus, Pertussis (Acellular, Component) and Poliomyelitis (Inactivated) Vaccine PoM
Injection, suspension of diphtheria toxoid, tetanus toxoid, acellular pertussis and inactivated poliomyelitis vaccine components adsorbed on a mineral carrier, net price 0.5-mL prefilled syringe = £17.56
**Excipients**   may include neomycin and polymyxin B
**Dose**
First booster dose
● **By intramuscular injection**
  **Child 3–10 years** 0.5 mL 3 years after primary immunisation; *see also* notes on booster doses, above

Available as part of childhood immunisation schedule, from health organisations or ImmForm
**Brands include** *Infanrix-IPV*®

### Adsorbed Diphtheria [low dose], Tetanus, Pertussis (Acellular, Component) and Poliomyelitis (Inactivated) Vaccine PoM
Injection, suspension of diphtheria toxoid [low dose], tetanus toxoid, acellular pertussis and inactivated poliomyelitis vaccine components adsorbed on a mineral carrier, net price 0.5-mL prefilled syringe = £11.98
**Excipients**   may include neomycin, polymyxin B and streptomycin
**Dose**
First booster dose
● **By intramuscular injection**
  **Child 3–10 years** 0.5 mL 3 years after primary immunisation; *see also* notes on booster doses, above

Available as part of childhood immunisation schedule from health organisations or ImmForm
**Brands include** *Repevax*®

*14   Immunological products and vaccines*

◢ **Diphtheria-containing vaccines for children over 10 years**

A low dose of diphtheria toxoid is sufficient to recall immunity in older children previously immunised against diphtheria but whose immunity may have diminished with time; it is insufficient to cause serious reactions in a child who is already immune. Preparations containing low dose diphtheria should be used for children *over 10 years*, both for primary immunisation and booster doses. For immunisation of pregnant women against pertussis see Diphtheria-containing Vaccines for Immunisation of Pregnant Women Against Pertussis, below.

**Adsorbed Diphtheria [low dose], Tetanus and Poliomyelitis (Inactivated) Vaccine** PoM

Injection, suspension of diphtheria toxoid [low dose], tetanus toxoid and inactivated poliomyelitis vaccine components adsorbed on a mineral carrier, net price 0.5-mL prefilled syringe = £6.35

**Excipients** may include neomycin, polymyxin B and streptomycin

**Dose**

Primary immunisation

● By intramuscular injection

**Child 10–18 years** 3 doses each of 0.5 mL separated by intervals of 1 month; second booster dose, 0.5 mL given 10 years after first booster dose (may also be used as first booster dose in those over 10 years who have received only 3 previous doses of a diphtheria-containing vaccine); see also notes on booster doses, above

Available as part of childhood schedule, from health organisations or ImmForm

**Brands include** *Revaxis*®

◢ **Diphtheria-containing vaccines for immunisation of pregnant women against pertussis**

For immunisation of children over 10 years against diphtheria see Diphtheria-containing Vaccines for Children Over 10 Years, above

**Adsorbed Diphtheria [low dose], Tetanus, Pertussis (Acellular, Component) and Poliomyelitis (Inactivated) Vaccine** PoM

Injection, suspension of diphtheria toxoid [low dose], tetanus toxoid, acellular pertussis and inactivated poliomyelitis vaccine components adsorbed on a mineral carrier, net price 0.5 mL prefilled syringe = £11.98

**Excipients** may include neomycin, polymyxin B and streptomycin

**Contra-indications** section 14.1; see also individual components of vaccine; also contra-indicated in pregnant women with a history of encephalopathy of unknown origin within 7 days of previous immunisation with a pertussis-containing vaccine

**Dose**

Vaccination of pregnant women against pertussis see p. 616

● By intramuscular injection

0.5 mL as a single dose

Available from ImmForm

**Brands include** *Repevax*®

◢ **Diphtheria antitoxin**

**Diphtheria antitoxin** is used for passive immunisation in suspected cases of diphtheria only (without waiting for bacteriological confirmation); tests for hypersensitivity should be first carried out. It is derived from horse serum, and reactions are common after administration; resuscitation facilities should be available immediately.

It is no longer used for prophylaxis because of the risk of hypersensitivity; unimmunised contacts should be promptly investigated and given antibacterial prophylaxis (Table 2, section 5.1) and vaccine (see Contacts above, p. 606).

**Diphtheria Antitoxin** PoM

Dip/Ser

**Dose**

**Prophylaxis**

Not recommended therefore no dose stated (see notes above)

**Treatment**

Consult product literature

Available from Centre for Infections (Tel (020) 8200 6868) or in Northern Ireland from Public Health Laboratory, Belfast City Hospital (Tel (028) 9032 9241).

# Haemophilus type b conjugate vaccine

**Haemophilus influenzae type b (Hib) vaccine** is made from capsular polysaccharide; it is conjugated with a protein such as tetanus toxoid to increase immunogenicity, especially in young children. Haemophilus influenzae type b vaccine is given in combination with diphtheria, tetanus, pertussis (acellular, component) and poliomyelitis (inactivated) vaccine, (see under Diphtheria containing Vaccines) as a component of the primary course of childhood immunisation (see Immunisation schedule, section 14.1). For infants under 1 year, the course consists of 3 doses of a vaccine containing *Haemophilus influenzae* type b component, with an interval of 1 month between doses. A booster dose of haemophilus influenzae type b vaccine (combined with meningococcal group C conjugate vaccine) should be given at around 12–13 months of age.

Children 1–10 years who have not been immunised against *Haemophilus influenzae* type b need to receive only 1 dose of the vaccine (combined with meningococcal group C conjugate vaccine). However, if a primary course of immunisation has not been completed, these children should be given 3 doses of diphtheria, tetanus, pertussis (acellular, component), poliomyelitis (inactivated) and haemophilus type b conjugate vaccine (adsorbed). The risk of infection falls sharply in older children and the vaccine is not normally required for children over 10 years.

Haemophilus influenzae type b vaccine may be given to those over 10 years who are considered to be at increased risk of invasive *H. influenzae* type b disease (such as those with sickle-cell disease or complement deficiency, or those receiving treatment for malignancy).

**Invasive *Haemophilus influenzae* type b disease** After recovery from infection, unimmunised and partially immunised index cases under 10 years of age should complete their age-specific course of immunisation. Previously vaccinated cases under 10 years of age should be given an additional dose of haemophilus influenzae type b vaccine (combined with meningococcal group C conjugate vaccine) if Hib antibody concentrations are low or if it is not possible to measure antibody concentrations. Index cases of any age with asplenia or splenic dysfunction should complete their immunisation according to the recommenda-

14

Immunological products and vaccines

tions below; fully vaccinated cases with asplenia or splenic dysfunction should be given an additional dose of haemophilus influenzae type b vaccine (combined with meningococcal group C conjugate vaccine) if they received their previous dose over 1 year ago.

For use of rifampicin in the prevention of secondary cases of *Haemophilus influenzae* type b disease, see Table 2, section 5.1

**Asplenia, splenic dysfunction, or complement deficiency**   Children diagnosed with asplenia, splenic dysfunction, or complement deficiency at:

- *under 2 years of age* should be vaccinated according to the Immunisation Schedule (section 14.1). The booster dose of haemophilus influenzae type b vaccine (combined with meningococcal group C conjugate vaccine), given at 12–13 months of age, should be followed at least 1 month later by one dose of meningococcal A, C, W135, and Y conjugate vaccine. An additional dose of haemophilus influenzae type b vaccine (combined with meningococcal group C conjugate vaccine) should be given after the second birthday;

- *over 2 years of age* should receive one dose of haemophilus influenzae type b vaccine (combined with meningococcal group C conjugate vaccine), followed 1 month later by one dose of meningococcal A, C, W135, and Y conjugate vaccine.

![icon] **HAEMOPHILUS TYPE B CONJUGATE VACCINE**

**Cautions**   see section 14.1

**Contra-indications**   see section 14.1

**Pregnancy**   see p. 601

**Breast-feeding**   see p. 601

**Side-effects**   see section 14.1; also, atopic dermatitis, hypotonia

**Licensed use**   *Menitorix*® is not licensed for use in children over 2 years

**Indications and dose**

See notes above and under preparation

   **Primary immunisation**, see under Diphtheria-containing vaccines

**Menitorix**® (GSK) [PoM]

Injection, powder for reconstitution, capsular polysaccharide of *Haemophilus influenzae* type b and capsular polysaccharide of *Neisseria meningitidis* group C (both conjugated to tetanus protein), net price single dose vial (with syringe containing 0.5 mL diluent) = £39.87

**Dose**

> - By intramuscular injection
>   **CHILD 1–10 year** 0.5 mL
>   **CHILD over 1 year** with asplenia or splenic dysfunction (see notes above), 0.5 mL

Available as part of the childhood immunisation schedule from ImmForm

◀ **Combined vaccines**

See also Diphtheria-containing vaccines

## Hepatitis A vaccine

**Hepatitis A vaccine** is prepared from formaldehyde-inactivated hepatitis A virus grown in human diploid cells.

Immunisation is recommended for:

- residents of homes for those with severe learning difficulties;

- children with haemophilia or other conditions treated with plasma-derived clotting factors;

- children with severe liver disease;

- children travelling to high-risk areas (see p. 627);

- adolescents who are at risk due to their sexual behaviour;

- parenteral drug abusers.

Immunisation should be considered for:

- children with chronic liver disease including chronic hepatitis B or chronic hepatitis C;

- prevention of secondary cases in close contacts of confirmed cases of hepatitis A, within 14 days of exposure to the primary case (within 8 weeks of exposure to the primary case where there is more than 1 contact in the household).

A booster dose of hepatitis A vaccine is usually given 6–12 months after the initial dose. A second booster dose can be given 20 years after the previous booster dose to those who continue to be at risk. Specialist advice should be sought on re-immunisation of immunocompromised individuals.

In children under 16 years, a single dose of the combined vaccine *Ambirix*® can be used to provide rapid protection against hepatitis A.

Intramuscular normal immunoglobulin (section 14.5.1) is recommended for use in addition to Hepatitis A vaccine for close contacts (of confirmed cases of hepatitis A) who have chronic liver disease or HIV infection, or who are immunosuppressed.

Post-exposure prophylaxis is not required for healthy children under 1 year of age, so long as all those involved in nappy changing are vaccinated against hepatitis A. However, children 2–12 months of age can be given a dose of hepatitis A vaccine if it is not possible to vaccinate their carers, or if the child becomes a source of infection to others [unlicensed use]; in these cases, if the child goes on to require long-term protection against hepatitis A after the first birthday, the full course of 2 doses should be given.

![icon] **HEPATITIS A VACCINE**

**Cautions**   section 14.1

**Contra-indications**   section 14.1

**Pregnancy**   see p. 601

**Breast-feeding**   see p. 601

**Side-effects**   section 14.1; for combination vaccines, see also Typhoid vaccines, p. 621

**Indications and dose**

   **Immunisation against hepatitis A infection**

      For dose, see under preparations

## Single component

**Avaxim®** (Sanofi Pasteur) PoM

Injection, suspension of formaldehyde-inactivated hepatitis A virus (GBM grown in human diploid cells) 320 antigen units/mL adsorbed onto aluminium hydroxide, net price 0.5-mL prefilled syringe = £18.10

Excipients include neomycin

**Dose**

- **By intramuscular injection**

  (see note below)

  **Child 16–18 years** 0.5 mL as a single dose; booster dose 0.5 mL 6–12 months after initial dose

  **Note** Booster dose may be delayed by up to 3 years if not given after recommended interval following primary dose with *Avaxim®*. The deltoid region is the preferred site of injection; not to be injected into the buttock (vaccine efficacy reduced). The subcutaneous route may be used for children with bleeding disorders

**Epaxal®** (Crucell) PoM

Injection, suspension of formaldehyde-inactivated hepatitis A virus (RG-SB grown in human diploid cells) at least 48 units/mL, net price 0.5-mL prefilled syringe = £23.81

**Dose**

- **By intramuscular injection**

  (see note below)

  **Child 1–18 years** 0.5 mL as a single dose; booster dose 0.5 mL 6–12 months after initial dose (1–6 months if splenectomised)

  **Note** Booster dose may be delayed by up to 4 years if not given after recommended interval following primary dose. The deltoid region is the preferred site of injection. The subcutaneous route may be used for children with bleeding disorders

**Important** *Epaxal®* contains influenza virus haemagglutinin grown in the allantoic cavity of chick embryos, and is therefore contra-indicated in those hypersensitive to eggs or chicken protein.

**Havrix Monodose®** (GSK) PoM

Injection, suspension of formaldehyde-inactivated hepatitis A virus (HM 175 grown in human diploid cells) 1440 ELISA units/mL adsorbed onto aluminium hydroxide, net price 1-mL prefilled syringe = £22.14, 0.5-mL (720 ELISA units) prefilled syringe (*Havrix Junior Monodose®*) = £16.77

Excipients include neomycin

**Dose**

- **By intramuscular injection**

  (see note below)

  **Child 1–15 years** 0.5 mL as a single dose; booster dose 0.5 mL 6–12 months after initial dose

  **Child 16–18 years** 1 mL as a single dose; booster dose 1 mL 6–12 months after initial dose

  **Note** Booster dose may be delayed by up to 3 years if not given after recommended interval following primary dose with *Havrix Monodose®*. The deltoid region is the preferred site of injection. The subcutaneous route may be used for children with bleeding disorders

**Vaqta® Paediatric** (Sanofi Pasteur) PoM

Injection, suspension of formaldehyde-inactivated hepatitis A virus (grown in human diploid cells) 50 antigen units/mL adsorbed onto aluminium hydroxyphosphate sulfate, net price 0.5-mL prefilled syringe = £14.74

Excipients include neomycin

**Dose**

- **By intramuscular injection**

  (see note below)

  **Child 1–18 years** 0.5 mL as a single dose; booster dose 0.5 mL 6–18 months after initial dose

  **Note** The deltoid region is the preferred site of injection. The subcutaneous route may be used for children with bleeding disorders (but immune response may be reduced)

## With hepatitis B vaccine

**Ambirix®** (GSK) PoM

Injection, suspension of inactivated hepatitis A virus (grown in human diploid cells) 720 ELISA units/mL absorbed onto aluminium hydroxide, and recombinant (DNA) hepatitis B surface antigen (grown in yeast cells) 20 micrograms/mL adsorbed onto aluminium hydroxide and aluminium phosphate, net price 1-mL prefilled syringe = £31.18

Excipients include neomycin

**Dose**

- **By intramuscular injection**

  (see note below)

  **Child 1–15 years** primary course, 2 doses of 1 mL, the second 6–12 months after initial dose

  **Note** Primary course should be completed with *Ambirix®* (single component vaccines given at appropriate intervals may be used for booster dose); the deltoid region is the preferred site of injection in older children; anterolateral thigh is the preferred site in infants; not to be injected into the buttock (vaccine efficacy reduced); subcutaneous route used for children with bleeding disorders (but immune response may be reduced)

  **Important** *Ambirix®* not recommended for post-exposure prophylaxis following percutaneous (needle-stick), ocular, or mucous membrane exposure to hepatitis B virus

**Twinrix®** (GSK) PoM

Injection, inactivated hepatitis A virus (grown in human diploid cells) 720 ELISA units/mL adsorbed onto aluminium hydroxide, and recombinant (DNA) hepatitis B surface antigen (grown in yeast cells) 20 micrograms/mL adsorbed onto aluminium phosphate, net price 1-mL prefilled syringe (*Twinrix® Adult*) = £27.76, 1-mL vial (*Twinrix® Adult*) = £24.44, 0.5-mL prefilled syringe (*Twinrix® Paediatric*) = £20.79

Excipients include neomycin

**Dose**

- **By intramuscular injection**

  (see note below)

  **Child 1–15 years** primary course 3 doses of 0.5 mL (*Twinrix® Paediatric*), the second 1 month and the third 6 months after first dose

  **Child 16–18 years** primary course, 3 doses of 1 mL (*Twinrix® Adult*), the second 1 month and the third 6 months after first dose

  Accelerated schedule (e.g. for travellers departing within 1 month) for child over 16 years, second dose given 7 days after first dose, third dose after further 14 days and fourth dose 12 months after the first dose

  **Note** Primary course should be completed with *Twinrix®* (single component vaccines given at appropriate intervals may be used for booster dose); the deltoid region is the preferred site of injection in older children; anterolateral thigh is the preferred site in infants; not to be injected into the buttock (vaccine efficacy reduced); subcutaneous route used for children with bleeding disorders (but immune response may be reduced).

  **Important** *Twinrix®* not recommended for post-exposure prophylaxis following percutaneous (needle-stick), ocular or mucous membrane exposure to hepatitis B virus.

**14** Immunological products and vaccines

◢With typhoid vaccine

## Hepatyrix® (GSK) PoM

Injection, suspension of inactivated hepatitis A virus (grown in human diploid cells) 1440 ELISA units/mL adsorbed onto aluminium hydroxide, combined with typhoid vaccine containing 25 micrograms/mL virulence polysaccharide antigen of *Salmonella typhi*, net price 1-mL prefilled syringe = £32.08

**Excipients** include neomycin

**Note** May be difficult to obtain

**Dose**

- **By intramuscular injection**
  (see note below)
  **Child 15–18 years** 1 mL as a single dose; booster doses, see under single component hepatitis A vaccine (above) and under polysaccharide typhoid vaccine, p. 621
  **Note** The deltoid region is the preferred site of injection; not to be injected into the buttock (vaccine efficacy reduced). The subcutaneous route may be used for children with bleeding disorders

## ViATIM® (Sanofi Pasteur) PoM

Injection, suspension of inactivated hepatitis A virus (grown in human diploid cells) 160 antigen units/mL adsorbed onto aluminium hydroxide, combined with typhoid vaccine containing 25 micrograms/mL virulence polysaccharide antigen of *Salmonella typhi*, net price 1-mL prefilled syringe = £29.80

**Dose**

- **By intramuscular injection**
  (see note below)
  **Child 16–18 years** 1 mL as a single dose; booster doses, see under single component hepatitis A vaccine (above) and under polysaccharide typhoid vaccine, p. 621
  **Note** The deltoid region is the preferred site of injection; not to be injected into the buttock (vaccine efficacy reduced). The subcutaneous route may be used for children with bleeding disorders

## Hepatitis B vaccine

**Hepatitis B vaccine** contains inactivated hepatitis B virus surface antigen (HBsAg) adsorbed on to aluminium hydroxide adjuvant. It is made biosynthetically using recombinant DNA technology. The vaccine is used in individuals at high risk of contracting hepatitis B.

In the UK, high-risk groups include:

- parenteral drug misusers, their sexual partners, and household contacts; other drug misusers who are likely to 'progress' to injecting;

- adolescents who are at risk from their sexual behaviour;

- close family contacts of an individual with chronic hepatitis B infection;

- babies whose mothers have had acute hepatitis B during pregnancy *or* are positive for hepatitis B surface antigen (regardless of e-antigen markers); hepatitis B vaccination is started immediately on delivery and *hepatitis B immunoglobulin* (see p. 625) given at the same time (but at a different site). Babies whose mothers are positive for hepatitis B surface antigen and for e-antigen antibody should receive the vaccine only (but babies weighing 1.5 kg or less should also receive the immunoglobulin regardless of the mother's e-antigen antibody status);

- children with haemophilia, those receiving regular blood transfusions or blood products, and carers responsible for the administration of such products;

- children with chronic renal failure including those on haemodialysis. Children receiving haemodialysis should be monitored for antibodies annually and re-immunised if necessary. Home carers (of dialysis patients) should be vaccinated;

- children with chronic liver disease;

- patients of day-care or residential accommodation for those with severe learning difficulties;

- children in custodial institutions;

- children travelling to areas of high or intermediate prevalence who are at increased risk or who plan to remain there for lengthy periods (see p. 627);

- families adopting children from countries with a high or intermediate prevalence of hepatitis B;

- foster carers and their families.

Different immunisation schedules for hepatitis B vaccine are recommended for specific circumstances (see under individual preparations); an 'accelerated schedule' is recommended for pre-exposure prophylaxis in high–risk groups where rapid protection is required, and for post-exposure prophylaxis (see below). Generally, three or four doses are required for primary immunisation. Immunisation may take up to 6 months to confer adequate protection; the duration of immunity is not known precisely, but a single booster 5 years after the primary course may be sufficient to maintain immunity for those who continue to be at risk.

Immunisation does not eliminate the need for commonsense precautions for avoiding the risk of infection from known carriers by the routes of infection which have been clearly established, consult *Guidance for Clinical Health Care Workers: Protection against Infection with Blood-borne Viruses* (available at www.dh.gov.uk). Accidental inoculation of hepatitis B virus-infected blood into a wound, incision, needle-prick, or abrasion may lead to infection, whereas it is unlikely that indirect exposure to a carrier will do so.

Following significant exposure to hepatitis B, an accelerated schedule, with the second dose given 1 month, and the third dose 2 months after the initial dose, is recommended. For those at continued risk, a fourth dose should be given 12 months after the first dose. More detailed guidance is given in the *Immunisation against Infectious Disease* handbook, see p. 600.

Specific **hepatitis B immunoglobulin** ('HBIG') is available for use with the vaccine in those accidentally inoculated and in neonates at special risk of infection (section 14.5.2).

A combined hepatitis A and hepatitis B vaccine is also available.

## ◢ HEPATITIS B VACCINE

**Cautions** section 14.1
**Contra-indications** section 14.1
**Pregnancy** see p. 601
**Breast-feeding** see p. 601
**Side-effects** section 14.1
**Indications and dose**
> Immunisation against hepatitis B infection
>> For dose see under preparations

## ◢Single component

**Engerix B®** (GSK) PoM

Injection, suspension of hepatitis B surface antigen (prepared from yeast cells by recombinant DNA technique) 20 micrograms/mL adsorbed onto aluminium hydroxide, net price 0.5-mL (paediatric) prefilled syringe = £9.67, 1-mL vial = £12.34, 1-mL prefilled syringe = £12.99

**Dose**

• **By intramuscular injection**

(see note below)

**Neonate** (except if born to hepatitis B surface antigen-positive mother, see below), 3 doses of 10 micrograms, second dose 1 month and third dose 6 months after first dose

**Child 1 month–16 years** 3 doses of 10 micrograms, second dose 1 month and third dose 6 months after first dose

**Child 16–18 years** 3 doses of 20 micrograms, second dose 1 month and third dose 6 months after first dose

Accelerated schedule (all age groups), second dose 1 month after first dose, third dose 2 months after first dose and fourth dose 12 months after first dose
Alternative schedule for Child 11–15 years, 2 doses of 20 micrograms, the second dose 6 months after the first dose (this schedule not suitable if high risk of infection between doses or if compliance with second dose uncertain)

**Infant born to hepatitis B surface antigen-positive mother** (see also notes above)

• **By intramuscular injection**

(see note below)

**Neonate** 4 doses of 10 micrograms, first dose at birth with hepatitis B immunoglobulin injection (separate site) the second 1 month, the third 2 months and the fourth 12 months after first dose

**Renal insufficiency (including haemodialysis patients)**

• **By intramuscular injection**

(see note below)

**Neonate** (except if born to hepatitis B surface antigen positive mother, see above), 3 doses of 10 micrograms, second dose 1 month and third dose 6 months after first dose *or* accelerated schedule, 4 doses of 10 micrograms, second dose 1 month, third dose 2 months, and fourth dose 12 months after first dose; immunisation schedule and booster doses may need to be adjusted in those with low antibody concentration

**Child 1 month–16 years** 3 doses of 10 micrograms, second dose 1 month and third dose 6 months after first dose *or* accelerated schedule, 4 doses of 10 micrograms, second dose 1 month, third dose 2 months, and fourth dose 12 months after first dose; immunisation schedule and booster doses may need to be adjusted in those with low antibody concentration

**Child 16–18 years** 4 doses of 40 micrograms, the second 1 month, the third 2 months and the fourth 6 months after the first dose; immunisation schedule and booster doses may need to be adjusted in those with low antibody concentration

**Note** Deltoid muscle is preferred site of injection in older children; anterolateral thigh is preferred site in neonates, infants and young children; not to be injected into the buttock (vaccine efficacy reduced)

**Fendrix®** (GSK) PoM

Injection, suspension of hepatitis B surface antigen (prepared from yeast cells by recombinant DNA technique) 40 micrograms/mL adsorbed onto aluminium phosphate, net price 0.5-mL prefilled syringe = £38.10

**Excipients** include traces of thiomersal

**Dose**

**Renal insufficiency patients (including pre-haemodialysis and haemodialysis patients)**

• **By intramuscular injection**

(see note below)

**Child 15–18 years** 4 doses of 20 micrograms, the second 1 month, the third 2 months and the fourth 6 months after the first dose; immunisation schedule and booster doses may need to be adjusted in those with low antibody concentration

**Note** Deltoid muscle is preferred site of injection; not to be injected into the buttock (vaccine efficacy reduced)

**HBvaxPRO®** (Sanofi Pasteur) PoM

Injection, suspension of hepatitis B surface antigen (prepared from yeast cells by recombinant DNA technique) 10 micrograms/mL adsorbed onto aluminium hydroxyphosphate sulfate, net price 0.5-mL (5-microgram) prefilled syringe = £8.95, 1-mL (10-microgram) prefilled syringe = £12.20; 40 micrograms/mL, 1-mL (40-microgram) vial = £27.60

**Dose**

• **By intramuscular injection**

(see note below)

**Neonate** (except if born to hepatitis B surface antigen-positive mother, see below), 3 doses of 5 micrograms, second dose 1 month and third dose 6 months after first dose

**Child 1 month–16 years** 3 doses of 5 micrograms, second dose 1 month and third dose 6 months after first dose

**Child 16–18 years** 3 doses of 10 micrograms, second dose 1 month and third dose 6 months after first dose

Accelerated schedule (all age groups), second dose 1 month after first dose, third dose 2 months after first dose with fourth dose at 12 months
Booster doses may be required in immunocompromised patients with low antibody concentration

**Infant born to hepatitis B surface antigen-positive mother** (see also notes above)

• **By intramuscular injection**

(see note below)

**Neonate** 4 doses of 5 micrograms, first dose at birth with hepatitis B immunoglobulin injection (separate site), the second 1 month, the third 2 months and the fourth 12 months after the first dose

**Chronic haemodialysis patients**

• **By intramuscular injection**

(see note below)

**Child 16–18 years** 3 doses of 40 micrograms, second dose 1 month and third dose 6 months after first dose; booster doses may be required in those with low antibody concentration

**Note** Deltoid muscle is preferred site of injection in older children; anterolateral thigh is preferred site in neonates and infants; not to be injected into the buttock (vaccine efficacy reduced)

## ◢With hepatitis A vaccine

See Hepatitis A Vaccine

# Human papillomavirus vaccines

**Human papillomavirus vaccine** is available as a bivalent vaccine (*Cervarix®*) or a quadrivalent vaccine (*Gardasil®*). *Cervarix®* is licensed for use in females for the prevention of cervical cancer and other pre-cancerous lesions caused by human papillomavirus types 16 and 18. *Gardasil®* is licensed for use in females for the prevention of cervical cancer, genital warts and pre-cancerous lesions caused by human papillomavirus types 6, 11, 16 and 18. The vaccines may also provide limited protection against disease caused by other types of human papillomavirus. The two vaccines are not interchangeable and one vaccine product should be used for an entire course.

Human papillomavirus vaccine will be most effective if given before sexual activity starts. The first dose is given to females aged 12 to 13 years, the second and third doses are given 1 and 4–6 months after the first dose (see Immunisation schedule, section 14.1); all 3 doses should be given within a 12-month period. If the course is interrupted, it should be resumed but not repeated, allowing the appropriate interval between the remaining doses. Where the second dose was given late and there are significant challenges in scheduling vaccination, or a high likelihood that the third dose will not be given, in exceptional circumstances, the third dose can be given at least 1 month after the second dose. Under the national programme in England, females remain eligible to receive the vaccine up to the age of 18 years if they did not receive the vaccine when scheduled. Where appropriate, immunisation with human papillomavirus vaccine should be offered to females coming into the UK as they may not have been offered protection in their country of origin. The duration of protection has not been established, but current studies suggest that protection is maintained for at least 6 years after completion of the primary course.

## HUMAN PAPILLOMAVIRUS VACCINES

**Cautions**    see section 14.1
**Contra-indications**    see section 14.1
**Pregnancy**    not known to be harmful, but vaccination should be postponed until completion of pregnancy
**Breast-feeding**    see p. 601
**Side-effects**    see section 14.1
**Indications and dose**

> See notes above and under preparations
> **Note**  To avoid confusion, prescribers should specify the brand to be dispensed

**Cervarix®** (GSK) [PoM]
Injection, suspension of virus-like particles of human papillomavirus type 16 (40 micrograms/mL), type 18 (40 micrograms/mL) capsid protein (prepared by recombinant DNA technique using a Baculovirus expression system) in monophosphoryl lipid A adjuvant adsorbed onto aluminium hydroxide, net price 0.5-mL prefilled syringe = £80.50
**Note**  To avoid confusion, prescribers should specify the brand to be dispensed

**Dose**
> **Prevention of premalignant genital lesions and cervical cancer (see notes above)**
> ● By intramuscular injection into deltoid region
> **Child 9–18 years** 3 doses of 0.5 mL, the second 1 month and the third 6 months after the first dose
> Alternative schedule for **Child 9–18 years**, 3 doses of 0.5 mL, the second 1–2.5 months, and the third 5–12 months after the first dose

**Gardasil®** (Sanofi Pasteur) ▼ [PoM]
Injection, suspension of virus-like particles of human papillomavirus type 6 (40 micrograms/mL), type 11 (80 micrograms/mL), type 16 (80 micrograms/mL), type 18 (40 micrograms/mL) capsid protein (prepared from yeast cells by recombinant DNA techni-

que) adsorbed onto aluminium hydroxyphosphate sulfate, net price 0.5-mL prefilled syringe = £86.50
**Note**  To avoid confusion, prescribers should specify the brand to be dispensed

**Dose**
> **Prevention of premalignant genital lesions, cervical cancer and genital warts (see notes above)**
> ● By intramuscular injection preferably into deltoid region or higher anterolateral thigh
> **Child 9–18 years** 3 doses of 0.5 mL, the second 2 months and the third 6 months after the first dose
> Alternative schedule for **Child 9–18 years**, 3 doses of 0.5 mL, the second at least 1 month and the third at least 4 months after the first dose; schedule should be completed within 12 months

## Influenza vaccine

While most viruses are antigenically stable, the influenza viruses A and B (especially A) are constantly altering their antigenic structure as indicated by changes in the haemagglutinins (H) and neuraminidases (N) on the surface of the viruses. It is essential that influenza vaccines in use contain the H and N components of the prevalent strain or strains recommended each year by the World Health Organization.

Seasonal influenza vaccines will not control epidemics — immunisation is recommended *only for persons at high risk*. Annual immunisation is strongly recommended for children (including infants that were preterm or low birth-weight) aged over 6 months with the following conditions:

- chronic respiratory disease (includes asthma treated with continuous or repeated use of inhaled or systemic corticosteroids or asthma with previous exacerbations requiring hospital admission);

- chronic heart disease;

- chronic liver disease;

- chronic renal disease;

- chronic neurological disease;

- diabetes mellitus;

- immunosuppression because of disease (including asplenia or splenic dysfunction) or treatment (including prolonged systemic corticosteroid treatment [for over 1 month at dose equivalents of prednisolone: *child under 20 kg*, 1 mg/kg or more daily; *child over 20 kg*, 20 mg or more daily] and chemotherapy);

- HIV infection (regardless of immune status).

Seasonal influenza vaccine is also recommended for all pregnant women, for children living in long-stay facilities, and for carers of children whose welfare may be at risk if the carer falls ill. Influenza immunisation should also be considered for household contacts of immunocompromised individuals.

Further information on pandemic influenza, avian influenza, and swine influenza may be found at www.dh.gov.uk/pandemicflu and at www.hpa.org.uk.

## INFLUENZA VACCINES

**Cautions**    see section 14.1; increased risk of fever in child under 5 years with *Viroflu®* and *Inflexal® V*, and in child 5–9 years with *Enzira®* or preparations marketed by Pfizer or CSL Biotherapies; **interactions:** Appendix 1 (vaccines)

**Contra-indications** see section 14.1 and also under *Fluenz*® below; avoid *Enzira*® or preparations marketed by Pfizer or CSL Biotherapies in child under 5 years—increased risk of febrile convulsions

**Pregnancy** see section 14.1; inactivated vaccines not known to be harmful; avoid *Fluenz*®

**Breast-feeding** see section 14.1; inactivated vaccines not known to be harmful; avoid *Fluenz*®

**Side-effects** see section 14.1; also reported, febrile convulsions and transient thrombocytopenia; *with intranasal spray*, rhinorrhoea

**Licensed use** Inactivated Influenza Vaccine (Surface Antigen) and *Fluvirin*® are not licensed for use in children under 4 years

**Indications and dose**

> **Annual immunisation against seasonal influenza**
>
> • By intramuscular injection
>
>   **Child 6 months–9 years** 0.5 mL (repeated after at least 4 weeks in children who have not received seasonal influenza vaccine previously)
>
>   **Child 9–18 years** 0.5 mL as a single dose
>
> • Intranasally
>
>   See under *Fluenz*® below

◀ **Seasonal influenza vaccines**

**Inactivated Influenza Vaccine (Split Virion)** PoM
Flu
Injection, suspension of formaldehyde-inactivated influenza virus (split virion) grown in fertilised hens' eggs, net price 0.25-mL prefilled syringe = £6.29, 0.5-mL prefilled syringe = £6.29
Excipients may include neomycin and polymyxin
Available from Sanofi Pasteur
Cautions increased risk of fever in child 5–9 years with preparations marketed by Pfizer or CSL Biotherapies—use alternative influenza vaccine if available
Contra-indications avoid preparations marketed by Pfizer or CSL Biotherapies in child under 5 years—increased risk of febrile convulsions

**Inactivated Influenza Vaccine (Surface Antigen)** PoM
Flu or Flu(adj)
Injection, suspension of propiolactone-inactivated influenza virus (surface antigen) grown in fertilised hens' eggs, net price 0.5-mL prefilled syringe = £4.15
Excipients may include neomycin, polymyxin B and traces of thiomersal
Available from Novartis Vaccines

**Agrippal**® (Novartis Vaccines) PoM
Injection, suspension of formaldehyde-inactivated influenza virus (surface antigen) grown in fertilised hens' eggs, net price 0.5-mL prefilled syringe = £5.85
Excipients include kanamycin and neomycin

**Enzira**® (Pfizer) PoM
Injection, suspension of inactivated influenza virus (split virion) grown in fertilised hens' eggs, net price 0.5-mL prefilled syringe = £6.33
Excipients include neomycin and polymyxin B
Cautions child 5–9 years (increased risk of fever)—use alternative influenza vaccine if available
Contra-indications child under 5 years—increased risk of febrile convulsions

**Fluarix**® (GSK) PoM
Injection, suspension of formaldehyde-inactivated influenza virus (split virion) grown in fertilised hens' eggs, net price 0.5-mL prefilled syringe = £5.39
Excipients include gentamicin
Note Ovalbumin content less than 100 nanograms/mL

**Fluvirin**® (Novartis Vaccines) PoM
Injection, suspension of formaldehyde-inactivated influenza virus (surface antigen) grown in fertilised hens' eggs, net price 0.5 mL prefilled syringe = £5.55
Excipients include neomycin, polymyxin B, and traces of thiomersal

**Imuvac**® (Abbott Healthcare) PoM
Injection, suspension of formaldehyde-inactivated influenza virus (surface antigen) grown in fertilised hens' eggs, net price 0.5-mL prefilled syringe = £6.59
Excipients include gentamicin

**Influvac Sub-unit**® (Abbott Healthcare) PoM
Injection, suspension of formaldehyde-inactivated influenza virus (surface antigen) grown in fertilised hens' eggs, net price 0.5-mL prefilled syringe = £5.22
Excipients include gentamicin

**Viroflu**® (Janssen) PoM
Injection, suspension of inactivated influenza virus (surface antigen, virosome) grown in fertilised hens' eggs, net price 0.5-mL prefilled syringe = £6.33
Excipients include neomycin and polymyxin B
Cautions child under 5 years (increased risk of fever)—use only if a safer alternative influenza vaccine is not available
Note Ovalbumin content less than 100 nanograms/mL
Note Also available as *Inflexal*® V

◀ **Seasonal influenza vaccine for intranasal use**

**Fluenz**® (AstraZeneca) ▼ PoM
Nasal spray, suspension of live, attenuated influenza virus (produced in vero cells and grown in fertilised hens' eggs), net price 0.2 mL nasal applicator = £14.00
Excipients include gelatin and gentamicin
Contra-indications see section 14.1; also severe asthma; avoid close contact with severely immunocompromised patients for 1–2 weeks after vaccination; concomitant use with antiviral therapy for influenza (avoid antivirals for at least 2 weeks after *Fluenz*®; avoid *Fluenz*® for at least 48 hours after stopping the antiviral); concomitant use with salicylates in children
Dose

> **Annual immunisation against seasonal influenza**
>
>   **Child 2–18 years** 0.1 mL into each nostril as a single dose; for children who have not received seasonal influenza vaccine previously, repeat after 4 weeks

## Measles vaccine

**Measles vaccine** has been replaced by a combined live measles, mumps and rubella vaccine (MMR vaccine).

MMR vaccine may be used in the control of outbreaks of measles (see under MMR Vaccine).

◀ **Single antigen vaccine**

No longer available in the UK

◀ **Combined vaccines**

See MMR vaccine, p. 614

14

Immunological products and vaccines

## Measles, Mumps and Rubella (MMR) vaccine

A combined live **measles, mumps, and rubella vaccine** (MMR vaccine) aims to eliminate measles, mumps and rubella (and congenital rubella syndrome). Every child should receive two doses of MMR vaccine by entry to primary school, unless there is a valid contra-indication (see section 14.1). MMR vaccine should be given irrespective of previous measles, mumps, or rubella infection or vaccination.

The first dose of MMR vaccine is given to children aged 12–13 months. A second dose is given before starting school at 3–5 years of age (see Immunisation schedule, section 14.1).

When protection against measles is required urgently (e.g. during a measles outbreak), the second dose of MMR vaccine can be given 1 month after the first dose; if the second dose is given before 18 months of age, then children should still receive the routine dose before starting school at 3–5 years of age.

Children presenting for pre-school booster who have not received the first dose of MMR vaccine should be given a dose of MMR vaccine followed 3 months later by a second dose. At school-leaving age or at entry into further education, MMR immunisation should be offered to individuals of both sexes who have not received 2 doses during childhood. In a young adult who has received only a single dose of MMR in childhood, a second dose is recommended to achieve full protection. If 2 doses of MMR vaccine are required, the second dose should be given one month after the initial dose.

MMR vaccine should be used to protect against rubella in *seronegative females of child-bearing age* (see Immunisation schedule, section 14.1). MMR vaccine may also be offered to previously *unimmunised and seronegative post-partum* mothers—vaccination a few days after delivery is important because about 60% of congenital abnormalities from rubella infection occur in babies of mothers who have borne more than one child. Immigrants arriving after the age of school immunisation are particularly likely to require immunisation.

**Contacts**    MMR vaccine may also be used in the control of outbreaks of measles and should be offered to susceptible children including babies aged over 6 months who are contacts of a case, within 3 days of exposure to infection; these children should still receive routine MMR vaccinations at the recommended ages. Children aged under 9 months for whom avoidance of measles infection is particularly important (such as those with history of recent severe illness) can be given normal immunoglobulin (section 14.5, p. 623) after exposure to measles; routine MMR immunisation should then be given after at least 3 months at the appropriate age.

MMR vaccine is **not suitable** for prophylaxis following exposure to mumps or rubella since the antibody response to the mumps and rubella components is too slow for effective prophylaxis.

Children with impaired immune response should not receive live vaccines (for advice on HIV see section 14.1). If they have been exposed to measles infection they should be given normal immunoglobulin (section 14.5).

**Travel**    Unimmunised children over 6 months of age travelling to areas where measles is endemic or epidemic should receive MMR vaccine. Children immunised before 12 months of age should still receive two doses of MMR at the recommended ages. If one dose of MMR has already been given to a child, then the second dose should be brought forward to at least one month after the first, to ensure complete protection. If the child is under 18 months of age and the second dose is given within 3 months of the first, then the routine dose, before starting school at 3–5 years, should still be given.

**Side-effects**    See section 14.1. Also malaise, fever, or a rash can occur after the first dose of MMR vaccine, most commonly about a week after vaccination and lasting about 2 to 3 days. Leaflets are available for parents on advice for reducing fever (including the use of paracetamol). Febrile seizures occur rarely 6 to 11 days after MMR vaccination; the incidence of febrile seizures is lower than that following measles infection. Parotid swelling occurs occasionally, usually in the third week, and rarely, arthropathy 2 to 3 weeks after immunisation. Adverse reactions are considerably less frequent after the second dose of MMR vaccine than after the first dose.

Idiopathic thrombocytopenic purpura has occurred rarely following MMR vaccination, usually within 6 weeks of the first dose. The risk of idiopathic thrombocytopenic purpura after MMR vaccine is much less than the risk after infection with wild measles or rubella virus. Children who develop idiopathic thrombocytopenic purpura within 6 weeks of the first dose of MMR should undergo serological testing before the second dose is due; if the results suggest incomplete immunity against measles, mumps or rubella then a second dose of MMR is recommended. The Specialist and Reference Microbiology Division, Health Protection Agency offers free serological testing for children who develop idiopathic thrombocytopenic purpura *within 6 weeks* of the first dose of MMR.

Post-vaccination aseptic meningitis was reported (rarely and with complete recovery) following vaccination with MMR vaccine containing Urabe mumps vaccine, which has now been discontinued; no cases have been confirmed in association with the currently used Jeryl Lynn mumps vaccine. Children with post-vaccination symptoms are not infectious.

> Reviews undertaken on behalf of the CSM, the Medical Research Council, and the Cochrane Collaboration, have not found any evidence of a link between MMR vaccination and bowel disease or autism. The Chief Medical Officers have advised that the MMR vaccine is the safest and best way to protect children against measles, mumps, and rubella. Information (including fact sheets and a list of references) may be obtained from:
> www.dh.gov.uk/immunisation

## MEASLES, MUMPS AND RUBELLA VACCINE, LIVE

**Cautions**    see section 14.1; also after immunoglobulin administration or blood transfusion, leave an interval of at least 3 months before MMR immunisation as antibody response to measles component may be reduced; **interactions:** Appendix 1 (vaccines)
**Hypersensitivity to egg**    MMR vaccine can be given safely even when the child has had an anaphylactic reaction to food

containing egg. Dislike of eggs, refusal to eat egg, or confirmed anaphylactic reactions to egg-containing food is not a contra-indication to MMR vaccination. Children with a confirmed anaphylactic reaction to the MMR vaccine should be assessed by a specialist.

**Contra-indications**   see section 14.1

**Pregnancy**   avoid pregnancy for at least 1 month after vaccination; see also, p. 601

**Breast-feeding**   see p. 601

**Side-effects**   see section 14.1 and notes above; also *less commonly* sleep disturbance, unusual crying in infants, also reported peripheral and optic neuritis.

**Licensed use**   not licensed for use in children under 9 months

**Indications and dose**

> **Immunisation against measles, mumps, and rubella**
>
> - **By intramuscular or deep subcutaneous injection**
>   **CHILD 6 months–18 years** primary immunisation, 2 doses each of 0.5 mL, see Immunisation schedule, section 14.1, p. 603; see also notes above for use in outbreaks, for contacts of cases, and for travel

◀**Combined vaccines**

**MMRvaxPro®** (Sanofi Pasteur) [PoM]
Injection, powder for reconstitution, live attenuated, measles virus (Enders' Edmonston strain) and mumps virus (Jeryl Lynn [Level B] strain) prepared in chick embryo cells, and rubella virus (Wistar RA 27/3 strain); single-dose vial (with syringe containing solvent)
**Excipients** include gelatin and neomycin
Only available as part of childhood immunisation schedule from health organisations or ImmForm

**Priorix®** (GSK) [PoM]
Injection, powder for reconstitution, live attenuated, measles virus (Schwarz strain) and mumps virus (RIT 4385 strain) prepared in chick embryo cells, and rubella virus (Wistar RA 27/3 strain), net price single-dose vial (with syringe containing solvent) = £6.37
**Excipients** include neomycin
Also available as part of childhood immunisation schedule from health organisations or ImmForm

## Meningococcal vaccines

Almost all childhood meningococcal disease in the UK is caused by *Neisseria meningitidis* serogroups B and C. **Meningococcal Group C conjugate vaccine** protects only against infection by serogroup C. The risk of meningococcal disease declines with age—immunisation is not generally recommended after the age of 25 years.

Tetravalent meningococcal vaccines that cover serotypes A, C, W135, and Y are available. Although the duration of protection has not been established, the **meningococcal A, C, W135, and Y conjugate vaccine** is likely to provide longer-lasting protection than the unconjugated meningococal polysaccharide vaccine. The antibody response to serotype C in unconjugated meningococcal polysaccharide vaccines in young children may be suboptimal.

**Childhood immunisation**   Meningococcal Group C conjugate vaccine provides long-term protection against infection by serogroup C of *Neisseria meningitidis*. Immunisation consists of 2 doses given at 3 months

and 4 months of age; a booster dose should be given at 12–13 months of age, usually combined with haemophilus influenzae type b vaccine (see Immunisation Schedule, section 14.1, p. 603).

It is recommended that meningococcal group C conjugate vaccine be given to anyone aged under 25 years who has not been vaccinated previously with this vaccine; those over 1 year receive a single dose. Children with confirmed serogroup C disease, who have previously been immunised with meningococcal group C vaccine, should be offered meningococcal group C conjugate vaccine before discharge from hospital.

**Asplenia, splenic dysfunction, or complement deficiency**   See p. 608.

**Travel**   Individuals travelling to countries of risk (see below) should be immunised with **meningococcal A, C, W135, and Y conjugate vaccine**, even if they have previously received meningitis C conjugate vaccine. If an individual has recently received meningococcal group C conjugate vaccine, an interval of at least 4 weeks should be allowed before administration of the tetravalent (A, C, W135, and Y) vaccine.

Vaccination is particularly important for those living with local people or visiting an area of risk during outbreaks.

Immunisation recommendations and requirements for visa entry for individual countries should be checked before travelling, particularly to countries in Sub-Saharan Africa, Asia, and the Indian sub-continent where outbreaks and epidemics of meningococcal infection are reported. Country-by-country information is available from the National Travel Health Network and Centre (www.nathnac.org).

Proof of vaccination with the tetravalent (A, C, W135 and Y) meningococcal vaccine is required for those travelling to Saudi Arabia during the Hajj and Umrah pilgrimages (where outbreaks of the W135 strain have occurred).

**Contacts**   For advice on the immunisation of *laboratory workers and close contacts* of cases of meningococcal disease in the UK and on the role of the vaccine in the control of *local outbreaks*, consult Guidelines for Public Health Management of Meningococcal Disease in the UK at www.hpa.org.uk. See Table 2, section 5.1 for antibacterial prophylaxis for prevention of secondary cases of meningococcal meningitis.

## ■ MENINGOCOCCAL VACCINES

**Cautions**   see section 14.1

**Contra-indications**   see section 14.1

**Pregnancy**   see p. 601

**Breast-feeding**   see p. 601

**Side-effects**   see section 14.1; also *rarely* symptoms of meningitis reported (but no evidence that vaccine causes meningococcal C meningitis)

**Licensed use**   Menveo® not licensed for use in children under 11 years

**Indications and dose**

> **Immunisation against *Neisseria meningitidis*** for dose, see under preparations

◀Meningococcal Group C conjugate vaccine

**Meningitec®** (Pfizer) PoM

Injection, suspension of capsular polysaccharide antigen of *Neisseria meningitidis* group C (conjugated to *Corynebacterium diphtheriae* protein), adsorbed onto aluminium phosphate, net price 0.5-mL pre-filled syringe = £7.50

**Dose**

* **By intramuscular injection**

    **Child 2 months–1 year** for routine immunisation, 0.5 mL, see notes above and Immunisation schedule, section 14.1

    **Child 1–18 years** 0.5 mL as a single dose

    **Note** Subcutaneous route used for children with bleeding disorders

Available as part of childhood immunisation schedule from ImmForm

**Menjugate Kit®** (Sanofi Pasteur) PoM

Injection, powder for reconstitution, capsular polysaccharide antigen of *Neisseria meningitidis* group C (conjugated to *Corynebacterium diphtheriae* protein), adsorbed onto aluminium hydroxide, single-dose vials

**Dose**

* **By intramuscular injection**

    **Child 2 months–1 year** for routine immunisation, 0.5 mL, see notes above and Immunisation schedule, section 14.1

    **Child 1–18 years** 0.5 mL as a single dose

    **Note** Subcutaneous route used for children with bleeding disorders

Available as part of childhood immunisation schedule from ImmForm

**NeisVac-C®** (Baxter) PoM

Injection, suspension of polysaccharide antigen of *Neisseria meningitidis* group C (conjugated to tetanus toxoid protein), adsorbed onto aluminium hydroxide, 0.5-mL prefilled syringe

**Dose**

* **By intramuscular injection**

    **Child 2 months–1 year** for routine immunisation, 0.5 mL, see notes above and Immunisation schedule, section 14.1

    **Child 1–18 years** 0.5 mL as a single dose

Available as part of childhood immunisation schedule from ImmForm

◀Meningococcal Group C conjugate vaccine with Haemophilus Influenzae type B vaccine

See *Haemophilus Influenzae* type B vaccine

◀Meningococcal A, C, W135, and Y conjugate vaccine

**Menveo®** (Novartis Vaccines) ▼ PoM

Injection, powder for reconstitution, capsular oligosaccharide antigens of *Neisseria meningitidis* groups A, C, W135, and Y (conjugated to *Corynebacterium diphtheriae* protein), net price single-dose vial (with syringe containing diluent) = £40.01

**Dose**

* **By intramuscular injection preferably into deltoid region**

    **Child 3 months–1 year** 2 doses of 0.5 mL separated by an interval of 1 month

    **Child 1–18 years** 0.5 mL as a single dose

**Nimenrix®** (GSK) ▼ PoM

Injection, powder for reconstitution, capsular polysaccharide antigens of *Neisseria meningitidis* groups A, C, W135, and Y (conjugated to tetanus toxoid protein), net price single-dose vial (with syringe containing diluent) = £30.00

**Dose**

* **By intramuscular injection preferably into deltoid region (or anterolateral thigh in child 1–2 years)**

    **Child 1–18 years** 0.5 mL as a single dose; a second dose may be considered after 1 year in those who continue to be at risk of *Neisseria meningitidis* serogroup A infection

◀Meningococcal polysaccharide A, C, W135 and Y vaccine

**ACWY Vax®** (GSK) PoM

Injection, powder for reconstitution, capsular polysaccharide antigens of *Neisseria meningitidis* groups A, C, W135 and Y, net price single-dose vial (with syringe containing diluent) = £16.73

**Dose**

* **By deep subcutaneous injection**

    **Child 5–18 years** 0.5 mL as a single dose; booster dose for those at continued risk, 0.5 mL every 5 years

# Mumps vaccine

◀**Single antigen vaccine**

No longer available in the UK

◀**Combined vaccines**

See MMR Vaccine, p. 614

# Pertussis vaccine

**Pertussis vaccine** is given as a combination preparation containing other vaccines (see Diphtheria Vaccines). Acellular vaccines are derived from highly purified components of *Bordetella pertussis*. Primary immunisation against pertussis (whooping cough) requires 3 doses of an acellular pertussis-containing vaccine (see Immunisation schedule, section 14.1, p. 603), given at intervals of 1 month from the age of 2 months.

All children up to the age of 10 years should receive primary immunisation with diphtheria, tetanus, pertussis (acellular, component), poliomyelitis (inactivated) and haemophilus type b conjugate vaccine (adsorbed).

A booster dose of an acellular pertussis-containing vaccine should ideally be given 3 years after the primary course, although, the interval can be reduced to 1 year if the primary course was delayed.

Children aged 1–10 years who have not received a *pertussis-containing* vaccine as part of their primary immunisation schedule should be offered 1 dose of a suitable pertussis-containing vaccine; after an interval of at least 1 year, a booster dose of a suitable pertussis-containing vaccine should be given. Immunisation against pertussis is not routinely recommended in individuals over 10 years of age.

**Vaccination of pregnant women against pertussis (October 2012)** In response to the current outbreak, the UK health departments have introduced a temporary programme to vaccinate pregnant women against pertussis. The aim of the programme is to boost the levels of pertussis–specific antibodies that are transferred, through the placenta, from the mother to the fetus, so that the newborn is protected before routine immunisation begins at 2 months of age.

Pregnant women should be offered a single dose of acellular pertussis-containing vaccine (as adsorbed diphtheria [low dose], tetanus, pertussis (acellular, component) and poliomyelitis (inactivated) vaccine; *Repevax*®) between 28 to 38 weeks of pregnancy; the optimal time for vaccination is between 28–32 weeks of pregnancy. Pregnant women should be offered a single dose of acellular pertussis-containing vaccine up to the onset of labour if they missed the opportunity for vaccination at 28–38 weeks of pregnancy. A single dose of acellular pertussis-containing vaccine may also be offered to new mothers, who have never previously been vaccinated against pertussis, until the child receives the first vaccination.

While this programme is in place, women who become pregnant again should be offered vaccination during each pregnancy to maximise transplacental transfer of antibody.

**Contacts** Vaccination against pertussis should be considered for close contacts of cases with pertussis who have been offered antibacterial prophylaxis (Table 2, section 5.1). Unimmunised or partially immunised contacts under 10 years of age should complete their vaccination against pertussis. A booster dose of an acellular pertussis-containing vaccine is recommended for contacts aged 10–18 years who have not received a pertussis-containing vaccine in the last 10 years and who have not received adsorbed diphtheria [low dose], tetanus, and poliomyelitis (inactivated) vaccine in the last month.

**Cautions**   Section 14.1

**Contra-indications**   Section 14.1

**Pregnancy**   see p. 601 and also Vaccination of Pregnant Women Against Pertussis above

**Breast-feeding**   see p. 601

**Side effects**   See also section 14.1. The incidence of local and systemic effects is generally lower with vaccines containing acellular pertussis components than with the whole-cell pertussis vaccine used. However, compared with primary vaccination, booster doses with vaccines containing acellular pertussis are reported to increase the risk of injection-site reactions (some of which affect the entire limb); local reactions do not contra-indicate further doses (see below).

The vaccine should not be withheld from children with a history to a preceding dose of:

* fever, irrespective of severity;
* persistent crying or screaming for more than 3 hours;
* severe local reaction, irrespective of extent.

◢**Combined vaccines**

Combined vaccines, see under Diphtheria vaccines

---

# Pneumococcal vaccines

Pneumococcal vaccines protect against infection with *Streptococcus pneumoniae* (pneumococcus); the vaccines contain polysaccharide from capsular pneumococci, **Pneumococcal polysaccharide vaccine** contains purified polysaccharide from 23 capsular types of pneumococci, whereas **pneumococcal polysaccharide conju-**

gate vaccine (adsorbed) contains polysaccharide from either 10 capsular types (*Synflorix*®) or 13 capsular types (*Prevenar* 13®) with the polysaccharide being conjugated to protein.

The 13-valent conjugate vaccine is used for childhood immunisation. The recommended schedule consists of 3 doses, the first at 2 months of age, the second at 4 months, and the third at 12–13 months (see Immunisation Schedule, section 14.1).

Pneumococcal vaccination is recommended for individuals at increased risk of pneumococcal infection as follows:

* child under 5 years with a history of invasive pneumococcal disease;
* asplenia or splenic dysfunction (including homozygous sickle cell disease and coeliac disease which could lead to splenic dysfunction);
* chronic respiratory disease (includes asthma treated with continuous or frequent use of a systemic corticosteroid);
* chronic heart disease;
* chronic renal disease;
* chronic liver disease;
* diabetes mellitus;
* immune deficiency because of disease (e.g. HIV infection) or treatment (including prolonged systemic corticosteroid treatment for over 1 month at dose equivalents of prednisolone: *child under 20 kg*, 1 mg/kg or more daily; *child over 20 kg*, 20 mg or more daily);
* presence of cochlear implant;
* conditions where leakage of cerebrospinal fluid could occur.

Where possible, the vaccine should be given at least 2 weeks before splenectomy, cochlear implant surgery, chemotherapy, or radiotherapy; children and carers should be given advice about increased risk of pneumococcal infection. If it is not practical to vaccinate at least 2 weeks before splenectomy, chemotherapy, or radiotherapy, the vaccine should be given at least 2 weeks after the splenectomy or, where possible, at least 3 months after completion of chemotherapy or radiotherapy. Prophylactic antibacterial therapy against pneumococcal infection (Table 2, section 5.1, p. 257) should not be stopped after immunisation. A patient card and information leaflet for patients with asplenia are available from the Department of Health or in Scotland from the Scottish Executive, Public Health Division 1 (Tel (0131) 244 2501).

**Choice of vaccine**   Children under 2 years at increased risk of pneumococcal infection (see list above) should receive the 13-valent pneumococcal polysaccharide conjugate vaccine (adsorbed) at the recommended ages, followed by a single dose of the 23-valent pneumococcal polysaccharide vaccine after their second birthday (see below). Children at increased risk of pneumococcal infection presenting late for vaccination should receive 2 doses (separated by at least 1 month) of the 13-valent pneumococcal polysaccharide conjugate vaccine (adsorbed) before the age of 12 months, and a third dose at 12–13 months. Children over 12 months and under 5 years (who have not been vaccinated or not completed the primary course) should receive a single dose of 13-valent

Immunological products and vaccines

pneumococcal polysaccharide conjugate vaccine (adsorbed) (2 doses separated by an interval of 2 months in the immunocompromised or those with asplenia or splenic dysfunction). All children under 5 years at increased risk of pneumococcal infection should receive a single dose of the 23-valent pneumococcal polysaccharide vaccine after their second birthday and at least 2 months after the final dose of the 13-valent pneumococcal polysaccharide conjugate vaccine (adsorbed).

Children over 5 years who are at increased risk of pneumococcal disease should receive a single dose of the 23-valent unconjugated pneumococcal polysaccharide vaccine.

**Revaccination**    In individuals with higher concentrations of antibodies to pneumococcal polysaccharides, revaccination with the 23-valent pneumococcal polysaccharide vaccine more commonly produces adverse reactions. Revaccination is therefore not recommended, except every 5 years in individuals in whom the antibody concentration is likely to decline rapidly (e.g. asplenia, splenic dysfunction and nephrotic syndrome). If there is doubt, the need for revaccination should be discussed with a haematologist, immunologist, or microbiologist.

## ◼ PNEUMOCOCCAL VACCINES

**Cautions**   see section 14.1
**Contra-indications**   see section 14.1
**Pregnancy**   see p. 601
**Breast-feeding**   see p. 601
**Side-effects**   see section 14.1; *also* Revaccination, above
**Indications and dose**

> Immunisation against pneumococcal infection
>    For dose see under preparations

### ◢ Pneumococcal polysaccharide vaccines

**Pneumovax® II** (Sanofi Pasteur)  PoM
Injection, polysaccharide from each of 23 capsular types of pneumococcus, net price 0.5-mL vial = £8.32
**Dose**

> • By subcutaneous or intramuscular injection
>    **Child 2–18 years** 0.5 mL; revaccination, see notes above

### ◢ Pneumococcal polysaccharide conjugate vaccine (adsorbed)

**Prevenar 13®** (Pfizer)  ▼ PoM
Injection, polysaccharide from each of 13 capsular types of pneumococcus (conjugated to carrier protein) adsorbed onto aluminium phosphate, net price 0.5-mL prefilled syringe = £49.10
**Dose**

> • By intramuscular injection
>    **Child 2 months–5 years** 0.5 mL (see notes above and Immunisation schedule, section 14.1)
>    **Note** Deltoid muscle is preferred site of injection in young children; anterolateral thigh is preferred site in infants

The dose in *BNF for Children* may differ from that in product literature

Available as part of childhood immunisation schedule from ImmForm

**Synflorix®** (GSK)  ▼ PoM
Injection, polysaccharide from each of 10 capsular types of pneumococcus (conjugated to carrier proteins) adsorbed onto aluminium phosphate, net price 0.5-mL prefilled syringe = £27.60
**Dose**

> • By intramuscular injection
>    **Child 6 weeks–5 years** consult product literature
>    **Note** Deltoid muscle is preferred site of injection in young children; anterolateral thigh is preferred site in infants

## Poliomyelitis vaccines

Two types of poliomyelitis vaccine (containing strains of poliovirus types 1, 2, and 3) are available, inactivated poliomyelitis vaccine (for injection) and live (oral) poliomyelitis vaccine. **Inactivated poliomyelitis vaccine**, only available in combined preparation (see under Diphtheria vaccines, combined), is recommended for routine immunisation; it is given by injection and contains inactivated strains of human poliovirus types 1, 2 and 3.

A course of primary immunisation consists of 3 doses of a combined preparation containing inactivated poliomyelitis vaccine starting at 2 months of age with intervals of 1 month between doses (see Immunisation schedule, section 14.1). A course of 3 doses should also be given to all unimmunised children; no child should remain unimmunised against poliomyelitis.

Two booster doses of a preparation containing inactivated poliomyelitis vaccine are recommended, the first before school entry and the second before leaving school (see Immunisation schedule, section 14.1). Further booster doses should be given every 10 years only to individuals at special risk.

**Live (oral) poliomyelitis vaccine** is no longer available for routine use; its use may be considered during large outbreaks, but advice should be sought from Public Health England. The live (oral) vaccine poses a very rare risk of vaccine-associated paralytic polio because the attenuated strain of the virus can revert to a virulent form. For this reason the live (oral) vaccine must **not** be used for immunosuppressed individuals or their household contacts. The use of inactivated poliomyelitis vaccine removes the risk of vaccine-associated paralytic polio altogether.

**Travel**   Unimmunised travellers to areas with a high incidence of poliomyelitis should receive a full 3–dose course of a preparation containing inactivated poliomyelitis vaccine. Those who have not been vaccinated in the last 10 years should receive a booster dose of adsorbed diphtheria [low dose], tetanus and poliomyelitis (inactivated) vaccine. Information about countries with a high incidence of poliomyelitis can be obtained from www.travax.nhs.uk or from the National Travel Health Network and Centre, p. 628 (www.nathnac.org).

## ◼ POLIOMYELITIS VACCINES

**Cautions**   see section 14.1; *also for live vaccine*, interactions: Appendix 1 (vaccines)
**Contra-indications**   see notes above and section 14.1
**Pregnancy**   see p. 601
**Breast-feeding**   see p. 601
**Side-effects**   see notes above and section 14.1
**Indications and dose**

> See under preparations

◢**Combined vaccines**

See under Diphtheria-containing Vaccines

◢**Inactivated (Salk) Vaccine**

See under Diphtheria-containing Vaccines

# Rabies vaccine

Rabies vaccine contains inactivated rabies virus culti-vated in either human diploid cells or purified chick embryo cells; vaccines are used for pre- and post-exposure prophylaxis.

**Pre-exposure prophylaxis**   Immunisation should be offered to children at high risk of exposure to rabies—where there is limited access to prompt medical care for those living in areas where rabies is enzootic, for those travelling to such areas for longer than 1 month, and for those on shorter visits who may be exposed to unusual risk. Transmission of rabies by humans has not been recorded but it is advised that those caring for children with the disease should be vaccinated.

Immunisation against rabies is indicated during pregnancy if there is substantial risk of exposure to rabies and rapid access to post-exposure prophylaxis is likely to be limited.

Up-to-date country-by-country information on the inci-dence of rabies can be obtained from the National Travel Health Network and Centre (www.nathnac.org) and, in Scotland, from Health Protection Scotland (www.hps.scot.nhs.uk).

Immunisation against rabies requires 3 doses of rabies vaccine, with further booster doses for those who remain at continued risk.

**Post-exposure management**   Following potential exposure to rabies, the wound or site of exposure (e.g. mucous membrane) should be cleansed under running water and washed for several minutes with soapy water as soon as possible after exposure. Disinfectant and a simple dressing can be applied, but suturing should be delayed because it may increase the risk of introducing rabies virus into the nerves.

Post-exposure prophylaxis against rabies depends on the level of risk in the country, the nature of exposure, and the individual's immunity. In each case, expert risk assessment and advice on appropriate management should be obtained from the local Public Health England Centre or Public Health England's Virus Reference Department, Colindale (tel. (020) 8200 4400) or the PHE Colindale Duty Doctor (tel. (020) 8200 6868), in Wales from the Public Health Wales local Health Pro-tection Team or Public Health Wales Virus Reference Laboratory (tel. (029) 2074 7747), in Scotland from the local on-call infectious diseases consultant, and in Northern Ireland from the Public Health Agency Duty Room (tel (028) 9055 3997/(028) 9063 2662) or the Regional Virology Service (tel. (028) 9024 0503).

There are no specific contra-indications to the use of rabies vaccine for post-exposure prophylaxis and its use should be considered whenever a child has been attacked by an animal in a country where rabies is enzootic, even if there is no direct evidence of rabies in the attacking animal. Because of the potential con-sequences of untreated rabies exposure and because rabies vaccination has not been associated with fetal abnormalities, pregnancy is not considered a contra-indication to post-exposure prophylaxis.

For post-exposure prophylaxis of *fully immunised* indivi-duals (who have previously received pre-exposure or post-exposure prophylaxis with cell-derived rabies vaccine), 2 doses of cell-derived vaccine, given on day 0 and day 3, are likely to be sufficient. Rabies immuno-globulin is not necessary in such cases.

Post-exposure treatment for *unimmunised individuals* (or those whose prophylaxis is possibly incomplete) com-prises 5 doses of rabies vaccine given over 1 month (on days 0, 3, 7, 14, and 30); also, depending on the level of risk (determined by factors such as the nature of the bite and the country where it was sustained), rabies immunoglobulin (section 14.5.2) is given on day 0. The immunisation course can be discontinued if it is proved that the child was not at risk.

## ◼ RABIES VACCINE

**Cautions**   see section 14.1

**Contra-indications**   see section 14.1; but see also Post-exposure Management in notes above

**Pregnancy**   see p. 601

**Breast-feeding**   see p. 601

**Side-effects**   see section 14.1; also reported paresis

**Indications and dose**

> **Pre-exposure immunisation against rabies**
>
> • By intramuscular injection in deltoid region or anterolateral thigh in infants
>
>    **Child 1 month–18 years** 1 mL on days 0, 7, and 21 or 28; for those at continued risk give a single reinforcing dose 1 year after the primary course is completed and booster doses every 3–5 years; for those at intermittent risk give booster doses every 2–5 years

> **Post-exposure immunisation against rabies**
>
> • By intramuscular injection in deltoid region or anterolateral thigh in infants
>
>    **Child 1 month–18 years** 1 mL (see notes above)

**Rabies Vaccine** (Sanofi Pasteur) [PoM]

Rab

Injection, powder for reconstitution, freeze-dried inactivated Wistar rabies virus strain PM/WI 38 1503-3M cultivated in human diploid cells, net price single-dose vial with syringe containing diluent = £31.90

Excipients   include neomycin

**Rabipur®** (Novartis Vaccines) [PoM]

Injection, powder for reconstitution, freeze-dried inactivated Flury LEP rabies virus strain cultivated in chick embryo cells, net price single-dose vial = £28.80

Excipients   include neomycin

# Rotavirus vaccine

**Rotavirus vaccine** is a live, oral vaccine licensed for immunisation of infants over 6 weeks of age for protec-tion against gastro-enteritis caused by rotavirus infec-tion. The vaccine is not included in the childhood immunisation schedule.

The rotavirus vaccine virus is excreted in the stool and may be transmitted to close contacts; the vaccine should be used with caution in those with immunosup-pressed close contacts. Carers of a recently vaccinated

Immunological products and vaccines

baby should be advised of the need to wash their hands after changing the baby's nappies.

# ROTAVIRUS VACCINE

**Cautions** see section 14.1; *also* diarrhoea or vomiting (postpone vaccination); immunosuppressed close contacts (see notes above); **interactions**: Appendix 1 (vaccines)

**Contra-indications** see section 14.1; also predisposition to, or history of, intussusception

**Side-effects** see section 14.1

**Indications and dose**

> Immunisation against gastro-enteritis caused by rotavirus infection
>
> • By mouth
>
> > **Child over 6 weeks** 2 doses of 1.5 mL, separated by an interval of at least 4 weeks; course should be completed before 24 weeks of age (preferably before 16 weeks)

**Rotarix®** (GSK) ▼ PoM
Oral suspension, live attenuated rotavirus (RIX4414 strain), net price 1.5 mL prefilled oral syringe = £41.38

## Rubella vaccine

A combined measles, mumps and rubella vaccine (MMR vaccine) aims to eliminate rubella (German measles) and congenital rubella syndrome. MMR vaccine is used for childhood vaccination as well as for vaccinating adults (including women of child-bearing age) who do not have immunity against rubella the combined live measles, mumps and rubella vaccine is a suitable alternative.

◀ **Single antigen vaccine**

No longer available in the UK; see MMR vaccine, p. 614

◀ **Combined vaccines**

see MMR vaccine

## Smallpox vaccine

Limited supplies of **smallpox vaccine** are held at the Specialist and Reference Microbiology Division, Public Health England Colindale (Tel. (020) 8200 4400) for the exclusive use of workers in laboratories where pox viruses (such as vaccinia) are handled.

If a wider use of the vaccine is being considered, *Guidelines for smallpox response and management in the post-eradication era* should be consulted at www.hpa.org.uk.

## Tetanus vaccines

**Tetanus vaccine** contains a cell-free purified toxin of *Clostridium tetani* adsorbed on aluminium hydroxide or aluminium phosphate to improve antigenicity.

Primary immunisation for children under 10 years consists of 3 doses of a combined preparation containing adsorbed tetanus vaccine (see Diphtheria-containing Vaccines), with an interval of 1 month between doses. Following routine childhood vaccination, 2 booster doses of a preparation containing adsorbed tetanus vaccine are recommended, the first before school entry and the second before leaving school. (see Immunisation schedule, section 14.1).

The recommended schedule of tetanus vaccination not only gives protection against tetanus in childhood but also gives the basic immunity for subsequent booster doses. In most circumstances, a total number of 5 doses of tetanus vaccine is considered sufficient for long-term protection.

For primary immunisation of children over 10 years previously unimmunised against tetanus, 3 doses of **adsorbed diphtheria [low dose], tetanus and polio-myelitis (inactivated) vaccine** are given with an interval of 1 month between doses (see Diphtheria-containing Vaccines).

**Cautions** See also Section 14.1. When a child presents for a booster dose but has been vaccinated following a tetanus-prone wound, the vaccine preparation administered at the time of injury should be determined. If this is not possible, the booster should still be given to ensure adequate protection against all antigens in the booster vaccine.

Very rarely, tetanus has developed after abdominal surgery; carers of children awaiting elective surgery should be asked about the child's tetanus immunisation status and the child should be immunised if necessary.

Parenteral drug abuse is also associated with tetanus; those abusing drugs by injection should be vaccinated if unimmunised—booster doses should be given if there is any doubt about their immunisation status.

Travel recommendations see section 14.6.

**Contra-indications** See section 14.1

**Pregnancy** see p. 601

**Breast-feeding** see p. 601

**Side-effects** See section 14.1

**Wounds** Wounds are considered to be tetanus-prone if they are sustained more than 6 hours before surgical treatment *or* at any interval after injury and are puncture-type (particularly if contaminated with soil or manure) *or* show much devitalised tissue *or* are septic *or* are compound fractures *or* contain foreign bodies. All wounds should receive thorough cleansing.

• For *clean wounds*: fully immunised individuals (those who have received a total of 5 doses of a tetanus-containing vaccine at appropriate intervals) and those whose primary immunisation is complete (with boosters up to date), do not require tetanus vaccine; individuals whose primary immunisation is incomplete or whose boosters are not up to date require a reinforcing dose of a tetanus-containing vaccine (followed by further doses as required to complete the schedule); non-immunised individuals (or those whose immunisation status is not known or who have been fully immunised but are now immunocompromised) should be given a dose of the appropriate tetanus-containing vaccine immediately (followed by completion of the full course of the vaccine if records confirm the need).

• For *tetanus-prone wounds*: management is as for clean wounds with the addition of a dose of tetanus immunoglobulin (section 14.5.2) given at a different site; in fully immunised individuals and those whose primary immunisation is complete (with boosters up to date) the immunoglobulin is needed only if the risk of infection is especially high (e.g. contamination with manure). Antibacterial prophylaxis (with benzylpenicillin, co-amoxiclav, or metronidazole) may also be required for tetanus-prone wounds.

**Combined vaccines**

See Diphtheria-containing Vaccines

## Tick-borne encephalitis vaccine

Tick-borne encephalitis vaccine contains inactivated tick-borne encephalitis virus cultivated in chick embyro cells. It is recommended for immunisation of those living in or visiting high-risk areas (see International Travel, section 14.6). Children walking or camping in warm forested areas of Central and Eastern Europe, Scandinavia, Northern and Eastern China, and some parts of Japan, particularly from April to November when ticks are most prevalent, are at greatest risk of tick-borne encephalitis. For full protection, 3 doses of the vaccine are required; booster doses are required every 3–5 years for those still at risk. Ideally, immunisation should be completed at least one month before travel.

### TICK-BORNE ENCEPHALITIS VACCINE, INACTIVATED

**Cautions** see section 14.1
**Contra-indications** see section 14.1
**Pregnancy** see p. 601
**Breast-feeding** see p. 601
**Side-effects** see section 14.1
**Indications and dose**

Immunisation against tick-borne encephalitis

- By intramuscular injection in deltoid region or anterolateral thigh in infants

  **Child 1–16 years** initial immunisation, 3 doses of 0.25 mL, second dose after 1–3 months and third dose after a further 5–12 months

  **Child 16–18 years** 3 doses each of 0.5 mL, second dose after 1–3 months and third dose after further 5–12 months

  Immunocompromised (including those receiving immunosuppressants), antibody concentration may be measured 4 weeks after second dose and dose repeated if protective levels not achieved

  **Note** To achieve more rapid protection, second dose may be given 14 days after first dose.

Booster doses, give first dose within 3 years after initial course, then every 3–5 years

**TicoVac®** (MASTA) PoM

Injection, suspension, formaldehyde-inactivated Neudörfl tick-borne encephalitis virus strain, (cultivated in chick embryo cells) adsorbed onto hydrated aluminium hydroxide, net price 0.25-mL prefilled syringe (*TicoVac Junior®*) = £28.00, 0.5-mL prefilled syringe = £32.00

**Excipients** include gentamicin and neomycin

## Typhoid vaccines

Typhoid vaccine is available as Vi capsular polysaccharide injectable vaccine (from *Salmonella typhi*) for injection; and as live attenuated *Salmonella typhi* vaccine for oral use.

Typhoid immunisation is advised for children travelling to:

- areas where typhoid is endemic, especially if staying with or visiting local people
- endemic areas where frequent or prolonged exposure to poor sanitation and poor food hygiene is likely

Typhoid vaccination is not a substitute for scrupulous personal hygiene (see p. 628).

Capsular **polysaccharide typhoid vaccine** is usually given by *intramuscular* injection. Children under 2 years may respond suboptimally to the vaccine, but children aged between 1–2 years should be immunised if the risk of typhoid fever is considered high (immunisation is not recommended for infants under 12 months). Booster doses are needed every 3 years on continued exposure.

**Oral typhoid vaccine** is a **live attenuated** vaccine contained in an enteric-coated capsule. One capsule taken on alternate days for a total of 3 doses, provides protection 7–10 days after the last dose. Protection may persist for up to 3 years in those constantly (or repeatedly) exposed to *Salmonella typhi*, but occasional travellers require further courses at intervals of 1 year.

**interactions** Oral typhoid vaccine is inactivated by concomitant administration of antibacterials or antimalarials:

- Antibacterials should be avoided for 3 days before and after oral typhoid vaccination;
- Mefloquine should be avoided for at least 12 hours before or after oral typhoid;
- For other antimalarials, vaccination with oral typhoid vaccine should be completed at least 3 days before the first dose of the antimalarial (except proguanil hydrochloride with atovaquone, which may be given concomitantly).

### TYPHOID VACCINE

**Cautions** section 14.1; **interactions**: see above and Appendix 1 (vaccines)
**Contra-indications** section 14.1; also for *oral* vaccine, acute gastro-intestinal illness
**Pregnancy** see p. 601
**Breast-feeding** see p. 601
**Side-effects** section 14.1
**Indications and dose**

Immunisation against typhoid fever

For dose see under preparations

**Typhoid polysaccharide vaccine for injection**

**Typherix®** (GSK) PoM

Injection, Vi capsular polysaccharide typhoid vaccine, 50 micrograms/mL virulence polysaccharide antigen of *Salmonella typhi*, net price 0.5-mL prefilled syringe = £9.93

**Note** May be difficult to obtain

**Dose**

- By intramuscular injection

  **Child under 2 years** [unlicensed use], 0.5 mL, at least 2 weeks before potential exposure to typhoid infection; response may be suboptimal (see notes above)

  **Child 2–18 years** 0.5 mL, at least 2 weeks before potential exposure to typhoid infection

**Typhim Vi®** (Sanofi Pasteur) [PoM]

Injection, Vi capsular polysaccharide typhoid vaccine, 50 micrograms/mL virulence polysaccharide antigen of formaldehyde-inactivated *Salmonella typhi*, net price 0.5-mL prefilled syringe = £9.00

**Dose**

- **By intramuscular injection**

  **Child under 2 years** [unlicensed use], 0.5 mL, at least 2 weeks before potential exposure to typhoid infection; response may be suboptimal (see notes above)

  **Child 2–18 years** 0.5 mL, at least 2 weeks before potential exposure to typhoid infection

◢**Polysaccharide vaccine with hepatitis A vaccine**

See Hepatitis A Vaccine

◢**Typhoid vaccine, live (oral)**

**Vivotif®** (Crucell) [PoM]

Capsules, e/c, live attenuated *Salmonella typhi* (Ty21a), net price 3-cap pack = £14.77. Label: 25, counselling, administration

**Dose**

- **By mouth**

  **Child 6–18 years** 1 capsule on days 1, 3, and 5

  **Counselling** Take one hour before a meal. Swallow as soon as possible after placing in mouth with a cold or lukewarm drink; it is important to store capsules in a refrigerator

## Varicella–zoster vaccine

Varicella–zoster vaccine (live) is licensed for immunisation against varicella in seronegative individuals. It is not recommended for routine use in children but can be given to seronegative healthy children over 1 year who come into close contact with individuals at high risk of severe varicella infections.

Rarely, the varicella–zoster vaccine virus has been transmitted from the vaccinated individual to close contacts. Therefore, contact with the following should be avoided if a vaccine-related cutaneous rash develops within 4–6 weeks of the first or second dose:

- varicella-susceptible pregnant females;

- individuals at high risk of severe varicella, including those with immunodeficiency or those receiving immunosuppressive therapy.

**Varicella–zoster immunoglobulin** is used to protect susceptible children at increased risk of varicella infection, see p. 626.

### ▮ VARICELLA–ZOSTER VACCINES

**Cautions** see section 14.1; also post-vaccination close-contact with susceptible individuals (see notes above): **interactions**: Appendix 1 (vaccines)

**Contra-indications** see section 14.1

**Pregnancy** avoid pregnancy for 3 months after vaccination; see also p. 601

**Breast-feeding** see p. 601

**Side-effects** see section 14.1; *also* varicella-like rash; *rarely* thrombocytopenia

**Indications and dose**

 Immunisation against varicella infection (see notes above)

  For dose, see under preparations

**Varilrix®** (GSK) [PoM]

Injection, powder for reconstitution, live attenuated varicella–zoster virus (Oka strain) propagated in human diploid cells, net price 0.5-mL vial (with diluent) = £27.31

**Excipients** include neomycin

**Dose**

- **By subcutaneous injection preferably into deltoid region**

  **Child 1–18 years** (see notes above), 2 doses of 0.5 mL separated by an interval of at least 6 weeks (minimum 4 weeks)

**Varivax®** (Sanofi Pasteur) ▼ [PoM]

Injection powder for reconstitution, live attenuated varicella-zoster virus (Oka/Merck strain) propagated in human diploid cells, net price 0.5-mL vial (with diluent) = £30.28

**Excipients** include gelatin and neomycin

**Dose**

- **By intramuscular or subcutaneous injection into deltoid region (or higher anterolateral thigh in young children)**

  **Child 1–13 years** (see notes above) 2 doses of 0.5 mL separated by an interval of at least 4 weeks (2 doses separated by 12 weeks in children with asymptomatic HIV infection)

  **Child 13–18 years** 2 doses of 0.5 mL separated by 4–8 weeks

## Yellow fever vaccine

Live yellow fever vaccine is indicated for those travelling to or living in areas where infection is endemic (see p. 627). Infants under 6 months of age should not be vaccinated because there is a small risk of encephalitis; infants aged 6–9 months should be vaccinated only if the risk of yellow fever is high and unavoidable (seek expert advice). The immunity which probably lasts for life is officially accepted for 10 years starting from 10 days after primary immunisation and for a further 10 years immediately after revaccination.

Very rarely vaccine-associated adverse effects have been reported, such as viscerotropic disease (yellow fever vaccine-associated viscerotropic disease, YEL-AVD), a syndrome which may include metabolic acidosis, muscle and liver cytolysis, and multi-organ failure. Neurological disorders (yellow fever vaccine-associated neurotropic disease, YEL-AND) such as encephalitis have also been reported. These *very rare* adverse effects have usually occured after the first dose of yellow fever vaccine in those with no previous immunity.

**Pregnancy** Live yellow fever vaccine should not be given during pregnancy, but if a significant risk of exposure cannot be avoided then vaccination should be delayed to the third trimester if possible (but the need for immunisation usually outweighs risk to the fetus).

**Breast-feeding** Vaccination should be considered in breast-feeding women when there is a real risk to the mother from yellow fever disease.

### ▮ YELLOW FEVER VACCINE

**Cautions** see section 14.1; also see **interactions**: Appendix 1 (vaccines)

**Contra-indications** see section 14.1 and notes above; also children under 6 months; history of thymus dysfunction

**Pregnancy** see notes above

**Breast-feeding** see notes above

**Side-effects** see section 14.1; *also* reported neurotropic disease, and viscerotropic disease (see notes above)

**Indications and dose**

**Immunisation against yellow fever**

- **By deep subcutaneous injection**

  **Child 9 months–18 years** 0.5 mL (see also notes above)

**Yellow Fever Vaccine, Live** [PoM]

Yel(live)

Injection, powder for reconstitution, live, attenuated 17D-204 strain of yellow fever virus, cultivated in chick embryos; single dose vial with syringe containing 0.5 mL diluent

Available (only to designated Yellow Fever Vaccination centres) as *Stamaril®*

# 14.5  Immunoglobulins

14.5.1  Normal Immunoglobulin

14.5.2  Disease-specific immunoglobulins

14.5.3  Anti-D (Rh$_0$) immunoglobulin

Two types of human immunoglobulin preparation are available, **normal immunoglobulin** and **disease-specific immunoglobulins**.

Human immunoglobulin is a sterile preparation of concentrated antibodies (immune globulins) recovered from pooled human plasma or serum obtained from outside the UK, tested and found non-reactive for hepatitis B surface antigen and for antibodies against hepatitis C virus and human immunodeficiency virus (types 1 and 2). A global shortage of human immunoglobulin and the rapidly increasing range of clinical indications for treatment with immunoglobulins has resulted in the need for a Demand Management programme in the UK (for further information consult www.ivig.nhs.uk and *Clinical Guidelines for Immunoglobulin Use*, www.gov.uk/dh).

Immunoglobulins of animal origin (antisera) were frequently associated with hypersensitivity reactions and are no longer used.

Further information on the use of immunoglobulins is included in the Health Protection Agency's *Immunoglobulin Handbook*: www.hpa.org.uk and in the Department of Health's publication, *Immunisation against Infectious Disease*, www.gov.uk/dh.

**Availability** Normal immunoglobulin for intramuscular administration is available from some regional Public Health laboratories for protection of contacts and the control of outbreaks of hepatitis A, measles, and rubella only. For other indications, subcutaneous or intravenous normal immunoglobulin should be purchased from the manufacturer.

**Disease-specific immunoglobulins** (section 14.5.2) are available from some regional Public Health laboratories with the exception of **tetanus immunoglobulin** which is available from BPL, hospital pharmacies, or blood transfusion departments. **Rabies immunoglobulin** is available from the Specialist and Reference Microbiology Division, Public Health England, Colindale. **Hepatitis B immunoglobulin** required by transplant centres should be obtained commercially.

In Scotland all immunoglobulins are available from the *Scottish National Blood Transfusion Service* (SNBTS).

In Wales all immunoglobulins are available from the *Welsh Blood Service* (WBS).

In Northern Ireland all immunoglobulins are available from the *Northern Ireland Blood Transfusion Service* (NIBTS).

## 14.5.1  Normal Immunoglobulin

Human **normal immunoglobulin** ('HNIG') is prepared from pools of at least 1000 donations of human plasma; it contains immunoglobulin G (IgG) and antibodies to hepatitis A, measles, mumps, rubella, varicella, and other viruses that are currently prevalent in the general population.

Normal immunoglobulin may **interfere with the immune response to live virus vaccines** which should therefore only be given **at least 3 weeks before or 3 months after** an injection of normal immunoglobulin (this does not apply to yellow fever vaccine since normal immunoglobulin does not contain antibody to this virus).

**Uses** Normal immunoglobulin (containing 10–18% protein) is administered by *intramuscular injection* for the protection of susceptible contacts against **hepatitis A** virus (infectious hepatitis), **measles** and, to a lesser extent, **rubella**. Injection of immunoglobulin produces immediate protection lasting for several weeks.

Normal immunoglobulin (containing 3–12% protein) for *intravenous administration* is used as *replacement therapy* for children with congenital agammaglobulinaemia and hypogammaglobulinaemia, and for the short-term treatment of idiopathic thrombocytopenic purpura and Kawasaki syndrome; it is also used for the prophylaxis of infection following bone-marrow transplantation and in children with symptomatic HIV infection who have recurrent bacterial infections. Normal immunoglobulin for replacement therapy may also be given intramuscularly or subcutaneously, but intravenous formulations are normally preferred. Intravenous immunoglobulin is also used in the treatment of Guillain-Barré syndrome as an alternative to plasma exchange.

The dose of normal immunoglobulin used as replacement therapy in patients with immunodeficiencies is **not the same** as the dose required for treatment of acute conditions. For Kawasaki syndrome a single dose of 2 g/kg by intravenous infusion should be given with concomitant aspirin (see section 2.9) within 10 days of onset of symptoms (but children with a delayed diagnosis may also benefit).

For guidance on the use of intravenous normal immunoglobulins and alternative therapies for other conditions, consult *Clinical Guidelines for Immunoglobulin Use* (www.gov.uk/dh).

**Hepatitis A** Hepatitis A vaccine is preferred for children at risk of infection (see p. 608) including those visiting areas where the disease is highly endemic (all countries excluding Northern and Western Europe, North America, Japan, Australia, and New Zealand). In unimmunised children, transmission of hepatitis A is reduced by good hygiene. Intramuscular normal immunoglobulin is no longer recommended for routine prophylaxis in travellers, but it may be indicated for

**14**

Immunological products and vaccines

immunocompromised patients if their antibody response to the vaccine is unlikely to be adequate.

Intramuscular normal immunoglobulin is recommended for prevention of infection in close contacts (of confirmed cases of hepatitis A) who have chronic liver disease or HIV infection, or who are immunosuppressed; normal immunoglobulin should be given as soon as possible, preferably within 14 days of exposure to the primary case. However, normal immunoglobulin can still be given to contacts at risk of severe disease up to 28 days after exposure to the primary case. Hepatitis A vaccine can be given at the same time, but it should be given at a separate injection site.

**Measles**   Intravenous or subcutaneous normal immunoglobulin may be given to prevent or attenuate an attack of measles in children with compromised immunity. Children with compromised immunity who have come into contact with measles should receive intravenous or subcutaneous normal immunoglobulin as soon as possible after exposure. It is most effective if given within 72 hours but can be effective if given within 6 days.

Subcutaneous or intramuscular normal immunoglobulin should also be considered for the following individuals if they have been in contact with a confirmed case of measles or with a person associated with a local outbreak:

- non-immune pregnant women
- infants under 9 months

Further advice should be sought from the Centre for Infections, Public Health England (tel. (020) 8200 6868).

Children with normal immunity who are not in the above categories and who have not been fully immunised against measles, can be given MMR vaccine (section 14.4) for prophylaxis following exposure to measles.

**Rubella**   Intramuscular immunoglobulin after exposure to rubella does **not** prevent infection in non-immune contacts and is **not** recommended for protection of pregnant females exposed to rubella. It may, however, reduce the likelihood of a clinical attack which may possibly reduce the risk to the fetus. Risk of intrauterine transmission is greatest in the first 11 weeks of pregnancy, between 16 and 20 weeks there is a minimal risk of deafness only, after 20 weeks there is no increased risk. Intramuscular normal immunoglobulin should be used only if termination of pregnancy would be unacceptable to the pregnant individual—it should be given as soon as possible after exposure. Serological follow-up of recipients is essential.

For routine prophylaxis, see MMR vaccine (p. 614).

## ▌ NORMAL IMMUNOGLOBULIN

**Cautions**   hypo- or agammaglobulinaemia with or without IgA deficiency; interference with live virus vaccines—see p. 623
   **Intravenous use** Thrombophilic disorders, or risk factors for arterial or venous thromboembolic events; obesity; ensure adequate hydration, renal insufficiency

**Contra-indications**   patients with selective IgA deficiency who have known antibody against IgA

**Renal impairment**   monitor for acute renal failure; consider discontinuation if renal function deteriorates. Intravenous preparations with added sucrose

have been associated with cases of renal dysfunction and acute renal failure

**Side-effects**   nausea, diarrhoea, chills, fever, headache, dizziness, arthralgia, myalgia, muscle spasms, low back pain; *rarely* hypotension, anaphylaxis, cutaneous skin reactions, aseptic meningitis, acute renal failure; also reported with *intravenous use*, injection site reactions, abdominal pain and distension, blood pressure fluctuations, haemolytic anaemia, thromboembolic events including myocardial infarction, stroke, pulmonary embolism, and deep vein thrombosis
   **Note** Adverse reactions are more likely to occur in patients receiving normal immunoglobulin for the first time, or following a prolonged period between treatments, or when a different brand of normal immunoglobulin is administered.

**Indications and dose**

   See under preparations

   **Note** Antibody titres can vary widely between normal immunoglobulin preparations from different manufacturers—formulations are **not interchangeable**; patients should be maintained on the same formulation throughout long-term treatment to avoid adverse effects

### ◀ For intramuscular use

**Normal Immunoglobulin** PoM
Normal immunoglobulin injection. 250-mg vial; 750-mg vial
**Dose**

> **To control outbreaks of hepatitis A** (see notes above)
>
> - By deep intramuscular injection
>   **Child under 10 years** 250 mg
>   **Child 10–18 years** 500 mg

> **Rubella in pregnancy, prevention of clinical attack**
>
> - By deep intramuscular injection
>   750 mg

Available from the Centre for Infections and other regional Health Protection Agency offices (for contacts and control of outbreaks only, see above)

### ◀ For subcutaneous use

**Note** Preparations for subcutaneous use may be administered by intramuscular injection if subcutaneous route not possible; intramuscular route not recommended for patients with thrombocytopenia or other bleeding disorders

**Gammanorm**® (Octapharma) ▼ PoM
Normal immunoglobulin (protein 16.5%) injection, net price 1.65 g (10 mL) = £113.85, 3.3 g (20 mL) = £227.70
**Electrolytes**   Na+ 1.09 mmol/10-mL vial
**Dose**

> **Antibody deficiency syndromes**
>
> - By subcutaneous infusion
>   Consult product literature

**Hizentra**® (CSL Behring) ▼ PoM
Normal immunoglobulin (protein 20%) injection, net price 1 g (5 mL) = £54.00, 2 g (10 mL) = £108.00, 3 g (15 mL) = £162.00, 4 g (20 mL) = £216.00
**Note** Contains L-proline; contra-indicated in patients with hyperprolinaemia
**Dose**

> **Antibody deficiency syndromes**
>
> - By subcutaneous infusion
>   Consult product literature

14   Immunological products and vaccines

**Subcuvia**® (Baxter) PoM

Normal immunoglobulin (protein 16%) injection, net price 800 mg (5 mL) = £32.56, 1.6 g (10 mL) = £65.12

**Dose**

**Antibody deficiency syndromes**

- **By subcutaneous infusion**
  Consult product literature (not licensed for use in children under 12 years)

**Subgam**® (BPL) PoM

Normal immunoglobulin (protein 14–18%) injection, net price 250-mg vial = £11.20, 750-mg vial = £28.50, 1.5-g vial = £57.00

**Dose**

**Antibody deficiency syndromes**

- **By subcutaneous infusion**
  Consult product literature

**Hepatitis A prophylaxis** (see also notes above)

- **By intramuscular injection**
  **Child under 10 years** 500 mg
  **Child 10–18 years** 750 mg

**Rubella prophylaxis in pregnancy** (see also notes above)

- **By intramuscular injection**
  750 mg

**Note** *Subgam*® is not licensed for prophylactic use, but due to difficulty in obtaining suitable immunoglobulin products, the Health Protection Agency recommends intramuscular use for prophylaxis against Hepatitis A, or rubella

◀ **For intravenous use**

**Note** Dose recommendation for Kawasaki Sydrome, see section 14.5.1; other indications—consult product literature for dosage regimens

**Aragam**® (Oxbridge) ▼ PoM

Intravenous infusion, human normal immunoglobulin (protein 5%), net price 2.5 g (50 mL) = £145.00, 5 g (100 mL) = £290.00, 10 g (200 mL) = £580.00, 20 g (400 mL) = £1160.00

**Excipients** include glucose 50 mg/mL

**Flebogamma**® **DIF** (Grifols) PoM

Intravenous infusion, human normal immunoglobulin, protein 5%, net price 0.5 g (10 mL) = £30.00, 2.5 g (50 mL) = £150.00, 5 g (100 mL) = £300.00, 10 g (200 mL) = £600.00, 20 g (400 mL) = £1200.00; protein 10%, 5 g (50 mL) = £300.00, 10 g (100 mL) = £600.00, 20 g (200 mL) = £1200.00

**Note** Both strengths contain sorbitol 50 mg/mL; contra-indicated in patients with hereditary fructose intolerance

**Gammagard S/D**® (Baxter) PoM

Intravenous infusion, powder for reconstitution, human normal immunoglobulin (providing protein 5% or 10%), net price 5 g (with diluent) = £200.50, 10 g (with diluent) = £401.00

**Gammaplex**® (BPL) ▼ PoM

Intravenous infusion, human normal immunoglobulin (protein 5%), net price 2.5 g (50 mL) = £85.00, 5 g (100 mL) = £170.00, 10 g (200 mL) = £340.00

**Note** Contains sorbitol 50 mg/mL; contra-indicated in patients with hereditary fructose intolerance

**Gamunex**® (Grifols) ▼ PoM

Intravenous infusion, human normal immunoglobulin (protein 10%), net price 5 g (50 mL) = £250.00, 10 g (100 mL) = £500.00, 20 g (200 mL) = £1000.00

**Note** Use Glucose 5% intravenous infusion if dilution prior to infusion required

**Intratect**® (Biotest UK) PoM

Intravenous infusion, human normal immunoglobulin (protein 5%), net price 1 g (20 mL) = £45.00, 2.5 g (50 mL) = £112.50, 5 g (100 mL) = £225.00, 10 g (200 mL) = £450.00

**Kiovig**® (Baxter) PoM

Intravenous infusion, human normal immunoglobulin (protein 10%), net price 1 g (10 mL) = £49.00, 2.5 g (25 mL) = £122.50, 5 g (50 mL) = £245.00, 10 g (100 mL) = £490.00, 20 g (200 mL) = £980.00, 30 g (300 mL) = £1470.00

**Note** Use Glucose 5% intravenous infusion, if dilution prior to administration is required

**Octagam**® (Octapharma) PoM

Intravenous infusion, human normal immunoglobulin, protein 5%, net price 2.5 g (50 mL) = £120.00, 5 g (100 mL) = £240.00, 10 g (200 mL) = £480.00; protein 10%, 2 g (20 mL) = £138.00, 5 g (50 mL) = £345.00, 10 g (100 mL) = £690.00, 20 g (200 mL) = £1380.00

**Note** Contains maltose (may cause falsely elevated results with blood glucose testing systems)

**Privigen**® (CSL Behring) PoM

Intravenous infusion, human normal immunoglobulin (protein 10%), net price 2.5 g (25 mL) = £135.00, 5 g (50 mL) = £270.00, 10 g (100 mL) = £540.00, 20 g (200 mL) = £1080.00

**Note** Contains L-proline; contra-indicated in patients with hyperprolinaemia

**Vigam**® (BPL) ▼ PoM

Intravenous infusion, human normal immunoglobulin (protein 5%), net price 2.5 g (50 mL) = £95.00, 5 g (100 mL) = £190.00, 10 g (200 mL) = £380.00

**Note** Contains sucrose (see Renal Impairment above)

## 14.5.2 Disease-specific immunoglobulins

Specific immunoglobulins are prepared by pooling the plasma of selected human donors with high levels of the specific antibody required. For further information, see *Immunoglobulin Handbook* (www.hpa.org.uk).

There are no specific immunoglobulins for hepatitis A, measles, or rubella—normal immunoglobulin, section 14.5.1 is used in certain circumstances. There is no specific immunoglobulin for mumps; neither normal immunoglobulin nor MMR vaccine is effective as post-exposure prophylaxis.

### Hepatitis B

Disease-specific **hepatitis B immunoglobulin** ('HBIG') is available for use in association with hepatitis B vaccine for the prevention of infection in infants born to mothers who have become infected with this virus in pregnancy or who are high-risk carriers (see Hepatitis B Vaccine, p. 610). Hepatitis B immunoglobulin will not inhibit the antibody response when given at the same time as hepatitis B vaccine, but should be given at different sites.

An intravenous preparation of hepatitis B-specific immunoglobulin is licensed for the prevention of hepatitis B recurrence in HBV-DNA negative patients who have undergone liver transplantation for liver failure caused by the virus.

Immunological products and vaccines

14 Immunological products and vaccines

# ■ HEPATITIS B IMMUNOGLOBULIN

**Cautions** IgA deficiency; interference with live virus vaccines—see under Normal Immunoglobulin, p. 623

**Side-effects** injection site swelling and pain, arthralgia; *rarely* anaphylaxis chest tightness, dyspnoea; also reported tremor, dizziness, facial oedema, glossitis, and buccal ulceration; for side-effects associated with *intravenous* immunoglobulins, see section 14.5.1

**Indications and dose**

See under preparations and see also notes above

**Hepatitis B Immunoglobulin** PoM
Injection, hepatitis B-specific immunoglobulin, 100 units/mL. Vials containing 200 units or 500 units, available from selected Health Protection Agency and NHS laboratories (except for Transplant Centres, see p. 623), also available from BPL

**Dose**

> **Prophylaxis against hepatitis B infection**
>
> • By intramuscular injection
>
> (as soon as possible after exposure; ideally within 48 hours, but no later than 7 days after exposure)
>
> **Child 1 month–5 years** 200 units
>
> **Child 5–10 years** 300 units
>
> **Child 10–18 years** 500 units

> **Prevention of transmitted infection at birth**
>
> • By intramuscular injection
>
> **Neonate** 200 units as soon as possible after birth; for full details consult *Immunisation against Infectious Disease* (www.dh.gov.uk)

**Hepatect® CP** (Biotest UK) PoM
Intravenous infusion, hepatitis B-specific immunoglobulin 50 units/mL, net price 500 units (10 mL) = £300.00, 2000 units (40 mL) = £1100.00, 5000 units (100 mL) = £3000.00

**Dose**

> Following exposure to hepatitis B virus-contaminated material (as soon as possible after exposure, but no later than 72 hours); prevention of transmitted infection at birth; prophylaxis against re-infection of transplanted liver
>
> Consult product literature

## Rabies

Following exposure of an unimmunised child to an animal in or from a country where the risk of rabies is high, the site of the bite should be washed with soapy water and specific **rabies immunoglobulin** of human origin should be administered. All of the dose should be injected around the site of the wound; if this is difficult or the wound has completely healed it can be given in the anterolateral thigh (remote from the site used for vaccination). Rabies vaccine should also be given intramuscularly at a different site (for details see Rabies Vaccine, p. 619).

# ■ RABIES IMMUNOGLOBULIN

**Cautions** IgA deficiency; interference with live virus vaccines—see p. 623 under Normal Immunoglobulin

**Side-effects** injection site swelling and pain; *rarely* anaphylaxis; buccal ulceration, glossitis, chest tightness, dyspnoea, tremor, dizziness, arthralgia, and facial oedema also reported

**Indications and dose**

> **Post-exposure prophylaxis against rabies infection**
>
> • By intramuscular injection
>
> 20 units/kg, *by infiltration* in and around the cleansed wound; if the wound not visible or healed or if infiltration of whole volume not possible, give remainder *by intramuscular injection* into anterolateral thigh (remote from vaccination site)

**Note** The potency of individual batches of rabies immunoglobulin from the manufacturer may vary; potency may also be described differently by different manufacturers. It is therefore critical to know the potency of the batch to be used and the weight of the patient in order to calculate the specific volume required to provide the necessary dose

**Rabies Immunoglobulin** PoM
(Antirabies Immunoglobulin Injection)
See notes above
Available from Specialist and Reference Microbiology Division, Public Health England (see section 14.5 under Availability) (also from BPL)

## Tetanus

Tetanus immunoglobulin, together with metronidazole (section 5.1.11) and wound cleansing, should also be used for the treatment of established cases of tetanus.

For the management of tetanus-prone wounds, **tetanus immunoglobulin** of human origin should be used in addition to wound cleansing and, where appropriate, antibacterial prophylaxis and a tetanus-containing vaccine (see Diphtheria-containing Vaccines, section 14.4).

# ■ TETANUS IMMUNOGLOBULIN

**Cautions** IgA deficiency; interference with live virus vaccines—see, p. 623

**Side-effects** injection site swelling and pain; *rarely* anaphylaxis; buccal ulceration; glossitis, chest tightness, dyspnoea, tremor, dizziness, arthralgia, and facial oedema also reported

**Indications and dose**

> **Post-exposure prophylaxis**
>
> • By intramuscular injection
>
> 250 units, increased to 500 units if more than 24 hours have elapsed or there is risk of heavy contamination or following burns

> **Treatment of tetanus infection**
>
> • By intramuscular injection
>
> 150 units/kg (multiple sites)

**Tetanus Immunoglobulin** PoM
(Antitetanus Immunoglobulin Injection)

Available from BPL
**Note** May be difficult to obtain

## Varicella–zoster

Varicella–zoster immunoglobulin (VZIG) is recommended for individuals who are at increased risk of severe varicella *and* who have no antibodies to varicella–zoster virus *and* who have significant exposure to chickenpox or herpes zoster. Those at increased risk include:

- neonates whose mothers develop chickenpox in the period 7 days before to 7 days after delivery;

- susceptible neonates exposed in the first 7 days of life;

- susceptible neonates or infants exposed whilst requiring intensive or prolonged special care nursing;

- susceptible women exposed at any stage of pregnancy (but when supplies of VZIG are short, may only be issued to those exposed in the first 20 weeks' gestation or to those near term) providing VZIG is given within 10 days of contact;

- immunocompromised individuals including those who have received corticosteroids in the previous 3 months at the following dose equivalents of prednisolone: *children* 2 mg/kg daily (or more than 40 mg) for at least 1 week or 1 mg/kg daily for 1 month.

**Important:** for full details consult *Immunisation against Infectious Disease.* **Varicella–zoster vaccine** is available—see section 14.4.

For treatment of varicella–zoster infections and attenuation of infection if varicella–zoster immunoglobulin not indicated, see section 5.3.2.1

## VARICELLA–ZOSTER IMMUNOGLOBULIN

**Cautions** IgA deficiency; interference with live virus vaccines—see p. 623 under Normal Immunoglobulins

**Side-effects** injection site swelling and pain; *rarely* anaphylaxis

**Indications and dose**

**Prophylaxis against varicella infection (as soon as possible—not later than 10 days after exposure)**
- By deep intramuscular injection

    **Neonate** 250 mg

    **Child 1 month–6 years** 250 mg

    **Child 6–11 years** 500 mg

    **Child 11–15 years** 750 mg

    **Child 15–18 years** 1 g

    Give second dose if further exposure occurs more than 3 weeks after first dose

**Note** No evidence that effective in treatment of severe disease.
Normal immunoglobulin for intravenous use (section 14.5.1) may be used in those unable to receive intramuscular injection.

**Varicella–Zoster Immunoglobulin** [PoM]
(Antivaricella–zoster Immunoglobulin)
Available from selected Health Protection Agency and NHS laboratories (see section 14.5 under Availability) (also from BPL)

## 14.5.3 Anti-D (Rh$_0$) immunoglobulin

This section is not included in *BNF for Children*. See BNF for use of Anti-D (Rh$_0$) immunoglobulin

## 14.6 International travel

**Note** For advice on **malaria chemoprophylaxis**, see section 5.4.1.

No special immunisation is required for travellers to the United States, Europe, Australia, or New Zealand although all travellers should have immunity to tetanus and poliomyelitis (and childhood immunisations should be up to date); see also Tick-borne Encephalitis, p. 621. Certain precautions are required in Non-European areas surrounding the Mediterranean, in Africa, the Middle East, Asia, and South America.

Travellers to areas that have a high incidence of **poliomyelitis** or **tuberculosis** should be immunised with the appropriate vaccine; in the case of poliomyelitis previously immunised adults may be given a booster dose of a preparation containing inactivated poliomyelitis vaccine. BCG immunisation is recommended for travellers aged under 16 years proposing to stay for longer than 3 months (or in close contact with the local population) in countries with an incidence[1] of tuberculosis greater than 40 per 100 000; it should preferably be given three months or more before departure.

**Yellow fever** immunisation is recommended for travel to the endemic zones of Africa and South America. Many countries require an International Certificate of Vaccination from individuals arriving from, or who have been travelling through, endemic areas, whilst other countries require a certificate from all entering travellers (consult the Department of Health handbook, *Health Information for Overseas Travel*, www.dh.gov.uk).

Immunisation against **meningococcal meningitis** is recommended for a number of areas of the world (for details, see p. 615).

Protection against **hepatitis A** is recommended for travellers to high-risk areas outside Northern and Western Europe, North America, Japan, Australia and New Zealand. Hepatitis A vaccine (see p. 608) is preferred and it is likely to be effective even if given shortly before departure; normal immunoglobulin is no longer given routinely but may be indicated in the immunocompromised (see p. 623). Special care must also be taken with food hygiene (see below).

**Hepatitis B** vaccine (see p. 610) is recommended for those travelling to areas of high prevalence who plan to remain there for lengthy periods and who may therefore be at increased risk of acquiring infection as the result of medical or dental procedures carried out in those countries. Short-term tourists are not generally at increased risk of infection but may place themselves at risk by their sexual behaviour when abroad.

Prophylactic immunisation against **rabies** (see p. 619) is recommended for travellers to enzootic areas on long journeys or to areas out of reach of immediate medical attention.

Travellers who have not had a **tetanus** booster in the last 10 years and are visiting areas where medical attention may not be accessible should receive a booster dose of adsorbed diphtheria [low dose], tetanus and inactivated poliomyelitis vaccine (see p. 605), even if they have received 5 doses of a tetanus-containing vaccine previously.

1. List of countries where the incidence of tuberculosis is greater than 40 cases per 100 000 is available at www.hpa.org.uk

Immunological products and vaccines

**Typhoid vaccine** is indicated for travellers to countries where typhoid is endemic, but the vaccine is no substitute for personal precautions (see below).

There is no requirement for cholera vaccination as a condition for entry into any country, but **oral cholera vaccine** (see p. 605) should be considered for backpackers and those travelling to situations where the risk is greatest (e.g. refugee camps). Regardless of vaccination, travellers to areas where cholera is endemic should take special care with food hygiene (see below).

Advice on **diphtheria**, on **Japanese encephalitis**[1] (vaccine available on named-patient basis from MASTA) and on **tick-borne encephalitis** is included in *Health Information for Overseas Travel*, see below.

**Food hygiene**   In areas where sanitation is poor, good food hygiene is important to help prevent hepatitis A, typhoid, cholera, and other diarrhoeal diseases (including travellers' diarrhoea). Food should be freshly prepared and hot, and uncooked vegetables (including green salads) should be avoided; only fruits which can be peeled should be eaten. Only suitable bottled water, or tap water that has been boiled, or treated with sterilising tablets should be used for drinking.

---

**Information on health advice for travellers**

Health professionals and travellers can find the latest information on immunisation requirements and precautions for avoiding disease while travelling from: www.nathnac.org

The handbook, *Health Information for Overseas Travel* (2010), which draws together essential information *for healthcare professionals* regarding health advice for travellers, can also be obtained from this website.

---

Immunisation requirements change from time to time, and information on the current requirements for any particular country may be obtained from the embassy or legation of the appropriate country or from:

National Travel Health Network and Centre
UCLH NHS Foundation trust
5th Floor West
250 Euston Road
London, NW1 2PG
Tel: 0845 602 6712
(9 a.m.–noon, 2–4.30 p.m. weekdays for healthcare professionals only)
www.nathnac.org

Travel Medicine Team
Health Protection Scotland
Clifton House
Clifton Place
Glasgow, G3 7LN
Tel: (0141) 300 1130
(2 p.m.–4 p.m. weekdays)
www.travax.nhs.uk (registration required; annual fee may be payable for users outside NHS Scotland)

Welsh Assembly Government
Tel: (029) 2082 5397
(9 a.m.–5.30 p.m. weekdays)

Department of Health and Social Services
Castle Buildings
Belfast
Stormont, BT4 3PP
Tel: (028) 9052 2118
(weekdays)

---

1. Japanese encephalitis vaccine not prescribable on the NHS; health authorities may investigate circumstances under which vaccine prescribed

# 15 Anaesthesia

## 15.1 General anaesthesia

**15.1.1** Intravenous anaesthetics

**15.1.2** Inhalational anaesthetics

**15.1.3** Antimuscarinic drugs

**15.1.4** Sedative and analgesic peri-operative drugs

**15.1.5** Neuromuscular blocking drugs

**15.1.6** Drugs for reversal of neuromuscular blockade

**15.1.7** Antagonists for central and respiratory depression

**15.1.8** Drugs for malignant hyperthermia

> **Important**
>
> The drugs in section 15.1 should only be administered by, or under the direct supervision of, personnel experienced in their use, with adequate training in anaesthesia and airway management, and when resuscitation equipment is available.

Several different types of drug are given together during general anaesthesia. Anaesthesia is induced with either a volatile drug given by inhalation (section 15.1.2) or with an intravenously administered drug (section 15.1.1); anaesthesia is maintained with an intravenous or inhalational anaesthetic. Analgesics (section 15.1.4), usually short-acting opioids, are also used. The use of neuromuscular blocking drugs (section 15.1.5) necessitates intermittent positive-pressure ventilation. Following surgery, anticholinesterases (section 15.1.6) can be given to reverse the effects of neuromuscular blocking drugs; specific antagonists (section 15.1.7) can be used to reverse central and respiratory depression caused by some drugs used in surgery. A topical local anaesthetic (section 15.2) can be used to reduce pain at the injection site.

Individual requirements vary considerably and the recommended doses are only a guide. Smaller doses are indicated in ill, shocked, or debilitated children and in significant hepatic impairment, while robust individuals may require larger doses. The required dose of induction agent may be less if the patient has been premedicated with a sedative agent (section 15.1.4) or if an opioid analgesic has been used.

**Surgery and long-term medication** The risk of losing disease control on stopping long-term medication before surgery is often greater than the risk posed by continuing it during surgery. It is vital that the anaesthetist knows about **all** drugs that a child is (or has been) taking.

Children with adrenal atrophy resulting from long-term corticosteroid use (section 6.3.2) may suffer a precipitous fall in blood pressure unless corticosteroid cover is

15 Anaesthesia

provided during anaesthesia and in the immediate postoperative period. Anaesthetists must therefore know whether a child is, or has been, receiving corticosteroids (including high-dose inhaled corticosteroids).

Other drugs that should normally not be stopped before surgery include drugs for epilepsy, asthma, immunosuppression, and metabolic, endocrine and cardiovascular disorders (but see potassium sparing diuretics, below). Expert advice is required for children receiving antivirals for HIV infection. For general advice on surgery in children with diabetes, see section 6.1.1.

Children taking antiplatelet medication or an oral anticoagulant present an increased risk for surgery. In these circumstances, the anaesthetist and surgeon should assess the relative risks and decide jointly whether the antiplatelet or the anticoagulant drug should be stopped or replaced with unfractionated or low molecular weight heparin therapy.

Drugs that should be stopped before surgery include combined oral contraceptives (see Surgery, section 7.3.1 for details). If antidepressants need to be stopped, they should be withdrawn gradually to avoid withdrawal symptoms. Tricyclic antidepressants need not be stopped, but there may be an increased risk of arrhythmias and hypotension (and dangerous interactions with vasopressor drugs); therefore, the anaesthetist should be informed if they are not stopped. Lithium should be stopped 24 hours before major surgery but the normal dose can be continued for minor surgery (with careful monitoring of fluids and electrolytes). Potassium-sparing diuretics may need to be withheld on the morning of surgery because hyperkalaemia may develop if renal perfusion is impaired or if there is tissue damage. Herbal medicines may be associated with adverse effects when given with anaesthetic drugs and consideration should be given to stopping them before surgery.

**Anaesthesia and skilled tasks**  Children and their carers should be very carefully warned about the risk of undertaking skilled tasks after the use of sedatives and analgesics during minor outpatient procedures. For intravenous benzodiazepines and for a short general anaesthetic the risk extends to **at least 24 hours** after administration. Responsible persons should be available to take children home. The dangers of taking **alcohol** should also be emphasised.

**Prophylaxis of acid aspiration**  Regurgitation and aspiration of gastric contents (Mendelson's syndrome) can be a complication of general anaesthesia, particularly in obstetrics and in gastro-oesophageal reflux disease; prophylaxis against acid aspiration is not routinely used in children but may be required in high-risk cases.

An $H_2$-receptor antagonist (section 1.3.1) or a **proton pump inhibitor** (section 1.3.5), such as omeprazole, can be used before surgery to increase the pH and reduce the volume of gastric fluid. They do not affect the pH of fluid already in the stomach and this limits their value in emergency procedures; oral $H_2$-receptor antagonists can be given 1–2 hours before the procedure, but omeprazole must be given at least 12 hours earlier.

## Anaesthesia, sedation, and resuscitation in dental practice

> For details see *A Conscious Decision: A review of the use of general anaesthesia and conscious sedation in primary dental care*; report by a group chaired by the Chief Medical Officer and Chief Dental Officer, July 2000 and associated documents. Further details can also be found in *Conscious Sedation in the Provision of Dental Care*; report of an Expert Group on Sedation for Dentistry (commissioned by the Department of Health), 2003. Both documents are available at www.dh.gov.uk.
>
> Guidance is also included in *Standards for Dental Professionals*, London, General Dental Council, May 2005 (and as amended subsequently) and *Conscious Sedation in Dentistry: Dental Clinical Guidance*, Scottish Dental Clinical Effectiveness Programme, May 2006 (www.sdcep.org.uk).

## 15.1.1  Intravenous anaesthetics

> **Important**
> The drugs in this section should only be administered by, or under the direct supervision of, personnel experienced in their use, with adequate training in anaesthesia and airway management, and when resuscitation equipment is available.

Intravenous anaesthetics may be used either to induce anaesthesia or for maintenance of anaesthesia throughout surgery. Intravenous anaesthetics nearly all produce their effect in one arm-brain circulation time and can cause apnoea and hypotension, and so adequate resuscitative facilities **must** be available. They are **contraindicated** if the anaesthetist is not confident of being able to maintain the airway. Extreme care is required in surgery of the mouth, pharynx, or larynx and in children with acute circulatory failure (shock) or fixed cardiac output.

To facilitate tracheal intubation, induction is usually followed by a neuromuscular blocking drug (section 15.1.5) or a short-acting opioid (section 15.1.4.3).

The doses of all intravenous anaesthetic drugs should be titrated according to response (except when using 'rapid sequence induction'). The doses and rates of administration should be reduced in those with hypovolaemia or cardiovascular disease; reduced doses may also be required in premedicated children.

**Total intravenous anaesthesia**  This is a technique in which surgery is carried out with all drugs given intravenously. Respiration can be spontaneous, or controlled with oxygen-enriched air. Neuromuscular blocking drugs can be used to provide relaxation and prevent reflex muscle movements. The main problem to be overcome is the assessment of depth of anaesthesia. Target Controlled Infusion (TCI) systems can be used to titrate intravenous anaesthetic infusions to predicted plasma-drug concentrations; specific models with paediatric pharmacokinetic data should be used for children.

**Anaesthesia and skilled tasks**  See section 15.1.

**Drugs used for intravenous anaesthesia**  Propofol, the most widely used intravenous anaesthetic, can be used for induction or maintenance of anaesthesia in children, but it is not commonly used in neonates.

Propofol is associated with rapid recovery and less hangover effect than other intravenous anaesthetics. It causes pain on intravenous injection which can be reduced by intravenous lidocaine. Significant extraneous muscle movements can occur. Rarely, convulsions, anaphylaxis, and delayed recovery from anaesthesia can occur after propofol administration; the onset of convulsions can be delayed. Propofol is associated with bradycardia, occasionally profound; intravenous administration of an antimuscarinic drug is used to treat this.

Propofol can be used for sedation during diagnostic procedures but is contra-indicated in children under 16 years receiving intensive care because of the risk of propofol infusion syndrome (potentially fatal effects, including metabolic acidosis, cardiac failure, rhabdomyolysis, hyperlipidaemia, and hepatomegaly).

**Thiopental sodium** is a barbiturate that is used for induction of anaesthesia, but it has no analgesic properties. Induction is generally smooth and rapid, but dose-related cardiorespiratory depression can occur. Awakening from a moderate dose of thiopental is rapid because the drug redistributes into other tissues, particularly fat. However, metabolism is slow and sedative effects can persist for 24 hours. Repeated doses have a cumulative effect particularly in neonates, and recovery is much slower.

**Etomidate** is an intravenous agent associated with rapid recovery without a hangover effect. Etomidate causes less hypotension than thiopental and propofol during induction. It produces a high incidence of extraneous muscle movements, which can be minimised by an opioid analgesic or a short-acting benzodiazepine given just before induction. Pain on injection can be reduced by injecting into a larger vein or by giving an opioid analgesic just before induction. Etomidate suppresses adrenocortical function, particularly on continuous administration, and it should not be used for maintenance of anaesthesia. It should be used with caution in patients with underlying adrenal insufficiency, for example, those with sepsis.

**Ketamine** causes less hypotension than thiopental and propofol during induction. It is sometimes used in children requiring repeat anaesthesia (such as for serial burns dressings), however recovery is relatively slow and there is a high incidence of extraneous muscle movements. Ketamine can cause hallucinations, nightmares, and other transient psychotic effects; these can be reduced by a benzodiazepine, such as diazepam or midazolam.

## ◤ ETOMIDATE

**Cautions**  see notes above; avoid in acute porphyria (section 9.8.2); **interactions:** Appendix 1 (anaesthetics, general)

**Contra-indications**  see notes above

**Hepatic impairment**  reduce dose in liver cirrhosis

**Pregnancy**  may depress neonatal respiration if used during delivery

**Breast-feeding**  breast-feeding can be resumed as soon as mother has recovered sufficiently from anaesthesia

**Side-effects**  see notes above; also nausea, vomiting, hypotension, apnoea, hyperventilation, stridor, rash;

*less commonly* hypersalivation, bradycardia, arrhythmias, hypertension, hiccups, cough, phlebitis; AV block, cardiac arrest, respiratory depression, seizures, shivering, and Stevens-Johnson syndrome also reported

**Indications and dose**

See under preparations

**Etomidate-Lipuro®** (B. Braun) ⒫ᴼᴹ
Injection (emulsion), etomidate 2 mg/mL, net price 10-mL amp = £1.53
Dose

**Induction of anaesthesia**

- By slow intravenous injection
  **Child 1 month–18 years** 150–300 micrograms/kg; child under 10 years may need up to 400 micrograms/kg

**Hypnomidate®** (Janssen) ⒫ᴼᴹ
Injection, etomidate 2 mg/mL, net price 10-mL amp = £1.38
**Excipients**  include propylene glycol (see Excipients, p. 2)
Dose

**Induction of anaesthesia**

- By slow intravenous injection
  **Child 1 month–18 years** 300 micrograms/kg (max. total dose 60 mg)

## ◤ KETAMINE

**Cautions**  see notes above; dehydration; hypertension; respiratory tract infection; increased cerebrospinal fluid pressure; predisposition to seizures, hallucinations, or nightmares; psychotic disorders; head injury or intracranial mass lesions; thyroid dysfunction; raised intraocular pressure; **interactions:** Appendix 1 (anaesthetics, general)

**Contra-indications**  see notes above; hypertension, pre-eclampsia or eclampsia, severe cardiac disease, stroke; raised intracranial pressure; head trauma; acute porphyria (section 9.8.2)

**Hepatic impairment**  consider dose reduction

**Pregnancy**  may depress neonatal respiration if used during delivery

**Breast-feeding**  avoid for at least 12 hours after last dose

**Side-effects**  see notes above; also nausea, vomiting, tachycardia, hypertension, diplopia, nystagmus, rash; *less commonly* arrhythmias, hypotension, bradycardia, respiratory depression, laryngospasm; *rarely* hypersalivation, apnoea, insomnia, cystitis (including haemorrhagic); *also reported* raised intra-ocular pressure

**Indications and dose**

**Sedation prior to invasive or painful procedures**

- By intravenous injection
  **Child 1 month–18 years** 1–2 mg/kg as a single dose

**Induction and maintenance of anaesthesia (short procedures)**

- By intravenous injection over at least 60 seconds
  **Neonate** 1–2 mg/kg produces 5–10 minutes of surgical anaesthesia, adjusted according to response
  **Child 1 month–12 years** 1–2 mg/kg produces 5–10 minutes of surgical anaesthesia, adjusted according to response

**15**
**Anaesthesia**

**Child 12–18 years** 1–4.5 mg/kg adjusted according to response (2 mg/kg usually produces 5–10 minutes of surgical anaesthesia)

- By intramuscular injection

**Neonate** 4 mg/kg usually produces 15 minutes of surgical anaesthesia, adjusted according to response

**Child 1 month–18 years** 4–13 mg/kg (4 mg/kg sufficient for some diagnostic procedures), adjusted according to response; 10 mg/kg usually produces 12–25 minutes of surgical anaesthesia

### Induction and maintenance of anaesthesia (longer procedures)

- By intravenous administration

**Neonate** initially 0.5–2 mg/kg by *intravenous injection*, followed by a *continuous intravenous infusion* of 8 micrograms/kg/minute adjusted according to response; up to 30 micrograms/kg/minute may be used to produce deep anaesthesia

**Child 1 month–18 years** initially 0.5–2 mg/kg by *intravenous injection* followed by a *continuous intravenous infusion* of 10–45 micrograms/kg/minute adjusted according to response

**Administration** for *continuous intravenous infusion*, dilute to a concentration of 1 mg/mL with Glucose 5% *or* Sodium Chloride 0.9%; use microdrip infusion for maintenance of anaesthesia

For *intravenous injection*, dilute 100 mg/mL strength to a concentration of not more than 50 mg/mL with Glucose 5% *or* Sodium Chloride 0.9%

**Ketalar®** (Pfizer) CD4-1
Injection, ketamine (as hydrochloride) 10 mg/mL, net price 20-mL vial = £5.06; 50 mg/mL, 10-mL vial = £8.77; 100 mg/mL, 10-mL vial = £16.10
**Note** 100 mg/mL, 10-mL vial may be difficult to obtain

## ▌ PROPOFOL

**Cautions** see notes above; cardiac impairment; respiratory impairment; hypovolaemia; epilepsy; hypotension; raised intracranial pressure; monitor blood-lipid concentration if risk of fat overload or if sedation longer than 3 days; **interactions:** Appendix 1 (anaesthetics, general)

**Contra-indications** see notes above

**Hepatic impairment** use with caution

**Renal impairment** use with caution

**Pregnancy** may depress neonatal respiration if used during delivery; max. dose for maintenance of anaesthesia, 6 mg/kg/hour

**Breast-feeding** breast-feeding can be resumed as soon as mother has recovered sufficiently from anaesthesia

**Side-effects** see notes above; also hypotension, tachycardia, flushing; transient apnoea, hyperventilation, coughing, and hiccup during induction; headache; *less commonly* thrombosis, phlebitis; *rarely* arrhythmia, headache, vertigo, shivering, euphoria; *very rarely* pancreatitis, pulmonary oedema, sexual disinhibition, and discoloration of urine; serious and sometimes fatal side-effects reported with prolonged infusion of doses exceeding 5 mg/kg/hour, including metabolic acidosis, rhabdomyolysis, hyperkalaemia, and cardiac failure, dystonia and dyskinesia also reported

### Indications and dose

#### Induction of anaesthesia using 0.5% *or* 1% injection

- By slow intravenous injection or by intravenous infusion

**Child 1 month–18 years** adjust dose according to age, body-weight, and response; usual dose in child 1 month–17 years 2.5–4 mg/kg; usual dose in child 17–18 years 1.5–2.5 mg/kg at a rate of 20–40 mg every 10 seconds until response

#### Induction of anaesthesia using 2% injection

- By intravenous infusion

**Child 3–18 years** adjust dose according to age, body-weight, and response; usual dose in child 3–17 years 2.5–4 mg/kg; usual dose in child 17–18 years 1.5–2.5 mg/kg at a rate of 20–40 mg every 10 seconds until response

#### Maintenance of anaesthesia using 1% injection

- By continuous intravenous infusion

**Child 1 month–18 years** adjust dose according to age, body-weight, and response; usual dose in child 1 month–17 years 9–15 mg/kg/hour; usual dose in child 17–18 years 4–12 mg/kg/hour, adjusted according to response

#### Maintenance of anaesthesia using 2% injection

- By continuous intravenous infusion

**Child 3–18 years** adjust dose according to age, body-weight, and response; usual dose in child 3–17 years 9–15 mg/kg/hour; usual dose in child 17–18 years 4–12 mg/kg/hour, adjusted according to response

#### Sedation of ventilated children in intensive care using 1% *or* 2% injection

- By continuous intravenous infusion

**Child 16–18 years** 0.3–4 mg/kg/hour, adjusted according to response

#### Induction of sedation for surgical and diagnostic procedures using 0.5% *or* 1% injection

- By slow intravenous injection

**Child 1 month–18 years** dose and rate of administration adjusted according to desired level of sedation and response; usual dose in child 1 month–17 years 1–2 mg/kg; usual dose in child 17–18 years 0.5–1 mg/kg over 1–5 minutes

#### Maintenance of sedation for surgical and diagnostic procedures using 0.5% injection

- By intravenous infusion

**Child 17–18 years** dose and rate of administration adjusted according to desired level of sedation and response; usual dose 1.5–4.5 mg/kg/hour (additionally, if rapid increase in sedation required, *by slow intravenous injection* 10–20 mg)

#### Maintenance of sedation for surgical and diagnostic procedures using 1% injection

- By intravenous infusion

**Child 1 month–18 years** dose and rate of administration adjusted according to desired level of sedation and response; usual dose in child 1 month–17 years 1.5–9 mg/kg/hour (additionally, if rapid increase in sedation required, *by slow intravenous injection*, max. 1 mg/kg); usual dose in child 17–18 years 1.5–4.5 mg/kg/hour (additionally, if rapid increase in sedation required, *by slow intravenous injection*, 10–20 mg)

**Maintenance of sedation for surgical and diagnostic procedures using 2% injection**

- **By intravenous infusion**

  **Child 3–18 years** dose and rate of administration adjusted according to desired level of sedation and response; usual dose in child 3–17 years 1.5–9 mg/kg/hour; usual dose in child 17–18 years 1.5–4.5 mg/kg/hour (additionally, if rapid increase in sedation required, *by slow intravenous injection* using 0.5% or 1% injection, 10–20 mg)

**Administration** shake before use; microbiological filter not recommended; may be administered via a Y-piece close to injection site co-administered with Glucose 5% *or* Sodium chloride 0.9%

**0.5% emulsion** for injection or infusion; may be administered undiluted, or diluted with Glucose 5% *or* Sodium chloride 0.9%; dilute to a concentration not less than 1 mg/mL

**1% emulsion** for injection or infusion; may be administered undiluted, or diluted with Glucose 5% (*Diprivan*® or *Propofol-Lipuro*®) *or* Sodium chloride 0.9% (*Propofol-Lipuro*® only); dilute to a concentration not less than 2 mg/mL; use within 6 hours of preparation

**2% emulsion** for infusion; do not dilute

**Propofol** (Non-proprietary) PoM
　0.5% injection (emulsion), propofol 5 mg/mL, net price 20-mL amp = £3.46
　**Brands include** *Propofol-Lipuro*®
　1% injection (emulsion), propofol 10 mg/mL, net price 20-mL amp = £4.18, 50-mL bottle = £10.10, 100-mL bottle = £19.40
　**Brands include** *Propofol-Lipuro*®, *Propoven*®
　2% injection (emulsion), propofol 20 mg/mL, net price 50-mL vial = £21.30
　**Brands include** *Propofol-Lipuro*®, *Propoven*®

**Diprivan**® (AstraZeneca) PoM
　1% injection (emulsion), propofol 10 mg/mL, net price 20-mL amp = £1.07, 50-mL prefilled syringe (for use with *Diprifusor*® TCI system) = £4.72
　2% injection (emulsion), propofol 20 mg/mL, net price 50-mL prefilled syringe (for use with *Diprifusor*® TCI system) = £5.27

---

## THIOPENTAL SODIUM
(Thiopentone sodium)

**Cautions** see notes above; cardiovascular disease; reconstituted solution is highly alkaline—extravasation causes tissue necrosis and severe pain; avoid intra-arterial injection; **interactions:** Appendix 1 (anaesthetics, general)

**Contra-indications** see notes above; acute porphyria (section 9.8.2); myotonic dystrophy

**Hepatic impairment** use with caution—reduce dose

**Renal impairment** caution in severe impairment

**Pregnancy** may depress neonatal respiration when used during delivery

**Breast-feeding** breast-feeding can be resumed as soon as mother has recovered sufficiently from anaesthesia

**Side-effects** hypotension, arrhythmias, myocardial depression, laryngeal spasm, cough, headache, sneezing, hypersensitivity reactions, rash

**Licensed use** not licensed for use in status epilepticus; not licensed for use by intravenous infusion

**Indications and dose**

### Induction of anaesthesia

- **By slow intravenous injection**

  **Neonate** initially up to 2 mg/kg, then 1 mg/kg repeated as necessary (max. total dose 4 mg/kg)

  **Child 1 month–18 years** initially up to 4 mg/kg, then 1 mg/kg repeated as necessary (max. total dose 7 mg/kg)

### Prolonged status epilepticus

- **By slow intravenous injection and intravenous infusion**

  **Neonate** initially up to 2 mg/kg *by intravenous injection*, then up to 8 mg/kg/hour *by continuous intravenous infusion*, adjusted according to response

  **Child 1 month–18 years** initially up to 4 mg/kg *by intravenous injection*, then up to 8 mg/kg/hour *by continuous intravenous infusion*, adjusted according to response

**Administration** For *intravenous injection*, dilute to a concentration of 25 mg/mL with Water for Injections, and give over at least 10–15 seconds; for *intravenous infusion* dilute to a concentration of 2.5 mg/mL with Sodium Chloride 0.9%

**Thiopental** (Archimedes) PoM
　Injection, powder for reconstitution, thiopental sodium, net price 500-mg vial = £3.68

---

## 15.1.2　Inhalational anaesthetics

> **Important**
> The drugs in this section should only be administered by, or under the direct supervision of, personnel experienced in their use, with adequate training in anaesthesia and airway management, and when resuscitation equipment is available.

Inhalational anaesthetics include gases and volatile liquids. *Gaseous anaesthetics* require suitable equipment for administration. *Volatile liquid anaesthetics* are administered using calibrated vaporisers, using air, oxygen, or nitrous oxide-oxygen mixtures as the carrier gas. To prevent hypoxia, the inspired gas mixture should contain a minimum of 25% oxygen at all times. Higher concentrations of oxygen (greater than 30%) are usually required during inhalational anaesthesia with nitrous oxide, see Nitrous Oxide, p. 635.

**Anaesthesia and skilled tasks** See section 15.1.

## Volatile liquid anaesthetics

Volatile liquid anaesthetics can be used for induction and maintenance of anaesthesia, and following induction with an intravenous anaesthetic (section 15.1.1).

Volatile liquid anaesthetics can trigger malignant hyperthermia (section 15.1.8) and are contra-indicated in those susceptible to malignant hyperthermia. They can increase cerebrospinal pressure and should be used with caution in those with raised intracranial pressure. They can also cause hepatotoxicity in those who are sensitised to halogenated anaesthetics. In children with neuromuscular disease, inhalational anaesthetics are very rarely associated with hyperkalaemia, resulting in cardiac arrhythmias and death. Cardiorespiratory depression, hypotension, and arrhythmias are common side-effects of volatile liquid anaesthetics.

**Isoflurane** is a volatile liquid anaesthetic. Heart rhythm is generally stable during isoflurane anaesthesia, but heart-rate can rise. Systemic arterial pressure and cardiac output can fall, owing to a decrease in systemic vascular resistance. Muscle relaxation occurs and the effects of muscle relaxant drugs are potentiated. Isoflurane can irritate mucous membranes, causing cough, breath-holding, and laryngospasm. Isoflurane is the preferred inhalational anaesthetic for use in obstetrics.

**Desflurane** is a rapid-acting volatile liquid anaesthetic; it is reported to have about one-fifth the potency of isoflurane. Emergence and recovery from anaesthesia are particularly rapid because of its low solubility. Desflurane is not recommended for induction of anaesthesia as it is irritant to the upper respiratory tract; cough, breath-holding, apnoea, laryngospasm, and increased secretions can occur.

**Sevoflurane** is a rapid-acting volatile liquid anaesthetic and is more potent than desflurane. Emergence and recovery are particularly rapid but slower than desflurane. Sevoflurane is non-irritant and is therefore used for inhalational induction of anaesthesia. Sevoflurane can interact with carbon dioxide absorbents to form compound A, a potentially nephrotoxic vinyl ether. However, in spite of extensive use, no cases of sevoflurane-induced permanent renal injury have been reported and the carbon dioxide absorbents used in the UK produce very low concentrations of compound A, even in low-flow anaesthetic systems.

## ▌ DESFLURANE

**Cautions** see notes above; **interactions**: Appendix 1 (anaesthetics, general)

**Contra-indications** see notes above

**Pregnancy** may depress neonatal respiration if used during delivery

**Breast-feeding** breast-feeding can be resumed as soon as mother has recovered sufficiently from anaesthesia

**Side-effects** see notes above

### Indications and dose

#### Induction of anaesthesia

● By inhalation through specifically calibrated vaporiser

> **Child 12–18 years** 4–11%, but **not** recommended (see notes above)

#### Maintenance of anaesthesia

● By inhalation through specifically calibrated vaporiser

> **Neonate** 2–6% in nitrous oxide-oxygen; 2.5–8.5% in oxygen or oxygen-enriched air
>
> **Child 1 month–18 years** 2–6% in nitrous oxide-oxygen; 2.5–8.5% in oxygen or oxygen-enriched air

## ▌ ISOFLURANE

**Cautions** see notes above; **interactions**: Appendix 1 (anaesthetics, general)

**Contra-indications** see notes above

**Pregnancy** may depress neonatal respiration if used during delivery

**Breast-feeding** breast-feeding can be resumed as soon as mother has recovered sufficiently from anaesthesia

**Side-effects** see notes above

### Indications and dose

#### Induction of anaesthesia

● By inhalation through specifically calibrated vaporiser

> **Neonate** increased gradually according to response from 0.5–3% in oxygen or nitrous oxide-oxygen
>
> **Child 1 month–18 years** increased gradually according to response from 0.5–3% in oxygen or nitrous oxide-oxygen

#### Maintenance of anaesthesia

● By inhalation through specifically calibrated vaporiser

> **Neonate** 1–2.5% in nitrous oxide-oxygen; additional 0.5–1% may be required if given with oxygen alone
>
> **Child 1 month–18 years** 1–2.5% in nitrous oxide-oxygen; additional 0.5–1% may be required if given with oxygen alone; caesarean section, 0.5–0.75% in nitrous oxide-oxygen

## ▌ SEVOFLURANE

**Cautions** see notes above; susceptibility to QT-interval prolongation; **interactions**: Appendix 1 (anaesthetics, general)

**Contra-indications** see notes above

**Renal impairment** use with caution

**Pregnancy** may depress neonatal respiration if used during delivery

**Breast-feeding** breast-feeding can be resumed as soon as mother has recovered sufficiently from anaesthesia

**Side-effects** see notes above; also urinary retention, leucopenia, agitation; cardiac arrest, torsade de pointes, dystonia, and seizures also reported

### Indications and dose

#### Induction of anaesthesia

● By inhalation through specifically calibrated vaporiser

> **Neonate** up to 4% in oxygen or nitrous oxide-oxygen, according to response
>
> **Child 1 month–18 years** initially 0.5–1% then increased gradually up to 8% in oxygen or nitrous oxide-oxygen, according to response

#### Maintenance of anaesthesia

● By inhalation through specifically calibrated vaporiser

> **Neonate** 0.5–2% in oxygen or nitrous oxide-oxygen, according to response
>
> **Child 1 month–18 years** 0.5–3% in oxygen or nitrous oxide-oxygen, according to response

Anaesthesia

## Nitrous oxide

Nitrous oxide is used for maintenance of anaesthesia and, in sub-anaesthetic concentrations, for analgesia. For *anaesthesia* it is commonly used in a concentration of 50 to 66% in oxygen as part of a balanced technique in association with other inhalational or intravenous agents. Nitrous oxide is unsatisfactory as a sole anaesthetic owing to lack of potency, but is useful as part of a combination of drugs since it allows a significant reduction in dosage.

For *analgesia* (without loss of consciousness) a mixture of nitrous oxide and oxygen containing 50% of each gas (*Entonox*®, *Equanox*®) is used. Self-administration using a demand valve may be used in children who are able to self-regulate their intake (usually over 5 years of age) for painful dressing changes, as an aid to postoperative physiotherapy, for wound debridement and in emergency ambulances.

Nitrous oxide may have a deleterious effect if used in children with an air-containing closed space since nitrous oxide diffuses into such a space with a resulting increase in pressure. This effect may be dangerous in the presence of a pneumothorax, which may enlarge to compromise respiration, or in the presence of intracranial air after head injury. Hypoxia can occur immediately following the administration of nitrous oxide; additional oxygen should always be given for several minutes after stopping the flow of nitrous oxide.

Exposure of children to nitrous oxide for prolonged periods, either by continuous or by intermittent administration, may result in megaloblastic anaemia owing to interference with the action of vitamin $B_{12}$; neurological toxic effects can occur without preceding overt haematological changes. For the same reason, exposure of theatre staff to nitrous oxide should be minimised. Depression of white cell formation may also occur.

Assessment of plasma-vitamin $B_{12}$ concentration should be considered before nitrous oxide anaesthesia in children at risk of deficiency, including children who have a poor or vegetarian diet and children with a history of anaemia. Nitrous oxide should **not** be given continuously for longer than 24 hours or more frequently than every 4 days without close supervision and haematological monitoring.

### ▮ NITROUS OXIDE

**Cautions**  see notes above; **interactions:** Appendix 1 (anaesthetics, general)

**Pregnancy**  may depress neonatal respiration if used during delivery

**Breast-feeding**  breast-feeding can be resumed as soon as mother has recovered sufficiently from anaesthesia

**Side-effects**  see notes above

**Indications and dose**

> **Maintenance of anaesthesia in conjunction with other anaesthetic agents**
> * By inhalation using suitable anaesthetic apparatus
>    **Neonate** 50–66% in oxygen
>    **Child 1 month–18 years** 50–66% in oxygen

**Analgesia**
* By inhalation using suitable anaesthetic apparatus

(see also notes above)

> **Neonate** up to 50% in oxygen, according to the child's needs
> **Child 1 month–18 years** up to 50% in oxygen, according to the child's needs

## 15.1.3  Antimuscarinic drugs

**Important**
The drugs in this section should only be administered by, or under the direct supervision of, personnel experienced in their use.

Antimuscarinic drugs are used (less commonly nowadays) as premedicants to dry bronchial and salivary secretions which are increased by intubation, upper airway surgery, or some inhalational anaesthetics, but they should not be used for this indication in children with cystic fibrosis. Antimuscarinics are also used before or with neostigmine (section 15.1.6) to prevent bradycardia, excessive salivation, and other muscarinic actions of neostigmine. They also prevent bradycardia and hypotension associated with drugs such as propofol and suxamethonium.

**Atropine sulfate** is now rarely used for premedication but still has an emergency role in the treatment of vagotonic side-effects. For its role in cardiopulmonary resuscitation, see section 2.7.3.

**Hyoscine hydrobromide** reduces secretions and also provides a degree of amnesia, sedation, and anti-emesis. Unlike atropine it may produce bradycardia rather than tachycardia. In some children hyoscine may cause the central anticholinergic syndrome (excitement, ataxia, hallucinations, behavioural abnormalities, and drowsiness).

**Glycopyrronium bromide** reduces salivary secretions. When given intravenously it produces less tachycardia than atropine. It is widely used with neostigmine for reversal of non-depolarising muscle relaxants (section 15.1.5).

Glycopyrronium or hyoscine hydrobromide are also used to control excessive secretions in upper airways or hypersalivation in palliative care and in children unable to control posture or with abnormal swallowing reflex; effective dose varies and tolerance may develop. The intramuscular route should be avoided if possible. Hyoscine transdermal patches may also be used (section 4.6).

### ▮ ATROPINE SULFATE

**Cautions**  see notes in section 1.2

> **Duration of action**  Since atropine has a shorter duration of action than neostigmine, late unopposed bradycardia may result; close monitoring of the patient is necessary

**Contra-indications**  see notes in section 1.2

**Pregnancy**  not known to be harmful; manufacturer advises caution

**Breast-feeding**  small amount present in milk—manufacturer advises caution

**Side-effects**  see notes in section 1.2

**Licensed use** not licensed for use by oral route; not licensed for use in children under 12 years for intra-operative bradycardia; not licensed for use in children under 12 years by intravenous route for premedication; not licensed for the control of muscarinic side-effects of edrophonium in reversal of competitive neuromuscular block

### Indications and dose

**Premedication**

● **By mouth 1–2 hours before induction of anaesthesia**

**Neonate** 20–40 micrograms/kg

**Child 1 month–18 years** 20–40 micrograms/kg (max. 900 micrograms)

● **By intravenous injection immediately before induction of anaesthesia**

**Neonate** 10 micrograms/kg

**Child 1 month–12 years** 20 micrograms/kg (minimum 100 micrograms, max. 600 micrograms)

**Child 12–18 years** 300–600 micrograms

● **By subcutaneous or intramuscular injection 30–60 minutes before induction of anaesthesia**

**Neonate** 10 micrograms/kg

**Child 1 month–12 years** 10–30 micrograms/kg (minimum 100 micrograms, max. 600 micrograms)

**Child 12–18 years** 300–600 micrograms

**Intra-operative bradycardia**

● **By intravenous injection**

**Neonate** 10–20 micrograms/kg

**Child 1 month–12 years** 10–20 micrograms/kg

**Child 12–18 years** 300–600 micrograms (larger doses in emergencies)

**Control of muscarinic side-effects of neostigmine 50 micrograms/kg in reversal of competitive neuromuscular block**

● **By intravenous injection**

**Neonate** 20 micrograms/kg

**Child 1 month–12 years** 20 micrograms/kg (max. 1.2 mg)

**Child 12–18 years** 0.6–1.2 mg

**Control of muscarinic side-effects of edrophonium in reversal of competitive neuromuscular block**

● **By intravenous injection**

**Child 1 month–18 years** 7 micrograms/kg (max. 600 micrograms)

**Cycloplegia, anterior uveitis** (section 11.5)

**Administration** for administration *by mouth*, injection solution may be given orally

**¹Atropine** (Non-proprietary) PoM

Injection, atropine sulfate 600 micrograms/mL, net price 1-mL amp = 62p

**Note** Other strengths also available

Injection, prefilled disposable syringe, atropine sulfate 100 micrograms/mL, net price 5 mL = £4.58, 10 mL = £5.39, 30 mL = £8.95

Injection, prefilled disposable syringe, atropine sulfate 200 micrograms/mL, net price 5 mL = £5.91; 300 micrograms/mL, 10 mL = £5.91; 600 micrograms/mL, 1 mL = £5.91

Oral solution, atropine sulfate 100 micrograms/mL available from 'special-order' manufacturers or specialist importing companies, see p. 823

Tablets◢, atropine sulfate 600 micrograms, net price 28-tab pack = £17.59

**¹Minijet® Atropine** (UCB Pharma) PoM

Injection, atropine sulfate 100 micrograms/mL, net price 5 mL = £5.04, 10 mL = £5.93, 30 mL = £9.85

---

## ▌ GLYCOPYRRONIUM BROMIDE
### (Glycopyrrolate)

**Cautions** see notes in section 1.2 (Antimuscarinics)

**Contra-indications** see notes in section 1.2 (Antimuscarinics)

**Side-effects** see notes in section 1.2 (Antimuscarinics)

**Licensed use** not licensed for use in control of upper airways secretion and hypersalivation

### Indications and dose

**Premedication at induction**

● **By intravenous or intramuscular injection**

**Neonate** 5 micrograms/kg

**Child 1 month–12 years** 4–8 micrograms/kg (max. 200 micrograms)

**Child 12–18 years** 200–400 micrograms *or* 4–5 micrograms/kg (max. 400 micrograms)

**Intra-operative bradycardia**

● **By intravenous injection**

**Neonate** 10 micrograms/kg, repeated if necessary

**Child 1 month–18 years** 4–8 micrograms/kg (max. 200 micrograms), repeated if necessary

**Control of muscarinic side-effects of neostigmine in reversal of competitive neuromuscular block**

● **By intravenous injection**

**Neonate** 10 micrograms/kg

**Child 1 month–12 years** 10 micrograms/kg (max. 500 micrograms)

**Child 12–18 years** 200 micrograms per 1 mg of neostigmine, *or* 10–15 micrograms/kg

**Control of upper airways secretion and hypersalivation**

● **By mouth**

**Child 1 month–18 years** 40–100 micrograms/kg (max. 2 mg) 3–4 times daily, adjusted according to response

● **By subcutaneous infusion**

**Child 1 month–12 years** 12–40 micrograms/kg/24 hours (max. 1.2 mg)

**Child 12–18 years** 0.6–1.2 mg/24 hours

● **By subcutaneous injection or intramuscular injection or intravenous injection (but see notes above)**

**Child 1 month–12 years** 4–10 micrograms/kg (max. 200 micrograms) 4 times a day when required

---

1. PoM restriction does not apply where administration is for saving life in emergency

**Child 12–18 years** 200 micrograms every 4 hours when required

**Administration** for administration *by mouth*, injection solution may be given or crushed tablets suspended in water

**Glycopyrronium bromide** (Non-proprietary)
Injection, glycopyrronium bromide 200 micrograms/mL, net price 1-mL amp = 54p, 3-mL amp = 91p
Tablets, glycopyrronium bromide 1 mg and 2 mg
Available on a named-patient basis from specialist importing companies, p. 823

◢With neostigmine metilsulfate
Section 15.1.6

## HYOSCINE HYDROBROMIDE
(Scopolamine hydrobromide)

**Cautions** see notes in section 1.2 and notes above; also epilepsy

**Contra-indications** see notes in section 1.2

**Hepatic impairment** see Hyoscine Hydrobromide, section 4.6

**Renal impairment** see Hyoscine Hydrobromide, section 4.6

**Pregnancy** see Hyoscine Hydrobromide, section 4.6

**Breast-feeding** see Hyoscine Hydrobromide, section 4.6

**Side-effects** see notes in section 1.2

**Indications and dose**

Premedication

● By subcutaneous or intramuscular injection 30–60 minutes before induction
  **Child 1–12 years** 15 micrograms/kg (max. 600 micrograms)
  **Child 12–18 years** 200–600 micrograms

**Note** Same dose may be given by intravenous injection immediately before induction

Motion sickness, excessive respiratory secretions, hypersalivation associated with clozapine therapy section 4.6

**Hyoscine** (Non-proprietary) PoM
Injection, hyoscine hydrobromide 400 micrograms/mL, net price 1-mL amp = £2.80; 600 micrograms/mL, 1-mL amp = £2.94

◢Preparations
For transdermal and oral preparations see section 4.6

## 15.1.4 Sedative and analgesic peri-operative drugs

15.1.4.1   Benzodiazepines
15.1.4.2   Non-opioid analgesics
15.1.4.3   Opioid analgesics
15.1.4.4   Other drugs for sedation

Important
The drugs in this section should only be administered by, or under the direct supervision of, personnel experienced in their use, with adequate training in anaesthesia and airway management.

**Premedication**    Fear and anxiety before a procedure (including the night before) can be minimised by using a sedative drug, usually a **benzodiazepine**. Pre-

medication may also augment the action of anaesthetics and provide some degree of pre-operative amnesia. The choice of drug depends on the individual child, the nature of the procedure, the anaesthetic to be used, and other prevailing circumstances such as outpatients, obstetrics, and recovery facilities. The choice also varies between elective and emergency procedures. Oral administration is preferred if possible; the rectal route should only be used in exceptional circumstances. Sedative premedication with benzodiazepines should be avoided in children with a compromised airway, CNS depression, or a history of sleep apnoea.

Premedicants can be given the night before major surgery; a further, smaller dose may be required the following morning if any delay in starting surgery is anticipated. Alternatively, the first dose may be given on the day of procedure.

Oral **midazolam** is the most common premedicant for children; **temazepam** may be used in older children. The antihistamine **alimemazine** (section 3.4.1) is occasionally used orally, but when given alone it may cause postoperative restlessness in the presence of pain.

**Sedation for clinical procedures**    Sedation of children during diagnostic and therapeutic procedures is used to reduce fear and anxiety, to control pain, and to minimise excessive movement. The choice of sedative drug will depend upon the intended procedure and whether the child is cooperative; some procedures are safer and more successful under anaesthesia. The child should be **monitored carefully**; monitoring should begin as soon as the sedative is given or when the child becomes drowsy, and should be continued until the child wakes up.

**Midazolam** and **chloral hydrate** (section 4.1.1) are suitable for sedating children for painless procedures, such as imaging. For painful procedures, alternative choices include **nitrous oxide** (section 15.1.2), **local anaesthesia** (section 15.2), **ketamine** (section 15.1.1), or concomitant use of sedation with **opioid** or **non-opioid analgesia** (section 4.7).

**Dental procedures**    Sedation for dental procedures should be limited to conscious sedation whenever possible. **Nitrous oxide** (section 15.1.2) alone and **midazolam** are effective for many children. For further information on hypnotics used for dental procedures, see p. 169.

**Anaesthesia and skilled tasks**    See section 15.1.

## 15.1.4.1 Benzodiazepines

Benzodiazepines possess useful properties for premedication including relief of anxiety, sedation, and amnesia; short-acting benzodiazepines taken by mouth are the most common premedicants. Benzodiazepines are also used for sedation prior to clinical procedures and for sedation in intensive care.

Benzodiazepines may occasionally cause marked respiratory depression and facilities for its treatment are essential; flumazenil (section 15.1.7) is used to antagonise the effects of benzodiazepines.

**Midazolam**, a water-soluble benzodiazepine, is the preferred benzodiazepine for premedication and for sedation for clinical procedures in children. It has a fast onset of action, and recovery is faster than for other benzodiazepines. Recovery may be longer in

15 Anaesthesia

children with a low cardiac output, or after repeated dosing.

Midazolam can be given by mouth [unlicensed], but its bitter acidic taste may need to be disguised. It can also be given buccally [unlicensed indication] or intranasally [unlicensed]. Midazolam is associated with profound sedation when high doses are given or when it is used with certain other drugs. It can cause severe disinhibition and restlessness in some children. Midazolam is not recommended for prolonged sedation in neonates; drug accumulation is likely to occur

### Overdosage with midazolam

There have been reports of overdosage in adults when high strength midazolam injection has been used for conscious sedation. The use of high strength midazolam (5 mg/mL in 2 mL and 10 mL ampoules, or 2 mg/mL in 5 mL ampoules) should be restricted to general anaesthesia, intensive care, palliative care, or other situations where the risk has been assessed. It is advised that flumazenil (section 15.1.7) is available where midazolam is used, to reverse the effects if necessary.

**Temazepam** is given by mouth for premedication in older children and has a short duration of action. Anxiolytic and sedative effects last about 90 minutes, although there may be residual drowsiness. Temazepam is rarely used for dental procedures in children.

**Lorazepam** produces more prolonged sedation than temazepam and it has marked amnesic effects.

Peri-operative use of **diazepam** is not recommended in children; onset and magnitude of response are unreliable, and paradoxical effects may occur. Diazepam is not used for dental procedures in children.

## ▌ LORAZEPAM

**Cautions** see notes above and section 4.8.2; **interactions**: Appendix 1 (anxiolytics and hypnotics)
**Contra-indications** see Diazepam, section 4.8.2
**Hepatic impairment** see Benzodiazepines, section 4.8.1
**Renal impairment** see Benzodiazepines, section 4.8.1
**Pregnancy** see Benzodiazepines, section 4.8.1
**Breast-feeding** see Benzodiazepines, section 4.8.1
**Side-effects** see notes above and Diazepam, section 4.8.2
**Licensed use** not licensed for use in children under 5 years by mouth; not licensed for use in children under 12 years by intravenous injection

### Indications and dose

#### Premedication

- **By mouth**

  **Child 1 month–12 years** 50–100 micrograms/kg (max. 4 mg) at least 1 hour before procedure

  **Child 12–18 years** 1–4 mg at least 1 hour before procedure

  **Note** Same dose may be given the night before procedure in addition to, or to replace, dose before procedure

- **By intravenous injection**

  **Child 1 month–18 years** 50–100 micrograms/kg (max. 4 mg)

  **Note** Give intravenous injection 30–45 minutes before procedure

#### Status epilepticus section 4.8.2

**Administration** for *intravenous injection*, dilute injection solution with an equal volume of Sodium Chloride 0.9%; give over 3–5 minutes; max. rate 50 micrograms/kg over 3 minutes

**Lorazepam** (Non-proprietary) CD4-1
Tablets, lorazepam 1 mg, net price 28-tab pack = £5.42; 2.5 mg, 28-tab pack = £7.11. Label: 2 or 19

Injection, lorazepam 4 mg/mL, net price 1-mL amp = 35p
**Excipients** include benzyl alcohol (avoid in neonates unless there is no safer alternative available, see Excipients, p. 2), propylene glycol
**Brands** include *Ativan*®

## ▌ MIDAZOLAM

**Cautions** see notes above; cardiac disease; respiratory disease; myasthenia gravis; neonates; history of drug or alcohol abuse; reduce dose if debilitated; risk of severe hypotension in children with hypovolaemia, vasoconstriction, hypothermia; avoid prolonged use (and abrupt withdrawal thereafter); **interactions**: Appendix 1 (anxiolytics and hypnotics)
**Contra-indications** marked neuromuscular respiratory weakness including unstable myasthenia gravis; severe respiratory depression; acute pulmonary insufficiency; sleep apnoea syndrome
**Hepatic impairment** use with caution; can precipitate coma
**Renal impairment** use with caution in chronic renal failure—increased cerebral sensitivity
**Pregnancy** avoid regular use (risk of neonatal withdrawal symptoms); use only if clear indication such as seizure control (high doses during late pregnancy or labour may cause neonatal hypothermia, hypotonia, and respiratory depression)
**Breast-feeding** small amount present in milk—avoid breast-feeding for 24 hours after administration (although amount probably too small to be harmful after single doses)
**Side-effects** see notes above; gastro-intestinal disturbances, dry mouth, hiccups, increased appetite, jaundice; hypotension, cardiac arrest, heart rate changes, anaphylaxis, thrombosis; laryngospasm, bronchospasm, respiratory depression and respiratory arrest (particularly with high doses or on rapid injection); drowsiness, confusion, ataxia, amnesia, headache, euphoria, hallucinations, convulsions (more common in neonates), fatigue, dizziness, vertigo, involuntary movements, paradoxical excitement and aggression, dysarthria; urinary retention, incontinence; blood disorders; muscle weakness; visual disturbances; salivation changes; skin reactions; injection-site reactions; with *intranasal administration* burning sensation, lacrimation, and severe irritation of nasal mucosa
**Licensed use** not licensed for use in children under 6 months for premedication and conscious sedation; not licensed for use by mouth; not licensed for use by buccal administration for conscious sedation

**Indications and dose**

Conscious sedation for procedures (but see notes above)

● By mouth

Child 1 month–18 years 500 micrograms/kg (max. 20 mg) 30–60 minutes before procedure

● By buccal administration

Child 6 months–10 years 200–300 micrograms/kg (max. 5 mg)

Child 10–18 years 6–7 mg (max. 8 mg if 70 kg or over)

● By rectum

Child 6 months–12 years 300–500 micrograms/kg 15–30 minutes before procedure

● By intravenous injection over 2–3 minutes 5–10 minutes before procedure

Child 1 month–6 years initially 25–50 micrograms/kg, increased if necessary in small steps (max. total dose 6 mg)

Child 6–12 years initially 25–50 micrograms/kg, increased if necessary in small steps (max. total dose 10 mg)

Child 12–18 years initially 25–50 micrograms/kg, increased if necessary in small steps (max. total dose 7.5 mg)

Premedication (but see notes above)

● By mouth

Child 1 month–18 years 500 micrograms/kg (max. 20 mg) 15–30 minutes before the procedure

● By rectum

Child 6 months–12 years 300–500 micrograms/kg 15–30 minutes before induction

Induction of anaesthesia (but rarely used)

● By slow intravenous injection

Child 7–18 years initially 150 micrograms/kg (max. 7.5 mg) given in steps of 50 micrograms/kg (max. 2.5 mg) over 2–5 minutes; wait for 2–5 minutes then give additional doses of 50 micrograms/kg (max. 2.5 mg) every 2 minutes if necessary; max. total dose 500 micrograms/kg (not exceeding 25 mg)

Sedation in intensive care

● By intravenous injection and continuous intravenous infusion

Neonate less than 32 weeks postmenstrual age 60 micrograms/kg/hour *by continuous intravenous infusion*, reduced after 24 hours to 30 micrograms/kg/hour; adjusted according to response; max. treatment duration 4 days

Neonate over 32 weeks postmenstrual age 60 micrograms/kg/hour *by continuous intravenous infusion* adjusted according to response; max. treatment duration 4 days

Child 1–6 months 60 micrograms/kg/hour *by continuous intravenous infusion* adjusted according to response

Child 6 months–12 years initially 50–200 micrograms/kg *by slow intravenous injection* over at least 3 minutes followed by 30–120 micrograms/kg/hour *by continuous intravenous infusion* adjusted according to response

Child 12–18 years initially 30–300 micrograms/kg *by slow intravenous injection* given in steps of 1–2.5 mg every 2 minutes followed by 30–200 micrograms/kg/hour *by continuous intravenous infusion* adjusted according to response

Note Initial dose may not be required and lower maintenance doses needed if opioid analgesics also used; reduce dose (or reduce or omit initial dose) in hypovolaemia, vasoconstriction, or hypothermia

Status epilepticus section 4.8.2

**Administration** for administration *by mouth*, injection solution may be diluted with apple or black currant juice, chocolate sauce, or cola

For *buccal administration*, administer half of the dose between the upper lip and gum on each side of the mouth using an oral syringe; retain in the mouth for at least 5 minutes then swallow

For *continuous intravenous infusion*, dilute with Glucose 5% *or* Sodium Chloride 0.9%

*Neonatal intensive care*, dilute 15 mg/kg body-weight to a final volume of 50 mL with infusion fluid; an intravenous infusion rate of 0.1 mL/hour provides a dose of 30 micrograms/kg/hour

For *rectal administration* of the injection solution, attach a plastic applicator onto the end of a syringe; if the volume to be given rectally is too small, dilute with Water for Injections

**Midazolam** (Non-proprietary) [CD3]

Oral liquid, midazolam 2.5 mg/mL, 100 mL Available from 'special-order' manufacturers or specialist importing companies, see p. 823

Injection, midazolam (as hydrochloride) 1 mg/mL, net price 2-mL amp = 50p, 5-mL amp = 60p, 50-mL vial = £7.87; 2 mg/mL, 5-mL amp = 65p; 5 mg/mL, 2-mL amp = 58p, 10-mL amp = £2.50

**Hypnovel**® (Roche) [CD3]

Injection, midazolam (as hydrochloride) 5 mg/mL, 2-mL amp = 72p

◢Buccal preparation

Section 4.8.2

---

▌ **TEMAZEPAM**

**Cautions** see notes above and Diazepam, section 4.8.2; **interactions**: Appendix 1 (anxiolytics and hypnotics)

**Contra-indications** see Diazepam, section 4.8.2

**Hepatic impairment** see Benzodiazepines, section 4.8.1

**Renal impairment** see Benzodiazepines, section 4.8.1

**Pregnancy** see Benzodiazepines, section 4.8.1

**Breast-feeding** see Benzodiazepines, section 4.8.1

**Side-effects** see notes above and Diazepam, section 4.8.2

**Licensed use** tablets not licensed for use in children

**Indications and dose**

Premedication

● By mouth

Child 12–18 years 10–20 mg 1 hour before procedure

15 Anaesthesia

**Temazepam** (Non-proprietary) CD3

Tablets, temazepam 10 mg, net price 28-tab pack = £3.42; 20 mg, 28-tab pack = £2.24. Label: 19
**Dental prescribing on NHS** Temazepam Tablets may be prescribed

Oral solution, temazepam 10 mg/5 mL, net price 300 mL = £33.44. Label: 19
Note Sugar-free versions are available and can be ordered by specifying 'sugar-free' on the prescription
**Dental prescribing on NHS** Temazepam Oral Solution may be prescribed
Note See p. 8 for prescribing requirements of controlled drugs

### 15.1.4.2 Non-opioid analgesics

Since non-steroidal anti-inflammatory drugs (NSAIDs) do not depress respiration, do not impair gastro-intestinal motility, and do not cause dependence, they may be useful alternatives or adjuncts to opioids for the relief of postoperative pain. NSAIDs may be inadequate for the relief of severe pain.

Diclofenac, ibuprofen (section 10.1.1), **paracetamol** (section 4.7.1), and **ketorolac** are used to relieve postoperative pain in children; diclofenac and paracetamol can be given parenterally and rectally as well as by mouth. Ketorolac is given by intravenous injection.

### ◼ KETOROLAC TROMETAMOL

**Cautions**   section 10.1.1; avoid in acute porphyria (section 9.8.2); **interactions**: Appendix 1 (NSAIDs)
**Contra-indications**   section 10.1.1; also complete or partial syndrome of nasal polyps; haemorrhagic diatheses (including coagulation disorders) and following operations with high risk of haemorrhage or incomplete haemostasis; confirmed or suspected cerebrovascular bleeding; hypovolaemia or dehydration
**Hepatic impairment**   section 10.1.1
**Renal impairment**   max. 60 mg daily by intravenous injection; avoid if serum creatinine greater than 160 micromol/litre; see also section 10.1.1
**Pregnancy**   section 10.1.1
**Breast-feeding**   amount too small to be harmful
**Side-effects**   section 10.1.1; also gastro-intestinal disturbances, taste disturbances, dry mouth; flushing, bradycardia, palpitation, chest pain, hypertension, pallor; dyspnoea, asthma; malaise, euphoria, psychosis, paraesthesia, convulsions, abnormal dreams, hyperkinesia, confusion, hallucinations, urinary frequency, thirst, sweating; hyponatraemia, hyperkalaemia, myalgia; visual disturbances (including optic neuritis); purpura, pain at injection site
**Licensed use**   not licensed for use in children under 16 years

#### Indications and dose

> **Short-term management of moderate to severe acute postoperative pain only**
> - **By intravenous injection over at least 15 seconds**
>   **Child 6 months–16 years** initially 0.5–1 mg/kg (max. 15 mg), then 500 micrograms/kg (max. 15 mg) every 6 hours as required; max. 60 mg daily; max. duration of treatment 2 days

> - **By intravenous injection over at least 15 seconds**
>   **Child 16–18 years** initially 10 mg, then 10–30 mg every 4–6 hours as required (up to every 2 hours during initial postoperative period); max. 90 mg daily (children weighing less than 50 kg max. 60 mg daily); max. duration of treatment 2 days

**Ketorolac** (Non-proprietary) PoM

Injection, ketorolac trometamol 30 mg/mL, net price 1-mL amp = £1.10

**Toradol®** (Roche) PoM

Injection, ketorolac trometamol 30 mg/mL, net price 1-mL amp = £1.08

### 15.1.4.3 Opioid analgesics

Opioid analgesics are now rarely used as premedicants; they are more likely to be administered at induction. Pre-operative use of opioid analgesics is generally limited to children who require control of existing pain. The main side-effects of opioid analgesics are respiratory depression, cardiovascular depression, nausea, and vomiting; for general notes on opioid analgesics and their use in postoperative pain, see section 4.7.2.

For the management of opioid-induced respiratory depression, see section 15.1.7.

**Intra-operative analgesia**   Opioid analgesics given in small doses before or with induction reduce the dose requirement of some drugs used during anaesthesia.

**Alfentanil, fentanyl**, and **remifentanil** are particularly useful because they act within 1–2 minutes and have short durations of action. The initial doses of alfentanil or fentanyl are followed either by successive intravenous injections or by an intravenous infusion; prolonged infusions increase the duration of effect. Repeated intra-operative doses of alfentanil or fentanyl should be given with care since the resulting respiratory depression can persist postoperatively and occasionally it may become apparent for the first time postoperatively when monitoring of the child might be less intensive. Alfentanil, fentanyl, and remifentanil can cause muscle rigidity, particularly of the chest wall muscle or jaw muscle, which can be managed by the use of neuromuscular blocking drugs.

In contrast to other opioids which are metabolised in the liver, remifentanil undergoes rapid metabolism by nonspecific blood and tissue esterases; its short duration of action allows prolonged administration at high dosage, without accumulation, and with little risk of residual postoperative respiratory depression. Remifentanil should not be given by intravenous injection intraoperatively, but it is well suited to continuous infusion; a supplementary analgesic is given before stopping the infusion of remifentanil.

**Neonates**   The half-life of fentanyl and alfentanil is prolonged in neonates and accumulation is likely with prolonged use.

### ◼ ALFENTANIL

**Cautions**   section 4.7.2 and notes above
**Contra-indications**   section 4.7.2
**Hepatic impairment**   section 4.7.2
**Renal impairment**   section 4.7.2

**Pregnancy**  section 4.7.2

**Breast-feeding**  present in milk—withhold breast-feeding for 24 hours

**Side-effects**  section 4.7.2 and notes above; also hypertension, myoclonic movements; *less commonly* arrhythmias, hiccup, laryngospasm; *rarely* epistaxis; also reported cardiac arrest, cough, convulsions, and pyrexia

### Indications and dose

> To avoid excessive dosage in obese children, dose may need to be calculated on the basis of ideal weight for height

---

Analgesia especially during short procedures; enhancement of anaesthesia

- **By intravenous injection over 30 seconds (with assisted ventilation)**

  **Neonate** initially 5–20 micrograms/kg; supplemental doses up to 10 micrograms/kg

  **Child 1 month–18 years** initially 10–20 micrograms/kg; supplemental doses up to 10 micrograms/kg

- **By intravenous infusion (with assisted ventilation)**

  **Neonate** initially 10–50 micrograms/kg over 10 minutes followed by 0.5–1 micrograms/kg/minute

  **Child 1 month–18 years** initially 50–100 micrograms/kg over 10 minutes followed by 0.5–1 micrograms/kg/minute

**Administration**  for *continuous or intermittent intravenous infusion* dilute in Glucose 5% *or* Sodium Chloride 0.9%

**Alfentanil** (Non-proprietary) CD2
  Injection, alfentanil (as hydrochloride) 500 micrograms/mL, net price 2-mL amp = 70p, 10-mL amp = £3.20

  Injection, alfentanil (as hydrochloride) 5 mg/mL, net price 1-mL amp = £2.50
  **Note** To be diluted before use

**Rapifen®** (Janssen) CD2
  Injection, alfentanil (as hydrochloride) 500 micrograms/mL, net price 2-mL amp = 64p; 10-mL amp = £2.90

  Intensive care injection, alfentanil (as hydrochloride) 5 mg/mL, net price 1-mL amp = £2.32
  **Note** To be diluted before use

## ◗ FENTANYL

**Cautions**  see Fentanyl, section 4.7.2 and notes above
**Contra-indications**  see notes in section 4.7.2
**Hepatic impairment**  see notes in section 4.7.2
**Renal impairment**  see notes in section 4.7.2
**Pregnancy**  see notes in section 4.7.2
**Breast-feeding**  see Fentanyl, section 4.7.2
**Side-effects**  see Fentanyl, section 4.7.2 and notes above; also myoclonic movements; *less commonly* laryngospasm; *rarely* asystole, insomnia

**Licensed use**  not licensed for use in children under 2 years; infusion not licensed for use in children under 12 years

### Indications and dose

> To avoid excessive dosage in obese children, dose may need to be calculated on the basis of ideal weight for height

---

Spontaneous respiration: analgesia during operation, enhancement of anaesthesia

- **By intravenous injection over at least 30 seconds**

  **Child 1 month–12 years** initially 1–3 micrograms/kg, then 1 microgram/kg as required

  **Child 12–18 years** initially 50–100 micrograms (max. 200 micrograms on specialist advice), then 25–50 micrograms as required

Assisted ventilation: analgesia during operation, enhancement of anaesthesia

- **By intravenous injection over at least 30 seconds**

  **Neonate** initially 1–5 micrograms/kg, then 1–3 micrograms/kg as required

  **Child 1 month–12 years** initially 1–5 micrograms/kg, then 1–3 micrograms/kg as required

  **Child 12–18 years** initially 1–5 micrograms/kg, then 50–200 micrograms as required

Assisted ventilation: analgesia and respiratory depression in intensive care

- **By intravenous administration**

  **Neonate** initially by *intravenous injection* 1–5 micrograms/kg, then by *intravenous infusion*, 1.5 micrograms/kg/hour adjusted according to response

  **Child 1 month–18 years** initially by *intravenous injection* 1–5 micrograms/kg, then by *intravenous infusion*, 1–6 micrograms/kg/hour adjusted according to response

Analgesia in other situations  section 4.7.2

---

**Administration**  for *intravenous infusion*, injection solution may be diluted in Glucose 5% *or* Sodium Chloride 0.9%

**Fentanyl** (Non-proprietary) CD2
  Injection, fentanyl (as citrate) 50 micrograms/mL, net price 2-mL amp = 30p, 10-mL amp = 64p

**Sublimaze®** (Janssen) CD2
  Injection, fentanyl (as citrate) 50 micrograms/mL, net price 10-mL amp = £1.31

## ◗ REMIFENTANIL

**Cautions**  section 4.7.2 and notes above
**Contra-indications**  section 4.7.2 and notes above; analgesia in conscious patients
**Hepatic impairment**  section 4.7.2
**Pregnancy**  no information available; see also section 4.7.2
**Breast-feeding**  avoid breast-feeding for 24 hours after administration—present in milk in *animal* studies
**Side-effects**  section 4.7.2 and notes above; also hypertension; *less commonly* hypoxia; *rarely* asystole; AV block and convulsions also reported
**Licensed use**  not licensed for use in children under 1 year

**15**
**Anaesthesia**

**Indications and dose**

> To avoid excessive dosage in obese children, dose should be calculated on the basis of ideal weight for height

**Enhancement and maintenance of anaesthesia in ventilated patients**

● **By intravenous administration**

**Neonate** by *intravenous infusion* 0.4–1 micrograms/kg/minute; additional doses of 1 microgram/kg can be given by *intravenous injection* during the intravenous infusion

**Child 1 month–12 years** initially by *intravenous injection* 0.1–1 micrograms/kg over at least 30 seconds (omitted if not required) then by *intravenous infusion* 0.05–1.3 micrograms/kg/minute according to anaesthetic technique and adjusted according to response; additional doses can be given by *intravenous injection* during the intravenous infusion

**Child 12–18 years** initially by *intravenous injection* 0.1–1 micrograms/kg over at least 30 seconds (omitted if not required) then by *intravenous infusion* 0.05–2 micrograms/kg/minute according to anaesthetic technique and adjusted according to response; additional doses can be given by *intravenous injection* during the intravenous infusion

**Administration**   for *intravenous injection*, reconstitute to a concentration of 1 mg/mL; for *continuous intravenous infusion*, dilute further with Glucose 5% or Sodium Chloride 0.9% to a concentration of 20–25 micrograms/mL for Child 1–12 years or 20–250 micrograms/mL (usually 50 micrograms/mL) for Child 12–18 years

**Remifentanil** (Non-proprietary) CD2
Injection, powder for reconstitution, remifentanil (as hydrochloride), net price 1-mg vial = £4.60; 2-mg vial = £9.20; 5-mg vial = £23.00

**Ultiva®** (GSK) CD2
Injection, powder for reconstitution, remifentanil (as hydrochloride), net price 1-mg vial = £5.12; 2-mg vial = £10.23; 5-mg vial = £25.58

### 15.1.4.4   Other drugs for sedation

This section is not included in *BNF for Children*.

### 15.1.5   Neuromuscular blocking drugs

**Important**
The drugs in this section should only be administered by, or under the direct supervision of, personnel experienced in their use, with adequate training in anaesthesia and airway management.

Neuromuscular blocking drugs used in anaesthesia are also known as **muscle relaxants**. By specific blockade of the neuromuscular junction they enable light anaesthesia to be used with adequate relaxation of the muscles of the abdomen and diaphragm. They also relax the vocal cords and allow the passage of a tracheal tube.

Their action differs from the muscle relaxants used in musculoskeletal disorders (section 10.2.2) that act on the spinal cord or brain.

Children who have received a neuromuscular blocking drug should **always** have their respiration assisted or controlled until the drug has been inactivated or antagonised (section 15.1.6). They should also receive sufficient concomitant inhalational or intravenous anaesthetic or sedative drugs to prevent awareness.

## Non-depolarising neuromuscular blocking drugs

Non-depolarising neuromuscular blocking drugs (also known as competitive muscle relaxants) compete with acetylcholine for receptor sites at the neuromuscular junction and their action can be reversed with anticholinesterases, such as neostigmine (section 15.1.6). Non-depolarising neuromuscular blocking drugs can be divided into the **aminosteroid** group, comprising pancuronium, rocuronium, and vecuronium, and the **benzylisoquinolinium** group, which includes atracurium, cisatracurium, and mivacurium.

Non-depolarising neuromuscular blocking drugs have a slower onset of action than suxamethonium. These drugs can be classified by their duration of action as short-acting (15–30 minutes), intermediate-acting (30–40 minutes), and long-acting (60–120 minutes), although duration of action is dose-dependent. Drugs with a shorter or intermediate duration of action, such as atracurium and vecuronium, are more widely used than those with a longer duration of action, such as pancuronium.

Non-depolarising neuromuscular blocking drugs have no sedative or analgesic effects and are not considered to trigger malignant hyperthermia.

For children receiving intensive care and who require tracheal intubation and mechanical ventilation, a non-depolarising neuromuscular blocking drug is chosen according to its onset of effect, duration of action, and side-effects. Rocuronium, with a rapid onset of effect, may facilitate intubation. Atracurium or cisatracurium may be suitable for long-term neuromuscular blockade since their duration of action is not dependent on elimination by the liver or the kidneys.

**Cautions**   Allergic cross-reactivity between neuromuscular blocking drugs has been reported; caution is advised in cases of hypersensitivity to these drugs. Their activity is prolonged in children with myasthenia gravis and in hypothermia, therefore lower doses are required. Non-depolarising neuromuscular blocking drugs should be used with great care in those with other neuromuscular disorders and those with fluid and electrolyte disturbances, as response in these children is unpredictable. Resistance may develop in children with burns who may require increased doses; low plasma cholinesterase activity in these children requires dose titration for mivacurium. The rate of administration of neuromuscular blocking drugs should be reduced in children with cardiovascular disease. **Interactions:** Appendix 1 (muscle relaxants).

**Pregnancy**   Non-depolarising neuromuscular blocking drugs are highly ionised at physiological pH and are therefore unlikely to cross the placenta in significant amounts.

**Breast-feeding** Because they are ionised at physiological pH, non-depolarising neuromuscular blocking drugs are unlikely to be present in milk in significant amounts. Breast-feeding may be resumed once the mother has recovered from neuromuscular block.

**Side-effects** Benzylisoquinolinium non-depolarising neuromuscular blocking drugs (except cisatracurium) are associated with histamine release, which can cause skin flushing, hypotension, tachycardia, bronchospasm, and very rarely, anaphylactoid reactions. Most aminosteroid neuromuscular blocking drugs produce minimal histamine release. Drugs with vagolytic activity can counteract any bradycardia that occurs during surgery. Acute myopathy has also been reported after prolonged use in intensive care.

**Atracurium**, a mixture of 10 isomers, is a benzylisoquinolinium neuromuscular blocking drug with an intermediate duration of action. It undergoes non-enzymatic metabolism which is independent of liver and kidney function, thus allowing its use in children with hepatic or renal impairment. Cardiovascular effects are associated with significant histamine release; histamine release can be minimised by administering slowly or in divided doses over at least 1 minute. Neonates may be more sensitive to the effects of atracurium and lower doses may be required.

**Cisatracurium** is a single isomer of atracurium. It is more potent and has a slightly longer duration of action than atracurium and provides greater cardiovascular stability because cisatracurium lacks histamine-releasing effects. In children aged 1 month to 12 years, cisatracurium has a shorter duration of action and produces faster spontaneous recovery.

**Mivacurium**, a benzylisoquinolinium neuromuscular blocking drug, has a short duration of action. It is metabolised by plasma cholinesterase and muscle paralysis is prolonged in individuals deficient in this enzyme. It is not associated with vagolytic activity or ganglionic blockade although histamine release can occur, particularly with rapid injection. In children under 12 years mivacurium has a faster onset, shorter duration of action, and produces more rapid spontaneous recovery.

**Pancuronium**, an aminosteroid neuromuscular blocking drug, has a long duration of action and is often used in children receiving long-term mechanical ventilation in intensive care units. It lacks a histamine-releasing effect, but vagolytic and sympathomimetic effects can cause tachycardia and hypertension. The half-life of pancuronium is prolonged in neonates; neonates should receive postoperative intermittent positive pressure ventilation.

**Rocuronium** exerts an effect within 2 minutes and has the most rapid onset of any of the non-depolarising neuromuscular blocking drugs. It is an aminosteroid neuromuscular blocking drug with an intermediate duration of action. It is reported to have minimal cardiovascular effects; high doses produce mild vagolytic activity. In most children, the duration of action of rocuronium may be shorter than in adults; however, in neonates and children under 2 years, usual doses may produce a more prolonged action.

**Vecuronium**, an aminosteroid neuromuscular blocking drug, has an intermediate duration of action. It does not generally produce histamine release and lacks cardiovascular effects. In most children, the duration of action of vecuronium may be shorter than in adults; however, in neonates and children under 2 years, usual doses may produce a more prolonged action.

## ATRACURIUM BESILATE
(Atracurium besylate)

**Cautions** see notes above
**Pregnancy** see notes above
**Breast-feeding** see notes above
**Side-effects** see notes above; seizures also reported
**Licensed use** not licensed for use in neonates
**Indications and dose**

> To avoid excessive dosage in obese children, dose should be calculated on the basis of ideal weight for height

**Neuromuscular blockade (short to intermediate duration) for surgery**
- **By intravenous administration**

  **Neonate** initially by *intravenous injection* 300–500 micrograms/kg followed *either* by *intravenous injection*, 100–200 micrograms/kg repeated as necessary *or* by *intravenous infusion*, 300–400 micrograms/kg/hour adjusted according to response

  **Child 1 month–18 years** initially by *intravenous injection* 300–600 micrograms/kg then 100–200 micrograms/kg repeated as necessary *or* initially by *intravenous injection* 200–600 micrograms/kg followed by *intravenous infusion*, 300–600 micrograms/kg/hour adjusted according to response

**Neuromuscular blockade during intensive care**
- **By intravenous administration**

  **Neonate** initially by *intravenous injection* 300–500 micrograms/kg followed *either* by *intravenous injection*, 100–200 micrograms/kg repeated as necessary *or* by *intravenous infusion*, 300–400 micrograms/kg/hour adjusted according to response; higher doses may be necessary

  **Child 1 month–18 years** initially by *intravenous injection* 300–600 micrograms/kg (optional) then by *intravenous infusion*, 270–1770 micrograms/kg/hour (usual dose 650–780 micrograms/kg/hour)

**Administration** for *continuous intravenous infusion*, dilute to a concentration of 0.5–5 mg/mL with Glucose 5% *or* Sodium Chloride 0.9%; stability varies with diluent.

*Neonatal intensive care*, dilute 60 mg/kg body-weight to a final volume of 50 mL with Glucose 5% or Sodium Chloride 0.9%; minimum concentration of 500 micrograms/mL, max. concentration of 5 mg/mL; an intravenous infusion rate of 0.1 mL/hour provides a dose of 120 micrograms/kg/hour

**Atracurium** (Non-proprietary) ᴾᵒᴹ
Injection, atracurium besilate 10 mg/mL, net price 2.5-mL amp = £1.85; 5-mL amp = £3.37; 25-mL vial = £14.45

**Tracrium**® (GSK) ᴾᵒᴹ
Injection, atracurium besilate 10 mg/mL, net price 2.5-mL amp = £1.66; 5-mL amp = £3.00; 25-mL vial = £12.91

**15**

**Anaesthesia**

## CISATRACURIUM

**Cautions**   see notes above
**Pregnancy**   see notes above
**Breast-feeding**   see notes above
**Side-effects**   see notes above; also bradycardia
**Indications and dose**

> To avoid excessive dosage in obese children, dose should be calculated on the basis of ideal weight for height

### Neuromuscular blockade (intermediate duration) during surgery

- **By intravenous injection**

  **Child 1 month–2 years** initially 150 micrograms/kg, then 30 micrograms/kg repeated approx. every 20 minutes as necessary

  **Child 2–12 years** initially 150 micrograms/kg (80–100 micrograms/kg if not for intubation), then 20 micrograms/kg repeated approx. every 10 minutes as necessary

  **Child 12–18 years** initially 150 micrograms/kg, then 30 micrograms/kg repeated approx. every 20 minutes as necessary

- **By intravenous administration**

  **Child 2–18 years** initially 150 micrograms/kg by *intravenous injection*, then by *intravenous infusion* 180 micrograms/kg/hour, reduced to 60–120 micrograms/kg/hour according to response

**Administration**   for *continuous intravenous infusion*, dilute to a concentration of 0.1–2 mg/mL with Glucose 5% or Sodium Chloride 0.9%; solutions of 2 mg/mL and 5 mg/mL may be infused undiluted

**Cisatracurium** (Non-proprietary) PoM
Injection, cisatracurium (as besilate) 2 mg/mL, net price 10-mL vial = £7.55; 5 mg/mL, 30-mL vial = £31.09

**Nimbex®** (GSK) PoM
Injection, cisatracurium (as besilate) 2 mg/mL, net price 10-mL amp = £7.55

Forte injection, cisatracurium (as besilate) 5 mg/mL, net price 30-mL vial = £31.09

## MIVACURIUM

**Cautions**   see notes above; low plasma cholinesterase activity
**Hepatic impairment**   reduce dose in severe impairment
**Renal impairment**   clinical effect prolonged in renal failure—reduce dose according to response
**Pregnancy**   see notes above
**Breast-feeding**   see notes above
**Side-effects**   see notes above
**Indications and dose**

> To avoid excessive dosage in obese children, dose should be calculated on the basis of ideal weight for height

### Neuromuscular blockade (short duration) during surgery

- **By intravenous administration**

  **Child 2–6 months** by *intravenous injection* initially 150 micrograms/kg, then *either* by *intravenous injection* 100 micrograms/kg repeated every 6–9 minutes as necessary *or* by *intravenous infusion*, 8–10 micrograms/kg/minute, adjusted if necessary every 3 minutes by 1 microgram/kg/minute to usual dose 11–14 micrograms/kg/minute

  **Child 6 months–12 years** by *intravenous injection* initially 200 micrograms/kg, then *either* by *intravenous injection* 100 micrograms/kg repeated every 6–9 minutes as necessary *or* by *intravenous infusion*, 8–10 micrograms/kg/minute, adjusted if necessary every 3 minutes by 1 microgram/kg/minute to usual dose 11–14 micrograms/kg/minute

  **Child 12–18 years** by *intravenous injection* initially 70–250 micrograms/kg, then *either* by *intravenous injection* 100 micrograms/kg repeated every 15 minutes as necessary *or* by *intravenous infusion*, 8–10 micrograms/kg/minute, adjusted if necessary every 3 minutes by 1 microgram/kg/minute to usual dose of 6–7 micrograms/kg/minute

**Administration**   for *intravenous injection*, give undiluted or dilute in Glucose 5% or Sodium Chloride 0.9%. Doses up to 150 micrograms/kg may be given over 5–15 seconds, higher doses should be given over 30 seconds. In asthma, cardiovascular disease or in those sensitive to reduced arterial blood pressure, give over 60 seconds.

**Mivacron®** (GSK) PoM
Injection, mivacurium (as chloride) 2 mg/mL, net price 5-mL amp = £2.79; 10-mL amp = £4.51

## PANCURONIUM BROMIDE

**Cautions**   see notes above
**Hepatic impairment**   possibly slower onset, higher dose requirement, and prolonged recovery time
**Renal impairment**   use with caution; prolonged duration of block
**Pregnancy**   see notes above
**Breast-feeding**   see notes above
**Side-effects**   see notes above
**Indications and dose**

> To avoid excessive dosage in obese children, dose should be calculated on the basis of ideal weight for height

### Neuromuscular blockade (long duration) during surgery

- **By intravenous injection**

  **Neonate** initially 100 micrograms/kg, then 50 micrograms/kg repeated as necessary

  **Child 1 month–18 years** initially 100 micrograms/kg, then 20 micrograms/kg repeated as necessary

**Administration**   for *intravenous injection*, give undiluted or dilute in Glucose 5% or Sodium Chloride 0.9%

**Pancuronium** (Non-proprietary) PoM
Injection, pancuronium bromide 2 mg/mL, net price 2-mL amp = £1.20

15   Anaesthesia

## ROCURONIUM BROMIDE

**Cautions** see notes above

**Hepatic impairment** reduce dose

**Renal impairment** reduce maintenance dose; prolonged paralysis

**Pregnancy** see notes above

**Breast-feeding** see notes above

**Side-effects** see notes above

**Licensed use** not licensed for use in children for assisted ventilation in intensive care

**Indications and dose**

> To avoid excessive dosage in obese children, dose should be calculated on the basis of ideal weight for height

### Neuromuscular blockade (intermediate duration) during surgery

• **By intravenous administration**

**Neonate** initially by *intravenous injection* 600 micrograms/kg, then *either* by *intravenous injection*, 150 micrograms/kg repeated as required *or* by *intravenous infusion*, 300–600 micrograms/kg/hour adjusted according to reponse

**Child 1 month–18 years** initially by *intravenous injection* 600 micrograms/kg, then *either* by *intravenous injection*, 150 micrograms/kg repeated as required *or* by *intravenous infusion*, 300–600 micrograms/kg/hour adjusted according to response

### Assisted ventilation in intensive care

• **By intravenous administration**

**Child 1 month–18 years** initially by *intravenous injection* 600 micrograms/kg (optional), then by *intravenous infusion*, 300–600 micrograms/kg/hour for first hour, then adjusted according to response

**Administration** for *continuous intravenous infusion* or via drip tubing, may be diluted with Glucose 5% *or* Sodium Chloride 0.9%

**Rocuronium** (Non-proprietary) [PoM]
Injection, rocuronium bromide 10 mg/mL, net price 5-mL vial = £3.00, 10-mL vial = £6.00

**Esmeron®** (MSD) [PoM]
Injection, rocuronium bromide 10 mg/mL, net price 5-mL vial = £2.90, 10-mL vial = £5.79

## VECURONIUM BROMIDE

**Cautions** see notes above

**Hepatic impairment** caution in significant impairment

**Renal impairment** caution in renal failure

**Pregnancy** see notes above

**Breast-feeding** see notes above

**Side-effects** see notes above

**Licensed use** not licensed for assisted ventilation in intensive care

**Indications and dose**

> To avoid excessive dosage in obese children, dose should be calculated on the basis of ideal weight for height

### Neuromuscular blockade (intermediate duration) during surgery

• **By intravenous administration**

**Neonate** by *intravenous injection* initially 80 micrograms/kg, then 30–50 micrograms/kg adjusted according to response

**Child 1 month–18 years** by *intravenous injection* initially 80–100 micrograms/kg, then *either* by *intravenous injection*, 20–30 micrograms/kg repeated as required *or* by *intravenous infusion*, 0.8–1.4 micrograms/kg/minute, adjusted according to response

### Assisted ventilation in intensive care

• **By intravenous injection**

**Neonate** initially 80 micrograms/kg, then 30–50 micrograms/kg adjusted according to response

• **By intravenous administration**

**Neonate** by *intravenous injection* 80 micrograms/kg, then by *intravenous infusion*, 0.8–1.4 micrograms/kg/minute, adjusted according to response (risk of accumulation—consider interruption of infusion)

**Child 1 month–18 years** initially by *intravenous injection* 80–100 micrograms/kg (optional), then by *intravenous infusion* 0.8–1.4 micrograms/kg/minute, adjusted according to response; up to 3 micrograms/kg/minute may be required

**Administration** reconstitute each vial with 5 mL Water for Injections to give 2 mg/mL solution; *alternatively* reconstitute with up to 10 mL Glucose 5% *or* Sodium Chloride 0.9% *or* Water for Injections—unsuitable for further dilution if not reconstituted with Water for Injections.

For *continuous intravenous infusion*, dilute reconstituted solution to a concentration up to 40 micrograms/mL with Glucose 5% *or* Sodium Chloride 0.9%; reconstituted solution can also be given via drip tubing.

*Neonatal intensive care*, reconstitute each vial with 5 mL Water for Injections to give a 2 mg/mL solution. Dilute 5 mg/kg body-weight to a final volume of 50 mL with Glucose 5% or Sodium Chloride 0.9%; an intravenous infusion rate of 0.5 mL/hour provides a dose of 50 micrograms/kg/hour; minimum concentration of 40 micrograms/mL

**Norcuron®** (Organon) [PoM]
Injection, powder for reconstitution, vecuronium bromide, net price 10-mg vial = £3.38 (with water for injections)

# Depolarising neuromuscular blocking drugs

**Suxamethonium** has the most rapid onset of action of any of the neuromuscular blocking drugs and is ideal if fast onset and brief duration of action are required e.g. with tracheal intubation. Neonates and young children are less sensitive to suxamethonium and a higher dose may be required.

Suxamethonium acts by mimicking acetylcholine at the neuromuscular junction but hydrolysis is much slower than for acetylcholine; depolarisation is therefore prolonged, resulting in neuromuscular blockade. Unlike the non-depolarising neuromuscular blocking drugs, its action cannot be reversed and recovery is spontaneous;

**15 Anaesthesia**

anticholinesterases such as neostigmine potentiate the neuromuscular block.

Suxamethonium should be given after anaesthetic induction because paralysis is usually preceded by painful muscle fasciculations. Bradycardia may occur; premedication with atropine (section 15.1.3) reduces bradycardia as well as the excessive salivation associated with suxamethonium use.

Prolonged paralysis may occur in **dual block**, which occurs with high or repeated doses of suxamethonium and is caused by the development of a non-depolarising block following the initial depolarising block; edrophonium (section 15.1.6) may be used to confirm the diagnosis of dual block. Children with myasthenia gravis are resistant to suxamethonium but can develop dual block resulting in delayed recovery. Prolonged paralysis may also occur in those with low or atypical plasma cholinesterase. Assisted ventilation should be continued until muscle function is restored.

### SUXAMETHONIUM CHLORIDE
(Succinylcholine chloride)

**Cautions** see notes above; hypersensitivity to other neuromuscular blocking drugs; patients with cardiac, respiratory or neuromuscular disease; raised intraocular pressure (avoid in penetrating eye injury); severe sepsis (risk of hyperkalaemia); **interactions:** Appendix 1 (muscle relaxants)

**Contra-indications** family history of malignant hyperthermia, hyperkalaemia; major trauma, severe burns, neurological disease involving acute wasting of major muscle, prolonged immobilisation—risk of hyperkalaemia; personal or family history of congenital myotonic disease, Duchenne muscular dystrophy; low plasma-cholinesterase activity (including severe liver disease, see below)

**Hepatic impairment** prolonged apnoea may occur in severe liver disease because of reduced hepatic synthesis of pseudocholinesterase

**Pregnancy** mildly prolonged neuromuscular blockade may occur

**Breast-feeding** unlikely to be present in breast milk in significant amounts (ionised at physiological pH); breast-feeding may be resumed once the mother recovered from neuromuscular block

**Side-effects** see notes above; also increased gastric pressure; hyperkalaemia; postoperative muscle pain, myoglobinuria, myoglobinaemia; increased intraocular pressure; flushing, rash; *rarely* arrhythmias, cardiac arrest; bronchospasm, apnoea, prolonged respiratory depression; limited jaw mobility; *very rarely* anaphylactic reactions, malignant hyperthermia; *also reported* hypertension, hypotension, rhabdomyolysis

**Indications and dose**

> **Neuromuscular blockade (short duration) during surgery**
> * By intravenous injection
>   > **Neonate** 2 mg/kg produces 5–10 minutes neuromuscular blockade
>   > **Child 1 month–1 year** 2 mg/kg
>   > **Child 1–18 years** 1 mg/kg
> * By intramuscular injection (onset in 2–3 minutes)
>   > **Neonate** up to 4 mg/kg produces 10–30 minutes neuromuscular blockade
>   > **Child 1 month–1 year** up to 4–5 mg/kg
>   > **Child 1–12 years** up to 4 mg/kg; max. 150 mg

**Administration** for *intravenous injection*, give undiluted *or* dilute with Glucose 5% *or* Sodium Chloride 0.9%

**Suxamethonium Chloride** (Non-proprietary) [PoM]
Injection, suxamethonium chloride 50 mg/mL, net price 2-mL amp = 58p, 2-mL prefilled syringe = £8.45

**Anectine®** (GSK) [PoM]
Injection, suxamethonium chloride 50 mg/mL, net price 2-mL amp = 71p

---

### 15.1.6 Drugs for reversal of neuromuscular blockade

> **Important**
> The drugs in this section should only be administered by, or under the direct supervision of, personnel experienced in their use.

## Anticholinesterases

Anticholinesterases reverse the effects of the non-depolarising (competitive) neuromuscular blocking drugs such as pancuronium, but they prolong the action of the depolarising neuromuscular blocking drug suxamethonium.

**Edrophonium** has a transient action and may be used in the diagnosis of suspected dual block due to suxamethonium. Atropine (section 15.1.3) is given before or with edrophonium to prevent muscarinic effects of edrophonium; it is also used in the diagnosis of myasthenia gravis (section 10.2.1).

**Neostigmine** has a longer duration of action than edrophonium and is used specifically for reversal of non-depolarising (competitive) blockade. It acts within one minute of intravenous injection and its effects last for 20 to 30 minutes; a second dose may then be necessary. Glycopyrronium or alternatively atropine (section 15.1.3), given before or with neostigmine, prevent bradycardia, excessive salivation, and other muscarinic effects of neostigmine.

### EDROPHONIUM CHLORIDE

**Cautions** section 10.2.1; atropine should also be given
**Contra-indications** section 10.2.1
**Pregnancy** section 10.2.1
**Breast-feeding** section 10.2.1
**Side-effects** section 10.2.1
**Indications and dose**

> **Brief reversal of non-depolarising neuromuscular blockade**
> * By intravenous injection over several minutes
>   > **Child 1 month–18 years** 500–700 micrograms/kg (after or with atropine)
>
> **Myasthenia gravis** section 10.2.1

**Edrophonium** (Non-proprietary) [PoM]
Injection, edrophonium chloride 10 mg/mL, net price 1-mL amp = £19.50

## NEOSTIGMINE METILSULFATE
(Neostigmine methylsulfate)

**Cautions** section 10.2.1; glycopyrronium or atropine should also be given

**Contra-indications** section 10.2.1

**Renal impairment** section 10.2.1

**Pregnancy** section 10.2.1

**Breast-feeding** section 10.2.1

**Side-effects** section 10.2.1

**Indications and dose**

Reversal of non-depolarising muscle block

- By intravenous injection over 1 minute

    **Neonate** 50 micrograms/kg, after or with glyco-pyrronium or atropine; a further dose of 25 micro-grams/kg may be required

    **Child 1 month–12 years** 50 micrograms/kg (max. 2.5 mg) after or with glycopyrronium or atropine; a further dose of 25 micrograms/kg may be required

    **Child 12–18 years** 50 micrograms/kg (max. 2.5 mg) after or with glycopyrronium or atropine; a further dose of 25 micrograms/kg (max. 2.5 mg) may be required

    Myasthenia gravis section 10.2.1

**Administration** for *intravenous injection*, give undiluted *or* dilute with Glucose 5% *or* Sodium Chloride 0.9%

**Neostigmine** (Non-proprietary) PoM
Injection, neostigmine metilsulfate 2.5 mg/mL, net price 1-mL amp = 58p

◀With glycopyrronium

**Glycopyrronium-Neostigmine** (Non-proprietary) PoM
Injection, neostigmine metilsulfate 2.5 mg, glyco-pyrronium bromide 500 micrograms/mL, net price 1-mL amp = 91p

Dose

Reversal of non-depolarising neuromuscular blockade

- By intravenous injection over 10–30 seconds

    **Child 1 month–18 years** 0.02 mL/kg (or 0.2 mL/kg of a 1 in 10 dilution), dose may be repeated if required (total max. 2 mL)

    **Administration** for *intravenous injection*, may be diluted with Sodium Chloride 0.9%

## Other drugs for reversal of neuromuscular blockade

**Sugammadex** is a modified gamma cyclodextrin that can be used for rapid reversal of neuromuscular blockade induced by rocuronium (section 15.1.5). In practice, sugammadex is used mainly for rapid reversal of neuromuscular blockade in an emergency.

The *Scottish Medicines Consortium*, p. 3 has advised (February 2013) that sugammadex (*Bridion®*) is accepted for restricted use within NHS Scotland for the routine reversal of neuromuscular blockade in high-risk patients only, or where prompt reversal of neuromuscular block is required.

## SUGAMMADEX

**Cautions** recurrence of neuromuscular blockade—monitor respiratory function until fully recovered; recovery may be delayed in cardiovascular disease;

pre-existing coagulation disorders or use of anticoagulants (unrelated to surgery); wait 24 hours before re-administering rocuronium; **interactions:** Appendix 1 (sugammadex)

**Renal impairment** avoid if estimated glomerular filtration rate less then 30 mL/minute/1.73 m$^2$

**Pregnancy** use with caution—no information available

**Side-effects** taste disturbances; *less commonly* allergic reactions; bronchospasm also reported

**Indications and dose**

Routine reversal of neuromuscular blockade induced by rocuronium

- By intravenous injection

    **Child 2–18 years** 2 mg/kg (consult product literature)

**Administration** for *intravenous injection* dose may be diluted to a concentration of 10 mg/mL with Sodium Chloride 0.9%

**Bridion®** (Schering-Plough) PoM
Injection, sugammadex (as sodium salt) 100 mg/mL, net price 2-mL amp = £59.64, 5-mL amp = £149.10
**Electrolytes** Na$^+$ 0.42 mmol/mL

## 15.1.7  Antagonists for central and respiratory depression

> **Important**
> The drugs in this section should only be administered by, or under the direct supervision of, personnel experienced in their use.

Respiratory depression is a major concern with opioid analgesics and it may be treated by artificial ventilation or be reversed by an opioid antagonist. **Naloxone** given intravenously immediately reverses opioid-induced respiratory depression but the dose may have to be repeated because of its **short duration of action**. Intramuscular injection of naloxone produces a more gradual and prolonged effect but absorption may be erratic. Care is required in children requiring pain relief because naloxone also antagonises the analgesic effect of opioids.

**Neonates**  Naloxone is used in newborn infants to reverse respiratory depression and sedation resulting from the use of opioids by the mother, usually for pain during labour. In neonates the effects of opioids may persist for up to 48 hours and in such cases naloxone is often given by intramuscular injection for its prolonged effect. In severe respiratory depression after birth, breathing should first be established (using artificial means if necessary) and naloxone administered only if use of opioids by the mother is thought to cause the respiratory depression; the infant should be monitored closely and further doses of naloxone administered as necessary.

**Flumazenil** is a benzodiazepine antagonist for the reversal of the central sedative effects of benzodiazepines after anaesthetic and similar procedures. Flumazenil has a shorter half-life and duration of action than diazepam and midazolam, so children may become resedated.

15 Anaesthesia

## FLUMAZENIL

**Cautions** short-acting (repeat doses may be necessary—benzodiazepine effects may persist for at least 24 hours); benzodiazepine dependence (may precipitate withdrawal symptoms); prolonged benzodiazepine therapy for epilepsy (risk of convulsions); history of panic disorders (risk of recurrence); ensure neuromuscular blockade cleared before giving; avoid rapid injection in high-risk or anxious children and following major surgery; head injury (rapid reversal of benzodiazepine sedation may cause convulsions)

**Contra-indications** life-threatening condition (e.g. raised intracranial pressure, status epilepticus) controlled by benzodiazepines

**Hepatic impairment** carefully titrate dose

**Pregnancy** not known to be harmful

**Breast-feeding** avoid breast-feeding for 24 hours

**Side-effects** nausea and vomiting; *less commonly* palpitation, anxiety, fear; *also reported* transient hypertension, tachycardia, flushing, agitation, convulsions (particularly in those with epilepsy), dizziness, sensory disturbance, chills, sweating

**Licensed use** not licensed for use in children under 1 year; not licensed for use by intravenous infusion in children; not licensed for use in children in intensive care

**Indications and dose**

> **Reversal of sedative effects of benzodiazepines**
> * **By intravenous injection over 15 seconds**
>> **Neonate** 10 micrograms/kg, repeat at 1-minute intervals if required
>> **Child 1 month–18 years** 10 micrograms/kg (max. 200 micrograms), repeated at 1-minute intervals if required; max. total dose of 50 micrograms/kg (1 mg) (2 mg in intensive care)
> * **By intravenous infusion, if drowsiness recurs after injection**
>> **Neonate** 2–10 micrograms/kg/hour, adjusted according to response
>> **Child 1 month–18 years** 2–10 micrograms/kg/hour, adjusted according to response; max. 400 micrograms/hour

> **Overdosage with benzodiazepines** see Emergency Treatment of Poisoning p. 29

**Administration** for *continuous intravenous infusion*, dilute with Glucose 5% *or* Sodium Chloride 0.9%

**Flumazenil** (Non-proprietary) [PoM]
Injection, flumazenil 100 micrograms/mL, net price 5-mL amp = £14.49

**Anexate**® (Roche) [PoM]
Injection, flumazenil 100 micrograms/mL, net price 5-mL amp = £13.66

## NALOXONE HYDROCHLORIDE

**Cautions** cardiovascular disease or those receiving cardiotoxic drugs (serious adverse cardiovascular effects reported); maternal physical dependence on opioids (may precipitate withdrawal in newborn); pain (see also under Titration of Dose, below); has short duration of action (see notes above)

**Titration of dose** In postoperative use, the dose should be titrated for each child in order to obtain sufficient respiratory response; however, naloxone antagonises analgesia

**Pregnancy** use only if potential benefit outweighs risk

**Breast-feeding** not orally bioavailable

**Side-effects** nausea, vomiting; hypotension, hypertension, ventricular tachycardia and fibrillation, cardiac arrest; hyperventilation, dyspnoea, pulmonary oedema; headache, dizziness; *less commonly* diarrhoea, dry mouth, agitation, excitement, paraesthesia, tremor, sweating; *very rarely* seizures and erythema multiforme

**Indications and dose**

> **Reversal of respiratory and CNS depression in neonate following maternal opioid use during labour**
> * **By intramuscular injection**
>> **Neonate** 200 micrograms (60 micrograms/kg) as a single dose at birth
> * **By intravenous or subcutaneous injection**
>> **Neonate** 10 micrograms/kg, repeated every 2–3 minutes if required

> **Reversal of postoperative respiratory depression**
> * **By intravenous injection**
>> **Neonate** 1 microgram/kg, repeated every 2–3 minutes if required
>> **Child 1 month–12 years** 1 microgram/kg, repeated every 2–3 minutes if required
>> **Child 12–18 years** 1.5–3 micrograms/kg; if response inadequate, give subsequent doses of 100 micrograms every 2 minutes

> **Overdosage with opioids** see Emergency Treatment of Poisoning, p. 27

◢ **Preparation**
See Emergency Treatment of Poisoning, p. 28

## 15.1.8 Drugs for malignant hyperthermia

> **Important**
> The drugs in this section should only be administered by, or under the direct supervision of, personnel experienced in their use.

Malignant hyperthermia is a rare but potentially lethal complication of anaesthesia. It is characterised by a rapid rise in temperature, increased muscle rigidity, tachycardia, and acidosis. The most common triggers of malignant hyperthermia are the volatile anaesthetics. Suxamethonium has also been implicated, but malignant hyperthermia is more likely if it is given following a volatile anaesthetic. Volatile anaesthetics and suxamethonium should be avoided during anaesthesia in children at high risk of malignant hyperthermia.

**Dantrolene** is used in the treatment of malignant hyperthermia. It acts on skeletal muscle cells by interfering with calcium efflux, thereby stopping the contractile process.

## DANTROLENE SODIUM

**Cautions** avoid extravasation (risk of tissue necrosis); **interactions:** Appendix 1 (muscle relaxants)

**Pregnancy** use only if potential benefit outweighs risk

**Breast-feeding** present in milk—use only if potential benefit outweighs risk

**Side-effects** hepatotoxicity, pulmonary oedema, dizziness, weakness, and injection-site reactions including erythema, rash, swelling, and thrombophlebitis

**Licensed use** not licensed for use in children

**Indications and dose**

> **Malignant hyperthermia**
> - By rapid intravenous injection
>     **Child 1 month–18 years** initially 2–3 mg/kg, then 1 mg/kg repeated as required (total max. dose 10 mg/kg)

> **Chronic severe spasticity of voluntary muscle** see section 10.2.2

**Dantrium Intravenous**® (SpePharm) PoM

Injection, powder for reconstitution, dantrolene sodium, net price 20-mg vial = £51.00 (hosp. only)

# 15.2 Local anaesthesia

> **Important**
>
> The drugs in section 15.2 should only be administered by, or under the direct supervision of, personnel experienced in their use, with adequate training in anaesthesia and airway management, and should not be administered parenterally unless adequate resuscitation equipment is available.

The use of local anaesthetics by injection or by application to mucous membranes to produce local analgesia is discussed in this section.

See also section 1.7 (anus), section 11.7 (eye), section 12.3 (oropharynx), and section 13.3 (skin).

**Use of local anaesthetics** Local anaesthetic drugs act by causing a reversible block to conduction along nerve fibres. They vary widely in their potency, toxicity, duration of action, stability, solubility in water, and ability to penetrate mucous membranes. These factors determine their application, e.g. topical (surface), infiltration, peripheral nerve block, intravenous regional anaesthesia (Bier's block), plexus, epidural (extradural), or spinal (intrathecal or subarachnoid) block. Local anaesthetics may also be used for postoperative pain relief, thereby reducing the need for analgesics such as opioids.

**Administration** The dose of local anaesthetic depends on the injection site and the procedure used. In determining the safe dosage, it is important to take account of the rate of absorption and excretion, and of the potency. The child's age, weight, physique, and clinical condition, and the vascularity of the administration site and the duration of administration, must also be considered.

Uptake of local anaesthetics into the systemic circulation determines their duration of action and produces toxicity.

Great care must be taken to avoid accidental intravascular injection; local anaesthetic injections should be given slowly in order to detect inadvertent intravascular administration. When prolonged analgesia is required, a long-acting local anaesthetic is preferred to minimise the likelihood of cumulative systemic toxicity. Local anaesthesia around the oral cavity may impair swallowing and therefore increases the risk of aspiration.

Following most regional anaesthetic procedures, maximum arterial plasma concentration of anaesthetic develops within about 10 to 25 minutes, so **careful surveillance** for toxic effects (see Toxicity and Side-effects, p. 650) is necessary during the first 30 minutes after injection.

Epidural anaesthesia is combined with general anaesthesia for certain surgical procedures in children.

**Use of vasoconstrictors** Local anaesthetics cause dilatation of blood vessels. The addition of a vasoconstrictor such as **adrenaline (epinephrine)** to the local anaesthetic preparation diminishes local blood flow, slowing the rate of absorption and thereby prolonging the anaesthetic effect. Great care should be taken to avoid inadvertent intravenous administration of a preparation containing adrenaline, and it is **not** advisable to give adrenaline with a local anaesthetic injection in digits or appendages because of the risk of ischaemic necrosis.

Adrenaline must be used in a low concentration when administered with a local anaesthetic (but see also Dental Anaesthesia, below). The total dose of adrenaline should **not** exceed 5 micrograms/kg (1 mL/kg of a 1 in 200 000 solution) and it is essential not to exceed a concentration of 1 in 200 000 (5 micrograms/mL) if more than 50 mL of the mixture is to be injected. Care must also be taken to calculate a safe maximum dose of local anaesthetic when using combination products. For prescribing information on adrenaline, see section 2.7.2. For drug interactions of adrenaline, see Appendix 1 (sympathomimetics).

In children with severe hypertension or unstable cardiac rhythm, the use of adrenaline with a local anaesthetic may be hazardous. For these children an anaesthetic without adrenaline should be used.

**Dental anaesthesia** Lidocaine is widely used in dental procedures; it is most often used in combination with **adrenaline** (epinephrine). Lidocaine 2% combined with adrenaline 1 in 80 000 (12.5 micrograms/mL) is a safe and effective preparation; there is no justification for using higher concentrations of adrenaline. See also Use of Vasoconstrictors, above.

The local anaesthetics **articaine** and **mepivacaine** are also used in dentistry; they are available in cartridges suitable for dental use. Mepivacaine is available with or without adrenaline, and articaine is available with adrenaline.

In children with severe hypertension or unstable cardiac rhythm, mepivacaine without adrenaline may be used. Alternatively, **prilocaine** with or without felypressin can be used but there is no evidence that it is any safer. Felypressin can cause coronary vasoconstriction when used at high doses; limit dose in children with coronary artery disease.

**Cautions of local anaesthetics** Local anaesthetics should be administered with caution in children, especially if debilitated (consider dose reduction) or those with impaired cardiac conduction, cardiovascular disease, hypovolaemia, shock, impaired respiratory function, epilepsy, or myasthenia gravis. See also Administration and Use of Vasoconstrictors, above.

**Contra-indications of local anaesthetics** Local anaesthetics should not be injected into inflamed or infected tissues nor should they be applied to damaged skin. In such circumstances, increased absorption into the blood increases the possibility of systemic side-effects, and the local anaesthetic effect may also be reduced by altered local pH. See also Use of Vaso-constrictors, p. 649.

Local anaesthetic preparations containing preservatives should not be used for caudal, epidural, or spinal block, or for intravenous regional anaesthesia (Bier's block).

Local anaesthetics can cause ototoxicity and should not be applied to the middle ear. They are also contra-indicated in children with complete heart block.

**Toxicity and side-effects**  A single application of a topical lidocaine preparation does not generally cause systemic side-effects. Toxic effects after administration of local anaesthetics are a result of excessively high plasma concentrations; severe toxicity usually results from inadvertent intravascular injection or too rapid injection.

The systemic toxicity of local anaesthetics mainly involves the central nervous and cardiovascular systems. CNS effects include a feeling of inebriation and lightheadedness followed by drowsiness, numbness of the tongue and perioral region, restlessness, paraesthesia (including sensations of hot and cold), dizziness, blurred vision, tinnitus, nausea and vomiting, muscle twitching, tremors, and convulsions. Transient excitation may also occur, followed by depression with drowsiness, respiratory failure, unconsciousness, and coma. Effects on the cardiovascular system include myocardial depression and peripheral vasodilatation resulting in hypotension and bradycardia; arrhythmias and cardiac arrest can occur.

Hypersensitivity reactions occur mainly with the ester-type local anaesthetics, such as tetracaine; reactions are less frequent with the amide types, such as articaine, bupivacaine, levobupivacaine, lidocaine, mepivacaine, prilocaine, and ropivacaine. Cross-sensitivity reactions may be avoided by using the alternative chemical type.

## Articaine

**Articaine** is an amide-type local anaesthetic used for dental anaesthesia (see Dental Anaesthesia, p. 649). It is available in a preparation that also contains adrenaline (see Use of Vasoconstrictors, p. 649).

### ▌ ARTICAINE HYDROCHLORIDE WITH ADRENALINE
(Carticaine hydrochloride with adrenaline)

**Cautions**  see Cautions of Local Anaesthetics, p. 649 and Adrenaline, section 2.7.2

**Contra-indications**  see Contra-indications of Local Anaesthetics, p. 649 and Adrenaline, section 2.7.2

**Hepatic impairment**  use with caution; increased risk of side-effects in severe impairment

**Renal impairment**  see Adrenaline, section 2.7.2

**Pregnancy**  use only if potential benefit outweighs risk—no information available

**Breast-feeding**  avoid breast-feeding for 48 hours after administration

**Side-effects**  see Toxicity and Side-effects, above and Adrenaline, section 2.7.2; also methaemoglobinaemia (see Prilocaine (p. 653) for treatment)

**Indications and dose**

> To avoid excessive dosage in obese children, dose should be calculated on the basis of ideal weight for height

---

**Infiltration anaesthesia in dentistry**

> **Child 4–18 years** consult expert dental sources; **important**: see also Administration, p. 649

**Septanest®** (Septodont) ▢PoM▢
Injection, articaine hydrochloride 40 mg/mL, adrenaline 1 in 200 000 (5 micrograms/mL), net price 2.2-mL cartridge = 41p
**Excipients**  include sulfites

Injection, articaine hydrochloride 40 mg/mL, adrenaline 1 in 100 000 (10 micrograms/mL), net price 2.2-mL cartridge = 41p
**Excipients**  include sulfites

---

## Bupivacaine

**Bupivacaine** has a longer duration of action than other local anaesthetics. It has a slow onset of action, taking up to 30 minutes for full effect. It is often used in lumbar epidural blockade and is particularly suitable for continuous epidural analgesia in labour, or for postoperative pain relief. It is the principal drug used for spinal anaesthesia. Hyperbaric solutions containing glucose may be used for spinal block.

### ▌ BUPIVACAINE HYDROCHLORIDE

**Cautions**  see Cautions of Local Anaesthetics, p. 649; myocardial depression may be more severe and more resistant to treatment; cardiovascular disease; hypertension; hypotension; cerebral atheroma; **interactions**: Appendix 1 (bupivacaine)

**Contra-indications**  see Contra-indications of Local Anaesthetics, p. 649

**Hepatic impairment**  use with caution in severe impairment

**Renal impairment**  use with caution in severe impairment

**Pregnancy**  large doses during delivery can cause neonatal respiratory depression, hypotonia, and bradycardia after paracervical or epidural block; use lower doses for intrathecal use during late pregnancy

**Breast-feeding**  amount too small to be harmful

**Side-effects**  see Toxicity and Side-effects, above

**Indications and dose**

> To avoid excessive dosage in obese children, dose should be calculated on the basis of ideal weight for height

> Adjusted according to child's physical status and nature of procedure, seek expert advice—**important**: see also under Administration, p. 649

**Bupivacaine** (Non-proprietary) PoM

Injection, anhydrous bupivacaine hydrochloride 2.5 mg/mL (0.25%), net price 10 mL = 82p; 5 mg/mL (0.5%), 10 mL = 94p

Infusion, anhydrous bupivacaine hydrochloride 1 mg/mL (0.1%), net price 100 mL = £8.41; 250 mL = £10.59; 1.25 mg/mL (0.125%), 250 mL = £10.80

**Marcain®** (AstraZeneca) PoM

Injection, anhydrous bupivacaine hydrochloride 2.5 mg/mL (*Marcain® 0.25%*), net price 10-mL *Polyamp®* = £1.06; 5 mg/mL (*Marcain® 0.5%*), 10-mL *Polyamp®* = £1.21

**Marcain Heavy®** (AstraZeneca) PoM

Injection, anhydrous bupivacaine hydrochloride 5 mg/mL (0.5%), glucose 80 mg/mL, net price 4-mL amp = £1.21

◢**With adrenaline**

For prescribing information on adrenaline, see section 2.7.2; see also Use of Vasoconstrictors, p. 649

**Bupivacaine and Adrenaline** (Non-proprietary) PoM

Injection, anhydrous bupivacaine hydrochloride 2.5 mg/mL (0.25%), adrenaline 1 in 200 000 (5 micrograms/mL), net price 10-mL amp = £1.40

Injection, anhydrous bupivacaine hydrochloride 5 mg/mL (0.5%), adrenaline 1 in 200 000 (5 micrograms/mL), net price 10-mL amp = £1.50

## Levobupivacaine

Levobupivacaine, an isomer of bupivacaine, has anaesthetic and analgesic properties similar to bupivacaine but is thought to have fewer adverse effects.

### ▊ LEVOBUPIVACAINE

**Note** Levobupivacaine is an isomer of bupivacaine

**Cautions** see Cautions of Local Anaesthetics, p. 649; cardiovascular disease; **interactions:** Appendix 1 (levobupivacaine)

**Contra-indications** see Contra-indications of Local Anaesthetics, p. 649

**Hepatic impairment** use with caution

**Pregnancy** large doses during delivery can cause neonatal respiratory depression, hypotonia, and bradycardia after epidural block; avoid if possible in first trimester—toxicity in *animal* studies; may cause fetal distress syndrome; do not use for paracervical block in obstetrics; do not use 7.5 mg/mL strength in obstetrics

**Breast-feeding** amount too small to be harmful

**Side-effects** see Toxicity and Side-effects, p. 650; also sweating, pyrexia, anaemia

**Licensed use** not licensed for use in children except for analgesia by ilioinguinal or iliohypogastric block

**Indications and dose**

> To avoid excessive dosage in obese children, dose should be calculated on the basis of ideal weight for height

> Adjusted according to child's physical status and nature of procedure, seek expert advice—**important: see also under Administration, p. 649**

**Chirocaine®** (AbbVie) PoM

Injection, levobupivacaine (as hydrochloride) 2.5 mg/mL, net price 10-mL amp = £1.42; 5 mg/mL, 10-mL amp = £1.62; 7.5 mg/mL, 10-mL amp = £2.43

**Note** For 1.25 mg/mL concentration dilute standard solutions with sodium chloride 0.9%

Infusion, levobupivacaine (as hydrochloride) 625 micrograms/mL, net price 100 mL = £6.63; 200 mL = £10.37; 1.25 mg/mL, net price 100 mL = £7.26, 200 mL = £12.20

---

## Lidocaine

Lidocaine is effectively absorbed from mucous membranes and is a useful surface anaesthetic in concentrations up to 10%. Except for surface anaesthesia and dental anaesthesia, solutions should **not** usually exceed 1% in strength. The duration of the block (with adrenaline) is about 90 minutes.

Application of a mixture of lidocaine and prilocaine (*EMLA®*) under an occlusive dressing provides surface anaesthesia for 1–2 hours. *EMLA®* does not appear to be effective in providing local anaesthesia for heel lancing in neonates.

---

### ▊ LIDOCAINE HYDROCHLORIDE
(Lignocaine hydrochloride)

**Cautions** see Cautions of Local Anaesthetics, p. 649 and section 2.3.2; hypertension; topical preparations can damage plastic cuffs of endotracheal tubes

**Contra-indications** see notes above, Contra-indications of Local Anaesthetics (p. 649), and section 2.3.2

**Hepatic impairment** section 2.3.2

**Renal impairment** section 2.3.2

**Pregnancy** large doses can cause fetal bradycardia; large doses during delivery can cause neonatal respiratory depression, hypotonia, or bradycardia after paracervical or epidural block

**Breast-feeding** section 2.3.2

**Side-effects** see Toxicity and Side-effects, p. 650 and section 2.3.2; also methaemoglobinaemia (see Prilocaine (p. 653) for treatment), nystagmus, rash; hypoglycaemia also reported following intrathecal or extradural administration

**Indications and dose**

> To avoid excessive dosage in obese children, dose should be calculated on the basis of ideal weight for height

#### Infiltration anaesthesia

● **By injection**

(see also Administration, p. 649, and *Important* warning below)

**Neonate** according to nature of procedure, up to 3 mg/kg (0.3 mL/kg of 1% solution), repeated not more often than every 4 hours

**Child 1 month–12 years** according to nature of procedure, up to 3 mg/kg (0.3 mL/kg of 1% solution), repeated not more often than every 4 hours

**Child 12–18 years** according to weight of child and nature of procedure, max. 200 mg, repeated not more often than every 4 hours

Surface anaesthesia see preparations below

Ventricular arrhythmias, neonatal seizures section 2.3.2

Intravenous regional anaesthesia and nerve blocks seek expert advice

Dental anaesthesia seek expert advice

> Important
> The licensed doses stated above may not be appropriate in some settings and expert advice should be sought

#### ◢Lidocaine hydrochloride injections

**Lidocaine** (Non-proprietary) [PoM]
Injection, lidocaine hydrochloride 5 mg/mL (0.5%), net price 10-mL amp = 35p; 10 mg/mL (1%), 2-mL amp = 25p, 5-mL amp = 26p, 10-mL amp = 39p, 10-mL prefilled syringe = £4.53, 20-mL amp = 75p; 20 mg/mL (2%), 2-mL amp = 32p, 5-mL amp = 31p

#### ◢With adrenaline

For prescribing information on adrenaline see section 2.7.2; see also Use of Vasoconstrictors, p. 649.

**Xylocaine**® (AstraZeneca) [PoM]
Injection, anhydrous lidocaine hydrochloride 10 mg/ mL (1%), adrenaline 1 in 200 000 (5 micrograms/ mL), net price 20-mL vial = 99p
Excipients  include sulfites

Injection, anhydrous lidocaine hydrochloride 20 mg/ mL (2%), adrenaline 1 in 200 000 (5 micrograms/ mL), net price 20-mL vial = £1.04
Excipients  include sulfites

#### ◢Lidocaine injections for dental use

A variety of lidocaine injections with adrenaline are available in dental cartridges; brand names include *Lignospan Special*®, *Rexocaine*®, and *Xylocaine*®.

For prescribing information on adrenaline see section 2.7.2; see also Use of Vasoconstrictors, p. 649.

Note  Consult expert dental sources for specific advice in relation to dose of lidocaine for dental anaesthesia

#### ◢Lidocaine for surface anaesthesia

**Lidocaine** (Non-proprietary)
Ointment, lidocaine 5%, net price 15 g = £4.95
Dose
> **Dental practice**
> **Child** rub gently into dry gum

> **Pain relief (in anal fissures, haemorrhoids, pruritus ani, pruritus vulvae, herpes zoster, or herpes labialis), lubricant in cystoscopy or proctoscopy**
> **Child** apply 1–2 mL when necessary; avoid long-term use

**Instillagel**® (CliniMed)
Gel, lidocaine hydrochloride 2%, chlorhexidine gluconate solution 0.25%, in a sterile lubricant basis in disposable syringe, net price 6-mL syringe = £1.41, 11-mL syringe = £1.58
Excipients  include hydroxybenzoates (parabens)

**Laryngojet**® (UCB Pharma) [PoM]
Solution, lidocaine hydrochloride 40 mg/mL (4%), net price per unit (4-mL vial and disposable sterile cannula with cover and vial injector) = £5.10
Dose
> **Anaesthesia of mucous membranes of oropharynx, trachea, and respiratory tract**
> **Child** up to 0.075 mL/kg (3 mg/kg) as a single dose sprayed, instilled (if a cavity) or applied with a swab; reduce dose according to size, age, and condition of child, max. 5 mL (200 mg)

**LMX 4**® (Ferndale)
Cream, lidocaine 4%, net price 5-g tube = £2.98; 5 × 5-g tube with 10 occlusive dressings = £16.90
Excipients  include benzyl alcohol and propylene glycol
Dose
> **Anaesthesia before venous cannulation or venepuncture**
> **Child 1 month–18 years** apply thick layer (1–2.5 g; child under 1 year max. 1 g) to small area (2.5 cm × 2.5 cm) of non-irritated skin at least 30 minutes before procedure; max. application time 5 hours (child 1–3 months, 60 minutes; child 3 months–1 year, 4 hours); remove cream with gauze and perform procedure after approximately 5 minutes

**Xylocaine**® (AstraZeneca)
Spray, lidocaine 10% (100 mg/g) supplying 10 mg lidocaine/dose; 500 spray doses per container, net price 50-mL bottle = £3.13
Dose
> **Bronchoscopy, laryngoscopy, oesophagoscopy, endotracheal intubation**
> **Child up to 18 years** up to 3 mg/kg

#### ◢With prilocaine

For prescribing information on prilocaine, see p. 653.

**EMLA**® (AstraZeneca)
Cream, lidocaine 2.5%, prilocaine 2.5%, net price 5-g tube = £1.73; 30-g tube (surgical pack) = £10.25; 5 × 5-g tube with 12 occlusive dressings (premedication pack) = £9.75
Dose
> **Anaesthesia before minor skin procedures including venepuncture**
> **Neonate** apply max. 1 g under occlusive dressing for max. 1 hour before procedure; max. 1 dose in 24 hours
> **Child 1–3 months** apply max. 1 g under occlusive dressing for max. 1 hour before procedure; max. 1 dose in 24 hours
> **Child 3 months–1 year** apply max. 2 g under occlusive dressing for max. 4 hours before procedure; max. 2 doses in 24 hours
> **Child 1–18 years** apply thick layer under occlusive dressing 1–5 hours before procedure (2–5 hours before procedures on large areas e.g. split skin grafting); max. 2 doses in 24 hours for child 1–12 years
> Note  Shorter application time of 15–30 minutes is recommended for children with atopic dermatitis (30 minutes before removal of mollusca)

#### ◢Lidocaine for ear, nose, and oropharyngeal use

For prescribing information on phenylephrine, see section 2.7.2.

**Lidocaine with phenylephrine** (Non-proprietary)
Topical solution, lidocaine hydrochloride 5%, phenylephrine hydrochloride 0.5%, net price 2.5 mL (with nasal applicator) = £9.98
Dose
> **Anaesthesia before nasal surgery, endoscopy, laryngoscopy, or removal of foreign bodies from the nose**
> **Child 12–18 years** up to max. 8 sprays

## Mepivacaine

Mepivacaine is an amide-type local anaesthetic used for dental anaesthesia (see Dental Anaesthesia, p. 649).

### ■ MEPIVACAINE HYDROCHLORIDE

**Cautions** see Cautions of Local Anaesthetics, p. 649

**Contra-indications** see Contra-indications of Local Anaesthetics, p. 649

**Hepatic impairment** use with caution; increased risk of side-effects in severe impairment

**Renal impairment** use with caution; increased risk of side-effects

**Pregnancy** use with caution in early pregnancy

**Breast-feeding** use with caution

**Side-effects** see Toxicity and Side-effects, p. 650

**Indications and dose**

> To avoid excessive dosage in obese children, dose should be calculated on the basis of ideal weight for height

> **Infiltration anaesthesia and nerve block in dentistry**
>
> **Child 3–18 years** consult expert dental sources

**Scandonest® 3% Plain** (Septodont) [PoM]
Injection, mepivacaine hydrochloride 30 mg/mL, net price 2.2-mL cartridge = 36p

**■ With adrenaline**

For prescribing information on adrenaline, see section 2.7.2; see Use of Vasoconstrictors, p. 649.

**Scandonest® 2% Special** (Septodont) [PoM]
Injection, mepivacaine hydrochloride 20 mg/mL, adrenaline 1 in 100 000 (10 micrograms/mL), net price 2.2-mL cartridge = 36p
Excipients include sulfites

## Prilocaine

Prilocaine is a local anaesthetic of low toxicity which is similar to lidocaine. If used in high doses, methaemoglobinaemia may occur, which can be treated with an intravenous injection of **methylthioninium chloride** (see Emergency Treatment of Poisoning, p. 24); neonates and infants under 6 months are particularly susceptible to methaemoglobinaemia.

### ■ PRILOCAINE HYDROCHLORIDE

**Cautions** see Cautions of Local Anaesthetics, p. 649; severe or untreated hypertension; concomitant drugs which cause methaemoglobinaemia; acute porphyria (section 9.8.2); **interactions**: Appendix 1 (prilocaine)

**Contra-indications** see Contra-indications of Local Anaesthetics, p. 649; anaemia, or congenital or acquired methaemoglobinaemia

**Hepatic impairment** use with caution; lower doses may be required for intrathecal anaesthesia

**Renal impairment** use with caution; lower doses may be required for intrathecal anaesthesia

**Pregnancy** large doses during delivery can cause neonatal respiratory depression, hypotonia, and bradycardia after epidural block; avoid paracervical or pudendal block in obstetrics (neonatal methaemo-

globinaemia reported); use lower doses for intrathecal use during late pregnancy

**Breast-feeding** present in milk but not known to be harmful

**Side-effects** see notes above and Toxicity and Side-effects, p. 650; also hypertension

**Indications and dose**

> To avoid excessive dosage in obese children, dose should be calculated on the basis of ideal weight for height

> **Infiltration anaesthesia (higher strengths for dental use only), nerve block**
>
> See under preparations below, seek expert advice—**important**: see also under Administration, p. 649

**Citanest 1%®** (AstraZeneca) [PoM]
Injection, prilocaine hydrochloride 10 mg/mL, net price 50-mL multidose vial = £2.01
Dose

> **Child 6 months–12 years** up to 5 mg/kg adjusted according to site of administration and response; max. 400 mg
>
> **Child 12–18 years** 100–200 mg/minute, or in incremental doses, to max. total dose 400 mg (adjusted according to site of administration and response)

**■ With lidocaine**

See Lidocaine, p. 652

**■ For dental use**

Note Consult expert dental sources for specific advice in relation to dose of prilocaine for dental anaesthesia

**Citanest 3% with Octapressin®** (Dentsply) [PoM]
Injection, prilocaine hydrochloride 30 mg/mL, felypressin 0.03 unit/mL, net price 2.2-mL cartridge and self-aspirating cartridge (both) = 47p

## Ropivacaine

Ropivacaine is an amide-type local anaesthetic agent similar to bupivacaine. It is less cardiotoxic than bupivacaine, but also less potent.

### ■ ROPIVACAINE HYDROCHLORIDE

**Cautions** see Cautions of Local Anaesthetics, p. 649; also acute porphyria (section 9.8.2); **interactions**: Appendix 1 (ropivacaine)

**Contra-indications** see Contra-indications of Local Anaesthetics, p. 649

**Hepatic impairment** use with caution in severe impairment

**Renal impairment** use with caution in severe impairment; increased risk of systemic toxicity in chronic renal failure

**Pregnancy** not known to be harmful; do not use for paracervical block in obstetrics

**Breast-feeding** not known to be harmful

**Side-effects** see Toxicity and Side-effects, p. 650; also hypertension, pyrexia; *less commonly* syncope and hypothermia

**Licensed use** 2 mg/mL strength not licensed for use in children under 12 years except for acute pain management by caudal epidural block and continuous epidural infusion; 7.5 mg/mL and 10 mg/mL

**15**

**Anaesthesia**

strengths not licensed for use in children under 12 years

**Indications and dose**

> To avoid excessive dosage in obese children, dose should be calculated on the basis of ideal weight for height

> Adjust according to child's physical status and nature of procedure, seek expert advice—**important**: see also under Administration, p. 649

**Ropivacaine** (Non-proprietary) PoM
Infusion, ropivacaine hydrochloride 2 mg/mL, net price 200 mL = £14.45

**Naropin**® (AstraZeneca) PoM
Injection, ropivacaine hydrochloride 2 mg/mL, net price 10-mL *Polyamp*® = £1.78; 7.5 mg/mL, 10-mL *Polyamp*® = £2.65; 10 mg/mL, 10-mL *Polyamp*® = £3.20
**Electrolytes** $Na^+$<0.5 mmol/mL

Infusion, ropivacaine hydrochloride 2 mg/mL, net price 200-mL *Polybag*® = £14.45
**Electrolytes** $Na^+$<0.5 mmol/mL

## Tetracaine

**Tetracaine** is an effective local anaesthetic for topical application; a 4% gel is indicated for anaesthesia before venepuncture or venous cannulation. Tetracaine is effective for 4–6 hours after a single application in most children. It is not recommended prior to neonatal heel lancing.

Tetracaine is rapidly absorbed from mucous membranes and should **never** be applied to inflamed, traumatised, or highly vascular surfaces. It should **never** be used to provide anaesthesia for bronchoscopy or cystoscopy because lidocaine is a safer alternative.

### ▌TETRACAINE
(Amethocaine)

**Cautions** see Cautions of Local Anaesthetics, p. 649

**Contra-indications** see Contra-indications of Local Anaesthetics, p. 649

**Breast-feeding** not known to be harmful

**Side-effects** see Toxicity and Side-effects, p. 650
   **Important**. Rapid and extensive absorption may result in systemic side-effects (see also notes above)

**Licensed use** not licensed for use in neonates

**Indications and dose**

> **Anaesthesia before venepuncture or venous cannulation** see preparation below

> **Eye** section 11.7

**Ametop**® (S&N Hlth.)
Gel, tetracaine 4%, net price 1.5-g tube = £1.08
**Excipients** include hydroxybenzoates (parabens)
Dose

> **Neonate** apply contents of tube (or appropriate proportion) to site of venepuncture or venous cannulation and cover with occlusive dressing; remove gel and dressing after 30 minutes for venepuncture and after 45 minutes for venous cannulation
>
> **Child 1 month–18 years** apply contents of tube (or appropriate proportion) to site of venepuncture or venous cannulation and cover with occlusive dressing;

remove gel and dressing after 30 minutes for venepuncture and after 45 minutes for venous cannulation

> **Note** Child 5–18 years, contents of max. 5 tubes applied at separate sites at a single time, child 1 month–5 years, contents of max. 1 tube applied at separate sites at a single time

# A1 Interactions

Two or more drugs given at the same time may exert their effects independently or may interact. The interaction may be potentiation or antagonism of one drug by another, or occasionally some other effect. Adverse drug interactions should be reported to the Medicines and Healthcare products Regulatory Agency (MHRA), through the Yellow Card Scheme (see Adverse Reactions to Drugs, p. 11), as for other adverse drug reactions.

Drug interactions may be **pharmacodynamic** or **pharmacokinetic**.

## Pharmacodynamic interactions

These are interactions between drugs which have similar or antagonistic pharmacological effects or side-effects. They may be due to competition at receptor sites, or occur between drugs acting on the same physiological system. They are usually predictable from a knowledge of the pharmacology of the interacting drugs; in general, those demonstrated with one drug are likely to occur with related drugs. They occur to a greater or lesser extent in most patients who receive the interacting drugs.

## Pharmacokinetic interactions

These occur when one drug alters the absorption, distribution, metabolism, or excretion of another, thus increasing or reducing the amount of drug available to produce its pharmacological effects. They are not easily predicted and many of them affect only a small proportion of patients taking the combination of drugs. Pharmacokinetic interactions occurring with one drug cannot be assumed to occur with related drugs unless their pharmacokinetic properties are known to be similar.

Pharmacokinetic interactions are of several types:

**Affecting absorption**    The rate of absorption or the total amount absorbed can both be altered by drug interactions. Delayed absorption is rarely of clinical importance unless high peak plasma concentrations are required (e.g. when giving an analgesic). Reduction in the total amount absorbed, however, may result in ineffective therapy.

**Due to changes in protein binding**    To a variable extent most drugs are loosely bound to plasma proteins. Protein-binding sites are non-specific and one drug can displace another thereby increasing its proportion free to diffuse from plasma to its site of action. This only produces a detectable increase in effect if it is an extensively bound drug (more than 90%) that is not widely distributed throughout the body. Even so displacement rarely produces more than transient potentiation because this increased concentration of free drug results in an increased rate of elimination.

Displacement from protein binding plays a part in the potentiation of warfarin by sulfonamides, and tolbutamide but the importance of these interactions is due mainly to the fact that warfarin metabolism is also inhibited.

**Affecting metabolism**    Many drugs are metabolised in the liver. Induction of the hepatic microsomal enzyme system by one drug can gradually increase the rate of metabolism of another, resulting in lower plasma concentrations and a reduced effect. On withdrawal of the inducer plasma concentrations increase and toxicity may occur. Barbiturates, griseofulvin, many antiepileptics, and rifampicin are the most important enzyme inducers. Drugs affected include warfarin and the oral contraceptives.

Conversely when one drug inhibits the metabolism of another higher plasma concentrations are produced, rapidly resulting in an increased effect with risk of toxicity. Some drugs which potentiate warfarin and phenytoin do so by this mechanism.

Isoenzymes of the hepatic cytochrome P450 system interact with a wide range of drugs. Drugs may be substrates, inducers or inhibitors of the different isoenzymes. A great deal of *in-vitro* information is available on the effect of drugs on the isoenzymes; however, since drugs are eliminated by a number of different metabolic routes as well as renal excretion, the clinical effects of interactions cannot be predicted accurately from laboratory data on the cytochrome P450 isoenzymes. Except where a combination of drugs is specifically contra-indicated, the BNF presents only interactions that have been reported in clinical practice. In all cases the possibility of an interaction must be considered if toxic effects occur or if the activity of a drug diminishes.

**Affecting renal excretion**    Drugs are eliminated through the kidney both by glomerular filtration and by active tubular secretion. Competition occurs between those which share active transport mechanisms in the proximal tubule. For example, salicylates and some other NSAIDs delay the excretion of methotrexate; serious methotrexate toxicity is possible.

## Relative importance of interactions

Many drug interactions are harmless and many of those which are potentially harmful only occur in a small proportion of patients; moreover, the severity of an interaction varies from one patient to another. Drugs with a small therapeutic ratio (e.g. phenytoin) and those which require careful control of dosage (e.g. anticoagulants, antihypertensives, and antidiabetics) are most often involved.

Patients at increased risk from drug interactions include those with impaired renal or liver function.

**Serious interactions**    The symbol ● has been placed against interactions that are **potentially serious** and where concomitant administration of the drugs involved should be **avoided** (or only undertaken with caution and appropriate monitoring).

Appendix 1: Interactions

Interactions that have no symbol do not usually have serious consequences.

## List of drug interactions

The following is an alphabetical list of drugs and their interactions; to avoid excessive cross-referencing each drug or group is listed twice: in the alphabetical list and also against the drug or group with which it interacts. For explanation of symbol • see above

### Abacavir

Analgesics: abacavir possibly reduces plasma concentration of methadone

Antibacterials: plasma concentration of abacavir possibly reduced by rifampicin

Antiepileptics: plasma concentration of abacavir possibly reduced by phenobarbital and phenytoin

• Antivirals: abacavir possibly reduces effects of •ribavirin; plasma concentration of abacavir reduced by •tipranavir

### Abatacept

Adalimumab: increased risk of side-effects when abatacept given with adalimumab

• Certolizumab pegol: avoid concomitant use of abatacept with •certolizumab pegol

• Etanercept: avoid concomitant use of abatacept with •etanercept

• Golimumab: avoid concomitant use of abatacept with •golimumab

• Infliximab: avoid concomitant use of abatacept with •infliximab

• Vaccines: avoid concomitant use of abatacept with live •vaccines (see p. 600)

### Acarbose see Antidiabetics

### ACE Inhibitors

Alcohol: enhanced hypotensive effect when ACE inhibitors given with alcohol

Aldesleukin: enhanced hypotensive effect when ACE inhibitors given with aldesleukin

Allopurinol: manufacturers state possible increased risk of leucopenia and hypersensitivity reactions when ACE inhibitors given with allopurinol especially in renal impairment

Alpha-blockers: enhanced hypotensive effect when ACE inhibitors given with alpha-blockers

Anaesthetics, General: enhanced hypotensive effect when ACE inhibitors given with general anaesthetics

Analgesics: increased risk of renal impairment when ACE inhibitors given with NSAIDs, also hypotensive effect antagonised

Angiotensin-II Receptor Antagonists: increased risk of hyperkalaemia when ACE inhibitors given with angiotensin-II receptor antagonists

Antacids: absorption of ACE inhibitors possibly reduced by antacids; absorption of captopril, enalapril and fosinopril reduced by antacids

Antibacterials: plasma concentration of active metabolite of imidapril reduced by rifampicin (reduced antihypertensive effect); quinapril tablets reduce absorption of tetracyclines (quinapril tablets contain magnesium carbonate); possible increased risk of hyperkalaemia when ACE inhibitors given with trimethoprim

Anticoagulants: increased risk of hyperkalaemia when ACE inhibitors given with heparins

Antidepressants: hypotensive effect of ACE inhibitors possibly enhanced by MAOIs

Antidiabetics: ACE inhibitors possibly enhance hypoglycaemic effect of insulin, metformin and sulfonylureas

Antipsychotics: enhanced hypotensive effect when ACE inhibitors given with antipsychotics

### ACE Inhibitors (continued)

Anxiolytics and Hypnotics: enhanced hypotensive effect when ACE inhibitors given with anxiolytics and hypnotics

Azathioprine: increased risk of anaemia or leucopenia when captopril given with azathioprine especially in renal impairment; increased risk of anaemia when enalapril given with azathioprine especially in renal impairment

Beta-blockers: enhanced hypotensive effect when ACE inhibitors given with beta-blockers

Calcium-channel Blockers: enhanced hypotensive effect when ACE inhibitors given with calcium-channel blockers

Cardiac Glycosides: captopril possibly increases plasma concentration of digoxin

• Ciclosporin: increased risk of hyperkalaemia when ACE inhibitors given with •ciclosporin

Clonidine: enhanced hypotensive effect when ACE inhibitors given with clonidine; antihypertensive effect of captopril possibly delayed by previous treatment with clonidine

Corticosteroids: hypotensive effect of ACE inhibitors antagonised by corticosteroids

Diazoxide: enhanced hypotensive effect when ACE inhibitors given with diazoxide

• Diuretics: enhanced hypotensive effect when ACE inhibitors given with •diuretics; increased risk of severe hyperkalaemia when ACE inhibitors given with •potassium-sparing diuretics and aldosterone antagonists

Dopaminergics: enhanced hypotensive effect when ACE inhibitors given with levodopa

• Gold: flushing and hypotension reported when ACE inhibitors given with •sodium aurothiomalate

• Lithium: ACE inhibitors reduce excretion of •lithium (increased plasma concentration)

Methyldopa: enhanced hypotensive effect when ACE inhibitors given with methyldopa

Moxisylyte: enhanced hypotensive effect when ACE inhibitors given with moxisylyte

Moxonidine: enhanced hypotensive effect when ACE inhibitors given with moxonidine

Muscle Relaxants: enhanced hypotensive effect when ACE inhibitors given with baclofen or tizanidine

Nitrates: enhanced hypotensive effect when ACE inhibitors given with nitrates

Oestrogens: hypotensive effect of ACE inhibitors antagonised by oestrogens

• Potassium Salts: increased risk of severe hyperkalaemia when ACE inhibitors given with •potassium salts

Probenecid: excretion of captopril reduced by probenecid

Prostaglandins: enhanced hypotensive effect when ACE inhibitors given with alprostadil

Vasodilator Antihypertensives: enhanced hypotensive effect when ACE inhibitors given with hydralazine, minoxidil or sodium nitroprusside

### Acebutolol see Beta-blockers

### Aceclofenac see NSAIDs

### Acemetacin see NSAIDs

### Acenocoumarol see Coumarins

### Acetazolamide see Diuretics

### Aciclovir

Note Interactions do not apply to topical aciclovir preparations

Note Valaciclovir interactions as for aciclovir

Ciclosporin: increased risk of nephrotoxicity when aciclovir given with ciclosporin

Mycophenolate: plasma concentration of aciclovir increased by mycophenolate, also plasma concentration of inactive metabolite of mycophenolate increased

Probenecid: excretion of aciclovir reduced by probenecid (increased plasma concentration)

**Aciclovir** *(continued)*

Tacrolimus: possible increased risk of nephrotoxicity when aciclovir given with tacrolimus

Theophylline: aciclovir possibly increases plasma concentration of theophylline

**Acitretin** *see* Retinoids

**Acrivastine** *see* Antihistamines

**Adalimumab**

Abatacept: increased risk of side-effects when adalimumab given with abatacept

• Anakinra: avoid concomitant use of adalimumab with •anakinra

• Vaccines: avoid concomitant use of adalimumab with live •vaccines (see p. 600)

**Adefovir**

Antivirals: avoidance of adefovir advised by manufacturer of tenofovir

Interferons: manufacturer of adefovir advises caution with peginterferon alfa

**Adenosine**

Note Possibility of interaction with drugs tending to impair myocardial conduction

Anaesthetics, Local: increased myocardial depression when anti-arrhythmics given with bupivacaine, levobupivacaine, prilocaine or ropivacaine

• Anti-arrhythmics: increased myocardial depression when anti-arrhythmics given with other •anti-arrhythmics

• Antipsychotics: increased risk of ventricular arrhythmias when anti-arrhythmics that prolong the QT interval given with •antipsychotics that prolong the QT interval

• Beta-blockers: increased myocardial depression when anti-arrhythmics given with •beta-blockers

• Dipyridamole: effect of adenosine enhanced and extended by •dipyridamole (important risk of toxicity)

Nicotine: effects of adenosine possibly enhanced by nicotine

Theophylline: anti-arrhythmic effect of adenosine antagonised by theophylline

**Adrenaline (epinephrine)** *see* Sympathomimetics

**Adrenergic Neurone Blockers**

Alcohol: enhanced hypotensive effect when adrenergic neurone blockers given with alcohol

Alpha-blockers: enhanced hypotensive effect when adrenergic neurone blockers given with alpha-blockers

• Anaesthetics, General: enhanced hypotensive effect when adrenergic neurone blockers given with •general anaesthetics

Analgesics: hypotensive effect of adrenergic neurone blockers antagonised by NSAIDs

Angiotensin-II Receptor Antagonists: enhanced hypotensive effect when adrenergic neurone blockers given with angiotensin-II receptor antagonists

Antidepressants: enhanced hypotensive effect when adrenergic neurone blockers given with MAOIs; hypotensive effect of adrenergic neurone blockers antagonised by tricyclics

Antipsychotics: hypotensive effect of adrenergic neurone blockers antagonised by haloperidol; hypotensive effect of adrenergic neurone blockers antagonised by higher doses of chlorpromazine; enhanced hypotensive effect when adrenergic neurone blockers given with phenothiazines

Anxiolytics and Hypnotics: enhanced hypotensive effect when adrenergic neurone blockers given with anxiolytics and hypnotics

Beta-blockers: enhanced hypotensive effect when adrenergic neurone blockers given with beta-blockers

Calcium-channel Blockers: enhanced hypotensive effect when adrenergic neurone blockers given with calcium-channel blockers

Clonidine: enhanced hypotensive effect when adrenergic neurone blockers given with clonidine

**Adrenergic Neurone Blockers** *(continued)*

Corticosteroids: hypotensive effect of adrenergic neurone blockers antagonised by corticosteroids

Diazoxide: enhanced hypotensive effect when adrenergic neurone blockers given with diazoxide

Diuretics: enhanced hypotensive effect when adrenergic neurone blockers given with diuretics

Dopaminergics: enhanced hypotensive effect when adrenergic neurone blockers given with levodopa

Methyldopa: enhanced hypotensive effect when adrenergic neurone blockers given with methyldopa

Moxisylyte: enhanced hypotensive effect when adrenergic neurone blockers given with moxisylyte

Moxonidine: enhanced hypotensive effect when adrenergic neurone blockers given with moxonidine

Muscle Relaxants: enhanced hypotensive effect when adrenergic neurone blockers given with baclofen or tizanidine

Nitrates: enhanced hypotensive effect when adrenergic neurone blockers given with nitrates

Oestrogens: hypotensive effect of adrenergic neurone blockers antagonised by oestrogens

Pizotifen: hypotensive effect of adrenergic neurone blockers antagonised by pizotifen

Prostaglandins: enhanced hypotensive effect when adrenergic neurone blockers given with alprostadil

• Sympathomimetics: hypotensive effect of guanethidine antagonised by •dexamfetamine and •lisdexamfetamine; hypotensive effect of adrenergic neurone blockers antagonised by •ephedrine, •isometheptene, •metaraminol, •methylphenidate, •noradrenaline (norepinephrine), •oxymetazoline, •phenylephrine, •pseudoephedrine and •xylometazoline

Vasodilator Antihypertensives: enhanced hypotensive effect when adrenergic neurone blockers given with hydralazine, minoxidil or sodium nitroprusside

**Adsorbents** *see* Kaolin

**Agalsidase Alfa and Beta**

Anti-arrhythmics: effects of agalsidase alfa and beta possibly inhibited by amiodarone (manufacturers of agalsidase alfa and beta advise avoid concomitant use)

Antibacterials: effects of agalsidase alfa and beta possibly inhibited by gentamicin (manufacturers of agalsidase alfa and beta advise avoid concomitant use)

Antimalarials: effects of agalsidase alfa and beta possibly inhibited by chloroquine and hydroxychloroquine (manufacturers of agalsidase alfa and beta advise avoid concomitant use)

**Agomelatine**

• Antibacterials: manufacturer of agomelatine advises avoid concomitant use with •ciprofloxacin

• Antidepressants: metabolism of agomelatine inhibited by •fluvoxamine (increased plasma concentration)

• Antimalarials: avoidance of antidepressants advised by manufacturer of •artemether with lumefantrine and •piperaquine with artenimol

Atomoxetine: possible increased risk of convulsions when antidepressants given with atomoxetine

**Alcohol**

ACE Inhibitors: enhanced hypotensive effect when alcohol given with ACE inhibitors

Adrenergic Neurone Blockers: enhanced hypotensive effect when alcohol given with adrenergic neurone blockers

Alpha-blockers: increased sedative effect when alcohol given with indoramin; enhanced hypotensive effect when alcohol given with alpha-blockers

Analgesics: enhanced hypotensive and sedative effects when alcohol given with opioid analgesics

Angiotensin-II Receptor Antagonists: enhanced hypotensive effect when alcohol given with angiotensin-II receptor antagonists

**Alcohol** *(continued)*

- Antibacterials: disulfiram-like reaction when alcohol given with metronidazole; possibility of disulfiram-like reaction when alcohol given with tinidazole; increased risk of convulsions when alcohol given with ●cycloserine
- Anticoagulants: major changes in consumption of alcohol may affect anticoagulant control with ●coumarins or ●phenindione
- Antidepressants: some beverages containing alcohol and some dealcoholised beverages contain tyramine which interacts with ●MAOIs (hypertensive crisis)—if no tyramine, enhanced hypotensive effect; sedative effects possibly increased when alcohol given with SSRIs; increased sedative effect when alcohol given with ●mirtazapine, ●tricyclic-related antidepressants or ●tricyclics

Antidiabetics: alcohol enhances hypoglycaemic effect of antidiabetics; increased risk of lactic acidosis when alcohol given with metformin

Antiepileptics: alcohol possibly increases CNS side-effects of carbamazepine; increased sedative effect when alcohol given with phenobarbital; chronic heavy consumption of alcohol possibly reduces plasma concentration of phenytoin; increased risk of blurred vision when alcohol given with retigabine

Antifungals: effects of alcohol possibly enhanced by griseofulvin

Antihistamines: increased sedative effect when alcohol given with antihistamines (possibly less effect with non-sedating antihistamines)

Antimuscarinics: increased sedative effect when alcohol given with hyoscine

Antipsychotics: increased sedative effect when alcohol given with antipsychotics

Anxiolytics and Hypnotics: increased sedative effect when alcohol given with anxiolytics and hypnotics

Beta-blockers: enhanced hypotensive effect when alcohol given with beta-blockers

Calcium-channel Blockers: enhanced hypotensive effect when alcohol given with calcium-channel blockers; plasma concentration of alcohol possibly increased by verapamil

Clonidine: enhanced hypotensive effect when alcohol given with clonidine

Cytotoxics: disulfiram-like reaction when alcohol given with procarbazine

Diazoxide: enhanced hypotensive effect when alcohol given with diazoxide

Disulfiram: disulfiram reaction when alcohol given with disulfiram (see BNF section 4.10.1)

Diuretics: enhanced hypotensive effect when alcohol given with diuretics

Dopaminergics: alcohol reduces tolerance to bromocriptine

Levamisole: possibility of disulfiram-like reaction when alcohol given with levamisole

Lofexidine: increased sedative effect when alcohol given with lofexidine

Methyldopa: enhanced hypotensive effect when alcohol given with methyldopa

Metoclopramide: absorption of alcohol possibly increased by metoclopramide

Moxonidine: enhanced hypotensive effect when alcohol given with moxonidine

Muscle Relaxants: increased sedative effect when alcohol given with baclofen, methocarbamol or tizanidine

Nicorandil: alcohol possibly enhances hypotensive effect of nicorandil

Nitrates: enhanced hypotensive effect when alcohol given with nitrates

- Paraldehyde: increased sedative effect when alcohol given with ●paraldehyde

**Alcohol** *(continued)*

- Retinoids: presence of alcohol causes etretinate to be formed from ●acitretin (increased risk of teratogenicity in women of child-bearing potential)

Sympathomimetics: alcohol possibly enhances effects of methylphenidate

Vasodilator Antihypertensives: enhanced hypotensive effect when alcohol given with hydralazine, minoxidil or sodium nitroprusside

**Aldesleukin**

ACE Inhibitors: enhanced hypotensive effect when aldesleukin given with ACE inhibitors

Alpha-blockers: enhanced hypotensive effect when aldesleukin given with alpha-blockers

Angiotensin-II Receptor Antagonists: enhanced hypotensive effect when aldesleukin given with angiotensin-II receptor antagonists

Antivirals: aldesleukin possibly increases plasma concentration of indinavir

Beta-blockers: enhanced hypotensive effect when aldesleukin given with beta-blockers

Calcium-channel Blockers: enhanced hypotensive effect when aldesleukin given with calcium-channel blockers

Clonidine: enhanced hypotensive effect when aldesleukin given with clonidine

- Corticosteroids: manufacturer of aldesleukin advises avoid concomitant use with ●corticosteroids
- Cytotoxics: manufacturer of aldesleukin advises avoid concomitant use with ●cisplatin, ●dacarbazine and ●vinblastine

Diazoxide: enhanced hypotensive effect when aldesleukin given with diazoxide

Diuretics: enhanced hypotensive effect when aldesleukin given with diuretics

Methyldopa: enhanced hypotensive effect when aldesleukin given with methyldopa

Moxonidine: enhanced hypotensive effect when aldesleukin given with moxonidine

Nitrates: enhanced hypotensive effect when aldesleukin given with nitrates

Vasodilator Antihypertensives: enhanced hypotensive effect when aldesleukin given with hydralazine, minoxidil or sodium nitroprusside

**Alendronic Acid** *see* Bisphosphonates

**Alfentanil** *see* Opioid Analgesics

**Alfuzosin** *see* Alpha-blockers

**Alimemazine** *see* Antihistamines

**Aliskiren**

Analgesics: hypotensive effect of aliskiren possibly antagonised by NSAIDs

Angiotensin-II Receptor Antagonists: plasma concentration of aliskiren possibly reduced by irbesartan

Antibacterials: plasma concentration of aliskiren reduced by rifampicin

Anticoagulants: increased risk of hyperkalaemia when aliskiren given with heparins

- Antifungals: plasma concentration of aliskiren increased by ketoconazole; plasma concentration of aliskiren increased by ●itraconazole—avoid concomitant use

Calcium-channel Blockers: plasma concentration of aliskiren increased by verapamil

- Ciclosporin: plasma concentration of aliskiren increased by ●ciclosporin—avoid concomitant use

Diuretics: aliskiren reduces plasma concentration of furosemide; increased risk of hyperkalaemia when aliskiren given with potassium-sparing diuretics and aldosterone antagonists

- Grapefruit Juice: plasma concentration of aliskiren reduced by ●grapefruit juice—avoid concomitant use

Potassium Salts: increased risk of hyperkalaemia when aliskiren given with potassium salts

**Alitretinoin** *see* Retinoids

**Alkylating Drugs** *see* Bendamustine, Busulfan, Carmustine, Cyclophosphamide, Estramustine, Ifosfamide, Lomustine, Melphalan, and Thiotepa

**Allopurinol**

ACE Inhibitors: manufacturers state possible increased risk of leucopenia and hypersensitivity reactions when allopurinol given with ACE inhibitors especially in renal impairment

Antibacterials: increased risk of rash when allopurinol given with amoxicillin or ampicillin

Anticoagulants: allopurinol possibly enhances anticoagulant effect of coumarins

• Antivirals: allopurinol increases plasma concentration of ●didanosine (risk of toxicity)—avoid concomitant use

• Azathioprine: allopurinol enhances effects and increases toxicity of ●azathioprine (reduce dose of azathioprine to one quarter of usual dose)

Ciclosporin: allopurinol possibly increases plasma concentration of ciclosporin (risk of nephrotoxicity)

• Cytotoxics: allopurinol enhances effects and increases toxicity of ●mercaptopurine (reduce dose of mercaptopurine to one quarter of usual dose); avoidance of allopurinol advised by manufacturer of ●capecitabine

Diuretics: increased risk of hypersensitivity when allopurinol given with thiazides and related diuretics especially in renal impairment

Theophylline: allopurinol possibly increases plasma concentration of theophylline

**Almotriptan** *see* 5HT$_1$-receptor Agonists (under HT)

**Alpha$_2$-adrenoceptor Stimulants** *see* Apraclonidine, Brimonidine, Clonidine, and Methyldopa

**Alpha-blockers**

ACE Inhibitors: enhanced hypotensive effect when alpha-blockers given with ACE inhibitors

Adrenergic Neurone Blockers: enhanced hypotensive effect when alpha-blockers given with adrenergic neurone blockers

Alcohol: enhanced hypotensive effect when alpha-blockers given with alcohol; increased sedative effect when indoramin given with alcohol

Aldesleukin: enhanced hypotensive effect when alpha-blockers given with aldesleukin

• Anaesthetics, General: enhanced hypotensive effect when alpha-blockers given with ●general anaesthetics

Analgesics: hypotensive effect of alpha-blockers antagonised by NSAIDs

Angiotensin-II Receptor Antagonists: enhanced hypotensive effect when alpha-blockers given with angiotensin-II receptor antagonists

• Antidepressants: enhanced hypotensive effect when alpha-blockers given with MAOIs; manufacturer of indoramin advises avoid concomitant use with ●MAOIs

Antifungals: plasma concentration of alfuzosin possibly increased by ketoconazole

Antipsychotics: enhanced hypotensive effect when alpha-blockers given with antipsychotics

• Antivirals: plasma concentration of alfuzosin possibly increased by ●ritonavir—avoid concomitant use; avoidance of alfuzosin advised by manufacturer of ●telaprevir

Anxiolytics and Hypnotics: enhanced hypotensive and sedative effects when alpha-blockers given with anxiolytics and hypnotics

• Beta-blockers: enhanced hypotensive effect when alpha-blockers given with ●beta-blockers, also increased risk of first-dose hypotension with post-synaptic alpha-blockers such as prazosin

• Calcium-channel Blockers: enhanced hypotensive effect when alpha-blockers given with ●calcium-channel blockers, also increased risk of first-dose hypotension with post-synaptic alpha-blockers such as prazosin

**Alpha-blockers** *(continued)*

Cardiac Glycosides: prazosin increases plasma concentration of digoxin

Clonidine: enhanced hypotensive effect when alpha-blockers given with clonidine

Corticosteroids: hypotensive effect of alpha-blockers antagonised by corticosteroids

Diazoxide: enhanced hypotensive effect when alpha-blockers given with diazoxide

• Diuretics: enhanced hypotensive effect when alpha-blockers given with ●diuretics, also increased risk of first-dose hypotension with post-synaptic alpha-blockers such as prazosin

Dopaminergics: enhanced hypotensive effect when alpha-blockers given with levodopa

Methyldopa: enhanced hypotensive effect when alpha-blockers given with methyldopa

• Moxisylyte: possible severe postural hypotension when alpha-blockers given with ●moxisylyte

Moxonidine: enhanced hypotensive effect when alpha-blockers given with moxonidine

Muscle Relaxants: enhanced hypotensive effect when alpha-blockers given with baclofen or tizanidine

Nitrates: enhanced hypotensive effect when alpha-blockers given with nitrates

Oestrogens: hypotensive effect of alpha-blockers antagonised by oestrogens

Prostaglandins: enhanced hypotensive effect when alpha-blockers given with alprostadil

• Sildenafil: enhanced hypotensive effect when alpha-blockers given with ●sildenafil (avoid alpha-blockers for 4 hours after sildenafil)—see also under Phosphodiesterase type-5 inhibitors, BNF section 7.4.5

• Sympathomimetics: avoid concomitant use of tolazoline with ●adrenaline (epinephrine) or ●dopamine

• Tadalafil: enhanced hypotensive effect when alpha-blockers given with ●tadalafil—see also under Phosphodiesterase type-5 inhibitors, BNF section 7.4.5; enhanced hypotensive effect when doxazosin given with ●tadalafil—manufacturer of tadalafil advises avoid concomitant use

• Ulcer-healing Drugs: effects of tolazoline antagonised by ●cimetidine and ●ranitidine

• Vardenafil: enhanced hypotensive effect when alpha-blockers (excludes tamsulosin) given with ●vardenafil—separate doses by 6 hours—see also under Phosphodiesterase type-5 inhibitors, BNF section 7.4.5

Vasodilator Antihypertensives: enhanced hypotensive effect when alpha-blockers given with hydralazine, minoxidil or sodium nitroprusside

**Alpha-blockers (post-synaptic)** *see* Alpha-blockers

**Alprazolam** *see* Anxiolytics and Hypnotics

**Alprostadil** *see* Prostaglandins

**Aluminium Hydroxide** *see* Antacids

**Amantadine**

Antimalarials: plasma concentration of amantadine possibly increased by quinine

Antipsychotics: increased risk of extrapyramidal side-effects when amantadine given with antipsychotics

Bupropion: increased risk of side-effects when amantadine given with bupropion

• Memantine: increased risk of CNS toxicity when amantadine given with ●memantine (manufacturer of memantine advises avoid concomitant use); effects of dopaminergics possibly enhanced by memantine

Methyldopa: increased risk of extrapyramidal side-effects when amantadine given with methyldopa; antiparkinsonian effect of dopaminergics antagonised by methyldopa

Tetrabenazine: increased risk of extrapyramidal side-effects when amantadine given with tetrabenazine

**Ambrisentan**

Antibacterials: plasma concentration of ambrisentan possibly increased by rifampicin

**Ambrisentan** *(continued)*
- Ciclosporin: plasma concentration of ambrisentan increased by ●ciclosporin (see Dose under Ambrisentan, BNF section 2.5.1)

**Amikacin** *see* Aminoglycosides

**Amiloride** *see* Diuretics

**Aminoglycosides**
Agalsidase Alfa and Beta: gentamicin possibly inhibits effects of agalsidase alfa and beta (manufacturers of agalsidase alfa and beta advise avoid concomitant use)
Analgesics: plasma concentration of amikacin and gentamicin in neonates possibly increased by indometacin
- Antibacterials: neomycin reduces absorption of phenoxymethylpenicillin; increased risk of nephrotoxicity when aminoglycosides given with colistimethate sodium or polymyxins; increased risk of nephrotoxicity and ototoxicity when aminoglycosides given with capreomycin or ●vancomycin; possible increased risk of nephrotoxicity when aminoglycosides given with cephalosporins
- Anticoagulants: experience in anticoagulant clinics suggests that INR possibly altered when neomycin (given for local action on gut) is given with ●coumarins or ●phenindione
Antidiabetics: neomycin possibly enhances hypoglycaemic effect of acarbose, also severity of gastrointestinal effects increased
Antifungals: increased risk of nephrotoxicity when aminoglycosides given with amphotericin
Bisphosphonates: increased risk of hypocalcaemia when aminoglycosides given with bisphosphonates
Cardiac Glycosides: neomycin reduces absorption of digoxin; gentamicin possibly increases plasma concentration of digoxin
- Ciclosporin: increased risk of nephrotoxicity when aminoglycosides given with ●ciclosporin
- Cytotoxics: neomycin possibly reduces absorption of methotrexate; neomycin reduces bioavailability of sorafenib; increased risk of nephrotoxicity and possibly of ototoxicity when aminoglycosides given with ●platinum compounds
- Diuretics: increased risk of ototoxicity when aminoglycosides given with ●loop diuretics
- Muscle Relaxants: aminoglycosides enhance effects of ●non-depolarising muscle relaxants and ●suxamethonium
- Parasympathomimetics: aminoglycosides antagonise effects of ●neostigmine and ●pyridostigmine
- Tacrolimus: increased risk of nephrotoxicity when aminoglycosides given with ●tacrolimus
Vaccines: antibacterials inactivate oral typhoid vaccine—see p. 621
Vitamins: neomycin possibly reduces absorption of vitamin A

**Aminophylline** *see* Theophylline

**Aminosalicylates**
Azathioprine: possible increased risk of leucopenia when aminosalicylates given with azathioprine
Cardiac Glycosides: sulfasalazine possibly reduces absorption of digoxin
Cytotoxics: possible increased risk of leucopenia when aminosalicylates given with mercaptopurine
Folates: sulfasalazine possibly reduces absorption of folic acid

**Amiodarone**
Note Amiodarone has a long half-life; there is a potential for drug interactions to occur for several weeks (or even months) after treatment with it has been stopped
Agalsidase Alfa and Beta: amiodarone possibly inhibits effects of agalsidase alfa and beta (manufacturers of agalsidase alfa and beta advise avoid concomitant use)

**Amiodarone** *(continued)*
Anaesthetics, Local: increased myocardial depression when anti-arrhythmics given with bupivacaine, levobupivacaine, prilocaine or ropivacaine
- Anti-arrhythmics: increased myocardial depression when anti-arrhythmics given with other ●anti-arrhythmics; increased risk of ventricular arrhythmias when amiodarone given with ●disopyramide or ●dronedarone—avoid concomitant use; amiodarone increases plasma concentration of ●flecainide (halve dose of flecainide)
- Antibacterials: increased risk of ventricular arrhythmias when amiodarone given with *parenteral* ●erythromycin—avoid concomitant use; increased risk of ventricular arrhythmias when amiodarone given with ●levofloxacin or ●moxifloxacin—avoid concomitant use; possible increased risk of ventricular arrhythmias when amiodarone given with sulfamethoxazole and trimethoprim (as co-trimoxazole)—manufacturer of amiodarone advises avoid concomitant use of co-trimoxazole; possible increased risk of ventricular arrhythmias when amiodarone given with ●telithromycin
- Anticoagulants: amiodarone inhibits metabolism of ●coumarins and ●phenindione (enhanced anticoagulant effect); amiodarone increases plasma concentration of ●dabigatran etexilate (see Dose under Dabigatran etexilate, BNF section 2.8.2)
- Antidepressants: increased risk of ventricular arrhythmias when amiodarone given with ●tricyclics—avoid concomitant use
- Antiepileptics: amiodarone inhibits metabolism of ●phenytoin (increased plasma concentration)
- Antihistamines: increased risk of ventricular arrhythmias when amiodarone given with ●mizolastine—avoid concomitant use
- Antimalarials: avoidance of amiodarone advised by manufacturer of ●piperaquine with artenimol (possible risk of ventricular arrhythmias); avoidance of amiodarone advised by manufacturer of ●artemether with lumefantrine (risk of ventricular arrhythmias); increased risk of ventricular arrhythmias when amiodarone given with ●chloroquine and hydroxychloroquine, ●mefloquine or ●quinine—avoid concomitant use
- Antimuscarinics: increased risk of ventricular arrhythmias when amiodarone given with ●tolterodine
- Antipsychotics: increased risk of ventricular arrhythmias when anti-arrhythmics that prolong the QT interval given with ●antipsychotics that prolong the QT interval; increased risk of ventricular arrhythmias when amiodarone given with ●benperidol—manufacturer of benperidol advises avoid concomitant use; increased risk of ventricular arrhythmias when amiodarone given with ●amisulpride, ●droperidol, ●haloperidol, ●phenothiazines, ●pimozide or ●zuclopenthixol—avoid concomitant use; increased risk of ventricular arrhythmias when amiodarone given with ●sulpiride
- Antivirals: plasma concentration of amiodarone possibly increased by ●atazanavir; plasma concentration of amiodarone possibly increased by ●fosamprenavir (increased risk of ventricular arrhythmias—avoid concomitant use); plasma concentration of amiodarone possibly increased by ●indinavir—avoid concomitant use; plasma concentration of amiodarone increased by ●ritonavir (increased risk of ventricular arrhythmias—avoid concomitant use); increased risk of ventricular arrhythmias when amiodarone given with ●saquinavir—avoid concomitant use; avoidance of amiodarone advised by manufacturer of ●telaprevir (risk of ventricular arrhythmias)
- Atomoxetine: increased risk of ventricular arrhythmias when amiodarone given with ●atomoxetine

**Amiodarone** *(continued)*
- Beta-blockers: increased risk of bradycardia, AV block and myocardial depression when amiodarone given with ●beta-blockers; increased myocardial depression when anti-arrhythmics given with ●beta-blockers; increased risk of ventricular arrhythmias when amiodarone given with ●sotalol—avoid concomitant use
- Calcium-channel Blockers: increased risk of bradycardia, AV block and myocardial depression when amiodarone given with ●diltiazem or ●verapamil
- Cardiac Glycosides: amiodarone increases plasma concentration of ●digoxin (halve dose of digoxin)

  Ciclosporin: amiodarone possibly increases plasma concentration of ciclosporin
- Colchicine: amiodarone possibly increases risk of ●colchicine toxicity
- Cytotoxics: possible increased risk of ventricular arrhythmias when amiodarone given with ●vandetanib—avoid concomitant use; increased risk of ventricular arrhythmias when amiodarone given with ●arsenic trioxide

  Diuretics: increased cardiac toxicity with amiodarone if hypokalaemia occurs with acetazolamide, loop diuretics or thiazides and related diuretics; amiodarone increases plasma concentration of eplerenone (reduce dose of eplerenone)

  Fidaxomicin: avoidance of amiodarone advised by manufacturer of fidaxomicin
- Fingolimod: possible increased risk of bradycardia when amiodarone given with ●fingolimod

  Grapefruit Juice: plasma concentration of amiodarone increased by grapefruit juice
- Ivabradine: increased risk of ventricular arrhythmias when amiodarone given with ●ivabradine
- Lipid-regulating Drugs: increased risk of myopathy when amiodarone given with ●simvastatin (see Dose under Simvastatin, p. 126)
- Lithium: manufacturer of amiodarone advises avoid concomitant use with ●lithium (risk of ventricular arrhythmias)

  Orlistat: plasma concentration of amiodarone possibly reduced by orlistat
- Pentamidine Isetionate: increased risk of ventricular arrhythmias when amiodarone given with ●pentamidine isetionate—avoid concomitant use

  Thyroid Hormones: for concomitant use of amiodarone and thyroid hormones see p. 82

  Ulcer-healing Drugs: plasma concentration of amiodarone increased by cimetidine

**Amisulpride** *see* Antipsychotics
**Amitriptyline** *see* Antidepressants, Tricyclic
**Amlodipine** *see* Calcium-channel Blockers
**Amoxicillin** *see* Penicillins
**Amphotericin**

  Note Close monitoring required with concomitant administration of nephrotoxic drugs or cytotoxics

  Antibacterials: increased risk of nephrotoxicity when amphotericin given with aminoglycosides or polymyxins; possible increased risk of nephrotoxicity when amphotericin given with vancomycin

  Antifungals: amphotericin reduces renal excretion and increases cellular uptake of flucytosine (toxicity possibly increased); effects of amphotericin possibly antagonised by imidazoles and triazoles; plasma concentration of amphotericin possibly increased by micafungin
- Cardiac Glycosides: hypokalaemia caused by amphotericin increases cardiac toxicity with ●cardiac glycosides
- Ciclosporin: increased risk of nephrotoxicity when amphotericin given with ●ciclosporin
- Corticosteroids: increased risk of hypokalaemia when amphotericin given with ●corticosteroids—avoid concomitant use unless corticosteroids needed to control reactions

**Amphotericin** *(continued)*
- Cytotoxics: increased risk of ventricular arrhythmias when amphotericin given with ●arsenic trioxide

  Diuretics: increased risk of hypokalaemia when amphotericin given with loop diuretics or thiazides and related diuretics

  Pentamidine Isetionate: possible increased risk of nephrotoxicity when amphotericin given with pentamidine isetionate
- Sodium Stibogluconate: possible increased risk of arrhythmias when amphotericin given after ●sodium stibogluconate—manufacturer of sodium stibogluconate advises giving 14 days apart
- Tacrolimus: increased risk of nephrotoxicity when amphotericin given with ●tacrolimus

**Ampicillin** *see* Penicillins
**Anabolic Steroids**
- Anticoagulants: anabolic steroids enhance anticoagulant effect of ●coumarins and ●phenindione

  Antidiabetics: anabolic steroids possibly enhance hypoglycaemic effect of antidiabetics

**Anaesthetics, General**
  Note *See also* Surgery and Long-term Medication, p. 629

  ACE Inhibitors: enhanced hypotensive effect when general anaesthetics given with ACE inhibitors
- Adrenergic Neurone Blockers: enhanced hypotensive effect when general anaesthetics given with ●adrenergic neurone blockers
- Alpha-blockers: enhanced hypotensive effect when general anaesthetics given with ●alpha-blockers

  Analgesics: metabolism of etomidate inhibited by fentanyl (consider reducing dose of etomidate); effects of thiopental possibly enhanced by aspirin; effects of intravenous general anaesthetics and volatile liquid general anaesthetics possibly enhanced by opioid analgesics

  Angiotensin-II Receptor Antagonists: enhanced hypotensive effect when general anaesthetics given with angiotensin-II receptor antagonists

  Antibacterials: effects of thiopental enhanced by sulfonamides; hypersensitivity-like reactions can occur when general anaesthetics given with *intravenous* vancomycin

  Antidepressants: increased risk of arrhythmias and hypotension when general anaesthetics given with tricyclics
- Antipsychotics: enhanced hypotensive effect when general anaesthetics given with ●antipsychotics; effects of thiopental enhanced by droperidol

  Anxiolytics and Hypnotics: increased sedative effect when general anaesthetics given with anxiolytics and hypnotics

  Beta-blockers: enhanced hypotensive effect when general anaesthetics given with beta-blockers
- Calcium-channel Blockers: enhanced hypotensive effect when general anaesthetics or isoflurane given with calcium-channel blockers; general anaesthetics enhance hypotensive effect of ●verapamil (also AV delay)

  Clonidine: enhanced hypotensive effect when general anaesthetics given with clonidine
- Cytotoxics: nitrous oxide increases antifolate effect of ●methotrexate—avoid concomitant use

  Diazoxide: enhanced hypotensive effect when general anaesthetics given with diazoxide

  Diuretics: enhanced hypotensive effect when general anaesthetics given with diuretics
- Dopaminergics: increased risk of arrhythmias when volatile liquid general anaesthetics given with ●levodopa
- Doxapram: increased risk of arrhythmias when volatile liquid general anaesthetics given with ●doxapram (avoid doxapram for at least 10 minutes after volatile liquid general anaesthetics)

## Anaesthetics, General (continued)

- Memantine: increased risk of CNS toxicity when ketamine given with ●memantine (manufacturer of memantine advises avoid concomitant use)

  Methyldopa: enhanced hypotensive effect when general anaesthetics given with methyldopa

  Metoclopramide: effects of thiopental enhanced by metoclopramide

  Moxonidine: enhanced hypotensive effect when general anaesthetics given with moxonidine
- Muscle Relaxants: increased risk of myocardial depression and bradycardia when propofol given with ●suxamethonium; volatile liquid general anaesthetics enhance effects of non-depolarising muscle relaxants and suxamethonium; ketamine enhances effects of atracurium

  Nitrates: enhanced hypotensive effect when general anaesthetics given with nitrates

  Oxytocin: oxytocic effect possibly reduced, also enhanced hypotensive effect and risk of arrhythmias when volatile liquid general anaesthetics given with oxytocin

  Probenecid: effects of thiopental possibly enhanced by probenecid
- Sympathomimetics: increased risk of arrhythmias when volatile liquid general anaesthetics given with ●adrenaline (epinephrine); increased risk of hypertension when volatile liquid general anaesthetics given with ●methylphenidate

  Theophylline: increased risk of convulsions when ketamine given with theophylline

  Vasodilator Antihypertensives: enhanced hypotensive effect when general anaesthetics given with hydralazine, minoxidil or sodium nitroprusside

## Anaesthetics, General (intravenous) see Anaesthetics, General

## Anaesthetics, General (volatile liquids) see Anaesthetics, General

## Anaesthetics, Local see Bupivacaine, Levobupivacaine, Lidocaine, Prilocaine, and Ropivacaine

## Anagrelide

- Cilostazol: manufacturer of anagrelide advises avoid concomitant use with ●cilostazol
- Phosphodiesterase Type-3 Inhibitors: manufacturer of anagrelide advises avoid concomitant use with ●enoximone and ●milrinone

## Anakinra

- Adalimumab: avoid concomitant use of anakinra with ●adalimumab
- Certolizumab pegol: avoid concomitant use of anakinra with ●certolizumab pegol
- Etanercept: avoid concomitant use of anakinra with ●etanercept
- Golimumab: avoid concomitant use of anakinra with ●golimumab
- Infliximab: avoid concomitant use of anakinra with ●infliximab
- Vaccines: avoid concomitant use of anakinra with live ●vaccines (see p. 600)

## Analgesics see Aspirin, Nefopam, NSAIDs, Opioid Analgesics, and Paracetamol

## Angiotensin-II Receptor Antagonists

ACE Inhibitors: increased risk of hyperkalaemia when angiotensin-II receptor antagonists given with ACE inhibitors

Adrenergic Neurone Blockers: enhanced hypotensive effect when angiotensin-II receptor antagonists given with adrenergic neurone blockers

Alcohol: enhanced hypotensive effect when angiotensin-II receptor antagonists given with alcohol

Aldesleukin: enhanced hypotensive effect when angiotensin-II receptor antagonists given with aldesleukin

Aliskiren: irbesartan possibly reduces plasma concentration of aliskiren

## Angiotensin-II Receptor Antagonists (continued)

Alpha-blockers: enhanced hypotensive effect when angiotensin-II receptor antagonists given with alpha-blockers

Anaesthetics, General: enhanced hypotensive effect when angiotensin-II receptor antagonists given with general anaesthetics

Analgesics: increased risk of renal impairment when angiotensin-II receptor antagonists given with NSAIDs, also hypotensive effect antagonised

Antibacterials: plasma concentration of losartan and its active metabolite reduced by rifampicin; possible increased risk of hyperkalaemia when angiotensin-II receptor antagonists given with trimethoprim

Anticoagulants: increased risk of hyperkalaemia when angiotensin-II receptor antagonists given with heparins

Antidepressants: hypotensive effect of angiotensin-II receptor antagonists possibly enhanced by MAOIs

Antipsychotics: enhanced hypotensive effect when angiotensin-II receptor antagonists given with antipsychotics

Anxiolytics and Hypnotics: enhanced hypotensive effect when angiotensin-II receptor antagonists given with anxiolytics and hypnotics

Beta-blockers: enhanced hypotensive effect when angiotensin-II receptor antagonists given with beta-blockers

Calcium-channel Blockers: enhanced hypotensive effect when angiotensin-II receptor antagonists given with calcium-channel blockers
- Ciclosporin: increased risk of hyperkalaemia when angiotensin-II receptor antagonists given with ●ciclosporin

  Clonidine: enhanced hypotensive effect when angiotensin-II receptor antagonists given with clonidine

  Corticosteroids: hypotensive effect of angiotensin-II receptor antagonists antagonised by corticosteroids

  Diazoxide: enhanced hypotensive effect when angiotensin-II receptor antagonists given with diazoxide
- Diuretics: enhanced hypotensive effect when angiotensin-II receptor antagonists given with ●diuretics; increased risk of hyperkalaemia when angiotensin-II receptor antagonists given with ●potassium-sparing diuretics and aldosterone antagonists

  Dopaminergics: enhanced hypotensive effect when angiotensin-II receptor antagonists given with levodopa
- Lithium: angiotensin-II receptor antagonists reduce excretion of ●lithium (increased plasma concentration)

  Methyldopa: enhanced hypotensive effect when angiotensin-II receptor antagonists given with methyldopa

  Moxisylyte: enhanced hypotensive effect when angiotensin-II receptor antagonists given with moxisylyte

  Moxonidine: enhanced hypotensive effect when angiotensin-II receptor antagonists given with moxonidine

  Muscle Relaxants: enhanced hypotensive effect when angiotensin-II receptor antagonists given with baclofen or tizanidine

  Nitrates: enhanced hypotensive effect when angiotensin-II receptor antagonists given with nitrates

  Oestrogens: hypotensive effect of angiotensin-II receptor antagonists antagonised by oestrogens
- Potassium Salts: increased risk of hyperkalaemia when angiotensin-II receptor antagonists given with ●potassium salts

  Prostaglandins: enhanced hypotensive effect when angiotensin-II receptor antagonists given with alprostadil

  Tacrolimus: increased risk of hyperkalaemia when angiotensin-II receptor antagonists given with tacrolimus

**Angiotensin-II Receptor Antagonists** *(continued)*

Vasodilator Antihypertensives: enhanced hypotensive effect when angiotensin-II receptor antagonists given with hydralazine, minoxidil or sodium nitroprusside

## Antacids

**Note** Antacids should preferably not be taken at the same time as other drugs since they may impair absorption

ACE Inhibitors: antacids possibly reduce absorption of ACE inhibitors; antacids reduce absorption of captopril, enalapril and fosinopril

Analgesics: alkaline urine due to some antacids increases excretion of aspirin

Antibacterials: antacids reduce absorption of azithromycin, cefaclor, cefpodoxime, ciprofloxacin, isoniazid, levofloxacin, moxifloxacin, norfloxacin, ofloxacin, rifampicin and tetracyclines; avoid concomitant use of antacids with methenamine; oral magnesium salts (as magnesium trisilicate) reduce absorption of nitrofurantoin

Antiepileptics: antacids reduce absorption of gabapentin and phenytoin

Antifungals: antacids reduce absorption of itraconazole and ketoconazole

Antihistamines: antacids reduce absorption of fexofenadine

Antimalarials: antacids reduce absorption of chloroquine and hydroxychloroquine; oral magnesium salts (as magnesium trisilicate) reduce absorption of proguanil

Antipsychotics: antacids reduce absorption of phenothiazines and sulpiride

Antivirals: antacids possibly reduce plasma concentration of atazanavir; manufacturer of rilpivirine advises give antacids 2 hours before or 4 hours after rilpivirine; antacids reduce absorption of tipranavir

Bile Acids: antacids possibly reduce absorption of bile acids

Bisphosphonates: antacids reduce absorption of bisphosphonates

Cardiac Glycosides: antacids possibly reduce absorption of digoxin

Corticosteroids: antacids reduce absorption of deflazacort

• Cytotoxics: antacids possibly reduce plasma concentration of ●erlotinib—give antacids at least 4 hours before or 2 hours after erlotinib

Deferasirox: antacids containing aluminium possibly reduce absorption of deferasirox (manufacturer of deferasirox advises avoid concomitant use)

Dipyridamole: antacids possibly reduce absorption of dipyridamole

Eltrombopag: antacids reduce absorption of eltrombopag (give at least 4 hours apart)

Iron: oral magnesium salts (as magnesium trisilicate) reduce absorption of *oral* iron

Lipid-regulating Drugs: antacids reduce absorption of rosuvastatin

Lithium: sodium bicarbonate increases excretion of lithium (reduced plasma concentration)

Mycophenolate: antacids reduce absorption of mycophenolate

Penicillamine: antacids reduce absorption of penicillamine

Polystyrene Sulfonate Resins: risk of intestinal obstruction when aluminium hydroxide given with polystyrene sulfonate resins; risk of metabolic alkalosis when oral magnesium salts given with polystyrene sulfonate resins

Thyroid Hormones: antacids possibly reduce absorption of levothyroxine

Ulcer-healing Drugs: antacids possibly reduce absorption of lansoprazole

**Antacids** *(continued)*

• Ulipristal: avoidance of antacids advised by manufacturer of *high-dose* ●ulipristal (contraceptive effect of ulipristal possibly reduced)

**Antazoline** *see* Antihistamines

**Anti-arrhythmics** *see* Adenosine, Amiodarone, Disopyramide, Dronedarone, Flecainide, Lidocaine, and Propafenone

**Antibacterials** *see* individual drugs

**Antibiotics (cytotoxic)** *see* Bleomycin, Doxorubicin, Epirubicin, Idarubicin, Mitomycin, and Mitoxantrone

**Anticoagulants** *see* Apixaban, Coumarins, Dabigatran Etexilate, Heparins, Phenindione, and Rivaroxaban

**Antidepressants** *see* Agomelatine; Antidepressants, SSRI; Antidepressants, Tricyclic; Antidepressants, Tricyclic (related); MAOIs; Mirtazapine; Moclobemide; Reboxetine; St John's Wort; Tryptophan; Venlafaxine

**Antidepressants, Noradrenaline Re-uptake Inhibitors** *see* Reboxetine

## Antidepressants, SSRI

Alcohol: sedative effects possibly increased when SSRIs given with alcohol

Anaesthetics, Local: fluvoxamine inhibits metabolism of ropivacaine—avoid prolonged administration of ropivacaine

• Analgesics: increased risk of bleeding when SSRIs given with ●NSAIDs or ●aspirin; fluoxetine, fluvoxamine, paroxetine and sertraline possibly increase plasma concentration of methadone; increased risk of CNS toxicity when SSRIs given with ●tramadol

Anti-arrhythmics: fluoxetine increases plasma concentration of flecainide; fluoxetine and paroxetine possibly inhibit metabolism of propafenone

• Antibacterials: possible increased risk of ventricular arrhythmias when citalopram given with ●telithromycin

• Anticoagulants: SSRIs possibly enhance anticoagulant effect of ●coumarins; possible increased risk of bleeding when SSRIs given with ●dabigatran etexilate

• Antidepressants: avoidance of fluvoxamine advised by manufacturer of ●reboxetine; possible increased serotonergic effects when SSRIs given with duloxetine; fluvoxamine inhibits metabolism of ●duloxetine—avoid concomitant use; CNS effects of SSRIs increased by ●MAOIs (risk of serious toxicity); citalopram, escitalopram, fluvoxamine, paroxetine or sertraline should not be started until 2 weeks after stopping ●MAOIs, also MAOIs should not be started until at least 1 week after stopping citalopram, escitalopram, fluvoxamine, paroxetine or sertraline; fluoxetine should not be started until 2 weeks after stopping ●MAOIs, also MAOIs should not be started until at least 5 weeks after stopping fluoxetine; increased risk of CNS toxicity when escitalopram given with ●moclobemide, preferably avoid concomitant use; after stopping citalopram, fluvoxamine, paroxetine or sertraline do not start ●moclobemide for at least 1 week; after stopping fluoxetine do not start ●moclobemide for 5 weeks; increased serotonergic effects when SSRIs given with ●St John's wort—avoid concomitant use; fluvoxamine inhibits metabolism of ●agomelatine (increased plasma concentration); possible increased serotonergic effects when fluoxetine or fluvoxamine given with mirtazapine; SSRIs increase plasma concentration of some ●tricyclics; agitation and nausea may occur when SSRIs given with ●tryptophan; CNS toxicity reported when fluoxetine given with tryptophan

• Antiepileptics: SSRIs antagonise anticonvulsant effect of ●antiepileptics (convulsive threshold lowered); fluoxetine and fluvoxamine increase plasma concentration of ●carbamazepine; plasma concentra-

## Antidepressants, SSRI

- Antiepileptics *(continued)*
tion of paroxetine reduced by phenobarbital and phenytoin; fluoxetine and fluvoxamine increase plasma concentration of ●phenytoin; plasma concentration of sertraline possibly reduced by phenytoin, also plasma concentration of phenytoin possibly increased
Antihistamines: antidepressant effect of SSRIs possibly antagonised by cyproheptadine
- Antimalarials: avoidance of antidepressants advised by manufacturer of ●artemether with lumefantrine and ●piperaquine with artenimol
Antimuscarinics: paroxetine increases plasma concentration of darifenacin and procyclidine
- Antipsychotics: avoidance of fluoxetine, fluvoxamine or sertraline advised by manufacturer of ●droperidol (risk of ventricular arrhythmias); fluoxetine increases plasma concentration of ●clozapine, ●haloperidol and risperidone; fluvoxamine possibly increases plasma concentration of asenapine and haloperidol; paroxetine inhibits metabolism of perphenazine (reduce dose of perphenazine); fluoxetine and paroxetine possibly inhibit metabolism of ●aripiprazole (reduce dose of aripiprazole); plasma concentration of paroxetine possibly increased by asenapine; citalopram possibly increases plasma concentration of clozapine (increased risk of toxicity); fluvoxamine, paroxetine and sertraline increase plasma concentration of ●clozapine; fluvoxamine increases plasma concentration of olanzapine; SSRIs possibly increase plasma concentration of ●pimozide (increased risk of ventricular arrhythmias—avoid concomitant use); paroxetine possibly increases plasma concentration of risperidone (increased risk of toxicity)
- Antivirals: plasma concentration of paroxetine and sertraline possibly reduced by darunavir; plasma concentration of SSRIs possibly increased by ●ritonavir; plasma concentration of paroxetine possibly reduced by ritonavir
- Anxiolytics and Hypnotics: fluoxetine increases plasma concentration of alprazolam; fluvoxamine increases plasma concentration of some benzodiazepines; fluvoxamine increases plasma concentration of ●melatonin—avoid concomitant use; sedative effects possibly increased when sertraline given with zolpidem
Atomoxetine: possible increased risk of convulsions when antidepressants given with atomoxetine; fluoxetine and paroxetine possibly inhibit metabolism of atomoxetine
Beta-blockers: citalopram and escitalopram increase plasma concentration of metoprolol; paroxetine possibly increases plasma concentration of metoprolol (enhanced effect); fluvoxamine increases plasma concentration of propranolol
Bupropion: plasma concentration of citalopram possibly increased by bupropion
Calcium-channel Blockers: fluoxetine possibly inhibits metabolism of nifedipine (increased plasma concentration)
- Clopidogrel: fluoxetine and fluvoxamine possibly reduce antiplatelet effect of ●clopidogrel
- Dopaminergics: fluoxetine should not be started until 2 weeks after stopping ●rasagiline, also rasagiline should not be started until at least 5 weeks after stopping fluoxetine; increased risk of CNS toxicity when SSRIs given with ●rasagiline; fluvoxamine should not be started until 2 weeks after stopping ●rasagiline; increased risk of hypertension and CNS excitation when fluvoxamine or sertraline given with ●selegiline (selegiline should not be started until 1 week after stopping fluvoxamine or sertraline, avoid fluvoxamine or sertraline for 2 weeks after stopping selegiline); increased risk of hypertension and CNS excitation when paroxetine given

## Antidepressants, SSRI

- Dopaminergics *(continued)*
with ●selegiline (selegiline should not be started until 2 weeks after stopping paroxetine, avoid paroxetine for 2 weeks after stopping selegiline); increased risk of hypertension and CNS excitation when fluoxetine given with ●selegiline (selegiline should not be started until 5 weeks after stopping fluoxetine, avoid fluoxetine for 2 weeks after stopping selegiline); avoidance of citalopram and escitalopram advised by manufacturer of selegiline
Grapefruit Juice: plasma concentration of sertraline possibly increased by grapefruit juice
- Hormone Antagonists: fluoxetine and paroxetine possibly inhibit metabolism of ●tamoxifen to active metabolite (avoid concomitant use)
- $5HT_1$-receptor Agonists: increased risk of CNS toxicity when citalopram given with ●$5HT_1$ agonists (manufacturer of citalopram advises avoid concomitant use); fluvoxamine inhibits the metabolism of frovatriptan; possible increased serotonergic effects when SSRIs given with naratriptan; CNS toxicity reported when sertraline given with sumatriptan; increased risk of CNS toxicity when citalopram, escitalopram, fluoxetine, fluvoxamine or paroxetine given with ●sumatriptan; fluvoxamine possibly inhibits metabolism of zolmitriptan (reduce dose of zolmitriptan)
- Lithium: Increased risk of CNS effects when SSRIs given with ●lithium (lithium toxicity reported)
- Methylthioninium: risk of CNS toxicity when SSRIs given with ●methylthioninium—avoid concomitant use (if avoidance not possible, use lowest possible dose of methylthioninium and observe patient for up to 4 hours after administration)
Metoclopramide: CNS toxicity reported when SSRIs given with metoclopramide
- Muscle Relaxants: fluvoxamine increases plasma concentration of ●tizanidine (increased risk of toxicity)—avoid concomitant use
Parasympathomimetics: paroxetine increases plasma concentration of galantamine
- Pirfenidone: fluvoxamine increases plasma concentration of ●pirfenidone—manufacturer of pirfenidone advises avoid concomitant use
Ranolazine: paroxetine increases plasma concentration of ranolazine
Roflumilast: fluvoxamine inhibits the metabolism of roflumilast
Sympathomimetics: metabolism of SSRIs possibly inhibited by methylphenidate
- Theophylline: fluvoxamine increases plasma concentration of ●theophylline (concomitant use should usually be avoided, but where not possible halve theophylline dose and monitor plasma-theophylline concentration)
Ticagrelor: possible increased risk of bleeding when citalopram, paroxetine or sertraline given with ticagrelor
Ulcer-healing Drugs: plasma concentration of citalopram, escitalopram and sertraline increased by cimetidine; fluvoxamine possibly increases plasma concentration of lansoprazole; plasma concentration of escitalopram increased by omeprazole

**Antidepressants, SSRI (related)** *see* Duloxetine and Venlafaxine

## Antidepressants, Tricyclic

Adrenergic Neurone Blockers: tricyclics antagonise hypotensive effect of adrenergic neurone blockers
- Alcohol: increased sedative effect when tricyclics given with ●alcohol
Alpha$_2$-adrenoceptor Stimulants: avoidance of tricyclics advised by manufacturer of apraclonidine and brimonidine

## Antidepressants, Tricyclic *(continued)*

Anaesthetics, General: increased risk of arrhythmias and hypotension when tricyclics given with general anaesthetics

- Analgesics: increased risk of CNS toxicity when tricyclics given with ●tramadol; side-effects possibly increased when tricyclics given with nefopam; sedative effects possibly increased when tricyclics given with opioid analgesics
- Anti-arrhythmics: increased risk of ventricular arrhythmias when tricyclics given with ●amiodarone—avoid concomitant use; increased risk of ventricular arrhythmias when tricyclics given with ●disopyramide or ●flecainide; avoidance of tricyclics advised by manufacturer of ●dronedarone (risk of ventricular arrhythmias); increased risk of arrhythmias when tricyclics given with ●propafenone
- Antibacterials: increased risk of ventricular arrhythmias when tricyclics given with ●moxifloxacin—avoid concomitant use; possible increased risk of ventricular arrhythmias when tricyclics given with ●telithromycin
- Anticoagulants: tricyclics may enhance or reduce anticoagulant effect of ●coumarins
- Antidepressants: possible increased serotonergic effects when amitriptyline or clomipramine given with duloxetine; increased risk of hypertension and CNS excitation when tricyclics given with ●MAOIs, tricyclics should not be started until 2 weeks after stopping MAOIs (3 weeks if starting clomipramine or imipramine), also MAOIs should not be started for at least 1–2 weeks after stopping tricyclics (3 weeks in the case of clomipramine or imipramine); after stopping tricyclics do not start ●moclobemide for at least 1 week; plasma concentration of some tricyclics increased by ●SSRIs; plasma concentration of amitriptyline reduced by St John's wort
- Antiepileptics: tricyclics antagonise anticonvulsant effect of ●antiepileptics (convulsive threshold lowered); metabolism of tricyclics accelerated by ●carbamazepine (reduced plasma concentration and reduced effect); metabolism of tricyclics possibly accelerated by ●phenobarbital (reduced plasma concentration); plasma concentration of tricyclics possibly reduced by ●phenytoin

Antifungals: plasma concentration of amitriptyline and nortriptyline possibly increased by fluconazole; plasma concentration of tricyclics possibly increased by terbinafine

Antihistamines: increased antimuscarinic and sedative effects when tricyclics given with antihistamines

- Antimalarials: avoidance of antidepressants advised by manufacturer of ●artemether with lumefantrine and ●piperaquine with artenimol

Antimuscarinics: increased risk of antimuscarinic side-effects when tricyclics given with antimuscarinics

- Antipsychotics: plasma concentration of tricyclics increased by ●antipsychotics—possible increased risk of ventricular arrhythmias; avoidance of tricyclics advised by manufacturer of ●droperidol (risk of ventricular arrhythmias); possible increased antimuscarinic side-effects when tricyclics given with clozapine; increased risk of antimuscarinic side-effects when tricyclics given with phenothiazines; increased risk of ventricular arrhythmias when tricyclics given with ●pimozide—avoid concomitant use
- Antivirals: plasma concentration of tricyclics possibly increased by ●ritonavir; increased risk of ventricular arrhythmias when tricyclics given with ●saquinavir—avoid concomitant use

Anxiolytics and Hypnotics: increased sedative effect when tricyclics given with anxiolytics and hypnotics

- Atomoxetine: increased risk of ventricular arrhythmias when tricyclics given with ●atomoxetine; possible

## Antidepressants, Tricyclic

- Atomoxetine *(continued)*
increased risk of convulsions when antidepressants given with atomoxetine
- Beta-blockers: plasma concentration of imipramine increased by labetalol and propranolol; increased risk of ventricular arrhythmias when tricyclics given with ●sotalol

Bupropion: plasma concentration of tricyclics possibly increased by bupropion (possible increased risk of convulsions)

Calcium-channel Blockers: plasma concentration of imipramine increased by diltiazem and verapamil; plasma concentration of tricyclics possibly increased by diltiazem and verapamil

Cannabis Extract: possible increased risk of hypertension and tachycardia when tricyclics given with cannabis extract

- Clonidine: tricyclics antagonise hypotensive effect of ●clonidine, also increased risk of hypertension on clonidine withdrawal
- Cytotoxics: increased risk of ventricular arrhythmias when amitriptyline or clomipramine given with ●arsenic trioxide

Disulfiram: metabolism of tricyclics inhibited by disulfiram (increased plasma concentration); concomitant amitriptyline reported to increase disulfiram reaction with alcohol

Diuretics: increased risk of postural hypotension when tricyclics given with diuretics

- Dopaminergics: caution with tricyclics advised by manufacturer of entacapone; increased risk of CNS toxicity when tricyclics given with ●rasagiline; CNS toxicity reported when tricyclics given with ●selegiline

Histamine: tricyclics theoretically antagonise effects of histamine—manufacturer of histamine advises avoid concomitant use

Lithium: risk of toxicity when tricyclics given with lithium

- Methylthioninium: risk of CNS toxicity when clomipramine given with ●methylthioninium—avoid concomitant use (if avoidance not possible, use lowest possible dose of methylthioninium and observe patient for up to 4 hours after administration)

Moxonidine: tricyclics possibly antagonise hypotensive effect of moxonidine (manufacturer of moxonidine advises avoid concomitant use)

Muscle Relaxants: tricyclics enhance muscle relaxant effect of baclofen

Nicorandil: tricyclics possibly enhance hypotensive effect of nicorandil

Nitrates: tricyclics reduce effects of sublingual tablets of nitrates (failure to dissolve under tongue owing to dry mouth)

Oestrogens: antidepressant effect of tricyclics antagonised by oestrogens (but side-effects of tricyclics possibly increased due to increased plasma concentration)

- Pentamidine Isetionate: increased risk of ventricular arrhythmias when tricyclics given with ●pentamidine isetionate

Sodium Oxybate: increased risk of side-effects when tricyclics given with sodium oxybate

- Sympathomimetics: increased risk of hypertension and arrhythmias when tricyclics given with ●adrenaline (epinephrine) (but local anaesthetics with adrenaline appear to be safe); metabolism of tricyclics possibly inhibited by methylphenidate; increased risk of hypertension and arrhythmias when tricyclics given with ●noradrenaline (norepinephrine)

Thyroid Hormones: effects of tricyclics possibly enhanced by thyroid hormones; effects of amitriptyline and imipramine enhanced by thyroid hormones

## Antidepressants, Tricyclic (continued)

Ulcer-healing Drugs: plasma concentration of tricyclics possibly increased by cimetidine; metabolism of amitriptyline, doxepin, imipramine and nortriptyline inhibited by cimetidine (increased plasma concentration)

## Antidepressants, Tricyclic (related)

- Alcohol: increased sedative effect when tricyclic-related antidepressants given with ●alcohol

Alpha$_2$-adrenoceptor Stimulants: avoidance of tricyclic-related antidepressants advised by manufacturer of apraclonidine and brimonidine

Antibacterials: plasma concentration of trazodone possibly increased by clarithromycin

Anticoagulants: trazodone may enhance or reduce anticoagulant effect of warfarin

- Antidepressants: tricyclic-related antidepressants should not be started until 2 weeks after stopping ●MAOIs, also MAOIs should not be started until at least 1–2 weeks after stopping tricyclic-related antidepressants; after stopping tricyclic-related antidepressants do not start ●moclobemide for at least 1 week

- Antiepileptics: tricyclic-related antidepressants possibly antagonise anticonvulsant effect of ●antiepileptics (convulsive threshold lowered); plasma concentration of mianserin and trazodone reduced by ●carbamazepine; metabolism of mianserin accelerated by ●phenobarbital (reduced plasma concentration); plasma concentration of mianserin reduced by ●phenytoin

Antihistamines: possible increased antimuscarinic and sedative effects when tricyclic-related antidepressants given with antihistamines

- Antimalarials: avoidance of antidepressants advised by manufacturer of ●artemether with lumefantrine and ●piperaquine with artenimol

Antimuscarinics: possible increased antimuscarinic side-effects when tricyclic-related antidepressants given with antimuscarinics

- Antivirals: plasma concentration of trazodone increased by ●ritonavir (increased risk of toxicity); increased risk of ventricular arrhythmias when trazodone given with ●saquinavir—avoid concomitant use; plasma concentration of trazodone possibly increased by telaprevir

Anxiolytics and Hypnotics: increased sedative effect when tricyclic-related antidepressants given with anxiolytics and hypnotics

Atomoxetine: possible increased risk of convulsions when antidepressants given with atomoxetine

Diazoxide: enhanced hypotensive effect when tricyclic-related antidepressants given with diazoxide

Nitrates: tricyclic-related antidepressants possibly reduce effects of sublingual tablets of nitrates (failure to dissolve under tongue owing to dry mouth)

Vasodilator Antihypertensives: enhanced hypotensive effect when tricyclic-related antidepressants given with hydralazine or sodium nitroprusside

## Antidiabetics

**Note** Other oral drugs may be taken at least 1 hour before or 4 hours after exenatide injection, or taken with a meal when exenatide is not administered, to minimise possible interference with absorption

ACE Inhibitors: hypoglycaemic effect of insulin, metformin and sulfonylureas possibly enhanced by ACE inhibitors

Alcohol: hypoglycaemic effect of antidiabetics enhanced by alcohol; increased risk of lactic acidosis when metformin given with alcohol

Anabolic Steroids: hypoglycaemic effect of antidiabetics possibly enhanced by anabolic steroids

- Analgesics: effects of sulfonylureas possibly enhanced by ●NSAIDs

## Antidiabetics (continued)

Anti-arrhythmics: hypoglycaemic effect of gliclazide, insulin and metformin possibly enhanced by disopyramide

- Antibacterials: hypoglycaemic effect of acarbose possibly enhanced by neomycin, also severity of gastro-intestinal effects increased; effects of repaglinide enhanced by clarithromycin; effects of glibenclamide possibly enhanced by norfloxacin; effects of linagliptin possibly reduced by rifampicin; plasma concentration of nateglinide reduced by rifampicin; hypoglycaemic effect of repaglinide possibly antagonised by rifampicin; effects of sulfonylureas enhanced by ●chloramphenicol; metabolism of tolbutamide accelerated by ●rifamycins (reduced effect); metabolism of sulfonylureas possibly accelerated by ●rifamycins (reduced effect); effects of sulfonylureas rarely enhanced by sulfonamides and trimethoprim; hypoglycaemic effect of sulfonylureas possibly enhanced by tetracyclines; hypoglycaemic effect of repaglinide possibly enhanced by trimethoprim—manufacturer advises avoid concomitant use

- Anticoagulants: exenatide possibly enhances anticoagulant effect of warfarin; hypoglycaemic effect of sulfonylureas possibly enhanced by ●coumarins, also possible changes to anticoagulant effect

Antidepressants: hypoglycaemic effect of antidiabetics possibly enhanced by MAOIs; hypoglycaemic effect of insulin, metformin and sulfonylureas enhanced by MAOIs

Antidiabetics: manufacturer of dapagliflozin advises avoid concomitant use with pioglitazone

Antiepileptics: tolbutamide transiently increases plasma concentration of phenytoin (possibility of toxicity); plasma concentration of glibenclamide possibly reduced by topiramate; plasma concentration of metformin possibly increased by topiramate

- Antifungals: plasma concentration of sulfonylureas increased by ●fluconazole and ●miconazole; hypoglycaemic effect of gliclazide and glipizide enhanced by ●miconazole—avoid concomitant use; hypoglycaemic effect of nateglinide possibly enhanced by fluconazole; hypoglycaemic effect of repaglinide possibly enhanced by itraconazole; hypoglycaemic effect of glipizide possibly enhanced by posaconazole; plasma concentration of sulfonylureas possibly increased by voriconazole

Antihistamines: thrombocyte count depressed when metformin given with ketotifen (manufacturer of ketotifen advises avoid concomitant use)

Antipsychotics: hypoglycaemic effect of sulfonylureas possibly antagonised by phenothiazines

Antivirals: plasma concentration of metformin possibly increased by rilpivirine; plasma concentration of tolbutamide possibly increased by ritonavir

Aprepitant: plasma concentration of tolbutamide reduced by aprepitant

Beta-blockers: warning signs of hypoglycaemia (such as tremor) with antidiabetics may be masked when given with beta-blockers; hypoglycaemic effect of insulin enhanced by beta-blockers

- Bosentan: increased risk of hepatotoxicity when glibenclamide given with ●bosentan—avoid concomitant use

Calcium-channel Blockers: glucose tolerance occasionally impaired when insulin given with nifedipine

Cardiac Glycosides: acarbose possibly reduces plasma concentration of digoxin; sitagliptin increases plasma concentration of digoxin

Ciclosporin: hypoglycaemic effect of repaglinide possibly enhanced by ciclosporin

Corticosteroids: hypoglycaemic effect of antidiabetics antagonised by corticosteroids

- Cytotoxics: avoidance of repaglinide advised by manufacturer of ●lapatinib

Antidiabetics *(continued)*

Deferasirox: plasma concentration of repaglinide increased by deferasirox

Diazoxide: hypoglycaemic effect of antidiabetics antagonised by diazoxide

Diuretics: hypoglycaemic effect of antidiabetics antagonised by loop diuretics and thiazides and related diuretics; dapagliflozin possibly enhances diuretic effect of loop diuretics and thiazides and related diuretics

Hormone Antagonists: requirements for insulin, metformin, repaglinide and sulfonylureas possibly reduced by lanreotide; requirements for insulin, metformin, repaglinide and sulfonylureas possibly reduced by octreotide; requirements for antidiabetics possibly reduced by pasireotide

Leflunomide: hypoglycaemic effect of tolbutamide possibly enhanced by leflunomide

• Lipid-regulating Drugs: absorption of glibenclamide reduced by colesevelam; hypoglycaemic effect of acarbose possibly enhanced by colestyramine; hypoglycaemic effect of nateglinide possibly enhanced by gemfibrozil; increased risk of severe hypoglycaemia when repaglinide given with •gemfibrozil—avoid concomitant use; plasma concentration of glibenclamide possibly increased by fluvastatin; may be improved glucose tolerance and an additive effect when insulin or sulfonylureas given with fibrates

Oestrogens: hypoglycaemic effect of antidiabetics antagonised by oestrogens

Orlistat: avoidance of acarbose advised by manufacturer of orlistat

Pancreatin: hypoglycaemic effect of acarbose antagonised by pancreatin

Progestogens: hypoglycaemic effect of antidiabetics antagonised by progestogens

• Sulfinpyrazone: effects of sulfonylureas enhanced by •sulfinpyrazone

Testosterone: hypoglycaemic effect of antidiabetics possibly enhanced by testosterone

Ulcer-healing Drugs: excretion of metformin reduced by cimetidine (increased plasma concentration); hypoglycaemic effect of sulfonylureas enhanced by cimetidine

Antiepileptics *see* Carbamazepine, Eslicarbazepine, Ethosuximide, Gabapentin, Lacosamide, Lamotrigine, Levetiracetam, Oxcarbazepine, Perampanel, Phenobarbital, Phenytoin, Pregabalin, Retigabine, Rufinamide, Stiripentol, Tiagabine, Topiramate, Valproate, Vigabatrin, and Zonisamide

Antifungals *see* Amphotericin; Antifungals, Imidazole; Antifungals, Triazole; Caspofungin; Flucytosine; Griseofulvin; Micafungin; Terbinafine

Antifungals, Imidazole

Aliskiren: ketoconazole increases plasma concentration of aliskiren

Alpha-blockers: ketoconazole possibly increases plasma concentration of alfuzosin

• Analgesics: ketoconazole inhibits metabolism of •buprenorphine (reduce dose of buprenorphine)

Antacids: absorption of ketoconazole reduced by antacids

• Anti-arrhythmics: increased risk of ventricular arrhythmias when ketoconazole given with •disopyramide—avoid concomitant use; ketoconazole increases plasma concentration of •dronedarone—avoid concomitant use

• Antibacterials: metabolism of ketoconazole accelerated by •rifampicin (reduced plasma concentration), also plasma concentration of rifampicin may be reduced by ketoconazole; plasma concentration of ketoconazole possibly reduced by isoniazid; avoidance of concomitant ketoconazole in severe renal and hepatic impairment advised by manufacturer of •telithromycin

Antifungals, Imidazole *(continued)*

• Anticoagulants: ketoconazole increases plasma concentration of •apixaban—manufacturer of apixaban advises avoid concomitant use; miconazole enhances anticoagulant effect of •coumarins (miconazole oral gel and possibly vaginal and topical formulations absorbed); ketoconazole enhances anticoagulant effect of •coumarins; ketoconazole increases plasma concentration of •dabigatran etexilate and •rivaroxaban—avoid concomitant use

• Antidepressants: avoidance of imidazoles advised by manufacturer of •reboxetine; ketoconazole increases plasma concentration of mirtazapine

• Antidiabetics: miconazole enhances hypoglycaemic effect of •gliclazide and •glipizide—avoid concomitant use; miconazole increases plasma concentration of •sulfonylureas

• Antiepileptics: ketoconazole and miconazole possibly increase plasma concentration of carbamazepine; ketoconazole increases plasma concentration of perampanel; plasma concentration of ketoconazole reduced by •phenytoin; miconazole enhances anticonvulsant effect of •phenytoin (plasma concentration of phenytoin increased)

Antifungals: imidazoles possibly antagonise effects of amphotericin

• Antihistamines: manufacturer of loratadine advises ketoconazole possibly increases plasma concentration of loratadine; imidazoles possibly inhibit metabolism of •mizolastine (avoid concomitant use); ketoconazole inhibits metabolism of •mizolastine—avoid concomitant use; ketoconazole increases plasma concentration of rupatadine

• Antimalarials: avoidance of imidazoles advised by manufacturer of •piperaquine with artenimol (possible risk of ventricular arrhythmias); avoidance of imidazoles advised by manufacturer of •artemether with lumefantrine; ketoconazole increases plasma concentration of mefloquine

Antimuscarinics: absorption of ketoconazole reduced by antimuscarinics; ketoconazole increases plasma concentration of darifenacin—avoid concomitant use; manufacturer of fesoterodine advises dose reduction when ketoconazole given with fesoterodine—consult fesoterodine product literature; ketoconazole increases plasma concentration of solifenacin; avoidance of ketoconazole advised by manufacturer of tolterodine

• Antipsychotics: ketoconazole inhibits metabolism of •aripiprazole (reduce dose of aripiprazole); increased risk of ventricular arrhythmias when imidazoles given with •pimozide—avoid concomitant use; imidazoles possibly increase plasma concentration of •quetiapine—manufacturer of quetiapine advises avoid concomitant use

• Antivirals: ketoconazole increases plasma concentration of •boceprevir and saquinavir; plasma concentration of both drugs increased when ketoconazole given with darunavir; plasma concentration of ketoconazole increased by fosamprenavir (also plasma concentration of fosamprenavir possibly increased); ketoconazole increases plasma concentration of •indinavir and •maraviroc (consider reducing dose of indinavir and maraviroc); plasma concentration of ketoconazole reduced by •nevirapine—avoid concomitant use; combination of ketoconazole with •ritonavir may increase plasma concentration of either drug (or both); imidazoles possibly increase plasma concentration of saquinavir; plasma concentration of both drugs possibly increased when ketoconazole given with •telaprevir (increased risk of ventricular arrhythmias)

• Anxiolytics and Hypnotics: ketoconazole increases plasma concentration of alprazolam; ketoconazole increases plasma concentration of •midazolam (risk of prolonged sedation)

**Antifungals, Imidazole** *(continued)*

Aprepitant: ketoconazole increases plasma concentration of aprepitant

Bosentan: ketoconazole increases plasma concentration of bosentan

- Calcium-channel Blockers: ketoconazole inhibits metabolism of ●felodipine (increased plasma concentration); avoidance of ketoconazole advised by manufacturer of lercanidipine; ketoconazole possibly inhibits metabolism of dihydropyridines (increased plasma concentration)
- Ciclosporin: ketoconazole inhibits metabolism of ●ciclosporin (increased plasma concentration); miconazole possibly inhibits metabolism of ●ciclosporin (increased plasma concentration)

Cilostazol: ketoconazole increases plasma concentration of cilostazol (consider reducing dose of cilostazol)

Cinacalcet: ketoconazole inhibits metabolism of cinacalcet (increased plasma concentration)

- Clopidogrel: ketoconazole possibly reduces antiplatelet effect of ●clopidogrel
- Colchicine: ketoconazole possibly increases risk of ●colchicine toxicity—suspend or reduce dose of colchicine (avoid concomitant use in hepatic or renal impairment)

Corticosteroids: ketoconazole possibly inhibits metabolism of corticosteroids; ketoconazole increases plasma concentration of *inhaled* and *oral* budesonide; ketoconazole increases plasma concentration of active metabolite of ciclesonide; ketoconazole increases plasma concentration of *inhaled* fluticasone and mometasone; ketoconazole inhibits the metabolism of methylprednisolone

- Cytotoxics: ketoconazole increases plasma concentration of axitinib (reduce dose of axitinib—consult axitinib product literature); ketoconazole increases plasma concentration of ●crizotinib, ●everolimus, ●lapatinib and ●nilotinib—avoid concomitant use; ketoconazole possibly increases plasma concentration of dasatinib; ketoconazole inhibits metabolism of erlotinib and sunitinib (increased plasma concentration); ketoconazole increases plasma concentration of bortezomib and imatinib; avoidance of ketoconazole advised by manufacturer of ●cabazitaxel and ●pazopanib; manufacturer of ruxolitinib advises dose reduction when ketoconazole given with ●ruxolitinib—consult ruxolitinib product literature; ketoconazole increases plasma concentration of active metabolite of ●temsirolimus—avoid concomitant use; *in vitro* studies suggest a possible interaction between ketoconazole and docetaxel (consult docetaxel product literature); possible increased risk of neutropenia when ketoconazole given with ●brentuximab vedotin; ketoconazole reduces plasma concentration of ●irinotecan (but concentration of active metabolite of irinotecan increased)—avoid concomitant use; ketoconazole increases plasma concentration of ●vinflunine—manufacturer of vinflunine advises avoid concomitant use
- Diuretics: ketoconazole increases plasma concentration of ●eplerenone—avoid concomitant use
- Domperidone: manufacturer of ketoconazole advises avoid concomitant use with ●domperidone (risk of ventricular arrhythmias)
- Ergot Alkaloids: increased risk of ergotism when imidazoles given with ●ergotamine and methysergide—avoid concomitant use

Fidaxomicin: avoidance of ketoconazole advised by manufacturer of fidaxomicin

- Fingolimod: ketoconazole increases plasma concentration of ●fingolimod
- 5HT$_1$-receptor Agonists: ketoconazole increases plasma concentration of almotriptan (increased risk of toxicity); ketoconazole increases plasma concen-

**Antifungals, Imidazole**

- 5HT$_1$-receptor Agonists *(continued)*
  tration of ●eletriptan (risk of toxicity)—avoid concomitant use
- Ivabradine: ketoconazole increases plasma concentration of ●ivabradine—avoid concomitant use

Lanthanum: absorption of ketoconazole possibly reduced by lanthanum (give at least 2 hours apart)

- Lenalidomide: ketoconazole possibly increases plasma concentration of ●lenalidomide (increased risk of toxicity)
- Lipid-regulating Drugs: possible increased risk of myopathy when imidazoles given with atorvastatin; increased risk of myopathy when ketoconazole given with ●simvastatin (avoid concomitant use); possible increased risk of myopathy when miconazole given with ●simvastatin

Mirabegron: when given with ketoconazole avoid or reduce dose of mirabegron in hepatic or renal impairment—see Mirabegron, BNF section 7.4.2

Oestrogens: anecdotal reports of contraceptive failure when imidazoles given with oestrogens

Parasympathomimetics: ketoconazole increases plasma concentration of galantamine

- Ranolazine: ketoconazole increases plasma concentration of ●ranolazine—avoid concomitant use
- Retinoids: ketoconazole increases plasma concentration of alitretinoin; ketoconazole possibly increases risk of ●tretinoin toxicity

Sildenafil: ketoconazole increases plasma concentration of sildenafil—reduce initial dose of sildenafil

- Sirolimus: ketoconazole increases plasma concentration of ●sirolimus—avoid concomitant use; miconazole increases plasma concentration of ●sirolimus

Sympathomimetics, Beta$_2$: ketoconazole inhibits metabolism of salmeterol (increased plasma concentration)

- Tacrolimus: imidazoles possibly increase plasma concentration of ●tacrolimus; ketoconazole increases plasma concentration of ●tacrolimus (consider reducing dose of tacrolimus)
- Tadalafil: ketoconazole increases plasma concentration of ●tadalafil—manufacturer of tadalafil advises avoid concomitant use
- Theophylline: ketoconazole possibly increases plasma concentration of ●theophylline
- Ticagrelor: ketoconazole increases plasma concentration of ●ticagrelor—manufacturer of ticagrelor advises avoid concomitant use

Tolvaptan: ketoconazole increases plasma concentration of tolvaptan

Ulcer-healing Drugs: absorption of ketoconazole reduced by histamine H$_2$-antagonists, proton pump inhibitors and sucralfate

- Vardenafil: ketoconazole increases plasma concentration of ●vardenafil—avoid concomitant use

Vitamins: ketoconazole possibly increases plasma concentration of paricalcitol

**Antifungals, Polyene** *see* Amphotericin

**Antifungals, Triazole**

Note In general, fluconazole interactions relate to multiple-dose treatment

- Aliskiren: itraconazole increases plasma concentration of ●aliskiren—avoid concomitant use
- Analgesics: fluconazole increases plasma concentration of celecoxib (halve dose of celecoxib); voriconazole increases plasma concentration of diclofenac, ibuprofen and ●oxycodone; fluconazole increases plasma concentration of flurbiprofen, ibuprofen and methadone; fluconazole increases plasma concentration of parecoxib (reduce dose of parecoxib); voriconazole increases plasma concentration of ●alfentanil and ●methadone (consider reducing dose of alfentanil and methadone); fluconazole inhibits metabolism of alfentanil (risk of prolonged or delayed respiratory depression);

## Antifungals, Triazole

- Analgesics *(continued)*
itraconazole possibly inhibits metabolism of alfentanil; triazoles possibly increase plasma concentration of ●fentanyl
Antacids: absorption of itraconazole reduced by antacids
- Anti-arrhythmics: manufacturer of itraconazole advises avoid concomitant use with ●disopyramide; avoidance of itraconazole, posaconazole and voriconazole advised by manufacturer of ●dronedarone
- Antibacterials: plasma concentration of itraconazole increased by clarithromycin; manufacturer of fluconazole advises avoid concomitant use with erythromycin; triazoles possibly increase plasma concentration of ●rifabutin (increased risk of uveitis—reduce rifabutin dose); posaconazole increases plasma concentration of ●rifabutin (also plasma concentration of posaconazole reduced); voriconazole increases plasma concentration of ●rifabutin, also rifabutin reduces plasma concentration of voriconazole (increase dose of voriconazole and also monitor for rifabutin toxicity); fluconazole increases plasma concentration of ●rifabutin (increased risk of uveitis—reduce rifabutin dose); plasma concentration of itraconazole reduced by ●rifabutin and ●rifampicin—manufacturer of itraconazole advises avoid concomitant use; plasma concentration of posaconazole reduced by ●rifampicin; plasma concentration of voriconazole reduced by ●rifampicin—avoid concomitant use; metabolism of fluconazole accelerated by ●rifampicin (reduced plasma concentration)
- Anticoagulants: avoidance of itraconazole, posaconazole and voriconazole advised by manufacturer of apixaban; fluconazole, itraconazole and voriconazole enhance anticoagulant effect of ●coumarins; itraconazole possibly increases plasma concentration of ●dabigatran etexilate—manufacturer of dabigatran etexilate advises avoid concomitant use; avoidance of itraconazole, posaconazole and voriconazole advised by manufacturer of rivaroxaban
- Antidepressants: avoidance of triazoles advised by manufacturer of ●reboxetine; fluconazole possibly increases plasma concentration of amitriptyline and nortriptyline; plasma concentration of voriconazole reduced by ●St John's wort—avoid concomitant use
- Antidiabetics: posaconazole possibly enhances hypoglycaemic effect of glipizide; fluconazole possibly enhances hypoglycaemic effect of nateglinide; itraconazole possibly enhances hypoglycaemic effect of repaglinide; voriconazole possibly increases plasma concentration of sulfonylureas; fluconazole increases plasma concentration of ●sulfonylureas
- Antiepileptics: plasma concentration of itraconazole and posaconazole possibly reduced by ●carbamazepine; fluconazole possibly increases plasma concentration of carbamazepine; plasma concentration of voriconazole possibly reduced by ●carbamazepine and ●phenobarbital—avoid concomitant use; plasma concentration of itraconazole and posaconazole possibly reduced by ●phenobarbital; voriconazole increases plasma concentration of ●phenytoin, also phenytoin reduces plasma concentration of voriconazole (increase dose of voriconazole and also monitor for phenytoin toxicity); plasma concentration of posaconazole reduced by ●phenytoin; plasma concentration of itraconazole reduced by ●phenytoin—avoid concomitant use; fluconazole increases plasma concentration of ●phenytoin (consider reducing dose of phenytoin)
Antifungals: triazoles possibly antagonise effects of amphotericin; monitoring for increased voriconazole side effects advised by manufacturer of fluconazole if voriconazole given after fluconazole; plasma

## Antifungals, Triazole

Antifungals *(continued)*
concentration of itraconazole increased by micafungin (consider reducing dose of itraconazole); plasma concentration of fluconazole increased by terbinafine
- Antihistamines: itraconazole inhibits metabolism of ●mizolastine—avoid concomitant use
- Antimalarials: avoidance of triazoles advised by manufacturer of ●piperaquine with artenimol (possible risk of ventricular arrhythmias); avoidance of triazoles advised by manufacturer of ●artemether with lumefantrine
Antimuscarinics: avoidance of itraconazole advised by manufacturer of darifenacin and tolterodine; manufacturer of fesoterodine advises dose reduction when itraconazole given with fesoterodine—consult fesoterodine product literature; itraconazole increases plasma concentration of solifenacin
- Antipsychotics: itraconazole possibly increases plasma concentration of haloperidol; itraconazole possibly inhibits metabolism of ●aripiprazole (reduce dose of aripiprazole); increased risk of ventricular arrhythmias when triazoles given with ●pimozide—avoid concomitant use; triazoles possibly increase plasma concentration of ●quetiapine—manufacturer of quetiapine advises avoid concomitant use
- Antivirals: posaconazole increases plasma concentration of ●atazanavir; plasma concentration of itraconazole and posaconazole reduced by ●efavirenz; plasma concentration of voriconazole reduced by ●efavirenz, also plasma concentration of efavirenz increased (increase voriconazole dose and reduce efavirenz dose); plasma concentration of posaconazole possibly reduced by fosamprenavir; plasma concentration of both drugs may increase when itraconazole given with fosamprenavir; itraconazole increases plasma concentration of ●indinavir (consider reducing dose of indinavir); fluconazole increases plasma concentration of ●nevirapine, ritonavir and tipranavir; plasma concentration of itraconazole possibly reduced by nevirapine—consider increasing dose of itraconazole; plasma concentration of voriconazole reduced by ●ritonavir—avoid concomitant use; combination of itraconazole with ●ritonavir may increase plasma concentration of either drug (or both); triazoles possibly increase plasma concentration of saquinavir; plasma concentration of itraconazole possibly increased by telaprevir; plasma concentration of voriconazole possibly affected by ●telaprevir (possible increased risk of ventricular arrhythmias); plasma concentration of posaconazole possibly increased by ●telaprevir (increased risk of ventricular arrhythmias); fluconazole increases plasma concentration of ●zidovudine (increased risk of toxicity)
- Anxiolytics and Hypnotics: itraconazole increases plasma concentration of alprazolam; fluconazole and voriconazole increase plasma concentration of ●diazepam (risk of prolonged sedation); fluconazole, itraconazole, posaconazole and voriconazole increase plasma concentration of ●midazolam (risk of prolonged sedation); itraconazole increases plasma concentration of buspirone (reduce dose of buspirone)
- Bosentan: fluconazole possibly increases plasma concentration of ●bosentan—avoid concomitant use; itraconazole possibly increases plasma concentration of bosentan
- Calcium-channel Blockers: negative inotropic effect possibly increased when itraconazole given with calcium-channel blockers; itraconazole inhibits metabolism of ●felodipine (increased plasma concentration); avoidance of itraconazole advised by manufacturer of lercanidipine; itraconazole possibly

## Antifungals, Triazole

- Calcium-channel Blockers *(continued)*
  inhibits metabolism of dihydropyridines (increased plasma concentration)
- Cardiac Glycosides: itraconazole increases plasma concentration of ●digoxin
- Ciclosporin: fluconazole, itraconazole, posaconazole and voriconazole inhibit metabolism of ●ciclosporin (increased plasma concentration)
- Clopidogrel: fluconazole, itraconazole and voriconazole possibly reduce antiplatelet effect of ●clopidogrel
- Colchicine: itraconazole possibly increases risk of ●colchicine toxicity—suspend or reduce dose of colchicine (avoid concomitant use in hepatic or renal impairment)

  Corticosteroids: itraconazole possibly inhibits metabolism of corticosteroids and methylprednisolone; itraconazole increases plasma concentration of *inhaled* budesonide and fluticasone
- Cytotoxics: itraconazole inhibits metabolism of busulfan (increased risk of toxicity); fluconazole and itraconazole possibly increase side-effects of cyclophosphamide; itraconazole possibly increases plasma concentration of axitinib (reduce dose of axitinib—consult axitinib product literature); itraconazole and voriconazole possibly increase plasma concentration of ●crizotinib—manufacturer of crizotinib advises avoid concomitant use; itraconazole, posaconazole and voriconazole possibly increase plasma concentration of ●everolimus—manufacturer of everolimus advises avoid concomitant use; itraconazole increases plasma concentration of gefitinib; avoidance of itraconazole, posaconazole and voriconazole advised by manufacturer of ●lapatinib; avoidance of itraconazole and voriconazole advised by manufacturer of ●nilotinib; avoidance of itraconazole and voriconazole advised by manufacturer of ●pazopanib; manufacturer of ruxolitinib advises dose reduction when fluconazole, itraconazole, posaconazole and voriconazole given with ●ruxolitinib—consult ruxolitinib product literature; avoidance of itraconazole and voriconazole advised by manufacturer of ●cabazitaxel; itraconazole possibly inhibits metabolism of ●vinblastine and ●vincristine (increased risk of neurotoxicity); itraconazole possibly inhibits metabolism of ●vincristine and ●vinorelbine (increased risk of neurotoxicity); itraconazole possibly increases plasma concentration of ●vinflunine—manufacturer of vinflunine advises avoid concomitant use
- Diuretics: fluconazole increases plasma concentration of eplerenone (reduce dose of eplerenone); itraconazole increases plasma concentration of ●eplerenone—avoid concomitant use; plasma concentration of fluconazole increased by hydrochlorothiazide
- Ergot Alkaloids: increased risk of ergotism when triazoles given with ●ergotamine and methysergide—avoid concomitant use
- 5HT$_1$-receptor Agonists: itraconazole increases plasma concentration of ●eletriptan (risk of toxicity)—avoid concomitant use
- Ivabradine: fluconazole increases plasma concentration of ivabradine—reduce initial dose of ivabradine; itraconazole possibly increases plasma concentration of ●ivabradine—avoid concomitant use
- Lenalidomide: itraconazole possibly increases plasma concentration of ●lenalidomide (increased risk of toxicity)
- Lipid-regulating Drugs: possible increased risk of myopathy when triazoles given with atorvastatin; increased risk of myopathy when posaconazole given with ●atorvastatin or ●simvastatin (avoid concomitant use); increased risk of myopathy when itraconazole given with ●atorvastatin; fluconazole

## Antifungals, Triazole

- Lipid-regulating Drugs *(continued)*
  increases plasma concentration of fluvastatin—possible increased risk of myopathy; possible increased risk of myopathy when fluconazole or voriconazole given with ●simvastatin; increased risk of myopathy when itraconazole given with ●simvastatin (avoid concomitant use)

  Mirabegron: when given with itraconazole avoid or reduce dose of mirabegron in hepatic or renal impairment—see Mirabegron, BNF section 7.4.2

  Oestrogens: plasma concentration of voriconazole increased by oestrogens

  Progestogens: plasma concentration of voriconazole possibly increased by progestogens
- Ranolazine: itraconazole, posaconazole and voriconazole possibly increase plasma concentration of ●ranolazine—manufacturer of ranolazine advises avoid concomitant use
- Retinoids: fluconazole and voriconazole possibly increase risk of ●tretinoin toxicity

  Sildenafil: itraconazole increases plasma concentration of sildenafil—reduce initial dose of sildenafil
- Sirolimus: fluconazole and posaconazole possibly increase plasma concentration of sirolimus; itraconazole and voriconazole increase plasma concentration of ●sirolimus—avoid concomitant use
- Tacrolimus: fluconazole, itraconazole, posaconazole and voriconazole increase plasma concentration of ●tacrolimus (consider reducing dose of tacrolimus)

  Tadalafil: itraconazole possibly increases plasma concentration of tadalafil
- Theophylline: fluconazole possibly increases plasma concentration of ●theophylline
- Ulcer-healing Drugs: plasma concentration of posaconazole reduced by ●cimetidine; voriconazole possibly increases plasma concentration of esomeprazole; voriconazole increases plasma concentration of omeprazole (consider reducing dose of omeprazole); manufacturer of posaconazole advises avoid concomitant use with histamine H$_2$-antagonists and proton pump inhibitors (plasma concentration of posaconazole possibly reduced); absorption of itraconazole reduced by histamine H$_2$-antagonists and proton pump inhibitors
- Vardenafil: itraconazole possibly increases plasma concentration of ●vardenafil—avoid concomitant use

## Antihistamines

**Note** Sedative interactions apply to a lesser extent to the non-sedating antihistamines. Interactions do not generally apply to antihistamines used for topical action (including inhalation)

Alcohol: increased sedative effect when antihistamines given with alcohol (possibly less effect with non-sedating antihistamines)
- Analgesics: sedative effects possibly increased when sedating antihistamines given with ●opioid analgesics

  Antacids: absorption of fexofenadine reduced by antacids
- Anti-arrhythmics: increased risk of ventricular arrhythmias when mizolastine given with ●amiodarone, ●disopyramide or ●flecainide—avoid concomitant use; manufacturer of mizolastine advises avoid concomitant use with propafenone (possible risk of ventricular arrhythmias)
- Antibacterials: plasma concentration of rupatadine increased by erythromycin; manufacturer of loratadine advises plasma concentration possibly increased by erythromycin; metabolism of mizolastine inhibited by ●erythromycin—avoid concomitant use; increased risk of ventricular arrhythmias when mizolastine given with ●moxifloxacin—avoid concomitant use; effects of fexofenadine possibly reduced by rifampicin; metabolism of mizolastine

## Antihistamines

- Antibacterials *(continued)*
  possibly inhibited by ●macrolides (avoid concomitant use)
  Antidepressants: manufacturer of promethazine advises avoid for 2 weeks after stopping MAOIs; increased antimuscarinic and sedative effects when antihistamines given with MAOIs or tricyclics; cyproheptadine possibly antagonises antidepressant effect of SSRIs; possible increased antimuscarinic and sedative effects when antihistamines given with tricyclic-related antidepressants
  Antidiabetics: thrombocyte count depressed when ketotifen given with metformin (manufacturer of ketotifen advises avoid concomitant use)
- Antifungals: plasma concentration of rupatadine increased by ketoconazole; manufacturer of loratadine advises plasma concentration possibly increased by ketoconazole; metabolism of mizolastine inhibited by ●itraconazole or ●ketoconazole—avoid concomitant use; metabolism of mizolastine possibly inhibited by ●imidazoles (avoid concomitant use)
- Antimalarials: avoidance of mizolastine advised by manufacturer of ●piperaquine with artenimol (possible risk of ventricular arrhythmias)
  Antimuscarinics: increased risk of antimuscarinic side-effects when antihistamines given with antimuscarinics
- Antivirals: plasma concentration of chlorphenamine possibly increased by lopinavir; plasma concentration of non-sedating antihistamines possibly increased by ritonavir; increased risk of ventricular arrhythmias when mizolastine given with ●saquinavir—avoid concomitant use
  Anxiolytics and Hypnotics: increased sedative effect when antihistamines given with anxiolytics and hypnotics
- Beta-blockers: increased risk of ventricular arrhythmias when mizolastine given with ●sotalol—avoid concomitant use
  Betahistine: antihistamines theoretically antagonise effect of betahistine
- Cytotoxics: possible increased risk of ventricular arrhythmias when mizolastine given with ●vandetanib—avoid concomitant use
- Grapefruit Juice: plasma concentration of bilastine reduced by grapefruit juice; plasma concentration of rupatadine increased by ●grapefruit juice—avoid concomitant use
  Histamine: antihistamines theoretically antagonise effects of histamine—manufacturer of histamine advises avoid concomitant use
  Ulcer-healing Drugs: manufacturer of loratadine advises plasma concentration possibly increased by cimetidine

## Antihistamines, Non-sedating *see* Antihistamines

## Antihistamines, Sedating *see* Antihistamines

## Antimalarials *see* Artemether with Lumefantrine, Chloroquine and Hydroxychloroquine, Mefloquine, Piperaquine with Artenimol, Primaquine, Proguanil, Pyrimethamine, and Quinine

## Antimetabolites *see* Cytarabine, Decitabine, Fludarabine, Fluorouracil, Gemcitabine, Mercaptopurine, Methotrexate, Pemetrexed, Raltitrexed, and Tioguanine

## Antimuscarinics

Note Many drugs have antimuscarinic effects; concomitant use of two or more such drugs can increase side-effects such as dry mouth, urine retention, and constipation; concomitant use can also lead to confusion in the elderly. Interactions do not generally apply to antimuscarinics used by inhalation
Alcohol: increased sedative effect when hyoscine given with alcohol
Analgesics: possible increased risk of antimuscarinic side-effects when antimuscarinics given with

## Antimuscarinics

Analgesics *(continued)*
  codeine; increased risk of antimuscarinic side-effects when antimuscarinics given with nefopam
- Anti-arrhythmics: increased risk of ventricular arrhythmias when tolterodine given with ●amiodarone, ●disopyramide or ●flecainide; increased risk of antimuscarinic side-effects when antimuscarinics given with disopyramide
  Antibacterials: manufacturer of fesoterodine advises dose reduction when fesoterodine given with clarithromycin and telithromycin—consult fesoterodine product literature; manufacturer of tolterodine advises avoid concomitant use with clarithromycin and erythromycin; plasma concentration of darifenacin possibly increased by erythromycin; plasma concentration of active metabolite of fesoterodine reduced by rifampicin
  Antidepressants: plasma concentration of darifenacin and procyclidine increased by paroxetine; increased risk of antimuscarinic side-effects when antimuscarinics given with MAOIs or tricyclics; possible increased antimuscarinic side-effects when antimuscarinics given with tricyclic-related antidepressants
  Antifungals: antimuscarinics reduce absorption of ketoconazole; manufacturer of fesoterodine advises dose reduction when fesoterodine given with itraconazole and ketoconazole—consult fesoterodine product literature; plasma concentration of darifenacin increased by ketoconazole—avoid concomitant use; plasma concentration of solifenacin increased by itraconazole and ketoconazole; manufacturer of tolterodine advises avoid concomitant use with itraconazole and ketoconazole; manufacturer of darifenacin advises avoid concomitant use with itraconazole
  Antihistamines: increased risk of antimuscarinic side-effects when antimuscarinics given with antihistamines
  Antipsychotics: antimuscarinics possibly reduce effects of haloperidol; increased risk of antimuscarinic side-effects when antimuscarinics given with clozapine; antimuscarinics reduce plasma concentration of phenothiazines, but risk of antimuscarinic side-effects increased
  Antivirals: manufacturer of darifenacin advises avoid concomitant use with atazanavir, fosamprenavir, indinavir, lopinavir, ritonavir, saquinavir and tipranavir; manufacturer of fesoterodine advises dose reduction when fesoterodine given with atazanavir, indinavir, ritonavir and saquinavir—consult fesoterodine product literature; manufacturer of tolterodine advises avoid concomitant use with fosamprenavir, indinavir, lopinavir, ritonavir and saquinavir; plasma concentration of solifenacin increased by ritonavir
- Beta-blockers: increased risk of ventricular arrhythmias when tolterodine given with ●sotalol
  Calcium-channel Blockers: manufacturer of darifenacin advises avoid concomitant use with verapamil
  Cardiac Glycosides: darifenacin possibly increases plasma concentration of digoxin
  Ciclosporin: manufacturer of darifenacin advises avoid concomitant use with ciclosporin
  Domperidone: antimuscarinics antagonise effects of domperidone on gastro-intestinal activity
  Dopaminergics: antimuscarinics possibly reduce absorption of levodopa
  Hormone Antagonists: possible increased risk of bradycardia when ipratropium or oxybutynin given with pasireotide
  Memantine: effects of antimuscarinics possibly enhanced by memantine
  Metoclopramide: antimuscarinics antagonise effects of metoclopramide on gastro-intestinal activity

## Antimuscarinics (continued)

Nitrates: antimuscarinics possibly reduce effects of sublingual tablets of nitrates (failure to dissolve under tongue owing to dry mouth)

Parasympathomimetics: antimuscarinics antagonise effects of parasympathomimetics

## Antipsychotics

**Note** Increased risk of toxicity with myelosuppressive drugs

**Note** Avoid concomitant use of clozapine with drugs that have a substantial potential for causing agranulocytosis

ACE Inhibitors: enhanced hypotensive effect when antipsychotics given with ACE inhibitors

Adrenergic Neurone Blockers: enhanced hypotensive effect when phenothiazines given with adrenergic neurone blockers; higher doses of chlorpromazine antagonise hypotensive effect of adrenergic neurone blockers; haloperidol antagonises hypotensive effect of adrenergic neurone blockers

Adsorbents: absorption of phenothiazines possibly reduced by kaolin

Alcohol: increased sedative effect when antipsychotics given with alcohol

Alpha-blockers: enhanced hypotensive effect when antipsychotics given with alpha-blockers

● Anaesthetics, General: droperidol enhances effects of thiopental; enhanced hypotensive effect when antipsychotics given with ●general anaesthetics

● Analgesics: possible severe drowsiness when haloperidol given with acemetacin or indometacin; increased risk of ventricular arrhythmias when antipsychotics that prolong the QT interval given with ●methadone; increased risk of ventricular arrhythmias when amisulpride given with ●methadone—avoid concomitant use; increased risk of convulsions when antipsychotics given with tramadol; enhanced hypotensive and sedative effects when antipsychotics given with opioid analgesics

Angiotensin-II Receptor Antagonists: enhanced hypotensive effect when antipsychotics given with angiotensin-II receptor antagonists

Antacids: absorption of phenothiazines and sulpiride reduced by antacids

● Anti-arrhythmics: increased risk of ventricular arrhythmias when antipsychotics that prolong the QT interval given with ●anti-arrhythmics that prolong the QT interval; increased risk of ventricular arrhythmias when amisulpride, droperidol, haloperidol, phenothiazines, pimozide or zuclopenthixol given with ●amiodarone—avoid concomitant use; increased risk of ventricular arrhythmias when benperidol given with ●amiodarone—manufacturer of benperidol advises avoid concomitant use; increased risk of ventricular arrhythmias when sulpiride given with ●amiodarone or ●disopyramide; increased risk of ventricular arrhythmias when amisulpride, droperidol, pimozide or zuclopenthixol given with ●disopyramide—avoid concomitant use; increased risk of ventricular arrhythmias when phenothiazines given with ●disopyramide; possible increased risk of ventricular arrhythmias when haloperidol given with ●disopyramide—avoid concomitant use; avoidance of phenothiazines advised by manufacturer of ●dronedarone (risk of ventricular arrhythmias); increased risk of arrhythmias when clozapine given with ●flecainide

● Antibacterials: increased risk of ventricular arrhythmias when pimozide given with ●clarithromycin, ●moxifloxacin or ●telithromycin—avoid concomitant use; plasma concentration of quetiapine possibly increased by ●clarithromycin—manufacturer of quetiapine advises avoid concomitant use; increased risk of ventricular arrhythmias when amisulpride given with ●erythromycin—avoid concomitant use; plasma concentration of clozapine possibly increased by ●erythromycin (possible increased risk of convulsions); possible increased risk of ventri-

## Antipsychotics

● Antibacterials (continued)

cular arrhythmias when pimozide given with ●erythromycin—avoid concomitant use; plasma concentration of quetiapine increased by ●erythromycin—manufacturer of quetiapine advises avoid concomitant use; increased risk of ventricular arrhythmias when sulpiride given with parenteral ●erythromycin; increased risk of ventricular arrhythmias when zuclopenthixol given with parenteral ●erythromycin—avoid concomitant use; plasma concentration of clozapine increased by ciprofloxacin; plasma concentration of olanzapine possibly increased by ciprofloxacin; increased risk of ventricular arrhythmias when droperidol, haloperidol, phenothiazines or zuclopenthixol given with ●moxifloxacin—avoid concomitant use; increased risk of ventricular arrhythmias when benperidol given with ●moxifloxacin—manufacturer of benperidol advises avoid concomitant use; plasma concentration of aripiprazole possibly reduced by ●rifabutin and ●rifampicin—increase dose of aripiprazole; plasma concentration of clozapine possibly reduced by rifampicin; metabolism of haloperidol accelerated by ●rifampicin (reduced plasma concentration); avoid concomitant use of clozapine with ●chloramphenicol or ●sulfonamides (increased risk of agranulocytosis); manufacturer of droperidol advises avoid concomitant use with ●macrolides (risk of ventricular arrhythmias); possible increased risk of ventricular arrhythmias when chlorpromazine given with ●telithromycin; plasma concentration of quetiapine possibly increased by telithromycin

● Antidepressants: plasma concentration of clozapine possibly increased by citalopram (increased risk of toxicity); metabolism of aripiprazole possibly inhibited by ●fluoxetine and ●paroxetine (reduce dose of aripiprazole); plasma concentration of clozapine, haloperidol and risperidone increased by ●fluoxetine; manufacturer of droperidol advises avoid concomitant use with ●fluoxetine, ●fluvoxamine, ●sertraline or ●tricyclics (risk of ventricular arrhythmias); plasma concentration of asenapine and haloperidol possibly increased by fluvoxamine; plasma concentration of clozapine and olanzapine increased by ●fluvoxamine; asenapine possibly increases plasma concentration of paroxetine; plasma concentration of clozapine increased by ●paroxetine, ●sertraline and ●venlafaxine; plasma concentration of risperidone possibly increased by paroxetine (increased risk of toxicity); metabolism of perphenazine inhibited by paroxetine (reduce dose of perphenazine); plasma concentration of haloperidol increased by venlafaxine; clozapine possibly increases CNS effects of ●MAOIs; plasma concentration of pimozide possibly increased by ●SSRIs (increased risk of ventricular arrhythmias—avoid concomitant use); plasma concentration of aripiprazole possibly reduced by ●St John's wort—increase dose of aripiprazole; increased risk of antimuscarinic side-effects when phenothiazines given with tricyclics; increased risk of ventricular arrhythmias when pimozide given with ●tricyclics—avoid concomitant use; possible increased antimuscarinic side-effects when clozapine given with tricyclics; antipsychotics increase plasma concentration of ●tricyclics—possible increased risk of ventricular arrhythmias

Antidiabetics: phenothiazines possibly antagonise hypoglycaemic effect of sulfonylureas

● Antiepileptics: antipsychotics antagonise anticonvulsant effect of ●antiepileptics (convulsive threshold lowered); plasma concentration of aripiprazole reduced by ●carbamazepine—increase dose of aripiprazole; plasma concentration of paliperi-

## Antipsychotics

- Antiepileptics *(continued)*
done reduced by carbamazepine; metabolism of haloperidol, olanzapine, quetiapine and risperidone accelerated by carbamazepine (reduced plasma concentration); metabolism of clozapine accelerated by •carbamazepine (reduced plasma concentration), also avoid concomitant use of drugs with substantial potential for causing agranulocytosis; metabolism of haloperidol accelerated by phenobarbital (reduced plasma concentration); plasma concentration of both drugs reduced when chlorpromazine given with phenobarbital; plasma concentration of clozapine possibly reduced by phenobarbital; plasma concentration of aripiprazole possibly reduced by •phenobarbital and •phenytoin—increase dose of aripiprazole; plasma concentration of haloperidol reduced by phenytoin; chlorpromazine possibly increases or decreases plasma concentration of phenytoin; metabolism of clozapine and quetiapine accelerated by phenytoin (reduced plasma concentration); plasma concentration of clozapine possibly increased or decreased by valproate; plasma concentration of quetiapine possibly increased by valproate; increased risk of side-effects including neutropenia when olanzapine given with •valproate

- Antifungals: metabolism of aripiprazole inhibited by •ketoconazole (reduce dose of aripiprazole); metabolism of aripiprazole possibly inhibited by •itraconazole (reduce dose of aripiprazole); plasma concentration of haloperidol possibly increased by itraconazole; increased risk of ventricular arrhythmias when pimozide given with •imidazoles or •triazoles—avoid concomitant use; plasma concentration of quetiapine possibly increased by •imidazoles and •triazoles—manufacturer of quetiapine advises avoid concomitant use

- Antimalarials: avoidance of droperidol, haloperidol, phenothiazines and pimozide advised by manufacturer of •piperaquine with artenimol (possible risk of ventricular arrhythmias); avoidance of antipsychotics advised by manufacturer of •artemether with lumefantrine; increased risk of ventricular arrhythmias when droperidol given with •chloroquine and hydroxychloroquine or •quinine—avoid concomitant use; increased risk of ventricular arrhythmias when pimozide given with •mefloquine or •quinine—avoid concomitant use; possible increased risk of ventricular arrhythmias when haloperidol given with •mefloquine or •quinine—avoid concomitant use

  Antimuscarinics: increased risk of antimuscarinic side-effects when clozapine given with antimuscarinics; plasma concentration of phenothiazines reduced by antimuscarinics, but risk of antimuscarinic side-effects increased; effects of haloperidol possibly reduced by antimuscarinics

- Antipsychotics: increased risk of ventricular arrhythmias when amisulpride, pimozide or sulpiride given with •droperidol—avoid concomitant use; increased risk of ventricular arrhythmias when phenothiazines that prolong the QT interval given with •droperidol—avoid concomitant use; avoid concomitant use of clozapine with depot formulation of •flupentixol, •fluphenazine, •haloperidol, •pipotiazine, •risperidone or •zuclopenthixol as cannot be withdrawn quickly if neutropenia occurs; increased risk of ventricular arrhythmias when sulpiride given with •haloperidol; chlorpromazine possibly increases plasma concentration of haloperidol; increased risk of ventricular arrhythmias when droperidol given with •haloperidol—avoid concomitant use; increased risk of ventricular arrhythmias when pimozide given with •phenothiazines—avoid conco-

## Antipsychotics

- Antipsychotics *(continued)*
mitant use; increased risk of ventricular arrhythmias when pimozide given with •sulpiride

- Antivirals: metabolism of aripiprazole possibly inhibited by •atazanavir, •fosamprenavir, •indinavir, •lopinavir, •ritonavir and •saquinavir (reduce dose of aripiprazole); plasma concentration of quetiapine possibly increased by •atazanavir, •boceprevir, •darunavir, •fosamprenavir, •indinavir, •lopinavir, •ritonavir, •saquinavir, •telaprevir and •tipranavir—manufacturer of quetiapine advises avoid concomitant use; plasma concentration of pimozide possibly increased by •atazanavir—avoid concomitant use; avoidance of pimozide advised by manufacturer of •boceprevir and •telaprevir; plasma concentration of pimozide possibly increased by •efavirenz, •indinavir and •saquinavir (increased risk of ventricular arrhythmias—avoid concomitant use); plasma concentration of aripiprazole possibly reduced by •efavirenz and •nevirapine—increase dose of aripiprazole; plasma concentration of pimozide increased by •fosamprenavir and •ritonavir (increased risk of ventricular arrhythmias—avoid concomitant use); plasma concentration of antipsychotics possibly increased by •ritonavir; plasma concentration of olanzapine reduced by ritonavir—consider increasing dose of olanzapine; avoidance of clozapine advised by manufacturer of •ritonavir (increased risk of toxicity); increased risk of ventricular arrhythmias when clozapine, haloperidol or phenothiazines given with •saquinavir—avoid concomitant use

- Anxiolytics and Hypnotics: increased sedative effect when antipsychotics given with anxiolytics and hypnotics; plasma concentration of haloperidol possibly increased by alprazolam; increased risk of hypotension, bradycardia and respiratory depression when *intramuscular* olanzapine given with *parenteral* •benzodiazepines; serious adverse events reported with concomitant use of clozapine and •benzodiazepines (causality not established); plasma concentration of haloperidol increased by buspirone

- Aprepitant: avoidance of pimozide advised by manufacturer of •aprepitant

- Atomoxetine: increased risk of ventricular arrhythmias when antipsychotics that prolong the QT interval given with •atomoxetine

- Beta-blockers: enhanced hypotensive effect when phenothiazines given with beta-blockers; plasma concentration of both drugs may increase when chlorpromazine given with •propranolol; increased risk of ventricular arrhythmias when amisulpride, phenothiazines, pimozide or sulpiride given with •sotalol; increased risk of ventricular arrhythmias when droperidol or zuclopenthixol given with •sotalol—avoid concomitant use; possible increased risk of ventricular arrhythmias when haloperidol given with •sotalol—avoid concomitant use

  Calcium-channel Blockers: enhanced hypotensive effect when antipsychotics given with calcium-channel blockers

  Clonidine: enhanced hypotensive effect when phenothiazines given with clonidine

- Cytotoxics: avoid concomitant use of clozapine with •cytotoxics (increased risk of agranulocytosis); caution with pimozide advised by manufacturer of •crizotinib; avoidance of pimozide advised by manufacturer of •lapatinib; possible increased risk of ventricular arrhythmias when amisulpride, chlorpromazine, haloperidol, pimozide, sulpiride or zuclopenthixol given with •vandetanib—avoid concomitant use; increased risk of ventricular arrhythmias when haloperidol given with •arsenic trioxide; increased risk of ventricular arrhythmias when

## Antipsychotics

- Cytotoxics *(continued)*
  antipsychotics that prolong the QT interval given with ●arsenic trioxide

  Deferasirox: avoidance of clozapine advised by manufacturer of deferasirox

  Desferrioxamine: manufacturer of levomepromazine advises avoid concomitant use with desferrioxamine; avoidance of prochlorperazine advised by manufacturer of desferrioxamine

  Diazoxide: enhanced hypotensive effect when phenothiazines given with diazoxide

- Diuretics: risk of ventricular arrhythmias with amisulpride increased by hypokalaemia caused by ●diuretics; risk of ventricular arrhythmias with pimozide increased by hypokalaemia caused by ●diuretics (avoid concomitant use); enhanced hypotensive effect when phenothiazines given with diuretics

  Dopaminergics: increased risk of extrapyramidal side-effects when antipsychotics given with amantadine; antipsychotics antagonise effects of apomorphine, levodopa and pergolide; antipsychotics antagonise hypoprolactinaemic and antiparkinsonian effects of bromocriptine and cabergoline; manufacturer of amisulpride advises avoid concomitant use of levodopa (antagonism of effect); avoidance of antipsychotics advised by manufacturer of pramipexole, ropinirole and rotigotine (antagonism of effect)

- Grapefruit Juice: plasma concentration of quetiapine possibly increased by ●grapefruit juice—manufacturer of quetiapine advises avoid concomitant use

  Histamine: antipsychotics theoretically antagonise effects of histamine—manufacturer of histamine advises avoid concomitant use

- Hormone Antagonists: manufacturer of droperidol advises avoid concomitant use with ●tamoxifen (risk of ventricular arrhythmias)

- Ivabradine: increased risk of ventricular arrhythmias when pimozide given with ●ivabradine

  Lithium: increased risk of extrapyramidal side-effects and possibly neurotoxicity when clozapine, flupentixol, haloperidol, phenothiazines or zuclopenthixol given with lithium; possible risk of toxicity when olanzapine given with lithium; increased risk of extrapyramidal side-effects when sulpiride given with lithium

  Memantine: effects of antipsychotics possibly reduced by memantine

  Methyldopa: enhanced hypotensive effect when antipsychotics given with methyldopa (also increased risk of extrapyramidal effects)

  Metoclopramide: increased risk of extrapyramidal side-effects when antipsychotics given with metoclopramide

  Moxonidine: enhanced hypotensive effect when phenothiazines given with moxonidine

  Muscle Relaxants: promazine possibly enhances effects of suxamethonium

  Nitrates: enhanced hypotensive effect when phenothiazines given with nitrates

- Penicillamine: avoid concomitant use of clozapine with ●penicillamine (increased risk of agranulocytosis)

- Pentamidine Isetionate: increased risk of ventricular arrhythmias when amisulpride or droperidol given with ●pentamidine isetionate—avoid concomitant use; increased risk of ventricular arrhythmias when phenothiazines given with ●pentamidine isetionate

  Sodium Benzoate: haloperidol possibly reduces effects of sodium benzoate

  Sodium Oxybate: antipsychotics possibly enhance effects of sodium oxybate

  Sodium Phenylbutyrate: haloperidol possibly reduces effects of sodium phenylbutyrate

  Sympathomimetics: antipsychotics antagonise hypertensive effect of sympathomimetics; antipsychotic

## Antipsychotics

Sympathomimetics *(continued)*
effects of chlorpromazine possibly antagonised by dexamfetamine; chlorpromazine possibly reduces effects of lisdexamfetamine; side-effects of risperidone possibly increased by methylphenidate

- Tacrolimus: manufacturer of droperidol advises avoid concomitant use with ●tacrolimus (risk of ventricular arrhythmias)

  Tetrabenazine: increased risk of extrapyramidal side-effects when antipsychotics given with tetrabenazine

  Ulcer-healing Drugs: effects of antipsychotics, chlorpromazine and clozapine possibly enhanced by cimetidine; plasma concentration of clozapine possibly reduced by omeprazole; absorption of sulpiride reduced by sucralfate

  Vasodilator Antihypertensives: enhanced hypotensive effect when phenothiazines given with hydralazine, minoxidil or sodium nitroprusside

## Antivirals *see* individual drugs

## Anxiolytics and Hypnotics

ACE Inhibitors: enhanced hypotensive effect when anxiolytics and hypnotics given with ACE inhibitors

Adrenergic Neurone Blockers: enhanced hypotensive effect when anxiolytics and hypnotics given with adrenergic neurone blockers

Alcohol: increased sedative effect when anxiolytics and hypnotics given with alcohol

Alpha-blockers: enhanced hypotensive and sedative effects when anxiolytics and hypnotics given with alpha-blockers

Anaesthetics, General: increased sedative effect when anxiolytics and hypnotics given with general anaesthetics

Analgesics: metabolism of midazolam possibly inhibited by fentanyl; increased sedative effect when anxiolytics and hypnotics given with opioid analgesics

Angiotensin-II Receptor Antagonists: enhanced hypotensive effect when anxiolytics and hypnotics given with angiotensin-II receptor antagonists

- Antibacterials: metabolism of midazolam inhibited by ●clarithromycin, ●erythromycin and ●telithromycin (increased plasma concentration with increased sedation); plasma concentration of buspirone increased by erythromycin (reduce dose of buspirone); metabolism of zopiclone inhibited by erythromycin; metabolism of benzodiazepines possibly accelerated by rifampicin (reduced plasma concentration); metabolism of diazepam and zaleplon accelerated by rifampicin (reduced plasma concentration); metabolism of buspirone possibly accelerated by rifampicin; metabolism of zolpidem accelerated by rifampicin (reduced plasma concentration and reduced effect); plasma concentration of zopiclone significantly reduced by rifampicin; metabolism of diazepam inhibited by isoniazid

  Anticoagulants: chloral may transiently enhance anticoagulant effect of coumarins

- Antidepressants: plasma concentration of alprazolam increased by fluoxetine; plasma concentration of melatonin increased by ●fluvoxamine—avoid concomitant use; plasma concentration of some benzodiazepines increased by fluvoxamine; sedative effects possibly increased when zolpidem given with sertraline; manufacturer of buspirone advises avoid concomitant use with MAOIs; avoidance of buspirone for 10 days after stopping tranylcypromine advised by manufacturer of tranylcypromine; plasma concentration of *oral* midazolam possibly reduced by St John's wort; increased sedative effect when anxiolytics and hypnotics given with mirtazapine, tricyclic-related antidepressants or tricyclics

**Anxiolytics and Hypnotics** (continued)

Antiepileptics: plasma concentration of clonazepam often reduced by **carbamazepine, phenobarbital** and **phenytoin**; plasma concentration of midazolam reduced by **carbamazepine** and **perampanel**; benzodiazepines possibly increase or decrease plasma concentration of **phenytoin**; diazepam increases or decreases plasma concentration of **phenytoin**; plasma concentration of clobazam increased by **stiripentol**; clobazam possibly increases plasma concentration of **valproate**; plasma concentration of diazepam and lorazepam possibly increased by **valproate**; increased risk of side-effects when clonazepam given with **valproate**

- Antifungals: plasma concentration of alprazolam increased by **itraconazole** and **ketoconazole**; plasma concentration of midazolam increased by ●**fluconazole**, ●**itraconazole**, ●**ketoconazole**, ●**posaconazole** and ●**voriconazole** (risk of prolonged sedation); plasma concentration of diazepam increased by ●**fluconazole** and ●**voriconazole** (risk of prolonged sedation); plasma concentration of buspirone increased by **itraconazole** (reduce dose of buspirone)

Antihistamines: increased sedative effect when anxiolytics and hypnotics given with **antihistamines**

- Antipsychotics: increased sedative effect when anxiolytics and hypnotics given with **antipsychotics**; alprazolam possibly increases plasma concentration of **haloperidol**; buspirone increases plasma concentration of **haloperidol**; serious adverse events reported with concomitant use of benzodiazepines and ●**clozapine** (causality not established); increased risk of hypotension, bradycardia and respiratory depression when *parenteral* benzodiazepines given with *intramuscular* ●**olanzapine**

- Antivirals: plasma concentration of midazolam possibly increased by ●**atazanavir**—avoid concomitant use of *oral* midazolam; plasma concentration of *oral* midazolam increased by ●**boceprevir**—manufacturer of boceprevir advises avoid concomitant use; increased risk of prolonged sedation when midazolam given with ●**efavirenz**—avoid concomitant use; plasma concentration of midazolam possibly increased by ●**fosamprenavir**, ●**indinavir**, ●**ritonavir** and ●**telaprevir** (risk of prolonged sedation—avoid concomitant use of *oral* midazolam); increased risk of prolonged sedation when alprazolam given with ●**indinavir**—avoid concomitant use; plasma concentration of alprazolam, diazepam, flurazepam and zolpidem possibly increased by ●**ritonavir** (risk of extreme sedation and respiratory depression—avoid concomitant use); plasma concentration of anxiolytics and hypnotics possibly increased by ●**ritonavir**; plasma concentration of buspirone increased by **ritonavir** (increased risk of toxicity); plasma concentration of midazolam increased by ●**saquinavir** (risk of prolonged sedation—avoid concomitant use of *oral* midazolam)

Aprepitant: plasma concentration of midazolam increased by **aprepitant** (risk of prolonged sedation)

Beta-blockers: enhanced hypotensive effect when anxiolytics and hypnotics given with **beta-blockers**

Calcium-channel Blockers: enhanced hypotensive effect when anxiolytics and hypnotics given with **calcium-channel blockers**; midazolam increases absorption of **lercanidipine**; plasma concentration of buspirone increased by **diltiazem** and **verapamil** (reduce dose of buspirone); metabolism of midazolam inhibited by **diltiazem** and **verapamil** (increased plasma concentration with increased sedation)

Cardiac Glycosides: alprazolam increases plasma concentration of **digoxin** (increased risk of toxicity)

Clonidine: enhanced hypotensive effect when anxiolytics and hypnotics given with **clonidine**

**Anxiolytics and Hypnotics** (continued)

- Cytotoxics: plasma concentration of midazolam increased by ●**crizotinib** and **nilotinib**

Deferasirox: plasma concentration of midazolam possibly reduced by **deferasirox**

Diazoxide: enhanced hypotensive effect when anxiolytics and hypnotics given with **diazoxide**

Disulfiram: metabolism of benzodiazepines inhibited by **disulfiram** (increased sedative effects); increased risk of temazepam toxicity when given with **disulfiram**

Diuretics: enhanced hypotensive effect when anxiolytics and hypnotics given with **diuretics**; administration of chloral with *parenteral* furosemide may displace thyroid hormone from binding sites

Dopaminergics: benzodiazepines possibly antagonise effects of **levodopa**

Grapefruit Juice: plasma concentration of *oral* midazolam possibly increased by **grapefruit juice**; plasma concentration of buspirone increased by **grapefruit juice**

Lipid-regulating Drugs: plasma concentration of midazolam possibly increased by **atorvastatin**

Lithium: increased risk of neurotoxicity when clonazepam given with **lithium**

Lofexidine: increased sedative effect when anxiolytics and hypnotics given with **lofexidine**

Methyldopa: enhanced hypotensive effect when anxiolytics and hypnotics given with **methyldopa**

- Methylthioninium: possible risk of CNS toxicity when buspirone given with ●**methylthioninium**—avoid concomitant use (if avoidance not possible, use lowest possible dose of methylthioninium and observe patient for up to 4 hours after administration)

Moxonidine: enhanced hypotensive effect when anxiolytics and hypnotics given with **moxonidine**; sedative effects possibly increased when benzodiazepines given with **moxonidine**

Muscle Relaxants: increased sedative effect when anxiolytics and hypnotics given with **baclofen** or **tizanidine**

Nitrates: enhanced hypotensive effect when anxiolytics and hypnotics given with **nitrates**

Oestrogens: plasma concentration of melatonin increased by **oestrogens**; plasma concentration of diazepam possibly increased by **oestrogens**

Probenecid: excretion of lorazepam reduced by **probenecid** (increased plasma concentration); excretion of nitrazepam possibly reduced by **probenecid** (increased plasma concentration)

Progestogens: plasma concentration of diazepam possibly increased by **progestogens**

- Sodium Oxybate: benzodiazepines enhance effects of ●**sodium oxybate** (avoid concomitant use)

Theophylline: effects of benzodiazepines possibly reduced by **theophylline**

Ulcer-healing Drugs: plasma concentration of melatonin increased by **cimetidine**; metabolism of benzodiazepines, clomethiazole and zaleplon inhibited by **cimetidine** (increased plasma concentration); metabolism of diazepam possibly inhibited by **esomeprazole** and **omeprazole** (increased plasma concentration)

Vasodilator Antihypertensives: enhanced hypotensive effect when anxiolytics and hypnotics given with **hydralazine, minoxidil** or **sodium nitroprusside**

**Apixaban**

- Analgesics: increased risk of haemorrhage when anticoagulants given with *intravenous* ●**diclofenac** (avoid concomitant use, including low-dose heparins); increased risk of haemorrhage when anticoagulants given with ●**ketorolac** (avoid concomitant use, including low-dose heparins)

Antibacterials: plasma concentration of apixaban reduced by **rifampicin**

**Apixaban** *(continued)*
- Anticoagulants: increased risk of haemorrhage when apixaban given with other ●anticoagulants (avoid concomitant use except when switching with other anticoagulants or using heparin to maintain catheter patency); increased risk of haemorrhage when other anticoagulants given with ●dabigatran etexilate and ●rivaroxaban (avoid concomitant use except when switching with other anticoagulants or using heparin to maintain catheter patency)
- Antifungals: plasma concentration of apixaban increased by ●ketoconazole—manufacturer of apixaban advises avoid concomitant use; manufacturer of apixaban advises avoid concomitant use with itraconazole, posaconazole and voriconazole
  Antivirals: manufacturer of apixaban advises avoid concomitant use with atazanavir, boceprevir, darunavir, fosamprenavir, indinavir, lopinavir, ritonavir, saquinavir, telaprevir and tipranavir
  Sulfinpyrazone: increased risk of bleeding when apixaban given with sulfinpyrazone

**Apomorphine**
  Antipsychotics: effects of apomorphine antagonised by antipsychotics
  Dopaminergics: effects of apomorphine possibly enhanced by entacapone
- 5HT$_3$-receptor Antagonists: possible increased hypotensive effect when apomorphine given with ●ondansetron—avoid concomitant use
  Memantine: effects of dopaminergics possibly enhanced by memantine
  Methyldopa: antiparkinsonian effect of dopaminergics antagonised by methyldopa

**Apraclonidine**
  Antidepressants: manufacturer of apraclonidine advises avoid concomitant use with MAOIs, tricyclic-related antidepressants and tricyclics
  Sympathomimetics: manufacturer of apraclonidine advises avoid concomitant use with sympathomimetics

**Aprepitant**
  Note Fosaprepitant is a prodrug of aprepitant
  Antibacterials: plasma concentration of aprepitant possibly increased by clarithromycin and telithromycin; plasma concentration of aprepitant reduced by rifampicin
  Anticoagulants: aprepitant possibly reduces anticoagulant effect of warfarin
- Antidepressants: manufacturer of aprepitant advises avoid concomitant use with ●St John's wort
  Antidiabetics: aprepitant reduces plasma concentration of tolbutamide
  Antiepileptics: plasma concentration of aprepitant possibly reduced by carbamazepine, phenobarbital and phenytoin
  Antifungals: plasma concentration of aprepitant increased by ketoconazole
- Antipsychotics: manufacturer of aprepitant advises avoid concomitant use with ●pimozide
  Antivirals: plasma concentration of aprepitant possibly increased by ritonavir
  Anxiolytics and Hypnotics: aprepitant increases plasma concentration of midazolam (risk of prolonged sedation)
  Calcium-channel Blockers: plasma concentration of both drugs may increase when aprepitant given with diltiazem
  Corticosteroids: aprepitant inhibits metabolism of dexamethasone and methylprednisolone (reduce dose of dexamethasone and methylprednisolone)
- Oestrogens: aprepitant possibly causes contraceptive failure of hormonal contraceptives containing ●oestrogens (alternative contraception recommended)
- Progestogens: aprepitant possibly causes contraceptive failure of hormonal contraceptives containing

**Aprepitant**
- Progestogens *(continued)*
  ●progestogens (alternative contraception recommended)

**Aripiprazole** *see* Antipsychotics
**Arsenic Trioxide**
- Anti-arrhythmics: increased risk of ventricular arrhythmias when arsenic trioxide given with ●amiodarone or ●disopyramide
- Antibacterials: increased risk of ventricular arrhythmias when arsenic trioxide given with ●erythromycin, ●levofloxacin or ●moxifloxacin
- Antidepressants: increased risk of ventricular arrhythmias when arsenic trioxide given with ●amitriptyline or ●clomipramine
- Antifungals: increased risk of ventricular arrhythmias when arsenic trioxide given with ●amphotericin
- Antimalarials: avoidance of arsenic trioxide advised by manufacturer of ●piperaquine with artenimol (possible risk of ventricular arrhythmias)
- Antipsychotics: increased risk of ventricular arrhythmias when arsenic trioxide given with ●antipsychotics that prolong the QT interval; increased risk of ventricular arrhythmias when arsenic trioxide given with ●haloperidol; avoid concomitant use of cytotoxics with ●clozapine (increased risk of agranulocytosis)
- Beta-blockers: increased risk of ventricular arrhythmias when arsenic trioxide given with ●sotalol
- Cytotoxics: possible increased risk of ventricular arrhythmias when arsenic trioxide given with ●vandetanib—avoid concomitant use
- Diuretics: risk of ventricular arrhythmias with arsenic trioxide increased by hypokalaemia caused by ●acetazolamide, ●loop diuretics or ●thiazides and related diuretics
- Lithium: increased risk of ventricular arrhythmias when arsenic trioxide given with ●lithium

**Artemether with Lumefantrine**
- Anti-arrhythmics: manufacturer of artemether with lumefantrine advises avoid concomitant use with ●amiodarone, ●disopyramide or ●flecainide (risk of ventricular arrhythmias)
- Antibacterials: manufacturer of artemether with lumefantrine advises avoid concomitant use with ●macrolides and ●quinolones
- Antidepressants: manufacturer of artemether with lumefantrine advises avoid concomitant use with ●antidepressants
- Antifungals: manufacturer of artemether with lumefantrine advises avoid concomitant use with ●imidazoles and ●triazoles
- Antimalarials: manufacturer of artemether with lumefantrine advises avoid concomitant use with ●antimalarials; increased risk of ventricular arrhythmias when artemether with lumefantrine given with ●quinine
- Antipsychotics: manufacturer of artemether with lumefantrine advises avoid concomitant use with ●antipsychotics
- Antivirals: manufacturer of artemether with lumefantrine advises caution with atazanavir, fosamprenavir, indinavir, lopinavir, ritonavir, saquinavir and tipranavir; avoidance of artemether with lumefantrine advised by manufacturer of ●boceprevir; plasma concentration of lumefantrine increased by darunavir
- Beta-blockers: manufacturer of artemether with lumefantrine advises avoid concomitant use with ●metoprolol and ●sotalol
- Cytotoxics: possible increased risk of ventricular arrhythmias when artemether with lumefantrine given with ●vandetanib—avoid concomitant use
  Grapefruit Juice: plasma concentration of artemether with lumefantrine possibly increased by grapefruit juice

**Artemether with Lumefantrine** (continued)

Histamine: avoidance of antimalarials advised by manufacturer of histamine
- Ulcer-healing Drugs: manufacturer of artemether with lumefantrine advises avoid concomitant use with ●cimetidine

Vaccines: antimalarials inactivate oral typhoid vaccine—see p. 621

**Ascorbic acid** *see* Vitamins

**Asenapine** *see* Antipsychotics

**Aspirin**

Adsorbents: absorption of aspirin possibly reduced by kaolin

Anaesthetics, General: aspirin possibly enhances effects of thiopental
- Analgesics: avoid concomitant use of aspirin with ●NSAIDs (increased side-effects); antiplatelet effect of aspirin possibly reduced by ibuprofen

Antacids: excretion of aspirin increased by alkaline urine due to some antacids
- Anticoagulants: increased risk of bleeding when aspirin given with ●coumarins or ●phenindione (due to antiplatelet effect); aspirin enhances anticoagulant effect of ●heparins
- Antidepressants: increased risk of bleeding when aspirin given with ●SSRIs or ●venlafaxine

Antiepileptics: aspirin enhances effects of phenytoin and valproate

Clopidogrel: increased risk of bleeding when aspirin given with clopidogrel

Corticosteroids: increased risk of gastro-intestinal bleeding and ulceration when aspirin given with corticosteroids, also corticosteroids reduce plasma concentration of salicylate
- Cytotoxics: aspirin reduces excretion of ●methotrexate (increased risk of toxicity)
- Diuretics: increased risk of toxicity when high-dose aspirin given with ●acetazolamide; aspirin antagonises diuretic effect of spironolactone; possible increased risk of toxicity when high-dose aspirin given with loop diuretics (also possible reduced effect of loop diuretics)

Iloprost: increased risk of bleeding when aspirin given with iloprost

Leukotriene Receptor Antagonists: aspirin increases plasma concentration of zafirlukast

Metoclopramide: rate of absorption of aspirin increased by metoclopramide (enhanced effect)

Probenecid: aspirin antagonises effects of probenecid

Sulfinpyrazone: aspirin antagonises effects of sulfinpyrazone

Vaccines: possible risk of Reyes syndrome when aspirin given with varicella-zoster vaccine—manufacturers advise avoid aspirin for 6 weeks after giving varicella-zoster vaccine

**Atazanavir**

Antacids: plasma concentration of atazanavir possibly reduced by antacids
- Anti-arrhythmics: atazanavir possibly increases plasma concentration of ●amiodarone and ●lidocaine
- Antibacterials: plasma concentration of both drugs increased when atazanavir given with clarithromycin; atazanavir increases plasma concentration of ●rifabutin (reduce dose of rifabutin); plasma concentration of atazanavir reduced by ●rifampicin—avoid concomitant use; avoidance of concomitant atazanavir in severe renal and hepatic impairment advised by manufacturer of ●telithromycin

Anticoagulants: atazanavir may enhance or reduce anticoagulant effect of warfarin; avoidance of atazanavir advised by manufacturer of apixaban and rivaroxaban
- Antidepressants: plasma concentration of atazanavir reduced by ●St John's wort—avoid concomitant use

**Atazanavir** (continued)
- Antifungals: plasma concentration of atazanavir increased by ●posaconazole
- Antimalarials: caution with atazanavir advised by manufacturer of artemether with lumefantrine; atazanavir possibly increases plasma concentration of ●quinine (increased risk of toxicity)

Antimuscarinics: avoidance of atazanavir advised by manufacturer of darifenacin; manufacturer of fesoterodine advises dose reduction when atazanavir given with fesoterodine—consult fesoterodine product literature
- Antipsychotics: atazanavir possibly inhibits metabolism of ●aripiprazole (reduce dose of aripiprazole); atazanavir possibly increases plasma concentration of ●pimozide—avoid concomitant use; atazanavir possibly increases plasma concentration of ●quetiapine—manufacturer of quetiapine advises avoid concomitant use
- Antivirals: plasma concentration of atazanavir reduced by ●boceprevir; manufacturer of atazanavir advises avoid concomitant use with ●efavirenz (plasma concentration of atazanavir reduced); avoid concomitant use of atazanavir with ●indinavir; atazanavir increases plasma concentration of ●maraviroc (consider reducing dose of maraviroc); plasma concentration of atazanavir possibly reduced by ●nevirapine—avoid concomitant use; increased risk of ventricular arrhythmias when atazanavir given with ●saquinavir—avoid concomitant use; atazanavir possibly reduces plasma concentration of telaprevir, also plasma concentration of atazanavir possibly increased; plasma concentration of atazanavir reduced by tenofovir, also plasma concentration of tenofovir possibly increased; atazanavir increases plasma concentration of tipranavir (also plasma concentration of atazanavir reduced)
- Anxiolytics and Hypnotics: atazanavir possibly increases plasma concentration of ●midazolam—avoid concomitant use of *oral* midazolam
- Calcium-channel Blockers: atazanavir increases plasma concentration of ●diltiazem (reduce dose of diltiazem); atazanavir possibly increases plasma concentration of verapamil
- Ciclosporin: atazanavir possibly increases plasma concentration of ●ciclosporin
- Colchicine: atazanavir possibly increases risk of ●colchicine toxicity—suspend or reduce dose of colchicine (avoid concomitant use in hepatic or renal impairment)
- Cytotoxics: atazanavir possibly increases plasma concentration of axitinib (reduce dose of axitinib—consult axitinib product literature); atazanavir possibly increases plasma concentration of ●crizotinib and ●everolimus—manufacturer of crizotinib and everolimus advises avoid concomitant use; avoidance of atazanavir advised by manufacturer of ●cabazitaxel and ●pazopanib; atazanavir possibly inhibits metabolism of ●irinotecan (increased risk of toxicity)
- Ergot Alkaloids: atazanavir possibly increases plasma concentration of ●ergot alkaloids—avoid concomitant use
- Lipid-regulating Drugs: possible increased risk of myopathy when atazanavir given with ●atorvastatin or pravastatin; possible increased risk of myopathy when atazanavir given with ●rosuvastatin—manufacturer of rosuvastatin advises avoid concomitant use; increased risk of myopathy when atazanavir given with ●simvastatin (avoid concomitant use)

Oestrogens: atazanavir increases plasma concentration of ethinylestradiol

Progestogens: atazanavir increases plasma concentration of norethisterone
- Ranolazine: atazanavir possibly increases plasma concentration of ●ranolazine—manufacturer of ranolazine advises avoid concomitant use

**Atazanavir** *(continued)*

- Sildenafil: atazanavir possibly increases side-effects of ●sildenafil
- Sirolimus: atazanavir possibly increases plasma concentration of ●sirolimus
- Tacrolimus: atazanavir possibly increases plasma concentration of ●tacrolimus
- Ticagrelor: atazanavir possibly increases plasma concentration of ●ticagrelor—manufacturer of ticagrelor advises avoid concomitant use
- Ulcer-healing Drugs: plasma concentration of atazanavir reduced by ●histamine H$_2$-antagonists; plasma concentration of atazanavir reduced by ●proton pump inhibitors—avoid or adjust dose of both drugs (consult product literature)

**Atenolol** *see* Beta-blockers

**Atomoxetine**

- Analgesics: increased risk of ventricular arrhythmias when atomoxetine given with ●methadone; possible increased risk of convulsions when atomoxetine given with tramadol
- Anti-arrhythmics: increased risk of ventricular arrhythmias when atomoxetine given with ●amiodarone or ●disopyramide
- Antibacterials: increased risk of ventricular arrhythmias when atomoxetine given with *parenteral* ●erythromycin; increased risk of ventricular arrhythmias when atomoxetine given with ●moxifloxacin
- Antidepressants: metabolism of atomoxetine possibly inhibited by fluoxetine and paroxetine; possible increased risk of convulsions when atomoxetine given with antidepressants; atomoxetine should not be started until 2 weeks after stopping ●MAOIs, also MAOIs should not be started until at least 2 weeks after stopping atomoxetine; increased risk of ventricular arrhythmias when atomoxetine given with ●tricyclics
- Antimalarials: increased risk of ventricular arrhythmias when atomoxetine given with ●mefloquine
- Antipsychotics: increased risk of ventricular arrhythmias when atomoxetine given with ●antipsychotics that prolong the QT interval
- Beta-blockers: increased risk of ventricular arrhythmias when atomoxetine given with ●sotalol
   Bupropion: possible increased risk of convulsions when atomoxetine given with bupropion
- Diuretics: risk of ventricular arrhythmias with atomoxetine increased by hypokalaemia caused by ●diuretics
   Sympathomimetics, Beta$_2$: Increased risk of cardiovascular side-effects when atomoxetine given with *parenteral* salbutamol

**Atorvastatin** *see* Statins

**Atovaquone**

- Antibacterials: manufacturer of atovaquone advises avoid concomitant use with rifabutin (plasma concentration of both drugs reduced); plasma concentration of atovaquone reduced by ●rifampicin (and concentration of rifampicin increased)—avoid concomitant use; plasma concentration of atovaquone reduced by tetracycline
- Antivirals: plasma concentration of atovaquone reduced by ●efavirenz—avoid concomitant use; atovaquone possibly reduces plasma concentration of indinavir; atovaquone increases plasma concentration of zidovudine (increased risk of toxicity)
   Cytotoxics: atovaquone possibly increases plasma concentration of etoposide
   Histamine: avoidance of atovaquone advised by manufacturer of histamine
   Metoclopramide: plasma concentration of atovaquone reduced by metoclopramide

**Atracurium** *see* Muscle Relaxants

**Atropine** *see* Antimuscarinics

**Axitinib**

   Antibacterials: plasma concentration of axitinib possibly increased by clarithromycin, erythromycin and telithromycin (reduce dose of axitinib—consult axitinib product literature); plasma concentration of axitinib possibly decreased by rifabutin (increase dose of axitinib—consult axitinib product literature); plasma concentration of axitinib decreased by rifampicin (increase dose of axitinib—consult axitinib product literature)
   Antidepressants: plasma concentration of axitinib possibly reduced by St John's wort—consider increasing dose of axitinib
   Antiepileptics: plasma concentration of axitinib possibly decreased by carbamazepine, phenobarbital and phenytoin (increase dose of axitinib—consult axitinib product literature)
   Antifungals: plasma concentration of axitinib increased by ketoconazole (reduce dose of axitinib—consult axitinib product literature); plasma concentration of axitinib possibly increased by itraconazole (reduce dose of axitinib—consult axitinib product literature)
- Antipsychotics: avoid concomitant use of cytotoxics with ●clozapine (increased risk of agranulocytosis)
   Antivirals: plasma concentration of axitinib possibly increased by atazanavir, indinavir, ritonavir and saquinavir (reduce dose of axitinib—consult axitinib product literature)
   Corticosteroids: plasma concentration of axitinib possibly decreased by dexamethasone (increase dose of axitinib—consult axitinib product literature)
   Grapefruit Juice: plasma concentration of axitinib possibly increased by grapefruit juice

**Azathioprine**

   ACE Inhibitors: increased risk of anaemia or leucopenia when azathioprine given with captopril especially in renal impairment; increased risk of anaemia when azathioprine given with enalapril especially in renal impairment
- Allopurinol: enhanced effects and increased toxicity of azathioprine when given with ●allopurinol (reduce dose of azathioprine to one quarter of usual dose)
   Aminosalicylates: possible increased risk of leucopenia when azathioprine given with aminosalicylates
- Antibacterials: increased risk of haematological toxicity when azathioprine given with ●sulfamethoxazole (as co-trimoxazole); increased risk of haematological toxicity when azathioprine given with ●trimethoprim (also with co-trimoxazole)
- Anticoagulants: azathioprine possibly reduces anticoagulant effect of ●coumarins
- Antivirals: myelosuppressive effects of azathioprine possibly enhanced by ●ribavirin
- Febuxostat: avoidance of azathioprine advised by manufacturer of ●febuxostat

**Azilsartan** *see* Angiotensin-II Receptor Antagonists

**Azithromycin** *see* Macrolides

**Aztreonam**

- Anticoagulants: aztreonam possibly enhances anticoagulant effect of ●coumarins
   Vaccines: antibacterials inactivate oral typhoid vaccine—see p. 621

**Baclofen** *see* Muscle Relaxants

**Balsalazide** *see* Aminosalicylates

**Bambuterol** *see* Sympathomimetics, Beta$_2$

**Beclometasone** *see* Corticosteroids

**Belimumab**

- Vaccines: avoid concomitant use of belimumab with live ●vaccines (see p. 600)

**Bendamustine**

- Antipsychotics: avoid concomitant use of cytotoxics with ●clozapine (increased risk of agranulocytosis)

**Bendroflumethiazide** *see* Diuretics

**Benperidol** *see* Antipsychotics
**Benzodiazepines** *see* Anxiolytics and Hypnotics
**Benzthiazide** *see* Diuretics
**Benzylpenicillin** *see* Penicillins
**Beta-blockers**

> **Note** Since systemic absorption may follow topical application of beta-blockers to the eye the possibility of interactions, in particular, with drugs such as verapamil should be borne in mind

ACE Inhibitors: enhanced hypotensive effect when beta-blockers given with ACE inhibitors

Adrenergic Neurone Blockers: enhanced hypotensive effect when beta-blockers given with adrenergic neurone blockers

Alcohol: enhanced hypotensive effect when beta-blockers given with alcohol

Aldesleukin: enhanced hypotensive effect when beta-blockers given with aldesleukin

- Alpha-blockers: enhanced hypotensive effect when beta-blockers given with ●alpha-blockers, also increased risk of first-dose hypotension with post-synaptic alpha-blockers such as prazosin

Anaesthetics, General: enhanced hypotensive effect when beta-blockers given with general anaesthetics

- Anaesthetics, Local: propranolol increases risk of ●bupivacaine toxicity

Analgesics: hypotensive effect of beta-blockers antagonised by NSAIDs; plasma concentration of esmolol possibly increased by morphine

Angiotensin-II Receptor Antagonists: enhanced hypotensive effect when beta-blockers given with angiotensin-II receptor antagonists

- Anti-arrhythmics: increased myocardial depression when beta-blockers given with ●anti-arrhythmics; increased risk of bradycardia, AV block and myocardial depression when beta-blockers given with ●amiodarone; increased risk of ventricular arrhythmias when sotalol given with ●amiodarone, ●disopyramide or ●dronedarone—avoid concomitant use; plasma concentration of metoprolol and propranolol possibly increased by dronedarone; increased risk of myocardial depression and bradycardia when beta-blockers given with ●flecainide; propranolol increases risk of ●lidocaine toxicity; plasma concentration of metoprolol and propranolol increased by propafenone

- Antibacterials: increased risk of ventricular arrhythmias when sotalol given with ●moxifloxacin—avoid concomitant use; metabolism of bisoprolol and propranolol accelerated by rifampicin (plasma concentration significantly reduced); plasma concentration of carvedilol, celiprolol and metoprolol reduced by rifampicin

- Antidepressants: plasma concentration of metoprolol increased by citalopram and escitalopram; plasma concentration of propranolol increased by fluvoxamine; plasma concentration of metoprolol possibly increased by paroxetine (enhanced effect); labetalol and propranolol increase plasma concentration of imipramine; enhanced hypotensive effect when beta-blockers given with MAOIs; increased risk of ventricular arrhythmias when sotalol given with ●tricyclics

Antidiabetics: beta-blockers may mask warning signs of hypoglycaemia (such as tremor) with antidiabetics; beta-blockers enhance hypoglycaemic effect of insulin

Antiepileptics: plasma concentration of propranolol possibly reduced by phenobarbital

- Antihistamines: increased risk of ventricular arrhythmias when sotalol given with ●mizolastine—avoid concomitant use

- Antimalarials: avoidance of sotalol advised by manufacturer of ●piperaquine with artenimol (possible risk of ventricular arrhythmias); avoidance of metoprolol and sotalol advised by manufacturer of

**Beta-blockers**
- Antimalarials *(continued)*
  ●artemether with lumefantrine; increased risk of bradycardia when beta-blockers given with mefloquine

- Antimuscarinics: increased risk of ventricular arrhythmias when sotalol given with ●tolterodine

- Antipsychotics: increased risk of ventricular arrhythmias when sotalol given with ●droperidol or ●zuclopenthixol—avoid concomitant use; possible increased risk of ventricular arrhythmias when sotalol given with ●haloperidol—avoid concomitant use; plasma concentration of both drugs may increase when propranolol given with ●chlorpromazine; increased risk of ventricular arrhythmias when sotalol given with ●amisulpride, ●phenothiazines, ●pimozide or ●sulpiride; enhanced hypotensive effect when beta-blockers given with phenothiazines

- Antivirals: increased risk of ventricular arrhythmias when sotalol given with ●saquinavir—avoid concomitant use; avoidance of sotalol advised by manufacturer of ●telaprevir (risk of ventricular arrhythmias); avoidance of metoprolol for heart failure advised by manufacturer of ●tipranavir

Anxiolytics and Hypnotics: enhanced hypotensive effect when beta-blockers given with anxiolytics and hypnotics

- Atomoxetine: increased risk of ventricular arrhythmias when sotalol given with ●atomoxetine

- Calcium-channel Blockers: enhanced hypotensive effect when beta-blockers given with calcium-channel blockers; possible severe hypotension and heart failure when beta-blockers given with ●nifedipine; increased risk of AV block and bradycardia when beta-blockers given with ●diltiazem; asystole, severe hypotension and heart failure when beta-blockers given with ●verapamil (see p. 107)

Cardiac Glycosides: increased risk of AV block and bradycardia when beta-blockers given with cardiac glycosides

- Ciclosporin: carvedilol increases plasma concentration of ●ciclosporin

- Clonidine: increased risk of withdrawal hypertension when beta-blockers given with ●clonidine (withdraw beta-blockers several days before slowly withdrawing clonidine)

Corticosteroids: hypotensive effect of beta-blockers antagonised by corticosteroids

- Cytotoxics: possible increased risk of bradycardia when beta-blockers given with crizotinib; possible increased risk of ventricular arrhythmias when sotalol given with ●vandetanib—avoid concomitant use; increased risk of ventricular arrhythmias when sotalol given with ●arsenic trioxide

Diazoxide: enhanced hypotensive effect when beta-blockers given with diazoxide

- Diuretics: enhanced hypotensive effect when beta-blockers given with diuretics; risk of ventricular arrhythmias with sotalol increased by hypokalaemia caused by ●loop diuretics or ●thiazides and related diuretics

Dopaminergics: enhanced hypotensive effect when beta-blockers given with levodopa

Ergot Alkaloids: increased peripheral vasoconstriction when beta-blockers given with ergotamine and methysergide

- Fingolimod: possible increased risk of bradycardia when beta-blockers given with ●fingolimod

Hormone Antagonists: possible increased risk of bradycardia when carteolol, metoprolol, propranolol or sotalol given with pasireotide

5HT₁-receptor Agonists: propranolol increases plasma concentration of rizatriptan (manufacturer of rizatriptan advises halve dose and avoid within 2 hours of propranolol)

## Beta-blockers *(continued)*

- Ivabradine: increased risk of ventricular arrhythmias when sotalol given with ●ivabradine
  Methyldopa: enhanced hypotensive effect when beta-blockers given with methyldopa
  Mirabegron: plasma concentration of metoprolol increased by mirabegron
- Moxisylyte: possible severe postural hypotension when beta-blockers given with ●moxisylyte
  Moxonidine: enhanced hypotensive effect when beta-blockers given with moxonidine
  Muscle Relaxants: propranolol enhances effects of muscle relaxants; enhanced hypotensive effect when beta-blockers given with baclofen; possible enhanced hypotensive effect and bradycardia when beta-blockers given with tizanidine
  Nitrates: enhanced hypotensive effect when beta-blockers given with nitrates
  Oestrogens: hypotensive effect of beta-blockers antagonised by oestrogens
  Parasympathomimetics: propranolol antagonises effects of neostigmine and pyridostigmine; increased risk of arrhythmias when beta-blockers given with pilocarpine
  Prostaglandins: enhanced hypotensive effect when beta-blockers given with alprostadil
- Ranolazine: avoidance of sotalol advised by manufacturer of ●ranolazine
- Sympathomimetics: increased risk of severe hypertension and bradycardia when non-cardioselective beta-blockers given with ●adrenaline (epinephrine), also reponse to adrenaline (epinephrine) may be reduced; increased risk of severe hypertension and bradycardia when non-cardioselective beta-blockers given with ●dobutamine; possible increased risk of severe hypertension and bradycardia when non-cardioselective beta-blockers given with ●noradrenaline (norepinephrine)
  Thyroid Hormones: metabolism of propranolol accelerated by levothyroxine
  Ulcer-healing Drugs: plasma concentration of labetalol, metoprolol and propranolol increased by cimetidine
  Vasodilator Antihypertensives: enhanced hypotensive effect when beta-blockers given with hydralazine, minoxidil or sodium nitroprusside

## Betahistine

Antihistamines: effect of betahistine theoretically antagonised by antihistamines

## Betamethasone *see* Corticosteroids

## Betaxolol *see* Beta-blockers

## Bethanechol *see* Parasympathomimetics

## Bexarotene

- Antipsychotics: avoid concomitant use of cytotoxics with ●clozapine (increased risk of agranulocytosis)
- Lipid-regulating Drugs: plasma concentration of bexarotene increased by ●gemfibrozil—avoid concomitant use

## Bezafibrate *see* Fibrates

## Bicalutamide

Anticoagulants: bicalutamide possibly enhances anticoagulant effect of coumarins

## Biguanides *see* Antidiabetics

## Bilastine *see* Antihistamines

## Bile Acid Sequestrants *see* Colesevelam, Colestipol, and Colestyramine

## Bile Acids

Antacids: absorption of bile acids possibly reduced by antacids
- Ciclosporin: ursodeoxycholic acid increases absorption of ●ciclosporin
  Lipid-regulating Drugs: absorption of bile acids possibly reduced by colestipol and colestyramine

## Bisoprolol *see* Beta-blockers

## Bisphosphonates

Antacids: absorption of bisphosphonates reduced by antacids
Antibacterials: increased risk of hypocalcaemia when bisphosphonates given with aminoglycosides
Calcium Salts: absorption of bisphosphonates reduced by calcium salts
- Cytotoxics: sodium clodronate increases plasma concentration of ●estramustine
  Iron: absorption of bisphosphonates reduced by *oral* iron

## Bleomycin

- Antipsychotics: avoid concomitant use of cytotoxics with ●clozapine (increased risk of agranulocytosis)
  Cardiac Glycosides: bleomycin possibly reduces absorption of digoxin *tablets*
- Cytotoxics: increased pulmonary toxicity when bleomycin given with ●cisplatin; increased risk of pulmonary toxicity when bleomycin given with ●brentuximab vedotin—avoid concomitant use

## Boceprevir

Analgesics: boceprevir possibly affects plasma concentration of methadone
- Antibacterials: manufacturer of boceprevir advises avoid concomitant use with ●rifampicin (plasma concentration of boceprevir possibly reduced)
  Anticoagulants: avoidance of boceprevir advised by manufacturer of apixaban
- Antiepileptics: manufacturer of boceprevir advises avoid concomitant use with ●carbamazepine, ●phenobarbital and ●phenytoin (plasma concentration of boceprevir possibly reduced)
- Antifungals: plasma concentration of boceprevir increased by ●ketoconazole
- Antimalarials: manufacturer of boceprevir advises avoid concomitant use with ●artemether with lumefantrine
- Antipsychotics: manufacturer of boceprevir advises avoid concomitant use with ●pimozide; boceprevir possibly increases plasma concentration of ●quetiapine—manufacturer of quetiapine advises avoid concomitant use
- Antivirals: boceprevir reduces plasma concentration of ●atazanavir; avoid concomitant use of boceprevir with ●darunavir; avoidance of boceprevir advised by manufacturer of ●fosamprenavir; manufacturers advise avoid concomitant use of boceprevir with ●lopinavir; plasma concentration of both drugs reduced when boceprevir given with ●ritonavir
- Anxiolytics and Hypnotics: boceprevir increases plasma concentration of *oral* ●midazolam—manufacturer of boceprevir advises avoid concomitant use
- Ciclosporin: boceprevir increases plasma concentration of ●ciclosporin
- Cytotoxics: manufacturer of boceprevir advises avoid concomitant use with ●dasatinib, ●erlotinib, ●gefitinib, ●imatinib, ●lapatinib, ●nilotinib, ●pazopanib, ●sorafenib and ●sunitinib; manufacturer of ruxolitinib advises dose reduction when boceprevir given with ●ruxolitinib—consult ruxolitinib product literature
- Ergot Alkaloids: manufacturer of boceprevir advises avoid concomitant use with ●ergot alkaloids
- Lipid-regulating Drugs: boceprevir enhances effects and increases toxicity of ●atorvastatin (reduce dose of atorvastatin); boceprevir increases plasma concentration of pravastatin; manufacturers advise avoid concomitant use of boceprevir with ●simvastatin
- Oestrogens: boceprevir possibly causes contraceptive failure of hormonal contraceptives containing ●oestrogens (alternative contraception recommended)
  Progestogens: boceprevir increases plasma concentration of drospirenone (increased risk of toxicity)

## Boceprevir *(continued)*
- Sirolimus: boceprevir possibly increases plasma concentration of ●sirolimus
- Tacrolimus: boceprevir increases plasma concentration of ●tacrolimus (reduce dose of tacrolimus)

## Bortezomib
Antifungals: plasma concentration of bortezomib increased by ketoconazole
- Antipsychotics: avoid concomitant use of cytotoxics with ●clozapine (increased risk of agranulocytosis)

## Bosentan
- Antibacterials: plasma concentration of bosentan reduced by ●rifampicin—avoid concomitant use
Anticoagulants: manufacturer of bosentan recommends monitoring anticoagulant effect of coumarins
- Antidiabetics: increased risk of hepatotoxicity when bosentan given with ●glibenclamide—avoid concomitant use
- Antifungals: plasma concentration of bosentan increased by ketoconazole; plasma concentration of bosentan possibly increased by ●fluconazole—avoid concomitant use; plasma concentration of bosentan possibly increased by itraconazole
- Antivirals: plasma concentration of bosentan increased by ●ritonavir; bosentan possibly reduces plasma concentration of telaprevir, also plasma concentration of bosentan possibly increased; avoidance of bosentan advised by manufacturer of tipranavir
- Ciclosporin: plasma concentration of bosentan increased by ●ciclosporin (also plasma concentration of ciclosporin reduced—avoid concomitant use)
Lipid-regulating Drugs: bosentan reduces plasma concentration of simvastatin
- Oestrogens: bosentan possibly causes contraceptive failure of hormonal contraceptives containing ●oestrogens (alternative contraception recommended)
- Progestogens: bosentan possibly causes contraceptive failure of hormonal contraceptives containing ●progestogens (alternative contraception recommended)
Sildenafil: bosentan reduces plasma concentration of sildenafil
Tadalafil: bosentan reduces plasma concentration of tadalafil

## Brentuximab vedotin
Antibacterials: effects of brentuximab vedotin possibly reduced by rifampicin
- Antifungals: possible increased risk of neutropenia when brentuximab vedotin given with ●ketoconazole
- Antipsychotics: avoid concomitant use of cytotoxics with ●clozapine (increased risk of agranulocytosis)
- Cytotoxics: increased risk of pulmonary toxicity when brentuximab vedotin given with ●bleomycin—avoid concomitant use

## Brimonidine
Antidepressants: manufacturer of brimonidine advises avoid concomitant use with MAOIs, tricyclic-related antidepressants and tricyclics

## Brinzolamide *see* Diuretics
## Bromocriptine
Alcohol: tolerance of bromocriptine reduced by alcohol
Antibacterials: plasma concentration of bromocriptine increased by erythromycin (increased risk of toxicity); plasma concentration of bromocriptine possibly increased by macrolides (increased risk of toxicity)
Antipsychotics: hypoprolactinaemic and antiparkinsonian effects of bromocriptine antagonised by antipsychotics
Domperidone: hypoprolactinaemic effect of bromocriptine possibly antagonised by domperidone

## Bromocriptine *(continued)*
Hormone Antagonists: plasma concentration of bromocriptine increased by octreotide
Memantine: effects of dopaminergics possibly enhanced by memantine
Methyldopa: antiparkinsonian effect of dopaminergics antagonised by methyldopa
Metoclopramide: hypoprolactinaemic effect of bromocriptine antagonised by metoclopramide
- Sympathomimetics: risk of toxicity when bromocriptine given with ●isometheptene

## Buclizine *see* Antihistamines
## Budesonide *see* Corticosteroids
## Bumetanide *see* Diuretics
## Bupivacaine
Anti-arrhythmics: increased myocardial depression when bupivacaine given with anti-arrhythmics
- Beta-blockers: increased risk of bupivacaine toxicity when given with ●propranolol

## Buprenorphine *see* Opioid Analgesics
## Bupropion
- Antidepressants: bupropion possibly increases plasma concentration of citalopram; manufacturer of bupropion advises avoid for 2 weeks after stopping ●MAOIs; manufacturer of bupropion advises avoid concomitant use with ●moclobemide; bupropion possibly increases plasma concentration of tricyclics (possible increased risk of convulsions)
Antiepileptics: plasma concentration of bupropion reduced by carbamazepine and phenytoin; metabolism of bupropion inhibited by valproate
Antivirals: metabolism of bupropion accelerated by efavirenz (reduced plasma concentration); plasma concentration of bupropion reduced by ritonavir
Atomoxetine: possible increased risk of convulsions when bupropion given with atomoxetine
Dopaminergics: increased risk of side-effects when bupropion given with amantadine or levodopa
- Hormone Antagonists: bupropion possibly inhibits metabolism of ●tamoxifen to active metabolite (avoid concomitant use)
- Methylthioninium: possible risk of CNS toxicity when bupropion given with ●methylthioninium—avoid concomitant use (if avoidance not possible, use lowest possible dose of methylthioninium and observe patient for up to 4 hours after administration)

## Buspirone *see* Anxiolytics and Hypnotics
## Busulfan
Analgesics: metabolism of *intravenous* busulfan possibly inhibited by paracetamol (manufacturer of *intravenous* busulfan advises caution within 72 hours of paracetamol)
- Antibacterials: plasma concentration of busulfan increased by ●metronidazole (increased risk of toxicity)
Antiepileptics: plasma concentration of busulfan possibly reduced by phenytoin
Antifungals: metabolism of busulfan inhibited by itraconazole (increased risk of toxicity)
- Antipsychotics: avoid concomitant use of cytotoxics with ●clozapine (increased risk of agranulocytosis)
Cytotoxics: increased risk of hepatotoxicity when busulfan given with tioguanine

## Butyrophenones *see* Antipsychotics
## Cabazitaxel
- Antibacterials: manufacturer of cabazitaxel advises avoid concomitant use with ●clarithromycin, ●rifabutin, ●rifampicin and ●telithromycin
- Antidepressants: manufacturer of cabazitaxel advises avoid concomitant use with ●St John's wort
- Antiepileptics: manufacturer of cabazitaxel advises avoid concomitant use with ●carbamazepine, ●phenobarbital and ●phenytoin

## Cabazitaxel (continued)

- Antifungals: manufacturer of cabazitaxel advises avoid concomitant use with ●itraconazole, ●ketoconazole and ●voriconazole
- Antipsychotics: avoid concomitant use of cytotoxics with ●clozapine (increased risk of agranulocytosis)
- Antivirals: manufacturer of cabazitaxel advises avoid concomitant use with ●atazanavir, ●indinavir, ●ritonavir and ●saquinavir

## Cabergoline

Antibacterials: plasma concentration of cabergoline increased by erythromycin (increased risk of toxicity); plasma concentration of cabergoline possibly increased by macrolides (increased risk of toxicity)

Antipsychotics: hypoprolactinaemic and antiparkinsonian effects of cabergoline antagonised by antipsychotics

Domperidone: hypoprolactinaemic effect of cabergoline possibly antagonised by domperidone

Memantine: effects of dopaminergics possibly enhanced by memantine

Methyldopa: antiparkinsonian effect of dopaminergics antagonised by methyldopa

Metoclopramide: hypoprolactinaemic effect of cabergoline antagonised by metoclopramide

## Calcium Salts

Note see also Antacids

Antibacterials: calcium salts reduce absorption of ciprofloxacin and tetracycline

Antivirals: manufacturer of rilpivirine advises give calcium salts 2 hours before or 4 hours after rilpivirine

Bisphosphonates: calcium salts reduce absorption of bisphosphonates

Cardiac Glycosides: large intravenous doses of calcium salts can precipitate arrhythmias when given with cardiac glycosides

Corticosteroids: absorption of calcium salts reduced by corticosteroids

Diuretics: increased risk of hypercalcaemia when calcium salts given with thiazides and related diuretics

Eltrombopag: calcium salts possibly reduce absorption of eltrombopag (give at least 4 hours apart)

Fluorides: calcium salts reduce absorption of fluorides

Iron: calcium salts reduce absorption of oral iron

Thyroid Hormones: calcium salts reduce absorption of levothyroxine

Zinc: calcium salts reduce absorption of zinc

## Calcium-channel Blockers

Note Dihydropyridine calcium-channel blockers include amlodipine, felodipine, isradipine, lacidipine, lercanidipine, nicardipine, nifedipine, and nimodipine

ACE Inhibitors: enhanced hypotensive effect when calcium-channel blockers given with ACE inhibitors

Adrenergic Neurone Blockers: enhanced hypotensive effect when calcium-channel blockers given with adrenergic neurone blockers

Alcohol: enhanced hypotensive effect when calcium-channel blockers given with alcohol; verapamil possibly increases plasma concentration of alcohol

Aldesleukin: enhanced hypotensive effect when calcium-channel blockers given with aldesleukin

Aliskiren: verapamil increases plasma concentration of aliskiren

- Alpha-blockers: enhanced hypotensive effect when calcium-channel blockers given with ●alpha-blockers, also increased risk of first-dose hypotension with post-synaptic alpha-blockers such as prazosin
- Anaesthetics, General: enhanced hypotensive effect when calcium-channel blockers given with general anaesthetics or isoflurane; hypotensive effect of verapamil enhanced by ●general anaesthetics (also AV delay)

Analgesics: hypotensive effect of calcium-channel blockers antagonised by NSAIDs; diltiazem inhibits metabolism of alfentanil (risk of prolonged or delayed respiratory depression)

## Calcium-channel Blockers (continued)

Angiotensin-II Receptor Antagonists: enhanced hypotensive effect when calcium-channel blockers given with angiotensin-II receptor antagonists

- Anti-arrhythmics: increased risk of bradycardia, AV block and myocardial depression when diltiazem or verapamil given with ●amiodarone; increased risk of myocardial depression and asystole when verapamil given with ●disopyramide or ●flecainide; increased risk of bradycardia and myocardial depression when diltiazem and verapamil given with ●dronedarone; nifedipine increases plasma concentration of ●dronedarone
- Antibacterials: metabolism of calcium-channel blockers possibly inhibited by ●clarithromycin, ●erythromycin and ●telithromycin (increased risk of side-effects); manufacturer of lercanidipine advises avoid concomitant use with erythromycin; metabolism of diltiazem, nifedipine, nimodipine and verapamil accelerated by ●rifampicin (plasma concentration significantly reduced); metabolism of isradipine and nicardipine possibly accelerated by ●rifampicin (possible significantly reduced plasma concentration)
- Anticoagulants: verapamil possibly increases plasma concentration of ●dabigatran etexilate (see Dose under Dabigatran etexilate, BNF section 2.8.2)
- Antidepressants: metabolism of nifedipine possibly inhibited by fluoxetine (increased plasma concentration); diltiazem and verapamil increase plasma concentration of imipramine; enhanced hypotensive effect when calcium-channel blockers given with MAOIs; plasma concentration of verapamil significantly reduced by ●St John's wort; plasma concentration of nifedipine reduced by St John's wort; plasma concentration of amlodipine possibly reduced by St John's wort; diltiazem and verapamil possibly increase plasma concentration of tricyclics

Antidiabetics: glucose tolerance occasionally impaired when nifedipine given with insulin

- Antiepileptics: diltiazem and verapamil enhance effects of ●carbamazepine; manufacturer of nimodipine advises avoid concomitant use with carbamazepine and phenytoin (plasma concentration of nimodipine possibly reduced); effects of dihydropyridines, nicardipine and nifedipine probably reduced by carbamazepine; effects of felodipine and isradipine reduced by carbamazepine; effects of calcium-channel blockers probably reduced by ●phenobarbital; manufacturer of nimodipine advises avoid concomitant use with ●phenobarbital (plasma concentration of nimodipine reduced); manufacturer of isradipine advises avoid concomitant use with phenobarbital and phenytoin; effects of felodipine and verapamil reduced by phenytoin; diltiazem increases plasma concentration of ●phenytoin but also effect of diltiazem reduced
- Antifungals: metabolism of dihydropyridines possibly inhibited by itraconazole and ketoconazole (increased plasma concentration); metabolism of felodipine inhibited by ●itraconazole and ●ketoconazole (increased plasma concentration); manufacturer of lercanidipine advises avoid concomitant use with itraconazole and ketoconazole; negative inotropic effect possibly increased when calcium-channel blockers given with itraconazole; plasma concentration of nifedipine increased by micafungin

Antimalarials: possible increased risk of bradycardia when calcium-channel blockers given with mefloquine

Antimuscarinics: avoidance of verapamil advised by manufacturer of darifenacin

Antipsychotics: enhanced hypotensive effect when calcium-channel blockers given with antipsychotics

- Antivirals: plasma concentration of verapamil possibly increased by atazanavir; plasma concentration of

## Calcium-channel Blockers

- Antivirals (continued)
  diltiazem increased by •atazanavir (reduce dose of diltiazem); plasma concentration of diltiazem reduced by efavirenz; plasma concentration of calcium-channel blockers possibly increased by •ritonavir; manufacturer of lercanidipine advises avoid concomitant use with ritonavir; caution with diltiazem, felodipine, nicardipine, nifedipine and verapamil advised by manufacturer of telaprevir; plasma concentration of amlodipine increased by telaprevir (consider reducing dose of amlodipine)

  Anxiolytics and Hypnotics: enhanced hypotensive effect when calcium-channel blockers given with anxiolytics and hypnotics; diltiazem and verapamil inhibit metabolism of midazolam (increased plasma concentration with increased sedation); absorption of lercanidipine increased by midazolam; diltiazem and verapamil increase plasma concentration of buspirone (reduce dose of buspirone)

  Aprepitant: plasma concentration of both drugs may increase when diltiazem given with aprepitant

- Beta-blockers: enhanced hypotensive effect when calcium-channel blockers given with beta-blockers; increased risk of AV block and bradycardia when diltiazem given with •beta-blockers; asystole, severe hypotension and heart failure when verapamil given with •beta-blockers (see p. 107); possible severe hypotension and heart failure when nifedipine given with •beta-blockers

  Calcium-channel Blockers: plasma concentration of both drugs may increase when diltiazem given with nifedipine

- Cardiac Glycosides: diltiazem, lercanidipine and nicardipine increase plasma concentration of •digoxin; verapamil increases plasma concentration of •digoxin, also increased risk of AV block and bradycardia; nifedipine possibly increases plasma concentration of •digoxin

- Ciclosporin: diltiazem, nicardipine and verapamil increase plasma concentration of •ciclosporin; combination of lercanidipine with •ciclosporin may increase plasma concentration of either drug (or both)—avoid concomitant use; plasma concentration of nifedipine possibly increased by ciclosporin (increased risk of toxicity including gingival hyperplasia)

  Cilostazol: diltiazem increases plasma concentration of cilostazol (consider reducing dose of cilostazol)

  Clonidine: enhanced hypotensive effect when calcium-channel blockers given with clonidine

- Colchicine: diltiazem and verapamil possibly increase risk of •colchicine toxicity—suspend or reduce dose of colchicine (avoid concomitant use in hepatic or renal impairment)

  Corticosteroids: hypotensive effect of calcium-channel blockers antagonised by corticosteroids; diltiazem increases plasma concentration of methylprednisolone

- Cytotoxics: verapamil possibly increases plasma concentration of doxorubicin; possible increased risk of bradycardia when diltiazem or verapamil given with crizotinib; plasma concentration of both drugs may increase when verapamil given with •everolimus; nifedipine possibly inhibits metabolism of vincristine

  Diazoxide: enhanced hypotensive effect when calcium-channel blockers given with diazoxide

  Diuretics: enhanced hypotensive effect when calcium-channel blockers given with diuretics; diltiazem and verapamil increase plasma concentration of eplerenone (reduce dose of eplerenone)

  Dopaminergics: enhanced hypotensive effect when calcium-channel blockers given with levodopa

  Fidaxomicin: avoidance of verapamil advised by manufacturer of fidaxomicin

## Calcium-channel Blockers (continued)

- Fingolimod: possible increased risk of bradycardia when diltiazem or verapamil given with •fingolimod

  Grapefruit Juice: plasma concentration of felodipine, isradipine, lacidipine, lercanidipine, nicardipine, nifedipine, nimodipine and verapamil increased by grapefruit juice; plasma concentration of amlodipine possibly increased by grapefruit juice

  Hormone Antagonists: diltiazem and verapamil increase plasma concentration of dutasteride; possible increased risk of bradycardia when diltiazem or verapamil given with pasireotide

- Ivabradine: diltiazem and verapamil increase plasma concentration of •ivabradine—avoid concomitant use

- Lenalidomide: verapamil possibly increases plasma concentration of •lenalidomide (increased risk of toxicity)

- Lipid-regulating Drugs: diltiazem increases plasma concentration of atorvastatin—possible increased risk of myopathy; possible increased risk of myopathy when amlodipine and diltiazem given with •simvastatin (see Dose under Simvastatin, p. 126); increased risk of myopathy when verapamil given with •simvastatin (see Dose under Simvastatin, p. 126)

  Lithium: neurotoxicity may occur when diltiazem or verapamil given with lithium without increased plasma concentration of lithium

- Magnesium (parenteral): profound hypotension reported with concomitant use of nifedipine and •parenteral magnesium in pre-eclampsia

  Methyldopa: enhanced hypotensive effect when calcium-channel blockers given with methyldopa

  Moxisylyte: enhanced hypotensive effect when calcium-channel blockers given with moxisylyte

  Moxonidine: enhanced hypotensive effect when calcium-channel blockers given with moxonidine

  Muscle Relaxants: verapamil enhances effects of non-depolarising muscle relaxants and suxamethonium; enhanced hypotensive effect when calcium-channel blockers given with baclofen or tizanidine; manufacturer of verapamil advises avoid concomitant use of *intravenous* dantrolene; possible increased risk of ventricular arrhythmias when diltiazem given with *intravenous* dantrolene—manufacturer of diltiazem advises avoid concomitant use; calcium-channel blockers possibly enhance effects of non-depolarising muscle relaxants

  Nitrates: enhanced hypotensive effect when calcium-channel blockers given with nitrates

  Oestrogens: hypotensive effect of calcium-channel blockers antagonised by oestrogens

  Prostaglandins: enhanced hypotensive effect when calcium-channel blockers given with alprostadil

  Ranolazine: diltiazem and verapamil increase plasma concentration of ranolazine (consider reducing dose of ranolazine)

  Sildenafil: enhanced hypotensive effect when amlodipine given with sildenafil

  Sirolimus: diltiazem increases plasma concentration of •sirolimus; plasma concentration of both drugs increased when verapamil given with •sirolimus

  Sulfinpyrazone: plasma concentration of verapamil reduced by sulfinpyrazone

- Tacrolimus: diltiazem and nifedipine increase plasma concentration of •tacrolimus; felodipine, nicardipine and verapamil possibly increase plasma concentration of tacrolimus

- Theophylline: calcium-channel blockers possibly increase plasma concentration of •theophylline (enhanced effect); diltiazem increases plasma concentration of theophylline; verapamil increases plasma concentration of •theophylline (enhanced effect)

**Calcium-channel Blockers** *(continued)*

Ticagrelor: diltiazem increases plasma concentration of ticagrelor

Ulcer-healing Drugs: metabolism of calcium-channel blockers possibly inhibited by cimetidine (increased plasma concentration); plasma concentration of isradipine increased by cimetidine (halve dose of isradipine)

Vardenafil: enhanced hypotensive effect when nifedipine given with vardenafil

Vasodilator Antihypertensives: enhanced hypotensive effect when calcium-channel blockers given with hydralazine, minoxidil or sodium nitroprusside

**Calcium-channel Blockers (dihydropyridines)** *see* Calcium-channel Blockers

**Candesartan** *see* Angiotensin-II Receptor Antagonists

**Cannabis Extract**

Antidepressants: possible increased risk of hypertension and tachycardia when cannabis extract given with tricyclics

**Capecitabine** *see* Fluorouracil

**Capreomycin**

Antibacterials: increased risk of nephrotoxicity when capreomycin given with colistimethate sodium or polymyxins; increased risk of nephrotoxicity and ototoxicity when capreomycin given with aminoglycosides or vancomycin

Cytotoxics: increased risk of nephrotoxicity and ototoxicity when capreomycin given with platinum compounds

Vaccines: antibacterials inactivate oral typhoid vaccine—see p. 621

**Captopril** *see* ACE Inhibitors

**Carbamazepine**

Alcohol: CNS side-effects of carbamazepine possibly increased by alcohol

● Analgesics: effects of carbamazepine enhanced by ●dextropropoxyphene; carbamazepine reduces plasma concentration of methadone; carbamazepine reduces effects of tramadol; carbamazepine possibly accelerates metabolism of paracetamol (also isolated reports of hepatotoxicity)

● Anti-arrhythmics: carbamazepine possibly reduces plasma concentration of ●dronedarone—avoid concomitant use

● Antibacterials: plasma concentration of carbamazepine increased by ●clarithromycin and ●erythromycin; plasma concentration of carbamazepine reduced by ●rifabutin; carbamazepine accelerates metabolism of doxycycline (reduced effect); plasma concentration of carbamazepine increased by ●isoniazid (also possibly increased isoniazid hepatotoxicity); carbamazepine reduces plasma concentration of ●telithromycin (avoid during and for 2 weeks after carbamazepine)

● Anticoagulants: carbamazepine accelerates metabolism of ●coumarins (reduced anticoagulant effect); carbamazepine possibly reduces plasma concentration of dabigatran etexilate—manufacturer of dabigatran etexilate advises avoid concomitant use

● Antidepressants: carbamazepine possibly reduces plasma concentration of reboxetine; plasma concentration of carbamazepine increased by ●fluoxetine and ●fluvoxamine; carbamazepine reduces plasma concentration of ●mianserin, mirtazapine and trazodone; manufacturer of carbamazepine advises avoid for 2 weeks after stopping ●MAOIs, also antagonism of anticonvulsant effect; anticonvulsant effect of antiepileptics possibly antagonised by MAOIs and ●tricyclic-related antidepressants (convulsive threshold lowered); anticonvulsant effect of antiepileptics antagonised by ●SSRIs and ●tricyclics (convulsive threshold lowered); avoid concomitant use of antiepileptics with ●St John's wort; carbamazepine accelerates metabolism of

**Carbamazepine**

● Antidepressants *(continued)*
●tricyclics (reduced plasma concentration and reduced effect)

● Antiepileptics: carbamazepine possibly reduces plasma concentration of eslicarbazepine but risk of side-effects increased; carbamazepine possibly reduces plasma concentration of ethosuximide and retigabine; carbamazepine often reduces plasma concentration of lamotrigine, also plasma concentration of an active metabolite of carbamazepine sometimes raised (but evidence is conflicting); possible increased risk of carbamazepine toxicity when given with levetiracetam; plasma concentration of carbamazepine sometimes reduced by oxcarbazepine (but concentration of an active metabolite of carbamazepine may be increased), also plasma concentration of an active metabolite of oxcarbazepine often reduced; carbamazepine reduces plasma concentration of ●perampanel (see Dose under Perampanel, p. 224); carbamazepine possibly increases plasma concentration of phenobarbital; plasma concentration of both drugs often reduced when carbamazepine given with phenytoin, also plasma concentration of phenytoin may be increased; plasma concentration of both drugs possibly reduced when carbamazepine given with rufinamide; plasma concentration of carbamazepine increased by ●stiripentol; carbamazepine reduces plasma concentration of tiagabine and zonisamide; carbamazepine often reduces plasma concentration of topiramate; carbamazepine reduces plasma concentration of valproate, also plasma concentration of active metabolite of carbamazepine increased

● Antifungals: plasma concentration of carbamazepine possibly increased by fluconazole, ketoconazole and miconazole; carbamazepine possibly reduces plasma concentration of itraconazole and ●posaconazole; carbamazepine possibly reduces plasma concentration of ●voriconazole—avoid concomitant use; carbamazepine possibly reduces plasma concentration of caspofungin—consider increasing dose of caspofungin

● Antimalarials: avoidance of carbamazepine advised by manufacturer of piperaquine with artenimol; anticonvulsant effect of antiepileptics antagonised by ●mefloquine

● Antipsychotics: anticonvulsant effect of antiepileptics antagonised by ●antipsychotics (convulsive threshold lowered); carbamazepine accelerates metabolism of haloperidol, olanzapine, quetiapine and risperidone (reduced plasma concentration); carbamazepine reduces plasma concentration of ●aripiprazole—increase dose of aripiprazole; carbamazepine accelerates metabolism of ●clozapine (reduced plasma concentration), also avoid concomitant use of drugs with substantial potential for causing agranulocytosis; carbamazepine reduces plasma concentration of paliperidone

● Antivirals: avoidance of carbamazepine advised by manufacturer of ●boceprevir and ●rilpivirine (plasma concentration of boceprevir and rilpivirine possibly reduced); carbamazepine possibly reduces plasma concentration of darunavir, fosamprenavir, lopinavir, saquinavir and tipranavir; plasma concentration of both drugs reduced when carbamazepine given with efavirenz; avoidance of carbamazepine advised by manufacturer of etravirine and ●telaprevir; carbamazepine possibly reduces plasma concentration of ●indinavir, also plasma concentration of carbamazepine possibly increased; carbamazepine reduces plasma concentration of nevirapine; plasma concentration of carbamazepine possibly increased by ●ritonavir

Anxiolytics and Hypnotics: carbamazepine often reduces plasma concentration of clonazepam;

## Carbamazepine

**Anxiolytics and Hypnotics** *(continued)*
carbamazepine reduces plasma concentration of midazolam

**Aprepitant:** carbamazepine possibly reduces plasma concentration of aprepitant

**Bupropion:** carbamazepine reduces plasma concentration of bupropion

- **Calcium-channel Blockers:** carbamazepine reduces effects of felodipine and isradipine; carbamazepine probably reduces effects of dihydropyridines, nicardipine and nifedipine; avoidance of carbamazepine advised by manufacturer of nimodipine (plasma concentration of nimodipine possibly reduced); effects of carbamazepine enhanced by ●diltiazem and ●verapamil

- **Ciclosporin:** carbamazepine accelerates metabolism of ●ciclosporin (reduced plasma concentration)

- **Clopidogrel:** carbamazepine possibly reduces antiplatelet effect of ●clopidogrel

- **Corticosteroids:** carbamazepine accelerates metabolism of ●corticosteroids (reduced effect)

- **Cytotoxics:** carbamazepine possibly decreases plasma concentration of axitinib (increase dose of axitinib—consult axitinib product literature); carbamazepine possibly reduces plasma concentration of crizotinib—manufacturer of crizotinib advises avoid concomitant use; avoidance of carbamazepine advised by manufacturer of ●cabazitaxel, gefitinib and vemurafenib; carbamazepine reduces plasma concentration of ●imatinib and ●lapatinib—avoid concomitant use; avoidance of carbamazepine advised by manufacturer of vandetanib (plasma concentration of vandetanib possibly reduced); carbamazepine possibly reduces plasma concentration of eribulin; carbamazepine reduces plasma concentration of irinotecan and its active metabolite

- **Diuretics:** increased risk of hyponatraemia when carbamazepine given with diuretics; plasma concentration of carbamazepine increased by ●acetazolamide; carbamazepine reduces plasma concentration of ●eplerenone—avoid concomitant use

- **Hormone Antagonists:** metabolism of carbamazepine inhibited by ●danazol (increased risk of toxicity); carbamazepine possibly accelerates metabolism of toremifene (reduced plasma concentration)

**5HT₃-receptor Antagonists:** carbamazepine accelerates metabolism of ondansetron (reduced effect)

- **Lipid-regulating Drugs:** carbamazepine reduces plasma concentration of ●simvastatin—consider increasing dose of simvastatin

**Lithium:** neurotoxicity may occur when carbamazepine given with lithium without increased plasma concentration of lithium

**Muscle Relaxants:** carbamazepine antagonises muscle relaxant effect of non-depolarising muscle relaxants (accelerated recovery from neuromuscular blockade)

- **Oestrogens:** carbamazepine accelerates metabolism of ●oestrogens (reduced contraceptive effect—see p. 398)

- **Orlistat:** possible increased risk of convulsions when antiepileptics given with ●orlistat

- **Progestogens:** carbamazepine accelerates metabolism of ●progestogens (reduced contraceptive effect—see p. 398)

**Retinoids:** plasma concentration of carbamazepine possibly reduced by isotretinoin

**Theophylline:** carbamazepine accelerates metabolism of theophylline (reduced effect)

**Thyroid Hormones:** carbamazepine accelerates metabolism of thyroid hormones (may increase requirements for thyroid hormones in hypothyroidism)

**Tibolone:** carbamazepine accelerates metabolism of tibolone (reduced plasma concentration)

## Carbamazepine *(continued)*

**Ticagrelor:** carbamazepine possibly reduces plasma concentration of ticagrelor

- **Ulcer-healing Drugs:** metabolism of carbamazepine inhibited by ●cimetidine (increased plasma concentration)

- **Ulipristal:** avoidance of carbamazepine advised by manufacturer of ●ulipristal (contraceptive effect of ulipristal possibly reduced)

**Vitamins:** carbamazepine possibly increases requirements for vitamin D

**Carbapenems** *see* Doripenem, Ertapenem, Imipenem with Cilastatin, and Meropenem

## Carbonic Anhydrase Inhibitors *see* Diuretics

## Carboplatin *see* Platinum Compounds

## Carboprost *see* Prostaglandins

## Cardiac Glycosides

**ACE Inhibitors:** plasma concentration of digoxin possibly increased by captopril

**Alpha-blockers:** plasma concentration of digoxin increased by prazosin

**Aminosalicylates:** absorption of digoxin possibly reduced by sulfasalazine

**Analgesics:** plasma concentration of cardiac glycosides possibly increased by NSAIDs, also possible exacerbation of heart failure and reduction of renal function

**Antacids:** absorption of digoxin possibly reduced by antacids

- **Anti-arrhythmics:** plasma concentration of digoxin increased by ●amiodarone, ●dronedarone and ●propafenone (halve dose of digoxin)

**Antibacterials:** plasma concentration of digoxin possibly increased by gentamicin, telithromycin and trimethoprim; absorption of digoxin reduced by neomycin; plasma concentration of digoxin possibly reduced by rifampicin; plasma concentration of digoxin increased by macrolides (increased risk of toxicity)

- **Antidepressants:** plasma concentration of digoxin reduced by ●St John's wort—avoid concomitant use

**Antidiabetics:** plasma concentration of digoxin possibly reduced by acarbose; plasma concentration of digoxin increased by sitagliptin

**Antiepileptics:** plasma concentration of digoxin possibly reduced by phenytoin

- **Antifungals:** increased cardiac toxicity with cardiac glycosides if hypokalaemia occurs with ●amphotericin; plasma concentration of digoxin increased by ●itraconazole

- **Antimalarials:** plasma concentration of digoxin possibly increased by ●chloroquine and hydroxychloroquine; possible increased risk of bradycardia when digoxin given with mefloquine; plasma concentration of digoxin increased by ●quinine

**Antimuscarinics:** plasma concentration of digoxin possibly increased by darifenacin

**Antivirals:** plasma concentration of digoxin increased by etravirine and telaprevir; plasma concentration of digoxin possibly increased by rilpivirine and ritonavir

**Anxiolytics and Hypnotics:** plasma concentration of digoxin increased by alprazolam (increased risk of toxicity)

**Beta-blockers:** increased risk of AV block and bradycardia when cardiac glycosides given with beta-blockers

**Calcium Salts:** arrhythmias can be precipitated when cardiac glycosides given with large *intravenous* doses of calcium salts

- **Calcium-channel Blockers:** plasma concentration of digoxin increased by ●diltiazem, ●lercanidipine and ●nicardipine; plasma concentration of digoxin possibly increased by ●nifedipine; plasma concentration

## Cardiac Glycosides

- Calcium-channel Blockers *(continued)* of digoxin increased by •verapamil, also increased risk of AV block and bradycardia
- Ciclosporin: plasma concentration of digoxin increased by •ciclosporin (increased risk of toxicity)
- Colchicine: possible increased risk of myopathy when digoxin given with •colchicine

  Corticosteroids: increased risk of hypokalaemia when cardiac glycosides given with corticosteroids

  Cytotoxics: absorption of digoxin *tablets* possibly reduced by bleomycin, carmustine, cyclophosphamide, cytarabine, doxorubicin, melphalan, methotrexate, procarbazine and vincristine; possible increased risk of bradycardia when digoxin given with crizotinib

- Diuretics: increased cardiac toxicity with cardiac glycosides if hypokalaemia occurs with •acetazolamide, •loop diuretics or •thiazides and related diuretics; plasma concentration of digoxin possibly increased by potassium canrenoate; plasma concentration of digoxin increased by •spironolactone

  Lenalidomide: plasma concentration of digoxin possibly increased by lenalidomide

  Lipid-regulating Drugs: absorption of cardiac glycosides possibly reduced by colestipol and colestyramine; plasma concentration of digoxin possibly increased by atorvastatin

  Mirabegron: plasma concentration of digoxin increased by mirabegron—reduce initial dose of digoxin

  Muscle Relaxants: risk of ventricular arrhythmias when cardiac glycosides given with suxamethonium; possible increased risk of bradycardia when cardiac glycosides given with tizanidine

  Penicillamine: plasma concentration of digoxin possibly reduced by penicillamine

  Ranolazine: plasma concentration of digoxin increased by ranolazine

  Sympathomimetics, Beta$_2$: plasma concentration of digoxin possibly reduced by salbutamol
- Ticagrelor: plasma concentration of digoxin increased by •ticagrelor

  Tolvaptan: plasma concentration of digoxin increased by tolvaptan (increased risk of toxicity)

  Ulcer-healing Drugs: plasma concentration of digoxin possibly slightly increased by proton pump inhibitors; absorption of cardiac glycosides possibly reduced by sucralfate

## Carmustine

- Antipsychotics: avoid concomitant use of cytotoxics with •clozapine (increased risk of agranulocytosis)

  Cardiac Glycosides: carmustine possibly reduces absorption of digoxin *tablets*

  Ulcer-healing Drugs: myelosuppressive effects of carmustine possibly enhanced by cimetidine

**Carteolol** *see* Beta-blockers

**Carvedilol** *see* Beta-blockers

## Caspofungin

  Antibacterials: plasma concentration of caspofungin initially increased and then reduced by rifampicin (consider increasing dose of caspofungin)

  Antiepileptics: plasma concentration of caspofungin possibly reduced by carbamazepine and phenytoin—consider increasing dose of caspofungin

  Antivirals: plasma concentration of caspofungin possibly reduced by efavirenz and nevirapine—consider increasing dose of caspofungin

- Ciclosporin: plasma concentration of caspofungin increased by •ciclosporin (manufacturer of caspofungin recommends monitoring liver enzymes)

  Corticosteroids: plasma concentration of caspofungin possibly reduced by dexamethasone—consider increasing dose of caspofungin

## Caspofungin *(continued)*

- Tacrolimus: caspofungin reduces plasma concentration of •tacrolimus

**Cefaclor** *see* Cephalosporins

**Cefadroxil** *see* Cephalosporins

**Cefalexin** *see* Cephalosporins

**Cefixime** *see* Cephalosporins

**Cefotaxime** *see* Cephalosporins

**Cefpodoxime** *see* Cephalosporins

**Cefradine** *see* Cephalosporins

**Ceftaroline** *see* Cephalosporins

**Ceftazidime** *see* Cephalosporins

**Ceftriaxone** *see* Cephalosporins

**Cefuroxime** *see* Cephalosporins

**Celecoxib** *see* NSAIDs

**Celiprolol** *see* Beta-blockers

## Cephalosporins

  Antacids: absorption of cefaclor and cefpodoxime reduced by antacids

  Antibacterials: possible increased risk of nephrotoxicity when cephalosporins given with aminoglycosides

- Anticoagulants: cephalosporins possibly enhance anticoagulant effect of •coumarins

  Probenecid: excretion of cephalosporins reduced by probenecid (increased plasma concentration)

  Ulcer-healing Drugs: absorption of cefpodoxime reduced by histamine H$_2$-antagonists

  Vaccines: antibacterials inactivate oral typhoid vaccine—see p. 621

## Certolizumab pegol

- Abatacept: avoid concomitant use of certolizumab pegol with •abatacept
- Anakinra: avoid concomitant use of certolizumab pegol with •anakinra
- Vaccines: avoid concomitant use of certolizumab pegol with live •vaccines (see p. 600)

**Cetirizine** *see* Antihistamines

**Chenodeoxycholic Acid** *see* Bile Acids

**Chloral** *see* Anxiolytics and Hypnotics

## Chloramphenicol

  Antibacterials: metabolism of chloramphenicol accelerated by rifampicin (reduced plasma concentration)

- Anticoagulants: chloramphenicol enhances anticoagulant effect of •coumarins
- Antidiabetics: chloramphenicol enhances effects of •sulfonylureas
- Antiepileptics: metabolism of chloramphenicol possibly accelerated by •phenobarbital (reduced plasma concentration); chloramphenicol increases plasma concentration of •phenytoin (increased risk of toxicity)
- Antipsychotics: avoid concomitant use of chloramphenicol with •clozapine (increased risk of agranulocytosis)
- Ciclosporin: chloramphenicol possibly increases plasma concentration of •ciclosporin
- Clopidogrel: chloramphenicol possibly reduces antiplatelet effect of •clopidogrel

  Hydroxocobalamin: chloramphenicol reduces response to hydroxocobalamin
- Tacrolimus: chloramphenicol possibly increases plasma concentration of •tacrolimus

  Vaccines: antibacterials inactivate oral typhoid vaccine—see p. 621

**Chlordiazepoxide** *see* Anxiolytics and Hypnotics

## Chloroquine and Hydroxychloroquine

  Adsorbents: absorption of chloroquine and hydroxychloroquine reduced by kaolin

  Agalsidase Alfa and Beta: chloroquine and hydroxychloroquine possibly inhibit effects of agalsidase alfa and beta (manufacturers of agalsidase alfa and beta advise avoid concomitant use)

**Chloroquine and Hydroxychloroquine** *(continued)*

Antacids: absorption of chloroquine and hydroxy-chloroquine reduced by antacids

• Anti-arrhythmics: increased risk of ventricular arrhythmias when chloroquine and hydroxychloroquine given with •amiodarone—avoid concomitant use

• Antibacterials: increased risk of ventricular arrhythmias when chloroquine and hydroxychloroquine given with •moxifloxacin—avoid concomitant use

• Antimalarials: avoidance of antimalarials advised by manufacturer of •artemether with lumefantrine; increased risk of convulsions when chloroquine and hydroxychloroquine given with •mefloquine

• Antipsychotics: increased risk of ventricular arrhythmias when chloroquine and hydroxychloroquine given with •droperidol—avoid concomitant use

• Cardiac Glycosides: chloroquine and hydroxychloroquine possibly increase plasma concentration of •digoxin

• Ciclosporin: chloroquine and hydroxychloroquine increase plasma concentration of •ciclosporin (increased risk of toxicity)

Histamine: avoidance of antimalarials advised by manufacturer of histamine

Lanthanum: absorption of chloroquine and hydroxy-chloroquine possibly reduced by lanthanum (give at least 2 hours apart)

Laronidase: chloroquine and hydroxychloroquine possibly inhibit effects of laronidase (manufacturer of laronidase advises avoid concomitant use)

Parasympathomimetics: chloroquine and hydroxy-chloroquine have potential to increase symptoms of myasthenia gravis and thus diminish effect of neostigmine and pyridostigmine

Ulcer-healing Drugs: metabolism of chloroquine and hydroxychloroquine inhibited by cimetidine (increased plasma concentration)

Vaccines: antimalarials inactivate oral typhoid vaccine—see p. 621

**Chlorothiazide** *see* Diuretics

**Chlorphenamine** *see* Antihistamines

**Chlorpromazine** *see* Antipsychotics

**Chlortalidone** *see* Diuretics

**Ciclesonide** *see* Corticosteroids

**Ciclosporin**

• ACE Inhibitors: increased risk of hyperkalaemia when ciclosporin given with •ACE inhibitors

• Aliskiren: ciclosporin increases plasma concentration of •aliskiren—avoid concomitant use

Allopurinol: plasma concentration of ciclosporin possibly increased by allopurinol (risk of nephrotoxicity)

• Ambrisentan: ciclosporin increases plasma concentration of •ambrisentan (see Dose under Ambrisentan, BNF section 2.5.1)

• Analgesics: increased risk of nephrotoxicity when ciclosporin given with •NSAIDs; ciclosporin increases plasma concentration of •diclofenac (halve dose of diclofenac)

• Angiotensin-II Receptor Antagonists: increased risk of hyperkalaemia when ciclosporin given with •angiotensin-II receptor antagonists

Anti-arrhythmics: plasma concentration of ciclosporin possibly increased by amiodarone and propafenone

• Antibacterials: metabolism of ciclosporin inhibited by •clarithromycin and •erythromycin (increased plasma concentration); metabolism of ciclosporin accelerated by •rifampicin (reduced plasma concentration); plasma concentration of ciclosporin possibly reduced by •sulfadiazine; increased risk of nephrotoxicity when ciclosporin given with •aminoglycosides, •polymyxins, •quinolones, •sulfonamides or •vancomycin; plasma concentration of ciclosporin possibly increased by •chloramphenicol and •telithromycin; increased risk of myopathy when ciclosporin given with •daptomycin (preferably avoid concomitant use); metabolism of ciclos-

**Ciclosporin**

• Antibacterials *(continued)*

porin possibly inhibited by •macrolides (increased plasma concentration); increased risk of nephrotoxicity when ciclosporin given with •trimethoprim, also plasma concentration of ciclosporin reduced by *intravenous* trimethoprim

• Anticoagulants: ciclosporin possibly increases plasma concentration of •dabigatran etexilate—manufacturer of dabigatran etexilate advises avoid concomitant use

• Antidepressants: plasma concentration of ciclosporin reduced by •St John's wort—avoid concomitant use

Antidiabetics: ciclosporin possibly enhances hypoglycaemic effect of repaglinide

• Antiepileptics: metabolism of ciclosporin accelerated by •carbamazepine, •phenobarbital and •phenytoin (reduced plasma concentration); plasma concentration of ciclosporin possibly reduced by oxcarbazepine

• Antifungals: metabolism of ciclosporin inhibited by •fluconazole, •itraconazole, •ketoconazole, •posaconazole and •voriconazole (increased plasma concentration); metabolism of ciclosporin possibly inhibited by •miconazole (increased plasma concentration); increased risk of nephrotoxicity when ciclosporin given with •amphotericin; ciclosporin increases plasma concentration of •caspofungin (manufacturer of caspofungin recommends monitoring liver enzymes); plasma concentration of ciclosporin possibly reduced by griseofulvin and terbinafine; plasma concentration of ciclosporin possibly increased by micafungin

• Antimalarials: plasma concentration of ciclosporin increased by •chloroquine and hydroxychloroquine (increased risk of toxicity)

Antimuscarinics: avoidance of ciclosporin advised by manufacturer of darifenacin

• Antivirals: increased risk of nephrotoxicity when ciclosporin given with aciclovir; plasma concentration of ciclosporin possibly increased by •atazanavir and •ritonavir; plasma concentration of ciclosporin increased by •boceprevir, •fosamprenavir and •indinavir; plasma concentration of ciclosporin possibly reduced by •efavirenz; plasma concentration of both drugs increased when ciclosporin given with •saquinavir; plasma concentration of both drugs increased when ciclosporin given with •telaprevir (reduce dose of ciclosporin)

• Beta-blockers: plasma concentration of ciclosporin increased by •carvedilol

• Bile Acids: absorption of ciclosporin increased by •ursodeoxycholic acid

• Bosentan: ciclosporin increases plasma concentration of •bosentan (also plasma concentration of ciclosporin reduced—avoid concomitant use)

• Calcium-channel Blockers: combination of ciclosporin with •lercanidipine may increase plasma concentration of either drug (or both)—avoid concomitant use; plasma concentration of ciclosporin increased by •diltiazem, •nicardipine and •verapamil; ciclosporin possibly increases plasma concentration of nifedipine (increased risk of toxicity including gingival hyperplasia)

• Cardiac Glycosides: ciclosporin increases plasma concentration of •digoxin (increased risk of toxicity)

• Colchicine: possible increased risk of nephrotoxicity and myotoxicity when ciclosporin given with •colchicine—suspend or reduce dose of colchicine (avoid concomitant use in hepatic or renal impairment)

• Corticosteroids: plasma concentration of ciclosporin increased by high-dose •methylprednisolone (risk of convulsions); ciclosporin increases plasma concentration of prednisolone

**Ciclosporin** *(continued)*

- Cytotoxics: increased risk of nephrotoxicity when ciclosporin given with ●melphalan; increased risk of neurotoxicity when ciclosporin given with ●doxorubicin; ciclosporin increases plasma concentration of ●epirubicin, ●everolimus and ●idarubicin; ciclosporin reduces excretion of mitoxantrone (increased plasma concentration); risk of toxicity when ciclosporin given with ●methotrexate; caution with ciclosporin advised by manufacturer of ●crizotinib; plasma concentration of ciclosporin possibly increased by imatinib; *in vitro* studies suggest a possible interaction between ciclosporin and docetaxel (consult docetaxel product literature); ciclosporin possibly increases plasma concentration of etoposide (increased risk of toxicity)
- Diuretics: plasma concentration of ciclosporin possibly increased by ●acetazolamide; increased risk of hyperkalaemia when ciclosporin given with ●potassium-sparing diuretics and aldosterone antagonists; increased risk of nephrotoxicity and possibly hypermagnesaemia when ciclosporin given with thiazides and related diuretics

  Fidaxomicin: avoidance of ciclosporin advised by manufacturer of fidaxomicin
- Grapefruit Juice: plasma concentration of ciclosporin increased by ●grapefruit juice (increased risk of toxicity)
- Hormone Antagonists: metabolism of ciclosporin inhibited by ●danazol (increased plasma concentration); plasma concentration of ciclosporin reduced by lanreotide and ●octreotide; plasma concentration of ciclosporin possibly reduced by ●pasireotide
- Lenalidomide: ciclosporin possibly increases plasma concentration of ●lenalidomide (increased risk of toxicity)
- Lipid-regulating Drugs: absorption of ciclosporin reduced by ●colesevelam; increased risk of renal impairment when ciclosporin given with bezafibrate or fenofibrate; increased risk of myopathy when ciclosporin given with ●atorvastatin (see Dose under Atorvastatin, p. 125); increased risk of myopathy when ciclosporin given with ●fluvastatin or ●pravastatin; increased risk of myopathy when ciclosporin given with ●rosuvastatin or ●simvastatin (avoid concomitant use); plasma concentration of both drugs may increase when ciclosporin given with ●ezetimibe

  Mannitol: possible increased risk of nephrotoxicity when ciclosporin given with mannitol
- Metoclopramide: plasma concentration of ciclosporin increased by ●metoclopramide

  Mifamurtide: avoidance of ciclosporin advised by manufacturer of mifamurtide
- Modafinil: plasma concentration of ciclosporin reduced by ●modafinil

  Oestrogens: plasma concentration of ciclosporin possibly increased by oestrogens
- Orlistat: absorption of ciclosporin possibly reduced by ●orlistat
- Potassium Salts: increased risk of hyperkalaemia when ciclosporin given with ●potassium salts

  Progestogens: plasma concentration of ciclosporin possibly increased by progestogens

  Ranolazine: plasma concentration of both drugs may increase when ciclosporin given with ranolazine

  Sevelamer: plasma concentration of ciclosporin possibly reduced by sevelamer

  Sirolimus: ciclosporin increases plasma concentration of sirolimus
- Sulfinpyrazone: plasma concentration of ciclosporin reduced by ●sulfinpyrazone
- Tacrolimus: plasma concentration of ciclosporin increased by ●tacrolimus (increased risk of nephrotoxicity)—avoid concomitant use

**Ciclosporin** *(continued)*

  Ticagrelor: plasma concentration of ciclosporin possibly increased by ticagrelor
- Ulcer-healing Drugs: plasma concentration of ciclosporin possibly increased by ●cimetidine; plasma concentration of ciclosporin possibly affected by omeprazole

  Vitamins: plasma concentration of ciclosporin possibly affected by vitamin E

**Cidofovir**

- Antivirals: manufacturers advise avoid concomitant use of cidofovir with ●tenofovir

**Cilazapril** *see* ACE Inhibitors

**Cilostazol**

- Anagrelide: avoidance of cilostazol advised by manufacturer of ●anagrelide

  Antibacterials: plasma concentration of cilostazol increased by erythromycin (consider reducing dose of cilostazol)

  Antifungals: plasma concentration of cilostazol increased by ketoconazole (consider reducing dose of cilostazol)

  Calcium-channel Blockers: plasma concentration of cilostazol increased by diltiazem (consider reducing dose of cilostazol)

  Ulcer-healing Drugs: plasma concentration of cilostazol increased by omeprazole (consider reducing dose of cilostazol)

**Cimetidine** *see* Histamine H$_2$-antagonists

**Cinacalcet**

  Antifungals: metabolism of cinacalcet inhibited by ketoconazole (increased plasma concentration)
- Hormone Antagonists: cinacalcet possibly inhibits metabolism of ●tamoxifen to active metabolite (avoid concomitant use)

**Cinnarizine** *see* Antihistamines

**Ciprofibrate** *see* Fibrates

**Ciprofloxacin** *see* Quinolones

**Cisatracurium** *see* Muscle Relaxants

**Cisplatin** *see* Platinum Compounds

**Citalopram** *see* Antidepressants, SSRI

**Clarithromycin** *see* Macrolides

**Clemastine** *see* Antihistamines

**Clindamycin**

- Muscle Relaxants: clindamycin enhances effects of ●non-depolarising muscle relaxants and ●suxamethonium

  Parasympathomimetics: clindamycin antagonises effects of neostigmine and pyridostigmine

  Vaccines: antibacterials inactivate oral typhoid vaccine—see p. 621

**Clobazam** *see* Anxiolytics and Hypnotics

**Clomethiazole** *see* Anxiolytics and Hypnotics

**Clomipramine** *see* Antidepressants, Tricyclic

**Clonazepam** *see* Anxiolytics and Hypnotics

**Clonidine**

  ACE Inhibitors: enhanced hypotensive effect when clonidine given with ACE inhibitors; previous treatment with clonidine possibly delays antihypertensive effect of captopril

  Adrenergic Neurone Blockers: enhanced hypotensive effect when clonidine given with adrenergic neurone blockers

  Alcohol: enhanced hypotensive effect when clonidine given with alcohol

  Aldesleukin: enhanced hypotensive effect when clonidine given with aldesleukin

  Alpha-blockers: enhanced hypotensive effect when clonidine given with alpha-blockers

  Anaesthetics, General: enhanced hypotensive effect when clonidine given with general anaesthetics

  Analgesics: hypotensive effect of clonidine antagonised by NSAIDs

**Clonidine** *(continued)*

Angiotensin-II Receptor Antagonists: enhanced hypotensive effect when clonidine given with angiotensin-II receptor antagonists

● Antidepressants: enhanced hypotensive effect when clonidine given with MAOIs; hypotensive effect of clonidine possibly antagonised by mirtazapine; hypotensive effect of clonidine antagonised by ●tricyclics, also increased risk of hypertension on clonidine withdrawal

Antipsychotics: enhanced hypotensive effect when clonidine given with phenothiazines

Anxiolytics and Hypnotics: enhanced hypotensive effect when clonidine given with anxiolytics and hypnotics

● Beta-blockers: increased risk of withdrawal hypertension when clonidine given with ●beta-blockers (withdraw beta-blockers several days before slowly withdrawing clonidine)

Calcium-channel Blockers: enhanced hypotensive effect when clonidine given with calcium-channel blockers

Corticosteroids: hypotensive effect of clonidine antagonised by corticosteroids

Cytotoxics: possible increased risk of bradycardia when clonidine given with crizotinib

Diazoxide: enhanced hypotensive effect when clonidine given with diazoxide

Diuretics: enhanced hypotensive effect when clonidine given with diuretics

Dopaminergics: enhanced hypotensive effect when clonidine given with levodopa

Histamine: avoidance of clonidine advised by manufacturer of histamine

Methyldopa: enhanced hypotensive effect when clonidine given with methyldopa

Moxisylyte: enhanced hypotensive effect when clonidine given with moxisylyte

Moxonidine: enhanced hypotensive effect when clonidine given with moxonidine

Muscle Relaxants: enhanced hypotensive effect when clonidine given with baclofen or tizanidine

Nitrates: enhanced hypotensive effect when clonidine given with nitrates

Oestrogens: hypotensive effect of clonidine antagonised by oestrogens

Prostaglandins: enhanced hypotensive effect when clonidine given with alprostadil

● Sympathomimetics: possible risk of hypertension when clonidine given with adrenaline (epinephrine) or noradrenaline (norepinephrine); serious adverse events reported with concomitant use of clonidine and ●methylphenidate (causality not established)

Vasodilator Antihypertensives: enhanced hypotensive effect when clonidine given with hydralazine, minoxidil or sodium nitroprusside

**Clopamide** *see* Diuretics

**Clopidogrel**

Analgesics: increased risk of bleeding when clopidogrel given with NSAIDs or aspirin

● Antibacterials: antiplatelet effect of clopidogrel possibly reduced by ●chloramphenicol, ●ciprofloxacin and ●erythromycin

● Anticoagulants: manufacturer of clopidogrel advises avoid concomitant use with ●warfarin; antiplatelet action of clopidogrel enhances anticoagulant effect of ●coumarins and ●phenindione; increased risk of bleeding when clopidogrel given with heparins

● Antidepressants: antiplatelet effect of clopidogrel possibly reduced by ●fluoxetine, ●fluvoxamine and ●moclobemide

● Antiepileptics: antiplatelet effect of clopidogrel possibly reduced by ●carbamazepine and ●oxcarbazepine

**Clopidogrel** *(continued)*

● Antifungals: antiplatelet effect of clopidogrel possibly reduced by ●fluconazole, ●itraconazole, ●ketoconazole and ●voriconazole

● Antivirals: antiplatelet effect of clopidogrel possibly reduced by ●etravirine

Dipyridamole: increased risk of bleeding when clopidogrel given with dipyridamole

Iloprost: increased risk of bleeding when clopidogrel given with iloprost

Prasugrel: possible increased risk of bleeding when clopidogrel given with prasugrel

● Ulcer-healing Drugs: antiplatelet effect of clopidogrel possibly reduced by ●cimetidine, lansoprazole, pantoprazole and rabeprazole; antiplatelet effect of clopidogrel reduced by ●esomeprazole and ●omeprazole

**Clozapine** *see* Antipsychotics

**Co-amoxiclav** *see* Penicillins

**Co-beneldopa** *see* Levodopa

**Co-careldopa** *see* Levodopa

**Codeine** *see* Opioid Analgesics

**Co-fluampicil** *see* Penicillins

**Colchicine**

● Anti-arrhythmics: possible increased risk of colchicine toxicity when given with ●amiodarone

● Antibacterials: possible increased risk of colchicine toxicity when given with ●azithromycin, ●clarithromycin, ●erythromycin and ●telithromycin—suspend or reduce dose of colchicine (avoid concomitant use in hepatic or renal impairment)

● Antifungals: possible increased risk of colchicine toxicity when given with ●itraconazole and ●ketoconazole—suspend or reduce dose of colchicine (avoid concomitant use in hepatic or renal impairment)

● Antivirals: possible increased risk of colchicine toxicity when given with ●atazanavir, ●indinavir, ●ritonavir and ●telaprevir—suspend or reduce dose of colchicine (avoid concomitant use in hepatic or renal impairment)

● Calcium-channel Blockers: possible increased risk of colchicine toxicity when given with ●diltiazem and ●verapamil—suspend or reduce dose of colchicine (avoid concomitant use in hepatic or renal impairment)

● Cardiac Glycosides: possible increased risk of myopathy when colchicine given with ●digoxin

● Ciclosporin: possible increased risk of nephrotoxicity and myotoxicity when colchicine given with ●ciclosporin—suspend or reduce dose of colchicine (avoid concomitant use in hepatic or renal impairment)

● Grapefruit Juice: possible increased risk of colchicine toxicity when given with ●grapefruit juice

● Lipid-regulating Drugs: possible increased risk of myopathy when colchicine given with ●fibrates or ●statins

**Colesevelam**

**Note** Other drugs should be taken at least 4 hours before or after colesevelam to reduce possible interference with absorption

Antidiabetics: colesevelam reduces absorption of glibenclamide

Antiepileptics: colesevelam possibly reduces absorption of phenytoin

● Ciclosporin: colesevelam reduces absorption of ●ciclosporin

Oestrogens: colesevelam reduces absorption of ethinylestradiol

Thyroid Hormones: colesevelam reduces absorption of levothyroxine

**Colestipol**

**Note** Other drugs should be taken at least 1 hour before or 4–6 hours after colestipol to reduce possible interference with absorption

Appendix 1: Interactions

## Colestipol *(continued)*

Antibacterials: colestipol possibly reduces absorption of tetracycline

Bile Acids: colestipol possibly reduces absorption of bile acids

Cardiac Glycosides: colestipol possibly reduces absorption of cardiac glycosides

Diuretics: colestipol reduces absorption of thiazides and related diuretics (give at least 2 hours apart)

Thyroid Hormones: colestipol reduces absorption of thyroid hormones

## Colestyramine

**Note** Other drugs should be taken at least 1 hour before or 4–6 hours after colestyramine to reduce possible interference with absorption

Analgesics: colestyramine increases the excretion of meloxicam; colestyramine reduces absorption of paracetamol

Antibacterials: colestyramine possibly reduces absorption of tetracycline; colestyramine antagonises effects of *oral* vancomycin

● Anticoagulants: colestyramine may enhance or reduce anticoagulant effect of ●coumarins and ●phenindione

Antidiabetics: colestyramine possibly enhances hypoglycaemic effect of acarbose

Antiepileptics: colestyramine possibly reduces absorption of valproate

Bile Acids: colestyramine possibly reduces absorption of bile acids

Cardiac Glycosides: colestyramine possibly reduces absorption of cardiac glycosides

Diuretics: colestyramine reduces absorption of thiazides and related diuretics (give at least 2 hours apart)

Leflunomide: colestyramine significantly decreases effect of leflunomide (enhanced elimination)—avoid unless drug elimination desired

Mycophenolate: colestyramine reduces absorption of mycophenolate

Raloxifene: colestyramine reduces absorption of raloxifene (manufacturer of raloxifene advises avoid concomitant administration)

Thyroid Hormones: colestyramine reduces absorption of thyroid hormones

## Colistimethate Sodium *see* Polymyxins

## Contraceptives, oral *see* Oestrogens and Progestogens

## Corticosteroids

**Note** Interactions do not generally apply to corticosteroids used for topical action (including inhalation) unless specified

ACE Inhibitors: corticosteroids antagonise hypotensive effect of ACE inhibitors

Adrenergic Neurone Blockers: corticosteroids antagonise hypotensive effect of adrenergic neurone blockers

● Aldesleukin: avoidance of corticosteroids advised by manufacturer of ●aldesleukin

Alpha-blockers: corticosteroids antagonise hypotensive effect of alpha-blockers

Analgesics: increased risk of gastro-intestinal bleeding and ulceration when corticosteroids given with NSAIDs; increased risk of gastro-intestinal bleeding and ulceration when corticosteroids given with aspirin, also corticosteroids reduce plasma concentration of salicylate

Angiotensin-II Receptor Antagonists: corticosteroids antagonise hypotensive effect of angiotensin-II receptor antagonists

Antacids: absorption of deflazacort reduced by antacids

● Antibacterials: plasma concentration of methylprednisolone possibly increased by clarithromycin; metabolism of corticosteroids possibly inhibited by erythromycin; metabolism of methylprednisolone inhibited by erythromycin; corticosteroids possibly reduce plasma concentration of isoniazid; metab-

## Corticosteroids

● Antibacterials *(continued)*
olism of corticosteroids accelerated by ●rifamycins (reduced effect)

● Anticoagulants: corticosteroids may enhance or reduce anticoagulant effect of ●coumarins (high-dose corticosteroids enhance anticoagulant effect); corticosteroids may enhance or reduce anticoagulant effect of phenindione

Antidiabetics: corticosteroids antagonise hypoglycaemic effect of antidiabetics

● Antiepileptics: metabolism of corticosteroids accelerated by ●carbamazepine, ●phenobarbital and ●phenytoin (reduced effect)

● Antifungals: metabolism of corticosteroids possibly inhibited by itraconazole and ketoconazole; plasma concentration of active metabolite of ciclesonide increased by ketoconazole; plasma concentration of *inhaled* fluticasone and mometasone increased by ketoconazole; plasma concentration of *inhaled* and *oral* budesonide increased by ketoconazole; metabolism of methylprednisolone inhibited by ketoconazole; increased risk of hypokalaemia when corticosteroids given with ●amphotericin—avoid concomitant use unless corticosteroids needed to control reactions; plasma concentration of *inhaled* budesonide and fluticasone increased by itraconazole; metabolism of methylprednisolone possibly inhibited by itraconazole; dexamethasone possibly reduces plasma concentration of caspofungin—consider increasing dose of caspofungin

● Antivirals: dexamethasone possibly reduces plasma concentration of indinavir, lopinavir, saquinavir and telaprevir; avoidance of dexamethasone (except when given as a single dose) advised by manufacturer of ●rilpivirine; plasma concentration of budesonide (including *inhaled, intranasal,* and *rectal* budesonide) possibly increased by ritonavir; plasma concentration of corticosteroids, dexamethasone and prednisolone possibly increased by ritonavir; plasma concentration of *inhaled* and *intranasal* fluticasone increased by ●ritonavir; plasma concentration of *inhaled* and *intranasal* budesonide and fluticasone possibly increased by telaprevir

Aprepitant: metabolism of dexamethasone and methylprednisolone inhibited by aprepitant (reduce dose of dexamethasone and methylprednisolone)

Beta-blockers: corticosteroids antagonise hypotensive effect of beta-blockers

Calcium Salts: corticosteroids reduce absorption of calcium salts

Calcium-channel Blockers: corticosteroids antagonise hypotensive effect of calcium-channel blockers; plasma concentration of methylprednisolone increased by diltiazem

Cardiac Glycosides: increased risk of hypokalaemia when corticosteroids given with cardiac glycosides

● Ciclosporin: high-dose methylprednisolone increases plasma concentration of ●ciclosporin (risk of convulsions); plasma concentration of prednisolone increased by ciclosporin

Clonidine: corticosteroids antagonise hypotensive effect of clonidine

Cytotoxics: dexamethasone possibly decreases plasma concentration of axitinib (increase dose of axitinib—consult axitinib product literature)

Diazoxide: corticosteroids antagonise hypotensive effect of diazoxide

Diuretics: corticosteroids antagonise diuretic effect of diuretics; increased risk of hypokalaemia when corticosteroids given with acetazolamide, loop diuretics or thiazides and related diuretics

Histamine: avoidance of corticosteroids advised by manufacturer of histamine

Methyldopa: corticosteroids antagonise hypotensive effect of methyldopa

**Corticosteroids** *(continued)*

Mifamurtide: avoidance of corticosteroids advised by manufacturer of mifamurtide

Mifepristone: effect of corticosteroids (including *inhaled* corticosteroids) may be reduced for 3–4 days after mifepristone

Moxonidine: corticosteroids antagonise hypotensive effect of moxonidine

Muscle Relaxants: corticosteroids possibly antagonise effects of pancuronium and vecuronium

Nitrates: corticosteroids antagonise hypotensive effect of nitrates

Oestrogens: plasma concentration of corticosteroids increased by oral contraceptives containing oestrogens

Sodium Benzoate: corticosteroids possibly reduce effects of sodium benzoate

Sodium Phenylbutyrate: corticosteroids possibly reduce effects of sodium phenylbutyrate

Somatropin: corticosteroids may inhibit growth-promoting effect of somatropin

Sympathomimetics: metabolism of dexamethasone accelerated by ephedrine

Sympathomimetics, Beta$_2$: increased risk of hypokalaemia when corticosteroids given with high doses of beta$_2$ sympathomimetics—see Hypokalaemia, p. 136

Theophylline: increased risk of hypokalaemia when corticosteroids given with theophylline

Ticagrelor: dexamethasone possibly reduces plasma concentration of ticagrelor

● Vaccines: high doses of corticosteroids impair immune response to ●vaccines, avoid concomitant use with live vaccines (see p. 600)

Vasodilator Antihypertensives: corticosteroids antagonise hypotensive effect of hydralazine, minoxidil and sodium nitroprusside

**Co-trimoxazole** *see* Trimethoprim and Sulfamethoxazole

**Coumarins**

Note Change in patient's clinical condition, particularly associated with liver disease, intercurrent illness, or drug administration, necessitates more frequent testing. Major changes in diet (especially involving salads and vegetables) and in alcohol consumption may also affect anticoagulant control

● Alcohol: anticoagulant control with coumarins may be affected by major changes in consumption of ●alcohol

Allopurinol: anticoagulant effect of coumarins possibly enhanced by allopurinol

● Anabolic Steroids: anticoagulant effect of coumarins enhanced by ●anabolic steroids

● Analgesics: anticoagulant effect of coumarins possibly enhanced by ●NSAIDs; increased risk of haemorrhage when anticoagulants given with *intravenous* ●diclofenac (avoid concomitant use, including low-dose heparins); increased risk of haemorrhage when anticoagulants given with ●ketorolac (avoid concomitant use, including low-dose heparins); anticoagulant effect of coumarins enhanced by ●tramadol; increased risk of bleeding when coumarins given with ●aspirin (due to antiplatelet action); anticoagulant effect of coumarins possibly enhanced by prolonged regular use of paracetamol

● Anti-arrhythmics: metabolism of coumarins inhibited by ●amiodarone (enhanced anticoagulant effect); anticoagulant effect of warfarin may be enhanced or reduced by disopyramide; anticoagulant effect of coumarins possibly enhanced by ●dronedarone; anticoagulant effect of coumarins enhanced by ●propafenone

● Antibacterials: experience in anticoagulant clinics suggests that INR possibly altered when coumarins are given with ●neomycin (given for local action on gut); anticoagulant effect of coumarins possibly

**Coumarins**

● Antibacterials *(continued)*

enhanced by ●azithromycin, ●aztreonam, ●cephalosporins, ciprofloxacin, levofloxacin, ●tetracyclines, tigecycline and trimethoprim; anticoagulant effect of coumarins enhanced by ●chloramphenicol, ●clarithromycin, ●erythromycin, ●metronidazole, ●nalidixic acid, ●norfloxacin, ●ofloxacin and ●sulfonamides; an interaction between coumarins and broad-spectrum penicillins has not been demonstrated in studies, but common experience in anticoagulant clinics is that INR can be altered; metabolism of coumarins accelerated by ●rifamycins (reduced anticoagulant effect)

● Anticoagulants: increased risk of haemorrhage when other anticoagulants given with ●apixaban, ●dabigatran etexilate and ●rivaroxaban (avoid concomitant use except when switching with other anticoagulants or using heparin to maintain catheter patency)

● Antidepressants: anticoagulant effect of warfarin possibly enhanced by ●venlafaxine; anticoagulant effect of warfarin may be enhanced or reduced by trazodone; anticoagulant effect of coumarins possibly enhanced by ●SSRIs; anticoagulant effect of coumarins reduced by ●St John's wort (avoid concomitant use); anticoagulant effect of warfarin enhanced by mirtazapine; anticoagulant effect of coumarins may be enhanced or reduced by ●tricyclics

● Antidiabetics: anticoagulant effect of warfarin possibly enhanced by exenatide; coumarins possibly enhance hypoglycaemic effect of ●sulfonylureas, also possible changes to anticoagulant effect

● Antiepileptics: metabolism of coumarins accelerated by ●carbamazepine and ●phenobarbital (reduced anticoagulant effect); plasma concentration of warfarin reduced by eslicarbazepine; metabolism of coumarins accelerated by ●phenytoin (possibility of reduced anticoagulant effect, but enhancement also reported); anticoagulant effect of coumarins possibly enhanced by valproate

● Antifungals: anticoagulant effect of coumarins enhanced by ●fluconazole, ●itraconazole, ●ketoconazole and ●voriconazole; anticoagulant effect of coumarins enhanced by ●miconazole (miconazole oral gel and possibly vaginal and topical formulations absorbed); anticoagulant effect of coumarins reduced by ●griseofulvin

Antimalarials: isolated reports that anticoagulant effect of warfarin may be enhanced by proguanil; plasma concentration of both drugs increased when warfarin given with quinine

● Antivirals: anticoagulant effect of warfarin may be enhanced or reduced by atazanavir, ●nevirapine and ●ritonavir; plasma concentration of coumarins possibly affected by ●efavirenz; anticoagulant effect of coumarins may be enhanced or reduced by fosamprenavir; anticoagulant effect of coumarins possibly enhanced by ●ritonavir; anticoagulant effect of warfarin possibly enhanced by saquinavir; plasma concentration of warfarin possibly affected by ●telaprevir

Anxiolytics and Hypnotics: anticoagulant effect of coumarins may transiently be enhanced by chloral

Aprepitant: anticoagulant effect of warfarin possibly reduced by aprepitant

● Azathioprine: anticoagulant effect of coumarins possibly reduced by ●azathioprine

Bosentan: monitoring anticoagulant effect of coumarins recommended by manufacturer of bosentan

● Clopidogrel: anticoagulant effect of coumarins enhanced due to antiplatelet action of ●clopidogrel; avoidance of warfarin advised by manufacturer of ●clopidogrel

**Coumarins** *(continued)*

- Corticosteroids: anticoagulant effect of coumarins may be enhanced or reduced by ●corticosteroids (high-dose corticosteroids enhance anticoagulant effect)
- Cranberry Juice: anticoagulant effect of coumarins possibly enhanced by ●cranberry juice—avoid concomitant use
- Cytotoxics: anticoagulant effect of coumarins possibly enhanced by ●etoposide, ●ifosfamide and ●sorafenib; anticoagulant effect of coumarins enhanced by ●fluorouracil; anticoagulant effect of warfarin possibly enhanced by ●gefitinib, gemcitabine and ●vemurafenib; anticoagulant effect of coumarins possibly reduced by ●mercaptopurine and ●mitotane; increased risk of bleeding when coumarins given with ●erlotinib; replacement of warfarin with a heparin advised by manufacturer of imatinib (possibility of enhanced warfarin effect)
- Dipyridamole: anticoagulant effect of coumarins enhanced due to antiplatelet action of ●dipyridamole
- Disulfiram: anticoagulant effect of coumarins enhanced by ●disulfiram
- Dopaminergics: anticoagulant effect of warfarin enhanced by ●entacapone
- Enteral Foods: anticoagulant effect of coumarins antagonised by vitamin K (present in some ●enteral feeds )
- Glucosamine: anticoagulant effect of warfarin enhanced by ●glucosamine (avoid concomitant use)
- Hormone Antagonists: anticoagulant effect of coumarins possibly enhanced by bicalutamide and ●toremifene; metabolism of coumarins inhibited by ●danazol (enhanced anticoagulant effect); anticoagulant effect of coumarins enhanced by ●flutamide and ●tamoxifen
  Iloprost: anticoagulant effect of coumarins possibly enhanced by iloprost
  Lactulose: anticoagulant effect of coumarins possibly enhanced by lactulose
  Leflunomide: anticoagulant effect of warfarin possibly enhanced by leflunomide
  Leukotriene Receptor Antagonists: anticoagulant effect of warfarin enhanced by zafirlukast
- Levamisole: anticoagulant effect of warfarin possibly enhanced by ●levamisole
- Lipid-regulating Drugs: anticoagulant effect of coumarins may be enhanced or reduced by ●colestyramine; anticoagulant effect of warfarin may be transiently reduced by atorvastatin; anticoagulant effect of coumarins enhanced by ●fibrates, ●fluvastatin and simvastatin; anticoagulant effect of coumarins possibly enhanced by ezetimibe and ●rosuvastatin
  Memantine: anticoagulant effect of warfarin possibly enhanced by memantine
  Oestrogens: anticoagulant effect of coumarins may be enhanced or reduced by oestrogens
  Orlistat: monitoring anticoagulant effect of coumarins recommended by manufacturer of orlistat
  Prasugrel: possible increased risk of bleeding when coumarins given with prasugrel
  Progestogens: anticoagulant effect of coumarins may be enhanced or reduced by progestogens
  Raloxifene: anticoagulant effect of coumarins antagonised by raloxifene
- Retinoids: anticoagulant effect of coumarins possibly reduced by ●acitretin
- Sulfinpyrazone: anticoagulant effect of coumarins enhanced by ●sulfinpyrazone
- Sympathomimetics: anticoagulant effect of coumarins possibly enhanced by ●methylphenidate
- Testolactone: anticoagulant effect of coumarins enhanced by ●testolactone
- Testosterone: anticoagulant effect of coumarins enhanced by ●testosterone

**Coumarins** *(continued)*

- Thyroid Hormones: anticoagulant effect of coumarins enhanced by ●thyroid hormones
  Ubidecarenone: anticoagulant effect of warfarin may be enhanced or reduced by ubidecarenone
- Ulcer-healing Drugs: metabolism of coumarins inhibited by ●cimetidine (enhanced anticoagulant effect); anticoagulant effect of coumarins possibly enhanced by ●esomeprazole, ●omeprazole and pantoprazole; absorption of coumarins possibly reduced by ●sucralfate (reduced anticoagulant effect)
  Vaccines: anticoagulant effect of warfarin possibly enhanced by influenza vaccine
- Vitamins: anticoagulant effect of coumarins possibly enhanced by ●vitamin E; anticoagulant effect of coumarins antagonised by ●vitamin K

**Cranberry Juice**

- Anticoagulants: cranberry juice possibly enhances anticoagulant effect of ●coumarins—avoid concomitant use

**Crizotinib**

- Analgesics: manufacturer of crizotinib advises caution with ●alfentanil and ●fentanyl
- Antibacterials: plasma concentration of crizotinib possibly increased by ●clarithromycin and ●telithromycin—manufacturer of crizotinib advises avoid concomitant use; plasma concentration of crizotinib possibly reduced by rifabutin—manufacturer of crizotinib advises avoid concomitant use; plasma concentration of crizotinib reduced by ●rifampicin—manufacturer of crizotinib advises avoid concomitant use
  Antidepressants: plasma concentration of crizotinib possibly reduced by St John's wort—manufacturer of crizotinib advises avoid concomitant use
  Antiepileptics: plasma concentration of crizotinib possibly reduced by carbamazepine, phenobarbital and phenytoin—manufacturer of crizotinib advises avoid concomitant use
- Antifungals: plasma concentration of crizotinib increased by ●ketoconazole—avoid concomitant use; plasma concentration of crizotinib possibly increased by ●itraconazole and ●voriconazole—manufacturer of crizotinib advises avoid concomitant use
  Antimalarials: possible increased risk of bradycardia when crizotinib given with mefloquine
- Antipsychotics: avoid concomitant use of cytotoxics with ●clozapine (increased risk of agranulocytosis); manufacturer of crizotinib advises caution with ●pimozide
- Antivirals: plasma concentration of crizotinib possibly increased by ●atazanavir, ●indinavir, ●ritonavir and ●saquinavir—manufacturer of crizotinib advises avoid concomitant use
- Anxiolytics and Hypnotics: crizotinib increases plasma concentration of ●midazolam
  Beta-blockers: possible increased risk of bradycardia when crizotinib given with beta-blockers
  Calcium-channel Blockers: possible increased risk of bradycardia when crizotinib given with diltiazem or verapamil
  Cardiac Glycosides: possible increased risk of bradycardia when crizotinib given with digoxin
- Ciclosporin: manufacturer of crizotinib advises caution with ●ciclosporin
  Clonidine: possible increased risk of bradycardia when crizotinib given with clonidine
- Ergot Alkaloids: manufacturer of crizotinib advises caution with ●ergot alkaloids
- Grapefruit Juice: plasma concentration of crizotinib possibly increased by ●grapefruit juice—manufacturer of crizotinib advises avoid concomitant use
- Oestrogens: manufacturer of crizotinib advises contraceptive effect of ●oestrogens possibly reduced

**Crizotinib** *(continued)*

Parasympathomimetics: possible increased risk of bradycardia when crizotinib given with pilocarpine

- Progestogens: manufacturer of crizotinib advises contraceptive effect of ●progestogens possibly reduced
- Sirolimus: manufacturer of crizotinib advises caution with ●sirolimus
- Tacrolimus: manufacturer of crizotinib advises caution with ●tacrolimus

**Cyclizine** *see* Antihistamines

**Cyclopenthiazide** *see* Diuretics

**Cyclopentolate** *see* Antimuscarinics

**Cyclophosphamide**

Antifungals: side-effects of cyclophosphamide possibly increased by fluconazole and itraconazole

- Antipsychotics: avoid concomitant use of cytotoxics with ●clozapine (increased risk of agranulocytosis)

Cardiac Glycosides: cyclophosphamide possibly reduces absorption of digoxin *tablets*

- Cytotoxics: increased toxicity when high-dose cyclophosphamide given with ●pentostatin—avoid concomitant use

Muscle Relaxants: cyclophosphamide enhances effects of suxamethonium

**Cycloserine**

- Alcohol: increased risk of convulsions when cycloserine given with ●alcohol

Antibacterials: increased risk of CNS toxicity when cycloserine given with isoniazid

Vaccines: antibacterials inactivate oral typhoid vaccine—see p. 621

**Cyproheptadine** *see* Antihistamines

**Cytarabine**

Antifungals: cytarabine possibly reduces plasma concentration of flucytosine

- Antipsychotics: avoid concomitant use of cytotoxics with ●clozapine (increased risk of agranulocytosis)

Cardiac Glycosides: cytarabine possibly reduces absorption of digoxin *tablets*

Cytotoxics: intracellular concentration of cytarabine increased by fludarabine

**Cytotoxics** *see* individual drugs

**Dabigatran Etexilate**

- Analgesics: possible increased risk of bleeding when dabigatran etexilate given with ●NSAIDs; increased risk of haemorrhage when anticoagulants given with *intravenous* ●diclofenac (avoid concomitant use, including low-dose heparins); increased risk of haemorrhage when anticoagulants given with ●ketorolac (avoid concomitant use, including low-dose heparins)
- Anti-arrhythmics: plasma concentration of dabigatran etexilate increased by ●amiodarone (see Dose under Dabigatran etexilate, BNF section 2.8.2); plasma concentration of dabigatran etexilate increased by ●dronedarone—avoid concomitant use
- Antibacterials: plasma concentration of dabigatran etexilate reduced by ●rifampicin—manufacturer of dabigatran etexilate advises avoid concomitant use
- Anticoagulants: increased risk of haemorrhage when dabigatran etexilate given with other ●anticoagulants (avoid concomitant use except when switching with other anticoagulants or using heparin to maintain catheter patency); increased risk of haemorrhage when other anticoagulants given with ●apixaban and ●rivaroxaban (avoid concomitant use except when switching with other anticoagulants or using heparin to maintain catheter patency)
- Antidepressants: possible increased risk of bleeding when dabigatran etexilate given with ●SSRI-related antidepressants or ●SSRIs; plasma concentration of dabigatran etexilate possibly reduced by St John's wort—manufacturer of dabigatran etexilate advises avoid concomitant use

**Dabigatran Etexilate** *(continued)*

Antiepileptics: plasma concentration of dabigatran etexilate possibly reduced by carbamazepine and phenytoin—manufacturer of dabigatran etexilate advises avoid concomitant use

- Antifungals: plasma concentration of dabigatran etexilate increased by ●ketoconazole—avoid concomitant use; plasma concentration of dabigatran etexilate possibly increased by ●itraconazole—manufacturer of dabigatran etexilate advises avoid concomitant use

Antivirals: plasma concentration of dabigatran etexilate possibly increased by rilpivirine and telaprevir

- Calcium-channel Blockers: plasma concentration of dabigatran etexilate possibly increased by ●verapamil (see Dose under Dabigatran etexilate, BNF section 2.8.2)
- Ciclosporin: plasma concentration of dabigatran etexilate possibly increased by ●ciclosporin—manufacturer of dabigatran etexilate advises avoid concomitant use
- Sulfinpyrazone: possible increased risk of bleeding when dabigatran etexilate given with ●sulfinpyrazone
- Tacrolimus: plasma concentration of dabigatran etexilate possibly increased by ●tacrolimus—manufacturer of dabigatran etexilate advises avoid concomitant use

**Dacarbazine**

- Aldesleukin: avoidance of dacarbazine advised by manufacturer of ●aldesleukin
- Antipsychotics: avoid concomitant use of cytotoxics with ●clozapine (increased risk of agranulocytosis)

**Dairy Products**

Antibacterials: dairy products reduce absorption of ciprofloxacin and norfloxacin; dairy products reduce absorption of tetracyclines (except doxycycline and minocycline)

Cytotoxics: dairy products possibly reduce plasma concentration of mercaptopurine—manufacturer of mercaptopurine advises give at least 1 hour before or 2 hours after dairy products

Eltrombopag: dairy products possibly reduce absorption of eltrombopag (give at least 4 hours apart)

**Dalteparin** *see* Heparins

**Danazol**

- Anticoagulants: danazol inhibits metabolism of ●coumarins (enhanced anticoagulant effect)
- Antiepileptics: danazol inhibits metabolism of ●carbamazepine (increased risk of toxicity)
- Ciclosporin: danazol inhibits metabolism of ●ciclosporin (increased plasma concentration)
- Lipid-regulating Drugs: possible increased risk of myopathy when danazol given with ●simvastatin—avoid concomitant use

Tacrolimus: danazol possibly increases plasma concentration of tacrolimus

**Dantrolene** *see* Muscle Relaxants

**Dapagliflozin** *see* Antidiabetics

**Dapsone**

Antibacterials: plasma concentration of dapsone reduced by rifamycins; plasma concentration of both drugs may increase when dapsone given with trimethoprim

- Antivirals: increased risk of ventricular arrhythmias when dapsone given with ●saquinavir—avoid concomitant use

Probenecid: excretion of dapsone reduced by probenecid (increased risk of side-effects)

Vaccines: antibacterials inactivate oral typhoid vaccine—see p. 621

**Daptomycin**

- Ciclosporin: increased risk of myopathy when daptomycin given with ●ciclosporin (preferably avoid concomitant use)

**Daptomycin** (continued)
- Lipid-regulating Drugs: increased risk of myopathy when daptomycin given with ●fibrates or ●statins (preferably avoid concomitant use)
  Vaccines: antibacterials inactivate oral typhoid vaccine—see p. 621

**Darifenacin** see Antimuscarinics

**Darunavir**
  Anti-arrhythmics: darunavir possibly increases plasma concentration of lidocaine—avoid concomitant use
- Antibacterials: darunavir increases plasma concentration of ●rifabutin (reduce dose of rifabutin); plasma concentration of darunavir significantly reduced by ●rifampicin—avoid concomitant use
  Anticoagulants: avoidance of darunavir advised by manufacturer of apixaban and rivaroxaban
- Antidepressants: darunavir possibly reduces plasma concentration of paroxetine and sertraline; plasma concentration of darunavir reduced by ●St John's wort—avoid concomitant use
  Antiepileptics: plasma concentration of darunavir possibly reduced by carbamazepine, phenobarbital and phenytoin
  Antifungals: plasma concentration of both drugs increased when darunavir given with ketoconazole
- Antimalarials: darunavir increases plasma concentration of lumefantrine; darunavir possibly increases plasma concentration of ●quinine (increased risk of toxicity)
- Antipsychotics: darunavir possibly increases plasma concentration of ●quetiapine—manufacturer of quetiapine advises avoid concomitant use
- Antivirals: avoid concomitant use of darunavir with ●boceprevir or ●telaprevir; Plasma concentration of darunavir reduced by ●efavirenz (adjust dose—consult product literature); plasma concentration of both drugs increased when darunavir given with indinavir; plasma concentration of darunavir reduced by ●lopinavir, also plasma concentration of lopinavir increased (avoid concomitant use); darunavir increases plasma concentration of ●maraviroc (consider reducing dose of maraviroc); increased risk of rash when darunavir given with raltegravir; plasma concentration of darunavir reduced by saquinavir
- Cytotoxics: darunavir possibly increases plasma concentration of ●everolimus—manufacturer of everolimus advises avoid concomitant use
- Lipid-regulating Drugs: possible increased risk of myopathy when darunavir given with atorvastatin; darunavir possibly increases plasma concentration of pravastatin; possible increased risk of myopathy when darunavir given with ●rosuvastatin—manufacturer of rosuvastatin advises avoid concomitant use
- Ranolazine: darunavir possibly increases plasma concentration of ●ranolazine—manufacturer of ranolazine advises avoid concomitant use

**Dasatinib**
- Antibacterials: metabolism of dasatinib accelerated by ●rifampicin (reduced plasma concentration—avoid concomitant use)
  Antifungals: plasma concentration of dasatinib possibly increased by ketoconazole
- Antipsychotics: avoid concomitant use of cytotoxics with ●clozapine (increased risk of agranulocytosis)
- Antivirals: avoidance of dasatinib advised by manufacturer of ●boceprevir
  Lipid-regulating Drugs: dasatinib possibly increases plasma concentration of simvastatin
  Ulcer-healing Drugs: plasma concentration of dasatinib possibly reduced by famotidine

**Decitabine**
- Antipsychotics: avoid concomitant use of cytotoxics with ●clozapine (increased risk of agranulocytosis)

**Deferasirox**
  Antacids: absorption of deferasirox possibly reduced by antacids containing aluminium (manufacturer of deferasirox advises avoid concomitant use)
  Antibacterials: plasma concentration of deferasirox reduced by rifampicin
  Antidiabetics: deferasirox increases plasma concentration of repaglinide
  Antipsychotics: manufacturer of deferasirox advises avoid concomitant use with clozapine
  Anxiolytics and Hypnotics: deferasirox possibly reduces plasma concentration of midazolam
  Muscle Relaxants: manufacturer of deferasirox advises avoid concomitant use with tizanidine
- Theophylline: deferasirox increases plasma concentration of ●theophylline (consider reducing dose of theophylline)

**Deflazacort** see Corticosteroids

**Demeclocycline** see Tetracyclines

**Desferrioxamine**
  Antipsychotics: avoidance of desferrioxamine advised by manufacturer of levomepromazine; manufacturer of desferrioxamine advises avoid concomitant use with prochlorperazine

**Desflurane** see Anaesthetics, General

**Desloratadine** see Antihistamines

**Desmopressin**
  Analgesics: effects of desmopressin enhanced by indometacin
  Loperamide: plasma concentration of oral desmopressin increased by loperamide

**Desogestrel** see Progestogens

**Dexamethasone** see Corticosteroids

**Dexamfetamine** see Sympathomimetics

**Dexibuprofen** see NSAIDs

**Dexketoprofen** see NSAIDs

**Dextromethorphan** see Opioid Analgesics

**Dextropropoxyphene** see Opioid Analgesics

**Diamorphine** see Opioid Analgesics

**Diazepam** see Anxiolytics and Hypnotics

**Diazoxide**
  ACE Inhibitors: enhanced hypotensive effect when diazoxide given with ACE inhibitors
  Adrenergic Neurone Blockers: enhanced hypotensive effect when diazoxide given with adrenergic neurone blockers
  Alcohol: enhanced hypotensive effect when diazoxide given with alcohol
  Aldesleukin: enhanced hypotensive effect when diazoxide given with aldesleukin
  Alpha-blockers: enhanced hypotensive effect when diazoxide given with alpha-blockers
  Anaesthetics, General: enhanced hypotensive effect when diazoxide given with general anaesthetics
  Analgesics: hypotensive effect of diazoxide antagonised by NSAIDs
  Angiotensin-II Receptor Antagonists: enhanced hypotensive effect when diazoxide given with angiotensin-II receptor antagonists
  Antidepressants: enhanced hypotensive effect when diazoxide given with MAOIs or tricyclic-related antidepressants
  Antidiabetics: diazoxide antagonises hypoglycaemic effect of antidiabetics
  Antiepileptics: diazoxide reduces plasma concentration of phenytoin, also effect of diazoxide may be reduced
  Antipsychotics: enhanced hypotensive effect when diazoxide given with phenothiazines
  Anxiolytics and Hypnotics: enhanced hypotensive effect when diazoxide given with anxiolytics and hypnotics
  Beta-blockers: enhanced hypotensive effect when diazoxide given with beta-blockers

**Diazoxide** (continued)

Calcium-channel Blockers: enhanced hypotensive effect when diazoxide given with calcium-channel blockers

Clonidine: enhanced hypotensive effect when diazoxide given with clonidine

Corticosteroids: hypotensive effect of diazoxide antagonised by corticosteroids

Diuretics: enhanced hypotensive and hyperglycaemic effects when diazoxide given with diuretics

Dopaminergics: enhanced hypotensive effect when diazoxide given with levodopa

Methyldopa: enhanced hypotensive effect when diazoxide given with methyldopa

Moxisylyte: enhanced hypotensive effect when diazoxide given with moxisylyte

Moxonidine: enhanced hypotensive effect when diazoxide given with moxonidine

Muscle Relaxants: enhanced hypotensive effect when diazoxide given with baclofen or tizanidine

Nitrates: enhanced hypotensive effect when diazoxide given with nitrates

Prostaglandins: enhanced hypotensive effect when diazoxide given with alprostadil

Vasodilator Antihypertensives: enhanced hypotensive effect when diazoxide given with hydralazine, minoxidil or sodium nitroprusside

**Diclofenac** see NSAIDs

**Dicycloverine** see Antimuscarinics

**Didanosine**

**Note** Antacids in tablet formulation may affect absorption of other drugs

- Allopurinol: plasma concentration of didanosine increased by ●allopurinol (risk of toxicity)—avoid concomitant use

Analgesics: plasma concentration of didanosine possibly reduced by methadone

Antibacterials: manufacturer of norfloxacin advises give didanosine at least 2 hours before or after norfloxacin

- Antivirals: plasma concentration of didanosine possibly increased by ganciclovir; increased risk of side-effects when didanosine given with ●ribavirin—avoid concomitant use; manufacturer of rilpivirine advises give didanosine 2 hours before or 4 hours after rilpivirine; increased risk of side-effects when didanosine given with ●stavudine; plasma concentration of didanosine increased by ●tenofovir (increased risk of toxicity)—avoid concomitant use; plasma concentration of didanosine reduced by ●tipranavir

- Cytotoxics: increased risk of toxicity when didanosine given with ●hydroxycarbamide—avoid concomitant use

**Dienogest** see Progestogens

**Digoxin** see Cardiac Glycosides

**Dihydrocodeine** see Opioid Analgesics

**Diltiazem** see Calcium-channel Blockers

**Dimethyl sulfoxide**

- Analgesics: avoid concomitant use of dimethyl sulfoxide with ●sulindac

**Dinoprostone** see Prostaglandins

**Diphenoxylate** see Opioid Analgesics

**Dipipanone** see Opioid Analgesics

**Dipyridamole**

Antacids: absorption of dipyridamole possibly reduced by antacids

- Anti-arrhythmics: dipyridamole enhances and extends the effects of ●adenosine (important risk of toxicity)

- Anticoagulants: antiplatelet action of dipyridamole enhances anticoagulant effect of ●coumarins and ●phenindione; dipyridamole enhances anticoagulant effect of heparins

Clopidogrel: increased risk of bleeding when dipyridamole given with clopidogrel

**Dipyridamole** (continued)

Cytotoxics: dipyridamole possibly reduces effects of fludarabine

**Disodium Etidronate** see Bisphosphonates

**Disodium Pamidronate** see Bisphosphonates

**Disopyramide**

Anaesthetics, Local: increased myocardial depression when anti-arrhythmics given with bupivacaine, levobupivacaine, prilocaine or ropivacaine

- Anti-arrhythmics: increased myocardial depression when anti-arrhythmics given with other ●anti-arrhythmics; increased risk of ventricular arrhythmias when disopyramide given with ●amiodarone or ●dronedarone—avoid concomitant use

- Antibacterials: plasma concentration of disopyramide possibly increased by ●azithromycin and ●clarithromycin (increased risk of toxicity); plasma concentration of disopyramide increased by ●erythromycin (increased risk of toxicity); increased risk of ventricular arrhythmias when disopyramide given with ●moxifloxacin—avoid concomitant use; metabolism of disopyramide accelerated by ●rifamycins (reduced plasma concentration); possible increased risk of ventricular arrhythmias when disopyramide given with ●telithromycin

Anticoagulants: disopyramide may enhance or reduce anticoagulant effect of warfarin

- Antidepressants: increased risk of ventricular arrhythmias when disopyramide given with ●tricyclics

Antidiabetics: disopyramide possibly enhances hypoglycaemic effect of gliclazide, insulin and metformin

Antiepileptics: metabolism of disopyramide accelerated by phenobarbital (reduced plasma concentration); plasma concentration of disopyramide reduced by phenytoin

- Antifungals: increased risk of ventricular arrhythmias when disopyramide given with ●ketoconazole—avoid concomitant use; avoidance of disopyramide advised by manufacturer of ●itraconazole

- Antihistamines: increased risk of ventricular arrhythmias when disopyramide given with ●mizolastine—avoid concomitant use

- Antimalarials: avoidance of disopyramide advised by manufacturer of ●piperaquine with artenimol (possible risk of ventricular arrhythmias); avoidance of disopyramide advised by manufacturer of ●artemether with lumefantrine (risk of ventricular arrhythmias)

- Antimuscarinics: increased risk of antimuscarinic side-effects when disopyramide given with antimuscarinics; increased risk of ventricular arrhythmias when disopyramide given with ●tolterodine

- Antipsychotics: increased risk of ventricular arrhythmias when anti-arrhythmics that prolong the QT interval given with ●antipsychotics that prolong the QT interval; increased risk of ventricular arrhythmias when disopyramide given with ●amisulpride, ●droperidol, ●pimozide or ●zuclopenthixol—avoid concomitant use; possible increased risk of ventricular arrhythmias when disopyramide given with ●haloperidol—avoid concomitant use; increased risk of ventricular arrhythmias when disopyramide given with ●phenothiazines or ●sulpiride

- Antivirals: plasma concentration of disopyramide possibly increased by ●ritonavir (increased risk of toxicity); increased risk of ventricular arrhythmias when disopyramide given with ●saquinavir—avoid concomitant use; avoidance of disopyramide advised by manufacturer of ●telaprevir (risk of ventricular arrhythmias)

- Atomoxetine: increased risk of ventricular arrhythmias when disopyramide given with ●atomoxetine

- Beta-blockers: increased myocardial depression when anti-arrhythmics given with ●beta-blockers; increased risk of ventricular arrhythmias when

## Disopyramide

- Beta-blockers *(continued)*
  disopyramide given with ●sotalol—avoid concomitant use
- Calcium-channel Blockers: increased risk of myocardial depression and asystole when disopyramide given with ●verapamil
- Cytotoxics: possible increased risk of ventricular arrhythmias when disopyramide given with ●vandetanib—avoid concomitant use; increased risk of ventricular arrhythmias when disopyramide given with ●arsenic trioxide
- Diuretics: increased cardiac toxicity with disopyramide if hypokalaemia occurs with ●acetazolamide, ●loop diuretics or ●thiazides and related diuretics
- Fingolimod: possible increased risk of bradycardia when disopyramide given with ●fingolimod
- Ivabradine: increased risk of ventricular arrhythmias when disopyramide given with ●ivabradine
  Nitrates: disopyramide reduces effects of sublingual tablets of nitrates (failure to dissolve under tongue owing to dry mouth)
- Pentamidine Isetionate: possible increased risk of ventricular arrhythmias when disopyramide given with ●pentamidine isetionate
- Ranolazine: avoidance of disopyramide advised by manufacturer of ●ranolazine
  Sildenafil: manufacturer of disopyramide advises avoid concomitant use with sildenafil (risk of ventricular arrhythmias)
  Tadalafil: manufacturer of disopyramide advises avoid concomitant use with tadalafil (risk of ventricular arrhythmias)
  Vardenafil: manufacturer of disopyramide advises avoid concomitant use with vardenafil (risk of ventricular arrhythmias)

## Disulfiram

  Alcohol: disulfiram reaction when disulfiram given with alcohol (see BNF section 4.10.1)
  Antibacterials: psychotic reaction reported when disulfiram given with metronidazole; CNS effects of disulfiram possibly increased by isoniazid
- Anticoagulants: disulfiram enhances anticoagulant effect of ●coumarins
  Antidepressants: increased disulfiram reaction with alcohol reported with concomitant amitriptyline; disulfiram inhibits metabolism of tricyclics (increased plasma concentration)
- Antiepileptics: disulfiram inhibits metabolism of ●phenytoin (increased risk of toxicity)
  Anxiolytics and Hypnotics: disulfiram increases risk of temazepam toxicity; disulfiram inhibits metabolism of benzodiazepines (increased sedative effects)
- Paraldehyde: risk of toxicity when disulfiram given with ●paraldehyde
  Theophylline: disulfiram inhibits metabolism of theophylline (increased risk of toxicity)

## Diuretics

  **Note** Since systemic absorption may follow topical application of brinzolamide to the eye, the possibility of interactions should be borne in mind
  **Note** Since systemic absorption may follow topical application of dorzolamide to the eye, the possibility of interactions should be borne in mind
- ACE Inhibitors: enhanced hypotensive effect when diuretics given with ●ACE inhibitors; increased risk of severe hyperkalaemia when potassium-sparing diuretics and aldosterone antagonists given with ●ACE inhibitors
  Adrenergic Neurone Blockers: enhanced hypotensive effect when diuretics given with adrenergic neurone blockers
  Alcohol: enhanced hypotensive effect when diuretics given with alcohol
  Aldesleukin: enhanced hypotensive effect when diuretics given with aldesleukin

## Diuretics *(continued)*

  Aliskiren: plasma concentration of furosemide reduced by aliskiren; increased risk of hyperkalaemia when potassium-sparing diuretics and aldosterone antagonists given with aliskiren
  Allopurinol: increased risk of hypersensitivity when thiazides and related diuretics given with allopurinol especially in renal impairment
- Alpha-blockers: enhanced hypotensive effect when diuretics given with ●alpha-blockers, also increased risk of first-dose hypotension with post-synaptic alpha-blockers such as prazosin
  Anaesthetics, General: enhanced hypotensive effect when diuretics given with general anaesthetics
- Analgesics: diuretics increase risk of nephrotoxicity of NSAIDs, also antagonism of diuretic effect; Diuretic effect of potassium canrenoate possibly antagonised by NSAIDs; possible increased risk of hyperkalaemia when potassium-sparing diuretics and aldosterone antagonists given with NSAIDs; effects of diuretics antagonised by indometacin and ketorolac; increased risk of hyperkalaemia when potassium-sparing diuretics and aldosterone antagonists given with indometacin; occasional reports of reduced renal function when triamterene given with ●indometacin—avoid concomitant use; diuretic effect of spironolactone antagonised by aspirin; possible increased risk of toxicity when loop diuretics given with high-dose aspirin (also possible reduced effect of loop diuretics); increased risk of toxicity when acetazolamide given with high-dose ●aspirin
- Angiotensin-II Receptor Antagonists: enhanced hypotensive effect when diuretics given with ●angiotensin-II receptor antagonists; increased risk of hyperkalaemia when potassium-sparing diuretics and aldosterone antagonists given with ●angiotensin-II receptor antagonists
- Anti-arrhythmics: plasma concentration of eplerenone increased by amiodarone (reduce dose of eplerenone); hypokalaemia caused by acetazolamide, loop diuretics or thiazides and related diuretics increases cardiac toxicity with amiodarone; hypokalaemia caused by acetazolamide, loop diuretics or thiazides and related diuretics increases cardiac toxicity with ●disopyramide; hypokalaemia caused by acetazolamide, loop diuretics or thiazides and related diuretics increases cardiac toxicity with ●flecainide; hypokalaemia caused by acetazolamide, loop diuretics or thiazides and related diuretics antagonises action of ●lidocaine
- Antibacterials: plasma concentration of eplerenone increased by ●clarithromycin and ●telithromycin—avoid concomitant use; plasma concentration of eplerenone increased by erythromycin (reduce dose of eplerenone); plasma concentration of eplerenone reduced by ●rifampicin—avoid concomitant use; avoidance of diuretics advised by manufacturer of lymecycline; increased risk of ototoxicity when loop diuretics given with ●aminoglycosides, ●polymyxins or ●vancomycin; acetazolamide antagonises effects of ●methenamine; possible increased risk of hyperkalaemia when spironolactone given with trimethoprim; increased risk of hyperkalaemia when eplerenone given with trimethoprim
- Antidepressants: possible increased risk of hypokalaemia when loop diuretics or thiazides and related diuretics given with reboxetine; enhanced hypotensive effect when diuretics given with MAOIs; plasma concentration of eplerenone reduced by ●St John's wort—avoid concomitant use; increased risk of postural hypotension when diuretics given with tricyclics
  Antidiabetics: loop diuretics and thiazides and related diuretics antagonise hypoglycaemic effect of antidiabetics; diuretic effect of loop diuretics and thi-

**Appendix 1: Interactions** *(side tab)*

## Diuretics

**Antidiabetics** *(continued)*
azides and related diuretics possibly enhanced by dapagliflozin

- **Antiepileptics:** increased risk of hyponatraemia when diuretics given with carbamazepine; acetazolamide increases plasma concentration of •carbamazepine; plasma concentration of eplerenone reduced by •carbamazepine, •phenobarbital and •phenytoin—avoid concomitant use; increased risk of osteomalacia when carbonic anhydrase inhibitors given with phenobarbital or phenytoin; effects of furosemide antagonised by phenytoin; acetazolamide possibly increases plasma concentration of •phenytoin; hydrochlorothiazide possibly increases plasma concentration of topiramate
- **Antifungals:** plasma concentration of eplerenone increased by •itraconazole and •ketoconazole—avoid concomitant use; increased risk of hypokalaemia when loop diuretics or thiazides and related diuretics given with amphotericin; hydrochlorothiazide increases plasma concentration of fluconazole; plasma concentration of eplerenone increased by fluconazole (reduce dose of eplerenone)
- **Antipsychotics:** hypokalaemia caused by diuretics increases risk of ventricular arrhythmias with •amisulpride; enhanced hypotensive effect when diuretics given with phenothiazines; hypokalaemia caused by diuretics increases risk of ventricular arrhythmias with •pimozide (avoid concomitant use)
- **Antivirals:** plasma concentration of eplerenone increased by •ritonavir—avoid concomitant use; plasma concentration of eplerenone increased by saquinavir (reduce dose of eplerenone)
- **Anxiolytics and Hypnotics:** enhanced hypotensive effect when diuretics given with anxiolytics and hypnotics; administration of *parenteral* furosemide with chloral may displace thyroid hormone from binding sites
- **Atomoxetine:** hypokalaemia caused by diuretics increases risk of ventricular arrhythmias with •atomoxetine
- **Beta-blockers:** enhanced hypotensive effect when diuretics given with beta-blockers; hypokalaemia caused by loop diuretics or thiazides and related diuretics increases risk of ventricular arrhythmias with •sotalol
- **Calcium Salts:** increased risk of hypercalcaemia when thiazides and related diuretics given with calcium salts
- **Calcium-channel Blockers:** enhanced hypotensive effect when diuretics given with calcium-channel blockers; plasma concentration of eplerenone increased by diltiazem and verapamil (reduce dose of eplerenone)
- **Cardiac Glycosides:** hypokalaemia caused by acetazolamide, loop diuretics or thiazides and related diuretics increases cardiac toxicity with •cardiac glycosides; potassium canrenoate possibly increases plasma concentration of digoxin; spironolactone increases plasma concentration of •digoxin
- **Ciclosporin:** increased risk of nephrotoxicity and possibly hypermagnesaemia when thiazides and related diuretics given with ciclosporin; increased risk of hyperkalaemia when potassium-sparing diuretics and aldosterone antagonists given with •ciclosporin; acetazolamide possibly increases plasma concentration of •ciclosporin
- **Clonidine:** enhanced hypotensive effect when diuretics given with clonidine
- **Corticosteroids:** diuretic effect of diuretics antagonised by corticosteroids; increased risk of hypokalaemia when acetazolamide, loop diuretics or thiazides and related diuretics given with corticosteroids

## Diuretics *(continued)*

- **Cytotoxics:** alkaline urine due to acetazolamide increases excretion of methotrexate; hypokalaemia caused by acetazolamide, loop diuretics or thiazides and related diuretics increases risk of ventricular arrhythmias with •arsenic trioxide; avoidance of spironolactone advised by manufacturer of mitotane (antagonism of effect); increased risk of nephrotoxicity and ototoxicity when diuretics given with platinum compounds
- **Diazoxide:** enhanced hypotensive and hyperglycaemic effects when diuretics given with diazoxide
- **Diuretics:** increased risk of hypokalaemia when loop diuretics or thiazides and related diuretics given with acetazolamide; profound diuresis possible when metolazone given with furosemide; increased risk of hypokalaemia when thiazides and related diuretics given with loop diuretics
- **Dopaminergics:** enhanced hypotensive effect when diuretics given with levodopa
- **Hormone Antagonists:** increased risk of hypercalcaemia when thiazides and related diuretics given with toremifene
- **Lipid-regulating Drugs:** absorption of thiazides and related diuretics reduced by colestipol and colestyramine (give at least 2 hours apart)
- **Lithium:** loop diuretics and thiazides and related diuretics reduce excretion of •lithium (increased plasma concentration and risk of toxicity)—loop diuretics safer than thiazides; potassium-sparing diuretics and aldosterone antagonists reduce excretion of •lithium (increased plasma concentration and risk of toxicity); acetazolamide increases the excretion of •lithium
- **Methyldopa:** enhanced hypotensive effect when diuretics given with methyldopa
- **Moxisylyte:** enhanced hypotensive effect when diuretics given with moxisylyte
- **Moxonidine:** enhanced hypotensive effect when diuretics given with moxonidine
- **Muscle Relaxants:** enhanced hypotensive effect when diuretics given with baclofen or tizanidine
- **Nitrates:** enhanced hypotensive effect when diuretics given with nitrates
- **Oestrogens:** diuretic effect of diuretics antagonised by oestrogens
- **Potassium Salts:** increased risk of hyperkalaemia when potassium-sparing diuretics and aldosterone antagonists given with •potassium salts
- **Progestogens:** risk of hyperkalaemia when potassium-sparing diuretics and aldosterone antagonists given with drospirenone (monitor serum potassium during first cycle)
- **Prostaglandins:** enhanced hypotensive effect when diuretics given with alprostadil
- **Sympathomimetics, Beta₂:** increased risk of hypokalaemia when acetazolamide, loop diuretics or thiazides and related diuretics given with high doses of beta₂ sympathomimetics—see Hypokalaemia, p. 136
- **Tacrolimus:** increased risk of hyperkalaemia when potassium-sparing diuretics and aldosterone antagonists given with •tacrolimus
- **Theophylline:** increased risk of hypokalaemia when acetazolamide, loop diuretics or thiazides and related diuretics given with theophylline
- **Vasodilator Antihypertensives:** enhanced hypotensive effect when diuretics given with hydralazine, minoxidil or sodium nitroprusside
- **Vitamins:** increased risk of hypercalcaemia when thiazides and related diuretics given with vitamin D

**Diuretics, Loop** *see* Diuretics
**Diuretics, Potassium-sparing and Aldosterone Antagonists** *see* Diuretics
**Diuretics, Thiazide and related** *see* Diuretics
**Dobutamine** *see* Sympathomimetics

## Docetaxel

Antibacterials: *in vitro* studies suggest a possible interaction between docetaxel and erythromycin (consult docetaxel product literature)

Antifungals: *in vitro* studies suggest a possible interaction between docetaxel and ketoconazole (consult docetaxel product literature)

- Antipsychotics: avoid concomitant use of cytotoxics with •clozapine (increased risk of agranulocytosis)
- Antivirals: plasma concentration of docetaxel possibly increased by •ritonavir (increased risk of toxicity)

Ciclosporin: *in vitro* studies suggest a possible interaction between docetaxel and ciclosporin (consult docetaxel product literature)

Cytotoxics: possible increased risk of neutropenia when docetaxel given with lapatinib; plasma concentration of docetaxel increased by sorafenib

## Domperidone

Analgesics: effects of domperidone on gastro-intestinal activity antagonised by opioid analgesics

- Antibacterials: possible increased risk of ventricular arrhythmias when domperidone given with •erythromycin
- Antifungals: avoidance of domperidone advised by manufacturer of •ketoconazole (risk of ventricular arrhythmias)
- Antimalarials: avoidance of domperidone advised by manufacturer of •piperaquine with artenimol (possible risk of ventricular arrhythmias)

Antimuscarinics: effects of domperidone on gastro-intestinal activity antagonised by antimuscarinics

- Antivirals: plasma concentration of domperidone possibly increased by •telaprevir—manufacturer of telaprevir advises avoid concomitant use

Dopaminergics: domperidone possibly antagonises hypoprolactinaemic effects of bromocriptine and cabergoline

## Donepezil *see* Parasympathomimetics

## Dopamine *see* Sympathomimetics

## Dopaminergics *see* Amantadine, Apomorphine, Bromocriptine, Cabergoline, Entacapone, Levodopa, Pergolide, Pramipexole, Quinagolide, Rasagiline, Ropinirole, Rotigotine, Selegiline, and Tolcapone

## Dopexamine *see* Sympathomimetics

## Doripenem

- Antiepileptics: carbapenems reduce plasma concentration of •valproate—avoid concomitant use

Probenecid: excretion of doripenem reduced by probenecid (manufacturers of doripenem advise avoid concomitant use)

Vaccines: antibacterials inactivate oral typhoid vaccine—see p. 621

## Dorzolamide *see* Diuretics

## Dosulepin *see* Antidepressants, Tricyclic

## Doxapram

- Anaesthetics, General: increased risk of arrhythmias when doxapram given with •volatile liquid general anaesthetics (avoid doxapram for at least 10 minutes after volatile liquid general anaesthetics)

Antidepressants: effects of doxapram enhanced by MAOIs

Sympathomimetics: increased risk of hypertension when doxapram given with sympathomimetics

Theophylline: increased CNS stimulation when doxapram given with theophylline

## Doxazosin *see* Alpha-blockers

## Doxepin *see* Antidepressants, Tricyclic

## Doxorubicin

- Antipsychotics: avoid concomitant use of cytotoxics with •clozapine (increased risk of agranulocytosis)

Antivirals: doxorubicin possibly inhibits effects of stavudine

Calcium-channel Blockers: plasma concentration of doxorubicin possibly increased by verapamil

## Doxorubicin *(continued)*

Cardiac Glycosides: doxorubicin possibly reduces absorption of digoxin *tablets*

- Ciclosporin: increased risk of neurotoxicity when doxorubicin given with •ciclosporin

Cytotoxics: plasma concentration of doxorubicin possibly increased by sorafenib

## Doxycycline *see* Tetracyclines

## Dronedarone

Anaesthetics, Local: increased myocardial depression when anti-arrhythmics given with bupivacaine, levobupivacaine, prilocaine or ropivacaine

- Anti-arrhythmics: increased myocardial depression when anti-arrhythmics given with •anti-arrhythmics; increased risk of ventricular arrhythmias when dronedarone given with •amiodarone or •disopyramide—avoid concomitant use
- Antibacterials: manufacturer of dronedarone advises avoid concomitant use with •clarithromycin (risk of ventricular arrhythmias); plasma concentration of dronedarone increased by •erythromycin (increased risk of ventricular arrhythmias—avoid concomitant use); plasma concentration of dronedarone reduced by •rifampicin—avoid concomitant use; increased risk of ventricular arrhythmias when dronedarone given with •telithromycin—avoid concomitant use
- Anticoagulants: dronedarone possibly enhances anticoagulant effect of •coumarins and •phenindione; dronedarone increases plasma concentration of •dabigatran etexilate—avoid concomitant use; avoidance of dronedarone advised by manufacturer of rivaroxaban
- Antidepressants: plasma concentration of dronedarone possibly reduced by •St John's wort—avoid concomitant use; manufacturer of dronedarone advises avoid concomitant use with •tricyclics (risk of ventricular arrhythmias)
- Antiepileptics: plasma concentration of dronedarone possibly reduced by •carbamazepine, •phenobarbital and •phenytoin—avoid concomitant use
- Antifungals: plasma concentration of dronedarone increased by •ketoconazole—avoid concomitant use; manufacturer of dronedarone advises avoid concomitant use with •itraconazole, •posaconazole and •voriconazole
- Antipsychotics: increased risk of ventricular arrhythmias when anti-arrhythmics that prolong the QT interval given with •antipsychotics that prolong the QT interval; manufacturer of dronedarone advises avoid concomitant use with •phenothiazines (risk of ventricular arrhythmias)
- Antivirals: manufacturer of dronedarone advises avoid concomitant use with •ritonavir; increased risk of ventricular arrhythmias when dronedarone given with •saquinavir—avoid concomitant use
- Beta-blockers: increased myocardial depression when anti-arrhythmics given with •beta-blockers; dronedarone possibly increases plasma concentration of metoprolol and propranolol; increased risk of ventricular arrhythmias when dronedarone given with •sotalol—avoid concomitant use
- Calcium-channel Blockers: plasma concentration of dronedarone increased by •nifedipine; increased risk of bradycardia and myocardial depression when dronedarone given with •diltiazem and •verapamil
- Cardiac Glycosides: dronedarone increases plasma concentration of •digoxin (halve dose of digoxin)

Fidaxomicin: avoidance of dronedarone advised by manufacturer of fidaxomicin

- Fingolimod: possible increased risk of bradycardia when dronedarone given with •fingolimod
- Grapefruit Juice: plasma concentration of dronedarone increased by •grapefruit juice—avoid concomitant use

**Dronedarone** *(continued)*
- Lipid-regulating Drugs: dronedarone possibly increases plasma concentration of atorvastatin and rosuvastatin; increased risk of myopathy when dronedarone given with •simvastatin

Sirolimus: manufacturer of dronedarone advises caution with sirolimus

Tacrolimus: manufacturer of dronedarone advises caution with tacrolimus

**Droperidol** *see* Antipsychotics

**Drospirenone** *see* Progestogens

**Duloxetine**

Analgesics: possible increased serotonergic effects when duloxetine given with pethidine or tramadol
- Antibacterials: metabolism of duloxetine inhibited by •ciprofloxacin—avoid concomitant use
- Anticoagulants: possible increased risk of bleeding when SSRI-related antidepressants given with •dabigatran etexilate
- Antidepressants: metabolism of duloxetine inhibited by •fluvoxamine—avoid concomitant use; possible increased serotonergic effects when duloxetine given with SSRIs, St John's wort, amitriptyline, clomipramine, •moclobemide, tryptophan or venlafaxine; duloxetine should not be started until 2 weeks after stopping •MAOIs, also MAOIs should not be started until at least 5 days after stopping duloxetine; after stopping SSRI-related antidepressants do not start •moclobemide for at least 1 week
- Antimalarials: avoidance of antidepressants advised by manufacturer of •artemether with lumefantrine and •piperaquine with artenimol

Atomoxetine: possible increased risk of convulsions when antidepressants given with atomoxetine

5HT$_1$-receptor Agonists: possible increased serotonergic effects when duloxetine given with 5HT$_1$ agonists
- Methylthioninium: risk of CNS toxicity when SSRI-related antidepressants given with •methylthioninium—avoid concomitant use (if avoidance not possible, use lowest possible dose of methylthioninium and observe patient for up to 4 hours after administration)

**Dutasteride**

Calcium-channel Blockers: plasma concentration of dutasteride increased by diltiazem and verapamil

**Dydrogesterone** *see* Progestogens

**Edrophonium** *see* Parasympathomimetics

**Efavirenz**

Analgesics: efavirenz reduces plasma concentration of methadone

Antibacterials: increased risk of rash when efavirenz given with clarithromycin; efavirenz reduces plasma concentration of rifabutin—increase dose of rifabutin; plasma concentration of efavirenz reduced by rifampicin—increase dose of efavirenz
- Anticoagulants: efavirenz possibly affects plasma concentration of •coumarins
- Antidepressants: plasma concentration of efavirenz reduced by •St John's wort—avoid concomitant use

Antiepileptics: plasma concentration of efavirenz reduced when efavirenz given with carbamazepine
- Antifungals: efavirenz reduces plasma concentration of itraconazole and •posaconazole; efavirenz reduces plasma concentration of •voriconazole, also plasma concentration of efavirenz increased (increase voriconazole dose and reduce efavirenz dose); efavirenz possibly reduces plasma concentration of caspofungin—consider increasing dose of caspofungin

Antimalarials: efavirenz possibly affects plasma concentration of proguanil
- Antipsychotics: efavirenz possibly reduces plasma concentration of •aripiprazole—increase dose of aripiprazole; efavirenz possibly increases plasma

**Efavirenz**
- Antipsychotics *(continued)* concentration of •pimozide (increased risk of ventricular arrhythmias—avoid concomitant use)
- Antivirals: avoidance of efavirenz advised by manufacturer of •atazanavir (plasma concentration of atazanavir reduced); efavirenz reduces plasma concentration of •darunavir (adjust dose—consult product literature); efavirenz possibly reduces plasma concentration of •etravirine—avoid concomitant use; efavirenz reduces plasma concentration of indinavir; efavirenz reduces plasma concentration of •lopinavir—consider increasing dose of lopinavir; efavirenz possibly reduces plasma concentration of •maraviroc—consider increasing dose of maraviroc; plasma concentration of efavirenz reduced by nevirapine; toxicity of efavirenz increased by ritonavir, monitor liver function tests; efavirenz significantly reduces plasma concentration of saquinavir; efavirenz reduces plasma concentration of •telaprevir—increase dose of telaprevir
- Anxiolytics and Hypnotics: increased risk of prolonged sedation when efavirenz given with •midazolam—avoid concomitant use
- Atovaquone: efavirenz reduces plasma concentration of •atovaquone—avoid concomitant use

Bupropion: efavirenz accelerates metabolism of bupropion (reduced plasma concentration)

Calcium-channel Blockers: efavirenz reduces plasma concentration of diltiazem
- Ciclosporin: efavirenz possibly reduces plasma concentration of •ciclosporin
- Ergot Alkaloids: increased risk of ergotism when efavirenz given with •ergot alkaloids—avoid concomitant use

Grapefruit Juice: plasma concentration of efavirenz possibly increased by grapefruit juice

Lipid-regulating Drugs: efavirenz reduces plasma concentration of atorvastatin, pravastatin and simvastatin
- Progestogens: efavirenz possibly reduces contraceptive effect of •progestogens
- Tacrolimus: efavirenz possibly affects plasma concentration of •tacrolimus

**Eletriptan** *see* 5HT$_1$-receptor Agonists (under HT)

**Eltrombopag**

Antacids: absorption of eltrombopag reduced by antacids (give at least 4 hours apart)

Antivirals: plasma concentration of eltrombopag possibly reduced by lopinavir

Calcium Salts: absorption of eltrombopag possibly reduced by calcium salts (give at least 4 hours apart)

Dairy Products: absorption of eltrombopag possibly reduced by dairy products (give at least 4 hours apart)

Iron: absorption of eltrombopag possibly reduced by *oral* iron (give at least 4 hours apart)
- Lipid-regulating Drugs: eltrombopag increases plasma concentration of •rosuvastatin (consider reducing dose of rosuvastatin)

Selenium: absorption of eltrombopag possibly reduced by selenium (give at least 4 hours apart)

Zinc: absorption of eltrombopag possibly reduced by zinc (give at least 4 hours apart)

**Emtricitabine**

Antivirals: manufacturer of emtricitabine advises avoid concomitant use with lamivudine

**Enalapril** *see* ACE Inhibitors

**Enoxaparin** *see* Heparins

**Enoximone** *see* Phosphodiesterase Inhibitors

**Entacapone**
- Anticoagulants: entacapone enhances anticoagulant effect of •warfarin

**Entacapone** *(continued)*
- Antidepressants: manufacturer of entacapone advises caution with moclobemide, tricyclics and venlafaxine; avoid concomitant use of entacapone with non-selective ●MAOIs
  Dopaminergics: entacapone possibly enhances effects of apomorphine; entacapone possibly reduces plasma concentration of rasagiline; manufacturer of entacapone advises max. dose of 10mg selegiline if used concomitantly
  Iron: absorption of entacapone reduced by *oral* iron
  Memantine: effects of dopaminergics possibly enhanced by memantine
  Methyldopa: entacapone possibly enhances effects of methyldopa; antiparkinsonian effect of dopaminergics antagonised by methyldopa
  Sympathomimetics: entacapone possibly enhances effects of adrenaline (epinephrine), dobutamine, dopamine and noradrenaline (norepinephrine)

**Enteral Foods**
- Anticoagulants: the presence of vitamin K in some enteral feeds can antagonise the anticoagulant effect of ●coumarins and ●phenindione
  Antiepileptics: enteral feeds possibly reduce absorption of phenytoin

**Ephedrine** *see* Sympathomimetics

**Epinephrine (adrenaline)** *see* Sympathomimetics

**Epirubicin**
- Antipsychotics: avoid concomitant use of cytotoxics with ●clozapine (increased risk of agranulocytosis)
- Ciclosporin: plasma concentration of epirubicin increased by ●ciclosporin
- Ulcer-healing Drugs: plasma concentration of epirubicin increased by ●cimetidine

**Eplerenone** *see* Diuretics

**Eprosartan** *see* Angiotensin-II Receptor Antagonists

**Eptifibatide**
  Iloprost: increased risk of bleeding when eptifibatide given with iloprost

**Ergometrine** *see* Ergot Alkaloids

**Ergot Alkaloids**
- Antibacterials: increased risk of ergotism when ergotamine and methysergide given with ●macrolides or ●telithromycin—avoid concomitant use; increased risk of ergotism when ergotamine and methysergide given with tetracyclines
  Antidepressants: possible risk of hypertension when ergotamine and methysergide given with reboxetine
- Antifungals: increased risk of ergotism when ergotamine and methysergide given with ●imidazoles or ●triazoles—avoid concomitant use
- Antivirals: plasma concentration of ergot alkaloids possibly increased by ●atazanavir—avoid concomitant use; avoidance of ergot alkaloids advised by manufacturer of ●boceprevir and ●telaprevir; increased risk of ergotism when ergot alkaloids given with ●efavirenz—avoid concomitant use; increased risk of ergotism when ergotamine and methysergide given with ●fosamprenavir, ●indinavir, ●ritonavir or ●saquinavir—avoid concomitant use
  Beta-blockers: increased peripheral vasoconstriction when ergotamine and methysergide given with beta-blockers
- Cytotoxics: caution with ergot alkaloids advised by manufacturer of ●crizotinib
- 5HT₁-receptor Agonists: increased risk of vasospasm when ergotamine and methysergide given with ●almotriptan, ●rizatriptan, ●sumatriptan or ●zolmitriptan (avoid ergotamine and methysergide for 6 hours after almotriptan, rizatriptan, sumatriptan or zolmitriptan, avoid almotriptan, rizatriptan, sumatriptan or zolmitriptan for 24 hours after ergotamine and methysergide); increased risk of vasospasm when ergotamine and methysergide given with

**Ergot Alkaloids**
- 5HT₁-receptor Agonists *(continued)*
  ●eletriptan, ●frovatriptan or ●naratriptan (avoid ergotamine and methysergide for 24 hours after eletriptan, frovatriptan or naratriptan, avoid eletriptan, frovatriptan or naratriptan for 24 hours after ergotamine and methysergide)
  Sympathomimetics: increased risk of ergotism when ergotamine and methysergide given with sympathomimetics
- Ticagrelor: plasma concentration of ergot alkaloids possibly increased by ●ticagrelor
- Ulcer-healing Drugs: increased risk of ergotism when ergotamine and methysergide given with ●cimetidine—avoid concomitant use

**Ergotamine and Methysergide** *see* Ergot Alkaloids

**Eribulin**
  Antibacterials: plasma concentration of eribulin possibly reduced by rifampicin
  Antidepressants: plasma concentration of eribulin possibly reduced by St John's wort
  Antiepileptics: plasma concentration of eribulin possibly reduced by carbamazepine and phenytoin
- Antipsychotics: avoid concomitant use of cytotoxics with ●clozapine (increased risk of agranulocytosis)

**Erlotinib**
- Analgesics: increased risk of bleeding when erlotinib given with ●NSAIDs
- Antacids: plasma concentration of erlotinib possibly reduced by ●antacids—give antacids at least 4 hours before or 2 hours after erlotinib
  Antibacterials: plasma concentration of erlotinib increased by ciprofloxacin; metabolism of erlotinib accelerated by rifampicin (reduced plasma concentration)
- Anticoagulants: increased risk of bleeding when erlotinib given with ●coumarins
  Antifungals: metabolism of erlotinib inhibited by ketoconazole (increased plasma concentration)
- Antipsychotics: avoid concomitant use of cytotoxics with ●clozapine (increased risk of agranulocytosis)
- Antivirals: avoidance of erlotinib advised by manufacturer of ●boceprevir
  Cytotoxics: plasma concentration of erlotinib possibly increased by capecitabine
- Ulcer-healing Drugs: manufacturer of erlotinib advises avoid concomitant use with ●cimetidine, ●esomeprazole, ●famotidine, ●lansoprazole, ●nizatidine, ●pantoprazole and ●rabeprazole; plasma concentration of erlotinib reduced by ●ranitidine—manufacturer of erlotinib advises give at least 2 hours before or 10 hours after ranitidine; plasma concentration of erlotinib reduced by ●omeprazole—manufacturer of erlotinib advises avoid concomitant use

**Ertapenem**
- Antiepileptics: carbapenems reduce plasma concentration of ●valproate—avoid concomitant use
  Vaccines: antibacterials inactivate oral typhoid vaccine—see p. 621

**Erythromycin** *see* Macrolides

**Escitalopram** *see* Antidepressants, SSRI

**Eslicarbazepine**
  Anticoagulants: eslicarbazepine reduces plasma concentration of warfarin
- Antidepressants: anticonvulsant effect of antiepileptics possibly antagonised by MAOIs and ●tricyclic-related antidepressants (convulsive threshold lowered); anticonvulsant effect of antiepileptics antagonised by ●SSRIs and ●tricyclics (convulsive threshold lowered); avoid concomitant use of antiepileptics with ●St John's wort
  Antiepileptics: plasma concentration of eslicarbazepine possibly reduced by carbamazepine but risk of side-effects increased; manufacturer of eslicarbaze-

## Eslicarbazepine

Antiepileptics *(continued)*
pine advises avoid concomitant use with oxcarbazepine; plasma concentration of eslicarbazepine reduced by phenytoin, also plasma concentration of phenytoin increased

* Antimalarials: anticonvulsant effect of antiepileptics antagonised by •mefloquine
* Antipsychotics: anticonvulsant effect of antiepileptics antagonised by •antipsychotics (convulsive threshold lowered)

Lipid-regulating Drugs: eslicarbazepine reduces plasma concentration of simvastatin—consider increasing dose of simvastatin

* Oestrogens: eslicarbazepine accelerates metabolism of •oestrogens (reduced contraceptive effect—see p. 398)
* Orlistat: possible increased risk of convulsions when antiepileptics given with •orlistat
* Progestogens: eslicarbazepine accelerates metabolism of •progestogens (reduced contraceptive effect—see p. 398)

## Esmolol *see* Beta-blockers

## Esomeprazole *see* Proton Pump Inhibitors

## Estradiol *see* Oestrogens

## Estramustine

* Antipsychotics: avoid concomitant use of cytotoxics with •clozapine (increased risk of agranulocytosis)
* Bisphosphonates: plasma concentration of estramustine increased by •sodium clodronate

## Estriol *see* Oestrogens

## Estrone *see* Oestrogens

## Etanercept

* Abatacept: avoid concomitant use of etanercept with •abatacept
* Anakinra: avoid concomitant use of etanercept with •anakinra
* Vaccines: avoid concomitant use of etanercept with live •vaccines (see p. 600)

## Ethinylestradiol *see* Oestrogens

## Ethosuximide

* Antibacterials: metabolism of ethosuximide inhibited by •isoniazid (increased plasma concentration and risk of toxicity)
* Antidepressants: anticonvulsant effect of antiepileptics possibly antagonised by MAOIs and •tricyclic-related antidepressants (convulsive threshold lowered); anticonvulsant effect of antiepileptics antagonised by •SSRIs and •tricyclics (convulsive threshold lowered); avoid concomitant use of antiepileptics with •St John's wort
* Antiepileptics: plasma concentration of ethosuximide possibly reduced by carbamazepine and phenobarbital; plasma concentration of ethosuximide possibly reduced by •phenytoin, also plasma concentration of phenytoin possibly increased; plasma concentration of ethosuximide possibly increased by valproate
* Antimalarials: anticonvulsant effect of antiepileptics antagonised by •mefloquine
* Antipsychotics: anticonvulsant effect of antiepileptics antagonised by •antipsychotics (convulsive threshold lowered)
* Orlistat: possible increased risk of convulsions when antiepileptics given with •orlistat

## Etodolac *see* NSAIDs

## Etomidate *see* Anaesthetics, General

## Etonogestrel *see* Progestogens

## Etoposide

* Anticoagulants: etoposide possibly enhances anticoagulant effect of •coumarins

Antiepileptics: plasma concentration of etoposide possibly reduced by phenobarbital and phenytoin

* Antipsychotics: avoid concomitant use of cytotoxics with •clozapine (increased risk of agranulocytosis)

## Etoposide *(continued)*

Atovaquone: plasma concentration of etoposide possibly increased by atovaquone
Ciclosporin: plasma concentration of etoposide possibly increased by ciclosporin (increased risk of toxicity)

## Etoricoxib *see* NSAIDs

## Etravirine

* Antibacterials: plasma concentration of etravirine increased by •clarithromycin, also plasma concentration of clarithromycin reduced; plasma concentration of both drugs reduced when etravirine given with •rifabutin; manufacturer of etravirine advises avoid concomitant use with rifampicin

Antidepressants: manufacturer of etravirine advises avoid concomitant use with St John's wort

Antiepileptics: manufacturer of etravirine advises avoid concomitant use with carbamazepine, phenobarbital and phenytoin

* Antivirals: plasma concentration of etravirine possibly reduced by •efavirenz and •nevirapine—avoid concomitant use; etravirine increases plasma concentration of •fosamprenavir (consider reducing dose of fosamprenavir); etravirine possibly reduces plasma concentration of •indinavir—avoid concomitant use; etravirine possibly reduces plasma concentration of maraviroc; plasma concentration of etravirine reduced by •tipranavir, also plasma concentration of tipranavir increased (avoid concomitant use)

Cardiac Glycosides: etravirine increases plasma concentration of digoxin

* Clopidogrel: etravirine possibly reduces antiplatelet effect of •clopidogrel

Lipid-regulating Drugs: etravirine possibly reduces plasma concentration of atorvastatin
Sildenafil: etravirine reduces plasma concentration of sildenafil

## Etynodiol *see* Progestogens

## Everolimus

* Antibacterials: plasma concentration of everolimus possibly increased by •clarithromycin and •telithromycin—manufacturer of everolimus advises avoid concomitant use; plasma concentration of everolimus increased by •erythromycin; plasma concentration of everolimus reduced by •rifampicin

Antidepressants: plasma concentration of everolimus possibly reduced by St John's wort—manufacturer of everolimus advises avoid concomitant use

* Antifungals: plasma concentration of everolimus increased by •ketoconazole—avoid concomitant use; plasma concentration of everolimus possibly increased by •itraconazole, •posaconazole and •voriconazole—manufacturer of everolimus advises avoid concomitant use
* Antipsychotics: avoid concomitant use of cytotoxics with •clozapine (increased risk of agranulocytosis)
* Antivirals: plasma concentration of everolimus possibly increased by •atazanavir, •darunavir, •indinavir, •ritonavir and •saquinavir—manufacturer of everolimus advises avoid concomitant use
* Calcium-channel Blockers: plasma concentration of both drugs may increase when everolimus given with •verapamil
* Ciclosporin: plasma concentration of everolimus increased by •ciclosporin

Grapefruit Juice: manufacturer of everolimus advises avoid concomitant use with grapefruit juice

## Exemestane

Antibacterials: plasma concentration of exemestane possibly reduced by rifampicin

## Exenatide *see* Antidiabetics

## Ezetimibe

Anticoagulants: ezetimibe possibly enhances anticoagulant effect of coumarins

**Ezetimibe** *(continued)*
- Ciclosporin: plasma concentration of both drugs may increase when ezetimibe given with ●ciclosporin
  Lipid-regulating Drugs: increased risk of cholelithiasis and gallbladder disease when ezetimibe given with fibrates—discontinue if suspected

**Famciclovir**
  Probenecid: excretion of famciclovir possibly reduced by probenecid (increased plasma concentration)

**Famotidine** *see* Histamine H₂-antagonists

**Fampridine**
- Ulcer-healing Drugs: manufacturer of fampridine advises avoid concomitant use with ●cimetidine

**Febuxostat**
- Azathioprine: manufacturer of febuxostat advises avoid concomitant use with ●azathioprine
- Cytotoxics: manufacturer of febuxostat advises avoid concomitant use with ●mercaptopurine
- Theophylline: manufacturer of febuxostat advises caution with ●theophylline

**Felodipine** *see* Calcium-channel Blockers

**Fenofibrate** *see* Fibrates

**Fenoprofen** *see* NSAIDs

**Fentanyl** *see* Opioid Analgesics

**Ferrous Salts** *see* Iron

**Fesoterodine** *see* Antimuscarinics

**Fexofenadine** *see* Antihistamines

**Fibrates**
- Antibacterials: increased risk of myopathy when fibrates given with ●daptomycin (preferably avoid concomitant use)
- Anticoagulants: fibrates enhance anticoagulant effect of ●coumarins and ●phenindione
- Antidiabetics: fibrates may improve glucose tolerance and have an additive effect with insulin or sulfonylureas; gemfibrozil possibly enhances hypoglycaemic effect of nateglinide; increased risk of severe hypoglycaemia when gemfibrozil given with ●repaglinide—avoid concomitant use
  Ciclosporin: increased risk of renal impairment when bezafibrate or fenofibrate given with ciclosporin
- Colchicine: possible increased risk of myopathy when fibrates given with ●colchicine
- Cytotoxics: gemfibrozil increases plasma concentration of ●bexarotene—avoid concomitant use
  Leukotriene Receptor Antagonists: gemfibrozil increases plasma concentration of montelukast
- Lipid-regulating Drugs: increased risk of myopathy when gemfibrozil given with ●atorvastatin, ●fluvastatin or ●pravastatin (preferably avoid concomitant use); increased risk of myopathy when fibrates given with ●rosuvastatin (see Dose under Rosuvastatin, p. 126); possible increased risk of myopathy when bezafibrate and ciprofibrate given with ●simvastatin (see Dose under Simvastatin, p. 126); increased risk of myopathy when gemfibrozil given with ●simvastatin (avoid concomitant use); increased risk of cholelithiasis and gallbladder disease when fibrates given with ezetimibe—discontinue if suspected; increased risk of myopathy when fibrates given with ●statins

**Fidaxomicin**
  Anti-arrhythmics: manufacturer of fidaxomicin advises avoid concomitant use with amiodarone and dronedarone
  Antibacterials: manufacturer of fidaxomicin advises avoid concomitant use with clarithromycin and erythromycin
  Antifungals: manufacturer of fidaxomicin advises avoid concomitant use with ketoconazole
  Calcium-channel Blockers: manufacturer of fidaxomicin advises avoid concomitant use with verapamil
  Ciclosporin: manufacturer of fidaxomicin advises avoid concomitant use with ciclosporin

**Filgrastim**
  **Note** Pegfilgrastim interactions as for filgrastim
  Cytotoxics: neutropenia possibly exacerbated when filgrastim given with fluorouracil

**Fingolimod**
- Anti-arrhythmics: possible increased risk of bradycardia when fingolimod given with ●amiodarone, ●disopyramide or ●dronedarone
- Antifungals: plasma concentration of fingolimod increased by ●ketoconazole
- Beta-blockers: possible increased risk of bradycardia when fingolimod given with ●beta-blockers
- Calcium-channel Blockers: possible increased risk of bradycardia when fingolimod given with ●diltiazem or ●verapamil

**Flavoxate** *see* Antimuscarinics

**Flecainide**
  Anaesthetics, Local: increased myocardial depression when anti-arrhythmics given with bupivacaine, levobupivacaine, prilocaine or ropivacaine
- Anti-arrhythmics: increased myocardial depression when anti-arrhythmics given with other ●anti-arrhythmics; plasma concentration of flecainide increased by ●amiodarone (halve dose of flecainide)
- Antidepressants: plasma concentration of flecainide increased by fluoxetine; increased risk of ventricular arrhythmias when flecainide given with ●tricyclics
- Antihistamines: increased risk of ventricular arrhythmias when flecainide given with ●mizolastine—avoid concomitant use
- Antimalarials: avoidance of flecainide advised by manufacturer of ●artemether with lumefantrine (risk of ventricular arrhythmias); plasma concentration of flecainide increased by ●quinine
- Antimuscarinics: increased risk of ventricular arrhythmias when flecainide given with ●tolterodine
- Antipsychotics: increased risk of ventricular arrhythmias when anti-arrhythmics that prolong the QT interval given with ●antipsychotics that prolong the QT interval; increased risk of arrhythmias when flecainide given with ●clozapine
- Antivirals: plasma concentration of flecainide possibly increased by ●fosamprenavir, ●indinavir, ●lopinavir and ●ritonavir (increased risk of ventricular arrhythmias—avoid concomitant use); increased risk of ventricular arrhythmias when flecainide given with ●saquinavir—avoid concomitant use; caution with flecainide advised by manufacturer of ●telaprevir (risk of ventricular arrhythmias)
- Beta-blockers: increased risk of myocardial depression and bradycardia when flecainide given with ●beta-blockers; increased myocardial depression when anti-arrhythmics given with ●beta-blockers
- Calcium-channel Blockers: increased risk of myocardial depression and asystole when flecainide given with ●verapamil
- Diuretics: increased cardiac toxicity with flecainide if hypokalaemia occurs with ●acetazolamide, ●loop diuretics or ●thiazides and related diuretics
  Ulcer-healing Drugs: metabolism of flecainide inhibited by cimetidine (increased plasma concentration)

**Flucloxacillin** *see* Penicillins

**Fluconazole** *see* Antifungals, Triazole

**Flucytosine**
  Antifungals: renal excretion of flucytosine decreased and cellular uptake increased by amphotericin (toxicity possibly increased)
  Cytotoxics: plasma concentration of flucytosine possibly reduced by cytarabine

**Fludarabine**
- Antipsychotics: avoid concomitant use of cytotoxics with ●clozapine (increased risk of agranulocytosis)
- Cytotoxics: fludarabine increases intracellular concentration of cytarabine; increased pulmonary toxicity when fludarabine given with ●pentostatin (unacceptably high incidence of fatalities)

**Fludarabine** (continued)

Dipyridamole: effects of fludarabine possibly reduced by dipyridamole

**Fludrocortisone** see Corticosteroids

**Flunisolide** see Corticosteroids

**Fluorides**

Calcium Salts: absorption of fluorides reduced by calcium salts

**Fluorouracil**

**Note** Capecitabine is a prodrug of fluorouracil

**Note** Tegafur is a prodrug of fluorouracil

- Allopurinol: manufacturer of capecitabine advises avoid concomitant use with ●allopurinol

Antibacterials: metabolism of fluorouracil inhibited by metronidazole (increased toxicity)

- Anticoagulants: fluorouracil enhances anticoagulant effect of ●coumarins

Antiepileptics: fluorouracil possibly inhibits metabolism of phenytoin (increased risk of toxicity)

- Antipsychotics: avoid concomitant use of cytotoxics with ●clozapine (increased risk of agranulocytosis)

Cytotoxics: capecitabine possibly increases plasma concentration of erlotinib

Filgrastim: neutropenia possibly exacerbated when fluorouracil given with filgrastim

- Temoporfin: increased skin photosensitivity when topical fluorouracil used with ●temoporfin

Ulcer-healing Drugs: metabolism of fluorouracil inhibited by cimetidine (increased plasma concentration)

**Fluoxetine** see Antidepressants, SSRI

**Flupentixol** see Antipsychotics

**Fluphenazine** see Antipsychotics

**Flurazepam** see Anxiolytics and Hypnotics

**Flurbiprofen** see NSAIDs

**Flutamide**

- Anticoagulants: flutamide enhances anticoagulant effect of ●coumarins

**Fluticasone** see Corticosteroids

**Fluvastatin** see Statins

**Fluvoxamine** see Antidepressants, SSRI

**Folates**

Aminosalicylates: absorption of folic acid possibly reduced by sulfasalazine

Antiepileptics: folates possibly reduce plasma concentration of phenobarbital and phenytoin

- Cytotoxics: avoidance of folates advised by manufacturer of ●raltitrexed

**Folic Acid** see Folates

**Folinic Acid** see Folates

**Formoterol** see Sympathomimetics, Beta$_2$

**Fosamprenavir**

**Note** Fosamprenavir is a prodrug of amprenavir

Analgesics: fosamprenavir reduces plasma concentration of methadone

- Anti-arrhythmics: fosamprenavir possibly increases plasma concentration of ●amiodarone, ●flecainide and ●propafenone (increased risk of ventricular arrhythmias—avoid concomitant use); fosamprenavir possibly increases plasma concentration of ●lidocaine—avoid concomitant use
- Antibacterials: fosamprenavir increases plasma concentration of ●rifabutin (reduce dose of rifabutin); plasma concentration of fosamprenavir significantly reduced by ●rifampicin—avoid concomitant use; avoidance of concomitant fosamprenavir in severe renal and hepatic impairment advised by manufacturer of ●telithromycin

Anticoagulants: avoidance of fosamprenavir advised by manufacturer of apixaban and rivaroxaban; fosamprenavir may enhance or reduce anticoagulant effect of coumarins

- Antidepressants: plasma concentration of fosamprenavir reduced by ●St John's wort—avoid concomitant use

**Fosamprenavir** (continued)

Antiepileptics: plasma concentration of fosamprenavir possibly reduced by carbamazepine and phenobarbital

Antifungals: fosamprenavir increases plasma concentration of ketoconazole (also plasma concentration of fosamprenavir possibly increased); plasma concentration of both drugs may increase when fosamprenavir given with itraconazole; fosamprenavir possibly reduces plasma concentration of posaconazole

- Antimalarials: caution with fosamprenavir advised by manufacturer of artemether with lumefantrine; fosamprenavir possibly increases plasma concentration of ●quinine (increased risk of toxicity)

Antimuscarinics: avoidance of fosamprenavir advised by manufacturer of darifenacin and tolterodine

- Antipsychotics: fosamprenavir possibly inhibits metabolism of ●aripiprazole (reduce dose of aripiprazole); fosamprenavir increases plasma concentration of ●pimozide (increased risk of ventricular arrhythmias—avoid concomitant use); fosamprenavir possibly increases plasma concentration of ●quetiapine—manufacturer of quetiapine advises avoid concomitant use
- Antivirals: manufacturer of fosamprenavir advises avoid concomitant use with ●boceprevir and ●raltegravir; plasma concentration of fosamprenavir increased by ●etravirine (consider reducing dose of fosamprenavir); plasma concentration of fosamprenavir reduced by lopinavir, effect on lopinavir plasma concentration not predictable—avoid concomitant use; plasma concentration of fosamprenavir reduced by ●maraviroc—avoid concomitant use; plasma concentration of fosamprenavir possibly reduced by nevirapine; manufacturers advise avoid concomitant use of fosamprenavir with ●telaprevir; plasma concentration of fosamprenavir reduced by ●tipranavir
- Anxiolytics and Hypnotics: fosamprenavir possibly increases plasma concentration of ●midazolam (risk of prolonged sedation—avoid concomitant use of oral midazolam)
- Ciclosporin: fosamprenavir increases plasma concentration of ●ciclosporin
- Ergot Alkaloids: increased risk of ergotism when fosamprenavir given with ●ergotamine and methysergide—avoid concomitant use
- Lipid-regulating Drugs: possible increased risk of myopathy when fosamprenavir given with atorvastatin; possible increased risk of myopathy when fosamprenavir given with ●rosuvastatin—manufacturer of rosuvastatin advises avoid concomitant use; possible increased risk of myopathy when fosamprenavir given with ●simvastatin—avoid concomitant use
- Ranolazine: fosamprenavir possibly increases plasma concentration of ●ranolazine—manufacturer of ranolazine advises avoid concomitant use

Sildenafil: fosamprenavir possibly increases plasma concentration of sildenafil

- Tacrolimus: fosamprenavir increases plasma concentration of ●tacrolimus

Tadalafil: fosamprenavir possibly increases plasma concentration of tadalafil

Vardenafil: fosamprenavir possibly increases plasma concentration of vardenafil

**Fosaprepitant** see Aprepitant

**Foscarnet**

- Pentamidine Isetionate: increased risk of hypocalcaemia when foscarnet given with parenteral ●pentamidine isetionate

**Fosinopril** see ACE Inhibitors

**Fosphenytoin** see Phenytoin

**Framycetin** see Aminoglycosides

**Frovatriptan** see 5HT$_1$-receptor Agonists (under HT)

**Furosemide** see Diuretics

## Fusidic Acid

- Antivirals: plasma concentration of both drugs increased when fusidic acid given with •ritonavir— avoid concomitant use; plasma concentration of both drugs may increase when fusidic acid given with saquinavir
- Lipid-regulating Drugs: risk of myopathy and rhabdomyolysis when fusidic acid given with •statins— avoid concomitant use and for 7 days after last fusidic acid dose

Sugammadex: fusidic acid possibly reduces response to sugammadex

Vaccines: antibacterials inactivate oral typhoid vaccine—see p. 621

## Gabapentin

Analgesics: bioavailability of gabapentin increased by morphine

Antacids: absorption of gabapentin reduced by antacids

- Antidepressants: anticonvulsant effect of antiepileptics possibly antagonised by MAOIs and •tricyclic-related antidepressants (convulsive threshold lowered); anticonvulsant effect of antiepileptics antagonised by •SSRIs and •tricyclics (convulsive threshold lowered); avoid concomitant use of antiepileptics with •St John's wort
- Antimalarials: anticonvulsant effect of antiepileptics antagonised by •mefloquine
- Antipsychotics: anticonvulsant effect of antiepileptics antagonised by •antipsychotics (convulsive threshold lowered)
- Orlistat: possible increased risk of convulsions when antiepileptics given with •orlistat

Galantamine see Parasympathomimetics

## Ganciclovir

Note Increased risk of myelosuppression with other myelosuppressive drugs—consult product literature

Note Valganciclovir interactions as for ganciclovir

- Antibacterials: increased risk of convulsions when ganciclovir given with •imipenem with cilastatin
- Antivirals: ganciclovir possibly increases plasma concentration of didanosine; profound myelosuppression when ganciclovir given with •zidovudine (if possible avoid concomitant administration, particularly during initial ganciclovir therapy)

Mycophenolate: plasma concentration of ganciclovir possibly increased by mycophenolate, also plasma concentration of inactive metabolite of mycophenolate possibly increased

Probenecid: excretion of ganciclovir reduced by probenecid (increased plasma concentration and risk of toxicity)

Tacrolimus: possible increased risk of nephrotoxicity when ganciclovir given with tacrolimus

## Gefitinib

- Antibacterials: plasma concentration of gefitinib reduced by •rifampicin—avoid concomitant use
- Anticoagulants: gefitinib possibly enhances anticoagulant effect of •warfarin

Antidepressants: manufacturer of gefitinib advises avoid concomitant use with St John's wort

Antiepileptics: manufacturer of gefitinib advises avoid concomitant use with carbamazepine, phenobarbital and phenytoin

Antifungals: plasma concentration of gefitinib increased by itraconazole

- Antipsychotics: avoid concomitant use of cytotoxics with •clozapine (increased risk of agranulocytosis)
- Antivirals: avoidance of gefitinib advised by manufacturer of •boceprevir
- Ulcer-healing Drugs: plasma concentration of gefitinib reduced by •ranitidine

## Gemcitabine

Anticoagulants: gemcitabine possibly enhances anticoagulant effect of warfarin

## Gemcitabine (continued)

- Antipsychotics: avoid concomitant use of cytotoxics with •clozapine (increased risk of agranulocytosis)

Gemeprost see Prostaglandins

Gemfibrozil see Fibrates

Gentamicin see Aminoglycosides

Gestodene see Progestogens

Glibenclamide see Antidiabetics

Gliclazide see Antidiabetics

Glimepiride see Antidiabetics

Glipizide see Antidiabetics

## Glucosamine

- Anticoagulants: glucosamine enhances anticoagulant effect of •warfarin (avoid concomitant use)

Glyceryl Trinitrate see Nitrates

Glycopyrronium see Antimuscarinics

Gold see Sodium Aurothiomalate

## Golimumab

- Abatacept: avoid concomitant use of golimumab with •abatacept
- Anakinra: avoid concomitant use of golimumab with •anakinra
- Vaccines: avoid concomitant use of golimumab with live •vaccines (see p. 600)

## Grapefruit Juice

- Aliskiren: grapefruit juice reduces plasma concentration of •aliskiren—avoid concomitant use
- Anti-arrhythmics: grapefruit juice increases plasma concentration of amiodarone; grapefruit juice increases plasma concentration of •dronedarone— avoid concomitant use

Antidepressants: grapefruit juice possibly increases plasma concentration of sertraline

- Antihistamines: grapefruit juice reduces plasma concentration of bilastine; grapefruit juice increases plasma concentration of •rupatadine—avoid concomitant use

Antimalarials: avoidance of grapefruit juice advised by manufacturer of piperaquine with artenimol; grapefruit juice possibly increases plasma concentration of artemether with lumefantrine

- Antipsychotics: grapefruit juice possibly increases plasma concentration of •quetiapine—manufacturer of quetiapine advises avoid concomitant use

Antivirals: grapefruit juice possibly increases plasma concentration of efavirenz

Anxiolytics and Hypnotics: grapefruit juice possibly increases plasma concentration of oral midazolam; grapefruit juice increases plasma concentration of buspirone

Calcium-channel Blockers: grapefruit juice possibly increases plasma concentration of amlodipine; grapefruit juice increases plasma concentration of felodipine, isradipine, lacidipine, lercanidipine, nicardipine, nifedipine, nimodipine and verapamil

- Ciclosporin: grapefruit juice increases plasma concentration of •ciclosporin (increased risk of toxicity)
- Colchicine: grapefruit juice possibly increases risk of •colchicine toxicity
- Cytotoxics: grapefruit juice possibly increases plasma concentration of axitinib; grapefruit juice possibly increases plasma concentration of •crizotinib and vinflunine—manufacturer of crizotinib and vinflunine advises avoid concomitant use; avoidance of grapefruit juice advised by manufacturer of everolimus, •lapatinib, •nilotinib and •pazopanib

Ivabradine: grapefruit juice increases plasma concentration of ivabradine

- Lipid-regulating Drugs: grapefruit juice possibly increases plasma concentration of atorvastatin; grapefruit juice increases plasma concentration of •simvastatin—avoid concomitant use

Pirfenidone: avoidance of grapefruit juice advised by manufacturer of pirfenidone

### Grapefruit Juice *(continued)*

- Ranolazine: grapefruit juice possibly increases plasma concentration of ●ranolazine—manufacturer of ranolazine advises avoid concomitant use

  Sildenafil: grapefruit juice possibly increases plasma concentration of sildenafil

- Sirolimus: grapefruit juice increases plasma concentration of ●sirolimus—avoid concomitant use

- Tacrolimus: grapefruit juice increases plasma concentration of ●tacrolimus

  Tadalafil: grapefruit juice possibly increases plasma concentration of tadalafil

- Tolvaptan: grapefruit juice increases plasma concentration of ●tolvaptan—avoid concomitant use

- Vardenafil: grapefruit juice possibly increases plasma concentration of ●vardenafil—avoid concomitant use

### Griseofulvin

  Alcohol: griseofulvin possibly enhances effects of alcohol

- Anticoagulants: griseofulvin reduces anticoagulant effect of ●coumarins

  Antiepileptics: absorption of griseofulvin reduced by phenobarbital (reduced effect)

  Ciclosporin: griseofulvin possibly reduces plasma concentration of ciclosporin

  Oestrogens: anecdotal reports of contraceptive failure and menstrual irregularities when griseofulvin given with oestrogens

  Progestogens: anecdotal reports of contraceptive failure and menstrual irregularities when griseofulvin given with progestogens

**Guanethidine** *see* Adrenergic Neurone Blockers

**Haloperidol** *see* Antipsychotics

**Heparin** *see* Heparins

### Heparins

  ACE Inhibitors: increased risk of hyperkalaemia when heparins given with ACE inhibitors

  Aliskiren: increased risk of hyperkalaemia when heparins given with aliskiren

- Analgesics: possible increased risk of bleeding when heparins given with NSAIDs; increased risk of haemorrhage when anticoagulants given with *intravenous* ●diclofenac (avoid concomitant use, including low-dose heparins); increased risk of haemorrhage when anticoagulants given with ●ketorolac (avoid concomitant use, including low-dose heparins); anticoagulant effect of heparins enhanced by ●aspirin

  Angiotensin-II Receptor Antagonists: increased risk of hyperkalaemia when heparins given with angiotensin-II receptor antagonists

- Anticoagulants: increased risk of haemorrhage when other anticoagulants given with ●apixaban, ●dabigatran etexilate and ●rivaroxaban (avoid concomitant use except when switching with other anticoagulants or using heparin to maintain catheter patency)

  Clopidogrel: increased risk of bleeding when heparins given with clopidogrel

  Dipyridamole: anticoagulant effect of heparins enhanced by dipyridamole

  Iloprost: anticoagulant effect of heparins possibly enhanced by iloprost

- Nitrates: anticoagulant effect of heparins reduced by *infusion* of ●glyceryl trinitrate

### Histamine

  Antidepressants: manufacturer of histamine advises avoid concomitant use with MAOIs; effects of histamine theoretically antagonised by tricyclics—manufacturer of histamine advises avoid concomitant use

  Antihistamines: effects of histamine theoretically antagonised by antihistamines—manufacturer of histamine advises avoid concomitant use

### Histamine *(continued)*

  Antimalarials: manufacturer of histamine advises avoid concomitant use with antimalarials

  Antipsychotics: effects of histamine theoretically antagonised by antipsychotics—manufacturer of histamine advises avoid concomitant use

  Atovaquone: manufacturer of histamine advises avoid concomitant use with atovaquone

  Clonidine: manufacturer of histamine advises avoid concomitant use with clonidine

  Corticosteroids: manufacturer of histamine advises avoid concomitant use with corticosteroids

  Ulcer-healing Drugs: effects of histamine theoretically antagonised by histamine $H_2$-antagonists—manufacturer of histamine advises avoid concomitant use

### Histamine $H_2$-antagonists

- Alpha-blockers: cimetidine and ranitidine antagonise effects of ●tolazoline

  Analgesics: cimetidine inhibits metabolism of opioid analgesics (increased plasma concentration)

- Anti-arrhythmics: cimetidine increases plasma concentration of amiodarone and ●propafenone; cimetidine inhibits metabolism of flecainide (increased plasma concentration); cimetidine increases plasma concentration of ●lidocaine (increased risk of toxicity)

  Antibacterials: histamine $H_2$-antagonists reduce absorption of cefpodoxime; cimetidine increases plasma concentration of erythromycin (increased risk of toxicity, including deafness); cimetidine inhibits metabolism of metronidazole (increased plasma concentration); metabolism of cimetidine accelerated by rifampicin (reduced plasma concentration)

- Anticoagulants: cimetidine inhibits metabolism of ●coumarins (enhanced anticoagulant effect)

  Antidepressants: cimetidine increases plasma concentration of citalopram, escitalopram, mirtazapine and sertraline; cimetidine inhibits metabolism of amitriptyline, doxepin, imipramine and nortriptyline (increased plasma concentration); cimetidine increases plasma concentration of moclobemide (halve dose of moclobemide); cimetidine possibly increases plasma concentration of tricyclics

  Antidiabetics: cimetidine reduces excretion of metformin (increased plasma concentration); cimetidine enhances hypoglycaemic effect of sulfonylureas

- Antiepileptics: cimetidine inhibits metabolism of ●carbamazepine, ●phenytoin and ●valproate (increased plasma concentration)

- Antifungals: histamine $H_2$-antagonists reduce absorption of itraconazole and ketoconazole; avoidance of histamine $H_2$-antagonists advised by manufacturer of posaconazole (plasma concentration of posaconazole possibly reduced); cimetidine reduces plasma concentration of ●posaconazole; cimetidine increases plasma concentration of terbinafine

  Antihistamines: manufacturer of loratadine advises cimetidine possibly increases plasma concentration of loratadine

- Antimalarials: avoidance of cimetidine advised by manufacturer of ●artemether with lumefantrine; cimetidine inhibits metabolism of chloroquine and hydroxychloroquine and quinine (increased plasma concentration)

  Antipsychotics: cimetidine possibly enhances effects of antipsychotics, chlorpromazine and clozapine

- Antivirals: histamine $H_2$-antagonists reduce plasma concentration of ●atazanavir; famotidine increases plasma concentration of raltegravir; avoidance of histamine $H_2$-antagonists for 12 hours before or 4 hours after rilpivirine advised by manufacturer of rilpivirine—consult product literature; cimetidine possibly increases plasma concentration of saquinavir

  Anxiolytics and Hypnotics: cimetidine inhibits metabolism of benzodiazepines, clomethiazole and

## Histamine H$_2$-antagonists

Anxiolytics and Hypnotics *(continued)*
zaleplon (increased plasma concentration); cimetidine increases plasma concentration of melatonin

Beta-blockers: cimetidine increases plasma concentration of labetalol, metoprolol and propranolol

Calcium-channel Blockers: cimetidine possibly inhibits metabolism of calcium-channel blockers (increased plasma concentration); cimetidine increases plasma concentration of isradipine (halve dose of isradipine)

- Ciclosporin: cimetidine possibly increases plasma concentration of ●ciclosporin
- Clopidogrel: cimetidine possibly reduces antiplatelet effect of ●clopidogrel
- Cytotoxics: cimetidine possibly enhances myelosuppressive effects of carmustine and lomustine; cimetidine increases plasma concentration of ●epirubicin; cimetidine inhibits metabolism of fluorouracil (increased plasma concentration); famotidine possibly reduces plasma concentration of dasatinib; avoidance of cimetidine, famotidine and nizatidine advised by manufacturer of ●erlotinib; ranitidine reduces plasma concentration of ●erlotinib—manufacturer of erlotinib advises give at least 2 hours before or 10 hours after ranitidine; ranitidine reduces plasma concentration of ●gefitinib; histamine H$_2$-antagonists possibly reduce absorption of lapatinib; histamine H$_2$-antagonists possibly reduce absorption of pazopanib—manufacturer of pazopanib advises give at least 2 hours before or 10 hours after histamine H$_2$-antagonists

Dopaminergics: cimetidine reduces excretion of pramipexole (increased plasma concentration)

- Ergot Alkaloids: increased risk of ergotism when cimetidine given with ●ergotamine and methysergide—avoid concomitant use
- Fampridine: avoidance of cimetidine advised by manufacturer of ●fampridine

Histamine: histamine H$_2$-antagonists theoretically antagonise effects of histamine—manufacturer of histamine advises avoid concomitant use

Hormone Antagonists: absorption of cimetidine possibly delayed by octreotide

5HT$_1$-receptor Agonists: cimetidine inhibits metabolism of zolmitriptan (reduce dose of zolmitriptan)

Mebendazole: cimetidine possibly inhibits metabolism of mebendazole (increased plasma concentration)

Roflumilast: cimetidine inhibits the metabolism of roflumilast

Sildenafil: cimetidine increases plasma concentration of sildenafil (consider reducing dose of sildenafil)

- Theophylline: cimetidine inhibits metabolism of ●theophylline (increased plasma concentration)

Thyroid Hormones: cimetidine reduces absorption of levothyroxine

- Uliprista: avoidance of histamine H$_2$-antagonists advised by manufacturer of *high-dose* ●ulipristal (contraceptive effect of ulipristal possibly reduced)

**Homatropine** *see* Antimuscarinics

**Hormone Antagonists** *see* Abiraterone Acetate, Bicalutamide, Danazol, Dutasteride, Exemestane, Flutamide, Lanreotide, Octreotide, Pasireotide, Tamoxifen, and Toremifene

## 5HT$_1$-receptor Agonists

- Antibacterials: plasma concentration of eletriptan increased by ●clarithromycin and ●erythromycin (risk of toxicity)—avoid concomitant use; metabolism of zolmitriptan possibly inhibited by quinolones (reduce dose of zolmitriptan)
- Antidepressants: increased risk of CNS toxicity when 5HT$_1$ agonists given with ●citalopram (manufacturer of citalopram advises avoid concomitant use); increased risk of CNS toxicity when sumatriptan given with ●citalopram, ●escitalopram, ●fluoxetine, ●fluvoxamine or ●paroxetine; metabolism of frova-

## 5HT$_1$-receptor Agonists

- Antidepressants *(continued)*
triptan inhibited by fluvoxamine; metabolism of zolmitriptan possibly inhibited by fluvoxamine (reduce dose of zolmitriptan); CNS toxicity reported when sumatriptan given with sertraline; possible increased serotonergic effects when 5HT$_1$ agonists given with duloxetine or venlafaxine; risk of CNS toxicity when rizatriptan or sumatriptan given with ●MAOIs (avoid rizatriptan or sumatriptan for 2 weeks after MAOIs); increased risk of CNS toxicity when zolmitriptan given with ●MAOIs; risk of CNS toxicity when rizatriptan or sumatriptan given with ●moclobemide (avoid rizatriptan or sumatriptan for 2 weeks after moclobemide); risk of CNS toxicity when zolmitriptan given with ●moclobemide (reduce dose of zolmitriptan); possible increased serotonergic effects when naratriptan given with SSRIs; increased serotonergic effects when 5HT$_1$ agonists given with ●St John's wort—avoid concomitant use
- Antifungals: plasma concentration of eletriptan increased by ●itraconazole and ●ketoconazole (risk of toxicity)—avoid concomitant use; plasma concentration of almotriptan increased by ketoconazole (increased risk of toxicity)
- Antivirals: plasma concentration of eletriptan increased by ●indinavir and ●ritonavir (risk of toxicity)—avoid concomitant use

Beta-blockers: plasma concentration of rizatriptan increased by propranolol (manufacturer of rizatriptan advises halve dose and avoid within 2 hours of propranolol)

Dopaminergics: avoidance of 5HT$_1$ agonists advised by manufacturer of selegiline

- Ergot Alkaloids: increased risk of vasospasm when eletriptan, frovatriptan or naratriptan given with ●ergotamine and methysergide (avoid ergotamine and methysergide 24 hours after eletriptan, frovatriptan or naratriptan, avoid eletriptan, frovatriptan or naratriptan for 24 hours after ergotamine and methysergide); increased risk of vasospasm when almotriptan, rizatriptan, sumatriptan or zolmitriptan given with ●ergotamine and methysergide (avoid ergotamine and methysergide for 6 hours after almotriptan, rizatriptan, sumatriptan or zolmitriptan, avoid almotriptan, rizatriptan, sumatriptan or zolmitriptan for 24 hours after ergotamine and methysergide)

Lithium: possible risk of toxicity when sumatriptan given with lithium

Ulcer-healing Drugs: metabolism of zolmitriptan inhibited by cimetidine (reduce dose of zolmitriptan)

## 5HT$_3$-receptor Antagonists

Analgesics: ondansetron possibly antagonises effects of tramadol

Antibacterials: metabolism of ondansetron accelerated by rifampicin (reduced effect)

Antiepileptics: metabolism of ondansetron accelerated by carbamazepine and phenytoin (reduced effect)

- Cytotoxics: increased risk of ventricular arrhythmias when ondansetron given with ●vandetanib—avoid concomitant use
- Dopaminergics: possible increased hypotensive effect when ondansetron given with ●apomorphine—avoid concomitant use

**Hydralazine** *see* Vasodilator Antihypertensives

**Hydrochlorothiazide** *see* Diuretics

**Hydrocortisone** *see* Corticosteroids

**Hydroflumethiazide** *see* Diuretics

**Hydromorphone** *see* Opioid Analgesics

**Hydrotalcite** *see* Antacids

**Hydroxocobalamin**

Antibacterials: response to hydroxocobalamin reduced by chloramphenicol

## Hydroxycarbamide
- Antipsychotics: avoid concomitant use of cytotoxics with •clozapine (increased risk of agranulocytosis)
- Antivirals: increased risk of toxicity when hydroxycarbamide given with •didanosine and •stavudine—avoid concomitant use

**Hydroxychloroquine** see Chloroquine and Hydroxychloroquine

**Hydroxyzine** see Antihistamines

**Hyoscine** see Antimuscarinics

**Ibandronic Acid** see Bisphosphonates

**Ibuprofen** see NSAIDs

## Idarubicin
- Antipsychotics: avoid concomitant use of cytotoxics with •clozapine (increased risk of agranulocytosis)
- Ciclosporin: plasma concentration of idarubicin increased by •ciclosporin

## Ifosfamide
- Anticoagulants: ifosfamide possibly enhances anticoagulant effect of •coumarins
- Antipsychotics: avoid concomitant use of cytotoxics with •clozapine (increased risk of agranulocytosis)
  Cytotoxics: increased risk of otoxicity when ifosfamide given with cisplatin

## Iloprost
Analgesics: increased risk of bleeding when iloprost given with NSAIDs or aspirin
Anticoagulants: iloprost possibly enhances anticoagulant effect of coumarins and heparins; increased risk of bleeding when iloprost given with phenindione
Clopidogrel: increased risk of bleeding when iloprost given with clopidogrel
Eptifibatide: increased risk of bleeding when iloprost given with eptifibatide
Tirofiban: increased risk of bleeding when iloprost given with tirofiban

## Imatinib
Analgesics: manufacturer of imatinib advises caution with paracetamol
- Antibacterials: plasma concentration of imatinib reduced by •rifampicin—avoid concomitant use
  Anticoagulants: manufacturer of imatinib advises replacement of warfarin with a heparin (possibility of enhanced warfarin effect)
- Antidepressants: plasma concentration of imatinib reduced by •St John's wort—avoid concomitant use
- Antiepileptics: plasma concentration of imatinib reduced by •carbamazepine, •oxcarbazepine and •phenytoin—avoid concomitant use
  Antifungals: plasma concentration of imatinib increased by ketoconazole
- Antipsychotics: avoid concomitant use of cytotoxics with •clozapine (increased risk of agranulocytosis)
- Antivirals: avoidance of imatinib advised by manufacturer of •boceprevir
  Ciclosporin: imatinib possibly increases plasma concentration of ciclosporin
  Lipid-regulating Drugs: imatinib increases plasma concentration of simvastatin
  Tacrolimus: imatinib increases plasma concentration of tacrolimus
  Thyroid Hormones: imatinib possibly reduces plasma concentration of levothyroxine

**Imidapril** see ACE Inhibitors

## Imipenem with Cilastatin
- Antiepileptics: carbapenems reduce plasma concentration of •valproate—avoid concomitant use
- Antivirals: increased risk of convulsions when imipenem with cilastatin given with •ganciclovir
  Vaccines: antibacterials inactivate oral typhoid vaccine—see p. 621

**Imipramine** see Antidepressants, Tricyclic

## Immunoglobulins
Note For advice on immunoglobulins and live virus vaccines, see under Normal Immunoglobulin, p. 623

**Indacaterol** see Sympathomimetics, Beta$_2$

**Indapamide** see Diuretics

## Indinavir
Aldesleukin: plasma concentration of indinavir possibly increased by aldesleukin
- Anti-arrhythmics: indinavir possibly increases plasma concentration of •amiodarone—avoid concomitant use; indinavir possibly increases plasma concentration of •flecainide (increased risk of ventricular arrhythmias—avoid concomitant use)
- Antibacterials: indinavir increases plasma concentration of •rifabutin—avoid concomitant use; metabolism of indinavir accelerated by •rifampicin (reduced plasma concentration—avoid concomitant use); avoidance of concomitant indinavir in severe renal and hepatic impairment advised by manufacturer of •telithromycin
  Anticoagulants: avoidance of indinavir advised by manufacturer of apixaban and rivaroxaban
- Antidepressants: plasma concentration of indinavir reduced by •St John's wort—avoid concomitant use
- Antiepileptics: plasma concentration of indinavir possibly reduced by •carbamazepine and •phenytoin, also plasma concentration of carbamazepine and phenytoin possibly increased; plasma concentration of indinavir possibly reduced by •phenobarbital
- Antifungals: plasma concentration of indinavir increased by •itraconazole and •ketoconazole (consider reducing dose of indinavir)
- Antimalarials: caution with indinavir advised by manufacturer of artemether with lumefantrine; indinavir possibly increases plasma concentration of •quinine (increased risk of toxicity)
  Antimuscarinics: avoidance of indinavir advised by manufacturer of darifenacin and tolterodine; manufacturer of fesoterodine advises dose reduction when indinavir given with fesoterodine—consult fesoterodine product literature
- Antipsychotics: indinavir possibly inhibits metabolism of •aripiprazole (reduce dose of aripiprazole); indinavir possibly increases plasma concentration of •pimozide (increased risk of ventricular arrhythmias—avoid concomitant use); indinavir possibly increases plasma concentration of •quetiapine—manufacturer of quetiapine advises avoid concomitant use
- Antivirals: avoid concomitant use of indinavir with •atazanavir; plasma concentration of both drugs increased when indinavir given with darunavir; plasma concentration of indinavir reduced by efavirenz and nevirapine; plasma concentration of indinavir possibly reduced by •etravirine—avoid concomitant use; indinavir increases plasma concentration of •maraviroc (consider reducing dose of maraviroc); plasma concentration of indinavir increased by ritonavir; indinavir increases plasma concentration of saquinavir
- Anxiolytics and Hypnotics: increased risk of prolonged sedation when indinavir given with •alprazolam—avoid concomitant use; indinavir possibly increases plasma concentration of •midazolam (risk of prolonged sedation—avoid concomitant use of *oral* midazolam)
  Atovaquone: plasma concentration of indinavir possibly reduced by atovaquone
- Ciclosporin: indinavir increases plasma concentration of •ciclosporin
- Colchicine: indinavir possibly increases risk of •colchicine toxicity—suspend or reduce dose of colchicine (avoid concomitant use in hepatic or renal impairment)

**Indinavir** *(continued)*

Corticosteroids: plasma concentration of indinavir possibly reduced by dexamethasone

- Cytotoxics: indinavir possibly increases plasma concentration of axitinib (reduce dose of axitinib—consult axitinib product literature); indinavir possibly increases plasma concentration of •crizotinib and •everolimus—manufacturer of crizotinib and everolimus advises avoid concomitant use; avoidance of indinavir advised by manufacturer of •cabazitaxel and •pazopanib; manufacturer of ruxolitinib advises dose reduction when indinavir given with •ruxolitinib—consult ruxolitinib product literature

- Ergot Alkaloids: increased risk of ergotism when indinavir given with •ergotamine and methysergide—avoid concomitant use

- 5HT$_1$-receptor Agonists: indinavir increases plasma concentration of •eletriptan (risk of toxicity)—avoid concomitant use

- Lipid-regulating Drugs: possible increased risk of myopathy when indinavir given with atorvastatin; possible increased risk of myopathy when indinavir given with •rosuvastatin—manufacturer of rosuvastatin advises avoid concomitant use; increased risk of myopathy when indinavir given with •simvastatin (avoid concomitant use)

- Ranolazine: indinavir possibly increases plasma concentration of •ranolazine—manufacturer of ranolazine advises avoid concomitant use

- Sildenafil: indinavir increases plasma concentration of •sildenafil—reduce initial dose of sildenafil

Tadalafil: indinavir possibly increases plasma concentration of tadalafil

- Vardenafil: indinavir increases plasma concentration of •vardenafil—avoid concomitant use

**Indometacin** *see* NSAIDs

**Indoramin** *see* Alpha-blockers

**Infliximab**

- Abatacept: avoid concomitant use of infliximab with •abatacept

- Anakinra: avoid concomitant use of infliximab with •anakinra

- Vaccines: avoid concomitant use of infliximab with live •vaccines (see p. 600)

**Influenza Vaccine** *see* Vaccines

**Insulin** *see* Antidiabetics

**Interferon Alfa** *see* Interferons

**Interferon Gamma** *see* Interferons

**Interferons**

Note Peginterferon alfa interactions as for interferon alfa

- Antivirals: caution with peginterferon alfa advised by manufacturer of adefovir; increased risk of peripheral neuropathy when interferon alfa given with •telbivudine

- Theophylline: interferon alfa inhibits metabolism of •theophylline (consider reducing dose of theophylline)

Vaccines: manufacturer of interferon gamma advises avoid concomitant use with vaccines

**Ipratropium** *see* Antimuscarinics

**Irbesartan** *see* Angiotensin-II Receptor Antagonists

**Irinotecan**

- Antidepressants: metabolism of irinotecan accelerated by •St John's wort (reduced plasma concentration—avoid concomitant use)

Antiepileptics: plasma concentration of irinotecan and its active metabolite reduced by carbamazepine, phenobarbital and phenytoin

- Antifungals: plasma concentration of irinotecan reduced by •ketoconazole (but concentration of active metabolite of irinotecan increased)—avoid concomitant use

- Antipsychotics: avoid concomitant use of cytotoxics with •clozapine (increased risk of agranulocytosis)

**Irinotecan** *(continued)*

- Antivirals: metabolism of irinotecan possibly inhibited by •atazanavir (increased risk of toxicity)

- Cytotoxics: plasma concentration of active metabolite of irinotecan increased by •lapatinib—consider reducing dose of irinotecan; plasma concentration of irinotecan possibly increased by sorafenib

**Iron**

Antacids: absorption of *oral* iron reduced by oral magnesium salts (as magnesium trisilicate)

Antibacterials: *oral* iron reduces absorption of ciprofloxacin, levofloxacin, moxifloxacin and ofloxacin; *oral* iron reduces absorption of norfloxacin (give at least 2 hours apart); *oral* iron reduces absorption of tetracyclines, also absorption of *oral* iron reduced by tetracyclines

Bisphosphonates: *oral* iron reduces absorption of bisphosphonates

Calcium Salts: absorption of *oral* iron reduced by calcium salts

Dopaminergics: *oral* iron reduces absorption of entacapone; *oral* iron possibly reduces absorption of levodopa

Eltrombopag: *oral* iron possibly reduces absorption of eltrombopag (give at least 4 hours apart)

Methyldopa: *oral* iron antagonises hypotensive effect of methyldopa

Mycophenolate: *oral* iron reduces absorption of mycophenolate

Penicillamine: *oral* iron reduces absorption of penicillamine

Thyroid Hormones: *oral* iron reduces absorption of levothyroxine (give at least 2 hours apart)

Trientine: absorption of *oral* iron reduced by trientine

Zinc: *oral* iron reduces absorption of zinc, also absorption of *oral* iron reduced by zinc

**Isocarboxazid** *see* MAOIs

**Isoflurane** *see* Anaesthetics, General

**Isometheptene** *see* Sympathomimetics

**Isoniazid**

Antacids: absorption of isoniazid reduced by antacids

- Antibacterials: increased risk of hepatotoxicity when isoniazid given with •rifampicin; increased risk of CNS toxicity when isoniazid given with cycloserine

- Antiepileptics: isoniazid increases plasma concentration of •carbamazepine (also possibly increased isoniazid hepatotoxicity); isoniazid inhibits metabolism of •ethosuximide (increased plasma concentration and risk of toxicity); isoniazid possibly inhibits metabolism of phenytoin (increased risk of toxicity)

Antifungals: isoniazid possibly reduces plasma concentration of ketoconazole

Anxiolytics and Hypnotics: isoniazid inhibits the metabolism of diazepam

Corticosteroids: plasma concentration of isoniazid possibly reduced by corticosteroids

Disulfiram: isoniazid possibly increases CNS effects of disulfiram

Dopaminergics: isoniazid possibly reduces effects of levodopa

Theophylline: isoniazid possibly increases plasma concentration of theophylline

Vaccines: antibacterials inactivate oral typhoid vaccine—see p. 621

**Isosorbide Dinitrate** *see* Nitrates

**Isosorbide Mononitrate** *see* Nitrates

**Isotretinoin** *see* Retinoids

**Isradipine** *see* Calcium-channel Blockers

**Itraconazole** *see* Antifungals, Triazole

**Ivabradine**

- Anti-arrhythmics: increased risk of ventricular arrhythmias when ivabradine given with •amiodarone or •disopyramide

- Antibacterials: plasma concentration of ivabradine possibly increased by •clarithromycin and •telithro-

## Ivabradine

- Antibacterials *(continued)*
  mycin—avoid concomitant use; increased risk of
  ventricular arrhythmias when ivabradine given with
  ●erythromycin—avoid concomitant use
  Antidepressants: plasma concentration of ivabradine
  reduced by St John's wort—avoid concomitant use
- Antifungals: plasma concentration of ivabradine
  increased by ●ketoconazole—avoid concomitant
  use; plasma concentration of ivabradine increased
  by fluconazole—reduce initial dose of ivabradine;
  plasma concentration of ivabradine possibly
  increased by ●itraconazole—avoid concomitant use
- Antimalarials: increased risk of ventricular arrhythmias when ivabradine given with ●mefloquine
- Antipsychotics: increased risk of ventricular arrhythmias when ivabradine given with ●pimozide
- Antivirals: plasma concentration of ivabradine possibly
  increased by ●ritonavir—avoid concomitant use
- Beta-blockers: increased risk of ventricular arrhythmias when ivabradine given with ●sotalol
- Calcium-channel Blockers: plasma concentration of
  ivabradine increased by ●diltiazem and ●verap-
  amil—avoid concomitant use
  Grapefruit Juice: plasma concentration of ivabradine
  increased by grapefruit juice
- Pentamidine Isetionate: increased risk of ventricular
  arrhythmias when ivabradine given with ●pent-
  amidine isetionate

## Kaolin

  Analgesics: kaolin possibly reduces absorption of
  aspirin
  Antibacterials: kaolin possibly reduces absorption of
  tetracyclines
  Antimalarials: kaolin reduces absorption of chloroquine and hydroxychloroquine
  Antipsychotics: kaolin possibly reduces absorption of
  phenothiazines

**Ketamine** *see* Anaesthetics, General
**Ketoconazole** *see* Antifungals, Imidazole
**Ketoprofen** *see* NSAIDs
**Ketorolac** *see* NSAIDs
**Ketotifen** *see* Antihistamines
**Labetalol** *see* Beta-blockers
**Lacidipine** *see* Calcium-channel Blockers

## Lacosamide

- Antidepressants: anticonvulsant effect of antiepileptics
  possibly antagonised by MAOIs and ●tricyclic-
  related antidepressants (convulsive threshold lowered); anticonvulsant effect of antiepileptics antagonised by ●SSRIs and ●tricyclics (convulsive threshold lowered); avoid concomitant use of
  antiepileptics with ●St John's wort
- Antimalarials: anticonvulsant effect of antiepileptics
  antagonised by ●mefloquine
- Antipsychotics: anticonvulsant effect of antiepileptics
  antagonised by ●antipsychotics (convulsive threshold lowered)
- Orlistat: possible increased risk of convulsions when
  antiepileptics given with ●orlistat

## Lactulose

  Anticoagulants: lactulose possibly enhances anticoagulant effect of coumarins

## Lamivudine

  Antibacterials: plasma concentration of lamivudine
  increased by trimethoprim (as co-trimoxazole)—
  avoid concomitant use of high-dose co-trimoxazole
  Antivirals: avoidance of lamivudine advised by manufacturer of emtricitabine

## Lamotrigine

- Antibacterials: plasma concentration of lamotrigine
  reduced by ●rifampicin
- Antidepressants: anticonvulsant effect of antiepileptics
  possibly antagonised by MAOIs and ●tricyclic-
  related antidepressants (convulsive threshold low-

## Lamotrigine

- Antidepressants *(continued)*
  ered); anticonvulsant effect of antiepileptics antagonised by ●SSRIs and ●tricyclics (convulsive threshold lowered); avoid concomitant use of antiepileptics with ●St John's wort
- Antiepileptics: plasma concentration of lamotrigine
  often reduced by carbamazepine, also plasma concentration of an active metabolite of carbamazepine
  sometimes raised (but evidence is conflicting);
  plasma concentration of lamotrigine reduced by
  phenobarbital and phenytoin; plasma concentration
  of lamotrigine increased by ●valproate (increased
  risk of toxicity—reduce lamotrigine dose)
- Antimalarials: anticonvulsant effect of antiepileptics
  antagonised by ●mefloquine
- Antipsychotics: anticonvulsant effect of antiepileptics
  antagonised by ●antipsychotics (convulsive threshold lowered)
  Antivirals: plasma concentration of lamotrigine possibly reduced by ritonavir
- Oestrogens: plasma concentration of lamotrigine
  reduced by ●oestrogens—consider increasing dose
  of lamotrigine
- Orlistat: possible increased risk of convulsions when
  antiepileptics given with ●orlistat
  Progestogens: plasma concentration of lamotrigine
  possibly increased by desogestrel

## Lanreotide

  Antidiabetics: lanreotide possibly reduces requirements for insulin, metformin, repaglinide and sulfonylureas
  Ciclosporin: lanreotide reduces plasma concentration
  of ciclosporin

**Lansoprazole** *see* Proton Pump Inhibitors

## Lanthanum

  Antibacterials: lanthanum possibly reduces absorption
  of quinolones (give at least 2 hours before or 4
  hours after lanthanum)
  Antifungals: lanthanum possibly reduces absorption of
  ketoconazole (give at least 2 hours apart)
  Antimalarials: lanthanum possibly reduces absorption
  of chloroquine and hydroxychloroquine (give at
  least 2 hours apart)
  Thyroid Hormones: lanthanum reduces absorption of
  levothyroxine (give at least 2 hours apart)

## Lapatinib

- Antibacterials: manufacturer of lapatinib advises avoid
  concomitant use with ●rifabutin, ●rifampicin and
  ●telithromycin
- Antidepressants: manufacturer of lapatinib advises
  avoid concomitant use with ●St John's wort
- Antidiabetics: manufacturer of lapatinib advises avoid
  concomitant use with ●repaglinide
- Antiepileptics: plasma concentration of lapatinib
  reduced by ●carbamazepine—avoid concomitant
  use; manufacturer of lapatinib advises avoid concomitant use with ●phenytoin
- Antifungals: plasma concentration of lapatinib
  increased by ●ketoconazole—avoid concomitant
  use; manufacturer of lapatinib advises avoid concomitant use with ●itraconazole, ●posaconazole and
  ●voriconazole
- Antipsychotics: avoid concomitant use of cytotoxics
  with ●clozapine (increased risk of agranulocytosis);
  manufacturer of lapatinib advises avoid concomitant use with ●pimozide
- Antivirals: avoidance of lapatinib advised by manufacturer of ●boceprevir; manufacturer of lapatinib
  advises avoid concomitant use with ●ritonavir and
  ●saquinavir
- Cytotoxics: lapatinib increases plasma concentration
  of pazopanib; possible increased risk of neutropenia
  when lapatinib given with docetaxel; increased risk
  of neutropenia when lapatinib given with ●paclitax-
  el; lapatinib increases plasma concentration of

## Lapatinib

- Cytotoxics *(continued)*
  active metabolite of ●irinotecan—consider reducing dose of irinotecan
- Grapefruit Juice: manufacturer of lapatinib advises avoid concomitant use with ●grapefruit juice
  Ulcer-healing Drugs: absorption of lapatinib possibly reduced by histamine $H_2$-antagonists and proton pump inhibitors

## Laronidase

Antimalarials: effects of laronidase possibly inhibited by chloroquine and hydroxychloroquine (manufacturer of laronidase advises avoid concomitant use)

## Leflunomide

**Note** Increased risk of toxicity with other haematotoxic and hepatotoxic drugs

Antibacterials: plasma concentration of active metabolite of leflunomide possibly increased by rifampicin

Anticoagulants: leflunomide possibly enhances anticoagulant effect of warfarin

Antidiabetics: leflunomide possibly enhances hypoglycaemic effect of tolbutamide

Antiepileptics: leflunomide possibly increases plasma concentration of phenytoin

- Cytotoxics: risk of toxicity when leflunomide given with ●methotrexate
  Lipid-regulating Drugs: the effect of leflunomide is significantly decreased by colestyramine (enhanced elimination)—avoid unless drug elimination desired
- Vaccines: avoid concomitant use of leflunomide with live ●vaccines (see p. 600)

## Lenalidomide

- Antibacterials: plasma concentration of lenalidomide possibly increased by ●clarithromycin (increased risk of toxicity)
- Antifungals: plasma concentration of lenalidomide possibly increased by ●itraconazole and ●ketoconazole (increased risk of toxicity)
- Calcium-channel Blockers: plasma concentration of lenalidomide possibly increased by ●verapamil (increased risk of toxicity)
  Cardiac Glycosides: lenalidomide possibly increases plasma concentration of digoxin
- Ciclosporin: plasma concentration of lenalidomide possibly increased by ●ciclosporin (increased risk of toxicity)

## Lercanidipine *see* Calcium-channel Blockers

## Leukotriene Receptor Antagonists

Analgesics: plasma concentration of zafirlukast increased by aspirin

Antibacterials: plasma concentration of zafirlukast reduced by erythromycin

Anticoagulants: zafirlukast enhances anticoagulant effect of warfarin

Antiepileptics: plasma concentration of montelukast reduced by phenobarbital

Lipid-regulating Drugs: plasma concentration of montelukast increased by gemfibrozil

Theophylline: zafirlukast possibly increases plasma concentration of theophylline, also plasma concentration of zafirlukast reduced

## Levamisole

Alcohol: possibility of disulfiram-like reaction when levamisole given with alcohol

- Anticoagulants: levamisole possibly enhances anticoagulant effect of ●warfarin
  Antiepileptics: levamisole possibly increases plasma concentration of phenytoin

## Levetiracetam

- Antidepressants: anticonvulsant effect of antiepileptics possibly antagonised by MAOIs and ●tricyclic-related antidepressants (convulsive threshold lowered); anticonvulsant effect of antiepileptics antagonised by ●SSRIs and ●tricyclics (convulsive thresh-

## Levetiracetam

- Antidepressants *(continued)*
  old lowered); avoid concomitant use of antiepileptics with ●St John's wort
  Antiepileptics: levetiracetam possibly increases risk of carbamazepine toxicity
- Antimalarials: anticonvulsant effect of antiepileptics antagonised by ●mefloquine
- Antipsychotics: anticonvulsant effect of antiepileptics antagonised by ●antipsychotics (convulsive threshold lowered)
- Orlistat: possible increased risk of convulsions when antiepileptics given with ●orlistat

## Levobunolol *see* Beta-blockers

## Levobupivacaine

Anti-arrhythmics: increased myocardial depression when levobupivacaine given with anti-arrhythmics

## Levocetirizine *see* Antihistamines

## Levodopa

ACE Inhibitors: enhanced hypotensive effect when levodopa given with ACE inhibitors

Adrenergic Neurone Blockers: enhanced hypotensive effect when levodopa given with adrenergic neurone blockers

Alpha-blockers: enhanced hypotensive effect when levodopa given with alpha-blockers

- Anaesthetics, General: increased risk of arrhythmias when levodopa given with ●volatile liquid general anaesthetics

Angiotensin-II Receptor Antagonists: enhanced hypotensive effect when levodopa given with angiotensin-II receptor antagonists

Antibacterials: effects of levodopa possibly reduced by isoniazid

- Antidepressants: risk of hypertensive crisis when levodopa given with ●MAOIs, avoid levodopa for at least 2 weeks after stopping MAOIs; increased risk of side-effects when levodopa given with moclobemide

Antiepileptics: effects of levodopa possibly reduced by phenytoin

Antimuscarinics: absorption of levodopa possibly reduced by antimuscarinics

Antipsychotics: effects of levodopa antagonised by antipsychotics; avoidance of levodopa advised by manufacturer of amisulpride (antagonism of effect)

Anxiolytics and Hypnotics: effects of levodopa possibly antagonised by benzodiazepines

Beta-blockers: enhanced hypotensive effect when levodopa given with beta-blockers

Bupropion: increased risk of side-effects when levodopa given with bupropion

Calcium-channel Blockers: enhanced hypotensive effect when levodopa given with calcium-channel blockers

Clonidine: enhanced hypotensive effect when levodopa given with clonidine

Diazoxide: enhanced hypotensive effect when levodopa given with diazoxide

Diuretics: enhanced hypotensive effect when levodopa given with diuretics

Dopaminergics: enhanced effects and increased toxicity of levodopa when given with selegiline (reduce dose of levodopa)

Iron: absorption of levodopa possibly reduced by *oral* iron

Memantine: effects of dopaminergics possibly enhanced by memantine

Methyldopa: enhanced hypotensive effect when levodopa given with methyldopa; antiparkinsonian effect of dopaminergics antagonised by methyldopa

Moxonidine: enhanced hypotensive effect when levodopa given with moxonidine

Muscle Relaxants: possible agitation, confusion and hallucinations when levodopa given with baclofen

**Levodopa** *(continued)*
Nitrates: enhanced hypotensive effect when levodopa given with nitrates
Vasodilator Antihypertensives: enhanced hypotensive effect when levodopa given with hydralazine, minoxidil or sodium nitroprusside
Vitamins: effects of levodopa reduced by pyridoxine when given without dopa-decarboxylase inhibitor

**Levofloxacin** *see* Quinolones

**Levofolinic Acid** *see* Folates

**Levomepromazine** *see* Antipsychotics

**Levonorgestrel** *see* Progestogens

**Levothyroxine** *see* Thyroid Hormones

**Lidocaine**
**Note** Interactions less likely when lidocaine used topically
Anaesthetics, Local: increased myocardial depression when anti-arrhythmics given with bupivacaine, levobupivacaine, prilocaine or ropivacaine
● Anti-arrhythmics: increased myocardial depression when anti-arrhythmics given with other ●anti-arrhythmics
● Antipsychotics: increased risk of ventricular arrhythmias when anti-arrhythmics that prolong the QT interval given with ●antipsychotics that prolong the QT interval
● Antivirals: plasma concentration of lidocaine possibly increased by ●atazanavir and lopinavir; plasma concentration of lidocaine possibly increased by darunavir and ●fosamprenavir—avoid concomitant use; increased risk of ventricular arrhythmias when lidocaine given with ●saquinavir—avoid concomitant use; caution with *intravenous* lidocaine advised by manufacturer of telaprevir
● Beta-blockers: increased myocardial depression when anti-arrhythmics given with ●beta-blockers; increased risk of lidocaine toxicity when given with ●propranolol
● Diuretics: action of lidocaine antagonised by hypokalaemia caused by ●acetazolamide, ●loop diuretics or ●thiazides and related diuretics
Muscle Relaxants: neuromuscular blockade enhanced and prolonged when lidocaine given with suxamethonium
● Ulcer-healing Drugs: plasma concentration of lidocaine increased by ●cimetidine (increased risk of toxicity)

**Linagliptin** *see* Antidiabetics

**Linezolid**
**Note** Linezolid is a reversible, non-selective MAO inhibitor—see interactions of MAOIs
Antibacterials: plasma concentration of linezolid reduced by rifampicin (possible therapeutic failure of linezolid)
Vaccines: antibacterials inactivate oral typhoid vaccine—see p. 621

**Liothyronine** *see* Thyroid Hormones

**Lipid-regulating Drugs** *see* Colesevelam, Colestipol, Colestyramine, Ezetimibe, Fibrates, Nicotinic Acid, and Statins

**Liraglutide** *see* Antidiabetics

**Lisdexamfetamine** *see* Sympathomimetics

**Lisinopril** *see* ACE Inhibitors

**Lithium**
● ACE Inhibitors: excretion of lithium reduced by ●ACE inhibitors (increased plasma concentration)
● Analgesics: excretion of lithium reduced by ●NSAIDs (increased risk of toxicity); excretion of lithium reduced by ●ketorolac (increased risk of toxicity)—avoid concomitant use
● Angiotensin-II Receptor Antagonists: excretion of lithium reduced by ●angiotensin-II receptor antagonists (increased plasma concentration)
Antacids: excretion of lithium increased by sodium bicarbonate (reduced plasma concentration)

**Lithium** *(continued)*
● Anti-arrhythmics: avoidance of lithium advised by manufacturer of ●amiodarone (risk of ventricular arrhythmias)
Antibacterials: increased risk of lithium toxicity when given with metronidazole
● Antidepressants: possible increased serotonergic effects when lithium given with venlafaxine; increased risk of CNS effects when lithium given with ●SSRIs (lithium toxicity reported); risk of toxicity when lithium given with tricyclics
Antiepileptics: neurotoxicity may occur when lithium given with carbamazepine or phenytoin without increased plasma concentration of lithium; plasma concentration of lithium possibly affected by topiramate
Antipsychotics: increased risk of extrapyramidal side-effects and possibly neurotoxicity when lithium given with clozapine, flupentixol, haloperidol, phenothiazines or zuclopenthixol; possible risk of toxicity when lithium given with olanzapine; increased risk of extrapyramidal side-effects when lithium given with sulpiride
Anxiolytics and Hypnotics: increased risk of neurotoxicity when lithium given with clonazepam
Calcium-channel Blockers: neurotoxicity may occur when lithium given with diltiazem or verapamil without increased plasma concentration of lithium
● Cytotoxics: increased risk of ventricular arrhythmias when lithium given with ●arsenic trioxide
● Diuretics: excretion of lithium increased by ●acetazolamide; excretion of lithium reduced by ●loop diuretics and ●thiazides and related diuretics (increased plasma concentration and risk of toxicity)—loop diuretics safer than thiazides; excretion of lithium reduced by ●potassium-sparing diuretics and aldosterone antagonists (increased plasma concentration and risk of toxicity)
$5HT_1$-receptor Agonists: possible risk of toxicity when lithium given with sumatriptan
● Methyldopa: neurotoxicity may occur when lithium given with ●methyldopa without increased plasma concentration of lithium
Muscle Relaxants: lithium enhances effects of muscle relaxants; hyperkinesis caused by lithium possibly aggravated by baclofen
Parasympathomimetics: lithium antagonises effects of neostigmine
Theophylline: excretion of lithium increased by theophylline (reduced plasma concentration)

**Lofepramine** *see* Antidepressants, Tricyclic

**Lofexidine**
Alcohol: increased sedative effect when lofexidine given with alcohol
Anxiolytics and Hypnotics: increased sedative effect when lofexidine given with anxiolytics and hypnotics

**Lomustine**
● Antipsychotics: avoid concomitant use of cytotoxics with ●clozapine (increased risk of agranulocytosis)
Ulcer-healing Drugs: myelosuppressive effects of lomustine possibly enhanced by cimetidine

**Loperamide**
Desmopressin: loperamide increases plasma concentration of oral desmopressin

**Lopinavir**
**Note** In combination with ritonavir as *Kaletra*® (ritonavir is present to inhibit lopinavir metabolism and increase plasma-lopinavir concentration)—see also Ritonavir
● Anti-arrhythmics: lopinavir possibly increases plasma concentration of ●flecainide (increased risk of ventricular arrhythmias—avoid concomitant use); lopinavir possibly increases plasma concentration of lidocaine
● Antibacterials: plasma concentration of lopinavir reduced by ●rifampicin—avoid concomitant use;

**Lopinavir**

- Antibacterials *(continued)*
  avoidance of concomitant lopinavir in severe renal and hepatic impairment advised by manufacturer of ●telithromycin

  Anticoagulants: avoidance of lopinavir advised by manufacturer of apixaban; manufacturers advise avoid concomitant use of lopinavir with rivaroxaban

- Antidepressants: plasma concentration of lopinavir reduced by ●St John's wort—avoid concomitant use

- Antiepileptics: plasma concentration of lopinavir possibly reduced by carbamazepine, ●phenobarbital and phenytoin

  Antihistamines: lopinavir possibly increases plasma concentration of chlorphenamine

  Antimalarials: caution with lopinavir advised by manufacturer of artemether with lumefantrine

  Antimuscarinics: avoidance of lopinavir advised by manufacturer of darifenacin and tolterodine

- Antipsychotics: lopinavir possibly inhibits metabolism of ●aripiprazole (reduce dose of aripiprazole); lopinavir possibly increases plasma concentration of ●quetiapine—manufacturer of quetiapine advises avoid concomitant use

- Antivirals: manufacturers advise avoid concomitant use of lopinavir with ●boceprevir and ●telaprevir; lopinavir reduces plasma concentration of ●darunavir, also plasma concentration of lopinavir increased (avoid concomitant use); plasma concentration of lopinavir reduced by ●efavirenz—consider increasing dose of lopinavir; lopinavir reduces plasma concentration of fosamprenavir, effect on lopinavir plasma concentration not predictable—avoid concomitant use; lopinavir increases plasma concentration of ●maraviroc (consider reducing dose of maraviroc); plasma concentration of lopinavir possibly reduced by ●nevirapine—consider increasing dose of lopinavir; increased risk of ventricular arrhythmias when lopinavir given with ●saquinavir—avoid concomitant use; lopinavir increases plasma concentration of tenofovir; plasma concentration of lopinavir reduced by ●tipranavir

  Corticosteroids: plasma concentration of lopinavir possibly reduced by dexamethasone

- Cytotoxics: manufacturer of ruxolitinib advises dose reduction when lopinavir given with ●ruxolitinib—consult ruxolitinib product literature

  Eltrombopag: lopinavir possibly reduces plasma concentration of eltrombopag

- Lipid-regulating Drugs: possible increased risk of myopathy when lopinavir given with atorvastatin; possible increased risk of myopathy when lopinavir given with ●rosuvastatin—manufacturer of rosuvastatin advises avoid concomitant use; possible increased risk of myopathy when lopinavir given with ●simvastatin—avoid concomitant use

- Ranolazine: lopinavir possibly increases plasma concentration of ●ranolazine—manufacturer of ranolazine advises avoid concomitant use

  Sirolimus: lopinavir possibly increases plasma concentration of sirolimus

  Sympathomimetics, Beta$_2$: manufacturer of lopinavir advises avoid concomitant use with salmeterol

**Loprazolam** *see* Anxiolytics and Hypnotics

**Loratadine** *see* Antihistamines

**Lorazepam** *see* Anxiolytics and Hypnotics

**Lormetazepam** *see* Anxiolytics and Hypnotics

**Losartan** *see* Angiotensin-II Receptor Antagonists

**Lumefantrine** *see* Artemether with Lumefantrine

**Lymecycline** *see* Tetracyclines

**Macrolides**

  Note *See also* Telithromycin

**Macrolides** *(continued)*

  Note Interactions do not apply to small amounts of erythromycin used topically

  Analgesics: erythromycin increases plasma concentration of alfentanil

  Antacids: absorption of azithromycin reduced by antacids

- Anti-arrhythmics: increased risk of ventricular arrhythmias when *parenteral* erythromycin given with ●amiodarone—avoid concomitant use; erythromycin increases plasma concentration of ●disopyramide (increased risk of toxicity); azithromycin and clarithromycin possibly increase plasma concentration of ●disopyramide (increased risk of toxicity); avoidance of clarithromycin advised by manufacturer of ●dronedarone (risk of ventricular arrhythmias); erythromycin increases plasma concentration of ●dronedarone (increased risk of ventricular arrhythmias—avoid concomitant use)

- Antibacterials: increased risk of ventricular arrhythmias when *parenteral* erythromycin given with ●moxifloxacin—avoid concomitant use; increased risk of side-effects including neutropenia when azithromycin given with ●rifabutin; clarithromycin increases plasma concentration of ●rifabutin (increased risk of toxicity—reduce rifabutin dose); erythromycin possibly increases plasma concentration of ●rifabutin (increased risk of toxicity—reduce rifabutin dose); plasma concentration of clarithromycin reduced by rifamycins

- Anticoagulants: clarithromycin and erythromycin enhance anticoagulant effect of ●coumarins; azithromycin possibly enhances anticoagulant effect of ●coumarins

- Antidepressants: avoidance of macrolides advised by manufacturer of ●reboxetine; clarithromycin possibly increases plasma concentration of trazodone

  Antidiabetics: clarithromycin enhances effects of repaglinide

- Antiepileptics: clarithromycin and erythromycin increase plasma concentration of ●carbamazepine; clarithromycin inhibits metabolism of phenytoin (increased plasma concentration); erythromycin possibly inhibits metabolism of valproate (increased plasma concentration)

  Antifungals: avoidance of erythromycin advised by manufacturer of fluconazole; clarithromycin increases plasma concentration of itraconazole

- Antihistamines: manufacturer of loratadine advises erythromycin possibly increases plasma concentration of loratadine; macrolides possibly inhibit metabolism of ●mizolastine (avoid concomitant use); erythromycin inhibits metabolism of ●mizolastine—avoid concomitant use; erythromycin increases plasma concentration of rupatadine

- Antimalarials: avoidance of macrolides advised by manufacturer of ●piperaquine with artenimol (possible risk of ventricular arrhythmias); avoidance of macrolides advised by manufacturer of ●artemether with lumefantrine

  Antimuscarinics: erythromycin possibly increases plasma concentration of darifenacin; manufacturer of fesoterodine advises dose reduction when clarithromycin given with fesoterodine—consult fesoterodine product literature; avoidance of clarithromycin and erythromycin advised by manufacturer of tolterodine

- Antipsychotics: avoidance of macrolides advised by manufacturer of ●droperidol (risk of ventricular arrhythmias); increased risk of ventricular arrhythmias when *parenteral* erythromycin given with ●zuclopenthixol—avoid concomitant use; increased risk of ventricular arrhythmias when erythromycin given with ●amisulpride—avoid concomitant use; erythromycin possibly increases plasma concentration of ●clozapine (possible increased risk of con-

## Macrolides

- Antipsychotics *(continued)*
vulsions); increased risk of ventricular arrhythmias when clarithromycin given with ●pimozide—avoid concomitant use; possible increased risk of ventricular arrhythmias when erythromycin given with ●pimozide—avoid concomitant use; clarithromycin possibly increases plasma concentration of ●quetiapine—manufacturer of quetiapine advises avoid concomitant use; erythromycin increases plasma concentration of ●quetiapine—manufacturer of quetiapine advises avoid concomitant use; increased risk of ventricular arrhythmias when *parenteral* erythromycin given with ●sulpiride

- Antivirals: plasma concentration of both drugs increased when clarithromycin given with atazanavir; increased risk of rash when clarithromycin given with efavirenz; clarithromycin increases plasma concentration of ●etravirine, also plasma concentration of clarithromycin reduced; clarithromycin possibly increases plasma concentration of ●maraviroc (consider reducing dose of maraviroc); plasma concentration of clarithromycin reduced by nevirapine (but concentration of an active metabolite increased), also plasma concentration of nevirapine increased; avoidance of clarithromycin and erythromycin advised by manufacturer of ●rilpivirine (plasma concentration of rilpivirine possibly increased); plasma concentration of azithromycin and erythromycin possibly increased by ritonavir; plasma concentration of clarithromycin increased by ●ritonavir (reduce dose of clarithromycin in renal impairment); increased risk of ventricular arrhythmias when clarithromycin or erythromycin given with ●saquinavir—avoid concomitant use; plasma concentration of both drugs possibly increased when clarithromycin and erythromycin given with ●telaprevir (increased risk of ventricular arrhythmias); plasma concentration of clarithromycin increased by ●tipranavir (reduce dose of clarithromycin in renal impairment), also clarithromycin increases plasma concentration of tipranavir; clarithromycin tablets reduce absorption of zidovudine (give at least 2 hours apart)

- Anxiolytics and Hypnotics: clarithromycin and erythromycin inhibit metabolism of ●midazolam (increased plasma concentration with increased sedation); erythromycin increases plasma concentration of buspirone (reduce dose of buspirone); erythromycin inhibits the metabolism of zopiclone

  Aprepitant: clarithromycin possibly increases plasma concentration of aprepitant

- Atomoxetine: increased risk of ventricular arrhythmias when *parenteral* erythromycin given with ●atomoxetine

- Calcium-channel Blockers: clarithromycin and erythromycin possibly inhibit metabolism of ●calcium-channel blockers (increased risk of side-effects); avoidance of erythromycin advised by manufacturer of lercanidipine

  Cardiac Glycosides: macrolides increase plasma concentration of digoxin (increased risk of toxicity)

- Ciclosporin: macrolides possibly inhibit metabolism of ●ciclosporin (increased plasma concentration); clarithromycin and erythromycin inhibit metabolism of ●ciclosporin (increased plasma concentration)

  Cilostazol: erythromycin increases plasma concentration of cilostazol (consider reducing dose of cilostazol)

- Clopidogrel: erythromycin possibly reduces antiplatelet effect of ●clopidogrel

- Colchicine: azithromycin, clarithromycin and erythromycin possibly increase risk of ●colchicine toxicity—suspend or reduce dose of colchicine (avoid concomitant use in hepatic or renal impairment)

## Macrolides *(continued)*

  Corticosteroids: erythromycin possibly inhibits metabolism of corticosteroids; erythromycin inhibits the metabolism of methylprednisolone; clarithromycin possibly increases plasma concentration of methylprednisolone

- Cytotoxics: clarithromycin and erythromycin possibly increase plasma concentration of axitinib (reduce dose of axitinib—consult axitinib product literature); clarithromycin possibly increases plasma concentration of ●crizotinib and ●everolimus—manufacturer of crizotinib and everolimus advises avoid concomitant use; erythromycin increases plasma concentration of ●everolimus; avoidance of clarithromycin advised by manufacturer of ●cabazitaxel, ●nilotinib and ●pazopanib; manufacturer of ruxolitinib advises dose reduction when clarithromycin given with ●ruxolitinib—consult ruxolitinib product literature; possible increased risk of ventricular arrhythmias when *parenteral* erythromycin given with ●vandetanib—avoid concomitant use; *in vitro* studies suggest a possible interaction between erythromycin and docetaxel (consult docetaxel product literature); increased risk of ventricular arrhythmias when erythromycin given with ●arsenic trioxide; erythromycin increases toxicity of ●vinblastine—avoid concomitant use; possible increased risk of neutropenia when clarithromycin given with ●vinorelbine

- Diuretics: clarithromycin increases plasma concentration of ●eplerenone—avoid concomitant use; erythromycin increases plasma concentration of eplerenone (reduce dose of eplerenone)

- Domperidone: possible increased risk of ventricular arrhythmias when erythromycin given with ●domperidone

  Dopaminergics: erythromycin increases plasma concentration of bromocriptine and cabergoline (increased risk of toxicity); macrolides possibly increase plasma concentration of bromocriptine and cabergoline (increased risk of toxicity)

- Ergot Alkaloids: increased risk of ergotism when macrolides given with ●ergotamine and methysergide—avoid concomitant use

  Fidaxomicin: avoidance of clarithromycin and erythromycin advised by manufacturer of fidaxomicin

- 5HT$_1$-receptor Agonists: clarithromycin and erythromycin increase plasma concentration of ●eletriptan (risk of toxicity)—avoid concomitant use

- Ivabradine: clarithromycin possibly increases plasma concentration of ●ivabradine—avoid concomitant use; increased risk of ventricular arrhythmias when erythromycin given with ●ivabradine—avoid concomitant use

- Lenalidomide: clarithromycin possibly increases plasma concentration of ●lenalidomide (increased risk of toxicity)

  Leukotriene Receptor Antagonists: erythromycin reduces plasma concentration of zafirlukast

- Lipid-regulating Drugs: clarithromycin increases plasma concentration of ●atorvastatin and pravastatin; possible increased risk of myopathy when erythromycin given with atorvastatin; erythromycin increases plasma concentration of pravastatin; erythromycin reduces plasma concentration of rosuvastatin; increased risk of myopathy when clarithromycin or erythromycin given with ●simvastatin (avoid concomitant use)

  Mirabegron: when given with clarithromycin avoid or reduce dose of mirabegron in hepatic or renal impairment—see Mirabegron, BNF section 7.4.2

  Oestrogens: erythromycin increases plasma concentration of estradiol

  Parasympathomimetics: erythromycin increases plasma concentration of galantamine

## Macrolides (continued)

- Pentamidine Isetionate: increased risk of ventricular arrhythmias when *parenteral* erythromycin given with •pentamidine isetionate

  Progestogens: erythromycin increases plasma concentration of dienogest

- Ranolazine: clarithromycin possibly increases plasma concentration of •ranolazine—manufacturer of ranolazine advises avoid concomitant use

  Sildenafil: clarithromycin possibly increases plasma concentration of sildenafil—reduce initial dose of sildenafil; erythromycin increases plasma concentration of sildenafil—reduce initial dose of sildenafil

- Sirolimus: clarithromycin increases plasma concentration of •sirolimus—avoid concomitant use; plasma concentration of both drugs increased when erythromycin given with •sirolimus

- Tacrolimus: clarithromycin and erythromycin increase plasma concentration of •tacrolimus

  Tadalafil: clarithromycin and erythromycin possibly increase plasma concentration of tadalafil

- Theophylline: clarithromycin possibly increases plasma concentration of theophylline; erythromycin increases plasma concentration of •theophylline (also theophylline may reduce absorption of *oral* erythromycin)

- Ticagrelor: clarithromycin possibly increases plasma concentration of •ticagrelor—manufacturer of ticagrelor advises avoid concomitant use; erythromycin possibly increases plasma concentration of ticagrelor

  Ulcer-healing Drugs: plasma concentration of erythromycin increased by cimetidine (increased risk of toxicity, including deafness); plasma concentration of both drugs increased when clarithromycin given with omeprazole

  Vaccines: antibacterials inactivate oral typhoid vaccine—see p. 621

  Vardenafil: erythromycin increases plasma concentration of vardenafil (reduce dose of vardenafil)

## Magnesium (parenteral)

- Calcium-channel Blockers: profound hypotension reported with concomitant use of parenteral magnesium and •nifedipine in pre-eclampsia

  Muscle Relaxants: parenteral magnesium enhances effects of non-depolarising muscle relaxants and suxamethonium

## Magnesium Salts (oral) *see* Antacids

## Mannitol

  Ciclosporin: possible increased risk of nephrotoxicity when mannitol given with ciclosporin

## MAOIs

  Note For interactions of reversible MAO-A inhibitors (RIMAs) see Moclobemide, and for interactions of MAO-B inhibitors see Rasagiline and Selegiline; the antibacterial Linezolid is a reversible, non-selective MAO inhibitor

  ACE Inhibitors: MAOIs possibly enhance hypotensive effect of ACE inhibitors

  Adrenergic Neurone Blockers: enhanced hypotensive effect when MAOIs given with adrenergic neurone blockers

- Alcohol: MAOIs interact with tyramine found in some beverages containing •alcohol and some dealcoholised beverages (hypertensive crisis)—if no tyramine, enhanced hypotensive effect

  Alpha₂-adrenoceptor Stimulants: avoidance of MAOIs advised by manufacturer of apraclonidine and brimonidine

- Alpha-blockers: avoidance of MAOIs advised by manufacturer of •indoramin; enhanced hypotensive effect when MAOIs given with alpha-blockers

- Analgesics: CNS excitation or depression (hypertension or hypotension) when MAOIs given with •pethidine—avoid concomitant use and for 2 weeks after stopping MAOIs; possible increased serotonergic effects and increased risk of convulsions when

## MAOIs

- Analgesics (continued)

  MAOIs given with •tramadol—some manufacturers advise avoid concomitant use and for 2 weeks after stopping MAOIs; avoidance of MAOIs advised by manufacturer of •nefopam; possible CNS excitation or depression (hypertension or hypotension) when MAOIs given with •opioid analgesics—some manufacturers advise avoid concomitant use and for 2 weeks after stopping MAOIs

  Angiotensin-II Receptor Antagonists: MAOIs possibly enhance hypotensive effect of angiotensin-II receptor antagonists

- Antidepressants: increased risk of hypertension and CNS excitation when MAOIs given with •reboxetine (MAOIs should not be started until 1 week after stopping reboxetine, avoid reboxetine for 2 weeks after stopping MAOIs); after stopping MAOIs do not start •citalopram, •escitalopram, •fluvoxamine, •paroxetine or •sertraline for 2 weeks, also MAOIs should not be started until at least 1 week after stopping citalopram, escitalopram, fluvoxamine, paroxetine or sertraline; after stopping MAOIs do not start •fluoxetine for 2 weeks, also MAOIs should not be started until at least 5 weeks after stopping fluoxetine; after stopping MAOIs do not start •duloxetine for 2 weeks, also MAOIs should not be started until at least 5 days after stopping duloxetine; enhanced CNS effects and toxicity when MAOIs given with •venlafaxine (venlafaxine should not be started until 2 weeks after stopping MAOIs, avoid MAOIs for 1 week after stopping venlafaxine); increased risk of hypertension and CNS excitation when MAOIs given with other •MAOIs (avoid for at least 2 weeks after stopping previous MAOIs and then start at a reduced dose); after stopping MAOIs do not start •moclobemide for at least 1 week; MAOIs increase CNS effects of •SSRIs (risk of serious toxicity); after stopping MAOIs do not start •mirtazapine for 2 weeks, also MAOIs should not be started until at least 2 weeks after stopping mirtazapine; after stopping MAOIs do not start •tricyclic-related antidepressants for 2 weeks, also MAOIs should not be started until at least 1–2 weeks after stopping tricyclic-related antidepressants; increased risk of hypertension and CNS excitation when MAOIs given with •tricyclics, tricyclics should not be started until 2 weeks after stopping MAOIs (3 weeks if starting clomipramine or imipramine), also MAOIs should not be started for at least 1–2 weeks after stopping tricyclics (3 weeks in the case of clomipramine or imipramine); CNS excitation and confusion when MAOIs given with •tryptophan (reduce dose of tryptophan)

  Antidiabetics: MAOIs possibly enhance hypoglycaemic effect of antidiabetics; MAOIs enhance hypoglycaemic effect of insulin, metformin and sulfonylureas

- Antiepileptics: MAOIs possibly antagonise anticonvulsant effect of antiepileptics (convulsive threshold lowered); avoidance for 2 weeks after stopping MAOIs advised by manufacturer of •carbamazepine, also antagonism of anticonvulsant effect

  Antihistamines: avoidance of promethazine for 2 weeks after stopping MAOIs advised by manufacturer of promethazine; increased antimuscarinic and sedative effects when MAOIs given with antihistamines

- Antimalarials: avoidance of antidepressants advised by manufacturer of •artemether with lumefantrine and •piperaquine with artenimol

  Antimuscarinics: increased risk of antimuscarinic side-effects when MAOIs given with antimuscarinics

**MAOIs** *(continued)*
- Antipsychotics: CNS effects of MAOIs possibly increased by ●clozapine

Anxiolytics and Hypnotics: manufacturer of tranylcypromine advises avoid buspirone for 10 days after stopping tranylcypromine; avoidance of MAOIs advised by manufacturer of buspirone
- Atomoxetine: after stopping MAOIs do not start ●atomoxetine for 2 weeks, also MAOIs should not be started until at least 2 weeks after stopping atomoxetine; possible increased risk of convulsions when antidepressants given with atomoxetine

Beta-blockers: enhanced hypotensive effect when MAOIs given with beta-blockers
- Bupropion: avoidance of bupropion for 2 weeks after stopping MAOIs advised by manufacturer of ●bupropion

Calcium-channel Blockers: enhanced hypotensive effect when MAOIs given with calcium-channel blockers

Clonidine: enhanced hypotensive effect when MAOIs given with clonidine

Diazoxide: enhanced hypotensive effect when MAOIs given with diazoxide

Diuretics: enhanced hypotensive effect when MAOIs given with diuretics
- Dopaminergics: avoid concomitant use of non-selective MAOIs with ●entacapone; risk of hypertensive crisis when MAOIs given with ●levodopa, avoid levodopa for at least 2 weeks after stopping MAOIs; risk of hypertensive crisis when MAOIs given with ●rasagiline, avoid MAOIs for at least 2 weeks after stopping rasagiline; enhanced hypotensive effect when MAOIs given with ●selegiline—manufacturer of selegiline advises avoid concomitant use; avoid concomitant use of MAOIs with tolcapone

Doxapram: MAOIs enhance effects of doxapram

Histamine: avoidance of MAOIs advised by manufacturer of histamine
- 5HT₁-receptor Agonists: risk of CNS toxicity when MAOIs given with ●rizatriptan or ●sumatriptan (avoid rizatriptan or sumatriptan for 2 weeks after MAOIs); increased risk of CNS toxicity when MAOIs given with ●zolmitriptan
- Methyldopa: avoidance of MAOIs advised by manufacturer of ●methyldopa

Moxonidine: enhanced hypotensive effect when MAOIs given with moxonidine

Muscle Relaxants: phenelzine enhances effects of suxamethonium

Nicorandil: enhanced hypotensive effect when MAOIs given with nicorandil

Nitrates: enhanced hypotensive effect when MAOIs given with nitrates

Pholcodine: avoidance of pholcodine for 2 weeks after stopping MAOIs advised by manufacturer of pholcodine
- Sympathomimetics: risk of hypertensive crisis when MAOIs given with ●sympathomimetics; risk of hypertensive crisis when MAOIs given with ●methylphenidate, some manufacturers advise avoid methylphenidate for at least 2 weeks after stopping MAOIs
- Tetrabenazine: risk of CNS toxicity when MAOIs given with ●tetrabenazine (avoid tetrabenazine for 2 weeks after MAOIs)

Vasodilator Antihypertensives: enhanced hypotensive effect when MAOIs given with hydralazine, minoxidil or sodium nitroprusside

**MAOIs, reversible** *see* Moclobemide
**Maraviroc**
- Antibacterials: plasma concentration of maraviroc possibly increased by ●clarithromycin and ●telithromycin (consider reducing dose of maraviroc); plasma concentration of maraviroc reduced by ●rifampicin—consider increasing dose of maraviroc

**Maraviroc** *(continued)*
- Antidepressants: plasma concentration of maraviroc possibly reduced by ●St John's wort—avoid concomitant use
- Antifungals: plasma concentration of maraviroc increased by ●ketoconazole (consider reducing dose of maraviroc)
- Antivirals: plasma concentration of maraviroc increased by ●atazanavir, ●darunavir, ●indinavir, ●lopinavir and ●saquinavir (consider reducing dose of maraviroc); plasma concentration of maraviroc possibly reduced by ●efavirenz—consider increasing dose of maraviroc; plasma concentration of maraviroc possibly reduced by etravirine; maraviroc reduces plasma concentration of ●fosamprenavir—avoid concomitant use; plasma concentration of maraviroc increased by ritonavir

**Mebendazole**
Ulcer-healing Drugs: metabolism of mebendazole possibly inhibited by cimetidine (increased plasma concentration)

**Medroxyprogesterone** *see* Progestogens
**Mefenamic Acid** *see* NSAIDs
**Mefloquine**
- Anti-arrhythmics: increased risk of ventricular arrhythmias when mefloquine given with ●amiodarone—avoid concomitant use
- Antibacterials: increased risk of ventricular arrhythmias when mefloquine given with ●moxifloxacin—avoid concomitant use; plasma concentration of mefloquine reduced by ●rifampicin—avoid concomitant use
- Antiepileptics: mefloquine antagonises anticonvulsant effect of ●antiepileptics

Antifungals: plasma concentration of mefloquine increased by ketoconazole
- Antimalarials: avoidance of antimalarials advised by manufacturer of ●artemether with lumefantrine; increased risk of convulsions when mefloquine given with ●chloroquine and hydroxychloroquine; increased risk of convulsions when mefloquine given with ●quinine (but should not prevent the use of *intravenous* quinine in severe cases)
- Antipsychotics: possible increased risk of ventricular arrhythmias when mefloquine given with ●haloperidol—avoid concomitant use; increased risk of ventricular arrhythmias when mefloquine given with ●pimozide—avoid concomitant use
- Atomoxetine: increased risk of ventricular arrhythmias when mefloquine given with ●atomoxetine

Beta-blockers: increased risk of bradycardia when mefloquine given with beta-blockers

Calcium-channel Blockers: possible increased risk of bradycardia when mefloquine given with calcium-channel blockers

Cardiac Glycosides: possible increased risk of bradycardia when mefloquine given with digoxin

Cytotoxics: possible increased risk of bradycardia when mefloquine given with crizotinib

Histamine: avoidance of antimalarials advised by manufacturer of histamine
- Ivabradine: increased risk of ventricular arrhythmias when mefloquine given with ●ivabradine

Vaccines: antimalarials inactivate oral typhoid vaccine—see p. 621

**Megestrol** *see* Progestogens
**Melatonin** *see* Anxiolytics and Hypnotics
**Meloxicam** *see* NSAIDs
**Melphalan**
Antibacterials: increased risk of melphalan toxicity when given with nalidixic acid
- Antipsychotics: avoid concomitant use of cytotoxics with ●clozapine (increased risk of agranulocytosis)

Cardiac Glycosides: melphalan possibly reduces absorption of digoxin *tablets*

**Melphalan** *(continued)*
- Ciclosporin: increased risk of nephrotoxicity when melphalan given with ●ciclosporin

**Memantine**
- Anaesthetics, General: increased risk of CNS toxicity when memantine given with ●ketamine (manufacturer of memantine advises avoid concomitant use)
- Analgesics: increased risk of CNS toxicity when memantine given with ●dextromethorphan (manufacturer of memantine advises avoid concomitant use)

Anticoagulants: memantine possibly enhances anticoagulant effect of warfarin

Antimuscarinics: memantine possibly enhances effects of antimuscarinics

Antipsychotics: memantine possibly reduces effects of antipsychotics
- Dopaminergics: memantine possibly enhances effects of dopaminergics and selegiline; increased risk of CNS toxicity when memantine given with ●amantadine (manufacturer of memantine advises avoid concomitant use)

Muscle Relaxants: memantine possibly modifies effects of baclofen and dantrolene

**Mepacrine**
Antimalarials: mepacrine increases plasma concentration of primaquine (increased risk of toxicity)

**Meprobamate** *see* Anxiolytics and Hypnotics

**Meptazinol** *see* Opioid Analgesics

**Mercaptopurine**
- Allopurinol: enhanced effects and increased toxicity of mercaptopurine when given with ●allopurinol (reduce dose of mercaptopurine to one quarter of usual dose)

Aminosalicylates: possible increased risk of leucopenia when mercaptopurine given with aminosalicylates
- Antibacterials: increased risk of haematological toxicity when mercaptopurine given with ●sulfamethoxazole (as co-trimoxazole); increased risk of haematological toxicity when mercaptopurine given with ●trimethoprim (also with co-trimoxazole)
- Anticoagulants: mercaptopurine possibly reduces anticoagulant effect of ●coumarins
- Antipsychotics: avoid concomitant use of cytotoxics with ●clozapine (increased risk of agranulocytosis)

Dairy Products: plasma concentration of mercaptopurine possibly reduced by dairy products—manufacturer of mercaptopurine advises give at least 1 hour before or 2 hours after dairy products
- Febuxostat: avoidance of mercaptopurine advised by manufacturer of ●febuxostat

**Meropenem**
- Antiepileptics: carbapenems reduce plasma concentration of ●valproate—avoid concomitant use

Probenecid: excretion of meropenem reduced by probenecid

Vaccines: antibacterials inactivate oral typhoid vaccine—see p. 621

**Mesalazine** *see* Aminosalicylates

**Mestranol** *see* Oestrogens

**Metaraminol** *see* Sympathomimetics

**Metformin** *see* Antidiabetics

**Methadone** *see* Opioid Analgesics

**Methenamine**
Antacids: avoid concomitant use of methenamine with antacids
- Antibacterials: increased risk of crystalluria when methenamine given with ●sulfonamides
- Diuretics: effects of methenamine antagonised by ●acetazolamide

Potassium Salts: avoid concomitant use of methenamine with potassium citrate

Sodium Citrate: avoid concomitant use of methenamine with sodium citrate

**Methenamine** *(continued)*
Vaccines: antibacterials inactivate oral typhoid vaccine—see p. 621

**Methocarbamol** *see* Muscle Relaxants

**Methotrexate**
- Anaesthetics, General: antifolate effect of methotrexate increased by ●nitrous oxide—avoid concomitant use
- Analgesics: excretion of methotrexate probably reduced by ●NSAIDs (increased risk of toxicity); excretion of methotrexate reduced by ●aspirin, ●diclofenac, ●ibuprofen, ●indometacin, ●ketoprofen, ●meloxicam and ●naproxen (increased risk of toxicity)
- Antibacterials: absorption of methotrexate possibly reduced by neomycin; excretion of methotrexate possibly reduced by ciprofloxacin (increased risk of toxicity); increased risk of haematological toxicity when methotrexate given with ●sulfamethoxazole (as co-trimoxazole); increased risk of methotrexate toxicity when given with doxycycline, sulfonamides or tetracycline; excretion of methotrexate reduced by penicillins (increased risk of toxicity); increased risk of haematological toxicity when methotrexate given with ●trimethoprim (also with co-trimoxazole)

Antiepileptics: antifolate effect of methotrexate increased by phenytoin
- Antimalarials: antifolate effect of methotrexate increased by ●pyrimethamine
- Antipsychotics: avoid concomitant use of cytotoxics with ●clozapine (increased risk of agranulocytosis)

Cardiac Glycosides: methotrexate possibly reduces absorption of digoxin *tablets*
- Ciclosporin: risk of toxicity when methotrexate given with ●ciclosporin
- Cytotoxics: increased pulmonary toxicity when methotrexate given with ●cisplatin

Diuretics: excretion of methotrexate increased by alkaline urine due to acetazolamide
- Leflunomide: risk of toxicity when methotrexate given with ●leflunomide
- Probenecid: excretion of methotrexate reduced by ●probenecid (increased risk of toxicity)
- Retinoids: plasma concentration of methotrexate increased by ●acitretin (also increased risk of hepatotoxicity)—avoid concomitant use

Theophylline: methotrexate possibly increases plasma concentration of theophylline

Ulcer-healing Drugs: excretion of methotrexate possibly reduced by proton pump inhibitors (increased risk of toxicity)

**Methoxamine** *see* Sympathomimetics

**Methyldopa**
ACE Inhibitors: enhanced hypotensive effect when methyldopa given with ACE inhibitors

Adrenergic Neurone Blockers: enhanced hypotensive effect when methyldopa given with adrenergic neurone blockers

Alcohol: enhanced hypotensive effect when methyldopa given with alcohol

Aldesleukin: enhanced hypotensive effect when methyldopa given with aldesleukin

Alpha-blockers: enhanced hypotensive effect when methyldopa given with alpha-blockers

Anaesthetics, General: enhanced hypotensive effect when methyldopa given with general anaesthetics

Analgesics: hypotensive effect of methyldopa antagonised by NSAIDs

Angiotensin-II Receptor Antagonists: enhanced hypotensive effect when methyldopa given with angiotensin-II receptor antagonists
- Antidepressants: manufacturer of methyldopa advises avoid concomitant use with ●MAOIs

Antipsychotics: enhanced hypotensive effect when methyldopa given with antipsychotics (also increased risk of extrapyramidal effects)

**Methyldopa** *(continued)*

Anxiolytics and Hypnotics: enhanced hypotensive effect when methyldopa given with anxiolytics and hypnotics

Beta-blockers: enhanced hypotensive effect when methyldopa given with beta-blockers

Calcium-channel Blockers: enhanced hypotensive effect when methyldopa given with calcium-channel blockers

Clonidine: enhanced hypotensive effect when methyldopa given with clonidine

Corticosteroids: hypotensive effect of methyldopa antagonised by corticosteroids

Diazoxide: enhanced hypotensive effect when methyldopa given with diazoxide

Diuretics: enhanced hypotensive effect when methyldopa given with diuretics

Dopaminergics: methyldopa antagonises antiparkinsonian effect of dopaminergics; increased risk of extrapyramidal side-effects when methyldopa given with amantadine; effects of methyldopa possibly enhanced by entacapone; enhanced hypotensive effect when methyldopa given with levodopa

Iron: hypotensive effect of methyldopa antagonised by *oral* iron

• Lithium: neurotoxicity may occur when methyldopa given with ●lithium without increased plasma concentration of lithium

Moxisylyte: enhanced hypotensive effect when methyldopa given with moxisylyte

Moxonidine: enhanced hypotensive effect when methyldopa given with moxonidine

Muscle Relaxants: enhanced hypotensive effect when methyldopa given with baclofen or tizanidine

Nitrates: enhanced hypotensive effect when methyldopa given with nitrates

Oestrogens: hypotensive effect of methyldopa antagonised by oestrogens

Prostaglandins: enhanced hypotensive effect when methyldopa given with alprostadil

• Sympathomimetics, Beta₂: acute hypotension reported when methyldopa given with *infusion of* ●salbutamol

Vasodilator Antihypertensives: enhanced hypotensive effect when methyldopa given with hydralazine, minoxidil or sodium nitroprusside

**Methylphenidate** *see* Sympathomimetics

**Methylprednisolone** *see* Corticosteroids

**Methylthioninium**

• Antidepressants: risk of CNS toxicity when methylthioninium given with ●SSRI-related antidepressants, ●SSRIs and ●clomipramine—avoid concomitant use (if avoidance not possible, use lowest possible dose of methylthioninium and observe patient for up to 4 hours after administration); possible risk of CNS toxicity when methylthioninium given with ●mirtazapine—avoid concomitant use (if avoidance not possible, use lowest possible dose of methylthioninium and observe patient for up to 4 hours after administration)

• Anxiolytics and Hypnotics: possible risk of CNS toxicity when methylthioninium given with ●buspirone—avoid concomitant use (if avoidance not possible, use lowest possible dose of methylthioninium and observe patient for up to 4 hours after administration)

• Bupropion: possible risk of CNS toxicity when methylthioninium given with ●bupropion—avoid concomitant use (if avoidance not possible, use lowest possible dose of methylthioninium and observe patient for up to 4 hours after administration)

**Methysergide** *see* Ergot Alkaloids

**Metoclopramide**

Alcohol: metoclopramide possibly increases absorption of alcohol

**Metoclopramide** *(continued)*

Anaesthetics, General: metoclopramide enhances effects of thiopental

Analgesics: metoclopramide increases rate of absorption of aspirin (enhanced effect); effects of metoclopramide on gastro-intestinal activity antagonised by opioid analgesics; metoclopramide increases rate of absorption of paracetamol

Antidepressants: CNS toxicity reported when metoclopramide given with SSRIs

Antimuscarinics: effects of metoclopramide on gastro-intestinal activity antagonised by antimuscarinics

Antipsychotics: increased risk of extrapyramidal side-effects when metoclopramide given with antipsychotics

Atovaquone: metoclopramide reduces plasma concentration of atovaquone

• Ciclosporin: metoclopramide increases plasma concentration of ●ciclosporin

Dopaminergics: metoclopramide antagonises hypoprolactinaemic effects of bromocriptine and cabergoline; metoclopramide antagonises antiparkinsonian effect of pergolide; avoidance of metoclopramide advised by manufacturer of ropinirole and rotigotine (antagonism of effect)

Muscle Relaxants: metoclopramide enhances effects of suxamethonium

Tetrabenazine: increased risk of extrapyramidal side-effects when metoclopramide given with tetrabenazine

**Metolazone** *see* Diuretics

**Metoprolol** *see* Beta-blockers

**Metronidazole**

**Note** Interactions do not apply to topical metronidazole preparations

Alcohol: disulfiram-like reaction when metronidazole given with alcohol

• Anticoagulants: metronidazole enhances anticoagulant effect of ●coumarins

Antiepileptics: metabolism of metronidazole accelerated by phenobarbital (reduced effect); metronidazole possibly inhibits metabolism of phenytoin (increased plasma concentration)

• Cytotoxics: metronidazole increases plasma concentration of ●busulfan (increased risk of toxicity); metronidazole inhibits metabolism of fluorouracil (increased toxicity)

Disulfiram: psychotic reaction reported when metronidazole given with disulfiram

Lithium: metronidazole increases risk of lithium toxicity

Mycophenolate: metronidazole possibly reduces bioavailability of mycophenolate

Ulcer-healing Drugs: metabolism of metronidazole inhibited by cimetidine (increased plasma concentration)

Vaccines: antibacterials inactivate oral typhoid vaccine—see p. 621

**Mianserin** *see* Antidepressants, Tricyclic (related)

**Micafungin**

Antifungals: micafungin possibly increases plasma concentration of amphotericin; micafungin increases plasma concentration of itraconazole (consider reducing dose of itraconazole)

Calcium-channel Blockers: micafungin increases plasma concentration of nifedipine

Ciclosporin: micafungin possibly increases plasma concentration of ciclosporin

Sirolimus: micafungin increases plasma concentration of sirolimus

**Miconazole** *see* Antifungals, Imidazole

**Midazolam** *see* Anxiolytics and Hypnotics

**Mifamurtide**

Analgesics: manufacturer of mifamurtide advises avoid concomitant use with high doses of NSAIDs

**Mifamurtide** *(continued)*

Ciclosporin: manufacturer of mifamurtide advises avoid concomitant use with ciclosporin

Corticosteroids: manufacturer of mifamurtide advises avoid concomitant use with corticosteroids

Tacrolimus: manufacturer of mifamurtide advises avoid concomitant use with tacrolimus

**Mifepristone**

Corticosteroids: mifepristone may reduce effect of corticosteroids (including *inhaled* corticosteroids) for 3–4 days

**Milrinone** *see* Phosphodiesterase Inhibitors

**Minocycline** *see* Tetracyclines

**Minoxidil** *see* Vasodilator Antihypertensives

**Mirabegron**

Antibacterials: avoid or reduce dose of mirabegron in hepatic or renal impairment when given with clarithromycin—see Mirabegron, BNF section 7.4.2

Antifungals: avoid or reduce dose of mirabegron in hepatic or renal impairment when given with itraconazole and ketoconazole—see Mirabegron, BNF section 7.4.2

Antivirals: avoid or reduce dose of mirabegron in hepatic or renal impairment when given with ritonavir—see Mirabegron, BNF section 7.4.2

Beta-blockers: mirabegron increases plasma concentration of metoprolol

Cardiac Glycosides: mirabegron increases plasma concentration of digoxin—reduce initial dose of digoxin

**Mirtazapine**

• Alcohol: increased sedative effect when mirtazapine given with •alcohol

Analgesics: possible increased serotonergic effects when mirtazapine given with tramadol

Anticoagulants: mirtazapine enhances anticoagulant effect of warfarin

• Antidepressants: possible increased serotonergic effects when mirtazapine given with fluoxetine, fluvoxamine or venlafaxine; mirtazapine should not be started until 2 weeks after stopping •MAOIs, also MAOIs should not be started until at least 2 weeks after stopping mirtazapine; after stopping mirtazapine do not start •moclobemide for at least 1 week

Antiepileptics: plasma concentration of mirtazapine reduced by carbamazepine and phenytoin

Antifungals: plasma concentration of mirtazapine increased by ketoconazole

• Antimalarials: avoidance of antidepressants advised by manufacturer of •artemether with lumefantrine and •piperaquine with artenimol

Anxiolytics and Hypnotics: increased sedative effect when mirtazapine given with anxiolytics and hypnotics

Atomoxetine: possible increased risk of convulsions when antidepressants given with atomoxetine

Clonidine: mirtazapine possibly antagonises hypotensive effect of clonidine

• Methylthioninium: possible risk of CNS toxicity when mirtazapine given with •methylthioninium—avoid concomitant use (if avoidance not possible, use lowest possible dose of methylthioninium and observe patient for up to 4 hours after administration)

Ulcer-healing Drugs: plasma concentration of mirtazapine increased by cimetidine

**Mitomycin**

• Antipsychotics: avoid concomitant use of cytotoxics with •clozapine (increased risk of agranulocytosis)

**Mitotane**

• Anticoagulants: mitotane possibly reduces anticoagulant effect of •coumarins

• Antipsychotics: avoid concomitant use of cytotoxics with •clozapine (increased risk of agranulocytosis)

Diuretics: manufacturer of mitotane advises avoid concomitant use of spironolactone (antagonism of effect)

**Mitoxantrone**

• Antipsychotics: avoid concomitant use of cytotoxics with •clozapine (increased risk of agranulocytosis)

Ciclosporin: excretion of mitoxantrone reduced by ciclosporin (increased plasma concentration)

**Mivacurium** *see* Muscle Relaxants

**Mizolastine** *see* Antihistamines

**Moclobemide**

• Analgesics: possible CNS excitation or depression (hypertension or hypotension) when moclobemide given with •dextromethorphan or •pethidine—avoid concomitant use; possible CNS excitation or depression (hypertension or hypotension) when moclobemide given with •opioid analgesics—manufacturer of moclobemide advises consider reducing dose of opioid analgesics

• Antidepressants: moclobemide should not be started for at least 1 week after stopping •MAOIs, •SSRI-related antidepressants, •citalopram, •fluvoxamine, •mirtazapine, •paroxetine, •sertraline, •tricyclic-related antidepressants or •tricyclics; increased risk of CNS toxicity when moclobemide given with •escitalopram, preferably avoid concomitant use; moclobemide should not be started until 5 weeks after stopping •fluoxetine; possible increased serotonergic effects when moclobemide given with •duloxetine

• Antimalarials: avoidance of antidepressants advised by manufacturer of •artemether with lumefantrine and •piperaquine with artenimol

Atomoxetine: possible increased risk of convulsions when antidepressants given with atomoxetine

• Bupropion: avoidance of moclobemide advised by manufacturer of •bupropion

• Clopidogrel: moclobemide possibly reduces antiplatelet effect of •clopidogrel

• Dopaminergics: caution with moclobemide advised by manufacturer of entacapone; increased risk of side-effects when moclobemide given with levodopa; avoid concomitant use of moclobemide with •selegiline

• 5HT₁-receptor Agonists: risk of CNS toxicity when moclobemide given with •rizatriptan or •sumatriptan (avoid rizatriptan or sumatriptan for 2 weeks after moclobemide); risk of CNS toxicity when moclobemide given with •zolmitriptan (reduce dose of zolmitriptan)

• Sympathomimetics: risk of hypertensive crisis when moclobemide given with •sympathomimetics

Ulcer-healing Drugs: plasma concentration of moclobemide increased by cimetidine (halve dose of moclobemide)

**Modafinil**

Antiepileptics: modafinil possibly increases plasma concentration of phenytoin

• Ciclosporin: modafinil reduces plasma concentration of •ciclosporin

• Oestrogens: modafinil accelerates metabolism of •oestrogens (reduced contraceptive effect—see p. 398)

**Moexipril** *see* ACE Inhibitors

**Mometasone** *see* Corticosteroids

**Monobactams** *see* Aztreonam

**Montelukast** *see* Leukotriene Receptor Antagonists

**Morphine** *see* Opioid Analgesics

**Moxifloxacin** *see* Quinolones

**Moxisylyte**

ACE Inhibitors: enhanced hypotensive effect when moxisylyte given with ACE inhibitors

Adrenergic Neurone Blockers: enhanced hypotensive effect when moxisylyte given with adrenergic neurone blockers

• Alpha-blockers: possible severe postural hypotension when moxisylyte given with •alpha-blockers

**Moxisylyte** *(continued)*

Angiotensin-II Receptor Antagonists: enhanced hypotensive effect when moxisylyte given with angiotensin-II receptor antagonists

• Beta-blockers: possible severe postural hypotension when moxisylyte given with ●beta-blockers

Calcium-channel Blockers: enhanced hypotensive effect when moxisylyte given with calcium-channel blockers

Clonidine: enhanced hypotensive effect when moxisylyte given with clonidine

Diazoxide: enhanced hypotensive effect when moxisylyte given with diazoxide

Diuretics: enhanced hypotensive effect when moxisylyte given with diuretics

Methyldopa: enhanced hypotensive effect when moxisylyte given with methyldopa

Moxonidine: enhanced hypotensive effect when moxisylyte given with moxonidine

Nitrates: enhanced hypotensive effect when moxisylyte given with nitrates

Vasodilator Antihypertensives: enhanced hypotensive effect when moxisylyte given with hydralazine, minoxidil or sodium nitroprusside

**Moxonidine**

ACE Inhibitors: enhanced hypotensive effect when moxonidine given with ACE inhibitors

Adrenergic Neurone Blockers: enhanced hypotensive effect when moxonidine given with adrenergic neurone blockers

Alcohol: enhanced hypotensive effect when moxonidine given with alcohol

Aldesleukin: enhanced hypotensive effect when moxonidine given with aldesleukin

Alpha-blockers: enhanced hypotensive effect when moxonidine given with alpha-blockers

Anaesthetics, General: enhanced hypotensive effect when moxonidine given with general anaesthetics

Analgesics: hypotensive effect of moxonidine antagonised by NSAIDs

Angiotensin-II Receptor Antagonists: enhanced hypotensive effect when moxonidine given with angiotensin-II receptor antagonists

Antidepressants: enhanced hypotensive effect when moxonidine given with MAOIs; hypotensive effect of moxonidine possibly antagonised by tricyclics (manufacturer of moxonidine advises avoid concomitant use)

Antipsychotics: enhanced hypotensive effect when moxonidine given with phenothiazines

Anxiolytics and Hypnotics: enhanced hypotensive effect when moxonidine given with anxiolytics and hypnotics; sedative effects possibly increased when moxonidine given with benzodiazepines

Beta-blockers: enhanced hypotensive effect when moxonidine given with beta-blockers

Calcium-channel Blockers: enhanced hypotensive effect when moxonidine given with calcium-channel blockers

Clonidine: enhanced hypotensive effect when moxonidine given with clonidine

Corticosteroids: hypotensive effect of moxonidine antagonised by corticosteroids

Diazoxide: enhanced hypotensive effect when moxonidine given with diazoxide

Diuretics: enhanced hypotensive effect when moxonidine given with diuretics

Dopaminergics: enhanced hypotensive effect when moxonidine given with levodopa

Methyldopa: enhanced hypotensive effect when moxonidine given with methyldopa

Moxisylyte: enhanced hypotensive effect when moxonidine given with moxisylyte

Muscle Relaxants: enhanced hypotensive effect when moxonidine given with baclofen or tizanidine

**Moxonidine** *(continued)*

Nitrates: enhanced hypotensive effect when moxonidine given with nitrates

Oestrogens: hypotensive effect of moxonidine antagonised by oestrogens

Prostaglandins: enhanced hypotensive effect when moxonidine given with alprostadil

Vasodilator Antihypertensives: enhanced hypotensive effect when moxonidine given with hydralazine, minoxidil or sodium nitroprusside

**Muscle Relaxants**

ACE Inhibitors: enhanced hypotensive effect when baclofen or tizanidine given with ACE inhibitors

Adrenergic Neurone Blockers: enhanced hypotensive effect when baclofen or tizanidine given with adrenergic neurone blockers

Alcohol: increased sedative effect when baclofen, methocarbamol or tizanidine given with alcohol

Alpha-blockers: enhanced hypotensive effect when baclofen or tizanidine given with alpha-blockers

• Anaesthetics, General: effects of atracurium enhanced by ketamine; increased risk of myocardial depression and bradycardia when suxamethonium given with ●propofol; effects of non-depolarising muscle relaxants and suxamethonium enhanced by volatile liquid general anaesthetics

Analgesics: excretion of baclofen possibly reduced by NSAIDs (increased risk of toxicity); excretion of baclofen reduced by ibuprofen (increased risk of toxicity); increased sedative effect when baclofen given with fentanyl or morphine

Angiotensin-II Receptor Antagonists: enhanced hypotensive effect when baclofen or tizanidine given with angiotensin-II receptor antagonists

Anti-arrhythmics: neuromuscular blockade enhanced and prolonged when suxamethonium given with lidocaine

• Antibacterials: effects of non-depolarising muscle relaxants and suxamethonium enhanced by piperacillin; plasma concentration of tizanidine increased by ●ciprofloxacin (increased risk of toxicity)—avoid concomitant use; plasma concentration of tizanidine possibly increased by norfloxacin (increased risk of toxicity); plasma concentration of tizanidine possibly reduced by rifampicin; effects of non-depolarising muscle relaxants and suxamethonium enhanced by ●aminoglycosides; effects of non-depolarising muscle relaxants and suxamethonium enhanced by ●clindamycin; effects of non-depolarising muscle relaxants and suxamethonium enhanced by ●polymyxins; effects of suxamethonium enhanced by ●vancomycin

• Antidepressants: plasma concentration of tizanidine increased by ●fluvoxamine (increased risk of toxicity)—avoid concomitant use; effects of suxamethonium enhanced by phenelzine; muscle relaxant effect of baclofen enhanced by tricyclics

• Antiepileptics: muscle relaxant effect of non-depolarising muscle relaxants antagonised by carbamazepine (accelerated recovery from neuromuscular blockade); effects of non-depolarising muscle relaxants reduced by *long-term use* of ●phenytoin (but effects of non-depolarising muscle relaxants might be increased by *acute use* of phenytoin)

Antimalarials: effects of suxamethonium possibly enhanced by quinine

Antipsychotics: effects of suxamethonium possibly enhanced by promazine

Anxiolytics and Hypnotics: increased sedative effect when baclofen or tizanidine given with anxiolytics and hypnotics

Beta-blockers: enhanced hypotensive effect when baclofen given with beta-blockers; possible enhanced hypotensive effect and bradycardia when tizanidine given with beta-blockers; effects of muscle relaxants enhanced by propranolol

**Muscle Relaxants** *(continued)*

Calcium-channel Blockers: enhanced hypotensive effect when baclofen or tizanidine given with calcium-channel blockers; effects of non-depolarising muscle relaxants possibly enhanced by calcium-channel blockers; possible increased risk of ventricular arrhythmias when *intravenous* dantrolene given with diltiazem—manufacturer of diltiazem advises avoid concomitant use; effects of non-depolarising muscle relaxants and suxamethonium enhanced by verapamil; avoidance of *intravenous* dantrolene advised by manufacturer of verapamil

Cardiac Glycosides: possible increased risk of bradycardia when tizanidine given with cardiac glycosides; risk of ventricular arrhythmias when suxamethonium given with cardiac glycosides

Clonidine: enhanced hypotensive effect when baclofen or tizanidine given with clonidine

Corticosteroids: effects of pancuronium and vecuronium possibly antagonised by corticosteroids

Cytotoxics: effects of suxamethonium enhanced by cyclophosphamide and thiotepa

Deferasirox: avoidance of tizanidine advised by manufacturer of deferasirox

Diazoxide: enhanced hypotensive effect when baclofen or tizanidine given with diazoxide

Diuretics: enhanced hypotensive effect when baclofen or tizanidine given with diuretics

Dopaminergics: possible agitation, confusion and hallucinations when baclofen given with levodopa

Lithium: effects of muscle relaxants enhanced by lithium; baclofen possibly aggravates hyperkinesis caused by lithium

Magnesium (parenteral): effects of non-depolarising muscle relaxants and suxamethonium enhanced by parenteral magnesium

Memantine: effects of baclofen and dantrolene possibly modified by memantine

Methyldopa: enhanced hypotensive effect when baclofen or tizanidine given with methyldopa

Metoclopramide: effects of suxamethonium enhanced by metoclopramide

Moxonidine: enhanced hypotensive effect when baclofen or tizanidine given with moxonidine

Nitrates: enhanced hypotensive effect when baclofen or tizanidine given with nitrates

Oestrogens: plasma concentration of tizanidine possibly increased by oestrogens (increased risk of toxicity)

Parasympathomimetics: effects of non-depolarising muscle relaxants possibly antagonised by donepezil; effects of suxamethonium possibly enhanced by donepezil; effects of non-depolarising muscle relaxants antagonised by edrophonium, neostigmine, pyridostigmine and rivastigmine; effects of suxamethonium enhanced by edrophonium, galantamine, neostigmine, pyridostigmine and rivastigmine

Progestogens: plasma concentration of tizanidine possibly increased by progestogens (increased risk of toxicity)

Sympathomimetics, Beta$_2$: effects of suxamethonium enhanced by bambuterol

Vasodilator Antihypertensives: enhanced hypotensive effect when baclofen or tizanidine given with hydralazine; enhanced hypotensive effect when baclofen or tizanidine given with minoxidil; enhanced hypotensive effect when baclofen or tizanidine given with sodium nitroprusside

**Muscle Relaxants, depolarising** *see* Muscle Relaxants

**Muscle Relaxants, non-depolarising** *see* Muscle Relaxants

**Mycophenolate**

Antacids: absorption of mycophenolate reduced by antacids

**Mycophenolate** *(continued)*

● Antibacterials: bioavailability of mycophenolate possibly reduced by metronidazole and norfloxacin; plasma concentration of active metabolite of mycophenolate reduced by ●rifampicin

Antivirals: mycophenolate increases plasma concentration of aciclovir, also plasma concentration of inactive metabolite of mycophenolate increased; mycophenolate possibly increases plasma concentration of ganciclovir, also plasma concentration of inactive metabolite of mycophenolate possibly increased

Iron: absorption of mycophenolate reduced by *oral* iron

Lipid-regulating Drugs: absorption of mycophenolate reduced by colestyramine

Sevelamer: plasma concentration of mycophenolate possibly reduced by sevelamer

**Mycophenolate Mofetil** *see* Mycophenolate

**Mycophenolate Sodium** *see* Mycophenolate

**Mycophenolic Acid** *see* Mycophenolate

**Nabumetone** *see* NSAIDs

**Nadolol** *see* Beta-blockers

**Nalidixic Acid** *see* Quinolones

**Nandrolone** *see* Anabolic Steroids

**Naproxen** *see* NSAIDs

**Naratriptan** *see* 5HT$_1$-receptor Agonists (under HT)

**Nateglinide** *see* Antidiabetics

**Nebivolol** *see* Beta-blockers

**Nefopam**

● Antidepressants: manufacturer of nefopam advises avoid concomitant use with ●MAOIs; side-effects possibly increased when nefopam given with tricyclics

Antimuscarinics: increased risk of antimuscarinic side-effects when nefopam given with antimuscarinics

**Neomycin** *see* Aminoglycosides

**Neostigmine** *see* Parasympathomimetics

**Nevirapine**

Analgesics: nevirapine possibly reduces plasma concentration of methadone

● Antibacterials: nevirapine reduces plasma concentration of clarithromycin (but concentration of an active metabolite increased), also plasma concentration of nevirapine increased; nevirapine possibly increases plasma concentration of rifabutin; plasma concentration of nevirapine reduced by ●rifampicin—avoid concomitant use

● Anticoagulants: nevirapine may enhance or reduce anticoagulant effect of ●warfarin

● Antidepressants: plasma concentration of nevirapine reduced by ●St John's wort—avoid concomitant use

Antiepileptics: plasma concentration of nevirapine reduced by carbamazepine

● Antifungals: nevirapine reduces plasma concentration of ●ketoconazole—avoid concomitant use; plasma concentration of nevirapine increased by ●fluconazole; nevirapine possibly reduces plasma concentration of caspofungin and itraconazole—consider increasing dose of caspofungin and itraconazole

● Antipsychotics: nevirapine possibly reduces plasma concentration of ●aripiprazole—increase dose of aripiprazole

● Antivirals: nevirapine possibly reduces plasma concentration of ●atazanavir and ●etravirine—avoid concomitant use; nevirapine reduces plasma concentration of efavirenz and indinavir; nevirapine possibly reduces plasma concentration of fosamprenavir; nevirapine possibly reduces plasma concentration of ●lopinavir—consider increasing dose of lopinavir

● Oestrogens: nevirapine accelerates metabolism of ●oestrogens (reduced contraceptive effect—see p. 398)

**Nevirapine** *(continued)*
- Progestogens: nevirapine accelerates metabolism of •progestogens (reduced contraceptive effect—see p. 398)

**Nicardipine** *see* Calcium-channel Blockers

**Nicorandil**
  Alcohol: hypotensive effect of nicorandil possibly enhanced by alcohol
  Antidepressants: enhanced hypotensive effect when nicorandil given with MAOIs; hypotensive effect of nicorandil possibly enhanced by tricyclics
- Sildenafil: hypotensive effect of nicorandil significantly enhanced by •sildenafil (avoid concomitant use)
- Tadalafil: hypotensive effect of nicorandil significantly enhanced by •tadalafil (avoid concomitant use)
- Vardenafil: possible increased hypotensive effect when nicorandil given with •vardenafil—avoid concomitant use
  Vasodilator Antihypertensives: possible enhanced hypotensive effect when nicorandil given with hydralazine, minoxidil or sodium nitroprusside

**Nicotine**
  Anti-arrhythmics: nicotine possibly enhances effects of adenosine

**Nicotinic Acid**
  **Note** Interactions apply to lipid-regulating doses of nicotinic acid
- Lipid-regulating Drugs: increased risk of myopathy when nicotinic acid given with •statins (applies to lipid regulating doses of nicotinic acid)

**Nifedipine** *see* Calcium-channel Blockers

**Nilotinib**
- Antibacterials: manufacturer of nilotinib advises avoid concomitant use with •clarithromycin and •telithromycin; plasma concentration of nilotinib reduced by •rifampicin—avoid concomitant use
- Antifungals: plasma concentration of nilotinib increased by •ketoconazole—avoid concomitant use; manufacturer of nilotinib advises avoid concomitant use with •itraconazole and •voriconazole
- Antipsychotics: avoid concomitant use of cytotoxics with •clozapine (increased risk of agranulocytosis)
- Antivirals: avoidance of nilotinib advised by manufacturer of •boceprevir; plasma concentration of nilotinib possibly increased by ritonavir—manufacturer of nilotinib advises avoid concomitant use
  Anxiolytics and Hypnotics: nilotinib increases plasma concentration of midazolam
- Grapefruit Juice: manufacturer of nilotinib advises avoid concomitant use with •grapefruit juice

**Nimodipine** *see* Calcium-channel Blockers

**Nitrates**
  ACE Inhibitors: enhanced hypotensive effect when nitrates given with ACE inhibitors
  Adrenergic Neurone Blockers: enhanced hypotensive effect when nitrates given with adrenergic neurone blockers
  Alcohol: enhanced hypotensive effect when nitrates given with alcohol
  Aldesleukin: enhanced hypotensive effect when nitrates given with aldesleukin
  Alpha-blockers: enhanced hypotensive effect when nitrates given with alpha-blockers
  Anaesthetics, General: enhanced hypotensive effect when nitrates given with general anaesthetics
  Analgesics: hypotensive effect of nitrates antagonised by NSAIDs
  Angiotensin-II Receptor Antagonists: enhanced hypotensive effect when nitrates given with angiotensin-II receptor antagonists
  Anti-arrhythmics: effects of sublingual tablets of nitrates reduced by disopyramide (failure to dissolve under tongue owing to dry mouth)
- Anticoagulants: *infusion* of glyceryl trinitrate reduces anticoagulant effect of •heparins

**Nitrates** *(continued)*
  Antidepressants: enhanced hypotensive effect when nitrates given with MAOIs; effects of sublingual tablets of nitrates possibly reduced by tricyclic-related antidepressants (failure to dissolve under tongue owing to dry mouth); effects of sublingual tablets of nitrates reduced by tricyclics (failure to dissolve under tongue owing to dry mouth)
  Antimuscarinics: effects of sublingual tablets of nitrates possibly reduced by antimuscarinics (failure to dissolve under tongue owing to dry mouth)
  Antipsychotics: enhanced hypotensive effect when nitrates given with phenothiazines
  Anxiolytics and Hypnotics: enhanced hypotensive effect when nitrates given with anxiolytics and hypnotics
  Beta-blockers: enhanced hypotensive effect when nitrates given with beta-blockers
  Calcium-channel Blockers: enhanced hypotensive effect when nitrates given with calcium-channel blockers
  Clonidine: enhanced hypotensive effect when nitrates given with clonidine
  Corticosteroids: hypotensive effect of nitrates antagonised by corticosteroids
  Diazoxide: enhanced hypotensive effect when nitrates given with diazoxide
  Diuretics: enhanced hypotensive effect when nitrates given with diuretics
  Dopaminergics: enhanced hypotensive effect when nitrates given with levodopa
  Methyldopa: enhanced hypotensive effect when nitrates given with methyldopa
  Moxisylyte: enhanced hypotensive effect when nitrates given with moxisylyte
  Moxonidine: enhanced hypotensive effect when nitrates given with moxonidine
  Muscle Relaxants: enhanced hypotensive effect when nitrates given with baclofen or tizanidine
  Oestrogens: hypotensive effect of nitrates antagonised by oestrogens
  Prostaglandins: enhanced hypotensive effect when nitrates given with alprostadil
- Sildenafil: hypotensive effect of nitrates significantly enhanced by •sildenafil (avoid concomitant use)
- Tadalafil: hypotensive effect of nitrates significantly enhanced by •tadalafil (avoid concomitant use)
- Vardenafil: possible increased hypotensive effect when nitrates given with •vardenafil—avoid concomitant use
  Vasodilator Antihypertensives: enhanced hypotensive effect when nitrates given with hydralazine, minoxidil or sodium nitroprusside

**Nitrazepam** *see* Anxiolytics and Hypnotics

**Nitrofurantoin**
  Antacids: absorption of nitrofurantoin reduced by oral magnesium salts (as magnesium trisilicate)
  Antibacterials: nitrofurantoin possibly antagonises effects of nalidixic acid
  Probenecid: excretion of nitrofurantoin reduced by probenecid (increased risk of side-effects)
  Sulfinpyrazone: excretion of nitrofurantoin reduced by sulfinpyrazone (increased risk of toxicity)
  Vaccines: antibacterials inactivate oral typhoid vaccine—see p. 621

**Nitroimidazoles** *see* Metronidazole and Tinidazole
**Nitrous Oxide** *see* Anaesthetics, General
**Nizatidine** *see* Histamine H₂-antagonists
**Noradrenaline (norepinephrine)** *see* Sympathomimetics
**Norelgestromin** *see* Progestogens
**Norepinephrine (noradrenaline)** *see* Sympathomimetics
**Norethisterone** *see* Progestogens
**Norfloxacin** *see* Quinolones

**Norgestimate** *see* Progestogens
**Norgestrel** *see* Progestogens
**Nortriptyline** *see* Antidepressants, Tricyclic
**NSAIDs**

**Note** *See also* Aspirin. Interactions do not generally apply to topical NSAIDs

ACE Inhibitors: increased risk of renal impairment when NSAIDs given with ACE inhibitors, also hypotensive effect antagonised

Adrenergic Neurone Blockers: NSAIDs antagonise hypotensive effect of adrenergic neurone blockers

Aliskiren: NSAIDs possibly antagonise hypotensive effect of aliskiren

Alpha-blockers: NSAIDs antagonise hypotensive effect of alpha-blockers

• Analgesics: avoid concomitant use of NSAIDs with •NSAIDs or •aspirin (increased side-effects); avoid concomitant use of NSAIDs with •ketorolac (increased side-effects and haemorrhage); ibuprofen possibly reduces antiplatelet effect of aspirin

Angiotensin-II Receptor Antagonists: increased risk of renal impairment when NSAIDs given with angiotensin-II receptor antagonists, also hypotensive effect antagonised

• Antibacterials: indometacin possibly increases plasma concentration of amikacin and gentamicin in neonates; plasma concentration of celecoxib, diclofenac and etoricoxib reduced by rifampicin; possible increased risk of convulsions when NSAIDs given with •quinolones

• Anticoagulants: increased risk of haemorrhage when *intravenous* diclofenac given with •anticoagulants (avoid concomitant use, including low-dose heparins); increased risk of haemorrhage when ketorolac given with •anticoagulants (avoid concomitant use, including low-dose heparins); NSAIDs possibly enhance anticoagulant effect of •coumarins and •phenindione; possible increased risk of bleeding when NSAIDs given with •dabigatran etexilate or heparins

• Antidepressants: increased risk of bleeding when NSAIDs given with •SSRIs or •venlafaxine

• Antidiabetics: NSAIDs possibly enhance effects of •sulfonylureas

Antifungals: plasma concentration of parecoxib increased by fluconazole (reduce dose of parecoxib); plasma concentration of celecoxib increased by fluconazole (halve dose of celecoxib); plasma concentration of flurbiprofen and ibuprofen increased by fluconazole; plasma concentration of diclofenac and ibuprofen increased by voriconazole

Antipsychotics: possible severe drowsiness when acemetacin or indometacin given with haloperidol

• Antivirals: plasma concentration of piroxicam increased by •ritonavir (risk of toxicity)—avoid concomitant use; plasma concentration of NSAIDs possibly increased by ritonavir; increased risk of haematological toxicity when NSAIDs given with zidovudine

Beta-blockers: NSAIDs antagonise hypotensive effect of beta-blockers

Calcium-channel Blockers: NSAIDs antagonise hypotensive effect of calcium-channel blockers

Cardiac Glycosides: NSAIDs possibly increase plasma concentration of cardiac glycosides, also possible exacerbation of heart failure and reduction of renal function

• Ciclosporin: increased risk of nephrotoxicity when NSAIDs given with •ciclosporin; plasma concentration of diclofenac increased by •ciclosporin (halve dose of diclofenac)

Clonidine: NSAIDs antagonise hypotensive effect of clonidine

Clopidogrel: increased risk of bleeding when NSAIDs given with clopidogrel

**NSAIDs** *(continued)*

Corticosteroids: increased risk of gastro-intestinal bleeding and ulceration when NSAIDs given with corticosteroids

• Cytotoxics: NSAIDs probably reduce excretion of •methotrexate (increased risk of toxicity); diclofenac, ibuprofen, indometacin, ketoprofen, meloxicam and naproxen reduce excretion of •methotrexate (increased risk of toxicity); increased risk of bleeding when NSAIDs given with •erlotinib

Desmopressin: indometacin enhances effects of desmopressin

Diazoxide: NSAIDs antagonise hypotensive effect of diazoxide

• Dimethyl sulfoxide: avoid concomitant use of sulindac with •dimethyl sulfoxide

• Diuretics: risk of nephrotoxicity of NSAIDs increased by diuretics, also antagonism of diuretic effect; indometacin and ketorolac antagonise effects of diuretics; NSAIDs possibly antagonise diuretic effect of potassium canrenoate; occasional reports of reduced renal function when indometacin given with •triamterene—avoid concomitant use; possible increased risk of hyperkalaemia when NSAIDs given with potassium-sparing diuretics and aldosterone antagonists; increased risk of hyperkalaemia when indometacin given with potassium-sparing diuretics and aldosterone antagonists

Iloprost: increased risk of bleeding when NSAIDs given with iloprost

Lipid-regulating Drugs: excretion of meloxicam increased by colestyramine

• Lithium: NSAIDs reduce excretion of •lithium (increased risk of toxicity); ketorolac reduces excretion of •lithium (increased risk of toxicity)—avoid concomitant use

Methyldopa: NSAIDs antagonise hypotensive effect of methyldopa

Mifamurtide: avoidance of high doses of NSAIDs advised by manufacturer of mifamurtide

Moxonidine: NSAIDs antagonise hypotensive effect of moxonidine

Muscle Relaxants: ibuprofen reduces excretion of baclofen (increased risk of toxicity); NSAIDs possibly reduce excretion of baclofen (increased risk of toxicity)

Nitrates: NSAIDs antagonise hypotensive effect of nitrates

Oestrogens: etoricoxib increases plasma concentration of ethinylestradiol

Penicillamine: possible increased risk of nephrotoxicity when NSAIDs given with penicillamine

• Pentoxifylline: possible increased risk of bleeding when NSAIDs given with pentoxifylline; increased risk of bleeding when ketorolac given with •pentoxifylline (avoid concomitant use)

Prasugrel: possible increased risk of bleeding when NSAIDs given with prasugrel

• Probenecid: excretion of acemetacin, dexketoprofen, indometacin, ketoprofen and naproxen reduced by •probenecid (increased plasma concentration); excretion of ketorolac reduced by •probenecid (increased plasma concentration)—avoid concomitant use

• Tacrolimus: possible increased risk of nephrotoxicity when NSAIDs given with tacrolimus; increased risk of nephrotoxicity when ibuprofen given with •tacrolimus

Vasodilator Antihypertensives: NSAIDs antagonise hypotensive effect of hydralazine, minoxidil and sodium nitroprusside

**Octreotide**

Antidiabetics: octreotide possibly reduces requirements for insulin, metformin, repaglinide and sulfonylureas

## Octreotide *(continued)*

- Ciclosporin: octreotide reduces plasma concentration of ●ciclosporin

    Dopaminergics: octreotide increases plasma concentration of bromocriptine

    Ulcer-healing Drugs: octreotide possibly delays absorption of cimetidine

## Oestrogens

> **Note** Interactions of combined oral contraceptives may also apply to combined contraceptive patches and vaginal rings, see p. 398

ACE Inhibitors: oestrogens antagonise hypotensive effect of ACE inhibitors

Adrenergic Neurone Blockers: oestrogens antagonise hypotensive effect of adrenergic neurone blockers

Alpha-blockers: oestrogens antagonise hypotensive effect of alpha-blockers

Analgesics: plasma concentration of ethinylestradiol increased by etoricoxib

Angiotensin-II Receptor Antagonists: oestrogens antagonise hypotensive effect of angiotensin-II receptor antagonists

- Antibacterials: plasma concentration of estradiol increased by erythromycin; metabolism of oestrogens accelerated by ●rifamycins (reduced contraceptive effect—see p. 398)

- Anticoagulants: oestrogens may enhance or reduce anticoagulant effect of coumarins; oestrogens antagonise anticoagulant effect of ●phenindione

- Antidepressants: contraceptive effect of oestrogens reduced by ●St John's wort (avoid concomitant use); oestrogens antagonise antidepressant effect of tricyclics (but side-effects of tricyclics possibly increased due to increased plasma concentration)

    Antidiabetics: oestrogens antagonise hypoglycaemic effect of antidiabetics

- Antiepileptics: metabolism of oestrogens accelerated by ●carbamazepine, ●eslicarbazepine, ●oxcarbazepine, ●phenobarbital, ●phenytoin, ●rufinamide and ●topiramate (reduced contraceptive effect—see p. 398); oestrogens reduce plasma concentration of ●lamotrigine—consider increasing dose of lamotrigine; ethinylestradiol possibly reduces plasma concentration of valproate

    Antifungals: oestrogens increase plasma concentration of voriconazole; anecdotal reports of contraceptive failure and menstrual irregularities when oestrogens given with griseofulvin; anecdotal reports of contraceptive failure when oestrogens given with imidazoles; occasional reports of breakthrough bleeding when oestrogens (used for contraception) given with terbinafine

- Antivirals: plasma concentration of ethinylestradiol increased by atazanavir; possible contraceptive failure of hormonal contraceptives containing oestrogens when given with ●boceprevir (alternative contraception recommended); metabolism of oestrogens accelerated by ●nevirapine and ●ritonavir (reduced contraceptive effect—see p. 398); plasma concentration of ethinylestradiol possibly reduced by ●telaprevir—manufacturer of telaprevir advises additional contraceptive precautions

    Anxiolytics and Hypnotics: oestrogens possibly increase plasma concentration of diazepam; oestrogens increase plasma concentration of melatonin

- Aprepitant: possible contraceptive failure of hormonal contraceptives containing oestrogens when given with ●aprepitant (alternative contraception recommended)

    Beta-blockers: oestrogens antagonise hypotensive effect of beta-blockers

- Bosentan: possible contraceptive failure of hormonal contraceptives containing oestrogens when given with ●bosentan (alternative contraception recommended)

## Oestrogens *(continued)*

Calcium-channel Blockers: oestrogens antagonise hypotensive effect of calcium-channel blockers

Ciclosporin: oestrogens possibly increase plasma concentration of ciclosporin

Clonidine: oestrogens antagonise hypotensive effect of clonidine

Corticosteroids: oral contraceptives containing oestrogens increase plasma concentration of corticosteroids

- Cytotoxics: possible reduction in contraceptive effect of oestrogens advised by manufacturer of ●crizotinib and ●vemurafenib

    Diuretics: oestrogens antagonise diuretic effect of diuretics

- Dopaminergics: oestrogens increase plasma concentration of ropinirole; oestrogens increase plasma concentration of ●selegiline—manufacturer of selegiline advises avoid concomitant use

    Lipid-regulating Drugs: absorption of ethinylestradiol reduced by colesevelam; plasma concentration of ethinylestradiol increased by atorvastatin and rosuvastatin

    Methyldopa: oestrogens antagonise hypotensive effect of methyldopa

- Modafinil: metabolism of oestrogens accelerated by ●modafinil (reduced contraceptive effect—see p. 398)

    Moxonidine: oestrogens antagonise hypotensive effect of moxonidine

    Muscle Relaxants: oestrogens possibly increase plasma concentration of tizanidine (increased risk of toxicity)

    Nitrates: oestrogens antagonise hypotensive effect of nitrates

    Somatropin: oestrogens (when used as oral replacement therapy) may increase dose requirements of somatropin

    Tacrolimus: ethinylestradiol possibly increases plasma concentration of tacrolimus

    Theophylline: oestrogens increase plasma concentration of theophylline (consider reducing dose of theophylline)

    Thyroid Hormones: oestrogens may increase requirements for thyroid hormones in hypothyroidism

    Vasodilator Antihypertensives: oestrogens antagonise hypotensive effect of hydralazine, minoxidil and sodium nitroprusside

**Oestrogens, conjugated** *see* Oestrogens

**Ofloxacin** *see* Quinolones

**Olanzapine** *see* Antipsychotics

**Olmesartan** *see* Angiotensin-II Receptor Antagonists

**Olsalazine** *see* Aminosalicylates

**Omeprazole** *see* Proton Pump Inhibitors

**Ondansetron** *see* 5HT$_3$-receptor Antagonists (under HT)

## Opioid Analgesics

Alcohol: enhanced hypotensive and sedative effects when opioid analgesics given with alcohol

Anaesthetics, General: fentanyl inhibits metabolism of etomidate (consider reducing dose of etomidate); opioid analgesics possibly enhance effects of intravenous general anaesthetics and volatile liquid general anaesthetics

- Antibacterials: plasma concentration of alfentanil increased by erythromycin; metabolism of alfentanil, codeine, fentanyl, methadone and morphine accelerated by rifampicin (reduced effect); metabolism of oxycodone possibly accelerated by rifampicin; metabolism of oxycodone inhibited by telithromycin; possible increased risk of ventricular arrhythmias when methadone given with ●telithromycin

- Anticoagulants: tramadol enhances anticoagulant effect of ●coumarins

## Opioid Analgesics *(continued)*

- Antidepressants: plasma concentration of methadone possibly increased by fluoxetine, fluvoxamine, paroxetine and sertraline; possible increased serotonergic effects when pethidine or tramadol given with duloxetine; possible increased serotonergic effects when tramadol given with mirtazapine or venlafaxine; possible CNS excitation or depression (hypertension or hypotension) when opioid analgesics given with ●MAOIs—some manufacturers advise avoid concomitant use and for 2 weeks after stopping MAOIs; possible increased serotonergic effects and increased risk of convulsions when tramadol given with ●MAOIs—some manufacturers advise avoid concomitant use and for 2 weeks after stopping MAOIs; CNS excitation or depression (hypertension or hypotension) when pethidine given with ●MAOIs—avoid concomitant use and for 2 weeks after stopping MAOIs; possible CNS excitation or depression (hypertension or hypotension) when opioid analgesics given with ●moclobemide—manufacturer of moclobemide advises consider reducing dose of opioid analgesics; possible CNS excitation or depression (hypertension or hypotension) when dextromethorphan or pethidine given with ●moclobemide—avoid concomitant use; increased risk of CNS toxicity when tramadol given with ●SSRIs or ●tricyclics; plasma concentration of methadone possibly reduced by St John's wort; sedative effects possibly increased when opioid analgesics given with tricyclics
- Antiepileptics: dextropropoxyphene enhances effects of ●carbamazepine; effects of tramadol reduced by carbamazepine; plasma concentration of methadone reduced by carbamazepine and phenobarbital; morphine increases bioavailability of gabapentin; metabolism of methadone accelerated by phenytoin (reduced effect and risk of withdrawal effects)
- Antifungals: metabolism of buprenorphine inhibited by ●ketoconazole (reduce dose of buprenorphine); metabolism of alfentanil inhibited by fluconazole (risk of prolonged or delayed respiratory depression); plasma concentration of methadone increased by fluconazole; metabolism of alfentanil possibly inhibited by itraconazole; plasma concentration of alfentanil and methadone increased by ●voriconazole (consider reducing dose of alfentanil and methadone); plasma concentration of oxycodone increased by ●voriconazole; plasma concentration of fentanyl possibly increased by ●triazoles
- Antihistamines: sedative effects possibly increased when opioid analgesics given with ●sedating antihistamines
- Antimalarials: avoidance of methadone advised by manufacturer of ●piperaquine with artenimol (possible risk of ventricular arrhythmias)
- Antimuscarinics: possible increased risk of antimuscarinic side-effects when codeine given with antimuscarinics
- Antipsychotics: enhanced hypotensive and sedative effects when opioid analgesics given with antipsychotics; increased risk of ventricular arrhythmias when methadone given with ●antipsychotics that prolong the QT interval; increased risk of convulsions when tramadol given with antipsychotics; increased risk of ventricular arrhythmias when methadone given with ●amisulpride—avoid concomitant use
- Antivirals: plasma concentration of methadone possibly reduced by abacavir, nevirapine and rilpivirine; plasma concentration of methadone possibly affected by boceprevir; methadone possibly reduces plasma concentration of didanosine; plasma concentration of methadone reduced by efavirenz, fosamprenavir and ritonavir; plasma concentration of alfentanil and fentanyl increased by ●ritonavir;

## Opioid Analgesics

- Antivirals *(continued)*
  plasma concentration of dextropropoxyphene increased by ●ritonavir (risk of toxicity)—avoid concomitant use; plasma concentration of buprenorphine possibly increased by ritonavir; plasma concentration of pethidine reduced by ●ritonavir, but plasma concentration of toxic pethidine metabolite increased (avoid concomitant use); plasma concentration of morphine possibly reduced by ritonavir; increased risk of ventricular arrhythmias when alfentanil, fentanyl or methadone given with ●saquinavir—avoid concomitant use; caution with methadone advised by manufacturer of ●telaprevir (risk of ventricular arrhythmias); buprenorphine possibly reduces plasma concentration of tipranavir; methadone possibly increases plasma concentration of zidovudine
- Anxiolytics and Hypnotics: increased sedative effect when opioid analgesics given with anxiolytics and hypnotics; fentanyl possibly inhibits metabolism of midazolam
- Atomoxetine: increased risk of ventricular arrhythmias when methadone given with ●atomoxetine; possible increased risk of convulsions when tramadol given with atomoxetine
- Beta-blockers: morphine possibly increases plasma concentration of esmolol
- Calcium-channel Blockers: metabolism of alfentanil inhibited by diltiazem (risk of prolonged or delayed respiratory depression)
- Cytotoxics: caution with alfentanil and fentanyl advised by manufacturer of ●crizotinib; possible increased risk of ventricular arrhythmias when methadone given with ●vandetanib—avoid concomitant use
- Domperidone: opioid analgesics antagonise effects of domperidone on gastro-intestinal activity
- Dopaminergics: avoid concomitant use of dextromethorphan with ●rasagiline; risk of CNS toxicity when pethidine given with ●rasagiline (avoid pethidine for 2 weeks after rasagiline); avoidance of opioid analgesics advised by manufacturer of selegiline; hyperpyrexia and CNS toxicity reported when pethidine given with ●selegiline (avoid concomitant use)
- 5HT₃-receptor Antagonists: effects of tramadol possibly antagonised by ondansetron
- Memantine: increased risk of CNS toxicity when dextromethorphan given with ●memantine (manufacturer of memantine advises avoid concomitant use)
- Metoclopramide: opioid analgesics antagonise effects of metoclopramide on gastro-intestinal activity
- Muscle Relaxants: increased sedative effect when fentanyl or morphine given with baclofen
- Sodium Oxybate: opioid analgesics enhance effects of ●sodium oxybate (avoid concomitant use)
- Ulcer-healing Drugs: metabolism of opioid analgesics inhibited by cimetidine (increased plasma concentration)

## Orlistat

- Anti-arrhythmics: orlistat possibly reduces plasma concentration of amiodarone
- Anticoagulants: manufacturer of orlistat recommends monitoring anticoagulant effect of coumarins
- Antidiabetics: manufacturer of orlistat advises avoid concomitant use with acarbose
- Antiepileptics: possible increased risk of convulsions when orlistat given with ●antiepileptics
- Ciclosporin: orlistat possibly reduces absorption of ●ciclosporin
- Thyroid Hormones: possible increased risk of hypothyroidism when orlistat given with levothyroxine

## Orphenadrine *see* Antimuscarinics

Oxaliplatin *see* Platinum Compounds
Oxandrolone *see* Anabolic Steroids
Oxazepam *see* Anxiolytics and Hypnotics
**Oxcarbazepine**
- Antidepressants: anticonvulsant effect of antiepileptics possibly antagonised by MAOIs and •tricyclic-related antidepressants (convulsive threshold lowered); anticonvulsant effect of antiepileptics antagonised by •SSRIs and •tricyclics (convulsive threshold lowered); avoid concomitant use of antiepileptics with •St John's wort
- Antiepileptics: oxcarbazepine sometimes reduces plasma concentration of carbamazepine (but concentration of an active metabolite of carbamazepine may be increased), also plasma concentration of an active metabolite of oxcarbazepine often reduced; avoidance of oxcarbazepine advised by manufacturer of eslicarbazepine; oxcarbazepine reduces plasma concentration of •perampanel (see Dose under Perampanel, p. 224); oxcarbazepine increases plasma concentration of phenobarbital and phenytoin, also plasma concentration of an active metabolite of oxcarbazepine reduced; plasma concentration of an active metabolite of oxcarbazepine sometimes reduced by valproate
- Antimalarials: anticonvulsant effect of antiepileptics antagonised by •mefloquine
- Antipsychotics: anticonvulsant effect of antiepileptics antagonised by •antipsychotics (convulsive threshold lowered)
- Antivirals: avoidance of oxcarbazepine advised by manufacturer of •rilpivirine (plasma concentration of rilpivirine possibly reduced)
  Ciclosporin: oxcarbazepine possibly reduces plasma concentration of ciclosporin
- Clopidogrel: oxcarbazepine possibly reduces antiplatelet effect of •clopidogrel
- Cytotoxics: oxcarbazepine reduces plasma concentration of •imatinib—avoid concomitant use
- Oestrogens: oxcarbazepine accelerates metabolism of •oestrogens (reduced contraceptive effect—see p. 398)
- Orlistat: possible increased risk of convulsions when antiepileptics given with •orlistat
- Progestogens: oxcarbazepine accelerates metabolism of •progestogens (reduced contraceptive effect—see p. 398)

Oxprenolol *see* Beta-blockers
Oxybutynin *see* Antimuscarinics
Oxycodone *see* Opioid Analgesics
Oxymetazoline *see* Sympathomimetics
Oxytetracycline *see* Tetracyclines
**Oxytocin**
  Anaesthetics, General: oxytocic effect possibly reduced, also enhanced hypotensive effect and risk of arrhythmias when oxytocin given with volatile liquid general anaesthetics
  Prostaglandins: uterotonic effect of oxytocin potentiated by prostaglandins
  Sympathomimetics: risk of hypertension when oxytocin given with vasoconstrictor sympathomimetics (due to enhanced vasopressor effect)
**Paclitaxel**
- Antipsychotics: avoid concomitant use of cytotoxics with •clozapine (increased risk of agranulocytosis)
  Antivirals: plasma concentration of paclitaxel increased by ritonavir
- Cytotoxics: increased risk of neutropenia when paclitaxel given with •lapatinib

Paliperidone *see* Antipsychotics
**Pancreatin**
  Antidiabetics: pancreatin antagonises hypoglycaemic effect of acarbose

Pancuronium *see* Muscle Relaxants
Pantoprazole *see* Proton Pump Inhibitors

Papaveretum *see* Opioid Analgesics
**Paracetamol**
  Anticoagulants: prolonged regular use of paracetamol possibly enhances anticoagulant effect of coumarins
  Antiepileptics: metabolism of paracetamol possibly accelerated by carbamazepine, phenobarbital and phenytoin (also isolated reports of hepatotoxicity)
  Cytotoxics: paracetamol possibly inhibits metabolism of *intravenous* busulfan (manufacturer of *intravenous* busulfan advises caution within 72 hours of paracetamol); caution with paracetamol advised by manufacturer of imatinib
  Lipid-regulating Drugs: absorption of paracetamol reduced by colestyramine
  Metoclopramide: rate of absorption of paracetamol increased by metoclopramide
**Paraldehyde**
- Alcohol: increased sedative effect when paraldehyde given with •alcohol
- Disulfiram: risk of toxicity when paraldehyde given with •disulfiram
**Parasympathomimetics**
  Anti-arrhythmics: effects of neostigmine and pyridostigmine possibly antagonised by propafenone
- Antibacterials: plasma concentration of galantamine increased by erythromycin; effects of neostigmine and pyridostigmine antagonised by •aminoglycosides; effects of neostigmine and pyridostigmine antagonised by clindamycin; effects of neostigmine and pyridostigmine antagonised by •polymyxins
  Antidepressants: plasma concentration of galantamine increased by paroxetine
  Antifungals: plasma concentration of galantamine increased by ketoconazole
  Antimalarials: effects of neostigmine and pyridostigmine may be diminished because of potential for chloroquine and hydroxychloroquine to increase symptoms of myasthenia gravis
  Antimuscarinics: effects of parasympathomimetics antagonised by antimuscarinics
  Beta-blockers: increased risk of arrhythmias when pilocarpine given with beta-blockers; effects of neostigmine and pyridostigmine antagonised by propranolol
  Cytotoxics: possible increased risk of bradycardia when pilocarpine given with crizotinib
  Lithium: effects of neostigmine antagonised by lithium
  Muscle Relaxants: donepezil possibly enhances effects of suxamethonium; edrophonium, galantamine, neostigmine, pyridostigmine and rivastigmine enhance effects of suxamethonium; donepezil possibly antagonises effects of non-depolarising muscle relaxants; edrophonium, neostigmine, pyridostigmine and rivastigmine antagonise effects of non-depolarising muscle relaxants

Parecoxib *see* NSAIDs
Paricalcitol *see* Vitamins
Paroxetine *see* Antidepressants, SSRI
**Pasireotide**
  Antidiabetics: pasireotide possibly reduces requirements for antidiabetics
  Antimuscarinics: possible increased risk of bradycardia when pasireotide given with ipratropium or oxybutynin
  Beta-blockers: possible increased risk of bradycardia when pasireotide given with carteolol, metoprolol, propranolol or sotalol
  Calcium-channel Blockers: possible increased risk of bradycardia when pasireotide given with diltiazem or verapamil
- Ciclosporin: pasireotide possibly reduces plasma concentration of •ciclosporin
**Pazopanib**
- Antibacterials: manufacturer of pazopanib advises avoid concomitant use with •clarithromycin, •rifampicin and •telithromycin

**Pazopanib** *(continued)*
- Antifungals: manufacturer of pazopanib advises avoid concomitant use with ●itraconazole, ●ketoconazole and ●voriconazole
- Antipsychotics: avoid concomitant use of cytotoxics with ●clozapine (increased risk of agranulocytosis)
- Antivirals: manufacturer of pazopanib advises avoid concomitant use with ●atazanavir, ●indinavir, ●ritonavir and ●saquinavir; avoidance of pazopanib advised by manufacturer of ●boceprevir

Cytotoxics: plasma concentration of pazopanib increased by lapatinib
- Grapefruit Juice: manufacturer of pazopanib advises avoid concomitant use with ●grapefruit juice

Ulcer-healing Drugs: absorption of pazopanib possibly reduced by histamine H$_2$-antagonists—manufacturer of pazopanib advises give at least 2 hours before or 10 hours after histamine H$_2$-antagonists; absorption of pazopanib possibly reduced by proton pump inhibitors—manufacturer of pazopanib advises give at the same time as proton pump inhibitors

**Pegfilgrastim** *see* Filgrastim

**Peginterferon Alfa** *see* Interferons

**Pemetrexed**
- Antimalarials: antifolate effect of pemetrexed increased by ●pyrimethamine
- Antipsychotics: avoid concomitant use of cytotoxics with ●clozapine (increased risk of agranulocytosis)

**Penicillamine**

Analgesics: possible increased risk of nephrotoxicity when penicillamine given with NSAIDs

Antacids: absorption of penicillamine reduced by antacids
- Antipsychotics: avoid concomitant use of penicillamine with ●clozapine (increased risk of agranulocytosis)

Cardiac Glycosides: penicillamine possibly reduces plasma concentration of digoxin

Gold: manufacturer of penicillamine advises avoid concomitant use with sodium aurothiomalate (increased risk of toxicity)

Iron: absorption of penicillamine reduced by *oral* iron

Zinc: penicillamine reduces absorption of zinc, also absorption of penicillamine reduced by zinc

**Penicillins**

Allopurinol: increased risk of rash when amoxicillin or ampicillin given with allopurinol

Antibacterials: absorption of phenoxymethylpenicillin reduced by neomycin; effects of penicillins possibly antagonised by tetracyclines

Anticoagulants: an interaction between broad-spectrum penicillins and coumarins and phenindione has not been demonstrated in studies, but common experience in anticoagulant clinics is that INR can be altered
- Antiepileptics: manufacturer of pivmecillinam advises avoid concomitant use with ●valproate

Cytotoxics: penicillins reduce excretion of methotrexate (increased risk of toxicity)

Muscle Relaxants: piperacillin enhances effects of non-depolarising muscle relaxants and suxamethonium

Probenecid: excretion of penicillins reduced by probenecid (increased plasma concentration)

Sulfinpyrazone: excretion of penicillins reduced by sulfinpyrazone

Vaccines: antibacterials inactivate oral typhoid vaccine—see p. 621

**Pentamidine Isetionate**
- Anti-arrhythmics: increased risk of ventricular arrhythmias when pentamidine isetionate given with ●amiodarone—avoid concomitant use; possible increased risk of ventricular arrhythmias when pentamidine isetionate given with ●disopyramide

**Pentamidine Isetionate** *(continued)*
- Antibacterials: increased risk of ventricular arrhythmias when pentamidine isetionate given with *parenteral* ●erythromycin; increased risk of ventricular arrhythmias when pentamidine isetionate given with ●moxifloxacin—avoid concomitant use; possible increased risk of ventricular arrhythmias when parenteral pentamidine isetionate given with ●telithromycin
- Antidepressants: increased risk of ventricular arrhythmias when pentamidine isetionate given with ●tricyclics

Antifungals: possible increased risk of nephrotoxicity when pentamidine isetionate given with amphotericin
- Antimalarials: avoidance of pentamidine isetionate advised by manufacturer of ●piperaquine with artenimol (possible risk of ventricular arrhythmias)
- Antipsychotics: increased risk of ventricular arrhythmias when pentamidine isetionate given with ●amisulpride or ●droperidol—avoid concomitant use; increased risk of ventricular arrhythmias when pentamidine isetionate given with ●phenothiazines
- Antivirals: increased risk of hypocalcaemia when *parenteral* pentamidine isetionate given with ●foscarnet; increased risk of ventricular arrhythmias when pentamidine isetionate given with ●saquinavir—avoid concomitant use
- Cytotoxics: possible increased risk of ventricular arrhythmias when pentamidine isetionate given with ●vandetanib—avoid concomitant use
- Ivabradine: increased risk of ventricular arrhythmias when pentamidine isetionate given with ●ivabradine

**Pentazocine** *see* Opioid Analgesics

**Pentostatin**
- Antipsychotics: avoid concomitant use of cytotoxics with ●clozapine (increased risk of agranulocytosis)
- Cytotoxics: increased toxicity when pentostatin given with high-dose ●cyclophosphamide—avoid concomitant use; increased pulmonary toxicity when pentostatin given with ●fludarabine (unacceptably high incidence of fatalities)

**Pentoxifylline**
- Analgesics: possible increased risk of bleeding when pentoxifylline given with NSAIDs; increased risk of bleeding when pentoxifylline given with ●ketorolac (avoid concomitant use)

Theophylline: pentoxifylline increases plasma concentration of theophylline

**Perampanel**
- Antidepressants: anticonvulsant effect of antiepileptics possibly antagonised by MAOIs and ●tricyclic-related antidepressants (convulsive threshold lowered); anticonvulsant effect of antiepileptics antagonised by ●SSRIs and ●tricyclics (convulsive threshold lowered); avoid concomitant use of antiepileptics with ●St John's wort
- Antiepileptics: plasma concentration of perampanel reduced by ●carbamazepine, ●oxcarbazepine and ●phenytoin (see Dose under Perampanel, p. 224); plasma concentration of perampanel reduced by topiramate

Antifungals: plasma concentration of perampanel increased by ketoconazole
- Antimalarials: anticonvulsant effect of antiepileptics antagonised by ●mefloquine
- Antipsychotics: anticonvulsant effect of antiepileptics antagonised by ●antipsychotics (convulsive threshold lowered)

Anxiolytics and Hypnotics: perampanel reduces plasma concentration of midazolam
- Orlistat: possible increased risk of convulsions when antiepileptics given with ●orlistat
- Progestogens: perampanel accelerates metabolism of ●progestogens (reduced contraceptive effect—see p. 398)

## Pergolide

Antipsychotics: effects of pergolide antagonised by antipsychotics

Memantine: effects of dopaminergics possibly enhanced by memantine

Methyldopa: antiparkinsonian effect of dopaminergics antagonised by methyldopa

Metoclopramide: antiparkinsonian effect of pergolide antagonised by metoclopramide

**Pericyazine** see Antipsychotics

**Perindopril** see ACE Inhibitors

**Perphenazine** see Antipsychotics

**Pethidine** see Opioid Analgesics

**Phenelzine** see MAOIs

## Phenindione

Note Change in patient's clinical condition particularly associated with liver disease, intercurrent illness, or drug administration, necessitates more frequent testing. Major changes in diet (especially involving salads and vegetables) and in alcohol consumption may also affect anticoagulant control

- Alcohol: anticoagulant control with phenindione may be affected by major changes in consumption of •alcohol
- Anabolic Steroids: anticoagulant effect of phenindione enhanced by •anabolic steroids
- Analgesics: anticoagulant effect of phenindione possibly enhanced by •NSAIDs; increased risk of haemorrhage when anticoagulants given with *intravenous* •diclofenac (avoid concomitant use, including low-dose heparins); increased risk of haemorrhage when anticoagulants given with •ketorolac (avoid concomitant use, including low-dose heparins); increased risk of bleeding when phenindione given with •aspirin (due to antiplatelet effect)
- Anti-arrhythmics: metabolism of phenindione inhibited by •amiodarone (enhanced anticoagulant effect); anticoagulant effect of phenindione possibly enhanced by •dronedarone
- Antibacterials: experience in anticoagulant clinics suggests that INR possibly altered when phenindione is given with •neomycin (given for local action on gut); anticoagulant effect of phenindione possibly enhanced by levofloxacin and •tetracyclines; an interaction between phenindione and broad-spectrum penicillins has not been demonstrated in studies, but common experience in anticoagulant clinics is that INR can be altered; metabolism of phenindione possibly inhibited by sulfonamides
- Anticoagulants: increased risk of haemorrhage when other anticoagulants given with •apixaban, •dabigatran etexilate and •rivaroxaban (avoid concomitant use except when switching with other anticoagulants or using heparin to maintain catheter patency)
- Antivirals: anticoagulant effect of phenindione possibly enhanced by •ritonavir
- Clopidogrel: anticoagulant effect of phenindione enhanced due to antiplatelet action of •clopidogrel

Corticosteroids: anticoagulant effect of phenindione may be enhanced or reduced by corticosteroids

- Dipyridamole: anticoagulant effect of phenindione enhanced due to antiplatelet action of •dipyridamole
- Enteral Foods: anticoagulant effect of phenindione antagonised by vitamin K (present in some •enteral feeds )

Iloprost: increased risk of bleeding when phenindione given with iloprost

- Lipid-regulating Drugs: anticoagulant effect of phenindione may be enhanced or reduced by •colestyramine; anticoagulant effect of phenindione possibly enhanced by •rosuvastatin; anticoagulant effect of phenindione enhanced by •fibrates
- Oestrogens: anticoagulant effect of phenindione antagonised by •oestrogens

## Phenindione *(continued)*

Prasugrel: possible increased risk of bleeding when phenindione given with prasugrel

- Progestogens: anticoagulant effect of phenindione antagonised by •progestogens
- Testolactone: anticoagulant effect of phenindione enhanced by •testolactone
- Testosterone: anticoagulant effect of phenindione enhanced by •testosterone
- Thyroid Hormones: anticoagulant effect of phenindione enhanced by •thyroid hormones
- Vitamins: anticoagulant effect of phenindione antagonised by •vitamin K

## Phenobarbital

Note Primidone interactions as for phenobarbital

Alcohol: increased sedative effect when phenobarbital given with alcohol

Analgesics: phenobarbital reduces plasma concentration of methadone; phenobarbital possibly accelerates metabolism of paracetamol (also isolated reports of hepatotoxicity)

- Anti-arrhythmics: phenobarbital accelerates metabolism of disopyramide (reduced plasma concentration); phenobarbital possibly reduces plasma concentration of •dronedarone—avoid concomitant use; phenobarbital possibly accelerates metabolism of propafenone
- Antibacterials: phenobarbital accelerates metabolism of metronidazole (reduced effect); phenobarbital possibly reduces plasma concentration of rifampicin; phenobarbital accelerates metabolism of doxycycline (reduced plasma concentration); phenobarbital possibly accelerates metabolism of •chloramphenicol (reduced plasma concentration); phenobarbital reduces plasma concentration of •telithromycin (avoid during and for 2 weeks after phenobarbital)
- Anticoagulants: phenobarbital accelerates metabolism of •coumarins (reduced anticoagulant effect)
- Antidepressants: phenobarbital possibly reduces plasma concentration of reboxetine; phenobarbital reduces plasma concentration of paroxetine; phenobarbital accelerates metabolism of •mianserin (reduced plasma concentration); anticonvulsant effect of antiepileptics possibly antagonised by MAOIs and •tricyclic-related antidepressants (convulsive threshold lowered); anticonvulsant effect of antiepileptics antagonised by •SSRIs and •tricyclics (convulsive threshold lowered); avoid concomitant use of antiepileptics with •St John's wort; phenobarbital possibly accelerates metabolism of •tricyclics (reduced plasma concentration)
- Antiepileptics: plasma concentration of phenobarbital possibly increased by carbamazepine; phenobarbital possibly reduces plasma concentration of ethosuximide, rufinamide and topiramate; phenobarbital reduces plasma concentration of lamotrigine, tiagabine and zonisamide; plasma concentration of phenobarbital increased by oxcarbazepine, also plasma concentration of an active metabolite of oxcarbazepine reduced; plasma concentration of phenobarbital often increased by phenytoin, plasma concentration of phenytoin often reduced but may be increased; plasma concentration of phenobarbital increased by •stiripentol; plasma concentration of phenobarbital increased by valproate (also plasma concentration of valproate reduced)
- Antifungals: phenobarbital possibly reduces plasma concentration of itraconazole and •posaconazole; phenobarbital possibly reduces plasma concentration of •voriconazole—avoid concomitant use; phenobarbital reduces absorption of griseofulvin (reduced effect)
- Antimalarials: avoidance of phenobarbital advised by manufacturer of piperaquine with artenimol;

**Phenobarbital**

- Antimalarials (continued)
  anticonvulsant effect of antiepileptics antagonised by •mefloquine
- Antipsychotics: anticonvulsant effect of antiepileptics antagonised by •antipsychotics (convulsive threshold lowered); phenobarbital accelerates metabolism of haloperidol (reduced plasma concentration); plasma concentration of both drugs reduced when phenobarbital given with chlorpromazine; phenobarbital possibly reduces plasma concentration of •aripiprazole—increase dose of aripiprazole; phenobarbital possibly reduces plasma concentration of clozapine
- Antivirals: phenobarbital possibly reduces plasma concentration of abacavir, darunavir, fosamprenavir, •indinavir, •lopinavir and •saquinavir; avoidance of phenobarbital advised by manufacturer of •boceprevir and •rilpivirine (plasma concentration of boceprevir and rilpivirine possibly reduced); avoidance of phenobarbital advised by manufacturer of etravirine and •telaprevir

Anxiolytics and Hypnotics: phenobarbital often reduces plasma concentration of clonazepam

Aprepitant: phenobarbital possibly reduces plasma concentration of aprepitant

Beta-blockers: phenobarbital possibly reduces plasma concentration of propranolol

- Calcium-channel Blockers: phenobarbital probably reduces effects of •calcium-channel blockers; avoidance of phenobarbital advised by manufacturer of isradipine; avoidance of phenobarbital advised by manufacturer of •nimodipine (plasma concentration of nimodipine reduced)
- Ciclosporin: phenobarbital accelerates metabolism of •ciclosporin (reduced plasma concentration)
- Corticosteroids: phenobarbital accelerates metabolism of •corticosteroids (reduced effect)
- Cytotoxics: phenobarbital possibly decreases plasma concentration of axitinib (increase dose of axitinib—consult axitinib product literature); phenobarbital possibly reduces plasma concentration of crizotinib—manufacturer of crizotinib advises avoid concomitant use; avoidance of phenobarbital advised by manufacturer of •cabazitaxel and gefitinib; avoidance of phenobarbital advised by manufacturer of vandetanib (plasma concentration of vandetanib possibly reduced); phenobarbital possibly reduces plasma concentration of etoposide; phenobarbital reduces plasma concentration of irinotecan and its active metabolite
- Diuretics: phenobarbital reduces plasma concentration of •eplerenone—avoid concomitant use; increased risk of osteomalacia when phenobarbital given with carbonic anhydrase inhibitors

Folates: plasma concentration of phenobarbital possibly reduced by folates

Hormone Antagonists: phenobarbital accelerates metabolism of toremifene (reduced plasma concentration)

Leukotriene Receptor Antagonists: phenobarbital reduces plasma concentration of montelukast

- Oestrogens: phenobarbital accelerates metabolism of •oestrogens (reduced contraceptive effect—see p. 398)
- Orlistat: possible increased risk of convulsions when antiepileptics given with •orlistat
- Progestogens: phenobarbital accelerates metabolism of •progestogens (reduced contraceptive effect—see p. 398)

Sodium Oxybate: avoidance of phenobarbital advised by manufacturer of sodium oxybate

Sympathomimetics: plasma concentration of phenobarbital possibly increased by methylphenidate

- Tacrolimus: phenobarbital reduces plasma concentration of •tacrolimus

**Phenobarbital** (continued)

- Theophylline: phenobarbital accelerates metabolism of •theophylline (reduced effect)

Thyroid Hormones: phenobarbital accelerates metabolism of thyroid hormones (may increase requirements for thyroid hormones in hypothyroidism)

Ticagrelor: phenobarbital possibly reduces plasma concentration of ticagrelor

- Ulipristal: avoidance of phenobarbital advised by manufacturer of •ulipristal (contraceptive effect of ulipristal possibly reduced)

Vitamins: phenobarbital possibly increases requirements for vitamin D

**Phenothiazines** see Antipsychotics

**Phenoxybenzamine** see Alpha-blockers

**Phenoxymethylpenicillin** see Penicillins

**Phentolamine** see Alpha-blockers

**Phenylephrine** see Sympathomimetics

**Phenytoin**

Note Fosphenytoin interactions as for phenytoin

Alcohol: plasma concentration of phenytoin possibly reduced by chronic heavy consumption of alcohol

Analgesics: phenytoin accelerates metabolism of methadone (reduced effect and risk of withdrawal effects); effects of phenytoin enhanced by aspirin; phenytoin possibly accelerates metabolism of paracetamol (also isolated reports of hepatotoxicity)

Antacids: absorption of phenytoin reduced by antacids

- Anti-arrhythmics: metabolism of phenytoin inhibited by •amiodarone (increased plasma concentration); phenytoin reduces plasma concentration of disopyramide; phenytoin possibly reduces plasma concentration of •dronedarone—avoid concomitant use
- Antibacterials: metabolism of phenytoin inhibited by clarithromycin (increased plasma concentration); metabolism of phenytoin possibly inhibited by metronidazole (increased plasma concentration); plasma concentration of phenytoin increased or decreased by ciprofloxacin; phenytoin accelerates metabolism of doxycycline (reduced plasma concentration); plasma concentration of phenytoin increased by •chloramphenicol (increased risk of toxicity); metabolism of phenytoin possibly inhibited by isoniazid (increased risk of toxicity); metabolism of phenytoin accelerated by •rifamycins (reduced plasma concentration); plasma concentration of phenytoin possibly increased by sulfonamides; phenytoin reduces plasma concentration of •telithromycin (avoid during and for 2 weeks after phenytoin); plasma concentration of phenytoin increased by •trimethoprim (also increased antifolate effect)
- Anticoagulants: phenytoin accelerates metabolism of •coumarins (possibility of reduced anticoagulant effect, but enhancement also reported); phenytoin possibly reduces plasma concentration of dabigatran etexilate—manufacturer of dabigatran etexilate advises avoid concomitant use
- Antidepressants: plasma concentration of phenytoin increased by •fluoxetine and •fluvoxamine; phenytoin reduces plasma concentration of •mianserin, mirtazapine and paroxetine; plasma concentration of phenytoin possibly increased by sertraline, also plasma concentration of sertraline possibly reduced; anticonvulsant effect of antiepileptics possibly antagonised by MAOIs and •tricyclic-related antidepressants (convulsive threshold lowered); anticonvulsant effect of antiepileptics antagonised by •SSRIs and •tricyclics (convulsive threshold lowered); avoid concomitant use of antiepileptics with •St John's wort; phenytoin possibly reduces plasma concentration of •tricyclics

Antidiabetics: plasma concentration of phenytoin transiently increased by tolbutamide (possibility of toxicity)

**Phenytoin** (continued)

- Antiepileptics: plasma concentration of both drugs often reduced when phenytoin given with carbamazepine, also plasma concentration of phenytoin may be increased; phenytoin reduces plasma concentration of eslicarbazepine, also plasma concentration of phenytoin increased; plasma concentration of phenytoin possibly increased by •ethosuximide, also plasma concentration of ethosuximide possibly reduced; phenytoin reduces plasma concentration of lamotrigine, tiagabine and zonisamide; plasma concentration of phenytoin increased by oxcarbazepine, also plasma concentration of an active metabolite of oxcarbazepine reduced; phenytoin reduces plasma concentration of •perampanel (see Dose under Perampanel, p. 224); phenytoin often increases plasma concentration of phenobarbital, plasma concentration of phenytoin often reduced but may be increased; phenytoin possibly reduces plasma concentration of retigabine; phenytoin possibly reduces plasma concentration of rufinamide, also plasma concentration of phenytoin possibly increased; plasma concentration of phenytoin increased by •stiripentol; plasma concentration of phenytoin increased by •topiramate (also plasma concentration of topiramate reduced); plasma concentration of phenytoin increased or possibly reduced when given with valproate, also plasma concentration of valproate reduced; plasma concentration of phenytoin reduced by vigabatrin
- Antifungals: phenytoin reduces plasma concentration of •ketoconazole and •posaconazole; anticonvulsant effect of phenytoin enhanced by •miconazole (plasma concentration of phenytoin increased); plasma concentration of phenytoin increased by •fluconazole (consider reducing dose of phenytoin); phenytoin reduces plasma concentration of •itraconazole—avoid concomitant use; plasma concentration of phenytoin increased by •voriconazole, also phenytoin reduces plasma concentration of voriconazole (increase dose of voriconazole and also monitor for phenytoin toxicity); phenytoin possibly reduces plasma concentration of caspofungin—consider increasing dose of caspofungin
- Antimalarials: avoidance of phenytoin advised by manufacturer of piperaquine with artenimol; anticonvulsant effect of antiepileptics antagonised by •mefloquine; anticonvulsant effect of phenytoin antagonised by •pyrimethamine, also increased antifolate effect
- Antipsychotics: anticonvulsant effect of antiepileptics antagonised by •antipsychotics (convulsive threshold lowered); phenytoin reduces plasma concentration of haloperidol; plasma concentration of phenytoin possibly increased or decreased by chlorpromazine; phenytoin possibly reduces plasma concentration of •aripiprazole—increase dose of aripiprazole; phenytoin accelerates metabolism of clozapine and quetiapine (reduced plasma concentration)
- Antivirals: phenytoin possibly reduces plasma concentration of abacavir, darunavir, lopinavir and saquinavir; avoidance of phenytoin advised by manufacturer of •boceprevir and •rilpivirine (plasma concentration of boceprevir and rilpivirine possibly reduced); avoidance of phenytoin advised by manufacturer of etravirine and •telaprevir; phenytoin possibly reduces plasma concentration of •indinavir, also plasma concentration of phenytoin possibly increased; phenytoin possibly reduces plasma concentration of ritonavir, also plasma concentration of phenytoin possibly affected; plasma concentration of phenytoin increased or decreased by zidovudine

**Phenytoin** (continued)

Anxiolytics and Hypnotics: phenytoin often reduces plasma concentration of clonazepam; plasma concentration of phenytoin increased or decreased by diazepam; plasma concentration of phenytoin possibly increased or decreased by benzodiazepines

Aprepitant: phenytoin possibly reduces plasma concentration of aprepitant

Bupropion: phenytoin reduces plasma concentration of bupropion

- Calcium-channel Blockers: phenytoin reduces effects of felodipine and verapamil; avoidance of phenytoin advised by manufacturer of isradipine; avoidance of phenytoin advised by manufacturer of nimodipine (plasma concentration of nimodipine possibly reduced); plasma concentration of phenytoin increased by •diltiazem but also effect of diltiazem reduced

Cardiac Glycosides: phenytoin possibly reduces plasma concentration of digoxin

- Ciclosporin: phenytoin accelerates metabolism of •ciclosporin (reduced plasma concentration)
- Corticosteroids: phenytoin accelerates metabolism of •corticosteroids (reduced effect)
- Cytotoxics: phenytoin possibly reduces plasma concentration of busulfan, eribulin and etoposide; metabolism of phenytoin possibly inhibited by fluorouracil (increased risk of toxicity); phenytoin increases antifolate effect of methotrexate; plasma concentration of phenytoin possibly reduced by cisplatin; phenytoin possibly decreases plasma concentration of axitinib (increase dose of axitinib—consult axitinib product literature); phenytoin possibly reduces plasma concentration of crizotinib—manufacturer of crizotinib advises avoid concomitant use; avoidance of phenytoin advised by manufacturer of •cabazitaxel, gefitinib, •lapatinib and vemurafenib; phenytoin reduces plasma concentration of •imatinib—avoid concomitant use; phenytoin reduces plasma concentration of irinotecan and its active metabolite

Diazoxide: plasma concentration of phenytoin reduced by diazoxide, also effect of diazoxide may be reduced

- Disulfiram: metabolism of phenytoin inhibited by •disulfiram (increased risk of toxicity)
- Diuretics: plasma concentration of phenytoin possibly increased by •acetazolamide; phenytoin antagonises effects of furosemide; phenytoin reduces plasma concentration of •eplerenone—avoid concomitant use; increased risk of osteomalacia when phenytoin given with carbonic anhydrase inhibitors

Dopaminergics: phenytoin possibly reduces effects of levodopa

Enteral Foods: absorption of phenytoin possibly reduced by enteral feeds

Folates: plasma concentration of phenytoin possibly reduced by folates

Hormone Antagonists: phenytoin possibly accelerates metabolism of toremifene

5HT$_3$-receptor Antagonists: phenytoin accelerates metabolism of ondansetron (reduced effect)

Leflunomide: plasma concentration of phenytoin possibly increased by leflunomide

Levamisole: plasma concentration of phenytoin possibly increased by levamisole

Lipid-regulating Drugs: absorption of phenytoin possibly reduced by colesevelam; combination of phenytoin with fluvastatin may increase plasma concentration of either drug (or both)

Lithium: neurotoxicity may occur when phenytoin given with lithium without increased plasma concentration of lithium

Modafinil: plasma concentration of phenytoin possibly increased by modafinil

**Phenytoin** *(continued)*

- Muscle Relaxants: *long-term use* of phenytoin reduces effects of ●non-depolarising muscle relaxants (but *acute use* of phenytoin might increase effects of non-depolarising muscle relaxants)
- Oestrogens: phenytoin accelerates metabolism of ●oestrogens (reduced contraceptive effect—see p. 398)
- Orlistat: possible increased risk of convulsions when antiepileptics given with ●orlistat
- Progestogens: phenytoin accelerates metabolism of ●progestogens (reduced contraceptive effect—see p. 398)
- Sulfinpyrazone: plasma concentration of phenytoin increased by ●sulfinpyrazone
  Sympathomimetics: plasma concentration of phenytoin increased by methylphenidate
  Tacrolimus: phenytoin reduces plasma concentration of tacrolimus, also plasma concentration of phenytoin possibly increased
- Theophylline: plasma concentration of both drugs reduced when phenytoin given with ●theophylline
  Thyroid Hormones: phenytoin accelerates metabolism of thyroid hormones (may increase requirements in hypothyroidism), also plasma concentration of phenytoin possibly increased
  Tibolone: phenytoin accelerates metabolism of tibolone
  Ticagrelor: phenytoin possibly reduces plasma concentration of ticagrelor
- Ulcer-healing Drugs: metabolism of phenytoin inhibited by ●cimetidine (increased plasma concentration); effects of phenytoin enhanced by ●esomeprazole; effects of phenytoin possibly enhanced by omeprazole; absorption of phenytoin reduced by ●sucralfate
- Ulipristal: avoidance of phenytoin advised by manufacturer of ●ulipristal (contraceptive effect of ulipristal possibly reduced)
  Vaccines: effects of phenytoin enhanced by influenza vaccine
  Vitamins: phenytoin possibly increases requirements for vitamin D

**Pholcodine**

  Antidepressants: manufacturer of pholcodine advises avoid for 2 weeks after stopping MAOIs

**Phosphodiesterase Type-3 Inhibitors**

- Anagrelide: avoidance of enoximone and milrinone advised by manufacturer of ●anagrelide

**Physostigmine** *see* Parasympathomimetics
**Pilocarpine** *see* Parasympathomimetics
**Pimozide** *see* Antipsychotics
**Pindolol** *see* Beta-blockers
**Pioglitazone** *see* Antidiabetics
**Piperacillin** *see* Penicillins
**Piperaquine** *see* Piperaquine with Artenimol

**Piperaquine with Artenimol**

  **Note** Piperaquine has a long half-life; there is a potential for drug interactions to occur for up to 3 months after treatment has been stopped

- Analgesics: manufacturer of piperaquine with artenimol advises avoid concomitant use with ●methadone (possible risk of ventricular arrhythmias)
- Anti-arrhythmics: manufacturer of piperaquine with artenimol advises avoid concomitant use with ●amiodarone and ●disopyramide (possible risk of ventricular arrhythmias)
- Antibacterials: manufacturer of piperaquine with artenimol advises avoid concomitant use with ●macrolides and ●moxifloxacin (possible risk of ventricular arrhythmias); manufacturer of piperaquine with artenimol advises avoid concomitant use with rifampicin
- Antidepressants: manufacturer of piperaquine with artenimol advises avoid concomitant use with ●antidepressants

**Piperaquine with Artenimol** *(continued)*

  Antiepileptics: manufacturer of piperaquine with artenimol advises avoid concomitant use with carbamazepine, phenobarbital and phenytoin

- Antifungals: manufacturer of piperaquine with artenimol advises avoid concomitant use with ●imidazoles and ●triazoles (possible risk of ventricular arrhythmias)
- Antihistamines: manufacturer of piperaquine with artenimol advises avoid concomitant use with ●mizolastine (possible risk of ventricular arrhythmias)
- Antimalarials: avoidance of antimalarials advised by manufacturer of ●artemether with lumefantrine
- Antipsychotics: manufacturer of piperaquine with artenimol advises avoid concomitant use with ●droperidol, ●haloperidol, ●phenothiazines and ●pimozide (possible risk of ventricular arrhythmias)
- Antivirals: manufacturer of piperaquine with artenimol advises avoid concomitant use with ●saquinavir (possible risk of ventricular arrhythmias)
- Beta-blockers: manufacturer of piperaquine with artenimol advises avoid concomitant use with ●sotalol (possible risk of ventricular arrhythmias)
- Cytotoxics: manufacturer of piperaquine with artenimol advises avoid concomitant use with ●arsenic trioxide (possible risk of ventricular arrhythmias); manufacturer of piperaquine with artenimol advises avoid concomitant use with ●vinblastine, ●vincristine, ●vinflunine and ●vinorelbine
- Domperidone: manufacturer of piperaquine with artenimol advises avoid concomitant use with ●domperidone (possible risk of ventricular arrhythmias)
  Grapefruit Juice: manufacturer of piperaquine with artenimol advises avoid concomitant use with grapefruit juice
  Histamine: avoidance of antimalarials advised by manufacturer of histamine
- Pentamidine Isetionate: manufacturer of piperaquine with artenimol advises avoid concomitant use with ●pentamidine isetionate (possible risk of ventricular arrhythmias)
  Vaccines: antimalarials inactivate oral typhoid vaccine—see p. 621

**Pipotiazine** *see* Antipsychotics
**Pirfenidone**

- Antidepressants: plasma concentration of pirfenidone increased by ●fluvoxamine—manufacturer of pirfenidone advises avoid concomitant use
  Grapefruit Juice: manufacturer of pirfenidone advises avoid concomitant use with grapefruit juice

**Piroxicam** *see* NSAIDs
**Pivmecillinam** *see* Penicillins
**Pizotifen**

  Adrenergic Neurone Blockers: pizotifen antagonises hypotensive effect of adrenergic neurone blockers

**Platinum Compounds**

- Aldesleukin: avoidance of cisplatin advised by manufacturer of ●aldesleukin
- Antibacterials: increased risk of nephrotoxicity and possibly of ototoxicity when platinum compounds given with ●aminoglycosides or ●polymyxins; increased risk of nephrotoxicity and ototoxicity when platinum compounds given with capreomycin; increased risk of nephrotoxicity and possibly of ototoxicity when cisplatin given with vancomycin
  Antiepileptics: cisplatin possibly reduces plasma concentration of phenytoin
- Antipsychotics: avoid concomitant use of cytotoxics with ●clozapine (increased risk of agranulocytosis)
- Cytotoxics: increased risk of ototoxicity when cisplatin given with ifosfamide; increased pulmonary toxicity when cisplatin given with ●bleomycin and ●methotrexate
  Diuretics: increased risk of nephrotoxicity and ototoxicity when platinum compounds given with diuretics

**Polymyxin B** *see* Polymyxins
**Polymyxins**
 Antibacterials: increased risk of nephrotoxicity when colistimethate sodium or polymyxins given with aminoglycosides; increased risk of nephrotoxicity when colistimethate sodium or polymyxins given with capreomycin; increased risk of nephrotoxicity when polymyxins given with vancomycin; increased risk of nephrotoxicity and ototoxicity when colistimethate sodium given with vancomycin
 Antifungals: increased risk of nephrotoxicity when polymyxins given with amphotericin
- Ciclosporin: increased risk of nephrotoxicity when polymyxins given with ●ciclosporin
- Cytotoxics: increased risk of nephrotoxicity and possibly of ototoxicity when polymyxins given with ●platinum compounds
- Diuretics: increased risk of otoxicity when polymyxins given with ●loop diuretics
- Muscle Relaxants: polymyxins enhance effects of ●non-depolarising muscle relaxants and ●suxamethonium
- Parasympathomimetics: polymyxins antagonise effects of ●neostigmine and ●pyridostigmine
 Vaccines: antibacterials inactivate oral typhoid vaccine—see p. 621

**Polystyrene Sulfonate Resins**
 Antacids: risk of intestinal obstruction when polystyrene sulfonate resins given with aluminium hydroxide; risk of metabolic alkalosis when polystyrene sulfonate resins given with oral magnesium salts
 Thyroid Hormones: polystyrene sulfonate resins reduce absorption of levothyroxine

**Posaconazole** *see* Antifungals, Triazole
**Potassium Canrenoate** *see* Diuretics
**Potassium Aminobenzoate**
 Antibacterials: potassium aminobenzoate inhibits effects of sulfonamides

**Potassium Bicarbonate** *see* Potassium Salts
**Potassium Chloride** *see* Potassium Salts
**Potassium Citrate** *see* Potassium Salts
**Potassium Salts**
 **Note** Includes salt substitutes
- ACE Inhibitors: increased risk of severe hyperkalaemia when potassium salts given with ●ACE inhibitors
- Aliskiren: increased risk of hyperkalaemia when potassium salts given with aliskiren
- Angiotensin-II Receptor Antagonists: increased risk of hyperkalaemia when potassium salts given with ●angiotensin-II receptor antagonists
 Antibacterials: avoid concomitant use of potassium citrate with methenamine
- Ciclosporin: increased risk of hyperkalaemia when potassium salts given with ●ciclosporin
- Diuretics: increased risk of hyperkalaemia when potassium salts given with ●potassium-sparing diuretics and aldosterone antagonists
- Tacrolimus: increased risk of hyperkalaemia when potassium salts given with ●tacrolimus

**Pramipexole**
 Antipsychotics: manufacturer of pramipexole advises avoid concomitant use of antipsychotics (antagonism of effect)
 Memantine: effects of dopaminergics possibly enhanced by memantine
 Methyldopa: antiparkinsonian effect of dopaminergics antagonised by methyldopa
 Ulcer-healing Drugs: excretion of pramipexole reduced by cimetidine (increased plasma concentration)

**Prasugrel**
 Analgesics: possible increased risk of bleeding when prasugrel given with NSAIDs

**Prasugrel** *(continued)*
 Anticoagulants: possible increased risk of bleeding when prasugrel given with coumarins or phenindione
 Clopidogrel: possible increased risk of bleeding when prasugrel given with clopidogrel

**Pravastatin** *see* Statins
**Prazosin** *see* Alpha-blockers
**Prednisolone** *see* Corticosteroids
**Prednisone** *see* Corticosteroids
**Pregabalin**
- Antidepressants: anticonvulsant effect of antiepileptics possibly antagonised by MAOIs and ●tricyclic-related antidepressants (convulsive threshold lowered); anticonvulsant effect of antiepileptics antagonised by ●SSRIs and ●tricyclics (convulsive threshold lowered); avoid concomitant use of antiepileptics with ●St John's wort
- Antimalarials: anticonvulsant effect of antiepileptics antagonised by ●mefloquine
- Antipsychotics: anticonvulsant effect of antiepileptics antagonised by ●antipsychotics (convulsive threshold lowered)
- Orlistat: possible increased risk of convulsions when antiepileptics given with ●orlistat

**Prilocaine**
 Anti-arrhythmics: increased myocardial depression when prilocaine given with anti-arrhythmics
 Antibacterials: increased risk of methaemoglobinaemia when prilocaine given with sulfonamides

**Primaquine**
- Antimalarials: avoidance of antimalarials advised by manufacturer of ●artemether with lumefantrine
 Histamine: avoidance of antimalarials advised by manufacturer of histamine
 Mepacrine: plasma concentration of primaquine increased by mepacrine (increased risk of toxicity)
 Vaccines: antimalarials inactivate oral typhoid vaccine—see p. 621

**Primidone** *see* Phenobarbital
**Probenecid**
 ACE Inhibitors: probenecid reduces excretion of captopril
 Anaesthetics, General: probenecid possibly enhances effects of thiopental
- Analgesics: probenecid reduces excretion of ●acemetacin, ●dexketoprofen, ●indometacin, ●ketoprofen and ●naproxen (increased plasma concentration); probenecid reduces excretion of ●ketorolac (increased plasma concentration)—avoid concomitant use; effects of probenecid antagonised by aspirin
 Antibacterials: probenecid reduces excretion of doripenem (manufacturers of doripenem advise avoid concomitant use); probenecid reduces excretion of meropenem; probenecid reduces excretion of cephalosporins, ciprofloxacin, nalidixic acid, norfloxacin and penicillins (increased plasma concentration); probenecid reduces excretion of dapsone and nitrofurantoin (increased risk of side-effects); effects of probenecid antagonised by pyrazinamide
- Antivirals: probenecid reduces excretion of aciclovir (increased plasma concentration); probenecid possibly reduces excretion of famciclovir (increased plasma concentration); probenecid reduces excretion of ganciclovir and ●zidovudine (increased plasma concentration and risk of toxicity)
 Anxiolytics and Hypnotics: probenecid reduces excretion of lorazepam (increased plasma concentration); probenecid possibly reduces excretion of nitrazepam (increased plasma concentration)
- Cytotoxics: probenecid reduces excretion of ●methotrexate (increased risk of toxicity)
 Sodium Benzoate: probenecid possibly reduces excretion of conjugate formed by sodium benzoate

**Probenecid** *(continued)*
    Sodium Phenylbutyrate: probenecid possibly reduces excretion of conjugate formed by sodium phenylbutyrate

**Procarbazine**
    Alcohol: disulfiram-like reaction when procarbazine given with alcohol
- Antipsychotics: avoid concomitant use of cytotoxics with ●clozapine (increased risk of agranulocytosis)
    Cardiac Glycosides: procarbazine possibly reduces absorption of digoxin *tablets*

**Prochlorperazine** *see* Antipsychotics

**Procyclidine** *see* Antimuscarinics

**Progesterone** *see* Progestogens

**Progestogens**

    **Note** Interactions of combined oral contraceptives may also apply to combined contraceptive patches and vaginal rings, see p. 398. For further information on interactions of oral progestogen-only contraceptives, see also p. 403; parenteral progestogen-only contraceptives, see also p. 404; the intra-uterine progestogen-only device, see also p. 405; hormonal emergency contraception, see also p. 409

- Antibacterials: plasma concentration of dienogest increased by erythromycin; metabolism of progestogens accelerated by ●rifamycins (reduced contraceptive effect—see p. 398)
- Anticoagulants: progestogens may enhance or reduce anticoagulant effect of coumarins; progestogens antagonise anticoagulant effect of ●phenindione
- Antidepressants: contraceptive effect of progestogens reduced by ●St John's wort (avoid concomitant use)
    Antidiabetics: progestogens antagonise hypoglycaemic effect of antidiabetics
- Antiepileptics: metabolism of progestogens accelerated by ●carbamazepine, ●eslicarbazepine, ●oxcarbazepine, ●perampanel, ●phenobarbital, ●phenytoin, ●rufinamide and ●topiramate (reduced contraceptive effect—see p. 398); desogestrel possibly increases plasma concentration of lamotrigine
    Antifungals: progestogens possibly increase plasma concentration of voriconazole; anecdotal reports of contraceptive failure and menstrual irregularities when progestogens given with griseofulvin; occasional reports of breakthrough bleeding when progestogens (used for contraception) given with terbinafine
- Antivirals: plasma concentration of norethisterone increased by atazanavir; plasma concentration of drospirenone increased by boceprevir (increased risk of toxicity); contraceptive effect of progestogens possibly reduced by ●efavirenz; metabolism of progestogens accelerated by ●nevirapine (reduced contraceptive effect—see p. 398)
    Anxiolytics and Hypnotics: progestogens possibly increase plasma concentration of diazepam
- Aprepitant: possible contraceptive failure of hormonal contraceptives containing progestogens when given with ●aprepitant (alternative contraception recommended)
- Bosentan: possible contraceptive failure of hormonal contraceptives containing progestogens when given with ●bosentan (alternative contraception recommended)
    Ciclosporin: progestogens possibly increase plasma concentration of ciclosporin
- Cytotoxics: possible reduction in contraceptive effect of progestogens advised by manufacturer of ●crizotinib and ●vemurafenib
    Diuretics: risk of hyperkalaemia when drospirenone given with potassium-sparing diuretics and aldosterone antagonists (monitor serum potassium during first cycle)
- Dopaminergics: progestogens increase plasma concentration of ●selegiline—manufacturer of selegiline advises avoid concomitant use

**Progestogens** *(continued)*
    Lipid-regulating Drugs: plasma concentration of norethisterone increased by atorvastatin; plasma concentration of active metabolite of norgestimate increased by rosuvastatin; plasma concentration of norgestrel increased by rosuvastatin
    Muscle Relaxants: progestogens possibly increase plasma concentration of tizanidine (increased risk of toxicity)
    Sugammadex: plasma concentration of progestogens possibly reduced by sugammadex—manufacturer of sugammadex advises additional contraceptive precautions
- Ulipristal: contraceptive effect of progestogens possibly reduced by ●ulipristal

**Proguanil**
    Antacids: absorption of proguanil reduced by oral magnesium salts (as magnesium trisilicate)
    Anticoagulants: isolated reports that proguanil may enhance anticoagulant effect of warfarin
- Antimalarials: avoidance of antimalarials advised by manufacturer of ●artemether with lumefantrine; increased antifolate effect when proguanil given with pyrimethamine
    Antivirals: plasma concentration of proguanil possibly affected by efavirenz
    Histamine: avoidance of antimalarials advised by manufacturer of histamine
    Vaccines: antimalarials inactivate oral typhoid vaccine—see p. 621

**Promazine** *see* Antipsychotics

**Promethazine** *see* Antihistamines

**Propafenone**
    Anaesthetics, Local: increased myocardial depression when anti-arrhythmics given with bupivacaine, levobupivacaine, prilocaine or ropivacaine
- Anti-arrhythmics: increased myocardial depression when anti-arrhythmics given with other ●anti-arrhythmics
- Antibacterials: metabolism of propafenone accelerated by ●rifampicin (reduced effect)
- Anticoagulants: propafenone enhances anticoagulant effect of ●coumarins
- Antidepressants: metabolism of propafenone possibly inhibited by fluoxetine and paroxetine; increased risk of arrhythmias when propafenone given with ●tricyclics
    Antiepileptics: metabolism of propafenone possibly accelerated by phenobarbital
    Antihistamines: avoidance of propafenone advised by manufacturer of mizolastine (possible risk of ventricular arrhythmias)
- Antipsychotics: increased risk of ventricular arrhythmias when anti-arrhythmics that prolong the QT interval given with ●antipsychotics that prolong the QT interval
- Antivirals: plasma concentration of propafenone possibly increased by ●fosamprenavir (increased risk of ventricular arrhythmias—avoid concomitant use); plasma concentration of propafenone increased by ●ritonavir (increased risk of ventricular arrhythmias—avoid concomitant use); increased risk of ventricular arrhythmias when propafenone given with ●saquinavir—avoid concomitant use; caution with propafenone advised by manufacturer of ●telaprevir (risk of ventricular arrhythmias)
- Beta-blockers: increased myocardial depression when anti-arrhythmics given with ●beta-blockers; propafenone increases plasma concentration of metoprolol and propranolol
- Cardiac Glycosides: propafenone increases plasma concentration of ●digoxin (halve dose of digoxin)
    Ciclosporin: propafenone possibly increases plasma concentration of ciclosporin
    Parasympathomimetics: propafenone possibly antagonises effects of neostigmine and pyridostigmine

**Propafenone** (continued)

Theophylline: propafenone increases plasma concentration of theophylline

• Ulcer-healing Drugs: plasma concentration of propafenone increased by ●cimetidine

**Propantheline** see Antimuscarinics

**Propiverine** see Antimuscarinics

**Propofol** see Anaesthetics, General

**Propranolol** see Beta-blockers

**Prostaglandins**

ACE Inhibitors: enhanced hypotensive effect when alprostadil given with ACE inhibitors

Adrenergic Neurone Blockers: enhanced hypotensive effect when alprostadil given with adrenergic neurone blockers

Alpha-blockers: enhanced hypotensive effect when alprostadil given with alpha-blockers

Angiotensin-II Receptor Antagonists: enhanced hypotensive effect when alprostadil given with angiotensin-II receptor antagonists

Beta-blockers: enhanced hypotensive effect when alprostadil given with beta-blockers

Calcium-channel Blockers: enhanced hypotensive effect when alprostadil given with calcium-channel blockers

Clonidine: enhanced hypotensive effect when alprostadil given with clonidine

Diazoxide: enhanced hypotensive effect when alprostadil given with diazoxide

Diuretics: enhanced hypotensive effect when alprostadil given with diuretics

Methyldopa: enhanced hypotensive effect when alprostadil given with methyldopa

Moxonidine: enhanced hypotensive effect when alprostadil given with moxonidine

Nitrates: enhanced hypotensive effect when alprostadil given with nitrates

Oxytocin: prostaglandins potentiate uterotonic effect of oxytocin

Vasodilator Antihypertensives: enhanced hypotensive effect when alprostadil given with hydralazine, minoxidil or sodium nitroprusside

**Protein Kinase Inhibitors** see Axitinib, Crizotinib, Dasatinib, Erlotinib, Everolimus, Gefitinib, Imatinib, Lapatinib, Nilotinib, Pazopanib, Ruxolitinib, Sorafenib, Sunitinib, Temsirolimus, Vandetanib, and Vemurafenib

**Proton Pump Inhibitors**

Antacids: absorption of lansoprazole possibly reduced by antacids

Antibacterials: plasma concentration of both drugs increased when omeprazole given with clarithromycin

• Anticoagulants: esomeprazole, omeprazole and pantoprazole possibly enhance anticoagulant effect of ●coumarins

Antidepressants: omeprazole increases plasma concentration of escitalopram; plasma concentration of lansoprazole possibly increased by fluvoxamine; plasma concentration of omeprazole possibly reduced by St John's wort

• Antiepileptics: omeprazole possibly enhances effects of phenytoin; esomeprazole enhances effects of ●phenytoin

Antifungals: proton pump inhibitors reduce absorption of itraconazole and ketoconazole; avoidance of proton pump inhibitors advised by manufacturer of posaconazole (plasma concentration of posaconazole possibly reduced); plasma concentration of esomeprazole possibly increased by voriconazole; plasma concentration of omeprazole increased by voriconazole (consider reducing dose of omeprazole)

Antipsychotics: omeprazole possibly reduces plasma concentration of clozapine

**Proton Pump Inhibitors** (continued)

• Antivirals: proton pump inhibitors reduce plasma concentration of ●atazanavir—avoid or adjust dose of both drugs (consult product literature); omeprazole increases plasma concentration of raltegravir; avoidance of esomeprazole, lansoprazole, pantoprazole and rabeprazole advised by manufacturer of rilpivirine (plasma concentration of rilpivirine possibly reduced); omeprazole reduces plasma concentration of ●rilpivirine—avoid concomitant use; esomeprazole, lansoprazole, pantoprazole and rabeprazole possibly increase plasma concentration of ●saquinavir—manufacturer of saquinavir advises avoid concomitant use; omeprazole increases plasma concentration of ●saquinavir—manufacturer of saquinavir advises avoid concomitant use; plasma concentration of esomeprazole and omeprazole reduced by ●tipranavir

Anxiolytics and Hypnotics: esomeprazole and omeprazole possibly inhibit metabolism of diazepam (increased plasma concentration)

Cardiac Glycosides: proton pump inhibitors possibly slightly increase plasma concentration of digoxin

Ciclosporin: omeprazole possibly affects plasma concentration of ciclosporin

Cilostazol: omeprazole increases plasma concentration of cilostazol (consider reducing dose of cilostazol)

• Clopidogrel: esomeprazole and omeprazole reduce antiplatelet effect of ●clopidogrel; lansoprazole, pantoprazole and rabeprazole possibly reduce antiplatelet effect of clopidogrel

• Cytotoxics: proton pump inhibitors possibly reduce excretion of methotrexate (increased risk of toxicity); avoidance of esomeprazole, lansoprazole, pantoprazole and rabeprazole advised by manufacturer of ●erlotinib; omeprazole reduces plasma concentration of ●erlotinib—manufacturer of erlotinib advises avoid concomitant use; proton pump inhibitors possibly reduce absorption of lapatinib; proton pump inhibitors possibly reduce absorption of pazopanib—manufacturer of pazopanib advises give at the same time as proton pump inhibitors; avoidance of proton pump inhibitors advised by manufacturer of vandetanib (absorption of vandetanib possibly reduced)

Tacrolimus: omeprazole possibly increases plasma concentration of tacrolimus

Ulcer-healing Drugs: absorption of lansoprazole possibly reduced by sucralfate

• Ulipristal: avoidance of proton pump inhibitors advised by manufacturer of high-dose ●ulipristal (contraceptive effect of ulipristal possibly reduced)

**Pseudoephedrine** see Sympathomimetics

**Pyrazinamide**

Probenecid: pyrazinamide antagonises effects of probenecid

Sulfinpyrazone: pyrazinamide antagonises effects of sulfinpyrazone

Vaccines: antibacterials inactivate oral typhoid vaccine—see p. 621

**Pyridostigmine** see Parasympathomimetics

**Pyridoxine** see Vitamins

**Pyrimethamine**

• Antibacterials: increased antifolate effect when pyrimethamine given with ●sulfonamides or ●trimethoprim

• Antiepileptics: pyrimethamine antagonises anticonvulsant effect of ●phenytoin, also increased antifolate effect

• Antimalarials: avoidance of antimalarials advised by manufacturer of ●artemether with lumefantrine; increased antifolate effect when pyrimethamine given with proguanil

Antivirals: increased antifolate effect when pyrimethamine given with zidovudine

**Pyrimethamine** (continued)

- Cytotoxics: pyrimethamine increases antifolate effect of ●methotrexate and ●pemetrexed

  Histamine: avoidance of antimalarials advised by manufacturer of histamine

  Vaccines: antimalarials inactivate oral typhoid vaccine—see p. 621

**Quetiapine** see Antipsychotics

**Quinagolide**

  Memantine: effects of dopaminergics possibly enhanced by memantine

  Methyldopa: antiparkinsonian effect of dopaminergics antagonised by methyldopa

**Quinapril** see ACE Inhibitors

**Quinine**

- Anti-arrhythmics: increased risk of ventricular arrhythmias when quinine given with ●amiodarone—avoid concomitant use; quinine increases plasma concentration of ●flecainide
- Antibacterials: increased risk of ventricular arrhythmias when quinine given with ●moxifloxacin—avoid concomitant use; plasma concentration of quinine reduced by ●rifampicin

  Anticoagulants: plasma concentration of both drugs increased when quinine given with warfarin

- Antimalarials: avoidance of antimalarials advised by manufacturer of ●artemether with lumefantrine; increased risk of ventricular arrhythmias when quinine given with ●artemether with lumefantrine; increased risk of convulsions when quinine given with ●mefloquine (but should not prevent the use of *intravenous* quinine in severe cases)
- Antipsychotics: increased risk of ventricular arrhythmias when quinine given with ●droperidol or ●pimozide—avoid concomitant use; possible increased risk of ventricular arrhythmias when quinine given with ●haloperidol—avoid concomitant use
- Antivirals: plasma concentration of quinine possibly increased by ●atazanavir, ●darunavir, ●fosamprenavir, ●indinavir and ●tipranavir (increased risk of toxicity); plasma concentration of quinine increased by ●ritonavir (increased risk of toxicity); increased risk of ventricular arrhythmias when quinine given with ●saquinavir—avoid concomitant use
- Cardiac Glycosides: quinine increases plasma concentration of ●digoxin

  Dopaminergics: quinine possibly increases plasma concentration of amantadine

  Histamine: avoidance of antimalarials advised by manufacturer of histamine

  Muscle Relaxants: quinine possibly enhances effects of suxamethonium

  Ulcer-healing Drugs: metabolism of quinine inhibited by cimetidine (increased plasma concentration)

  Vaccines: antimalarials inactivate oral typhoid vaccine—see p. 621

**Quinolones**

- Analgesics: possible increased risk of convulsions when quinolones given with ●NSAIDs

  Antacids: absorption of ciprofloxacin, levofloxacin, moxifloxacin, norfloxacin and ofloxacin reduced by antacids

- Anti-arrhythmics: increased risk of ventricular arrhythmias when levofloxacin or moxifloxacin given with ●amiodarone—avoid concomitant use; increased risk of ventricular arrhythmias when moxifloxacin given with ●disopyramide—avoid concomitant use
- Antibacterials: increased risk of ventricular arrhythmias when moxifloxacin given with *parenteral* ●erythromycin—avoid concomitant use; effects of nalidixic acid possibly antagonised by nitrofurantoin; possible increased risk of ventricular arrhythmias when moxifloxacin given with ●telithromycin

**Quinolones** (continued)

- Anticoagulants: ciprofloxacin and levofloxacin possibly enhance anticoagulant effect of coumarins; nalidixic acid, norfloxacin and ofloxacin enhance anticoagulant effect of ●coumarins; levofloxacin possibly enhances anticoagulant effect of phenindione
- Antidepressants: ciprofloxacin inhibits metabolism of ●duloxetine—avoid concomitant use; avoidance of ciprofloxacin advised by manufacturer of ●agomelatine; increased risk of ventricular arrhythmias when moxifloxacin given with ●tricyclics—avoid concomitant use

  Antidiabetics: norfloxacin possibly enhances effects of glibenclamide

  Antiepileptics: ciprofloxacin increases or decreases plasma concentration of phenytoin

- Antihistamines: increased risk of ventricular arrhythmias when moxifloxacin given with ●mizolastine—avoid concomitant use
- Antimalarials: avoidance of moxifloxacin advised by manufacturer of ●piperaquine with artenimol (possible risk of ventricular arrhythmias); avoidance of quinolones advised by manufacturer of ●artemether with lumefantrine; increased risk of ventricular arrhythmias when moxifloxacin given with ●chloroquine and hydroxychloroquine, ●mefloquine or ●quinine—avoid concomitant use
- Antipsychotics: increased risk of ventricular arrhythmias when moxifloxacin given with ●benperidol—manufacturer of benperidol advises avoid concomitant use; increased risk of ventricular arrhythmias when moxifloxacin given with ●droperidol, ●haloperidol, ●phenothiazines, ●pimozide or ●zuclopenthixol—avoid concomitant use; ciprofloxacin increases plasma concentration of clozapine; ciprofloxacin possibly increases plasma concentration of olanzapine
- Antivirals: manufacturer of norfloxacin advises give didanosine at least 2 hours before or after norfloxacin; increased risk of ventricular arrhythmias when moxifloxacin given with ●saquinavir—avoid concomitant use
- Atomoxetine: increased risk of ventricular arrhythmias when moxifloxacin given with ●atomoxetine
- Beta-blockers: increased risk of ventricular arrhythmias when moxifloxacin given with ●sotalol—avoid concomitant use

  Calcium Salts: absorption of ciprofloxacin reduced by calcium salts

- Ciclosporin: increased risk of nephrotoxicity when quinolones given with ●ciclosporin
- Clopidogrel: ciprofloxacin possibly reduces antiplatelet effect of ●clopidogrel
- Cytotoxics: nalidixic acid increases risk of melphalan toxicity; ciprofloxacin possibly reduces excretion of methotrexate (increased risk of toxicity); ciprofloxacin increases plasma concentration of erlotinib; possible increased risk of ventricular arrhythmias when moxifloxacin given with ●vandetanib—avoid concomitant use; increased risk of ventricular arrhythmias when levofloxacin or moxifloxacin given with ●arsenic trioxide

  Dairy Products: absorption of ciprofloxacin and norfloxacin reduced by dairy products

  Dopaminergics: ciprofloxacin increases plasma concentration of rasagiline; ciprofloxacin inhibits metabolism of ropinirole (increased plasma concentration)

  5HT$_1$-receptor Agonists: quinolones possibly inhibit metabolism of zolmitriptan (reduce dose of zolmitriptan)

  Iron: absorption of ciprofloxacin, levofloxacin, moxifloxacin and ofloxacin reduced by *oral* iron; absorption of norfloxacin reduced by *oral* iron (give at least 2 hours apart)

**Quinolones** *(continued)*

Lanthanum: absorption of quinolones possibly reduced by lanthanum (give at least 2 hours before or 4 hours after lanthanum)

● Muscle Relaxants: norfloxacin possibly increases plasma concentration of tizanidine (increased risk of toxicity); ciprofloxacin increases plasma concentration of ●tizanidine (increased risk of toxicity)—avoid concomitant use

Mycophenolate: norfloxacin possibly reduces bioavailability of mycophenolate

● Pentamidine Isetionate: increased risk of ventricular arrhythmias when moxifloxacin given with ●pentamidine isetionate—avoid concomitant use

Probenecid: excretion of ciprofloxacin, nalidixic acid and norfloxacin reduced by probenecid (increased plasma concentration)

Sevelamer: bioavailability of ciprofloxacin reduced by sevelamer

Strontium Ranelate: absorption of quinolones reduced by strontium ranelate (manufacturer of strontium ranelate advises avoid concomitant use)

● Theophylline: possible increased risk of convulsions when quinolones given with ●theophylline; ciprofloxacin and norfloxacin increase plasma concentration of ●theophylline

Ulcer-healing Drugs: absorption of ciprofloxacin, levofloxacin, moxifloxacin and ofloxacin reduced by sucralfate; absorption of norfloxacin reduced by sucralfate (give at least 2 hours apart)

Vaccines: antibacterials inactivate oral typhoid vaccine—see p. 621

Zinc: absorption of ciprofloxacin, levofloxacin, moxifloxacin and ofloxacin reduced by zinc; absorption of norfloxacin reduced by zinc (give at least 2 hours apart)

**Rabeprazole** *see* Proton Pump Inhibitors

**Raloxifene**

Anticoagulants: raloxifene antagonises anticoagulant effect of coumarins

Lipid-regulating Drugs: absorption of raloxifene reduced by colestyramine (manufacturer of raloxifene advises avoid concomitant administration)

**Raltegravir**

● Antibacterials: plasma concentration of raltegravir reduced by ●rifampicin—consider increasing dose of raltegravir

● Antivirals: increased risk of rash when raltegravir given with darunavir; avoidance of raltegravir advised by manufacturer of ●fosamprenavir

Ulcer-healing Drugs: plasma concentration of raltegravir increased by famotidine and omeprazole

**Raltitrexed**

● Antipsychotics: avoid concomitant use of cytotoxics with ●clozapine (increased risk of agranulocytosis)

● Folates: manufacturer of raltitrexed advises avoid concomitant use with ●folates

**Ramipril** *see* ACE Inhibitors

**Ranitidine** *see* Histamine H₂-antagonists

**Ranolazine**

● Anti-arrhythmics: manufacturer of ranolazine advises avoid concomitant use with ●disopyramide

● Antibacterials: plasma concentration of ranolazine possibly increased by ●clarithromycin and ●telithromycin—manufacturer of ranolazine advises avoid concomitant use; plasma concentration of ranolazine reduced by ●rifampicin—manufacturer of ranolazine advises avoid concomitant use

Antidepressants: plasma concentration of ranolazine increased by paroxetine

● Antifungals: plasma concentration of ranolazine increased by ●ketoconazole—avoid concomitant use; plasma concentration of ranolazine possibly increased by ●itraconazole, ●posaconazole and ●voriconazole—manufacturer of ranolazine advises avoid concomitant use

**Ranolazine** *(continued)*

● Antivirals: plasma concentration of ranolazine possibly increased by ●atazanavir, ●darunavir, ●fosamprenavir, ●indinavir, ●lopinavir, ●ritonavir, ●saquinavir and ●tipranavir—manufacturer of ranolazine advises avoid concomitant use

● Beta-blockers: manufacturer of ranolazine advises avoid concomitant use with ●sotalol

Calcium-channel Blockers: plasma concentration of ranolazine increased by diltiazem and verapamil (consider reducing dose of ranolazine)

Cardiac Glycosides: ranolazine increases plasma concentration of digoxin

Ciclosporin: plasma concentration of both drugs may increase when ranolazine given with ciclosporin

● Grapefruit Juice: plasma concentration of ranolazine possibly increased by ●grapefruit juice—manufacturer of ranolazine advises avoid concomitant use

● Lipid-regulating Drugs: ranolazine increases plasma concentration of ●simvastatin (see Dose under Simvastatin, BNF section 2.12)

● Tacrolimus: ranolazine increases plasma concentration of ●tacrolimus

**Rasagiline**

Note Rasagiline is a MAO-B inhibitor

● Analgesics: avoid concomitant use of rasagiline with ●dextromethorphan; risk of CNS toxicity when rasagiline given with ●pethidine (avoid pethidine for 2 weeks after rasagiline)

Antibacterials: plasma concentration of rasagiline increased by ciprofloxacin

● Antidepressants: after stopping rasagiline do not start ●fluoxetine for 2 weeks, also rasagiline should not be started until at least 5 weeks after stopping fluoxetine; after stopping rasagiline do not start ●fluvoxamine for 2 weeks; risk of hypertensive crisis when rasagiline given with ●MAOIs, avoid MAOIs for at least 2 weeks after stopping rasagiline; increased risk of CNS toxicity when rasagiline given with ●SSRIs or ●tricyclics

Dopaminergics: plasma concentration of rasagiline possibly reduced by entacapone

Memantine: effects of dopaminergics possibly enhanced by memantine

Methyldopa: antiparkinsonian effect of dopaminergics antagonised by methyldopa

● Sympathomimetics: avoid concomitant use of rasagiline with ●sympathomimetics

**Reboxetine**

● Antibacterials: manufacturer of reboxetine advises avoid concomitant use with ●macrolides

● Antidepressants: manufacturer of reboxetine advises avoid concomitant use with ●fluvoxamine; increased risk of hypertension and CNS excitation when reboxetine given with ●MAOIs (MAOIs should not be started until 1 week after stopping reboxetine, avoid reboxetine for 2 weeks after stopping MAOIs)

Antiepileptics: plasma concentration of reboxetine possibly reduced by carbamazepine and phenobarbital

● Antifungals: manufacturer of reboxetine advises avoid concomitant use with ●imidazoles and ●triazoles

● Antimalarials: avoidance of antidepressants advised by manufacturer of ●artemether with lumefantrine and ●piperaquine with artenimol

Atomoxetine: possible increased risk of convulsions when antidepressants given with atomoxetine

Diuretics: possible increased risk of hypokalaemia when reboxetine given with loop diuretics or thiazides and related diuretics

Ergot Alkaloids: possible risk of hypertension when reboxetine given with ergotamine and methysergide

**Remifentanil** *see* Opioid Analgesics

**Repaglinide** *see* Antidiabetics

## Retigabine

Alcohol: increased risk of blurred vision when retigabine given with alcohol

- Antidepressants: anticonvulsant effect of antiepileptics possibly antagonised by MAOIs and •tricyclic-related antidepressants (convulsive threshold lowered); anticonvulsant effect of antiepileptics antagonised by •SSRIs and •tricyclics (convulsive threshold lowered); avoid concomitant use of antiepileptics with •St John's wort

Antiepileptics: plasma concentration of retigabine possibly reduced by carbamazepine and phenytoin

- Antimalarials: anticonvulsant effect of antiepileptics antagonised by •mefloquine

- Antipsychotics: anticonvulsant effect of antiepileptics antagonised by •antipsychotics (convulsive threshold lowered)

- Orlistat: possible increased risk of convulsions when antiepileptics given with •orlistat

## Retinoids

- Alcohol: etretinate formed from acitretin in presence of •alcohol (increased risk of teratogenecity in women of child-bearing potential)

- Antibacterials: possible increased risk of benign intracranial hypertension when retinoids given with •tetracyclines (avoid concomitant use)

- Anticoagulants: acitretin possibly reduces anticoagulant effect of •coumarins

Antiepileptics: isotretinoin possibly reduces plasma concentration of carbamazepine

- Antifungals: plasma concentration of alitretinoin increased by ketoconazole; possible increased risk of tretinoin toxicity when given with •fluconazole, •ketoconazole and •voriconazole

- Cytotoxics: acitretin increases plasma concentration of •methotrexate (also increased risk of hepatotoxicity)—avoid concomitant use

Lipid-regulating Drugs: alitretinoin reduces plasma concentration of simvastatin

- Vitamins: risk of hypervitaminosis A when retinoids given with •vitamin A—avoid concomitant use

## Ribavirin

- Antivirals: effects of ribavirin possibly reduced by •abacavir; increased risk of side-effects when ribavirin given with •didanosine—avoid concomitant use; increased risk of toxicity when ribavirin given with •stavudine; increased risk of anaemia when ribavirin given with •zidovudine—avoid concomitant use

- Azathioprine: ribavirin possibly enhances myelosuppressive effects of •azathioprine

**Rifabutin** see Rifamycins

**Rifampicin** see Rifamycins

## Rifamycins

Note Interactions do not apply to rifaximin

ACE Inhibitors: rifampicin reduces plasma concentration of active metabolite of imidapril (reduced antihypertensive effect)

Aliskiren: rifampicin reduces plasma concentration of aliskiren

Ambrisentan: rifampicin possibly increases plasma concentration of ambrisentan

Analgesics: rifampicin reduces plasma concentration of celecoxib, diclofenac and etoricoxib; rifampicin accelerates metabolism of alfentanil, codeine, fentanyl, methadone and morphine (reduced effect); rifampicin possibly accelerates metabolism of oxycodone

Angiotensin-II Receptor Antagonists: rifampicin reduces plasma concentration of losartan and its active metabolite

Antacids: absorption of rifampicin reduced by antacids

- Anti-arrhythmics: rifamycins accelerate metabolism of •disopyramide (reduced plasma concentration); rifampicin reduces plasma concentration of •drone-

## Rifamycins

- Anti-arrhythmics (continued)

darone—avoid concomitant use; rifampicin accelerates metabolism of •propafenone (reduced effect)

- Antibacterials: increased risk of side-effects including neutropenia when rifabutin given with •azithromycin; rifamycins reduce plasma concentration of clarithromycin and dapsone; plasma concentration of rifabutin increased by •clarithromycin (increased risk of toxicity—reduce rifabutin dose); plasma concentration of rifabutin possibly increased by •erythromycin (increased risk of toxicity—reduce rifabutin dose); rifampicin possibly reduces plasma concentration of tinidazole and trimethoprim; rifampicin reduces plasma concentration of doxycycline—consider increasing dose of doxycycline; rifampicin accelerates metabolism of chloramphenicol (reduced plasma concentration); increased risk of hepatotoxicity when rifampicin given with •isoniazid; rifampicin reduces plasma concentration of linezolid (possible therapeutic failure of linezolid); rifampicin reduces plasma concentration of •telithromycin (avoid during and for 2 weeks after rifampicin)

- Anticoagulants: rifampicin reduces plasma concentration of apixaban and rivaroxaban; rifamycins accelerate metabolism of •coumarins (reduced anticoagulant effect); rifampicin reduces plasma concentration of •dabigatran etexilate—manufacturer of dabigatran etexilate advises avoid concomitant use

- Antidiabetics: rifamycins accelerate metabolism of •tolbutamide (reduced effect); rifampicin possibly reduces effects of linagliptin; rifampicin reduces plasma concentration of nateglinide; rifampicin possibly antagonises hypoglycaemic effect of repaglinide; rifamycins possibly accelerate metabolism of •sulfonylureas (reduced effect)

- Antiepileptics: rifabutin reduces plasma concentration of •carbamazepine; rifampicin reduces plasma concentration of •lamotrigine; plasma concentration of rifampicin possibly reduced by phenobarbital; rifamycins accelerate metabolism of •phenytoin (reduced plasma concentration)

- Antifungals: rifampicin accelerates metabolism of •ketoconazole (reduced plasma concentration), also plasma concentration of rifampicin may be reduced by ketoconazole; plasma concentration of rifabutin increased by •fluconazole (increased risk of uveitis—reduce rifabutin dose); rifampicin accelerates metabolism of •fluconazole (reduced plasma concentration); rifabutin and rifampicin reduce plasma concentration of •itraconazole—manufacturer of itraconazole advises avoid concomitant use; plasma concentration of rifabutin increased by •posaconazole (also plasma concentration of posaconazole reduced); rifampicin reduces plasma concentration of •posaconazole and •terbinafine; plasma concentration of rifabutin increased by •voriconazole, also rifabutin reduces plasma concentration of voriconazole (increase dose of voriconazole and also monitor for rifabutin toxicity); rifampicin reduces plasma concentration of •voriconazole—avoid concomitant use; rifampicin initially increases and then reduces plasma concentration of caspofungin (consider increasing dose of caspofungin); plasma concentration of rifabutin possibly increased by •triazoles (increased risk of uveitis—reduce rifabutin dose)

Antihistamines: rifampicin possibly reduces effects of fexofenadine

- Antimalarials: avoidance of rifampicin advised by manufacturer of piperaquine with artenimol; rifampicin reduces plasma concentration of •mefloquine—avoid concomitant use; rifampicin reduces plasma concentration of •quinine

## Rifamycins *(continued)*

Antimuscarinics: rifampicin reduces plasma concentration of active metabolite of fesoterodine

- Antipsychotics: rifampicin accelerates metabolism of ●haloperidol (reduced plasma concentration); rifabutin and rifampicin possibly reduce plasma concentration of ●aripiprazole—increase dose of aripiprazole; rifampicin possibly reduces plasma concentration of clozapine

- Antivirals: rifampicin possibly reduces plasma concentration of abacavir and ritonavir; rifampicin reduces plasma concentration of ●atazanavir, ●lopinavir, ●nevirapine and ●rilpivirine—avoid concomitant use; plasma concentration of rifabutin increased by ●atazanavir, ●darunavir, ●fosamprenavir and ●tipranavir (reduce dose of rifabutin); avoidance of rifampicin advised by manufacturer of ●boceprevir (plasma concentration of boceprevir possibly reduced); rifampicin significantly reduces plasma concentration of ●darunavir, ●fosamprenavir and ●telaprevir—avoid concomitant use; rifampicin reduces plasma concentration of efavirenz—increase dose of efavirenz; plasma concentration of rifabutin reduced by efavirenz—increase dose of rifabutin; plasma concentration of both drugs reduced when rifampicin given with ●etravirine; avoidance of rifampicin advised by manufacturer of etravirine and zidovudine; rifampicin accelerates metabolism of ●indinavir (reduced plasma concentration—avoid concomitant use); plasma concentration of rifabutin increased by ●indinavir—avoid concomitant use; rifampicin reduces plasma concentration of ●maraviroc and ●raltegravir—consider increasing dose of maraviroc and raltegravir; plasma concentration of rifabutin possibly increased by nevirapine; rifabutin reduces plasma concentration of ●rilpivirine—avoid concomitant use; plasma concentration of rifabutin increased by ●ritonavir (increased risk of toxicity—reduce rifabutin dose); plasma concentration of rifabutin increased by ●saquinavir (also plasma concentration of saquinavir reduced)—reduce rifabutin dose; rifampicin significantly reduces plasma concentration of ●saquinavir, also risk of hepatotoxicity—avoid concomitant use; avoidance of rifabutin advised by manufacturer of ●telaprevir; rifampicin possibly reduces plasma concentration of ●tipranavir—avoid concomitant use

Anxiolytics and Hypnotics: rifampicin accelerates metabolism of diazepam and zaleplon (reduced plasma concentration); rifampicin possibly accelerates metabolism of benzodiazepines (reduced plasma concentration); rifampicin possibly accelerates metabolism of buspirone; rifampicin accelerates metabolism of zolpidem (reduced plasma concentration and reduced effect); rifampicin significantly reduces plasma concentration of zopiclone

Aprepitant: rifampicin reduces plasma concentration of aprepitant

- Atovaquone: avoidance of concomitant rifabutin advised by manufacturer of atovaquone (plasma concentration of both drugs reduced); rifampicin reduces plasma concentration of ●atovaquone (and concentration of rifampicin increased)—avoid concomitant use

Beta-blockers: rifampicin accelerates metabolism of bisoprolol and propranolol (plasma concentration significantly reduced); rifampicin reduces plasma concentration of carvedilol, celiprolol and metoprolol

- Bosentan: rifampicin reduces plasma concentration of ●bosentan—avoid concomitant use

- Calcium-channel Blockers: rifampicin possibly accelerates metabolism of ●isradipine and ●nicardipine (possible significantly reduced plasma concentra-

## Rifamycins

- Calcium-channel Blockers *(continued)* tion); rifampicin accelerates metabolism of ●diltiazem, ●nifedipine, ●nimodipine and ●verapamil (plasma concentration significantly reduced)

Cardiac Glycosides: rifampicin possibly reduces plasma concentration of digoxin

- Ciclosporin: rifampicin accelerates metabolism of ●ciclosporin (reduced plasma concentration)

- Corticosteroids: rifamycins accelerate metabolism of ●corticosteroids (reduced effect)

- Cytotoxics: rifabutin possibly decreases plasma concentration of axitinib (increase dose of axitinib—consult axitinib product literature); rifampicin decreases plasma concentration of axitinib (increase dose of axitinib—consult axitinib product literature); rifabutin possibly reduces plasma concentration of crizotinib—manufacturer of crizotinib advises avoid concomitant use; rifampicin reduces plasma concentration of ●crizotinib—manufacturer of crizotinib advises avoid concomitant use; rifampicin accelerates metabolism of ●dasatinib (reduced plasma concentration—avoid concomitant use); rifampicin accelerates metabolism of erlotinib and sunitinib (reduced plasma concentration); rifampicin reduces plasma concentration of ●everolimus, ruxolitinib and sorafenib; rifampicin reduces plasma concentration of ●gefitinib, ●imatinib and ●nilotinib—avoid concomitant use; avoidance of rifabutin and rifampicin advised by manufacturer of ●lapatinib; avoidance of rifampicin advised by manufacturer of ●cabazitaxel, ●pazopanib and vemurafenib; rifampicin reduces plasma concentration of active metabolite of ●temsirolimus—avoid concomitant use; avoidance of rifampicin advised by manufacturer of vandetanib (plasma concentration of vandetanib reduced); avoidance of rifabutin advised by manufacturer of ●cabazitaxel and vemurafenib; rifampicin possibly reduces effects of brentuximab vedotin; rifampicin possibly reduces plasma concentration of eribulin; rifampicin possibly reduces plasma concentration of ●vinflunine—manufacturer of vinflunine advises avoid concomitant use

Deferasirox: rifampicin reduces plasma concentration of deferasirox

- Diuretics: rifampicin reduces plasma concentration of ●eplerenone—avoid concomitant use

Hormone Antagonists: rifampicin possibly reduces plasma concentration of exemestane; rifampicin accelerates metabolism of tamoxifen (reduced plasma concentration)

$5HT_3$-receptor Antagonists: rifampicin accelerates metabolism of ondansetron (reduced effect)

Leflunomide: rifampicin possibly increases plasma concentration of active metabolite of leflunomide

Lipid-regulating Drugs: rifampicin possibly reduces plasma concentration of atorvastatin and simvastatin; rifampicin accelerates metabolism of fluvastatin (reduced effect)

Muscle Relaxants: rifampicin possibly reduces plasma concentration of tizanidine

- Mycophenolate: rifampicin reduces plasma concentration of active metabolite of ●mycophenolate

- Oestrogens: rifamycins accelerate metabolism of ●oestrogens (reduced contraceptive effect—see p. 398)

- Progestogens: rifamycins accelerate metabolism of ●progestogens (reduced contraceptive effect—see p. 398)

- Ranolazine: rifampicin reduces plasma concentration of ●ranolazine—manufacturer of ranolazine advises avoid concomitant use

Roflumilast: rifampicin reduces plasma concentration of roflumilast—consider increasing dose of roflumilast

**Rifamycins** (continued)
- Sirolimus: rifabutin and rifampicin reduce plasma concentration of ●sirolimus—avoid concomitant use
- Tacrolimus: rifabutin possibly reduces plasma concentration of tacrolimus; rifampicin reduces plasma concentration of ●tacrolimus
- Tadalafil: rifampicin reduces plasma concentration of ●tadalafil—manufacturer of tadalafil advises avoid concomitant use

Theophylline: rifampicin accelerates metabolism of theophylline (reduced plasma concentration)

Thyroid Hormones: rifampicin accelerates metabolism of levothyroxine (may increase requirements for levothyroxine in hypothyroidism)

Tibolone: rifampicin accelerates metabolism of tibolone (reduced plasma concentration)

Ticagrelor: rifampicin reduces plasma concentration of ●ticagrelor

Tolvaptan: rifampicin reduces plasma concentration of tolvaptan

Ulcer-healing Drugs: rifampicin accelerates metabolism of cimetidine (reduced plasma concentration)
- Ulipristal: avoidance of rifampicin advised by manufacturer of ●ulipristal (contraceptive effect of ulipristal possibly reduced)

Vaccines: antibacterials inactivate oral typhoid vaccine—see p. 621

**Rilpivirine**

Analgesics: rilpivirine possibly reduces plasma concentration of methadone

Antacids: manufacturer of rilpivirine advises give antacids 2 hours before or 4 hours after rilpivirine
- Antibacterials: manufacturer of rilpivirine advises avoid concomitant use with ●clarithromycin and ●erythromycin (plasma concentration of rilpivirine possibly increased); plasma concentration of rilpivirine reduced by ●rifabutin and ●rifampicin—avoid concomitant use

Anticoagulants: rilpivirine possibly increases plasma concentration of dabigatran etexilate
- Antidepressants: manufacturer of rilpivirine advises avoid concomitant use with ●St John's wort (plasma concentration of rilpivirine possibly reduced)

Antidiabetics: rilpivirine possibly increases plasma concentration of metformin
- Antiepileptics: manufacturer of rilpivirine advises avoid concomitant use with ●carbamazepine, ●oxcarbazepine, ●phenobarbital and ●phenytoin (plasma concentration of rilpivirine reduced)

Antivirals: manufacturer of rilpivirine advises give didanosine 2 hours before or 4 hours after rilpivirine

Calcium Salts: manufacturer of rilpivirine advises give calcium salts 2 hours before or 4 hours after rilpivirine

Cardiac Glycosides: rilpivirine possibly increases plasma concentration of digoxin
- Corticosteroids: manufacturer of rilpivirine advises avoid concomitant use with ●dexamethasone (except when given as a single dose)
- Ulcer-healing Drugs: manufacturer of rilpivirine advises avoid concomitant use with esomeprazole, lansoprazole, pantoprazole and rabeprazole (plasma concentration of rilpivirine possibly reduced); plasma concentration of rilpivirine reduced by ●omeprazole—avoid concomitant use; manufacturer of rilpivirine advises avoid histamine $H_2$-antagonists for 12 hours before or 4 hours after rilpivirine—consult product literature

**Risedronate Sodium** see Bisphosphonates
**Risperidone** see Antipsychotics
**Ritonavir**
- Alpha-blockers: ritonavir possibly increases plasma concentration of ●alfuzosin—avoid concomitant use

**Ritonavir** (continued)
- Analgesics: ritonavir possibly increases plasma concentration of NSAIDs and buprenorphine; ritonavir increases plasma concentration of ●dextropropoxyphene and ●piroxicam (risk of toxicity)—avoid concomitant use; ritonavir increases plasma concentration of ●alfentanil and ●fentanyl; ritonavir reduces plasma concentration of methadone; ritonavir possibly reduces plasma concentration of morphine; ritonavir reduces plasma concentration of ●pethidine, but increases plasma concentration of toxic metabolite of pethidine (avoid concomitant use)
- Anti-arrhythmics: ritonavir increases plasma concentration of ●amiodarone and ●propafenone (increased risk of ventricular arrhythmias—avoid concomitant use); ritonavir possibly increases plasma concentration of ●disopyramide (increased risk of toxicity); avoidance of ritonavir advised by manufacturer of ●dronedarone; ritonavir possibly increases plasma concentration of ●flecainide (increased risk of ventricular arrhythmias—avoid concomitant use)
- Antibacterials: ritonavir possibly increases plasma concentration of azithromycin and erythromycin; ritonavir increases plasma concentration of ●clarithromycin (reduce dose of clarithromycin in renal impairment); ritonavir increases plasma concentration of ●rifabutin (increased risk of toxicity—reduce rifabutin dose); plasma concentration of ritonavir possibly reduced by rifampicin; plasma concentration of both drugs increased when ritonavir given with ●fusidic acid—avoid concomitant use; avoidance of concomitant ritonavir in severe renal and hepatic impairment advised by manufacturer of ●telithromycin
- Anticoagulants: ritonavir may enhance or reduce anticoagulant effect of ●warfarin; avoidance of ritonavir advised by manufacturer of apixaban; ritonavir possibly enhances anticoagulant effect of ●coumarins and ●phenindione; ritonavir increases plasma concentration of ●rivaroxaban—avoid concomitant use

Antidepressants: ritonavir possibly reduces plasma concentration of paroxetine; ritonavir increases plasma concentration of ●trazodone (increased risk of toxicity); ritonavir possibly increases plasma concentration of ●SSRIs and ●tricyclics; plasma concentration of ritonavir reduced by ●St John's wort—avoid concomitant use

Antidiabetics: ritonavir possibly increases plasma concentration of tolbutamide
- Antiepileptics: ritonavir possibly increases plasma concentration of ●carbamazepine; ritonavir possibly reduces plasma concentration of lamotrigine and valproate; plasma concentration of ritonavir possibly reduced by phenytoin, also plasma concentration of phenytoin possibly affected
- Antifungals: combination of ritonavir with ●itraconazole or ●ketoconazole may increase plasma concentration of either drug (or both); plasma concentration of ritonavir increased by fluconazole; ritonavir reduces plasma concentration of ●voriconazole—avoid concomitant use

Antihistamines: ritonavir possibly increases plasma concentration of non-sedating antihistamines
- Antimalarials: caution with ritonavir advised by manufacturer of artemether with lumefantrine; ritonavir increases plasma concentration of ●quinine (increased risk of toxicity)

Antimuscarinics: avoidance of ritonavir advised by manufacturer of darifenacin and tolterodine; manufacturer of fesoterodine advises dose reduction when ritonavir given with fesoterodine—consult fesoterodine product literature; ritonavir increases plasma concentration of solifenacin
- Antipsychotics: ritonavir possibly increases plasma concentration of ●antipsychotics; ritonavir possibly

## Ritonavir

- Antipsychotics *(continued)*
  inhibits metabolism of ●aripiprazole (reduce dose of aripiprazole); manufacturer of ritonavir advises avoid concomitant use with ●clozapine (increased risk of toxicity); ritonavir reduces plasma concentration of olanzapine—consider increasing dose of olanzapine; ritonavir increases plasma concentration of ●pimozide (increased risk of ventricular arrhythmias—avoid concomitant use); ritonavir possibly increases plasma concentration of ●quetiapine—manufacturer of quetiapine advises avoid concomitant use
- Antivirals: plasma concentration of both drugs reduced when ritonavir given with ●boceprevir; ritonavir increases toxicity of efavirenz, monitor liver function tests; ritonavir increases plasma concentration of indinavir, maraviroc and ●saquinavir; ritonavir possibly reduces plasma concentration of telaprevir
- Anxiolytics and Hypnotics: ritonavir possibly increases plasma concentration of ●anxiolytics and hypnotics; ritonavir possibly increases plasma concentration of ●alprazolam, ●diazepam, ●flurazepam and ●zolpidem (risk of extreme sedation and respiratory depression—avoid concomitant use); ritonavir possibly increases plasma concentration of ●midazolam (risk of prolonged sedation—avoid concomitant use of *oral* midazolam); ritonavir increases plasma concentration of buspirone (increased risk of toxicity)
  Aprepitant: ritonavir possibly increases plasma concentration of aprepitant
- Bosentan: ritonavir increases plasma concentration of ●bosentan
  Bupropion: ritonavir reduces plasma concentration of bupropion
- Calcium-channel Blockers: ritonavir possibly increases plasma concentration of ●calcium-channel blockers; avoidance of ritonavir advised by manufacturer of lercanidipine
  Cardiac Glycosides: ritonavir possibly increases plasma concentration of digoxin
- Ciclosporin: ritonavir possibly increases plasma concentration of ●ciclosporin
- Colchicine: ritonavir possibly increases risk of ●colchicine toxicity—suspend or reduce dose of colchicine (avoid concomitant use in hepatic or renal impairment)
- Corticosteroids: ritonavir possibly increases plasma concentration of corticosteroids, dexamethasone and prednisolone; ritonavir possibly increases plasma concentration of budesonide (including *inhaled*, *intranasal*, and *rectal* budesonide); ritonavir increases plasma concentration of *inhaled* and *intranasal* ●fluticasone
- Cytotoxics: ritonavir possibly increases plasma concentration of axitinib (reduce dose of axitinib—consult axitinib product literature); ritonavir possibly increases plasma concentration of ●crizotinib, ●everolimus, nilotinib and ●vinflunine—manufacturer of crizotinib, everolimus, nilotinib and vinflunine advises avoid concomitant use; avoidance of ritonavir advised by manufacturer of ●cabazitaxel, ●lapatinib and ●pazopanib; manufacturer of ruxolitinib advises dose reduction when ritonavir given with ●ruxolitinib—consult ruxolitinib product literature; ritonavir possibly increases plasma concentration of ●docetaxel (increased risk of toxicity); ritonavir increases plasma concentration of paclitaxel; ritonavir possibly increases plasma concentration of vinblastine
- Diuretics: ritonavir increases plasma concentration of ●eplerenone—avoid concomitant use
- Ergot Alkaloids: increased risk of ergotism when ritonavir given with ●ergotamine and methysergide—avoid concomitant use

## Ritonavir *(continued)*

- 5HT$_1$-receptor Agonists: ritonavir increases plasma concentration of ●eletriptan (risk of toxicity)—avoid concomitant use
- Ivabradine: ritonavir possibly increases plasma concentration of ●ivabradine—avoid concomitant use
- Lipid-regulating Drugs: possible increased risk of myopathy when ritonavir given with atorvastatin; possible increased risk of myopathy when ritonavir given with ●rosuvastatin—manufacturer of rosuvastatin advises avoid concomitant use; increased risk of myopathy when ritonavir given with ●simvastatin (avoid concomitant use)
  Mirabegron: when given with ritonavir avoid or reduce dose of mirabegron in hepatic or renal impairment—see Mirabegron, BNF section 7.4.2
- Oestrogens: ritonavir accelerates metabolism of ●oestrogens (reduced contraceptive effect—see p. 398)
- Ranolazine: ritonavir possibly increases plasma concentration of ●ranolazine—manufacturer of ranolazine advises avoid concomitant use
- Sildenafil: ritonavir significantly increases plasma concentration of ●sildenafil—avoid concomitant use
  Sympathomimetics: ritonavir possibly increases plasma concentration of dexamfetamine
  Sympathomimetics, Beta$_2$: manufacturer of ritonavir advises avoid concomitant use with salmeterol
- Tacrolimus: ritonavir possibly increases plasma concentration of ●tacrolimus
- Tadalafil: ritonavir increases plasma concentration of ●tadalafil—manufacturer of tadalafil advises avoid concomitant use
- Theophylline: ritonavir accelerates metabolism of ●theophylline (reduced plasma concentration)
- Ticagrelor: ritonavir possibly increases plasma concentration of ●ticagrelor—manufacturer of ticagrelor advises avoid concomitant use
- Ulipristal: avoidance of ritonavir advised by manufacturer of ●ulipristal (contraceptive effect of ulipristal possibly reduced)
- Vardenafil: ritonavir increases plasma concentration of ●vardenafil—avoid concomitant use

## Rivaroxaban

- Analgesics: increased risk of haemorrhage when anticoagulants given with *intravenous* ●diclofenac (avoid concomitant use, including low-dose heparins); increased risk of haemorrhage when anticoagulants given with ●ketorolac (avoid concomitant use, including low-dose heparins)
  Anti-arrhythmics: manufacturer of rivaroxaban advises avoid concomitant use with dronedarone
  Antibacterials: plasma concentration of rivaroxaban reduced by rifampicin
- Anticoagulants: increased risk of haemorrhage when rivaroxaban given with other ●anticoagulants (avoid concomitant use except when switching with other anticoagulants or using heparin to maintain catheter patency); increased risk of haemorrhage when other anticoagulants given with ●apixaban and ●dabigatran etexilate (avoid concomitant use except when switching with other anticoagulants or using heparin to maintain catheter patency)
- Antifungals: plasma concentration of rivaroxaban increased by ●ketoconazole—avoid concomitant use; manufacturer of rivaroxaban advises avoid concomitant use with itraconazole, posaconazole and voriconazole
- Antivirals: manufacturer of rivaroxaban advises avoid concomitant use with atazanavir, darunavir, fosamprenavir, indinavir, saquinavir and tipranavir; manufacturers advise avoid concomitant use of rivaroxaban with lopinavir; plasma concentration of rivaroxaban increased by ●ritonavir—avoid concomitant use

**Rivastigmine** *see* Parasympathomimetics

**Rizatriptan** see 5HT$_1$-receptor Agonists (under HT)

**Rocuronium** see Muscle Relaxants

**Roflumilast**

Antibacterials: plasma concentration of roflumilast reduced by rifampicin—consider increasing dose of roflumilast

Antidepressants: metabolism of roflumilast inhibited by fluvoxamine

Theophylline: manufacturer of roflumilast advises avoid concomitant use with theophylline

Ulcer-healing Drugs: metabolism of roflumilast inhibited by cimetidine

**Ropinirole**

Antibacterials: metabolism of ropinirole inhibited by ciprofloxacin (increased plasma concentration)

Antipsychotics: manufacturer of ropinirole advises avoid concomitant use of antipsychotics (antagonism of effect)

Memantine: effects of dopaminergics possibly enhanced by memantine

Methyldopa: antiparkinsonian effect of dopaminergics antagonised by methyldopa

Metoclopramide: manufacturer of ropinirole advises avoid concomitant use of metoclopramide (antagonism of effect)

Oestrogens: plasma concentration of ropinirole increased by oestrogens

**Ropivacaine**

Anti-arrhythmics: increased myocardial depression when ropivacaine given with anti-arrhythmics

Antidepressants: metabolism of ropivacaine inhibited by fluvoxamine—avoid prolonged administration of ropivacaine

**Rosuvastatin** see Statins

**Rotigotine**

Antipsychotics: manufacturer of rotigotine advises avoid concomitant use of antipsychotics (antagonism of effect)

Memantine: effects of dopaminergics possibly enhanced by memantine

Methyldopa: antiparkinsonian effect of dopaminergics antagonised by methyldopa

Metoclopramide: manufacturer of rotigotine advises avoid concomitant use of metoclopramide (antagonism of effect)

**Rufinamide**

• Antidepressants: anticonvulsant effect of antiepileptics possibly antagonised by MAOIs and •tricyclic-related antidepressants (convulsive threshold lowered); anticonvulsant effect of antiepileptics antagonised by •SSRIs and •tricyclics (convulsive threshold lowered); avoid concomitant use of antiepileptics with •St John's wort

Antiepileptics: plasma concentration of both drugs possibly reduced when rufinamide given with carbamazepine; plasma concentration of rufinamide possibly reduced by phenobarbital; plasma concentration of rufinamide possibly reduced by phenytoin, also plasma concentration of phenytoin possibly increased; plasma concentration of rufinamide possibly increased by valproate (reduce dose of rufinamide)

• Antimalarials: anticonvulsant effect of antiepileptics antagonised by •mefloquine

• Antipsychotics: anticonvulsant effect of antiepileptics antagonised by •antipsychotics (convulsive threshold lowered)

• Oestrogens: rufinamide accelerates metabolism of •oestrogens (reduced contraceptive effect—see p. 398)

• Orlistat: possible increased risk of convulsions when antiepileptics given with •orlistat

• Progestogens: rufinamide accelerates metabolism of •progestogens (reduced contraceptive effect—see p. 398)

**Rupatadine** see Antihistamines

**Ruxolitinib**

• Antibacterials: manufacturer of ruxolitinib advises dose reduction when ruxolitinib given with •clarithromycin and •telithromycin—consult ruxolitinib product literature; plasma concentration of ruxolitinib reduced by rifampicin

• Antifungals: manufacturer of ruxolitinib advises dose reduction when ruxolitinib given with •fluconazole, •itraconazole, •ketoconazole, •posaconazole and •voriconazole—consult ruxolitinib product literature

• Antipsychotics: avoid concomitant use of cytotoxics with •clozapine (increased risk of agranulocytosis)

• Antivirals: manufacturer of ruxolitinib advises dose reduction when ruxolitinib given with •boceprevir, •indinavir, •lopinavir, •ritonavir, •saquinavir and •telaprevir—consult ruxolitinib product literature

**St John's Wort**

Analgesics: St John's wort possibly reduces plasma concentration of methadone

• Anti-arrhythmics: St John's wort possibly reduces plasma concentration of •dronedarone—avoid concomitant use

• Antibacterials: St John's wort reduces plasma concentration of •telithromycin (avoid during and for 2 weeks after St John's wort)

• Anticoagulants: St John's wort reduces anticoagulant effect of •coumarins (avoid concomitant use); St John's wort possibly reduces plasma concentration of dabigatran etexilate—manufacturer of dabigatran etexilate advises avoid concomitant use

• Antidepressants: possible increased serotonergic effects when St John's wort given with duloxetine or venlafaxine; St John's wort reduces plasma concentration of amitriptyline; increased serotonergic effects when St John's wort given with •SSRIs—avoid concomitant use

• Antiepileptics: avoid concomitant use of St John's wort with •antiepileptics

• Antifungals: St John's wort reduces plasma concentration of •voriconazole—avoid concomitant use

• Antimalarials: avoidance of antidepressants advised by manufacturer of •artemether with lumefantrine and •piperaquine with artenimol

• Antipsychotics: St John's wort possibly reduces plasma concentration of •aripiprazole—increase dose of aripiprazole

• Antivirals: St John's wort reduces plasma concentration of •atazanavir, •darunavir, •efavirenz, •fosamprenavir, •indinavir, •lopinavir, •nevirapine, •ritonavir and •saquinavir—avoid concomitant use; avoidance of St John's wort advised by manufacturer of etravirine and •telaprevir; St John's wort possibly reduces plasma concentration of •maraviroc and •tipranavir—avoid concomitant use; avoidance of St John's wort advised by manufacturer of •rilpivirine (plasma concentration of rilpivirine possibly reduced)

Anxiolytics and Hypnotics: St John's wort possibly reduces plasma concentration of oral midazolam

• Aprepitant: avoidance of St John's wort advised by manufacturer of •aprepitant

Atomoxetine: possible increased risk of convulsions when antidepressants given with atomoxetine

• Calcium-channel Blockers: St John's wort possibly reduces plasma concentration of amlodipine; St John's wort reduces plasma concentration of nifedipine; St John's wort significantly reduces plasma concentration of •verapamil

• Cardiac Glycosides: St John's wort reduces plasma concentration of •digoxin—avoid concomitant use

• Ciclosporin: St John's wort reduces plasma concentration of •ciclosporin—avoid concomitant use

• Cytotoxics: St John's wort possibly reduces plasma concentration of axitinib—consider increasing dose of axitinib; St John's wort possibly reduces plasma

## St John's Wort

- Cytotoxics *(continued)*
  concentration of crizotinib, everolimus and ●vinflu-nine—manufacturer of crizotinib, everolimus and vinflunine advises avoid concomitant use; avoid-ance of St John's wort advised by manufacturer of ●cabazitaxel, gefitinib, ●lapatinib and vemurafenib; St John's wort reduces plasma concentration of ●imatinib—avoid concomitant use; avoidance of St John's wort advised by manufacturer of vandetanib (plasma concentration of vandetanib possibly reduced); St John's wort possibly reduces plasma concentration of eribulin; St John's wort accelerates metabolism of ●irinotecan (reduced plasma concen-tration—avoid concomitant use)
- Diuretics: St John's wort reduces plasma concentra-tion of ●eplerenone—avoid concomitant use
- 5HT$_1$-receptor Agonists: increased serotonergic effects when St John's wort given with ●5HT$_1$ agonists—avoid concomitant use
  Ivabradine: St John's wort reduces plasma concentra-tion of ivabradine—avoid concomitant use
  Lipid-regulating Drugs: St John's wort reduces plasma concentration of simvastatin
- Oestrogens: St John's wort reduces contraceptive effect of ●oestrogens (avoid concomitant use)
- Progestogens: St John's wort reduces contraceptive effect of ●progestogens (avoid concomitant use)
- Tacrolimus: St John's wort reduces plasma concentra-tion of ●tacrolimus—avoid concomitant use
  Theophylline: St John's wort possibly reduces plasma concentration of theophylline
  Ulcer-healing Drugs: St John's wort possibly reduces plasma concentration of omeprazole
- Ulipristal: avoidance of St John's wort advised by manufacturer of ●ulipristal (contraceptive effect of ulipristal possibly reduced)

**Salbutamol** *see* Sympathomimetics, Beta$_2$

**Salmeterol** *see* Sympathomimetics, Beta$_2$

## Saquinavir

- Analgesics: increased risk of ventricular arrhythmias when saquinavir given with ●alfentanil, ●fentanyl or ●methadone—avoid concomitant use
- Anti-arrhythmics: increased risk of ventricular arrhyth-mias when saquinavir given with ●amiodarone, ●disopyramide, ●dronedarone, ●flecainide, ●lido-caine or ●propafenone—avoid concomitant use
- Antibacterials: increased risk of ventricular arrhyth-mias when saquinavir given with ●clarithromycin, ●dapsone, ●erythromycin or ●moxifloxacin—avoid concomitant use; saquinavir increases plasma con-centration of ●rifabutin (also plasma concentration of saquinavir reduced)—reduce rifabutin dose; plasma concentration of saquinavir significantly reduced by ●rifampicin, also risk of hepatotoxi-city—avoid concomitant use; plasma concentration of both drugs may increase when saquinavir given with fusidic acid; avoidance of saquinavir advised by manufacturer of ●telithromycin (risk of ventri-cular arrhythmias)
  Anticoagulants: saquinavir possibly enhances anti-coagulant effect of warfarin; avoidance of saquinavir advised by manufacturer of apixaban and rivaroxa-ban
- Antidepressants: increased risk of ventricular arrhyth-mias when saquinavir given with ●trazodone or ●tri-cyclics—avoid concomitant use; plasma concentra-tion of saquinavir reduced by ●St John's wort—avoid concomitant use
- Antiepileptics: plasma concentration of saquinavir possibly reduced by carbamazepine, ●phenobarbital and phenytoin
  Antifungals: plasma concentration of saquinavir increased by ketoconazole; plasma concentration of

## Saquinavir

Antifungals *(continued)*
saquinavir possibly increased by imidazoles and triazoles
- Antihistamines: increased risk of ventricular arrhyth-mias when saquinavir given with ●mizolastine—avoid concomitant use
- Antimalarials: avoidance of saquinavir advised by manufacturer of ●piperaquine with artenimol (possi-ble risk of ventricular arrhythmias); caution with saquinavir advised by manufacturer of artemether with lumefantrine; increased risk of ventricular arrhythmias when saquinavir given with ●quinine—avoid concomitant use
  Antimuscarinics: avoidance of saquinavir advised by manufacturer of darifenacin and tolterodine; manu-facturer of fesoterodine advises dose reduction when saquinavir given with fesoterodine—consult fesoterodine product literature
- Antipsychotics: increased risk of ventricular arrhyth-mias when saquinavir given with ●clozapine, ●halo-peridol or ●phenothiazines—avoid concomitant use; saquinavir possibly inhibits metabolism of ●aripipra-zole (reduce dose of aripiprazole); saquinavir possi-bly increases plasma concentration of ●pimozide (increased risk of ventricular arrhythmias—avoid concomitant use); saquinavir possibly increases plasma concentration of ●quetiapine—manufacturer of quetiapine advises avoid concomitant use
- Antivirals: increased risk of ventricular arrhythmias when saquinavir given with ●atazanavir or ●lopina-vir—avoid concomitant use; saquinavir reduces plasma concentration of darunavir; plasma concen-tration of saquinavir significantly reduced by efavir-enz; plasma concentration of saquinavir increased by indinavir and ●ritonavir; saquinavir increases plasma concentration of ●maraviroc (consider redu-cing dose of maraviroc); plasma concentration of saquinavir reduced by ●tipranavir
- Anxiolytics and Hypnotics: saquinavir increases plasma concentration of ●midazolam (risk of pro-longed sedation—avoid concomitant use of *oral* midazolam)
- Beta-blockers: increased risk of ventricular arrhyth-mias when saquinavir given with ●sotalol—avoid concomitant use
- Ciclosporin: plasma concentration of both drugs increased when saquinavir given with ●ciclosporin
  Corticosteroids: plasma concentration of saquinavir possibly reduced by dexamethasone
- Cytotoxics: saquinavir possibly increases plasma con-centration of axitinib (reduce dose of axitinib—con-sult axitinib product literature); saquinavir possibly increases plasma concentration of ●crizotinib and ●everolimus—manufacturer of crizotinib and evero-limus advises avoid concomitant use; avoidance of saquinavir advised by manufacturer of ●cabazitaxel, ●lapatinib and ●pazopanib; manufacturer of ruxoliti-nib advises dose reduction when saquinavir given with ●ruxolitinib—consult ruxolitinib product litera-ture
  Diuretics: saquinavir increases plasma concentration of eplerenone (reduce dose of eplerenone)
- Ergot Alkaloids: increased risk of ergotism when saquinavir given with ●ergotamine and methy-sergide—avoid concomitant use
- Lipid-regulating Drugs: possible increased risk of myo-pathy when saquinavir given with atorvastatin; pos-sible increased risk of myopathy when saquinavir given with ●rosuvastatin—manufacturer of rosuvas-tatin advises avoid concomitant use; increased risk of myopathy when saquinavir given with ●simva-statin (avoid concomitant use)
- Pentamidine Isetionate: increased risk of ventricular arrhythmias when saquinavir given with ●pent-amidine isetionate—avoid concomitant use

**Saquinavir** *(continued)*
- Ranolazine: saquinavir possibly increases plasma concentration of ●ranolazine—manufacturer of ranolazine advises avoid concomitant use
- Sildenafil: increased risk of ventricular arrhythmias when saquinavir given with ●sildenafil—avoid concomitant use
- Tacrolimus: saquinavir increases plasma concentration of ●tacrolimus (consider reducing dose of tacrolimus)
- Tadalafil: increased risk of ventricular arrhythmias when saquinavir given with ●tadalafil—avoid concomitant use
- Ulcer-healing Drugs: plasma concentration of saquinavir possibly increased by cimetidine; plasma concentration of saquinavir possibly increased by ●esomeprazole, ●lansoprazole, ●pantoprazole and ●rabeprazole—manufacturer of saquinavir advises avoid concomitant use; plasma concentration of saquinavir increased by ●omeprazole—manufacturer of saquinavir advises avoid concomitant use
- Vardenafil: increased risk of ventricular arrhythmias when saquinavir given with ●vardenafil—avoid concomitant use

**Saxagliptin** *see* Antidiabetics

**Selegiline**
Note Selegiline is a MAO-B inhibitor
- Analgesics: hyperpyrexia and CNS toxicity reported when selegiline given with ●pethidine (avoid concomitant use); manufacturer of selegiline advises avoid concomitant use with opioid analgesics
- Antidepressants: manufacturer of selegiline advises avoid concomitant use with citalopram and escitalopram; increased risk of hypertension and CNS excitation when selegiline given with ●fluoxetine (selegiline should not be started until 5 weeks after stopping fluoxetine, avoid fluoxetine for 2 weeks after stopping selegiline); increased risk of hypertension and CNS excitation when selegiline given with ●fluvoxamine, ●sertraline or ●venlafaxine (selegiline should not be started until 1 week after stopping fluvoxamine, sertraline or venlafaxine, avoid fluvoxamine, sertraline or venlafaxine for 2 weeks after stopping selegiline); increased risk of hypertension and CNS excitation when selegiline given with ●paroxetine (selegiline should not be started until 2 weeks after stopping paroxetine, avoid paroxetine for 2 weeks after stopping selegiline); enhanced hypotensive effect when selegiline given with ●MAOIs—manufacturer of selegiline advises avoid concomitant use; avoid concomitant use of selegiline with ●moclobemide; CNS toxicity reported when selegiline given with ●tricyclics
- Dopaminergics: max. dose of 10mg daily advised by manufacturer of entacapone if used concomitantly; selegiline enhances effects and increases toxicity of levodopa (reduce dose of levodopa)
- 5HT$_1$-receptor Agonists: manufacturer of selegiline advises avoid concomitant use with 5HT$_1$ agonists
- Memantine: effects of dopaminergics and selegiline possibly enhanced by memantine
- Methyldopa: antiparkinsonian effect of dopaminergics antagonised by methyldopa
- Oestrogens: plasma concentration of selegiline increased by ●oestrogens—manufacturer of selegiline advises avoid concomitant use
- Progestogens: plasma concentration of selegiline increased by ●progestogens—manufacturer of selegiline advises avoid concomitant use
- Sympathomimetics: manufacturer of selegiline advises avoid concomitant use with sympathomimetics; risk of hypertensive crisis when selegiline given with ●dopamine

**Selenium**
- Eltrombopag: selenium possibly reduces absorption of eltrombopag (give at least 4 hours apart)

**Selenium** *(continued)*
- Vitamins: absorption of selenium possibly reduced by ascorbic acid (give at least 4 hours apart)

**Sertraline** *see* Antidepressants, SSRI

**Sevelamer**
- Antibacterials: sevelamer reduces bioavailability of ciprofloxacin
- Ciclosporin: sevelamer possibly reduces plasma concentration of ciclosporin
- Mycophenolate: sevelamer possibly reduces plasma concentration of mycophenolate
- Tacrolimus: sevelamer possibly reduces plasma concentration of tacrolimus
- Thyroid Hormones: sevelamer possibly reduces absorption of levothyroxine

**Sevoflurane** *see* Anaesthetics, General

**Sildenafil**
- Alpha-blockers: enhanced hypotensive effect when sildenafil given with ●alpha-blockers (avoid alpha-blockers for 4 hours after sildenafil)—see also under Phosphodiesterase type-5 inhibitors, BNF section 7.4.5
- Anti-arrhythmics: avoidance of sildenafil advised by manufacturer of disopyramide (risk of ventricular arrhythmias)
- Antibacterials: plasma concentration of sildenafil possibly increased by clarithromycin and telithromycin—reduce initial dose of sildenafil; plasma concentration of sildenafil increased by erythromycin—reduce initial dose of sildenafil
- Antifungals: plasma concentration of sildenafil increased by itraconazole and ketoconazole—reduce initial dose of sildenafil
- Antivirals: side-effects of sildenafil possibly increased by ●atazanavir; plasma concentration of sildenafil reduced by etravirine; plasma concentration of sildenafil possibly increased by fosamprenavir; plasma concentration of sildenafil increased by ●indinavir—reduce initial dose of sildenafil; plasma concentration of sildenafil significantly increased by ●ritonavir—avoid concomitant use; increased risk of ventricular arrhythmias when sildenafil given with ●saquinavir—avoid concomitant use; avoidance of sildenafil advised by manufacturer of ●telaprevir
- Bosentan: plasma concentration of sildenafil reduced by bosentan
- Calcium-channel Blockers: enhanced hypotensive effect when sildenafil given with amlodipine
- Grapefruit Juice: plasma concentration of sildenafil possibly increased by grapefruit juice
- Nicorandil: sildenafil significantly enhances hypotensive effect of ●nicorandil (avoid concomitant use)
- Nitrates: sildenafil significantly enhances hypotensive effect of ●nitrates (avoid concomitant use)
- Ulcer-healing Drugs: plasma concentration of sildenafil increased by cimetidine (consider reducing dose of sildenafil)

**Simvastatin** *see* Statins

**Sirolimus**
- Anti-arrhythmics: caution with sirolimus advised by manufacturer of dronedarone
- Antibacterials: plasma concentration of sirolimus increased by ●clarithromycin and ●telithromycin—avoid concomitant use; plasma concentration of both drugs increased when sirolimus given with ●erythromycin; plasma concentration of sirolimus reduced by ●rifabutin and ●rifampicin—avoid concomitant use
- Antifungals: plasma concentration of sirolimus increased by ●itraconazole, ●ketoconazole and ●voriconazole—avoid concomitant use; plasma concentration of sirolimus increased by micafungin and ●miconazole; plasma concentration of sirolimus possibly increased by fluconazole and posaconazole
- Antivirals: plasma concentration of sirolimus possibly increased by ●atazanavir, ●boceprevir and lopinavir;

## Sirolimus

- Antivirals *(continued)*
  plasma concentration of both drugs increased when sirolimus given with ●telaprevir (reduce dose of sirolimus)
- Calcium-channel Blockers: plasma concentration of sirolimus increased by ●diltiazem; plasma concentration of both drugs increased when sirolimus given with ●verapamil
  Ciclosporin: plasma concentration of sirolimus increased by ciclosporin
- Cytotoxics: caution with sirolimus advised by manufacturer of ●crizotinib
- Grapefruit Juice: plasma concentration of sirolimus increased by ●grapefruit juice—avoid concomitant use

**Sitagliptin** *see* Antidiabetics

## Sodium Aurothiomalate

- ACE Inhibitors: flushing and hypotension reported when sodium aurothiomalate given with ●ACE inhibitors
  Penicillamine: avoidance of sodium aurothiomalate advised by manufacturer of penicillamine (increased risk of toxicity)

## Sodium Benzoate

  Antiepileptics: effects of sodium benzoate possibly reduced by valproate
  Antipsychotics: effects of sodium benzoate possibly reduced by haloperidol
  Corticosteroids: effects of sodium benzoate possibly reduced by corticosteroids
  Probenecid: excretion of conjugate formed by sodium benzoate possibly reduced by probenecid

**Sodium Bicarbonate** *see* Antacids

## Sodium Citrate

  Antibacterials: avoid concomitant use of sodium citrate with methenamine

**Sodium Clodronate** *see* Bisphosphonates

**Sodium Nitroprusside** *see* Vasodilator Antihypertensives

## Sodium Oxybate

- Analgesics: effects of sodium oxybate enhanced by ●opioid analgesics (avoid concomitant use)
  Antidepressants: increased risk of side-effects when sodium oxybate given with tricyclics
  Antiepileptics: manufacturer of sodium oxybate advises avoid concomitant use with phenobarbital
  Antipsychotics: effects of sodium oxybate possibly enhanced by antipsychotics
- Anxiolytics and Hypnotics: effects of sodium oxybate enhanced by ●benzodiazepines (avoid concomitant use)

## Sodium Phenylbutyrate

  Antiepileptics: effects of sodium phenylbutyrate possibly reduced by valproate
  Antipsychotics: effects of sodium phenylbutyrate possibly reduced by haloperidol
  Corticosteroids: effects of sodium phenylbutyrate possibly reduced by corticosteroids
  Probenecid: excretion of conjugate formed by sodium phenylbutyrate possibly reduced by probenecid

## Sodium Stibogluconate

- Antifungals: possible increased risk of arrhythmias when sodium stibogluconate given before ●amphotericin—manufacturer of sodium stibogluconate advises giving 14 days apart

**Sodium Valproate** *see* Valproate

**Solifenacin** *see* Antimuscarinics

## Somatropin

  Corticosteroids: growth-promoting effect of somatropin may be inhibited by corticosteroids
  Oestrogens: increased doses of somatropin may be needed when given with oestrogens (when used as oral replacement therapy)

## Sorafenib

  Antibacterials: bioavailability of sorafenib reduced by neomycin; plasma concentration of sorafenib reduced by rifampicin
- Anticoagulants: sorafenib possibly enhances anticoagulant effect of ●coumarins
- Antipsychotics: avoid concomitant use of cytotoxics with ●clozapine (increased risk of agranulocytosis)
- Antivirals: avoidance of sorafenib advised by manufacturer of ●boceprevir
  Cytotoxics: sorafenib possibly increases plasma concentration of doxorubicin and irinotecan; sorafenib increases plasma concentration of docetaxel

**Sotalol** *see* Beta-blockers

**Spironolactone** *see* Diuretics

## Statins

  Antacids: absorption of rosuvastatin reduced by antacids
- Anti-arrhythmics: increased risk of myopathy when simvastatin given with ●amiodarone (see Dose under Simvastatin, p. 126); increased risk of myopathy when simvastatin given with ●dronedarone; plasma concentration of atorvastatin and rosuvastatin possibly increased by dronedarone
- Antibacterials: plasma concentration of atorvastatin and pravastatin increased by ●clarithromycin; increased risk of myopathy when simvastatin given with ●clarithromycin, ●erythromycin or ●telithromycin (avoid concomitant use); plasma concentration of rosuvastatin reduced by erythromycin; possible increased risk of myopathy when atorvastatin given with erythromycin; plasma concentration of pravastatin increased by erythromycin; plasma concentration of atorvastatin and simvastatin possibly reduced by rifampicin; metabolism of fluvastatin accelerated by rifampicin (reduced effect); increased risk of myopathy when statins given with ●daptomycin (preferably avoid concomitant use); risk of myopathy and rhabdomyolysis when statins given with ●fusidic acid—avoid concomitant use and for 7 days after last fusidic acid dose; possible increased risk of myopathy when pravastatin given with telithromycin; increased risk of myopathy when atorvastatin given with ●telithromycin (avoid concomitant use)
- Anticoagulants: atorvastatin may transiently reduce anticoagulant effect of warfarin; fluvastatin and simvastatin enhance anticoagulant effect of ●coumarins; rosuvastatin possibly enhances anticoagulant effect of ●coumarins and ●phenindione
  Antidepressants: plasma concentration of simvastatin reduced by St John's wort
  Antidiabetics: fluvastatin possibly increases plasma concentration of glibenclamide
- Antiepileptics: plasma concentration of simvastatin reduced by ●carbamazepine and eslicarbazepine—consider increasing dose of simvastatin; combination of fluvastatin with phenytoin may increase plasma concentration of either drug (or both)
- Antifungals: increased risk of myopathy when simvastatin given with ●itraconazole, ●ketoconazole or ●posaconazole (avoid concomitant use); possible increased risk of myopathy when simvastatin given with ●fluconazole, ●miconazole or voriconazole; plasma concentration of fluvastatin increased by fluconazole—possible increased risk of myopathy; increased risk of myopathy when atorvastatin given with ●itraconazole; increased risk of myopathy when atorvastatin given with ●posaconazole (avoid concomitant use); possible increased risk of myopathy when atorvastatin given with imidazoles or triazoles
- Antivirals: possible increased risk of myopathy when rosuvastatin given with ●atazanavir, ●darunavir, ●fosamprenavir, ●indinavir, ●lopinavir, ●ritonavir and ●saquinavir—manufacturer of rosuvastatin

**Statins**

- Antivirals *(continued)*

   advises avoid concomitant use; increased risk of myopathy when simvastatin given with ●atazanavir, ●indinavir, ●ritonavir or ●saquinavir (avoid concomitant use); possible increased risk of myopathy when atorvastatin or pravastatin given with ●atazanavir; manufacturers advise avoid concomitant use of simvastatin with ●boceprevir and ●telaprevir; plasma concentration of pravastatin increased by boceprevir; enhanced effects and increased toxicity of atorvastatin when given with ●boceprevir (reduce dose of atorvastatin); plasma concentration of pravastatin possibly increased by darunavir; possible increased risk of myopathy when atorvastatin given with darunavir, fosamprenavir, indinavir, lopinavir, ritonavir or saquinavir; plasma concentration of atorvastatin, pravastatin and simvastatin reduced by efavirenz; plasma concentration of atorvastatin possibly reduced by etravirine; possible increased risk of myopathy when simvastatin given with ●fosamprenavir or ●lopinavir—avoid concomitant use; avoidance of atorvastatin advised by manufacturer of ●telaprevir; increased risk of myopathy when atorvastatin given with ●tipranavir (see Dose under Atorvastatin, p. 125); plasma concentration of rosuvastatin possibly increased by ●tipranavir—manufacturer of rosuvastatin advises avoid concomitant use; plasma concentration of simvastatin possibly increased by ●tipranavir—avoid concomitant use

   Anxiolytics and Hypnotics: atorvastatin possibly increases plasma concentration of midazolam

   Bosentan: plasma concentration of simvastatin reduced by bosentan

- Calcium-channel Blockers: possible increased risk of myopathy when simvastatin given with ●amlodipine and diltiazem (see Dose under Simvastatin, p. 126); plasma concentration of atorvastatin increased by diltiazem—possible increased risk of myopathy; increased risk of myopathy when simvastatin given with ●verapamil (see Dose under Simvastatin, p. 126)

   Cardiac Glycosides: atorvastatin possibly increases plasma concentration of digoxin

- Ciclosporin: increased risk of myopathy when rosuvastatin or simvastatin given with ●ciclosporin (avoid concomitant use); increased risk of myopathy when atorvastatin given with ●ciclosporin (see Dose under Atorvastatin, p. 125); increased risk of myopathy when fluvastatin or pravastatin given with ●ciclosporin

- Colchicine: possible increased risk of myopathy when statins given with ●colchicine

   Cytotoxics: plasma concentration of simvastatin possibly increased by dasatinib; plasma concentration of simvastatin increased by imatinib

- Eltrombopag: plasma concentration of rosuvastatin increased by ●eltrombopag (consider reducing dose of rosuvastatin)

- Grapefruit Juice: plasma concentration of atorvastatin possibly increased by grapefruit juice; plasma concentration of simvastatin increased by ●grapefruit juice—avoid concomitant use

- Hormone Antagonists: possible increased risk of myopathy when simvastatin given with ●danazol—avoid concomitant use

- Lipid-regulating Drugs: possible increased risk of myopathy when simvastatin given with ●bezafibrate and ●ciprofibrate (see Dose under Simvastatin, p. 126); increased risk of myopathy when atorvastatin, fluvastatin or pravastatin given with ●gemfibrozil (preferably avoid concomitant use); increased risk of myopathy when simvastatin given with ●gemfibrozil (avoid concomitant use); increased risk of myopathy

**Statins**

- Lipid-regulating Drugs *(continued)*

   when rosuvastatin given with ●fibrates (see Dose under Rosuvastatin, p. 126); increased risk of myopathy when statins given with ●fibrates; increased risk of myopathy when statins given with ●nicotinic acid (applies to lipid regulating doses of nicotinic acid)

   Oestrogens: atorvastatin and rosuvastatin increase plasma concentration of ethinylestradiol

   Progestogens: atorvastatin increases plasma concentration of norethisterone; rosuvastatin increases plasma concentration of active metabolite of norgestimate; rosuvastatin increases plasma concentration of norgestrel

- Ranolazine: plasma concentration of simvastatin increased by ●ranolazine (see Dose under Simvastatin, BNF section 2.12)

   Retinoids: plasma concentration of simvastatin reduced by alitretinoin

- Ticagrelor: plasma concentration of simvastatin increased by ●ticagrelor (increased risk of toxicity)

**Stavudine**

- Antivirals: increased risk of side-effects when stavudine given with ●didanosine; increased risk of toxicity when stavudine given with ●ribavirin; effects of stavudine possibly inhibited by ●zidovudine (manufacturers advise avoid concomitant use)

- Cytotoxics: effects of stavudine possibly inhibited by doxorubicin; increased risk of toxicity when stavudine given with ●hydroxycarbamide—avoid concomitant use

**Stiripentol**

- Antidepressants: anticonvulsant effect of antiepileptics possibly antagonised by MAOIs and ●tricyclic-related antidepressants (convulsive threshold lowered); anticonvulsant effect of antiepileptics antagonised by ●SSRIs and ●tricyclics (convulsive threshold lowered); avoid concomitant use of antiepileptics with ●St John's wort

- Antiepileptics: stiripentol increases plasma concentration of ●carbamazepine, ●phenobarbital and ●phenytoin

- Antimalarials: anticonvulsant effect of antiepileptics antagonised by ●mefloquine

- Antipsychotics: anticonvulsant effect of antiepileptics antagonised by ●antipsychotics (convulsive threshold lowered)

   Anxiolytics and Hypnotics: stiripentol increases plasma concentration of clobazam

- Orlistat: possible increased risk of convulsions when antiepileptics given with ●orlistat

**Streptomycin** *see* Aminoglycosides

**Strontium Ranelate**

   Antibacterials: strontium ranelate reduces absorption of quinolones and tetracyclines (manufacturer of strontium ranelate advises avoid concomitant use)

**Sucralfate**

   Antibacterials: sucralfate reduces absorption of ciprofloxacin, levofloxacin, moxifloxacin, ofloxacin and tetracyclines; sucralfate reduces absorption of norfloxacin (give at least 2 hours apart)

- Anticoagulants: sucralfate possibly reduces absorption of ●coumarins (reduced anticoagulant effect)

- Antiepileptics: sucralfate reduces absorption of ●phenytoin

   Antifungals: sucralfate reduces absorption of ketoconazole

   Antipsychotics: sucralfate reduces absorption of sulpiride

   Cardiac Glycosides: sucralfate possibly reduces absorption of cardiac glycosides

   Theophylline: sucralfate possibly reduces absorption of theophylline (give at least 2 hours apart)

**Sucralfate** *(continued)*
  Thyroid Hormones: sucralfate reduces absorption of levothyroxine
  Ulcer-healing Drugs: sucralfate possibly reduces absorption of lansoprazole

**Sugammadex**
  Antibacterials: response to sugammadex possibly reduced by fusidic acid
  Progestogens: sugammadex possibly reduces plasma concentration of progestogens—manufacturer of sugammadex advises additional contraceptive precautions

**Sulfadiazine** *see* Sulfonamides

**Sulfadoxine** *see* Sulfonamides

**Sulfamethoxazole** *see* Sulfonamides

**Sulfasalazine** *see* Aminosalicylates

**Sulfinpyrazone**
  Analgesics: effects of sulfinpyrazone antagonised by aspirin
  Antibacterials: sulfinpyrazone reduces excretion of nitrofurantoin (increased risk of toxicity); sulfinpyrazone reduces excretion of penicillins; effects of sulfinpyrazone antagonised by pyrazinamide
● Anticoagulants: increased risk of bleeding when sulfinpyrazone given with apixaban; sulfinpyrazone enhances anticoagulant effect of ●coumarins; possible increased risk of bleeding when sulfinpyrazone given with ●dabigatran etexilate
● Antidiabetics: sulfinpyrazone enhances effects of ●sulfonylureas
● Antiepileptics: sulfinpyrazone increases plasma concentration of ●phenytoin
  Calcium-channel Blockers: sulfinpyrazone reduces plasma concentration of verapamil
● Ciclosporin: sulfinpyrazone reduces plasma concentration of ●ciclosporin
  Theophylline: sulfinpyrazone reduces plasma concentration of theophylline

**Sulfonamides**
  Anaesthetics, General: sulfonamides enhance effects of thiopental
  Anaesthetics, Local: increased risk of methaemoglobinaemia when sulfonamides given with prilocaine
  Anti-arrhythmics: possible increased risk of ventricular arrhythmias when sulfamethoxazole (as co-trimoxazole) given with amiodarone—manufacturer of amiodarone advises avoid concomitant use of co-trimoxazole
● Antibacterials: increased risk of crystalluria when sulfonamides given with ●methenamine
● Anticoagulants: sulfonamides enhance anticoagulant effect of ●coumarins; sulfonamides possibly inhibit metabolism of phenindione
  Antidiabetics: sulfonamides rarely enhance the effects of sulfonylureas
  Antiepileptics: sulfonamides possibly increase plasma concentration of phenytoin
● Antimalarials: increased antifolate effect when sulfonamides given with ●pyrimethamine
● Antipsychotics: avoid concomitant use of sulfonamides with ●clozapine (increased risk of agranulocytosis)
● Azathioprine: increased risk of haematological toxicity when sulfamethoxazole (as co-trimoxazole) given with ●azathioprine
● Ciclosporin: increased risk of nephrotoxicity when sulfonamides given with ●ciclosporin; sulfadiazine possibly reduces plasma concentration of ●ciclosporin
● Cytotoxics: increased risk of haematological toxicity when sulfamethoxazole (as co-trimoxazole) given with ●mercaptopurine or ●methotrexate; sulfonamides increase risk of methotrexate toxicity
  Potassium Aminobenzoate: effects of sulfonamides inhibited by potassium aminobenzoate

**Sulfonamides** *(continued)*
  Vaccines: antibacterials inactivate oral typhoid vaccine—see p. 621

**Sulfonylureas** *see* Antidiabetics

**Sulindac** *see* NSAIDs

**Sulpiride** *see* Antipsychotics

**Sumatriptan** *see* 5HT₁-receptor Agonists (under HT)

**Sunitinib**
  Antibacterials: metabolism of sunitinib accelerated by rifampicin (reduced plasma concentration)
  Antifungals: metabolism of sunitinib inhibited by ketoconazole (increased plasma concentration)
● Antipsychotics: avoid concomitant use of cytotoxics with ●clozapine (increased risk of agranulocytosis)
● Antivirals: avoidance of sunitinib advised by manufacturer of ●boceprevir

**Suxamethonium** *see* Muscle Relaxants

**Sympathomimetics**
● Adrenergic Neurone Blockers: ephedrine, isometheptene, metaraminol, methylphenidate, noradrenaline (norepinephrine), oxymetazoline, phenylephrine, pseudoephedrine and xylometazoline antagonise hypotensive effect of ●adrenergic neurone blockers; dexamfetamine and lisdexamfetamine antagonise hypotensive effect of ●guanethidine
  Alcohol: effects of methylphenidate possibly enhanced by alcohol
  Alpha₂-adrenoceptor Stimulants: avoidance of sympathomimetics advised by manufacturer of apraclonidine
● Alpha-blockers: avoid concomitant use of adrenaline (epinephrine) or dopamine with ●tolazoline
● Anaesthetics, General: increased risk of arrhythmias when adrenaline (epinephrine) given with ●volatile liquid general anaesthetics; increased risk of hypertension when methylphenidate given with ●volatile liquid general anaesthetics
● Anticoagulants: methylphenidate possibly enhances anticoagulant effect of ●coumarins
● Antidepressants: risk of hypertensive crisis when methylphenidate given with ●MAOIs, some manufacturers advise avoid methylphenidate for at least 2 weeks after stopping MAOIs; risk of hypertensive crisis when sympathomimetics given with ●MAOIs or ●moclobemide; methylphenidate possibly inhibits metabolism of SSRIs and tricyclics; increased risk of hypertension and arrhythmias when noradrenaline (norepinephrine) given with ●tricyclics; increased risk of hypertension and arrhythmias when adrenaline (epinephrine) given with ●tricyclics (but local anaesthetics with adrenaline appear to be safe)
  Antiepileptics: methylphenidate possibly increases plasma concentration of phenobarbital; methylphenidate increases plasma concentration of phenytoin
  Antipsychotics: hypertensive effect of sympathomimetics antagonised by antipsychotics; effects of lisdexamfetamine possibly reduced by chlorpromazine; dexamfetamine possibly antagonises antipsychotic effects of chlorpromazine; methylphenidate possibly increases side-effects of risperidone
  Antivirals: plasma concentration of dexamfetamine possibly increased by ritonavir
● Beta-blockers: increased risk of severe hypertension and bradycardia when adrenaline (epinephrine) given with non-cardioselective ●beta-blockers, also response to adrenaline (epinephrine) may be reduced; increased risk of severe hypertension and bradycardia when dobutamine given with non-cardioselective ●beta-blockers; possible increased risk of severe hypertension and bradycardia when noradrenaline (norepinephrine) given with non-cardioselective ●beta-blockers
● Clonidine: possible risk of hypertension when adrenaline (epinephrine) or noradrenaline (norepinephrine)

## Sympathomimetics

- Clonidine *(continued)*
  given with clonidine; serious adverse events reported with concomitant use of methylphenidate and ●clonidine (causality not established)

  Corticosteroids: ephedrine accelerates metabolism of dexamethasone

- Dopaminergics: risk of toxicity when isometheptene given with ●bromocriptine; effects of adrenaline (epinephrine), dobutamine, dopamine and noradrenaline (norepinephrine) possibly enhanced by entacapone; avoid concomitant use of sympathomimetics with ●rasagiline; risk of hypertensive crisis when dopamine given with ●selegiline; avoidance of sympathomimetics advised by manufacturer of selegiline

  Doxapram: increased risk of hypertension when sympathomimetics given with doxapram

  Ergot Alkaloids: increased risk of ergotism when sympathomimetics given with ergotamine and methysergide

  Oxytocin: risk of hypertension when vasoconstrictor sympathomimetics given with oxytocin (due to enhanced vasopressor effect)

- Sympathomimetics: effects of adrenaline (epinephrine) possibly enhanced by ●dopexamine; dopexamine possibly enhances effects of ●noradrenaline (norepinephrine)

  Theophylline: avoidance of ephedrine in children advised by manufacturer of theophylline

## Sympathomimetics, Beta$_2$

Antifungals: metabolism of salmeterol inhibited by ketoconazole (increased plasma concentration)

- Antivirals: avoidance of salmeterol advised by manufacturer of lopinavir, ritonavir and tipranavir; avoidance of salmeterol advised by manufacturer of ●telaprevir (risk of ventricular arrhythmias)

  Atomoxetine: Increased risk of cardiovascular side-effects when *parenteral* salbutamol given with atomoxetine

  Cardiac Glycosides: salbutamol possibly reduces plasma concentration of digoxin

  Corticosteroids: increased risk of hypokalaemia when high doses of beta$_2$ sympathomimetics given with corticosteroids—see Hypokalaemia, p. 136

  Diuretics: increased risk of hypokalaemia when high doses of beta$_2$ sympathomimetics given with acetazolamide, loop diuretics or thiazides and related diuretics—see Hypokalaemia, p. 136

- Methyldopa: acute hypotension reported when *infusion* of salbutamol given with ●methyldopa

  Muscle Relaxants: bambuterol enhances effects of suxamethonium

  Theophylline: increased risk of hypokalaemia when high doses of beta$_2$ sympathomimetics given with theophylline—see Hypokalaemia, p. 136

## Tacrolimus

**Note** Interactions do not generally apply to tacrolimus used topically; risk of facial flushing and skin irritation with alcohol consumption (p. 576) does not apply to tacrolimus taken systemically

- Analgesics: possible increased risk of nephrotoxicity when tacrolimus given with NSAIDs; increased risk of nephrotoxicity when tacrolimus given with ●ibuprofen

  Angiotensin-II Receptor Antagonists: increased risk of hyperkalaemia when tacrolimus given with angiotensin-II receptor antagonists

  Anti-arrhythmics: caution with tacrolimus advised by manufacturer of dronedarone

- Antibacterials: plasma concentration of tacrolimus increased by ●clarithromycin and ●erythromycin; plasma concentration of tacrolimus possibly reduced by rifabutin; plasma concentration of tacrolimus reduced by ●rifampicin; increased risk of nephrotoxicity when tacrolimus given with ●amino-

## Tacrolimus

- Antibacterials *(continued)*
  glycosides; plasma concentration of tacrolimus possibly increased by ●chloramphenicol and ●telithromycin; possible increased risk of nephrotoxicity when tacrolimus given with vancomycin

- Anticoagulants: tacrolimus possibly increases plasma concentration of ●dabigatran etexilate—manufacturer of dabigatran etexilate advises avoid concomitant use

- Antidepressants: plasma concentration of tacrolimus reduced by ●St John's wort—avoid concomitant use

- Antiepileptics: plasma concentration of tacrolimus reduced by ●phenobarbital; plasma concentration of tacrolimus reduced by phenytoin, also plasma concentration of phenytoin possibly increased

- Antifungals: plasma concentration of tacrolimus increased by ●fluconazole, ●itraconazole, ●ketoconazole, ●posaconazole and ●voriconazole (consider reducing dose of tacrolimus); increased risk of nephrotoxicity when tacrolimus given with ●amphotericin; plasma concentration of tacrolimus reduced by ●caspofungin; plasma concentration of tacrolimus possibly increased by ●imidazoles

- Antipsychotics: avoidance of tacrolimus advised by manufacturer of ●droperidol (risk of ventricular arrhythmias)

- Antivirals: possible increased risk of nephrotoxicity when tacrolimus given with aciclovir or ganciclovir; plasma concentration of tacrolimus possibly increased by ●atazanavir and ●ritonavir; plasma concentration of tacrolimus increased by ●boceprevir (reduce dose of tacrolimus); plasma concentration of tacrolimus possibly affected by ●efavirenz; plasma concentration of tacrolimus increased by ●fosamprenavir; plasma concentration of tacrolimus increased by ●saquinavir (consider reducing dose of tacrolimus); plasma concentration of both drugs increased when tacrolimus given with ●telaprevir (reduce dose of tacrolimus)

- Calcium-channel Blockers: plasma concentration of tacrolimus possibly increased by felodipine, nicardipine and verapamil; plasma concentration of tacrolimus increased by ●diltiazem and ●nifedipine

- Ciclosporin: tacrolimus increases plasma concentration of ●ciclosporin (increased risk of nephrotoxicity)—avoid concomitant use

- Cytotoxics: caution with tacrolimus advised by manufacturer of ●crizotinib; plasma concentration of tacrolimus increased by imatinib

- Diuretics: increased risk of hyperkalaemia when tacrolimus given with ●potassium-sparing diuretics and aldosterone antagonists

- Grapefruit Juice: plasma concentration of tacrolimus increased by ●grapefruit juice

  Hormone Antagonists: plasma concentration of tacrolimus possibly increased by danazol

  Mifamurtide: avoidance of tacrolimus advised by manufacturer of mifamurtide

  Oestrogens: plasma concentration of tacrolimus possibly increased by ethinylestradiol

- Potassium Salts: increased risk of hyperkalaemia when tacrolimus given with ●potassium salts

- Ranolazine: plasma concentration of tacrolimus increased by ●ranolazine

  Sevelamer: plasma concentration of tacrolimus possibly reduced by sevelamer

  Ulcer-healing Drugs: plasma concentration of tacrolimus possibly increased by omeprazole

## Tadalafil

- Alpha-blockers: enhanced hypotensive effect when tadalafil given with ●doxazosin—manufacturer of tadalafil advises avoid concomitant use; enhanced hypotensive effect when tadalafil given with ●alpha-

## Tadalafil

- Alpha-blockers *(continued)*
  blockers—see also under Phosphodiesterase type-5 inhibitors, BNF section 7.4.5

  Anti-arrhythmics: avoidance of tadalafil advised by manufacturer of disopyramide (risk of ventricular arrhythmias)

- Antibacterials: plasma concentration of tadalafil possibly increased by clarithromycin and erythromycin; plasma concentration of tadalafil reduced by ●rifampicin—manufacturer of tadalafil advises avoid concomitant use

- Antifungals: plasma concentration of tadalafil increased by ●ketoconazole—manufacturer of tadalafil advises avoid concomitant use; plasma concentration of tadalafil possibly increased by itraconazole

- Antivirals: plasma concentration of tadalafil possibly increased by fosamprenavir and indinavir; plasma concentration of tadalafil increased by ●ritonavir—manufacturer of tadalafil advises avoid concomitant use; increased risk of ventricular arrhythmias when tadalafil given with ●saquinavir—avoid concomitant use; avoidance of high doses of tadalafil advised by manufacturer of ●telaprevir—consult product literature

  Bosentan: plasma concentration of tadalafil reduced by bosentan

  Grapefruit Juice: plasma concentration of tadalafil possibly increased by grapefruit juice

- Nicorandil: tadalafil significantly enhances hypotensive effect of ●nicorandil (avoid concomitant use)

- Nitrates: tadalafil significantly enhances hypotensive effect of ●nitrates (avoid concomitant use)

## Tamoxifen

  Antibacterials: metabolism of tamoxifen accelerated by rifampicin (reduced plasma concentration)

- Anticoagulants: tamoxifen enhances anticoagulant effect of ●coumarins

- Antidepressants: metabolism of tamoxifen to active metabolite possibly inhibited by ●fluoxetine and ●paroxetine (avoid concomitant use)

- Antipsychotics: avoidance of tamoxifen advised by manufacturer of ●droperidol (risk of ventricular arrhythmias)

- Bupropion: metabolism of tamoxifen to active metabolite possibly inhibited by ●bupropion (avoid concomitant use)

- Cinacalcet: metabolism of tamoxifen to active metabolite possibly inhibited by ●cinacalcet (avoid concomitant use)

## Tamsulosin *see* Alpha-blockers

## Tapentadol *see* Opioid Analgesics

## Taxanes *see* Cabazitaxel, Docetaxel, and Paclitaxel

## Tegafur *see* Fluorouracil

## Teicoplanin

  Vaccines: antibacterials inactivate oral typhoid vaccine—see p. 621

## Telaprevir

- Alpha-blockers: manufacturer of telaprevir advises avoid concomitant use with ●alfuzosin

- Analgesics: manufacturer of telaprevir advises caution with ●methadone (risk of ventricular arrhythmias)

- Anti-arrhythmics: manufacturer of telaprevir advises avoid concomitant use with ●amiodarone or ●disopyramide (risk of ventricular arrhythmias); manufacturer of telaprevir advises caution with ●flecainide and ●propafenone (risk of ventricular arrhythmias); manufacturer of telaprevir advises caution with *intravenous* lidocaine

- Antibacterials: plasma concentration of both drugs possibly increased when telaprevir given with ●clarithromycin, ●erythromycin and ●telithromycin (increased risk of ventricular arrhythmias); manufacturer of telaprevir advises avoid concomitant use

## Telaprevir

- Antibacterials *(continued)*
  with ●rifabutin; plasma concentration of telaprevir significantly reduced by ●rifampicin—avoid concomitant use

- Anticoagulants: telaprevir possibly affects plasma concentration of ●warfarin; avoidance of telaprevir advised by manufacturer of apixaban; telaprevir possibly increases plasma concentration of dabigatran etexilate

- Antidepressants: telaprevir possibly increases plasma concentration of trazodone; manufacturer of telaprevir advises avoid concomitant use with ●St John's wort

- Antiepileptics: manufacturer of telaprevir advises avoid concomitant use with ●carbamazepine, ●phenobarbital and ●phenytoin

- Antifungals: plasma concentration of both drugs possibly increased when telaprevir given with ●ketoconazole (increased risk of ventricular arrhythmias); telaprevir possibly increases plasma concentration of itraconazole; telaprevir possibly increases plasma concentration of ●posaconazole (increased risk of ventricular arrhythmias); telaprevir possibly affects plasma concentration of ●voriconazole (possible increased risk of ventricular arrhythmias)

- Antipsychotics: manufacturer of telaprevir advises avoid concomitant use with ●pimozide; telaprevir possibly increases plasma concentration of ●quetiapine—manufacturer of quetiapine advises avoid concomitant use

- Antivirals: plasma concentration of telaprevir possibly reduced by atazanavir, also plasma concentration of atazanavir possibly increased; avoid concomitant use of telaprevir with ●darunavir; plasma concentration of telaprevir reduced by ●efavirenz—increase dose of telaprevir; manufacturers advise avoid concomitant use of telaprevir with ●fosamprenavir and ●lopinavir; plasma concentration of telaprevir possibly reduced by ritonavir; telaprevir increases plasma concentration of tenofovir

- Anxiolytics and Hypnotics: telaprevir possibly increases plasma concentration of ●midazolam (risk of prolonged sedation—avoid concomitant use of *oral* midazolam)

- Beta-blockers: manufacturer of telaprevir advises avoid concomitant use with ●sotalol (risk of ventricular arrhythmias)

  Bosentan: plasma concentration of telaprevir possibly reduced by bosentan, also plasma concentration of bosentan possibly increased

  Calcium-channel Blockers: telaprevir increases plasma concentration of amlodipine (consider reducing dose of amlodipine); manufacturer of telaprevir advises caution with diltiazem, felodipine, nicardipine, nifedipine and verapamil

  Cardiac Glycosides: telaprevir increases plasma concentration of digoxin

- Ciclosporin: plasma concentration of both drugs increased when telaprevir given with ●ciclosporin (reduce dose of ciclosporin)

- Colchicine: telaprevir possibly increases risk of ●colchicine toxicity—suspend or reduce dose of colchicine (avoid concomitant use in hepatic or renal impairment)

  Corticosteroids: telaprevir possibly increases plasma concentration of *inhaled* and *intranasal* budesonide and fluticasone; plasma concentration of telaprevir possibly reduced by dexamethasone

- Cytotoxics: manufacturer of ruxolitinib advises dose reduction when telaprevir given with ●ruxolitinib—consult ruxolitinib product literature

- Domperidone: telaprevir possibly increases plasma concentration of ●domperidone—manufacturer of telaprevir advises avoid concomitant use

*Appendix 1: Interactions*

**Telaprevir** *(continued)*
- Ergot Alkaloids: manufacturer of telaprevir advises avoid concomitant use with ●ergot alkaloids
- Lipid-regulating Drugs: manufacturer of telaprevir advises avoid concomitant use with ●atorvastatin; manufacturers advise avoid concomitant use of telaprevir with ●simvastatin
- Oestrogens: telaprevir possibly reduces plasma concentration of ●ethinylestradiol—manufacturer of telaprevir advises additional contraceptive precautions
- Sildenafil: manufacturer of telaprevir advises avoid concomitant use with ●sildenafil
- Sirolimus: plasma concentration of both drugs increased when telaprevir given with ●sirolimus (reduce dose of sirolimus)
- Sympathomimetics, Beta₂: manufacturer of telaprevir advises avoid concomitant use with ●salmeterol (risk of ventricular arrhythmias)
- Tacrolimus: plasma concentration of both drugs increased when telaprevir given with ●tacrolimus (reduce dose of tacrolimus)
- Tadalafil: manufacturer of telaprevir advises avoid concomitant use with high doses of ●tadalafil—consult product literature
- Vardenafil: manufacturer of telaprevir advises avoid concomitant use with ●vardenafil

**Telbivudine**
- Interferons: increased risk of peripheral neuropathy when telbivudine given with ●interferon alfa

**Telithromycin**
- Analgesics: possible increased risk of ventricular arrhythmias when telithromycin given with ●methadone; telithromycin inhibits the metabolism of oxycodone
- Anti-arrhythmics: possible increased risk of ventricular arrhythmias when telithromycin given with ●amiodarone and ●disopyramide; increased risk of ventricular arrhythmias when telithromycin given with ●dronedarone—avoid concomitant use
- Antibacterials: possible increased risk of ventricular arrhythmias when telithromycin given with ●moxifloxacin; plasma concentration of telithromycin reduced by ●rifampicin (avoid during and for 2 weeks after rifampicin)
- Antidepressants: possible increased risk of ventricular arrhythmias when telithromycin given with ●citalopram and ●tricyclics; plasma concentration of telithromycin reduced by ●St John's wort (avoid during and for 2 weeks after St John's wort)
- Antiepileptics: plasma concentration of telithromycin reduced by ●carbamazepine, ●phenobarbital and ●phenytoin (avoid during and for 2 weeks after carbamazepine, phenobarbital and phenytoin)
- Antifungals: manufacturer of telithromycin advises avoid concomitant use with ●ketoconazole in severe renal and hepatic impairment
  Antimuscarinics: manufacturer of fesoterodine advises dose reduction when telithromycin given with fesoterodine—consult fesoterodine product literature
- Antipsychotics: possible increased risk of ventricular arrhythmias when telithromycin given with ●chlorpromazine; increased risk of ventricular arrhythmias when telithromycin given with ●pimozide—avoid concomitant use; telithromycin possibly increases plasma concentration of quetiapine
- Antivirals: manufacturer of telithromycin advises avoid concomitant use with ●atazanavir, ●fosamprenavir, ●indinavir, ●lopinavir, ●ritonavir and ●tipranavir in severe renal and hepatic impairment; telithromycin possibly increases plasma concentration of ●maraviroc (consider reducing dose of maraviroc); manufacturer of telithromycin advises avoid concomitant use with ●saquinavir (risk of ventricular arrhythmias); plasma concentration of both drugs possibly increased when telithromycin

**Telithromycin**
- Antivirals *(continued)*
  given with ●telaprevir (increased risk of ventricular arrhythmias)
- Anxiolytics and Hypnotics: telithromycin inhibits metabolism of ●midazolam (increased plasma concentration with increased sedation)
  Aprepitant: telithromycin possibly increases plasma concentration of aprepitant
- Calcium-channel Blockers: telithromycin possibly inhibits metabolism of ●calcium-channel blockers (increased risk of side-effects)
  Cardiac Glycosides: telithromycin possibly increases plasma concentration of digoxin
- Ciclosporin: telithromycin possibly increases plasma concentration of ●ciclosporin
- Colchicine: telithromycin possibly increases risk of ●colchicine toxicity—suspend or reduce dose of colchicine (avoid concomitant use in hepatic or renal impairment)
- Cytotoxics: telithromycin possibly increases plasma concentration of axitinib (reduce dose of axitinib—consult axitinib product literature); telithromycin possibly increases plasma concentration of ●crizotinib and ●everolimus—manufacturer of crizotinib and everolimus advises avoid concomitant use; avoidance of telithromycin advised by manufacturer of ●cabazitaxel, ●lapatinib, ●nilotinib and ●pazopanib; manufacturer of ruxolitinib advises dose reduction when telithromycin given with ●ruxolitinib—consult ruxolitinib product literature
- Diuretics: telithromycin increases plasma concentration of ●eplerenone—avoid concomitant use
- Ergot Alkaloids: increased risk of ergotism when telithromycin given with ●ergotamine and methysergide—avoid concomitant use
- Ivabradine: telithromycin possibly increases plasma concentration of ●ivabradine—avoid concomitant use
- Lipid-regulating Drugs: increased risk of myopathy when telithromycin given with ●atorvastatin or ●simvastatin (avoid concomitant use); possible increased risk of myopathy when telithromycin given with pravastatin
- Pentamidine Isetionate: possible increased risk of ventricular arrhythmias when telithromycin given with parenteral ●pentamidine isetionate
- Ranolazine: telithromycin possibly increases plasma concentration of ●ranolazine—manufacturer of ranolazine advises avoid concomitant use
  Sildenafil: telithromycin possibly increases plasma concentration of sildenafil—reduce initial dose of sildenafil
- Sirolimus: telithromycin increases plasma concentration of ●sirolimus—avoid concomitant use
- Tacrolimus: telithromycin possibly increases plasma concentration of ●tacrolimus
  Vaccines: antibacterials inactivate oral typhoid vaccine—see p. 621

**Telmisartan** *see* Angiotensin-II Receptor Antagonists
**Temazepam** *see* Anxiolytics and Hypnotics
**Temocillin** *see* Penicillins
**Temoporfin**
- Cytotoxics: increased skin photosensitivity when temoporfin given with *topical* ●fluorouracil
**Temozolomide**
  Antiepileptics: plasma concentration of temozolomide increased by valproate
- Antipsychotics: avoid concomitant use of cytotoxics with ●clozapine (increased risk of agranulocytosis)
**Temsirolimus**
  **Note** The main active metabolite of temsirolimus is sirolimus—*see also* interactions of sirolimus and consult product literature

**Temsirolimus** *(continued)*
- Antibacterials: plasma concentration of active metabolite of temsirolimus reduced by ●rifampicin—avoid concomitant use
- Antifungals: plasma concentration of active metabolite of temsirolimus increased by ●ketoconazole—avoid concomitant use
- Antipsychotics: avoid concomitant use of cytotoxics with ●clozapine (increased risk of agranulocytosis)

**Tenofovir**
- Antivirals: manufacturer of tenofovir advises avoid concomitant use with adefovir; tenofovir reduces plasma concentration of atazanavir, also plasma concentration of tenofovir possibly increased; manufacturers advise avoid concomitant use of tenofovir with ●cidofovir; tenofovir increases plasma concentration of ●didanosine (increased risk of toxicity)—avoid concomitant use; plasma concentration of tenofovir increased by lopinavir and telaprevir

**Tenoxicam** *see* NSAIDs

**Terazosin** *see* Alpha-blockers

**Terbinafine**
- Antibacterials: plasma concentration of terbinafine reduced by ●rifampicin
  Antidepressants: terbinafine possibly increases plasma concentration of tricyclics
  Antifungals: terbinafine increases plasma concentration of fluconazole
  Ciclosporin: terbinafine possibly reduces plasma concentration of ciclosporin
  Oestrogens: occasional reports of breakthrough bleeding when terbinafine given with oestrogens (when used for contraception)
  Progestogens: occasional reports of breakthrough bleeding when terbinafine given with progestogens (when used for contraception)
  Ulcer-healing Drugs: plasma concentration of terbinafine increased by cimetidine

**Terbutaline** *see* Sympathomimetics, Beta$_2$

**Testolactone**
- Anticoagulants: testolactone enhances anticoagulant effect of ●coumarins and ●phenindione

**Testosterone**
- Anticoagulants: testosterone enhances anticoagulant effect of ●coumarins and ●phenindione
  Antidiabetics: testosterone possibly enhances hypoglycaemic effect of antidiabetics

**Tetrabenazine**
- Antidepressants: risk of CNS toxicity when tetrabenazine given with ●MAOIs (avoid tetrabenazine for 2 weeks after MAOIs)
  Antipsychotics: increased risk of extrapyramidal side-effects when tetrabenazine given with antipsychotics
  Dopaminergics: increased risk of extrapyramidal side-effects when tetrabenazine given with amantadine
  Metoclopramide: increased risk of extrapyramidal side-effects when tetrabenazine given with metoclopramide

**Tetracosactide** *see* Corticosteroids

**Tetracycline** *see* Tetracyclines

**Tetracyclines**
  ACE Inhibitors: absorption of tetracyclines reduced by quinapril tablets (quinapril tablets contain magnesium carbonate)
  Adsorbents: absorption of tetracyclines possibly reduced by kaolin
  Antacids: absorption of tetracyclines reduced by antacids
  Antibacterials: plasma concentration of doxycycline reduced by rifampicin—consider increasing dose of doxycycline; tetracyclines possibly antagonise effects of penicillins

**Tetracyclines** *(continued)*
- Anticoagulants: tetracyclines possibly enhance anticoagulant effect of ●coumarins and ●phenindione
  Antidiabetics: tetracyclines possibly enhance hypoglycaemic effect of sulfonylureas
  Antiepileptics: metabolism of doxycycline accelerated by carbamazepine (reduced effect); metabolism of doxycycline accelerated by phenobarbital and phenytoin (reduced plasma concentration)
  Atovaquone: tetracycline reduces plasma concentration of atovaquone
  Calcium Salts: absorption of tetracycline reduced by calcium salts
  Cytotoxics: doxycycline or tetracycline increase risk of methotrexate toxicity
  Dairy Products: absorption of tetracyclines (except doxycycline and minocycline) reduced by dairy products
  Diuretics: manufacturer of lymecycline advises avoid concomitant use with diuretics
  Ergot Alkaloids: increased risk of ergotism when tetracyclines given with ergotamine and methysergide
  Iron: absorption of tetracyclines reduced by *oral* iron, also absorption of *oral* iron reduced by tetracyclines
  Lipid-regulating Drugs: absorption of tetracycline possibly reduced by colestipol and colestyramine
- Retinoids: possible increased risk of benign intracranial hypertension when tetracyclines given with ●retinoids (avoid concomitant use)
  Strontium Ranelate: absorption of tetracyclines reduced by strontium ranelate (manufacturer of strontium ranelate advises avoid concomitant use)
  Ulcer-healing Drugs: absorption of tetracyclines reduced by sucralfate and tripotassium dicitratobismuthate
  Vaccines: antibacterials inactivate oral typhoid vaccine—see p. 621
  Zinc: absorption of tetracyclines reduced by zinc, also absorption of zinc reduced by tetracyclines

**Theophylline**
  Allopurinol: plasma concentration of theophylline possibly increased by allopurinol
  Anaesthetics, General: increased risk of convulsions when theophylline given with ketamine
  Anti-arrhythmics: theophylline antagonises anti-arrhythmic effect of adenosine; plasma concentration of theophylline increased by propafenone
- Antibacterials: plasma concentration of theophylline possibly increased by clarithromycin and isoniazid; plasma concentration of theophylline increased by ●erythromycin (also theophylline may reduce absorption of *oral* erythromycin); plasma concentration of theophylline increased by ●ciprofloxacin and ●norfloxacin; metabolism of theophylline accelerated by rifampicin (reduced plasma concentration); possible increased risk of convulsions when theophylline given with ●quinolones
- Antidepressants: plasma concentration of theophylline increased by ●fluvoxamine (concomitant use should usually be avoided, but where not possible halve theophylline dose and monitor plasma-theophylline concentration); plasma concentration of theophylline possibly reduced by St John's wort
- Antiepileptics: metabolism of theophylline accelerated by carbamazepine and ●phenobarbital (reduced effect); plasma concentration of both drugs reduced when theophylline given with ●phenytoin
- Antifungals: plasma concentration of theophylline possibly increased by ●fluconazole and ●ketoconazole
- Antivirals: plasma concentration of theophylline possibly increased by aciclovir; metabolism of theophylline accelerated by ●ritonavir (reduced plasma concentration)
  Anxiolytics and Hypnotics: theophylline possibly reduces effects of benzodiazepines

## Theophylline (continued)

- Calcium-channel Blockers: plasma concentration of theophylline possibly increased by ●calcium-channel blockers (enhanced effect); plasma concentration of theophylline increased by diltiazem; plasma concentration of theophylline increased by ●verapamil (enhanced effect)

  Corticosteroids: increased risk of hypokalaemia when theophylline given with corticosteroids

  Cytotoxics: plasma concentration of theophylline possibly increased by methotrexate

- Deferasirox: plasma concentration of theophylline increased by ●deferasirox (consider reducing dose of theophylline)

  Disulfiram: metabolism of theophylline inhibited by disulfiram (increased risk of toxicity)

  Diuretics: increased risk of hypokalaemia when theophylline given with acetazolamide, loop diuretics or thiazides and related diuretics

  Doxapram: increased CNS stimulation when theophylline given with doxapram

- Febuxostat: caution with theophylline advised by manufacturer of ●febuxostat

- Interferons: metabolism of theophylline inhibited by ●interferon alfa (consider reducing dose of theophylline)

  Leukotriene Receptor Antagonists: plasma concentration of theophylline possibly increased by zafirlukast, also plasma concentration of zafirlukast reduced

  Lithium: theophylline increases excretion of lithium (reduced plasma concentration)

  Oestrogens: plasma concentration of theophylline increased by oestrogens (consider reducing dose of theophylline)

  Pentoxifylline: plasma concentration of theophylline increased by pentoxifylline

  Roflumilast: avoidance of theophylline advised by manufacturer of roflumilast

  Sulfinpyrazone: plasma concentration of theophylline reduced by sulfinpyrazone

  Sympathomimetics: manufacturer of theophylline advises avoid concomitant use with ephedrine in children

  Sympathomimetics, Beta$_2$: increased risk of hypokalaemia when theophylline given with high doses of beta$_2$ sympathomimetics—see Hypokalaemia, p. 136

- Ulcer-healing Drugs: metabolism of theophylline inhibited by ●cimetidine (increased plasma concentration); absorption of theophylline possibly reduced by sucralfate (give at least 2 hours apart)

  Vaccines: plasma concentration of theophylline possibly increased by influenza vaccine

## Thiazolidinediones see Antidiabetics

## Thiopental see Anaesthetics, General

## Thiotepa

- Antipsychotics: avoid concomitant use of cytotoxics with ●clozapine (increased risk of agranulocytosis)

  Muscle Relaxants: thiotepa enhances effects of suxamethonium

## Thioxanthenes see Antipsychotics

## Thyroid Hormones

  Antacids: absorption of levothyroxine possibly reduced by antacids

  Anti-arrhythmics: for concomitant use of thyroid hormones and amiodarone see p. 82

  Antibacterials: metabolism of levothyroxine accelerated by rifampicin (may increase requirements for levothyroxine in hypothyroidism)

- Anticoagulants: thyroid hormones enhance anticoagulant effect of ●coumarins and ●phenindione

  Antidepressants: thyroid hormones enhance effects of amitriptyline and imipramine; thyroid hormones possibly enhance effects of tricyclics

## Thyroid Hormones (continued)

  Antiepileptics: metabolism of thyroid hormones accelerated by carbamazepine and phenobarbital (may increase requirements for thyroid hormones in hypothyroidism); metabolism of thyroid hormones accelerated by phenytoin (may increase requirements in hypothyroidism), also plasma concentration of phenytoin possibly increased

  Beta-blockers: levothyroxine accelerates metabolism of propranolol

  Calcium Salts: absorption of levothyroxine reduced by calcium salts

  Cytotoxics: plasma concentration of levothyroxine possibly reduced by imatinib

  Iron: absorption of levothyroxine reduced by oral iron (give at least 2 hours apart)

  Lanthanum: absorption of levothyroxine reduced by lanthanum (give at least 2 hours apart)

  Lipid-regulating Drugs: absorption of levothyroxine reduced by colesevelam; absorption of thyroid hormones reduced by colestipol and colestyramine

  Oestrogens: requirements for thyroid hormones in hypothyroidism may be increased by oestrogens

  Orlistat: possible increased risk of hypothyroidism when levothyroxine given with orlistat

  Polystyrene Sulfonate Resins: absorption of levothyroxine reduced by polystyrene sulfonate resins

  Sevelamer: absorption of levothyroxine possibly reduced by sevelamer

  Ulcer-healing Drugs: absorption of levothyroxine reduced by cimetidine and sucralfate

## Tiagabine

- Antidepressants: anticonvulsant effect of antiepileptics possibly antagonised by MAOIs and ●tricyclic-related antidepressants (convulsive threshold lowered); anticonvulsant effect of antiepileptics antagonised by ●SSRIs and ●tricyclics (convulsive threshold lowered); avoid concomitant use of antiepileptics with ●St John's wort

  Antiepileptics: plasma concentration of tiagabine reduced by carbamazepine, phenobarbital and phenytoin

- Antimalarials: anticonvulsant effect of antiepileptics antagonised by ●mefloquine

- Antipsychotics: anticonvulsant effect of antiepileptics antagonised by ●antipsychotics (convulsive threshold lowered)

- Orlistat: possible increased risk of convulsions when antiepileptics given with ●orlistat

## Tiaprofenic Acid see NSAIDs

## Tibolone

  Antibacterials: metabolism of tibolone accelerated by rifampicin (reduced plasma concentration)

  Antiepileptics: metabolism of tibolone accelerated by carbamazepine (reduced plasma concentration); metabolism of tibolone accelerated by phenytoin

## Ticagrelor

- Antibacterials: plasma concentration of ticagrelor possibly increased by ●clarithromycin—manufacturer of ticagrelor advises avoid concomitant use; plasma concentration of ticagrelor possibly increased by erythromycin; plasma concentration of ticagrelor reduced by ●rifampicin

  Antidepressants: possible increased risk of bleeding when ticagrelor given with citalopram, paroxetine or sertraline

  Antiepileptics: plasma concentration of ticagrelor possibly reduced by carbamazepine, phenobarbital and phenytoin

- Antifungals: plasma concentration of ticagrelor increased by ●ketoconazole—manufacturer of ticagrelor advises avoid concomitant use

- Antivirals: plasma concentration of ticagrelor possibly increased by ●atazanavir and ●ritonavir—manufacturer of ticagrelor advises avoid concomitant use

**Ticagrelor** *(continued)*
Calcium-channel Blockers: plasma concentration of ticagrelor increased by diltiazem
● Cardiac Glycosides: ticagrelor increases plasma concentration of ●digoxin
Ciclosporin: ticagrelor possibly increases plasma concentration of ciclosporin
Corticosteroids: plasma concentration of ticagrelor possibly reduced by dexamethasone
● Ergot Alkaloids: ticagrelor possibly increases plasma concentration of ●ergot alkaloids
● Lipid-regulating Drugs: ticagrelor increases plasma concentration of ●simvastatin (increased risk of toxicity)

**Ticarcillin** *see* Penicillins
**Tigecycline**
Anticoagulants: tigecycline possibly enhances anticoagulant effect of coumarins
Vaccines: antibacterials inactivate oral typhoid vaccine—see p. 621

**Timolol** *see* Beta-blockers
**Tinidazole**
Alcohol: possibility of disulfiram-like reaction when tinidazole given with alcohol
Antibacterials: plasma concentration of tinidazole possibly reduced by rifampicin
Vaccines: antibacterials inactivate oral typhoid vaccine—see p. 621

**Tinzaparin** *see* Heparins
**Tioguanine**
● Antipsychotics: avoid concomitant use of cytotoxics with ●clozapine (increased risk of agranulocytosis)
Cytotoxics: increased risk of hepatotoxicity when tioguanine given with busulfan

**Tiotropium** *see* Antimuscarinics
**Tipranavir**
Analgesics: plasma concentration of tipranavir possibly reduced by buprenorphine
Antacids: absorption of tipranavir reduced by antacids
● Antibacterials: tipranavir increases plasma concentration of ●clarithromycin (reduce dose of clarithromycin in renal impairment), also plasma concentration of tipranavir increased by clarithromycin; tipranavir increases plasma concentration of ●rifabutin (reduce dose of rifabutin); plasma concentration of tipranavir possibly reduced by ●rifampicin—avoid concomitant use; avoidance of concomitant tipranavir in severe renal and hepatic impairment advised by manufacturer of ●telithromycin
Anticoagulants: avoidance of tipranavir advised by manufacturer of apixaban and rivaroxaban
● Antidepressants: plasma concentration of tipranavir possibly reduced by ●St John's wort—avoid concomitant use
Antiepileptics: plasma concentration of tipranavir possibly reduced by carbamazepine
Antifungals: plasma concentration of tipranavir increased by fluconazole
● Antimalarials: caution with tipranavir advised by manufacturer of artemether with lumefantrine; tipranavir possibly increases plasma concentration of ●quinine (increased risk of toxicity)
Antimuscarinics: avoidance of tipranavir advised by manufacturer of darifenacin
● Antipsychotics: tipranavir possibly increases plasma concentration of ●quetiapine—manufacturer of quetiapine advises avoid concomitant use
● Antivirals: tipranavir reduces plasma concentration of ●abacavir, ●didanosine, ●fosamprenavir, ●lopinavir, ●saquinavir and ●zidovudine; plasma concentration of tipranavir increased by atazanavir (also plasma concentration of atazanavir reduced); tipranavir reduces plasma concentration of ●etravirine, also plasma concentration of tipranavir increased (avoid concomitant use)

**Tipranavir** *(continued)*
● Beta-blockers: manufacturer of tipranavir advises avoid concomitant use with ●metoprolol for heart failure
Bosentan: manufacturer of tipranavir advises avoid concomitant use with bosentan
● Lipid-regulating Drugs: increased risk of myopathy when tipranavir given with ●atorvastatin (see Dose under Atorvastatin, p. 125); tipranavir possibly increases plasma concentration of ●rosuvastatin—manufacturer of rosuvastatin advises avoid concomitant use; tipranavir possibly increases plasma concentration of ●simvastatin—avoid concomitant use
● Ranolazine: tipranavir possibly increases plasma concentration of ●ranolazine—manufacturer of ranolazine advises avoid concomitant use
Sympathomimetics, Beta$_2$: manufacturer of tipranavir advises avoid concomitant use with salmeterol
● Ulcer-healing Drugs: tipranavir reduces plasma concentration of ●esomeprazole and ●omeprazole
Vardenafil: manufacturer of tipranavir advises caution with vardenafil
Vitamins: increased risk of bleeding when tipranavir given with high doses of vitamin E

**Tirofiban**
Iloprost: increased risk of bleeding when tirofiban given with iloprost

**Tizanidine** *see* Muscle Relaxants
**Tobramycin** *see* Aminoglycosides
**Tocilizumab**
● Vaccines: avoid concomitant use of tocilizumab with live ●vaccines (see p. 600)

**Tolazoline** *see* Alpha-blockers
**Tolbutamide** *see* Antidiabetics
**Tolcapone**
Antidepressants: avoid concomitant use of tolcapone with MAOIs
Memantine: effects of dopaminergics possibly enhanced by memantine
Methyldopa: antiparkinsonian effect of dopaminergics antagonised by methyldopa

**Tolfenamic Acid** *see* NSAIDs
**Tolterodine** *see* Antimuscarinics
**Tolvaptan**
Antibacterials: plasma concentration of tolvaptan reduced by rifampicin
Antifungals: plasma concentration of tolvaptan increased by ketoconazole
Cardiac Glycosides: tolvaptan increases plasma concentration of digoxin (increased risk of toxicity)
● Grapefruit Juice: plasma concentration of tolvaptan increased by ●grapefruit juice—avoid concomitant use

**Topiramate**
● Antidepressants: anticonvulsant effect of antiepileptics possibly antagonised by MAOIs and ●tricyclic-related antidepressants (convulsive threshold lowered); anticonvulsant effect of antiepileptics antagonised by ●SSRIs and ●tricyclics (convulsive threshold lowered); avoid concomitant use of antiepileptics with ●St John's wort
Antidiabetics: topiramate possibly increases plasma concentration of metformin; topiramate possibly reduces plasma concentration of glibenclamide
● Antiepileptics: plasma concentration of topiramate often reduced by carbamazepine; topiramate reduces plasma concentration of perampanel; plasma concentration of topiramate possibly reduced by phenobarbital; topiramate increases plasma concentration of ●phenytoin (also plasma concentration of topiramate reduced); hyperammonaemia and CNS toxicity reported when topiramate given with valproate

## Topiramate *(continued)*

- Antimalarials: anticonvulsant effect of antiepileptics antagonised by ●mefloquine
- Antipsychotics: anticonvulsant effect of antiepileptics antagonised by ●antipsychotics (convulsive threshold lowered)

  Diuretics: plasma concentration of topiramate possibly increased by hydrochlorothiazide

  Lithium: topiramate possibly affects plasma concentration of lithium
- Oestrogens: topiramate accelerates metabolism of ●oestrogens (reduced contraceptive effect—see p. 398)
- Orlistat: possible increased risk of convulsions when antiepileptics given with ●orlistat
- Progestogens: topiramate accelerates metabolism of ●progestogens (reduced contraceptive effect—see p. 398)

## Torasemide *see* Diuretics

## Toremifene

- Anticoagulants: toremifene possibly enhances anticoagulant effect of ●coumarins

  Antiepileptics: metabolism of toremifene possibly accelerated by carbamazepine (reduced plasma concentration); metabolism of toremifene accelerated by phenobarbital (reduced plasma concentration); metabolism of toremifene possibly accelerated by phenytoin
- Cytotoxics: possible increased risk of ventricular arrhythmias when toremifene given with ●vandetanib—avoid concomitant use

  Diuretics: increased risk of hypercalcaemia when toremifene given with thiazides and related diuretics

## Trabectedin

- Antipsychotics: avoid concomitant use of cytotoxics with ●clozapine (increased risk of agranulocytosis)

## Tramadol *see* Opioid Analgesics

## Trandolapril *see* ACE Inhibitors

## Tranylcypromine *see* MAOIs

## Trazodone *see* Antidepressants, Tricyclic (related)

## Tretinoin *see* Retinoids

## Triamcinolone *see* Corticosteroids

## Triamterene *see* Diuretics

## Trientine

Iron: trientine reduces absorption of *oral* iron

Zinc: trientine reduces absorption of zinc, also absorption of trientine reduced by zinc

## Trifluoperazine *see* Antipsychotics

## Trihexyphenidyl *see* Antimuscarinics

## Trimethoprim

ACE Inhibitors: possible increased risk of hyperkalaemia when trimethoprim given with ACE inhibitors

Angiotensin-II Receptor Antagonists: possible increased risk of hyperkalaemia when trimethoprim given with angiotensin-II receptor antagonists

Anti-arrhythmics: possible increased risk of ventricular arrhythmias when trimethoprim (as co-trimoxazole) given with amiodarone—manufacturer of amiodarone advises avoid concomitant use of co-trimoxazole

Antibacterials: plasma concentration of trimethoprim possibly reduced by rifampicin; plasma concentration of both drugs may increase when trimethoprim given with dapsone

Anticoagulants: trimethoprim possibly enhances anticoagulant effect of coumarins

Antidiabetics: trimethoprim possibly enhances hypoglycaemic effect of repaglinide—manufacturer advises avoid concomitant use; trimethoprim rarely enhances the effects of sulfonylureas
- Antiepileptics: trimethoprim increases plasma concentration of ●phenytoin (also increased antifolate effect)

## Trimethoprim *(continued)*

- Antimalarials: increased antifolate effect when trimethoprim given with ●pyrimethamine

  Antivirals: trimethoprim (as co-trimoxazole) increases plasma concentration of lamivudine—avoid concomitant use of high-dose co-trimoxazole
- Azathioprine: increased risk of haematological toxicity when trimethoprim (also with co-trimoxazole) given with ●azathioprine

  Cardiac Glycosides: trimethoprim possibly increases plasma concentration of digoxin
- Ciclosporin: increased risk of nephrotoxicity when trimethoprim given with ●ciclosporin, also plasma concentration of ciclosporin reduced by *intravenous* trimethoprim
- Cytotoxics: increased risk of haematological toxicity when trimethoprim (also with co-trimoxazole) given with ●mercaptopurine or ●methotrexate

  Diuretics: increased risk of hyperkalaemia when trimethoprim given with eplerenone; possible increased risk of hyperkalaemia when trimethoprim given with spironolactone

  Vaccines: antibacterials inactivate oral typhoid vaccine—see p. 621

## Trimipramine *see* Antidepressants, Tricyclic

## Tripotassium Dicitratobismuthate

Antibacterials: tripotassium dicitratobismuthate reduces absorption of tetracyclines

## Tropicamide *see* Antimuscarinics

## Trospium *see* Antimuscarinics

## Tryptophan

- Antidepressants: CNS toxicity reported when tryptophan given with fluoxetine; possible increased serotonergic effects when tryptophan given with duloxetine; CNS excitation and confusion when tryptophan given with ●MAOIs (reduce dose of tryptophan); agitation and nausea may occur when tryptophan given with ●SSRIs
- Antimalarials: avoidance of antidepressants advised by manufacturer of ●artemether with lumefantrine and ●piperaquine with artenimol

  Atomoxetine: possible increased risk of convulsions when antidepressants given with atomoxetine

## Typhoid Vaccine (oral) *see* Vaccines

## Typhoid Vaccine (parenteral) *see* Vaccines

## Ubidecarenone

Anticoagulants: ubidecarenone may enhance or reduce anticoagulant effect of warfarin

## Ulcer-healing Drugs *see* Histamine H₂-antagonists, Proton Pump Inhibitors, Sucralfate, and Tripotassium Dicitratobismuthate

## Ulipristal

- Antacids: manufacturer of *high-dose* ulipristal advises avoid concomitant use with ●antacids (contraceptive effect of ulipristal possibly reduced)
- Antibacterials: manufacturer of ulipristal advises avoid concomitant use with ●rifampicin (contraceptive effect of ulipristal possibly reduced)
- Antidepressants: manufacturer of ulipristal advises avoid concomitant use with ●St John's wort (contraceptive effect of ulipristal possibly reduced)
- Antiepileptics: manufacturer of ulipristal advises avoid concomitant use with ●carbamazepine, ●phenobarbital and ●phenytoin (contraceptive effect of ulipristal possibly reduced)
- Antivirals: manufacturer of ulipristal advises avoid concomitant use with ●ritonavir (contraceptive effect of ulipristal possibly reduced)
- Progestogens: ulipristal possibly reduces contraceptive effect of ●progestogens
- Ulcer-healing Drugs: manufacturer of *high-dose* ulipristal advises avoid concomitant use with ●histamine H₂-antagonists and ●proton pump inhibitors (contraceptive effect of ulipristal possibly reduced)

## Ursodeoxycholic Acid *see* Bile Acids

## Ustekinumab

- Vaccines: avoid concomitant use of ustekinumab with live ●vaccines (see p. 600)

## Vaccines

**Note** For a general warning on live vaccines and high doses of corticosteroids or other immunosuppressive drugs, see p. 600; for advice on live vaccines and immunoglobulins, see under Normal Immunoglobulin, p. 623

- Abatacept: avoid concomitant use of live vaccines with ●abatacept (see p. 600)
- Adalimumab: avoid concomitant use of live vaccines with ●adalimumab (see p. 600)
- Anakinra: avoid concomitant use of live vaccines with ●anakinra (see p. 600)

Analgesics: possible risk of Reyes syndrome when varicella-zoster vaccine given with aspirin—manufacturers advise avoid aspirin for 6 weeks after giving varicella-zoster vaccine

Antibacterials: oral typhoid vaccine inactivated by antibacterials—see p. 621

Anticoagulants: influenza vaccine possibly enhances anticoagulant effect of warfarin

Antiepileptics: influenza vaccine enhances effects of phenytoin

Antimalarials: oral typhoid vaccine inactivated by antimalarials—see p. 621

- Belimumab: avoid concomitant use of live vaccines with ●belimumab (see p. 600)
- Certolizumab pegol: avoid concomitant use of live vaccines with ●certolizumab pegol (see p. 600)
- Corticosteroids: immune response to vaccines impaired by high doses of ●corticosteroids, avoid concomitant use with live vaccines (see p. 600)
- Etanercept: avoid concomitant use of live vaccines with ●etanercept (see p. 600)
- Golimumab: avoid concomitant use of live vaccines with ●golimumab (see p. 600)
- Infliximab: avoid concomitant use of live vaccines with ●infliximab (see p. 600)

Interferons: avoidance of vaccines advised by manufacturer of interferon gamma

- Leflunomide: avoid concomitant use of live vaccines with ●leflunomide (see p. 600)

Theophylline: influenza vaccine possibly increases plasma concentration of theophylline

- Tocilizumab: avoid concomitant use of live vaccines with ●tocilizumab (see p. 600)
- Ustekinumab: avoid concomitant use of live vaccines with ●ustekinumab (see p. 600)

## Valaciclovir *see* Aciclovir

## Valganciclovir *see* Ganciclovir

## Valproate

Analgesics: effects of valproate enhanced by aspirin

- Antibacterials: metabolism of valproate possibly inhibited by erythromycin (increased plasma concentration); avoidance of valproate advised by manufacturer of ●pivmecillinam; plasma concentration of valproate reduced by ●carbapenems—avoid concomitant use

Anticoagulants: valproate possibly enhances anticoagulant effect of coumarins

- Antidepressants: anticonvulsant effect of antiepileptics possibly antagonised by MAOIs and ●tricyclic-related antidepressants (convulsive threshold lowered); anticonvulsant effect of antiepileptics antagonised by ●SSRIs and ●tricyclics (convulsive threshold lowered); avoid concomitant use of antiepileptics with ●St John's wort
- Antiepileptics: plasma concentration of valproate reduced by carbamazepine, also plasma concentration of active metabolite of carbamazepine increased; valproate possibly increases plasma concentration of ethosuximide; valproate increases plasma concentration of ●lamotrigine (increased risk of toxicity—reduce lamotrigine dose); valproate sometimes reduces plasma concentration of an

## Valproate

- Antiepileptics *(continued)*
  active metabolite of oxcarbazepine; valproate increases plasma concentration of phenobarbital (also plasma concentration of valproate reduced); valproate increases or possibly decreases plasma concentration of phenytoin, also plasma concentration of valproate reduced; valproate possibly increases plasma concentration of rufinamide (reduce dose of rufinamide); hyperammonaemia and CNS toxicity reported when valproate given with topiramate
- Antimalarials: anticonvulsant effect of antiepileptics antagonised by ●mefloquine
- Antipsychotics: anticonvulsant effect of antiepileptics antagonised by ●antipsychotics (convulsive threshold lowered); valproate possibly increases or decreases plasma concentration of clozapine; increased risk of side-effects including neutropenia when valproate given with ●olanzapine; valproate possibly increases plasma concentration of quetiapine

Antivirals: plasma concentration of valproate possibly reduced by ritonavir; valproate possibly increases plasma concentration of zidovudine (increased risk of toxicity)

Anxiolytics and Hypnotics: plasma concentration of valproate possibly increased by clobazam; increased risk of side-effects when valproate given with clonazepam; valproate possibly increases plasma concentration of diazepam and lorazepam

Bupropion: valproate inhibits the metabolism of bupropion

Cytotoxics: valproate increases plasma concentration of temozolomide

Lipid-regulating Drugs: absorption of valproate possibly reduced by colestyramine

Oestrogens: plasma concentration of valproate possibly reduced by ethinylestradiol

- Orlistat: possible increased risk of convulsions when antiepileptics given with ●orlistat

Sodium Benzoate: valproate possibly reduces effects of sodium benzoate

Sodium Phenylbutyrate: valproate possibly reduces effects of sodium phenylbutyrate

- Ulcer-healing Drugs: metabolism of valproate inhibited by ●cimetidine (increased plasma concentration)

## Valsartan *see* Angiotensin-II Receptor Antagonists

## Vancomycin

Anaesthetics, General: hypersensitivity-like reactions can occur when *intravenous* vancomycin given with general anaesthetics

- Antibacterials: increased risk of nephrotoxicity and ototoxicity when vancomycin given with ●aminoglycosides, capreomycin or colistimethate sodium; increased risk of nephrotoxicity when vancomycin given with polymyxins

Antifungals: possible increased risk of nephrotoxicity when vancomycin given with amphotericin

- Ciclosporin: increased risk of nephrotoxicity when vancomycin given with ●ciclosporin

Cytotoxics: increased risk of nephrotoxicity and possibly of ototoxicity when vancomycin given with cisplatin

- Diuretics: increased risk of otoxicity when vancomycin given with ●loop diuretics

Lipid-regulating Drugs: effects of *oral* vancomycin antagonised by colestyramine

- Muscle Relaxants: vancomycin enhances effects of ●suxamethonium

Tacrolimus: possible increased risk of nephrotoxicity when vancomycin given with tacrolimus

Vaccines: antibacterials inactivate oral typhoid vaccine—see p. 621

## Vandetanib

- Analgesics: possible increased risk of ventricular arrhythmias when vandetanib given with ●methadone—avoid concomitant use
- Anti-arrhythmics: possible increased risk of ventricular arrhythmias when vandetanib given with ●amiodarone or ●disopyramide—avoid concomitant use
- Antibacterials: possible increased risk of ventricular arrhythmias when vandetanib given with *parenteral* ●erythromycin—avoid concomitant use; possible increased risk of ventricular arrhythmias when vandetanib given with ●moxifloxacin—avoid concomitant use; manufacturer of vandetanib advises avoid concomitant use with rifampicin (plasma concentration of vandetanib reduced)
- Antidepressants: manufacturer of vandetanib advises avoid concomitant use with St John's wort (plasma concentration of vandetanib possibly reduced)
- Antiepileptics: manufacturer of vandetanib advises avoid concomitant use with carbamazepine and phenobarbital (plasma concentration of vandetanib possibly reduced)
- Antihistamines: possible increased risk of ventricular arrhythmias when vandetanib given with ●mizolastine—avoid concomitant use
- Antimalarials: possible increased risk of ventricular arrhythmias when vandetanib given with ●artemether with lumefantrine—avoid concomitant use
- Antipsychotics: possible increased risk of ventricular arrhythmias when vandetanib given with ●amisulpride, ●chlorpromazine, ●haloperidol, ●pimozide, ●sulpiride or ●zuclopenthixol—avoid concomitant use; avoid concomitant use of cytotoxics with ●clozapine (increased risk of agranulocytosis)
- Beta-blockers: possible increased risk of ventricular arrhythmias when vandetanib given with ●sotalol—avoid concomitant use
- Cytotoxics: possible increased risk of ventricular arrhythmias when vandetanib given with ●arsenic trioxide—avoid concomitant use
- Hormone Antagonists: possible increased risk of ventricular arrhythmias when vandetanib given with ●toremifene—avoid concomitant use
- 5HT$_3$-receptor Antagonists: increased risk of ventricular arrhythmias when vandetanib given with ●ondansetron—avoid concomitant use
- Pentamidine Isetionate: possible increased risk of ventricular arrhythmias when vandetanib given with ●pentamidine isetionate—avoid concomitant use
- Ulcer-healing Drugs: manufacturer of vandetanib advises avoid concomitant use with proton pump inhibitors (absorption of vandetanib possibly reduced)

## Vardenafil

- Alpha-blockers: enhanced hypotensive effect when vardenafil given with ●alpha-blockers (excludes tamsulosin)—separate doses by 6 hours—see also under Phosphodiesterase type-5 inhibitors, BNF section 7.4.5
- Anti-arrhythmics: avoidance of vardenafil advised by manufacturer of disopyramide (risk of ventricular arrhythmias)
- Antibacterials: plasma concentration of vardenafil increased by erythromycin (reduce dose of vardenafil)
- Antifungals: plasma concentration of vardenafil increased by ●ketoconazole—avoid concomitant use; plasma concentration of vardenafil possibly increased by ●itraconazole—avoid concomitant use
- Antivirals: plasma concentration of vardenafil possibly increased by fosamprenavir; plasma concentration of vardenafil increased by ●indinavir and ●ritonavir—avoid concomitant use; increased risk of ventricular arrhythmias when vardenafil given with ●saquinavir—avoid concomitant use; avoidance of

## Vardenafil

- Antivirals *(continued)*
  vardenafil advised by manufacturer of ●telaprevir; caution with vardenafil advised by manufacturer of tipranavir
- Calcium-channel Blockers: enhanced hypotensive effect when vardenafil given with nifedipine
- Grapefruit Juice: plasma concentration of vardenafil possibly increased by ●grapefruit juice—avoid concomitant use
- Nicorandil: possible increased hypotensive effect when vardenafil given with ●nicorandil—avoid concomitant use
- Nitrates: possible increased hypotensive effect when vardenafil given with ●nitrates—avoid concomitant use

## Varicella-zoster Vaccine *see* Vaccines

## Vasodilator Antihypertensives

ACE Inhibitors: enhanced hypotensive effect when hydralazine, minoxidil or sodium nitroprusside given with ACE inhibitors

Adrenergic Neurone Blockers: enhanced hypotensive effect when hydralazine, minoxidil or sodium nitroprusside given with adrenergic neurone blockers

Alcohol: enhanced hypotensive effect when hydralazine, minoxidil or sodium nitroprusside given with alcohol

Aldesleukin: enhanced hypotensive effect when hydralazine, minoxidil or sodium nitroprusside given with aldesleukin

Alpha-blockers: enhanced hypotensive effect when hydralazine, minoxidil or sodium nitroprusside given with alpha-blockers

Anaesthetics, General: enhanced hypotensive effect when hydralazine, minoxidil or sodium nitroprusside given with general anaesthetics

Analgesics: hypotensive effect of hydralazine, minoxidil and sodium nitroprusside antagonised by NSAIDs

Angiotensin-II Receptor Antagonists: enhanced hypotensive effect when hydralazine, minoxidil or sodium nitroprusside given with angiotensin-II receptor antagonists

Antidepressants: enhanced hypotensive effect when hydralazine, minoxidil or sodium nitroprusside given with MAOIs; enhanced hypotensive effect when hydralazine or sodium nitroprusside given with tricyclic-related antidepressants

Antipsychotics: enhanced hypotensive effect when hydralazine, minoxidil or sodium nitroprusside given with phenothiazines

Anxiolytics and Hypnotics: enhanced hypotensive effect when hydralazine, minoxidil or sodium nitroprusside given with anxiolytics and hypnotics

Beta-blockers: enhanced hypotensive effect when hydralazine, minoxidil or sodium nitroprusside given with beta-blockers

Calcium-channel Blockers: enhanced hypotensive effect when hydralazine, minoxidil or sodium nitroprusside given with calcium-channel blockers

Clonidine: enhanced hypotensive effect when hydralazine, minoxidil or sodium nitroprusside given with clonidine

Corticosteroids: hypotensive effect of hydralazine, minoxidil and sodium nitroprusside antagonised by corticosteroids

Diazoxide: enhanced hypotensive effect when hydralazine, minoxidil or sodium nitroprusside given with diazoxide

Diuretics: enhanced hypotensive effect when hydralazine, minoxidil or sodium nitroprusside given with diuretics

Dopaminergics: enhanced hypotensive effect when hydralazine, minoxidil or sodium nitroprusside given with levodopa

**Vasodilator Antihypertensives** *(continued)*

Methyldopa: enhanced hypotensive effect when hydralazine, minoxidil or sodium nitroprusside given with methyldopa

Moxisylyte: enhanced hypotensive effect when hydralazine, minoxidil or sodium nitroprusside given with moxisylyte

Moxonidine: enhanced hypotensive effect when hydralazine, minoxidil or sodium nitroprusside given with moxonidine

Muscle Relaxants: enhanced hypotensive effect when hydralazine, minoxidil or sodium nitroprusside given with baclofen; enhanced hypotensive effect when hydralazine, minoxidil or sodium nitroprusside given with tizanidine

Nicorandil: possible enhanced hypotensive effect when hydralazine, minoxidil or sodium nitroprusside given with nicorandil

Nitrates: enhanced hypotensive effect when hydralazine, minoxidil or sodium nitroprusside given with nitrates

Oestrogens: hypotensive effect of hydralazine, minoxidil and sodium nitroprusside antagonised by oestrogens

Prostaglandins: enhanced hypotensive effect when hydralazine, minoxidil or sodium nitroprusside given with alprostadil

Vasodilator Antihypertensives: enhanced hypotensive effect when hydralazine given with minoxidil or sodium nitroprusside; enhanced hypotensive effect when minoxidil given with sodium nitroprusside

**Vecuronium** *see* Muscle Relaxants

**Vemurafenib**

Antibacterials: manufacturer of vemurafenib advises avoid concomitant use with rifabutin and rifampicin

• Anticoagulants: vemurafenib possibly enhances anticoagulant effect of ●warfarin

Antidepressants: manufacturer of vemurafenib advises avoid concomitant use with St John's wort

Antiepileptics: manufacturer of vemurafenib advises avoid concomitant use with carbamazepine and phenytoin

• Antipsychotics: avoid concomitant use of cytotoxics with ●clozapine (increased risk of agranulocytosis)

• Oestrogens: manufacturer of vemurafenib advises contraceptive effect of ●oestrogens possibly reduced

• Progestogens: manufacturer of vemurafenib advises contraceptive effect of ●progestogens possibly reduced

**Venlafaxine**

• Analgesics: increased risk of bleeding when venlafaxine given with ●NSAIDs or ●aspirin; possible increased serotonergic effects when venlafaxine given with tramadol

• Anticoagulants: venlafaxine possibly enhances anticoagulant effect of ●warfarin; possible increased risk of bleeding when SSRI-related antidepressants given with ●dabigatran etexilate

• Antidepressants: possible increased serotonergic effects when venlafaxine given with St John's wort, duloxetine or mirtazapine; enhanced CNS effects and toxicity when venlafaxine given with ●MAOIs (venlafaxine should not be started until 2 weeks after stopping MAOIs, avoid MAOIs for 1 week after stopping venlafaxine); after stopping SSRI-related antidepressants do not start ●moclobemide for at least 1 week

• Antimalarials: avoidance of antidepressants advised by manufacturer of ●artemether with lumefantrine and ●piperaquine with artenimol

• Antipsychotics: venlafaxine increases plasma concentration of ●clozapine and haloperidol

Atomoxetine: possible increased risk of convulsions when antidepressants given with atomoxetine

**Venlafaxine** *(continued)*

• Dopaminergics: caution with venlafaxine advised by manufacturer of entacapone; increased risk of hypertension and CNS excitation when venlafaxine given with ●selegiline (selegiline should not be started until 1 week after stopping venlafaxine, avoid venlafaxine for 2 weeks after stopping selegiline)

$5HT_1$-receptor Agonists: possible increased serotonergic effects when venlafaxine given with $5HT_1$ agonists

Lithium: possible increased serotonergic effects when venlafaxine given with lithium

• Methylthioninium: risk of CNS toxicity when SSRI-related antidepressants given with ●methylthioninium—avoid concomitant use (if avoidance not possible, use lowest possible dose of methylthioninium and observe patient for up to 4 hours after administration)

**Verapamil** *see* Calcium-channel Blockers

**Vigabatrin**

• Antidepressants: anticonvulsant effect of antiepileptics possibly antagonised by MAOIs and ●tricyclic-related antidepressants (convulsive threshold lowered); anticonvulsant effect of antiepileptics antagonised by ●SSRIs and ●tricyclics (convulsive threshold lowered); avoid concomitant use of antiepileptics with ●St John's wort

Antiepileptics: vigabatrin reduces plasma concentration of phenytoin

• Antimalarials: anticonvulsant effect of antiepileptics antagonised by ●mefloquine

• Antipsychotics: anticonvulsant effect of antiepileptics antagonised by ●antipsychotics (convulsive threshold lowered)

• Orlistat: possible increased risk of convulsions when antiepileptics given with ●orlistat

**Vildagliptin** *see* Antidiabetics

**Vinblastine**

• Aldesleukin: avoidance of vinblastine advised by manufacturer of ●aldesleukin

• Antibacterials: toxicity of vinblastine increased by ●erythromycin—avoid concomitant use

• Antifungals: metabolism of vinblastine possibly inhibited by ●posaconazole (increased risk of neurotoxicity)

• Antimalarials: avoidance of vinblastine advised by manufacturer of ●piperaquine with artenimol

• Antipsychotics: avoid concomitant use of cytotoxics with ●clozapine (increased risk of agranulocytosis)

Antivirals: plasma concentration of vinblastine possibly increased by ritonavir

**Vincristine**

• Antifungals: metabolism of vincristine possibly inhibited by ●itraconazole and ●posaconazole (increased risk of neurotoxicity)

• Antimalarials: avoidance of vincristine advised by manufacturer of ●piperaquine with artenimol

• Antipsychotics: avoid concomitant use of cytotoxics with ●clozapine (increased risk of agranulocytosis)

Calcium-channel Blockers: metabolism of vincristine possibly inhibited by nifedipine

Cardiac Glycosides: vincristine possibly reduces absorption of digoxin *tablets*

**Vinflunine**

• Antibacterials: plasma concentration of vinflunine possibly reduced by ●rifampicin—manufacturer of vinflunine advises avoid concomitant use

• Antidepressants: plasma concentration of vinflunine possibly reduced by ●St John's wort—manufacturer of vinflunine advises avoid concomitant use

• Antifungals: plasma concentration of vinflunine increased by ●ketoconazole—manufacturer of vinflunine advises avoid concomitant use; plasma concentration of vinflunine possibly increased by

## Vinflunine
- Antifungals *(continued)*
  - •itraconazole—manufacturer of vinflunine advises avoid concomitant use
- Antimalarials: avoidance of vinflunine advised by manufacturer of •piperaquine with artenimol
- Antipsychotics: avoid concomitant use of cytotoxics with •clozapine (increased risk of agranulocytosis)
- Antivirals: plasma concentration of vinflunine possibly increased by •ritonavir—manufacturer of vinflunine advises avoid concomitant use

  Grapefruit Juice: plasma concentration of vinflunine possibly increased by grapefruit juice—manufacturer of vinflunine advises avoid concomitant use

## Vinorelbine
- Antibacterials: possible increased risk of neutropenia when vinorelbine given with •clarithromycin
- Antifungals: metabolism of vinorelbine possibly inhibited by •itraconazole (increased risk of neurotoxicity)
- Antimalarials: avoidance of vinorelbine advised by manufacturer of •piperaquine with artenimol
- Antipsychotics: avoid concomitant use of cytotoxics with •clozapine (increased risk of agranulocytosis)

**Vitamin A** *see* Vitamins

**Vitamin D** *see* Vitamins

**Vitamin E** *see* Vitamins

**Vitamin K (Phytomenadione)** *see* Vitamins

## Vitamins
Antibacterials: absorption of vitamin A possibly reduced by neomycin
- Anticoagulants: vitamin K antagonises anticoagulant effect of •coumarins and •phenindione; vitamin E possibly enhances anticoagulant effect of •coumarins

  Antiepileptics: vitamin D requirements possibly increased when given with carbamazepine, phenobarbital or phenytoin

  Antifungals: plasma concentration of paricalcitol possibly increased by ketoconazole

  Antivirals: increased risk of bleeding when high doses of vitamin E given with tipranavir

  Ciclosporin: vitamin E possibly affects plasma concentration of ciclosporin

  Diuretics: increased risk of hypercalcaemia when vitamin D given with thiazides and related diuretics

  Dopaminergics: pyridoxine reduces effects of levodopa when given without dopa-decarboxylase inhibitor
- Retinoids: risk of hypervitaminosis A when vitamin A given with •retinoids—avoid concomitant use

  Selenium: ascorbic acid possibly reduces absorption of selenium (give at least 4 hours apart)

**Voriconazole** *see* Antifungals, Triazole

**Warfarin** *see* Coumarins

**Xipamide** *see* Diuretics

**Xylometazoline** *see* Sympathomimetics

**Zafirlukast** *see* Leukotriene Receptor Antagonists

**Zaleplon** *see* Anxiolytics and Hypnotics

## Zidovudine
**Note** Increased risk of toxicity with nephrotoxic and myelosuppressive drugs—for further details consult product literature

Analgesics: increased risk of haematological toxicity when zidovudine given with NSAIDs; plasma concentration of zidovudine possibly increased by methadone

## Zidovudine *(continued)*
Antibacterials: absorption of zidovudine reduced by clarithromycin tablets (give at least 2 hours apart); manufacturer of zidovudine advises avoid concomitant use with rifampicin

Antiepileptics: zidovudine increases or decreases plasma concentration of phenytoin; plasma concentration of zidovudine possibly increased by valproate (increased risk of toxicity)
- Antifungals: plasma concentration of zidovudine increased by •fluconazole (increased risk of toxicity)

  Antimalarials: increased antifolate effect when zidovudine given with pyrimethamine
- Antivirals: profound myelosuppression when zidovudine given with •ganciclovir (if possible avoid concomitant administration, particularly during initial ganciclovir therapy); increased risk of anaemia when zidovudine given with •ribavirin—avoid concomitant use; zidovudine possibly inhibits effects of •stavudine (manufacturers advise avoid concomitant use); plasma concentration of zidovudine reduced by •tipranavir

  Atovaquone: plasma concentration of zidovudine increased by atovaquone (increased risk of toxicity)
- Probenecid: excretion of zidovudine reduced by •probenecid (increased plasma concentration and risk of toxicity)

## Zinc
Antibacterials: zinc reduces absorption of ciprofloxacin, levofloxacin, moxifloxacin and ofloxacin; zinc reduces absorption of norfloxacin (give at least 2 hours apart); zinc reduces absorption of tetracyclines, also absorption of zinc reduced by tetracyclines

Calcium Salts: absorption of zinc reduced by calcium salts

Eltrombopag: zinc possibly reduces absorption of eltrombopag (give at least 4 hours apart)

Iron: absorption of zinc reduced by *oral* iron, also absorption of *oral* iron reduced by zinc

Penicillamine: absorption of zinc reduced by penicillamine, also absorption of penicillamine reduced by zinc

Trientine: absorption of zinc reduced by trientine, also absorption of trientine reduced by zinc

**Zoledronic Acid** *see* Bisphosphonates

**Zolmitriptan** *see* 5HT$_1$-receptor Agonists (under HT)

**Zolpidem** *see* Anxiolytics and Hypnotics

## Zonisamide
- Antidepressants: anticonvulsant effect of antiepileptics possibly antagonised by MAOIs and •tricyclic-related antidepressants (convulsive threshold lowered); anticonvulsant effect of antiepileptics antagonised by •SSRIs and •tricyclics (convulsive threshold lowered); avoid concomitant use of antiepileptics with •St John's wort

  Antiepileptics: plasma concentration of zonisamide reduced by carbamazepine, phenobarbital and phenytoin
- Antimalarials: anticonvulsant effect of antiepileptics antagonised by •mefloquine
- Antipsychotics: anticonvulsant effect of antiepileptics antagonised by •antipsychotics (convulsive threshold lowered)
- Orlistat: possible increased risk of convulsions when antiepileptics given with •orlistat

**Zopiclone** *see* Anxiolytics and Hypnotics

**Zuclopenthixol** *see* Antipsychotics

# A2 Borderline substances

General Practitioners are reminded that the ACBS recommends products on the basis that they may be regarded as drugs for the management of specified conditions. Doctors should satisfy themselves that the products can safely be prescribed, that patients are adequately monitored and that, where necessary, expert hospital supervision is available.

**Foods which may be prescribed on FP10, GP10 (Scotland), or WP10 (Wales)** All the food products listed in this appendix have ACBS approval. The clinical condition for which the product has been approved is included with each entry.

**Note** Foods included in this appendix may contain cariogenic sugars and appropriate oral hygiene measures should be taken.

**Enteral feeds and nutritional supplements** For most enteral feeds and nutritional supplements, the main source of **carbohydrate** is either maltodextrin or glucose syrup; other carbohydrate sources are listed in the relevant table, below. Feeds containing residual lactose (less than 1 g lactose/100 mL formula) are described as 'clinically lactose-free' or 'lactose-free' by some manufacturers. The presence of lactose (including residual lactose) in feeds is indicated in the relevant table, below. The primary sources of **protein** or **amino acids** are included with each product entry. The **fat** or **oil** content is derived from a variety of sources such as vegetables, soya bean, corn, palm nuts, and seeds; where the fat content is derived from animal or fish sources, this information is included in the relevant table, below. The presence of medium chain triglycerides (MCT) is also noted where the quantity exceeds 30% of the fat content.

Enteral feeds and nutritional supplements can contain varying amounts of **vitamins**, **minerals**, and **trace elements**—the manufacturer's product literature should be consulted for more detailed information. For further information on enteral nutrition, see section 9.4.2. Feeds containing vitamin K may affect the INR in children receiving warfarin; see **interactions**: Appendix 1 (vitamins).

The suitability of food products for patients requiring a vegan, kosher, halal, or other compliant diet should be confirmed with individual manufacturers.

**Note** Feeds containing more than 6 g/100 mL protein or 2 g/100 mL fibre should be avoided in children unless recommended by an appropriate specialist or dietician.

**Standard ACBS indications:**

Disease-related malnutrition, intractable malabsorption, pre-operative preparation of malnourished patients, dysphagia, proven inflammatory bowel disease, following total gastrectomy, short-bowel syndrome, bowel fistula

**Paediatric ACBS indications:**

Disease-related malnutrition, intractable malabsorption, growth failure, pre-operative preparation of malnourished patients, dysphagia, short-bowel syndrome, bowel fistula

In certain conditions some foods (and toilet preparations) have characteristics of drugs and the Advisory Committee on Borderline Substances (ACBS) advises as to the circumstances in which such substances may be regarded as drugs. Prescriptions issued in accordance with the Committee's advice and endorsed 'ACBS' will normally not be investigated.

Appendix 2: Borderline substances

Appendix 2: Borderline substances

## A2.1 Enteral feeds (non-disease specific)

### A2.1.1 Enteral feeds: 1 kcal/mL and less than 5 g protein/100 mL

**A2.1.1.1 Enteral feeds (non-disease specific): less than 5 g protein/100 mL**

Not suitable for use in child under 1 year unless otherwise stated; not recommended for child 1–6 years

| Product | Formulation | Energy | Protein | Carbohydrate | Fat | Fibre | Special Characteristics | ACBS Indications | Presentation & Flavour |
|---|---|---|---|---|---|---|---|---|---|
| Fresubin® Original (Fresenius Kabi) | Liquid (sip or tube feed) **per 100 mL** | 420 kJ (100 kcal) | 3.8 g cows' milk soya | 13.8 g (sugars 3.5 g[1]) | 3.4 g | Nil | Gluten-free Residual lactose Contains fish gelatin Feed in flexible pack contains fish oil and fish gelatin | Standard, p. 757 | Bottle: 200 mL = £1.78 Black currant, chocolate, nut, peach, vanilla Flexible pack: 500 mL = £3.45 1000 mL = £6.81 1500 mL = £10.23 |
| Fresubin® Original Fibre (Fresenius Kabi) | Liquid (tube feed) **per 100 mL** | 420 kJ (100 kcal) | 3.8 g cows' milk soya | 13 g (sugars 0.9 g) | 3.4 g | 1.5 g | Gluten-free Residual lactose Contains fish oil | Standard, p. 757 except bowel fistula and pre-operative preparation of malnourished patients. Not suitable for child under 2 years | Flexible pack: 500 mL = £3.90 1000 mL = £7.78 |
| Fresubin® 1500 Complete (Fresenius Kabi) | Liquid (tube feed) **per 100 mL** | 420 kJ (100 kcal) | 3.8 g cows' milk soya | 13 g (sugars 0.9 g) | 3.4 g | 1.5 g | Gluten-free Residual lactose Contains fish oil | Standard, p. 757 except bowel fistula and pre-operative preparation of malnourished patients. Not suitable for child under 2 years | Flexible pack: 1500 mL = £11.94 |
| Jevity® (Abbott) | Liquid (tube feed) **per 100 mL** | 449 kJ (107 kcal) | 4 g caseinates | 14.1 g (sugars 470 mg) | 3.47 g | 1.76 g | Gluten-free Residual lactose | Standard, p. 757 except bowel fistula. Not suitable for child under 2 years | Flexible pack: 500 mL = £4.16 1000 mL = £7.81 1500 mL = £11.73 |
| Novasource® GI Control (Nestlé) | Liquid (tube feed) **per 100 mL** | 444 kJ (106 kcal) | 4.1 g cows' milk | 14.4 g (sugars 500 mg) | 3.5 g (MCT 40 %) | 2.2 g | Gluten-free Residual lactose | Standard, p. 757 | Flexible pack: 500 mL = £4.78 |
| Nutrison® (Nutricia Clinical) | Liquid (tube feed) **per 100 mL** | 420 kJ (100 kcal) | 4 g cows' milk | 12.3 g (sugars 1 g) | 3.9 g | Nil | Gluten-free Residual lactose | Standard, p. 757 | Bottle: 500 mL = £3.76 Flexible pack: 500 mL = £4.17 1000 mL = £7.32 1500 mL = £10.97 |

1. Sugar content varies with flavour

**Appendix 2: Borderline substances**

| Product (Manufacturer) | Formulation | Energy | Protein | Carbohydrate | Fat | | Special characteristics | ACBS indications | Presentation and price |
|---|---|---|---|---|---|---|---|---|---|
| Nutrison Multi Fibre (Nutricia Clinical) | Liquid (tube feed) per 100 mL | 420 kJ (100 kcal) | 4 g cows' milk | 12.3 g (sugars 1 g) | 3.9 g | 1.5 g | Gluten-free, Residual lactose | Standard, p. 757 except bowel fistula | Bottle: 500 mL = £4.09; Flexible pack: 500 mL = £4.51, 1000 mL = £8.16, 1500 mL = £12.25 |
| Osmolite (Abbott) | Liquid (tube feed) per 100 mL | 424 kJ (100 kcal) | 4 g caseinates soy isolate | 13.6 g (sugars 630 mg) | 3.4 g | Nil | Gluten-free, Residual lactose | Standard, p. 757 | Can: 250 mL = £1.88; Bottle: 500 mL = £3.57, 1000 mL = £6.81, 1500 mL = £10.22 |

## Soya protein formula (see also section A2.3.1)

| Product (Manufacturer) | Formulation | Energy | Protein | Carbohydrate | Fat | | Special characteristics | ACBS indications | Presentation and price |
|---|---|---|---|---|---|---|---|---|---|
| Fresubin Soya Fibre (Fresenius Kabi) | Liquid (tube feed) per 100 mL | 420 kJ (100 kcal) | 3.8 g soya protein | 13.3 g (sugars 4.1 g) | 3.6 g | 2 g | Gluten-free, Lactose-free, Contains fish oil | Standard, p. 757; also cows' milk protein intolerance, lactose intolerance | Flexible pack: 500 mL = £4.03 |
| Nutrison Soya (Nutricia Clinical) | Liquid (tube feed) per 100 mL | 420 kJ (100 kcal) | 4 g soy isolate | 12.3 g (sugars 1 g) | 3.9 g | Nil | Gluten-free, Residual lactose, Milk protein-free | Standard, p. 757; also cows' milk protein and lactose intolerance | Bottle: 500 mL = £4.34; Flexible pack: 1000 mL = £8.69 |
| Nutrison Soya Multi Fibre (Nutricia Clinical) | Liquid (tube feed) per 100 mL | 420 kJ (100 kcal) | 4 g soy isolate | 12.3 g (sugars 700 mg) | 3.9 g | 1.5 g | Gluten-free, Residual lactose, Milk protein-free | Standard, p. 757 except bowel fistula; also cows' milk protein and lactose intolerance | Flexible pack: 1500 mL = £14.46 |

## Peptide-based formula

| Product (Manufacturer) | Formulation | Energy | Protein | Carbohydrate | Fat | | Special characteristics | ACBS indications | Presentation and price |
|---|---|---|---|---|---|---|---|---|---|
| Peptamen (Nestlé) | Liquid (sip or tube feed) per 100 mL | 420 kJ (100 kcal) | 4 g whey peptides | 12.7 g (sugars 480 mg[1]) | 3.7 g (MCT 70%) | Nil | Gluten-free, Residual lactose | Short bowel syndrome, intractable malabsorption, proven inflammatory bowel disease, bowel fistula | Bottle: 200 mL = £2.83 Vanilla; Flexible pack: 500 mL = £5.86, 1000 mL = £11.00 |
| Peptisorb (Nutricia Clinical) | Liquid (tube feed) per 100 mL | 425 kJ (100 kcal) | 4 g whey protein hydrolysate | 17.6 g (sugars 1.7 g) | 1.7 g (MCT 47%) | Nil | Gluten-free, Residual lactose | Short bowel syndrome, intractable malabsorption, proven inflammatory bowel disease, bowel fistula | Bottle: 500 mL = £5.76; Flexible pack: 500 mL = £6.31, 1000 mL = £11.41 |
| Survimed OPD (Fresenius Kabi) | Liquid (tube feed) per 100 mL | 420 kJ (100 kcal) | 4.5 g whey protein hydrolysate | 14.3 g (sugars 1.1 g) | 2.8 g (MCT 51%) | 100 mg | Gluten-free, Residual lactose, Contains fish oil | Standard, p. 757; also growth failure | Flexible pack: 500 mL = £5.75, 1000 mL = £12.52 |

1. Sugar content varies with flavour

Appendix 2: Borderline substances

## A2.1.1.2 Enteral feeds: less than 1 kcal/mL and less than 5 g protein/100 mL
Not suitable for use in child under 1 year unless otherwise stated; not recommended for child 1–6 years

### Amino acid formula (essential and non-essential amino acids)

| Product | Formulation | Energy | Protein | Carbohydrate | Fat | Fibre | Special Characteristics | ACBS Indications | Presentation & Flavour |
|---|---|---|---|---|---|---|---|---|---|
| Elemental 028® Extra (Nutricia Clinical) | Liquid (sip feed) **per 100 mL** | 360 kJ (86 kcal) | 2.5 g (protein equivalent) | 11 g (sugars 4.7 g) | 3.5 g (MCT 35 %) | Nil | Short bowel syndrome, intractable malabsorption, proven inflammatory bowel disease, bowel fistula | | Carton: 250 mL = £3.19 Grapefruit, orange and pineapple, summer fruits |
| | Standard dilution (20 %) of powder (sip or tube feed) **per 100 mL** | 374 kJ (89 kcal)[1] | 2.5 g (protein equivalent) | 11.8 g (sugars 1.8 g) | 3.5 g (MCT 35 %) | Nil | | | Sachet: 100 g = £6.01 Banana, citrus, orange, unflavoured[2] |

Powder provides protein equivalent 12.5 g, carbohydrate 59 g, fat 17.45 g, energy 1871 kJ (443 kcal)/100 g

1. Nutritional values vary with flavour—consult product literature
2. Flavouring: see *Modjul*® Flavour System, p. 791

## A2.1.2 Enteral feeds (non-disease specific); 5 g (or more) protein/100 mL

### A2.1.2.1 Enteral feeds: 1.5 kcal/mL and 5 g (or more) protein/100 mL
Not suitable for use in child under 1 year unless otherwise stated; not recommended for child 1–6 years

| Product | Formulation | Energy | Protein | Carbohydrate | Fat | Fibre | Special Characteristics | ACBS Indications | Presentation & Flavour |
|---|---|---|---|---|---|---|---|---|---|
| Fresubin® 2250 Complete (Fresenius Kabi) | Liquid (tube feed) **per 100 mL** | 630 kJ (150 kcal) | 5.6 g cows' milk | 18.8 g (sugars 1.5 g) | 5.8 g | 2 g | Gluten-free Residual lactose Contains fish oil and fish gelatin | Standard, p. 757 | Flexible pack: 1500 mL = £12.25 |
| Fresubin® Energy (Fresenius Kabi) | Liquid (sip feed) **per 100 mL** | 630 kJ (150 kcal) | 5.6 g cows' milk | 18.8 g (sugars[1]) | 5.8 g | Nil | Gluten-free[2] Residual lactose Contains fish gelatin | Standard, p. 757 | Bottle: 200 mL = £1.78 Banana, black currant, cappuccino, chocolate, lemon, neutral, strawberry, tropical fruits, vanilla |
| | Liquid (tube feed) **per 100 mL** | 630 kJ (150 kcal) | 5.6 g cows' milk | 18.8 g (sugars 1.4 g) | 5.8 g | Nil | Gluten-free Residual lactose Contains fish oil and fish gelatin | Standard, p. 757 | Flexible pack: 500 mL = £4.21 1000 mL = £8.28 1500 mL = £11.10 |

1. Sugar content varies with flavour
2. Strawberry flavour may contain traces of wheat starch and egg

| Product | Formulation per 100 mL | Energy | Protein | Carbohydrate | Fat | Fibre | Notes | Reference | Presentation |
|---|---|---|---|---|---|---|---|---|---|
| Fresubin® Energy Fibre (Fresenius Kabi) | Liquid (sip feed) **per 100 mL** | 630 kJ (150 kcal) | 5.6 g cows' milk | 18.8 g (sugars¹) | 5.8 g | 2 g | Gluten-free, Residual lactose, Contains fish gelatin | Standard, p. 757 | Bottle: 200 mL = £1.87, Banana, caramel, cherry, chocolate, strawberry, vanilla |
|  | Liquid (tube feed) **per 100 mL** | 630 kJ (150 kcal) | 5.6 g cows' milk | 18.8 g (sugars 1.5 g) | 5.8 g | 2 g | Gluten-free, Residual lactose, Contains fish oil and fish gelatin | Standard, p. 757 | Flexible pack: 500 mL = £4.63, 1000 mL = £8.82 |
| Fresubin® HP Energy (Fresenius Kabi) | Liquid (tube feed) **per 100 mL** | 630 kJ (150 kcal) | 7.5 g cows' milk | 17 g (sugars 1 g) | 5.8 g (MCT 57%) | Nil | Gluten-free, Residual lactose, Contains fish oil and fish gelatin | Standard, p. 757; also CAPD and haemodialysis | Flexible pack: 500 mL = £4.29, 1000 mL = £8.60 |
| Jevity® 1.5 kcal (Abbott) | Liquid (tube feed) **per 100 mL** | 649 kJ (154 kcal) | 6.38 g caseinates and soy isolate | 20.1 g (sugars 1.47 g) | 4.9 g | 2.2 g | Gluten-free, Residual lactose | Standard, p. 757. Not suitable for child under 2 years; not recommended for child 2–10 years | Flexible pack: 500 mL = £4.92, 1000 mL = £9.40, 1500 mL = £14.67 |
| Novasource® GI Forte (Nestlé) | Liquid (tube feed) **per 100 mL** | 631 kJ (150 kcal) | 6 g cows' milk | 18.3 g (sugars 1.8 g) | 5.9 g | 2.2 g | Gluten-free, Residual lactose | Standard, p. 757 | Flexible pack: 500 mL = £4.75, 1000 mL = £9.50 |
| Nutrison® Energy (Nutricia Clinical) | Liquid (tube feed) **per 100 mL** | 630 kJ (150 kcal) | 6 g cows' milk | 18.5 g (sugars 1.5 g) | 5.8 g | Nil | Gluten-free, Residual lactose | Standard, p. 757 | Bottle: 500 mL = £4.38, Flexible pack: 500 mL = £4.86, 1000 mL = £8.81, 1500 mL = £13.18 |
| Nutrison® Energy Multi Fibre (Nutricia Clinical) | Liquid (tube feed) **per 100 mL** | 630 kJ (150 kcal) | 6 g cows' milk | 18.5 g (sugars 1.5 g) | 5.8 g | 1.5 g | Gluten-free, Residual lactose | Standard, p. 757 | Bottle: 500 mL = £4.90, Flexible pack: 500 mL = £5.39, 1000 mL = £9.77, 1500 mL = £15.66 |

1. Sugar content varies with flavour

**Appendix 2: Borderline substances**

## A2.1.2.1 Enteral feeds: 1.5 kcal/mL and 5 g (or more) protein/100 mL (product list continued)

Not suitable for use in child under 1 year unless otherwise stated; not recommended for child 1–6 years

| Product | Formulation | Energy | Protein | Carbohydrate | Fat | Fibre | Special Characteristics | ACBS Indications | Presentation & Flavour |
|---|---|---|---|---|---|---|---|---|---|
| Osmolite® 1.5 kcal (Abbott) | Liquid (tube feed) **per 100 mL** | 632 kJ (150 kcal) | 6.25 g cows' milk soya protein isolate | 20 g (sugars 4.9 g) | 5 g | Nil | Gluten-free Residual lactose | Standard, p. 757 | Flexible pack: 500 mL = £4.37 1000 mL = £8.54 1500 mL = £12.79 |
| Resource® Energy (Nestlé) | Liquid (sip feed) **per 100 mL** | 630 kJ (150 kcal) | 5.6 g cows' milk | 21 g (sugars 5.2 g[1]) | 5 g | less than 500 mg | Gluten-free Residual lactose | Standard, p. 757 Not suitable for use in child under 3 years | Bottle: 4 × 200 mL = £6.97 Apricot, banana, chocolate, coffee, strawberry-raspberry, vanilla |

1. Sugar content varies with flavour

## A2.1.2.2 Enteral feeds: Less than 1.5 kcal/mL and 5 g (or more) protein/100 mL

Not suitable for use in child under 1 year unless otherwise stated; not recommended for child 1–6 years

| Product | Formulation | Energy | Protein | Carbohydrate | Fat | Fibre | Special Characteristics | ACBS Indications | Presentation & Flavour |
|---|---|---|---|---|---|---|---|---|---|
| Fresubin® 1000 Complete (Fresenius Kabi) | Liquid (tube feed) **per 100 mL** | 420 kJ (100 kcal) | 5.5 g cows' milk | 12.5 g (sugars 1.1 g) | 3.1 g | 2 g | Gluten-free Residual lactose Contains fish oil | Standard, p. 757 | Flexible pack: 1000 mL = £8.82 |
| Fresubin® 1200 Complete (Fresenius Kabi) | Liquid (tube feed) **per 100 mL** | 500 kJ (120 kcal) | 6 g cows' milk | 15 g (sugars 1.22 g) | 4.1 g | 2 g | Gluten-free Residual lactose Contains fish oil | Standard, p. 757 | Flexible pack: 1000 mL = £11.41 |
| Fresubin® 1800 Complete (Fresenius Kabi) | Liquid (tube feed) **per 100 mL** | 500 kJ (120 kcal) | 6 g cows' milk | 15 g (sugars 1.22 g) | 4.1 g | 2 g | Gluten-free Residual lactose Contains fish oil | Standard, p. 757 | Flexible pack: 1500 mL = £11.23 |
| Jevity® Plus (Abbott) | Liquid (tube feed) **per 100 mL** | 514 kJ (122 kcal) | 5.5 g caseinates soy isolates | 15.1 g (sugars 890 mg) | 3.93 g | 2.2 g | Gluten-free Residual lactose | Standard, p. 757 Not suitable for child under 2 years; not recommended for child 2–10 years | Flexible pack: 500 mL = £4.48 1000 mL = £9.16 1500 mL = £13.75 |
| Jevity® Plus HP (Abbott) | Liquid (tube feed) **per 100 mL** | 551 kJ (131 kcal) | 8.13 g cows' milk soy isolates | 14.2 g (sugars 950 mg) | 4.33 g | 1.5 g | Gluten-free Residual lactose | Standard, p. 757; also CAPD, haemodialysis Not suitable for child under 2 years; not recommended for child 2–10 years | Flexible pack: 500 mL = £4.57 |
| Jevity® Promote (Abbott) | Liquid (tube feed) **per 100 mL** | 434 kJ (103 kcal) | 5.55 g caseinates soy isolates | 12 g (sugars 670 mg) | 3.32 g | 1.7 g | Gluten-free Residual lactose | Standard, p. 757 Not suitable for child under 2 years; not recommended for child 2–10 years | Flexible pack: 1000 mL = £8.95 |

| Product | Formulation | Energy | Protein | Carbohydrate | Fat | Fibre | Special characteristics | Presentation / indications | Flexible pack |
|---|---|---|---|---|---|---|---|---|---|
| Nutrison® MCT (Nutricia Clinical) | Liquid (tube feed) per 100 mL | 420 kJ (100 kcal) | 5 g cows' milk | 12.6 g (sugars 1 g) | 3.3 g (MCT 61%) | Nil | Gluten-free Residual lactose | Standard, p. 757 | Flexible pack: 1000 mL = £8.15 |
| Nutrison® Protein Plus (Nutricia Clinical) | Liquid (tube feed) per 100 mL | 525 kJ (125 kcal) | 6.3 g cows' milk | 14.2 g (sugars 1.1 g) | 4.9 g | Nil | Gluten-free Residual lactose | Standard, p. 757 | Flexible pack: 1000 mL = £8.39 |
| Nutrison® Protein Plus Multi Fibre (Nutricia Clinical) | Liquid (tube feed) per 100 mL | 525 kJ (125 kcal) | 6.3 g cow's milk | 14.1 g (sugars 1.1 g) | 4.9 g | 1.5 g | Gluten-free Residual lactose | Disease related malnutrition | Flexible pack: 1000 mL = £9.34 |
| Nutrison® 800 Complete Multi Fibre (Nutricia Clinical) | Liquid (tube feed) per 100 mL | 345 kJ (83 kcal) | 5.5 g cows' milk pea protein soya protein | 8.8 g (sugars 600 mg) | 2.5 g | 1.5 g | Gluten-free Residual lactose Contains fish oil | Standard, p. 757 except bowel fistula Not suitable for child under 6 years; not recommended for child 6–12 years | Flexible pack: 1000 mL = £9.32 |
| Nutrison® 1000 Complete Multi Fibre (Nutricia Clinical) | Liquid (tube feed) per 100 mL | 420 kJ (100 kcal) | 5.5 g cows' milk | 11.3 g (sugars 700 mg) | 3.7 g | 2 g | Gluten-free Residual lactose | Disease related malnutrition in patients with low energy and/or low fluid requirements | Flexible pack: 1000 mL = £8.85 |
| Nutrison® 1200 Complete Multi Fibre (Nutricia Clinical) | Liquid (tube feed) per 100 mL | 505 kJ (120 kcal) | 5.5 g cows' milk | 15 g (sugars 1.2 g) | 4.3 g | 2 g | Gluten-free Residual lactose | Standard, p. 757 except bowel fistula | Flexible pack: 1000 mL = £9.59 1500 mL = £14.41 |
| Osmolite® Plus (Abbott) | Liquid (tube feed) per 100 mL | 508 kJ (121 kcal) | 5.55 g caseinates | 15.8 g (sugars 730 mg) | 3.93 g | Nil | Gluten-free Residual lactose | Standard, p. 757 Not suitable for child under 10 years | Flexible pack: 500 mL = £4.18 1000 mL = £8.06 1500 mL = £12.07 |
| Peptamen® HN (Nestlé) | Liquid (tube feed) per 100 mL | 556 kJ (133 kcal) | 6.6 g whey protein hydrolysates | 15.6 g (sugars 1.4 g) | 4.9 g (MCT 70%) | Nil | Gluten-free Residual lactose Hydrolysed with pork trypsin | Short bowel syndrome, intractable malabsorption, proven inflammatory bowel disease, bowel fistula Not suitable for child under 3 years | Flexible pack: 500 mL = £6.32 |
| Perative® (Abbott) | Liquid (sip or tube feed) per 100 mL | 552 kJ (131 kcal) | 6.7 g caseinate whey protein hydrolysates | 17.7 g (sugars 660 mg) | 3.7 g (MCT 42%) | Nil | Gluten-free Residual lactose | Standard, p. 757 Not suitable for child under 5 years | Flexible pack: 500 mL = £5.82 1000 mL = £11.65 |

Appendix 2: Borderline substances

**Appendix 2: Borderline substances**

## A2.1.2.3 Enteral feeds: More than 1.5 kcal/mL and 5 g (or more) protein/100 mL

Not suitable for use in child under 1 year unless otherwise stated; not recommended for child 1–6 years

| Product | Formulation | Energy | Protein | Carbohydrate | Fat | Fibre | Special Characteristics | ACBS Indications | Presentation & Flavour |
|---------|-------------|--------|---------|--------------|-----|-------|-------------------------|------------------|------------------------|
| Ensure® Twocal (Abbott) | Liquid (sip or tube feed) **per 100 mL** | 838 kJ (200 kcal) | 8.4 g cows' milk | 21 g (sugars 4.5 g) | 8.9 g | 1 g | Gluten-free Residual lactose | Standard, p. 757; *also* haemodialysis and CAPD | Bottle: 200 mL = £2.14 Banana, neutral, strawberry, vanilla |

## A2.1.3 Enteral feeds (non-disease specific): Child under 12 years

### A2.1.3.1 Enteral feeds, Child: Less than 1 kcal/mL and less than 4 g protein/100 mL

| Product | Formulation | Energy | Protein | Carbohydrate | Fat | Fibre | Special Characteristics | ACBS Indications | Presentation & Flavour |
|---------|-------------|--------|---------|--------------|-----|-------|-------------------------|------------------|------------------------|
| Nutrini® Low Energy Multi Fibre (Nutricia Clinical) | Liquid (tube feed) **per 100 mL** | 315 kJ (75 kcal) | 2.1 g whey protein and caseinate | 9.3 g (sugars 600 mg) | 3.3 g | 800 mg | Gluten-free Residual lactose Contains fish oil | Paediatric, p. 757 except bowel fistula, in child 1–6 years, body-weight 8–20 kg | Bottle: 200 mL = £2.16 Flexible pack: 500 mL = £5.47 |
| Nutriprem® 1 (Cow & Gate) | Liquid (sip feed) **per 100 mL** | 335 kJ (80 kcal) | 2.5 g whey protein and casein | 7.6 g (lactose 6.3 g) | 4.4 g | 800 mg | Contains soya, fish oil and egg lipid | Low birth-weight formula | Bottle: 60 mL Hospital supply only |
| Nutriprem® 2 (Cow & Gate) | Liquid (sip feed) **per 100 mL** | 310 kJ (75 kcal) | 2 g whey protein and casein | 7.4 g (lactose 5.8 g) | 4 g | 600 mg | Contains soya, fish oil and egg lipid | Catch-up growth in pre-term infants (less than 35 weeks at birth) and small for gestational-age infants up to 6 months corrected age | Carton: 200 mL = £1.59 (Bottle: 100 mL Hospital supply only |
| | Standard dilution (15.3%) of powder (sip feed) **per 100 mL** | 315 kJ (75 kcal) | 2 g whey protein and casein | 7.4 g (lactose 5.9 g) | 4 g (including MCT oil) | 600 mg | | | Can: 900 g = £10.64 (5.1-g measuring scoop provided) |

Powder provides: protein 13 g, carbohydrate 48.3 g, fat 26.7 g, fibre 5.2 g, energy 2030 kJ (485 kcal)/100 g

| Product | Formulation | Energy | Protein | Carbohydrate | Fat | Fibre | Special Characteristics | ACBS Indications | Presentation & Flavour |
|---------|-------------|--------|---------|--------------|-----|-------|-------------------------|------------------|------------------------|
| SMA® Gold Prem 2 (SMA Nutrition) | Standard dilution (14%) of powder (sip feed) **per 100 mL** | 305 kJ (73 kcal) | 1.9 g cows' milk | 7.5 g sugars 6.4 g | 3.9 g | Nil | Contains lactose | Catch-up growth in preterm and small for gestational age infants on discharge from hospital, up to 6 months corrected age | Can: 400 g = £4.57 (4.7-g measuring scoop provided) |

Powder provides: protein 14 g, carbohydrate 54 g, fat 28 g, energy 2180 kJ (524 kcal)/100 g

| SMA® High Energy (SMA Nutrition) | Liquid (sip feed) **per 100 mL** | 382 kJ (91 kcal) | 2 g whey protein and casein | 9.8 g lactose | 4.9 g | Nil | Contains lactose | Disease related malnutrition and malabsorption, and growth failure in child from birth to 18 months | Carton: 250 mL = £2.08 |

## Amino acid formula (essential and non-essential amino acids)

| Emsogen® (SHS) | Standard dilution (20 %) of powder (sip or tube feed) **per 100 mL** | 368 kJ (88 kcal)[1] | 2.5 g protein equivalent (essential and non-essential amino acids) | 12 g (sugars 1.6 g) | 3.3 g[2] (MCT 83 %) | Nil | Lactose-free | Short-bowel syndrome, intractable malabsorption, proven inflammatory bowel disease, bowel fistula. Not suitable for child under 1 year or as sole source of nutrition in child 1–5 years | Sachet: 100 g = £6.18 Orange, unflavoured[3] |

Powder provides: protein equivalent 12.5 g, carbohydrate 60 g, fat 16.4 g, energy 1839 kJ (438 kcal)/100 g

1. Nutritional values vary with flavour—consult product literature
2. Additional source of alpha linolenic acid needed if used as sole source of nutrition
3. Flavouring: see *Modjul*® Flavour System, p. 791

## A2.1.3.2 Enteral feeds, Child: 1 kcal/mL and less than 4 g protein/100 mL

Not suitable for use in child under 1 year unless otherwise stated

| Product | Formulation | Energy | Protein | Carbohydrate | Fat | Fibre | Special Characteristics | ACBS Indications | Presentation & Flavour |
|---|---|---|---|---|---|---|---|---|---|
| Clinutren® Junior (Nestlé) | Standard dilution (22%) of powder (sip or tube feed) **per 100 mL** | 420 kJ (100 kcal) | 2.97 g whey protein and caseinate | 13.3 g | 3.9 g | Nil | Gluten-free Residual lactose | Standard, p. 757, and growth failure in child 1–10 years | Can: 400 g = £10.57 Vanilla (7.85-g measuring scoop provided) |

Powder provides: protein 13.9 g, carbohydrate 62.2 g, fat 18.3 g, energy 1950 kJ (467 kcal)/100 g

| Frebini® Original (Fresenius Kabi) | Liquid (tube feed) **per 100 mL** | 420 kJ (100 kcal) | 2.5 g cows' milk | 12.5 g (sugars 700 mg) | 4.4 g | Nil | Gluten-free Residual lactose Contains fish oils and fish gelatin | Standard, p. 757, and growth failure in child 1–10 years, body-weight 8–30 kg | Flexible pack: 500 mL = £5.09 |
| Frebini® Original Fibre (Fresenius Kabi) | Liquid (tube feed) **per 100 mL** | 420 kJ (100 kcal) | 2.5 g cows' milk | 12.5 g (sugars 700 mg) | 4.4 g | 750 mg | Gluten-free Residual lactose Contains fish oils and fish gelatin | Standard, p. 757, and growth failure in child 1–10 years, body-weight 8–30 kg | Flexible pack: 500 mL = £5.65 |
| Infatrini® (Nutricia Clinical) | Liquid (sip or tube feed) **per 100 mL** | 415 kJ (100 kcal) | 2.6 g cows' milk | 10.3 g (lactose 5.2 g) | 5.4 g | 800 mg | Gluten-free Contains fish oil | Failure to thrive, disease-related malnutrition and malabsorption, in child from birth up to body-weight 8 kg | Bottle: 100 mL = £1.03 200 mL = £1.94 Flexible pack: 500 mL = £5.25 |

Appendix 2: Borderline substances

Appendix 2: Borderline substances

## A2.1.3.2 Enteral feeds: Child: 1 kcal/mL and less than 4 g protein/100 mL (product list continued)

Not suitable for use in child under 1 year unless otherwise stated

| Product | Formulation | Energy | Protein | Carbohydrate | Fat | Fibre | Special Characteristics | ACBS Indications | Presentation & Flavour |
|---|---|---|---|---|---|---|---|---|---|
| Nutrini® (Nutricia Clinical) | Liquid (tube feed) per 100 mL | 420 kJ (100 kcal) | 2.8 g cows' milk | 12.3 g (sugars 1 g) | 4.4 g | Nil | Gluten-free Residual lactose | Standard, p. 757, and growth failure in child 1–6 years, body-weight 8–20 kg | Bottle: 200 mL = £2.58 Flexible pack: 500 mL = £5.80 |
| Nutrini® Multi Fibre (Nutricia Clinical) | Liquid (tube feed) per 100 mL | 420 kJ (100 kcal) | 2.8 g whey protein and caseinate | 12.3 g (sugars 800 mg) | 4.4 g | 800 mg | Gluten-free Residual lactose Contains fish oil | Standard, p. 757, and growth failure in child 1–6 years, body-weight 8–20 kg | Bottle: 200 mL = £2.58 Flexible pack: 500 mL = £6.45 |
| Paediasure® (Abbott) | Liquid (sip or tube feed) per 100 mL | 422 kJ (100 kcal)[1] | 2.8 g cows' milk | 11.2 g (sugars 3.92 g) | 4.98 g | Nil | Gluten-free Residual lactose | Paediatric, p. 757 in child 1–10 years, body-weight 8–30 kg | Bottle: 200 mL = £2.10 Banana, chocolate, strawberry, vanilla Flexible pack: 500 mL = £5.24 Vanilla |
| Paediasure® Fibre (Abbott) | Liquid (sip or tube feed) per 100 mL | 424 kJ (101 kcal)[1] | 2.8 g caseinates and whey protein | 10.9 g (sugars 3.84 g) | 4.98 g | 730 mg | Gluten-free Residual lactose | Paediatric, p. 757 in child 1–10 years, body-weight 8–30 kg | Bottle: 200 mL = £2.30 Banana, strawberry, vanilla Flexible pack: 500 mL = £5.82 Vanilla |
| Paediasure® Peptide (Abbott) | Liquid (sip or tube feed) per 100 mL | 420 kJ (100 kcal) | 3 g whey protein and caseinate | 13 g (sugars 2.98 g) | 4 g (MCT 50%) | Nil | Gluten-free Residual lactose | Standard, p. 757, and growth failure in child 1–10 years, body-weight 8–30 kg | Bottle: 200 mL = £3.56 Vanilla Flexible pack: 500 mL = £8.89 Vanilla |
| Similac® High Energy (Abbott) | Liquid (sip or tube feed) per 100 mL | 419 kJ (100 kcal)[2] | 2.6 g cows' milk and whey protein | 10.1 g (sugars 5.6 g) | 5.2 g | 400 mg | Gluten-free Contains lactose and soy oil | Increased energy requirements, faltering growth, and/or need for fluid restriction, in child body-weight up to 8 kg | Bottle: 120 mL = £1.23 200 mL = £2.06 |
| Tentrini® (Nutricia Clinical) | Liquid (tube feed) per 100 mL | 420 kJ (100 kcal) | 3.3 g whey protein and caseinate | 12.3 g (sugars 800 mg) | 4.2 g | Nil | Gluten-free Residual lactose Contains fish oil | Standard, p. 757, and growth failure in child 7–12 years, body-weight 21–45 kg | Flexible pack: 500 mL = £5.57 |
| Tentrini® Multi Fibre (Nutricia Clinical) | Liquid (tube feed) per 100 mL | 420 kJ (100 kcal) | 3.3 g whey protein and caseinate | 12.3 g (sugars 800 mg) | 4.2 g | 1.1 g | Gluten-free Residual lactose Contains fish oil | Standard, p. 757, except bowel fistula, and growth failure in child 7–12 years body-weight 21–45 kg | Bottle or Flexible pack: 500 mL = £5.40 |

1. Nutritional values vary with flavour—consult product literature
2. Nutritional values vary with pack size—consult product literature

## Hydrolysate Formula See also Infant Formula (Hydrolysate), section 2.3.1

| | Formulation | Energy | Protein | Carbohydrate | Fat | Fibre | Special Characteristics | ACBS Indications | Presentation & Flavour |
|---|---|---|---|---|---|---|---|---|---|
| Nutrini® Peptisorb (Nutricia Clinical) | Liquid (tube feed) per 100 mL | 420 kJ (100 kcal) | 2.8 g whey protein hydrolysate | 13.7 g (sugars 800 mg) | 3.9 g (MCT 46 %) | Nil | Gluten-free Residual lactose | Standard, p. 757, and growth failure in child 1–6 years, body-weight 8–20 kg | Flexible pack: 500 mL = £8.71 |
| Peptamen® Junior (Nestlé) | Liquid (tube feed) per 100 mL | 420 kJ (100 kcal) | 3 g whey protein hydrolysate | 13.2 g | 4 g (MCT 60 %) | Nil | Gluten-free Residual lactose Hydrolysed with pork trypsin | Short bowel syndrome, intractable malabsorption, proven inflammatory bowel disease, bowel fistula, in child 1–10 years | Can: 400 g = £15.36 Vanilla (7.86-g measuring scoop provided) |
| | Standard dilution (22%) of powder (sip or tube feed) per 100 mL | 420 kJ (100 kcal) | 3 g whey protein hydrolysate | 13.8 g | 3.85 g (MCT 60 %) | Nil | Gluten-free Residual lactose Hydrolysed with bacterial trypsin | | |

Powder provides: protein 13.7 g, carbohydrate 62.9 g, fat 17.5 g, energy 1910 kJ (457 kcal)/100 g

## A2.1.3.3 Enteral feeds, Child: More than 1 kcal/mL and less than 4 g protein/100 mL
Not suitable for use in child under 1 year unless otherwise stated

| Product | Formulation | Energy | Protein | Carbohydrate | Fat | Fibre | Special Characteristics | ACBS Indications | Presentation & Flavour |
|---|---|---|---|---|---|---|---|---|---|
| Fortini® (Nutricia Clinical) | Liquid (sip feed) per 100 mL | 630 kJ (150 kcal) | 3.4 g cows' milk | 18.8 g (sugars 7.4 g) | 6.8 g | Nil | Gluten-free Residual lactose | Disease-related malnutrition and growth failure in child 1–6 years, body-weight 8–20 kg | Bottle: 200 mL = £2.77 Strawberry, vanilla |
| Fortini® Multifibre (Nutricia Clinical) | Liquid (sip feed) per 100 mL | 630 kJ (150 kcal) | 3.4 g cows' milk | 18.8 g (sugars 7.4 g) | 6.8 g | 1.5 g | Gluten-free Residual lactose | Disease-related malnutrition and growth failure in child 1–6 years, body-weight 8–20 kg | Bottle: 200 mL = £2.91 Banana, chocolate, strawberry, vanilla, and unflavoured |
| Fortini® Smoothie Multifibre (Nutricia Clinical) | Liquid (sip feed) per 100 mL | 625 kJ (150 kcal) | 3.4 g cows' milk | 19 g (sugars 11.5 g) | 6.4 g | 1.4 g | Gluten-free Residual lactose | Disease-related malnutrition and growth failure in child 1–6 years, body-weight 8–20 kg | Bottle: 200 mL = £2.91 Berry fruit, summer fruit |
| Frebini® Energy Drink (Fresenius Kabi) | Liquid (sip feed) per 100 mL | 630 kJ (150 kcal) | 3.8 g cows' milk | 18.7 g (sugars 4.5 g) | 6.7 g | Nil | Gluten-free Residual lactose | Disease-related malnutrition and growth failure in child 1–10 years, body-weight 8–30 kg | Bottle: 200 mL = £2.42 Banana, strawberry |
| Frebini® Energy (Fresenius Kabi) | Liquid (tube feed) per 100 mL | 630 kJ (150 kcal) | 3.75 g cows' milk | 18.75 g (sugars 830 mg) | 6.7 g | Nil | Gluten-free Residual lactose Contains fish oil and fish gelatin | Standard, p. 757, and failure in child 1–10 years, body-weight 8–30 kg | Flexible pack: 500 mL = £6.21 |

**Appendix 2: Borderline substances**

## Appendix 2: Borderline substances

### A2.1.3.3 Enteral feeds, Child: More than 1 kcal/mL and less than 4 g protein/100 mL (product list continued)

Not suitable for use in child under 1 year unless otherwise stated

| Product | Formulation | Energy | Protein | Carbohydrate | Fat | Fibre | Special Characteristics | ACBS Indications | Presentation & Flavour |
|---|---|---|---|---|---|---|---|---|---|
| Frebini® Energy Fibre Drink (Fresenius Kabi) | Liquid (sip feed) per 100 mL | 630 kJ (150 kcal) | 3.8 g cows' milk | 18.75 g (sugars 4.5 g[1]) | 6.7 g | 1.1 g | Gluten-free Residual lactose | Disease-related malnutrition and growth failure in child 1–10 years, body-weight 8–30 kg | Bottle: 200 mL = £2.47 Chocolate, vanilla |
| Frebini® Energy Fibre (Fresenius Kabi) | Liquid (tube feed) per 100 mL | 630 kJ (150 kcal) | 3.75 g cows' milk | 18.75 g (sugars 830 mg) | 6.7 g | 1.13 g | Gluten-free Residual lactose Contains fish oils and fish gelatin | Standard, p. 757, and growth failure in child 1–10 years, body-weight 8–30 kg | Flexible pack: 500 mL = £6.82 |
| Resource® Junior (Nestlé) | Liquid (sip feed) per 100 mL | 630 kJ (150 kcal)[2] | 3 g cows' milk | 20.6 g (sugars 4.9 g) | 6.2 g | Nil | Gluten-free Residual lactose | Standard, p. 757 in child 1–10 years | Bottle: 200 mL = £1.84 Chocolate, strawberry, vanilla |

1. Sugar content varies with flavour
2. Nutritional values vary with flavour—consult product literature

### A2.1.3.4 Enteral feeds, Child: 1.5 kcal/mL and more than 4 g protein/100 mL

Not suitable for use in child under 1 year unless otherwise stated

| Product | Formulation | Energy | Protein | Carbohydrate | Fat | Fibre | Special Characteristics | ACBS Indications | Presentation & Flavour |
|---|---|---|---|---|---|---|---|---|---|
| Nutrini® Energy (Nutricia Clinical) | Liquid (tube feed) per 100 mL | 630 kJ (150 kcal) | 4.1 g caseinate whey protein | 18.5 g (sugars 1.1 g) | 6.7 g | Nil | Gluten-free Residual lactose Contains fish oil | Standard, p. 757, and growth failure in child 1–6 years, body-weight 8–20 kg | Bottle: 200 mL = £2.84 Flexible pack: 500 mL = £7.28 |
| Nutrini® Energy Multi Fibre (Nutricia Clinical) | Liquid (tube feed) per 100 mL | 630 kJ (150 kcal) | 4.1 g caseinate whey protein | 18.5 g (sugars 1.1 g) | 6.7 g | 800 mg | Gluten-free Residual lactose Contains fish oil | Paediatric, p. 757 except bowel fistula; also total gastrectomy, in child 1–6 years, body-weight 8–20 kg | Bottle: 200 mL = £3.01 Flexible pack: 500 mL = £7.50 |
| Paediasure® Plus (Abbott) | Liquid (sip or tube feed) per 100 mL | 632 kJ (151 kcal) | 4.2 g caseinates whey protein | 16.7 g[1] | 7.47 g | Nil | Gluten-free Residual lactose | Paediatric, p. 757 in child 1–10 years, body-weight 8–30 kg | Bottle: 200 mL = £2.56 Banana, strawberry, vanilla, unflavoured Flexible pack: 500 mL = £6.57 Vanilla |

1. Sugar content varies with presentation

| Product | Formulation | Energy | Protein | Carbohydrate | Fat | Fibre | Special Characteristics | ACBS Indications | Presentation & Flavour |
|---|---|---|---|---|---|---|---|---|---|
| Paediasure® Plus Fibre (Abbott) | Liquid (sip or tube feed) **per 100 mL** | 635 kJ (152 kcal)[1] | 4.2 g caseinates whey protein | 16.4 g (sugars 5.3 g[2]) | 7.47 g | 1.1 g | Gluten-free Residual lactose | Paediatric, p. 757 in child 1–10 years, body-weight 8–30 kg | Bottle: 200 mL = £2.79 Banana, strawberry, vanilla Flexible pack: 500 mL = £7.00 Vanilla |
| Peptamen® junior Advance (Nestlé) | Liquid (tube feed) **per 100 mL** | 630 kJ (150 kcal) | 4.5 g whey protein | 18 g (sugars 2.1 g) | 6.6 g (MCT 61%) | 540 mg | Gluten-free Residual lactose Hydrolysed with pork trypsin Contains fish oil | Intractable malabsorption, short-bowel syndrome, bowel fistula, and proven inflammatory bowel disease in child 1–10 years | Flexible pack: 500 mL = £7.00 |
| Tentrini® Energy (Nutricia Clinical) | Liquid (tube feed) **per 100 mL** | 630 kJ (150 kcal) | 4.9 g whey protein and caseinate | 18.5 g (sugars 1.1 g) | 6.3 g | Nil | Gluten-free Residual lactose Contains fish oil | Standard, p. 757, and growth failure, in child 7–12 years, body-weight 21–45 kg | Flexible pack: 500 mL = £6.07 |
| Tentrini® Energy Multi Fibre (Nutricia Clinical) | Liquid (tube feed) **per 100 mL** | 630 kJ (150 kcal) | 4.9 g whey protein and caseinate | 18.5 g (sugars 1.1 g) | 6.3 g | 1.1 g | Gluten-free Residual lactose Contains fish oil | Paediatric, p. 757, and proven inflammatory bowel disease, in child 7–12 years, body-weight 21–45 kg | Bottle or Flexible pack: 500 mL = £6.70 |

1. Nutritional values vary with flavour—consult product literature
2. Sugar content varies with presentation

## A2.2 Nutritional supplements (non-disease specific)

### A2.2.1 Nutritional supplements: less than 5 g protein/100 mL

### A2.2.1.1 Nutritional supplements: 1 kcal/mL and less than 5 g protein/100 mL
Not suitable for use in child under 1 year; use with caution in child 1–5 years unless otherwise stated

| Product | Formulation | Energy | Protein | Carbohydrate | Fat | Fibre | Special Characteristics | ACBS Indications | Presentation & Flavour |
|---|---|---|---|---|---|---|---|---|---|
| Ensure® (Abbott) | Liquid (sip or tube feed) **per 100 mL** | 423 kJ (100 kcal)[1] | 4 g caseinates soy isolate | 13.6 g (sugars 3.93 g) | 3.36 g | Nil | Gluten-free Residual lactose | Standard, p. 757 | Can: 250 mL = £2.07 Chocolate, coffee, vanilla |

1. Nutritional values vary with flavour—consult product literature

Appendix 2: Borderline substances

**Appendix 2: Borderline substances**

## A2.2.1.2 Nutritional supplements: More than 1 kcal/mL and less than 5 g protein/100 mL

Not suitable for use in child under 1 year; use with caution in child 1–5 years unless otherwise stated

| Product | Formulation | Energy | Protein | Carbohydrate | Fat | Fibre | Special Characteristics | ACBS Indications | Presentation & Flavour |
|---|---|---|---|---|---|---|---|---|---|
| Ensure® Plus Juce (Abbott) | Liquid (sip feed) **per 100 mL** | 638 kJ (150 kcal) | 4.8 g whey protein isolate | 32.7 g (sugars 9.4 g[1]) | Nil | Nil | Gluten-free Residual lactose Non-milk taste | Standard, p. 757 | Bottle: 220 mL = £1.80 Apple, fruit punch, lemon-lime, orange, peach, strawberry |
| Fortijuce® (Nutricia Clinical) | Liquid (sip feed) **per 100 mL** | 640 kJ (150 kcal) | 4.0 g cows' milk | 33.5 g (sugars 13.1 g[1]) | Nil | Nil | Gluten-free Residual lactose Non-milk taste | Standard, p. 757 Not suitable for child under 3 years | Bottle: 200 mL = £1.85 Apple, black currant, forest fruits, lemon, orange, strawberry, tropical; Starter pack (mixed) 4 × 200 mL = £7.40 |
| Fresubin® Jucy Drink (Fresenius Kabi) | Liquid (sip feed) **per 100 mL** | 630 kJ (150 kcal) | 4 g whey protein | 33.5 g (sugars 8 g) | Nil | Nil | Gluten-free Residual lactose | Standard, p. 757; *also* CAPD, haemodialysis | Bottle: 4 × 200 mL = £7.28 Apple, black currant, cherry, orange, pineapple |
| Paediasure® Plus Juce (Abbott) | Liquid (sip feed) **per 100 mL** | 638 kJ (150 kcal)[2] | 4.2 g cows' milk | 33.3 g (sugars 9.4 g) | Nil | Nil | Gluten-free Residual lactose Non-milk taste | Nutritional supplement in child 1–10 years, body-weight 8–30 kg with disease-related malnutrition and, or growth failure | Bottle: 200 mL = £2.77 Apple, very berry |
| ProvideXtra® Juce Drink (Fresenius Kabi) | Liquid (sip feed) **per 100 mL** | 630 kJ (150 kcal) | 4.0 g pea and soya protein hydrolysates | 33.5 g[1] | Nil | Nil[3] | Gluten-free Lactose-free Non-milk taste Sweet-flavoured products contain fish gelatin | Standard, p. 757 | Bottle: 200 mL = £1.75 Apple, black currant, cherry, lemon-lime, orange-pineapple |
| Resource® Dessert Energy (Nestlé) | Semi-solid **per 100 g** | 671 kJ (160 kcal) | 4.8 g cows' milk | 21.2 g (sugars 9.9 g[1]) | 6.2 g | Nil | Gluten-free Contains lactose | Standard, p. 757; also CAPD, haemodialysis | Cup: 125 g = £1.47 Caramel, chocolate, vanilla |
| Resource® Fruit (Nestlé) | Liquid (sip feed) **per 100 mL** | 520 kJ (125 kcal) | 4 g whey protein hydrolysate | 27 g (sugars 9.5 g[1]) | less than 200 mg | less than 200 mg[3] | Gluten-free Residual lactose Non-milk taste | Standard, p. 757 Not suitable for child under 3 years | Bottle: 4 × 200 mL = £7.02 Apple, orange, pear-cherry, raspberry-black currant |

1. Sugar content varies with flavour
2. Nutritional values vary with flavour—consult product literature
3. Fibre content varies with flavour

## A2.2.2 Nutritional supplements: 5 g (or more) protein/100 mL

### A2.2.2.1 Nutritional supplements: 1.5 kcal/mL and 5 g (or more) protein/100 mL

Not suitable for use in child under 1 year; use with caution in child 1–5 years unless otherwise stated

| Product | Formulation | Energy | Protein | Carbohydrate | Fat | Fibre | Special Characteristics | ACBS Indications | Presentation & Flavour |
|---|---|---|---|---|---|---|---|---|---|
| Ensure® Plus Fibre (Abbott) | Liquid (sip or tube feed) **per 100 mL** | 652 kJ (155 kcal)[1] | 6.25 g cows' milk soya protein isolate | 20.2 g (sugars 5.5 g) | 4.92 g | 2.5 g | Gluten-free Residual lactose | Standard, p. 757; *also* CAPD, haemodialysis | Bottle: 200 mL = £1.85 Banana, chocolate, raspberry, strawberry, vanilla |
| Ensure® Plus Milkshake style (Abbott) | Liquid (sip or tube feed) **per 100 mL** | 632 kJ (150 kcal)[1] | 6.25 g cows' milk soya protein isolate | 20.2 g (sugars 5.6 g incl. sucrose) | 4.92 g | Nil | Gluten-free Residual lactose | Standard, p. 757; *also* CAPD, haemodialysis | Bottle: 220 mL = £1.98 Banana, black currant, caramel, chocolate, coffee, fruits of the forest, orange, peach, raspberry, strawberry, vanilla, neutral |
| Ensure® Plus Savoury (Abbott) | Liquid (sip or tube feed) **per 100 mL** | 632 kJ (150 kcal)[1] | 6.25 g cows' milk soy protein isolate | 20.2 g (sugars 1.13 g) | 4.92 g | Nil | Gluten-free Residual lactose | Standard, p. 757; *also* CAPD, haemodialysis | Bottle: 220 mL = £1.98 Chicken, mushroom |
| Ensure® Plus Yoghurt style (Abbott) | Liquid (sip feed) **per 100 mL** | 632 kJ (150 kcal)[1] | 6.25 g cows' milk | 20.2 g (sugars 11.7 g) | 4.92 g | Nil | Gluten-free Residual lactose | Standard, p. 757; *also* CAPD, haemodialysis | Bottle: 220 mL = £1.85 Peach, strawberry |
| Ensure® Plus Commence (Abbott) | Starter pack (5–10 day's supply), contains: *Ensure® Plus Milkshake Style* (various flavours), 1 pack (10 × 220-mL) = £18.52. | | | | | | | | |
| Fortisip® Bottle (Nutricia Clinical) | Liquid (sip feed) **per 100 mL** | 630 kJ (150 kcal) | 6 g cows' milk | 18.4 g[2] | 5.8 g | Nil | Gluten-free Residual lactose | Standard, p. 757 Not suitable for child under 3 years | Bottle: 200 mL = £1.85 Banana, chocolate, neutral, orange, strawberry, toffee, tropical fruits, vanilla |
| Fortisip® Multi Fibre (Nutricia Clinical) | Liquid (sip feed) **per 100 mL** | 630 kJ (150 kcal) | 6 g cows' milk | 18.4 g (sugars 7.0 g) | 5.8 g | 2.3 g | Gluten-free Residual lactose | Standard, p. 757 Not suitable for child under 3 years | Bottle: 200 mL = £1.91 Vanilla |
| Fortisip® Yoghurt Style (Nutricia Clinical) | Liquid (sip feed) **per 100 mL** | 630 kJ (150 kcal) | 6 g cows' milk | 18.7 g (sugars 10.8 g) | 5.8 g | 200 mg | Gluten-free Contains lactose | Standard, p. 757 Not suitable for child under 3 years | Bottle: 200 mL = £1.85 Peach-orange, raspberry, vanilla-lemon |

1. Nutritional values vary with flavour—consult product literature
2. Sugar content varies with flavour

Appendix 2: Borderline substances

**Appendix 2: Borderline substances**

### A2.2.2.1 Nutritional supplements: 1.5 kcal/mL and 5 g (or more) protein/100 mL (product list continued)

Not suitable for use in child under 1 year; use with caution in child 1–5 years unless otherwise stated

| Product | Formulation | Energy | Protein | Carbohydrate | Fat | Fibre | Special Characteristics | ACBS Indications | Presentation & Flavour |
|---|---|---|---|---|---|---|---|---|---|
| Fortisip® Range (Nutricia Clinical) | Starter pack contains 4 × Fortisip® Bottle, 4 × Fortijuce®, 2 × Fortisip® Yogurt Style, 1 pack (10 × 200 mL) = £18.50. | | | | | | | | |
| Fresubin® Protein Energy Drink (Fresenius Kabi) | Liquid (sip feed) per 100 mL | 630 kJ (150 kcal) | 10 g cows' milk | 12.4 g (sugars 6.4 g[1]) | 6.7 g | Nil[2] | Gluten-free Residual lactose Contains fish gelatin | Standard, p. 757; also CAPD, haemodialysis | Bottle: 200 mL = £1.82 Cappuccino, chocolate, strawberry, tropical fruits, vanilla |
| Fresubin® Thickened (Fresenius Kabi) | Liquid (sip feed) per 100 mL | 630 kJ (150 kcal) | 10 g cows' milk | 12.2 g (sugars 7.1 g[3]) | 6.7 g | 480 mg[4] | Gluten-free Residual lactose | Dysphagia or disease-related malnutrition Not suitable for child under 3 years. | Bottle: 200 mL = £2.10 Syrup (Stage 1) and custard (Stage 2) consistencies Strawberry, vanilla |
| Fresubin® YOcrème (Fresenius Kabi) | Semi-solid per 100 g | 630 kJ (150 kcal) | 7.5 g whey protein | 19.5 g (sugars 16.8 g) | 4.7 g | Nil | Gluten-free Contains lactose | Dysphagia, or presence or risk of malnutrition Not suitable for child under 3 years | Pot: 4 × 125 g = £7.48 Apricot-peach, biscuit, lemon, raspberry |

1. Sugar content varies with flavour
2. Fibre content varies with flavour
3. Sugar content varies with consistency
4. Fibre content varies with consistency

### A2.2.2.2 Nutritional supplements: Less than 1.5 kcal/mL and 5 g (or more) protein/100 mL

Not suitable for use in child under 1 year; use with caution in child 1–5 years unless otherwise stated

| Product | Formulation | Energy | Protein | Carbohydrate | Fat | Fibre | Special Characteristics | ACBS Indications | Presentation & Flavour |
|---|---|---|---|---|---|---|---|---|---|
| Clinutren® Dessert (Nestlé) | Semi-solid per 100 g | 520 kJ (125 kcal) | 9.5 g cows' milk | 15.5 g (sugars 14 g[1]) | 2.6 g | 500 mg[2] | Gluten-free Contains lactose | Standard, p. 757; also CAPD, haemodialysis Not suitable for child under 3 years | Pot: 4 × 125 g = £5.88 Caramel, chocolate, peach, vanilla |
| Ensure® Plus Crème (Abbott) | Semi-solid per 100 g | 574 kJ (137 kcal)[3] | 5.68 g cow's milk and soy protein isolates | 18.4 g (sugars 12.4 g) | 4.47 g | Nil | Gluten-free Residual lactose Contains soya | Standard, p. 757; also CAPD, haemodialysis Not suitable for child under 3 years | Pot: 125 g = £1.72 Banana, chocolate, neutral, vanilla |
| Fortimel® Regular (Nutricia Clinical) | Liquid (sip feed) per 100 mL | 420 kJ (100 kcal) | 10 g cows' milk | 10.3 g (sugars 8.1 g[1]) | 2.1 g | Nil | Gluten-free Contains lactose | Standard, p. 757 Not suitable for child under 3 years | Bottle: 200 mL = £1.57 Chocolate, forest fruits, strawberry, vanilla |

1. Sugar content varies with flavour
2. Fibre content varies with flavour

| Product | Formulation | Energy | Protein | Carbohydrate | Fat | Fibre | Special Characteristics | ACBS Indications | Presentation & Flavour |
|---|---|---|---|---|---|---|---|---|---|
| Nutilis® Fruit Stage 3 (Nutricia Clinical) | Semi-Solid **per 100 g** | 560 kJ (133 kcal) | 7 g whey isolate | 16.7 g (sugars 11.3 g) | 4 g | 2.6 g | Gluten-free Residual lactose | Standard, p. 757 except bowel fistula; *also* CAPD, haemodialysis Not suitable for child under 3 years | Pot: 3 × 150 g = £7.08 Apple, strawberry |
| Oral Impact® (Nestlé) | Standard dilution of powder (74 g in 250 mL water) (sip feed) **per 100 mL** | 425 kJ (101 kcal)[1] | 5.6 g cows' milk | 13.4 g (sugars 7.4 g) | 2.8 g | 1 g | Residual lactose Contains fish oil | Pre-operative nutritional supplement for malnourished patients or patients at risk of malnourishment Not suitable for child under 3 years | Sachet: 5 × 74 g = £15.41 Citrus, coffee, tropical |

Powder provides: protein 16.8 g, carbohydrate 40.2 g, fat 8.3 g, fibre 3 g, energy 1276 kJ (303 kcal)/74 g

| Product | Formulation | Energy | Protein | Carbohydrate | Fat | Fibre | Special Characteristics | ACBS Indications | Presentation & Flavour |
|---|---|---|---|---|---|---|---|---|---|
| Resource® Protein (Nestlé) | Liquid (sip feed) **per 100 mL** | 530 kJ (125 kcal)[1] | 9.4 g cows' milk | 14 g (sugars 4.5 g) | 3.5 g | Nil | Gluten-free Contains lactose | Standard, p. 757 Not suitable for child under 3 years | Bottle: 200 mL = £1.45 Apricot, chocolate, forest fruits, strawberry, vanilla |

1. Nutritional values vary with flavour—consult product literature

## A2.2.3 Nutritional supplements: More than 1.5 kcal/mL and 5 g (or more) protein/100 mL

Not suitable for use in child under 1 year; use with caution in child 1–5 years unless otherwise stated

| Product | Formulation | Energy | Protein | Carbohydrate | Fat | Fibre | Special Characteristics | ACBS Indications | Presentation & Flavour |
|---|---|---|---|---|---|---|---|---|---|
| Complan® Shake (Complan Foods) | Powder **per 57 g** | 1057 kJ (251 kcal)[1] | 8.8 g cows' milk | 35.2 g (sugars 22.7 g) | 8.4 g | Trace | Gluten-free Contains lactose | Standard, p. 757 | Sachet: 4 × 57 g = £3.44 Banana, chocolate, original, strawberry, vanilla Starter pack: 5 × 57 g = £5.07 |

Powder 57 g reconstituted with 200 mL whole milk provides: protein 15.6 g, carbohydrate 44.5 g, fat 16.4 g, energy 1621 kJ (387 kcal)

| Product | Formulation | Energy | Protein | Carbohydrate | Fat | Fibre | Special Characteristics | ACBS Indications | Presentation & Flavour |
|---|---|---|---|---|---|---|---|---|---|
| Foodlink® Complete (Foodlink) | Powder **per 100 g** | 1838 kJ (437 kcal)[1] | 21.9 g cows' milk | 57.3 g | 13.3 g | Nil | Contains lactose | Standard, p. 757 | Carton: 450 g = £3.29 Banana, chocolate, neutral, strawberry |

Recommended serving = 3 heaped tablespoonfuls in 250 mL water provides: protein 12.5 g, carbohydrate 32.7 g, fat 7.6 g, energy 1048 kJ (249 kcal)[1]

| Product | Formulation | Energy | Protein | Carbohydrate | Fat | Fibre | Special Characteristics | ACBS Indications | Presentation & Flavour |
|---|---|---|---|---|---|---|---|---|---|
| Foodlink® Complete with Fibre (Foodlink) | Powder **per 100 g** | 1804 kJ (428 kcal)[1] | 19.5 g cows' milk | 57.1 g (sugars 36.8 g) | 12.3 g | 8 g | Contains lactose | Standard, p. 757 | Sachet: 10 × 63 g = £6.67 Vanilla + fibre |

Recommended serving = 4 heaped tablespoonfuls in 250 mL water provides: protein 12.3 g, carbohydrate 38 g, fat 7.5 g, fibre 5 g, energy 1137 kJ (270 kcal)[1]

1. Nutritional values vary with flavour—consult product literature

Appendix 2: Borderline substances

**Appendix 2: Borderline substances**

## A2.2.2.3 Nutritional supplements: More than 1.5 kcal/mL and 5 g (or more) protein/100 mL *(product list continued)*

Not suitable for use in child under 1 year; use with caution in child 1–5 years unless otherwise stated

| Product | Formulation | Energy | Protein | Carbohydrate | Fat | Fibre | Special Characteristics | ACBS Indications | Presentation & Flavour |
|---|---|---|---|---|---|---|---|---|---|
| Forticreme® Complete (Nutricia Clinical) | Semi-solid **per 100 g** | 675 kJ (160 kcal) | 9.5 g cows' milk | 19.2 g (sugars 10.6 g) | 5 g | 100 mg[1] | Gluten-free Residual lactose | Standard, p. 757; *also* CAPD, haemodialysis Not suitable for child under 3 years | Pot: 4 × 125 g = £7.20 Banana, chocolate, forest fruits, vanilla |
| Fortisip® Compact (Nutricia Clinical) | Liquid (sip feed) **per 100 mL** | 1010 kJ (240 kcal) | 9.6 g cows' milk | 29.7 g (sugars 15 g) | 9.3 g | Nil | Residual lactose | Standard, p. 757 Not suitable for child under 3 years | Bottle: 125 mL = £1.85 Apricot, banana, chocolate, forest fruits, mocha, strawberry, vanilla Starter pack: 6 × 125 mL = £11.10 |
| Fortisip® Compact Fibre (Nutricia Clinical) | Liquid (sip feed) **per 100 mL** | 1000 kJ (240 kcal) | 9.4 g cows' milk | 25.2 g (sugars 13.9 g) | 10.4 g | 3.6 g | Gluten-free Residual lactose | Standard, p. 757 Not suitable for child under 3 years | Bottle: 125 mL = £1.91 Mocha, strawberry, vanilla |
| Fortisip® Compact Protein (Nutricia Clinical) | Liquid (sip feed) **per 100 mL** | 1010 kJ (240 kcal)[2] | 14.4 g cows' milk | 24.4 g (sugars 13.3 g) | 9.4 g | Nil | Gluten-free Residual lactose | Standard, p. 757 Not suitable for child under 3 years | Bottle: 4 × 125 mL = £7.76 Banana, mocha, strawberry, vanilla |
| Fortisip® Extra (Nutricia Clinical) | Liquid (sip feed) **per 100 mL** | 675 kJ (160 kcal) | 10 g cows' milk | 18.1 g (sugars 9 g) | 5.3 g | Nil[1] | Gluten-free Contains lactose | Standard, p. 757 Not suitable for child under 3 years | Bottle: 200 mL = £1.85 Chocolate, forest fruits, mocha, strawberry, vanilla Starter pack: forest fruits, 4 × 200 mL = £7.58 |
| Fresubin® 2 kcal (Fresenius Kabi) | Liquid (sip feed) **per 100 mL** | 840 kJ (200 kcal) | 10 g cows' milk | 22.5 g (sugars 5.8 g[3]) | 7.8 g | Nil | Gluten-free Residual lactose | Standard, p. 757; *also* CAPD, haemodialysis | Bottle: 200 mL = £1.73 Apricot-peach, cappuccino, fruits of the forest, neutral, toffee, vanilla |
| Fresubin® 2 kcal Fibre (Fresenius Kabi) | Liquid (sip feed) **per 100 mL** | 840 kJ (200 kcal)[2] | 10 g cows' milk | 22.5 g (sugars 5.8 g) | 7.8 g | 1.6 g | Gluten-free Residual lactose | Standard, p. 757; *also* CAPD, haemodialysis | Bottle: 200 mL = £1.73 Apricot-peach, cappuccino, chocolate, lemon, neutral, vanilla |
| Fresubin® Crème (Fresenius Kabi) | Semi-solid **per 100 g** | 775 kJ (185 kcal)[2] | 10 g cows' milk | 19 g (sugars 14.4 g) | 7.2 g | 2 g | Gluten-free Residual lactose | Standard, p. 757; *also* CAPD, haemodialysis Not suitable for child under 3 years | Pot: 4 × 125 g = £7.08 Cappuccino, chocolate, praline, strawberry, vanilla |
| Fresubin® Powder Extra (Fresenius Kabi) | Powder **per 100 g** | 1764 kJ (420 kcal)[2] | 17.5 g cows' milk whey protein | 63 g (sugars 24.7 g) | 10.9 g | Nil | Gluten-free Contains lactose | Standard, p. 757 | Sachet: 7 × 62 g = £5.60 Chocolate, neutral, strawberry, vanilla |

Powder 62 g reconstituted with 200 mL whole milk provides: protein 17.7 g, carbohydrate 48.5 g, fat 14.8 g, energy 1658 kJ (397 kcal)

1. Fibre content varies with flavour
2. Nutritional values vary with flavour—consult product literature

| Product | Formulation | Energy | Protein (source) | Carbohydrate | Fat | Fibre | Special characteristics | Prescribing notes | Presentation / flavours / price |
|---|---|---|---|---|---|---|---|---|---|
| Nutilis® Complete Stage 1 (Nutricia Clinical) | Liquid (pre-thickened) **per 100 mL** | 1010 kJ (240 kcal) | 9.6 g cows' milk | 29.1 g (sugars 5.4 g) | 9.3 g | 3.2 g | Residual lactose | Standard, p. 757 Not suitable for child under 3 years | Bottle: 125 mL = £2.10 Strawberry, vanilla |
| Renilon® 7.5 (Nutricia Clinical) | Liquid (sip feed) **per 100 mL** | 840 kJ (200 kcal) | 7.5 g cows' milk | 20 g (sugars 4.8 g) | 10 g | Nil | Gluten-free Residual lactose | Standard, p. 757 Not suitable for child under 3 years | Carton: 125 mL = £1.85 Apricot, caramel |
| Resource® 2.0 Fibre (Nestlé) | Liquid (sip feed) **per 100 mL** | 836 kJ (200 kcal)[1] | 9 g cows' milk | 21.4 g (sugars 5.5 g) | 8.7 g | 2.5 g | Gluten-free Residual lactose | Standard, p. 757 Not suitable for child under 6 years; caution in child 6–10 years | Carton: 200 mL = £1.80 Apricot, coffee, neutral, strawberry, summer fruits, vanilla |
| Resource® Dessert Fruit (Nestlé) | Semi-solid **per 100 g** | 678 kJ (160 kcal)[1] | 5 g cows' milk | 24 g (sugars 16.4 g) | 5 g | 1.4 g | Gluten-free Residual lactose | Standard, p. 757; also CAPD, haemodialysis | Cup: 3 × 125 g = £4.41 Apple, apple-peach, apple-strawberry[2] |
| Vegenat-med® Balanced Protein (Vegenat) | Powder **per 110 g serving** | 1924 kJ (458 kcal)[1] | 18 g cows' milk | 62 g | 15.35 g | 5.8 g | Gluten-free Residual lactose | Standard, p. 757 except bowel fistula Not suitable for child under 14 years | Sachet: 12 × 110 g = £36.26 Apple, chocolate, honey, orange |
| Vegenat-med® High Protein (Vegenat) | Powder **per 110 g serving** | 1940 kJ (463 kcal)[1] | 23.3 g cows' milk | 57.2 g | 15.6 g | 6 g | Gluten-free Residual lactose | Standard, p. 757 except bowel fistula Not suitable for child under 14 years | Sachet: 12 × 110 g = £50.76 Chicken, chickpea, fish, fish-vegetable, ham, lentil, veal, vegetable, winter vegetable 12 × 110 g = £48.95 Curry chicken 12 × 110 g = £48.22 Lemon, rice with lemon 24 × 55 g = £46.50 Rice with apple |

1. Nutritional values vary with flavour—consult product literature
2. Flavour not suitable for child under 3 years

**Appendix 2: Borderline substances**

## A2.3 Specialised formulas

### A2.3.1 Specialised formulas: Infant and child

Specialised formulas are suitable for infants from birth unless otherwise indicated (see also A2.1.3.1 Enteral feeds (non-disease specific); Child under 12 years)

#### Specialised formulas: Infant and child: Amino acid-based formula

**ACBS Indications:** Proven whole protein intolerance, short bowel syndrome, intractable malabsorption, or other gastro-intestinal disorders where an elemental diet is indicated

| Product | Formulation | Energy | Protein | Carbohydrate | Fat | Fibre | Special Characteristics | ACBS Indications | Presentation & Flavour |
|---|---|---|---|---|---|---|---|---|---|
| Neocate® Active (SHS) | Standard dilution (21%) of powder **per 300 mL serving** (63-g sachet made up to 300 mL with water) | 1255 kJ (300 kcal) | 8.3 g protein equivalent (essential and non-essential amino acids) | 34 g (sugars 3.1 g[1]) | 14.5 g | Nil | Milk protein-free | See above / Nutritional supplement only / Not suitable for child under 1 year | Sachet: 15 × 63 g = £56.04 / Black currant, unflavoured[2] |
| Powder provides: protein equivalent 13.1 g, carbohydrate 54 g, fat 23 g, energy 1992 kJ (475 kcal)/100 g | | | | | | | | | |
| Neocate® Advance (SHS) | Standard dilution (25%) of powder **per 100 mL** | 420 kJ (100 kcal) | 2.5 g protein equivalent (essential and non-essential amino acids) | 14.6 g (sugars 1.3 g[1]) | 3.5 g (MCT 35 %) | Nil | Milk protein-free | See above / Not suitable for child under 1 year | Sachet: 100 g = £4.94 / Unflavoured[2] / 15 × 50 g = £38.99 / Banana-vanilla |
| Powder provides: protein equivalent 10 g, carbohydrate 58.5 g, fat 14 g, energy 1683 kJ (400 kcal)/100 g | | | | | | | | | |
| Neocate® LCP (SHS) | Standard dilution (14.7%) of powder **per 100 mL** | 293 kJ (70 kcal) | 1.9 g protein equivalent (essential and non-essential amino acids) | 7.9 g (sugars 720 mg) | 3.4 g | Nil | Milk protein-free | Cows' milk allergy, multiple food protein intolerance, and conditions requiring an elemental diet | Can: 400 g = £23.83 (4.9 g measuring scoop provided) |
| Powder provides: protein equivalent 13 g, carbohydrate 54 g, fat 23 g, energy 1990 kJ (475 kcal)/100 g | | | | | | | | | |
| Neocate® Spoon (Nutricia Clinical) | Standard dilution (38 %) of powder **per 97 g serving** (37-g sachet diluted with 60 mL water) | 733 kJ (175 kcal) | 3 g protein equivalent (essential and non-essential amino acids) | 24.9 g (sugars 4.6 g) | 7 g | Nil | Milk protein-free | Cows' milk allergy, multiple food protein intolerance, and conditions requiring an elemental diet / Not suitable for child under 6 months | Sachet: 15 × 37 g = £36.38 |
| Powder provides protein equivalent 8.2 g, carbohydrate 67.4 g, fat 18.8 g, energy 1981 kJ (472 kcal)/100 g | | | | | | | | | |

1. Sugar content varies with flavour

| Product | Preparation | Energy | Protein | Carbohydrate | Fat | | Special characteristics | Indications | Presentation |
|---|---|---|---|---|---|---|---|---|---|
| Nutramigen® AA (Mead Johnson) | Standard dilution (13.6%) of powder **per 100 mL** | 286 kJ (68 kcal) | 1.89 g essential and non-essential amino acids | 7 g | 3.6 g | Nil | Gluten-free Lactose-free | Severe cows' milk protein intolerance, or multiple food intolerance, and other gastro-intestinal disorders where an elemental diet is specifically indicated | Can: 400 g = £22.89 (4.5-g measuring scoop provided) |

Powder provides: protein 13.9 g, carbohydrate 51 g, fat 26 g, energy 2092 kJ (498 kcal)/100 g

## Specialised formulas: Infant and child: Hydrolysate formula

| Product | Preparation | Energy | Protein | Carbohydrate | Fat | | Special characteristics | Indications | Presentation |
|---|---|---|---|---|---|---|---|---|---|
| Aptamil Pepti® 1 (Allergy) (Milupa) | Standard dilution (13.6%) of powder **per 100 mL** | 280 kJ (67 kcal) | 1.6 g whey hydrolysed | 7.1 g (sugars 3.5 g) | 3.5 g | 600 mg | Contains lactose and fish oil | Established cows' milk protein intolerance, with or without secondary lactose intolerance | Can: 400 g = £8.62 900 g = £19.39 (4.5-g measuring scoop provided) |

Formerly Aptamil Pepti®
Powder provides: protein 11.6 g, carbohydrate 52 g, fat 25.6 g, energy 2025 kJ (484 kcal)/100 g

| Product | Preparation | Energy | Protein | Carbohydrate | Fat | | Special characteristics | Indications | Presentation |
|---|---|---|---|---|---|---|---|---|---|
| Aptamil Pepti® 2 (Allergy) (Milupa) | Standard dilution (14.3%) of powder **per 100 mL** | 285 kJ (68 kcal) | 1.6 g whey hydrolysed | 8 g (sugars 3.6 g) | 3.1 g | 600 mg | Contains lactose and fish oil | Established cows' milk protein allergy or intolerance Not suitable for child under 6 months | Can: 900 g = £19.39 (4.8-g measuring scoop provided) |

Powder provides: protein 11.2 g, carbohydrate 56.1 g, fat 21.8 g, energy 1985 kJ (473 kcal)/100 g

| Product | Preparation | Energy | Protein | Carbohydrate | Fat | | Special characteristics | Indications | Presentation |
|---|---|---|---|---|---|---|---|---|---|
| Cow & Gate Pepti-Junior® (Cow & Gate) | Standard dilution (12.8%) of powder **per 100 mL** | 275 kJ (66 kcal) | 1.8 g whey hydrolysed | 6.8 g (sugars 1.1 g) | 3.5 g | Nil | Residual lactose Contains fish oil | Disaccharide and/or whole protein intolerance, or where amino acids and peptides are indicated in conjunction with medium chain triglycerides | Can: 450 g = £11.01 (4.3-g measuring scoop provided) |

Powder provides: protein 14 g, carbohydrate 53.4 g, fat 27.3 g, energy 2155 kJ (515 kcal)/100 g

| Product | Preparation | Energy | Protein | Carbohydrate | Fat | | Special characteristics | Indications | Presentation |
|---|---|---|---|---|---|---|---|---|---|
| Infatrini® Peptisorb (Nutricia Clinical) | Liquid (sip or tube feed) **per 100 mL** | 420 kJ (100 kcal) | 2.6 g whey protein hydrolysate | 10.3 g (sugars 2.7 g) | 5.4 g (MCT 50%) | Nil | Gluten-free Residual lactose Contains fish oil | Disease-related malnutrition, intractable malabsorption, proven inflammatory bowel disease, short bowel syndrome, bowel fistula, and intolerance to whole protein feeds in child from birth to 18 months or body-weight up to 9 kg | Bottle: 200 mL = £3.22 |

| Product | Preparation | Energy | Protein | Carbohydrate | Fat | | Special characteristics | Indications | Presentation |
|---|---|---|---|---|---|---|---|---|---|
| Nutramigen® Lipil 1 (Mead Johnson) | Standard dilution (13.5%) of powder **per 100 mL** | 280 kJ (68 kcal) | 1.9 g casein hydrolysed | 7.5 g | 3.4 g | Nil | Gluten-free Lactose-free | Disaccharide and/or whole protein intolerance where additional medium chain triglycerides are not included | Can: 400 g = £9.29 (4.5-g measuring scoop provided) |

Powder provides: protein 14 g, carbohydrate 55 g, fat 25 g, energy 2100 kJ (500 kcal)/100 g

**Appendix 2: Borderline substances**

Appendix 2: Borderline substances

## A2.3.1 Specialised formulas: Infant and child *(product list continued)*

Specialised formulas are suitable for infants from birth unless otherwise indicated *(see also* A2.1.3.1 Enteral feeds (non-disease specific); Child under 12 years)

| Product | Formulation | Energy | Protein | Carbohydrate | Fat | Fibre | Special Characteristics | ACBS Indications | Presentation & Flavour |
|---|---|---|---|---|---|---|---|---|---|
| Nutramigen® Lipil 2 (Mead Johnson) | Standard dilution (14.6%) of powder **per 100 mL** | 285 kJ (68 kcal) | 1.7 g casein hydrolysed | 8.6 g | 2.9 g | Nil | Gluten-free Lactose-free | Established disaccharide and/or whole protein intolerance (where additional chain triglycerides are not indicated) Not suitable for child under 6 months | Can: 400 g = £8.95 (4.9-g measuring scoop provided) |
| Powder provides: protein 11.6 g, carbohydrate 59 g, fat 20 g, energy 1950 kJ (466 kcal)/100 g |
| Pepdite® (SHS) | Standard dilution (15%) of powder **per 100 mL** | 297 kJ (71 kcal) | 2.1 g protein equivalent (non-milk hydrolysate) | 7.8 g (sugars 700 mg) | 3.5 g | Nil | Lactose-free Contains meat (pork) and soya derivatives | Disaccharide and/or whole protein intolerance | Can: 400 g = £15.05 (5-g measuring scoop provided) |
| Powder provides: protein equivalent 13.8 g, carbohydrate 52 g, fat 23.2 g, energy 1977 kJ (472 kcal)/100 g |
| Pepdite® 1+ (SHS) | Standard dilution (22.8%) of powder **per 100 mL** | 423 kJ (100 kcal) | 3.1 g protein equivalent (non-milk hydrolysate, essential amino acids) | 13 g (sugars 1.2 g) | 3.9 g (MCT 35 %) | Nil | Lactose-free Contains meat (pork) and soya derivatives | Disaccharide and/or whole protein intolerance, or where amino acids or peptides are indicated in conjunction with medium chain triglycerides Not suitable for child under 1 year | Can: 400 g = £15.81 Unflavoured[1] |
| Powder provides: protein equivalent 13.8 g, carbohydrate 57 g, fat 17.3 g, energy 1844 kJ (439 kcal)/100 g |
| Pregestimil® Lipil (Mead Johnson) | Standard dilution (13.5%) of powder **per 100 mL** | 280 kJ (68 kcal) | 1.89 g casein hydrolysed | 6.9 g | 3.8 g (MCT 54 %) | Nil | Gluten-free Lactose-free | Disaccharide and/or whole protein intolerance, or where amino acids or peptides are indicated in conjunction with medium chain triglycerides | Can: 400 g = £10.18 (4.5-g measuring scoop provided) |
| Powder provides: protein 14 g, carbohydrate 51 g, fat 28 g, energy 2100 kJ (500 kcal)/100 g |

### Specialised formulas: Infant and child: Residual lactose formula

| Product | Formulation | Energy | Protein | Carbohydrate | Fat | Fibre | Special Characteristics | ACBS Indications | Presentation & Flavour |
|---|---|---|---|---|---|---|---|---|---|
| Enfamil® O-Lac (Mead Johnson) | Standard dilution (13%) of powder **per 100 mL** | 280 kJ (68 kcal) | 1.42 g cows' milk | 7.2 g | 3.7 g | Nil | Gluten-free Residual lactose | Proven lactose intolerance | Can: 400 g = £4.16 (4.3-g measuring scoop provided) |
| Powder provides: protein 10.9 g, carbohydrate 55 g, fat 28 g, energy 2200 kJ (524 kcal)/100 g |

1. Flavouring: see *Modjul®* Flavour System, p. 791

| Product | Preparation | Protein | Carbohydrate (sugars) | Fat (MCT) | Characteristics | Indication | Presentation |
|---|---|---|---|---|---|---|---|
| Galactomin 17® (SHS) | Standard dilution (13.6%) of powder per 100 mL | 1.7 g protein equivalent (cows' milk) | 7.5 g (sugars 1.4 g) | 3.7 g | Nil | Residual lactose | Proven lactose intolerance in pre-school children, galactosaemia, and galactokinase deficiency | Can: 400 g = £14.13 Unflavoured[1] (4.3-g measuring scoop provided) |
| SMA® LF (SMA Nutrition) | Standard dilution (13%) of powder per 100 mL | 1.5 g casein, whey | 7.2 g (sugars 2.6 g) | 3.6 g | Nil | Residual lactose | Proven lactose intolerance | Can: 430 g = £4.60. |

Powder provides: protein equivalent 12.3 g, carbohydrate 55.3 g, fat 27.2 g, energy 2155 kJ (515 kcal)/100 g

Powder provides: protein 12 g, carbohydrate 55.6 g, fat 28 g, energy 2185 kJ (522 kcal)/100 g

## Specialised formulas: Infant and child: MCT-enhanced formula

| Product | Preparation | Protein | Carbohydrate (sugars) | Fat (MCT) | Characteristics | Indication | Presentation |
|---|---|---|---|---|---|---|---|
| Caprilon® (SHS) | Standard dilution (12.7%) of powder per 100 mL | 1.5 g cows' milk | 7 g (sugars 1.3 g) | 3.6 g (MCT 75 %) | Nil | Contains lactose | Disorders in which a high intake of MCT is beneficial | Can: 420 g = £14.62 (4.2-g measuring scoop provided) |
| Lipistart® (Vitaflo) | Standard dilution (15%) of powder per 100 mL | 2.1 g protein equivalent (whey, soya) | 8.3 g (sugars 700 mg) | 3.1 g (MCT 81%) | Nil | Residual lactose | Dietary management of fat malabsorption, long-chain fatty acid oxidation disorders, and other disorders requiring a high MCT, low LCT formula | Can: 400 g = £18.09 (5-g measuring scoop provided) |

Powder provides: protein 11.8 g, carbohydrate 55.1 g, fat 28.3 g, energy 2184 kJ (522 kcal)/100 g

Powder provides: protein equivalent 13.7 g, carbohydrate 55.3 g, fat 20.6 g, energy 1883 kJ (450 kcal)/100 g

| Product | Preparation | Protein | Carbohydrate (sugars) | Fat (MCT) | Characteristics | Indication | Presentation |
|---|---|---|---|---|---|---|---|
| MCT Pepdite® (SHS) | Standard dilution (15%) of powder per 100 mL | 2 g protein equivalent (non-milk peptides, essential amino acids) | 8.8 g (sugars 1.2 g) | 2.7 g (MCT 75%) | Nil | Gluten-free Lactose-free Contains meat (pork) and soya derivatives | Disorders in which a high intake of MCT is beneficial | Can: 400 g = £16.39 (5-g measuring scoop provided) |
| MCT Pepdite® +1 (SHS) | Standard dilution (20%) of powder per 100 mL | 2.8 g protein equivalent (non-milk peptides, essential amino acids) | 11.8 g (sugars 1.6 g) | 3.6 g (MCT 75%) | Nil | Gluten-free Lactose-free Contains meat (pork) and soya derivatives | Disorders in which a high intake of MCT is beneficial Not suitable for child under 1 year | Can: 400 g = £16.39 Unflavoured[1] |

Powder provides: protein equivalent 13.8 g, carbohydrate 59 g, fat 18 g, energy 1903 kJ (453 kcal)/100 g

Powder provides: protein equivalent 13.8 g, carbohydrate 59 g, fat 18 g, energy 1903 kJ (453 kcal)/100 g

1. Flavouring: see Modjul® Flavour System, p. 791

Appendix 2: Borderline substances

**Appendix 2: Borderline substances**

## A2.3.1 Specialised formulas: Infant and child (product list continued)
Specialised formulas are suitable for infants from birth unless otherwise indicated (see also A2.1.3.1 Enteral feeds (non-disease specific); Child under 12 years)

| Product | Formulation | Energy | Protein | Carbohydrate | Fat | Fibre | Special Characteristics | ACBS Indications | Presentation & Flavour |
|---|---|---|---|---|---|---|---|---|---|
| Monogen® (SHS) | Standard dilution (17.5%) of powder **per 100 mL** | 313 kJ (74 kcal) | 2 g protein equivalent (whey) | 12 g (sugars 1.2 g) | 2.1 g (MCT 90 %) | Nil | Residual lactose Supplementation with essential fatty acids may be needed | Long-chain acyl-CoA dehydrogenase deficiency (LCAD), carnitine palmitoyl transferase deficiency (CPTD), primary and secondary lipoprotein lipase deficiency | Can: 400 g = £17.07 Unflavoured[1] (5-g measuring scoop provided) |

Powder provides: protein equivalent 11.4 g, carbohydrate 68 g, fat 11.8 g, energy 1786 kJ (424 kcal)/100 g

### Specialised formulas: Infant and child: Soya-based formula

| Product | Formulation | Energy | Protein | Carbohydrate | Fat | Fibre | Special Characteristics | ACBS Indications | Presentation & Flavour |
|---|---|---|---|---|---|---|---|---|---|
| InfaSoy® (Cow & Gate) | Standard dilution (12.8%) of powder **per 100 mL** | 275 kJ (66 kcal) | 1.6 g soya | 7 g (sugars 1 g) | 3.5 g | Nil | Lactose-free | Proven lactose and associated sucrose intolerance in pre-school children, galactokinase deficiency, galactosaemia, and proven whole cows' milk sensitivity | Can: 900 g = £7.47 (4.3-g measuring scoop provided) |

Powder provides: protein 12.8 g, carbohydrate 54.5 g, fat 27.3 g, energy 2150 kJ (514 kcal)/100 g

| Product | Formulation | Energy | Protein | Carbohydrate | Fat | Fibre | Special Characteristics | ACBS Indications | Presentation & Flavour |
|---|---|---|---|---|---|---|---|---|---|
| Wysoy® (Wyeth) | Standard dilution (13.2%) of powder **per 100 mL** | 280 kJ (67 kcal) | 1.8 g soya protein isolate | 6.9 g (sugars 2.5 g) | 3.6 g | Nil | Lactose-free | Proven lactose and associated sucrose intolerance in pre-school children, galactokinase deficiency, galactosaemia, and proven whole cows' milk sensitivity | Can: 430 g = £4.59 860 g = £8.75 |

Powder provides: protein 14 g, carbohydrate 54 g, fat 27 g, energy 2155 kJ (515 kcal)/100 g

### Specialised formulas: Infant and child: Low calcium formula

| Product | Formulation | Energy | Protein | Carbohydrate | Fat | Fibre | Special Characteristics | ACBS Indications | Presentation & Flavour |
|---|---|---|---|---|---|---|---|---|---|
| Locasol® (SHS) | Standard dilution (13.1%) of powder **per 100 mL** | 278 kJ (66 kcal) | 1.9 g cows' milk | 7 g (sugars 6.9 g) | 3.4 g | Nil | Contains lactose Calcium less than 7 mg/ 100 mL No added vitamin D | Conditions of calcium intolerance requiring restriction of calcium and vitamin D intake | Can: 400 g = £19.63 (4.4-g measuring scoop provided) |

Powder provides: protein 14.6 g, carbohydrate 53.7 g, fat 26.1 g, energy 2125 kJ (508 kcal)/100 g

### Specialised formulas: Infant and child: Fructose-based formula

| Product | Formulation | Energy | Protein | Carbohydrate | Fat | Fibre | Special Characteristics | ACBS Indications | Presentation & Flavour |
|---|---|---|---|---|---|---|---|---|---|
| Galactomin 19® (SHS) | Standard dilution (12.9%) of powder **per 100 mL** | 288 kJ (69 kcal) | 1.9 g protein equivalent (cows' milk) | 6.4 g (fructose 6.3 g) | 4 g | Nil | Residual lactose, galactose and glucose | Conditions of glucose plus galactose intolerance | Can: 400 g = £37.18 |

Powder provides: protein equivalent 14.6 g, carbohydrate 49.7 g, fat 30.8 g, energy 2233 kJ (534 kcal)/100 g

1. Flavouring: see Modjul® Flavour System, p. 791

## Specialised formulas: Infant and child: Pre-thickened infant feeds

Note: Not to be used for a period of more than 6 months; not to be used in conjunction with any other feed thickener or antacid products

| Product | Formulation | Energy | Protein | Carbohydrate | Fat | Fibre | Special Characteristics | ACBS Indications | Presentation & Flavour |
|---|---|---|---|---|---|---|---|---|---|
| Enfamil® AR (Mead Johnson) | Standard dilution (13.5%) of powder **per 100 mL** | 285 kJ (68 kcal) | 1.7 g cows' milk | 7.6 g (lactose 4.6 g) | 3.5 g | Nil | Contains lactose, pregelatinised rice starch | Significant gastro-oesophageal reflux | Can: 400 g = £3.12 (4.5-g measuring scoop provided) |

Powder provides: protein 12.5 g, carbohydrate 56 g, fat 26 g, energy 2093 kJ (500 kcal)/100 g

| | | | | | | | | | |
|---|---|---|---|---|---|---|---|---|---|
| SMA® Staydown (SMA Nutrition) | Standard dilution (12.9%) of powder **per 100 mL** | 279 kJ (67 kcal) | 1.6 g casein, whey | 7 g (lactose 5 g) | 3.6 g | Nil | Contains lactose, pre-cooked corn starch | Significant gastro-oesophageal reflux | Can: 900 g = £6.62 |

Powder provides: protein 12.4 g, carbohydrate 54.3 g, fat 28 g, energy 2166 kJ (518 kcal)/100 g

## A2.3.2 Specialised formulas for specific clinical conditions

| Product | Formulation | Energy | Protein | Carbohydrate | Fat | Fibre | Special Characteristics | ACBS Indications | Presentation & Flavour |
|---|---|---|---|---|---|---|---|---|---|
| Alicalm® (SHS) | Standard dilution (30%) of powder **per 100 mL** | 567 kJ (135 kcal) | 4.5 g caseinate whey | 17.4 g (sugars 3.2 g) | 5.3 g | Nil | Residual lactose | Crohn's disease Not suitable for child under 1 year; use as nutritional supplement only in children 1–6 years. | Powder: 400 g = £18.08 Vanilla |

Powder provides: protein 15 g, carbohydrate 58 g, fat 17.5 g, energy 1889 kJ (450 kcal)/100 g

| | | | | | | | | | |
|---|---|---|---|---|---|---|---|---|---|
| Forticare® (Nutricia Clinical) | Liquid (sip feed) **per 100 mL** | 675 kJ (160 kcal) | 9 g cows' milk | 19.1 g (sugars 13.6 g) | 5.3 g | 2.1 g | Gluten-free Residual lactose Contains fish oil | Nutritional supplement in patients with lung cancer undergoing chemotherapy, or with pancreatic cancer Not suitable in child under 3 years | Carton: 125 mL = £2.02 Cappuccino, orange-lemon, peach-ginger |
| Generaid® (SHS) | Powder **per 100 g** | 1586 kJ (374 kcal) | 76 g protein equivalent (whey protein, plus branched chain amino acids) | 5 g (sugars 5 g) | 5.5 g | Nil | Electrolytes/100 g: Na⁺ 6.1 mmol K⁺ 10.8 mmol Ca²⁺ 6.5 mmol P⁻ 6.45 mmol | Nutritional supplement for use in chronic liver disease and/or porto-hepatic encephalopathy | Tub: 400 g = £51.46 Unflavoured[1] |

1. Flavouring: see Modjul® Flavour System, p. 791

**Appendix 2: Borderline substances**

**Appendix 2: Borderline substances**

## A2.3.2 Specialised formulas for specific clinical conditions (product list continued)

| Product | Formulation | Energy | Protein | Carbohydrate | Fat | Fibre | Special Characteristics | ACBS Indications | Presentation & Flavour |
|---|---|---|---|---|---|---|---|---|---|
| Generaid® Plus (SHS) | Standard dilution (22 %) of powder **per 100 mL** | 428 kJ (102 kcal) | 2.4 g protein equivalent (whey protein, branched c-hain amino acids) | 13.6 g (sugars 1.4 g) | 4.2 g (MCT 32 %) | Nil | Electrolytes/100 mL: Na⁺ 0.7 mmol K⁺ 2.7 mmol Ca²⁺ 1.72 mmol P⁺ 1.67 mmol | Enteral feed or nutritional supplement in children over 1 year with hepatic disorders | Can: 400 g = £18.40 Unflavoured¹ (5-g measuring scoop provided) |
| *Powder provides: protein equivalent 11 g, carbohydrate 62 g, fat 19 g, energy 1944 kJ (463 kcal)/100 g* | | | | | | | | | |
| Heparon® Junior (SHS) | Standard dilution (18%) of powder **per 100 mL** | 363 kJ (86 kcal) | 2 g cows' milk | 11.6 g (sugars 2.9 g) | 3.6 g | Nil | Contains lactose Electrolytes/100 mL: Na⁺ 0.56 mmol K⁺ 1.9 mmol Ca²⁺ 2.3 mmol P⁺ 1.6 mmol | Enteral feed or nutritional supplement for children with acute or chronic liver failure | Can: 400 g = £18.20 (4.5-g measuring scoop provided) |
| *Powder provides: protein 11.1 g, carbohydrate 64.2 g, fat 19.9 g, energy 2016 kJ (480 kcal)/100 g* | | | | | | | | | |
| KetoCal® (SHS) | Standard dilution (20 %) of powder **per 100 mL** | 602 kJ (146 kcal) | 3.1 g cows' milk with additional amino acids | 600 mg (sugars 120 mg) | 14.6 g (LCT 100 %) | Nil | Electrolytes/100 mL: Na⁺ 4.3 mmol K⁺ 4.1 mmol Ca²⁺ 2.15 mmol P⁺ 2.77 mmol | Enteral feed or nutritional supplement as part of ketogenic diet in management of epilepsy resistant to drug therapy, in children over 1 year, only on the advice of secondary care physician with experience of ketogenic diet | Can: 300 g = £25.62 Vanilla, Unflavoured |
| *Powder provides: protein 15.25 g, carbohydrate 3 g, fat 73 g, energy 3011 kJ (730 kcal)/100 g* | | | | | | | | | |
| KetoCal® 4:1 LQ (SHS) | Liquid (sip or tube feed) **per 100 mL** | 620 kJ (150 kcal) | 3.09 g casein and whey with additional a-mino acids | 610 mg (sugars 230 mg) | 14.8 g (LCT 100 %) | 1.12 g | Residual lactose Electrolytes/100 mL: Na⁺ 4.9 mmol K⁺ 4.7 mmol Ca²⁺ 2.4 mmol P⁺ 3.1 mmol | Enteral feed or nutritional supplement as part of ketogenic diet in management of drug resistant epilepsy or other conditions for which a ketogenic diet is indicated in children 1–10 years; as a nutritional supplement in children over 10 years | Carton: 237 mL = £4.56 Vanilla |
| Kindergen® (SHS) | Standard dilution (20 %) of powder **per 100 mL** | 421 kJ (101 kcal) | 1.5 g whey protein | 11.8 mg (sugars 1.2 g) | 5.3 g (LCT 93 %) | Nil | Electrolytes/100 mL: Na⁺ 2 mmol K⁺ 0.6 mmol Ca²⁺ 2.8 mmol P⁺ 3 mmol Low Vitamin A | Enteral feed or nutritional supplement for children with chronic renal failure receiving peritoneal rapid overnight dialysis | Tub: 400 g = £24.44 (5-g measuring scoop provided) |
| *Powder provides: protein 7.5 g, carbohydrate 59 g, fat 26.3 g, energy 2104 kJ (504 kcal)/100 g* | | | | | | | | | |

1. Flavouring: see *Modjul® Flavour System*, p. 791

| Product | Form | Energy | Protein | Carbohydrate | Fat | | Special characteristics | Indications | Presentation |
|---|---|---|---|---|---|---|---|---|---|
| Modulen IBD® (Nestlé) | Standard dilution (20%) of powder (sip or tube feed) per 100 mL | 420 kJ (100 kcal) | 3.6 g casein | 11 g (sugars 3.98 g) | 4.7 g | Nil | Gluten-free Residual lactose | Crohn's disease active phase, and in remission if malnourished | Can: 400 g = £14.38 Unflavoured[1] (8.3-g measuring scoop provided) |
| | Powder provides: protein 18 g, carbohydrate 54 g, fat 23 g, 2070 kJ (500 kcal)/100 g | | | | | | | | |
| Nepro® (Abbott) | Liquid (sip or tube feed) per 100 mL | 838 kJ (200 kcal)[2] | 7 g cows' milk | 20.6 g (sugars 3.26 g) | 9.6 g | 1.56 g | Gluten-free. Residual lactose. Electrolytes/100 mL: $Na^+$ 3.67 mmol, $K^+$ 2.72 mmol, $Ca^{2+}$ 3.43 mmol, $P^+$ 2.23 mmol | Enteral feed or nutritional supplement in patients with chronic renal failure who are on haemodialysis or CAPD, or with cirrhosis, or other conditions requiring a high energy, low fluid, low electrolyte diet. Not suitable for child under 1 year; use with caution in child 1–5 years | Carton: 200 mL = £2.41 Strawberry, vanilla Flexible pack: 500 mL = £5.22 Vanilla |
| ProSure® (Abbott) | Liquid (sip or tube feed) per 100 mL | 536 kJ (127 kcal)[2] | 6.65 g cows' milk | 18.3 g (sugars 2.95 g) | 2.56 g | 2.07 g | Gluten-free. Residual lactose. Contains fish oil | Nutritional supplement for patients with pancreatic cancer. Not suitable for child under 1 year; use with caution in child 1–4 years | Carton: 240 mL = £2.85 Vanilla |
| Renamil® (KoRa) | Powder (sip or tube feed when reconstituted) per 100 g | 2003 kJ (477 kcal) | 4.6 g cows' milk | 70.8 g | 19.3 g | Nil | Contains lactose. Gluten-free. Electrolytes/100 g: $Na^+$ 1.04 mmol, $K^+$ 0.13 mmol, $Ca^{2+}$ 10.22 mmol, $P^+$ 1.06 mmol. Contains no vitamin A or vitamin D | Enteral feed or nutritional supplement for adults and children over 1 year with chronic renal failure | Sachet: 10 × 100 g = £25.40 |
| Renapro® (KoRa) | Powder per 100 g | 1580 kJ (372 kcal) | 90 g whey protein | 800 mg | 1 g | Nil | Gluten-free. Residual lactose. Electrolytes/100 g: $Na^+$ 23 mmol, $K^+$ 2 mmol, $Ca^{2+}$ 4.99 mmol, $P^+$ 4.84 mmol | Nutritional supplement for biochemically proven hypoproteinaemia and patients undergoing dialysis. Not suitable for child under 1 year | Sachet: 30 × 20 g = £69.60 |
| | Powder provides: protein 18 g, energy 316 kJ (74 kcal)/20-g sachet | | | | | | | | |

1. Flavouring: see Flavour Mix®, p. 791
2. Nutritional values vary with flavour—consult product literature

Appendix 2: Borderline substances

**Appendix 2: Borderline substances**

### A2.3.2 Specialised formulas for specific clinical conditions *(product list continued)*

| Product | Formulation | Energy | Protein | Carbohydrate | Fat | Fibre | Special Characteristics | ACBS Indications | Presentation & Flavour |
|---|---|---|---|---|---|---|---|---|---|
| Renastart® (Vitaflo) | Standard dilution (20%) of powder **per 100 mL** | 413 kJ (99 kcal) | 1.5 g cows' milk soya | 12.5 g (sugars 1.3 g) | 4.8 g | Nil | Contains lactose Electrolytes/100 mL: Na⁺ 2.1 mmol K⁺ 0.6 mmol Ca²⁺ 0.6 mmol P⁻ 0.6 mmol | Dietary management of renal failure in child from birth to 10 years | Sachet: 10 × 100 g = £63.54 Unflavoured (7-g measuring scoop provided) |

Powder provides: protein 7.5 g, carbohydrate 62.5 g, fat 23.8 g, energy 2066 kJ (494 kcal)/100 g

| Product | Formulation | Energy | Protein | Carbohydrate | Fat | Fibre | Special Characteristics | ACBS Indications | Presentation & Flavour |
|---|---|---|---|---|---|---|---|---|---|
| Suplena® (Abbott) | Liquid (sip or tube feed) **per 100 mL** | 840 kJ (200 kcal) | 3 g caseinates | 25.5 g (sugars 2.7 g) | 9.6 g | Nil | Gluten-free Residual lactose Electrolytes/100 mL: Na⁺ 3.39 mmol K⁺ 2.87 mmol Ca²⁺ 3.48 mmol P⁻ 2.39 mmol | Enteral feed or nutritional supplement in patients with chronic or acute renal failure who are not undergoing dialysis, or with chronic or acute liver disease with fluid restriction; other conditions requiring high energy, low protein, low electrolyte, low volume enteral feed Not suitable for child under 1 year; use with caution in child 1–5 years | Can: 237 mL = £2.47 Vanilla |

## A2.4 Feed supplements

### A2.4.1 High-energy supplements

#### A2.4.1.1 High-energy supplements: carbohydrate

Flavoured carbohydrate supplements are not suitable for child under 1 year; liquid supplements should be diluted before use in child under 5 years

**ACBS Indications:** disease-related malnutrition, malabsorption states, or other conditions requiring fortification with a high or readily available carbohydrate supplement

| Product | Formulation | Energy | Protein | Carbohydrate | Fat | Fibre | Special Characteristics | ACBS Indications | Presentation & Flavour |
|---|---|---|---|---|---|---|---|---|---|
| Caloreen® (Nestlé) | Powder **per 100 g** | 1640 kJ (390 kcal) | Nil | 96 g Maltodextrin | Nil | Nil | Gluten-free Lactose-free | See above Not suitable for child under 3 years | Powder: 500 g = £3.52 Unflavoured (10-g measuring scoop provided) |
| Maxijul® Super Soluble (SHS) | Powder **per 100 g** | 1615 kJ (380 kcal) | Nil | 95 g Glucose polymer (sugars 8.6 g) | Nil | Nil | Gluten-free Lactose-free | See above | Sachets: 4 × 132 g = £5.44 Can: 200 g = £2.19 2.5 kg = £19.25 25 kg = £130.76 Unflavoured |
| Maxijul® Liquid (SHS) | Liquid **per 100 mL** | 850 kJ (200 kcal) | Nil | 50 g Glucose polymer (sugars 4.5 g[1]) | Nil | Nil | Gluten-free Lactose-free | See above | Carton: 200 mL = £1.37 Orange, unflavoured |
| Polycal® (Nutricia Clinical) | Powder **per 100 g** | 1630 kJ (384 kcal) | Nil | 96 g Maltodextrin (sugars 6 g) | Nil | Nil | Gluten-free Lactose-free | See above | Can: 400 g = £3.75 Neutral (5-g measuring scoop provided) |
| | Liquid **per 100 mL** | 1050 kJ (247 kcal) | Nil | 61.9 g Maltodextrin (sugars 12.2 g) | Nil | Nil | | See above; liquid not suitable for child under 3 years | Bottle: 200 mL = £1.50 Neutral, orange |
| S.O.S.® (Vitaflo) | Powder **per 100 g** | 1590 kJ (380 kcal) | Nil | 95 g (sugars 9 g) | Nil | Nil | | For use as an emergency regimen in the dietary management of inborn errors of metabolism in adults and children from birth | Sachets:[2] 30 × 21 g (S.O.S. 10) = £6.83; 30 × 31 g (S.O.S. 15) = £10.08; 30 × 42 g (S.O.S. 20) = £13.65; 30 × 52 g (S.O.S. 25) = £16.90 |
| | | | | | | | | | Contents of each sachet should be reconstituted with water to a total volume of 200 mL |
| Vitajoule® (Vitaflo) | Powder **per 100 g** | 1590 kJ (380 kcal) | Nil | 95 g Dried glucose syrup (sugars 9 g) | Nil | Nil | Gluten-free Lactose-free | See above | Can: 500 g = £4.09 2.5 kg = £19.90 25 kg = £119.86 (10-g measuring scoop provided) |

1. Sugar content varies with flavour
2. S.O.S. products are age-range specific—consult product literature

**Appendix 2: Borderline substances**

Appendix 2: Borderline substances

## A2.4.1.2 High-energy supplements: fat

Liquid supplements should be diluted before use in child under 5 years

**ACBS indications:** disease-related malnutrition, malabsorption states, or other conditions requiring fortification with a high fat (or fat and carbohydrate) supplement

| Product | Formulation | Energy | Protein | Carbohydrate | Fat | Fibre | Special Characteristics | ACBS Indications | Presentation & Flavour |
|---|---|---|---|---|---|---|---|---|---|
| Calogen® (Nutricia Clinical) | Liquid (emulsion) **per 100 mL** | 1850 kJ (450 kcal)[1] | Nil | 100 mg | 50 g (LCT 100 %) | Nil | Gluten-free Lactose-free | See above | Bottle: 200 mL = £4.00 500 mL = £9.83 Banana[2], neutral, strawberry[2] |
| Fresubin® 5 kcal Shot (Fresenius Kabi) | Liquid (emulsion) **per 100 mL** | 2100 kJ (500 kcal) | Nil | 4.0 g (sucrose) | 53.8 g | 400 mg | Gluten-free Lactose-free | See above Not suitable for child under 3 years | Bottle: 120 mL = £2.55 Lemon, neutral |
| Liquigen® (SHS) | Liquid (emulsion) **per 100 mL** | 1850 kJ (450 kcal) | Nil | Nil | 50 g (MCT 97 %) Fractionated coconut oil | Nil | Gluten-free Lactose-free | Steatorrhoea associated with cystic fibrosis of the pancreas, intestinal lymphangiectasia, intestinal surgery, chronic liver disease, liver cirrhosis, other proven malabsorption syndromes, ketogenic diet in epilepsy, and in type 1 lipoproteinaemia Not suitable for child under 1 year | Bottle: 250 mL = £7.79 |
| Medium-chain Triglyceride (MCT) Oil (Nutricia Clinical) | Liquid **per 100 mL** | 3515 kJ (855 kcal) | Nil | Nil | MCT 100 % | Nil | | Nutritional supplement for steatorrhoea associated with cystic fibrosis of the pancreas, intestinal lymphangiectasia, intestinal surgery, chronic liver disease and liver cirrhosis, other proven malabsorption syndromes, ketogenic diet in management of epilepsy, type 1 hyperlipoproteinaemia | Bottle: 500 mL = £12.34 |
| **Fat and Carbohydrate** | | | | | | | | | |
| Duocal® (SHS) | Liquid **per 100 mL** | 695 kJ (166 kcal) | Nil | 23.7 g (sugars 2.1 g) | 7.9 g (MCT 30 %) | Nil | Contains vitamin E | See above | Bottle: 250 mL = £3.37 |

1. Nutritional values vary with flavour—consult product literature
2. Flavour not suitable for child under 3 years

| Product | Formulation | Energy | Protein | Carbohydrate | Fat | Fibre | Special Characteristics | ACBS Indications | Presentation & Flavour |
|---|---|---|---|---|---|---|---|---|---|
| Duocal® Super Soluble (SHS) | Powder **per 100 g** | 2061 kJ (492 kcal) | Nil | 72.7 g (sugars 6.5 g) | 22.3 g (MCT 35%) | Nil | Gluten-free Lactose-free | See above | Can: 400 g = £15.20 (5-g measuring scoop provided) |
| Energivit® (SHS) | Standard dilution (15%) of powder **per 100 mL** | 309 kJ (74 kcal) | Nil | 10 g (sugars 900 mg) | 3.75 g | Nil | Lactose-free With vitamins, minerals, and trace elements | For children requiring additional energy, vitamins, minerals, and trace elements following a protein-restricted diet | Can: 400 g = £18.49 (5-g measuring scoop provided) |

Powder provides: carbohydrate 66.7 g, fat 25 g, energy 2059 kJ (492 kcal)/100 g

| | | | | | | | | | |
|---|---|---|---|---|---|---|---|---|---|
| MCT Duocal® (SHS) | Powder **per 100 g** | 2082 kJ (497 kcal) | Nil | 72 g (sugars 10.1 g) | 23.2 g (MCT 83%) | Nil | | See above | Can: 400 g = £18.07 |

## A2.4.1.3 High-energy supplements: protein

**ACBS Indications:** disease-related malnutrition, malabsorption states, or other conditions requiring fortification with a high fat or carbohydrate (with protein) supplement

| Product | Formulation | Energy | Protein | Carbohydrate | Fat | Fibre | Special Characteristics | ACBS Indications | Presentation & Flavour |
|---|---|---|---|---|---|---|---|---|---|
| Casilan 90® (Heinz) | Powder **per 100 g** | 1572 kJ (370 kcal) | 90 g cows' milk | 300 mg | 1 g | Nil | Gluten-free Electrolytes/100 g: $Na^+$ 1.3 mmol $K^+$ 8.7 mmol $Ca^{2+}$ 35 mmol $P^-$ 22.6 mmol | Nutritional supplement for use in biochemically proven hypoproteinaemia | Can: 250 g = £6.49 |
| Protifar® (Nutricia Clinical) | Powder **per 100 g** | 1580 kJ (373 kcal) | 88.5 g cows' milk | less than 1.5 g | 1.6 g | Nil | Gluten-free Residual lactose Electrolytes/100 mL: $Na^+$ 1.3 mmol $K^+$ 1.28 mmol $Ca^{2+}$ 33.75 mmol $P^-$ 22.58 mmol | Nutritional supplement for use in biochemically proven hypoproteinaemia | Can: 225 g = £7.44 Unflavoured (2.5-g measuring scoop provided) |

Powder provides: protein 2.2 g per 2.5 g

| | | | | | | | | | |
|---|---|---|---|---|---|---|---|---|---|
| Vitapro® (Vitaflo) | Powder **per 100 g** | 1506 kJ (360 kcal) | 75 g whey protein isolate | 9 g | 6 g | Nil | Contains lactose | Biochemically proven hypoproteinaemia | Tub: 250 g = £7.47 2 kg = £58.69 (5-g measuring scoop provided) |

**Appendix 2: Borderline substances**

**Appendix 2: Borderline substances**

## A2.4.1.3 High-energy supplements: protein (product list continued)

ACBS indications: disease-related malnutrition, malabsorption states, or other conditions requiring fortification with a high fat or carbohydrate (with protein) supplement

| Product | Formulation | Energy | Protein | Carbohydrate | Fat | Fibre | Special Characteristics | ACBS Indications | Presentation & Flavour |
|---|---|---|---|---|---|---|---|---|---|
| **Protein and carbohydrate** | | | | | | | | | |
| Dialamine® (SHS) | Standard dilution (20%) of powder **per 100 mL** | 264 kJ (62 kcal) | 4.3 g protein equivalent (essential and non-essential amino acids) | 11.2 g (sugars 10.2 g) | Nil | Nil | Contains vitamin C | Hypoproteinaemia, chronic renal failure, wound fistula leakage with excessive protein loss, conditions requiring a controlled nitrogen intake, and haemodialysis Not suitable for child under 6 months | Can: 400 g = £61.74 Orange |
| Powder provides: protein equivalent 25 g, carbohydrate 65 g, vitamin C 125 mg, energy 1530 kJ (360 kcal)/100 g | | | | | | | | | |
| ProSource® (Nutrinovo) | Liquid **per 30 mL** | 420 kJ (100 kcal) | 10 g collagen protein whey protein isolate | 15 g (sugars 8 g) | Nil | Nil | Gluten-free Lactose-free May contain porcine derivatives | Biochemically proven hypoproteinaemia Not recommended for child under 3 years | Sachet: 100 × 30 mL = £83.36 Citrus-berry, neutral, orange creme |
| **Protein, fat, and carbohydrate** | | | | | | | | | |
| Calogen® Extra (Nutricia Clinical) | Liquid **per 100 mL** | 1650 kJ (400 kcal)[1] | 5 g cows' milk | 4.5 g (sugars 3.5 g) | 40.3 g | Nil | Gluten-free Residual lactose Contains vitamins and minerals | See above Not suitable for child under 3 years; use with caution in child 3–6 years May require dilution for child 3–5 years | Bottle: 200 mL = £4.56 Neutral, strawberry |
| Calogen® Extra Shots (Nutricia Clinical) | Liquid **per 100 mL** | 1650 kJ (400 kcal)[1] | 5 g cows' milk | 4.5 g (sugars 3.5 g) | 40.3 g | Nil | Gluten-free Residual lactose With vitamins and minerals | See above Not suitable for child under 3 years; use with caution in child 3–6 years May require dilution for child 3–5 years | Pot: 6 × 40 mL = £5.75 Neutral, strawberry |
| Calshake® (Fresenius Kabi) | Powder **per 87 g** | 1841 kJ (439 kcal)[1] | 4.1 g cows' milk | 56.4 g (sugars 20 g) | 22 g | Nil | Contains lactose Gluten-free | See above Not suitable for child under 1 year | Sachet: 87 g = £2.01 Banana, neutral, strawberry, vanilla 90 g = £2.01 Chocolate |

Powder: one sachet reconstituted with 240 mL whole milk provides approx. 2 kcal/mL and protein 12 g

1. Nutritional values vary with flavour—consult product literature

| Product | Form | Energy | Protein (source) | Carbohydrate | Fat | Fibre | Special characteristics | Notes | Presentation |
|---|---|---|---|---|---|---|---|---|---|
| Enshake® (Abbott) | Powder **per 100 g** | 1893 kJ (450 kcal)[1] | 8.4 g cows' milk, soy protein isolate | 69 g (sugars 14.5 g) | 15.6 g | Nil | Residual lactose Contains vitamins and minerals | See above Not suitable for child under 1 year; use with caution in child 1–6 years | Sachet: 96.5 g = £1.98 Banana, chocolate, strawberry, vanilla |

Powder: 96.5 g reconstituted with 240 mL whole milk provides approx. 2 kcal/mL and protein 16 g

| Product | Form | Energy | Protein (source) | Carbohydrate | Fat | Fibre | Special characteristics | Notes | Presentation |
|---|---|---|---|---|---|---|---|---|---|
| MCT Procal® (Vitaflo) | Powder **per 100 g** | 2742 kJ (657 kcal) | 12.5 g cows' milk | 20.6 g (sugars 3.1 g) | 63.1 g (MCT 99%) | Nil | Contains lactose | Dietary management of disorders of long-chain fatty acid oxidation, fat malabsorption, and other disorders requiring a low LCT, high MCT supplement. Not suitable for child under 1 year | Sachet: 30 × 16 g = £22.20 |

Powder 16 g provides: protein 2 g, carbohydrate 3.3 g, fat 10.1 g, energy 439 kJ (105 kcal)

| Product | Form | Energy | Protein (source) | Carbohydrate | Fat | Fibre | Special characteristics | Notes | Presentation |
|---|---|---|---|---|---|---|---|---|---|
| Pro-Cal® (Vitaflo) | Powder **per 100 g** | 2787 kJ (667 kcal) | 13.6 g cows' milk | 28.2 g (sugars 16 g) | 55.5 g | Nil | Contains lactose Gluten-free | See above Not suitable for child under 1 year; use with caution in child 1–5 years | Sachets: 25 × 15 g = £13.51 Tub: 510 g = £12.52 1.5 kg = £25.50 12.5 kg = £181.28 25 kg = £279.36 (15-g measuring scoop provided) |

Powder 15 g provides: protein 2 g, carbohydrate 4.2 g, fat 8.3 g, energy 418 kJ (100 kcal)

| Product | Form | Energy | Protein (source) | Carbohydrate | Fat | Fibre | Special characteristics | Notes | Presentation |
|---|---|---|---|---|---|---|---|---|---|
| Pro-Cal® Shot (Vitaflo) | Liquid **per 100 mL** | 1393 kJ (334 kcal) | 6.7 g cows' milk | 13.4 g | 28.2 g | Nil | Contains lactose Gluten-free | See above Not suitable for child under 1 year | Bottle: 6 × 250 mL = £26.76 Banana, neutral, strawberry[2] Starter pack: 3 × 250 mL = £13.39 |
| Pro-Cal® Singles (Vitaflo) | Liquid **per 100 mL** | 1395 kJ (333 kcal) | 6.7 g cows' milk soya | 13.3 g (sugars 13.3 g) | 28.3 g | Nil | Contains lactose Gluten-free | See above Not suitable for child under 1 year; use with caution in child 1–5 years | Pot: 60 × 30 mL = £38.45 |
| QuickCal® (Vitaflo) | Powder **per 100 g** | 3263 kJ (780 kcal) | 4.6 g cows' milk | 17 g | 77 g | Nil | Contains lactose | See above Not suitable for child under 1 year | Sachets: 25 × 13 g = £12.16 |

Powder 13 g provides: protein 600 mg, carbohydrate 2.2 g, fat 10 g, energy 418 kJ (100 kcal)

1. Nutritional values vary with flavour—consult product literature
2. Flavour not suitable for child under 3 years

Appendix 2: Borderline substances

### A2.4.1.3 High-energy supplements: protein (product list continued)

ACBS indications: disease-related malnutrition, malabsorption states, or other conditions requiring fortification with a high fat or carbohydrate (with protein) supplement

| Product | Formulation | Energy | Protein | Carbohydrate | Fat | Fibre | Special Characteristics | ACBS Indications | Presentation & Flavour |
|---|---|---|---|---|---|---|---|---|---|
| Scandishake® Mix (Nutricia Clinical) | Powder per 100 g | 2099 kJ (500 kcal)[1] | 4.7 g cows' milk | 65 g (sugars 14.3 g) | 24.7 g | Nil | Gluten-free Contains lactose | See above Not suitable for child under 3 years | Sachet: 85 g = £2.08 Banana, caramel, chocolate, strawberry, vanilla, unflavoured |
| | | | | | | | | Powder: 85 g reconstituted with 240 mL whole milk provides: protein 11.7 g, carbohydrate 66.8 g, fat 30.4 g, energy 2457 kJ (588 kcal) | |
| Vitasavoury® (Vitaflo) | Powder per 100 g | 2590 kJ (619 kcal)[1] | 12.7 g cows' milk | 23.5 g (sugars 1.5 g) | 52.3 g | 6.2 g | Contains lactose | See above Not suitable for child under 3 years | Cup (200 kcal): 24 × 33 g = £26.80 Sachet (300 kcal) 10 × 50 g = £16.35 Chicken, leek and potato, mushroom, vegetable |

1. Nutritional values vary with flavour—consult product literature

### A2.4.2 Fibre, vitamin, and mineral supplements

| Product | Formulation | Energy | Protein | Carbohydrate | Fat | Fibre | Special Characteristics | ACBS Indications | Presentation & Flavour |
|---|---|---|---|---|---|---|---|---|---|
| **High-fibre supplements** | | | | | | | | | |
| Resource® Optifibre® (Nestlé) | Powder per 100 g | 323 kJ (76 kcal) | Nil | 19 g guar gum, partially hydrolysed | Nil | 78 g | Gluten-free Lactose-free | Standard, p. 757 except dysphagia Not suitable for child under 5 years | Sachet: 16 × 10 g = £7.72 Can: 250 g = £9.51 (5-g measuring scoop provided) |
| **Vitamin and Mineral supplements** | | | | | | | | | |
| FruitiVits® (Vitaflo) | Powder per 100 g | 133 kJ (33 kcal) | Nil | 8.3 g (sugars 400 mg) | less than 100 mg | 3.3 g | | Vitamin, mineral, and trace element supplement in children 3–10 years with restrictive therapeutic diets | Sachets: 30 × 6 g = £60.00 Orange |
| Paediatric Seravit® (SHS) | Powder per 100 g | 1275 kJ (300 kcal) | Nil | 75 g (sugars 6.75 g[1]) | Nil | Nil | | Vitamin, mineral, and trace element supplement in infants and children with restrictive therapeutic diets | Tub: 200 g = £14.37 Unflavoured[2] 200 g = £15.30 Pineapple[3] (5-g measuring scoop provided) |

1. Sugar content varies with flavour
2. Flavouring: see Modjul® Flavour System, p. 791
3. Flavour not suitable for child under 6 months

## A2.5   Feed additives

### A2.5.1   Special additives for conditions of intolerance

**Colief**® (Forum)

Liquid, lactase 50 000 units/g, net price 7-mL dropper bottle = £8.40

For the relief of symptoms associated with lactose intolerance in infants, provided that lactose intolerance is confirmed by the presence of reducing substances and/or excessive acid in stools, a low concentration of the corresponding disaccharide enzyme on intestinal biopsy or by breath hydrogen test or lactose intolerance test. For dosage and administration details, consult product literature

**Fructose**

(Laevulose)

For proven glucose/galactose intolerance

### A2.5.2   Feed thickeners and pre-thickened drinks

**Carobel, Instant**® (Cow & Gate)

Powder, carob seed flour. Net price 135 g = £2.97

For thickening feeds in the treatment of vomiting

**Multi-thick**® (Abbott)

Powder, modified maize starch, gluten- and lactose-free, net price 250 g = £4.83

For thickening of liquids and foods in dysphagia. Not suitable for children under 1 year except in cases of failure to thrive

**Nutilis**® **Powder** (Nutricia Clinical)

Powder, carbohydrate 86 g, energy 1520 kJ (358 kcal)/100 g, modified maize starch, gluten- and lactose-free, net price 20 × 9-g sachets = £5.88, 225 g = £4.51

For thickening of foods in dysphagia. Not suitable for child under 1 year except in cases of failure to thrive

**Resource**® **Thickened Drink** (Nestlé)

Liquid, carbohydrate 22 g, energy: orange 382 kJ (90 kcal)/apple 376 kJ (89 kcal)/100 mL. Flavours; apple or orange, syrup or custard consistencies. Gluten- and lactose-free, net price 12 × 114-mL cups = £7.44

For dysphagia. Not suitable for children under 1 year

**Resource**® **ThickenUp**® (Nestlé)

Powder, modified maize starch. Gluten- and lactose-free, net price 227 g = £4.35; 74 × 4.5-g sachet = £16.66

For thickening of foods in dysphagia. Not suitable for children under 1 year

**Resource**® **ThickenUp**® **Clear** (Nestlé)

Powder, maltodextrin, xanthum gum, gluten- and lactose-free, net price 125 g = £8.46; 24 × 1.2-g sachets = £5.28

For thickening of liquids or foods in dysphagia. Not suitable for children under 3 years

**SLO Drinks**® (SLO Drinks)

Powder, carbohydrate content varies with flavour and chosen consistency (3 consistencies available), see product literature. Flavours: black currant, lemon, orange; (hot drinks) chocolate, white coffee, white tea, net price 25 × 115 mL = £7.50

Nutritional supplement for patient hydration in the dietary management of dysphagia. Not suitable for children under 3 years

**Thick and Easy**® (Fresenius Kabi)

Powder. Modified maize starch, net price 225-g can = £4.46; 100 × 9-g sachets = £26.35; 4.54 kg = £70.53

For thickening of foods in dysphagia. Not suitable for children under 1 year except in cases of failure to thrive

**Thicken Aid**® (M & A Pharmachem)

Powder, modified maize starch, maltodextrin, gluten- and lactose-free, net price 225 g = £4.15; 100 × 9-g sachets = £26.05

For thickening of foods in dysphagia. Not suitable for children under 1 year

**Thixo-D**® (Sutherland)

Powder, modified maize starch, gluten-free. Net price 375-g tub = £7.15

For thickening of foods in dysphagia. Not suitable for children under 1 year except in cases of failure to thrive

**Vitaquick**® (Vitaflo)

Powder. Modified maize starch. Net price 300 g = £6.66; 2 kg = £33.91; 6 kg = £87.83

For thickening of foods in dysphagia. Not suitable for children under 1 year except in cases of failure to thrive

### A2.5.3   Flavouring preparations

**Flavour Mix**® (Nestlé)

Powder, flavours: banana, chocolate, coffee, lemon-lime, or strawberry, net price 60 g = £6.85

**FlavourPac**® (Vitaflo)

Powder, flavours: black currant, lemon, orange, tropical or raspberry, net price 30 × 4-g sachets = £11.54

For use with Vitaflo's range of unflavoured protein substitutes for metabolic diseases; not suitable for child under 1 year

**Modjul**® **Flavour System** (SHS)

Powder, carbohydrate-based flavours, black currant, orange, pineapple, 100 g = £10.24; cherry-vanilla, grapefruit, lemon-lime, 20 × 5-g sachets = £10.24

For use with unflavoured SHS products based on peptides or amino acids; not suitable for child under 6 months

## A2.6   Foods for special diets

### A2.6.1   Gluten-free foods

> **ACBS indications:** established gluten-sensitive enteropathies including steatorrhoea due to gluten sensitivity, coeliac disease, and dermatitis herpetiformis.

## Bread

◀Loaves

**Barkat**® (Gluten Free Foods Ltd)

Gluten-free. Loaf, multigrain 500 g = £4.83. Loaf, sliced, wholemeal 500 g = £3.36. Loaf, sliced, part-baked, country-style 250 g = £3.69. Loaf, sliced, part-baked, white 300 g = £2.70, 550 g = £4.88. Rice bread, brown 500 g = £4.83; 500 g = £4.83

**Dietary Specials**® (Nutrition Point)
Gluten-free. Loaf, sliced, multigrain, brown 400 g = £3.01; white 400 g = £3.01

**Ener-G**® (General Dietary)
Gluten-free. Loaf, sliced Seattle brown 600 g = £5.28. Rice bread, sliced, brown 474 g = £4.59; white 456 g = £4.59. Rice loaf, sliced 612 g = £4.59. Tapioca bread, sliced 480 g = £4.59

**Genius Gluten Free**® (Genius Foods)
Gluten-free. Loaf, unsliced, brown 400 g = £2.59; white 400 g = £2.59. Loaf, sliced, brown 400 g = £2.59; white 400 g = £2.59

**Glutafin**® (Nutrition Point)
Gluten-free. Loaf, sliced, fibre 400 g = £3.41; white 400 g = £3.41

**Glutafin**® **Select** (Nutrition Point)
Gluten-free. Loaf, sliced, fresh, brown 400 g = £3.25; white 400 g = £3.25. Loaf, sliced, fibre 400 g = £3.12; white 400 g = £3.12. Loaf, seeded 400 g = £3.39

**Juvela**® (Juvela)
Gluten-free. Loaf, sliced, fresh, fibre 400 g = £2.97; white 400 g = £3.23. Loaf, sliced, white 400 g = £3.10; fibre 400 g = £3.10. Loaf, white 400 g = £3.10; fibre 400 g = £3.10. Loaf, part-baked, fibre 400 g = £3.33; white 400 g = £3.46

**Lifestyle**® (Ultrapharm)
Gluten-free. Loaf, sliced, brown 400 g = £2.82; high fibre 400 g = £2.82; white 400 g = £2.82. Loaf, brown 400 g = £2.82; high fibre 400 g = £2.82; white 400 g = £2.82

**Livwell**® (Livwell)
Gluten-free. Loaf, sliced, brown (seeded) 200 g = £2.25; white 200 g = £2.25

**Pasticely**® (GFF Trade)
Gluten-free. Loaf, sandwich, sliced, white 260 g = £3.29; rustic, sliced, white 260 g = £3.29

**Proceli**® (Proceli)
Gluten-free. Loaf, sliced, white 165 g = £2.30; sandwich 155 g = £2.32. Rice bread, brown 220 g = £2.30; sandwich 220 g = £2.30

**Sunnyvale**® (Everfresh)
Gluten-free. Loaf, mixed grain, sour dough 400 g = £1.91

**Ultra**® (Ultrapharm)
Gluten-free. Loaf, white 400 g = £2.46; high fibre 500 g = £3.35

**Warburtons**® (Warburtons)
Gluten-free. Loaf, brown 400 g = £2.99; white 400 g = £2.99

**Wellfoods**® (Wellfoods)
Gluten-free. Loaf, sliced 600 g = £4.95; unsliced 600 g = £4.85

◀**Baguettes, buns and rolls**

**Barkat**® (Gluten Free Foods Ltd)
Gluten-free. Baguette, part-baked 200 g = £3.69. Rolls, part-baked 2 x 100 g = £3.30; 6 x 50 g = £3.69

**Ener-G**® (General Dietary)
Gluten-free. Rolls, dinner × 6 = £3.11; white, long 4 × 55 g = £2.50; round 4 × 55 g = £2.50

**Glutafin**® (Nutrition Point)
Gluten-free. Baguette 2 × 175 g = £3.20. Rolls, fibre 4 × 50 g = £3.41; white 4 × 50 g = £3.41

**Glutafin**® **Select** (Nutrition Point)
Gluten-free. Rolls, part-baked, white 4 × 50 g = £3.35; long 2 × 75 g = £2.56

**Juvela**® (Juvela)
Gluten-free. Rolls, fresh, fibre 5 × 85 g = £4.17; white 5 × 85 g = £4.17. Rolls, fibre 5 × 85 g = £4.18; white 5 × 85 g = £4.18. Rolls, part-baked, fibre 5 × 75 g = £4.33; white 5 × 75 g = £4.33

**Lifestyle**® (Ultrapharm)
Gluten-free. Rolls, brown 5 × 80 g = £2.82; high fibre 5 × 80 g = £2.82; white 5 × 80 g = £2.82

**Livwell**® (Livwell)
Gluten-free. Baguette, white 250 g = £2.50. Buns, toasting 4 × 50 g = £2.50. Rolls, white 4 = £2.25. Rolls, part-baked, circle (bagel) 2 × 90 g = £2.50; dinner (square) 2 × 80 g = £2.09

**Pasticely**® (GFF Trade)
Gluten-free. Baguette, part–baked, white 160 g = £1.99. Rolls, part-baked, white 2 × 80 g = 2.39; rustic, part-baked, white 2 × 105 g = £2.39

**Proceli**® (Proceli)
Gluten-free. Baguette, part-baked 2 × 125 g = £3.24. Buns 4 × 50 g = £3.26. Lunch rolls, white 8 × 34 g = £3.26. Rolls, part-baked, white, dinner 4 × 35 g = £2.18; hotdog 3 × 35 g = £2.24

**Ultra**® (Ultrapharm)
Gluten-free. Baguette, 2 × 200 g = £2.46. Rolls, 4 × 70 g = £2.46

**Warburtons**® (Warburtons)
Gluten-free. Rolls, brown 3 × 100 g = £2.49; white 3 × 100 g = £2.49

**Wellfoods**® (Wellfoods)
Gluten-free. Burger buns 4 × 75 g = £3.95. Rolls 4 × 70 g = £3.65

◀**Speciality breads**

**Livwell**® (Livwell)
Gluten-free. Flat bread (pitta) 4 = £3.00. Tear-drop shape (naan) 2 × 90 g = £3.00

## Cereals

**Juvela**® (Juvela)
Gluten-free. Fibre flakes 300 g = £2.70; flakes 300 g = £2.70; pure oats 500 g = £2.70

**Nairns**® (Nairns)
Gluten-free. Oat porridge 500 g = £2.89

## Cookies and biscuits

**Barkat**® (Gluten Free Foods Ltd)
Gluten-free. Biscuits, coffee-style 200 g = £ 2.86; digestive 175 g = £2.20

**Ener-G**® (General Dietary)
Gluten-free. Cookies, vanilla 435 g = £5.23

**Glutafin**® (Nutrition Point)
Gluten-free. Biscuits, plain 200 g = £3.77; digestive 150 g = £1.94; savoury shorts 150 g = £2.65; shortbread 100 g = £1.60; sweet (without chocolate or sultanas) 150 g = £1.94; tea 150 g = £1.94

**Juvela**® (Juvela)
Gluten-free. Biscuits, digestive 150 g = £2.67; savoury 150 g = £3.35; sweet 150 g = £2.52, tea 150 g = £2.67

**Ultra**® (Ultrapharm)
Gluten-free. Biscuits, sweet 250 g = £2.93

## Crackers, crispbreads, and breadsticks

**Barkat**® (Gluten Free Foods Ltd)
Gluten-free. Crackers, round (matzo) 200 g = £2.97

**Dietary Specials**® (Nutrition Point)
Gluten-free. Cracker bread 150 g = £1.94

**Glutafin**® (Nutrition Point)
Gluten-free. Crackers, high fibre 200 g = £2.64; plain 200 g = £3.16; mini 175 g = £2.70

**Juvela**® (Juvela)
Gluten-free. Crispbread, plain 200 g = £4.06

**Ultra**® (Ultrapharm)
Gluten-free. Crackerbread 200 g = £1.77

## Flour mixes and xanthan gum

◢Flour mixes

**Barkat**® (Gluten Free Foods Ltd)
Gluten-free. Flour mix, bread 500 g = £5.74. Plain 750 g = £5.88

**Finax**® (Drossa)
Gluten-free. Flour mix, bread, fibre 1 kg = £9.92. Flour mix 900 g = £8.66; coarse 900 g = £8.66

**Glutafin**® (Nutrition Point)
Gluten-free. Flour mix, fibre 500 g = £5.91; white 500 g = £5.91

**Glutafin Select**® (Nutrition Point)
Gluten-free. Flour mix, bread, fibre 500 g = £6.06; white 500 g = £6.06. Fibre 500 g = £6.06; white 500 g = £5.91

**Heron Foods**® (Gluten Free Foods Ltd)
Gluten-free. Flour mix, organic, bread, standard 500 g = £8.30; high fibre 500 g = £8.30

**Il Pane di Anna**® (GFF Trade)
Gluten-free. Flour mix, bread, white 500 g = £5.25. Cake, white 500 g = £5.25. Pizza base 500 g = £5.25

**Juvela**® (Juvela)
Gluten-free. Flour mix, fibre 500 g = £6.44; plain 500 g = £6.44; harvest 500 g = £6.44

**Mrs Crimbles**® (Stiletto Foods)
Gluten-free. Bread mix, net price 275 g = £1.04. Pastry mix, net price 200 g = £1.04

**Orgran**® (Community)
Gluten-free. Flour mix, bread 450 g = £3.10. Self-raising 500 g = £3.10. Pastry and pizza 375 g = £3.80

**Proceli**® (Proceli)
Gluten-free. Flour mix, white 1 kg = £9.95

**Pure**® (Innovative)
Gluten-free. Flour mix, blended 1 kg = £3.90. Potato starch 500 g = £1.55. Rice, brown 500 g = £1.45; white 500 g = £1.55. Tapioca starch 500 g = £2.08. Teff, brown 1 kg = £4.40; white 1 kg = £4.40

**Tobia**® (Tobia Teff)
Gluten-free. Flour mix, teff, brown 1 kg = £2.95; white 1 kg = £2.95

**Tritamyl**® (Gluten Free Foods Ltd)
Gluten-free. Flour mix, bread, brown 1 kg = £6.60; white 2 kg = £13.20. Plain 2 kg = £13.20

**Wellfoods**® (Wellfoods)
Gluten-free. Flour mix, plain 1 kg = £7.65

◢Xanthan gum

**Ener-G**® (General Dietary)
Gluten-free. Xanthan gum 170 g = £7.25

**Pure**® (Innovative)
Gluten-free. Xanthan gum 100 g = £6.00

## Pasta

**Barkat**® (Gluten Free Foods Ltd)
Gluten-free. Pasta, animal shapes 500 g = £4.95; macaroni 500 g = £4.95; spaghetti 500 g = £4.95; spirals 500 g = £4.95; tagliatelle 500 g = £4.95. Buckwheat, penne 250 g = £2.48; spirals 250 g = £2.48

**BiAlimenta**® (Drossa)
Gluten-free. Pasta, acini di pepe 500 g = £5.97; formati misti 500 g = £5.97; penne 500 g = £5.97; sagnette 500 g = £5.97; spirali 500 g = £5.97; tubetti 500 g = £5.90; potato-based, gnocchi 500 g = £5.59; perle di gnocchi 500 g = £5.60

**Dietary Specials**® (Nutrition Point)
Gluten-free. Pasta, fusilli 500 g = £3.44; penne 500 g = £3.44; spaghetti 500 g = £3.44

**Ener-G**® (General Dietary)
Gluten-free. Pasta, rice-based, lasagne 454 g = £4.27; macaroni 454 g = £4.27; shells, small 454 g = £4.27 spaghetti 454 g = £4.27; vermicelli 300 g = £4.27

**Glutafin**® (Nutrition Point)
Gluten-free. Pasta, lasagne 250 g = £3.21; macaroni penne 500 g = £6.13; shells 500 g = £6.13; spirals 500 g = £6.13; spaghetti, long 500 g = £6.13; tagliatelle 250 g = £3.21

**Juvela**® (Juvela)
Gluten-free. Pasta, fusilli 500 g = £6.31; lasagne 250 g = £3.22; macaroni 500 g = £6.31; spaghetti 500 g = £6.31; tagliatelle 250 g = £3.04. Fibre, penne 500 g = £5.79

**Orgran®** (Community)
Gluten-free. Pasta, rice and corn, lasagne 200 g =
£3.03; macaroni 250 g = £2.35. Spirals, buckwheat
250 g = £2.35; corn 250 g = £2.35; brown rice 250 g
= £2.42; rice and corn 250 g = £2.35; rice and millet
250 g = £2.35

**Pasticely®** (GFF Trade)
Gluten-free. Pasta, macaroni 500 g = £2.99; elbow
500 g = £2.99; spaghetti 500 g = £2.99

**Proceli®** (Proceli)
Gluten-free. Pasta, macaroni penne 250 g = £2.95;
spaghetti, short 2 × 250 g = £5.90; spirals 250 g =
£2.59

**Rizopia®** (PGR Health Foods)
Gluten-free. Pasta, brown rice, fusilli 500 g = £2.60;
lasagne 375 g = £2.60; penne 500 g = £2.60;
spaghetti 500 g = £2.60

**Ultra®** (Ultrapharm)
Gluten-free. Pasta, fusilli 250 g = £2.95; penne 250 g
= £2.95; spaghetti 250 g = £2.95

## Pizza bases

**Barkat®** (Gluten Free Foods Ltd)
Gluten-free. Pizza crust, rice, brown 150 g = £4.21;
white 150 g = £4.21

**Dietary Specials®** (Nutrition Point)
Gluten-free. Pizza base 2 × 150 g = £5.27

**Glutafin®** (Nutrition Point)
Gluten-free. Pizza base 2 × 150 g = £5.98

**Juvela®** (Juvela)
Gluten-free. Pizza base 2 × 180 g = £7.70

**Pasticely®** (GFF Trade)
Gluten-free. Pizza base 165 g = £2.99

**Proceli®** (Proceli)
Gluten-free. Pizza base 2 × 250 g = £3.90

**Ultra®** (Ultrapharm)
Gluten-free. Pizza base 2 × 200 g = £2.65

**Wellfoods®** (Wellfoods)
Gluten-free. Pizza base 2 × 300 g = £8.95

### A2.6.1.1  Gluten- and wheat-free foods

ACBS indications: established gluten-sensitive
enteropathies with coexisting established wheat sensitivity only.

**Ener-G®** (General Dietary)
Gluten-free, wheat-free. Bread loaf, six flour 576 g =
£3.60. Rolls, Seattle brown, round (hamburger) 4 ×
119 g = £3.00; long (hot dog) 4 × 119 g = £3.00.
Pizza base, 3 × 124 g = £3.75

**Glutafin®** (Nutrition Point)
Gluten-free, wheat-free. Flour mix, bread 500 g =
£6.06; fibre 500 g = £6.06. Crispbread 150 g = £3.82

**Heron Foods®** (Gluten Free Foods Ltd)
Gluten-free, wheat-free. Flour mix, organic, bread,
fibre 500 g = £8.30. Bread and cake mix 500 g =
£6.33

### A2.6.2  Low-protein foods

ACBS indications: inherited metabolic disorders,
renal or liver failure, requiring a low-protein diet

## Bread

**Ener-G®** (General Dietary)
Low protein, Rice bread, 600 g = £4.71

**Juvela®** (Juvela)
Low protein. Loaf, sliced 400 g = £3.19. Rolls 5 ×
70 g = £3.96

**Loprofin®** (SHS)
Low protein. Loaf, part-baked, sliced 400 g = £3.35.
Rolls, part-baked 4 × 65 g = £3.52

**PK Foods®** (Gluten Free Foods Ltd)
Low protein. Loaf, white, sliced 550 g = £4.40

**Ultra PKU®** (Ultrapharm)
Low-protein. Loaf 400 g = £2.65

## Cake, biscuits, and snacks

**Harifen®** (Ultrapharm)
Low protein. Cracker toast, 200 g = £2.75

**Juvela®** (Juvela)
Low-protein. Cookies, cinnamon 125 g = £6.67;
chocolate chip 110 g = £6.67; orange 125 g = £6.67

**Loprofin®** (SHS)
Low-protein. Wafers, chocolate 100 g = £2.17;
vanilla 100 g = £2.17. Crackers 150 g = £3.05, herb
150 g = £3.05

**PK Foods®** (Gluten Free Foods Ltd)
Low-protein. *Aminex®* biscuits 200 g = £4.67;
cookies 150 g = £4.67. Cookies, chocolate chip
150 g = £4.67; cinnamon 150 g = £4.67; orange
150 g = £4.67. Rusks 200 g = £4.67. Cripsbread 75 g
= £2.24

**Promin®** (Firstplay Dietary)
Low-protein. Cooked and flavoured Pasta Snax,
ready-salted 12 × 25 g = £9.84; salt and vinegar 12
× 25 g = £9.84; cheese and onion 12 × 25 g =
£9.84; jalapeno 12 × 25 g = £9.84

**Taranis®** (Firstplay Dietary)
Low-protein. Cake bars, apricot 6 × 40 g = £5.77,
lemon 6 × 40 g = £5.51; pear 6 × 40 g = £5.77

**Vita Bite®** (Vitaflo)
Low protein. Bar, protein 30 mg (less than 2.5 mg
phenylalanine), carbohydrate 15.35 g, fat 8.4 g,
energy 572 kJ (137 kcal)/25 g. Chocolate flavoured,
25 g = £1.02
Not recommended for any child under 1 year

## Cereals

**Loprofin®** (SHS)
Low-protein. Breakfast cereal flakes, apple 375 g =
£6.70; chocolate 375 g = £6.70; strawberry 375 g =
£6.70. Cereal loops 375 g = £6.95

**Promin®** (Firstplay Dietary)
Low-protein. Hot breakfast (powder sachets), apple and cinnamon 6 × 57 g = £7.35, banana 6 × 57 g = £7.35, chocolate 6 × 57 g = £7.35; original 6 × 56 g = £7.35

## Desserts

**Loprofin®** (SHS)
Low-protein. Powder, chocolate 150 g = £4.10; strawberry 150 g = £4.10; vanilla 150 g = £4.10

**PK Foods®** (Gluten Free Foods Ltd)
Low-protein. Jelly, orange 4 × 80 g = £7.43, cherry 4 × 80 g = £7.43
ACBS Indications

**Promin®** (Firstplay Dietary)
Low-protein. Dessert mix, caramel 6 × 36.5 g = £5.77; custard 6 × 36.5 g = £5.77; chocolate and banana 6 × 36.5 g = £5.77; strawberry and vanilla 6 × 36.5 g = £5.77. Rice pudding imitation, apple 4 × 69 g = £5.77; banana 4 × 69 g = £5.77; original 4 × 69 g = £5.77; strawberry 4 × 69 g = £5.77

## Flour mixes and egg substitutes

**Ener-G®** (General Dietary)
Low-protein. Egg replacer 454 g = £4.34

**Fate®** (Fate)
Low protein. All purpose mix 500 g = £6.66. Cake mix, 2 × 250 g = £6.66; chocolate-flavour 2 × 250 g = £6.66

**Juvela®** (Juvela)
Low-protein. Mix 500 g = £6.82

**Loprofin®** (SHS)
Low-protein. Mix, plain 500 g = £7.09; chocolate 500 g = £7.50; lemon 500 g = £7.50. Egg replacer 2 × 250 g = £13.03. Egg-white replacer 100 g = £8.38

**PK Foods®** (Gluten Free Foods Ltd)
Low-protein. Flour mix 750 g = £9.91. Egg replacer 350 g = £4.67
ACBS Indications

## Pasta

**Loprofin®** (SHS)
Low-protein. Pasta, animal shapes 500 g = £7.13; spirals 500 g = £7.42; lasagne 250 g = £3.61; macaroni elbows 250 g = £3.56; penne 500 g = £7.42; spaghetti 500 g = £7.42; tagliatelle 250 g = £3.56; vermicelli 250 g = £3.69. Rice, imitation 500 g = £7.20

**Promin®** (Firstplay Dietary)
Low-protein. Pasta, alphabet shapes 500 g = £6.48; lasagne sheets 200 g = £2.76; macaroni 500 g = £6.48; noodles, flat 500 g = £6.48; shells 500 g = £6.48; spaghetti, short-cut 500 g = £6.48; spirals 500 g = £6.48. Rice, imitation 500 g = £6.48. Tricolour pasta, alphabet shapes 500 g = £6.48; shells 500 g = £6.48; spirals 500 g = £6.48

## Pizza bases

**Juvela®** (Juvela)
Low-protein. Pizza base 2 × 180 g = £7.55

**Ultra PKU®** (Ultrapharm)
Low-protein. Pizza base 5 × 80 g = £2.45

## Savoury meals and mixes

**Promin®** (Firstplay Dietary)
Low-protein. Burger mix 2 × 62 g = £5.77; lamb & mint 2 × 62 g = £5.77. Couscous 500 g = £6.48. Pasta elbows in cheese and broccoli sauce 4 × 66 g = £7.54. Pasta meal 500 g = £6.48. Pasta shells in tomato, pepper, and herb sauce 4 × 72 g = £7.54. Pasta spirals in Moroccan sauce 4 × 72 g = £7.54. Sausage mix, apple & sage 4 × 30 g = £6.49; original 4 × 30 g = £6.49; tomato & basil 4 × 30 g = £6.49. Xpot, all day scramble 4 × 60 g = £20.36; beef and tomato 4 × 60 g = £20.36; chip shop curry 4 × 60 g = £20.36; rogan style curry 4 × 60 g = £20.36

## Spreads

**Taranis®** (Firstplay Dietary)
Low-protein. Spread, hazelnut 230 g = £6.80

## A2.7 Nutritional supplements for metabolic diseases

### Glutaric aciduria (type 1)

**GA1 Anamix® Infant** (SHS)
Powder, protein equivalent (essential and non-essential amino acids except lysine, and low tryptophan) 13.1 g, carbohydrate 49.5 g, fat 23 g, fibre 5.3 g, energy 1915 kJ (457 kcal)/100 g, with vitamins, minerals, and trace elements; *standard dilution* (15%) provides protein equivalent 2 g, carbohydrate 7.4 g, fat 3.5 g, fibre 800 mg, energy 287 kJ (69 kcal)/100 mL. Unflavoured, net price 400 g = £32.70 (5-g measuring scoop provided)
Nutritional supplement for the dietary management of proven glutaric aciduria (type 1) in children from birth to 3 years

**GA Gel®** (Vitaflo)
Gel, protein equivalent (essential and non-essential amino acids except lysine, and low tryptophan) 10 g, carbohydrate 10.3 g, fat trace, energy 339 kJ (81 kcal)/24 g, with vitamins, minerals, and trace elements. Unflavoured (flavouring: see *FlavourPac®*, p. 791), net price 30 × 24-g sachets = £194.56
Nutritional supplement for dietary management of type 1 glutaric aciduria in children 6 months–10 years

**[1]XLYS, Low TRY, Maxamaid** (SHS)
Powder, protein equivalent (essential and non-essential amino acids except lysine, and low tryptophan) 25 g, carbohydrate 51 g, fat less than 500 mg, energy 1311 kJ (309 kcal)/100 g, with vitamins, minerals, and trace elements. Unflavoured, (flavouring: see *Modjul®* Flavour System, p. 791), net price 500 g = £82.57
Nutritional supplement for dietary management of type 1 glutaric aciduria

1. Maxamaid products are generally intended for use in children 1–8 years

**XLYS, TRY, Glutaridon** (SHS)
Powder, protein equivalent (essential and non-essential amino acids except lysine and tryptophan) 79 g, carbohydrate 4 g, energy 1411 kJ (332 kcal)/100 g, Lactose-free. Unflavoured, (flavouring: see *Modjul*® Flavour System, p. 791), net price 2 × 500 g = £312.84
Nutritional supplement for type 1 glutaric aciduria in children and adults; requires additional source of vitamins, minerals and trace elements

## Glycogen storage disease

**Corn flour and corn starch**
For hypoglycaemia associated with glycogen-storage disease

**Glucose**
(Dextrose monohydrate)
Net price 500 g = £1.18.
For glycogen storage disease and sucrose/isomaltose intolerance

**Glycosade**® (Vitaflo)
Powder, protein 200 mg, carbohydrate (maize starch) 47.6 g, fat 100 mg, fibre less than 600 mg, energy 803 kJ (192 kcal)/60 g, net price 30 × 60-g sachets = £92.03
A nutritional supplement for use in the dietary management of glycogen storage disease and other metabolic conditions where a constant supply of glucose is essential. Not suitable for use in children under 2 years

## Homocystinuria or hypermethioninaemia

**HCU Anamix**® **Infant** (SHS)
Powder, protein equivalent (essential and non-essential amino acids except methionine) 13.1 g, carbohydrate 49.5 g, fat 23 g, fibre 5.3 g, energy 1915 kJ (457 kcal)/100 g, with vitamins, minerals, and trace elements; *standard dilution* (15%) provides protein equivalent 2 g, carbohydrate 7.4 g, fat 3,5 g, fibre 800 mg, energy 287 kJ (69 kcal)/100 mL. Unflavoured, net price 400 g = £32.70 (5-g measuring scoop provided)
Nutritional supplement for the dietary management of proven vitamin $B_6$ non-responsive homocystinuria or hypermethioninaemia in children from birth to 3 years

**HCU cooler**® (Vitaflo)
Liquid, protein (essential and non-essential amino acids except methionine) 15 g, carbohydrate 7 g, fat 500 mg, energy 386 kJ (92 kcal)/130 mL, with vitamins, minerals and trace elements. Orange or red flavour, net price 30 × 130-mL pouch = £277.20
A methionine-free protein substitute for use as a nutritional supplement in children over 3 years with homocystinuria

**HCU Express**® **15** (Vitaflo)
Powder, protein (essential and non-essential amino acids except methionine) 15 g, carbohydrate 3.8 g, fat 30 mg, energy 315 kJ (75.3 kcal)/25 g with vitamins, minerals, and trace elements. Unflavoured, (flavouring: see *FlavourPac*®, p. 791), net price 30 × 25- g sachets = £277.88
A methionine-free protein substitute for use as a nutritional supplement in children over 8 years with homocystinuria

**HCU Express**® **20** (Vitaflo)
Powder, protein (essential and non-essential amino acids except methionine) 20 g, carbohydrate 4.7 g, fat 70 mg, energy 416 kJ (99 kcal)/34 g with vitamins, minerals, and trace elements. Unflavoured (flavouring: see *FlavourPac*®, p. 791), net price 30 × 34-g sachets = £398.15
A methionine-free protein substitute for use as a nutritional supplement in children over 8 years with homocystinuria

**HCU gel**® (Vitaflo)
Powder, protein (essential and non-essential amino acids except methionine) 10 g, carbohydrate 10.3 g, fat 20 mg, energy 339 kJ (81 kcal)/24 g with vitamins, minerals, and trace elements. Unflavoured, (flavouring: see *FlavourPac*®, p. 791), net price 30 × 24-g sachets = £194.51
A methionine-free protein substitute for use as a nutritional supplement for the dietary management of children 1–10 years with homocystinuria

**HCU Lophlex**® **LQ 20** (Nutricia Clinical)
Liquid, protein equivalent (essential and non-essential amino acids except methionine) 20 g, carbohydrate 8.8 g, fat 440 mg, energy 509 kJ (120 kcal)/125 mL, with vitamins, minerals, and trace elements. Juicy berries flavour, net price 125 mL = £14.80
Nutritional supplement for the dietary management of homocystinuria in children over 3 years

**HCU LV**® (SHS)
Powder, protein (essential and non-essential amino acids except methionine) 20 g, carbohydrate 2.5 g, fat 190 mg, energy 390 kJ (92 kcal)/27.8-g sachet, with vitamins, minerals, and trace elements. Unflavoured (flavouring: see *Modjul*® Flavour System, p. 791), or tropical flavour (formulation varies slightly), net price 30 × 27.8-g sachets = £434.40
Nutritional supplement for the dietary management of hypermethioninaemia or vitamin $B_6$ non-responsive homocystinuria in children over 8 years

**XMET Homidon** (SHS)
Powder, protein equivalent (essential and non-essential amino acids, except methionine) 77 g, carbohydrate 4.5 g, fat nil, energy 1386 kJ (326 kcal)/100 g. Unflavoured, (flavouring: see *Modjul*® Flavour System, p. 791), net price 500 g = £156.42
Nutritional supplement for the dietary management of hypermethioninaemia or homocystinuria in children

**[1]XMET Maxamaid** (SHS)
Powder, protein equivalent (essential and non-essential amino acids except methionine) 25 g, carbohydrate 51 g, fat less than 500 mg, energy 1311 kJ (309 kcal)/100 g, with vitamins, minerals, and trace elements. Unflavoured (flavouring: see *Modjul*® Flavour System, p. 791), net price 500 g = £82.57
Nutritional supplement for the dietary management of hypermethioninaemia or homocystinuria

---

1. Maxamaid products are generally intended for use in children 1–8 years

[1]**XMET Maxamum**® (SHS)
Powder, protein equivalent (essential and non-essential amino acids except methionine) 39 g, carbohydrate 34 g, fat less than 500 mg, energy 1260 kJ (297 kcal)/100 g, with vitamins, minerals, and trace elements. Unflavoured, (flavouring: see *Modjul*® Flavour System, p. 791), net price 500 g = £132.36
Nutritional supplement for the dietary management of hypermethioninaemi or homocystinuria

## Hyperlysinaemia

**HYPER LYS Anamix**® **Infant** (SHS)
Powder, protein equivalent (essential and non-essential amino acids except lysine) 13.1 g, carbohydrate 49.5 g, fat 23 g, fibre 5.3 g, energy 1915 kJ (457 kcal)/100 g, with vitamins, minerals, and trace elements; *standard dilution* (15%) provides protein equivalent 2 g, carbohydrate 7.4 g, fat 3.5 g, fibre 800 mg, energy 287 kJ (69 kcal)/100 mL. Unflavoured, net price 400 g = £32.70 (5-g measuring scoop provided)
Nutritional supplement for the dietary management of proven hyperlysinaemia in children from birth to 3 years

[2]**XLYS Maxamaid** (SHS)
Powder, protein equivalent (essential and non-essential amino acids except lysine) 25 g, carbohydrate 51 g, fat less than 500 mg, energy 1311 kJ (309 kcal)/100 g with vitamins, minerals, and trace elements. Unflavoured, (flavouring: see *Modjul*® Flavour System, p. 791), net price 500 g = £82.57
Nutritional supplement for the dietary management of hyperlysinaemia

## Isovaleric acidaemia

**IVA Anamix**® **Infant** (SHS)
Powder, protein equivalent (essential and non-essential amino acids except leucine) 13.1 g, carbohydrate 49.5 g, fat 23 g, fibre 5.3 g, energy 1915 kJ (457 kcal)/100 g, with vitamins, minerals, and trace elements; *standard dilution* (15%) provides protein equivalent 2 g, carbohydrate 7.4 g, fat 3.5 g, fibre 800 mg, energy 287 kJ (69 kcal)/100 mL. Unflavoured, net price 400 g = £32.70 (5-g measuring scoop provided)
Nutritional supplement for the dietary management of proven isovaleric acidaemia or other proven disorders of leucine metabolism in children from birth to 3 years

**XLEU Faladon** (SHS)
Powder, protein equivalent (essential and non-essential amino acids except leucine) 77 g, carbohydrate 4.5 g, fat nil, energy 1386 kJ (326 kcal)/100 g. Unflavoured, (flavouring: see *Modjul*® Flavour System, p. 791), net price 200 g = £62.55
Nutritional supplement for the dietary management of isovaleric acidaemia in children

---

1. Maxamum products are generally intended for use in children over 8 years
2. Maxamaid products are generally intended for use in children 1–8 years

[2]**XLEU Maxamaid** (SHS)
Powder, protein equivalent (essential and non-essential amino acids except leucine) 25 g, carbohydrate 51 g, fat less than 500 mg, energy 1311 kJ (309 kcal)/100 g with vitamins, minerals, and trace elements. Unflavoured, (flavouring: see *Modjul*® Flavour System, p. 791), net price 500 g = £82.57
Nutritional supplement for the dietary management of isovaleric acidaemia

## Maple syrup urine disease

**MSUD Aid III**® (SHS)
Powder, protein equivalent (essential and non-essential amino acids except isoleucine, leucine, and valine) 77 g, carbohydrate 4.5 g, fat nil, energy 1386 kJ (326 kcal)/100 g. Unflavoured, (flavouring: see *Modjul*® Flavour System, p. 791), net price 500 g = £156.42
Nutritional supplement for the dietary management of maple syrup urine disease and related conditions in children and adults where it is necessary to limit the intake of branched chain amino acids

**MSUD Anamix**® **Infant** (SHS)
Powder, protein equivalent (essential and non-essential amino acids except isoleucine, leucine, and valine) 13.1 g, carbohydrate 49.5 g, fat 23 g, fibre 5.3 g, energy 1915 kJ (457 kcal)/100 g, with vitamins, minerals, and trace elements; *standard dilution* (15%) provides protein equivalent 2 g, carbohydrate 7.4 g, fat 3.5 g, fibre 800 mg, energy 287 kJ (69 kcal)/100 mL. Unflavoured, net price 400 g = £32.70 (5-g measuring scoop provided)
Nutritional supplement for the dietary management of proven maple syrup urine disease in children from birth to 3 years

**MSUD Anamix**® **Junior** (SHS)
Powder, protein equivalent (essential and non-essential amino acids except isoleucine, leucine, and valine) 8.4 g, carbohydrate 11 g, fat 3.9 g, energy 474 kJ (113 kcal)/29-g sachet, with vitamins, minerals, and trace elements. Unflavoured, (flavouring: see *Modjul*® Flavour System, p. 791), net price 30 × 29-g sachets = £166.73
Nutritional supplement for the dietary management of maple syrup urine disease in children 1–10 years

**MSUD Anamix**® **Junior LQ** (SHS)
Liquid, protein equivalent (essential and non-essential amino acids except isoleucine, leucine, and valine) 10 g, carbohydrate 8.8 g, fat 4.8 g, fibre 310 mg, energy 497 kJ (118 kcal)/125 mL, with vitamins, minerals, and trace elements. Lactose-free. Orange flavour, net price 125-mL carton = £7.58
Nutritional supplement for the dietary management of maple syrup urine disease in children 1–10 years

**MSUD express**® **15** (Vitaflo)
Powder, protein equivalent (essential and non-essential amino acids except leucine, isoleucine, and valine) 15 g, carbohydrate 3.8 g, fat less than 100 mg, energy 315 kJ (75 kcal)/25 g, with vitamins, minerals, and trace elements. Unflavoured, (flavouring: see *FlavourPac*®, p. 791), net price 30 × 25-g sachets = £271.88
Nutritional supplement for the dietary management of maple syrup urine disease in children over 8 years and adults

**Appendix 2: Borderline substances**

**Appendix 2: Borderline substances**

### MSUD express® 20 (Vitaflo)

Powder, protein equivalent (essential and non-essential amino acids except leucine, isoleucine, and valine) 20 g, carbohydrate 4.7 g, fat less than 100 mg, energy 416 kJ (99 kcal)/34 g, with vitamins, minerals, and trace elements. Unflavoured, (flavouring: see *FlavourPac®*, p. 791), net price 30 × 34-g sachets = £398.15
Nutritional supplement for the dietary management of maple syrup urine disease in children over 8 years and adults

### MSUD cooler® (Vitaflo)

Liquid, protein equivalent (essential and non-essential amino acids except leucine, isoleucine, and valine) 15 g, carbohydrate 7 g, fat 500 mg, energy 386 kJ (92 kcal)/130-mL pouch, with vitamins, minerals, and trace elements. Orange or red flavour, net price 30 × 130-mL = £277.20
Nutritional supplement for the dietary management of maple syrup urine disease in children over 3 years and adults

### MSUD Gel® (Vitaflo)

Powder, protein equivalent (essential and non-essential amino acids except leucine, isoleucine, and valine) 10 g, carbohydrate 10.3 g, fat less than 100 mg, energy 339 kJ (81 kcal)/24 g, with vitamins, minerals, and trace elements. Unflavoured, (flavouring: see *FlavourPac®*, p. 791), net price 30 × 24-g sachets = £194.51
Nutritional supplement for the dietary management of maple syrup urine disease in children 1–10 years

### MSUD Lophlex® LQ 20 (Nutricia Clinical)

Liquid, protein equivalent (essential and non-essential amino acids except isoleucine, leucine, and valine) 20 g, carbohydrate 8.8 g, fat less than 500 mg, energy 509 kJ (120 kcal)/125 mL, with vitamins, minerals, and trace elements. Juicy berries flavour, net price 125 mL = £14.80
Nutritional supplement for the dietary management of maple syrup urine disease in children over 3 years

### [1]MSUD Maxamaid® (SHS)

Powder, protein equivalent (essential and non-essential amino acids except isoleucine, leucine, and valine) 25 g, carbohydrate 51 g, fat less than 500 mg, energy 1311 kJ (309 kcal)/100 g, with vitamins, minerals, and trace elements. Unflavoured, (flavouring: see *Modjul®* Flavour System, p. 791), net price 500 g = £82.57
Nutritional supplement for the dietary management of maple syrup urine disease

### [2]MSUD Maxamum® (SHS)

Powder, protein equivalent (essential and non-essential amino acids except isoleucine, leucine, and valine) 39 g, carbohydrate 34 g, fat less than 500 mg, energy 1260 kJ (297 kcal)/100 g, with vitamins, minerals, and trace elements. Orange flavour or unflavoured, (flavouring: see *Modjul®* Flavour System, p. 791), net price 500 g = £132.36
Nutritional supplement for the dietary management of maple syrup urine disease

1. Maxamaid products are generally intended for use in children 1–8 years
2. Maxamum products are generally intended for use in children over 8 years

## Methylmalonic propionic acidaemia

### MMA/PA Anamix® Infant (SHS)

Powder, protein equivalent (essential and non-essential amino acids except methionine, threonine, and valine, and low isoleucine) 13.1 g, carbohydrate 49.5 g, fat 23 g, fibre 5.3 g, energy 1915 kJ (457 kcal)/100 g, with vitamins, minerals, and trace elements; *standard dilution* (15%) provides protein equivalent 2 g, carbohydrate 7.4 g, fat 3.5 g, fibre 800 mg, energy 287 kJ (69 kcal)/100 mL. Unflavoured, net price 400 g = £32.70 (5-g measuring scoop provided)
Nutritional supplement for the dietary management of proven methylmalonic acidaemia or propionic acidaemia in children from birth to 3 years

### XMTVI Asadon (SHS)

Powder, protein equivalent (essential and non-essential amino acids except methionine, threonine, and valine, and low isoleucine) 77 g, carbohydrate 4.5 g, fat nil, energy 1386 kJ (326 kcal)/100 g. Unflavoured, (flavouring: see *Modjul®* Flavour System, p. 791), net price 200 g = £62.55
Nutritional supplement for the dietary management of methylmalonic acidaemia or propionic acidaemia in children and adults

### [1]XMTVI Maxamaid (SHS)

Powder, protein equivalent (essential and non-essential amino acids except methionine, threonine, and valine, and low isoleucine) 25 g, carbohydrate 51 g, fat less than 500 mg, energy 1311 kJ (309 kcal)/100 g, with vitamins, minerals, and trace elements. Unflavoured, (flavouring: see *Modjul®* Flavour System, p. 791), net price 500 g = £82.57
Nutritional supplement for the dietary management of methylmalonic acidaemia or propionic acidaemia

### [2]XMTVI Maxamum (SHS)

Powder, protein equivalent (essential and non-essential amino acids except methionine, threonine, and valine, and low isoleucine) 39 g, carbohydrate 34 g, fat less than 500 mg, energy 1260 kJ (297 kcal)/100 g, with vitamins, minerals, and trace elements. Unflavoured, (flavouring: see *Modjul®* Flavour System, p. 791), net price 500 g = £132.36
Nutritional supplement for the dietary management of methylmalonic acidaemia or propionic acidaemia

## Other inborn errors of metabolism

### Cystine500® (Vitaflo)

Powder, cystine 500 mg, carbohydrate 3.3 g, fat nil, energy 63 kJ (15 kcal)/4 g, net price 30 × 4-g sachets = £48.86
Nutritional supplement for the dietary management of inborn errors of amino acid metabolism in adults and children from birth

### DocOmega® (Vitaflo)

Powder, protein (cows' milk, soya) 100 mg, carbohydrate 3.2 g, fat 500 mg (of which docosahexaenoic acid 200 mg), fibre nil, energy 74 kJ (18 kcal)/4 g, with minerals, net price 30 x 4-g sachets = £32.20
Nutritional supplement for the dietary management of inborn errors of metabolism for adults and children from birth

**EAA® Supplement** (Vitaflo)
Powder, protein equivalent (essential amino acids)
5 g, carbohydrate 4 g, fat nil, energy 151 kJ
(36 kcal)/12.5 g, with vitamins, minerals, and trace
elements. Tropical flavour, net price 50 × 12.5-g
sachets = £174.48
Nutritional supplement for the dietary management of
disorders of protein metabolism including urea cycle
disorders in children over 3 years

**Isoleucine50®** (Vitaflo)
Powder, isoleucine 50 mg, carbohydrate 3.8 g, fat nil,
energy 63 kJ (15 kcal)/4 g, net price 30 × 4-g
sachets = £48.86
Nutritional supplement for use in the dietary management
of inborn errors of amino acid metabolism in adults and
children from birth

**KeyOmega®** (Vitaflo)
Powder, protein (cows' milk, soya) 170 mg,
carbohydrate 2.8 g, fat 800 mg (of which arachidonic
acid 200 mg, docosahexaenoic acid 100 mg), energy
80 kJ (19 kcal)/4 g, net price 30 × 4-g sachet =
£32.92
Nutritional supplement for the dietary management of
inborn errors of metabolism

**Leucine100®** (Vitaflo)
Powder, leucine 100 mg, carbohydrate 3.7 g, fat nil,
energy 63 kJ (15 kcal)/4 g, net price 30 × 4-g
sachets = £48.86
Nutritional supplement for the dietary management of
inborn errors of amino acid metabolism in adults and
children from birth

**Low protein drink** (Milupa )
Powder, protein (cows' milk) 4.5 g (phenylalanine
100 mg), carbohydrate 59.5 g, fat 29.9 g, fibre nil,
energy 2194 kJ (528 kcal)/100 g, with vitamins,
minerals, and trace elements. Contains lactose. Net
price 400 g = £7.76 (5-g measuring scoop provided)
Nutritional supplement for the dietary management of
inborn errors of amino acid metabolism in adults and
children over 1 year

**Note** Termed *Milupa® lp-drink* by manufacturer

**Phenylalanine50®** (Vitaflo)
Powder, phenylalanine 50 mg, carbohydrate 3.8 g, fat
nil, energy 63 kJ (15 kcal)/4 g, net price 30 × 4-g
sachets = £47.43
Nutritional supplement for use in the dietary management
of inborn errors of metabolism in adults and children from
birth

**ProZero®** (Vitaflo)
Liquid, carbohydrate 8.1 g (of which sugars 3.5 g),
fat 3.8 g, energy 278 kJ (66 kcal)/100 mL. Contains
lactose. Net price 18 × 250 mL = £22.50; 6 ×
1 litre = £30.00
A protein-free nutritional supplement for the dietary
management of inborn errors of metabolism in children
over 6 months and adults

**Tyrosine1000®** (Vitaflo)
Powder, tyrosine 1 g, carbohydrate 2.9 g, fat nil,
energy 63 kJ (15 kcal)/4-g sachet, net price 30 × 4-
g sachets = £4.48
Nutritional supplement for the dietary management of
inborn errors of amino acid metabolism in adults and
children from birth

**Valine50®** (Vitaflo)
Powder, valine 50 mg, carbohydrate 3.8 g, fat nil,
energy 63 kJ (15 kcal)/4 g, net price 30 × 4-g
sachets = £48.86
Nutritional supplement for the dietary management of
inborn errors of amino acid metabolism in adults and
children from birth

## Phenylketonuria

**Add-Ins®** (SHS)
Powder, protein equivalent (containing essential and
non-essential amino acids except phenylalanine)
10 g, carbohydrate nil, fat 5.1 g, energy 359 kJ
(86 kcal)/18.2-g sachet, with vitamins, minerals, and
trace elements. Unflavoured, net price 60 × 18.2-g
sachets = £315.60
Nutritional supplement for the dietary management of
proven phenylketonuria in children over 4 years

**Easiphen®** (SHS)
Liquid, protein equivalent (containing essential and
non-essential amino acids except phenylalanine)
6.7 g, carbohydrate 5.1 g, fat 2 g, energy 275 kJ
(65 kcal)/100 mL with vitamins, minerals, and trace
elements. Flavours: forest berries, orange, or
tropical fruit, net price 250-mL carton = £8.11
Nutritional supplement for the dietary management of
proven phenylketonuria in children over 8 years

**Lophlex®** (SHS)
Powder, protein equivalent (essential and non-
essential amino acids except phenylalanine) 20 g,
carbohydrate 2.5 g, fat 60 mg, fibre 220 mg, energy
385 kJ (91 kcal)/27.8-g sachet, with vitamins,
minerals, and trace elements. Flavours: berry,
orange, or unflavoured, net price 30 × 27.8-g
sachets = £243.60
Nutritional supplement for the dietary management of
proven phenylketonuria in children over 8 years and adults
including pregnant women

**Loprofin® PKU Drink** (SHS)
Liquid, protein (cows' milk) 400 mg (phenylalanine
10 mg), lactose 9.4 g, fat 2 g, energy 165 kJ
(40 kcal)/100 mL. Net price 200-mL carton = 61p
Nutritional supplement for the dietary management of
phenylketonuria in children over 1 year

**Loprofin® Sno-Pro** (SHS)
Liquid, protein (cows' milk) 220 mg (phenylalanine
12.5 mg), carbohydrate 8 g, fat 3.8 g, energy 273 kJ
(65 kcal)/100 mL. Contains lactose. Net price
200 mL = £1.05
Nutritional supplement for the dietary management of
phenylketonuria, chronic renal failure and other inborn
errors of amino acid metabolism

**Milupa PKU 2-prima®** (Milupa)
Powder, protein equivalent (essential and non-
essential amino acids except phenylalanine) 60 g,
carbohydrate 10 g, fat nil, energy 1190 kJ (280 kcal)/
100 g, with vitamins, minerals, and trace elements.
Vanilla flavour, net price 500 g = £131.68
Nutritional supplement for the dietary management of
phenylketonuria in children 1–8 years

**Milupa PKU 2-secunda®** (Milupa)
Powder, protein equivalent (essential and non-
essential amino acids except phenylalanine) 70 g,
carbohydrate 6.8 g, fat nil, energy 1306 kJ
(307 kcal)/100 g, with vitamins, minerals, and trace
elements. Vanilla flavour, net price 500 g = £153.62
Nutritional supplement for the dietary management of
phenylketonuria in children 9–15 years

Appendix 2: Borderline substances

**Milupa PKU 3-advanta®** (Milupa)

Powder, protein equivalent (essential and non-essential amino acids except phenylalanine) 70 g, carbohydrate 4.7 g, fat nil, energy 1270 kJ (299 kcal)/100 g, with vitamins, minerals, and trace elements. Vanilla flavour, net price 500 g = £153.62
Nutritional supplement for the dietary management of phenylketonuria in children over 15 years

**Phlexy-10® Exchange System** (SHS)

Capsules, protein equivalent (essential and non-essential amino acids except phenylalanine) 416.5 mg/capsule, net price 200-cap pack = £35.77

Tablets, protein equivalent (essential and non-essential amino acids except phenylalanine) 833 mg tablet, net price 75-tab pack = £23.17

Drink Mix, powder, protein equivalent (essential and non-essential amino acids except phenylalanine) 8.33 g, carbohydrate 8.8 g/20-g sachet. Apple-black currant, citrus, or tropical flavour, net price 30 × 20-g sachet = £107.86
Nutritional supplement for the dietary management of phenylketonuria

**Phlexy-Vits®** (SHS)

Powder, vitamins, minerals, and trace elements, net price 30 × 7-g sachets = £60.00

Tablets, vitamins, minerals, and trace elements, net price 180-tab pack = £68.26
For use as a vitamin and mineral component of restricted therapeutic diets in children over 11 years and adults with phenylketonuria and similar amino acid abnormalities

**PK Aid 4®** (SHS)

Powder, protein equivalent (essential and non-essential amino acids except phenylalanine) 79 g, carbohydrate 4.5 g, fat nil, energy 1420 kJ (334 kcal)/100 g. Unflavoured, (flavouring: see *Modjul®* Flavour System, p. 791), net price 500 g = £120.24 (5-g measuring scoop provided)
Nutritional supplement for the dietary management of phenylketonuria in children and adults

**PKU Anamix® First Spoon** (SHS)

Powder, protein equivalent (essential and non-essential amino acids except phenylalanine) 5 g, carbohydrate 4.8 g, fat 150 mg, fibre nil, energy 168 kJ (41 kcal)/12.5-g sachet, with vitamins, minerals, and trace elements, net price 30 × 12.5 g = £81.00
Nutritional supplement for the dietary management of proven phenylketonuria in children from 6 months to 5 years

**PKU Anamix® Infant** (SHS)

Powder, protein equivalent (essential and non-essential amino acids except phenylalanine) 13.1 g, carbohydrate 49.5 g, fat 23 g, fibre 5.3 g, energy 1915 kJ (457 kcal)/100 g, with vitamins, minerals, and trace elements; *standard dilution* (15%) provides protein equivalent 2 g, carbohydrate 7.4 g, fat 3.5 g, fibre 800 mg, energy 287 kJ (69 kcal)/100 mL. Unflavoured, net price 400 g = £29.72 (5-g measuring scoop provided)
Nutritional supplement for the dietary management of proven phenylketonuria in children from birth to 3 years

**PKU Anamix® Junior** (SHS)

Powder, protein equivalent (essential and non-essential amino acids except phenylalanine) 8.4 g, carbohydrate 9.9 g, fat 3.9 g, energy 455 kJ (108 kcal)/29-g sachet, with vitamins, minerals, and trace elements. Flavours: chocolate, pineapple-vanilla, or unflavoured (carbohydrate 11 g, energy 474 kJ (113 kcal)/29-g sachet), net price 30 × 29-g sachets = £106.20
Nutritional supplement for the dietary management of phenylketonuria in children 1–10 years

**PKU Anamix Junior LQ®** (SHS)

Liquid, protein equivalent (essential and non-essential amino acids except phenylalanine) 10 g, carbohydrate 8.8 g, fat 4.8 g, fibre 310 mg, energy 497 kJ (118 kcal)/125 mL, with vitamins, minerals, and trace elements. Lactose-free. Flavours: Berry, orange, or unflavoured, net price 125-mL carton = £4.72
Nutritional supplement for the dietary supplement of phenyketonuria in children 1–10 years

**PKU cooler10®** (Vitaflo)

Liquid, protein equivalent (essential and non-essential amino acids except phenylalanine) 10 g, carbohydrate 5.1 g, energy 258 kJ (62 kcal)/87-mL pouch, with vitamins, minerals, and trace elements. Unflavoured (white) or flavoured (orange, purple, or red), net price 30 × 87-mL = £112.80
Nutritional supplement for the dietary management of phenylketonuria in children over 3 years

**PKU cooler15®** (Vitaflo)

Liquid, protein equivalent (essential and non-essential amino acids except phenylalanine) 15 g, carbohydrate 7.8 g, energy 386 kJ (92 kcal)/130-mL pouch, with vitamins, minerals, and trace elements. Unflavoured (white) or flavoured (orange, purple, or red), net price 30 x 130 mL = £168.00
Nutritional supplement for the dietary management of phenylketonuria in children over 3 years

**PKU cooler20®** (Vitaflo)

Liquid, protein equivalent (essential and non-essential amino acids except phenylalanine) 20 g, carbohydrate 10.2 g, energy 517 kJ (124 kcal)/174-mL pouch, with vitamins, minerals, and trace elements. Unflavoured (white) or flavoured (orange, purple, or red), net price 30 × 174 mL = £225.60
Nutritional supplement for the dietary management of phenylketonuria in children over 3 years

**PKU express15®** (Vitaflo)

Powder, protein equivalent (essential and non-essential amino acids except phenylalanine) 15 g, carbohydrate 2.4 g, energy 293 kJ (70 kcal)/25 g, with vitamins, minerals, and trace elements. Lemon, orange, tropical, or unflavoured (carbohydrate 3.4 g, energy 310 kJ (74 kcal)/25 g), (flavouring: see *FlavourPac®*, p. 791), net price 30 x 25-g sachets = £164.84
Nutritional supplement for the dietary management of phenylketonuria in children over 3 years

**PKU express20®** (Vitaflo)
Powder, protein equivalent (essential and non-essential amino acids except phenylalanine) 20 g, carbohydrate 3.3 g, energy 389 kJ (93 kcal)/34 g, with vitamins, minerals, and trace elements. Lemon, orange, tropical, or unflavoured (carbohydrate 4.7 g, energy 416 kJ (99 kcal)/34 g), (flavouring: see *FlavourPac®*, p. 791), net price 30 × 34-g sachets = £241.38
Nutritional supplement for the dietary management of phenylketonuria in children over 3 years

**PKU gel®** (Vitaflo)
Powder, protein equivalent (essential and non-essential amino acids except phenylalanine) 10 g, carbohydrate 8.9 g, fat less than 100 mg, energy 318 kJ (76 kcal)/24 g, with vitamins, minerals, and trace elements. Orange, raspberry, or unflavoured (carbohydrate 10.3 g, energy 339 kJ (81 kcal)/24 g), (flavouring: see *FlavourPac®*, p. 791), net price 30 × 24-g sachets = £125.24
For use as part of the low-protein dietary management of phenylketonuria in children 1–10 years

**PKU Lophlex® LQ 10** (SHS)
Liquid, protein equivalent (essential and non-essential amino acids except phenylalanine) 10 g, carbohydrate 4.4 g, fibre 250 mg, energy 245 kJ (58 kcal)/62.5 mL, with vitamins, minerals, and trace elements. Flavours: berry, citrus, orange, or tropical, net price 62.5-mL carton = £4.77; juicy berries, juicy orange (energy 246 kJ (58 kcal)/62.5 mL), 62.5-mL carton = £3.96
Nutritional supplement for the dietary management of phenylketonuria in children over 4 years and adults including pregnant women

**PKU Lophlex® LQ 20** (SHS)
Liquid, protein equivalent (essential and non-essential amino acids except phenylalanine) 20 g, carbohydrate 8.8 g, fibre 340 mg, energy 490 kJ (115 kcal)/125 mL, with vitamins, minerals, and trace elements. Flavours: berry, citrus, orange, or tropical, net price 125-mL carton = £9.53; juicy berries, juicy orange (fibre 500 mg, energy 493 kJ (116 kcal)/125 mL), 125-mL carton = £9.12
Nutritional supplement for the dietary management of phenylketonuria in children over 4 years and adults including pregnant women

**PKU squeezie®** (Vitaflo)
Liquid, protein equivalent (essential and non-essential amino acids except phenylalanine) 10 g, carbohydrate 22.5 g, fat 500 mg, energy 565 kJ (135 kcal)/85 g, with vitamins, minerals, and trace elements. Flavour: apple-banana, net price 30 x 85-g pouch = £119.74
Nutritional supplement for the dietary management of phenylketonuria in children from 6 months to 10 years

**PKU Start®** (Vitaflo)
Liquid, protein equivalent (essential and non-essential amino acids except phenylalanine) 2 g, carbohydrate 8.3 g, fat 2.9 g, energy 286 kJ (68 kcal)/100 mL with vitamins, minerals, and trace elements. Contains lactose and fish oil. Net price 500-mL bottle = £5.58
For the dietary management of phenylketonuria in children under 12 months

**L-Tyrosine** (SHS)
Powder, L-tyrosine 20 g, carbohydrate 76.8 g, fat nil, energy 1612 kJ (379 kcal)/100 g, net price 100 g = £20.20
Nutritional supplement for the dietary management of phenylketonuria in pregnant women with low plasma tyrosine concentrations

**[1]XP Maxamaid** (SHS)
Powder, protein equivalent (essential and non-essential amino acids except phenylalanine) 25 g, carbohydrate 51 g, fat less than 500 mg, energy 1311 kJ (309 kcal)/100 g, with vitamins, minerals, and trace elements. Orange flavour, or unflavoured (flavouring; see *Modjul®* Flavour System, p. 791), net price 500 g = £48.85
Nutritional supplement for the dietary management of phenylketonuria in children 1–8 years

**[2]XP Maxamum®** (SHS)
Powder, protein equivalent (essential and non-essential amino acids except phenylalanine) 39 g, carbohydrate 34 g, fat less than 500 mg, energy 1260 kJ (297 kcal)/100 g, with vitamins, minerals, and trace elements. Orange, or unflavoured (flavouring; see *Modjul®* Flavour System, p. 791), net price 30 × 50-g sachets = £226.50, 500 g = £75.54
Nutritional supplement for the dietary management of phenylketonuria in children over 8 years

## Tyrosinaemia

**Methionine-free TYR Anamix® Infant** (SHS)
Powder, protein equivalent (essential and non-essential amino acids except methionine, phenylalanine, and tyrosine) 13.1 g, carbohydrate 49.5 g, fat 23 g, fibre 5.3 g, energy 1915 kJ (457 kcal)/100 g, with vitamins, minerals, and trace elements; *standard dilution* (15%) provides protein equivalent 2 g, carbohydrate 7.4 g, fat 3.5 g, fibre 800 mg, energy 287 kJ (69 kcal)/100 mL. Unflavoured, net price 400 g = £32.70 (5-g measuring scoop provided)
Nutritional supplement for the dietary management of proven tyrosinaemia type 1 in children from birth to 3 years

**TYR Anamix® Infant** (SHS)
Powder, protein equivalent (essential and non-essential amino acids except phenylalanine and tyrosine) 13.1 g, carbohydrate 49.5 g, fat 23 g, fibre 5.3 g, energy 1915 kJ (457 kcal)/100 g, with vitamins, minerals, and trace elements; *standard dilution* (15%) provides protein equivalent 2 g, carbohydrate 7.4 g, fat 3.5 g, fibre 800 mg, energy 287 kJ (69 kcal)/100 mL. Unflavoured, net price 400 g = £32.70 (5-g measuring scoop provided)
Nutritional supplement for the dietary management of proven tyrosinaemia where plasma-methionine concentrations are normal in children from birth to 3 years

---

1. Maxamaid products are generally intended for use in children 1–8 years
2. Maxamum products are generally intended for use in children over 8 years

**TYR Anamix® Junior** (SHS)

Powder, protein equivalent (essential and non-essential amino acids except phenylalanine and tyrosine) 8.4 g, carbohydrate 11 g, fat 3.9 g, energy 475 kJ (113 kcal)/29-g sachet, with vitamins, minerals, and trace elements. Unflavoured, net price 30 x 29-g sachets = £173.32

Nutritional supplement for the dietary management of proven tyrosinaemia in children 1–10 years

**TYR Anamix® Junior LQ** (SHS)

Liquid, protein equivalent (essential and non-essential amino acids except phenylalanine and tyrosine) 10 g, carbohydrate 8.8 g, fat 4.8 g, fibre 310 mg, energy 500 kJ (119 kcal)/125 mL, with vitamins, minerals and trace elements. Orange flavour, net price 36 x 125-mL bottle = £272.79

Nutritional supplement for the dietary management of tyrosinaemia type 1 (when nitisinone (NTBC) is used, see section 9.8.1), type II, and type III, in children over 1 year

**TYR cooler®** (Vitaflo)

Liquid, protein equivalent (essential and non-essential amino acids except tyrosine and phenylalanine) 15 g, carbohydrate 7 g, fat 500 mg, energy 386 kJ (92 kcal)/130 mL, with vitamins, minerals, and trace elements. Orange or red flavour, net price 30 × 130-mL pouch = £277.20

Nutritional supplement for the dietary management of tyrosinaemia in children over 8 years

**TYR express15®** (Vitaflo)

Powder, protein equivalent (essential and non-essential amino acids except tyrosine and phenylalanine) 15 g, carbohydrate 3.4 g, fat less than 100 mg, energy 310 kJ (74 kcal)/25 g, with vitamins, minerals, and trace elements. Unflavoured (flavouring: see *FlavourPac®*, p. 791), net price 30 × 25-g sachets = £271.88

Nutritional supplement for the dietary management of tyrosinaemia in children over 8 years

**TYR express20®** (Vitaflo)

Powder, protein equivalent (essential and non-essential amino acids except tyrosine and phenylalanine) 20 g, carbohydrate 4.7 g, fat less than 100 mg, energy 416 kJ (99 kcal)/34 g, with vitamins, minerals, and trace elements. Unflavoured (flavouring: see *FlavourPac®*, p. 791), net price 30 × 34-g sachets = £398.15

Nutritional supplement for the dietary management of tyrosinaemia in children over 8 years

**TYR Gel®** (Vitaflo)

Gel, protein equivalent (essential and non-essential amino acids except tyrosine and phenylalanine) 10 g, carbohydrate 10.3 g, fat less than 100 mg, energy 339 kJ (81 kcal)/24 g, with vitamins, minerals and trace elements. Unflavoured (flavouring: see *FlavourPac®*, p. 791), net price 30 × 24-g sachets = £194.51

Nutritional supplement for the dietary management of tyrosinaemia in children 1–10 years

**TYR Lophlex® LQ 20** (Nutricia Clinical)

Liquid, protein equivalent (essential and non-essential amino acids except phenylalanine and tyrosine) 20 g, carbohydrate 8.8 g, fat less than 500 mg, fibre 500 mg, energy 509 kJ (120 kcal)/125 mL, with vitamins, minerals, and trace elements. Juicy berries flavour, net price 125 mL = £14.80

Nutritional supplement for the dietary management of tyrosinaemia in children over 3 years

**[1]XPHEN TYR Maxamaid** (SHS)

Powder, protein equivalent (essential and non-essential amino acids except phenylalanine and tyrosine) 25 g, carbohydrate 51 g, fat less than 500 mg, energy 1311 kJ (309 kcal)/100 g, with vitamins, minerals, and trace elements. Unflavoured (flavouring: see *Modjul®* Flavour System, p. 791), net price 500 g = £82.57

Nutritional supplement for the dietary management of tyrosinaemia in children 1–8 years

**XPHEN TYR Tyrosidon** (SHS)

Powder, protein equivalent (essential and non-essential amino acids except phenylalanine and tyrosine) 77 g, carbohydrate 4.5 g, fat nil, energy 1386 kJ (326 kcal)/100 g. Unflavoured (flavouring: see *Modjul®* Flavour System, p. 791), net price 500 g = £156.42

Nutritional supplement for the management of tyrosinaemia in children and adults where plasma-methionine concentrations are normal

**XPTM Tyrosidon** (SHS)

Powder, protein equivalent (essential and non-essential amino acids except methionine, phenylalanine, and tyrosine) 77 g, carbohydrate 4.5 g, fat nil, energy 1386 kJ (326 kcal)/100 g. Unflavoured (flavouring: see *Modjul®* Flavour System, p. 791), net price 500 g = £156.42

Nutritional supplement for the dietary management of tyrosinaemia type I in children and adults where plasma-methionine concentrations are above normal

## Conditions for which ACBS products can be prescribed

**Note** This is a list of clinical conditions for which the ACBS has approved toilet preparations. For details of the preparations see Chapter 13.

### Birthmarks

See Disfiguring skin lesions, below

### Dermatitis

*Aveeno®* Bath Oil; *Aveeno®* Cream; *Aveeno®* lotion; *E45®* Emollient Bath Oil; *E45®* Emollient Wash Cream; *E45®* Lotion

### Dermatitis herpetiformis

See also Gluten-sensitive enteropathies, p. 791

### Disfiguring skin lesions (birthmarks, mutilating lesions, scars, vitiligo)

*Covermark®* classic foundation and finishing powder; *Dermablend®* Ultra corrective foundation; *Dermacolor®* Camouflage cream and fixing powder; *Keromask®* masking cream and finishing powder; *Veil®* Cover cream and Finishing Powder. (Cleansing Creams, Cleansing Milks, and Cleansing Lotions are excluded)

---

1. Maxamaid products are generally intended for use in children 1–8 years

### Disinfectants (antiseptics)

May be prescribed on an FP10 only when ordered in such quantities and with such directions as are appropriate for the treatment of patients, but not for general hygenic purposes

### Dry mouth (xerostomia)

For patients suffering from dry mouth as a result of having (or having undergone) radiotherapy, or sicca syndrome.

*AS Saliva Orthana®*; *Biotène Oralbalance®*; *BioXtra®*; *Glandosane®*; *Saliveze®*; *Salivix®*

For details of preparations see section 12.3.5, p. 550

### Eczema

See Dermatitis, above

### Photodermatoses (skin protection in)

*Anthelios®* XL SPF 50+ Melt-in cream; *Sunsense®* Ultra; *Uvistat®* Lipscreen SPF 50, *Uvistat®* Suncream SPF 30 and 50

For details of preparations see section 13.8.1, p. 584

### Pruritus

See Dermatitis, above

# A3 Cautionary and advisory labels for dispensed medicines

Preparations in the *BNF for Children* include code numbers of the cautionary labels that pharmacists are recommended to add when dispensing. It is also expected that, when necessary, pharmacists will counsel children or their carers.

Counselling needs to be related to the age, experience, background, and understanding of the child or carer. The pharmacist should ensure understanding of how to take or use the medicine and how to follow the correct dosage schedule. Any effects of the medicine on co-ordination, performance of skilled tasks, any foods or medicines to be avoided, and what to do if a dose is missed should also be explained. Other matters, such as the possibility of staining of the clothes or skin, or discoloration of urine or stools by a medicine should also be mentioned.

For some preparations there is a special need for counselling, such as an unusual method or time of administration or a potential interaction with a common food or domestic remedy, and this should be mentioned where necessary.

**Original packs** Most preparations are now dispensed in unbroken original packs that include further advice for the patient in the form of patient information leaflets. The advice in patient information leaflets may be less appropriate when the medicine is for a child, particularly for unlicensed medicines or indications. Pharmacists should explain discrepancies to carers, if necessary. The patient information leaflet should only be withheld in exceptional circumstances because it contains other information that should be provided. Label 10 may be of value where appropriate. More general leaflets advising on the administration of preparations such as eye drops, eye ointments, inhalers, and suppositories are also available.

**Scope of labels** In general, no label recommendations are provided for injections on the assumption that they will be administered by a healthcare professional or a well-instructed child or carer. The labelling is not exhaustive and pharmacists are recommended to use their professional discretion in labelling new preparations and those for which no labels are shown.

Individual labelling advice is not given on the administration of the large variety of antacids. In the absence of instructions from the prescriber, and if on enquiry the patient has had no verbal instructions, the directions given under 'Dose' should be used on the label.

It is recognised that there may be occasions when pharmacists will use their knowledge and professional discretion and decide to omit one or more of the recommended labels for a particular child. In this case counselling is of the utmost importance. There may also be an occasion when a prescriber does not wish additional cautionary labels to be used, in which case the prescription should be endorsed 'NCL' (no cautionary labels). The exact wording that is required instead should then be specified on the prescription.

Pharmacists label medicines with various wordings in addition to those directions specified on the prescription. Such labels include 'Shake the bottle', 'For external use only', and 'Store in a cool place', as well as 'Discard . . . . days after opening' and 'Do not use after . . . .', which apply particularly to antibiotic mixtures, diluted liquid and topical preparations, and to eye-drops. Although not listed in the *BNF for Children* these labels should continue to be used when appropriate; indeed, 'For external use only' is a legal requirement on external liquid preparations, while 'Keep out of the reach of children' is a legal requirement on all dispensed medicines. Care should be taken not to obscure other relevant information with adhesive labelling.

It is the usual practice for patients to take standard tablets with water or other liquid and for this reason no separate label has been recommended.

The label wordings recommended by the *BNF for Children* apply to medicines dispensed against a prescription. Children and carers should be made aware that a dispensed medicine should never be taken by, or shared with, anyone other than for whom the prescriber intended it. Therefore, the *BNF for Children* does not include warnings against the use of a dispensed medicine by persons other than for whom it was specifically prescribed.

The label or labels for each preparation are recommended after careful consideration of the information available. However, it is recognised that in some cases this information may be either incomplete or open to a different interpretation. The *BNF for Children* will therefore be grateful to receive any constructive comments on the labelling suggested for any preparation.

## Recommended label wordings

For *BNF for Children* 2011–2012, a revised set of cautionary and advisory labels has been introduced. All of the existing labels have been user-tested, and the revised wording selected reflects terminology that is better understood by patients.

Wordings which can be given as separate warnings are labels 1–19, 29–30, and 32. Wordings which can be incorporated in an appropriate position in the directions for dosage or administration are labels 21–28. A label has been omitted for number 20; labels 31 and 33 no longer apply to any medicines in the *BNF for children* and have therefore been deleted.

If separate labels are used it is recommended that the wordings be used without modification. If changes are made to suit computer requirements, care should be taken to retain the sense of the original.

**1      Warning: This medicine may make you sleepy**

To be used on *preparations for children* containing antihistamines, or other preparations given to children where the warnings of label 2 on driving or alcohol would not be appropriate.

**2      Warning: This medicine may make you sleepy. If this happens, do not drive or use tools or machines. Do not drink alcohol**

To be used on *preparations for adults that can cause drowsiness*, thereby affecting the ability to drive and operate hazardous machinery; label 1 is more appropriate for children. *It is an offence to drive while under the influence of drink or drugs.*

Some of these preparations only cause drowsiness in the first few days of treatment and some only cause drowsiness in higher doses.

In such cases the patient should be told that the advice applies until the effects have worn off. However many of these preparations can produce a slowing of reaction time and a loss of mental concentration that can have the same effects as drowsiness.

Avoidance of alcoholic drink is recommended because the effects of CNS depressants are enhanced by alcohol. Strict prohibition however could lead to some patients not taking the medicine. Pharmacists should therefore explain the risk and encourage compliance, particularly in patients who may think they already tolerate the effects of alcohol (see also label 3). Queries from patients with epilepsy regarding fitness to drive should be referred back to the patient's doctor.

Side-effects unrelated to drowsiness that may affect a patient's ability to drive or operate machinery safely include *blurred vision, dizziness, or nausea*. In general, no label has been recommended to cover these cases, but the patient should be suitably counselled.

**3      Warning: This medicine may make you sleepy. If this happens, do not drive or use tools or machines**

To be used on *preparations containing monoamine-oxidase inhibitors*; the warning to avoid alcohol and dealcoholised (low alcohol) drink is covered by the patient information leaflet.

Also to be used as for label 2 but where alcohol is not an issue.

**4      Warning: Do not drink alcohol**

To be used on *preparations where a reaction such as flushing may occur if alcohol is taken* (e.g. metronidazole). Alcohol may also enhance the hypoglycaemia produced by some oral antidiabetic drugs but routine application of a warning label is not considered necessary.

Patients should be advised not to drink alcohol for as long as they are receiving/using a course of medication, and in some cases for a period of time after the course is finished.

**5      Do not take indigestion remedies 2 hours before or after you take this medicine**

To be used with label 25 on *preparations coated to resist gastric acid* (e.g. enteric-coated tablets). This is to avoid the possibility of premature dissolution of the coating in the presence of an alkaline pH.

Label 5 also applies to drugs such as ketoconazole *where the absorption is significantly affected by antacids.*

Pharmacists will be aware (from a knowledge of physiology) that the usual time during which indigestion remedies should be avoided is at least 2 hours before and after the majority of medicines have been taken; where a manufacturer advises a different time period, this can be followed, and should be explained to the patient.

**6      Do not take indigestion remedies, or medicines containing iron or zinc, 2 hours before or after you take this medicine**

To be used on *preparations containing ofloxacin and some other quinolones, doxycycline, lymecycline, minocycline, and penicillamine*. These drugs chelate calcium, iron, and zinc and are less well absorbed when taken with calcium-containing antacids or preparations containing iron or zinc. Pharmacists will be aware (from a knowledge of physiology) that these incompatible preparations should

be taken at least 2 hours apart for the majority of medicines; where a manufacturer advises a different time period, this can be followed, and should be explained to the patient.

**7      Do not take milk, indigestion remedies, or medicines containing iron or zinc, 2 hours before or after you take this medicine**

To be used on *preparations containing ciprofloxacin, norfloxacin, or tetracyclines that chelate calcium, iron, magnesium, and zinc*, and are thus less available for absorption. Pharmacists will be aware (from a knowledge of physiology) that these incompatible preparations should be taken at least 2 hours apart for the majority of medicines; where a manufacturer advises a different time period, this can be followed, and should be explained to the patient. Doxycycline, lymecycline, and minocycline are less liable to form chelates and therefore only require label 6 (see above).

**8      Warning: Do not stop taking this medicine unless your doctor tells you to stop**

To be used on *preparations that contain a drug which is required to be taken over long periods without the patient necessarily perceiving any benefit* (e.g. antituberculous drugs).

Also to be used on *preparations that contain a drug whose withdrawal is likely to be a particular hazard* (e.g. clonidine for hypertension). Label 10 (see below) is more appropriate for corticosteroids.

**9      Space the doses evenly throughout the day. Keep taking this medicine until the course is finished, unless you are told to stop**

To be used on *preparations where a course of treatment should be completed* to reduce the incidence of relapse or failure of treatment.

The preparations are antimicrobial drugs given by mouth. Very occasionally, some may have severe side-effects (e.g. diarrhoea in patients receiving clindamycin) and in such cases the patient may need to be advised of reasons for stopping treatment quickly and returning to the doctor.

**10     Warning: Read the additional information given with this medicine**

To be used particularly on *preparations containing anticoagulants, lithium, and oral corticosteroids*. The appropriate treatment card should be given to the patient and any necessary explanations given.

This label may also be used on other preparations to remind the patient of the instructions that have been given.

**11     Protect your skin from sunlight—even on a bright but cloudy day. Do not use sunbeds**

To be used on *preparations that may cause phototoxic or photoallergic reactions* if the patient is exposed to ultraviolet radiation. Many drugs other than those listed (e.g. phenothiazines and sulfonamides) may on rare occasions cause reactions in susceptible patients. Exposure to high intensity ultraviolet radiation from sunray lamps and sunbeds is particularly likely to cause reactions.

**12     Do not take anything containing aspirin while taking this medicine**

To be used on *preparations containing probenecid and sulfinpyrazone* whose activity is reduced by aspirin. Label 12 should not be used for anticoagulants since label 10 is more appropriate.

**13     Dissolve or mix with water before taking**

To be used on *preparations that are intended to be dissolved in water* (e.g. soluble tablets) or *mixed with water* (e.g. powders, granules) before use. In a few cases other liquids such as fruit juice or milk may be used.

**14     This medicine may colour your urine. This is harmless**

To be used on *preparations that may cause the patient's urine to turn an unusual colour*. These include triamterene (blue under some lights), levodopa (dark reddish), and rifampicin (red).

**15     Caution: flammable. Keep your body away from fire or flames after you have put on the medicine**

To be used on *preparations containing sufficient flammable solvent to render them flammable if exposed to a naked flame.*

16 **Dissolve the tablet under your tongue—do not swallow. Store the tablets in this bottle with the cap tightly closed. Get a new supply 8 weeks after opening**

To be used on *glyceryl trinitrate tablets* to remind the patient not to transfer the tablets to plastic or less suitable containers.

17 **Do not take more than . . . in 24 hours**

To be used on *preparations for the treatment of acute migraine* except those containing ergotamine, for which label 18 is used. The dose form should be specified, e.g. tablets or capsules.

It may also be used on preparations for which no dose has been specified by the prescriber.

18 **Do not take more than . . . in 24 hours. Also, do not take more than . . . in any one week**

To be used on preparations containing ergotamine. The dose form should be specified, e.g. tablets or suppositories.

19 **Warning: This medicine makes you sleepy. If you still feel sleepy the next day, do not drive or use tools or machines. Do not drink alcohol**

To be used on *preparations containing hypnotics (or some other drugs with sedative effects) prescribed to be taken at night*. On the rare occasions (e.g. nitrazepam in epilepsy) when hypnotics are prescribed for daytime administration this label would clearly not be appropriate. Also to be used as an *alternative to the label 2 wording* (the choice being at the discretion of the pharmacist) *for anxiolytics prescribed to be taken at night*.

It is hoped that this wording will convey adequately the problem of residual morning sedation after taking 'sleeping tablets'.

21 **Take with or just after food, or a meal**

To be used on *preparations that are liable to cause gastric irritation, or those that are better absorbed with food*. Patients should be advised that a *small amount of food is sufficient*.

22 **Take 30 to 60 minutes before food**

To be used on some preparations *whose absorption is thereby improved*.

Most oral antibacterials require label 23 instead (see below).

23 **Take this medicine when your stomach is empty. This means an hour before food or 2 hours after food**

To be used on *oral antibacterials whose absorption may be reduced by the presence of food and acid in the stomach*.

24 **Suck or chew this medicine**

To be used on *preparations that should be sucked or chewed*. The pharmacist should use discretion as to which of these words is appropriate.

25 **Swallow this medicine whole. Do not chew or crush**

To be used on *preparations that are enteric-coated or designed for modified-release*.

Also to be used on *preparations that taste very unpleasant or may damage the mouth* if not swallowed whole.

Patients should be advised (where relevant) that some modified-release preparations can be broken in half, but that the halved tablet should still be swallowed whole, and not chewed or crushed.

26 **Dissolve this medicine under your tongue**

To be used on *preparations designed for sublingual use*. Patients should be advised to hold under the tongue and avoid swallowing until dissolved. The buccal mucosa between the gum and cheek is occasionally specified by the prescriber.

27 **Take with a full glass of water**

To be used on *preparations that should be well diluted* (e.g. chloral hydrate), *where a high fluid intake is required* (e.g. sulfonamides), or *where water is required to aid the action* (e.g. methylcellulose). The patient should be advised that 'a full glass' means at least 150 mL. In most cases fruit juice, tea, or coffee may be used.

28 **Spread thinly on the affected skin only**

To be used on *external preparations* that should be applied sparingly (e.g. corticosteroids, dithranol).

29 **Do not take more than 2 at any one time. Do not take more than 8 in 24 hours**

To be used on containers of dispensed *solid dose preparations containing paracetamol for adults when the instruction on the label indicates that the dose can be taken on an 'as required' basis*. The dose form should be specified, e.g. tablets or capsules.

This label has been introduced because of the serious consequences of overdosage with paracetamol.

30 **Contains paracetamol. Do not take anything else containing paracetamol while taking this medicine. Talk to a doctor at once if you take too much of this medicine, even if you feel well**

To be used on all containers of dispensed *preparations containing paracetamol*.

32 **Contains aspirin. Do not take anything else containing aspirin while taking this medicine**

To be used on containers of dispensed *preparations containing aspirin when the name on the label does not include the word 'aspirin'*.

# A4 Intravenous infusions for neonatal intensive care

**Intravenous policy** A local policy on the dilution of drugs with intravenous fluids should be drawn up by a multi-disciplinary team and issued as a document to the members of staff concerned.

Centralised additive services are provided in a number of hospital pharmacy departments and should be used in preference to making additions on wards.

The information that follows should be read in conjunction with local policy documents.

## Guidelines

1. Drugs should only be diluted with infusion fluid when constant plasma concentrations are needed or when the administration of a more concentrated solution would be harmful.

2. In general, only one drug should be mixed with an infusion fluid in a syringe and the components should be compatible. Ready-prepared solutions should be used whenever possible. Drugs should not normally be added to blood products, mannitol, or sodium bicarbonate. Only specially formulated additives should be used with fat emulsions or amino-acid solutions (section 9.3).

3. Solutions should be thoroughly mixed by shaking and checked for absence of particulate matter before use.

4. Strict asepsis should be maintained throughout and in general the giving set should not be used for more than 24 hours (for drug admixtures).

5. The infusion syringe should be labelled with the neonate's name and hospital number, the name and quantity of drug, the infusion fluid, and the expiry date and time. If a problem occurs during administration, containers should be retained for a period after use in case they are needed for investigation.

6. Administration using a suitable motorised syringe driver is advocated for preparations where strict control over administration is required.

7. It is good practice to examine intravenous infusions from time to time while they are running. If cloudiness, crystallisation, change of colour, or any other sign of interaction or contamination is observed the infusion should be discontinued.

## Problems

**Microbial contamination** The accidental entry and subsequent growth of micro-organisms converts the infusion fluid pathway into a potential vehicle for infection with micro-organisms, particularly species of Candida, Enterobacter, and Klebsiella. Ready-prepared infusions containing the additional drugs, or infusions prepared by an additive service (when available) should therefore be used in preference to making extemporaneous additions to infusion containers on wards etc. However, when this is necessary strict aseptic procedure should be followed.

**Incompatibility** Physical and chemical incompatibilities may occur with loss of potency, increase in toxicity, or other adverse effect. The solutions may become opalescent or precipitation may occur, but in many instances there is no visual indication of incompatibility. Interaction may take place at any point in the infusion fluid pathway, and the potential for incompatibility is increased when more than one substance is added to the infusion fluid.

**Common incompatibilities** Precipitation reactions are numerous and varied and may occur as a result of pH, concentration changes, 'salting-out' effects, complexation or other chemical changes. Precipitation or other particle formation must be avoided since, apart from lack of control of dosage on administration, it may initiate or exacerbate adverse effects. This is particularly important in the case of drugs which have been implicated in either thrombophlebitis (e.g. diazepam) or in skin sloughing or necrosis caused by extravasation (e.g. sodium bicarbonate and parenteral nutrition). It is also especially important to effect solution of colloidal drugs and to prevent their subsequent precipitation in order to avoid a pyrogenic reaction (e.g. amphotericin).

It is considered undesirable to mix beta-lactam antibiotics, such as semi-synthetic penicillins and cephalosporins, with proteinaceous materials on the grounds that immunogenic and allergenic conjugates could be formed.

A number of preparations undergo significant loss of potency when added singly or in combination to large volume infusions. Examples include ampicillin in infusions that contain glucose or lactates.

**Blood** Because of the large number of incompatibilities, drugs should not be added to blood and blood products for infusion purposes. Examples of incompatibility with blood include hypertonic mannitol solutions (irreversible crenation of red cells), dextrans (rouleaux formation and interference with cross-matching), glucose (clumping of red cells), and oxytocin (inactivated).

If the giving set is not changed after the administration of blood, but used for other infusion fluids, a fibrin clot may form which, apart from blocking the set, increases the likelihood of microbial growth.

**Intravenous fat emulsions** These may break down with coalescence of fat globules and separation of phases when additions such as antibacterials or electrolytes are made, thus increasing the possibility of embolism. Only specially formulated products such as *Vitlipid N®* (section 9.3) may be added to appropriate intravenous fat emulsions.

**Other infusions** Infusions that frequently give rise to incompatibility include amino acids, mannitol, and sodium bicarbonate.

## Method

Ready-prepared infusions should be used whenever available. When dilution of drugs is required to be made extemporaneously, any product reconstitution instructions such as those relating to concentration, vehicle, mixing, and handling precautions should be strictly followed using an aseptic technique throughout. Once the product has been reconstituted, further dilution with the infusion fluid should be made immediately in order to minimise microbial contamination and, with certain products, to prevent degradation or other formulation change which may occur; e.g. reconstituted ampicillin injection degrades rapidly on standing, and also may form polymers which could cause sensitivity reactions.

It is also important in certain instances that an infusion fluid of specific pH be used (e.g. **furosemide** injection requires dilution in infusions of pH greater than 5.5).

When drug dilutions are made it is important to mix thoroughly; additions should not be made to an infusion container that has been connected to a giving set, as mixing is hampered. If the solutions are not thoroughly mixed, a concentrated layer of the drug may form owing to differences in density. **Potassium chloride** is particularly prone to this 'layering' effect when added without adequate mixing to infusions; if such a mixture is administered it may have a serious effect on the heart.

A time limit between dilution and completion of administration must be imposed for certain admixtures to guarantee satisfactory drug potency and compatibility. For admixtures in which degradation occurs without the formation of toxic substances, an acceptable limit is the time taken for 10% decomposition of the drug. When toxic substances are produced stricter limits may be imposed. Because of the risk of microbial contamination a maximum time limit of 24 hours may be appropriate for additions made elsewhere than in hospital pharmacies offering central additive service.

Certain injections must be protected from light during continuous infusion to minimise oxidation, e.g. sodium nitroprusside.

## Table of drugs given by continuous intravenous infusion to neonates

The table lists key drugs given by continuous intravenous infusion to neonates.

> Covers dilution with *Glucose intravenous infusion* 5% and 10% and *Sodium chloride intravenous infusion* 0.9%. Compatibility with glucose 5% and with sodium chloride 0.9% indicates compatibility with *Sodium chloride and glucose intravenous infusion*. Infusion of a large volume of hypotonic solution should be avoided, therefore care should be taken if water for injections is used.

### Adrenaline/Epinephrine (p. 112)

Dilute 3 mg/kg body-weight to a final volume of 50 mL with Glucose 5% *or* Sodium Chloride 0.9%; an intravenous infusion rate of 0.1 mL/hour provides a dose of 100 nanograms/kg/minute; infuse through a central venous catheter. Incompatible with bicarbonate and alkaline solutions.
**Note** Usually made up with adrenaline 1 in 1000 (1 mg/mL) solution; this concentration of adrenaline is not licensed for intravenous administration

### Alprostadil (*Prostin VR®*) (p. 130)

Dilute 150 micrograms/kg body-weight to a final volume of 50 mL with Glucose 5% *or* Sodium Chloride 0.9%; an intravenous infusion rate of 0.1 mL/hour provides a dose of 5 nanograms/kg/minute. Undiluted solution must not come into contact with the barrel of the plastic syringe; add the required volume of alprostadil to a volume of infusion fluid in the syringe, and then make up to final volume

### Atracurium besilate (p. 643)

Dilute 60 mg/kg body-weight to a final volume of 50 mL with Glucose 5% *or* Sodium Chloride 0.9%; an intravenous infusion rate of 0.1 mL/hour provides a dose of 120 micrograms/kg/hour; minimum concentration of 500 micrograms/mL, max. concentration of 5 mg/mL

### Dobutamine (as hydrochloride) (p. 109)

Dilute 30 mg/kg body-weight to a final volume of 50 mL with Glucose 5% *or* Sodium Chloride 0.9%; an intravenous infusion rate of 0.5 mL/hour provides a dose of 5 micrograms/kg/minute; max. concentration of 5 mg/mL; infuse higher concentration solutions through central venous catheter only. Incompatible with bicarbonate and other strong alkaline solutions

> Intravenous infusion information for neonatal intensive care *only*; for information in other children, see individual drug monographs.

### Dopamine hydrochloride (p. 110)

Dilute 30 mg/kg body-weight to a final volume of 50 mL with Glucose 5% *or* Sodium Chloride 0.9%; an intravenous infusion rate of 0.3 mL/hour provides a dose of 3 micrograms/kg/minute; max. concentration of 3.2 mg/mL; infuse higher concentration solutions through central venous catheter. Incompatible with bicarbonate and other alkaline solutions

### Epoprostenol (*Flolan®*) (p. 95)

Reconstitute the 500-microgram vial using the glycine buffer diluent provided to make a 10 micrograms/mL concentrate (pH 10.5); filter the concentrate using the filter provided; the concentrate can be administered via a central venous catheter, or it may be diluted further.
*Neonate body-weight under 2 kg*, using the concentrate, dilute 150 micrograms/kg body-weight to a final volume of 50 mL with Sodium Chloride 0.9%; an intravenous infusion rate of 0.1 mL/hour provides a dose of 5 nanograms/kg/minute.
*Neonate body-weight over 2 kg*, using the concentrate, dilute 60 micrograms/kg body-weight to a final volume of 50 mL with Sodium Chloride 0.9%; an intravenous infusion rate of 0.1 mL/hour provides a dose of 2 nanograms/kg/minute.
**Note** Diluted solution stable for 12 hours at room temperature, although some units use for 24 hours and allow for loss of potency. Minimum concentration of 1.43 micrograms/mL

### Glyceryl trinitrate (p. 103)

Dilute 3 mg/kg body-weight to a final volume of 50 mL with Glucose 5% *or* Sodium Chloride 0.9%; an intravenous infusion rate of 1 mL/hour provides a dose of 1 microgram/kg/minute; max. concentration of 400 micrograms/mL (but concentration of 1 mg/mL has been used via a central venous catheter).

**Note** Glass or polyethylene apparatus is preferable; loss of potency will occur if PVC is used

### Heparin (as sodium) (p. 113)

*Maintenance of umbilical arterial catheter*, dilute 50 units to a final volume of 50 mL with Sodium Chloride 0.45% *or* use ready-made bag containing 500 units in 500 mL Sodium Chloride 0.9%; infuse at 0.5 mL/hour.

*Treatment of thrombosis*, dilute 1250 units/kg body-weight to a final volume of 50 mL with Glucose 5% *or* Sodium Chloride 0.9%; an intravenous infusion rate of 1 mL/hour provides a dose of 25 units/kg/hour

### Insulin (soluble) (p. 353)

Dilute 5 units to a final volume of 50 mL with Sodium Chloride 0.9% and mix thoroughly; an intravenous infusion rate of 0.1 mL/kg/hour provides a dose of 0.01 units/kg/hour.

**Note** Insulin may be absorbed by plastics, flush giving set with 5 mL of infusion fluid containing insulin

### Midazolam (p. 236 and p. 638)

Dilute 15 mg/kg body-weight to a final volume of 50 mL with Glucose 5% *or* Sodium Chloride 0.9%; an intravenous infusion rate of 0.1 mL/hour provides a dose of 30 micrograms/kg/hour

Intravenous infusion information for neonatal intensive care *only*; for information in other children, see individual drug monographs.

### Morphine sulfate (p. 208)

Dilute 2.5 mg/kg body-weight to a final volume of 50 mL with Glucose 5% *or* 10% *or* Sodium Chloride 0.9%; an intravenous infusion rate of 0.1 mL/hour provides a dose of 5 micrograms/kg/hour

### Noradrenaline/Norepinephrine (p. 111)

Dilute 600 micrograms (base)/kg body-weight to a final volume of 50 mL with Glucose 5% *or* Sodium Chloride and Glucose; an intravenous infusion rate of 0.1 mL/hour provides a dose of 20 nanograms (base)/kg/minute; infuse through central venous catheter; max. concentration of noradrenaline (base) 40 micrograms/mL (higher concentrations can be used if fluid restricted). Discard if discoloured. Incompatible with bicarbonate or alkaline solutions.

**Note** 500 micrograms of noradrenaline base is equivalent to 1 mg of acid tartrate. Dose expressed as the base

### Vecuronium (p. 645)

Reconstitute each vial with 5 mL Water for Injections to give a 2 mg/mL solution. Dilute 5 mg/kg body-weight to a final volume of 50 mL with Glucose 5% or Sodium Chloride 0.9%; an intravenous infusion rate of 0.5 mL/hour provides a dose of 50 micrograms/kg/hour; minimum concentration of 40 micrograms/mL

Appendix 4: Intravenous infusions for neonatal intensive care

# Dental Practitioners' Formulary

## List of Dental Preparations

The following list has been approved by the appropriate Secretaries of State, and the preparations therein may be prescribed by dental practitioners on form FP10D (GP14 in Scotland, WP10D in Wales).

Licensed **sugar-free** versions, where available, are preferred.

Licensed **alcohol-free** mouthwashes, where available, are preferred.

Aciclovir Cream, BP
Aciclovir Oral Suspension, BP, 200 mg/5 mL
Aciclovir Tablets, BP, 200 mg
Aciclovir Tablets, BP, 800 mg
Amoxicillin Capsules, BP
Amoxicillin Oral Powder, DPF
Amoxicillin Oral Suspension, BP
Ampicillin Capsules, BP
Ampicillin Oral Suspension, BP
Artificial Saliva Gel, DPF
Artificial Saliva Oral Spray, DPF
[1]Artificial Saliva Substitutes as listed below (to be prescribed only for indications approved by ACBS):
    AS Saliva Orthana®
    Glandosane®
    BioXtra® Gel Mouthspray
    BioXtra® Moisturising Gel
    Saliveze®
    Salivix®
[2]Aspirin Tablets, Dispersible, BP
Azithromycin Capsules, 250 mg, DPF
Azithromycin Oral Suspension, 200 mg/5 mL, DPF
Azithromycin Tablets, 250 mg, DPF
Azithromycin Tablets, 500 mg, DPF
Beclometasone Pressurised Inhalation, BP, 50 micrograms/metered inhalation, CFC-free, as:
    Clenil Modulite®
Benzydamine Mouthwash, BP 0.15%
Benzydamine Oromucosal Spray, BP 0.15%
Betamethasone Soluble Tablets, 500 micrograms, DPF
Carbamazepine Tablets, BP
Cefalexin Capsules, BP
Cefalexin Oral Suspension, BP
Cefalexin Tablets, BP
Cefradine Capsules, BP
Cetirizine Oral Solution, BP, 5 mg/5 mL
Cetirizine Tablets, BP, 10 mg
Chlorhexidine Gluconate Gel, BP
Chlorhexidine Mouthwash, BP
Chlorhexidine Oral Spray, DPF
Chlorphenamine Oral Solution, BP
Chlorphenamine Tablets, BP
Choline Salicylate Dental Gel, BP
Clarithromycin Oral Suspension, 125 mg/5 mL, DPF
Clarithromycin Oral Suspension, 250 mg/5 mL, DPF
Clarithromycin Tablets, BP

Clindamycin Capsules, BP
Co-amoxiclav Tablets, BP, 250/125 (amoxicillin 250 mg as trihydrate, clavulanic acid 125 mg as potassium salt)
Co-amoxiclav Oral Suspension, BP, 125/31 (amoxicillin 125 mg as trihydrate, clavulanic acid 31.25 mg as potassium salt)/5 mL
Co-amoxiclav Oral Suspension, BP, 250/62 (amoxicillin 250 mg as trihydrate, clavulanic acid 62.5 mg as potassium salt)/5 mL
Diazepam Oral Solution, BP, 2 mg/5 mL
Diazepam Tablets, BP
Diclofenac Sodium Tablets, Gastro-resistant, BP
Dihydrocodeine Tablets, BP, 30 mg
Doxycycline Tablets, Dispersible, BP
Doxycycline Capsules, BP, 100 mg
Doxycycline Tablets, 20 mg, DPF
Ephedrine Nasal Drops, BP
Erythromycin Ethyl Succinate Oral Suspension, BP
Erythromycin Ethyl Succinate Tablets, BP
Erythromycin Stearate Tablets, BP
Erythromycin Tablets, Gastro-resistant, BP
Fluconazole Capsules, 50 mg, DPF
Fluconazole Oral Suspension, 50 mg/5 mL, DPF
Hydrocortisone Cream, BP, 1%
Hydrocortisone Oromucosal Tablets, BP
Hydrogen Peroxide Mouthwash, BP, 6%
Ibuprofen Oral Suspension, BP, sugar-free
Ibuprofen Tablets, BP
Lansoprazole Capsules, Gastro-resistant, BP
Lidocaine Ointment, BP, 5%
Lidocaine Spray 10%, BP
Loratadine Syrup, 5 mg/5 mL, DPF
Loratadine Tablets, BP, 10 mg
[3]Menthol and Eucalyptus Inhalation, BP 1980
Metronidazole Oral Suspension, BP
Metronidazole Tablets, BP
Miconazole Cream, BP
Miconazole Oromucosal Gel, BP
Miconazole and Hydrocortisone Cream, BP
Miconazole and Hydrocortisone Ointment, BP
Mouthwash Solution-tablets, DPF
Nystatin Oral Suspension, BP
Omeprazole Capsules, Gastro-resistant, BP
Oxytetracycline Tablets, BP
[4]Paracetamol Oral Suspension, BP
Paracetamol Tablets, BP
Paracetamol Tablets, Soluble, BP
Penciclovir Cream, DPF
Phenoxymethylpenicillin Oral Solution, BP
Phenoxymethylpenicillin Tablets, BP
Promethazine Hydrochloride Tablets, BP
Promethazine Oral Solution, BP
Saliva Stimulating Tablets, DPF
Sodium Chloride Mouthwash, Compound, BP
Sodium Fluoride Mouthwash, BP

---

1. Indications approved by the ACBS are: patients suffering from dry mouth as a result of having (or having undergone) radiotherapy or sicca syndrome
2. The BP directs that when soluble aspirin tablets are prescribed, dispersible aspirin tablets should be dispensed

3. This preparation does not appear in subsequent editions of the BP
4. The BP directs that when Paediatric Paracetamol Oral Suspension or Paediatric Paracetamol Mixture is prescribed and no strength stated Paracetamol Oral Suspension 120 mg/5 mL should be dispensed

Sodium Fluoride Oral Drops, BP
Sodium Fluoride Tablets, BP
Sodium Fluoride Toothpaste 0.619%, DPF
Sodium Fluoride Toothpaste 1.1%, DPF
Sodium Fusidate Ointment, BP
Temazepam Oral Solution, BP
Temazepam Tablets, BP
Tetracycline Tablets, BP

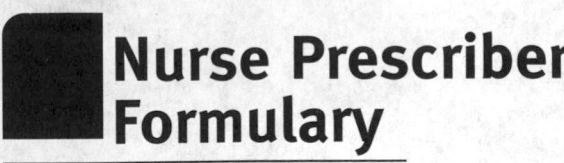

# Nurse Prescribers' Formulary

## Nurse Prescribers' Formulary for Community Practitioners

**Nurse Prescribers' Formulary Appendix** (Appendix NPF). List of preparations approved by the Secretary of State which may be prescribed on form FP10P (form HS21(N) in Northern Ireland, form GP10(N) in Scotland, forms FP10(CN) and FP10(PN) in Wales or, when available, WP10CN and WP10PN in Wales) by Nurses for National Health Service patients.

Community practitioners who have completed the necessary training may only prescribe items appearing in the nurse prescribers' list set out below. Community Practitioner Nurse Prescribers are recommended to prescribe generically, except where this would not be clinically appropriate or where there is no approved generic name.

## Medicinal Preparations
Almond Oil Ear Drops, BP
Arachis Oil Enema, NPF
[1]Aspirin Tablets, Dispersible, 300 mg, BP
Bisacodyl Suppositories, BP (includes 5-mg and 10-mg strengths)
Bisacodyl Tablets, BP
Catheter Maintenance Solution, Sodium Chloride, NPF
Catheter Maintenance Solution, 'Solution G', NPF
Catheter Maintenance Solution, 'Solution R', NPF
Chlorhexidine Gluconate Alcoholic Solutions containing at least 0.05%
Chlorhexidine Gluconate Aqueous Solutions containing at least 0.05%
Choline Salicylate Dental Gel, BP
Clotrimazole Cream 1%, BP
Co-danthramer Capsules, NPF
Co-danthramer Capsules, Strong, NPF
Co-danthramer Oral Suspension, NPF
Co-danthramer Oral Suspension, Strong, NPF
Co-danthrusate Capsules, BP
Co-danthrusate Oral Suspension, NPF
Crotamiton Cream, BP
Crotamiton Lotion, BP
Dimeticone barrier creams containing at least 10%
Dimeticone Lotion, NPF
Docusate Capsules, BP
Docusate Enema, NPF
Docusate Oral Solution, BP
Docusate Oral Solution, Paediatric, BP
Econazole Cream 1%, BP
Emollients as listed below:
    Aquadrate® 10% w/w Cream
    Arachis Oil, BP
    Balneum® Plus Cream
    Cetraben® Emollient Cream
    Dermamist®
    Diprobase® Cream
    Diprobase® Ointment
    Doublebase®
    Doublebase Dayleve® Gel

    E45® Cream
    E45® Itch Relief Cream
    Emulsifying Ointment, BP
    Eucerin® Intensive 10% w/w Urea Treatment Cream
    Eucerin® Intensive 10% w/w Urea Treatment Lotion
    Hydromol® Cream
    Hydromol® Intensive
    Hydrous Ointment, BP
    Lipobase®
    Liquid and White Soft Paraffin Ointment, NPF
    Neutrogena® Norwegian Formula Dermatological Cream
    Nutraplus® Cream
    Oilatum® Cream
    Oilatum® Junior Cream
    Paraffin, White Soft
    Paraffin, Yellow Soft, BP
    Ultrabase®
    Unguentum M®
Emollient Bath and Shower Preparations as listed below:
    Aqueous Cream, BP
    [2]Balneum®
    [2]Balneum Plus® Bath Oil
    Cetraben® Emollient Bath Additive
    Dermalo® Bath Emollient
    Diprobath®
    Doublebase® Emollient Bath Additive
    Doublebase® Emollient Shower Gel
    Doublebase® Emollient Wash Gel
    Hydromol® Bath and Shower Emollient
    Oilatum® Emollient
    Oilatum® Gel
    Oilatum® Junior Bath Additive
    Zerolatum® Emollient Medicinal Bath Oil
Folic Acid Tablets 400 micrograms, BP
Glycerol Suppositories, BP
[3]Ibuprofen Oral Suspension, BP
[3]Ibuprofen Tablets, BP
Ispaghula Husk Granules, BP
Ispaghula Husk Granules, Effervescent, BP
Ispaghula Husk Oral Powder, BP
Lactulose Solution, BP
Lidocaine Ointment, BP
Lidocaine and Chlorhexidine Gel, BP
Macrogol Oral Liquid, Compound, NPF
Macrogol Oral Powder, Compound, NPF
Macrogol Oral Powder, Compound, Half-strength, NPF
Magnesium Hydroxide Mixture, BP
Magnesium Sulfate Paste, BP
Malathion aqueous lotions containing at least 0.5%
Mebendazole Oral Suspension, NPF
Mebendazole Tablets, NPF
Methylcellulose Tablets, BP
Miconazole Cream 2%, BP
Miconazole Oromucosal Gel, BP

---

1. Max. 96 tablets; max. pack size 32 tablets
2. Except pack sizes that are not to be prescribed under the NHS (see Part XVIIIA of the Drug Tariff, Part XI of the Northern Ireland Drug Tariff)
3. Except for indications and doses that are [PoM]

Mouthwash Solution-tablets, NPF
Nicotine Inhalation Cartridge for Oromucosal Use, NPF
Nicotine Lozenge, NPF
Nicotine Medicated Chewing Gum, NPF
Nicotine Nasal Spray, NPF
Nicotine Oral Spray, NPF
Nicotine Sublingual Tablets, NPF
Nicotine Transdermal Patches, NPF
Nystatin Oral Suspension, BP
Olive Oil Ear Drops, BP
Paracetamol Oral Suspension, BP (includes 120 mg/
   5 mL and 250 mg/5 mL strengths—both of which are
   available as sugar-free formulations)
[1]Paracetamol Tablets, BP
[1]Paracetamol Tablets, Soluble, BP (includes 120-mg
   and 500-mg tablets)
Permethrin Cream, NPF
Phosphate Suppositories, NPF
Phosphates Enema, BP
Piperazine and Senna Powder, NPF
Povidone–Iodine Solution, BP
Senna Oral Solution, NPF
Senna Tablets, BP
Senna and Ispaghula Granules, NPF
Sodium Chloride Solution, Sterile, BP
Sodium Citrate Compound Enema, NPF
Sodium Picosulfate Capsules, NPF
Sodium Picosulfate Elixir, NPF
Spermicidal contraceptives as listed below:
   Gygel® Contraceptive Jelly
Sterculia Granules, NPF
Sterculia and Frangula Granules, NPF
Titanium Ointment, BP
Water for Injections, BP
Zinc and Castor Oil Ointment, BP
Zinc Oxide and Dimeticone Spray, NPF
Zinc Oxide Impregnated Medicated Bandage, NPF
Zinc Oxide Impregnated Medicated Stocking, NPF
Zinc Paste Bandage, BP 1993
Zinc Paste and Ichthammol Bandage, BP 1993

## Appliances and Reagents (including Wound Management Products)

Community Practitioner Nurse Prescribers in England, Wales and Northern Ireland can prescribe any appliance or reagent in the relevant Drug Tariff. In the Scottish Drug Tariff, Appliances and Reagents which may **not** be prescribed by Nurses are annotated **Nx**.

**Appliances** (including Contraceptive Devices[2]) as listed in Part IXA of the Drug Tariff (Part III of the Northern Ireland Drug Tariff, Part 3 (Appliances) and Part 2 (Dressings) of the Scottish Drug Tariff)

**Incontinence Appliances** as listed in Part IXB of the Drug Tariff (Part III of the Northern Ireland Drug Tariff, Part 5 of the Scottish Drug Tariff)

**Stoma Appliances and Associated Products** as listed in Part IXC of the Drug Tariff (Part III of the Northern Ireland Drug Tariff, Part 6 of the Scottish Drug Tariff)

**Chemical Reagents** as listed in Part IXR of the Drug Tariff (Part II of the Northern Ireland Drug Tariff, Part 9 of the Scottish Drug Tariff)

The Drug Tariffs can be accessed online at:
National Health Service Drug Tariff for England and Wales:
www.ppa.org.uk/ppa/edt_intro.htm
Health and Personal Social Services for Northern Ireland Drug Tariff:
www.dhsspsni.gov.uk/pas-tariff
Scottish Drug Tariff: www.isdscotland.org/Health-Topics/Prescribing-and-Medicines/Scottish-Drug-Tariff/

1. Max. 96 tablets; max. pack size 32 tablets
2. Nurse Prescribers in Family Planning Clinics—where it is not appropriate for nurse prescribers in family planning clinics to prescribe contraceptive devices using form FP10(P) (forms FP10(CN) and FP10(PN), or when available WP10CN and WP10PN, in Wales), they may prescribe using the same system as doctors in the clinic

# Non-medical prescribing

A range of non-medical healthcare professionals can prescribe medicines for patients as either Independent or Supplementary Prescribers.

Independent prescribers are practitioners responsible and accountable for the assessment of patients with previously undiagnosed or diagnosed conditions and for decisions about the clinical management required, including prescribing. They are recommended to prescribe generically, except where this would not be clinically appropriate or where there is no approved non-proprietary name.

Supplementary prescribing is a partnership between an independent prescriber (a doctor or a dentist) and a supplementary prescriber to implement an agreed Clinical Management Plan for an individual patient with that patient's agreement.

Independent and Supplementary Prescribers are identified by an annotation next to their name in the relevant professional register.

Information and guidance on non-medical prescribing is available on the Department of Health website at www. gov.uk/government/news/nurse-and-pharmacist-independent-prescribing-changes-announced.

For information on the mixing of medicines by Independent and Supplementary Prescribers, see *Mixing of medicines prior to administration in clinical practice—responding to legislative changes*, National Prescribing Centre, May 2010 (available at www.npc.nhs.uk/improving_safety/mixing_meds/resources/mixing_of_medicines.pdf).

For information on the supply and administration of medicines to groups of patients using Patient Group Directions, see p. 3.

## Nurses

Nurse Independent Prescribers (formerly known as Extended Formulary Nurse Prescribers) are able to prescribe any medicine for any medical condition.

Nurse Independent Prescribers are able to prescribe, administer, and give directions for the administration of Schedule 2, 3, 4, and 5 Controlled Drugs. This extends to diamorphine, dipipanone, or cocaine for treating organic disease or injury, but not for treating addiction.

Nurse Independent Prescribers must work within their own level of professional competence and expertise.

For information on prescribing from the Nurse Prescribers' Formulary for Community Practitioners, see Nurse Prescribers' Formulary for Community Practitioners p. 812.

## Pharmacists

Pharmacist Independent Prescribers can prescribe any medicine for any medical condition.

They are also able to prescribe, administer, and give directions for the administration of Schedule 2, 3, 4, and 5 Controlled Drugs. This extends to diamorphine, dipipanone, or cocaine for treating organic disease or injury, but not for treating addiction.

Pharmacist Independent Prescribers must work within their own level of professional competence and expertise.

## Optometrists

Optometrist Independent Prescribers can prescribe any licensed medicine for ocular conditions affecting the eye and the tissues surrounding the eye, except Controlled Drugs or medicines for parenteral administration. Optometrist Independent Prescribers must work within their own level of professional competence and expertise.

# Index of manufacturers

The following is an alphabetical list of manufacturers and other companies referenced in the BNF, with their medicines information or general contact details. For information on 'special-order' manufacturers and specialist importing companies see p. 823.

**3M**
3M Health Care Ltd
tel: (01509) 611 611

**A&H**
Allen & Hanburys Ltd
See GSK

**A1 Pharmaceuticals**
A1 Pharmaceuticals Plc
tel: (01708) 528 900
sales@a1plc.co.uk

**Abbott**
See AbbVie

**Abbott Healthcare**
Abbott Healthcare Products Ltd
tel: (023) 8046 7000
medinfo.shl@abbott.com

**AbbVie**
AbbVie Ltd
tel: (01628) 773 355
ukmedinfo@abbott.com

**Abraxis**
Abraxis BioScience Ltd
tel: (020) 7081 0850
abraxismedical@idispharma.com

**Acorus**
Acorus Therapeutics Ltd
tel: (01244) 625 152

**Actavis**
Actavis UK Ltd
tel: (01271) 311 257
medinfo@actavis.co.uk

**Actelion**
Actelion Pharmaceuticals UK Ltd
tel: (020) 8987 3333
medinfo_uk@actelion.com

**Activa**
Activa Healthcare
tel: 0845 060 6707
advice@activahealthcare.co.uk

**Adienne**
Adienne Pharma and Biotech
tel: 0039 (0) 335 873 8731

**ADI Medical**
ADI Medical UK
tel: (01628) 485159
info@adimedical.co.uk

**Advancis**
Advancis Medical Ltd
tel: (01623) 751 500
info@advancis.co.uk

**Advantech Surgical**
Advantech Surgical Ltd
tel: 0845 130 5866
customerservice@newgel.co.uk

**AgaMatrix**
AgaMatrix Europe Ltd
tel: (01235) 838 639
info@wavesense.co.uk

**Agepha**
Agepha GmbH
tel: (020) 3239 6241
uk@agepha.com

**Aguettant**
Aguettant Ltd
tel: (01934) 835 694
info@aguettant.co.uk

**Air Products**
Air Products plc
tel: 0800 373 580

**Alan Pharmaceuticals**
Alan Pharmaceuticals
tel: (020) 7284 2887

**Alcon**
Alcon Laboratories (UK) Ltd
tel: (01442) 341 234

**Alexion**
Alexion Pharma UK Ltd
tel: (01932) 359 220
alexion.uk@alxn.com

**Alissa**
Alissa Healthcare
tel: (01489) 780 759
enquiries@alissahealthcare.com

**ALK-Abelló**
ALK-Abelló (UK) Ltd
tel: (0118) 903 7940
info@uk.alk-abello.com

**Alkopharma**
Alkopharma Sarl
tel: (0041) 277 206 969
regulatory@alkopharma.com

**Allergan**
Allergan Ltd
tel: (01628) 494 026

**Allergy**
Allergy Therapeutics Ltd
tel: (01903) 844 702

**Alliance**
Alliance Pharmaceuticals Ltd
tel: (01249) 466 966
info@alliancepharma.co.uk

**Almirall**
Almirall Ltd
tel: 0800 008 7399
almirall@professionalinformation.co.uk

**Altacor**
Altacor Ltd
tel: (01223) 421 411
info@altacor-pharma.com

**Amdipharm**
Amdipharm plc
tel: 0870 777 7675
medinfo@amdipharm.com

**Amgen**
Amgen Ltd
tel: (01223) 420 305
gbinfoline@amgen.com

**Amred**
Amred Healthcare Ltd
tel: (0330) 333 0079
info@amredhealthcare.com

**Apollo Medical**
Apollo Medical Technologies Ltd
tel: (01636) 831 201
supercheck2@btinternet.com

**Archimed**
Archimed
tel: 0800 756 9951
enquiries@archimed.co.uk

**Archimedes**
Archimedes Pharma UK Ltd
tel: (0118) 931 5094
medicalinformationUK@archimedes-pharma.com

**Arctic Medical**
Arctic Medical Ltd
tel: (01303) 277 751
sales@arcticmedical.co.uk

**Ardana**
Ardana Bioscience Ltd
tel: (0131) 226 8550

**Ark Therapeutics**
Ark Therapeutics Group Plc
tel: (020) 7388 7722
info@arktherapeutics.com

**Aspen**
Aspen
tel: 0800 008 7392
aspenglobal@professionalinformation.co.uk

**Aspen Medical**
Aspen Medical Europe Ltd
tel: (01527) 587 728
customers@aspenmedicaleurope.com

**AS Pharma**
AS Pharma Ltd
tel: 0870 066 4117
info@aspharma.co.uk

**Aspire**
Aspire Pharma Ltd
tel: (01730) 231 148
info@aspirepharma.co.uk

**Astellas**
Astellas Pharma Ltd
tel: (020) 3379 8000
medinfo.gb@astellas.com

**AstraZeneca**
AstraZeneca UK Ltd
tel: 0800 783 0033
medical.informationuk@astrazeneca.com

**Auden Mckenzie**
Auden Mckenzie (Pharma Division) Ltd
tel: (01895) 627 420

**Axcan**
Axcan Pharma SA
tel: (0033) 130 461 900

**Crucell**
Crucell (UK) Ltd
tel: 0844 800 3907
info@crucell.co.uk

**CSL Behring**
CSL Behring UK Ltd
tel: (01444) 447 400
medinfo@cslbehring.com

**Daiichi Sankyo**
Daiichi Sankyo UK Ltd
tel: (01753) 482 771
medinfo@daiichi-sankyo.co.uk

**Danetre**
Danetre Health Products Ltd
tel: (01327) 310 909
enquiries@danetrehealthproducts.com

**DDD**
DDD Ltd
tel: (01923) 229 251

**Dee**
Dee Pharmaceuticals Ltd
tel: (01978) 661993
enquiries@deepharmaceuticalsltd.co.uk

**Dental Health**
Dental Health Products Ltd
tel: (01622) 749 222

**Dentsply**
Dentsply Ltd
tel: (01932) 837 279

**Dermal**
Dermal Laboratories Ltd
tel: (01462) 458 866

**Dermato Logical**
Dermato Logical Ltd
tel: (0208) 449 2931
enquiries@aqua-max.co.uk

**Dermatonics**
Dermatonics Ltd
tel: (01480) 462 910
sales@dermatonics.co.uk

**Derma UK**
Derma UK Ltd
tel: (01462) 733 500
info@dermauk.co.uk

**DeVilbiss**
DeVilbiss Healthcare UK Ltd
tel: (01384) 446 688

**Dexcel**
Dexcel-Pharma Ltd
tel: (01327) 312 266
office@dexcelpharma.co.uk

**DHP Healthcare**
DHP Healthcare Ltd
tel: (01622) 749 222
sales@dhphealthcare.co.uk

**DiME**
DiME
tel: (01483) 715 008
info@dime-med.com

**Dreamskin**
Dreamskin Health Ltd
tel: (01707) 228 688

**Dr Falk**
Dr Falk Pharma UK Ltd
tel: (01628) 536 600

**Drossa**
Drossa Ltd
tel: (020) 3393 0859
info@drossa.co.uk

**Durbin**
Durbin plc
tel: (020) 8869 6500
info@durbin.co.uk

**Eakin**
T G Eakin
tel: (028) 9187 1000
mail@eakin.co.uk

**Easigrip**
Easigrip Ltd
tel: (01926) 497 108
enquiry@easigrip.co.uk

**Ecolab**
Ecolab UK
tel: (0113) 232 0066
info.healthcare@ecolab.co.uk

**Egis**
Egis Pharmaceuticals UK Ltd
tel: (020) 7266 2669
enquiries@medimpexuk.com

**Eisai**
Eisai Ltd
tel: (020) 8600 1400
lmedinfo@eisai.net

**Encysive**
Encysive (UK) Ltd
tel: (01895) 876 168

**Entra Health**
Entra Health Systems
tel: (0113) 815 5108

**Espere**
Espere Healthcare Ltd
tel: (01234) 834 614
info@esperehealth.co.uk

**Essential**
Essential Pharmaceuticals Ltd
tel: (01784) 477 167
info@essentialpharmaceuticals.com

**Ethicon**
Ethicon Ltd
tel: (01506) 594 500

**Eumedica**
Eumedica S.A.
tel: (020) 8444 3377
enquiries@eumedica.com

**European Pharma**
European Pharma Group
tel: 0031 (0) 20 316 0140
info@insujet.com

**EUSA Pharma**
EUSA Pharma (Europe) Ltd
tel: (01438) 740 720
medinfo-uk@eusapharma.com

**Everfresh**
Everfresh Natural Foods
tel: (01296) 425 333

**Fabre**
Pierre Fabre Ltd
tel: (01962) 874 435
medicalinformation@pierre-fabre.co.uk

**Fate**
Fate Special Foods
tel: (01215) 224 433

**Fenton**
Fenton Pharmaceuticals Ltd
tel: (020) 7224 1388
mail@Fent-Pharm.co.uk

**Ferndale**
Ferndale Pharmaceuticals Ltd
tel: (01937) 541 122
info@ferndalepharma.co.uk

**Ferring**
Ferring Pharmaceuticals (UK)
tel: 0844 931 0050
medical@ferring.com

**Firstplay Dietary**
Firstplay Dietary Foods Ltd
tel: (0161) 474 7576

**Flynn**
Flynn Pharma Ltd
tel: (01438) 727 822
medinfo@flynnpharma.com

**Foodlink**
Foodlink (UK) Ltd
tel: (01752) 344 544
info@foodlinkltd.co.uk

**Ford**
Ford Medical Associates Ltd
tel: (01233) 633 224
enquiries@fordmedical.co.uk

**Forest**
Forest Laboratories UK Ltd
tel: (01322) 421 800
medinfo@forest-labs.co.uk

**Forum**
Forum Health Products Ltd
tel: (01737) 773 711

**Fox**
C. H. Fox Ltd
tel: (020) 7240 3111

**Fresenius Biotech**
Fresenius Biotech GmbH
tel: 0049 (0) 893 065 9311
med.info@fresenius-biotech.com

**Fresenius Kabi**
Fresenius Kabi Ltd
tel: (01928) 533 533
med.info-uk@fresenius-kabi.com

**Fresenius Medical Care**
Fresenius Medical Care UK Ltd
tel: (01623) 445 171
medinfo-uk@fmc-ag.com

**Frontier**
Frontier Multigate
tel: (01495) 233 050
multigate@frontier-group.co.uk

**Fyne Dynamics**
Fyne Dynamics Ltd
tel: (01279) 423 423
info@fyne-dynamics.com

**Galderma**
Galderma (UK) Ltd
tel: (01923) 208 950
medinfo.uk@galderma.com

**Galen**
Galen Ltd
tel: (028) 3833 4974
customer.services@galen.co.uk

**GE Healthcare**
GE Healthcare
tel: (01494) 544 000

**Geistlich**
Geistlich Pharma
tel: (01244) 347 534

**General Dietary**
General Dietary Ltd
tel: (020) 8336 2323

**Generics**
See Mylan

**Genius Foods**
Genius Foods Ltd
tel: 0845 874 4000
info@geniusglutenfree.com

**Genopharm**
Laboratoires Genopharm
tel: (0808) 234 2664
info@genopharm.eu

**Genus**
Genus Pharmaceuticals
tel: (01635) 568 400
info@genuspharma.com

**Genzyme**
Genzyme Therapeutics
tel: (01865) 405 200
ukmedinfo@genzyme.com

**GFF Trade**
GF Foods Ltd
tel: (01757) 289 207
admin@gffdirect.co.uk

**Gilead**
Gilead Sciences Ltd
tel: (01223) 897 555
ukmedinfo@gilead.com

**Glenwood**
Glenwood GmbH
tel: (0049) 815 199 8790
info@glenwood.de

**GlucoRx**
GlucoRx Ltd
tel: (01483) 755 133
info@glucorx.co.uk

**Gluten Free Foods Ltd**
Gluten Free Foods Ltd
tel: (020) 8953 4444
info@glutenfree-foods.co.uk

**Goldshield**
See Mercury

**GP Pharma**
See Derma UK

**Grifols**
Grifols UK Ltd
tel: (01223) 395 700
reception.uk@grifols.com

**Grünenthal**
Grünenthal Ltd
tel: 0870 351 8960
medicalinformationuk@grunenthal.com

**GSK**
GlaxoSmithKline
tel: 0800 221 441
customercontactuk@gsk.com

**GSK Consumer Healthcare**
GlaxoSmithKline Consumer Healthcare
tel: (020) 8047 2500
customer.relations@gsk.com

**H&R**
H&R Healthcare Ltd
tel: (01482) 631 606

**Hampton**
Hampton Pharmaceuticals Ltd
tel: (01923) 251 777

**Hartmann**
Paul Hartmann Ltd
tel: (01706) 363 200
info@uk.hartmann.info

**Heinz**
H. J. Heinz Company Ltd
tel: (020) 8573 7757
farleys_heinz@heinz.co.uk

**Henleys**
Henleys Medical Supplies Ltd
tel: (01707) 333 164

**HFA Healthcare**
HFA Healthcare Ltd
tel: 0844 335 8270

**HK Pharma**
HK Pharma Ltd
tel: (01438) 356 926

**Hollister**
Hollister Ltd
tel: (0118) 989 5000

**Hospira**
Hospira UK Ltd
tel: (01926) 834 400
medinfouk@hospira.com

**HRA Pharma**
HRA Pharma UK & Ireland Ltd
tel: 0800 917 9548
med.info.uk@hra-pharma.com

**Huntleigh**
Huntleigh Healthcare Ltd
tel: (01582) 413 104

**Idis**
Idis Ltd
tel: (01932) 824 000
mi@idispharma.com

**INCA-Pharm**
INCA-Pharm UK
tel: (01748) 828 812
info@inca-pharm.com

**Infai**
Infai UK Ltd
tel: (01904) 435 228
info@infai.co.uk

**Innovative**
Innovative Solutions UK Ltd
tel: (01706) 746 713
enquiries@innovative-solutions.org.uk

**Insight**
Insight Medical Products Ltd
tel: (01666) 500 055
info@insightmedical.net

**InterMune**
InterMune
tel: (03308) 080 960
med-info@intermune.co.uk

**Internis**
Internis Pharmaceuticals Ltd
tel: (020) 8346 5588
regulatory@jensongroup.com

**Intrapharm**
Intrapharm Laboratories Ltd
tel: (01628) 771 800
sales@intrapharmlabs.com

**Ipsen**
Ipsen Ltd
tel: (01753) 627 777
medical.information.uk@ipsen.com

**Iroko**
Iroko Cardio GmbH
tel: (020) 3002 8114
info@irokocardio.com

**IS Pharmaceuticals**
See Sinclair IS

**IVAX**
See TEVA UK

**J&J**
Johnson & Johnson Ltd
tel: (01628) 822 222
medinfo@congb.jnj.com

**Janssen**
Janssen-Cilag Ltd
tel: 0800 731 8450
medinfo@its.jnj.com

**Jobskin**
Jobskin Ltd
tel: (0115) 973 4300
dw@jobskin.co.uk

**Juvela**
Juvela (Hero UK) Ltd
tel: (0151) 432 5300
info@juvela.co.uk

**K/L**
K/L Pharmaceuticals Ltd
tel: (01294) 215 951

**Kappin**
Kappin Ltd
tel: (020) 8961 8511

**KCI Medical**
KCI Medical Ltd
tel: (01865) 840 600

**Kestrel Ophthalmics**
Kestrel Ophthalmics Ltd
tel: (01202) 658 444
info@kestrelophthalmics.co.uk

**King**
King Pharmaceuticals Ltd
tel: (01438) 356 924

**KoRa**
KoRa Healthcare Ltd
tel: 0845 303 8631
info@kora.ie

**Labopharm**
Labopharm Europe Ltd
tel: 0800 028 0037
medinfo@paladin-labs.com

**LaCorium**
LaCorium Health (UK) Ltd
tel: 0800 158 8233
ukinfo@flexitol.com

**Lantor**
Lantor UK Ltd
tel: (01204) 855 000
help@lantor.co.uk

**LEO**
LEO Laboratories Ltd
tel: (01844) 347 333
medical-info.uk@leo-pharma.com

**LifeScan**
LifeScan
tel: 0800 001 210

**Lilly**
Eli Lilly & Co Ltd
tel: (01256) 315 000
ukmedinfo@lilly.com

**Lincoln Medical**
Lincoln Medical Ltd
tel: (01722) 742 900
info@lincolnmedical.co.uk

**Linderma**
Linderma Ltd
tel: (01942) 816 184
linderma@virgin.net

**Lipomed**
Lipomed GmbH
tel: (0041) 6170 20200
save@lipomed.com

**Livwell**
Livwell Ltd
tel: 0845 120 0038
info@livwell.eu

**LogixX**
LogixX Pharma Solutions Ltd
tel: (01189) 011 747
medinfo@logixxpharma.com

**Lornamead**
Lornamead UK Ltd
tel: (01276) 674000
lornamead@dhl.com

**LPC**
LPC Pharmaceuticals Ltd
tel: (01582) 560 393
info@lpcpharma.com

**Lundbeck**
Lundbeck Ltd
tel: (01908) 638 972
ukmedicalinformation@lundbeck.com

**L'Oréal Active**
L'Oréal Active Cosmetics UK
tel: 0800 055 6822

**M & A Pharmachem**
M & A Pharmachem Ltd
tel: (01942) 816 184

**Manuka Medical**
Manuka Medical Ltd
tel: (01623) 600 669

**Manx**
Manx Healthcare
tel: (01926) 482 511
info@manxhealthcare.com

**Marlborough**
Marlborough Pharmaceuticals
tel: (01748) 828 789
info@marlborough-pharma.co.uk

**Martindale**
Martindale Pharma
tel: (01277) 266 600
medinfo@martindalepharma.co.uk

**MASTA**
MASTA
tel: (0113) 238 7500
medical@masta.org

**McNeil**
McNeil Products Ltd
tel: (01628) 822 222

**MDE**
Medical Diagnostics Europe Ltd
tel: 0845 370 8077
info@mdediagnostic.co.uk

**Mead Johnson**
Mead Johnson Nutritionals
tel: (01895) 523 764

**Meadow**
Meadow Laboratories Ltd
tel: (020) 8597 1203

**Meda**
Meda Pharmaceuticals Ltd
tel: (01748) 828 810
meda@professionalinformation.co.uk

**Medac**
Medac (UK)
tel: (01786) 458 086
info@medac-uk.co.uk

**Medical Developments**
Medical Developments UK Ltd
tel: 0870 850 1234
enquiries@ashfieldin2focus.com

**Medicare**
Medicare Plus International Ltd
tel: (020) 8810 8811
info@medicare-plus.com

**Medicom**
Medicom Healthcare Ltd
tel: (01489) 574 119
info@medicomhealthcare.com

**Medihoney**
Medihoney (Europe) Ltd
tel: 0800 071 3912

**Medisana**
Medisana
tel: +49 (0) 2131/36 68 0

**Medlock**
Medlock Medical Ltd
tel: (0161) 621 2100

**MedLogic**
MedLogic Global Ltd
tel: (01752) 209 955
enquiries@mlgl.co.uk

**Menarini**
A. Menarini Farmaceutica Internazionale SRL
tel: (01628) 856 400
menarini@medinformation.co.uk

**Menarini Diagnostics**
A. Menarini Diagnostics
tel: (0118) 944 4100

**Merck Serono**
Merck Serono Ltd
tel: (020) 8818 7200
medinfo.uk@merckserono.net

**Mercury**
Mercury Pharma Group
tel: 0870 070 3033
medicalinformation@mercurypharma.com

**Merz**
Merz Pharma UK Ltd
tel: (020) 8236 0000
info@merzpharma.co.uk

**Micro Medical**
Micro Medical Ltd
tel: (01634) 893 500

**Milupa**
Milupa Aptamil
tel: 0845 762 3676
careline@aptamil4hcps.co.uk

**Mitsubishi**
Mitsubishi Pharma
tel: (0207) 382 9000
medinfo@mitsubishi-pharma.eu

**Mölnlycke**
Mölnlycke Health Care Ltd
tel: (0161) 777 2628
info.uk@molnlycke.net

**Moorfields**
Moorfields Pharmaceuticals
tel: (020) 7684 9090

**Morningside**
Morningside Healthcare Ltd
tel: (0116) 204 5950

**Movianto**
Movianto UK
tel: (01234) 248 500
movianto.uk@movianto.com

**MSD**
Merck Sharp & Dohme Ltd
tel: (01992) 467 272
medicalinformationuk@merck.com

**Mylan**
Mylan
tel: (01707) 853 000
info@mylan.co.uk

**Nagor**
Nagor Ltd
tel: (01624) 625 556
enquiries@nagor.com

**Nairns**
Nairn's Oatcakes Ltd
tel: (0131) 620 7000

**Napp**
Napp Pharmaceuticals Ltd
tel: (01223) 424 444

**Neoceuticals**
Neoceuticals Ltd
tel: (01748) 828 865

**Neolab**
Neolab Ltd
tel: (01256) 704 110
info@neolab.co.uk

**Neomedic**
Neomedic Ltd
tel: (01923) 836 379
marketing@neomedic.co.uk

**Nestlé**
Nestlé Nutrition
tel: 00800 6887 4846
nestlehealthcarenutrition@uk.nestle.com

**Newport**
Newport Pharmaceuticals Ltd
tel: (00353) 1890 3011

**NIBTS**
Northern Ireland Blood Transfusion Service
tel: (028) 9032 1414
inet@nibts.hscni.net

**Nipro Diagnostics**
Nipro Diagnostics (UK) Ltd
tel: (01489) 569 469
info@homediagnostics-uk.com

**Nordic**
Nordic Pharma UK Ltd
tel: (0118) 929 8233
info@nordicpharma.co.uk

**Norgine**
Norgine Pharmaceuticals Ltd
tel: (01895) 826 600

**Nova**
Nova Laboratories Ltd
tel: 08707 120 655
xaluprine@aptivsolutions.com

**Novartis**
Novartis Pharmaceuticals UK Ltd
tel: (01276) 698 370
medinfo.uk@novartis.com

**Novartis Consumer Health**
Novartis Consumer Health
tel: (01276) 687 202
medicalaffairs.uk@novartis.com

**Novartis Vaccines**
Novartis Vaccines Ltd
tel: 0845 745 1500
service.uk@novartis.com

**Novo Nordisk**
Novo Nordisk Ltd
tel: (01293) 613 555

**nSPIRE Health**
nSPIRE Health Ltd
tel: (01992) 526 300
info@nspirehealth.com

**Nutricia Clinical**
Nutricia Clinical Care
tel: (01225) 711 688
resourcecentre@nutricia.com

**Nutrinovo**
Nutrinovo Ltd
tel: (01304) 829 068
info@nutrinovo.com

**Nutrition Point**
Nutrition Point Ltd
tel: (07041) 544 044
info@nutritionpoint.co.uk

**Nycomed**
Nycomed UK Ltd
tel: (01628) 646 4397
medinfo@nycomed.com

**OakMed**
OakMed Ltd
tel: 0800 592 786
orders@oakmed.co.uk

**Ocon Chemicals**
Ocon Chemicals Ltd
tel: (00353) 21 431 8555
info@oconchemicals.com

**Octapharma**
Octapharma Ltd
tel: (0161) 837 3770
octapharma@octapharma.co.uk

**Omega Pharma**
Omega Pharma
tel: (01748) 828 860
omega@professionalinformation.co.uk

**Omron**
Omron Healthcare (UK) Ltd
tel: 0870 750 2771
info.omronhealthcare.uk@eu.omron.com

**Organon**
See MSD

**Orion**
Orion Pharma (UK) Ltd
tel: (01635) 520 300
medicalinformation@orionpharma.com

**Orphan Europe**
Orphan Europe (UK) Ltd
tel: (01491) 414 333
infouk@orphan-europe.com

**Otsuka**
Otsuka Pharmaceuticals (UK) Ltd
tel: (020) 8756 3100
otsuka@medinformation.co.uk

**Ovation**
Ovation Healthcare International Ltd
tel: (00353) 1613 9707

**Owen Mumford**
Owen Mumford Ltd
tel: (01993) 812 021
customerservices@owenmumford.co.uk

**Oxbridge**
Oxbridge Pharma Ltd
tel: (020) 8335 4110
enquiries@oxbridgepharma.com

**Oxford Nutrition**
Oxford Nutrition Ltd
tel: (01626) 832 067
info@nutrinox.com

**Pari**
PARI Medical Ltd
tel: (01932) 341 122
infouk@pari.de

**Parkside**
Parkside Healthcare
tel: (0161) 795 2792

**Peckforton**
Peckforton Pharmaceuticals Ltd
tel: (01270) 582 255
info@peckforton.com

**Penn**
Penn Pharmaceuticals Services Ltd
tel: (01495) 711 222
penn@pennpharm.co.uk

**Pfizer**
Pfizer Ltd
tel: (01304) 616 161
EUMEDINFO@pfizer.com

**PGR Health Foods**
PGR Health Foods Ltd
tel: (01992) 581 715
info@pgrhealthfoods.co.uk

**Pharmacia**
See Pfizer

**Pharmacosmos**
Pharmacosmos UK Ltd
tel: (01844) 269 007
info@vitalineuk.co.uk

**Pharma Mar**
See Idis

**Pharma Nord**
Pharma Nord (UK) Ltd
tel: (01670) 519 989
uksales@pharmanord.co.uk

**Pharmasure**
Pharmasure Ltd
tel: (01923) 233 466
info@pharmasure.co.uk

**Pharmaxis**
Pharmaxis Pharmaceuticals Ltd
tel: (01628) 902 053
med.info@pharmaxis.com.au

**PharSafer**
PharSafer Associates Ltd
tel: (01483) 212151
medinfoenquiries@pharsafer.com

**Pinewood**
Pinewood Healthcare
tel: (00353) 523 6253
info@pinewood.ie

**Potters**
Potters Herbal Medicines
tel: (01942) 219 960

**Preglem UK**
Preglem UK, a Division of Gedeon Richter (UK) Ltd
tel: (0207) 604 8806
medinfo.uk.ie@preglem.com

**Proceli**
Proceli
tel: (01226) 713 044
admin@proceli.co.uk

**Procter & Gamble**
Procter & Gamble (Health and Beauty Care) Ltd
tel: (0191) 297 5000

**Profile**
Profile Pharma Ltd
tel: 0800 1300 855
info@profilepharma.com

**ProStrakan**
ProStrakan Ltd
tel: (01896) 664 000
medinfo@prostrakan.com

**Protex**
Protex Healthcare (UK) Ltd
tel: 0870 011 4112
orders@protexhealthcare.co.uk

**Ranbaxy**
Ranbaxy UK Ltd
tel: (020) 8280 1986
medinfoeurope@ranbaxy.com

**Ransom**
Ransom Consumer Healthcare
tel: (01462) 437 615
info@williamransom.com

**Ratiopharm UK**
Ratiopharm UK Ltd
tel: (023) 9231 3592
info@ratiopharm.co.uk

**Reckitt Benckiser**
Reckitt Benckiser Healthcare
tel: (01482) 326 151
info.MIU@reckittbenckiser.com

**Recordati**
Recordati Pharmaceuticals Ltd
tel: (01491) 576 336
medinfo@recordati.co.uk

**ReSource Medical**
ReSource Medical UK Ltd
tel: (01484) 531 489
info@resource-medical.co.uk

**Respironics**
Philips Respironics (UK) Ltd
tel: 0800 130 0840
rukmarketing@respironics.com

**RF Medical**
RF Medical Supplies Ltd
tel: (0151) 493 1473
enquiries@rfmedicalsupplies.co.uk

**Richardson**
Richardson Healthcare Ltd
tel: 0800 170 1126
info@richardsonhealthcare.com

**Riemser**
Riemser Arzneimittel AG
tel: (0049) 383 517 6679
info@RIEMSER.de

**RIS Products**
RIS Products Ltd
tel: (01438) 840 135

**Robinsons**
Robinson Healthcare Ltd
tel: (01909) 735 064
enquiry@robinsonhealthcare.com

**Roche**
Roche Products Ltd
tel: 0800 328 1629
medinfo.uk@roche.com

**Roche Diagnostics**
Roche Diagnostics Ltd
tel: (01444) 256 000

**Rosemont**
Rosemont Pharmaceuticals Ltd
tel: 0800 919 312
infodesk@rosemontpharma.com

**Rowa**
Rowa Pharmaceuticals Ltd
tel: (00353) 275 0077
rowa@rowa-pharma.ie

**S&N Hlth.**
Smith & Nephew Healthcare Ltd
tel: (01482) 222 200
advice@smith-nephew.com

**Sallis**
Sallis Healthcare Ltd
tel: (0115) 978 7841

**Sandoz**
Sandoz Ltd
tel: (01276) 698 020
sandoz@professionalinformation.co.uk

**Sanochemia**
Sanochemia Diagnostics UK Ltd
tel: (0117) 906 3562

**Sanofi-Aventis**
Sanofi-Aventis Ltd
tel: 0845 372 7101
uk-medicalinformation@sanofi-aventis.
com

**Sanofi Pasteur**
Sanofi Pasteur MSD Ltd
tel: (01628) 785 291

**SanoMed**
SanoMed Manufacturing bv
tel: +32 503 93627
info@sanomed.nl

**Schering-Plough**
See MSD

**Schuco**
Schuco International Ltd
tel: (020) 8368 1642
sales@schuco.co.uk

**Schülke**
Schülke UK
tel: (0114) 254 3500
mail.uk@schuelke.com

**Scope Ophthalmics**
Scope Ophthamics Ltd
tel: (01293) 897 209
info@scopeophthalmics.com

**SD Biosensor**
SD Biosensor, Inc.
tel: 0082 31 300 0475
sales@sdbiosensor.com

**SD Healthcare**
SD Healthcare
tel: (0161) 776 7626
sales@sdhealthcare.com

**Septodont**
Septodont Ltd
tel: (01622) 695 520

**Servier**
Servier Laboratories Ltd
tel: (01753) 666 409
medical.information@uk.netgrs.com

**Seven Seas**
Seven Seas Ltd
tel: (01482) 375 234

**Shermond**
Shermond
tel: 0870 242 7701
sales@shermond.com

**Shire**
Shire Pharmaceuticals Ltd
tel: 0800 055 6614
medinfouk@shire.com

**Shire HGT**
Shire Human Genetic Therapies
tel: (01256) 894 000
hgtmedcomm@shire.com

**SHS**
SHS International Ltd
tel: (0151) 228 8161

**Siemens**
Siemens Healthcare Diagnostics Ltd
tel: 0845 600 1966
dx-diag_sales-uk.med@siemens.com

**Sigma-Tau**
Sigma-Tau Pharma Ltd (UK)
tel: 0800 043 1268
medical.information@sigma-tau.co.uk

**SilDerm**
SilDerm Ltd
tel: (01260) 271 666

**Sinclair IS**
Sinclair IS Pharma
tel: (01244) 625 152
enquiries@ispharma.plc.uk

**Skin Camouflage Co.**
The Skin Camouflage Company Ltd
tel: (01507) 343 091
smjcovermark@aol.com

**Skinnies**
Skinnies UK
tel: (01562) 546 123
info@skinniesuk.com

**SLO Drinks**
SLO Drinks Ltd
tel: 0845 222 2205
info@slodrinks.com

**SMA Nutrition**
See Wyeth

**SNBTS**
Scottish National Blood Transfusion
Service
tel: (0131) 536 5700
contact.pfc@snbts.csa.scot.nhs.uk

**Sound Opinion**
Sound Opinion
tel: 0870 192 3283
enquiries@medinformation.co.uk

**Sovereign**
See Amdipharm

**Speciality European**
Speciality European Pharma Ltd
tel: (020) 7421 7400
info@spepharma.com

**Spectrum Thea**
Spectrum Thea Pharmaceuticals
tel: 0870 192 3283
theasupport@spectrum-thea.co.uk

**SpePharm**
SpePharm UK Ltd
tel: 0844 800 7579
medinfo.uk@spepharm.com

**Spirit**
Spirit Healthcare Ltd
tel: 0800 881 5423
cs@spirit-healthcare.co.uk

**Squibb**
See Bristol-Myers Squibb

**SSL**
SSL International plc
tel: 0870 122 2690
medical.information@ssl-international.
com

**Stanningley**
Stanningley Pharma Ltd
tel: (01159) 124 253
medinfo@stanningleypharma.co.uk

**STD Pharmaceutical**
STD Pharmaceutical Products Ltd
tel: (01432) 373 555
enquiries@stdpharm.co.uk

**Steraid**
Steraid (Gainsborough) Ltd
tel: (01427) 677 559

**Stiefel**
Stiefel Laboratories (UK) Ltd
tel: (01628) 612 000

**Stiletto Foods**
Stiletto Foods UK Ltd
tel: 0845 130 0869

**Stragen**
Stragen UK Ltd
tel: 0870 351 8744
info@stragenuk.com

**Su-Med**
Su-Med International UK Ltd
tel: (01457) 890 980
sales@sumed.co.uk

**Sutherland**
Sutherland Health Ltd
tel: (01635) 874 488

**Swedish Orphan**
Swedish Orphan Biovitrum Ltd
tel: (01638) 722 380

**Synergy Healthcare**
Synergy Healthcare (UK) Ltd
tel: (0161) 624 5641
healthcaresolutions@synergyhealthplc.
com

**Syner-Med**
Syner-Med (Pharmaceutical Products)
Ltd
tel: 0845 634 2100
mail@syner-med.com

**Systagenix**
Systagenix Wound Management
tel: (01344) 871 000

**Takeda**
Takeda UK Ltd
tel: (01628) 537 900
medinfo@takeda.co.uk

**Talley**
Talley Group Ltd
tel: (01794) 503 500

**Taro**
Taro Pharmaceuticals (UK) Ltd
tel: 0870 736 9544
customerservice@taropharma.co.uk

**Teofarma**
Teofarma S.r.l.
tel: (01748) 828 857
teofarma@professionalinformation.co.uk

**Teva**
Teva Pharmaceuticals Ltd
med.info@tevapharma.co.uk

**TEVA UK**
TEVA UK Ltd
tel: 0870 502 0304
medinfo@tevauk.com

**The Medicines Company**
The Medicines Company
tel: 00800 8436 3326
medical.information@themedco.com

**Therabel**
Therabel Pharma UK Ltd
tel: 0800 066 5446
info@therabel.co.uk

**The Urology Co.**
The Urology Company Ltd
tel: (020) 3077 5411
info@theurologyco.com

**Thomas Blake**
Thomas Blake Cosmetic Creams Ltd
tel: (01207) 279 432
sales@veilcover.com

**Thornton & Ross**
Thornton & Ross Ltd
tel: (01484) 842 217

**Tillomed**
Tillomed Laboratories Ltd
tel: (01480) 402 400
info@tillomed.co.uk

**Tillotts**
Tillotts Pharma UK Ltd
tel: 0845 034 4476

**TMC**
TMC Pharma Services Ltd
tel: (01252) 842 255
info@tmcpharma.com

**Tobia Teff**
Tobia Teff UK Ltd
tel: (020) 7328 2045
info@tobiateff.co.uk

**Torbet**
Torbet Laboratories Ltd
tel: (01953) 607 856
customerservices@cambridge-healthcare.co.uk

**Transdermal**
Transdermal Ltd
tel: (020) 8654 2251
info@transdermal.co.uk

**TRB Chemedica**
TRB Chemedica (UK) Ltd
tel: 0845 330 7556

**Typharm**
Typharm Ltd
tel: (01603) 735 200
customerservices@typharm.com

**UCB Pharma**
UCB Pharma Ltd
tel: (01753) 534 655
medicalinformationuk@ucb.com

**Ultrapharm**
Ultrapharm Ltd
tel: (01491) 578 016

**Univar**
Univar Ltd
tel: (01908) 362 200
trientine@univareurope.com

**Unomedical**
Unomedical Ltd
tel: (01527) 587 700

**Urgo**
Urgo Ltd
tel: (01509) 502 051
woundcare@uk.urgo.com

**Vegenat**
c/o Archaelis Ltd
tel: 0870 803 2484

**Vifor**
Vifor Pharma UK Ltd
tel: (01276) 853 633
medicalinfo_uk@viforpharma.com

**ViiV**
ViiV Healthcare UK Ltd
See GSK

**Viridian**
Viridian Pharma Ltd
tel: (01633) 400 335
info@viridianpharma.co.uk

**ViroPharma**
ViroPharma Ltd
tel: (020) 7572 1222

**Vitaflo**
Vitaflo International Ltd
tel: (0151) 709 9020
vitaflo@vitaflo.co.uk

**Vitalograph**
Vitalograph Ltd
tel: (01280) 827 110
sales@vitalograph.co.uk

**Wallace Cameron**
Wallace Cameron Ltd
tel: (01698) 354 600
sales@wallacecameron.com

**Wallace Mfg**
Wallace Manufacturing Chemists Ltd
tel: (01235) 538 700
info@alinter.co.uk

**Warburtons**
Warburtons
tel: (01204) 513 004

**Warner Chilcott**
Warner Chilcott UK Ltd
tel: (01932) 824 700

**WBS**
Welsh Blood Service
tel: (01443) 622 000
donor.care@wales.nhs.uk

**Wellfoods**
Wellfoods Ltd
tel: (01226) 381 712
wellfoods@wellfoods.co.uk

**Williams**
Williams Medical Supplies Ltd
tel: (01685) 844 739

**Winthrop**
Winthrop Pharmaceuticals UK Ltd
tel: (01483) 554 101
winthrop@professionalinformation.co.uk

**Wockhardt**
Wockhardt UK Ltd
tel: (01978) 661 261

**Wyeth**
Wyeth Pharmaceuticals
tel: (01628) 604 377
EUMEDINFO@pfizer.com

**Wynlit**
Wynlit Laboratories
tel: (07903) 370 130

**Wyvern**
Wyvern Medical Ltd
tel: (01531) 631 105

**Zentiva**
Zentiva
See Sanofi-Aventis

**Zeroderma**
Zeroderma Ltd
tel: (01858) 525 643

# Special-order Manufacturers

Unlicensed medicines are available from 'special-order' manufacturers and specialist-importing companies; the MHRA maintains a register of these companies at http://tinyurl.com/cdslke

Licensed **hospital manufacturing units** also manufacture 'special-order' products as unlicensed medicines, the principal NHS units are listed below. A database (*Pro-File*; www.pro-file.nhs.uk) provides information on medicines manufactured in the NHS; access is restricted to NHS pharmacy staff.

The Association of Pharmaceutical Specials Manufacturers may also be able to provide further information about commercial companies (www.apsm-uk.com).

> The MHRA recommends that an unlicensed medicine should only be used when a patient has special requirements that cannot be met by use of a licensed medicine

## England

### London

**Barts and the London NHS Trust**
Mr J. Singh
Head of PMU
Barts Health NHS Trust
Pathology and Pharmacy Building
Royal London Hospital
80 Newark St
Whitechapel
London, E1 2ES
tel: (020) 3246 0274 (order)
tel: (020) 3246 0399 (enquiry)
jasdeep.singh@bartshealth.nhs.uk

**Guy's and St. Thomas' NHS Foundation Trust**
Mr P. Forsey
Associate Chief Pharmacist
Guy's and St. Thomas' NHS Foundation Trust
Pharmacy Department
Guy's Hospital
Great Maze Pond
London, SE1 9RT
tel: (020) 7188 4992 (order)
tel: (020) 7188 5003 (enquiry)
fax: (020) 7188 5013
paul.forsey@gstt.nhs.uk

**Moorfields Pharmaceuticals**
Mr N. Precious
Technical Director
Moorfields Pharmaceuticals
34 Nile St
London, N1 7TP
tel: (020) 7684 9090 (order)
tel: (020) 7684 8574 (enquiry)
fax: (020) 7502 2332
nick.precious@moorfields.nhs.uk

**North West London Hospitals NHS Trust**
Dr K. Middleton
North West London Hospitals NHS Trust
Northwick Park Hospital
Watford Rd
Harrow
Middlesex, HA1 3UJ
tel: (020) 8869 2295 (order)
tel: (020) 8869 2204/2223 (enquiry)
keith.middleton@nwlh.nhs.uk

**Royal Free Hampstead NHS Trust**
Ms C. Trehane
Production Manager
Royal Free
Pond St
London, NW3 2QG
tel: (020) 7830 2424 (order)
tel: (020) 7830 2282 (enquiry)
fax: (020) 7794 1875
christine.trehane@nhs.net

**St George's Healthcare NHS Trust**
Mr V. Kumar
Assistant Chief Pharmacist
Technical Services
St George's Hospital
Blackshaw Rd
Tooting
London, SW17 0QT
tel: (020) 8725 1770/1768
fax: (020) 8725 3947
vinodh.kumar@stgeorges.nhs.uk

**University College Hospital NHS Foundation Trust**
Mr T. Murphy
Production Manager
University College Hospital
235 Euston Rd
London, NW1 2BU
tel: (020) 7380 9723 (order)
tel: (020) 7380 9472 (enquiry)
fax: (020) 7380 9726
tony.murphy@uclh.nhs.uk

### Midlands and Eastern

**Barking, Havering and Redbridge University Trust**
Mr N. Fisher
Senior Principal Pharmacist
Pharmacy Department
Queen's Hospital
Romford
Essex, RM7 0AG
tel: (01708) 435 463 (order)
tel: (01708) 435 042 (enquiry)
neil.fisher@bhrhospitals.nhs.uk

**Burton Hospitals NHS Trust**
Mr P. Williams
Pharmacy Technical and Support Services Manager
Pharmacy Manufacturing Unit
Queens Hospital
Burton Hospitals NHS Trust
Belvedere Rd
Burton-on-Trent, DE13 0RB
tel: (01283) 511 511 (or 566 333) ext: 5115 (order) 5138 (enquiry)
fax: (01283) 593 036
paul.williams@burtonh-tr.wmids.nhs.uk

**Colchester Hospital University NHS Foundation Trust**
Mrs A. Reynolds
Pharmacy Business Manager
Pharmacy Support Unit
Colchester General Hospital
Turner Rd
Colchester, CO4 5JL
tel: (01206) 742 007 (order)
tel: (01206) 746 148 (enquiry)
fax: (01206) 841 249
pharmacy.stores@colchesterhospital.nhs.uk (order)
psuenquiries@colchesterhospital.nhs.uk (enquiries)

**Ipswich Hospital NHS Trust**
Dr J. Harwood
Production Manager
Pharmacy Manufacturing Unit
Ipswich Hospital NHS Trust
Heath Rd
Ipswich, IP4 5PD
tel: (01473) 703 440 (order)
tel: (01473) 703 603 (enquiry)
fax: (01473) 703 609
john.harwood@ipswichhospital.nhs.uk

**Nottingham University Hospitals NHS Trust**
Ms J. Kendall
Assistant Head of Pharmacy, Technical and Logistical Services
Pharmacy Production Units
Nottingham University Hospitals NHS Trust
Queens Medical Centre Campus
Nottingham, NG7 2UH
tel: (0115) 875 4521 (order)
tel: (0115) 924 9924 ext: 64177 (enquiry)
fax: (0115) 970 9780
jeanette.kendall@nuh.nhs.uk

**University Hospital of North Staffordshire NHS Trust**
Ms K. Ferguson
Chief Technician
Pharmacy Technical Services
University Hospital of North Staffordshire NHS Trust
City General Site
Stoke-on-Trent, ST4 6QG
tel: (01782) 674 568 (order)
tel: (01782) 674 568 (enquiry)
fax: (01782) 674 575
caroline.ferguson@uhns.nhs.uk

## North East

**The Newcastle upon Tyne Hospitals NHS Foundation Trust**
Mr Y. Hunter-Blair
Production Manager
Newcastle Specials
Pharmacy Production Unit
Royal Victoria Infirmary
Queen Victoria Rd
Newcastle-upon-Tyne, NE1 4LP
tel: (0191) 282 0395 (order)
tel: (0191) 282 0389 (enquiry)
fax: (0191) 282 0469
yan.hunter-blair@nuth.nhs.uk

## North West

**Preston Pharmaceuticals**
Ms A. Nutman
Assistant Director of Pharmacy
Preston Pharmaceuticals
Royal Preston Hospital
Fulwood
Preston, PR2 9HT
tel: (01772) 523 617 (order)
tel: (01772) 522 593 (enquiry)
fax: (01772) 523 645
angela.nutman@lthtr.nhs.uk

**Stockport Pharmaceuticals**
Mrs S. Miller
Production Manager
Stockport Pharmaceuticals
Pharmacy Department
Stepping Hill Hospital
Stockport, SK2 7JE
tel: (0161) 419 5666 (order)
tel: (0161) 419 5657 (enquiry)
fax: (0161) 419 5426
sally.miller@stockport.nhs.uk

## South

**Portsmouth Hospitals NHS Trust**
Mr R. Lucas
Product Development Manager
Pharmacy Manufacturing Unit
Portsmouth Hospitals NHS Trust
Unit D2, Railway Triangle Industrial Estate
Walton Road
Farlington, Portsmouth, PO6 1TF
tel: (02392) 389 078 (order)
tel: (02392) 316 312 (enquiry)
fax: (02392) 316 316
robert.lucas@porthosp.nhs.uk

## South East

**East Sussex Healthcare NHS Trust**
Mr P. Keen
Business Manager
Eastbourne Pharmaceuticals
Eastbourne District General Hospital
East Sussex Hospitals NHS Trust
Kings Drive, Eastbourne, BN21 2UD
tel: (01323) 414 906 (order)
tel: (01323) 417 400 ext: 3076 (enquiry)
fax: (01323) 414 931
paul.keen@esht.nhs.uk

## South West

**Torbay PMU**
Mr P. Bendell
Pharmacy Manufacturing Services Manager
Torbay PMU
South Devon Healthcare NHS Foundation Trust
Kemmings Close, Long Rd
Paignton, TQ4 7TW
tel: (01803) 664 707
fax: (01803) 664 354
phil.bendell@nhs.net

## Yorkshire

**Calderdale and Huddersfield NHS Foundation Trust**
Dr S. Langford
Pharmacy Production Director
Pharmacy Manufacturing Unit
Huddersfield Royal Infirmary
Gate 2-Acre Mills, School St
Lindley
Huddersfield, HD3 3ET
tel: (01484) 355 388 (order)
tel: (01484) 355 371 (enquiry)
fax: (01484) 355 377
stephen.langford@cht.nhs.uk

## Northern Ireland

**Victoria Pharmaceuticals**
Ms C. McBride
Production Manager
Victoria Pharmaceuticals
Plenum Building
Royal Hospitals
Grosvenor Road
Belfast, BT12 6BA
tel: (028) 9263 0070 (order/enquiry)
fax: (028) 9063 5282 (order/enquiry)
colettemcbride@belfasttrust.hscni.net

## Scotland

**NHS Greater Glasgow and Clyde**
Mr G. Conkie
Production Manager
Western Infirmary
Dumbarton Rd
Glasgow, G11 6NT
tel: (0141) 211 2754 (order)
tel: (0141) 211 2882 (enquiry)
fax: (0141) 211 1967
graham.conkie@ggc.scot.nhs.uk

**Tayside Pharmaceuticals**
Dr B. Millar
General Manager
Tayside Pharmaceuticals
Ninewells Hospital
Dundee, DD1 9SY
tel: (01382) 632 052 (order)
tel: (01382) 632 183 (enquiry)
fax: (01382) 632 060
baxter.millar@nhs.net

## Wales

**Cardiff and Vale University Health Board**
Mr P. Spark
Principal Pharmacist (Production)
Cardiff and Vale University Health Board
20 Fieldway
Cardiff, CF14 4HY
tel: (029) 2074 8120
fax: (029) 2074 8130
paul.spark@wales.nhs.uk

# Index

Principal page references are
printed in **bold** type. Proprietary
(trade) names and names of organisms are printed in *italic* type;
where the BNF does not include a
full entry for a branded product, the
non-proprietary name is shown in
brackets

## A

*A2A Spacer*, 143
Abacavir, 312, **313**, 314
   lamivudine and zidovudine
     with, 314
   lamivudine with, 314
Abatacept, **511**, 512
Abbreviations
   latin, *inside back cover*
   symbols and, *inside back cover*
   units, 4
Abdominal surgery, antibacterial
   prophylaxis, 257
*Abelcet*, 308
Abetalipoproteinaemia, 485
*Abidec*, 488
*Abilify*, 178
*Able Spacer*, 143
Abscess, dental, 253
Absence seizures, 218
*Acanthamoeba* keratitis, 521
   contact lenses, 536
Acarbose, 360
Acaricides, 593
ACBS
   foods, 757
   toilet preparations, 802
*Accolate*, 151
*Accrete D3*, 485
*Accu-Chek* products, 364
*Accuhaler*
   *Flixotide*, 148
   *Seretide*, 149
   *Serevent*, 139
   *Ventolin*, 138
ACE inhibitors, 99
   diuretics with, 100
   heart failure, 99
   renal function, 99
*Acea*, 589
Acetaminophen *see* Paracetamol
Acetazolamide
   diuretic, 81
   epilepsy, 233, **529**
   glaucoma, 527, **529**
   intracranial pressure, raised,
    **529**
Acetic acid, otitis externa, 537
Acetylcholine, **534**, 535

Acetylcysteine
   cystic fibrosis, 164
   eye, 532
   meconium ileus, 164
   mucolytic, **164**
   paracetamol poisoning, 26, **27**
Acetylsalicylic acid *see* Aspirin
Aciclovir
   herpes simplex, **324**
     eye, 324, **523**
     genital, 395, 593
     labialis, 593
     skin, **593**
   herpes stomatitis, 547
   herpes zoster, **324**
   varicella-zoster, **324**
Acid aspiration, prophylaxis, 630
*Acidex*, 37
Acidosis
   lactic, 313
   metabolic, 462, 465
Acitretin, 570, **573**, 574
*Acnamino MR*, 278
Acne, 577
   infantile, 577, 581
   systemic treatment, 580
   topical treatment, 577
*Acnecide*, 577
*Acnocin* (co-cyprindiol), 581
Acrivastine, 151, **152**
Acrodermatitis enteropathica, 479
ACTH *see* Corticotropin, 382
*Actidose-Aqua Advance*, 25
*Actilyse* preparations, 120, 121
Actinic keratoses, 585
Actinomycin D *see* Dactinomycin,
   **421**
*Actiq*, 207
Activated charcoal, 24, **25**
*Active*, 364, 365
*Actonel*, 390
   Once a Week, *390*
*Actrapid*, 353
*Acular*, 535
*ACWY Vax*, 616
Acyclovir *see* Aciclovir
*Adalat* preparations, 106
Adalimumab, 510, **512**
Adapalene, **579**
   benzoyl peroxide with, 579
*Adcal*, 474
*Adcal-D₃* preparations, 485
*Adcortyl Intra-articular / Intradermal*,
   508
*Add-Ins*, 799
*Addiphos*, 469
Addison's disease, 369
Additives *see* Excipients
*Additrace*, 469
Adefovir, 328
*Adenocor*, 83
*Adenoscan*, 83
Adenosine, **82**, 83
Adenovirus, 330

ADH *see* Antidiuretic hormone,
   385
ADHD *see* Attention deficit
   hyperactivity disorder, 188
Adhesive, tissue, 595
*Adipine* preparations, 106
*Adoport*, 437
Adrenal function test, 382
Adrenal insufficiency, 369
Adrenal suppression
   metyrapone, 391
   surgery, 371
   systemic corticosteroids, 371
   topical corticosteroids, 560
Adrenaline
   anaphylaxis, 158, **159**, 160
   bradycardia, 81
   croup, 135
   hypotension, 112
   infusion table (neonatal), 808
   local anaesthesia, 649, 651
   palliative care, capillary
    bleeding, 17
   self administration, 159
Adrenergic neurone blocking
   drugs, 97
Adrenoceptor agonists, 135
Adsorbents
   gastro-intestinal, 46
   poisoning, 24
*Advagraf*, 439
*Advantage Plus*, 364
*Advate* (factor VIII fraction), 123
Adverse reactions
   prevention of, 12
   reporting, 11
Advisory Committee on
   Borderline Substances *see* ACBS
Advisory labels *see* Cautionary
   and advisory labels
*AeroChamber Plus*, 143
Agalsidase
   alfa, **490**, 491
   beta, **490**, 491
Agammaglobulinaemia,
   congenital, replacement therapy,
   623
*Agrippal*, 613
AIDS
   treatment, 312
   vaccines and, 601
*Airomir* preparations, 138
*AirSalb* (salbutamol), 138
*AirZone*, 142
*Aknemin* (minocycline), 278
*Aknemycin Plus*, 580
Albendazole
   hookworms, 347
   hydatid disease, 347
   larva migrans, 348
   strongyloidiasis, 348

Index

Index

Index

Index

Index

**Index**

Index

# E

Index

**Index**

# G

Index

Index

Index

Index

Index

**Index**

Index

Index

Index

Index

BNFC

# YellowCard® — It's easiest to report online at www.mhra.gov.uk/yellowcard

COMMISSION ON HUMAN MEDICINES (CHM)

MHRA

## SUSPECTED ADVERSE DRUG REACTIONS

If you suspect an adverse reaction may be related to one or more drugs/vaccines/complementary remedies, please complete this Yellow Card. See 'Adverse reactions to drugs' section in BNFC or www.mhra.gov.uk/yellowcard for guidance. Do not be put off reporting because some details are not known.

## PATIENT DETAILS

Patient Initials: _____  Sex: M / F  Ethnicity: _____  Weight if known (kg): _____

Age (at time of reaction): _____  Identification number (e.g. Your Practice or Hospital Ref): _____

## SUSPECTED DRUG(S)/VACCINE(S)

| Drug/Vaccine (Brand if known) | Batch | Route | Dosage | Date started | Date stopped | Prescribed for |
|---|---|---|---|---|---|---|
| | | | | | | |
| | | | | | | |
| | | | | | | |

## SUSPECTED REACTION(S)

Please describe the reaction(s) and any treatment given:

Date reaction(s) started: _____  Date reaction(s) stopped: _____

Do you consider the reactions to be serious?  Yes / No

If yes, please indicate why the reaction is considered to be serious (please tick all that apply):

Patient died due to reaction ☐

Life threatening ☐

Congenital abnormality ☐

Involved or prolonged inpatient hospitalisation ☐

Involved persistent or significant disability or incapacity ☐

Medically significant; please give details: _____

Outcome

Recovered ☐

Recovering ☐

Continuing ☐

Other ☐

# It's easiest to report online at www.mhra.gov.uk/yellowcard

## OTHER DRUG(S) (including self-medication and complementary remedies)

Did the patient take any other medicines/vaccines/complementary remedies in the last 3 months prior to the reaction? Yes / No

If yes, please give the following information if known:

| Drug/Vaccine (Brand if known) | Batch | Route | Dosage | Date started | Date stopped | Prescribed for |
|---|---|---|---|---|---|---|
| | | | | | | |
| | | | | | | |
| | | | | | | |
| | | | | | | |

**Additional relevant information** e.g. medical history, test results, known allergies, rechallenge (if performed), suspect drug interactions. For congenital abnormalities please state all other drugs taken during pregnancy and the last menstrual period.

Please list any medicines obtained from the internet: _____

---

## REPORTER DETAILS
Name and Professional Address: _____

Postcode: _____ Tel No: _____
Email: _____
Speciality: _____
Signature: _____ Date: _____

## CLINICIAN (if not the reporter)
Name and Professional Address: _____

Postcode: _____
Email: _____
Speciality: _____
Date: _____

Information on adverse drug reactions received by the MHRA can be downloaded at *www.mhra.gov.uk/daps*
Stay up-to-date on the latest advice for the safe use of medicines with our monthly bulletin *Drug Safety Update*, at *www.mhra.gov.uk/drugsafetyupdate*

Please attach additional pages if necessary.   Send to: FREEPOST YELLOW CARD (no other address details required)

BNFC

In Confidence

# YellowCard® It's easiest to report online at www.mhra.gov.uk/yellowcard

COMMISSION ON HUMAN MEDICINES (CHM)

MHRA

## SUSPECTED ADVERSE DRUG REACTIONS

If you suspect an adverse reaction may be related to one or more drugs/vaccines/complementary remedies, please complete this Yellow Card. See 'Adverse reactions to drugs' section in BNFC or www.mhra.gov.uk/yellowcard for guidance. Do not be put off reporting because some details are not known.

### PATIENT DETAILS
Patient Initials: _____  Sex: M / F  Ethnicity: _____  Weight if known (kg): _____

Age (at time of reaction): _____  Identification number (e.g. Your Practice or Hospital Ref): _____

### SUSPECTED DRUG(S)/VACCINE(S)

| Drug/Vaccine (Brand if known) | Batch | Route | Dosage | Date started | Date stopped | Prescribed for |
|---|---|---|---|---|---|---|
| | | | | | | |
| | | | | | | |
| | | | | | | |
| | | | | | | |

### SUSPECTED REACTION(S)
Please describe the reaction(s) and any treatment given:

Date reaction(s) started: _____  Date reaction(s) stopped: _____

Do you consider the reactions to be serious?  Yes / No

If yes, please indicate why the reaction is considered to be serious (please tick all that apply):

Patient died due to reaction ☐

Involved or prolonged inpatient hospitalisation ☐

Life threatening ☐

Involved persistent or significant disability or incapacity ☐

Congenital abnormality ☐

Medically significant; please give details: _____

Outcome

Recovered ☐
Recovering ☐
Continuing ☐
Other ☐

# It's easiest to report online at www.mhra.gov.uk/yellowcard

## OTHER DRUG(S) (including self-medication and complementary remedies)

Did the patient take any other medicines/vaccines/complementary remedies in the last 3 months prior to the reaction? Yes / No

If yes, please give the following information if known:

| Drug/Vaccine (Brand if known) | Batch | Route | Dosage | Date started | Date stopped | Prescribed for |
|---|---|---|---|---|---|---|
| | | | | | | |
| | | | | | | |
| | | | | | | |
| | | | | | | |

**Additional relevant information** e.g. medical history, test results, known allergies, rechallenge (if performed), suspect drug interactions. For congenital abnormalities please state all other drugs taken during pregnancy and the last menstrual period.

Please list any medicines obtained from the internet: _____

## REPORTER DETAILS
Name and Professional Address: _____

_____

Postcode: _____ Tel No: _____
Email: _____
Speciality: _____
Signature: _____ Date: _____

## CLINICIAN (if not the reporter)
Name and Professional Address: _____

_____

Postcode: _____
Email: _____
Speciality: _____
Date: _____ Tel No: _____

Information on adverse drug reactions received by the MHRA can be downloaded at *www.mhra.gov.uk/daps*
Stay up-to-date on the latest advice for the safe use of medicines with our monthly bulletin *Drug Safety Update*, at *www.mhra.gov.uk/drugsafetyupdate*

Please attach additional pages if necessary.   Send to: FREEPOST YELLOW CARD (no other address details required)

BNFC

# YellowCard® It's easiest to report online at www.mhra.gov.uk/yellowcard

MHRA

COMMISSION ON HUMAN MEDICINES (CHM)

## SUSPECTED ADVERSE DRUG REACTIONS

If you suspect an adverse reaction may be related to one or more drugs/vaccines/complementary remedies, please complete this Yellow Card. See 'Adverse reactions to drugs' section in BNFC or www.mhra.gov.uk/yellowcard for guidance. Do not be put off reporting because some details are not known.

### PATIENT DETAILS
Patient Initials: _____  Sex: M / F  Ethnicity: _____  Weight if known (kg): _____

Age (at time of reaction): _____  Identification number (e.g. Your Practice or Hospital Ref): _____

### SUSPECTED DRUG(S)/VACCINE(S)

| Drug/Vaccine (Brand if known) | Batch | Route | Dosage | Date started | Date stopped | Prescribed for |
|---|---|---|---|---|---|---|
| | | | | | | |
| | | | | | | |
| | | | | | | |

### SUSPECTED REACTION(S)
Please describe the reaction(s) and any treatment given:

Date reaction(s) started: _____  Date reaction(s) stopped: _____

Do you consider the reactions to be serious?  Yes / No

If yes, please indicate why the reaction is considered to be serious (please tick all that apply):

Patient died due to reaction ☐

Life threatening ☐

Congenital abnormality ☐

Involved or prolonged inpatient hospitalisation ☐

Involved persistent or significant disability or incapacity ☐

Medically significant; please give details: _____

**Outcome**

Recovered ☐

Recovering ☐

Continuing ☐

Other ☐

# It's easiest to report online at www.mhra.gov.uk/yellowcard

## OTHER DRUG(S) (including self-medication and complementary remedies)

Did the patient take any other medicines/vaccines/complementary remedies in the last 3 months prior to the reaction? Yes / No
If yes, please give the following information if known:

| Drug/Vaccine (Brand if known) | Batch | Route | Dosage | Date started | Date stopped | Prescribed for |
|---|---|---|---|---|---|---|
| | | | | | | |
| | | | | | | |
| | | | | | | |
| | | | | | | |

**Additional relevant information** e.g. medical history, test results, known allergies, rechallenge (if performed), suspect drug interactions. For congenital abnormalities please state all other drugs taken during pregnancy and the last menstrual period.

Please list any medicines obtained from the internet: _____

## REPORTER DETAILS
Name and Professional Address: _____

_____

Postcode: _____ Tel No: _____
Email: _____
Speciality: _____
Signature: _____ Date: _____

## CLINICIAN (if not the reporter)
Name and Professional Address: _____

_____

Postcode: _____ Tel No: _____
Email: _____
Speciality: _____
Date: _____

Information on adverse drug reactions received by the MHRA can be downloaded at *www.mhra.gov.uk/daps*
Stay up-to-date on the latest advice for the safe use of medicines with our monthly bulletin *Drug Safety Update*, at *www.mhra.gov.uk/drugsafetyupdate*

Please attach additional pages if necessary.  Send to: FREEPOST YELLOW CARD (no other address details required)

BNFC

In Confidence

# YellowCard® It's easiest to report online at www.mhra.gov.uk/yellowcard

COMMISSION ON HUMAN MEDICINES (CHM)

MHRA

## SUSPECTED ADVERSE DRUG REACTIONS

If you suspect an adverse reaction may be related to one or more drugs/vaccines/complementary remedies, please complete this Yellow Card. See 'Adverse reactions to drugs' section in BNFC or www.mhra.gov.uk/yellowcard for guidance. Do not be put off reporting because some details are not known.

## PATIENT DETAILS    Patient Initials: _____    Sex: M / F    Ethnicity: _____    Weight if known (kg): _____

Age (at time of reaction): _____    Identification number (e.g. Your Practice or Hospital Ref): _____

## SUSPECTED DRUG(S)/VACCINE(S)

| Drug/Vaccine (Brand if known) | Batch | Route | Dosage | Date started | Date stopped | Prescribed for |
|---|---|---|---|---|---|---|
| | | | | | | |
| | | | | | | |
| | | | | | | |

## SUSPECTED REACTION(S)    Please describe the reaction(s) and any treatment given:

Outcome

☐ Recovered
☐ Recovering
☐ Continuing
☐ Other

Date reaction(s) started: _____    Date reaction(s) stopped: _____

Do you consider the reactions to be serious?    Yes / No

If yes, please indicate why the reaction is considered to be serious (please tick all that apply):

☐ Patient died due to reaction
☐ Life threatening
☐ Congenital abnormality

☐ Involved or prolonged inpatient hospitalisation
☐ Involved persistent or significant disability or incapacity
☐ Medically significant; please give details: _____

## It's easiest to report online at www.mhra.gov.uk/yellowcard

## OTHER DRUG(S) (including self-medication and complementary remedies)

Did the patient take any other medicines/vaccines/complementary remedies in the last 3 months prior to the reaction? Yes / No
If yes, please give the following information if known:

| Drug/Vaccine (Brand if known) | Batch | Route | Dosage | Date started | Date stopped | Prescribed for |
|---|---|---|---|---|---|---|
| | | | | | | |
| | | | | | | |
| | | | | | | |
| | | | | | | |

**Additional relevant information** e.g. medical history, test results, known allergies, rechallenge (if performed), suspect drug interactions. For congenital abnormalities please state all other drugs taken during pregnancy and the last menstrual period.

Please list any medicines obtained from the internet: _____

### REPORTER DETAILS
Name and Professional Address: _____

Postcode: _____ Tel No: _____
Email: _____
Speciality: _____
Signature: _____ Date: _____

### CLINICIAN (if not the reporter)
Name and Professional Address: _____

Postcode: _____ Tel No: _____
Email: _____
Speciality: _____
Date: _____

Information on adverse drug reactions received by the MHRA can be downloaded at *www.mhra.gov.uk/daps*
Stay up-to-date on the latest advice for the safe use of medicines with our monthly bulletin *Drug Safety Update*, at *www.mhra.gov.uk/drugsafetyupdate*

Please attach additional pages if necessary. Send to: FREEPOST YELLOW CARD (no other address details required)

# NEWBORN LIFE SUPPORT

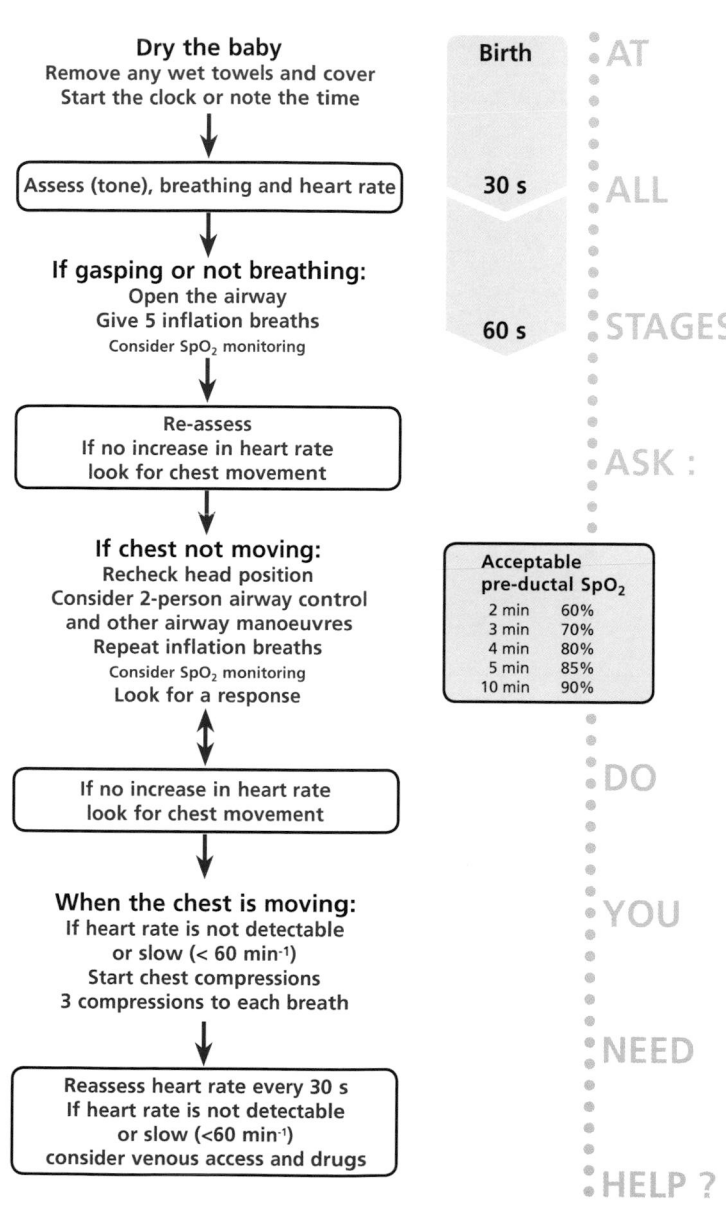

**Dry the baby**
Remove any wet towels and cover
Start the clock or note the time

**Birth**

Assess (tone), breathing and heart rate

**30 s**

**If gasping or not breathing:**
Open the airway
Give 5 inflation breaths
Consider SpO$_2$ monitoring

**60 s**

Re-assess
If no increase in heart rate
look for chest movement

**If chest not moving:**
Recheck head position
Consider 2-person airway control
and other airway manoeuvres
Repeat inflation breaths
Consider SpO$_2$ monitoring
Look for a response

**Acceptable pre-ductal SpO$_2$**

| | |
|---|---|
| 2 min | 60% |
| 3 min | 70% |
| 4 min | 80% |
| 5 min | 85% |
| 10 min | 90% |

If no increase in heart rate
look for chest movement

**When the chest is moving:**
If heart rate is not detectable
or slow (< 60 min$^{-1}$)
Start chest compressions
3 compressions to each breath

Reassess heart rate every 30 s
If heart rate is not detectable
or slow (<60 min$^{-1}$)
consider venous access and drugs

AT

ALL

STAGES

ASK :

DO

YOU

NEED

HELP ?

# PAEDIATRIC BASIC LIFE SUPPORT
## (Healthcare professionals with a duty to respond)

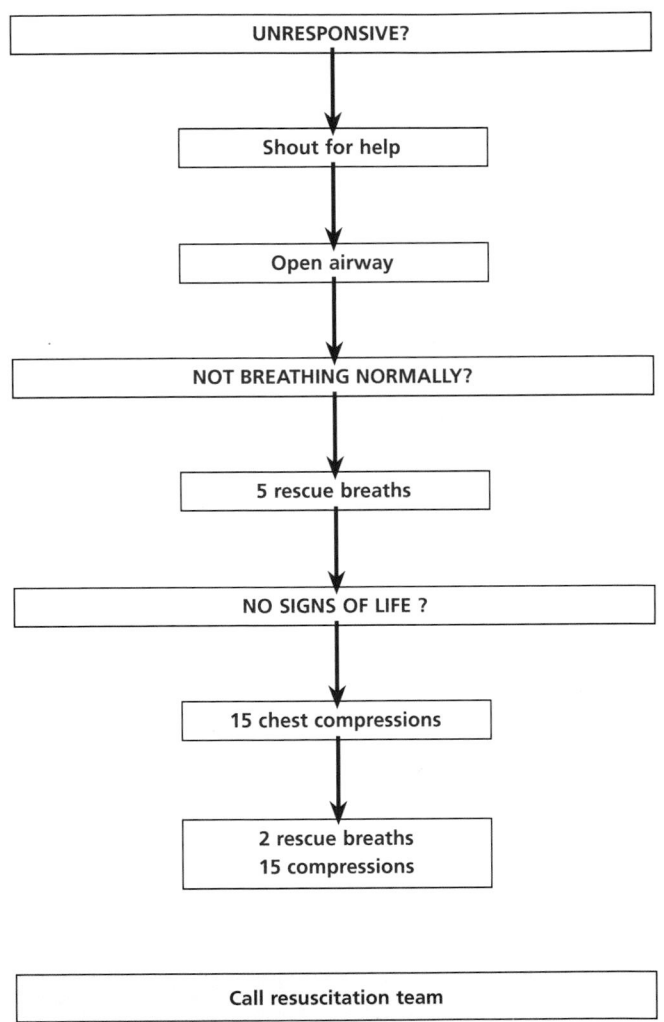

UNRESPONSIVE?

Shout for help

Open airway

NOT BREATHING NORMALLY?

5 rescue breaths

NO SIGNS OF LIFE ?

15 chest compressions

2 rescue breaths
15 compressions

Call resuscitation team

# PAEDIATRIC ADVANCED LIFE SUPPORT

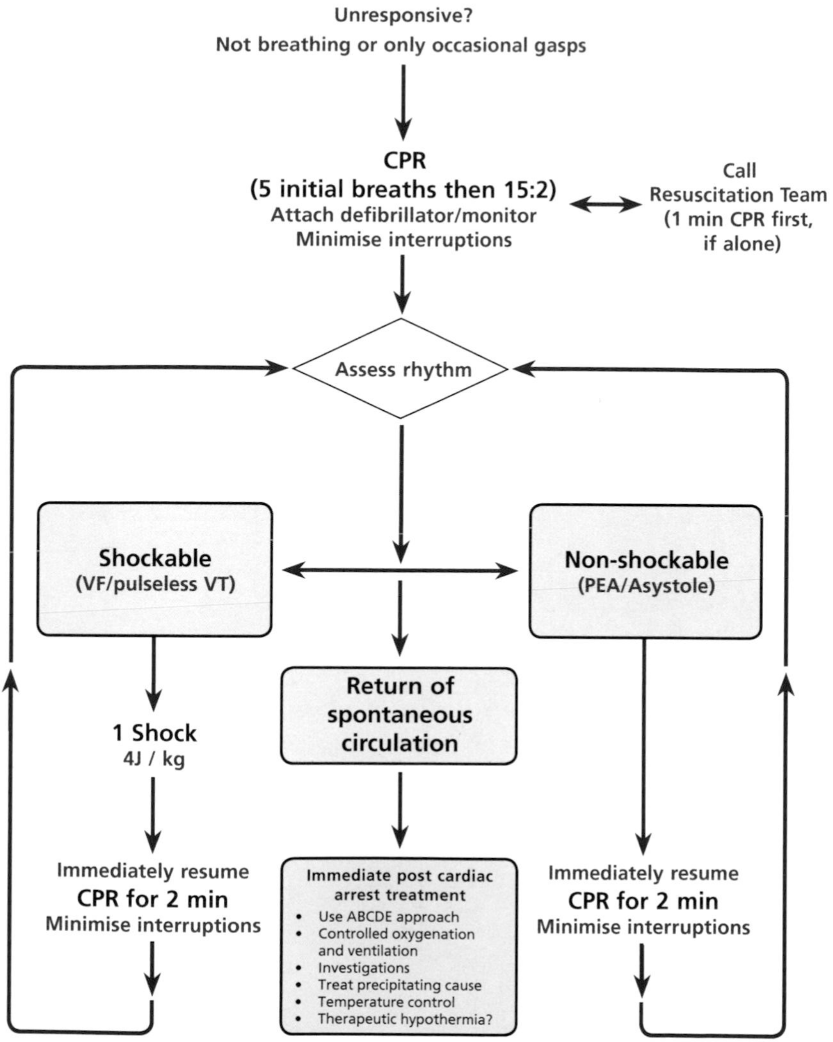

Unresponsive?
Not breathing or only occasional gasps

↓

**CPR**
**(5 initial breaths then 15:2)**
Attach defibrillator/monitor
Minimise interruptions

↔ Call
Resuscitation Team
(1 min CPR first,
if alone)

↓

**Assess rhythm**

**Shockable**
(VF/pulseless VT)

↔

**Non-shockable**
(PEA/Asystole)

**Return of spontaneous circulation**

**1 Shock**
4J / kg

↓

Immediately resume
**CPR for 2 min**
Minimise interruptions

**Immediate post cardiac arrest treatment**
- Use ABCDE approach
- Controlled oxygenation and ventilation
- Investigations
- Treat precipitating cause
- Temperature control
- Therapeutic hypothermia?

Immediately resume
**CPR for 2 min**
Minimise interruptions

---

**During CPR**
- Ensure high-quality CPR: rate, depth, recoil
- Plan actions before interrupting CPR
- Give oxygen
- Vascular access (intravenous, intraosseous)
- Give adrenaline every 3-5 min
- Consider advanced airway and capnography
- Continuous chest compressions when advanced airway in place
- Correct reversible causes

**Reversible causes**
- Hypoxia
- Hypovolaemia
- Hypo- / hyperkalaemia / metabolic
- Hypothermia
- Tension pneumothorax
- Toxins
- Tamponade - cardiac
- Thromboembolism

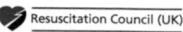
Resuscitation Council (UK)

# BODY SURFACE AREA IN CHILDREN
## Body-weight under 40kg

| Body-weight (kg) | Surface area (m²) | Body-weight (kg) | Surface area (m²) |
|---|---|---|---|
| 1 | 0.10 | 17 | 0.71 |
| 1.5 | 0.13 | 18 | 0.74 |
| 2 | 0.16 | 19 | 0.77 |
| 2.5 | 0.19 | 20 | 0.79 |
| 3 | 0.21 | 21 | 0.82 |
| 3.5 | 0.24 | 22 | 0.85 |
| 4 | 0.26 | 23 | 0.87 |
| 4.5 | 0.28 | 24 | 0.90 |
| 5 | 0.30 | 25 | 0.92 |
| 5.5 | 0.32 | 26 | 0.95 |
| 6 | 0.34 | 27 | 0.97 |
| 6.5 | 0.36 | 28 | 1.0 |
| 7 | 0.38 | 29 | 1.0 |
| 7.5 | 0.40 | 30 | 1.1 |
| 8 | 0.42 | 31 | 1.1 |
| 8.5 | 0.44 | 32 | 1.1 |
| 9 | 0.46 | 33 | 1.1 |
| 9.5 | 0.47 | 34 | 1.1 |
| 10 | 0.49 | 35 | 1.2 |
| 11 | 0.53 | 36 | 1.2 |
| 12 | 0.56 | 37 | 1.2 |
| 13 | 0.59 | 38 | 1.2 |
| 14 | 0.62 | 39 | 1.3 |
| 15 | 0.65 | 40 | 1.3 |
| 16 | 0.68 | | |

Values are calculated using the Boyd equation

**Note** Height is not required to estimate body surface area using these tables

Adapted by permission from Macmillan Publishers Ltd: Sharkey I et al, *British Journal of Cancer* 2001; **85** (1): 23–28, © 2001

# BODY SURFACE AREA IN CHILDREN
## Body-weight over 40kg

| Body-weight (kg) | Surface area (m²) | Body-weight (kg) | Surface area (m²) |
|---|---|---|---|
| 41 | 1.3 | 66 | 1.8 |
| 42 | 1.3 | 67 | 1.8 |
| 43 | 1.3 | 68 | 1.8 |
| 44 | 1.4 | 69 | 1.8 |
| 45 | 1.4 | 70 | 1.9 |
| 46 | 1.4 | 71 | 1.9 |
| 47 | 1.4 | 72 | 1.9 |
| 48 | 1.4 | 73 | 1.9 |
| 49 | 1.5 | 74 | 1.9 |
| 50 | 1.5 | 75 | 1.9 |
| 51 | 1.5 | 76 | 2.0 |
| 52 | 1.5 | 77 | 2.0 |
| 53 | 1.5 | 78 | 2.0 |
| 54 | 1.6 | 79 | 2.0 |
| 55 | 1.6 | 80 | 2.0 |
| 56 | 1.6 | 81 | 2.0 |
| 57 | 1.6 | 82 | 2.1 |
| 58 | 1.6 | 83 | 2.1 |
| 59 | 1.7 | 84 | 2.1 |
| 60 | 1.7 | 85 | 2.1 |
| 61 | 1.7 | 86 | 2.1 |
| 62 | 1.7 | 87 | 2.1 |
| 63 | 1.7 | 88 | 2.2 |
| 64 | 1.7 | 89 | 2.2 |
| 65 | 1.8 | 90 | 2.2 |

Values are calculated using the Boyd equation

**Note** Height is not required to estimate body surface area using these tables

# Medical emergencies in the community

Drug treatment outlined below is intended for use by community healthcare professionals. Only drugs that are used for immediate relief are shown; advice on supporting care is not given. Where the child's condition requires investigation and further treatment, the child should be transferred to hospital promptly.

## Anaphylaxis
(section 3.4.3)

**Adrenaline injection** (1 mg/mL (1 in 1000))

- By intramuscular injection
  Child under 6 years 150 micrograms (0.15 mL), repeated every 5 minutes if necessary
  Child 6–12 years 300 micrograms (0.3 mL), repeated every 5 minutes if necessary
  Child 12–18 years 500 micrograms (0.5 mL), repeated every 5 minutes if necessary; 300 micrograms (0.3 mL) should be given if child is small or prepubertal

High-flow **oxygen** (section 3.6) and **intravenous fluids** should be given as soon as available.

**Chlorphenamine injection** by intramuscular or intravenous injection (section 3.4.1) may help counter histamine-mediated vasodilation and bronchoconstriction.

**Hydrocortisone** (preferably as sodium succinate) by intravenous injection (section 6.3.2) has delayed action but it should be given to severely affected children to prevent further deterioration.

## Asthma: acute
(section 3.1)

Regard each emergency consultation as being for **severe acute asthma** until shown otherwise; failure to respond adequately **at any time** requires immediate transfer to hospital

*Either* **salbutamol** aerosol inhaler (100 micrograms/metered inhalation)

- By aerosol inhalation via large-volume spacer (and a close-fitting face mask if child under 3 years)
  Child under 18 years 2–10 puffs each inhaled separately, repeated at 10–20 minute intervals or as necessary

*or* **salbutamol** nebuliser solution (1 mg/mL, 2 mg/mL)

- By inhalation of nebulised solution (via oxygen-driven nebuliser if available)
  Child under 5 years 2.5 mg every 20–30 minutes or as necessary
  Child 5–12 years 2.5–5 mg every 20–30 minutes or as necessary
  Child 12–18 years 5 mg every 20–30 minutes or as necessary

*or* **terbutaline** nebulised solution (2.5 mg/mL)

- By inhalation of nebulised solution (via oxygen-driven nebuliser if available)
  Child under 5 years 5 mg every 20–30 minutes or as necessary

Child 5–12 years 5–10 mg every 20–30 minutes or as necessary
Child 12–18 years 10 mg every 20–30 minutes or as necessary

**Plus** (in all cases)

*Either* **prednisolone** tablets (*or* **prednisolone** soluble tablets) (5 mg)

- By mouth
  Child under 12 years 1–2 mg/kg (max. 40 mg) once daily for up to 3 days or longer if necessary; if the child has been taking an oral corticosteroid for more than a few days, give prednisolone 2 mg/kg (max. 60 mg) once daily
  Child 12–18 years 40–50 mg once daily for at least 5 days

*or* **hydrocortisone** (preferably as sodium succinate)

- By intravenous injection
  Child up to 18 years 4 mg/kg (max. 100 mg) every 6 hours, until conversion to oral prednisolone is possible; alternative dose if weight unavailable, Child under 2 years 25 mg, 2–5 years 50 mg, 5–18 years 100 mg

High-flow **oxygen** (section 3.6) should be given if available (via face mask)

Monitor response 15 to 30 minutes after nebulisation; if any signs of acute asthma persist, arrange hospital admission. While awaiting ambulance, repeat **nebulised beta$_2$ agonist** (as above) and give with

**ipratropium** nebuliser solution (250 micrograms/mL)

- By inhalation of nebulised solution (via oxygen-driven nebuliser if available)
  Child under 12 years 250 micrograms repeated every 20–30 minutes for the first 2 hours, then every 4–6 hours as necessary
  Child 12–18 years 500 micrograms every 4–6 hours as necessary

## Convulsive (including febrile) seizures lasting longer than 5 minutes
(section 4.8.2 and section 4.8.3)

**Midazolam** buccal solution

- By buccal administration, repeated once after 10 minutes if necessary
  Neonate 300 micrograms/kg
  Child 1–3 months 300 micrograms/kg (max. 2.5 mg)
  Child 3 months–1 year 2.5 mg
  Child 1–5 years 5 mg
  Child 5–10 years 7.5 mg
  Child 10–18 years 10 mg

*or* **diazepam** rectal solution (2 mg/mL, 4 mg/mL)

- By rectum, repeated once after 10 minutes if necessary
  Neonate 1.25–2.5 mg
  Child 1 month–2 years 5 mg
  Child 2–12 years 5–10 mg
  Child 12–18 years 10–20 mg

## Croup
(section 3.1)

**Dexamethasone** oral solution (2 mg/5 mL)

- By mouth
  Child 1 month–2 years 150 micrograms/kg as a single dose

## Diabetic hypoglycaemia
(section 6.1.4)

**Glucose** or **sucrose**

- By mouth
  Child 2–18 years approx. 10–20 g (55–110 mL *Lucozade®* Energy Original or 100–200 mL *Coca-Cola®*—both non-diet versions *or* 2–4 teaspoonfuls of sugar *or* 3–6 sugar lumps), repeated after 10–15 minutes if necessary

*or* if hypoglycaemia unresponsive *or* if oral route cannot be used

**Glucagon** injection (1 mg/mL)

- By subcutaneous, intramuscular or intravenous injection
  Child body-weight under 25 kg 500 micrograms (0.5 mL)
  Child body-weight over 25 kg 1 mg (1 mL)

*or* if hypoglycaemia prolonged *or* unresponsive to glucagon after 10 minutes

**Glucose** intravenous infusion (10%)

- By intravenous injection into large vein
  Child 1 month–18 years 5 mL/kg (glucose 500 mg/kg)

## Meningococcal disease
(Table 1, section 5.1)

**Benzylpenicillin sodium** injection (600 mg, 1.2 g)

- By intravenous injection (or by intramuscular injection if venous access not available)
  Neonate 300 mg
  Child 1 month–1 year 300 mg
  Child 1–10 years 600 mg
  Child 10–18 years 1.2 g
  **Note** A single dose should be given before urgent transfer to hospital, so long as this does not delay the transfer

*or* if history of allergy to penicillin

**Cefotaxime** injection (1 g)

- By intravenous injection (or by intramuscular injection if venous access not available)
  Neonate 50 mg/kg
  Child 1 month–12 years 50 mg/kg (max. 1 g)
  Child 12–18 years 1 g
  **Note** A single dose can be given before urgent transfer to hospital, so long as this does not delay the transfer

*or* if history of immediate hypersensitivity reaction (including anaphylaxis, angioedema, urticaria, or rash immediately after administration) to penicillin or to cephalosporins

**Chloramphenicol** injection (1 g)

- By intravenous injection
  Child 1 month–18 years 12.5–25 mg/kg
  **Note** A single dose can be given before urgent transfer to hospital, so long as this does not delay the transfer

## Approximate conversions and units

| lb | kg | stones | kg | mL | fl oz |
|----|------|--------|-------|------|-------|
| 1 | 0.45 | 1 | 6.35 | 50 | 1.8 |
| 2 | 0.91 | 2 | 12.70 | 100 | 3.5 |
| 3 | 1.36 | 3 | 19.05 | 150 | 5.3 |
| 4 | 1.81 | 4 | 25.40 | 200 | 7.0 |
| 5 | 2.27 | 5 | 31.75 | 500 | 17.6 |
| 6 | 2.72 | 6 | 38.10 | 1000 | 35.2 |
| 7 | 3.18 | 7 | 44.45 | | |
| 8 | 3.63 | 8 | 50.80 | | |
| 9 | 4.08 | 9 | 57.15 | | |
| 10 | 4.54 | 10 | 63.50 | | |
| 11 | 4.99 | 11 | 69.85 | | |
| 12 | 5.44 | 12 | 76.20 | | |
| 13 | 5.90 | 13 | 82.55 | | |
| 14 | 6.35 | 14 | 88.90 | | |
| | | 15 | 95.25 | | |

## Length

| | |
|---|---|
| 1 metre (m) | = 1000 millimetres (mm) |
| 1 centimetre (cm) | = 10 mm |
| 1 inch (in) | = 25.4 mm |
| 1 foot (ft) | = 12 inches |
| 12 inches | = 304.8 mm |

## Mass

| | |
|---|---|
| 1 kilogram (kg) | = 1000 grams (g) |
| 1 gram (g) | = 1000 milligrams (mg) |
| 1 milligram (mg) | = 1000 micrograms |
| 1 microgram | = 1000 nanograms |
| 1 nanogram | = 1000 picograms |

## Volume

| | |
|---|---|
| 1 litre | = 1000 millilitres (mL) |
| 1 millilitre (1 mL) | = 1000 microlitres |
| 1 pint | ≈ 568 mL |

## Other units

| | |
|---|---|
| 1 kilocalorie (kcal) | = 4186.8 joules (J) |
| 1000 kilocalories (kcal) | = 4.1868 megajoules (MJ) |
| 1 megajoule (MJ) | = 238.8 kilocalories (kcal) |
| 1 millimetre of mercury (mmHg) | = 133.3 pascals (Pa) |
| 1 kilopascal (kPa) | = 7.5 mmHg (pressure) |

> **Plasma-drug concentrations** in *BNF for Children* are expressed in mass units per litre (e.g. mg/litre). The approximate equivalent in terms of amount of substance units (e.g. micromol/litre) is given in brackets.

## Prescribing for children

### Weight, height, and gender

The table below shows the **mean values** for weight, height and gender by age; these values have been derived from the UK-WHO growth charts 2009 and UK1990 standard centile charts, by extrapolating the 50th centile, and may be used to calculate doses in the absence of actual measurements. However, the child's actual weight and height might vary considerably from the values in the table and it is important to see the child to ensure that the value chosen is appropriate. In most cases the child's actual measurement should be obtained as soon as possible and the dose re-calculated.

| Age | Weight kg | Height cm |
|-----|-----------|-----------|
| Full term neonate | 3.5 | 51 |
| 1 month | 4.3 | 55 |
| 2 months | 5.4 | 58 |
| 3 months | 6.1 | 61 |
| 4 months | 6.7 | 63 |
| 6 months | 7.6 | 67 |
| 1 year | 9 | 75 |
| 3 years | 14 | 96 |
| 5 years | 18 | 109 |
| 7 years | 23 | 122 |
| 10 years | 32 | 138 |
| 12 years | 39 | 149 |
| 14 year-old boy | 49 | 163 |
| 14 year-old girl | 50 | 159 |
| Adult male | 68 | 176 |
| Adult female | 58 | 164 |